C000140353

GRAINGER & ALLISON'S DIAGNOSTIC RADIOLOGY

A Textbook of Medical Imaging

Executive Content Strategist: Michael Houston
Content Development Specialist: Martin Mellor Publishing Services Ltd
Project Manager: Andrew Riley
Design: Ellen Zanolle
Illustration Manager: Jennifer Rose
Illustrator: Antbits, Ltd.
Marketing Manager: Veronica Short

GRAINGER & ALLISON'S DIAGNOSTIC RADIOLOGY

6TH EDITION

A Textbook of Medical Imaging

Volume 2

EDITED BY

Andreas Adam, CBE, MB, BS(Hons), PhD, FRCP, FRCR, FRCS, FFRRCSI(Hon), FRANZCR(Hon), FACR(Hon), FMedSci

Adrian K. Dixon, MD, MD(Hon caus), FRCP, FRCR, FRCS, FFRRCSI(Hon), FRANZCR(Hon), FACR(Hon), FMedSci

Jonathan H. Gillard, BSc, MA, MD, FRCP, FRCR, MBA

Cornelia M. Schaefer-Prokop, MD, PhD

For additional online content visit expertconsult.com

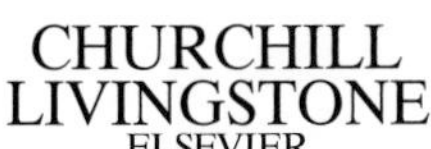

Edinburgh London New York Oxford Philadelphia St Louis Sydney Toronto

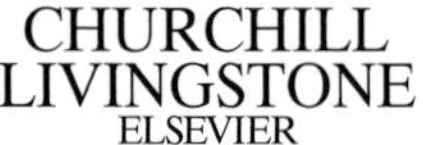

CHURCHILL LIVINGSTONE an imprint of Elsevier Limited

© 2015, Elsevier Limited. All rights reserved.

First edition 1986
Second edition 1991
Third edition 1997
Fourth edition 2001
Fifth edition 2008

The right of Andreas Adam, Adrian K. Dixon, Jonathan H. Gillard and Cornelia M. Schaefer-Prokop to be identified as editors of this work has been asserted by them in accordance with the Copyright, Designs and Patents Act 1988.

No part of this publication may be reproduced or transmitted in any form or by any means, electronic or mechanical, including photocopying, recording, or any information storage and retrieval system, without permission in writing from the publisher. Details on how to seek permission, further information about the Publisher's permissions policies and our arrangements with organizations such as the Copyright Clearance Center and the Copyright Licensing Agency, can be found at our website: www.elsevier.com/permissions.

This book and the individual contributions contained in it are protected under copyright by the Publisher (other than as may be noted herein).

Notices

Knowledge and best practice in this field are constantly changing. As new research and experience broaden our understanding, changes in research methods, professional practices, or medical treatment may become necessary.

Practitioners and researchers must always rely on their own experience and knowledge in evaluating and using any information, methods, compounds, or experiments described herein. In using such information or methods they should be mindful of their own safety and the safety of others, including parties for whom they have a professional responsibility.

With respect to any drug or pharmaceutical products identified, readers are advised to check the most current information provided (i) on procedures featured or (ii) by the manufacturer of each product to be administered, to verify the recommended dose or formula, the method and duration of administration, and contraindications. It is the responsibility of practitioners, relying on their own experience and knowledge of their patients, to make diagnoses, to determine dosages and the best treatment for each individual patient, and to take all appropriate safety precautions.

To the fullest extent of the law, neither the Publisher nor the authors, contributors, or editors, assume any liability for any injury and/or damage to persons or property as a matter of products liability, negligence or otherwise, or from any use or operation of any methods, products, instructions, or ideas contained in the material herein.

ISBN: 978-0-7020-4295-9

e-book ISBN: 978-0-7020-6128-8

Printed in China

Last digit is the print number: 9 8 7 6 5 4 3 2 1

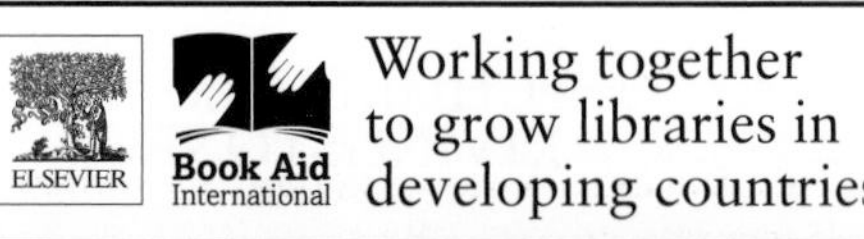

Contents

SECTION C ABDOMINAL IMAGING, 591

Section Editors: Michael M. Maher • Adrian K. Dixon

VOLUME 2

SECTION D THE MUSCULOSKELETAL SYSTEM, 1035

Section Editors: Andrew J. Grainger • Philip O'Connor

SECTION E THE SPINE, 1277

Section Editors: Jonathan H. Gillard • H. Rolf Jäger

SECTION F
NEUROIMAGING, 1391

Section Editors: H. Rolf Jäger • Jonathan H. Gillard

SECTION G
ONCOLOGICAL IMAGING, 1649

Section Editors: Vicky Goh • Andreas Adam

SECTION H
PAEDIATRIC IMAGING, 1769

Section Editors: Catherine M. Owens • Jonathan H. Gillard

SECTION I
INTERVENTIONAL RADIOLOGY, 2043

Section Editors: Anna-Maria Belli • Michael J. Lee • Andreas Adam

Preface

This sixth edition of the landmark Grainger and Allison textbook 'Diagnostic Radiology' is truly a cooperative venture. Two new active Lead Editors (Jonathan Gillard and Cornelia Schaefer-Prokop) have joined Andy Adam and Adrian Dixon. They bring with them considerable expertise in neuroradiology and chest radiology, respectively. Another new feature is the introduction of very energetic Section Editors, Michael Maher (abdomen), Cathy Owens (paediatrics), Phil O'Connor and Andrew Grainger (musculoskeletal), Rolf Jäger (neuroradiology), Vicky Goh (oncology), and Anna-Maria Belli and Michael Lee (intervention). The expectation is that these section editors will subsequently develop small niche spin-off educational/teaching books based on this material, but expanded in their chosen sub-specialties, in exactly the same way that Nyree Griffin and Lee Grant have done (2013) for the main textbook.

We hope that this new edition of this book will help to maintain its role as the leading general textbook for those pursuing radiological training in the UK, mainland Europe, Asia, Africa, Australia and New Zealand; certainly it has been written very much with qualifying examinations in those countries in mind (FRCR, FFRCSI, EDiR, FRANZCR, DNB, etc.). Radiologists in the American communities should find it helpful when preparing for their board examinations. It should also serve as a useful reference text for most radiological departments. We hope it will remain as a ready source of reference material for most radiological queries—even in the days of the internet. The support given to the editors and authors by the team at Elsevier has been exemplary. Michael Houston has now wholeheartedly supported this project for several decades. Martin Mellor has been the lynchpin in keeping authors (and editors!) up to the mark. Andrew Riley has been instrumental in the closing stages of typesetting and proofreading. Thank you gentlemen: we could not have done it without you! Nor could we have done it without the continued support of the cast of over 190 authors from around the world who have generously given of their time and expertise to this 'living' textbook, not only those who have helped in this edition but also those who have contributed to previous editions. Again we are very grateful.

Andreas Adam,
Adrian K. Dixon,
Jonathan H. Gillard,
Cornelia M. Schaefer-Prokop

List of Section Editors

Andreas Adam, CBE, MB, BS(Hons), PhD, FRCP, FRCR, FRCS, FFRRCSI(Hon), FRANZCR(Hon), FACR(Hon), FMedSci
Professor of Interventional Radiology, King's College London, London, UK (Section G: Oncological imaging; Section I: Interventional radiology)

Anna-Maria Belli, FRCR, EBIR
Professor of Interventional Radiology; Consultant Radiologist, Radiology Department, St George's Healthcare NHS Trust, London, UK (Section I: Interventional radiology)

Adrian K. Dixon, MD, MD(Hon caus), FRCP, FRCR, FRCS, FFRRCSI(Hon), FRANZCR(Hon), FACR(Hon), FMedSci
Professor Emeritus of Radiology; Master, Peterhouse, Cambridge, UK (Section A: Principles of imaging techniques and general issues; Section B: The chest and cardiovascular system; Section C: Abdominal imaging)

Jonathan H. Gillard, BSc, MA, MD, FRCP, FRCR, MBA
Professor of Neuroradiology, University of Cambridge, Addenbrooke's Hospital, Cambridge, UK (Section E: The spine; Section F: Neuroimaging; Section H: Paediatric imaging)

Vicky Goh, MA, MBBChir, MD, MRCP, FRCR
Chair of Clinical Cancer Imaging, Division of Imaging Sciences and Biomedical Engineering, King's College London; Honorary Consultant Radiologist, Guy's and St Thomas' Hospitals, London, UK (Section G: Oncological imaging)

Andrew J. Grainger, BM, BS, MRCP, FRCR
Consultant and Honorary Clinical Associate Professor, Musculoskeletal Radiology, Leeds Teaching Hospitals and Leeds Musculoskeletal Biomedical Research Centre, Leeds, UK (Section D: The musculoskeletal system)

H. Rolf Jäger, MD, FRCR
Reader in Neuroradiology, Department of Brain Repair and Rehabilitation, UCL Institute of Neurology, UCL Faculty of Brain Sciences; Consultant Neuroradiologist, Lysholm Department of Neuroradiology, National Hospital for Neurology and Neurosurgery, and Department of Imaging, University College London Hospitals, London, UK (Section E: The spine; Section F: Neuroimaging)

Michael J. Lee, MSc, FRCPI, FRCR, FFR (RCSI), FSIR, EBIR
Professor of Radiology, Royal College of Surgeons in Ireland; Consultant Interventional Radiologist, Beaumont Hospital, Dublin, Ireland (Section I: Interventional radiology)

Michael M. Maher, MD, FRCSI, FRCR, FFR (RCSI)
Professor of Radiology, University College Cork; Consultant Radiologist, Cork University Hospital and Mercy University Hospital, Cork, Ireland (Section C: Abdominal imaging)

Philip O'Connor, MBBS, MRCP, FRCR, FFSEM(UK)
Musculoskeletal Radiologist, Clinical Radiology, Leeds Teaching Hospitals Trust, The University of Leeds, West Yorkshire, UK (Section D: The musculoskeletal system)

Catherine M. Owens, BSc, MBBS, MRCP, FRCR
Consultant Radiologist and Honorary Reader, Department of Imaging, Great Ormond Street Hospital, London, UK (Section H: Paediatric imaging)

Cornelia M. Schaefer-Prokop, MD, PhD
Professor of Radiology, Meander Medical Centre, Amersfoort, The Netherlands (Section A: Principles of imaging techniques and general issues; Section B: The chest and cardiovascular system)

List of Contributors

Andreas Adam, CBE, MB, BS(Hons), PhD, FRCP, FRCR, FRCS, FFRRCSI(Hon), FRANZCR(Hon), FACR(Hon), FMedSci
Professor of Interventional Radiology, King's College London, London, UK

E. Jane Adam, MB, BS(Hons), MRCP, FRCR
Consultant Radiologist, St George's Healthcare NHS Trust, London, UK

Judith E. Adams, MBBS, FRCR, FRCP, FBIR
Professor of Clinical Radiology, Department of Radiology and Manchester Academic Health Science Centre, The Royal Infirmary, Central Manchester University Hospitals NHS Foundation Trust, Manchester, UK

Omar Agosto, MD
Clinical Assistant Professor, Diagnostic Radiology, Temple University School of Medicine; Director of Body MRI and Body CT, Diagnostic Radiology, Jeanes Hospital and Northeastern Ambulatory Care Center-Temple University Healthcare System, Philadelphia, PA, USA

Farah Alobeidi, MA, MB BChir, MRCS, FRCR
Neuroradiology Fellow, Lysholm Department of Neuroradiology, The National Hospital for Neurology and Neurosurgery, London, UK

Roberto Alonzi, BSc, MBBS, MRCP, FRCR, MD
Consultant in Clinical Oncology, Mount Vernon Cancer Centre, Northwood; Senior Lecturer, The Cancer Institute, University College London, London, UK

Allan C. Andi, BSc(Hons), MRCS(Ed), FRCR
Consultant Radiologist, The Hillingdon Hospitals NHS Foundation Trust, London, UK

Maria I. Argyropoulou, MD, PhD
Professor of Radiology, Department of Radiology, University of Ioannina, Greece

Owen Arthurs, MB, Bchir, PhD, FRCR
Consultant Paediatric Radiologist, Radiology, Great Ormond Street Hospital, London, UK

Susan M. Ascher, MD
Professor of Radiology, Georgetown University School of Medicine; Co-Director, Abdominal Imaging, Georgetown University Hospital, Washington, DC, USA

Norbert Avril, MD
Professor and Research Scholar, Department of Radiology, Case Western Reserve University, University Hospitals Case Medical Center, Cleveland, OH, USA

Zelena A. Aziz, MRCP, FRCR, MD
Consultant Chest Radiologist, London Chest Hospital, Barts Health NHS Trust, London, UK

Danielle Balériaux, MD
Professor Emeritus, Neuroradiology, Hôpital Erasme ULB, Brussels, Belgium

Jelle O. Barentsz, MD, PhD
Professor of Radiology, Department of Radiology, Prostate MR Reference Center, Radboud University Nijmegen Medical Center, Nijmegen, The Netherlands

Frederik Barkhof, MD, PhD
Professor of Neuroradiology, Alzheimer Center and Department of Radiology, VU University Medical Center, Amsterdam, The Netherlands

Sue J. Barter, MBBS, MRCP, DMRD, FRCR, FRCP
Consultant Radiologist, Department of Radiology, Cambridge University Hospitals NHS Foundation Trust, Cambridge, UK

Timothy Beale, MBBS, FRCS, FRCR
Consultant Head and Neck Radiologist, University College Hospital, Royal National Throat Nose and Ear Hospital, London, UK

Philip W.P. Bearcroft, MA, MB, BChir, FRCR, FRCP
Consultant Radiologist, Department of Radiology, Cambridge University Hospitals NHS Foundation, Cambridge, UK

Catherine Beigelman-Aubry, MD
Priva Docent-Maitre d'enseignement et recherche, Radiodiagnostic and Interventional Radiology, Centre Hospitalier Universitaire Vaudois, Lausanne, Switzerland

Anna-Maria Belli, FRCR, EBIR
Professor of Interventional Radiology; Consultant Radiologist, Radiology Department, St George's Healthcare NHS Trust, London, UK

Lol Berman, FRCP, FRCR
Lecturer and Honorary Consultant, University Department of Radiology, Addenbrooke's Hospital, Cambridge, UK

Sanjeev Bhalla, MD
Chief, Cardiothoracic Radiology, Mallinckrodt Institute of Radiology, Washington University in St Louis, St Louis, MO, USA

Joti Jonathan Bhattacharya, MBBS, MSc, FRCR
Consultant Neuroradiologist, Department of Neuroradiology, Institute of Neurological Sciences, Southern General Hospital, Glasgow, UK

Jan Bogaert, MD, PhD
Professor of Medicine, Department of Radiology, University Hospital Gasthuisberg, University of Leuven, Leuven, Belgium

Joyce G.R. Bomers, MSc PhD
Candidate, Department of Radiology, Radboud University Nijmegen Medical Centre, Nijmegen, The Netherlands

David J. Bowden, MA, VetMB, MB, BChir, FRCR
Senior Registrar, University of Cambridge, Addenbrooke's Hospital, Cambridge, UK

David J. Breen, MRCP, FRCR
Consultant Abdominal Radiologist; Honorary Senior Lecturer in Radiology, Department of Radiology, Southampton University Hospitals, Southampton, UK

Jackie Brown, BDS, MSc, FDSRCPS, DDRRCR
Consultant Dental and Maxillofacial Radiologist, Guy's and St Thomas' Hospitals Foundation Trust; Senior Lecturer at King's College London Dental Institute of Guy's, King's College and St Thomas' Hospitals, London, UK

Robert S.D. Campbell, MB, ChB, FRCR
Consultant Musculoskeletal Radiologist, Department of Radiology, Royal Liverpool University Hospital, Liverpool, UK

Dina F. Caroline, MD, PhD
Professor of Radiology, Temple University Hospital, Philadelphia, PA, USA

Jean-François Chateil, MD, PhD
Professor, CHU de Bordeaux, Service d'imagerie anténatale, de l'enfant et de la femme; University of Bordeaux, Bordeaux, France

W.K. 'Kling' Chong, BMedSci, MBChB, MD, MRCP, FRCR
Specialty Lead for Radiology/Imaging; Consultant Paediatric Neuroradiologist, Department of Radiology, Great Ormond Street Hospital, London, UK

Joo-Young Chun, MBBS, MSc, MRCS, FRCR
Consultant Interventional Radiologist, Royal London Hospital, Barts Health NHS Trust, London, UK

Richard H. Cohan, BA, MD, FACR
Professor of Radiology, Department of Radiology, University of Michigan Hospital, Ann Arbor, MI, USA

Susan J. Copley, MBBS, MD, FRCR, FRCP
Consultant Radiologist and Reader in Thoracic Imaging, Hammersmith Hospital, Imperial College NHS Trust, London, UK

David O. Cosgrove, MA, MSc, FRCP, FRCR
Emeritus Professor, Imaging Sciences, Imperial College, Hammersmith Hospital, London, UK

Nigel C. Cowan, MA, MB, Bchir, FRCP, FRCR
Consultant Radiologist, The Manor Hospital, Oxford, UK

Ahmed Daghir, MRCP, FRCR
Clinical Fellow, Department of Radiology, Nuffield Orthopaedic Centre, Oxford, UK

Maria Daskalogiannaki, MD, PhD
Consultant Radiologist, Radiology, University Hospital of Iraklion, Iraklion, Greece

Chandra Dass, MBBS, DMRD
Clinical Associate Professor, Department of Radiology, Temple University Hospital, Philadelphia, PA, USA

Indran Davangnanam, MB, BCh, BMedSci, FRCR
Consultant Neuroradiologist, National Hospital for Neurology and Neurosurgery, Lysholm Radiological Department; Radiology, Moorfields Eye Hospital; Honorary Research Associate, The Brain Repair and Rehabilitation Unit, Institute of Neurology, London, UK

A. Mark Davies, MBChB, DMRD, FRCR
Consultant Radiologist, MRI Centre, Royal Orthopaedic Hospital NHS Foundation Trust, Birmingham, UK

Albert de Roos, MD
Professor of Radiology, Department of Radiology, Leiden University Medical Center, Leiden, The Netherlands

Arthur M. De Schepper Sr., MD, PhD†
Former Radiologist, Department of Radiology, University Hospital Antwerp, Edegem, Belgium

Sujal R. Desai, MD, MRCP, FRCR
Consultant Radiologist, King's College Hospital, London, UK

Adrian K. Dixon, MD, FRCP, FRCR, FRCS, FFRRCSI(Hon), FRANZCR(Hon), FACR(Hon), FMedSci
Professor Emeritus of Radiology; Master, Peterhouse College, Cambridge, UK

Veronica Donoghue, FRCR, FFRRCSI
Consultant Paediatric Radiologist, Radiology Department, Children's University Hospital, Dublin, Ireland

Andrew J. Dunn, MBChB, FRCR
Consultant Musculoskeletal Radiologist, Department of Radiology, Royal Liverpool University Hospital, Liverpool, UK

Marina Easty, MBBS, BSc, MRCP, FRCR, PGCert Nuc Med
Consultant Paediatric Radiologist, Radiology Department, Great Ormond Street Hospital, London, UK

Robert J. Eckersley, PhD
Senior Lecturer, Division of Imaging Sciences, Biomedical Engineering Department, King's College London, St Thomas' Hospital, London, UK

Tarek El-Diasty, MD
Professor of Radiology, Radiology Department, Urology and Nephrology Center, Mansoura University, Mansoura, Egypt

Mohamed Abou El-Ghar, MD
Professor of Radiodiagnosis, Radiology Department, Urology and Nephrology Center, Mansoura University, Mansoura, Egypt

Christoph Engelke, MD
Geschäftsführender Oberarzt, Abteilung Diagnostische Radiologie, Universitätsmedizin Göttingen, Germany

Andrew J. Evans, MRCP, FRCR
Professor of Breast Imaging, University of Dundee, Hon Consultant Radiologist, NHS Tayside, Ninewells Hospital and Medical School, Dundee, UK

Rossella Fattori, MD
Professor of Radiology; Director, Invasive Cardiology, Emergency Department, San Salvatore Hospital, Pesaro, Italy

Kirsten Forbes, MB BChir, MD, MRCP, FRCR
Consultant Neuroradiologist, Department of Neuroradiology, Institute of Neurological Sciences, Southern General Hospital, Glasgow, UK

Tomás Franquet, MD
Chief Section of Thoracic Imaging, Department of Radiology, Hospital de Sant Pau; Associate Professor of Radiology, Universitat Autonoma de Barcelona, Barcelona, Spain

Alan H. Freeman, MBBS, FRCR
Consultant Radiologist, Department of Radiology, Addenbrooke's Hospital, Cambridge University Hospitals NHS Foundation Trust, Cambridge, UK

Susan Freeman, MRCP, FRCR
Consultant Radiologist, Department of Radiology, Cambridge University Hospitals NHS FoundationTrust, Cambridge, UK

Julia Frühwald-Pallamar, MD
Assistant Professor of Radiology, Medical University of Vienna, Department of Biomedical Imaging and Image-Guided Therapy, Subdivision of Neuroradiology and Musculoskeletal Radiology, Vienna, Austria

Ferdia Gallagher, MA, PhD, MRCP, FRCR
Cancer Research UK Clinician Scientist Fellow, CRUK Cambridge Research Institute; Honorary Consultant Radiologist, Addenbrooke's Hospital, Cambridge, UK

Massimo Gallucci, MD, PhD
Professor of Neuroradiology, Neuroradiology Service, San Salvatore University Hospital, L'Aquila, Italy

Bhaskar Ganai, BSc(MedSci) Hons, MBChB, MRCS, FRCR, EBIR
Lecturer in Interventional Radiology, Royal College of Surgeons in Ireland, Department of Radiology, Beaumont Hospital, Dublin, Ireland

Pilar Garcia-Peña, MD, PhD
Paediatric Radiologist, Hospital Materno-Infantil, Barcelona, Spain

Jacob Geleijns, PhD
Medical Physicist, Radiology Department, Leiden University Medical Center, Leiden, The Netherlands

Robert N. Gibson, MBBS, MD, FRANZCR, DDU
Professor, Department of Radiology, Royal Melbourne Hospital, Parkville, Victoria, Australia

Jonathan H. Gillard, BSc, MA, MD, FRCP, FRCR, MBA
Professor of Neuroradiology, University of Cambridge, Addenbrooke's Hospital, Cambridge, UK

†The editors were saddened to hear of the death of this outstanding author since submission of the typescript of this chapter.

Fergus Gleeson, MD
Radiologist, Department of Radiology, Churchill Hospital, Oxford, UK

Edmund M. Godfrey, MA, FRCR
Consultant Radiologist, Department of Radiology, Cambridge University Hospitals NHS Foundation Trust, Cambridge, UK

Vicky Goh, MA, MBBChir, MD, MRCP, FRCR
Chair of Clinical Cancer Imaging, Division of Imaging Sciences and Biomedical Engineering, King's College London; Honorary Consultant Radiologist, Guy's and St Thomas' Hospitals, London, UK

Beatriz Gomez Anson, MD, PhD, FRCR
Clinical Head of Neuroradiology, Unit of Neuroradiology, Department of Radiology, Hospital Santa Creu i Sant Pau, Universitat Autonoma, Barcelona, Spain

Nicholas Gourtsoyiannis, MD, PhD, FRCR(Hon), FRCSI(Hon)
Professor Emeritus, University of Crete, Medical School, Crete, Greece

Andrew J. Grainger, BM, BS, MRCP, FRCR
Consultant and Honorary Clinical Associate Professor, Musculoskeletal Radiology, Leeds Teaching Hospitals and Leeds Musculoskeletal Biomedical Research Centre, Leeds, UK

Claudio Granata, MD
Consultant Radiologist, Department of Radiology, IRCCS Giannina Gaslini, Italy

Martin J. Graves, PhD, Csci, FIPEM, FHEA
Consultant Clinical Scientist, Cambridge University Hospitals NHS Foundation Trust, Cambridge, UK

Philippe A. Grenier, MD
Professor, Radiology, Hôpital Pitié-Salpêtrière, Paris, France

Roxana S. Gunny, MBBS, MRCP, FRCR
Consultant Neuroradiologist, Department of Radiology, Great Ormond Street Hospital, London, UK

Christopher J. Hammond, BMBCh, MA, MRCS, FRCR
Consultant Vascular Radiologist, Department of Radiology, Leeds General Infirmary, Leeds, UK

David M. Hansell, MD, FRCP, FRCR, FRSM
Professor of Thoracic Imaging, Radiology, Royal Brompton Hospital, London, UK

Ieneke J.C. Hartmann, MD, PhD
Radiologist, Radiology, Maasstad Hospital, Rotterdam, The Netherlands

Christopher J. Harvey, MBBS, BSc, MRCP, FRCR
Consultant Radiologist, Department of Imaging, Hammersmith Hospital, London, UK

Melanie A. Hopper, MB ChB, MRCS, FRCR
Consultant Radiologist, Department of Radiology, Addenbrooke's Hospital, Cambridge University Hospitals NHS Foundation Trust, Cambridge, UK

Peter Hoskin, MD, FRCP, FRCR
Consultant in Clinical Oncology, Mount Vernon Cancer Centre, Northwood; Professor in Clinical Oncology, University College London, London, UK

Hedvig Hricak, MD, PhD, Dr(hc)
Chair, Department of Radiology, Memorial Sloan-Kettering Cancer Center, New York, NY, USA

Philip M. Hughes, MBBS, MRCP, FRCR
Consultant Radiologist, Radiology, Plymouth Hospitals Trust, Plymouth, Cornwall, UK

Paul Humphries, BSc, MBBS, MRCP, FRCR
Consultant Paediatric Radiologist, University College London Hospital NHS Trust and Great Ormond Street Hospital, London, UK

Brian F. Hutton, BSc, MSc, PhD
Professor of Medical Physics in Nuclear Medicine and Molecular Imaging Science, Institute of Nuclear Medicine, University College London, London, UK; Professor, Centre for Medical Radiation Physics, University of Wollongong, NSW, Australia

James E. Jackson, FRCP, FRCR
Consultant Radiologist, Department of Imaging, Hammersmith Hospital, London, UK

H. Rolf Jäger, MD, FRCR
Reader in Neuroradiology, Department of Brain Repair and Rehabilitation, UCL Institute of Neurology, UCL Faculty of Brain Sciences; Consultant Neuroradiologist, Lysholm Department of Neuroradiology, National Hospital for Neurology and Neurosurgery, and Department of Imaging, University College London Hospitals, London, UK

Jonathan J. James, BMBS, FRCR
Consultant Radiologist, Nottingham Breast Institute, City Hospital, Nottingham, UK

Steven L.J. James, MB, ChB, FRCR
Consultant Musculoskeletal Radiologist, The Royal Orthopaedic Hospital NHS Foundation Trust, Birmingham, UK

Cylen Javidan-Nejad, MD
Associate Professor of Cardiothoracic Radiology, Mallinckrodt Institute of Radiology, Washington University in St Louis, St Louis, MO, USA

Karl Johnson, BSc, MB ChB, MRCP, FRCR
Consultant Paediatric Radiologist, Birmingham Children's Hospital, Birmingham, UK

Brynmor P. Jones, BSc(Hons), MBBS, MRCP, FRCR
Consultant Neuroradiologist, Imperial College Healthcare NHS Trust, Charing Cross Hospital, London, UK

Hefin Jones, MRCP, FRCR
Radiologist, Department of Clinical Radiology, University Hospital Birmingham, New Queen Elizabeth Hospital, Birmingham, UK

Ruchi Kabra, MBBS, BSc, MRCS, FRCR
Neuroradiology Fellow, King's College Hospital, London, UK

Konstantinos Katsanos, MSc, MD, PhD, EBIR
Consultant Vascular and Interventional Radiologist, Endovascular, Spine and Interventional Oncology, Department of Interventional Radiology, Guy's and St Thomas' Hospitals, London, UK

Leonardo Kayat Bittencourt, MD
Radiologist, Department of Radiology, Federal University of Rio de Janeiro, Brazil

Aoife Keeling, FFRRCSI, MRCPI, MSc
Consultant Interventional Radiologist, Beaumont Hospital, Dublin, Ireland

Fleur Kilburn-Toppin, MA, MB, BChir, FRCR
Consultant Radiologist, West Suffolk Hospital, Bury St Edmunds, Suffolk, UK

Lucia J.M. Kroft, MD, PhD
Radiologist, Department of Radiology, Leiden University Medical Center, Leiden, The Netherlands

Olga Lazoura, MD, PhD
Consultant Radiologist, Royal Free Hospital, London, UK

Michael J. Lee, MSc, FRCPI, FRCR, FFRRCSI, FSIR, EBIR
Professor of Radiology, Royal College of Surgeons in Ireland; Consultant Interventional Radiologist, Beaumont Hospital, Dublin, Ireland

Adrian Lim, MD, FRCR
Adjunct Professor and Consultant Radiologist, Imperial College London Healthcare NHS Trust, London, UK

Thomas M. Link, MD, PhD
Professor of Radiology; Chief, Musculoskeletal Imaging; Clinical Director Musculoskeletal and Quantitative Imaging Research, Department of Radiology and Biomedical Imaging, University of California San Francisco, San Francisco, CA, USA

David J. Lomas, MA, MB, BChir, FRCR, FRCP
Professor of Clinical MRI, University Radiology Department, Addenbrooke's Hospital, Cambridge, UK

Luigi Lovato, MD
Radiologist, Cardiovascular Radiology Unit, Cardiothoracic Radiology, Cardiovascular-Thoracic Department, S. Orsola Hospital, Bologna, Italy

Patrick McLaughlin, MB BCh, BAO, BMedSc FFRRCSI
Lecturer in Radiology, Department of Radiology, University College Cork, Cork, Ireland

Eugene McNally, MB BCh, BAO, FRCPI, FRCR
Consultant Musculoskeletal Radiologist and Clinical Lead, Nuffield Orthopaedic Centre and University of Oxford, Oxford, UK

David MacVicar, MA, FRCP, FRCR, FBIR
Consultant Radiologist, Department of Diagnostic Radiology, Royal Marsden Hospital, Sutton, Surrey UK

Michael Maher, MD, FRCSI, FRCR, FFRRCSI
Professor of Radiology, University College Cork; Consultant Radiologist, Cork University Hospital and Mercy University Hospital, Cork, Ireland

Lorenzo Mannelli, MD, PhD
Radiologist, Department of Radiology, University of Washington, Seattle, WA, USA

Katharina Marten-Engelke, MD
Professor of Radiology, Diagnostic Breast Centre, Göttingen, Germany

Tomasz Matys, PhD, FRCR
Specialist Registrar in Clinical Radiology; Neuroradiology Fellow, Addenbrooke's Hospital, Cambridge University Hospitals NHS Foundation Trust, Cambridge, UK

James F.M. Meaney, FRCR
Consultant Radiologist; Director, Centre for Advanced Medical Imaging, St James's Hospital, Dublin, Ireland

Agostino Meduri, MD
Adjunct Professor, Bioimaging and Radiological Sciences, Catholic University of the Sacred Heart, Rome, Italy

Amrish Mehta, MBBS, BSc(Hons), FRCR
Consultant Neuroradiologist, Department of Imaging, Imperial College Healthcare NHS Trust, London, UK

Caroline Micallef, MD, FRCR
Consultant Neuroradiologist, National Hospital for Neurology and Neurosurgery, University College London Hospitals, London, UK

Kenneth A. Miles, MBBS, MD, MSc, FRCR, FRCP, FRANZCR
Professorial Research Associate, Institute of Nuclear Medicine, University College London, UK; Visiting Medical Officer, Department of Molecular Imaging, Princess Alexandra Hospital, Brisbane, Australia

Lisa A. Miller, MD
Assistant Professor, Department of Diagnostic Radiology and Nuclear Medicine, University of Maryland Medical School, Baltimore, MD, USA

Stuart E. Mirvis, MD, FACR
Professor of Diagnostic Radiology; Director, Division of Emergency Radiology, Department of Radiology and Nuclear Medicine, University of Maryland School of Medicine, Baltimore, MD, USA

Katherine Miszkiel, BM(Hons), MRCP, FRCR
Consultant Neuroradiologist, Lysholm Department of Neuroradiology, The National Hospital for Neuroradiology and Neurosurgery; Honorary Consultant Neuroradiologist, Moorfields Eye Hospital, London, UK

Robert A. Morgan, MB ChB, MRCP, FRCR, EBIR
Consultant Vascular and Interventional Radiologist, Radiology Department, St George's NHS Trust, London, UK

Iain D. Morrison, MBBS, MRCP, FRCR
Consultant Radiologist, Kent and Canterbury Hospital, East Kent Hospitals University NHS Foundation Trust, Canterbury, UK

Richard J. Morse, MBBS, MRCP, FRCR
Consultant Radiologist, Royal Cornwall Hospital, Truro, Cornwall, UK

Jonathan G. Moss, MB ChB, FRCS(Ed), FRCR
Professor of Interventional Radiology, Department of Radiology, North Glasgow University Hospitals, Gartnavel General Hospital, Glasgow, UK

Arjun Nair, MB ChB, MRCP, FRCR
Fellow in Thoracic Imaging, Department of Radiology, Royal Brompton Hospital, London, UK

Luigi Natale, MD
Researcher and Aggregate Professor of Radiology, Radiological Sciences Department, Catholic University of Sacred Heart, Rome, Italy

Anthony A. Nicholson, BSc, MSc, MB, ChB, FRCR, FFRRCSI(Hon), FCIRSE, EBIR
Consultant Vascular and Interventional Radiologist, Leeds Teaching Hospitals, Leeds, UK

Owen J. O'Connor, MD, FFRRCSI, MB, BCh, BAO, BMedSci
Inerventional Radiology Fellow, Radiology, Massachusetts General Hospital, Boston, MA, USA

Philip O'Connor, MBBS, MRCP, FRCR, FFSEM(UK)
Musculoskeletal Radiologist, Clinical Radiology, Leeds Teaching Hospitals Trust, The University of Leeds, West Yorkshire, UK

Paul O'Donnell, MBBS, MRCP, FRCR
Consultant Radiologist, Royal National Orthopaedic Hospital; Honorary Senior Lecturer, University College London, London, UK

Amaka C. Offiah, BSc, MBBS, MRCP, FRCR, PhD, HEFCE
Clinical Senior Lecturer, Academic Unit of Child Health, University of Sheffield; Consultant Paediatric Radiologist, Academic Unit of Child Health, Sheffield Children's NHS Foundation Trust, Sheffield, UK

Øystein E. Olsen, PhD
Consultant Radiologist, Radiology Department, Great Ormond Street Hospital, London, UK

Lil-Sofie Ording Müller, MD, PhD
Consultant Paediatric Radiologist, Section for Paediatric Radiology, Division of Diagnostics and Intervention, Oslo University Hospital, Ullevål, Oslo, Norway

Catherine M. Owens, BSc, MBBS, MRCP, FRCR
Consultant Radiologist and Honorary Reader, Department of Imaging, Great Ormond Street Hospital, London, UK

Simon P.G. Padley, MBBS, BSc, MRCP, FRCR
Consultant Radiologist, Chelsea and Westminster Hospital and Royal Brompton Hospital; Reader in Radiology, Imperial College School of Medicine, London, UK

Paul M. Parizel, MD, PhD
Professor and Chair, Department of Radiology, Antwerp University Hospital, University of Antwerp, Edegem, Belgium

Nadeem Parkar, MD
Fellow in Cardiothoracic Imaging, Mallinckrodt Institute of Radiology, Washington University in St Louis, St Louis, MO, USA

Uday Patel, MB ChB, MRCP, FRCR
Consultant Radiologist, Department of Radiology, St George's Hospital, London, UK

Anne Paterson, MBBS, MRCP, FRCR, FFRRCSI
Consultant Paediatric Radiologist, Department of Radiology, Royal Belfast Hospital for Sick Children, Belfast, UK

Andrew Plumb, BMBCh, MRCP, FRCR
Research Fellow in Gastrointestinal Radiology, University College London Hospitals, London, UK

Panos Prassopoulos, MD, PhD
Professor of Radiology, Department of Radiology, University Hospital of Alexandroupoli, Democritous University of Thrace, Alexandroupoli, Greece

Mathias Prokop, MD, PhD
Professor of Radiology; Chairman, Department of Radiology, Radboud University Medical Centre, Nijmegen, The Netherlands

Michael A. Quail, MSc, MB ChB(Hons), MRCPCH
British Heart Foundation Clinical Research Training Fellow, Centre for Cardiovascular Imaging, UCL Institute of Cardiovascular Science; Paediatric Cardiology Academic Clinical Fellow, Department of Cardiology, Great Ormond Street Hospital, London, UK

Nigel Raby, MB ChB, MRCP, FRCR
Consultant Radiologist, Department of Radiology, Western Infirmary, Glasgow, UK

Balashanmugam Rajashanker, MBBS, MRCP, FRCR
Consultant Radiologist, Clinical Radiology, Central Manchester Foundation Trust, Manchester, UK

James J. Rankine, MB ChB, MRCP, MRaD, FRCR, MD
Consultant Radiologist and Honorary Clinical Associate Professor, Department of Radiology, Leeds General Infirmary, Leeds, West Yorkshire, UK

Lakshmi Ratnam, MBChB, MRCP, FRCR
Consultant Interventional Radiologist, Radiology, St George's Hospital, London, UK

Jim A. Reekers, MD, PhD, EBIR
Professor of Radiology, Department of Radiology, Academic Medical Centre Amsterdam, University of Amsterdam, The Netherlands

Peter Reimer, MD, PhD
Professor, Institute of Diagnostic and Interventional Radiology, Klinikum Karlsruhe, Academic Teaching Hospital, Karlsruhe, Germany

John H. Reynolds, MMedSci, FRCR, DMRD
Consultant Radiologist, Department of Radiology, Birmingham Heartlands Hospital, Birmingham, UK

Rodney H. Reznek, MA, FRANZCR(Hon), FFRRCSI(Hon), FRCP, FRCR
Emeritus Professor of Cancer Imaging, Cancer Institute, Queen Mary's University London, St Bartholomew's Hospital, West Smithfield, London, UK

Michael Riccabona, OA
Professor, Department of Radiology, Division of Pediatric Radiology, Universitätsklinikum-LKH, Graz, Austria

James Ricketts, BMBS
Radiology Registrar, Derriford Hospital, Plymouth, UK

Karen Rosendahl, MD, PhD
Consultant Paediatric Radiologist, Haukeland University Hospital; Professor, Department of Clinical Medicine, University of Bergen, Norway

Andrea Rossi, MD
Head, Pediatric Neuroradiology Unit, Istituto Giannina Gaslini; Contract Professor of Neuroradiology, University of Genoa, Genoa, Italy

Giles Rottenberg, MBBS, MRCP, FRCR
Consultant Radiologist, Department of Radiology, Guy's and St Thomas' NHS Foundation Trust, London, UK

John Rout, BDS, FDSRCS, MDentSci, DDRRCR, FRCR
Consultant Oral and Maxillofacial Radiologist, Radiology Department, Birmingham Dental Hospital, Birmingham, UK

Alex Rovira, MD
Head of Magnetic Resonance Unit (IDI), Department of Radiology, Vall d'Hebron University Hospital, Barcelona, Spain

Elizabeth Rutherford, BMedSci, MBBS, MRCS, FRCR
Consultant Radiologist, University Hospitals Southampton NHS Trust, Southampton, UK

Tarun Sabarwal, FRCR, FRCRI, EBIR, FRSIR, FCIRSE
Consultant Interventional Radiologist, Clinical Lead Interventional Radiology, Guy's and St Thomas' Hospitals, London, UK

Anju Sahdev, MBBS, MRCP, FRCR
Consultant Uro-Gynae Radiologist, Department of Imaging, St Bartholomew's Hospital, Barts Health, West Smithfield, London, UK

Asif Saifuddin, BSc(Hons), MB ChB, MRCP, FRCR
Consultant Musculoskeletal Radiologist, Imaging Department, The Royal National Orthopaedic Hospital, Stanmore, Middlesex, UK

Evis Sala, MD, PhD, FRCR
University Lecturer and Honorary Consultant Radiologist, University Department of Radiology, Addenbrooke's Hospital, Cambridge, UK

Cornelia M. Schaefer-Prokop, MD, PhD
Professor of Radiology, Meander Medical Centre, Amersfoort, The Netherlands

Wolfgang Schima, MD, MSc
Professor, Department of Diagnostic and Interventional Radiology, KH Göttlicher Heiland Hospital; KH der Barmherzigen Schwestern Wien; Sankt Josef-Krankenhaus, Vienna, Austria

Daniel J. Scoffings, BSc(Hons), MBBS, MRCP(UK), FRCR
Consultant Neuroradiologist, Department of Radiology, Addenbrooke's Hospital, Cambridge, UK

Djilda Segerman, MA, MSc, MIPEM
Former Head of Nuclear Medicine Physics, Department of Nuclear Medicine, Brighton and Sussex University Hospitals NHS Trust, Brighton, UK

Eva Serrao, MD
Marie Curie Fellow, Cancer Research UK Cambridge Research Institute, University of Cambridge, Li Ka Shing Centre, Cambridge, UK

Nadeem Shaida, MRCP, FRCR, FHEA
Radiology Registrar, Department of Radiology, Cambridge University Hospitals NHS Foundation Trust, Cambridge, UK

Ashley S. Shaw, MB ChB, MRCP, FRCR, MA
Consultant and Associate Lecturer, Department of Radiology, Addenbrooke's Hospital, Cambridge, UK

John M. Stevens, MBBS, DRACR, FRCR
Consultant Radiologist (retired), formerly at Lyshom Department of Neuroradiology, Radiology Department, The National Hospital for Neurology and Neurosurgery, London, UK

Nasim Sheikh-Bahaei, MD, MRCP, FRCR
Clinical Lecturer, University Department of Radiology, Cambridge University Hospitals NHS Foundation Trust, Cambridge, UK

Beth Shepherd, MBBS, MA(Cantab), MRCS, FRCR
Radiology Registrar, University Hospital Southampton NHS Foundation Trust, Southampton, Hampshire, UK

Hans-Marc J. Siebelink, MD, PhD
Non-Invasive Imaging, Department of Cardiology, Leiden University Medical Center, Leiden, The Netherlands

Pia C. Sundgren, MD, PhD
Professor of Radiology; Head, Department of Diagnostic Radiology, Clinical Sciences Lund, Lund University; Center for Medical Imaging and Physiology, Skåne University Hospital, Lund, Sweden

Tom Sutherland, MBBS, MMed, FRANZCR
Radiologist, Medical Imaging Department, St Vincents Hospital, Melbourne, Victoria, Australia

Nicola Sverzellati, PhD
Researcher, Department of Surgical Sciences, Radiology Section, University of Parma, Parma, Italy

Denis Tack, MD, PhD
Radiologist, Department of Radiology, RHMS Clinique Louis Caty, Baudour; CHU de Charleroi, Charleroi, Belgium

Andrew M. Taylor, BA(Hons), BM BCh, MRCP, FRCR
Professor of Cardiovascular Imaging, Centre for Cardiovascular Imaging, UCL Institute of Cardiovascular Science and Great Ormond Street Hospital for Children, London, UK

Stuart A. Taylor, MBBS, BSc, MD, MRCP, FRCR
Professor of Medical Imaging, Centre for Medical Imaging, University College London, London, UK

Avnesh S. Thakor, BA, MA, MSc, MD, PhD, MB BChir, FHEA, FRCR
Fellow in Interventional Radiology, University of Cambridge, UK; Visiting Scholar, Molecular Imaging Program, Stanford University, CA, USA

Henrik S. Thomsen, MD, MSc
Professor of Radiology, Faculty of Health and Medical Sciences, University of Copenhagen and Consultant, Copenhagen University Hospital, Herlev, Denmark

Majda M. Thurnher, MD
Associate Professor of Radiology, Medical University Vienna, Department of Biomedical Imaging and Image-Guided Therapy, Vienna, Austria

Stefanie C. Thust, MD, FRCR
Neuroradiology Fellow, National Hospital of Neurorology and Neurosurgery, London, UK

Luc van den Hauwe, MD
Consultant Radiologist, Department of Radiology, University Hospital Antwerp, Edegem; Department of Radiology, AZ KLINA, Brasschaat, Belgium

Johan W. van Goethem, MD, PhD
Vice Departmental Head, Department of Radiology and Neuroradiology, Antwerp University Hospital, Edegem, Belgium

Thomas Van Thielen, MD
Resident, Department of Radiology, University Hospital Antwerp, Edegem, Belgium

Johny A. Verschakelen, MD, PhD
Director, Chest Radiology, Department of Radiology, University Hospitals Leuven, Leuven, Belgium

Geert M. Villeirs, MD, PhD
Radiologist, Division of Genitourinary Radiology, Ghent University Hospital, Ghent, Belgium

Zaid Viney, MBBS, MRCP, FRCR
Consultant Radiologist, Department of Radiology, Guy's and St Thomas' NHS Foundation Trust, London, UK

Sarah J. Vinnicombe, BSc(Hons), MRCP, FRCR
Clinical Senior Lecturer, Cancer Imaging; Honorary Consultant Radiologist, Division of Imaging and Technology, Medical Research Institute, Ninewells Hospital Medical School, Dundee, UK

Anthony Watkinson, BSc, MSc, MBBS, FRCS, FRCR, EBIR
Consultant Radiologist, The Royal Devon and Exeter Hospital; Honorary Professor of Interventional Radiology, The Peninsula Medical School, Exeter, UK

Tom A. Watson, MBChB, FRCR
Paediatric Radiology Fellow, Department of Imaging, Great Ormond Street Hospital, London, UK

Jos J.M. Westenberg, PhD
Assistant Professor, Department of Radiology, Leiden University Medical Center, Leiden, The Netherlands

Richard W. Whitehouse, MB, ChB, MD, FRCR
Consultant Radiologist, Clinical Radiology, Manchester Royal Infirmary, Manchester, UK

Iain D. Wilkinson, BSc, MSc, PhD
Professor of MR Physics, Academic Radiology, University of Sheffield, Sheffield, UK

A. Robin M. Wilson, FRCR, FRCP(E)
Consultant Radiologist, Department of Clinical Radiology, The Royal Marsden Hospital, Sutton, UK

Reddi Prasad Yadavali, MBBS, MRCS, FRCR, EBIR
Consultant Interventional Radiologist, Department of Radiology, Aberdeen Royal Infirmary; Honorary Senior Clinical Lecturer, School of Medicine and Dentistry, University of Aberdeen, Aberdeen, UK

Carolyn Young, HDCR
Radiographer, Radiology Department, Great Ormond Street Hospital, London, UK

Peter Zampakis, PhD, MSc, MD
Consultant Neuroradiologist, Radiology, University Hospital of Patras, Patras, Achaias, Greece

SECTION D

THE MUSCULOSKELETAL SYSTEM

Section Editors: Andrew J. Grainger • Philip O'Connor

CHAPTER 45

Imaging Techniques and Fundamental Observations for the Musculoskeletal System

Philip W.P. Bearcroft • Melanie A. Hopper

CHAPTER OUTLINE

INTRODUCTION

There are numerous imaging investigations available to clinicians and radiologists for the assessment of musculoskeletal disease. This chapter will describe the individual investigations, concentrating on the strengths and weaknesses of each technique. Variations will be discussed and recent imaging advances detailed. A working knowledge of the normal appearance of musculoskeletal structures is essential and these will then be described. Finally, three common imaging scenarios will be explained: calcification in soft tissues, gas in soft tissues and periosteal reaction.

IMAGING TECHNIQUES AVAILABLE

Radiography

Radiography has an important role in the preliminary evaluation of musculoskeletal disorders and for many conditions no further imaging is required. The technique relies upon the differing absorption of ionising radiation by tissues within the body. As a result, radiography provides excellent contrast between tissues such as fat and muscle and bone. It does not, however, provide contrast between soft tissues and has limited ability to demonstrate bone loss compared to cross-sectional techniques.

To aid diagnosis, two views of a body part are typically taken. Conventionally these are in the lateral plane and the anteroposterior (AP) plane, which is termed dorsopedal (DP) in the feet and dorsopalmar (DP) in the hands. Particularly in trauma, two views, preferably orthogonal, are important to minimise misinterpretation of overlapping structures (Fig. 45-1).

In complex anatomical areas or when specific information is needed, additional or alternative views are frequently obtained.

Benefits

Radiographs are readily available as an imaging technique. Traditionally viewed as hard copy film, technological advances now mean that in the majority of institutions radiographs are obtained, viewed and stored digitally. The picture archiving and communication system (PACS) provides immediate access to previous radiographs for comparison not just for radiography but for all imaging investigations.

Radiographs also provide initial soft-tissue assessment and can demonstrate soft-tissue swelling as well as joint effusions, which can be particularly useful in areas where bony abnormality may be radiographically occult (Fig. 45-2).

Disadvantages

An awareness of the limitations of radiographic evaluation is crucial. As in other areas of the body, artefact from external structures such as clothing and from overlapping structures can be misinterpreted as an abnormality. Some sites can be difficult to appreciate fully using radiographs. The medial end of the clavicle, for example, can be problematic due to multiple overlying structures and an abnormality may be more difficult to detect. It is important that radiographs, as with other imaging investigations, are interpreted in light of the clinical details and additional imaging should be undertaken if concern persists. The lack of radiographic soft-tissue evaluation is well recognised as the attenuation of X-rays by most soft-tissue structures lies within a narrow range and this limits the interrogation of soft-tissue structures.

One of the main drawbacks of radiography is its reliance upon ionising radiation and the potential resulting side effects. However, particularly in the extremities, the dose involved is minimal and although the hazards of

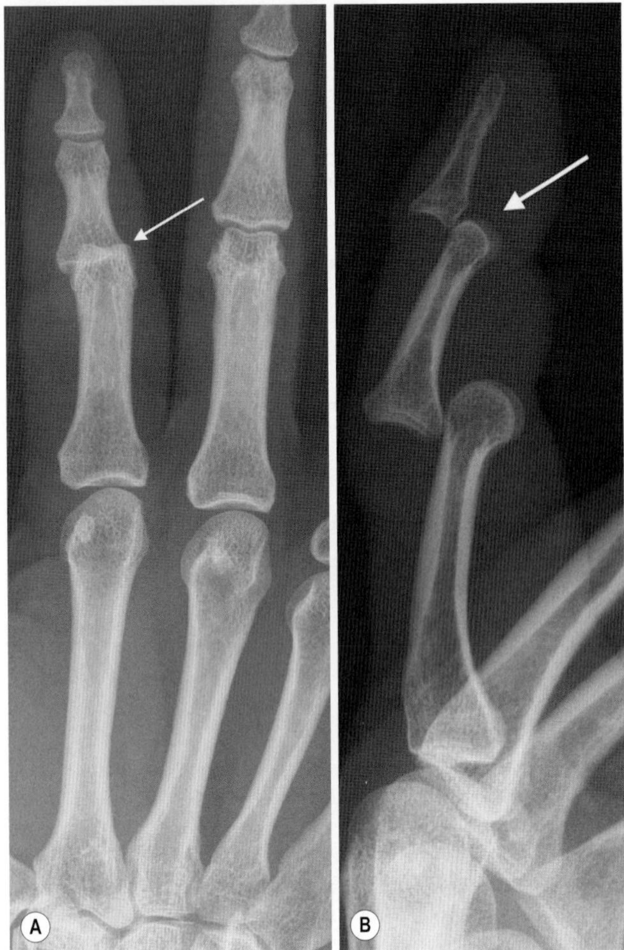

FIGURE 45-1 ■ (A) AP radiograph of index finger demonstrates dislocation of the proximal interphalangeal joint (arrow). (B) Dislocated distal interphalangeal joint is only evident on the orthogonal view (arrow).

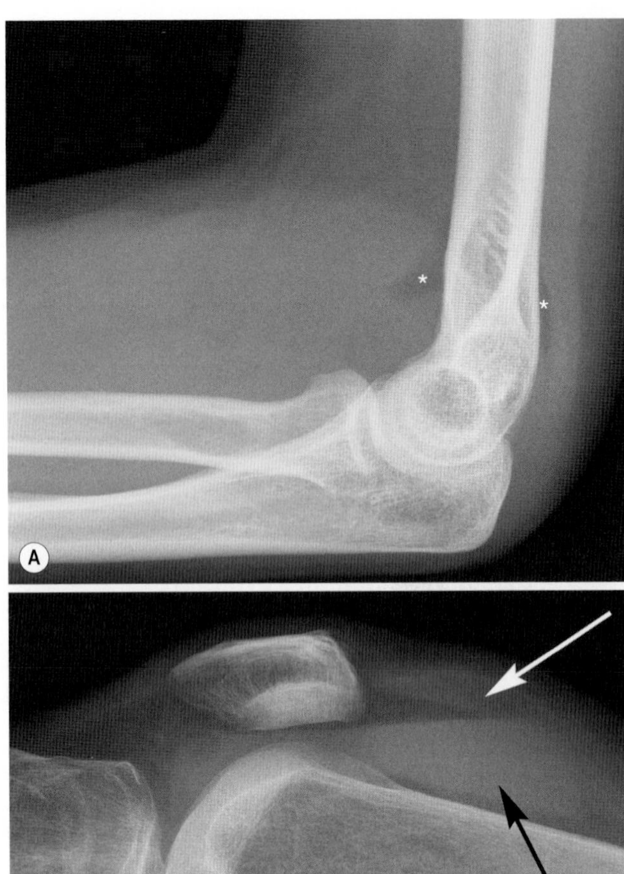

FIGURE 45-2 ■ (A) Lateral radiograph of the elbow shows joint effusion displacing the fat pads (*) indicating intra-articular injury. (B) Horizontal beam lateral radiograph of the knee shows lipohaemarthrosis due to occult fracture with a linear fat (white arrow)/fluid (black arrow) level.

ionising radiation should never be ignored, the diagnostic benefits generally outweigh the possible risk when radiographs are correctly used.

Advances and Variations

Stress Views. Standard radiographs allow static evaluation of musculoskeletal structures. Imaging a joint under passive or active stress may also provide indirect assessment of ligamentous injury.[1,2] For example, comparative flexion and extension views of the cervical spine provide valuable information regarding stability of the atlanto-axial joint (Fig. 45-3).

Fluoroscopy. Fluoroscopic techniques have a wide range of uses across radiological specialties. They utilise an X-ray source similar to standard radiographs but provide real-time dynamic video images that are typically used in the radiology department and in orthopaedic surgery to guide interventional procedures such as needle placement and fracture reduction. Images are viewed on a digital unit and are amplified to enable them to be seen in normal light, especially useful in the operating theatre.

Arthrography. The basic premise of arthrography is the injection of a radio-opaque contrast medium into a joint usually guided by fluoroscopy, although US guidance can be used as an alternative. Distension of the joint provides indirect information about the soft tissues which can be deduced from the distribution of the injected contrast medium (Fig. 45-4). Fluoroscopic evaluation also allows an element of dynamic assessment. With the advent of more sophisticated cross-sectional imaging which provides detailed and direct assessment of the internal joint structures, arthrography is now more frequently used in combination with MRI and, occasionally, CT following the injection of gadolinium-based or iodine-based contrast medium, respectively. Arthrography is frequently combined with the injection of local anaesthetic to

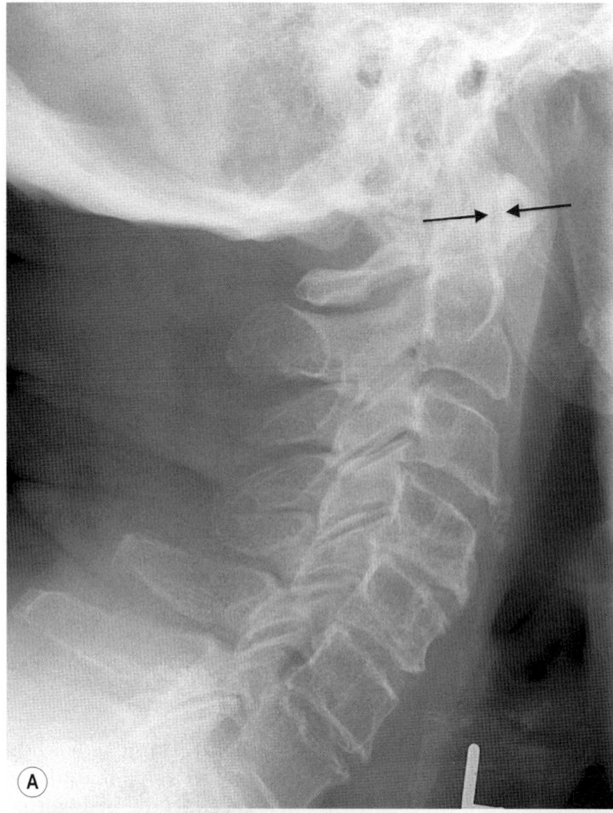

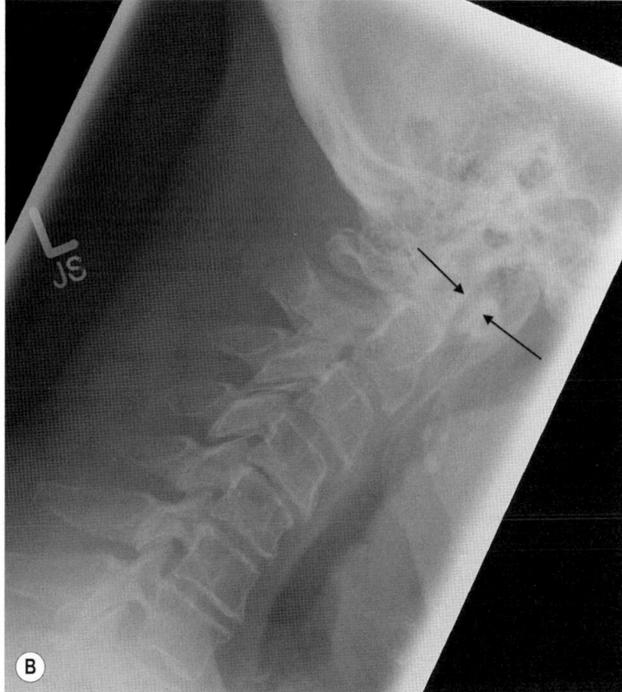

FIGURE 45-3 ■ Lateral radiographs of the cervical spine in (A) extension and (B) flexion. Atlantoaxial subluxation due to disruption of the transverse ligament is demonstrated on the view taken in flexion with widening of the atlantoaxial distance (black arrows).

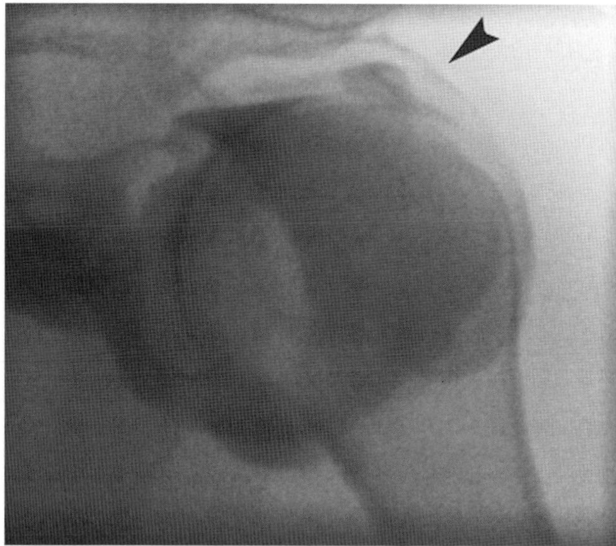

FIGURE 45-4 ■ Fluoroscopic image of the shoulder shows contrast medium within the glenohumeral joint extending into the subacromial bursa (arrowhead) indicating a rotator cuff tear.

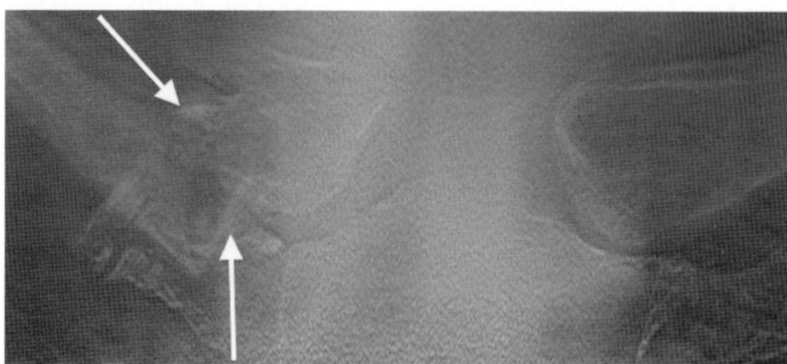

FIGURE 45-5 ■ Tomographic image of medial right medial clavicle fracture (arrows), normal left side.

provide additional diagnostic information in patients with possible joint symptoms, helping distinguish assymtpomatic and symptomatic abnormalities; corticosteroid may be introduced as a therapeutic agent.

Tomosynthesis. Digital tomosynthesis represents a modification of the conventional radiographic technique to acquire multiple low-dose images of a body part across a range of projection angles of the X-ray tube. Currently well established in breast imaging, interest in the application of tomosynthesis to other areas, including the musculoskeletal system, is growing.[3] The radiation dose is greater than that of conventional radiography but less than CT and preliminary studies suggest it has a role in the imaging of orthopaedic prostheses as the metallic-related streak artefacts encountered with CT is reduced.[4] Digital tomosynthesis also reduces the difficulty of composite shadow, showing promise in the assessment of anatomically complex areas (Fig. 45-5).

Ultrasound (US)

In current clinical practice US has an important role in the diagnosis and management of musculoskeletal disease,

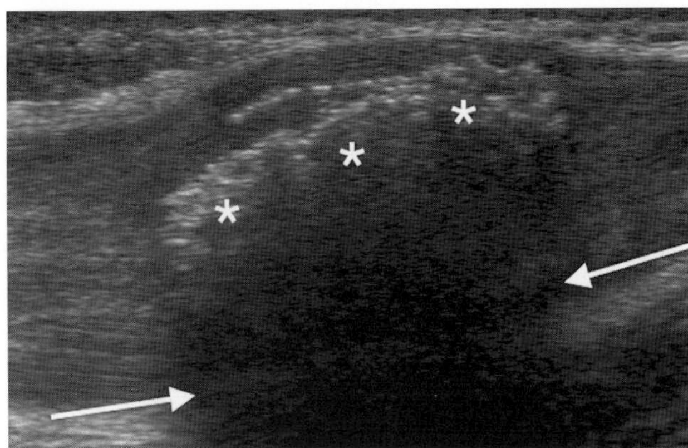

FIGURE 45-6 ■ Sonographic image of the medial thigh shows heterotopic calcification (*) and posterior acoustic shadowing (arrows) within the adductor musculature not evident on radiographic assessment.

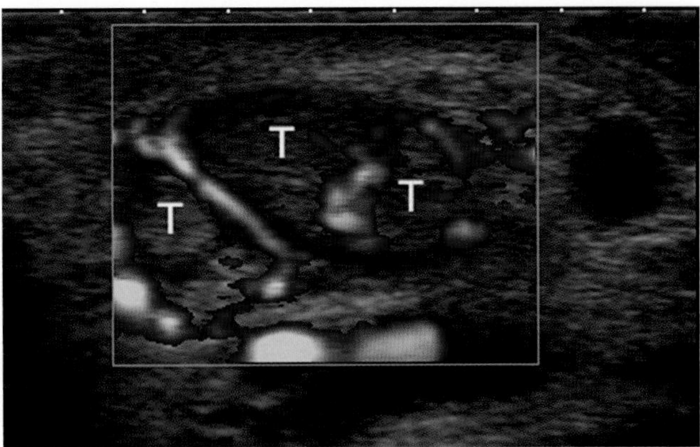

FIGURE 45-7 ■ Transverse PD sonogram of the first extensor compartment tendons (T) at the wrist. Abnormal vascularisation, particularly within the tendon sheath surrounding the tendons, indicates tenosynovitis.

providing high-resolution assessment of soft tissues. Evaluation of bone is limited, but US can afford information regarding the bony surface and periosteum. Typically, musculoskeletal US requires a linear array high-frequency probe of at least 7 MHz, and greater than 10 MHz is preferred. This is ideal for superficial abnormalities; deeper lesions necessitate a lower-frequency probe to provide adequate depth, albeit at reduced spatial resolution.

Benefits

US main benefits lie in its ability to give real-time, high-resolution and dynamic diagnostic information. In general the technique is fast and well tolerated by patients and allows direct clinical correlation of symptoms and abnormalites by the operator. Importantly, there is no ionising radiation. The ability of US to differentiate between solid and cystic structures is particularly useful in the musculoskeletal system. Soft-tissue calcification is evident earlier on US than on radiographs (Fig. 45-6).

Doppler assessment of vascularity is important in soft-tissue masses and also in the assessment of inflammatory and degenerative disorders where the presence of new blood vessel formation, known as neovascularisation, can be used to indicate disease activity and healing (Fig. 45-7). For the assessment of the majority of musculoskeletal conditions, the direction of vascular flow is not particularly useful and so the more sensitive power Doppler (PD) is favoured over colour Doppler techniques, as PD maximises spatial resolution and flow sensitivity at the expense of directional information.

The ability of US to demonstrate the movement of tissues in real time underpins one of its main advantages during review of musculoskeletal disorders. Abnormalities such as tendon subluxation and impingement may be clinically suspected but confirmation using real-time US can be invaluable diagnostically and as an aid to treatment. There is widespread use of US guidance for interventional techniques. The anatomy of the extremities in particular allows excellent needle visualisation as it is nearly always possible to position the needle parallel to the transducer, maximising the clarity with which a needle is seen.

Disadvantages

Ultrasound is operator dependent and there is a steep learning curve. Artefacts can be challenging in musculoskeletal scanning.[5] Anisotropy describes the artefactual loss of tissue reflectivity when the US beam is applied at an oblique course to the tissue fibres under examination. The highly structured and fibrillar arrangement of tissues such as tendons and muscle makes this a particular problem in musculoskeletal US (Fig. 45-8A) and the resultant hypoechogenicity can simulate an abnormality such as tendinosis or tearing of a muscle or tendon. Beam edge artefact is evident at the edge of larger tendons such as the Achilles, with loss of normal signal and posterior acoustic shadowing that can mimic or conceal abnormal findings.

Advances and Variations

Beam steering of the transducer array produces tilting of the beam electronically of up to 40° from the main beam direction. When utilised instead of, or in addition to, manual angulation of the probe, this allows image generation from differing angles and provides a reduction in or even elimination of anisotropic artefact (Fig. 45-8).

Extended field-of-view (EFOV) or panoramic ultrasound gives a continuous image greater than the size of the ultrasound probe and although this does not necessarily improve the diagnostic ability of US, it provides images which more readily demonstrate the relevant abnormal findings than on the static images obtained by the operator (Fig. 45-9).

Elastography. The US assessment of tissue elasticity as an aid to diagnosis is well established in other radiological sub-specialities such as breast imaging and early studies suggest that there will be a role for the technique in musculoskeletal scanning. Elastography provides an assessment of tissue stiffness and requires the operator to

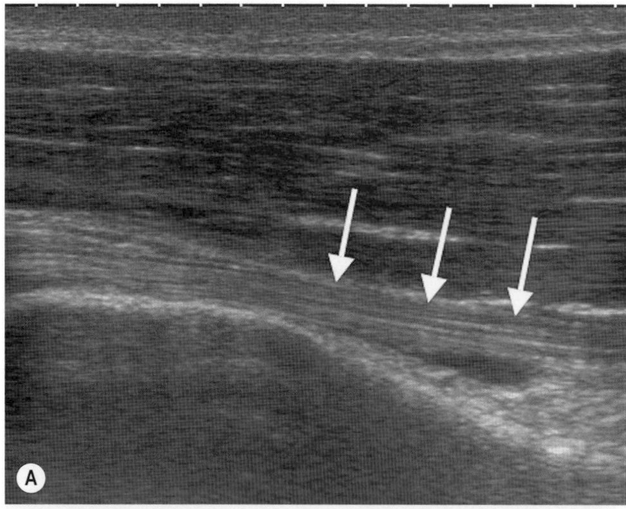

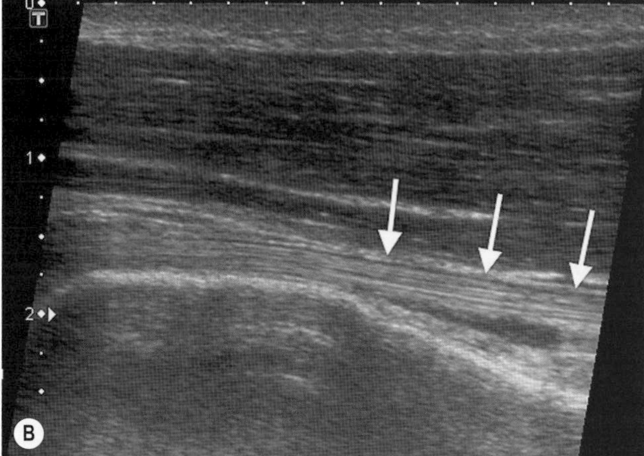

FIGURE 45-8 ■ Longitudinal ultrasound images of the long head of biceps tendon (arrows). (A) Distal anisotropic artefact. (B) Artefact eliminated using beam steer.

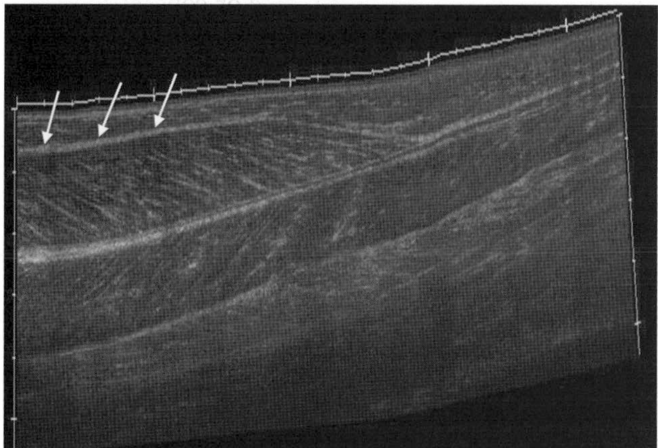

FIGURE 45-9 ■ EFOV sonogram of the lower calf shows hypoechoic fascicle bundles covered by hyperechoic perimysium. Echogenic epimysium surrounds each muscle (arrows).

gently compress the tissues under evaluation beneath the transducer. The strain or displacement of the tissues is determined by their hardness or softness. Normal ligaments and tendons are resistant to compression but tissue softening occurs in several conditions including degeneration and trauma.[6] The potential of elastography does not lie in the replacement of traditional B-mode US imaging but rather as a complementary technique. There is particular potential in the assessment of soft-tissue conditions which on B- mode imaging have an isoechoic appearance to the normal surrounding tissues such as early tendon degeneration or tearing (Fig. 45-10).

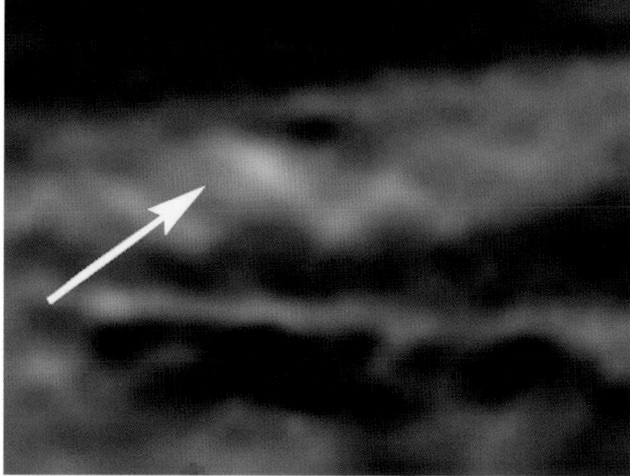

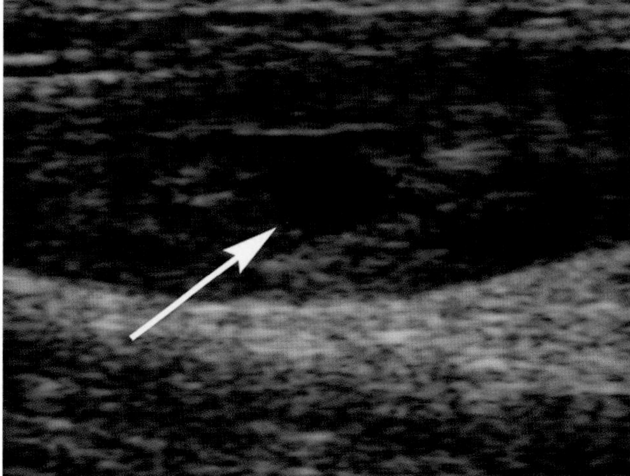

FIGURE 45-10 ■ Partial thickness tear of the Achilles tendon. B-mode US shows focal hypoechogenicity (lower arrow). Elastogram shows decreased tendon stiffness (upper arrow).

Contrast-enhanced US. Development of abnormal new blood vessels in musculoskeletal pathology is accompanied by the formation of abnormal nerves and there is good scientific correlation between these changes and pain.[7] Therefore, the early identification of new vessels is important in the diagnosis of disease and potentially provides a target for treatment (Fig. 45-7).

Contrast media-enhanced US (CEUS) detects low blood flow that may not be detectable by more traditional Doppler techniques. The intravenous injection of microbubble contrast media has been shown to allow more accurate assessment of synovial vascularity, which in turn correlates with disease activity in rheumatological disorders.[8] How this will influence patient management in the clinical setting is not fully understood and currently the use of CEUS in the assessment and follow-up of rheumatological disease remains at the research level.

Computed Tomography (CT)

Benefits

CT is ideally suited for the evaluation of bony structures and soft-tissue calcification and provides excellent spatial resolution and demarcation of bony structure and detail. Typically, images are acquired in the axial plane but it is a noteworthy strength that CT images can be reconstructed into any other plane. Surface 3D-rendered reformatting can also be a useful aid to surgical planning.

Despite its limitations in assessment of muscle and fat, CT has a role in imaging patients in whom MRI is contraindicated and can be combined with the injection of intra-articular iodinated contrast media in a similar way to the more widely utilised MR arthrography.

Disadvantages

As with radiography, CT relies upon ionising radiation. CT, even of an extremity, is associated with a radiation dose many times that of conventional radiography. This is more of a consideration in CT of the axial skeleton where radiation is also directed through the thoracic and abdominal organs. For the evaluation of musculoskeletal conditions, the main weakness of CT lies in the poor differentiation of soft-tissues structures as, even when abnormal, their attenuation values remain similar to adjacent normal structures and so are relatively poorly demonstrated. Despite the structural bony detail afforded, CT is not the optimum imaging investigation for infiltrative bone marrow disorders as alterations in the water/fat content are generally more usefully demonstrated using MRI. Artefact from metallic devices such as orthopaedic prostheses is arguably less problematic for CT than MRI but may still limit diagnostic performance.

Advances and Variations

Many advances in modern CT imaging are directed towards maintaining image quality whilst reducing dose and a variety of techniques such as multiplanar image acquisition and iterative reconstruction have been employed.[9] CT is widely used for detailed evaluation of bony trauma and fracture assessment. The exquisite bone detail it provides allows for review of focal bony metastases, be they lytic, sclerotic or mixed. These are generally more conspicuous on MR images but CT crucially provides important information regarding cortical breach and potential pathological fracture risk.

Dual-energy CT. Utilising two X-ray tubes positioned at 90° to each other with corresponding detectors allows the simultaneous acquisition of images with different energy levels. Analysis of the data sets can differentiate, for example, uric acid crystals from gout against calcium within soft tissues and thus reliably detect gouty tophi.[10,11] Dual-energy CT also has been shown to demonstrate post-traumatic bone bruising due to changes in marrow composition,[12] previously an area where CT has not been helpful.

The role of CT is continuously expanding; for example, in many centres radiographic skeletal surveys for multiple myeloma have been successfully replaced with vertex-to-knee low-dose CT.[13]

Magnetic Resonance Imaging (MRI)

The advent of MRI revolutionised the imaging of musculoskeletal structures, providing unequalled direct assessment of soft tissues and joints.

Benefits

MR images are generated by the effect of a strong magnetic field on the hydrogen nuclei in water molecules, thereby avoiding the potential risks of ionising radiation. Like CT, MRI provides excellent spatial resolution but its ability to distinguish between two similar tissues (contrast resolution) is far superior. MRI is a rapidly progressing technology; particular interest has evolved in functional MRI techniques, enabling the visualisation of physiological processes and their changes in different disease states.

Disadvantages

The contraindications of MRI apply to imaging musculoskeletal structures as to any body system. Because of the strong magnetic field strength, many implantable medical devices such as cardiac pacemakers are considered to be unsafe. Ferrous materials also cause significant difficulty for the radiologist due to susceptibility artefact from image distortion and signal voids. Modern orthopaedic prostheses produced from titanium and other non-ferrous materials are less problematic than older devices but can still provide a challenge. Much time has been invested in the development and improvement of metal artefact reduction sequences (MARS) to limit this problem.[14] MRI is highly sensitive but findings are not always specific. High signal within bone marrow on fluid-sensitive sequences, for example, may be due to a range of clinical entities from trauma to infection or tumour. It is therefore important to interpret imaging findings in the context of clinical history and examination. MR is not a stand-alone technique and correlation with other investigations is important.

Advances and Variations

MR Arthrography. Performing arthrography with gadolinium contrast medium and combining with MRI provides joint distension and additional information about the internal joint structures.[15] Used principally in the shoulder and hip, MR arthrography has a particular use for the assessment of labral injury.

Cartilage Imaging. MRI is an excellent investigation for non-invasive assessment of articular cartilage. As advances develop in the treatment of chondral injury, so the interest in accurate cartilage-specific sequences increases. As yet, no single sequence has proven to be perfect and advances have concentrated on assessment of morphological changes and biochemical alterations in early chondral damage.

Imaging sequences such as fluid-sensitive fast spin-echo (FSE) and 3D T1-weighted spoiled gradient-recalled echo (SPRG) provide excellent review of morphological changes such as surface fissuring and cartilage loss. Biochemical changes relate mainly to variation in cartilage water content and abnormalities of proteoglycan composition and distribution which have been shown to correlate with cartilage degeneration. Anomalies in water content can be assessed by T2 mapping and techniques such as delayed gadolinium-enhanced MR imaging cartilage (dGEMRIC) identify abnormality of chondral structure before morphological abnormalities become evident. Newer techniques assessing cartilage sodium content (Na MRI) show promise in the early identification of cartilage injury.[16]

MR Elastography (MRE). Changes in muscle structure and/or composition can occur in a range of conditions causing alteration of tissue stiffness. MRE gives a quantitative and non-invasive assessment of tissue stiffness by measuring the propagation of mechanical waves through the tissue. MRE has already proven useful in liver and breast disease. Studies have shown the technique can evaluate changes in the mechanical properties of muscle due to conditions such as neuromuscular disease and malignancy but the role of MRE in routine practice has yet to be established.[17]

Diffusion-weighted MRI. Diffusion-weighted MRI (DWI) provides tissue characterisation visualising the movement of water molecules. Diseased tissues demonstrate altered diffusion capacity and several studies have indicated improved sensitivity in the detection of skeletal metastases when comparing DWI to conventional MRI. MR can also assess the direction of water diffusion; this provides diffusion tensor imaging and tractography.[18] Initial results in musculoskeletal diseases have been promising as it is now possible to appreciate directly variations in fibre microarchitecture in, for example, muscles rather than secondary change.

Nuclear Medicine

All nuclear medicine scintigraphic procedures require the introduction of a radiopharmaceutical into the patient; the emitted radiation is then detected by a camera and displayed in much the same way as a standard radiograph. The skeletal scintogram is the most commonly encountered nuclear medicine technique for the evaluation of musculoskeletal abnormalities. This utilises technetium-99m-labelled methylene diphosphonate (^{99m}Tc-MDP), which identifies increased osteoblastic activity and therefore areas of high bone turnover (Fig. 45-11).

Benefits

Bone scintigraphy is widely available and is highly sensitive for a broad spectrum of osseous conditions as changes in bone metabolism predate alterations in morphology.

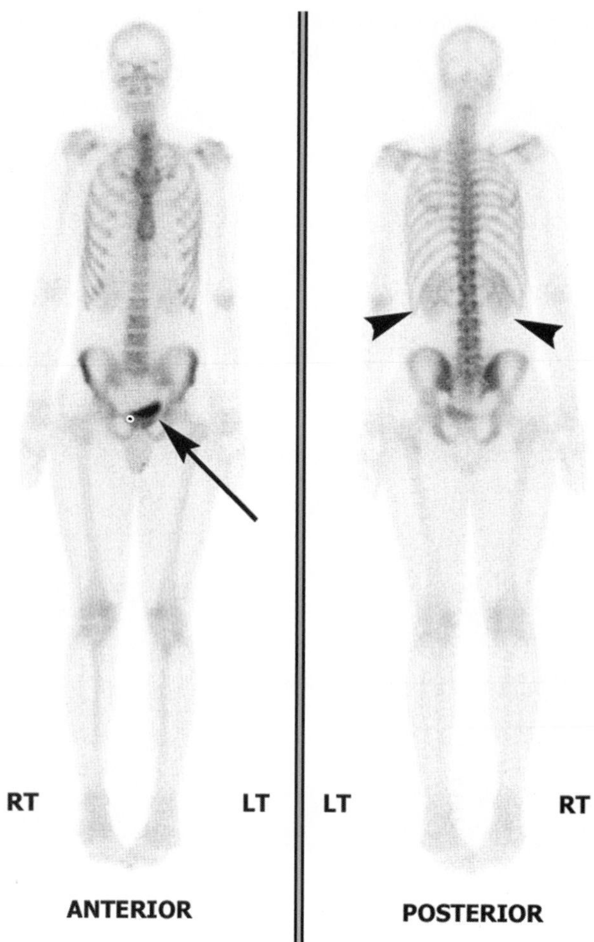

FIGURE 45-11 ■ ^{99m}Tc-MDP bone scintogram shows normal distribution of radiotracer within the skeleton and urinary tract. The renal outlines are visible (arrowhead) and radiotracer is evident within the urinary bladder (arrow).

It delivers a functional assessment of bone metabolism of the entire skeleton at the same time. Triple-phase scintigraphy obtains images at three different time periods after injection of the radiotracer and improves the differentiation of bony and soft-tissue disease.

Disadvantages

Although highly sensitive, bone scintigraphy has low specificity. Increased bone turnover is evident in a wide spectrum of bone disorders, including degeneration, infection, trauma and malignancy. Lytic lesions without increase in osteoblastic activity such as multiple myeloma are occult. Accurate localisation can be difficult, particularly in anatomically complex locations. The radiation dose of the injected radiotracer is high compared to radiography and is applied to the entire body rather than limited to the area under review. The spatial resolution of standard scintigraphy is several times less than other imaging investigations.

Advances and Variations

Single photon emission computed tomography (SPECT) can be utilised in musculoskeletal disease using similar

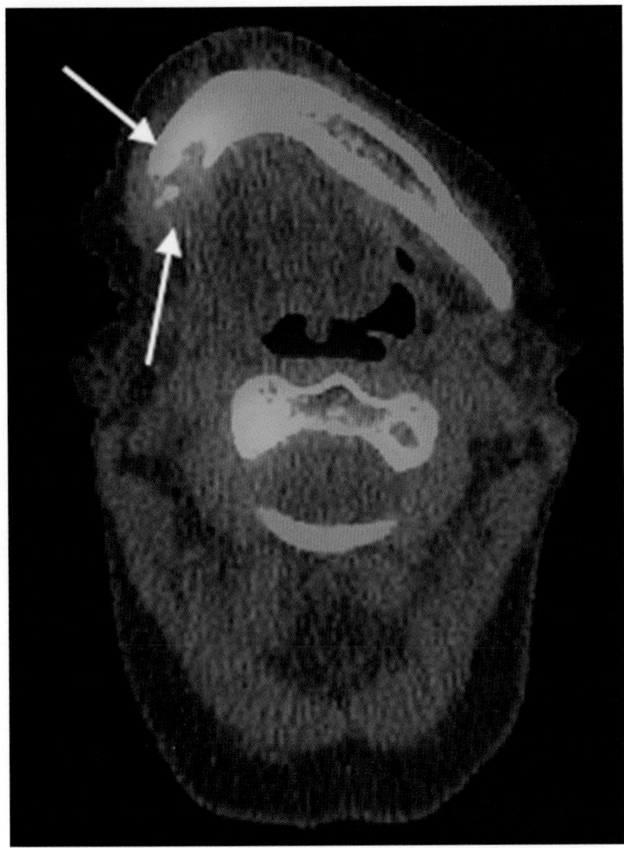

FIGURE 45-12 ■ **SPECT CT of the mandible.** Axial image shows increased radiotracer uptake (arrows) due to osteonecrosis of the jaw; increased uptake posteriorly is due to degeneration within the cervical spine.

radiopharmecuticals to traditional bone scintigraphy. The benefit lies in the multiplanar data acquired, which can be reformatted to provide 3D images. Side-by-side comparison with CT or overlying both data sets with software-based fusion can give anatomical correlation, but this is being superseded by hybrid SPECT CT superimposing the scintigraphic findings on high-resolution CT images to give functional anatomical mapping (Fig. 45-12). Studies suggest this may be useful in assessment of a range of musculoskeletal disorders such as infection, trauma and osteoarthrosis, particularly in areas such as the spine and other anatomically complex locations.[19]

NORMAL IMAGING APPEARANCES

Radiography

Bones and Joints

Radiographs provide an excellent primary assessment of bone and joint conditions. In the case of trauma, radiographs reliably identify fractures and dislocation. They provide useful assessment of painful bones and joints and are invaluable for the review of bony deformity and anatomical variation. Normal bone has a dense cortex of varying thickness. Radiographs demonstrate a distinct corticomedullary junction and within the medulla trabecular structure should be appreciated. Different bones have differing ratios of cortex and medullary cavity; this affects their radiographic appearance and how readily abnormality is radiographically visualised when diseased.

Soft Tissues

Air, fat and skeletal muscle have differing absorption characteristics for ionising radiation and it is possible to discriminate between them on radiographs. In general, however, radiographs have poor sensitivity for the detection of soft-tissue abnormalities.

Ultrasound

Bone and Joints

Ultrasound is unable to provide diagnostic information regarding internal bone structure but periosteal reaction may be seen and US can be used to confirm fractures of superficial bones such as metatarsal stress fractures or fractures in children. The growth plate can be identified as a distinct hypoechoic interruption to the hyperechoic cortex in the skeletally immature skeleton and should not be mistaken for a fracture.

There is increasing interest in the use of US as an aid to clinical assessment of joint disease.[20] US is highly sensitive for the detection of joint fluid. Simple joint fluid is hypoechoic and compressible and posterior acoustic enhancement can be appreciated. Internal echoes within joint fluid may be seen due to debris, proteinaceous fluid, crystal arthropathy and even loose bodies. Normal synovium is not visible at US. Abnormal synovium has a wide range of appearances from anechoic to hyperechoic intra-articular tissue. Internal vascularity can be helpful and, unlike joint fluid, thickened synovium may be deformed by probe pressure but is not displaced.

Hyaline cartilage has a uniform hypoechoic appearance similar to joint fluid. It may be necessary to displace adjacent joint fluid with probe pressure to fully appreciate the underlying cartilage. The bone cortex should be clearly evident as a continuous hyperechoic structure. Near the articular surfaces, in particular, normal grooves in the cortex should not be mistaken for bony erosions; this is particularly prominent over the dorsal aspect of the metacarpal heads.

Soft Tissues

Fat. Subcutaneous fat is clearly defined as a separate layer deep to the dermal tissues. Predominantly hypoechoic, there are multiple linear hyperechoic connective tissue septa within the fat. The majority of these lie parallel to the skin surface.

Muscle, Tendons and Ligaments. The majority of skeletal muscle is superficial and therefore readily assessed using a linear array high-frequency transducer.

A lower-frequency linear probe or even a curvilinear probe may be used for deeper structures such as the gluteal musculature. Skeletal muscle is generally less echogenic than subcutaneous fat with a highly organised configuration. Muscle fibres are arranged as separate hypoechoic fascicles wrapped by a thin connective tissue endomysium which is not readily visualised. Groups of fascicles are bundled together by a thicker, echogenic perimysial sheath, clearly distinguished at US. Each muscle is encompassed by a dense and irregular connective tissue echogenic epimysium; this layer forms a continuation with the tendon and with the endomysium and perimysium (Fig. 45-9). Finally there is a fascial integument covering the epimysium; this is not defined as a separate structure at imaging. The echogenicity of muscle can change, depending upon its state; relaxed muscle is often more echogenic than when contracted.

Muscle fibres frequently lie obliquely to the skin surface and this, combined with their linear arrangement, makes anisotropic artefact a consideration when evaluating for abnormality. It is important to appreciate the underlying muscle structure and to image transverse and longitudinal to the muscle not just to the limb.

Tendons possess a fibrillar arrangement of echogenic fascicles which lie parallel to the longitudinal axis of the tendon (Figs. 45-8 and 45-13). The surrounding tendon sheath can be identified as a highly echogenic thin line lying immediately adjacent. When present, the synovial sheath is usually anechoic and not identified as a separate layer. In certain areas such as the wrist and ankle a small amount of synovial fluid is normal and acts to cushion the tendon during movement. It is important to assess a tendon in both a relaxed state and under tension. Generally, under tension, the tendon becomes taut, reducing anisotropy and providing more reliable assessment of internal hypoechoic foci. However, this also temporarily obliterates small abnormal blood vessels within the tendon which are more fully appreciated with the tendon relaxed.

Dynamic assessment of the muscle tendon unit can provide useful diagnostic information. Injury to the tendon itself or to surrounding structures can allow the tendon to sublux or dislocate within the normal range of movement.

Ligaments. Similar to tendons, ligaments are composed of type 1 collagen fibres which are arrayed in an echogenic and fibrillar distribution. Normal ligaments vary in size and comparison with the contralateral side is often useful. Injury causes loss of the linear structure and disruption of fibres with hypoechoic foci. Evaluation with the ligament under tension is preferred.

Nerves. Even small distal neural structures are exquisitely demonstrated using US (Fig. 45-13). Each nerve is enveloped by its epineurium, a loose connective tissue matrix. The multiple hypoechoic neural fascicles are individually covered by echogenic layers of dense connective tissue, termed the perineurium. Imaging transverse to the nerve allows the operator to identify the fascicles as separate discreet round bundles. Longitudinal evaluation shows the parallel fascicular arrangement.

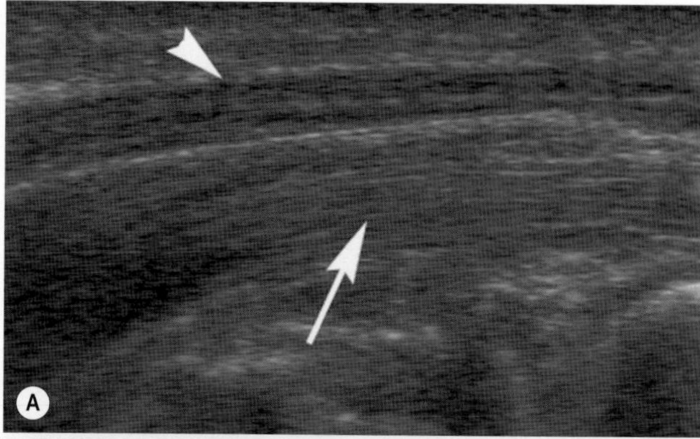

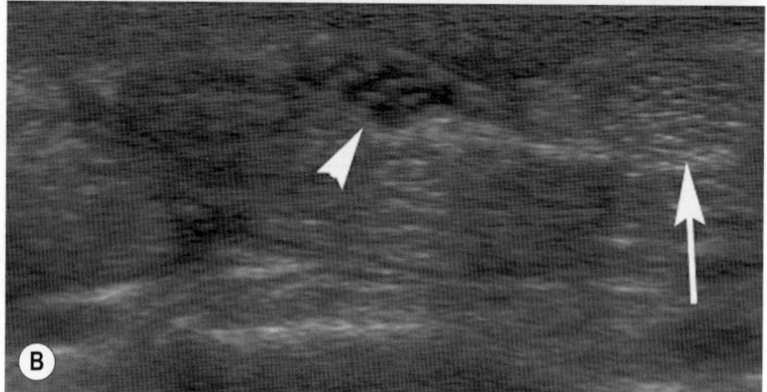

FIGURE 45-13 ■ (A) Longitudinal and (B) transverse ultrasound images of the median nerve (arrowheads) showing hypoechoic fascicles differing from the fibrillar pattern within adjacent tendons (arrows).

Computed Tomography

Bone

Bony cortex is a dense high-attenuation layer thinning at the metaphyses and epiphyses of long bones. Individual trabeculae can be appreciated within the medullary cavity on CT. Bone is a dynamic organ and alterations in bone morphology can indicate disease processes: for example, the presence of osteophytes in osteoarthrosis.

Soft Tissues

Even by adjusting the window and level parameters to maximise contrast between adjacent soft-tissue elements, it is not usually possible to differentiate normal from abnormal soft-tissue structures in musculoskeletal disease. Conversely, although the attenuation values of fat and skeletal muscle differ enough that they can be distinguished as separate tissues, this is seldom useful clinically.

MRI

Bone and Joints

With its ability to differentiate fatty and haematopoietic marrow, MRI is a valuable technique for non-invasive marrow assessment.

It is essential to remember that bone is a dynamic organ. Age-dependent variation in both composition and distribution of bone marrow is well recognised. At birth the entire skeleton contains red haematopoietic marrow

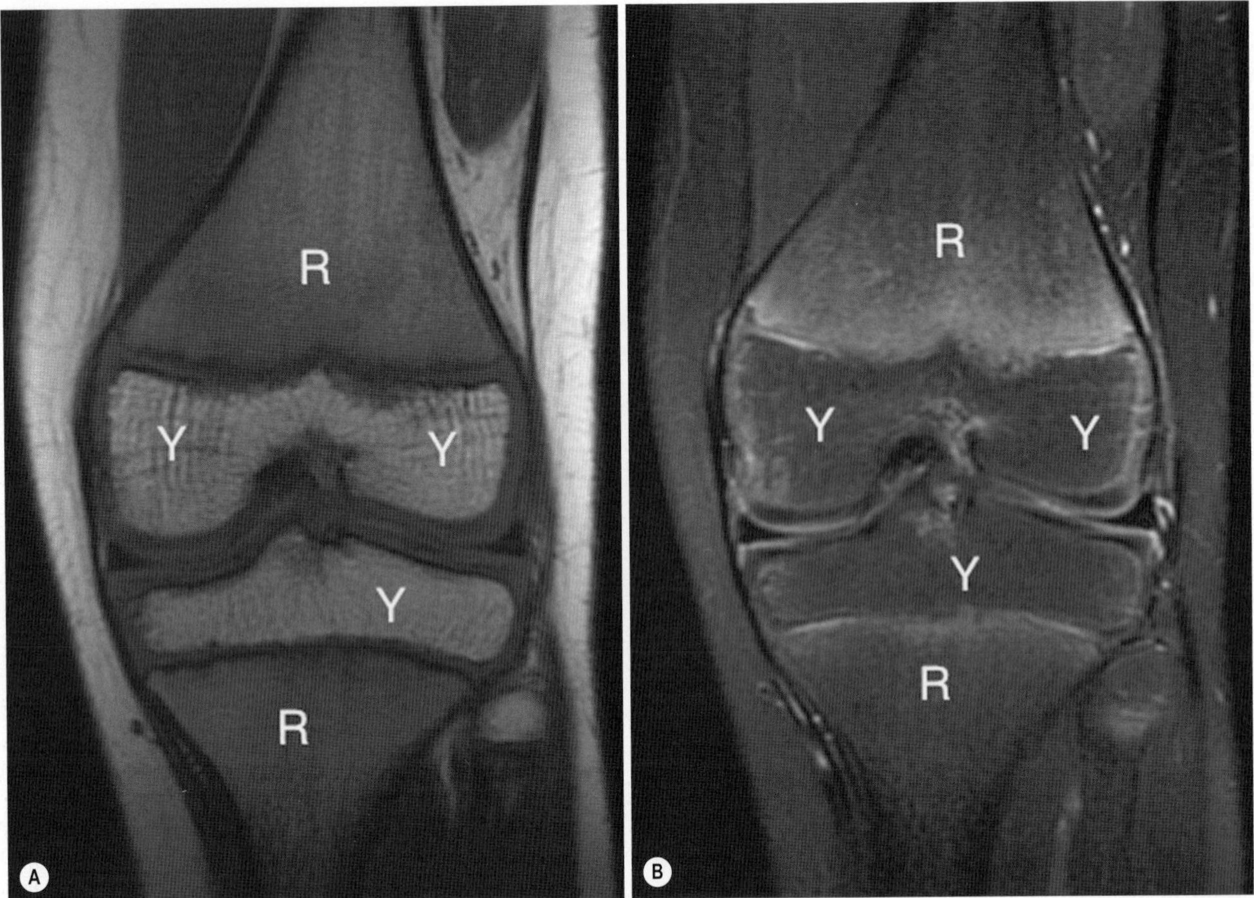

FIGURE 45-14 ■ Coronal MR images of a skeletally immature patient. (A) T1-weighted and (B) proton density fat-saturated images showing yellow marrow in the epiphyses (Y) and red marrow in the metadiaphyses (R).

and over the next two decades there is a predictable conversion to yellow fatty bone marrow. Conversion is a symmetrical process, beginning in the peripheral long bones, and follows a centripetal course to the axial skeleton. Within each bone, conversion starts around the vessels within the mid-diaphysis, expanding out towards the metaphyses. As the epiphyses and apophyses ossify, they contain yellow marrow (Fig. 45-14). By the end of the third decade conversion is complete and bone marrow has an adult distribution; the majority of the adult skeleton contains yellow marrow and red marrow persists only in the skull, spine, clavicles, scapulae, pelvis and proximal humeral and femoral metaphyses (hence the predilection of bloodborne metastases to these sites in adults).

An increase in functional demand can trigger reconversion of fatty to haematopoietic marrow. This process can arise secondary to benign conditions such as heavy smoking and is seen in chronic anaemia whatever the underlying cause. Reconversion occurs in a predictable pattern exactly reversing the conversion process occurring from axial to distal. Although this appears straightforward, the interpretation of marrow signal abnormalities is complex with a wide spectrum of normal variation; it can be difficult to differentiate red marrow hyperplasia from malignant infiltration.

The appearance of normal bone marrow on MRI is determined by the pulse sequence parameters and the marrow constituents, particularly the proportion of fat cells but also the relative quantities of water and trabecular matrix. Differentiation between fatty and haematopoietic marrow is best appreciated on T1-weighted sequences. Yellow or fatty marrow has signal characteristics similar to those of subcutaneous fat on T1-weighted imaging. On T2-weighted sequences fatty marrow signal intensity is typically higher than muscle and similar to or slightly lower than subcutaneous fat. The appearance of yellow marrow using gradient-echo sequences is variable and predominantly dependent upon the quantity of trabecular bone. Trabeculae produce susceptibility and the higher the density of trabeculae, the greater the artefact and signal loss seen on gradient-echo sequences.

On T1-weighted imaging, haematopoietic marrow signal is lower than yellow marrow but still higher than that of the intervertebral discs and muscle (Fig. 45-14A). Red marrow has a similar or slightly higher signal than skeletal muscle on both T1- and T2-weighted imaging. This is a useful comparison as, outside the neonatal period, decreased signal relative to muscle is a sensitive indicator of non-physiological marrow infiltration.

Red marrow returns intermediate signal similar to skeletal muscle, whereas yellow marrow signal is lower than muscle on fluid-sensitive, fat-suppression sequences such as STIR or fat-saturated T2 (T2fs) sequences (Fig. 45-14B). These sequences can be used to emphasise the conspicuity of abnormal processes as the majority will cause increased fluid signal. Use of gadolinium-based contrast medium can also be used to accentuate the presence of abnormalities, as normal adult marrow does not significantly enhance but many malignancies will demonstrate increased signal intensity. Care must be taken in interpretation of the paediatric skeleton following contrast medium as normal enhancement of the vertebral marrow in infants and even young children can be striking.

Unlike other imaging investigations, MRI allows direct evaluation of the internal joint soft-tissue structures. As techniques for the treatment of chondral injury improve, accurate assessment of cartilage becomes more important. Proton density fat-supressed and T2-weighted sequences are widely used in routine practice and show hyaline cartilage as a discreet intermediate signal layer separate to high signal fluid and low signal bony cortex (Fig. 45-14B). Increased cartilage signal indicates increased fluid content and is indicative of chondral softening or chondromalacia. More advanced injury such as fissuring, irregularity or cartilage defect can be assessed. Further sequences optimised for assessment of morphological and biochemical changes within articular cartilage have been developed and are discussed earlier in the chapter.

Soft Tissues

Normal fat returns returns high signal on both T1- and fast spin-echo (FSE) T2-weighted sequences and signal should be uniformly saturated (decreased) using fat suppression sequences such as STIR or spectral fat suppression (Fig. 45-15). Internal connective tissue septation can be appreciated but is less conspicuous than on US evaluation. The deep fascia is evident as a discrete low signal band demarcating subcutaneous fat from the underlying muscle compartments.

Generally, muscle abnormalities can be grouped into abnormal masses, muscle atrophy, disorders causing muscle oedema and anatomical variations. It is critical to employ sequences which will demonstrate these conditions and normally a combination of T1-weighted and fluid sensitive T2 fat-suppressed (T2fs) or STIR sequences are used.

Normal skeletal muscle signal is slightly higher than water and much lower than fat on T1-weighted sequences. On T2-weighted sequences skeletal muscle signal is much lower than both fat and fluid and on STIR or T2fs sequences normal muscle signal is higher than fat and lower than fluid (Fig. 45-15). Skeletal muscles are symmetrical when compared to the contralateral side; this is particularly useful when assessing for subtle findings such as focal scarring or anomalous muscles. The fat distribution within a muscle generally conforms to a predictable and often characteristic pattern. The musculotendinous junction does not represent a discreet cutoff between muscle fibres and the tendon; instead, there is a gradual coalescence of tendon fibres. Denervation and disuse fat

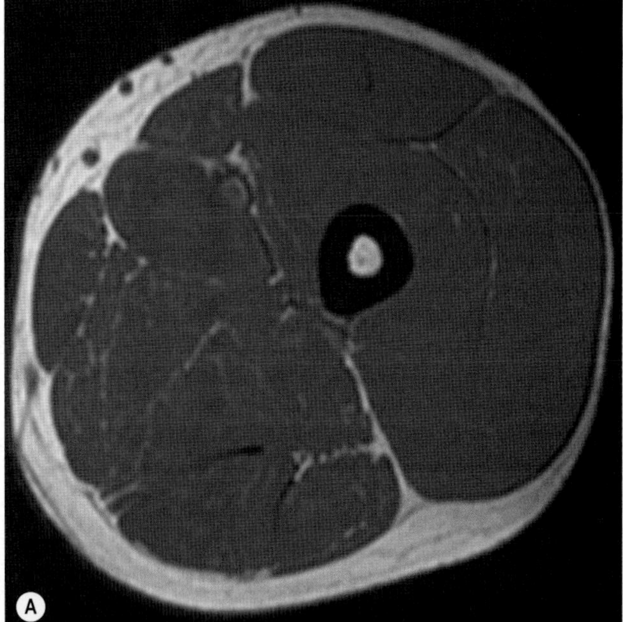

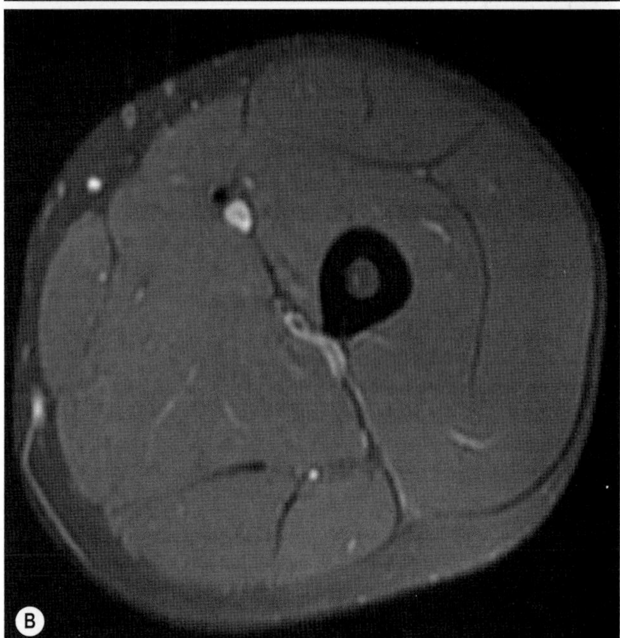

FIGURE 45-15 ■ Axial MR images through the mid-thigh. (A) T1- and (B) T2-weighted fat-saturated images showing skin, normal fat distribution, muscle and bone.

atrophy of a muscle begins first around this myotendinous junction.

Tendons and ligaments are both chiefly composed of type 1 collagen and have a similar MR appearance, being of low signal on all conventional sequences.

SPECIFIC RADIOLOGICAL SCENARIOS

Soft-tissue Calcification and Ossification

Soft-tissue mineralisation is frequently encountered in routine radiological practice. It is important to

TABLE 45-1 **Soft-Tissue Calcification**

Dystrophic calcification
Metabolic calcification
Calcium pyrophosphate deposition disease
Tumoral calcinosis
Malignant calcification

differentiate between calcification and ossification to aid with diagnosis, although this can be difficult in small lesions and calcification can progress to ossification over time.

Ossified foci have a cortex and internal medullary trabeculation mirroring normal bone structure. Soft-tissue calcification can occur in a myriad of abnormalities (Table 45-1); over 95% of lesions, however, are due to dystrophic calcification. Metabolic calcification, calcium hydroxyapatite deposition disease, tumoral calcinosis and malignant causes of calcification/ossification are much less common.

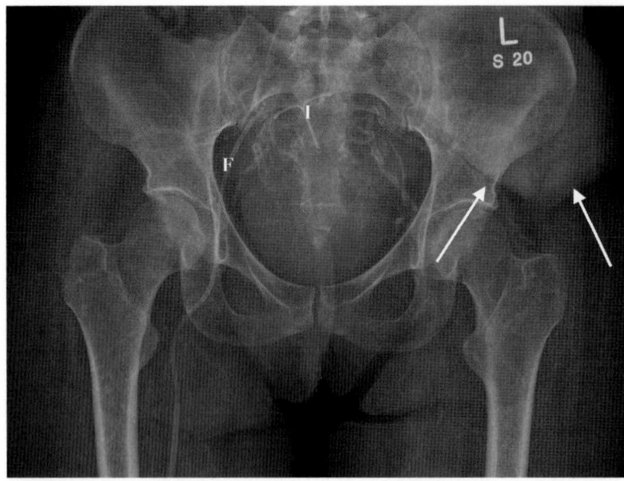

FIGURE 45-16 ■ **Pelvic radiograph of a patient with chronic renal failure.** Extensive vascular calcification and soft-tissue calcification. External artefact from ileostomy bag (arrows), IUCD (I) and right femoral line (F).

Dystrophic Calcification

By far the most common cause of soft-tissue calcification, dystrophic calcification occurs in damaged or devitalised tissues with formation of amorphous calcified deposits which may evolve into ossification. Importantly, dystrophic calcification is not related to abnormalities of serum calcium or phosphate. The misnomer myositis ossificans has previously been used to describe soft-tissue mineralisation particularly secondary to trauma. As this often does not occur in muscle, does not always have an inflammatory aetiology and may not always be ossified, the term has generally been replaced with heterotopic calcification or ossification.

Arterial Vascular Calcification. Although previously considered to be a passive process, recent studies have indicated that the underlying mechanisms of vascular calcification are active and highly regulated. Arterial calcification is a reliable clinical marker for atherosclerosis and the extent of calcification strongly correlates with the severity of arterial disease.[21] Vascular calcification models divide aetiology into two main categories. Subintimal lipid deposition occurring in atherosclerotic disease triggers a cascade similar to that occurring in soft-tissue calcification. The extent of arterial calcification ranges from irregular plaques to extensive tramline calcification predominantly affecting the aorta, pelvic and lower extremity arteries. Non-atherosclerotic calcification affects the media of the arterial wall and is believed to be triggered by interaction with toxins such as in diabetes, hyperparathyroidism and uraemia. This causes a finer and sometimes granular calcific pattern. In practice, the processes involved in medial calcification are also implicated in accelerated atherosclerosis and so there is considerable overlap in their radiological appearance (Fig. 45-16).

Venous Vascular Calcification. Calcification around a venous valve is relatively common and has the characteristic appearance of lamellation with central lucency visible when viewed en face. These phleboliths are most often encountered related to the pelvic venous plexus or lower limb veins (Fig. 45-17) but may also be seen in chronic varicosities and less frequently within soft-tissue haemangiomas. The combination of multiple enchondromas (Ollier's disease) and soft-tissue haemangiomas is seen in Maffucci's syndrome (Fig. 45-18).

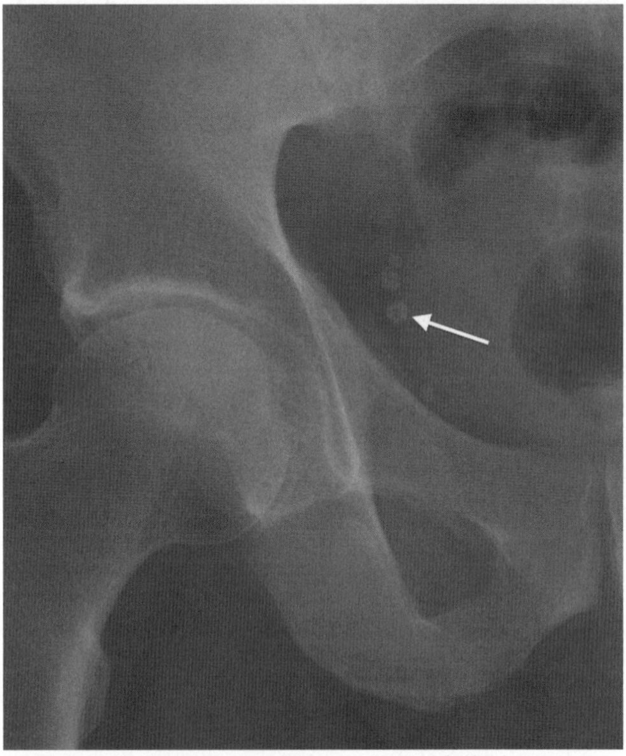

FIGURE 45-17 ■ **Hip radiograph shows phleboliths of the pelvis venous plexus.** One phlebolith is en face and so has a central lucency (arrow).

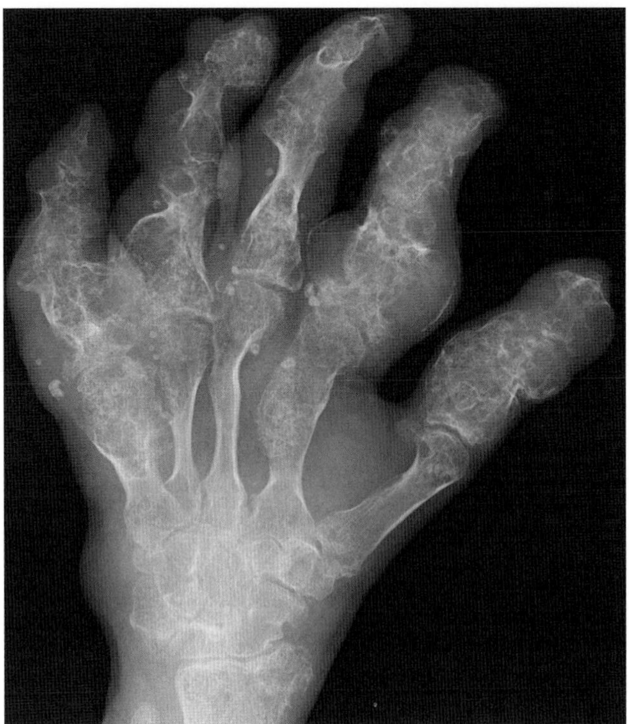

FIGURE 45-18 ■ **Hand radiograph of patient with Maffucci's syndrome shows extensive multiple enchondromas with phleboliths in soft-tissue haemangiomas.**

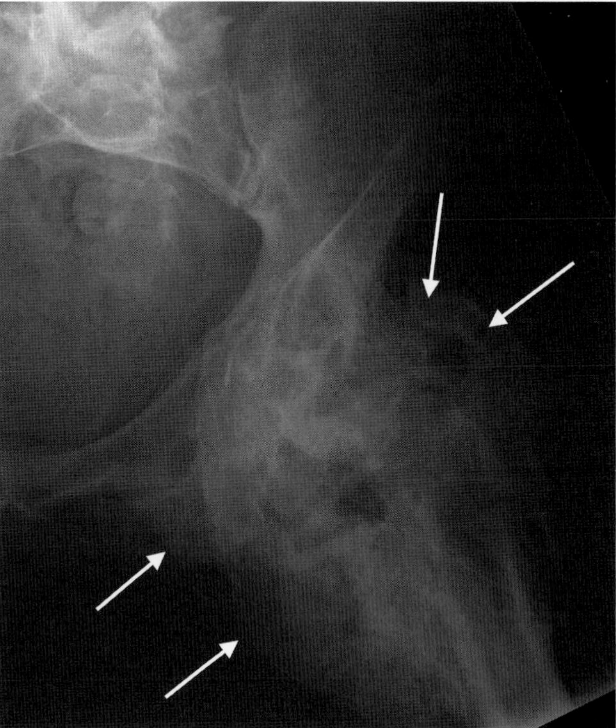

FIGURE 45-19 ■ **Extensive heterotopic ossification with ankylosis (arrows) of the left hip in a patient with post-traumatic quadriplegia.**

Trauma. Calcification is commonly seen related to previous soft-tissue injury. Even seemingly minor trauma such as subcutaneous or intramuscular injections can stimulate the development of dense calcifications occurring at the characteristic injection sites such as the upper arm and buttocks. Post-traumatic heterotopic mineralisation is recognised as a common complication following closed head injuries, burns and in paraplegia.[22] Ossification can be extensive and ankylosis is not infrequent if calcification bridges across the joint. Classically the shoulder and pelvic girdles and elbows are affected (Fig. 45-19). US can be a useful diagnostic tool for focal calcification as it will show calcification not yet visible on plain film (Fig. 45-6).

Calcium Hydroxyapatite Deposition Disease. Calcium hydroxyapatite deposition disease (HADD) should be differentiated from the other crystal deposition disorders, calcium pyrophosphate dihydrate deposition disease (CPPD) and monosodium urate crystal deposition disease (gout). HADD represents the formation of calcium hydroxyapatite crystals within the periarticular soft tissues and usually manifests as amorphous, dystrophic calcification within the tendons of the rotator cuff (Fig. 45-20). Typically affecting the middle-aged and elderly, HADD generally has a mono-articular presentation and can be very painful, mimicking infection or conditions such as frozen shoulder. The underlying aetiology is thought to be linked to minor repetitive trauma causing necrosis and inflammation. Over time the calcific deposits may regress, remain stable or mature. Ultrasound can be of value in assessing the maturity of these deposts; in general, dense fragmented deposits with distal acoustic shadowing are indicators of more long-standing calcification.

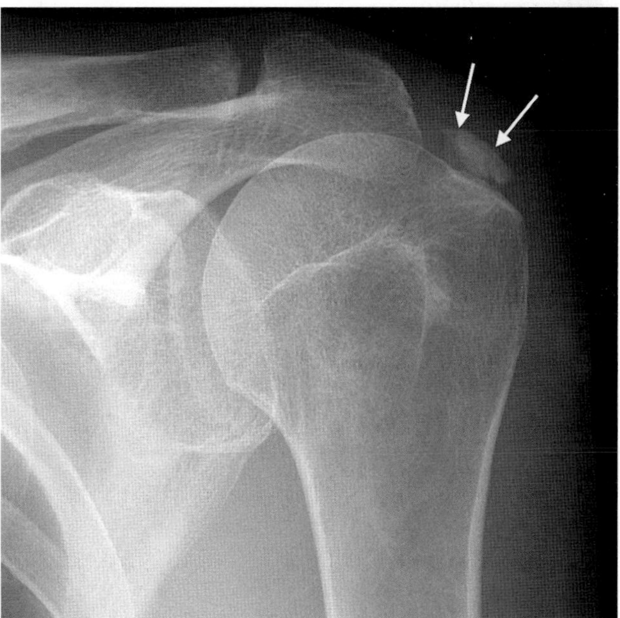

FIGURE 45-20 ■ **AP radiograph of shoulder showing dense hydroxyapatite deposit (arrows) in the superior rotator cuff in a patient with calcific tendinosis.**

Congenital Causes for Soft-tissue Calcification. Fibrodysplasia ossificans progressiva (FOP) is a rare, autosomal dominant disorder with variable penetrance causing replacement of normal muscle and connective tissue by profuse heterotopic ossification. The initial manifestation is swelling of the muscular fascial planes, usually affecting the neck and shoulder planes first. This is followed by multifocal calcification progressing into ossification. Over time, mobility becomes restricted and respiration is constrained by bands of extraseletal bone formation within the thorax. CT, MRI and scintigraphy can identify early changes.[23] FOP is associated with short first metacarpals and metatarsals along with small cervical vertebral bodies with relative prominence of the pedicles. The condition is usually fatal in early life.

Infection

Bacterial and Fungal Infection. Calcification is a rare feature of bacterial infection but may occur in the cavity of an abscess. Extensive calcified lymphadenitis is highly suggestive of previous tuberculous infection. A similar appearance is seen in fungal infection with histoplasmosis and coccidioidomycosis where these are endemic. Neural calcification is reported almost exclusively in leprosy and so is a significant finding.[24] Calcification most frequently occurs as linear opacification, typically of the ulnar nerve (Fig. 45-21).

Parasitic Infection. Soft-tissue calcification related to parasitic infection often has a distinctive morphology indicative of the pathogen involved. Most of these infections are rare in the developed world but are encountered occasionally in visitors or migrants from endemic areas. Cysticercosis can develop in the brain and skeletal muscle following exposure to the eggs of *Taenia solium* (pork tapeworm) and should be differentiated from infection by the adult tapeworm, which affects the gut. The disease is endemic in Central and South America, Africa, Asia and parts of Eastern Europe. Within muscle, cysticercosis is seen as multiple foci of intramuscular calcification, which are orientated longitudinally along the muscle fibres and measure up to 1 cm in length; these characteristically have the appearance of grains of rice (Fig. 45-22). *Dracunculus medinensis* (guinea worm) causes a parasitic infection (dracunculiasis) found throughout tropical Africa, the Middle East, India, the Far East and the northern countries of South America. Larvae are ingested in contaminated drinking water and pass through the intestinal wall to mature in the subcutaneous tissues where the calcification of the dead adult female guinea worm has a distinctive long coiled or curled appearance (Fig. 45-23). Infection with the filarial *Loa loa* may also give calcification of the adult worm within the subcutaneous soft tissues. In loiasis the calcification has a fine linear or coiled thread-like appearance and is best seen in the extremities. *Loa loa* is endemic in West and Central Africa. Infection occurs from a fly bite, with the larvae maturing into the adult worm within the subcutaneous tissues.

Autoimmune

Dermatomyositis. Dermatomyositis is an inflammatory muscle disorder of unknown aetiology modulated by

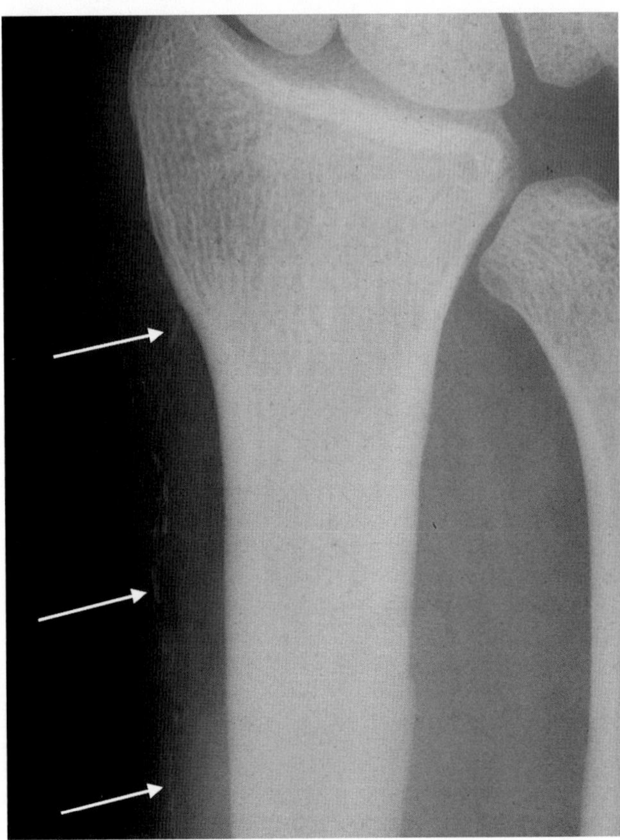

FIGURE 45-21 ■ Radiograph of the forearm shows neural calcification (arrows) in leprosy.

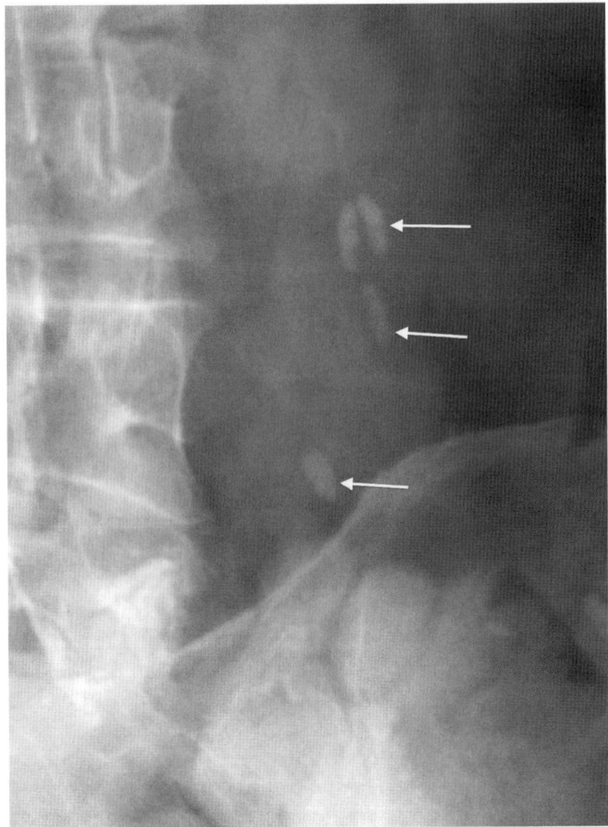

FIGURE 45-22 ■ Rice-like calcification of cysticercosis (arrows) affecting the psoas muscle.

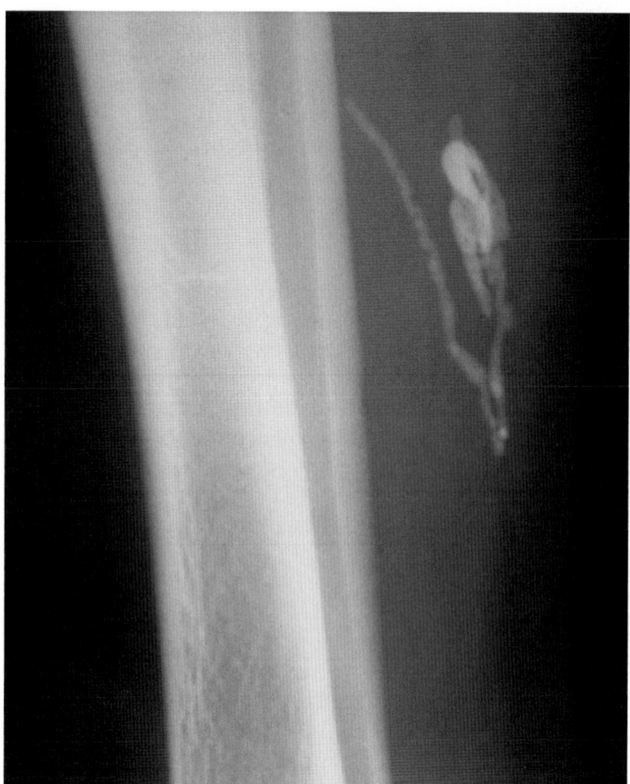

FIGURE 45-23 ■ Coiled calcification within the subcutaneous tissues of the lower leg in guinea worm infection.

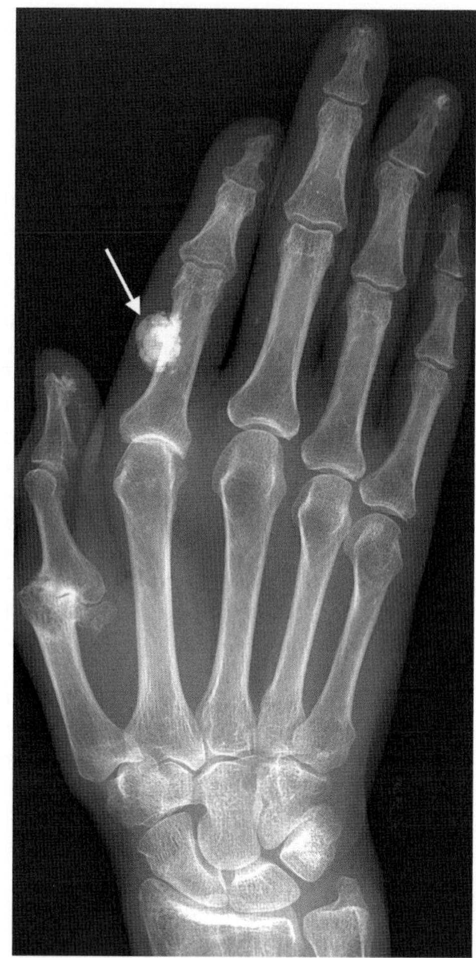

FIGURE 45-24 ■ Radiograph of the hand in a patient with progressive systemic sclerosis. Calcinosis circumscripta (arrow), soft-tissue loss of the tip of the index finger and thumb MCP joint arthritis are present.

the immune system. Several infectious agents such as Coxsackie virus and *Toxoplasma* have been implicated as possible triggers. The disorder can occur at any age and may affect either sex, but is most common in adult women, although there is a severe juvenile form. Skin and muscle involvement is typically seen but patients may also develop joint disease and debilitating oesophageal and cardiopulmonary disease. Dermatomyositis is frequently associated with non-specific subcutaneous calcinosis appreciated on radiographs; the formation of sheet-like calcification along muscle and fascial planes is characteristic but much less common. In the adult form, there is a strong association with malignancy, particularly of the bronchus, breast, stomach and ovary.[25]

Progressive Systemic Sclerosis (Scleroderma). This is a generalised autoimmune disorder of unknown cause which is characterised by extensive fibrosis and widespread small vessel vasculopathy. Scleroderma refers to the cutaneous manifestation but there is frequent visceral involvement, particularly of the oesophagus, kidneys, heart and lungs. Typical features in the hands are resorption of the terminal phalanges (acro-osteolysis), discrete soft-tissue calcification (calcinosis circumscripta) (Fig. 45-24) and occasionally intra-articular calcification. Erosions can occur due to overlap with rheumatoid arthritis and other connective tissue diseases.

Neoplastic. Dystrophic localised intratumoral calcification can be seen in both benign and malignant lesions due to haemorrhage and necrosis. In malignant disease this can occur due to treatment response. This differs from those tumours that mineralise due to the presence of osteoprogenitor cell populations; these are discussed later in the chapter. The pattern of soft-tissue mineralisation can point towards the underlying cause. Punctate or 'ring and arc' calcification is seen with soft-tissue chondromas; phleboliths are classically seen in haemangiomas. Lipomas, particularly when parosteal, can ossify.

Metabolic Calcification. Metabolic calcification, also known as metastatic calcification, is the accumulation of calcium salts in normal tissue and occurs as the result of elevated serum calcium-phosphate product. When the calcification is evident at radiography, there is a diffuse deposition of fine granular calcification. There are a range of causes, but chronic renal failure is the most common (Fig. 45-16). Other causes to consider include hyperparathyroidism, sarcoidosis and certain drugs. Metabolic calcification due to primary hyperparathyroidism is rarely encountered in modern medical practice as it is generally diagnosed and treated before the development of radiographic abnormality but it can cause arterial and periarticular calcification as well as chondrocalcinosis. Secondary hyperparathyroidism is typically seen in relation to chronic renal disease. Periarticular and soft-tissue calcification can be a prominent feature, particularly in association with long-term renal dialysis where it has a dramatic negative impact on prognosis.[26] Chondrocalcinosis is infrequently seen in secondary hyperparathyroidism.

Hypoparathyroid states such as hypoparathyroidism, pseudohypoparathyroidism and pseudopseudohypoparathyroidism can also cause abnormal soft-tissue calcification. Primary deficiency of parathormone (PTH) occurs usually due to surgical excision of, or trauma to, the parathyroid glands. Calcification, when it occurs, is typically subcutaneous. Premature closure of the epiphyses, osteosclerosis and basal ganglia calcification may also be evident. Pseudohypoparathyroidism has several subtypes but is an X-linked dominant disorder caused by intrinsic resistance to PTH. Radiographic features are similar to hypoparathyroidism but there are characteristic phenotypic changes including rounded facies, and short fourth and fifth metacarpals/metatarsals. Pseudopseudohypoparathyroidism is also an inherited disorder; the imaging appearances are identical to those of pseudohypoparathyroidism but the serum calcium and phosphate levels are normal.

Abnormal soft-tissue calcification related to drug excess is now rarely encountered as a solitary abnormality but metabolic calcification can occur with drugs which impact upon the complex inter-regulation of calcium, phosphate and vitamin D. Hypervitaminosis D is generally seen in chronic renal failure in those reliant on dialysis but is also seen due to the treatment of rickets and osteomalacia. The radiological features relate to the formation of smooth, lobulated masses of calcium hydroxyapatite within and around joints, and within tendon sheaths and bursae. In children hypervitaminosis D causes the development of dense metaphyseal bands and diffuse cortical thickening, which may be associated with generalised osteosclerosis. In the mature skeleton most of these features are absent and osteosclerosis may be the only skeletal manifestation.[27] Excessive intake of alkali, usually calcium carbonate and milk, is reported in patients with renal impairment and peptic ulcer disease can result in the deposition of soft-tissue calcification, which is similar in appearance to that seen in hypervitaminosis D and can mimic other disorders such as renal osteodystrophy, collagen vascular disorders and idiopathic tumoral calcinosis.

Calcium Pyrophosphate Dihydrate Deposition Disease (CPPD)

CPPD is the umbrella term for the abnormal accretion of calcium pyrophosphate dihydrate crystals in and around joints. There is thought to be an association between CPPD and many other conditions such as diabetes, hyperparathyroidism, haemachromatosis, hypomagnesaemia and gout. CPPD can manifest as acute intermittent synovitis (pseudogout), chronic pyrophosphate arthropathy or chondrocalcinosis. Pyrophosphate arthropathy is radiologically similar to osteoarthrosis (OA) and may be indistinguishable on imaging. Suggestive features include an unusual pattern of joint involvement such as the radiocapitellar articulation of the elbow, large subchondral cysts and a relative paucity of osteophytes. Pyrophosphate arthropathy can be rapidly destructive and bone fragmentation may be a feature. Chondrocalcinosis is most commonly seen in the knee and can affect hyaline (articular) cartilage and fibrocartilage (menisci, triangular fibrocartilage, symphysis pubis and annulus fibrosus).

Tumoral Calcinosis

Tumoral calcinosis is a rare hereditary dysfunction of phosphate metabolism occurring particularly in patients of African descent. Biochemistry shows normal serum calcium but there may be mild hyperphosphataemia. Radiologically there is deposition of characteristic large, globular soft-tissue calcification around joints, predominantly affecting the extensor surface where there is generally bursal involvement. CT may demonstrate the lesions to be cystic with internal layering of calcium.

Malignant Calcification

The soft-tissue malignancies that classically mineralise are extraskeletal osteosarcoma, extraskeletal chondrosarcoma and synovial sarcoma as well as metastases from bone-forming tumours (Fig. 45-25). In the latter, calcification is seen in up to 30% of cases and can range from fine non-specific calcified foci to dense eccentric calcification.

Rarely, disseminated malignancy such as leukaemia, myeloma or bony metastases can manifest with widespread soft-tissue calcification due to hypercalcaemia from extensive bone destruction.

Gas in the Soft Tissues

Air or gas within the soft tissues is indicated by radiolucency on radiographs or CT; this can take the form of locules or can be more linear, outlining the soft-tissue planes. Small locules of gas can be difficult to appreciate on MRI and returns low signal on all sequences (Fig. 45-26). Soft-tissue gas may form directly within the soft tissues or, more commonly, is seen following perforation of the skin or a body cavity.

Vacuum phenomenon occurs in synovial joints, intervertebral discs and vertebral bodies due to the accumulation of gas, mainly nitrogen, in the adjacent soft tissues. The appearances can be accentuated by traction on the effected joint: hence the term 'vacuum phenomonenon' despite no true vacuum being present. The gas appears as radiolucent lines that can be seen using radiography. The majority of cases are attributed to degeneration but more rarely vacuum phenomenon related to fracture non-union, infection or tumour is described.[28]

Soft-tissue gas occurring secondary to infection is most frequently seen in the extremities of patients with diabetes or peripheral vascular disease (Fig. 45-27). Gas is typically produced by anaerobic bacteria; the classic example is gas gangrene caused by several species of *Clostridium*. This can be life-threatening and in its most severe form causes critical sepsis, extensive oedema and soft-tissue necrosis with gas formation which may be palpable as subcutaneous crepitus. Other anaerobic

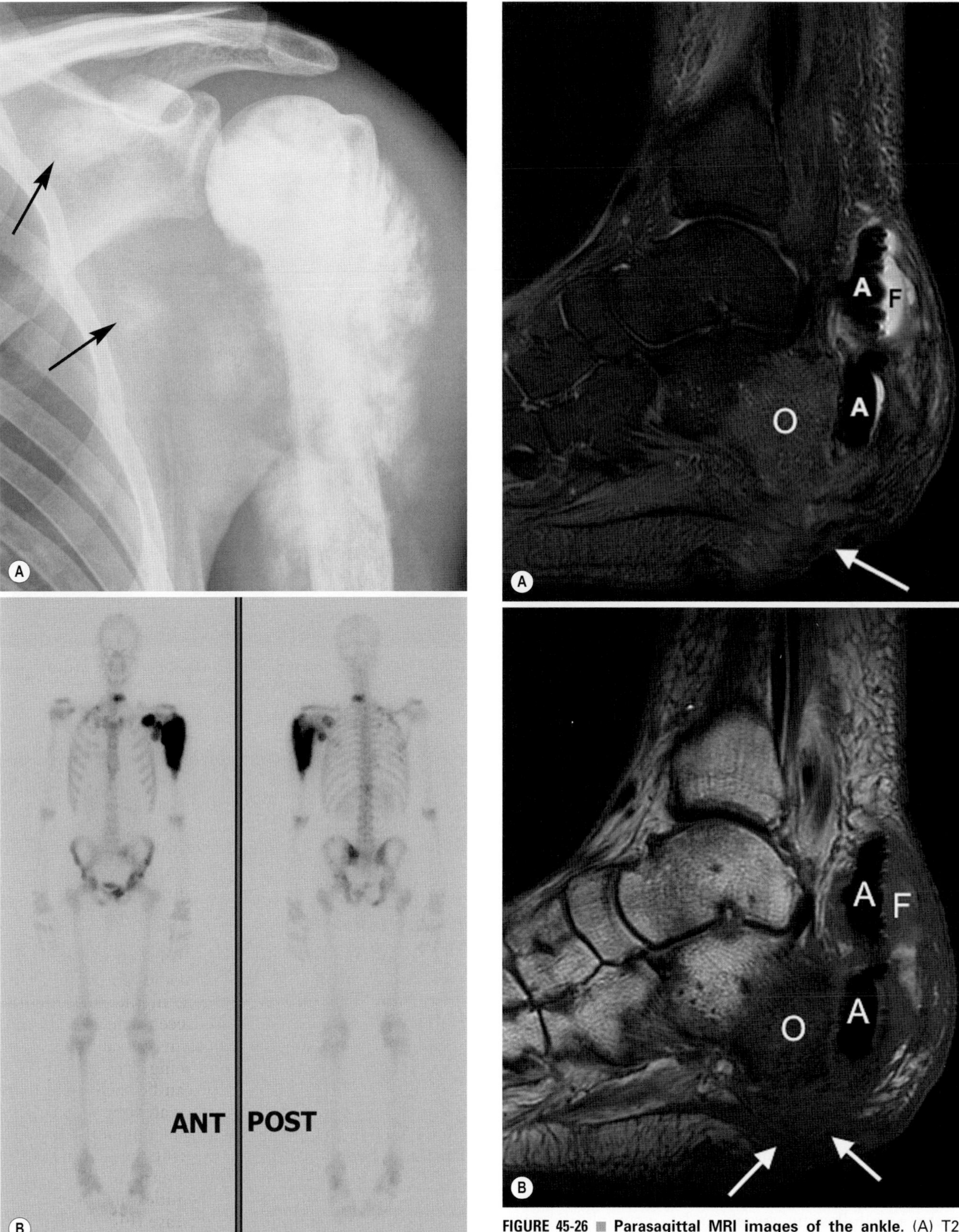

FIGURE 45-25 ■ Osteosarcoma of the proximal humerus. (A) Radiograph shows dense new bone formation and aggressive periosteal reaction. Ossified lymph node metastases (arrows). (B) ^{99m}Tc-MDP bone scintigraphy shows increased radiotracer uptake within the primary humeral lesion, malignant lymph nodes within the axilla and spinal and pelvic bone metastases.

FIGURE 45-26 ■ Parasagittal MRI images of the ankle. (A) T2-weighted fat-saturated and (B) T1-weighted images show fluid (F) and air (A) collections posteriorly tracking from a plantar ulcer (arrows). There is osteomyelitis within the calcaneus with intraosseous gas and surrounding bone oedema (O).

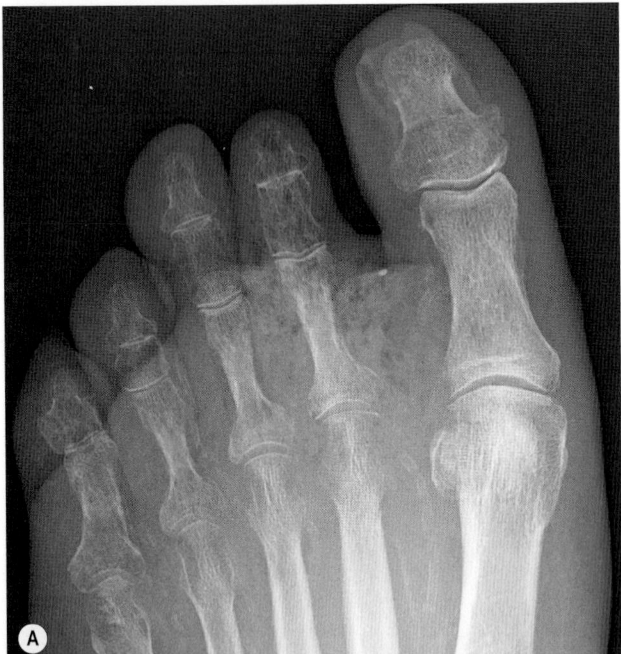

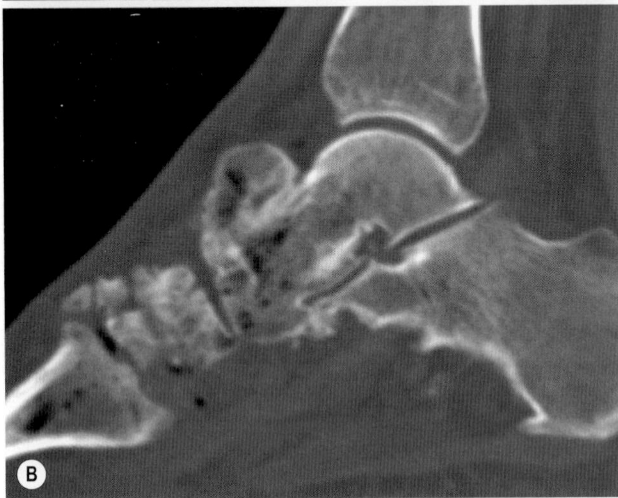

FIGURE 45-27 ■ Soft-tissue gas. (A) Radiograph of the forefoot in a diabetic patient with the dappled low-density appearances of gas in the soft tissues of the second toe; note vascular calcification and osteopenia. (B) Reformatted sagittal CT image shows extensive soft tissue, joint and intraosseous low-density gas due to infection in a different patient.

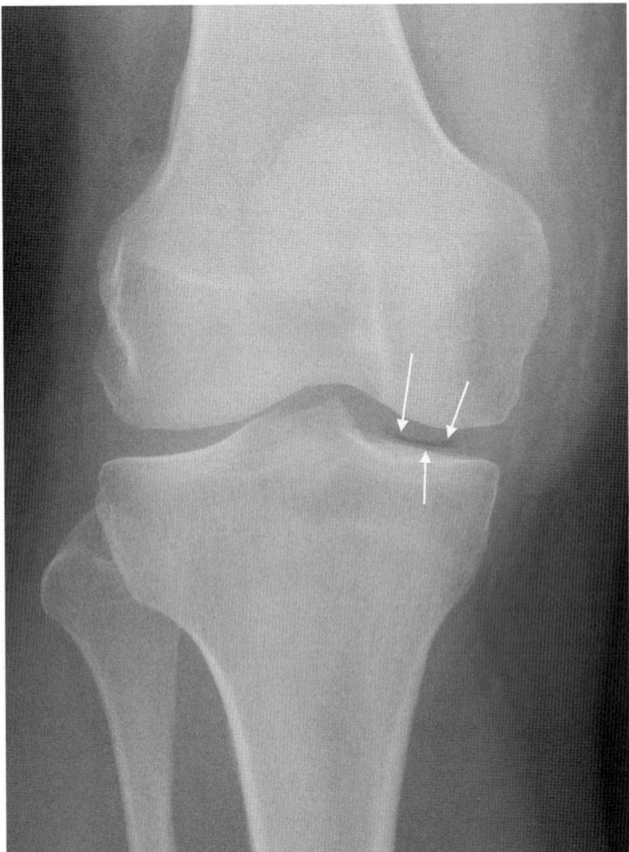

FIGURE 45-28 ■ Radiograph of the knee shows intra-articular gas (arrows) following penetrating injury.

bacteria such as coliforms, *Bacteroides*, anaerobic *Streptococcus* species and *Aerobacter aerogenes* may also produce gas, although these tend to be less severe, causing more localised infection than *Clostridium* spp.

Soft-tissue gas is frequently seen in conjunction with trauma. Breach of the respiratory or gastrointestinal tract may occur following blunt trauma, for example, and is also seen following surgery and as a complication following interventional procedures such as central line insertion. Gas within the soft tissues of the chest or retroperitoneum is termed surgical emphysema and locules of air may be palpated deep to the skin.

Air can be introduced into the soft tissues following penetrating injury through the skin. It is important to recognise breach of a joint capsule following a soft-tissue laceration as joint washout is indicated to prevent septic arthritis (Fig. 45-28). Associated foreign bodies can be diagnosed on radiographs when they are radio-opaque: for example, glass. Organic foreign bodies such as wood are better assessed using ultrasound.

Periosteal Reaction

The periosteum is a dense layer of specialised connective tissue which invests the outer bony cortex except at the articulating surfaces of synovial joints. The outer periosteal stratum is a dense, innervated and vascularised fibrous sheath providing nourishment and sensory innervation. The inner layer or cambium is more loosely arranged and contains osteoblasts and osteoprogenitor cells, which are essential for bone repair and growth. Compact Sharpey's fibres anchor the periosteum to the underlying bone lamellae. Functionally, the periosteum also provides attachment for ligaments and tendons.

Direct or indirect insult to the periosteal layer causes it to elevate from the underlying bony cortex. This causes a non-specific radiological finding termed periosteal reaction. The insult can take many forms, including trauma, infection, malignancy, arthritis and drug reaction (Table 45-2). There is considerable overlap in the different appearances of periosteal reaction; although it is not possible to discriminate between malignant and benign

TABLE 45-2 Differential Diagnosis of Periosteal Reaction

Congenital	Periosteal reaction of the newborn
Genetic	Caffey disease
	Pachydermoperiostosis
Arthritides	Psoriatic arthritis
	Reactive arthritis
Infection	
Trauma	Fracture
	Stress injury
Metabolic	Hypertrophic osteoarthropathy
	Thyroid acropachy
Drugs	Prostaglandins
	Fluorosis
	Hypervitaminosis A
Tumours	Primary bone malignancy
	Leukaemia and lymphoma
	Osteoid osteoma
	Eosinophilic granuloma
	Chondroblastoma
Vascular	Venous stasis

TABLE 45-3 Types of Periosteal Reaction

Non-aggressive	Thin
	Solid
	Thick and irregular
	Septated
Aggressive	Spiculated
	Hair-on-end
	Sunburst
	Laminated
	Disorganised
	Interrupted
	Codman triangle

conditions, certain features differentiate between non-aggressive and aggressive forms (Table 45-3).

Non-aggressive Periosteal Reaction

Congenital. Physiologic periosteal reaction of the newborn is a well-recognised radiological finding of unknown aetiology causing symmetrical continuous periosteal reaction, typically of the long bones. It is seen in term and pre-term neonates and is important to differentiate from non-accidental injury.

Genetic. Also known as infantile cortical hyperostosis, Caffey's disease is a rare and benign self-limiting genetic condition of early infancy which can be either familial or sporadic in terms of transmission. Developing as a triad of rapidly evolving cortical thickening, soft-tissue swelling and hyperirritability,[29] the disorder most commonly affects the mandible but can involve any bone and often more than one site is affected. Long bone involvement is confined to the diaphysis; there is marked cortical thickening with bony expansion and abnormality may persist for months or even years. Given the features, it is vital to exclude osteomyelitis, trauma and malignancy.

Pachydermoperiostosis or primary hypertrophic osteoarthropathy occurs in older children, classically in pubertal boys. This rare familial condition characteristically causes insidious thickening of the skin of the face and clubbing of the digits. Radiologically there is symmetrical development of often exuberant irregular periosteal reaction of the long bones. Unlike secondary hypertrophic osteoarthropathy, in pachydermoperiostosis the periosteal reaction extends to involve the epiphysis.

Arthritis. Psoriatic arthritis may develop before the dermatological manifestations are exhibited. Bone proliferation, enthesopathy and periosteal reaction, in addition to marginal erosions, are well-recognised features. The periosteal reaction can be exuberant and aggressive in appearance and is classically juxta-articular. As the periosteal reaction matures with time it progresses into solid new bone.

Reactive arthritis is a seronegative arthritis occurring as an autoimmune response to infection. There is a strong relationship to human leucocyte antigen (HLA) B27. A wide range of infectious agents have been described but the majority of cases relate to genitourinary infection, particularly *Chlamydia trachomatis* or gastrointestinal infection with *Campylobacter*, *Shigella* or *Salmonella* species. The resultant periosteal reaction is identical to that seen in psoriatic arthritis but typically affects the lower limbs.

Trauma. Subtle periosteal reaction at a site of pain may be the only radiographic feature of a stress fracture (Fig. 45-29A); it should be emphasised that up to 80% of stress fractures are radiographically occult at presentation and delayed or additional imaging may be warranted. Periosteal reaction occurring at a fracture site can have a variable appearance, ranging from smooth, solid periostitis to disorganised and aggressive periosteal reaction (Fig. 45-29).

Metabolic. Secondary hypertrophic osteoarthopathy (HOA) is a common manifestation of extraskeletal disease causing symmetric, generalised periosteal reaction of tubular bones. Unlike primary hypertrophic osteoarthopathy, there is sparing of the epiphyses. HOA is classically described related to pulmonary abnormalities when it may be termed hypertrophic pulmonary osteoarthopathy. Lung cancer, and non-small cell cancer in particular, is the most common cause but HOA is also recognised in conjunction with tumours of the pleura and mediastinum, suppurative lung disease (for example, bronchiectasis or empyema), pulmonary metastases and cystic fibrosis. Less commonly, HOA occurs due to gastrointestinal disease such as biliary cirrhosis or inflammatory bowel disease.

Developing as digital clubbing, swelling of the hands and feet and exophthalmos, thyroid acropachy is a rare complication of autoimmune thyroid disease. There is generalised and relatively symmetrical periosteal reaction which is irregular and may be spiculated that typically involves the mid-diaphyses of the metacarpals, metatarsals and phalanges.

Drugs. Several drugs are known to cause periosteal reaction. Excess intake of fluorine causes dental abnormalities when occurring in childhood. In adults excess fluorine intake results in increased bone density with reduced bone elasticity, giving an increased fracture risk. Osteosclerosis is accompanied by a thick and undulating periosteal reaction and widening of the diaphyses.

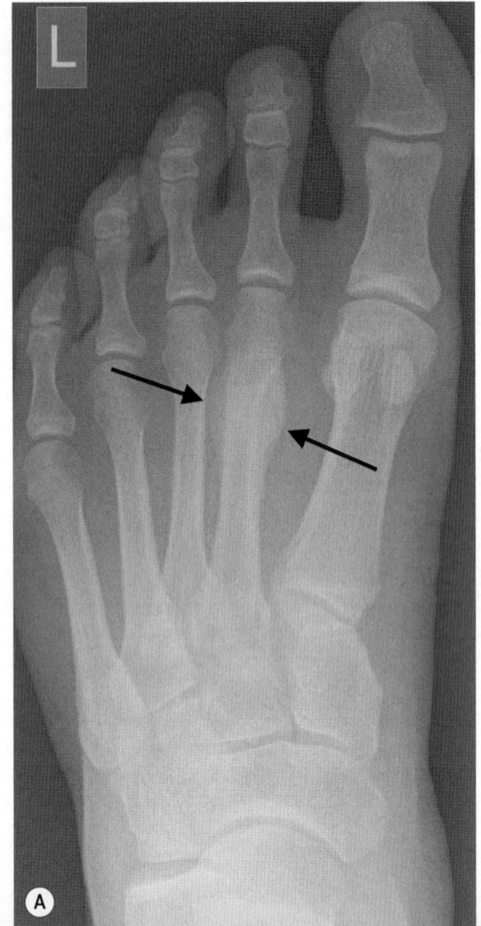

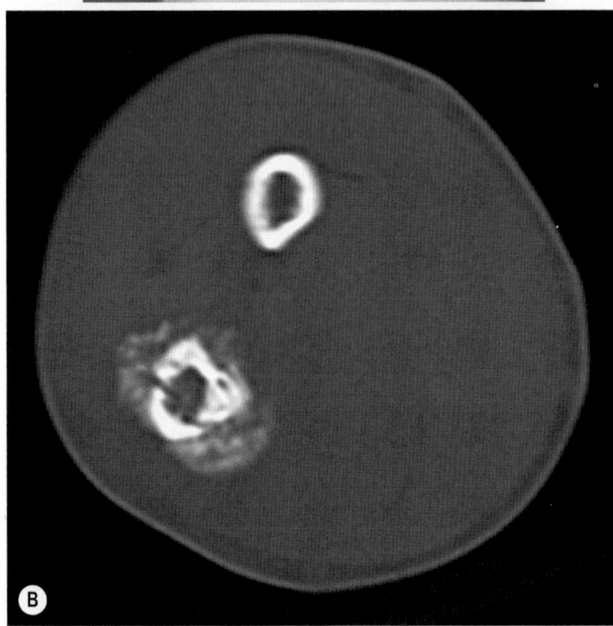

FIGURE 45-29 ■ **Different patients.** (A) Radiograph shows stress fracture of the second metatarsal with periosteal reaction (arrows). (B) Axial CT of healing ulna fracture. The fracture remains ununited with florid surrounding periosteal reaction and callus.

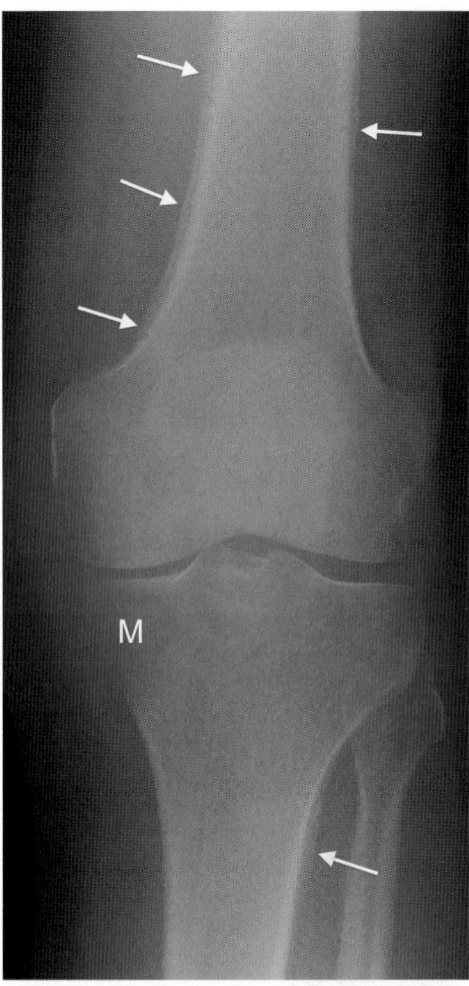

FIGURE 45-30 ■ **Hypertrophic osteoarthropathy in a patient with lung cancer.** Periosteal reaction of the distal femur and proximal tibia (arrows). Lytic metastasis (M) within the medial tibia with cortical destruction.

Calcification or ossification of ligaments, tendons and interosseous membranes is a distinctive feature. Fluorosis is endemic in areas such as China and India.

Prostaglandins are used in infants to maintain a patent ductus arteriosus in ductal-dependent congenital heart disease. They can produce a diffuse cortical proliferation believed to occur due to decreased osteoclast activity.[30] This is associated with limb swelling and pain which resolves following the cessation of treatment.

Chronic hypervitaminosis A may present with anorexia and dermatological symptoms in adults and children. Radiologically there is a smooth and solid periosteal reaction of the long bones, which in the immature skeleton can be associated with metaphyseal splaying, thinning of the growth plate and premature fusion. In the distal femur, in particular, the epiphysis may evolve into a conical shape invaginating into the metaphysis.

Tumours. Slow-growing bone tumours typically exhibit non-aggressive periosteal reaction. The most common example is the benign osteoid osteoma which develops as fusiform, smooth, focal and eccentric periosteal reaction with a central lucent nidus which may

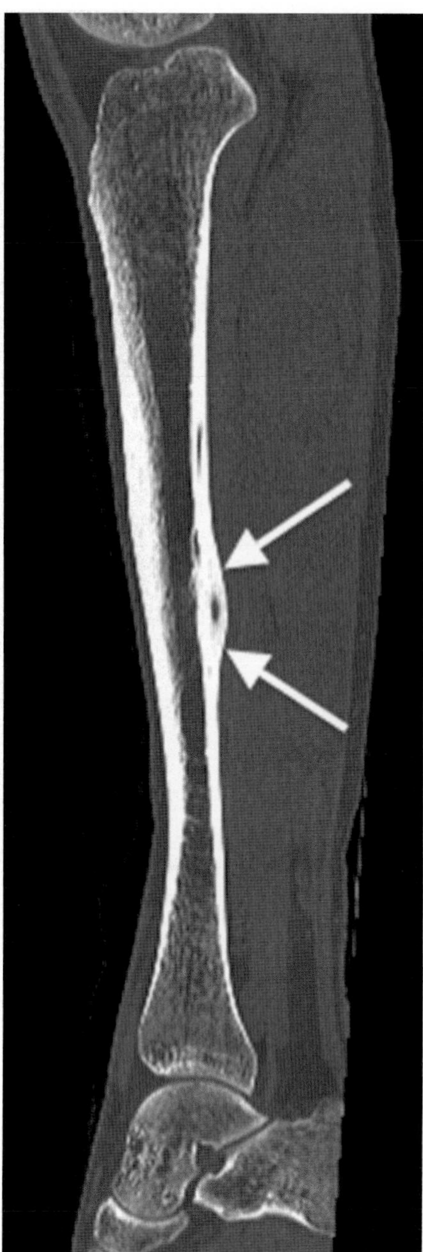

FIGURE 45-31 ■ Osteoid osteoma of the tibia. Reformatted sagittal CT shows smooth fusiform periosteal reaction and lucent nidus (arrows).

contain a dense calcified centre (Fig. 45-31). Occurring in the second and third decades, osteoid osteomas most often affect the femur, tibia and humerus. These tumours are chemically active, producing prostaglandins that stimulate new bone formation in the area around the lesion.

Vascular. Periosteal reaction due to chronic vascular insufficiency is commonly seen in the older population, almost exclusively affecting the tibia and fibula and occasionally the metatarsals and phalanges. Radiographs reveal a solid and undulating, non-aggressive periosteal reaction which initially is separate from the underlying cortex but blends with it over time. There may be other features of venous stasis such as phleboliths, and soft-tissue swelling is a common finding.

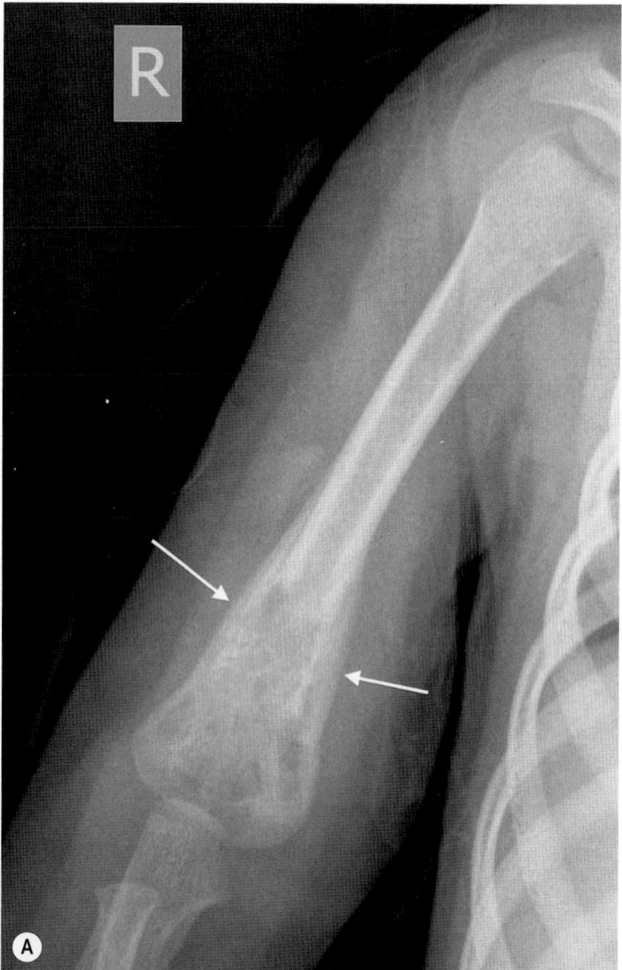

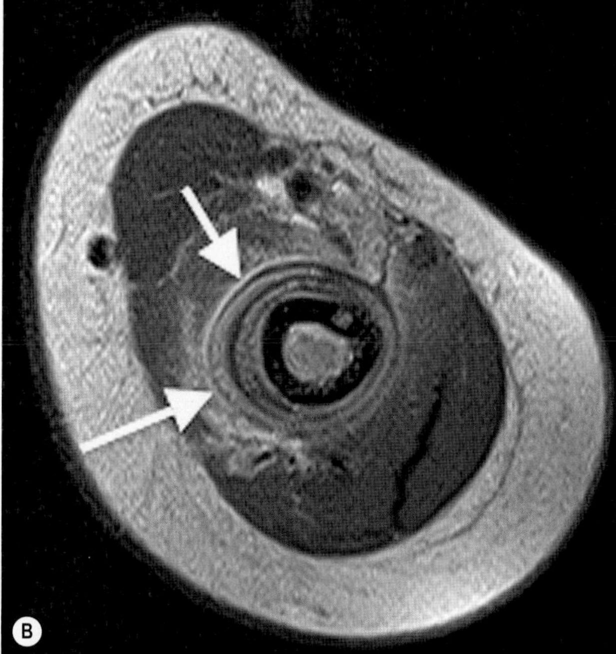

FIGURE 45-32 ■ Aggressive periosteal reaction in Langerhans cell histiocytosis in a paediatric patient. Bone destruction and lamellated periosteal reaction (arrows) shown on (A) AP radiograph and (B) axial T2 MRI.

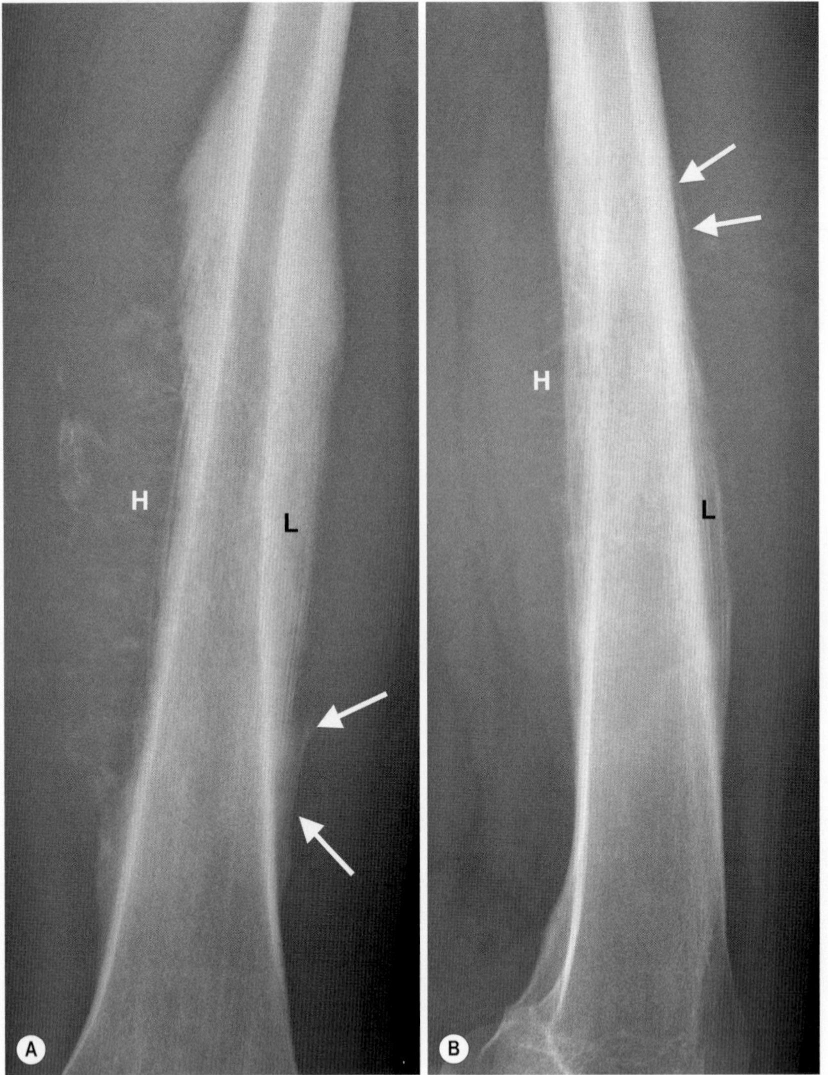

FIGURE 45-33 ■ **Ewing's sarcoma of the femur.** (A) AP and (B) lateral radiographs show lamellated (L) and hair-on-end (H) periosteal reaction with Codman triangle formation (arrows).

Aggressive Periosteal Reaction. Aggressive periosteal reaction occurs due to a rapidly progressive disease process, typically primary bone malignancy, osteomyelitis or metastatic bone disease. Some benign bone disorders such as aneurysmal bone cysts, however, are well recognised as having periosteal reaction with aggressive features. Several subtypes of aggressive periosteal reaction are described; although certain traits are more common with specific conditions, there is sizable overlap in appearance.

Lamellated periosteal reaction occurs parallel to the long axis of the bone and can be seen as multiple layers of concentric new bone formation. Sometimes referred to as 'onion-skin' periosteal reaction, this is described as a feature of Ewing's sarcoma but may also be seen in osteosarcoma, lymphoma and rarely infection (Figs. 45-32 and 45-33). Periosteal reaction with a radial orientation to the bone represents invasion of perforating vascular channels and along Sharpey's fibres. This can have the perpendicular 'hair-on-end' pattern (Fig. 45-33) seen in Ewing's sarcoma, osteosarcoma and rarely infection, or there may be a divergent 'sunburst' arrangement more typical of osteosarcoma, osteoblastoma and osteoblastic metastases (Fig. 45-25).

A Codman triangle is a zone of periosteal elevation seen in association with a soft-tissue mass or at the border of cortical destruction or tumour extension (Fig. 45-33A). It is a feature of primary bone tumours such as osteosarcoma and Ewing's sarcoma but can also be caused by metastases, infection or trauma.

For a full list of references, please see ExpertConsult.

FURTHER READING

6. Ophir J, Céspedes I, Ponnekanti H, et al. Elastography: a quantitative method for imaging the elasticity of biological tissues. Ultrason Imaging 1991;13(2):111–34.

7. Danielson P, Alfredson H, Forsgren S. Distribution of general (PGP 9.5) and sensory (substance P/CGRP) innervations in the human patellar tendon. Knee Surg Sports Traumatol Arthrosc 2006;14(2):125–32.
8. McNally EG. Ultrasound of the small joints of the hands and feet: current status. Skeletal Radiol 2008;37(2):99–113.
9. McCollough CH, Primak AN, Braun N, et al. Strategies for reducing radiation dose in CT. Radiol Clin North Am 2009;47(1): 27–40.
10. Choi HK, Al-Arfaj AM, Eftekhari A, et al. Dual energy computed tomography in tophaceous gout. Ann Rheum Dis 2009;68(10): 1609–12.
11. Nicolaou S, Yong-Hing CJ, Galea-Soler S, et al. Dual-energy CT as a potential new diagnostic tool in the management of gout in the acute setting. Am J Roentgenol 2010;194(4):1072–8.
12. Pache G, Krauss B, Strohm P, et al. Dual-energy CT virtual noncalcium technique: detecting posttraumatic bone marrow lesions—feasibility study. Radiology 2010;256(2):617–24.

CHAPTER 46

Internal Derangements of Joints: Upper and Lower Limbs

Robert S.D. Campbell • Andrew J. Dunn • Eugene McNally • Ahmed Daghir

CHAPTER OUTLINE

INTRODUCTION

Magnetic resonance imaging (MRI) and ultrasound now allow the radiologist to undertake detailed examinations of the soft tissues of joints including tendons, ligaments, cartilage and fibrocartilagenous structures such as the menisci. Injuries that previously had to be inferred from patterns of bone injury shown on conventional radiographs can now be assessed in great detail allowing prognosis for conservative management and planning for surgical decision making. While common features exist in terms of the appearance of tendon and ligament abnormalities, the individual biomechanical properties of the different joints and the varying requirements of these joints strongly influence the patterns of injury seen. Broadly, soft-tissue joint injury falls into two patterns: acute injuries such as an acute ligament tear or osteochondral injury and chronic injury. Chronic injury generally occurs as a result of chronic and repetitive microtrauma to the structure concerned. Examples include tendinopathy and impingement syndromes. In this chapter we have used the term 'tendinopathy' (sometimes also known as tendinosis) to refer to chronic degenerative change in tendons. This was previously referred to as tendinitis, but this term has fallen out of use as it implies an inflammatory process which is not a feature of the chronic pattern of tendon injury being described.

THE SHOULDER

The shoulder is the most mobile joint in the human body. Movement occurs primarily through the glenohumeral joint, but with a large contribution from the scapulothoracic articulation. The upper limb and scapula articulate with the trunk through the acromioclavicular and sternoclavicular joints. The wide range of movement that can occur at the shoulder is possible because of the shallow cup provided by the glenoid and relatively large humeral head. This configuration has been likened to a golf ball on a golf tee and is inherently unstable. Stability to the glenohumeral joint is provided through the soft tissues of the rotator cuff tendons and ligaments, which are susceptible to injury.

The glenoid fossa of the scapula articulates with the head of the humerus to form the glenohumeral joint (GHJ). The glenoid is shallow, pear shaped and anteverted in both the sagittal and axial planes. The fibrocartilaginous labrum runs circumferentially around the glenoid, increasing the overall surface area and contributing to the stability of the joint.

The GHJ is surrounded by a number of synovial-lined bursae that communicate with each other and provide lubrication for the motion of the rotator cuff tendons. The subscapularis bursa (SSB) lies anteriorly between the subscapularis tendon and the anterior deltoid muscle. The subacromial bursa (SAB) lies between the supraspinatus and infraspinatus tendons and the undersurface of the acromion, ACJ and lateral end of the clavicle. The subdeltoid bursa (SDB) is continuous with the lateral aspects of the SAB and SSB and continues posteriorly beneath the posterior belly of the deltoid muscle.

The rotator cuff muscles and tendons along with the long head of biceps are the dynamic stabilisers of the GHJ. The rotator cuff muscles arise from the scapula, passing laterally, to insert on the proximal humerus. They contribute to abduction as well as internal and external rotation of the humerus. The coracoacromial arch is formed by the coracoid, the acromion and the intervening coracoacromial ligament, under which the supraspinatus tendon (SST) passes. The rotator cuff comprises:

- Subscapularis: inserts on lesser tuberosity
- Supraspinatus: inserts anterior facet of greater tuberosity
- Infraspinatus: inserts middle facet of greater tuberosity
- Teres minor: inserts posterior facet of greater tuberosity.

The long head of biceps (LHB) tendon arises from the supraglenoid tubercle and superior labrum. The intra-articular component passes between the subscapularis and supraspinatus tendons in a region known as the rotator interval, and enters the bicipital groove on the anterior aspect of the humeral head. The LHB is stabilised within the rotator interval by the biceps pulley comprised of coracohumeral and superior glenohumeral ligaments.

The static stabilisers of the GHJ are the glenohumeral (G-H) ligaments which are condensations of the joint capsule. They comprise the superior, middle and inferior glenohumeral ligaments. The IGHL is the most important of the G-H ligaments. It is divided into anterior and posterior components, which act like a hammock to support the humeral head in abduction.

The commonest types of internal derangement of the shoulder relate to:

- rotator cuff disease
- GHJ instability
- superior labral tears.

Rotator Cuff Disease

The commonest cause of rotator cuff tendon tears is external impingement occurring mostly in patients over the age of 40 years. Acute injuries are uncommon in the younger population, except in athletes. Impingement of the rotator cuff tendons occurs between the humeral head and coracoacromial arch during abduction of the upper arm. Initially there is reversible oedema and haemorrhage in the tendons, which may lead to tendinopathy and eventually failure of the tendon.[1] The subacromial space may be reduced by bony abnormalities such as AC joint osteophytes and abnormalities of the shape of the acromion. Secondary impingement may occur through abnormal coordination of the rotator cuff muscles and abnormal scapulothoracic movement.

The impingement phenomenon is associated with the development of subacromial bursitis, and acromial bone spur formation. This further limits the subacromial space and aggravates the impingement process.[1]

Tendinopathy is defined as tendon injury on a cellular level that is most commonly age related and degenerative in nature but may also occur following trauma in younger individuals. The connective tissue that binds and organises the collagen bundles of the tendon undergoes microscopic tearing that leads to activation of inflammatory mediators and disorganised tendon healing. The tendon often thickens and may show features of delamination, mucoid degeneration and eventually partial tearing on imaging.[2] Calcific tendinopathy is characterised by intrasubstance deposition of calcium hydroxyapatite crystals of unknown aetiology. The calcific deposits may be asymptomatic but can become painful when they produce focal tendon swelling that may contribute to external impingement. Release of calcium from the tendon into the overlying SAB can produce an acute inflammatory bursal reaction.

Rotator cuff tendon tears are defined as partial or full thickness. A partial thickness tear (PTT) involves either the articular surface (commonest) or the bursal surface (less common), but does not extend all the way through the tendon.[2] A full thickness tear (FTT) extends from the articular surface to the bursal surface and creates an abnormal communication between the GHJ and SAB. The term full thickness only indicates that the tear extends through the full thickness of the tendon; it does not imply the tear extends from the anterior edge of the tendon to the posterior edge. However, as the tear size increases, the whole tendon may become torn (anterior to posterior) creating a massive tear with medial tendon retraction. The supraspinatus is most commonly affected, but tears may progress to involve both infraspinatus and subscapularis.

Tears of the LHB pulley and subscapularis tendon may lead to medial subluxation of the LHB tendon from the bicipital groove. The LHB may also show features on tendinopathy or may eventually rupture.

Radiography is useful for demonstrating bony abnormalities of the AC joint and acromion and excluding associated GHJ arthrosis (Fig. 46-1). Marked narrowing of the subacromial space is a specific but insensitive sign of a full thickness rotator cuff tear[3] (Fig. 46-2). MRI and ultrasound (US) directly visualise the rotator cuff tendons.

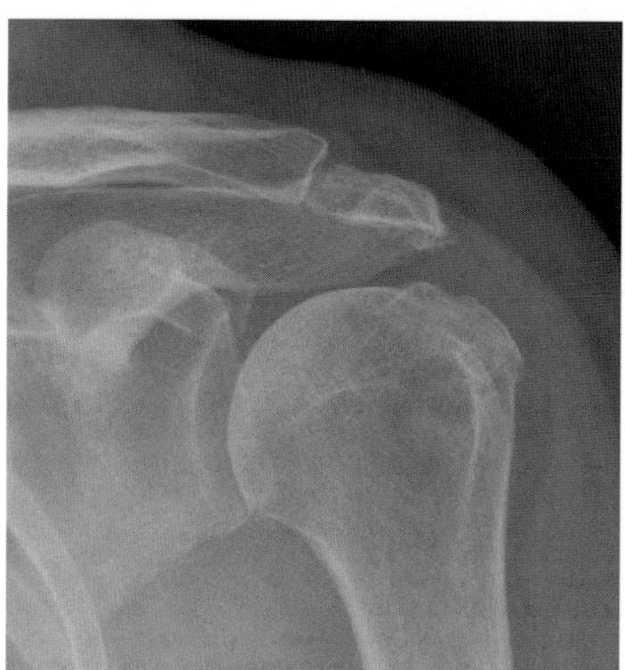

FIGURE 46-1 ■ AP radiograph of the shoulder demonstrating bony enthesophyte formation on the lateral margin of the acromion and the greater tuberosity secondary to external impingement.

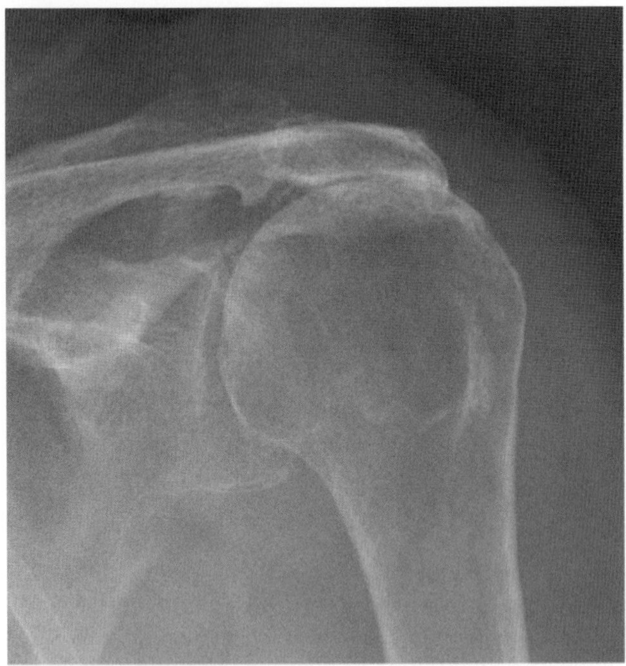

FIGURE 46-2 ■ AP radiograph of the shoulder demonstrating narrowing of the subacromial space and bony impingement of the humerus and acromion secondary to chronic rotator cuff tear.

Both techniques are capable of diagnosing tendinopathy (Fig. 46-3), and have nearly 100% accuracy rates for FTTs of the rotator cuff.[4] MR arthrography is not usually indicated for primary rotator cuff disease. The most important features to describe that help determine management include the following:

- size of cuff tear
- location of cuff tear
- presence of associated rotator cuff muscle atrophy
- dislocation or rupture of the LHB tendon
- bony abnormalities of the coracoacromial arch
- secondary arthrosis of the GHJ.

The primary sign of a rotator cuff FTT is a focal deficiency of the tendon (Figs. 46-4 and 46-5). This nearly always occurs at the tendon insertion on the tuberosity. The margins of the tear are best delineated when there is fluid within the tendon defect. Secondary signs of an FTT include the presence of fluid in both the GHJ and SAB, and flattening or concavity of the subacromial fat plane.

PTTs are less reliably demonstrated by both MRI and US, and it may be difficult to differentiate tendinopathy from partial tears. Focal clefts, tears, or tendon thinning affecting the articular margin of the footprint of the tuberosity are most common (Figs. 46-6 and 46-7). Tendon thickening is not always present. It is important not to mistake magic angle phenomenon on short TE MR sequences or anisotropy on US as evidence of tendinopathy.[2]

Calcific tendinopathy can be visualised on radiographs as discrete amorphous deposits of calcium density. On US they are echogenic and may or may not cast acoustic shadowing (Fig. 46-8). Small deposits of calcium may be

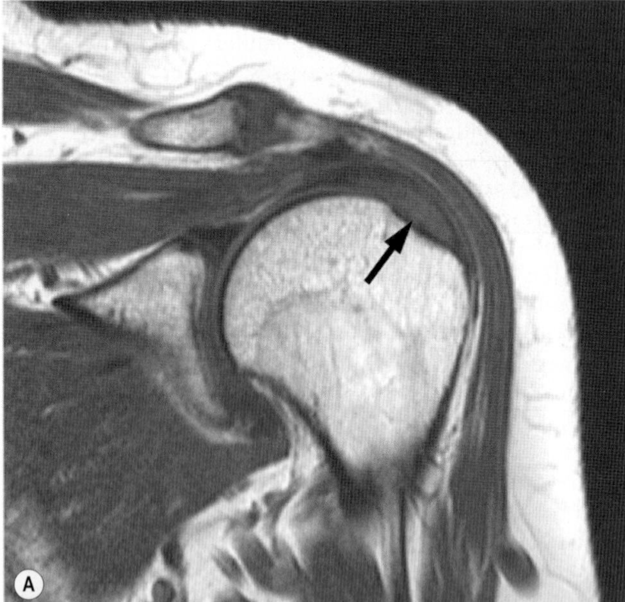

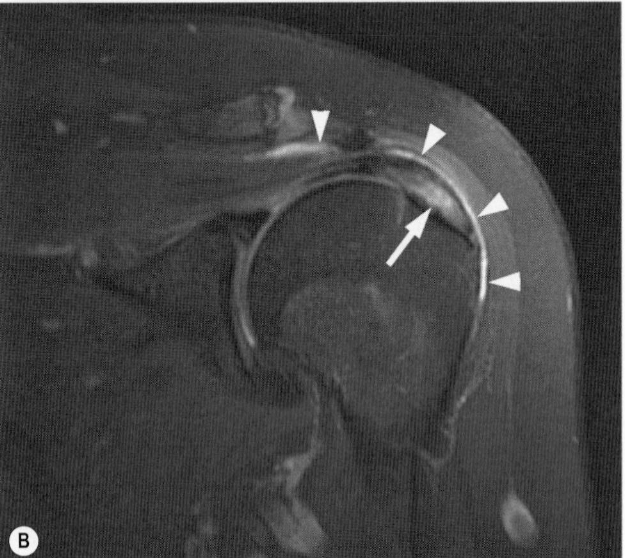

FIGURE 46-3 ■ Coronal oblique T1W (A) and T2FS (B) MR images of a patient with external impingement. High SI fluid is present in the subacromial bursa on the T2W image, indicating bursitis (arrowheads). The supraspinatus tendon is thickened with increased SI on both T1W and T2W sequences as a result of associated tendinopathy (arrows).

difficult to detect on MRI as both the calcification and surrounding tendon are of low SI.

GHJ Instability

The GHJ is an inherently unstable joint. Injury or abnormality of the static stabilisers renders the joint susceptible to recurrent dislocation, and further injury. Chronic GHJ instability may lead to secondary arthrosis if untreated. Imaging is used to document the extent of internal derangement in order to determine the therapeutic options.[5]

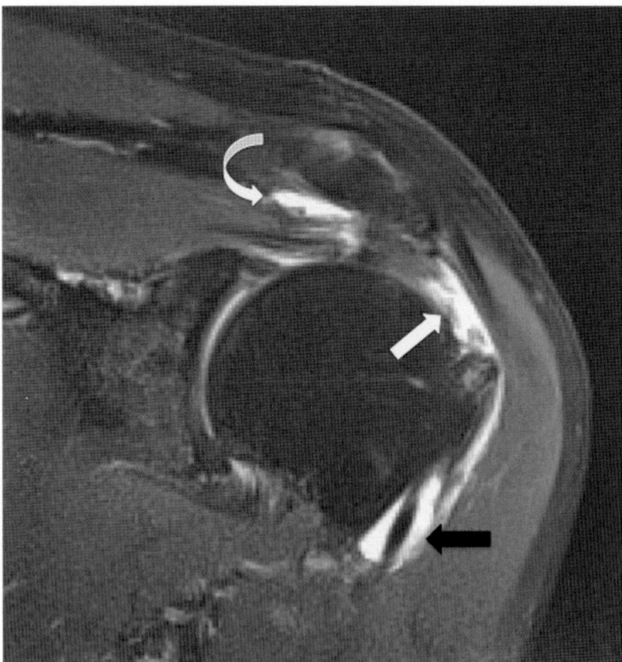

FIGURE 46-4 ■ **Coronal oblique T2FS image.** There is a partial thickness tear of the supraspinatus tendon which is filled by high SI fluid (white arrow). There is also fluid within the glenohumeral joint around the biceps tendon sheath (black arrow), and within the subacromial bursa (curved white arrow), indicating the abnormal communication between the two compartments created by the tendon tear.

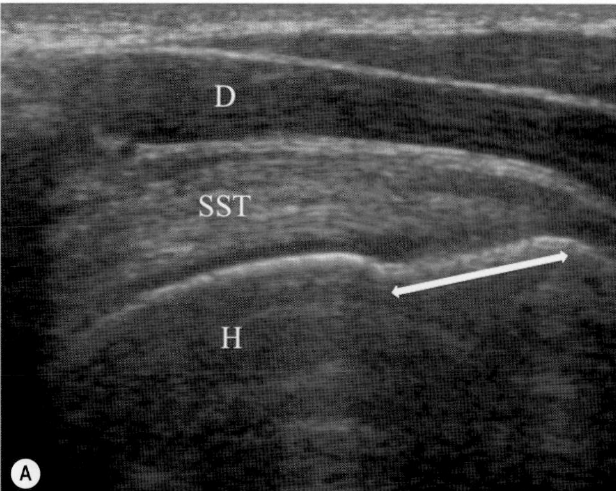

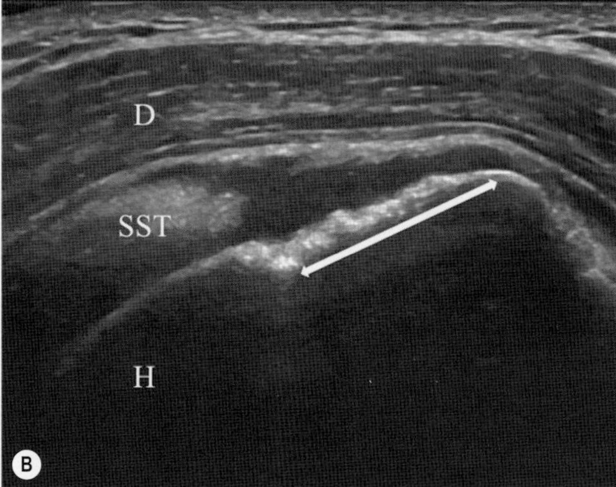

FIGURE 46-5 ■ Normal longitudinal US image of the supraspinatus tendon (A). The echogenic tendon inserts across the footprint of the greater tuberosity (double arrow). A full thickness tear of supraspinatus (B) is demonstrated as a focal deficiency of the tendon which is filled by low reflective joint fluid. D, deltoid muscle; H, humeral head; SST, supraspinatus tendon.

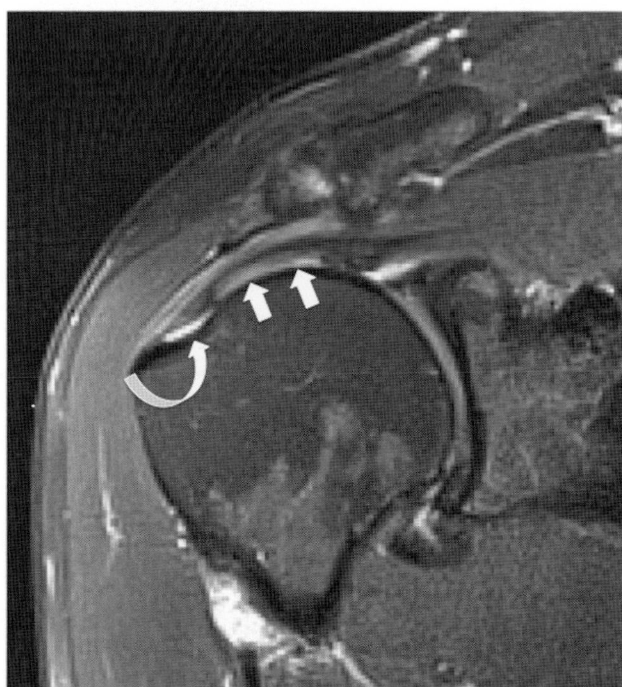

FIGURE 46-6 ■ **Coronal oblique T2FS image.** There is a partial thickness tear of the supraspinatus tendon, with a linear area of fluid SI tracking part way across the insertion point of the tendon on the footprint of the tuberosity (curved white arrow). There is also more extensive partial articular surface tearing of the proximal tendon (white arrows).

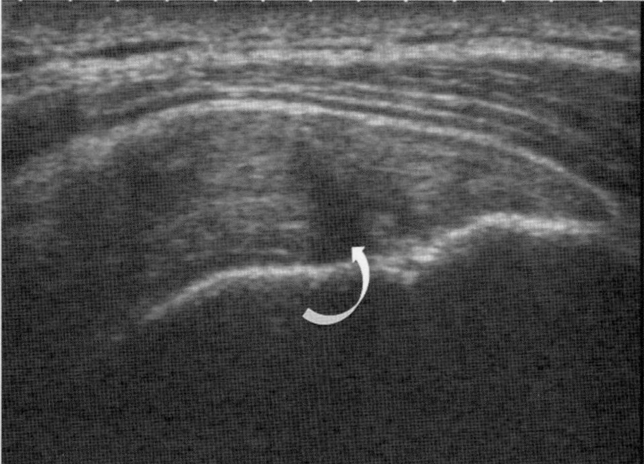

FIGURE 46-7 ■ **Longitudinal US images of a partial thickness tear of the supraspinatus tendon.** There is a focal low reflective area on the articular surface of the tendon (curved arrow). The tear does not extend across the whole of the tuberosity, and does not involve the full tendon width.

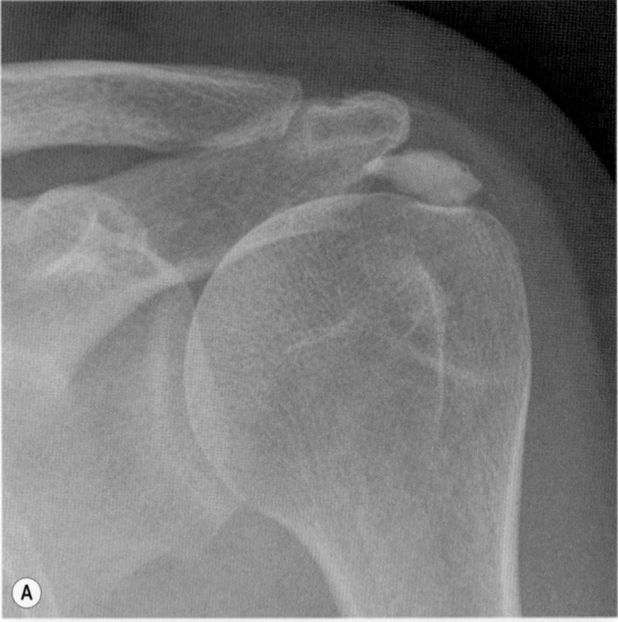

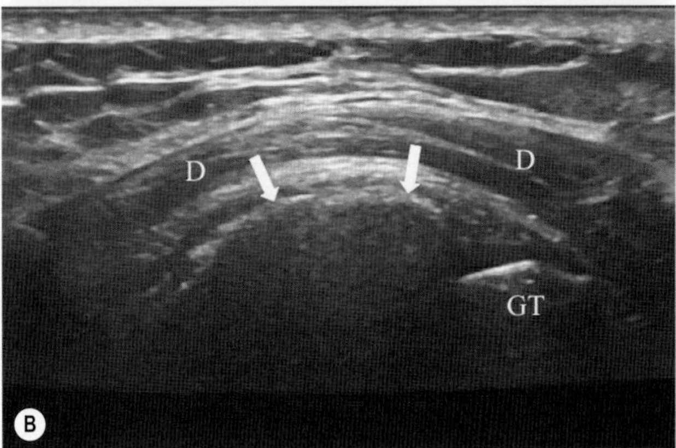

FIGURE 46-8 ■ AP radiograph of the shoulder (A) demonstrating calcific tendonitis with an amorphous deposit of calcium density overlying the greater tuberosity. The longitudinal US image (B) shows the calcific deposit within the suprasinatus tendon as a highly reflective curvilinear area (white arrows). There is posterior acoustic shadowing which partly obscures the underlying humeral head. D, deltoid muscle; GT, greater tuberosity.

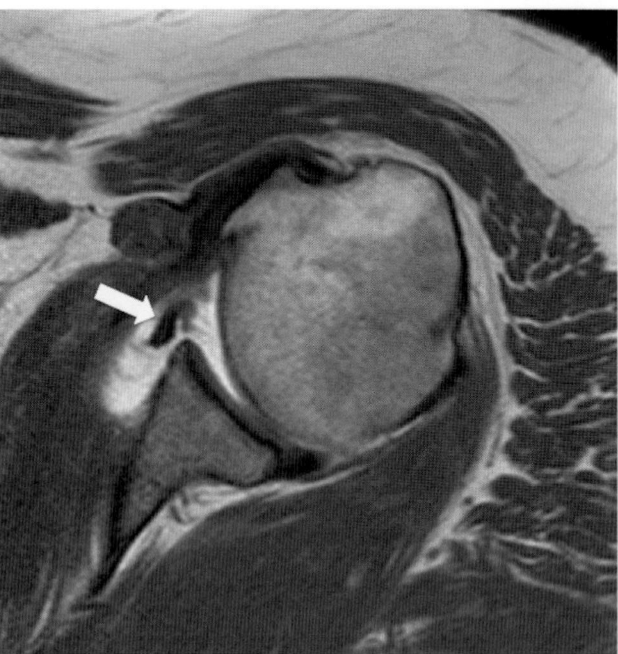

FIGURE 46-9 ■ **Axial T1W image from an MR arthrogram study acquired through the inferior glenoid below the level of the coracoid process.** There is high SI contrast medium extending deep to the low SI fibrocartilaginous labrum (white arrow) as a result of labral detachment (compare with the appearance of the posterior labrum). This is a typical Bankart lesion, with no associated bony defect of the glenoid rim.

Instability of the GHJ may be dependent on three factors, referred to as the Bayley triangle:

- traumatic structural
- atraumatic structural
- habitual non-structural (abnormal muscle patterning).

A combination of these factors may be present in any one patient, but trauma is the commonest cause of instability. Anteroinferior dislocation is the commonest presentation. Posterior dislocation is frequently encountered following epileptic seizures. Inferior dislocation is rare.

Radiographs are the primary imaging technique to confirm GHJ dislocation and establish joint congruity following reduction. Anteroposterior and axial views or a modified caudal angled axial are most appropriate. MRI, MR arthrography or CT arthrography are used in the non-acute setting to assess the static stabilisers.[6]

Anterior GHJ dislocation causes tearing and detachment of the anteroinferior glenoid labrum, known as a Bankart lesion. The location of the labral tear is described according to clockface terminology: 12 o'clock represents the biceps anchor, and 3 o'clock is anterior at the equator of the glenoid. Fluid signal intensity or contrast medium extending between the glenoid and labrum is the primary sign of a labral tear (Fig. 46-9). The labrum may become displaced, and it is important to assess the position of the labrum with respect to the face of the glenoid.

More severe injury may be associated with a bony injury of the glenoid rim, usually called a bony Bankart lesion (Fig. 46-10). Non-enhanced CT may occasionally be preferred to assess the size of the bony defect of the glenoid. There is usually associated impaction injury on the posterosuperior aspect of the humeral head called a Hill–Sachs defect (Figs. 46-11 and 46-12).

In posterior dislocation the location of labral and humeral injury is opposite to anterior dislocation, and are termed reverse Bankart lesions and reverse Hill–Sachs defects.

Injury to the joint capsule and glenohumeral ligaments is common. The anterior band of IGHL is the most important joint stabiliser. It may be torn at the humeral insertion or less commonly from its origin on the glenoid. Imaging with the arm in *ab*duction and *e*xternal *r*otation (ABER imaging) is sometimes used to assess the integrity of the ligament, to identify the degree of labral displacement and loss of joint congruity.[5]

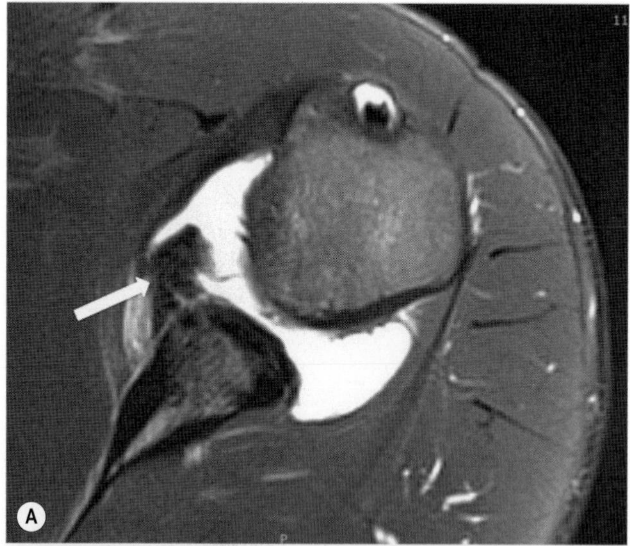

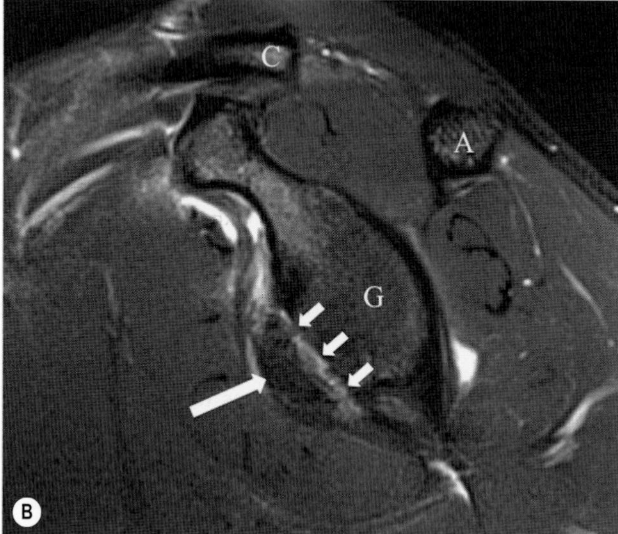

FIGURE 46-10 ■ Axial FS T1W (A) and sagittal oblique FS T1W (B) MR arthrogram images demonstrating a bony Bankart lesion resulting from anterior glenohumeral dislocation. The fibrocartilaginous anterior labrum and glenoid rim are separated from the remainder of the glenoid and displaced medially (white arrow). The fracture line is best seen on the sagittal image (small white arrows). A, acromion; C, clavicle; G, glenoid.

The most important features to describe that help determine management include:

- Location and extent of labral defect
  - use clockface terminology.
- Pattern of labral displacement.
- Presence of bony glenoid rim defects.
  - assess the cross-sectional area of involvement.
- Associated GHJ ligament deficiency.
- Glenoid version.
- Secondary arthrosis of the GHJ.
- Size and depth of the Hill–Sachs defect.

Superior Labral Tears

Tears of the superior labrum and biceps anchor are commonly encountered injuries in overhead throwing athletes. Abnormal traction on the biceps anchor and superior labrum results in tears that usually extend posteriorly. They are often referred to as *s*uperior *l*abral tears *a*nterior to *p*osterior (SLAP tears).[7] MRI, MR arthrography or CT arthrography may assess the glenoid labrum.

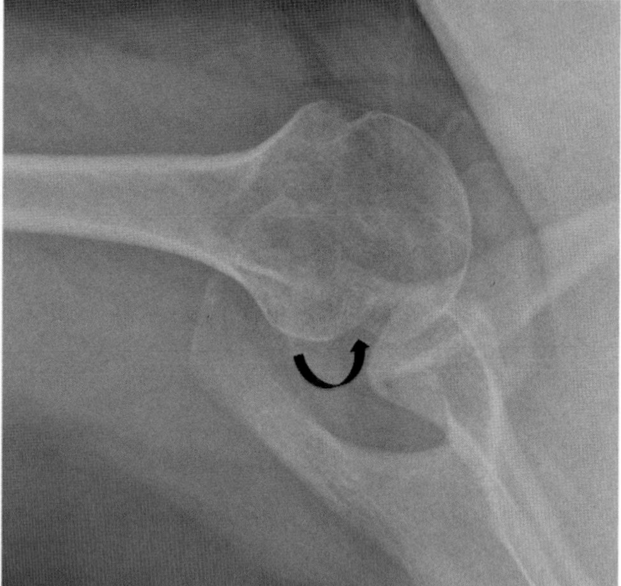

FIGURE 46-11 ■ Subaxial radiograph of the shoulder showing a Hill–Sachs deformity (curved black arrow) secondary to previous traumatic dislocation.

Contrast medium or fluid signal intensity extending into the substance of the labrum or through the chondrolabral junction is the primary sign of a SLAP tear (Fig. 46-13). Tears may be localised to the posterosuperior labrum, or may be more extensive. There may be tear extension into the LHB tendon. There are many grades of SLAP tears described but the extent of the tear and the structures involved are the most important features.[8]

The most important features to describe that help determine management include:

- Extent of labral tear
  - use clockface terminology.
- Involvement of biceps anchor and tendon.
- Presence of associated rotator cuff tears.

THE ACROMIOCLAVICULAR JOINT

The AC joint is a synovial plane joint. All the forces of glenohumeral and scapulothoracic movements are transmitted to the trunk through the ACJ and sternoclavicular joint. Osteoathritis (OA) of the ACJ is common and the associated capsular thickening and osteophyte formation is a contributor to external impingement of the shoulder.

The ACJ has strong capsular ligaments, and is also stabilised by the coracoclavicular (C-C) ligaments. Traumatic disruption and dislocation of the joint is described by the Rockwood classification:

Grade I: undisplaced injury with sprain of acromioclavicular ligaments.

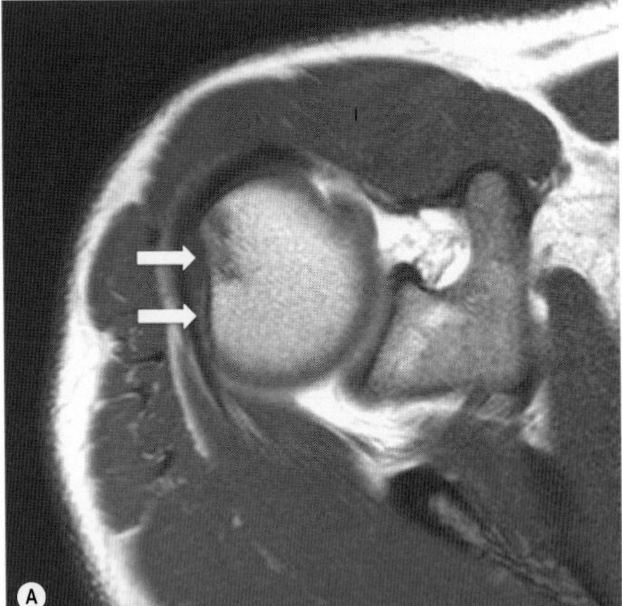

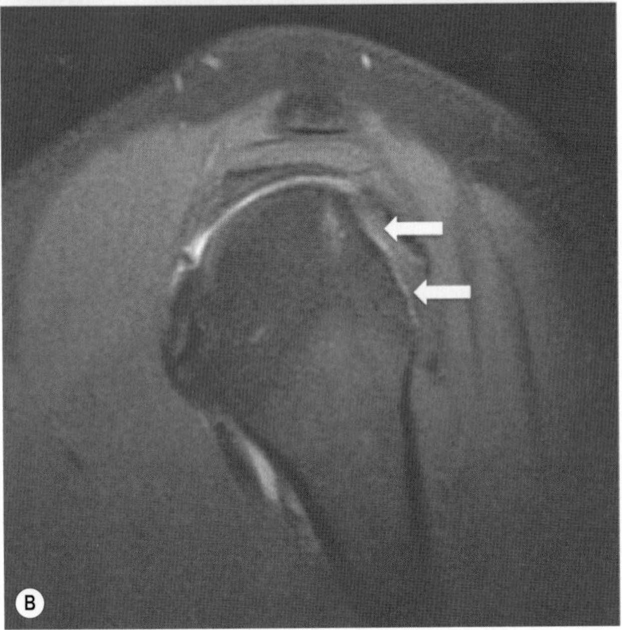

FIGURE 46-12 ■ Axial T1W image from an MR arthrogram study demonstrating a Hill–Sachs lesion (A). There is flattening of the posterolateral humeral head (white arrows), which should normally be approximately spherical at the level of the coracoid process. The same lesion is also seen on the corresponding sagittal oblique T2FS image (B).

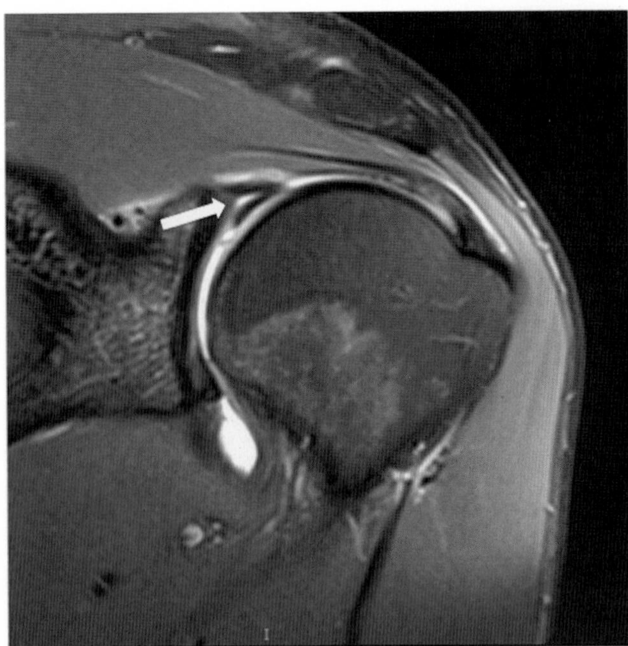

FIGURE 46-13 ■ **Coronal FS T2W MR arthrogram image.** There is high SI contrast medium extending into the substance of the superior labrum, indicating a superior labrum anterior to posterior (SLAP) tear.

Grade II: ACJ widening with <50% superior displacement of lateral clavicle.

Grade III: >100% superior displacement of lateral clavicle.

Grade IV: posterior displacement of lateral clavicle.

Grade III and IV injuries are associated with disruption of the C-C ligaments and above are treated surgically. Grade I and II injuries usually resolve spontaneously. However, some patients may present with persistent pain and instability. Ligament reconstruction may be required in the athletic population.[9] Weight-bearing radiographs may demonstrate abnormal joint widening, and the C-C ligaments can be visualised directly by MRI (Fig. 46-14).

Post-traumatic osteolysis of the lateral clavicle occurs in approximately 6% of ACJ disruptions and may also be seen with repetitive ACJ microtrauma such as weightlifting (Fig. 46-15).

THE STERNOCLAVICULAR JOINT

The sternoclavicular joint (SCJ) is a synovial saddle joint, with a cartilaginous articular disc. It has limited movement, but like the AC joint transmits the forces of shoulder movement to the trunk. It is very prone to osteoarthritis, which may be associated with chronic anterior subluxation. Radiographic evaluation of the SC joints may be difficult but CT or MRI readily demonstrate the features of arthrosis.[10]

Traumatic subluxation and dislocation usually occurs anteriorly. Posterior dislocation is a rare but important injury, as the displaced medial clavicle may be associated with vascular injury in the superior mediastinum.[11]

THE ELBOW

The elbow is a complex synovial hinge joint. It comprises the ulnotrochlear and radiocapitellar articulations which allow flexion and extension of the elbow. The proximal radioulnar joint (in conjuction with the distal radioulnar joint) enables pronation and supination of the forearm by rotation of the radius around the ulna.[12]

The primary flexors are biceps brachii, brachialis and brachoradialis. Triceps is the main extensor. Supination

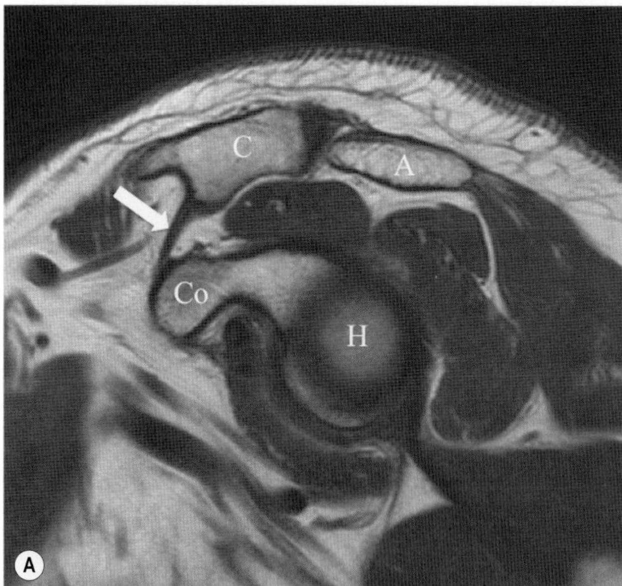

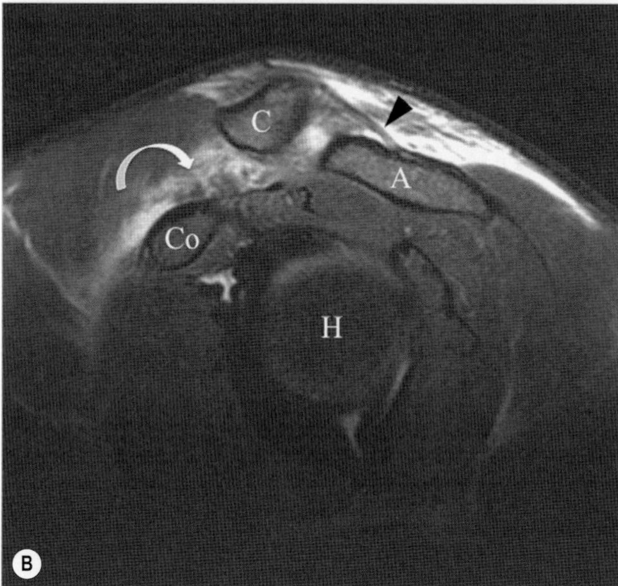

FIGURE 46-14 ■ Sagittal oblique T1W image (A) of the normal coracoclavicular (C-C) ligament. The FS T2W MR image (B) was acquired in a patient following traumatic disruption of the acromioclavicular joint. The joint is normally aligned, but there is fluid within the joint, there is stripping of the superior joint capsule (arrowhead) and there is high SI haemorrhage in the overlying soft tissues. In addition there is haemorrhage between the coracoid and clavicle secondary to C-C ligament disruption (white arrow). A, acromion; C, clavicle; Co, coracoid; H, humeral head.

of the forearm occurs through the action of biceps and supinator. Pronation is by pronator teres, and pronator quadratus (at the wrist). The common tendon for wrist and hand extension arises from the lateral humeral epicondyle, and the common flexor tendon from the medial epicondyle.

The joint is stabilised by the ulnar collateral and radial collateral ligaments. The radial collateral complex includes the annular ligament which supports the radial head.

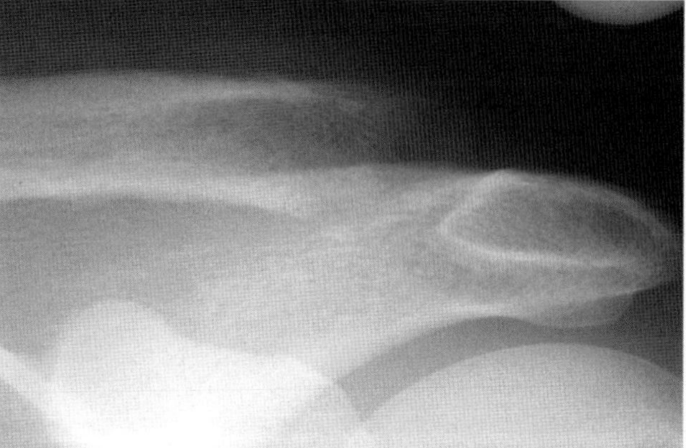

FIGURE 46-15 ■ **AP radiograph of the AC joint.** There is widening of the joint, with resorption and loss of the cortical margin of the lateral clavicle as a result of post-traumatic osteolysis.

Tendons

Insertional tendinopathy around the elbow joint most commonly affects:

- common extensor origin: tennis elbow
- common flexor origin: golfer's elbow
- distal biceps tendon.

The triceps and other tendons are rarely involved.

Tendinopathy of the common extensor and flexor tendons presents with localised pain over the distal humeral epicondyles. It is often a clinical diagnosis, although imaging may be performed in refractory cases to confirm the diagnosis and exclude a tear. Ultrasound is frequently used to guide injection therapy.

The affected tendon is thickened and hyporeflective on US, with neovascularisation on Doppler imaging (Fig. 46-16). High SI is demonstrated on fluid-sensitive MRI sequences (Fig. 46-17). Tendon tears are demonstrated as focal areas of deficiency.[13] In chronic cases, new bone formation may be seen on radiographs at the tendon enthesis. Calcific tendinopathy is much less common than in the rotator cuff of the shoulder.

The distal biceps tendon inserts on the tuberosity of the proximal radius. It does not have a tendon sheath, but surrounding connective tissue is known as a paratenon. It is surrounded near the insertion by the bicipitoradial bursa. Distal biceps tears are often clinically unrecognised, but may be amenable to surgery if diagnosed early. In the early stages the tendon is thickened and there may be an effusion in the bicipitoradial bursa (Fig. 46-18). In complete rupture the tendon retracts proximally. MRI and US may be used to confirm the diagnosis and locate the tendon end (Figs. 46-19 and 46-20).

Bone and Cartilage

The capitellum is the third most commonly affected site in osteochondritis dissecans (after the knee and ankle). It commonly affects teenagers and young adults. A focal osteochondral fragment or defect may be visualised on radiographs. Cross-sectional imaging with MRI, MR arthrography or CT arthrography is used to detect radiographically occult lesions and for grading osteochondral

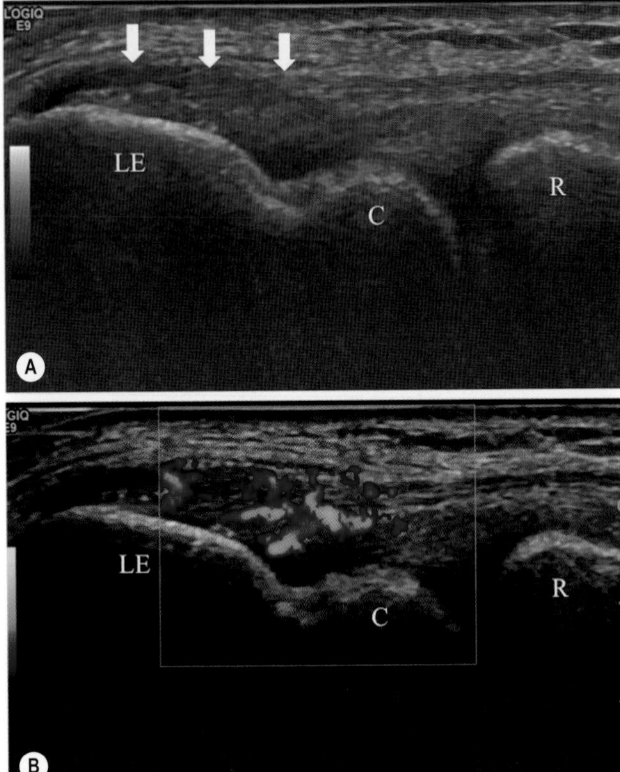

FIGURE 46-16 ■ **Longitudinal US images of tennis elbow.** The common extensor tendon is low reflective and thickened (white arrows) on the grey-scale image (A). The power Doppler image (B) demonstrates prominent neovascularisation. C, capitellum; LE, lateral epicondyle; R, radial head.

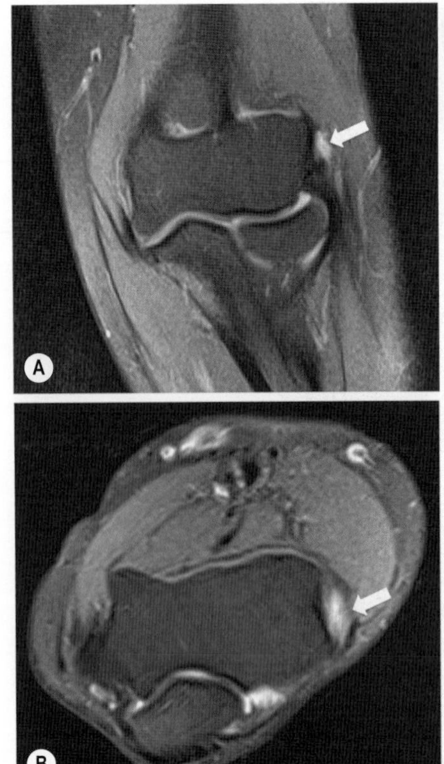

FIGURE 46-17 ■ Coronal (A) and axial (B) FS T2W MR images of the elbow. There is a focal area of high SI intensity tendinopathy in the common extensor tendon origin (white arrows) secondary to insertional tendinopathy (tennis elbow).

lesions (Fig. 46-21). The osteochondral fragment may remain in situ or lie remotely within the elbow joint. Fluid SI at the base of the osteochondral lesion on MRI, or contrast medium tracking around the fragment on arthrographic images, is a sign of an unstable lesion. Integrity of the overlying articular cartilage is a good sign of stability.

Reports should include:

- size and location of osteochondral defect;
- stability of the lesion and integrity of overlying cartilage; and
- presence of any remote intra-articular bodies.

Intra-articular bodies are also frequently encountered in OA of the elbow. They may be calcified, but non-calcified chondral bodies may also occur. CT is often utilised to assess the size and location of osteophytes before surgery, as well as identify small loose bodies. Chondral bodies are not visualised on radiographs or conventional CT. In some cases pre- and post-angiography CT may be performed (Fig. 46-22). Conventional MRI is less sensitive for detection of small intra-articular bodies.

Ligaments

The collateral ligaments of the elbow may be torn as the result of an elbow dislocation, and may require surgical repair. A coronoid process fracture is a sign of an

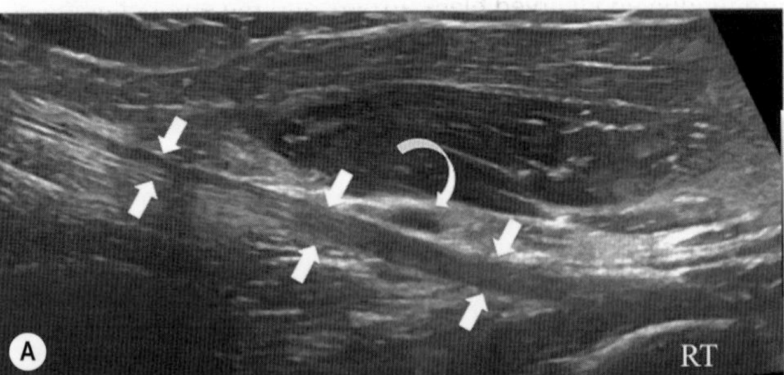

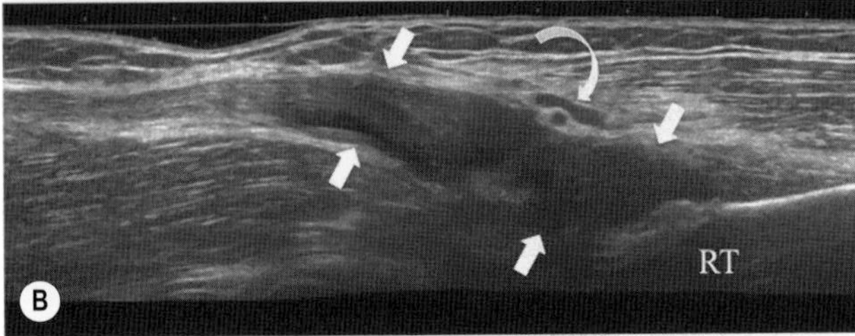

FIGURE 46-18 ■ Longitudinal US (A) of a normal distal biceps tendon (white arrows). The tendon is of uniform size and echotexture and inserts on the radial tuberosity. In a patient with elbow pain, severe tendinopathy is present, with marked tendon thickening and low reflective change (B). Note the relationship of the tendon to the brachial vessels (curved white arrows). RT, radial tuberosity.

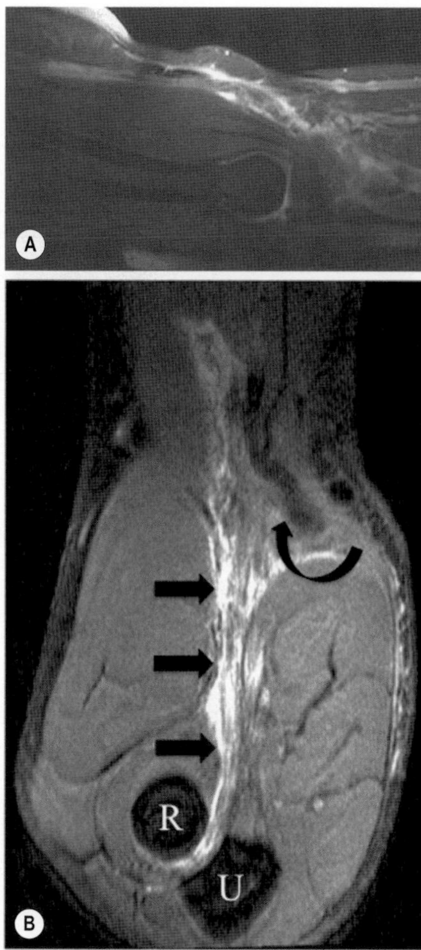

FIGURE 46-19 ■ FS T2W MR images of a complete distal biceps tendon tear. The sagittal image (A) demonstrates high SI haemorrhage around the poorly defined retracted tendon end (white arrows). The corresponding FABS image (B) acquired with the arm above the head with the elbow flexed demonstrates the torn tendon end (curved black arrow), and the empty fluid-filled tendon sheath extending down to the insertion on the radial tuberosity (black arrows). B, biceps muscle; R, radius; T, trochlea; U, ulna.

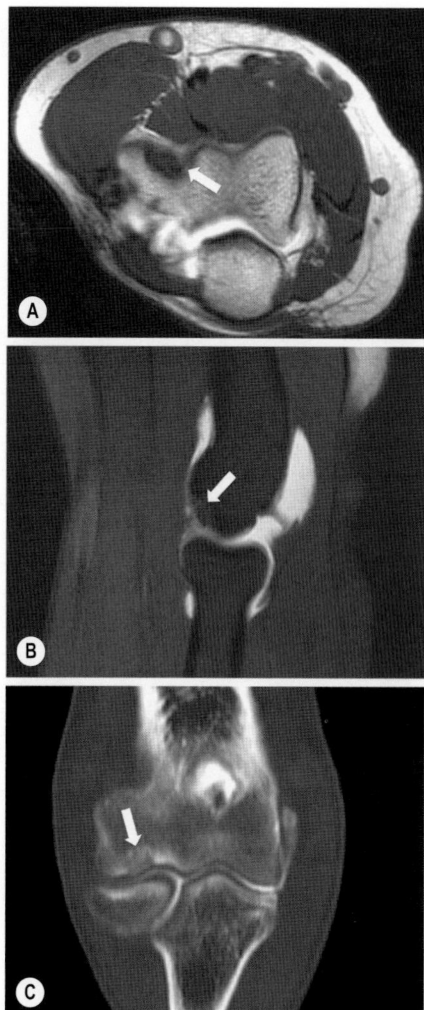

FIGURE 46-21 ■ Osteochondritis dissecans (OCD) of the capitellum. The OCD lesion is seen on the T1W (A) and FS T1W (B) MR arthrogram images as an area of low SI in the subchondral bone. There is no high SI contrast medium extending around of the base of the lesion, indicating the articular cartilage is intact, and the lesion is stable. The corresponding coronal CT arthrogram image (C) also confirms the integrity of the articular cartilage.

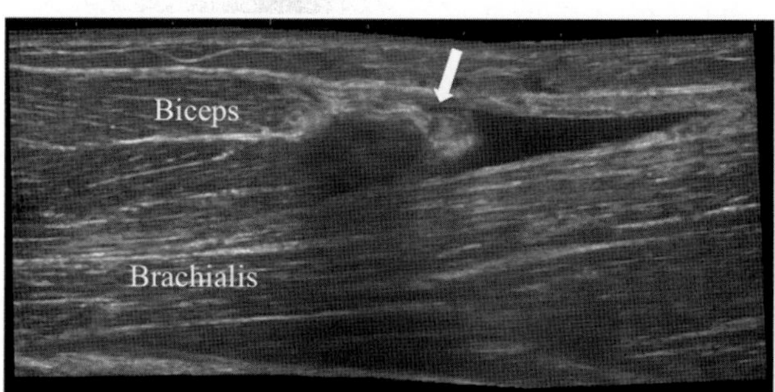

FIGURE 46-20 ■ Longitudinal US image of a distal biceps tendon tear. The torn retracted tendon end (white arrow) is accentuated by the presence of acoustic shadowing because of edge artefact and the low reflective fluid in the tendon sheath distally.

unrecognised elbow dislocation. Chronic tears of the ulnar collateral ligament are infrequently encountered in some throwing sports and in weightlifters.

In acute injuries MRI shows the presence of soft-tissue oedema and haemorrhage around the affected ligament. MR arthrography may be preferred for diagnosis of chronic tears. Acute ulnar collateral ligament (UCL) tears often occur at the proximal origin on the medial humeral epicondyle (Fig. 46-23). In chronic tears the defect is usually at the insertion on the sublime tubercle of the ulna.[14]

HAND AND WRIST

The wrist is a synovial joint, formed from the articulations between the radius and ulna, the eight carpal bones

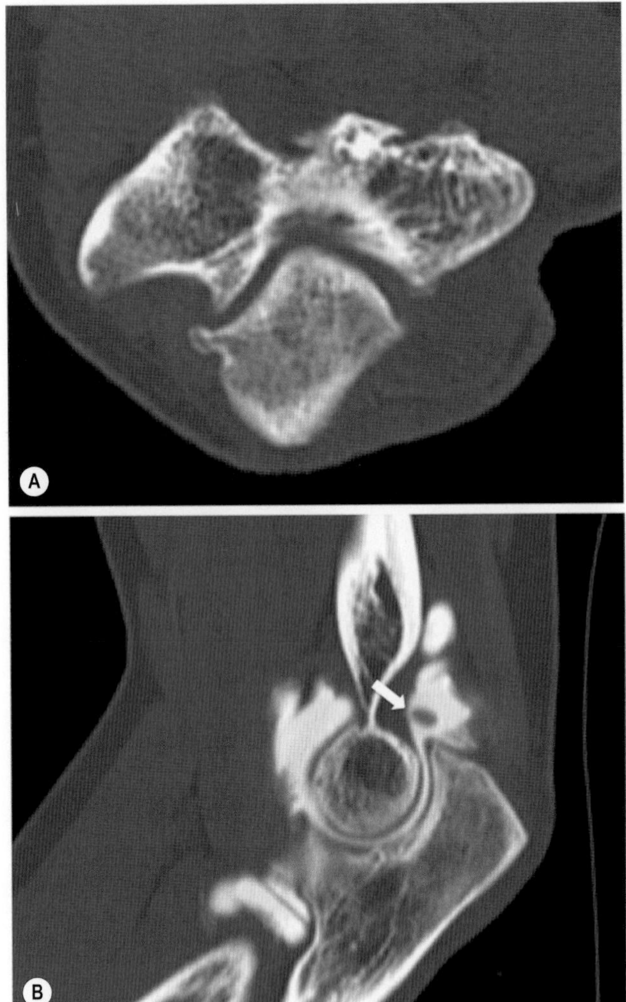

FIGURE 46-22 ■ Axial CT image (A) of early OA of the elbow. There is an osteophyte arising from the olecranon. The corresponding sagittal CT arthrogram image (B) demonstrates a non-radiopaque chondral body in the posterior joint recess (white arrow).

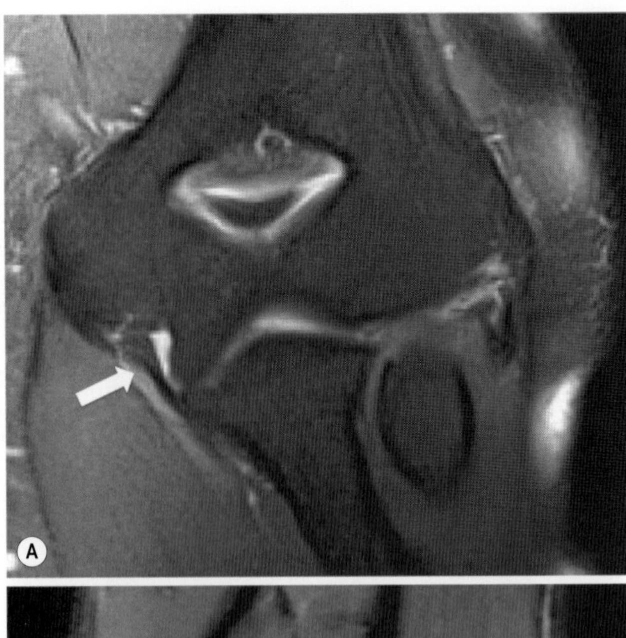

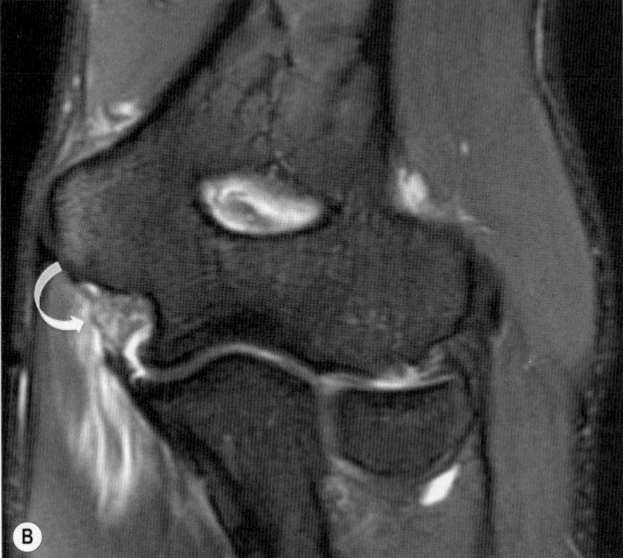

FIGURE 46-23 ■ Coronal FS T2W MR image (A) of a normal ulnar collateral ligament (UCL) of the elbow (white arrow). In a patient with an acute valgus strain injury (B), there is a tear of the UCL at the proximal origin on the lateral humeral epicondyle (curved white arrow), and there is surrounding soft-tissue haemorrhage.

and the metacarpal bones. The distal radioulnar joint allows supination and pronation of the forearm.

The mechanics of the wrist are complex, but movement occurs primarily through the proximal carpal row, comprising the scaphoid, lunate and triquetrum. This acts as a bridge between the forearm bones and the distal carpal row, which is relatively rigid. The proximal carpal row is referred to as the intercalated segment, and the lunate acts as the keystone. Stability between the segments of the proximal row is maintained by the intrinsic scapholunate and lunotriquetral ligaments. Stability between the radius and ulna, the proximal and distal carpal rows is maintained by multiple dorsal and volar extrinsic ligaments. Carpal alignment is assessed on PA radiographs, by identifying continuity of the articular surfaces of the carpal bones (known as the arcs of Gilula).

The first carpometacarpal joint between the trapezium and first metacarpal is more mobile than the other CMC joints to allow for the greater range of movements of the thumb. It has a separate synovial compartment.

The distal radioulnar joint and ulnocarpal joint are stabilised by the triangular fibrocartilage (TFC) complex. The TFC is a cartilaginous disc that arises from the ulnar border of the distal radius and attaches to the fovea of the ulnar styloid. Its margins blend with the dorsal and volar radioulnar ligaments, and the extensor carpi ulnaris (ECU) tendon sheath.

The flexor tendons of the fingers and thumb pass through the carpal tunnel, which is maintained superficially by the flexor retinaculum, which extends from the hook of hamate and pisiform to the scaphoid and trapezium. The median nerve passes through the carpal tunnel to enter the palm. The extensor tendons are stabilised by the extensor retinaculum on the dorsal aspect of the wrist at the level of the first carpal row.

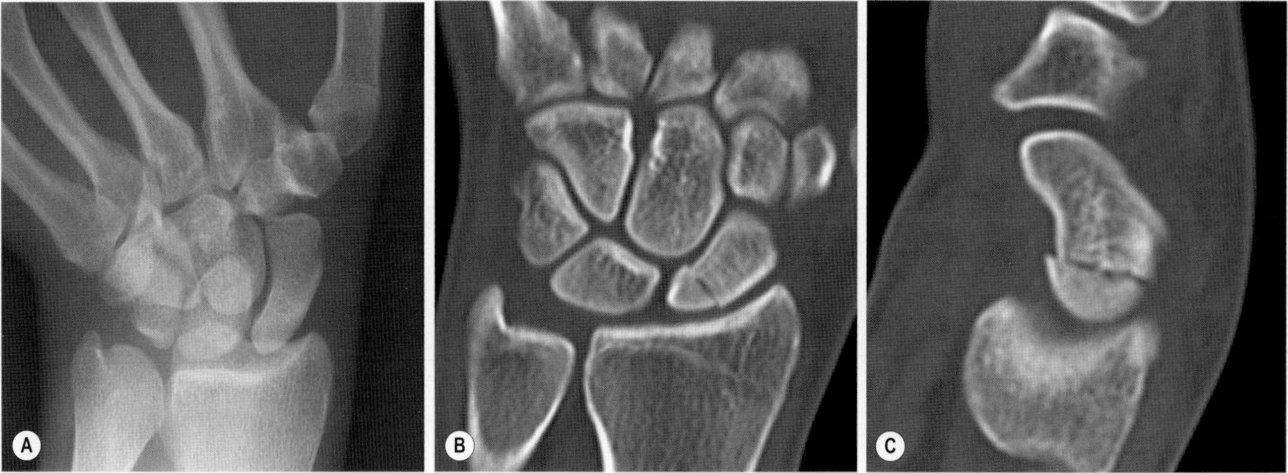

FIGURE 46-24 ■ Follow-up oblique radiograph (A) of the wrist in a patient with previous scaphoid fracture. There is an ill-defined sclerotic area in the proximal pole but there is no visible fracture line. However, the corresponding coronal (B) and sagittal oblique (C) CT MPRs clearly show fracture non-union.

Bone

Fractures around the wrist are common. Waist of scaphoid fractures may be associated with avascular necrosis of the proximal pole. The more proximal the fracture site, the higher the incidence of fracture non-union.

Radiological signs of avascular necrosis (AVN) include sclerosis of the proximal pole, which may progress to articular collapse and bone fragmentation. CT is used to assess the state of fracture union (Fig. 46-24). Signs of AVN on MRI include low SI sclerosis on T1-weighted (T1W) images and short T1 inversion recovery (STIR) images. Marrow oedema on STIR images is an indicator of persistent vascular perfusion in the proximal segment. The absence of enhancement with gadolinium contrast medium on fat-saturated T1W images in areas of sclerosis is a reliable indicator of lack of vascularity[15] (Fig. 46-25).

Spontaneous AVN of the lunate is known as Keinböck's disease. The radiographic and MRI features are the same as AVN of the scaphoid (Fig. 46-26). It may be associated with negative ulnar variance (short ulna). Advanced bony collapse in both proximal scaphoid fractures and AVN of the lunate results in late-stage secondary osteroarthritis.

Wrist Ligaments

Tears of the ligaments of the wrist can result in carpal instability. Disruption of the intrinsic ligaments results in intercalated segment instability. This is also termed dissociative carpal instability because there is dissociation between the segments of the proximal carpal row.

The scapholunate ligament is most frequently involved. Radiographs may show scapholunate diastasis (>3 mm). The lunate demonstrates dorsal rotation on lateral views and volar rotation of the scaphoid. This results in an increase in the scapholunate angle (>60°) known as dorsal intercalated segment instability (DISI) (Fig. 46-27). A DISI deformity of the carpus may also be associated with fractures of the scaphoid.

Disruption of the lunotriquetral ligament is less common. In this situation there is volar rotation of the lunate on lateral radiographs, with reduction of the scapholunate angle (<30°). On PA radiographs there may be an obvious step between the distal articular surface of the lunate and triquetrum. This is termed volar intercalated segment instability (VISI).

More subtle degrees of instability may be demonstrated by an instability series of radiographs acquired with radial and ulnar deviation and with a clenched fist view. Video fluoroscopy is also useful for assessing dynamic wrist instability.

Abnormal communication between the radiocarpal and midcarpal joints may be seen on arthrography (Fig. 46-28), which is usually combined with MRI or CT[16] (Figs. 46-29 and 46-30). However, direct visualisation of the ligaments is possible with conventional MRI. The most important features to describe that help determine management include the following:

- Carpal alignment
  - scapholunate angle
  - scapholunate diastasis
  - disruption of the arcs of Gilula.
- Integrity of the intrinsic ligaments.
- Presence of associated arthrosis.

Injuries to the extrinsic ligaments result in a variety of complex radiocarpal and midcarpal non-dissociative instabilities.

Lunate and perilunate dislocations are important injuries. In lunate dislocation, the lunate dislocates in a volar direction with loss of the articulation of the radius and other carpal bones. In perilunate dislocation, the lunate retains the articulation with the radius and the remainder of the carpus dislocates in a dorsal or volar direction. PA radiographs show an abnormal triangular appearance of the lunate. Differentiation of lunate versus perilunate dislocation is best made on a lateral radiograph. Both injuries may be associated with scaphoid (or other carpal) fractures, which indicates a greater degree of wrist instability.

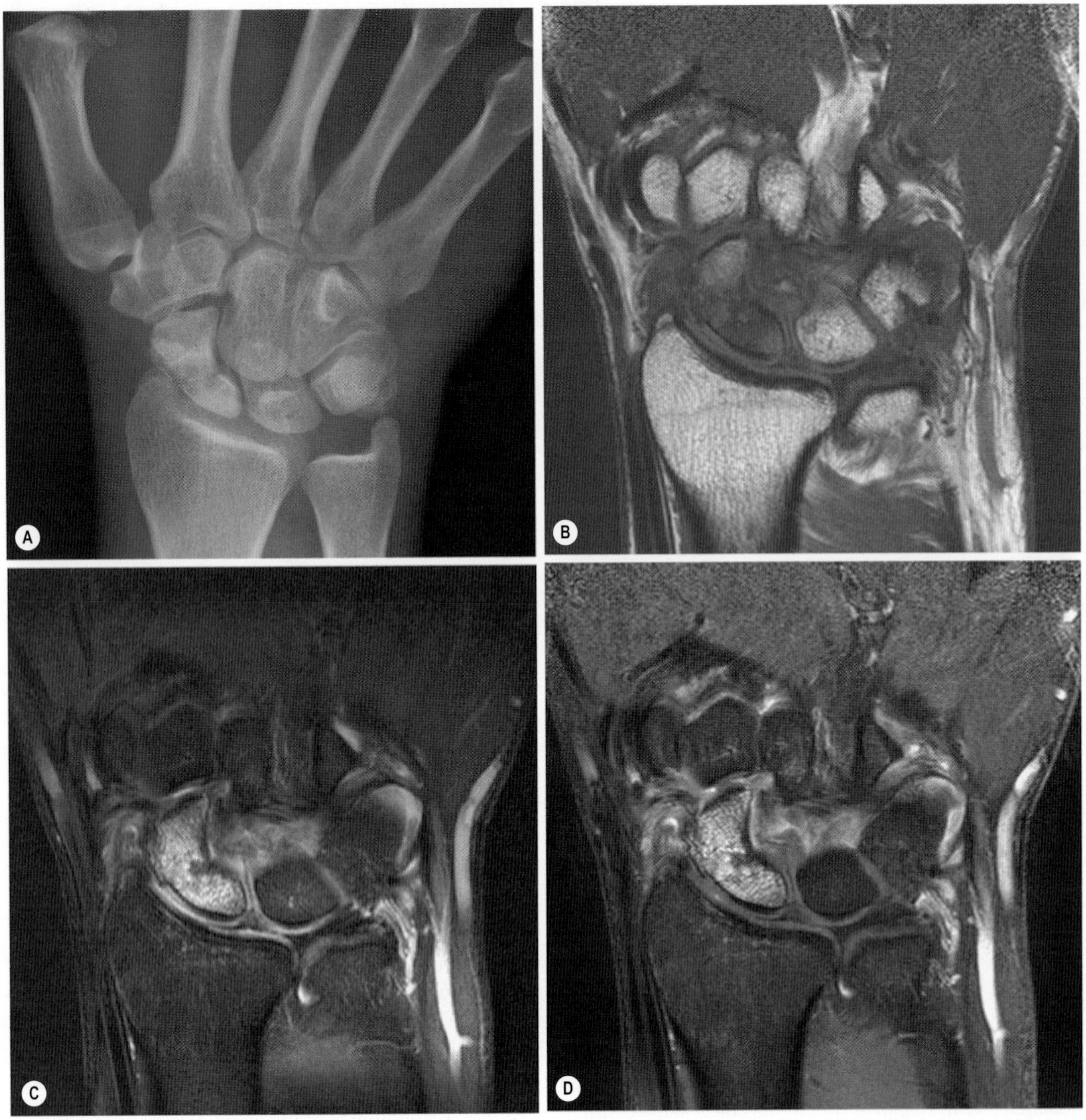

FIGURE 46-25 ■ PA radiograph of the wrist (A) showing non-union of a scaphoid fracture. There is sclerosis of the proximal pole segment indicating possible avascular necrosis (AVN). The corresponding coronal T1W MR image (B) demonstrates low SI within the marrow cavity, which is also consistent with AVN. However, there is high SI oedema on the T2FS image (C), and the post-contrast medium T1FS image (D) shows marked enhancement, indicating persistent vascularity of the scaphoid.

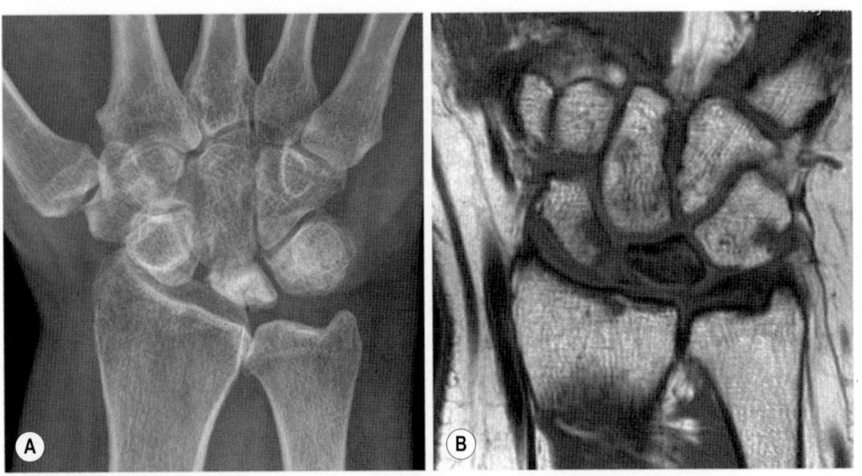

FIGURE 46-26 ■ AP radiograph (A) of the wrist with avascular necrosis of the lunate (Keinböck's disease). The lunate is small and sclerotic with features of early subchondral fragmentation. The coronal T1W image (B) shows the same features with low SI marrow indicating bone sclerosis. No marrow oedema was present on the T2FS images (not shown).

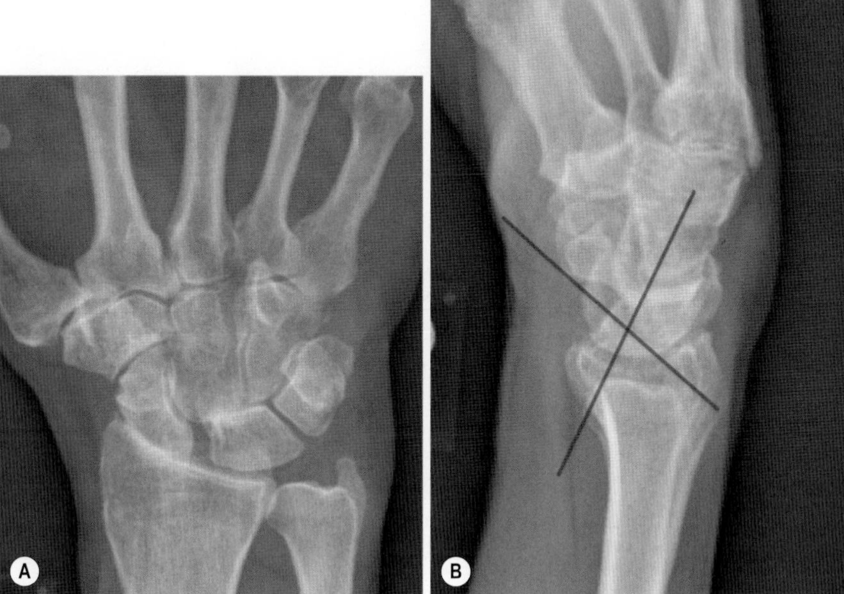

FIGURE 46-27 ■ AP (A) and lateral (B) radiographs of the wrist in a patient with scapholunate ligament rupture, dorsal intercalated segment instability (DISI), and secondary OA. There is scapholunate diastasis on the AP view, with widening of the joint space. The scapholunate angle (black lines) is increased above 60° on the lateral view with dorsal tilt of the lunate (normal scapholunate angle = 30–60°).

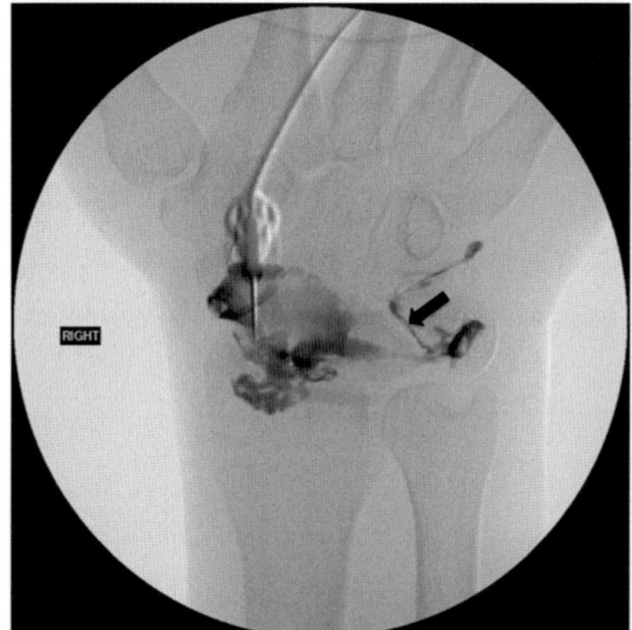

FIGURE 46-28 ■ **Fluoroscopic image acquired during digital subtraction arthrography of the wrist.** The radiocarpal joint has been injected and contrast medium fills the joint space. There is leak of contrast medium through the lunotriquetral joint into the midcarpal joint (black arrow), indicating ligament rupture.

Triangular Fibrocartilage

The TFC is composed of fibrocartilage and is normally low SI on all MRI pulse sequences (Fig. 46-31). Tears of the TFC complex may present as ulnar-sided wrist pain. They occur as either a degenerative phenomenon or as an acute injury. Degenerative tears frequently result in central perforation of the TFC (Fig. 46-32), and are associated with positive ulnar variance (long ulna). This in turn may lead to ulnar abutment on the triquetrum, which is another cause of ulnar-sided wrist pain.

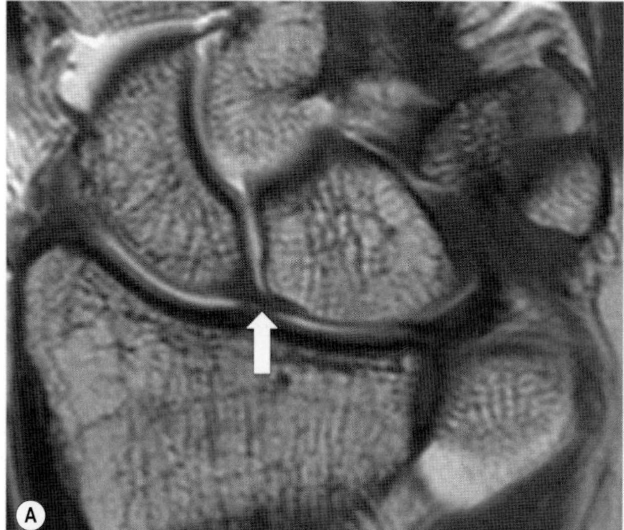

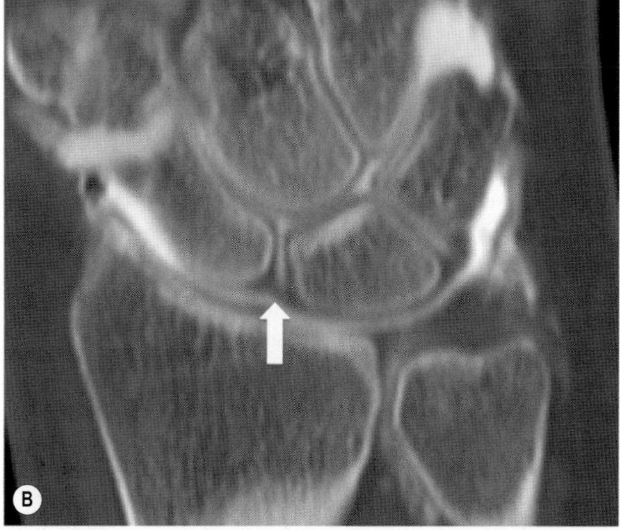

FIGURE 46-29 ■ Normal scapholunate ligament on coronal T1W MR arthrogram (A) and CT arthrogram (B) images (white arrows).

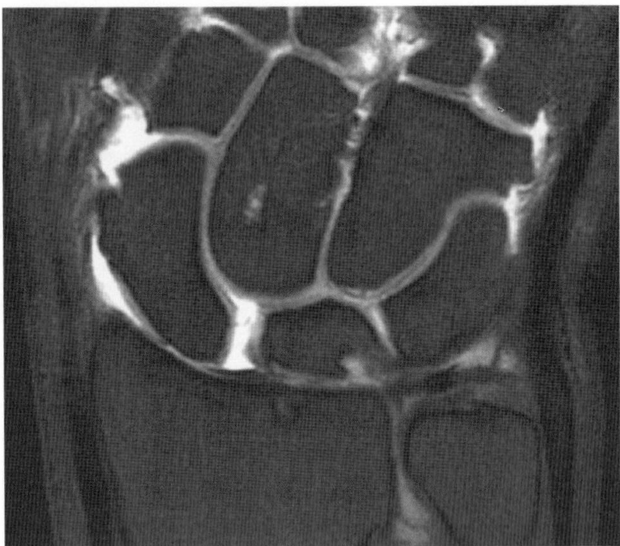

FIGURE 46-30 ■ **Scapholunate ligament disruption on an FS T1W MR arthrogram image.** The ligament is absent, and there is scapholunate diastasis. There are features of early secondary OA change with loss of articular cartilage on the scaphoid and lunate with a subchondral cyst in the lunate.

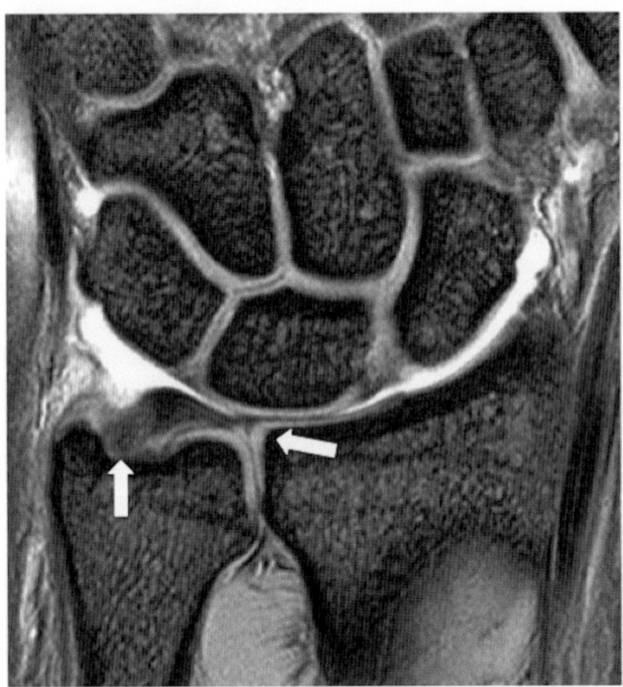

FIGURE 46-31 ■ Normal appearance of the low SI of the triangular fibrocartilage (TFC) on a coronal T2W gradient-echo MR arthrogram. The radial and ulnar attachments are well demonstrated (white arrows).

Traumatic TFC tears often affect the ulnar attachments and are associated with ulnar styloid fractures (Fig. 46-33). These injuries may also involve the dorsal and volar radioulnar ligaments and can lead to DRUJ instability.

Wrist Tendons

The tendons of the wrist are divided into extensor and flexor tendons. The extensor tendons form six groups with separate synovial sheaths, numbered from a radial to ulnar direction at the level of the radiocarpal joint.

Extensor tendinopathy is commonly seen in the extensor carpi ulnaris (ECU) tendon as it passes over the ulnar

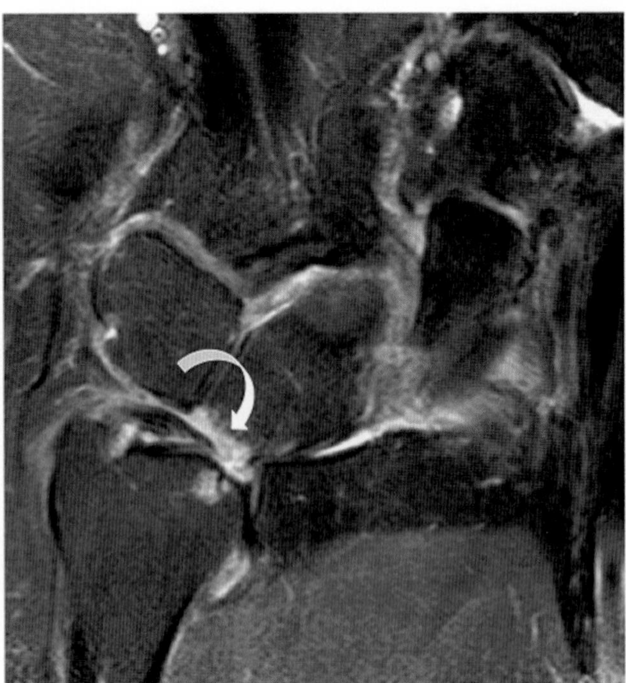

FIGURE 46-32 ■ **Degenerative TFC perforation on a coronal FS T1W MR arthrogram.** There is a large central defect of the TFC (curved white arrow), outlined by the high SI intra-articular contrast medium. There are associated OA changes in the wrist and DRUJ, with loss of articular cartilage and a subchondral cyst in the distal ulna.

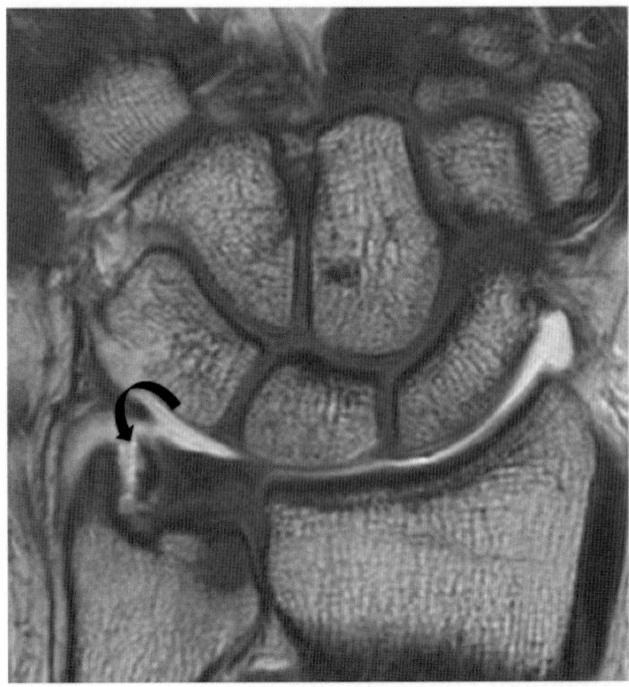

FIGURE 46-33 ■ **Traumatic TFC tear on a coronal T1W MR arthrogram.** There is avulsion of the ulnar styloid attachment of the TFC, with contrast medium extending between the TFC and styloid process (curved black arrow).

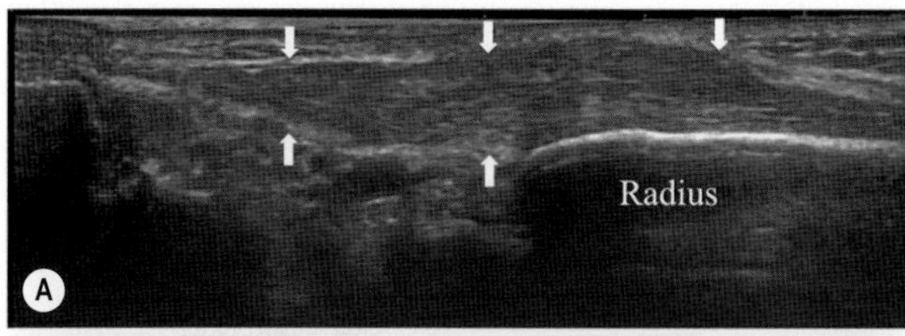

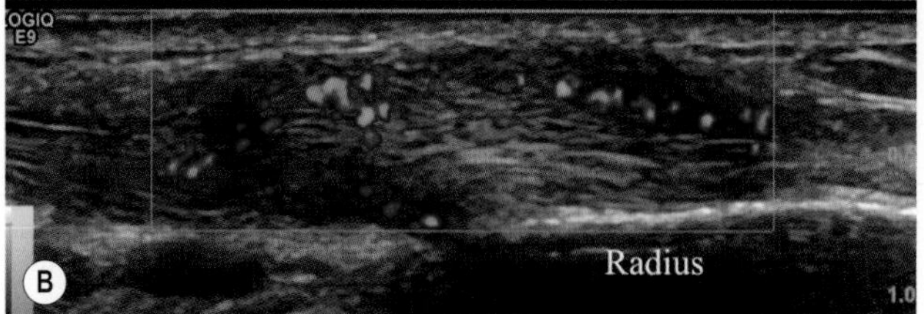

FIGURE 46-34 ■ Longitudinal grey-scale US image of the extensor group I tendons of the wrist (A). There is thickening of the tendon with echogenic thickening of the tendon sheath (white arrows) representing stenosing tenosynovitis (De Quervain's disease). There is associated tendon neovascularisation on the corresponding power Doppler image (B).

styloid. This is a common site for tenosynovitis in the setting of inflammatory arthropathy that may produce erosion of the ulnar styloid. Another commonly encountered extensor tendinopathy affects the extensor group I tendons of abductor pollicis longus and extensor pollicis brevis.[17] This is frequently associated with a stenosing tendosynovitis known as De Quervain's tenosynovitis (Fig. 46-34).

The flexor tendons are grouped within the carpal tunnel, with the exception of the flexor carpi ulnaris and radialis tendons. Isolated flexor tendinopathy is uncommon, though generalised flexor tenosynovitis may occur with rheumatoid arthritis. This increases the pressure within the carpal tunnel and may cause a secondary carpal tunnel syndrome by compression of the median nerve.

Median Nerve

Carpal tunnel syndrome is a neuropathy of the median nerve. It is usually idiopathic, or associated with pregnancy. Direct nerve compression may occur within the carpal tunnel in patients with synovitis of the wrist or flexor tendons. Lesions with mass effect arising from the tendon sheath or peripheral nerve sheath tumours are occasionally encountered.

Diagnosis is often made by a combination of clinical findings and nerve conduction studies. US or MRI may be required in cases with atypical features. Imaging is used to visualise abnormalities of the nerve, and to exclude secondary causes of carpal tunnel syndrome. The changes in the nerve are variable and include flattening of the nerve within the carpal tunnel, and proximal thickening. A cross-sectional area of > 10 mm^2 is suggestive of carpal tunnel syndrome. Qualitative changes within the nerve such as loss of normal fascicular pattern on US or increased SI on MRI are unreliable signs in isolation.[18]

UCL of Thumb

Tears of the ulnar collateral ligament of the thumb are common. They are often referred to as gamekeeper's thumb or skier's thumb. Undisplaced ligament tears can be treated conservatively, but displaced tears will not heal and require surgical repair.

In a displaced tear the ligament is torn from the distal insertion and retracts proximally around the aponeurosis of the adductor pollicis. This is known as a Stener lesion.[19] The displaced ligament can be demonstrated on both MRI and US (Fig. 46-35).

THE HIP

The hip is a large ball-and-socket joint which allows a wide range of movement while maintaining strong stability such that dislocation is much less frequent than in the shoulder. The cup-shaped acetabulum is formed at the junction of the ilial, ischial and pubic bones. The depth of the acetabulum is increased by the fibrocartilaginous labrum. Stability is further increased by the iliofemoral, ischiofemoral and pubofemoral ligaments which reinforce the joint capsule. The acetabulum and femoral head are lined by hyaline cartilage. The ligamentum teres is a weak ligament attaching to the fovea of the femoral head. It transmits the foveal artery, though in adults most of the blood supply of the femoral head is provided by the circumflex femoral arteries.

Labrum and Cartilage

The fibrocartilaginous labrum forms a ring at the margin of the acetabulum, increasing the stability of the joint by deepening the acetabular fossa. Lesions of the acetabular labrum constitute one of the most common internal derangements of the hip. Tears of the labrum may be traumatic or degenerative and are a cause of pain and mechanical symptoms. The gold standard imaging technique is MRI following injection of gadolinium contrast medium into the joint (MR arthrography). However, with modern high field strength systems some centres make use of conventional MRI without arthrographic contrast medium. The torn labrum may appear small, irregular, absent or may demonstrate linear penetration of contrast agent into the tear (Fig. 46-36). The anterosuperior and superior portions of the labrum are most frequently affected. Fluid tracking through the tear may form a paralabral cyst which is a useful indication of an underlying labral tear. Occasionally intra-articular contrast material can be seen communicating with the cyst on MR arthrographic images. Labral tears are often associated with adjacent articular cartilage damage and it is proposed that a labral tear is a precursor to the development of osteoarthritis. However, it is also important to recognise that labral degenerative tears are seen in association with osteoarthritis and the precise relationship between the two entities is as yet unclear.

Traumatic tears may arise from impingement between the femoral head and neck and the acetabular rim. This condition is known as femoroacetabular impingement.

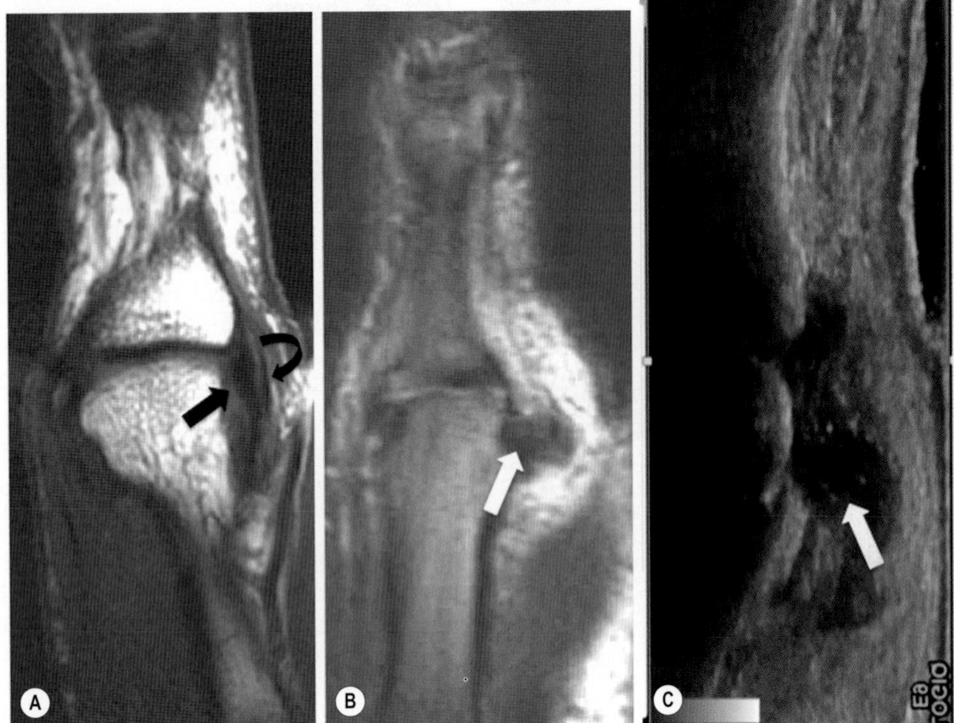

FIGURE 46-35 ■ Coronal T1W image (A) demonstrating the normal low SI ulnar collateral ligament (UCL) of the metacarpal joint of the thumb (black arrow), and the overlying adductor aponeurosis (curved black arrow). The coronal FS T2W MR image (B) and corresponding longitudinal US image (C) show a retracted UCL tear (Stener lesion) in a patient following a valgus strain injury (white arrows).

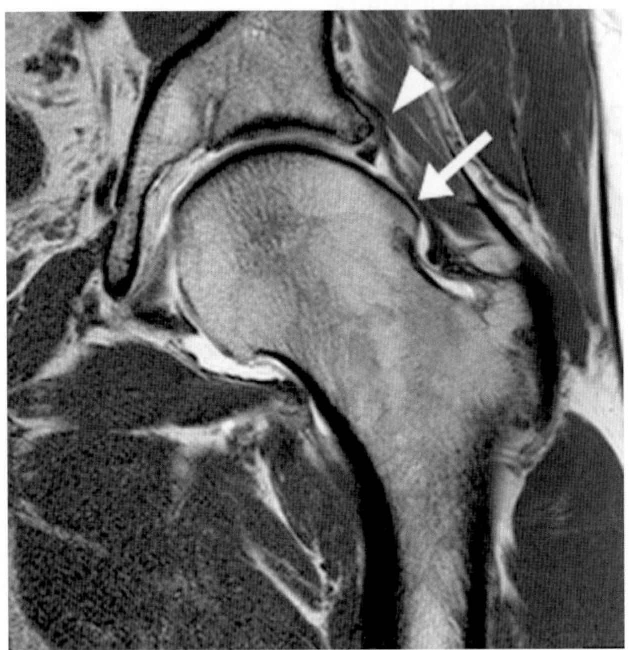

FIGURE 46-36 ■ **Cam deformity and labral tear.** Coronal T1-weighted MR arthrographic image. High signal intra-articular contrast medium is shown penetrating between the labrum and acetabulum (arrowhead) indicating a labral tear. There is an osseous bump, or cam deformity of the lateral femoral head (arrow).

Two kinds of femoroacetabular impingement are described, cam type and pincer type, though these often coexist.[20] Cam impingement is caused by the presence of an abnormal osseous 'bump' found on the anterior or lateral aspect of the femoral head–neck junction (Fig. 46-36). This produces abnormal contact between femur and acetabular rim in certain positions and typically presents in young athletic men. The α angle can be used to identify this loss of sphericity on a cross-table lateral radiograph or axial oblique MRI (Fig. 46-37). An α angle measuring greater than 50° may be taken as abnormal.[21] Repeated contact between the osseous bump and the anterior acetabulum during hip flexion results in a labral tear and/or cartilage damage. CT is an excellent technique for demonstrating the bone morphology in this condition, although MR arthrography is able to show the cartilage and labral damage. Acetabular cartilage delamination (separation of the cartilage from the underlying bone), sometimes termed a 'carpet lesion', is common in cam-type impingement and may be detected on MR arthrography.[22] The information provided by arthrographic MRI is important, as joint-sparing treatment (such as cam re-contouring) is unlikely to give effective symptom relief if there is established severe cartilage damage.

Pincer-type impingement, more common in middle-aged women, results from overcoverage of the femoral head by the acetabulum. This can be due to a deep acetabulum, bone hypertrophy at the acetabular rim or abnormal acetabular retroversion, the latter leading to an

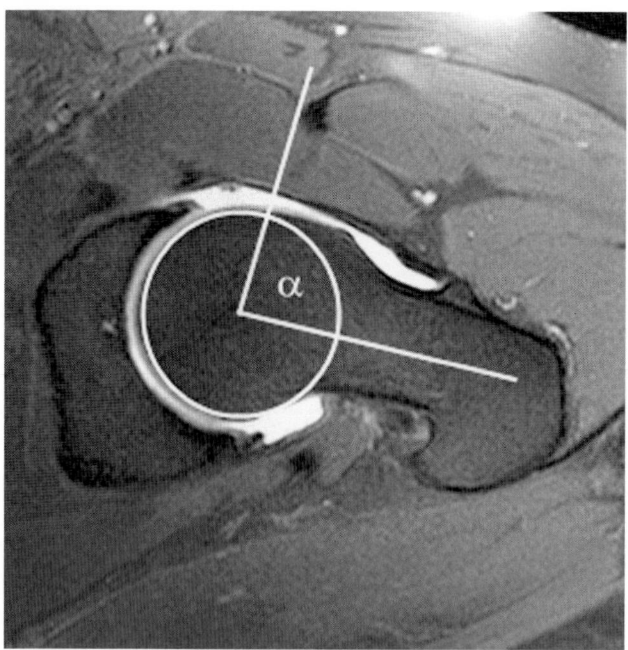

FIGURE 46-37 ■ The α angle measured on an axial oblique T1-weighted fat-saturated MR arthrographic image shows loss of sphericity of the femoral head (cam deformity). A circle of best fit is drawn around the femoral head. A line is drawn along the femoral neck axis. A second line is drawn from the centre of the femoral head to the point on the circle where the femoral head begins to protrude from it. The α angle is measured between the two lines.

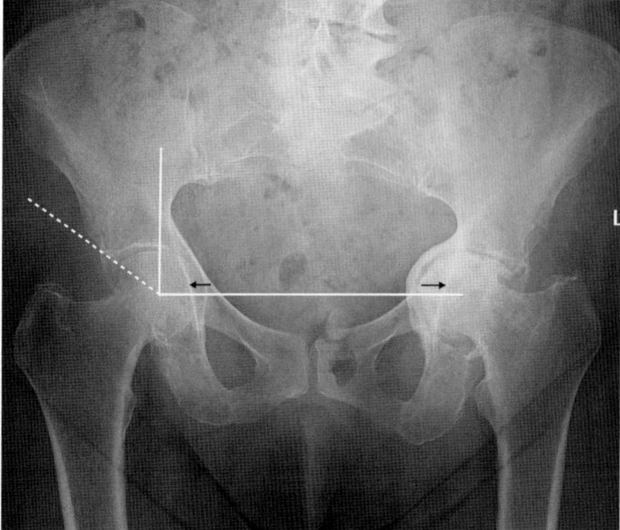

FIGURE 46-38 ■ **AP pelvic radiograph.** At both hips the femoral head is seen to overlap the ilioischial line (arrows) indicating bilateral protrusio acetabuli, which in this female patient was idiopathic. Note severe secondary degeneration in the left hip joint. The centre-edge angle detects overcoverage of the femoral head. A line is drawn perpendicular to an axis through both femoral head centres. A second line is drawn from the femoral head centre to the most lateral point of the acetabular roof. The centre-edge angle lies between the two lines.

effective overcoverage of the femoral head anteriorly. On hip flexion the abnormal morphology results in impingement between the acetabular rim and the femoral neck, leading to labral and cartilage damage. The centre-edge angle is a method to identify acetabular overcoverage on an AP radiograph of the pelvis (Fig. 46-38). A centre-edge angle greater than 40° may be considered abnormal.[23] Coxa profunda and protusio acetabuli are two types of deformity that predispose to pincer-type impingement. Coxa profunda is identified on an AP radiograph when the floor of the acetabular fossa overlaps the ilioischial line. Protrusio acetabuli, more severe, is present when the femoral head itself overlaps the ilioischial line (Fig. 46-38).

Muscle and Tendon

Muscle and tendon injury around the hip is common. This may result from acute trauma such as may be sustained in sporting activities or, particularly in the case of tendon injury, from chronic repetitive microtrauma. The hamstring and adductor origins are commonly affected in young athletes while gluteus medius tendon degeneration (tendinopathy) and tears are more common in the elderly. On MRI and ultrasound, the appearances vary depending on the severity of the injury. In the case of muscle injury, findings may range from minor muscle oedema to discontinuity of fibres and muscle retraction. In chronic cases there may be fatty atrophy or muscle ossification. Tendon disease in the form of tears or tendinopathic change may also be demonstrated; the latter is seen as loss of the normal tendon low signal on T1- and T2-weighted MR images along with thickening of the tendon. Ultrasound will also show tendon discontinuities and tendinopathy.

Avulsion of an unfused apophysis at a muscle attachment may occur in children undertaking athletic activities. The anterior superior iliac spine (sartorius muscle), the anterior inferior iliac spine (rectus femoris) and ischial tuberosity (hamstring) are common sites of involvement (Fig. 46-39). Because avulsed apophyses continue to form bone, this can lead to bizarre mass-like appearances on imaging when presentation is delayed. The location of the bone 'mass' and the age of the patient are key to making the correct diagnosis.

While mechanical snaps and clicks can arise from within the joint, for instance in the presence of a labral tear or loose body, such mechanical symptoms may also arise from extra-articular causes. The snapping hip describes a snap or clunk felt by the patient when undertaking a particular movement. It may be associated with pain and the snap may be audible. Two of the most common extra-articular varieties are the snapping iliotibial band (external type) and the snapping iliopsoas tendon (internal type). Both can be imaged using ultrasound, which allows continuous visualisation of the relevant structures while the patient reproduces the snapping. In the external type the gluteus maximus muscle can be shown initially lying over the greater trochanter before abruptly moving posteriorly to bring the iliotibial band into contact with the greater trochanter.[24] In the internal type the iliopsoas tendon rotates abnormally before abruptly reversing and forcefully striking the superior pubic ramus.[25]

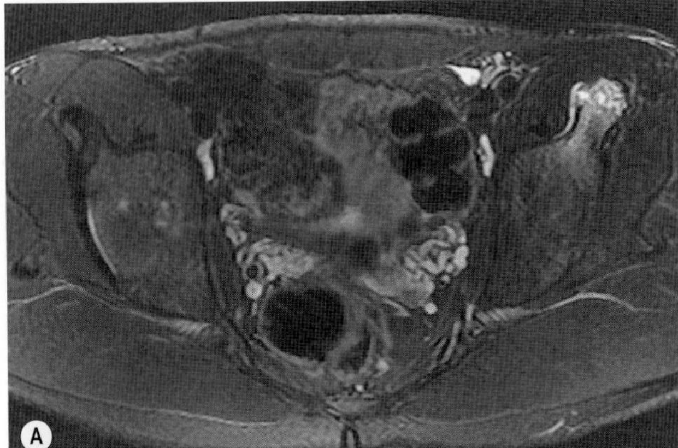

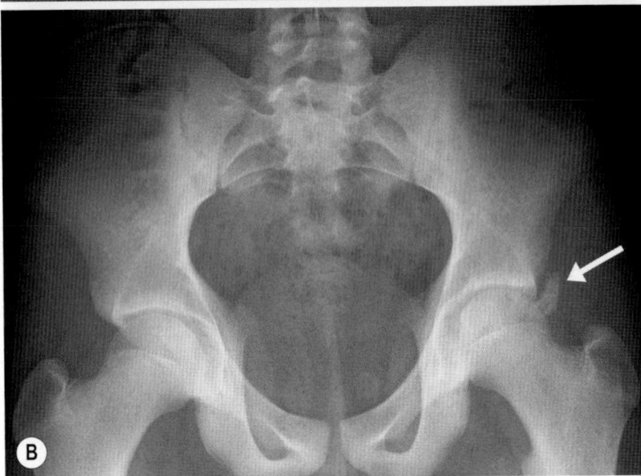

FIGURE 46-39 ■ Avulsion of the straight head of rectus femoris from the anterior inferior iliac spine (AIIS). (A) Axial T2-weighted fat-saturated image of the pelvis demonstrates oedema at the left AIIS and irregularity of the apophysis. (B) Plain radiograph taken 5 months later shows displacement of the apophysis from the AIIS.

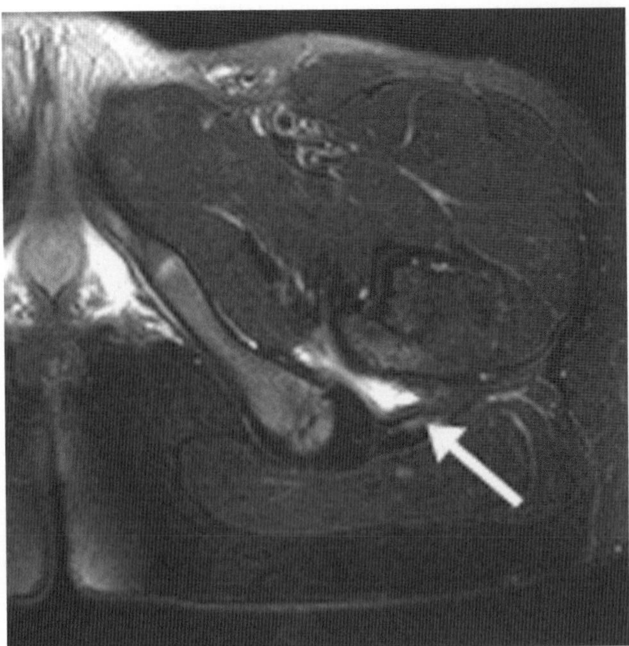

FIGURE 46-40 ■ Ischiofemoral impingement. Axial T2-weighted fat-saturated image shows bursa formation in a narrowed ischiofemoral space.

TABLE 46-1 Potential Causes of Hip AVN

- Idiopathic
- Trauma and vascular
  - Fracture (including complication of fracture fixation)
  - Radiotherapy
  - Dysbaric osteonecrosis (caisson disease)
  - Arteritis
- Inflammatory
  - Pancreatitis
  - Connective tissue disease
  - Rheumatoid arthritis
- Metabolic and endocrine
  - Pregnancy
  - Diabetes
  - Cushing's syndrome
  - Gaucher's disease
- Toxic
  - Steroids
  - Alcohol
  - Immunosuppressives
- Haematological disorders
  - Sickle cell anaemia
  - Polycythemia rubra vera
  - Haemophilia

Ischiofemoral impingement is a recently described condition predominantly affecting women associated with narrowing of the space between the ischial tuberosity and lesser trochanter of the femur. It is thought that the quadratus femoris muscle which passes through this space may be impinged during repetitive hip movement, giving rise to pain. MRI reveals narrowing of the space associated with oedema of the quadratus femoris muscle belly and adjacent free fluid (Fig. 46-40).[26] However, similar appearances may be found in asymptomatic individuals and the clinical significance of this has not yet been established.

Bone

Avascular necrosis of the femoral head has many potential underlying causes (Table 46-1). MRI is the preferred technique, allowing early detection of signal change in the subchondral region of the femoral head. The 'double line' sign on fluid-sensitive sequences, characteristic of AVN, describes a low signal sclerotic line next to a high signal hypervascular line which demarcates the extent of the lesion (Fig. 46-41). There may be accompanying bone marrow oedema in the femoral head and neck. The extent of involvement on MRI has prognostic value in determining the outcome after decompressive surgery.[27] Conventional radiographs are much less sensitive in the early stages of AVN, but as the process progresses they will typically show a linear subchondral lucency that progresses to articular collapse and sclerosis. Both hips should be imaged together, as bilateral involvement is common.

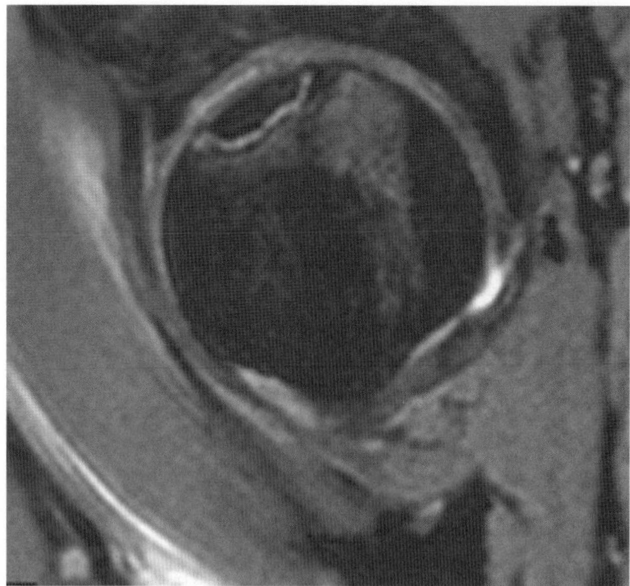

FIGURE 46-41 ■ Avascular necrosis (AVN) in the femoral head. Sagittal oblique T2-weighted fat-saturated image demonstrates a region of subchondral AVN demarcated by the characteristic 'double line' sign.

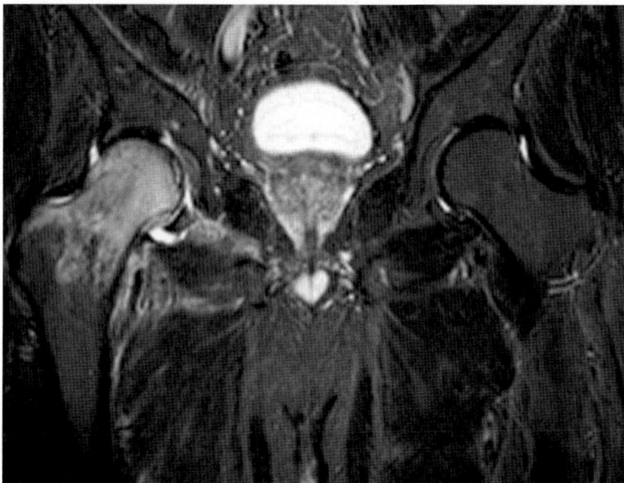

FIGURE 46-42 ■ Transient osteoporosis of the right hip. Coronal T2-weighted fat-saturated image shows extensive bone marrow oedema in the right femoral head and neck. See text for the differential diagnosis.

Transient osteoporosis of the hip (TOP), also known as bone marrow oedema syndrome, is a self-limiting painful condition of uncertain aetiology.[28] On MRI this appears as extensive bone marrow oedema signal involving the femoral head and/or neck (Fig. 46-42). Conventional radiographs may show reduced bone density but MRI is the most important tool in diagnosis. Following resolution in the hip, the condition may go on to involve other parts of the skeleton, in which case the condition is called regional migratory osteoporosis. Bone marrow high signal (oedema) seen in the femoral head and/or neck raises several possible diagnoses, including transient osteoporosis, that should also be considered (Table 46-2).

TABLE 46-2 Causes of Femoral Head/Neck Bone Marrow Oedema

- Transient osteoporosis
- Avascular necrosis
- Fracture
  - Including fatigue and insufficiency fractures
- Arthropathy (including joint sepsis)
  - Will normally involve both sides of the joint
- Osteoid osteoma
- Osteomyelitis
- Myeloma and metastases

Bursae

Bursae are synovial-lined structures found in many sites around the musculoskeletal system, and it is their normal function to facilitate the movement between muscles and adjacent structures. Bursal inflammation, or bursitis, may result from overuse injury or from involvement by systemic inflammatory conditions such as inflammatory arthritis. On imaging, a normal bursa will often be unseen, or appear as a thin layer of fluid between tissues. When inflamed (bursitis), imaging will show the bursa as a more substantial fluid-containing structure. There may be thickening of the bursal walls and adjacent soft-tissue oedema. Several bursae are recognised around the hip, but the most common to be associated with symptoms are the iliopsoas and the greater trochanteric bursae. The trochanteric bursae are a group of bursae found deep to the gluteus maximus, gluteus medius and gluteus minimus muscles.[29] 'Trochanteric bursitis' is a relatively common condition which may involve one or more of the bursae and typically occurs in middle-aged women. Trochanteric bursitis presents with lateral hip pain and may be associated with tendinopathy of gluteus medius (Fig. 46-43). The iliopsoas bursa is the largest bursa in the body and communicates with the hip joint in approximately 15% of individuals. It lies deep to the iliopsoas muscle and passes directly over the anterior hip joint capsule. Iliopsoas bursitis typically presents with anterior hip pain related to movement or with an anterior groin mass if large.

THE KNEE

The knee is the largest joint in the body and comprises three compartments, the medial and lateral femorotibial compartments and the patellofemoral compartment. The femoral condyles articulate with the tibial condyles, and the patella articulates with the femoral trochlea. The joint capsule encloses the articular surfaces, menisci and cruciate ligaments. The collateral ligaments and tendons are extra-articular, apart from the popliteus tendon, which has an intra-articular portion. The bony articular surfaces alone are inherently unstable, so these soft-tissue supporting structures are vital to the joint stability and are prone to injury. MRI remains the imaging technique of choice for evaluating most internal knee derangements. It is well suited for demonstrating the menisci,

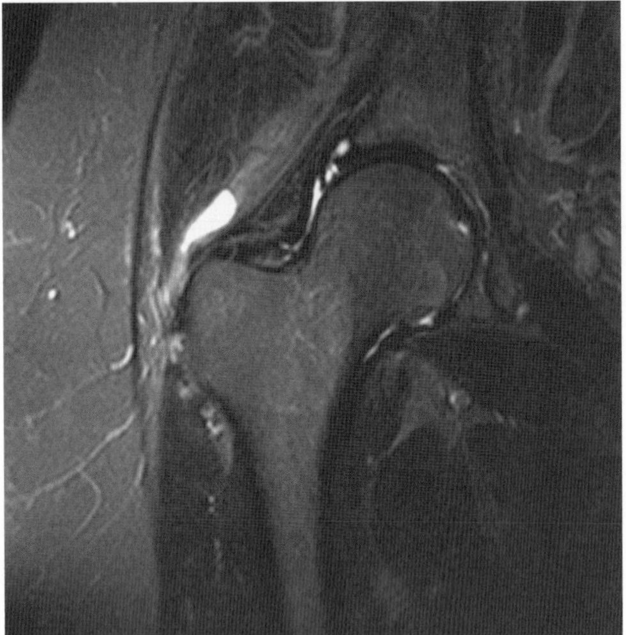

FIGURE 46-43 ■ **Trochanteric bursitis.** Coronal T2-weighted fat-saturated image shows fluid distension of the subgluteus medius bursa. There is associated thickening and oedema of the gluteus medius tendon insertion.

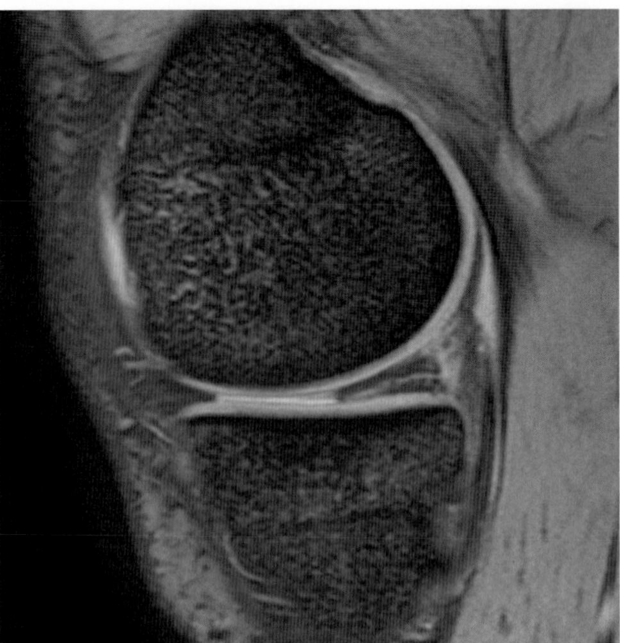

FIGURE 46-44 ■ **Horizontal tear of the medial meniscus.** Sagittal gradient-echo image shows linear high signal in the posterior meniscus extending to the free edge.

tendons and ligaments. However, ultrasound can be used to demonstrate the peripheral joint structures, showing the medial and lateral collateral ligaments and soft tissues of the extensor mechanism well.

Menisci

The menisci are two semilunar fibrocartilaginous structures located between the articular cartilage of the femoral and tibial condyles. They each have a crescent shape with an anterior and posterior horn and a body. The tips of the horns are attached to the tibial plateau adjacent to the intercondylar eminence. These attachments are known as the meniscal roots. The medial meniscus is larger than the lateral and has a larger posterior horn than anterior horn. In the case of the lateral meniscus, the horns are of similar size, but in approximately 5% of individuals the lateral meniscus has a discoid morphology. A discoid meniscus is associated with increased incidence of pathology from a young age. Sagittal MRI sequences of the normal meniscus show a bow-tie configuration at the periphery. On progressive images toward the intercondylar fossa the meniscus appears as two triangles representing the anterior and posterior horns. The normal menisci exhibit uniform low signal on all MRI sequences, although in children some increased signal is frequently identified in the posterior third. Degeneration may lead to intrameniscal high signal, or 'myxoid change', particularly in the posterior medial meniscus. A tear is diagnosed on MRI when high signal is demonstrated extending to the articular surface of the meniscus. Tears may be horizontal or vertical depending on whether they reach one meniscal surface or two. A complex tear is diagnosed when two or more tear configurations are present. The configuration of a meniscal tear has important implications for management. Horizontal tears are frequently degenerative in nature and may be asymptomatic (Fig. 46-44). Joint fluid may escape through a horizontal tear, forming a parameniscal cyst. Two types of vertical tear are recognised. Longitudinal tears lie within the substance of the meniscus, tracking circumferentially. They often involve the periphery of the meniscus where the blood supply is better and may therefore heal spontaneously. As the name suggests, radial tears extend radially into the meniscus from the free edge; they take several forms. A small oblique slit is a common form and is called a parrot beak tear (Fig. 46-45). If it traverses the full width, a radial tear may split the meniscus, leading to separation of the two parts. A 'ghost meniscus' describes the MRI appearance of a complete radial tear where the image section passes through the split (Fig. 46-46). This sign is most often found in tears involving the posterior root of the medial meniscus. Some tears have a fragment which may displace and cause locking; this is particularly common with longitudinal tears, which, in particular, can give rise to a 'bucket handle' tear. Here the meniscal fragment remaining attached at both ends flips into the intercondylar notch (Fig. 46-47). The 'double PCL sign' describes a sagittal view showing the posterior cruciate ligament (PCL) and a second parallel low signal structure representing the displaced bucket handle fragment of a torn meniscus (Fig. 46-48).

Anterior Cruciate Ligament

The anterior cruciate ligament (ACL) attaches proximally at the posteromedial margin of the lateral femoral condyle in the intercondylar fossa and distally at the anterior aspect of the tibial intercondylar eminence. The

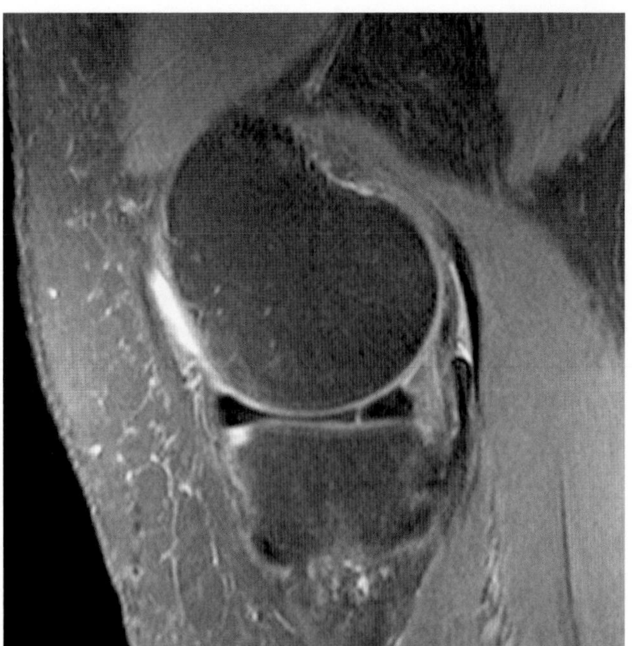

FIGURE 46-45 ■ Radial tear of the medial meniscus on a sagittal proton density fat-saturated image.

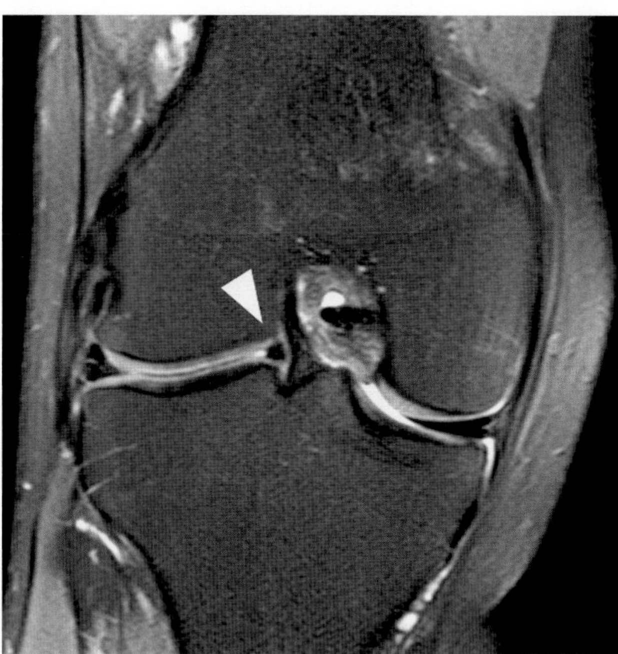

FIGURE 46-47 ■ 'Bucket handle' tear of the lateral meniscus. Coronal proton density fat-saturated image demonstrates a flipped fragment of the lateral meniscus (arrowhead) in the intercondylar fossa.

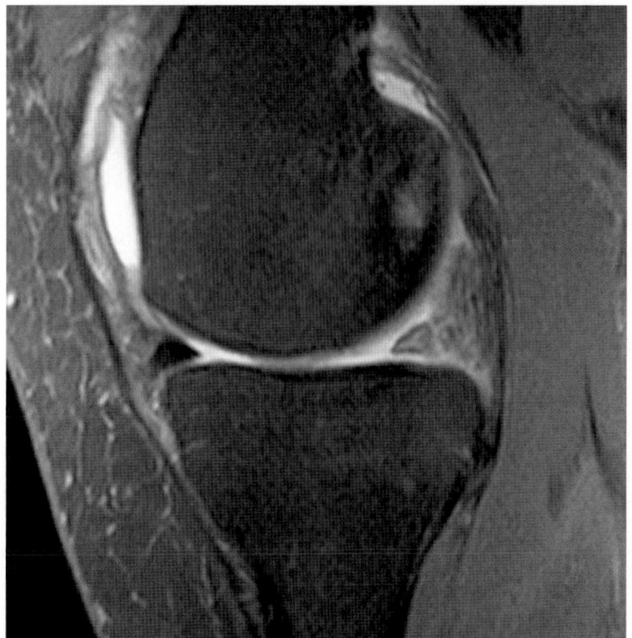

FIGURE 46-46 ■ 'Ghost meniscus'. Sagittal proton density fat-saturated image shows abnormal high signal of the posterior medial meniscus due to a complete radial tear.

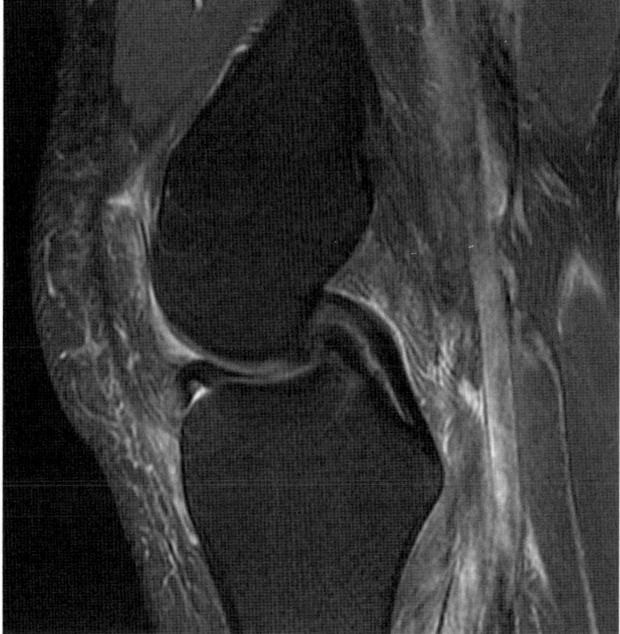

FIGURE 46-48 ■ Double PCL sign. Sagittal proton density fat-saturated image shows a flipped fragment of a 'bucket handle' meniscal tear that lies in the intercondylar fossa deep to the PCL.

ACL acts to restrain anterior translation and, to a lesser extent, internal rotation of the tibia relative to the femur. On MRI, the ligament is best visualised on sagittal images, appearing normally as fan-shaped bundles of taut fibres. Two bundles, the anteromedial and posterolateral, may be differentiated on the coronal and axial sequences. As fluid and loose connective tissue may be interspaced between the bundles, the ACL often appears larger and of more mixed signal intensity than the PCL.

ACL tears are common sporting injuries. On MRI, complete tears appear as discontinuity of the fibres, increased signal and/or laxity (Fig. 46-49). The

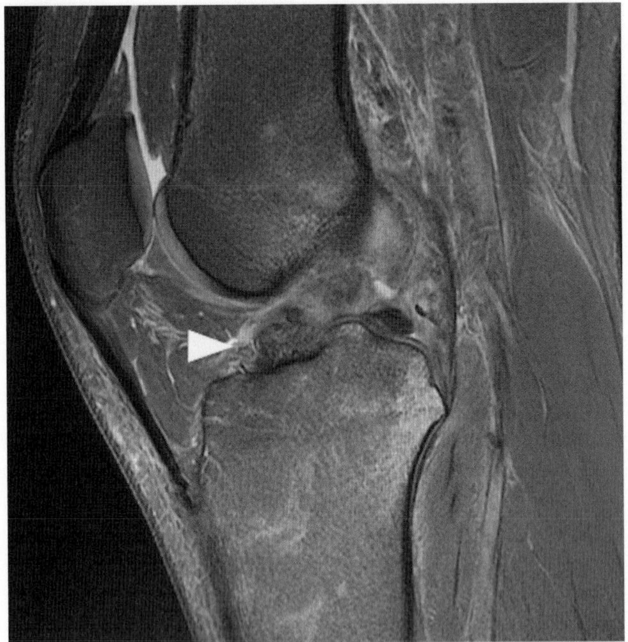

FIGURE 46-49 ■ Complete intrasubstance ACL tear. Sagittal proton density fat-saturated image reveals retracted ACL fibres (arrowhead) at the distal attachment and no intact proximal fibres. Note bone marrow oedema in a typical location in the posterior tibia.

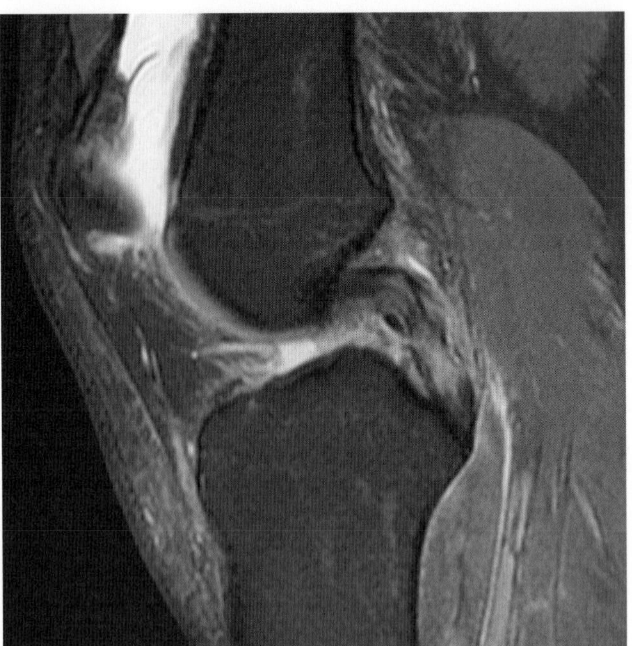

FIGURE 46-50 ■ PCL tear. Sagittal proton density fat-saturated image shows abnormal signal and thickening of the distal PCL.

mid-substance of the ligament is injured more frequently than the proximal or distal portions. Partial tears or sprains of the ACL are recognised on MRI by altered signal and/or laxity in the presence of continuity of some fibres. There are several secondary imaging signs associated with ACL injury. Typically there is microfracture in the posterior aspect of the lateral tibial plateau and the subarticular lateral femoral condyle, reflecting impaction between these sites during subluxation of the knee at the time of the injury (pivot shift injury). ACL tears may be accompanied by anterior translation of the tibia relative to the femur. This can be detected on sagittal images as it will cause buckling of the PCL. The lateral notch sign, which is specific but not very sensitive for ACL injury, describes abnormally deep indentation of the condylopatellar sulcus of the lateral femoral condyle on a lateral conventional radiograph.[30] ACL injuries are commonly associated with injury to other structures. O'Donaghue's triad describes tears of the ACL, MCL and medial meniscus. A Segond fracture, which has a high association with ACL injury, describes avulsion of a fracture fragment from the lateral margin of the lateral tibial condyle at the attachment of the joint capsule.

Posterior Cruciate Ligament

The posterior cruciate ligament (PCL) extends from the anterolateral margin of the medial femoral condyle to the posterior aspect of the tibial intercondylar eminence. It normally appears as a thick low signal bundle that is visualised well in all planes on MRI. Tears of the PCL, e.g. from a sporting or dashboard-type injury, may result in instability characterised by posterior translation of the tibia relative to the femur. Partial intrasubstance ruptures of the PCL are more common than complete tears and avulsions. Intrasubstance tears exhibit thickening and altered signal on MRI while usually maintaining the appearance of a continuous structure (Fig. 46-50).[31] Microfracture of the anterior aspect of the tibial plateau is typical. Associated soft-tissue injury is common, including tears of the ACL, medial collateral ligament and posterolateral corner.

Medial Collateral Ligament

The medial collateral ligament (MCL) has superficial and deep components; the former are more important for maintaining knee stability in the presence of valgus forces. The posterior oblique ligament is found more posteriorly and is formed by contributions from the superficial and deep MCL. Together with the semimembranosus tendon, it is an important stabiliser of the knee posteromedially. Coronal MRI sequences clearly identify the MCL as a thin low signal band, differentiating the superficial portion from the much shorter deep portion which has attachments to the middle third of the lateral meniscus. Injury to the MCL may be classified according to severity.[32] A Grade 1 sprain is a periligamentous injury characterised by oedema around the ligament which maintains low signal. A Grade 2 injury represents a partial tear with focal intraligamentous thickening and altered signal intensity as a result of oedema and/or haemorrhage. A Grade 3, or complete, tear shows complete discontinuity across the ligament. Chronic ossification of the proximal MCL following injury is known as a Pellegrini–Stieda lesion.

Lateral Collateral Ligament Complex and Posterolateral Corner

Lateral joint stability is provided by a number of structures including anteriorly, the iliotibial band, which attaches onto the proximal tibia. The lateral collateral ligament (LCL), or fibular collateral ligament, passes between the lateral femoral condyle and the fibular head. The biceps femoris tendon has a common attachment with the LCL to the fibular head known as the conjoint tendon. LCL tears may arise within the ligamentous substance or from avulsion at the fibular head.

The LCL is a component of the posterolateral corner complex of supporting structures which also includes the popliteus tendon, biceps tendon, arcuate ligament, popliteofibular ligament and posterior joint capsule. Injury to the posterolateral corner is often associated with damage to other ligamentous structures, most commonly tears of the ACL. Posterolateral corner injuries may lead to posterolateral instability which has implications for surgical management, particularly when associated with ACL injuries. While the LCL, biceps tendon and popliteus are seen well on MRI, it is often difficult to reliably evaluate the smaller components of the posterolateral corner individually because of their small size and orientation.

The Extensor Mechanism and Patellofemoral Joint

The patella is a sesamoid bone (the largest in the body) that lies between the quadriceps tendon proximally and the patellar tendon distally. The medial and lateral patellar retinacula also form part of the extensor mechanism. The patella articulates with the trochlea groove, or sulcus, of the femur. This groove is an important component in providing stability to the patella. Trochlea dysplasia describes a shallow sulcus (this can be measured on imaging) that predisposes to patellar dislocation. An abnormally high position of the patella (patella alta) may contribute to patellar maltracking and/or cartilage damage. The Insall–Salvati ratio assesses relative patella height and is given by the ratio of patellar tendon length to the length of the patella itself. It can be calculated from conventional radiographs or sagittal MRI images.[33,34] Axial MRI or CT images may be used to measure the tibial tubercle–trochlea groove distance (TTD) which identifies lateralisation of the patellar tendon insertion (which predisposes to lateral dislocation).[35] The patella is prone to dislocate laterally due to the valgus force of the quadriceps muscle group, although in the majority of cases this dislocation is transient and by the time of presentation to hospital the patella has reduced. Nevertheless there are characteristic MRI findings in acute patellar dislocation–relocation (Fig. 46-51). These include subcortical bone marrow oedema of the medial patella and lateral femoral condyle reflecting 'kissing contusions'. There is usually an associated tear of the medial patellar retinaculum and/or an osteochondral fracture of the patella.

Cartilage degeneration in the knee is common as a feature of osteoarthritis. Chondromalacia patellae describes cartilage damage occurring in adolescents and young adults which primarily involves the patellofemoral compartment. This may be associated with patellar misalignment or trauma. Cartilage damage can be graded according to severity. Early damage is demonstrated on MRI as signal abnormality and thinning. Progressive damage appears as full-thickness fissuring or a defect. The presence of subchondral oedema or cyst formation indicates the most severe damage.

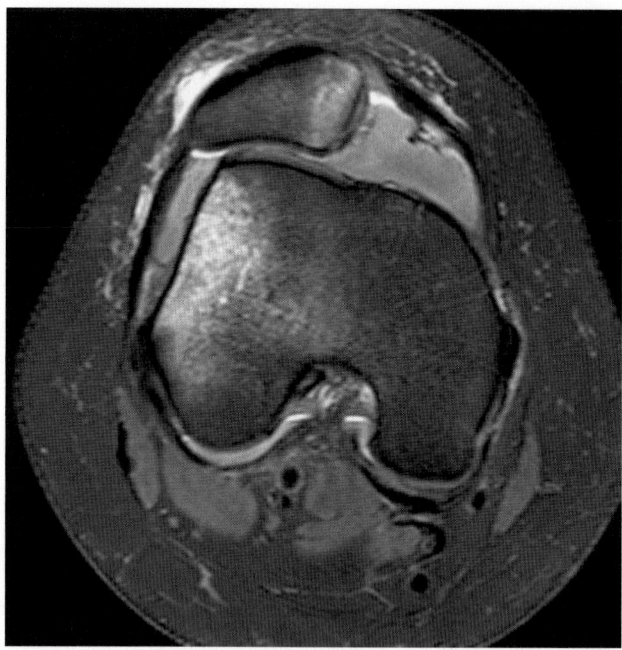

FIGURE 46-51 ■ Acute patellar dislocation–relocation. Axial proton density fat-saturated image shows typical bone marrow oedema reflecting 'kissing contusions' of the medial patella and lateral femoral condyle. Note the shallow trochlea sulcus and lateral patella tilt which predispose to dislocation.

Patellar tendinopathy involving the proximal tendon attachment is commonly referred to as 'jumper's knee' because of its association with athletic activities that involve jumping. It can be demonstrated on MRI and ultrasound where it typically appears as focal thickening of the central deep portion of the proximal tendon with increased Doppler vascularity (Fig. 46-52). On ultrasound the tendinopathic tendon shows low reflectivity and on MRI increased intrasubstance signal. Patellar tendinopathy may also involve the more distal tendon. Osgood–Schlatter disease is a common condition in children aged between 8 and 13 years and is characterised by distal patellar tendinopathy, tibial tubercle enlargement or fragmentation and thickening of the overlying soft tissues. The condition is thought to result from repetitive traction injury related to sporting activity. Tears of the patella or quadriceps tendons may occur, typically on the background of tendinopathy. They are readily evaluated with ultrasound or MRI.

Bone and Cartilage

Osteochondritis dissecans is a common condition of uncertain aetiology affecting children and adolescents. It is characterised by focal cartilage and subchondral bone

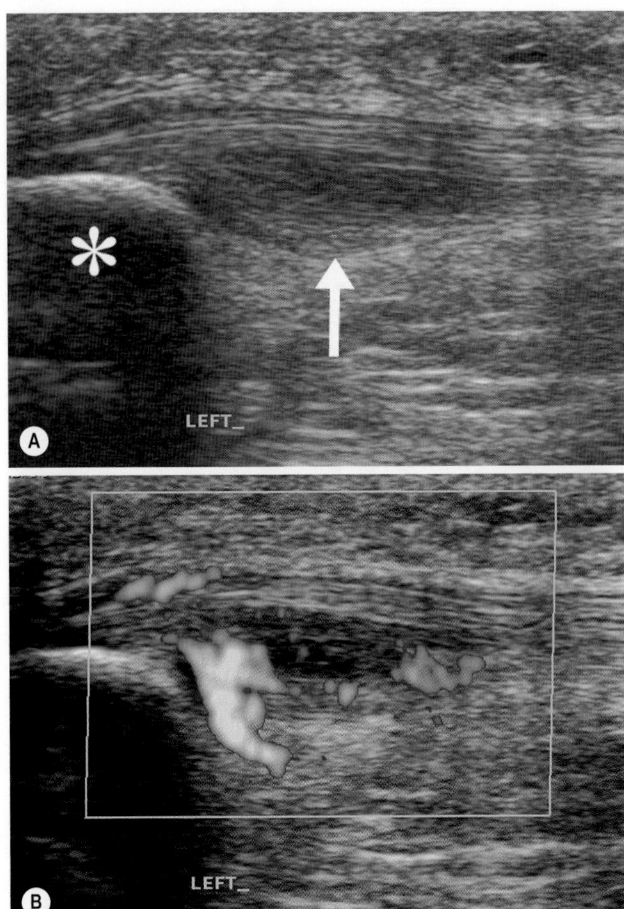

FIGURE 46-52 ■ **Jumper's knee.** Longitudinal ultrasound images of proximal patellar tendinopathy. (A) Note thickening and hypoechogenicity of the deep part of the proximal tendon (arrow); * indicates the patella. (B) Doppler interrogation reveals marked neovascularity of the proximal tendon (in orange).

abnormality, and most commonly involves the lateral aspect of the medial femoral condyle. Conventional radiographs may reveal linear subarticular lucency with adjacent sclerosis but they are not sensitive. MRI clearly demonstrates these lesions, allowing measurement and localisation. A rim of fluid signal which undercuts the involved bone implies the lesion has become detached and may go on to displace into the joint space.

Repeated mechanical trauma to the articular surfaces of the knee may lead to subchondral fractures. Often occult on conventional radiographs, these lesions are demonstrated on fluid-sensitive MRI sequences as focal linear subchondral low signal (indicating the fracture line) with intense surrounding oedema-like signal in the bone marrow. Cartilage and meniscal damage may predispose to such injuries. Normal forces in the absence of predisposing abnormality may cause subchondral fracture if the underlying bone is weak (insufficiency fracture). Subchondral insufficiency fracture was sometimes previously referred to as 'spontaneous osteonecrosis of the knee', a term that is incorrect and becoming archaic. Recent interest has focused on a condition called 'bone marrow oedema syndrome' or 'transient osteoporosis' which is believed to predispose to insufficiency fracture in the knee and elsewhere (Fig. 46-53).[28]

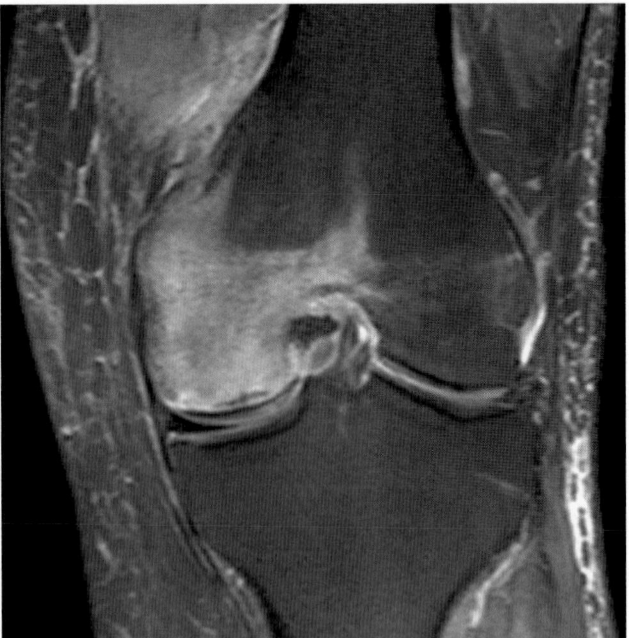

FIGURE 46-53 ■ **Transient osteoporosis of the knee.** Coronal proton density fat-saturated image shows extensive bone marrow oedema in the medial femoral condyle. Note there is subchondral linear low signal indicating associated insufficiency fracture.

Bursae

There are numerous anatomical bursae around the knee. Inflammation of a bursa, or bursitis, is commonly caused by friction from repetitive movement, though bursae may also be involved in systemic inflammatory conditions such as rheumatoid arthritis. Around the patellar tendon there are the superficial infrapatellar, deep infrapatellar and prepatellar bursae. Bursitis may affect any of these, and involvement of the last is called 'housemaid's knee'. Friction between the distal iliotibial band and lateral femoral condyle may give rise to bursitis known as 'runner's knee'. Inflammation of the pes anserine bursa gives rise to pain over the anteromedial aspect of the proximal tibia. The most commonly involved bursa in the popliteal region lies between the medial head of gastrocnemius and the semimembranosus tendon, the popliteal bursa. This communicates with the joint and distension of this bursa is called a popliteal or baker's cyst.

THE ANKLE AND FOOT

The ankle allows a wide range of movement, but also has to transmit considerable forces. It is the most commonly injured joint, with ligamentous injury in the form of sprains and tears particularly common. Patients typically present with pain and/or instability following such injury. The talar dome articulates with the tibial plafond and small facets on the medial and lateral malleoli. The malleoli contribute to the joint stability and provide attachments for the collateral ligaments, which are themselves important stabilisers of the ankle. The distal tibiofibular joint is a fibrous joint that contains a synovial recess extending from the ankle joint. Several tendons crossing the ankle joint are also prone to injury.

Ligaments

Injuries sustained to the ankle usually result from inversion or eversion. Inversion injuries are significantly more common than eversion injuries, with the result that the lateral ankle ligaments are torn more frequently than the medial. Three components of the lateral collateral ligament complex are recognised: the anterior and posterior talofibular ligaments and the calcaneofibular ligament. The anterior talofibular ligament is the most vulnerable to injury, followed by the calcaneofibular ligament. The posterior talofibular ligament is rarely injured except in the most severe cases. MRI or ultrasound may be used for assessment of these structures. On imaging, ligament damage may appear as altered signal/echogenicity, thickening, thinning, or absence (indicating a complete tear) (Fig. 46-54).[36] Damage to the lateral ligaments may lead to chronic anterolateral impingement in the absence of frank instability. Anterolateral impingement describes repetitive soft-tissue injury in the anterolateral gutter, causing synovitis and haemorrhage, which may be identified on MRI.[37]

The most important medial ankle ligaments include the anterior and posterior tibiotalar (also known as deltoid), tibio-spring and spring ligaments. The spring ligament extends from the calcaneus to the navicular and functions as an important stabiliser of the foot arch together with the posterior tibial tendon. The distal tibiotalar syndesmosis comprises anterior, interosseous and posterior tibiofibular ligaments. Strong forces are usually required to disrupt the syndesmotic ligaments such as those resulting in an ankle fracture. However, syndesmotic ligament injuries do occur, typically as a sports injury.

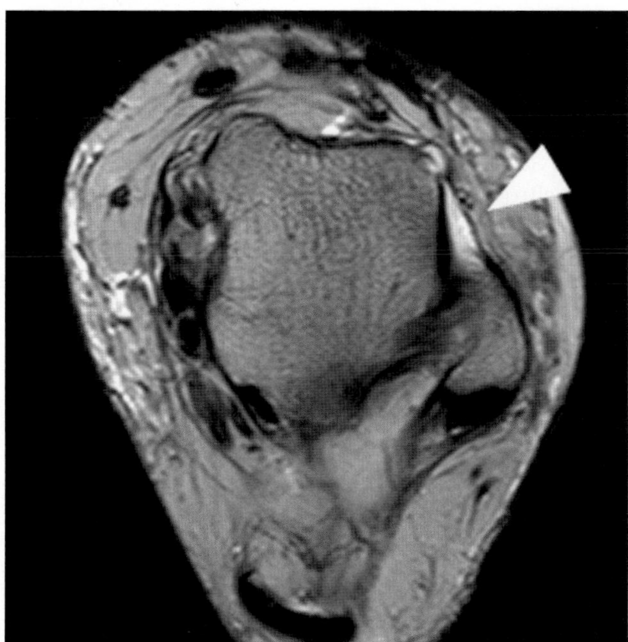

FIGURE 46-54 ■ **Anterior talofibular ligament tear.** Axial oblique T2-weighted image shows absence of ligament fibres in the usual position (arrowhead), indicating a chronic tear.

Tendons

Tendon abnormalities are common about the ankle. The tendons crossing the ankle anteriorly, medially and laterally do so in tendon sheaths and symptoms may relate to tenosynovitis as well as to tendinopathy if there is symptomatic intrinsic degeneration, tear, or subluxation/dislocation of the tendon itself. The last of these may occur if there is retinacular injury. The Achilles tendon is the largest tendon in the body. It is also vulnerable to tendinopathy and tears. Like the patellar tendon, the Achilles does not have a tendon sheath, but its surrounding tissues may still become inflamed. This is known as paratenonitis. Ultrasound and MRI are both excellent techniques for assessing the tendons. Ultrasound has the advantage of greater spatial resolution, Doppler flow to show inflammatory hyperaemia and dynamic imaging with ankle movement.

The posteromedial ankle tendons comprise the tibialis posterior (TP), flexor digitorum longus (FDL) and flexor hallucis longus (FHL) tendons. TP is the strongest of these, with approximately twice the cross-sectional area of FDL. It is also the most frequently affected by pathology. TP function is important in maintaining the medial arch of the foot (with the spring ligament) and tears of TP may lead to flat foot deformity. An os naviculare is a sesamoid bone located at the insertion of TP. Tenosynovitis appears as increased fluid in the tendon sheath, sometimes with altered appearance of the tendon itself. Ultrasound can help confirm the diagnosis by demonstrating hyperaemia on Doppler interrogation of the tendon or its sheath (Fig. 46-55). On MRI, a greater cross-sectional area of fluid than tendon is suggestive of tenosynovitis. The FHL and very occasionally the FDL tendon sheaths communicate with the ankle joint in a minority of individuals. Therefore fluid in these tendon sheaths may relate to an ankle joint effusion.

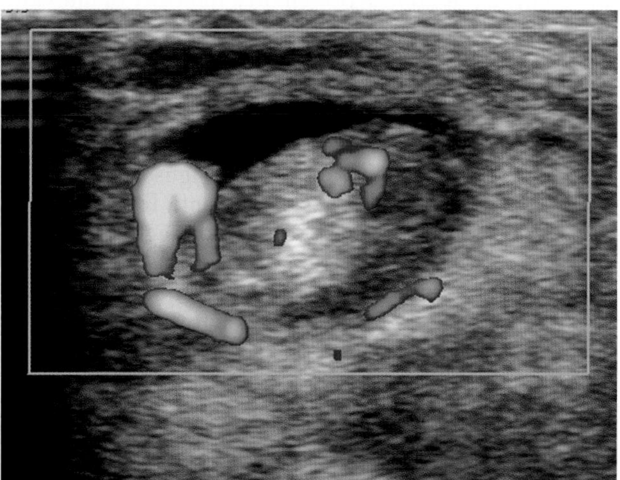

FIGURE 46-55 ■ **Tibialis posterior tenosynovitis.** Transverse ultrasound image reveals anechoic fluid in the tendon sheath and marked neovascularity of the tendon sheath (orange) on Doppler interrogation.

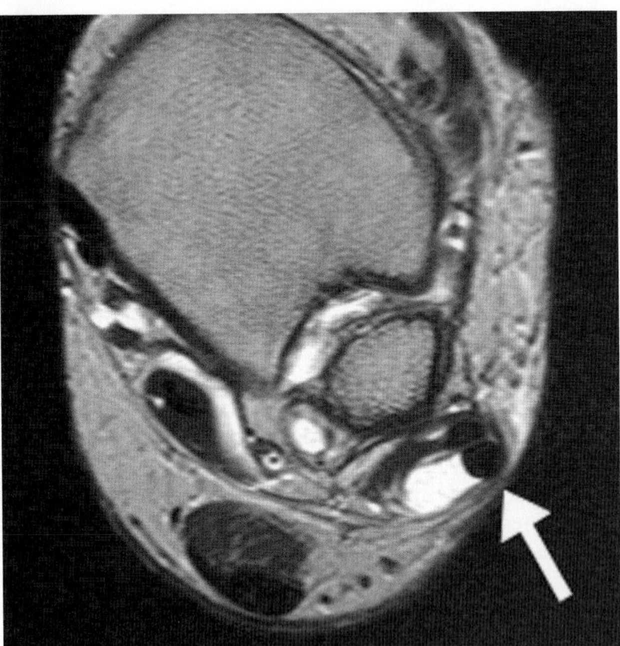

FIGURE 46-56 ■ Peroneal tendon dislocation. Axial oblique T2-weighted image shows anterolateral dislocation of the peroneal tendons (arrow). Note abnormal fluid in the tendon sheath.

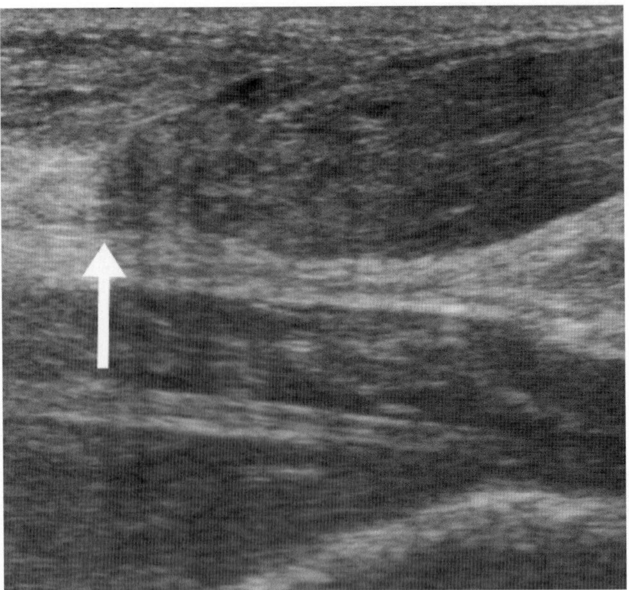

FIGURE 46-57 ■ Complete tear of Achilles tendon. Longitudinal ultrasound image reveals the position of the retracted proximal tendon end (arrow).

The peroneal tendons pass posterior to the lateral malleolus, where the peroneus brevis (PB) tendon is normally located between the peroneus longus (PL) tendon and the malleolus in the fibular groove. Both tendons are retained by the superior peroneal retinaculum (SPR). The SPR extends from the posterolateral fibular periostium to the Achilles tendon aponeurosis. The PB tendon is prone to longitudinal tears or 'splits'. In the early stages the PB tendon adopts a semilunar or boomerang shape which progresses to a split with inter-positioning of the PL tendon between the split fibres of PB. Tears of the SPR may lead to peroneal tendon dislocation (Fig. 46-56). Dynamic imaging with ultrasound shows lateral dislocation of the peroneal tendons from the fibular groove with provocative movements.[38] A sesamoid os peroneum within the PL tendon is present in a minority of individuals. The os peroneum may be associated with PL tendinopathy or may itself be fractured or inflamed, giving rise to pain. Tears of PL tend to occur at the level of the cuboid tunnel or just distal to an os perineum, if present. Pathology of the anterior ankle tendons, comprising the tibialis anterior, extensor hallucis longus and extensor digitorum longus tendons, is infrequent. Tears of tibialis anterior occur more commonly in older age groups particularly close to the insertion of the medial cuneiform.

Achilles tendinopathy is common and may be related to athletic activities in young adults. However, more typically it occurs in the middle aged. It results from chronic microtrauma to the tendon, leading to tendon degeneration. Typically there is focal fusiform thickening of the tendon involving the mid-portion, with increased signal on short and long TE MRI and low reflectivity and loss of normal tendon echotexture on US. The insertion is less often involved, although this can be affected by enthesopathy or by mechanical impingement from a prominent posterior calcaneal process (Haglund's bump). Ultrasound also demonstrates hyperaemia on Doppler interrogation of the tendon or deep fat pad (Kager's fat pad). The Achilles tendon lacks a tendon sheath. However, inflammation of the surrounding tissues or paratenon, (paratenonitis) may be seen, particularly in runners. The paratenon is found on the superficial, medial and lateral aspects of the tendon and when inflamed appears on MRI as a rim of ill-defined increased signal on these aspects of the tendon. On ultrasound the paratenon appears as a hyporeflective rim. Acute tears of the Achilles tendon may be partial or complete. Complete tears (which are much more common) exhibit no continuity of fibres and may show retraction (Fig. 46-57). Dynamic ultrasound imaging is useful for measuring the separation of the tendon ends for surgical planning.[39] The retrocalcaneal bursa is located deep to the insertion of the Achilles tendon. Inflammation of this bursa may be found in association with Achilles tendinopathy and usually results from chronic and repetitive microtrauma, frequently described as overuse injury. Systemic inflammatory disorders including rheumatoid and seronegative arthritis may also cause inflammation of the Achilles tendon insertion or retrocalcaneal bursa. Retro-Achilles bursitis involves the bursa superficial to the Achilles tendon.

Bone

Osteochondral lesion (OCL) of the talar dome is a common cause of persisting deep ankle pain. Most talar OCL occur following trauma, though some medial lesions arise without a history of injury.[40] OCL is easily missed on conventional radiographs of the ankle. MRI is very sensitive for OCL, allowing assessment of location and size (Fig. 46-58). The presence of fluid signal around the lesion helps to determine whether the lesion is partially detached, detached or displaced.

Impingement may occur in various locations around the ankle, the commonest types being anterolateral (see

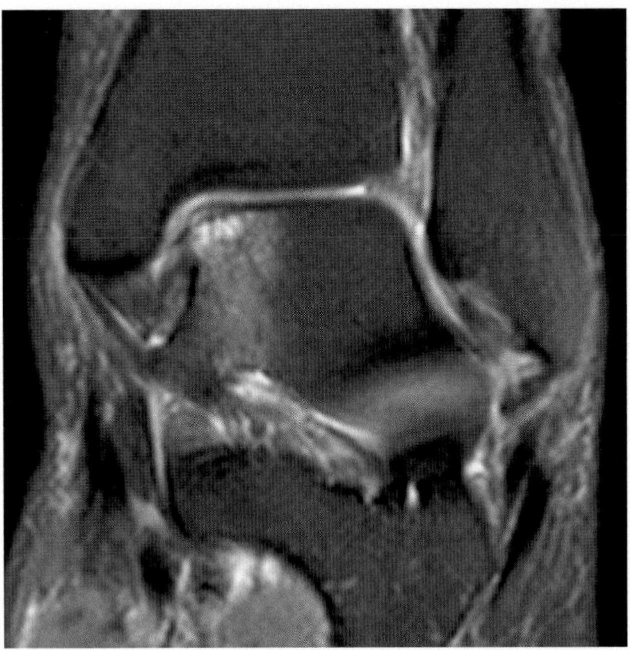

FIGURE 46-58 ■ Osteochondral lesion of the talar dome. Coronal T2-weighted fat-saturated image shows subchondral cyst formation in the medial talar dome and surrounding bone marrow oedema.

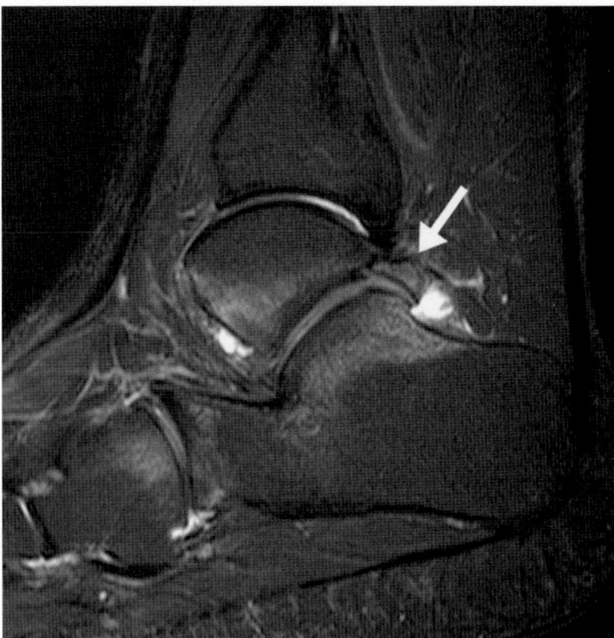

FIGURE 46-59 ■ Posterior ankle impingement. Sagittal T2-weighted fat-saturated image shows bone marrow oedema within a prominent os trigonum (arrow) and the posterior calcaneus.

above), anterior and posterior. Anterior impingement occurs between bony spurs on the dorsal talar neck and anterior tibial plafond, a condition associated with kicking activities like soccer. These spurs can be readily identified on lateral radiographs. MRI may additionally reveal synovitis and lateral ankle ligament damage.[41] Posterior impingement is most frequently associated with a large os trigonum or Stieda process of the talus (Fig. 46-59). These give rise to chronic compression of soft tissues against the posterior tibia in activities that involve repetitive forced plantar flexion as in ballet dancing.[42]

Tarsal Coalition

Tarsal coalition refers to developmental fusion of two (rarely three) bones in the hind-foot. Coalition may be osseous or non-osseous (the latter may be fibrous or cartilaginous). The most common type is calcaneonavicular followed by subtalar, other types being much less common. In calcaneonavicular coalition the navicular is fused to the calcaneus through an elongated anterior calcaneal process (Fig. 46-60). In subtalar coalition there is fusion between the talus and calcaneus at or adjacent to the middle subtalar joint. This results in a characteristic 'C-sign' on a lateral radiograph reflecting continuation of the bone contour through the coalition. MRI and CT are much more sensitive than plain radiographs for tarsal coalition. Stress changes may also be demonstrated at the site of coalition or in nearby structures.

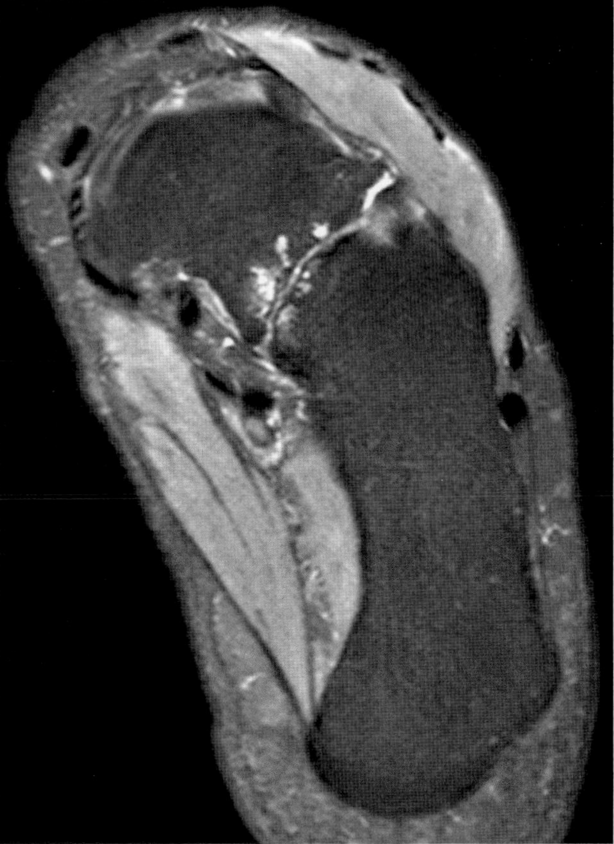

FIGURE 46-60 ■ Calcaneonavicular coalition. Axial T2-weighted fat-saturated image reveals abnormal articulation between the calcaneus and navicular without marrow continuity, indicating non-osseous coalition. Note there is subcortical cyst formation resulting from abnormal stresses.

Other Soft-Tissue Abnormalities

Plantar fasciitis is a common cause of heel pain thought to result from chronic microtrauma of the plantar fascia from biomechanical stress. The central band is most

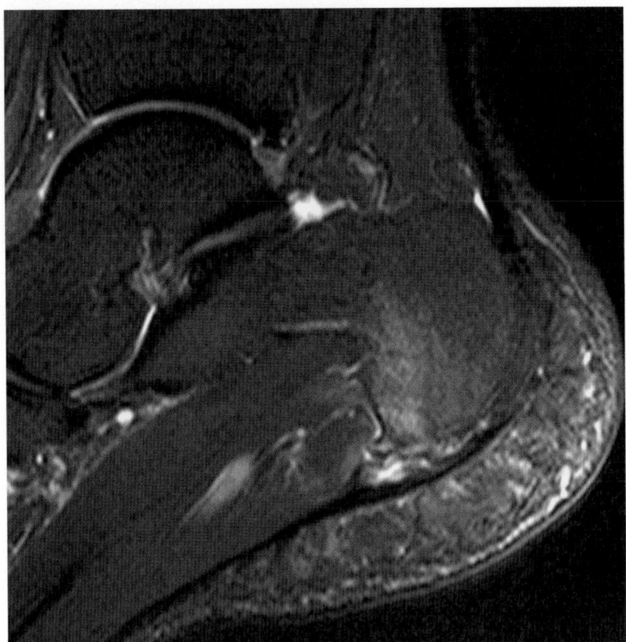

FIGURE 46-61 ■ **Plantar fasciitis.** Sagittal T2-weighted fat-saturated image demonstrates oedema and thickening of the origin of the plantar fascia. Note the presence of bone marrow oedema in the adjacent part of the calcaneus.

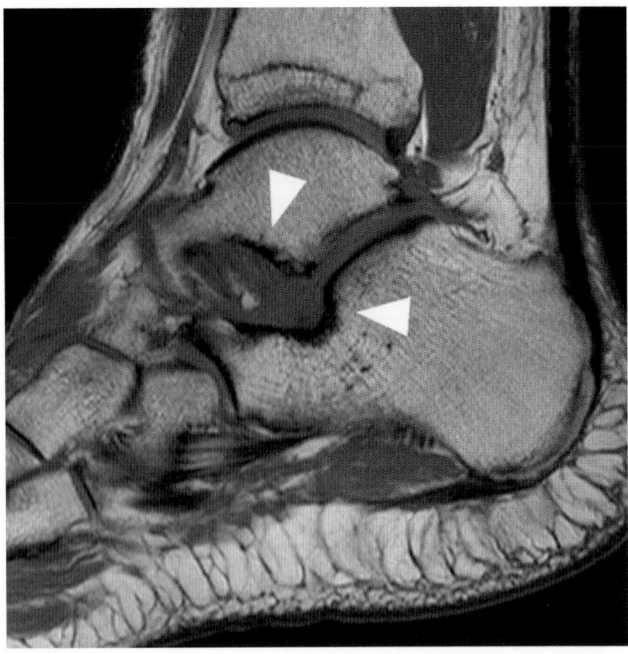

FIGURE 46-62 ■ **Sinus tarsi syndrome.** Sagittal T1-weighted image reveals replacement of the normal high signal of the fat in the sinus tarsi with intermediate signal (arrowheads), indicating inflammation.

frequently involved near its calcaneal origin. The diagnosis is made on ultrasound when there is thickening of the fascia (normally measuring up to 5 mm[43]) and loss of normal echogenic fibrillar texture. MRI reveals thickening and increased signal on fluid-sensitive sequences, indicating inflammation (Fig. 46-61). A calcaneal spur may be present but this is often found in the absence of plantar fasciitis and there is no role for conventional radiographs in the diagnosis of plantar fasciitis. Other less common causes of plantar fascia thickening to consider include seronegative arthropathy, plantar fibroma and hyperlipidaemia.

The sinus tarsi is a cone-shaped space between the anterior and posterior subtalar joints containing fat surrounding ligaments, small vessels and nerve endings. Sinus tarsi syndrome describes pain arising from this structure, typically occurring with a history of an ankle sprain. The exact aetiology is unclear and it may be that this syndrome has a number of different causes. The condition is identified on MRI as loss of the normal high T1 fat signal in the sinus tarsi (Fig. 46-62).[44]

Tarsal tunnel syndrome is an entrapment neuropathy of the posterior tibial nerve giving rise to pain/paraesthesia on the plantar aspect of the foot and a positive Tinel's sign. Muscle weakness is less common. The posterior tibial nerve is compressed within the tarsal tunnel, a compartment in the posteromedial ankle which is bounded by the flexor retinaculum. The tunnel transmits the posterior tibial nerve as part of a neurovascular bundle and the tendons of TP, FDL and FHL. MRI or ultrasound may be used to identify a lesion compressing the nerve such as a ganglion, bone fracture, nerve sheath tumour or accessory FDL. MRI may additionally reveal oedema in denervated muscles supplied by the nerve.

The plantar plate is a fibrocartilaginous structure extending from the metatarsal neck to the base of the proximal phalanx of each toe. Its function is to resist hyperextension of the MTP joint. Plantar plate rupture most commonly affects the great toe. It may be diagnosed with ultrasound or MRI. MRI with injection of contrast medium into the MTP joint dorsally demonstrates escape of the contrast agent through the torn plantar plate, leading to opacification of the flexor tendon sheath.

Morton neuroma is another cause of metatarsalgia, most commonly arising in the third web space. It is thought to result from repetitive compression of the plantar common digital nerve, leading to perineural fibrosis. On ultrasound a Morton's neuroma typically appears as a rounded hypoechoic mass. On MRI it appears as a low-to-intermediate signal intensity mass in a characteristic position. The advantage of ultrasound in this setting is to guide injection therapy after the diagnosis has been confirmed.

For a full list of references, please see ExpertConsult.

FURTHER READING

21. Tannast M, Siebenrock KA, Anderson SE. Femoroacetabular impingement: radiographic diagnosis—what the radiologist should know. Am J Roentgenol 2007;188(6):1540–52.
27. Lafforgue P, Dahan E, Chagnaud C, et al. Early-stage avascular necrosis of the femoral head: MR imaging for prognosis in 31 cases with at least 2 years of follow-up. Radiology 1993;187(1):199–204.
28. Korompilias AV, Karantanas AH, Lykissas MG, Beris AE. Bone marrow edema syndrome. Skeletal Radiol 2009;38(5):425–36.
36. Perrich KD, Goodwin DW, Hecht PJ, Cheung Y. Ankle ligaments on MRI: appearance of normal and injured ligaments. Am J Roentgenol 2009;193(3):687–95.

Bone Tumours (1): Benign Tumours and Tumour-Like Lesions of Bone

Asif Saifuddin

CHAPTER OUTLINE

GENERAL CHARACTERISTICS OF BONE TUMOURS

Bone tumours may be benign or malignant, and are currently classified according to the World Health Organisation Classification of 2002.[1] The pre-biopsy diagnosis of a bone tumour depends upon several features, including patient age, lesion location and finally the radiological characteristics. The latter allows an assessment of rate of growth (generally indicative of benignity or malignancy) and underlying histological subtype, based predominantly upon patterns of matrix mineralisation (Table 47-1).

Age at Presentation

Patient age is of huge importance in suggesting a differential diagnosis of a focal bone lesion. Primary bone tumours are rare below the age of 5 years and over the age of 40 years, with the exception of myeloma and chondrosarcoma. Metastases are the commonest lesions over the age of 40 years.

RADIOLOGICAL ASSESSMENT OF BONE TUMOURS[1]

Location

The location of the lesion within the skeleton (appendicular, axial) and within the individual bone (epiphysis, metaphysis, diaphysis; intramedullary, intracortical, surface) must be considered in detail when discussing individual tumours, since it has a considerable influence on differential diagnosis.

Rate of Growth

When considering rate of growth, the most important feature is the lesion margin. In benign and low-grade malignant neoplasms, this margin is sharp (geographical; Type 1). Type 1A has a rim of sclerosis between the lesion and the host bone (Fig. 47-1A), Type 1B is a very well defined lytic lesion but with no marginal sclerosis (Fig. 47-1B), while Type 1C has a slightly less sharp, non-sclerotic margin (Fig. 47-1C). Type 2 is moth-eaten destruction, which represents the next most aggressive pattern and is characterised by multiple lucent areas measuring 2–5 mm in diameter separated by bone which has yet to be destroyed (Fig. 47-2). Type 3 is permeative destruction, which is the most aggressive pattern and is composed of multiple coalescing small ill-defined lesions 1 mm or less in diameter with a zone of transition of several centimetres (Fig. 47-3). Radiographs inevitably underestimate the extent of medullary involvement, which is more clearly shown on magnetic resonance imaging (MRI).

Regions with apparently intact cortex may show extracortical tumour masses. This phenomenon often leads, in highly malignant tumours such as Ewing's sarcoma, to 'cortical saucerisation' as the tumour, temporarily restrained by the periosteum, erodes back through the cortical bone.

Benign or low-grade malignant neoplasms tend to remain within the medullary cavity until late in their development. Typically, the cortex is not destroyed, but slow erosion of its endosteal surface (endosteal scalloping) together with periosteal new bone formation results

TABLE 47-1 **Classification of Primary Benign Bone Tumours**

Cartilage tumours	Osteochondroma
	Chondroma
	• Enchondroma
	• Periosteal chondromas
	• Multiple chondromatosis
	Chondroblastoma
	Chondromyxoid fibroma
Osteogenic tumours	Osteoid osteoma
	Osteoblastoma
Fibrogenic tumours	Desmoplastic fibroma
Fibrohistiocytic tumours	Benign fibrous hystiocytoma
	• Fibrous cortical defect
	• Non-ossifying fibroma
Giant cell tumour	Giant cell tumour
Vascular tumours	Haemangioma
Smooth muscle tumours	Leiomyoma
Lipogenic tumours	Lipoma
Neural tumours	Neurilemmoma
Miscellaneous lesions	Aneurysmal bone cyst
	Solitary bone cyst
	Fibrous dysplasia
	Osteofibrous dysplasia
	Langerhans cell histiocytosis (eosinophilic granuloma)
	Erdheim–Chester disease
	Chest wall hamartoma

Modified from WHO 2002 Classification.[1]

in expansion of bone (Fig. 47-1A). Conversely, high-grade malignant tumours commonly extend through the cortex by the time of presentation, resulting in cortical destruction and an adjacent extraosseous mass (Fig. 47-3).

Periosteal Reaction[2]

Periosteal reaction is of various types with none being pathognomonic of any particular tumour: rather, the type helps to indicate the aggressiveness of the lesion. A thick, well-formed (solid) periosteal reaction (Fig. 47-4A) indicates a slow rate of growth but not necessarily a benign tumour, since it may be seen with chondrosarcoma. Laminated periosteal reaction (Fig. 47-4B) indicates subperiosteal extension of tumour, infection or haematoma. Lesions demonstrating periodic growth may show a multi-laminated pattern (Fig. 47-4C). A Codman's triangle indicates the limit of subperiosteal tumour in a longitudinal direction (Fig. 47-4B). Vertical (sunburst spiculation or 'hair-on-end') types of periosteal reaction are seen with the most aggressive tumours such as osteosarcoma (Fig. 47-4D) and Ewing's sarcoma. However, the most rapidly growing lesions may not be associated with any radiographically visible periosteal response, since mineralisation of the deep layer of periosteum can take 2 weeks.

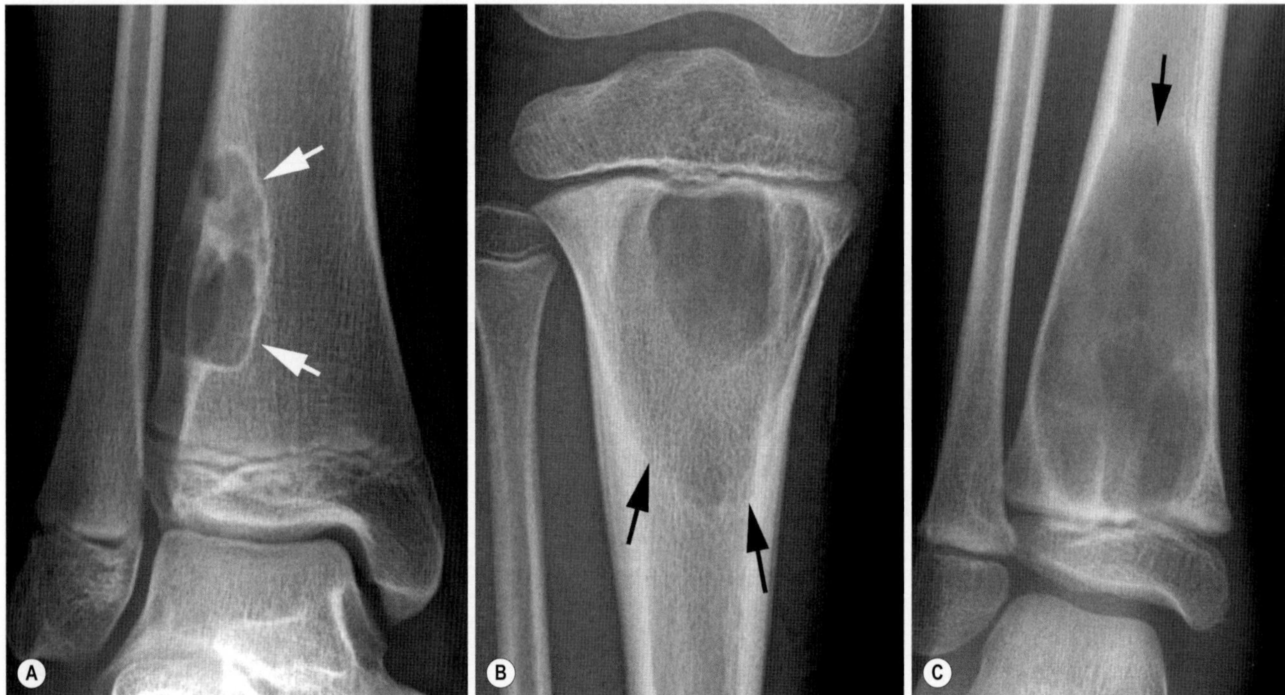

FIGURE 47-1 ■ **Patterns of bone destruction. Geographic.** (A) Type 1A AP radiograph of the distal tibia in a patient with non-ossifying fibroma (NOF), demonstrating the sharp, thin sclerotic margin (arrows). (B) Type 1B AP radiograph of the proximal tibia in a patient with an aneurysmal bone cyst (ABC) showing a well-defined, non-sclerotic margin (arrows). (C) Type 1C AP radiograph of the distal tibia in a patient with an ABC showing a slightly less well-defined, non-sclerotic margin (arrows).

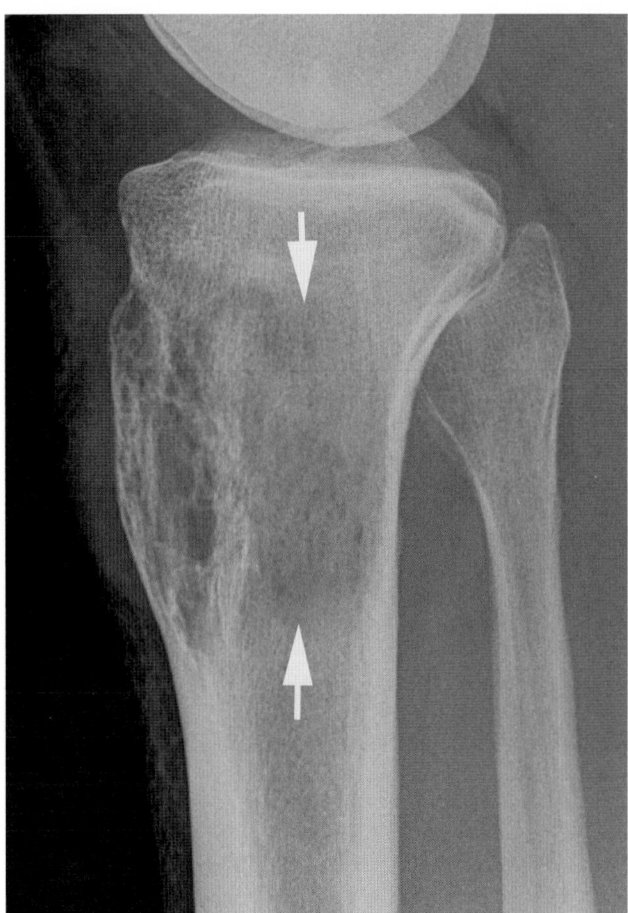

FIGURE 47-2 ■ Patterns of bone destruction. Moth-eaten. Lateral radiograph of the proximal tibia showing a 'moth-eaten' appearance (arrows) caused by the coalescence of multiple small lytic areas.

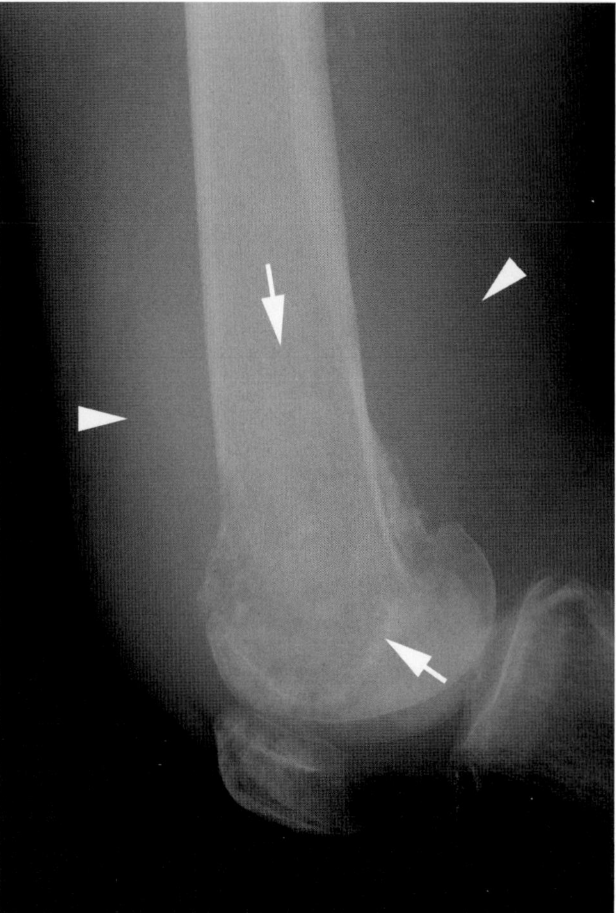

FIGURE 47-3 ■ Patterns of bone destruction. Permeative. Lateral radiograph of the distal femur showing a 'permeative' pattern of bone destruction (arrows). Note also the large circumferential extraosseous mass (arrowheads).

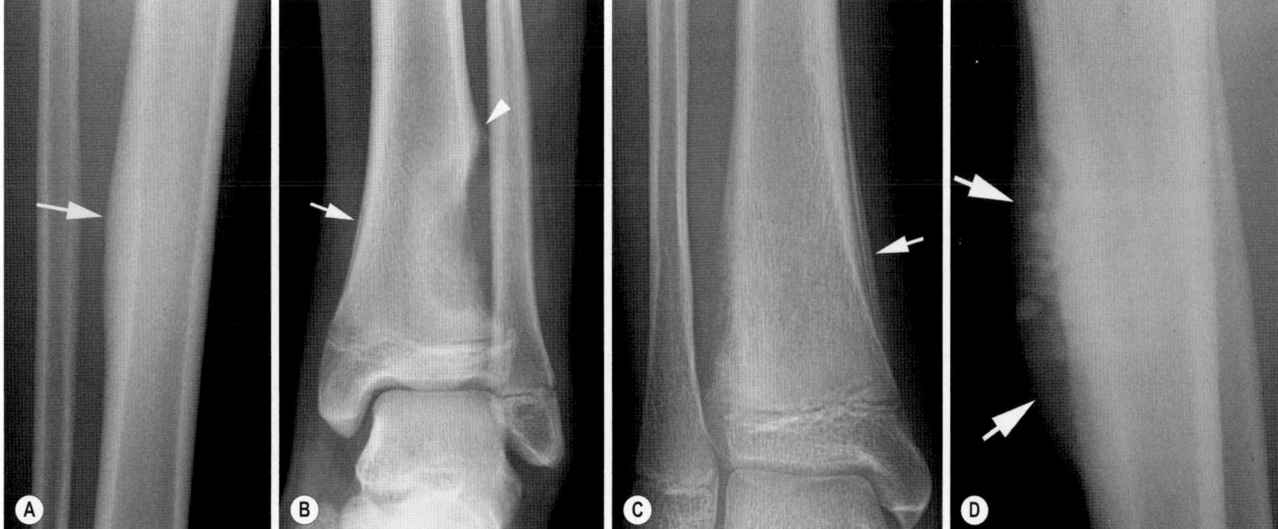

FIGURE 47-4 ■ Patterns of periosteal reaction. (A) Coned AP radiograph of the tibial diaphysis showing solid periosteal reaction (arrow) due to an occult osteoid osteoma. (B) AP radiograph of the distal tibia showing a single, laminated periosteal reaction (arrow) associated with an ABC. Note also the Codman's triangle (arrowhead). (C) AP radiograph of the distal tibia showing a multi-laminated periosteal reaction (arrow) associated with acute osteomyelitis. (D) Coned lateral radiograph of the proximal tibia showing a coarse 'sunburst'-type vertical periosteal reaction associated with osteosarcoma.

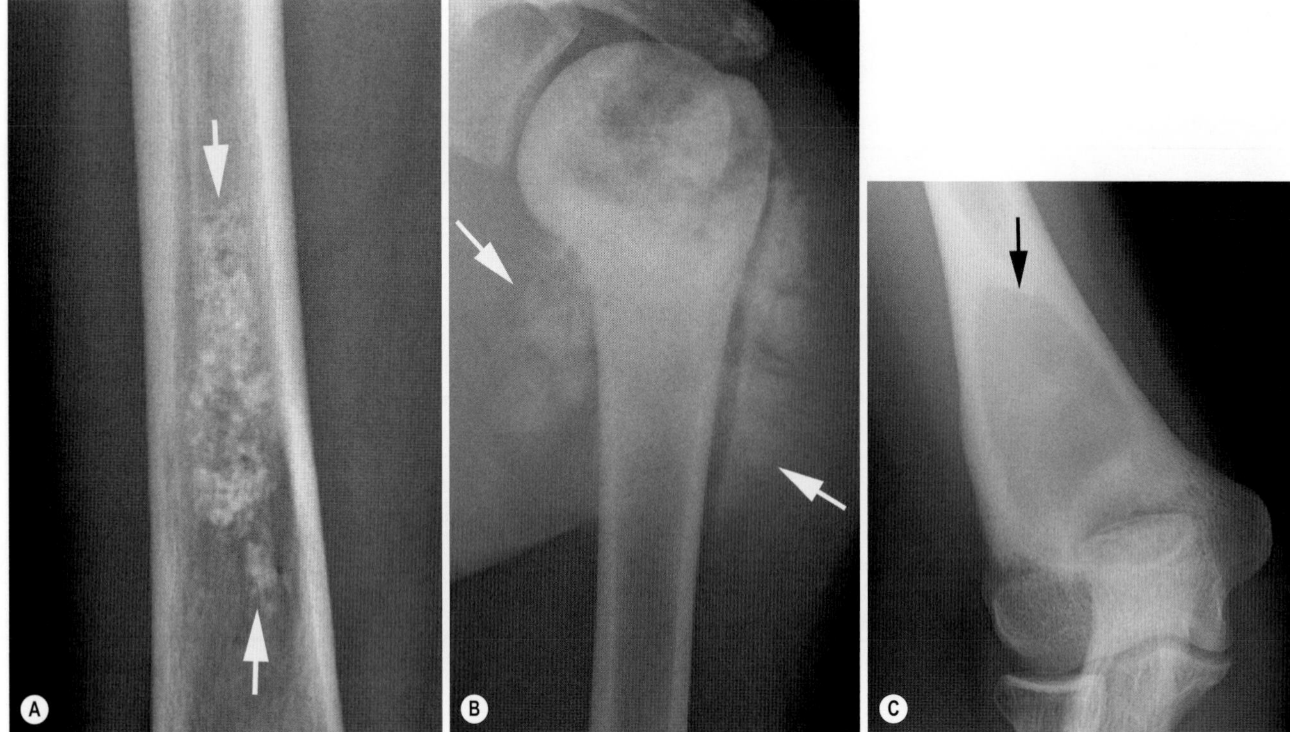

FIGURE 47-5 ■ Patterns of matrix mineralisation. (A) Coned AP radiograph of the femoral diaphysis in a patient with grade 2 chondrosarcoma, showing typical punctate chondral calcification. (B) AP radiograph of the proximal humerus in a patient with osteoblastic osteosarcoma showing typical 'cloud-like' osseous mineralisation (arrows). (C) AP radiograph of the distal humerus femur in a patient with fibrous dysplasia showing typical 'ground-glass' mineralisation (arrow).

Matrix Mineralisation

The matrix of a tumour represents the extracellular material produced by the tumour cells within which the cells lie. Certain tumours produce characteristic radiographically visible matrix mineralisation, which allows the histological cell type to be predicted. Chondral calcifications are typically linear, curvilinear, ring-like, punctate or nodular (Fig. 47-5A). Osseous mineralisation is cloud-like and poorly defined (Fig. 47-5B), whereas diffuse matrix mineralisation in benign fibrous tumours produces the characteristic 'ground-glass' appearance (Fig. 47-5C), seen most commonly in fibrous dysplasia. Some neoplasms, such as adenocarcinoma metastases, can provoke reactive mineralisation, whereas calcifications within an intraosseous lipoma are due to associated fat necrosis. Also, some bone sarcomas may develop on underlying calcified bone infarcts.

CT and MRI in Diagnosis and Staging

CT is excellent for demonstrating the presence of radiographically occult matrix mineralisation and the persistence of a thin cortical shell, indicating that the tumour still lies deep to the periosteum. CT also plays a major role in the investigation of cortical thickening, allowing the demonstration of the cause, such as the nidus of an osteoid osteoma or a stress fracture.

The major role of MRI is in local staging, particularly for high-grade malignant tumours such as osteosarcoma, where the intraosseous extent, identification of 'skip' lesions and relationship to the neurovascular bundle and adjacent joint can all be assessed with great accuracy.[3] Such information is vital for planning surgical management, be it limb salvage or amputation. Dynamic contrast-enhanced MRI has been advocated for determining chemotherapeutic response, but its role in routine patient management is unclear.

In the presence of a purely lytic lesion, several MRI features may help in further lesion characterisation.[4] The presence of profound low signal intensity (SI) on T2*-weighted gradient-echo images indicates chronic haemorrhage and may be seen with giant cell tumour. MRI is very sensitive to the presence of fluid–fluid levels (FFLs) and the degree of FFL change is related to histological diagnosis.[5] Lesions that are completely filled with FFLs are almost always aneurysmal bone cysts (ABCs). MRI can also demonstrate a fatty matrix, as seen with haemangioma and intraosseous lipoma. The vascular nature of renal metastases has been demonstrated by the presence of the 'flow-void' sign.[6] MRI is very sensitive to reactive medullary and soft-tissue oedema, which characterises certain lesions such as osteoid osteoma, osteoblastoma, chondroblastoma and Brodie's abscess.[7]

Bone scintigraphy plays little role in the diagnostic work-up of a suspected primary bone tumour, with the possible exception of osteoid osteoma or osteoblastoma, particularly in the spine. However, scintigraphy is still useful for the identification of skeletal metastases, although this role has recently been challenged by whole-body MRI.[8]

The position of techniques such as MR spectroscopy, positron emission tomography (PET) and computed tomography PET (CT-PET) in the management of suspected bone tumours is as yet unclear, while whole-body diffusion-weighted MRI (WBDWI) is highly sensitive for the identification of skeletal metastases.[9] Finally, the use of ultrasound[10] and CT[11] for image-guided needle biopsy is well established, while MR-guided biopsy has also been developed for targeting subtle marrow lesions.[12]

BENIGN BONE TUMOURS

Benign bone tumours are currently classified according to the 2002 World Health Organisation system based on their cell of origin[1] (Table 47-1).

CARTILAGE TUMOURS

Osteochondroma[13]

Recent genetic studies indicate that osteochondroma is a true neoplasm, which may also arise following radiotherapy and accounts for 20–50% of benign bone tumours. Osteochondromas present from 2 to 60 years, but the highest incidence is in the second decade, with a male-to-female ratio of 1.4–3.6 : 1.

Long bones are commonly affected, especially around the knee (~40%), the commonest locations being the distal femur, proximal humerus, proximal tibia and proximal femur. The commonest flat bones affected are the ilium and scapula. Lesions may be classified as either pedunculated, when they have a thin stalk that typically points away from the adjacent joint, or sessile when they arise from a broad base. They are typically metaphyseal in location.

Diaphyseal aclasis (hereditary multiple exostoses, HME) constitutes an uncommon autosomal dominant disorder in which the exostoses may be larger than the solitary variety and may lead to shortening or deformity of the affected limbs. The metaphyses in this condition are also typically widened and dysplastic (Fig. 47-6).

Osteochondromas present with mechanical problems such as an enlarging mass, pressure on adjoining structures (muscles, nerves, vessels), or rarely with fracture of the bony stem. Mechanical irritation of overlying soft tissues may result in adventitial bursa formation, which can mimic sarcomatous degeneration. MRI is highly accurate in the assessment of symptomatic osteochondromas.[14] The incidence of chondrosarcomatous change in the cartilage cap is very small in a solitary osteochondroma (probably <1%), while malignant degeneration in diaphyseal aclasis is approximated at 3–5%.

Radiological Features

The lesion appears as an outgrowth from the normal cortex, with which it is continuous. Pedunculated lesions have a long slim neck (Fig. 47-7A), whereas sessile lesions have a broad base from the bone of origin (Fig. 47-7B). Continuity between the medullary cavity of the lesion and that of the underlying bone is essential for the diagnosis and is best demonstrated on either CT or MRI (Fig. 47-8A). The cartilage cap is optimally demonstrated on axial proton density-weighted (PDW) or T2W fast spin-echo (FSE) MRI, when the hyperintense cartilage contrasts well against the adjacent iso-/hypointense muscle (Fig. 47-8A) and it should not exceed 2-cm thickness in adults. The cartilage cap can also be visualised and measured on ultrasound where it appears hypoechoic in contrast to the brightly reflective bone surfaces. Complications associated with OC include bursa formation

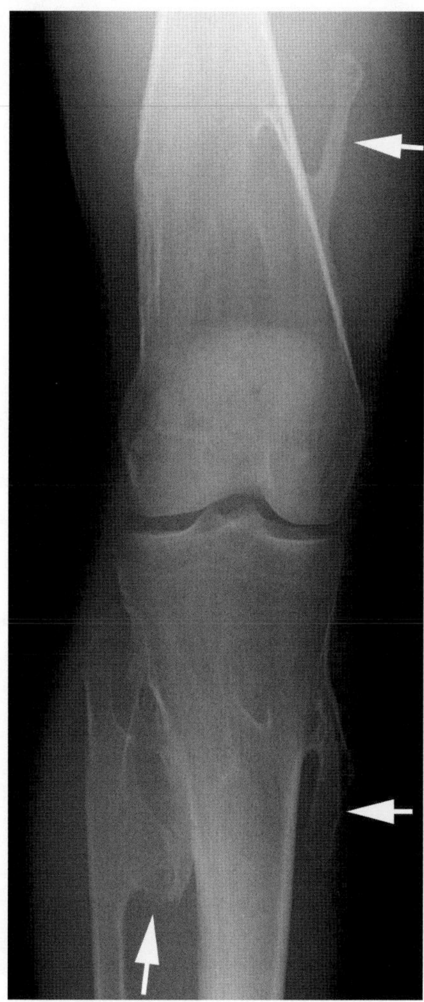

FIGURE 47-6 ■ **Diaphyseal aclasis.** AP radiograph of the right knee showing multiple osteochondromas (arrows) and associated widening of the distal femoral and proximal tibial metaphyses.

(Fig. 47-8B), neurovascular compromise and, rarely, pseudoaneurysm (Fig. 47-8C).

(En)Chondroma[13]

(En)Chondroma is an intramedullary neoplasm comprising lobules of benign hyaline cartilage and is the second commonest benign chondral lesion after osteochondroma, accounting for approximately 8% of all primary bone tumours and tumour-like lesion in a large biopsy series. However, the true prevalence of enchondromas is unknown since the majority are asymptomatic. Incidental enchondromas have been identified in approximately 3% of routine knee MRI studies. Enchondromas affect the tubular bones of the hands and feet in 40–65% of cases and present either when they become symptomatic due to increasing size, as pathological fracture (in 60% of cases) or as incidental findings. The majority arise in the proximal phalanges (40–50%), followed by the metacarpals (15–30%) and middle phalanges (20–30%). The small bones of the feet are involved in 7% of cases. Approximately 25% are found in the femur, tibia and humerus, while other sites are very rare. The age range is 10–80 years, with most presenting in the second to fourth decades. There is equal prevalence among both genders.

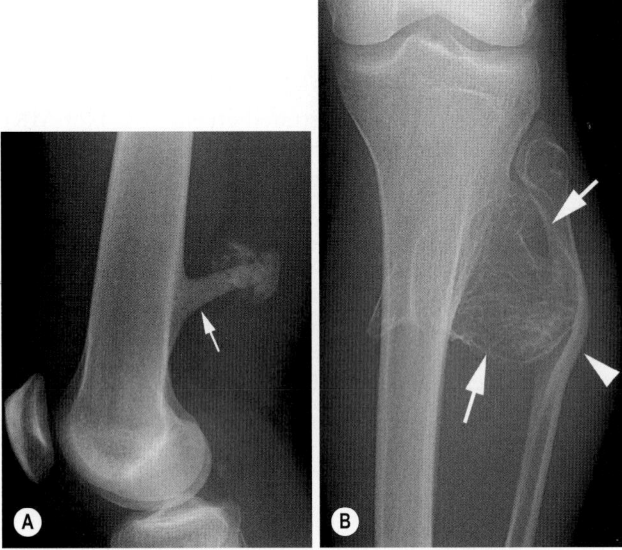

FIGURE 47-7 ■ Osteochondroma. (A) Lateral radiograph of the distal femur showing a typical pedunculated osteochondroma (arrow). (B) AP radiograph of the proximal tibia showing a sessile osteochondroma (arrows) with associated pressure deformity of the adjacent fibula (arrowhead).

Radiological Features

Most enchondromas arise centrally in the phalanges and metacarpals. Lesions are typically metaphyseal or diaphyseal, with epiphyseal location accounting for approximately 8%. Enchondromas are often eccentric and 75% are solitary. They are typically well-circumscribed, lobular or oval lytic lesions, which may expand the cortex (Fig. 47-9A). Size at presentation ranges from 10 to 50 mm. Chondral-type mineralisation may be identified within the matrix.

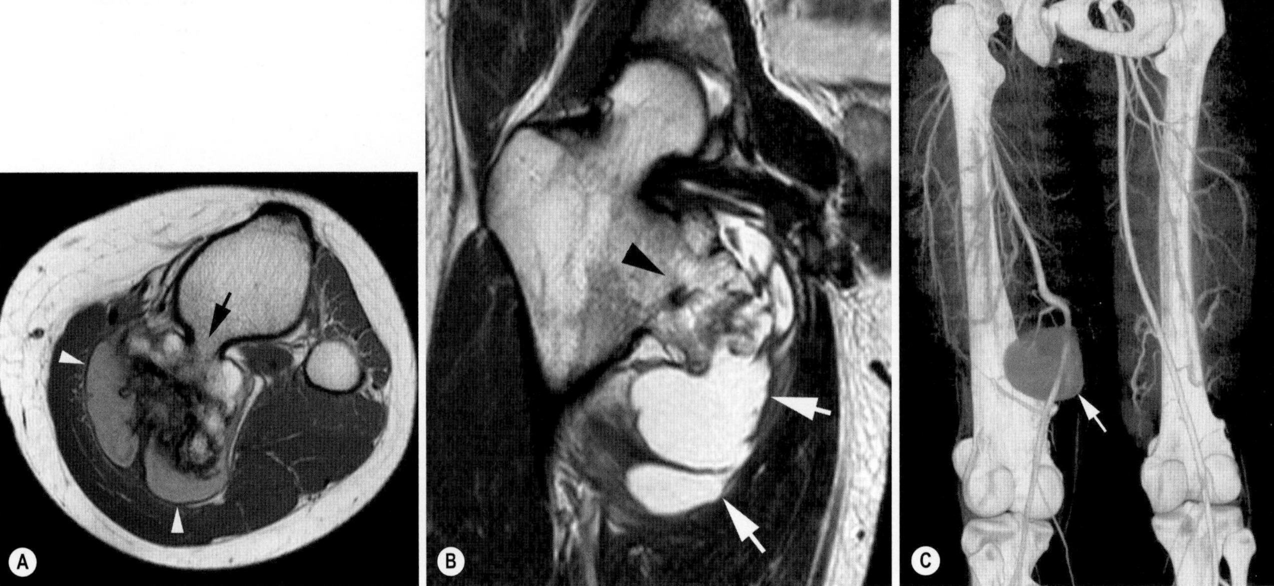

FIGURE 47-8 ■ Osteochondroma. MRI features. (A) Axial PDW FSE MRI through the proximal tibia showing medullary continuity (arrow) between the osteochondroma and host bone. The cartilage cap is mildly hyperintense and surrounded by a thin, hypointense perichondrium (arrowheads). (B) Coronal T2W FSE MRI of the hip showing a bursa (arrows) complicating a sessile osteochondroma (arrowhead) of the proximal femur. (C) Posterior view 3D CT maximum intensity projection (MIP) of the femora in a patient with diaphyseal aclasis showing a popliteal artery pseudoaneurysm (arrow).

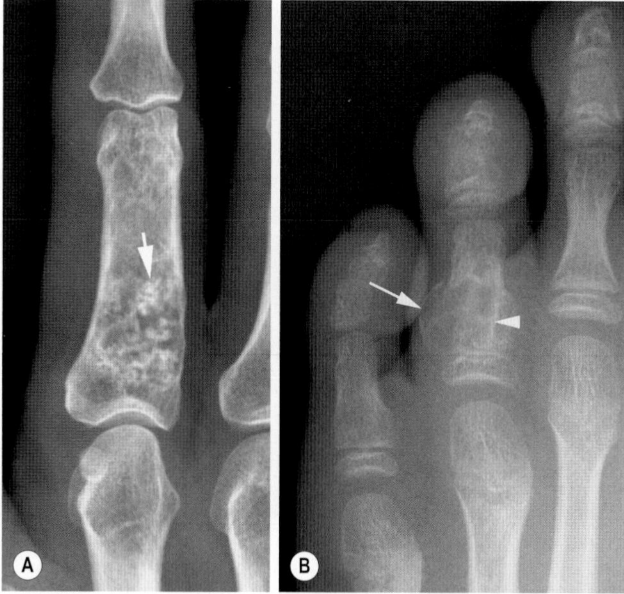

FIGURE 47-9 ■ Enchondroma. (A) AP radiograph of the index finger showing a lobular, mildly expansile lesion with typical chondral matrix mineralisation (arrow). (B) DP radiograph of the forefoot showing an eccentrically placed enchondroma of the fourth toe proximal phalanx (arrowhead) with an associated extraosseous component covered by a thin cortical shell (arrow).

The term 'enchondroma protuberans' has been used to describe an eccentrically placed enchondroma with an associated extraosseous component which is usually covered by a thin shell of intact cortical bone (Fig. 47-9B). Most cases arise in the fingers or toes and they may be difficult to distinguish from periosteal chondroma, although this may not be clinically relevant since both lesions have the same management.

The differentiation between a relatively large enchondroma and a grade 1 chondrosarcoma can be difficult. Lesion size above 5–6 cm and deep endosteal scalloping are suggestive of chondrosarcoma,[15] but prominent scalloping can also be seen with an eccentrically placed chondroma, which has been termed an 'endosteal chondroma'. However, this differentiation may not be of clinical relevance, since both can be treated in the same way, with either careful clinical and imaging follow-up, or curettage with cementation. Low-grade chondral tumours have characteristic MRI features, showing a lobular margin with intermediate T1-weighted signal intensity (T1W SI) (Fig. 47-10A) and T2-weighted/short tau inversion recovery (T2W/STIR) hyperintensity without surrounding reactive oedema (Fig. 47-10B). Matrix mineralisation manifests as punctate areas of signal void. A hypointense rim and septations may also be seen, the latter showing enhancement following IV gadolinium contrast medium.[13]

Less Common Varieties of Chondroma

Periosteal Chondroma.[16] These are rare lesions affecting children and young adults and are located in the metaphyses of tubular bones, most commonly the proximal humerus followed by the femur and tibia. They are also seen in the small bones of the hands and feet, in which

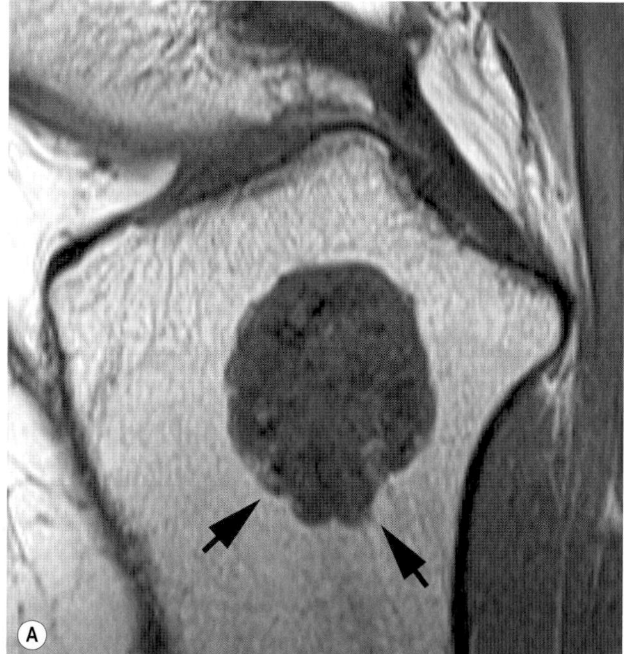

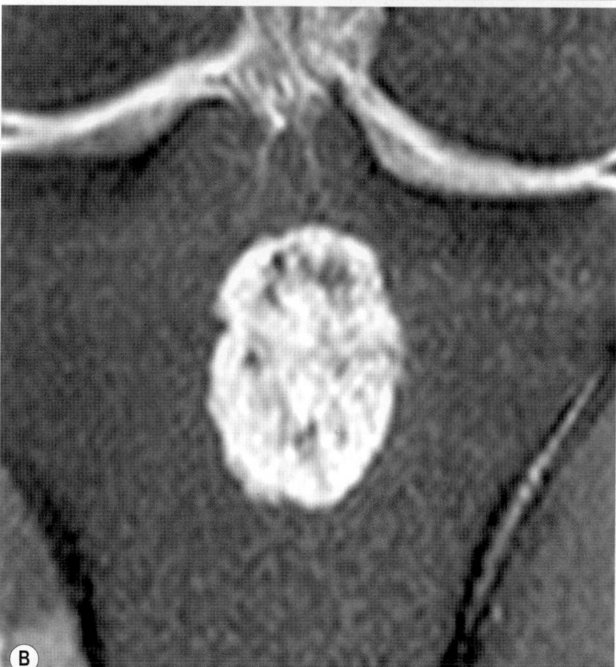

FIGURE 47-10 ■ Enchondroma. MRI features. (A) Sagittal T1W SE MRI showing classical appearances of a chondroma, with a lobular inferior margin (arrows). (B) Coronal fat-suppressed T2W FSE MRI showing the hyperintense lesion with matrix mineralisation manifest as punctate areas of signal void. Note the absence of surrounding reactive oedema-like SI.

case some extension into the underlying medullary cavity is commonly seen. Radiologically, each appears as a well-defined area of cortical erosion typically measuring 1–3 cm with mature periosteal reaction and sometimes a thin external shell of bone. Cartilaginous matrix mineralisation is observed in half the cases (Fig. 47-11A). MRI shows the features of a chondral lesion with a lobular hyperintense mass on T2-weighted images adjacent to the

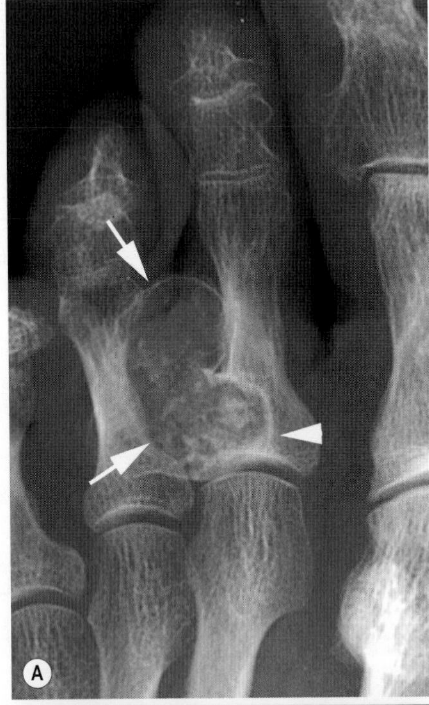

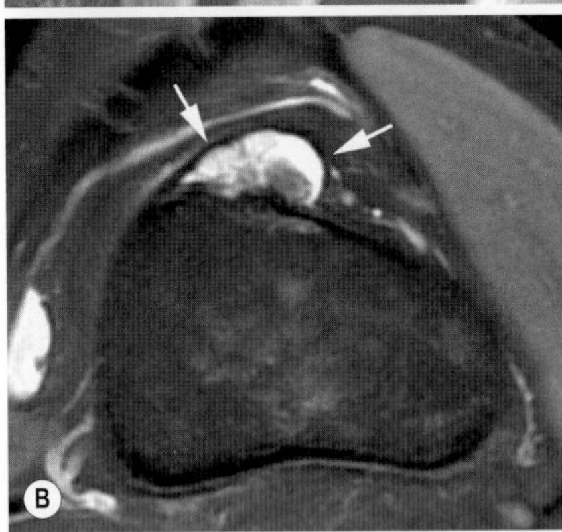

FIGURE 47-11 ■ Periosteal chondroma. (A) DP radiograph of the second toe showing a surface lesion with a thin surrounding calcified rim (arrows) and extension into the adjacent medullary cavity (arrowhead). (B) Axial fat-suppressed T2W FSE MRI showing a hyperintense lobular lesion (arrows) based on the anterior distal femoral cortex, without medullary infiltration.

cortex (Fig. 47-11B). The differential diagnosis includes periosteal chondrosarcoma and periosteal osteosarcoma. Malignant transformation has not been reported.

Enchondromatosis (Ollier's Disease). Rare disease. Prevalence is estimated at around 1 in 100,000. In addition to multiple enchondromas, flame-like rests of cartilage in the metaphyses impede bone growth and may result in bowing, angulation and bone enlargement (Fig. 47-12). Malignant change is reported in 5–30% of cases.

Enchondromatosis with Haemangiomas (Maffucci's Syndrome). This rare disorder combines multiple enchondromas and soft-tissue haemangiomas (occasionally lymphangiomas). The condition is unilateral in 50% of cases. Radiographically, the presence of phleboliths differentiates the disorder from Ollier's disease, while the

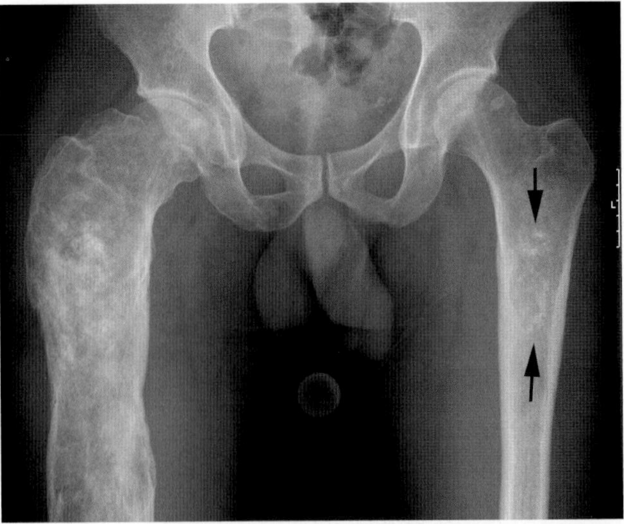

FIGURE 47-12 ■ Enchondromatosis. AP radiograph of the hips and proximal femora showing multiple enchondromas, with expansion of the proximal right femur and deformity consistent with Ollier's disease. A lesion is also seen on the left side (arrows).

haemangiomas are well demonstrated by MRI. The true incidence of chondrosarcomatous change is uncertain because of the rarity of the disease, but is reported in approximately 20% of cases, usually in patients over the age of 40 years.

Chondroblastoma[13,17]

Chondroblastoma accounts for approximately 1% of all bone neoplasms, with 80–90% occurring between the ages of 5 and 25 years (mean age ~20 years). However, lesions of the flat bones such as the talus commonly present later. The male : female ratio is almost 2.7 : 1. Chondroblastoma has rarely been associated with metastases (especially to the lung) and a rare variant termed 'aggressive' (atypical) chondroblastoma, associated with cortical destruction and soft-tissue extension, has also been described.

Chondroblastoma commonly presents as monoarthropathy, since it is typically located in the epiphysis of a long bone, and may promote a synovial reaction. Fifty per cent arise around the knee, while the proximal femur and humeral head are also commonly affected (~20% each). Chondroblastoma is classically located eccentrically in the epiphysis (40%), but with partial closure of the growth plate it usually extends into the metaphysis (55%). The apophyses and sesamoid bones can also be involved, accounting for involvement of the greater trochanter of the femur and the greater tuberosity of the humerus. Approximately 2% are located purely within the metaphysis or diaphysis.[18] In the feet, the calcaneus and talus are most commonly involved, while chondroblastoma is the commonest tumour of the patella.

Radiological Features

The lesion is usually spherical or lobular with a fine sclerotic margin, measuring 1–4 cm in size (Fig. 47-13A).

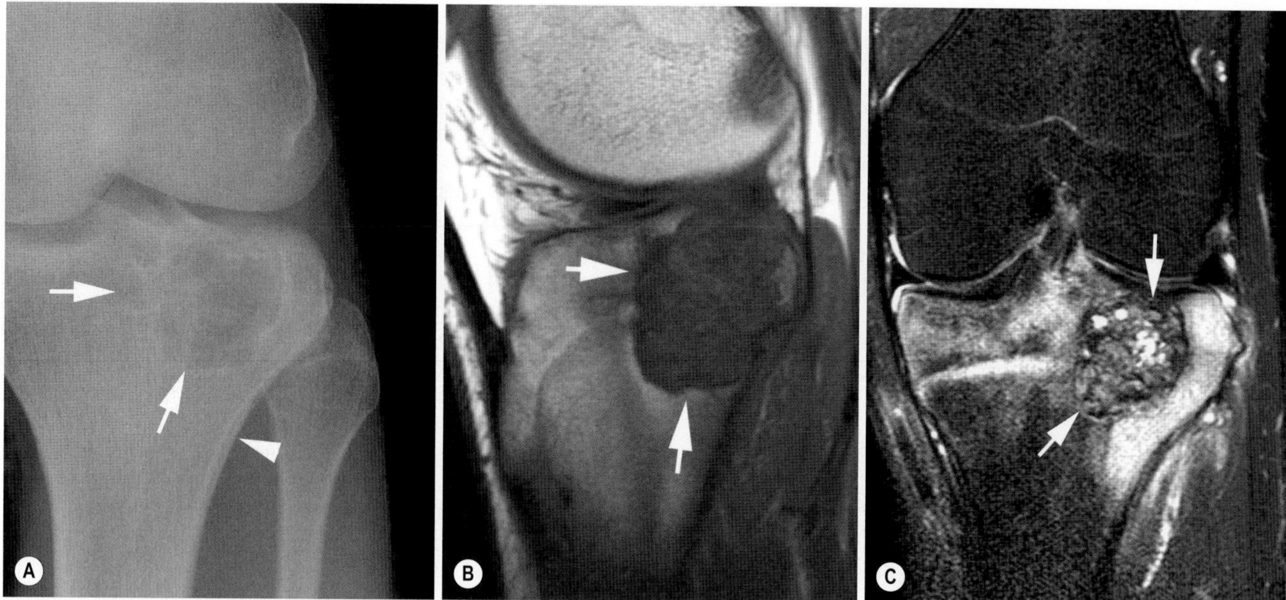

FIGURE 47-13 ■ **Chondroblastoma.** (A) AP radiograph of the knee showing a lobular, lytic lesion (arrows) in the proximal tibial epiphysis with extension into the metaphysis. A solid periosteal response (arrowhead) is also noted. (B) Sagittal T1W SE MRI showing an intermediate SI lesion (arrows). (C) Coronal STIR MRI demonstrates heterogeneous low SI (arrows) with prominent surrounding reactive marrow oedema-like SI.

Matrix mineralisation is demonstrated in ~30% radiographically. Linear metaphyseal periosteal reaction is present in almost 60% of long bone cases (Fig. 47-13A). MRI shows intermediate T1W SI (Fig. 47-13B) with variable SI on T2W images (Fig. 47-13C), including hypointensity and FFLs due to secondary aneurysmal bone cyst (ABC) change (~15% of cases). Associated marrow and soft-tissue oedema and reactive joint effusion are almost invariable (Fig. 47-13C). The differential diagnosis of lytic epiphyseal lesions in children includes Brodie's abscess. In adults, subchondral cysts and clear cell chondrosarcoma need to be considered.

Chondromyxoid Fibroma[13,19]

Chondromyxoid fibroma accounts for less than 0.5% of biopsied primary bone tumours, with 75% of cases occurring between 10 and 30 years of age (mean age 25 years). Most lesions are metaphyseal and eccentric within the medulla, resulting in thinning and expansion of the cortex. The long bones account for 60% of cases, with 40% arising in the flat bones (ilium 10%) or small tubular bones of the hands and feet (17%). The upper third of the tibia accounts for approximately 25% of all chondromyxoid fibromas. Juxtacortical lesions have also been reported.

Radiological Features

In the proximal tibia, chondromyxoid fibroma appears as an eccentric, lobular lesion with a sclerotic margin (Fig. 47-14). Periosteal reaction and soft-tissue extension are uncommon and matrix calcification is seen in only 12.5% of lesions. MRI shows no particular diagnostic features. Outside its classical location, it has no characteristic imaging appearances.

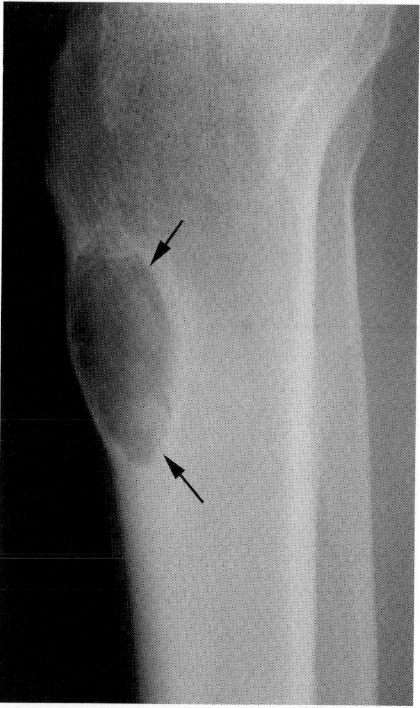

FIGURE 47-14 ■ **Chondromyxoid fibroma.** Lateral radiograph of the proximal tibia showing an eccentric lytic lesion with a sclerotic margin (arrows) and expansion of the anterior cortex.

OSTEOGENIC TUMOURS[20]

Osteoid Osteoma (OO)[21]

This small benign, vascular, osteoblastic tumour is often associated with a characteristic clinical picture of night pain relieved by aspirin and accounts for approximately

10% of all biopsied benign tumours. Most patients present in the second and third decades of life and the male : female ratio is 2–3 : 1.

OO is most common in the appendicular skeleton, with over 50% located in the diaphysis or metaphysis of the tibia or femur. However, almost no skeletal site is exempt. There are two classification systems describing the location of the lesion within bone, the first based on radiography where the nidus is either intracortical, medullary (cancellous) or subperiosteal. The second, based on CT findings, describes the nidus as being subperiosteal, intracortical, endosteal or intramedullary.[21] Approximately 13% of cases are intra-articular, causing synovitis and presenting as monoarthropathy.[22]

Radiological Features

The characteristic feature of OO is the nidus, which may appear lytic, sclerotic or most commonly of mixed density depending upon the degree of central mineralisation. The nidus measures up to15 mm in diameter and is commonly surrounded by a region of reactive medullary sclerosis and solid periosteal reaction (Fig. 47-15), the degree of which depends upon the age of the patient and the location within the bone (subperiosteal lesions and those in younger patients being more reactive than medullary or intra-articular lesions). Dense bony reactive changes may obscure a small nidus on plain radiographs (Fig. 47-4A). Rarely, a multifocal nidus is found.[23]

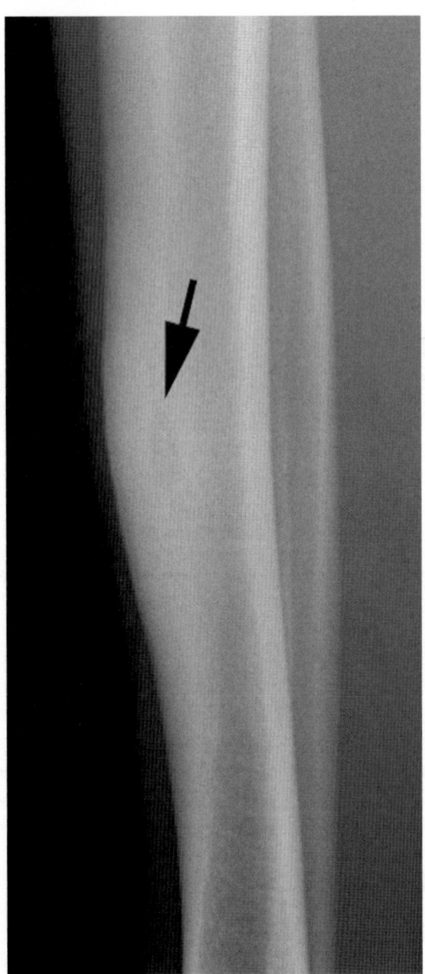

FIGURE 47-15 ■ **Osteoid osteoma.** Lateral radiograph of the tibial diaphysis shows solid thickening of the cortex, within which is a small calcified nidus (arrow).

Bone scintigraphy now plays little role in the diagnosis or management of the lesion, while CT demonstrates the classical features of a round or oval soft-tissue density nidus, which commonly shows central dense mineralisation (Fig. 47-16A).[24] The associated reactive bone changes are also well demonstrated. A recently described finding is the 'vascular groove sign', which is manifest by the presence of thin, serpentine channels in the thickened bone surrounding the nidus (Fig. 47-16A) and has sensitivity and specificity of approximately 75 and 95%, respectively, for the diagnosis of OO.[25]

With improvements in MR technology, the nidus of an OO is now commonly visualised (Fig. 47-16B), appearing as heterogenously low–intermediate SI on both T1W and T2W images and enhancing strongly following administration of intravenous contrast medium. In addition to the reactive bony changes, oedema-like marrow and soft-tissue SI is almost invariably seen adjacent to the nidus (Fig. 47-16C). High-resolution imaging and the use of dynamic contrast-enhanced gradient-echo techniques can further improve identification of the nidus.[26] However, a very small nidus may still be occult on MRI.

Periosteal reaction is typically absent with intra-articular lesions, lesions in the terminal phalanges and those deep in medullary bone or at tendinous or ligamentous insertions. Intra-articular lesions are most commonly seen in the hip and may present with local osteopenia due to disuse (Fig. 47-17A), while MRI will show reactive bone and soft-tissue oedema-like changes and a joint effusion (Fig. 47-17B). The nidus is usually demonstrated on CT (Fig. 47-17C).

OO in the ankle and foot region may be difficult to diagnose. The subperiosteal region of the talar neck is a classical site (Fig. 47-18), but cancellous lesions of the hindfoot bones are commonly radiologically occult. MRI will show the reactive oedema-like changes, which are usually limited to a single bone, but CT is usually required to demonstrate the nidus.[27]

The natural history of OO is one of spontaneous resolution, which may be promoted with the use of non-steroidal anti-inflammatory drugs.[28] However, the current treatment of choice is CT-guided radiofrequency ablation, which is minimally invasive and has a high success rate.[24] CT in successfully treated cases commonly shows complete ossification of the nidus (Fig. 47-19) or a minimal nidus rest, while MRI may continue to show reactive bone and soft-tissue changes even after clinically successful treatment.[29]

The differential diagnosis of OO includes small areas of chronic osteomyelitis, chondroblastoma, Langerhans cell histiocytosis (LCH) and fibrous dysplasia. However, these lesions, when small enough, can also be successfully treated by CT-guided radiofrequency ablation.[24]

Osteoblastoma[30]

Osteoblastoma (OB) possesses histological similarities to OO and is differentiated primarily by its size, being

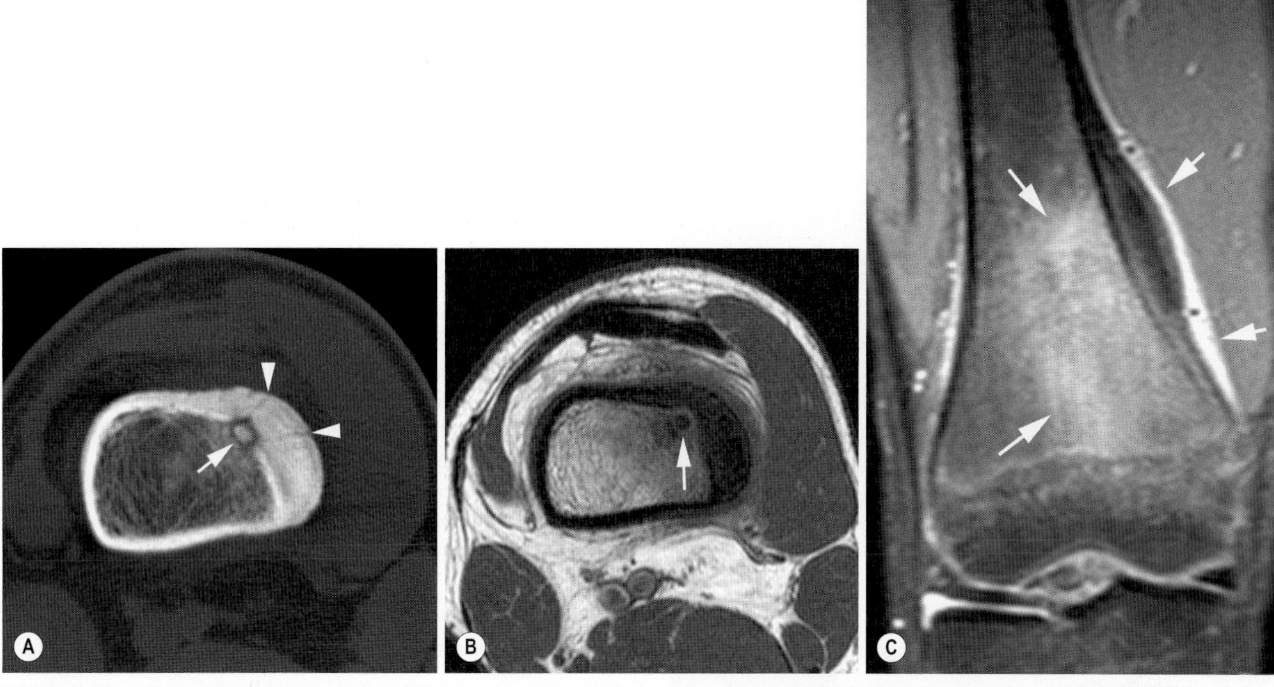

FIGURE 47-16 ■ **Osteoid osteoma.** (A) Axial CT shows a densely mineralised intracortical nidus (arrow), with solid adjacent periosteal thickening containing multiple vascular channels (arrowheads). (B) Axial T1W SE MRI clearly demonstrates the hypointense nidus (arrow) and the cortical thickening. (C) Coronal STIR MRI shows the reactive oedema-like SI changes (arrows).

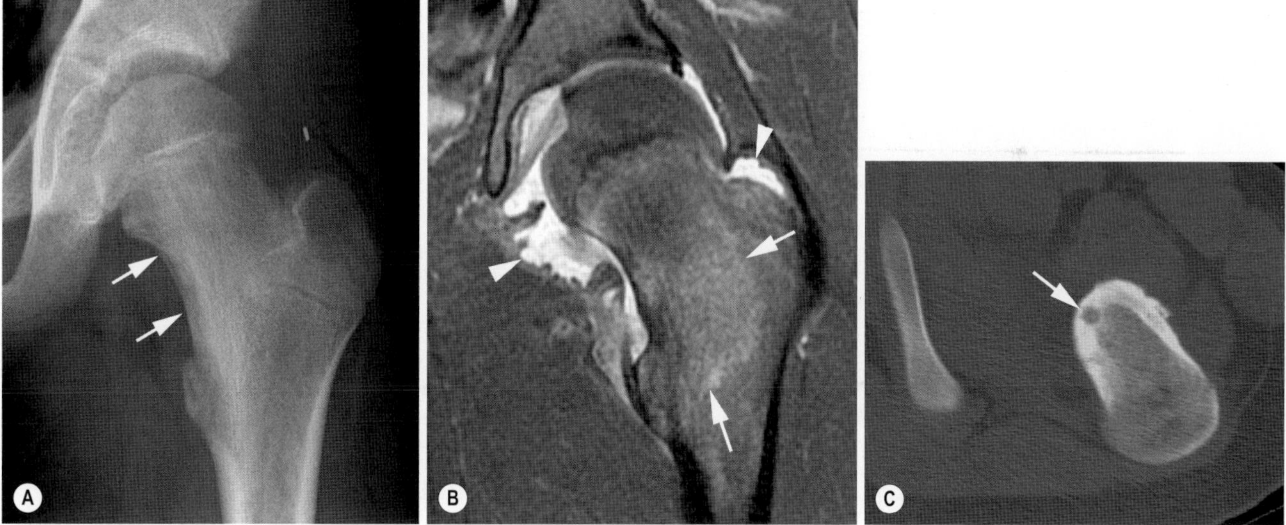

FIGURE 47-17 ■ **Intra-articular osteoid osteoma.** (A) AP radiograph of the left hip shows mild disuse osteopenia and some thickening of the calcar (arrows). (B) Coronal STIR MRI demonstrates reactive oedema-like marrow SI changes in the femoral neck (arrows) and a joint effusion (arrowheads). (C) Axial CT shows the small nidus (arrow) in the thickened calcar.

typically greater than 1.5 cm in diameter. It also shows a more aggressive growth pattern with potential for extra-osseous extension, and does not resolve spontaneously. OB is a rare tumour accounting for less than 1% of all primary bone neoplasms. Over 80% of patients are under the age of 30 years and the male: female ratio is 2–3 : 1. The presentation differs from OO in that pain is not usually acute or severe and is rarely relieved by aspirin. The humerus is the commonest location in the appendicular skeleton and the lesion arises in the medullary cavity, although a periosteal location has also been described.[31]

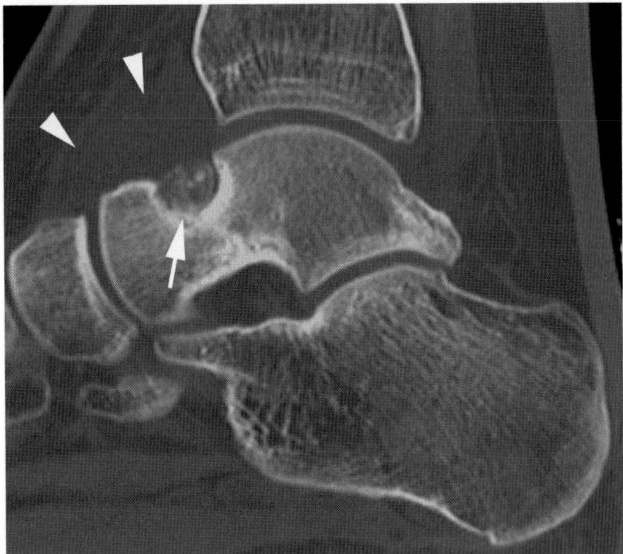

FIGURE 47-18 ■ **Osteoid osteoma of the foot.** Sagittal CT multiplanar reconstruction (MPR) showing a subperiosteal OO nidus (arrow) in the talar neck with associated reactive synovitis in the anterior recess of the joint (arrowheads).

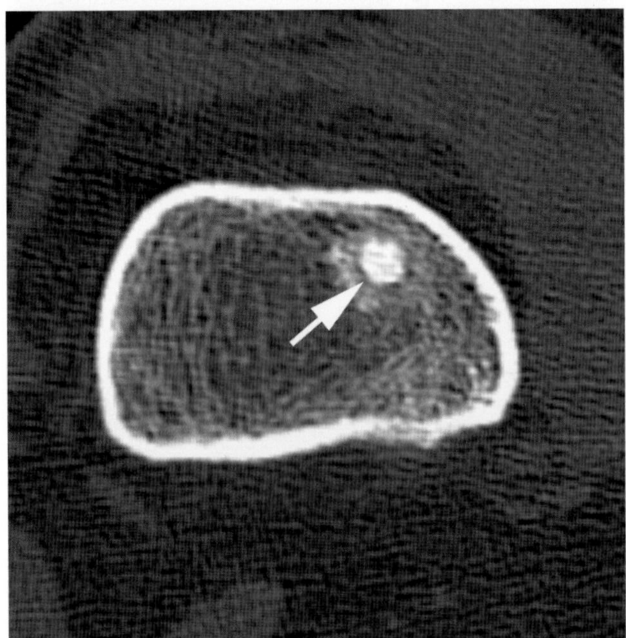

FIGURE 47-19 ■ **Radiofrequency ablation of osteoid osteoma.** Same case as described in the legend to Fig. 47-16. Axial CT shows complete ossification of the nidus (arrow) following successful CT-guided RF ablation.

Radiological Features

The lesion is predominantly lytic, measuring over 2 cm in diameter, with larger lesions showing a greater degree of matrix mineralisation (Fig. 47-20A). CT often reveals occult calcification, which can be punctate, nodular or generalised (Fig. 47-20B). Larger lesions may result in bone expansion with or without a surrounding shell of reactive bone. OB can also produce an extracortical mass, which may be reactive or due to tumour extension. As with OO, scintigraphy is always positive and MRI shows a low–intermediate SI lesion with associated reactive changes as seen with OO, but of a lesser intensity (Fig. 47-20C). Secondary ABC change may also be seen, manifest by the development of FFLs.

In the long bones, the differential diagnosis includes Brodie's abscess and Langerhans cell histiocytosis.

FIBROGENIC TUMOURS

Desmoplastic Fibroma[32]

Desmoplastic fibroma is a rare, locally aggressive benign neoplasm with similar histological features to soft-tissue fibromatosis. It accounts for 0.06% of all bone tumours and 0.3% of benign bone neoplasms. Seventy per cent of cases present between 10 and 30 years of age (mean age 21 years) with no particular predilection for men or women. Desmoplastic fibroma usually arises in the metaphyseal region of long bones (femur, humerus, tibia and radius constitute 56% of cases), the mandible (26%) and ilium (14%). It is rarely associated with fibrous dysplasia.

Radiological Features

Most lesions are metadiaphyseal and arise as either subperiosteal or intraosseous tumours. Many are large at presentation (over 5 cm in diameter) and two patterns are seen: an ill-defined moth-eaten or permeative lesion and an expanding, trabeculated lesion (Fig. 47-21).

The MRI features are non-specific, showing heterogeneous intermediate SI on T1W images and hyperintensity on T2W images with irregular enhancement following gadolinium.[33] When the soft tissues are invaded, it may be difficult to distinguish from bony invasion by soft-tissue fibromatosis. Although desmoplastic fibroma is considered a benign lesion, metastasis has been reported following local recurrence.

FIBROHISTIOCYTIC TUMOURS[34,35]

Fibrous cortical defect, non-ossifying fibroma and benign fibrous histiocytoma all share identical histological appearances but are differentiated by their clinical and radiological features.

Fibrous Cortical Defect

Fibrous cortical defect (FCD) is most commonly identified in the distal femoral and proximal tibial metaphyses as an incidental finding, appearing as a cortically based lytic lesion commonly with a thin sclerotic margin (Fig. 47-22). The lesion typically consolidates/fades with time.

Non-Ossifying Fibroma

Non-ossifying fibroma (NOF) is a benign neoplasm, which is commonly identified incidentally, or may present with pathological fracture when large enough. The lesion may also be painful when associated with a stress fracture,

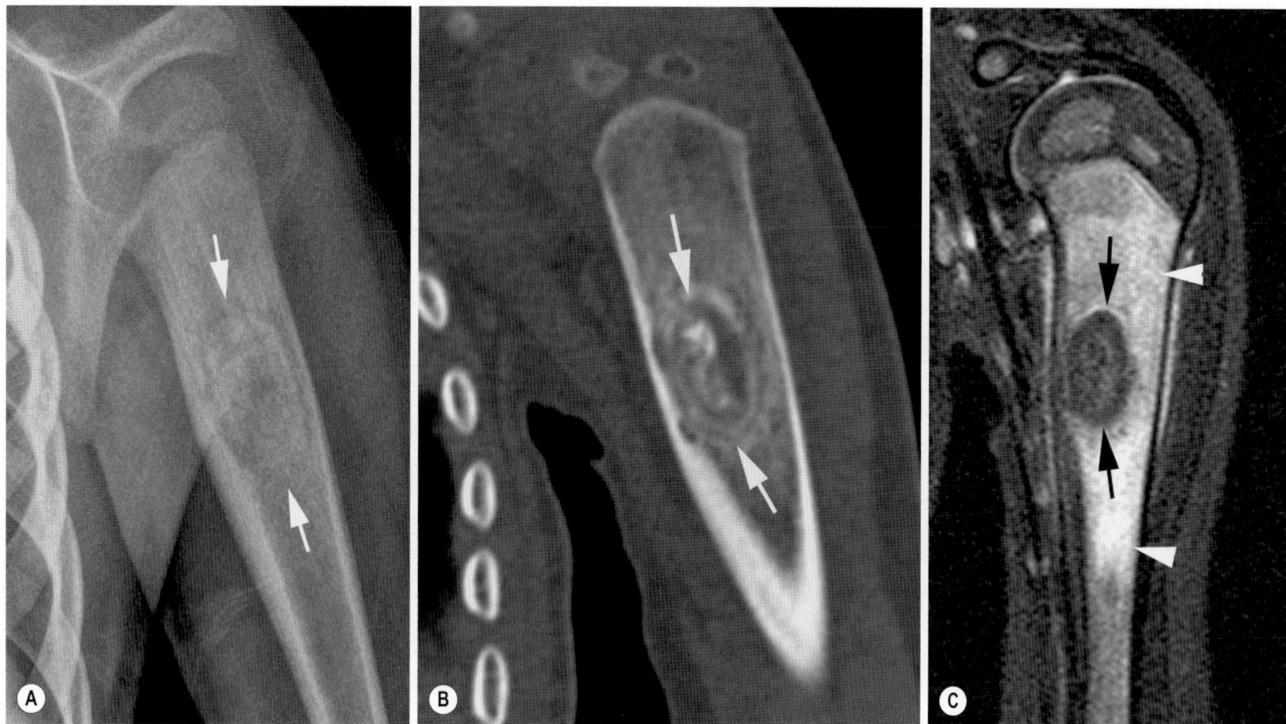

FIGURE 47-20 ■ Osteoblastoma. (A) AP radiograph of the left proximal humerus showing a large mixed lytic-sclerotic lesion (arrows) in the medullary cavity with associated periosteal thickening. (B) Coronal CT MPR shows the oval, mineralised lesion (arrows). (C) Coronal STIR MRI demonstrates a hypointense tumour (arrows) with extensive reactive oedema-like marrow changes (arrowheads).

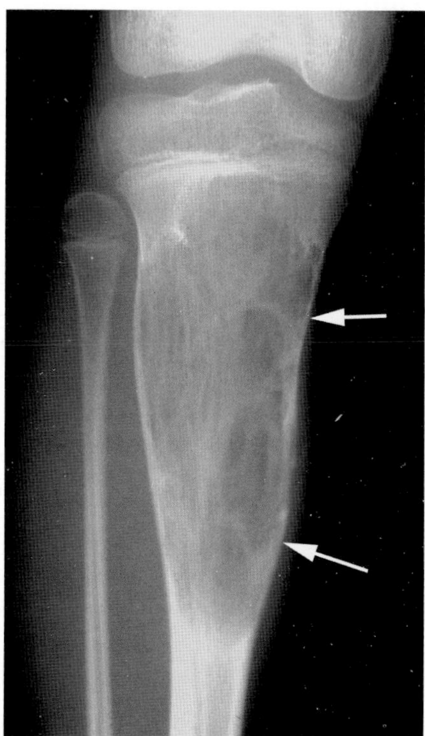

FIGURE 47-21 ■ Desmoplastic fibroma. AP radiograph of the proximal tibia showing an expansile aggressive metaphyseal lesion (arrows).

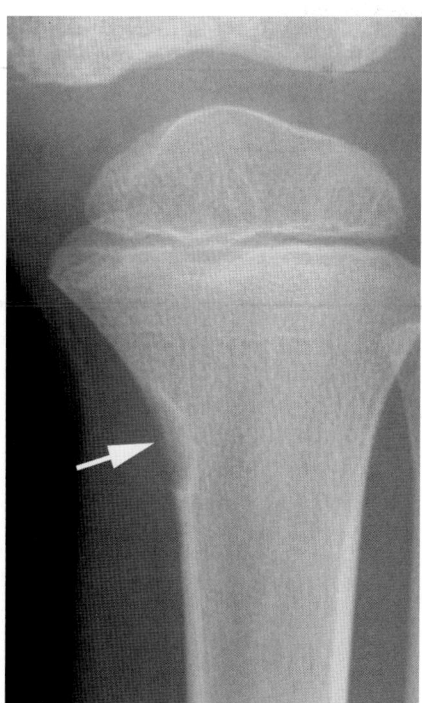

FIGURE 47-22 ■ Fibrous cortical defect. AP radiograph of the proximal tibia showing a small, elongated lytic lesion (arrow) in the medial proximal tibial metaphysis.

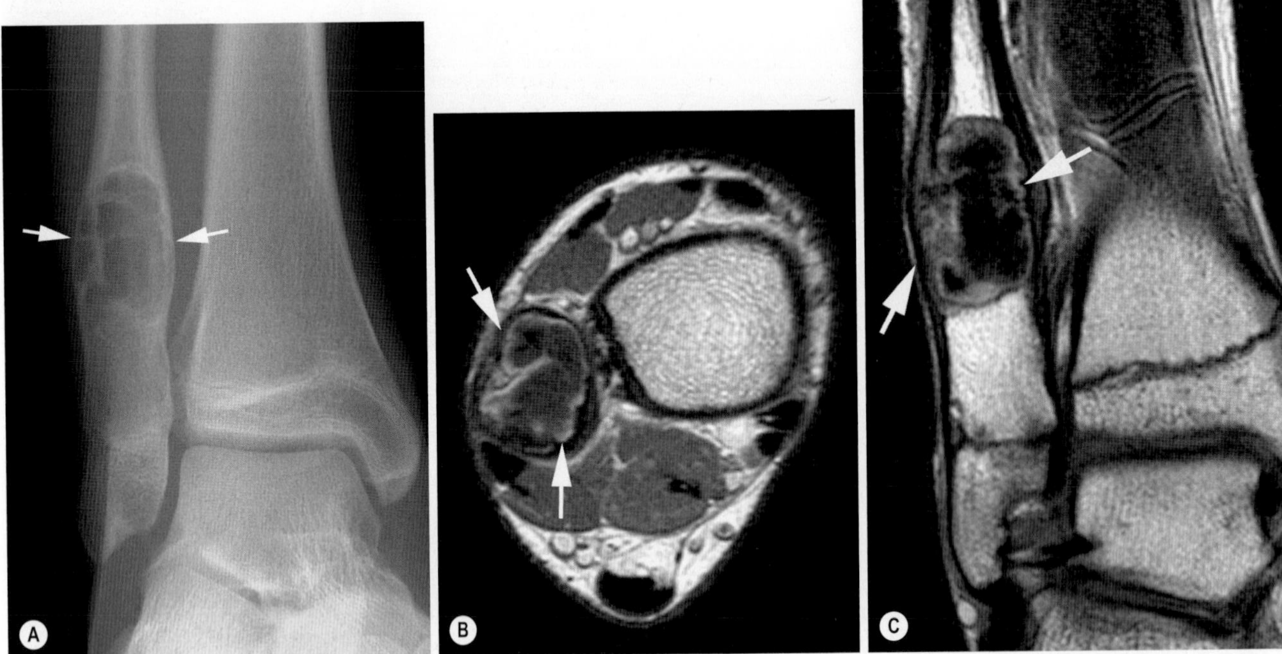

FIGURE 47-23 ■ **Non-ossifying fibroma.** (A) AP radiograph of the ankle showing a lobular lesion (arrows) expanding the distal fibular metadiaphysis. (B) Axial PDW FSE and (C) coronal T2W FSE MR images showing a lobular lesion (arrows) containing prominent areas of hypointensity due to its fibrous nature.

typically with proximal tibial lesions.[36] Patients usually present in the second decade of life and a slight male preponderance is recorded. The majority (~90%) involve the lower limbs, particularly the tibia and distal end of the femur. Multiple lesions are found and occasionally a familial incidence is reported, in which case an association with neurofibromatosis (5%) may be present. The Jaffe–Campanacci syndrome consists of multiple (usually unilateral) NOFs with café-au-lait spots but no other stigmata of neurofibromatosis. NOF can usually be diagnosed radiologically, in which case biopsy is unnecessary.

Radiological Features

The lesions are metaphyseal or diametaphyseal and essentially intracortical. A lobular appearance is classical, with the lesion usually enlarging into the medullary cavity. The tumour is oval with its long axis in the line of the bone (Fig. 47-1A). When NOF arises in a slim bone such as the fibula, it crosses the shaft readily and its characteristic intracortical origin is less obvious (Fig. 47-23A). It may then resemble other entities, such as ABC. Periosteal reaction is typically seen only after fracture.

On MRI, NOF shows low–intermediate SI on T1W and PDW images (Fig. 47-23B) and enhances following administration of intravenous gadolinium contrast medium. On T2W images, approximately 80% are hypointense (Fig. 47-23C), but with marginal or septal hyperintensity and the remainder are hyperintense. Marginal sclerosis appears as a hypointense rim.[37] Reactive marrow oedema may also be seen, particularly if the lesion is complicated by a stress or pathological fracture, while secondary ABC change manifests as the presence of FFLs.

Benign Fibrous Histiocytoma[38]

Benign fibrous histiocytoma (BFH) is an uncommon lesion occurring in an older age group and in a different location to NOF. BFH typically presents between 20 and 50 years, with a mean age in the third decade; the male:female ratio is equal.

Radiological Features

Most frequently the lesion resembles a giant cell tumour, occurring in an eccentric subarticular location, but with a well-defined sclerotic margin indicating slower growth. About one-third occur on either side of the knee. The MRI features are also similar to GCT.

GIANT CELL TUMOUR

Giant Cell Tumour[39,40]

Giant cell tumour (GCT) is an aggressive benign neoplasm accounting for approximately 20% of benign bone tumours. However, malignant change in GCT is recognised, being either primary or secondary,[41] and benign lesions may rarely metastasise to the lungs.[42] Multifocal, metachronous GCT has also been reported,[43] which is associated with hyperparathyroidism. Hyperparathyroidism should therefore be assessed for. GCT rarely complicates familial polyostotic Paget's disease of bone.[66]

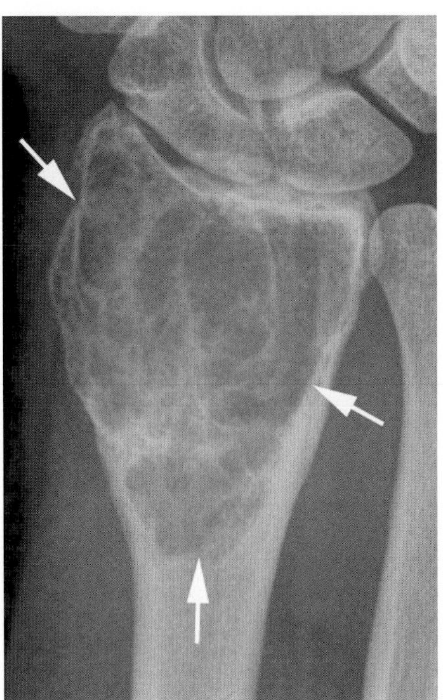

FIGURE 47-24 ■ **Giant cell tumour.** AP radiograph of the wrist showing a distal radial subarticular lytic lesion (arrows) with internal trabeculation.

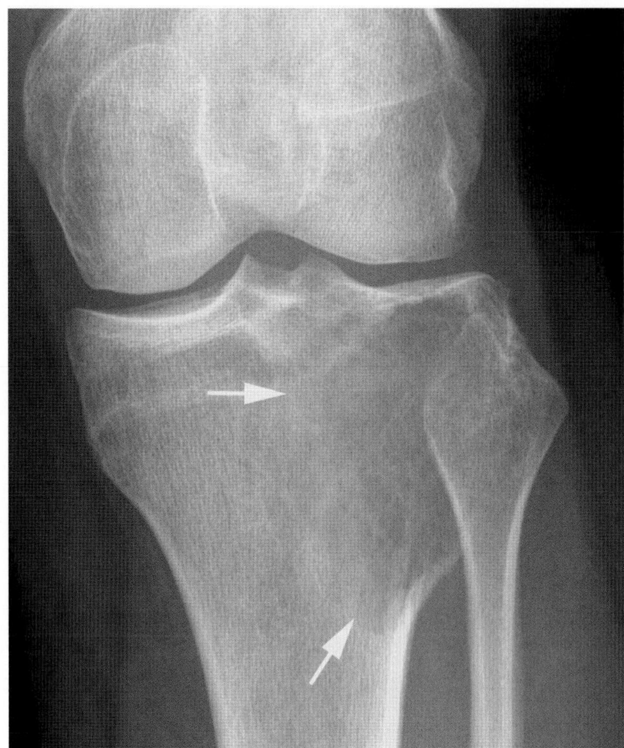

FIGURE 47-25 ■ **Giant cell tumour.** AP radiograph of the knee showing an eccentric, subarticular lytic lesion of the proximal tibia with a poorly defined margin (arrows) and destruction of the lateral cortex.

Approximately 80% occur between 18 and 45 years of age, with a male : female ratio of 2 : 3. The tumour nearly always occurs in a subarticular or subcortical region (adjacent to a fused apophysis) of a long bone, with the knee (distal femur/proximal tibia—55%), distal radius (10%) and proximal humerus (6%) being the commonest sites.

Radiological Features

GCT is classically a subarticular, eccentric, lytic lesion with a geographic, non-sclerotic margin (Fig. 47-24). However, a poorly defined margin indicative of a more aggressive lesion may be identified in 10–15% of cases (Fig. 47-25). Involvement of the subchondral or apophyseal bone is seen in 95–99% of GCTs at presentation, although lesions arising in the immature skeleton involve the metaphysis adjacent to the growth plate. The tumour usually measures 5–7 cm in size. Apparent trabeculation and cortical expansion are common features and periosteal reaction is seen in 10–15% of cases, indicating healing of a pathological fracture. Cortical destruction with extraosseous extension may occur in up to 50% of cases.

On MRI, the tumour is iso- or hypointense on T1W images (Fig. 47-26A) and shows heterogeneous hyperintensity on STIR. Areas of hyperintensity on T1W indicate the presence of subacute haemorrhage. Profound hypointensity on T2W images in solid areas of the tumour is seen in the majority of cases, being due to the deposition of haemosiderin from chronic recurrent haemorrhage (Fig. 47-26B). Marrow oedema is also demonstrated, while FFLs indicate the presence of secondary ABC change, which is reported in approximately 15% of cases. Malignant GCT has no characteristic distinguishing features.

The most important differential diagnostic considerations are lytic osteosarcoma and, in older patients, malignant fibrous histiocytoma or a subarticular lytic metastasis, particularly from a primary renal tumour.

VASCULAR TUMOURS[44]

Haemangioma[45]

Both single and multiple haemangiomas occur in bone and may be regarded as congenital vascular malformations. However, many present as isolated bone lesions and are therefore included in the differential diagnosis of a bone tumour. Haemangiomas are classified histologically as capillary, cavernous, arteriovenous or venous. Osseous capillary haemangiomas most commonly affect the vertebral body, whereas osseous cavernous haemangiomas affect the skull vault. Involvement of the appendicular skeleton is relatively rare.

Radiological Features

As in vertebral lesions, fine or coarse vertical trabeculation is seen with haemangioma involving the epiphyses and metaphyses of long bones, with the direction of the linear striations running along the axis of the bone.

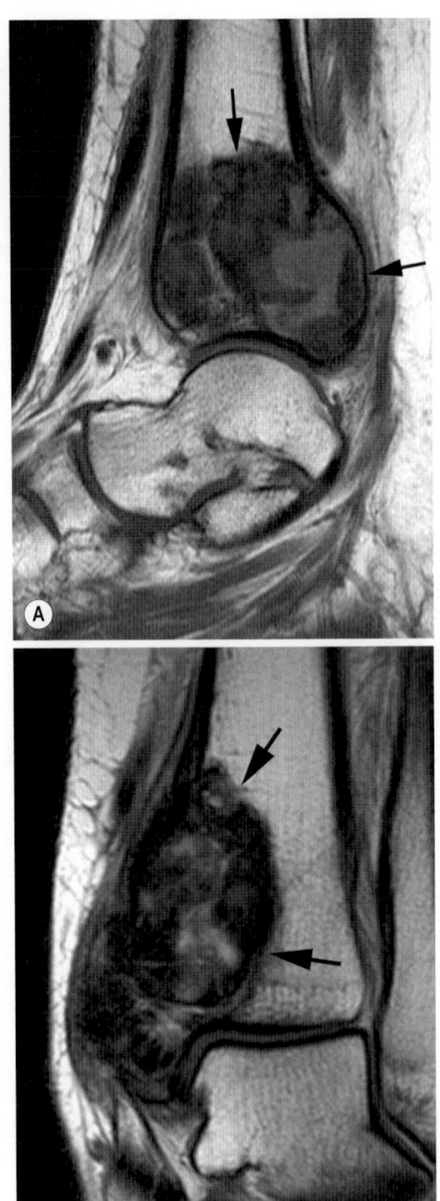

FIGURE 47-26 ■ **Giant cell tumour.** (A) Sagittal T1W and (B) coronal T2W FSE MRI of the ankle showing a distal tibial GCT (arrows), which demonstrates profound heterogeneous low SI due to the presence of haemosiderin from chronic haemorrhage.

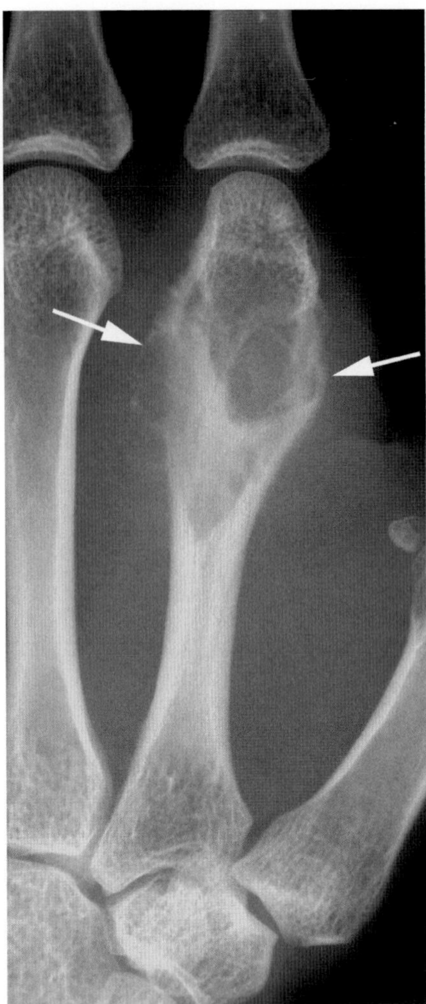

FIGURE 47-27 ■ **Haemangioma.** AP radiograph of the ring finger metacarpal showing an expansile lytic lesion (arrows) containing coarse trabeculation.

Occasionally, well-defined vascular channels may be evident. Bone expansion and extraosseous extension are also recognised features (Fig. 47-27). Scintigraphy typically shows triple-phase uptake due to the vascular nature of the lesion, while CT demonstrates the thickened trabeculae as dense 'dots' within a fatty matrix (Fig. 47-28). On MRI, long and flat bone haemangiomas are typically of intermediate SI on T1W and hyperintense on T2W, only occasionally having a predominantly fatty matrix. The thickened trabeculae may be evident as linear areas of signal void.

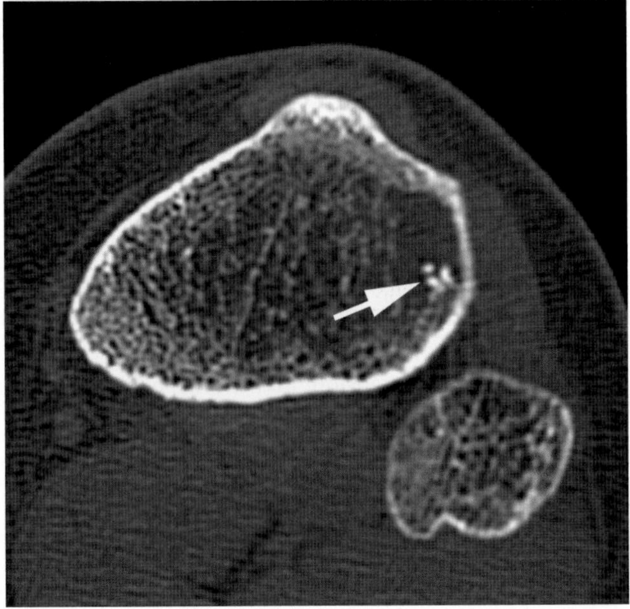

FIGURE 47-28 ■ **Haemangioma.** Axial CT through the proximal tibia showing a poorly defined lytic lesion containing multiple, dense thickened trabeculae (arrow).

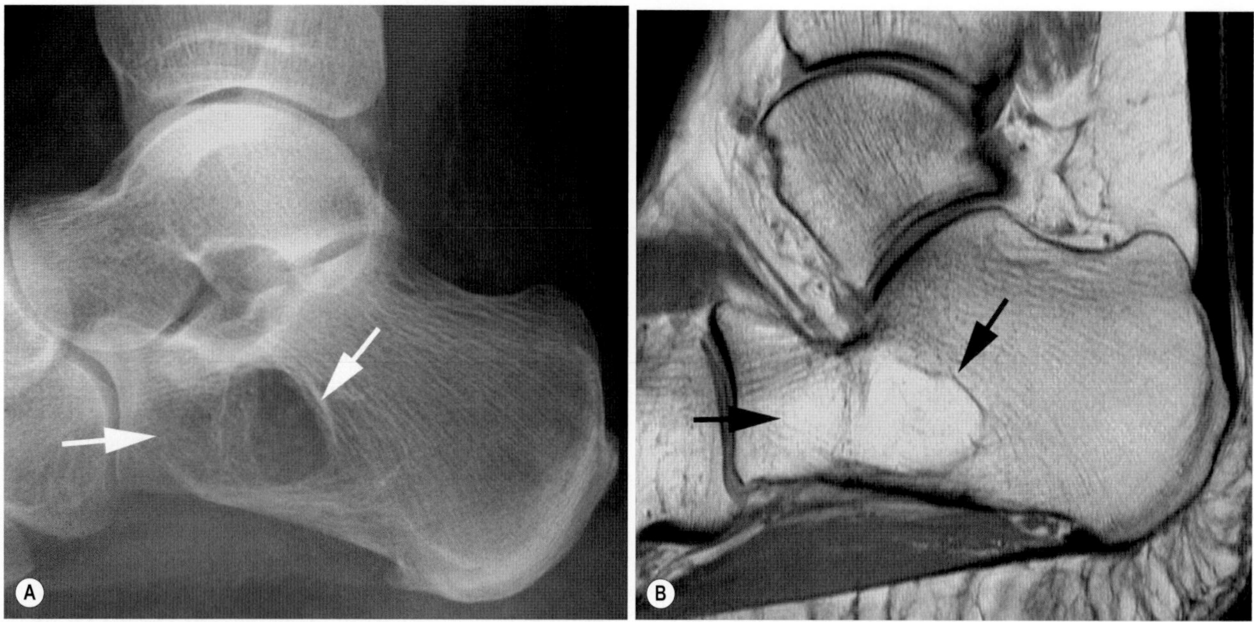

FIGURE 47-29 ■ **Intraosseous lipoma.** (A) Lateral radiograph of the calcaneus showing a well-defined lytic lesion (arrows) in the calcaneal body. (B) Sagittal T1W SE MRI shows the lesion to be hyperintense (arrows) consistent with a fatty matrix.

SMOOTH MUSCLE TUMOURS

Leiomyoma[46]

Intraosseous leiomyoma is an exceedingly rare tumour with less than 20 reported cases. It may present with non-specific pain and appears as a unilocular or multilocular lytic lesion with a sclerotic rim, mimicking a NOF. The CT and MRI features are non-specific.

LIPOGENIC TUMOURS[47]

Intraosseous Lipoma

Intraosseous lipoma[48] arises in the medulla and produces expansion, sometimes with endosteal scalloping and trabeculation, resembling a cyst or even fibrous dysplasia. Calcification is also seen. Most affect the lower limb, with a predilection for the calcaneus (Fig. 47-29A) and femur. CT and MRI (Fig. 47-29B) establish the diagnosis by demonstrating the fatty nature of the matrix. Calcification and cystic degeneration due to fat necrosis can also be identified.

Parosteal Lipoma

Parosteal lipoma is a rare lesion which is most frequently encountered around the proximal radius, where it may cause posterior interosseous nerve palsy. It may result in pressure erosion of the bone and the formation of circumferential juxtacortical new bone. The combination of such peripheral ossification with a tumour of otherwise fatty matrix, demonstrated either by CT (Fig. 47-30) or MRI,[49] establishes the radiological diagnosis.

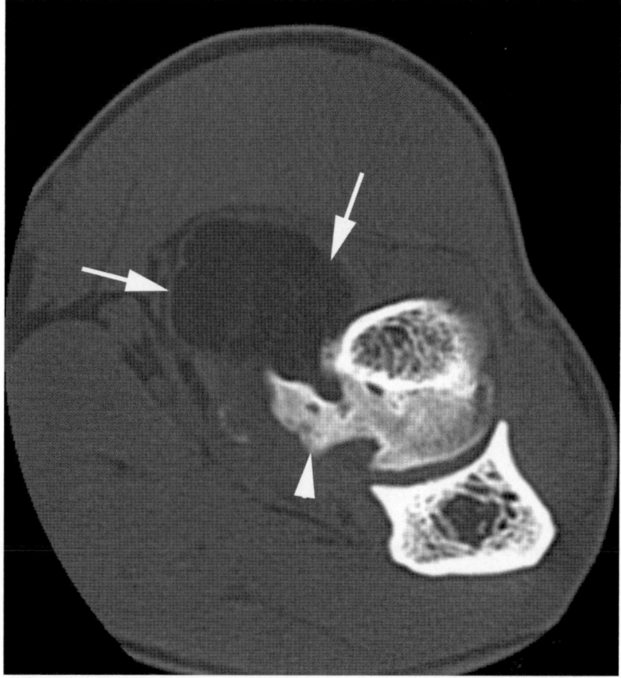

FIGURE 47-30 ■ **Parosteal lipoma.** Axial CT of the elbow showing a fatty mass (arrows) arising in association with a parosteal bony lesion (arrowhead) from the proximal radius.

NEURAL TUMOURS

Schwannoma of Bone[50]

Primary schwannomas of bone are defined as arising within the medullary cavity and are extremely rare lesions, which are usually sporadic but may be associated with the

Carney complex (myxomas of the heart and skin, hyperpigmentation of the skin and endocrine overactivity). Most occur in the long bones and present with pain. The radiological features are non-specific, being those of a benign lytic bone lesion and the tumour is successfully treated by local excision.

MISCELLANEOUS LESIONS

Aneurysmal Bone Cyst[51,52]

Primary Aneurysmal bone cyst (ABC) accounts for 1–2% of all primary bone lesions and usually presents in the second decade, with 70–80% occurring between 5 and 20 years of age; the male : female ratio is equal. ABC can involve many sites, but the long bones (>50% of cases) and spine (20% of cases) are most common. Involvement of flat bones is most common in the pelvis.

Secondary ABC change can develop in a variety of benign or malignant lesions, including non-ossifying fibroma, chondroblastoma, giant cell tumour, fibrous dysplasia, osteoblastoma and osteosarcoma.

Radiological Features[53]

The classical lesion (accounting for 75–80%) is a purely lytic, expansile intramedullary lesion in the metaphysis of a long bone extending to the growth plate, which may be centrally (Fig. 47-1B, C) or, more commonly eccentrically (Figs. 47-4B, 47-31A) placed. Twenty per cent of long bone ABCs involve the diaphysis. A thin 'egg-shell' covering of expanded cortex is often identified, particularly with CT, which may also demonstrate fine septal ossification. Apparent trabeculation due to ridging of the endosteal cortex is also a feature, as is marginal periosteal reaction. Intracortical or subperiosteal ABC (Fig. 47-31B) is also observed.[54]

The lesion shows heterogeneous intermediate SI on T1W images (Fig. 47-31C) and a thin sclerotic margin with internal hypointense internal septa may be seen, which may enhance following administration of gadolinium contrast medium. T2 or PDW images almost invariably demonstrate multiple FFLs (Fig. 47-31D), which commonly fill the whole of the lesion. Reactive medullary oedema is also a frequent feature. The absence of fluid levels may indicate a 'solid' variant of ABC, which is most commonly reported in the long bones.[55]

The most important differential diagnosis of ABC is telangiectatic osteosarcoma.

Simple Bone Cyst[51,56]

Simple bone cyst (SBC) or unicameral bone cyst usually presents between the ages of 5 and 15 years, with less than 15% reported over the age of 20 years. The male : female ratio is 2.5 : 1 and presentation with pathological fracture is classical, especially with humeral lesions.

The proximal humerus is by far the commonest site (>60% of cases), followed by the proximal femur (approximately 30% of cases). Other sites tend to affect adults and include the calcaneus and the posterior iliac blade.

Radiological Features

Initially, SBCs are located in the proximal metaphysis of the humerus or femur and progress toward the diaphysis with skeletal growth, eventually reaching the mid-diaphysis, by which time they are usually healed. Occasionally, the cyst adheres to the growth plate and extension into the epiphysis/apophysis is reported in 2% of lesions. SBC usually lies centrally in the shaft, expanding the bone symmetrically and thinning the cortex. The lesion is typically 6–8 cm in size. Apparent trabeculation is common, but periosteal reaction is not seen without fracture, which may result in a fragment of cortex penetrating the cyst lining, resulting in the fallen fragment sign (Fig. 47-32).

MRI demonstrates the fluid content of the lesion, homogeneous low-to-intermediate SI on T1W images and marked hyperintensity on T2W or STIR images. These appearances are altered by the presence of fracture, in which case haemorrhage may result in the presence of FFLs and pericystic oedema.[57] Following administration of intravenous contrast medium, rim enhancement is observed.

The major differential diagnosis includes ABC and fibrous dysplasia.

Fibrous Dysplasia[58]

Fibrous dysplasia (FD) accounts for approximately 7% of benign bone tumours and may either be monostotic (70–85%) or polyostotic. FD is usually painless unless a fracture has occurred. Seventy-five per cent of cases present before the age of 30 years and there is no gender predilection. The commonest sites of monostotic FD are the ribs (28%), proximal femur (23%) and craniofacial bones (20%).

Polyostotic FD may range from the involvement of two bones to more than 75% of the skeleton. Approximately 30–50% of patients with polyostotic disease have café au lait spots. FD may be associated with a variety of syndromes. McCune–Albright's *syndrome* consists of polyostotic FD (typically unilateral), ipsilateral café au lait spots and endocrine disturbance, most commonly precocious puberty in girls. Mazabraud's *syndrome* consists of FD (most commonly polyostotic) and soft-tissue myxomata.[59]

Radiological Features

Radiologically, FD presents as a geographic lesion that may cause bone expansion and deformity with diffuse ground-glass matrix mineralisation (Fig. 47-33). A thick sclerotic margin ('rind' sign) is characteristic (Fig. 47-34). Purely lytic lesions are also seen, indicating extensive cystic degeneration. The metadiaphyseal region is typically affected in long bones. Periosteal reaction is not a

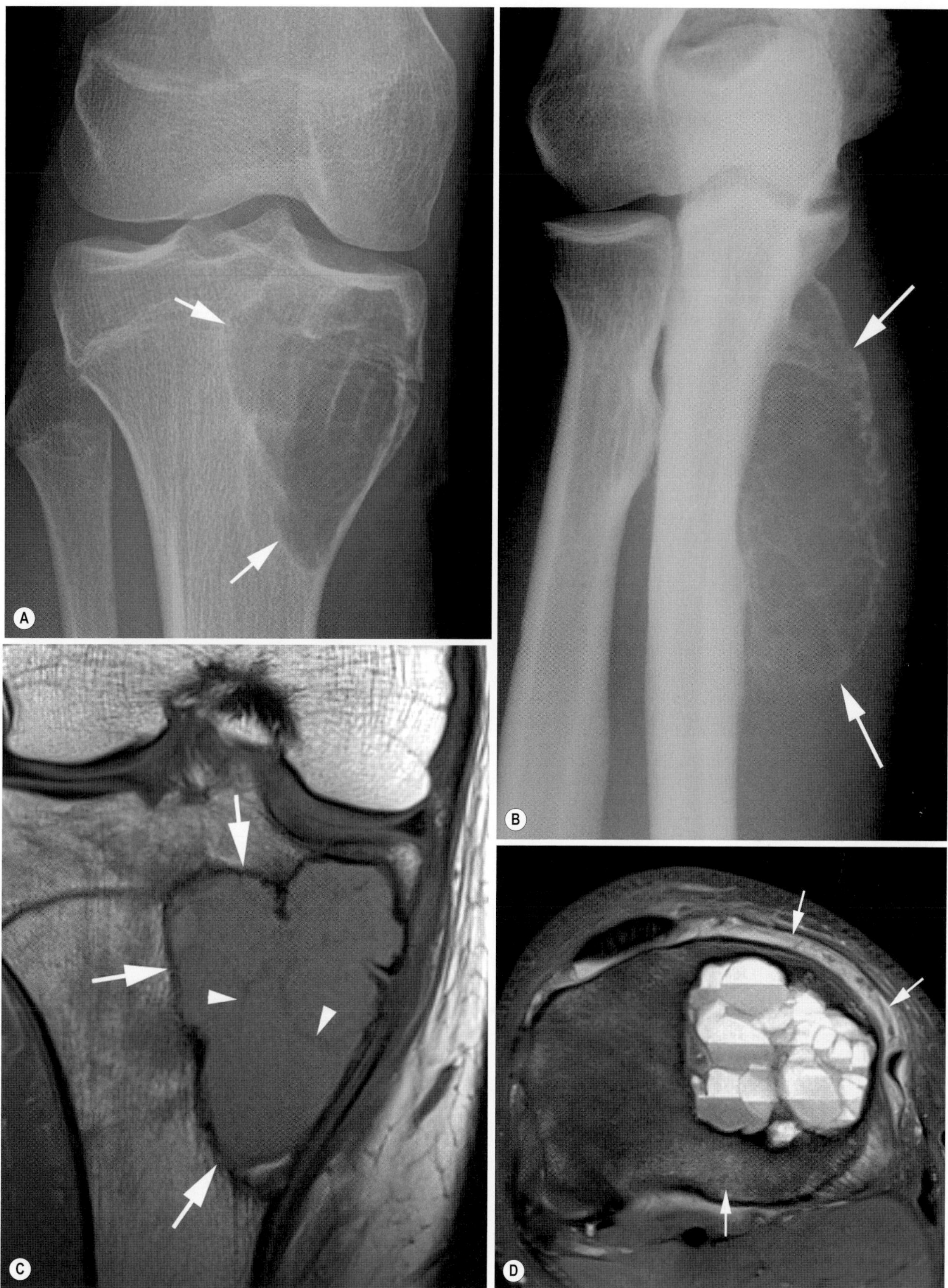

FIGURE 47-31 ■ **Aneurysmal bone cyst.** (A) AP radiograph showing a mildly expansile lytic lesion with a thin sclerotic margin (arrows) located eccentrically within the proximal tibial metaphysis. (B) AP radiograph of the proximal forearm showing an expansile lesion with a thin sclerotic margin (arrows) arising from the surface of the proximal ulna. (C) Coronal T1W SE MRI showing an intermediate SI lesion (arrows) with thin internal septae (arrowheads). (D) Axial fat-suppressed T2W FSE MRI demonstrates multiple fluid–fluid levels filling the lesion with mild surrounding reactive medullary and soft-tissue oedema (arrows).

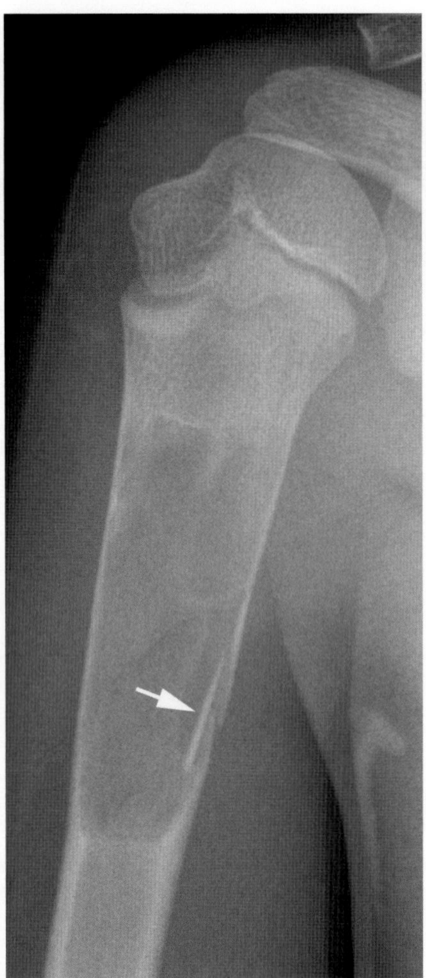

FIGURE 47-32 ■ **Simple bone cyst.** AP radiograph of the right proximal humerus showing a fractured simple bone cyst with a 'fallen fragment' (arrow).

feature in the absence of fracture. Varus deformity of the proximal femur ('shepherd's crook' deformity) is a characteristic late finding.

Skeletal scintigraphy is the best technique for identifying polyostotic disease (Fig. 47-35), although whole-body MRI may also be used. CT beautifully demonstrates the ground-glass matrix (Fig. 47-36), which may not be evident radiologically, helping to establish the diagnosis without the need for biopsy. On MRI,[60] lesions are usually isointense on T1W but may show areas of mild hyperintensity due to haemorrhage (Fig. 47-37A). Lesions may be of intermediate SI or hyperintense on T2W, depending upon whether the tumour is mainly fibrous or has undergone cystic change. Internal septa and FFLs may also be seen (Fig. 47-37B). Following administration of intravenous contrast medium, either uniform or septal enhancement is described.

The identification of associated chondroid calcification indicates a diagnosis of fibrocartilaginous dysplasia. Malignant change in fibrous dysplasia is rare, being reported in 0.5% of cases. It is more common in polyostotic disease and may follow prior radiotherapy.

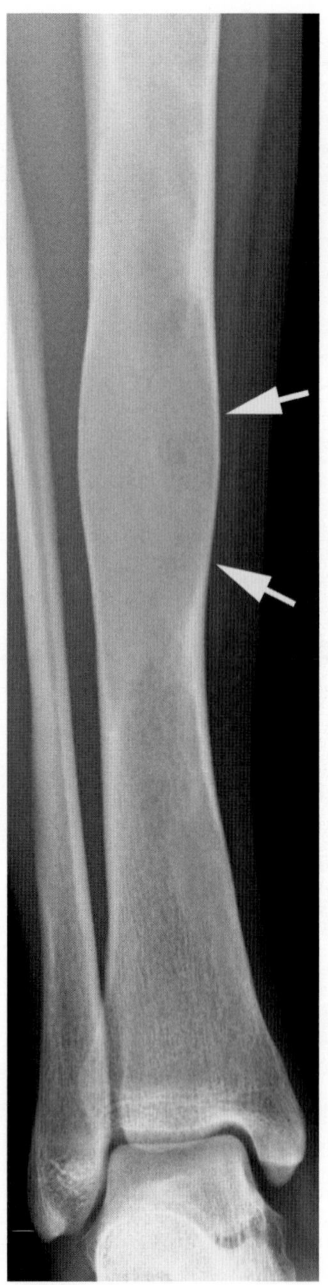

FIGURE 47-33 ■ **Fibrous dysplasia**. AP radiograph of the tibia showing a mildly expansile lesion (arrows) with diffuse 'ground-glass' matrix mineralisation.

Osteofibrous Dysplasia[61]

Osteofibrous dysplasia (OFD) is a rare lesion that histologically resembles fibrous dysplasia and the stroma of adamantinoma. However, it has a specific clinical and radiological picture. Presentation is from birth to 40 years, with almost 50% occurring under the age of 10 years; the male:female ratio is equal. The tibia is affected in over 90% of cases and in two-thirds of these the anterior mid-diaphyseal cortex is involved. Multiple lesions may occur in the same bone, but the ipsilateral fibula is also affected in 20% of cases. Bilateral involvement may occur.

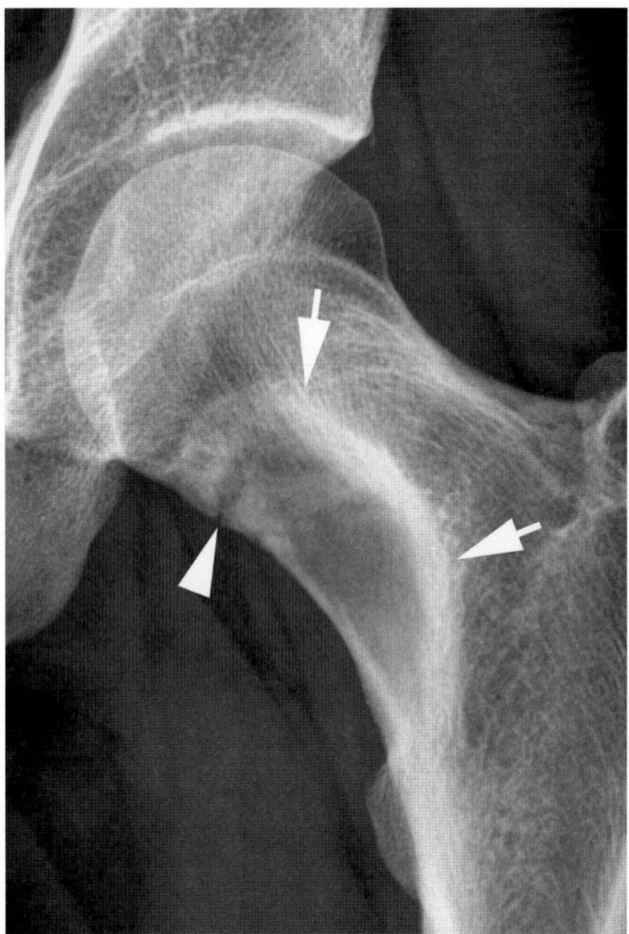

FIGURE 47-34 ■ Fibrous dysplasia. AP radiograph of the hip showing a lesion in the medial femoral neck with a thick sclerotic border (arrows) and a complicating insufficiency fracture (arrowhead).

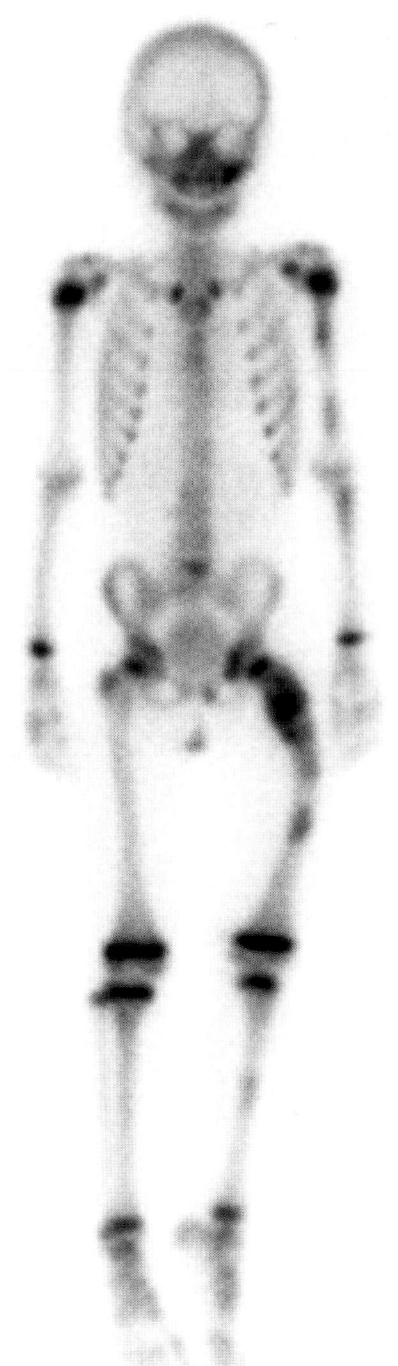

FIGURE 47-35 ■ Fibrous dysplasia. Whole-body bone scintigram showing polyostotic disease involving the left side of the body.

Radiological Features

In early infancy the lesion expands and bows the tibia with a sclerotic rim. After 3 months of age, the lesion is eccentric, multilocular and may be purely lytic (Fig. 47-38) or show ground-glass matrix mineralisation similar to that of FD. Cross-sectional imaging confirms its intracortical origin, but otherwise it shows no characteristic features, although MRI may be of value in the differentiation from osteofibous dysplasia-like adamantinoma and adamantinoma.[62]

Langerhans Cell Histiocytosis (LCH)[63]

LCH represents a spectrum of disorders characterised by the idiopathic proliferation of histiocytes (Langerhans cells), which can involve virtually any organ and present either as focal/multifocal lesions or as a multi-organ systemic disease. Three forms of the disease were classically described: eosinophilic granuloma, Letterer–Siwe disease and Hand–Schüller–Christian disease, these having different clinical and radiological manifestations. Currently, the disorder is classified as being localised (single-system disease) or disseminated (multi-system disease), the latter cases further categorised as being either 'low risk' or 'risk'.[64]

Localised skeletal disease accounts for approximately 70% of cases of LCH and is classically seen in children between the ages of 5 and 15 years who present with focal bone pain, but lesions may also be asymptomatic. LCH can involve any bone, but most lesions involve the skull, pelvis, spine, mandible and ribs. The long bones are involved in 25–35% of cases of monostotic disease, with

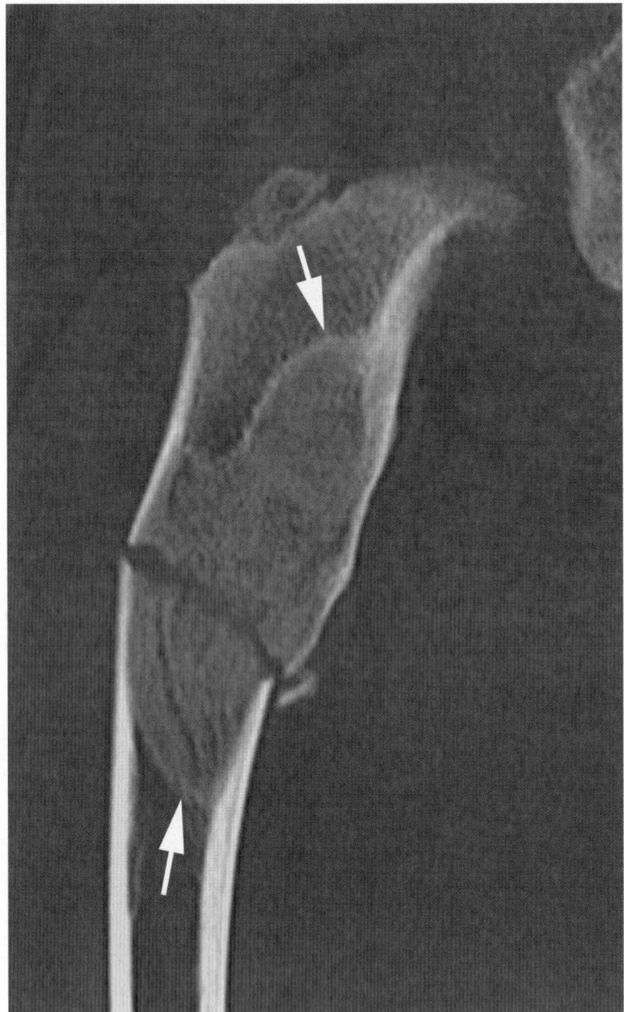

FIGURE 47-36 ■ Fibrous dysplasia. Coronal CT MPR of the proximal femur showing a well-defined lesion with a 'ground-glass' matrix (arrows), through which there has been a pathological fracture.

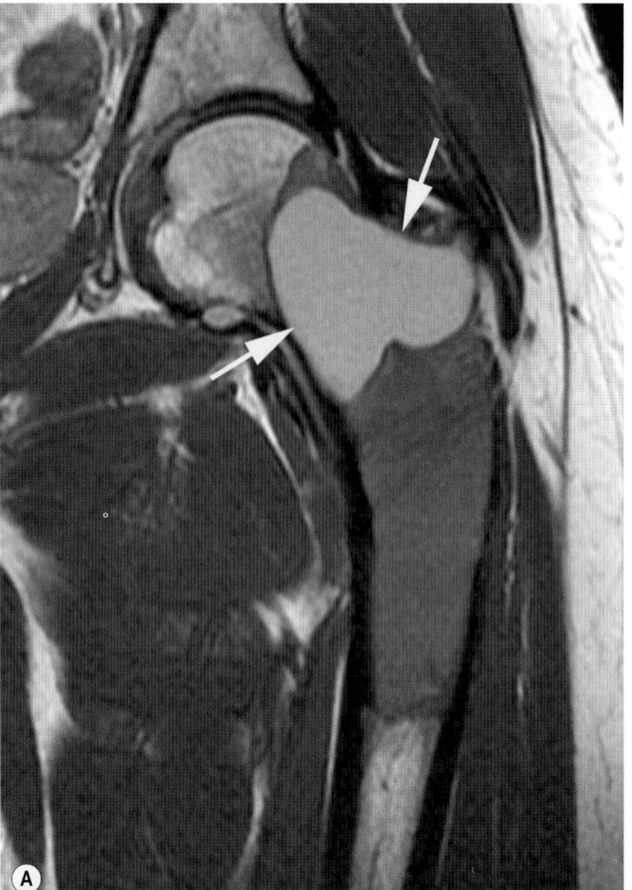

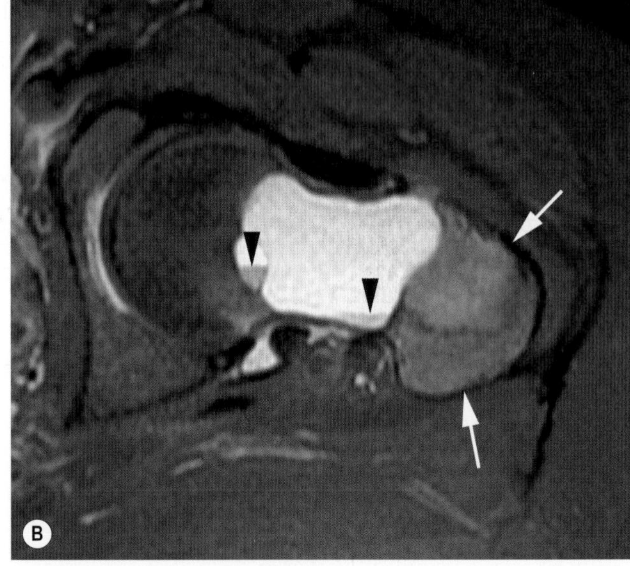

FIGURE 47-37 ■ Fibrous dysplasia. (A) Coronal T1W SE MRI showing a lesion in the left femoral neck with combined intermediate and increased SI (arrows), the latter due to haemorrhage. (B) Axial fat-suppressed T2W FSE MRI shows the fibrous component of the tumour to have intermediate SI (arrows), while the haemorrhagic component is hyperintense. Note also the FFLs (arrowheads).

the femur, tibia and humerus being the most common locations. Multiple lesions are seen in 10% of cases at presentation.

Radiological Features

Long bone lesions are usually located centrally within the diaphysis (~60%), followed by the metaphysis/metadiaphysis. Epiphyseal involvement is rare (~2%). The lesions are lytic, showing a fairly aggressive pattern of bone destruction (Fig. 47-39A) with occasional reactive medullary sclerosis. A multi-laminated periosteal response is commonly seen, while endosteal scalloping and mild bone expansion are also features.

MRI shows a poorly defined lesion with intermediate signal intensity. Active lesions are almost invariably associated with reactive marrow and soft-tissue oedema and periostitis (Fig. 47-39B). Cortical destruction and soft-tissue masses have rarely been described in adults with

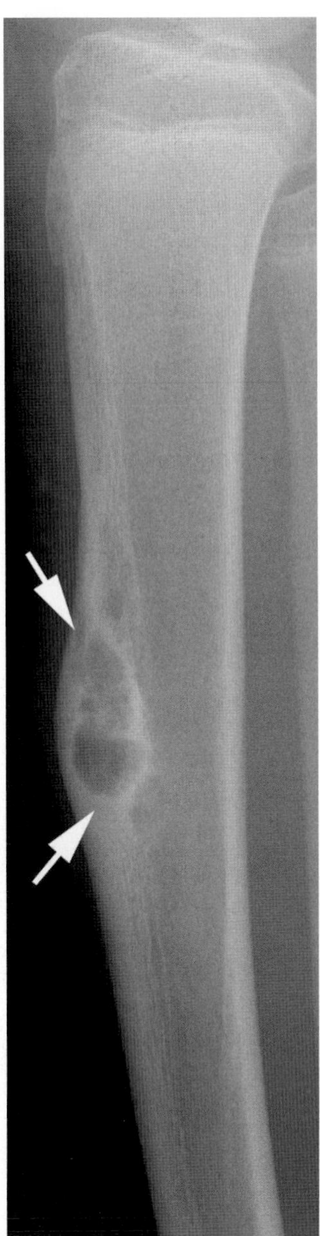

FIGURE 47-38 ■ **Osteofibrous dysplasia.** Lateral radiograph of the proximal tibia showing a lobular lesion (arrows) within the anterior cortex.

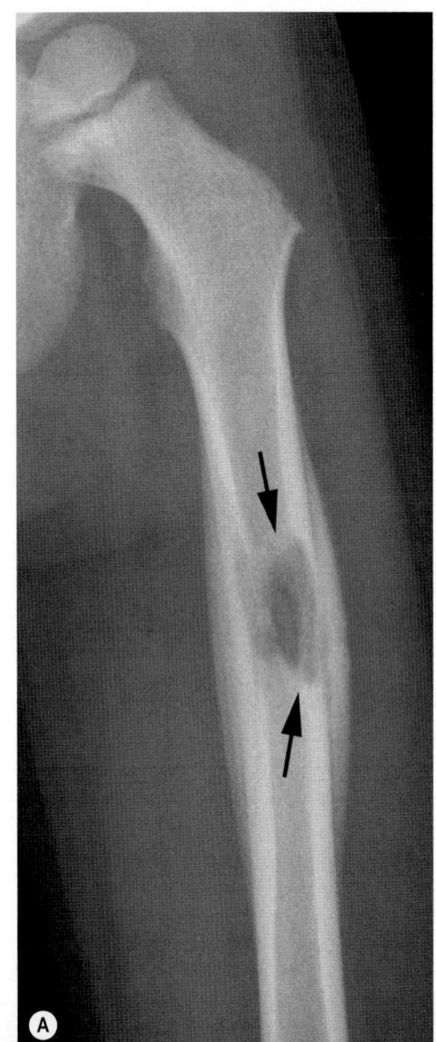

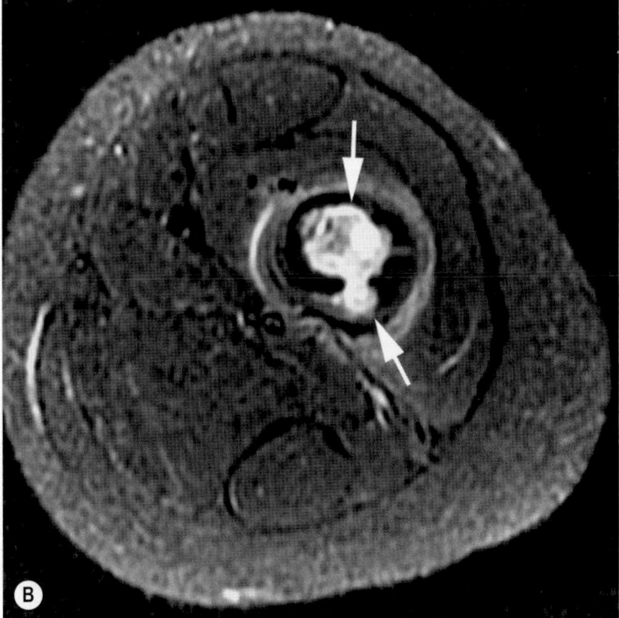

FIGURE 47-39 ■ **LCH.** (A) AP radiograph of the left proximal femur showing an irregular lytic lesion (arrows) with a multi-laminated periosteal response. (B) Axial fat-suppressed T2W FSE MRI showing an irregular hyperintense lesion (arrows) with associated periosteal response and soft-tissue oedema.

LCH.[64] Whole-body MRI may replace scintigraphy for the assessment of multifocal disease.

Erdheim–Chester's Disease[65]

Erdheim–Chester's disease is a rare form of histiocytosis characterised by the medullary infiltration of foamy, lipid-laden histiocytes. It usually presents in adults over the age of 40 years with bone pain most commonly related to the knees and ankles. Radiographs classically demonstrate bilateral, symmetrical metaphyseal and diaphyseal medullary sclerosis with sparing of the epiphyses.

For a full list of references, please see ExpertConsult.

FURTHER READING

3. Saifuddin A. The accuracy of imaging in the local staging of appendicular osteosarcoma. Skeletal Radiol 2002;31:191–201.
4. Alyas F, James SL, Davies AM, Saifuddin A. The role of MR imaging in the diagnostic characterisation of appendicular bone tumours and tumour-like conditions. Eur Radiol 2007;17:2675–86.
7. James SL, Panicek DM, Davies AM. Bone marrow oedema associated with benign and malignant bone tumours. Eur J Radiol 2008;67:11–21.
9. Khoo MM, Tyler PA, Saifuddin A, Padhani AR. Diffusion-weighted imaging (DWI) in musculoskeletal MRI: a critical review. Skeletal Radiol 2011;40:665–81.
13. Douis H, Saifuddin A. The Imaging of cartilaginous bone tumours: Part 1—benign lesions. Skel Radiol 2012;41(10):1195–212.
21. Chai JW, Hong SH, Choi JY, et al. Radiologic diagnosis of osteoid osteoma: from simple to challenging findings. Radiographics 2010;30:737–49.
34. Smith SE, Kransdorf MJ. Primary musculoskeletal tumors of fibrous origin. Semin Musculoskelet Radiol 2000;4:73–88.
39. Murphy MD, Nomikos GC, Flemming DJ, et al. From the archives of AFIP. Imaging of giant cell tumor and giant cell reparative granuloma of bone: radiologic-pathologic correlation. Radiographics 2001;21:1283–309.
44. Wenger DE, Wold LE. Benign vascular lesions of bone: radiologic and pathologic features. Skeletal Radiol 2000;29:63–74.
53. Mahnken AH, Nolte-Ernsting CC, Wildberger JE, et al. Aneurysmal bone cyst: value of MR imaging and conventional radiography. Eur Radiol 2003;13:1118–24.
60. Jee WH, Choi KH, Choe BY, et al. Fibrous dysplasia: MR imaging characteristics with radiopathologic correlation. Am J Roentgenol 1996;167:1523–7.

CHAPTER 48

Bone Tumours (2): Malignant Bone Tumours

A. Mark Davies • Steven L.J. James • Asif Saifuddin

CHAPTER OUTLINE

INTRODUCTION

Bone tumours can be generally divided into two groups: benign, including tumour-like lesions (see Chapter 47), and malignant. The malignant category can be subclassified into primary, secondary and metastatic. In common parlance the terms secondary and metastatic are frequently used interchangeably. In the context of this chapter, however, the term secondary is reserved for those tumours arising from malignant transformation of a pre-existing benign bone condition.

BONE METASTASES

Bone metastasis or metastatic disease refers to the spread of a malignant tumour from its primary site to a non-adjacent part of the skeletal system. They are relatively common, frequently found on imaging to be multiple and are the commonest bone malignancy over 40 years of age. Approximately, 10% of carcinoma metastases will present as a solitary bone lesion. A solitary lesion in a middle-aged or elderly patient is, therefore, still more likely to be a metastasis than a primary malignant bone tumour. Post-mortem studies have shown that bone is the third commonest site of metastatic spread after the lung and liver.

Metastases are assumed to arise from venous tumour emboli, from the primary tumour or from prior disease spread to the regional lymph nodes or other metastases, e.g. in the lung. Venous embolisation of malignant cells is multifactorial but is particularly related to the vascularity of the primary tumour and/or access to a valveless venous plexus, e.g. Batson's vertebral plexus.

Bone metastasis is a relatively late occurrence in the natural history of malignant disease because the lungs trap most tumour emboli. It is recognised that bone metastases may occur without obvious evidence of pulmonary involvement due to:

1. Pulmonary lesions that are present but occult;
2. Transpulmonary spread of malignant cells;
3. Paradoxical embolisation via a patent foremen ovale; and
4. Retrograde venous embolism with involvement of the vertebral column.

Arguably, the incidence of truly occult pulmonary metastases is less these days due to the superior sensitivity of multidetector CT of the chest routinely used in cancer staging as compared with standard radiography or single slice CT employed in the past.

The most common primary malignancies metastasising to bone are carcinoma of the breast, bronchus, prostate, kidney and thyroid, making up over 80% of all patients with bone metastases. The overall incidence of bone metastases during life is uncertain and will depend on the sensitivity of the imaging technique employed. At the time of death the prevalence of bone metastases is approximately 80–85% for breast and prostate cancer, more variable for lung cancer with a quoted range of between 40 and 80%, 50–60% for thyroid cancer and 20–35% for renal cancer. With modern improved cancer management leading to longer survival times, bone metastases have become a fairly common occurrence in everyday medical practice.

Distribution of Bone Metastases

The commonest sites of metastatic involvement are those containing red bone marrow, explaining why the axial skeleton is affected more commonly than the appendicular skeleton in adults; hence, the predilection for the spine, pelvis, proximal femora and humeri, ribs, sternum and skull (Fig. 48-1). Spinal metastases occur most commonly in the thoracic vertebrae, but carcinomas arising

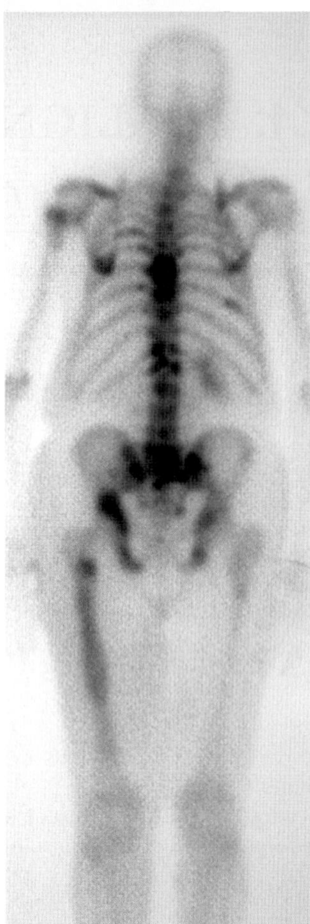

FIGURE 48-1 ■ Whole-body ^{99m}Tc-MDP (methylene diphosphonate) bone scintigram (posterior view) showing multiple regions of increased uptake due to prostatic carcinoma metastases. Involvement typically occurs in the spine, pelvis and ribs.

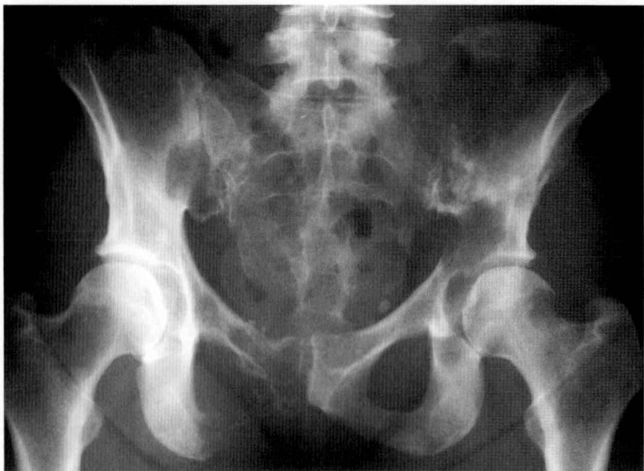

FIGURE 48-2 ■ **AP radiograph of the pelvis showing multiple lytic breast metastases.**

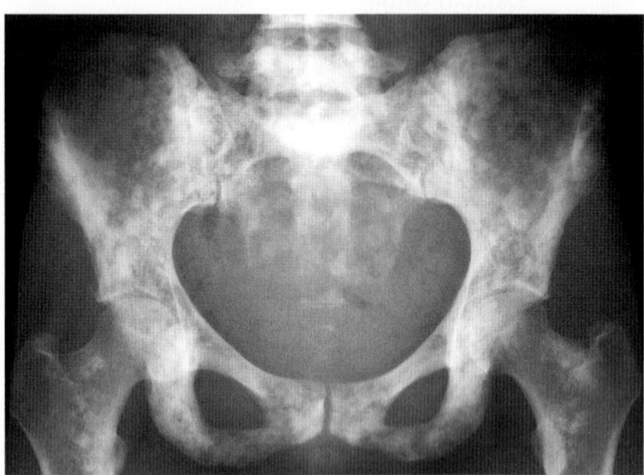

FIGURE 48-3 ■ **AP radiograph of the pelvis showing multiple sclerotic breast metastases.**

within the pelvis, particularly prostatic carcinoma, show a predilection for the lumbosacral spine.

Diagnosis of Bone Metastases

Clinical

Unexplained back or limb pain in a patient with a history of carcinoma may indicate a skeletal metastasis. Non-mechanical pain (i.e. bone pain at rest) is highly suggestive of tumour, be it primary or metastatic. A metastasis may present with a pathological fracture following minor trauma. Radiographs are necessary to reveal the pre-existing lesion. Elevation of the serum alkaline phosphatase is a non-specific finding and typically is not seen until multiple bone metastases have developed.

Radiological Features

Bone metastases may be lytic (most common) (Fig. 48-2), mixed lytic and sclerotic and predominantly sclerotic (Fig. 48-3). Small lytic lesions confined to the medullary bone can be difficult to identify on radiographs, particularly in complex anatomical areas such as the pelvis and spine or where there is reduced bone density (osteopenia). It is much easier to detect a metastasis as and when there is evidence of cortical destruction. It is for this reason that vertebral metastases are frequently first detected on radiographs as showing destruction of the cortex of a pedicle even though cross-sectional imaging may reveal fairly extensive destruction of the medullary bone in the adjacent vertebral body (Fig. 48-4). As the destructive process increases, a soft-tissue mass may develop. A periosteal reaction may be seen but this is usually less pronounced than those seen in primary bone malignancies. Exceptions include some prostatic metastases and mucinous adenocarcinoma metastases from the colon. Some carcinomas, such as renal, almost always produce lytic metastases. Others, such as prostate, are most commonly osoteoblastic, while breast metastases may show a mixed appearance. It should be noted that the osteoblastic reaction reflects the response of the host bone to the metastasis rather than the production of tumour bone, which is a characteristic of osteosarcoma. Cortical-based metastases are less common than

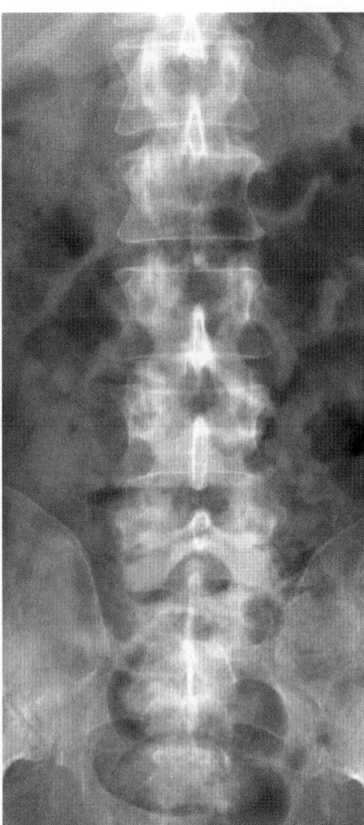

FIGURE 48-4 ■ AP radiograph of the lumbar spine. There is a renal metastasis destroying the left pedicle of the L1 vertebra.

medullary and tend to arise along the diaphyses of the long bones from lung, kidney and breast primaries (Fig. 48-5).

The importance of identifying multiple lesions cannot be overemphasised, as an individual metastasis may be indistinguishable from a primary malignant bone tumour. For this purpose, ^{99m}Tc-MDP bone scintigraphy is the most cost-effective method, although both whole-body MRI and ^{18}F-fluoride PET/CT are considered more sensitive. A variety of scintigraphic abnormalities are seen, with the most common being multiple foci of increased skeletal activity, predominantly in the axial skeleton (Fig. 48-1). Abnormal increased activity relies on an intact local blood supply and increased host bone osteoblastic activity. Metastases that have infarcted or stimulate no host osteoblastic response may appear as photopenic areas or 'cold spots', most commonly seen with larger renal metastases. Occasionally a combination of 'hot' and 'cold' lesions occurs. Diffuse osteoblastic metastatic disease, typically from breast or prostate carcinoma, may result in a 'superscan' appearance where there is generalised increase in skeletal activity with a relative paucity of renal activity.

It is important to recognise that not all foci of abnormally increased activity on bone scintigraphy, in a patient being investigated for suspected metastatic disease, need necessarily be due to metastases. Foci of activity in the ribs, particularly if contiguous, suggest old fractures, linear foci peripherally in the sacrum suggest insufficiency fractures and intense expanded foci of activity extending up to a joint margin may indicate Paget's disease. Any area of unexplained abnormal uptake should be correlated with further up-to-date imaging. Generally, MRI is utilised as it is more sensitive than radiography, and more specific than scintigraphy. Most metastases are located within the medulla and show reduced signal intensity (SI) on T1-weighted sequences, with increased SI on T2-weighted or fat-suppressed sequences. The identification of a hyperintense 'halo' around a lesion is a feature highly suggestive of a metastasis on fluid-sensitive images. Both whole-body MRI and FDG-PET are being increasingly utilised in the detection and monitoring of bone metastases.[1,2] The efficacy of PET can be increased with fused anatomical imaging, e.g. PET/CT.[3]

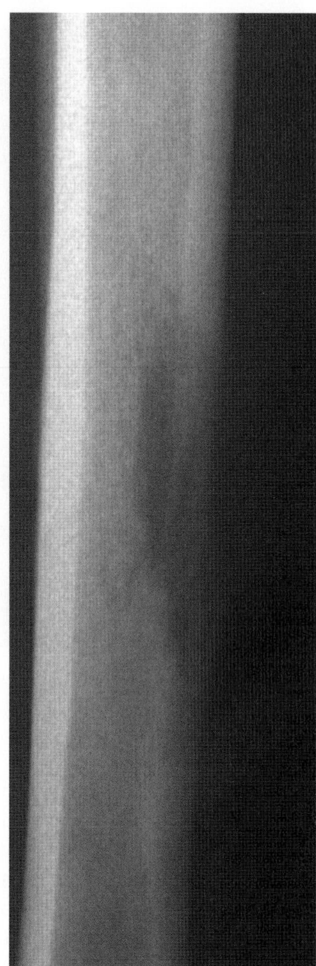

FIGURE 48-5 ■ Detail of an AP radiograph of the tibia showing a cortically based metastasis from carcinoma of the bronchus.

Prostate. Prostatic metastases are typically osteoblastic (sclerotic) (Fig. 48-6) or mixed, with purely lytic lesions being very rare. Occasionally, long bone metastases may exhibit a prominent 'sunburst' periosteal reaction mimicking an osteosarcoma, a rare disease in this age group in the absence of Paget's disease or previous radiotherapy. Disseminated prostatic metastases may produce confluent sclerosis on radiographs, simulating other disorders such as myelofibrosis and Paget's disease, although the latter condition can usually be excluded by noting the absence of bony expansion. Assessment of the prostate serum antigen (PSA) level can be useful in determining the value of performing bone scintigraphy. If the PSA

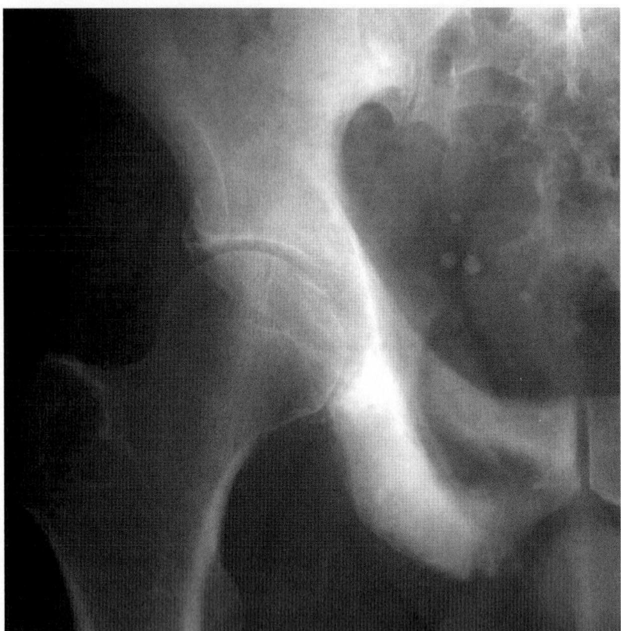

FIGURE 48-6 ■ AP radiograph of the hip showing a sclerotic prostatic metastasis in the ischium.

level is <10 ng/mL the likelihood of positive bone scintigraphy is <1%. This increases to approximately 10% if the PSA level is 10–50 ng/mL and 50% with a PSA level >50 ng/mL. While ^{99m}Tc-MDP bone scintigraphy may be adequate for the initial identification of prostatic metastases, FDG-PET is preferred after treatment for distinguishing persistent active metastases from healing bone.

Breast. Most breast bone metastases are lytic (Fig. 48-2) but breast carcinoma is the commonest cause of osteoblastic metastases in women (Fig. 48-3). About 10% of metastases are purely osteoblastic and 10% mixed. Diffuse marrow infiltration may occur and only become radiographically visible when sclerosis develops after therapy. In this situation the sclerosis may be mistaken for disease progression rather than a response to treatment. Breast metastases have a predilection for the spine, pelvis and ribs. Patients may present with acute-onset vertebral collapse at one or more levels and positive neurology. In this clinical situation the differential diagnosis would include benign causes such as osteoporotic collapse and malignant causes such as metastases from other primaries, lymphoma and myeloma. Further investigation with MRI ± diffusion-weighted imaging would be mandatory. Bone scintigraphy is usually sufficient to confirm/exclude bone metastases when clinical or laboratory parameters are suspicious but after treatment, follow-up studies may show increased activity due to the 'flare phenomenon' secondary to the normal healing response of bone. Again, in this context FDG-PET may be preferred with increasing activity indicating a lack of response to treatment.

Lung. Lung metastasis to bone is common. Most spread to the axial skeleton and are typically lytic. Metastases to the hands and feet (acrometastases), although rare, originate from a lung primary in approximately half of cases (Fig. 48-7).[4] Bronchogenic carcinoma is the commonest source of cortical-based metastases with large lesions showing the so-called 'cookie-bite' appearance (Fig. 48-5). It is also the commonest disorder associated with hypertrophic osteoarthropathy, formerly known as hypertrophic pulmonary osteoarthropathy. A single or multiple layer periosteal reaction along the distal long bones, including the hands and feet, characterises this condition. Bone scintigraphy will reveal symmetrical increased linear activity along the long bones, known as 'double stripe' or 'parallel tract' sign.

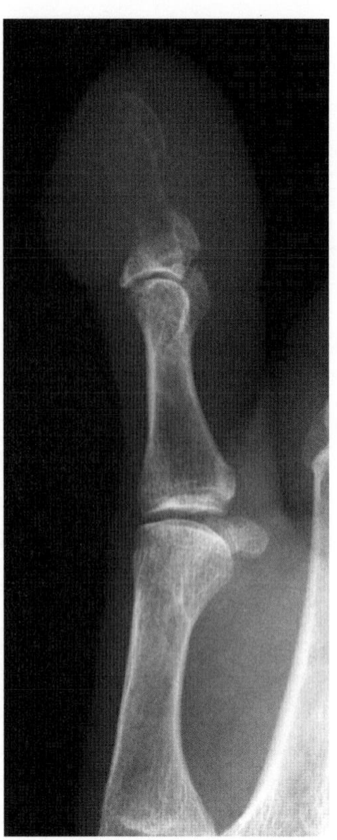

FIGURE 48-7 ■ Lateral radiograph of the thumb showing destruction of the terminal phalanx due to a bronchial carcinoma metastasis (acrometastasis).

Kidney. Renal carcinoma is the commonest primary malignancy associated with solitary bone metastases. Solitary or multiple lesions are invariably lytic and may be expansile (blowout) and trabeculated. So-called expansile metastases may also be typically seen in thyroid metastases (Fig. 48-8) and less commonly in breast and lung. A similar radiographic appearance may be seen with plasmacytoma and, if subarticular, in a younger age group, giant cell tumour of bone. Renal metastases tend to be hypervascular, exhibiting multiple serpiginous signal voids within and around the periphery of the lesion on MRI.[5]

Melanoma. After extension to locoregional lymph nodes, malignant melanoma can spread to almost any part of the body, including the axial skeleton. It is important to appreciate that melanoma metastases may be

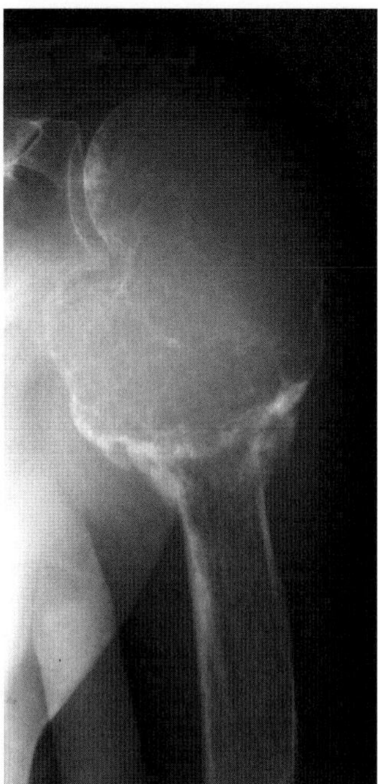

FIGURE 48-8 ■ **AP radiograph of the proximal humerus showing an expansile thyroid metastasis.**

clinically silent and that there can be a long latent period between treatment of the primary lesion and the development of the metastasis. Most bone metastases from melanoma are lytic. Melanin is paramagnetic and, depending on the concentration, the metastasis may show mild hyperintensity on T1-weighted MR images.

Radiological Investigation of Bone Metastases

When a known primary malignancy is established, the presence or absence of metastases is part of the routine surgical staging process. This will vary, depending on the nature of the primary and local/national guidelines. In most situations bone scintigraphy is adequate for assessing the whole skeleton (Fig. 48-1). Combining the study with SPECT may increase the sensitivity in detecting small lesions in anatomically complex areas such as the spine. Whole-body MRI may be preferred because of its increased sensitivity but it should be noted that if only coronal sequences are obtained both rib and spinal lesions may be overlooked.

When there is no history of prior malignancy then, in patients over 40 years of age, a CT study of the chest, abdomen and pelvis should be performed. Should the staging studies show the bone lesion to be solitary, then an image-guided needle biopsy will be required, irrespective of whether there is a documented prior history or current imaging evidence of a primary malignancy elsewhere. This is because the bone lesion need not necessarily be related to that other tumour and failure to establish the correct diagnosis could lead to inappropriate management prejudicial to the long-term prognosis for the patient. This biopsy should be performed so as to

TABLE 48-1 Mirels' Rating System for Prediction of Pathological Fracture Risk of Metastases in Long Bones as Measured on Radiographs[6]

Score	Site	Nature	Size[a]	Pain
1	Upper extremity	Blastic	$<\frac{1}{3}$	Mild
2	Lower extremity[b]	Mixed[c]	$\frac{1}{3}$–$\frac{2}{3}$	Moderate
3	Peritrochanteric	Lytic	$>\frac{2}{3}$	Severe

[a]Relative proportion of bone width involved with tumour.
[b]Non-perithrochanteric lower extremity.
[c]Mixed lytic and blastic.

avoid contamination of uninvolved anatomical compartments in case the histology reveals a primary malignancy of bone rather than a metastasis. In cases with disseminated metastases to multiple organ systems, where palliative care is the only reasonable management, needle biopsy is arguably unnecessary. In patients with a suspected primary malignancy and bone metastases, a needle biopsy of the most accessible bone lesion may be the quickest and easiest way to establish a definitive tissue diagnosis.

An important cause of morbidity in patients with bone metastases is the development of pathological fractures. This is most common in the spine, with or without neurological compromise, and in the lower limbs because of weight-bearing. It is clearly advantageous for the patient if these debilitating fractures can be prevented with prophylactic fixation. In the long bones the Mirels' scoring system is widely employed to assess fracture risk (Table 48-1).[6]

In the past the identification of bone metastases usually meant an early demise for the patient; but nowadays modern therapies and improved surgical techniques are leading to longer survival times. Therefore, follow-up imaging to assess response of bone metastases to treatments is not uncommon. Such imaging can be difficult to interpret: while disease progression is usually obvious, it can be more problematic to confirm lack of progression. The 'flare phenomenon' on bone scintigraphy is an example where a good response to therapy may be misinterpreted as disease progression. It is also important to recognise that new bone lesions may not be further metastases but actually caused by the drugs administered. This includes bone infarction after chemotherapy and/or steroids and necrosis of the mandible and atypical stress fractures in the femora after bisphosphonate therapy.[7] It is likely that FDG-PET will have an increasing role in the assessment of the response of bone metastases to therapy.

Bone Metastases in Children

This is a distinctly less common occurrence than in adults. In the younger child the commonest disseminated neoplasms affecting bone are neuroblastoma and leukaemia, which may have identical radiographic appearances. The commonest paediatric soft-tissue sarcoma and also the commonest to metastasise to bone is rhabdomyosarcoma, with a 10% incidence identified at time of initial diagnosis. Retinoblastoma may involve bone by direct spread and blood-borne metastases. It is also one of a number of conditions associated with an increased incidence of osteosarcoma. Both osteosarcoma and Ewing sarcoma may present or develop local (skip) or distant bone metastases. The commonest intracranial neoplasm to metastasise to bone outside the skull is cerebellar medulloblastoma, typically after surgery to the primary tumour.

PRIMARY MALIGNANT NEOPLASMS OF BONE

Primary malignant tumours of the skeleton are rare, accounting for only 0.2% of all neoplasms, with an annual incidence of new diagnoses of approximately 1/100,000 population. Major advances in the past 40 years in chemotherapy and limb-salvage surgery have vastly improved the outcome, such that in specialist centres, the 5-year survival for appendicular osteosarcoma now exceeds 60%. The classification of these tumours, as described by the World Health Organisation, is based on their histopathological characteristics.[8] While the tumours themselves have remained unchanged over the years, the nomenclature has metamorphosed as successive generations of pathologists have attempted to refine and reclassify these disorders.

Radiographs remain of fundamental importance in the detection and diagnosis of a primary bone tumour, be it benign or malignant. Radiographic features suggestive of an aggressive and therefore more likely to be malignant lesion include a wide zone of transition (permeative or moth-eaten), an aggressive periosteal reaction (onion-skin, Codman angle or spiculated), cortical destruction and a soft-tissue mass.[9] Matrix mineralisation does not help to distinguish benign from malignant disorders but can be an indicator of the underlying histopathological origin, be it osteoid (i.e. bone-forming) or chondroid (i.e. cartilage-forming).

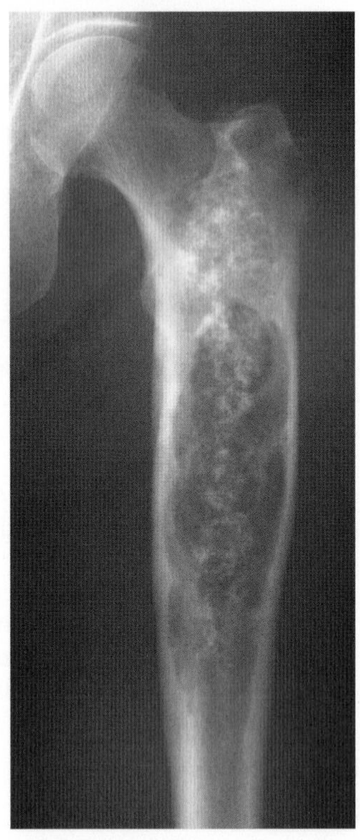

FIGURE 48-9 ■ AP radiograph of the femur showing an extensive central chondrosarcoma with typical chondroid matrix, cortical expansion and thickening with endosteal scalloping.

CHONDROID ORIGIN

Chondrosarcoma

Chondrosarcoma is a malignant cartilage-forming tumour accounting for 8–17% of all biopsied primary bone tumours and 20–25% of all biopsied malignant bone tumours. It is classified as central if arising within medullary bone (Fig. 48-9) and peripheral if arising from the surface of bone. It is further subclassified as primary if arising de novo or secondary if arising from a pre-existing bony lesion, usually an enchondroma (central type) or osteochondroma (peripheral type) either as a solitary occurrence or as part of the bone dysplasias of Ollier's disease (multiple enchondromatosis), Maffucci's syndrome (multiple enchondromatosis and soft-tissue angiomas) and hereditary multiple exostoses (diaphyseal aclasis) (Fig. 48-10). The incidence of malignant change in solitary enchondroma and osteochondroma is <1% and in hereditary multiple exostoses <5%. The incidence is somewhat higher, at approximately 20% in Ollier's disease and 30% in Maffucci's syndrome.

Chondrosarcoma is also classified according to its histological grade. These are defined as low grade (grade 1; 45–50% of cases), intermediate grade (grade 2; 30–40% of cases), high grade (grade 3; 10–25% of cases) and dedifferentiated, which refers to the development of areas of high-grade non-cartilaginous sarcoma within the chondrosarcoma (10% of cases), typically osteosarcoma or spindle cell sarcoma (Fig. 48-11).[10] Other distinct variants include mesenchymal and clear-cell chondrosarcoma.

Clinical Presentation

Most patients are above the age of 50 years, with the peak incidence in the fifth to seventh decades. Secondary chondrosarcoma tends to present at a slightly younger age in the fourth and fifth decades. Chondrosarcoma is sufficiently rare in children that the diagnosis should be seriously questioned if proffered by a pathologist based

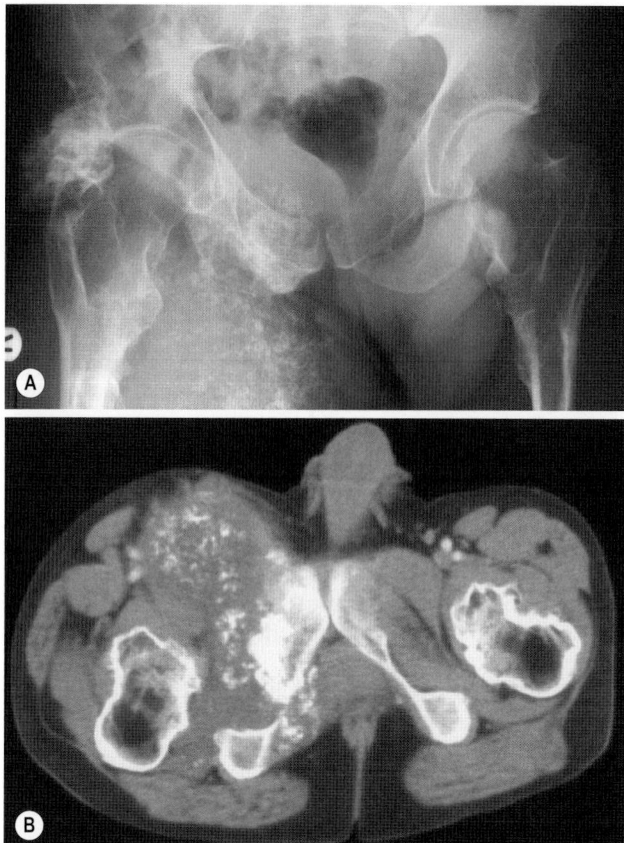

FIGURE 48-10 ■ (A) AP radiograph and (B) CT of the hips in a patient with hereditary multiple exostoses (diaphyseal aclasis). There is a large peripheral chondrosarcoma arising from the right pubis.

on a needle biopsy specimen. There is a minor male preponderance and the commonest site of occurrence is the pelvis (Fig. 48-10), proximal femur (Fig. 48-9) and proximal humerus. Approximately 9% of chondrosarcomas occur in the ribs, making this the most common primary malignancy, other than myeloma, to arise at this location. Chondrosarcomas in the hands and feet are rare in contradistinction to the high incidence of enchondromas at both these sites.

Imaging Features

The radiographic features of central chondrosarcoma are those of a lytic lesion, well-defined in low-grade cases and progressively increasingly ill-defined in higher-grade cases.[11,12] Chondroid calcification is visible in 75% cases, variously described as ring-and-arc, punctate, stippled or popcorn in appearance (Fig. 48-9). The relatively slow growth of the tumour allows for reactive change to occur in the adjacent normal bone. There is a combination of endosteal resorption producing endosteal scalloping and periosteal new bone formation. In time this leads to bony expansion with varying thickness of the replacement cortex. In the higher-grade cases, cortical destruction and soft-tissue extension reveal the aggressive nature of the process (Figs. 48.11A, 48.12A). CT can be helpful in

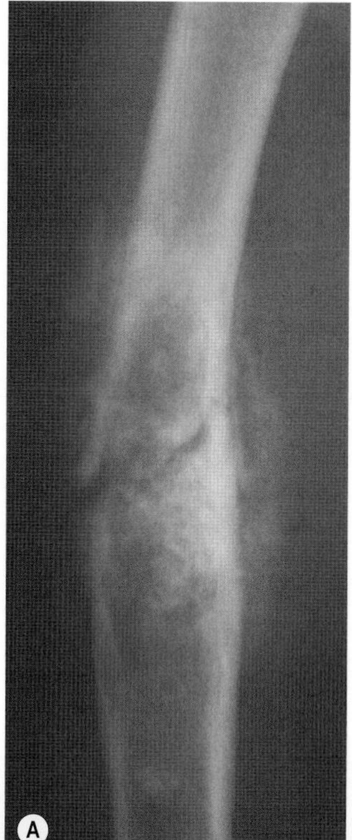

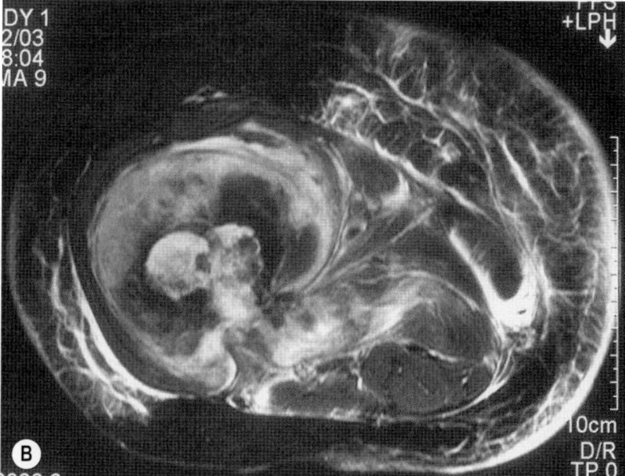

FIGURE 48-11 ■ (A) AP radiograph of the femur showing a pathological fracture through a dedifferentiated chondrosarcoma. (B) Axial T2-weighted fat-suppressed image showing soft-tissue extension with areas of low signal intensity indicative of malignant osteoid.

identifying occult chondroid matrix not visible on radiographs. MR imaging shows a typical hyperintense multilobular pattern on fluid-sensitive sequences with low signal intensity foci representing chondroid calcification on all pulse sequences (Fig. 48-12B). Most chondrosarcomas are poorly vacularised and enhancement after intravenous administration of a gadolinium chelate is limited, typically showing a peripheral or septal pattern. The identification on T2-weighted images of a mass of intermediate signal intensity adjacent to the hyperintense multilobular tumour is highly suggestive of dedifferentiation. Such areas should be targeted for image-guided

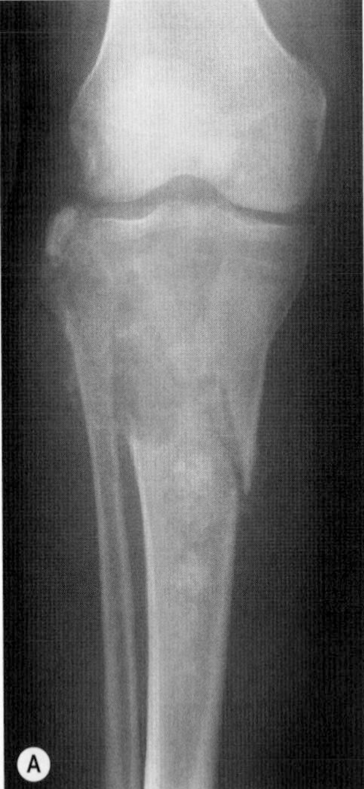

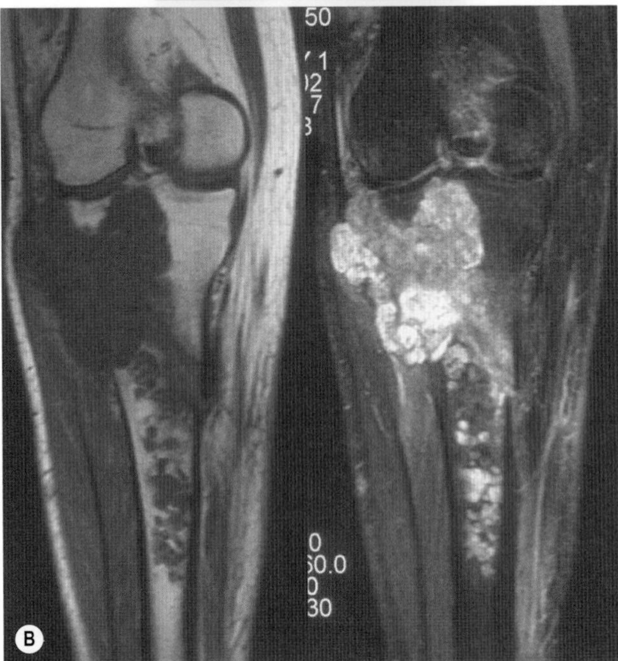

FIGURE 48-12 ■ (A) AP radiograph and (B) coronal T1-weighted and STIR images of the proximal tibia in a patient with Ollier's disease (multiple enchondromatosis). Typical features of benign enchondroma distally with an aggressive tumour destroying the cortex and soft-tissue extension proximally due to malignant transformation into a secondary central chondrosarcoma.

biopsy. A common diagnostic dilemma is the distinction of a low-grade chondrosarcoma from an enchondroma. This is an increasing problem with improved access to MR imaging. The incidence of 'incidental' central cartilage tumours around the knee in adults undergoing routine knee imaging is approximately 3%. There are no hard-and-fast-rules in this respect and the issue is compounded by the fact that pathologists often have as much difficulty in the diagnosis of these borderline lesions as do the radiologists. Lesions in excess of 5 cm in length and with deep endosteal cortical scalloping (greater than two-thirds) are suggestive of chondrosarcoma as opposed to enchondroma. Bone scintigraphy cannot be reliably used to distinguish benign from malignant lesions, as up to 30% of enchondromas in adults may show some increased activity due to persistent endochondral ossification. However, as over 80% of chondrosarcomas show increased activity, normal background skeletal activity favours the diagnosis of enchondroma. Unenhanced and static contrast-enhanced MRI is also of limited value. Both dynamic contrast-enhanced MRI[13–15] and FDG-PET imaging have been claimed to be useful but many remain sceptical when the histological diagnosis, at least in low-grade lesions, remains somewhat subjective.

Identification of a secondary peripheral chondrosarcoma from an osteochondroma should be clinically suspected if pain develops or there is continued growth after skeletal maturity. Radiographic features of malignant change consist of destruction of part of the calcified cap or ossified stem of the osteochondroma with dispersal of the calcifications within a soft-tissue mass. The thickness of the cartilage cap cannot be reliably measured on radiographs but can be determined with ultrasound, CT or MRI. If the cartilage cap is less than 2 cm in thickness, then malignancy is unlikely. If it is greater than 2 cm, the likelihood of malignancy increases (Fig. 48-10B).[16] It is important that any measurement is made perpendicular to the bony component of the osteochondroma as tangential measurements from cross-sectional imaging may overestimate the thickness of the cartilage cap. Malignant transformation of an osteochondroma may be mimicked by other complications that are associated with the development of an overlying soft-tissue mass, including inflammatory bursa and pseudoaneurysm formation.[17,18]

Other Chondrosarcoma Variants

Periosteal Chondrosarcoma

Periosteal chondrosarcoma, also known as juxtacortical chondrosarcoma, is a rare tumour arising on the outer surface of long bones, commonly the metaphysis of the proximal humerus and distal femur. It is characterised by a cartilaginous mass usually greater than 5 cm in length with a variable degree of cartilage calcification. It can be distinguished from the other surface form of chondrosarcoma, the peripheral chondrosarcoma, by the lack of continuity with the underlying medullary bone.

Mesenchymal Chondrosarcoma

Mesenchymal chondrosarcoma occurs at a younger age than conventional chondrosarcoma, most commonly in the second and third decades. It is a high-grade malignancy comprising approximately 5% of all chondrosarcomas. It contains well-differentiated hyaline cartilage with more cellular malignant matrix than conventional chondrosarcoma. Radiographically, it is indistinguishable from central chondrosarcoma but there is a predilection for the mandible and ribs. Local recurrence and

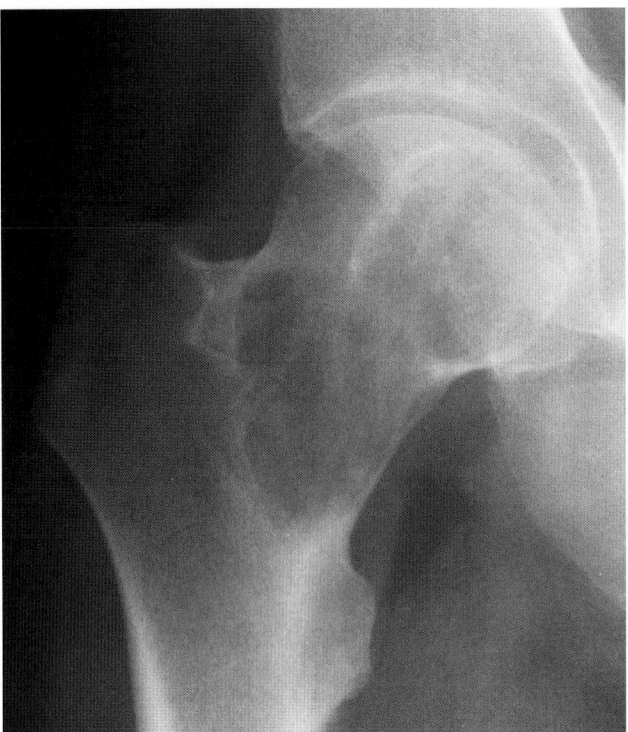

FIGURE 48-13 ■ AP radiograph of the hip showing a clear-cell chondrosarcoma as a well-defined lytic lesion extending up to the articular margin.

disseminated metastases occur early and more frequently than with conventional chondrosarcoma.

Clear Cell Chondrosarcoma

Clear cell chondrosarcoma accounts for approximately 2% of all chondrosarcomas. Most cases arise in the third to fifth decades. Radiographically, it appears as a well-defined, lytic subarticular lesion (Fig. 48-13). Matrix calcification is uncommon. It can mimic a chondroblastoma although the age group tends to be older. Growth tends to be slow and so it can be mistaken for a subchondral cyst/intraosseous ganglion.

OSTEOID ORIGIN

Osteosarcoma

Osteosarcoma is the commonest non-haematological primary bone malignancy, with an estimated annual incidence of approximately 4 per million population. Sixty per cent of cases present under the age of 25 years, with a minor male preponderance, and 75% of all cases are the high-grade medullary type frequently referred to as conventional osteosarcoma. The remainder are made up of other variants distinguished by site and histological grade.[19,20] Osteosarcoma may also occur secondary to Paget's disease, radiotherapy or as the dedifferentiated component of a lower-grade sarcoma such as chondrosarcoma and parosteal osteosarcoma. An association with several rare clinical syndromes is recognised. These include Li–Fraumeni syndrome, Rothmund–Thomson syndrome and familial retinoblastoma.

Central Osteosarcomas

Conventional Central Osteosarcoma

Clinical Presentation. This high-grade tumour is the commonest form of osteosarcoma. Approximately 80% present before 30 years of age, but it is uncommon under the age of 10 years and rare under 5 years. In the 10% of cases occurring over 40 years of age it is frequently secondary to a pre-existing disorder of bone, such as Paget's disease.

Presentation is typically with pain and a palpable mass not infrequently attributed to an unrelated previous incident of trauma. Osteosarcoma classically arises in the metaphyseal region of the growing end of long bones and about 50–75% are found in the distal femur or proximal tibia (Fig. 48-14). Diaphyseal osteosarcoma accounts for less than 10% cases. Other commonly affected sites include the proximal humerus and femur. Rarer sites include the ilium, ribs, scapula, vertebrae and jaw.

Imaging Features. Conventional osteosarcoma typically presents as a metaphyseal lesion with a moth-eaten or permeative pattern of bone destruction. The medullary component is lytic with a spectrum of tumour osteoid. This can produce mineralisation variously described as solid, amorphous, 'cloud-like' and 'ivory-like' (Fig. 48-14C). There is a spectrum of radiographic appearances from the entirely lytic (13% cases) through to the entirely sclerotic. Cortical destruction is common, resulting in the development of an eccentric extra-osseous soft-tissue mass, which commonly shows typical osseous amorphous matrix mineralisation. The density of the extraosseous mass is increased by periosteal new bone formation that is frequently complex, comprising perpendicular/spiculated, 'sunburst', lamellated/onion-skin with reactive Codman's angles at the margin of the tumour (Fig. 48-14).

Although MR imaging contributes little to the imaging diagnosis, it is mandatory for local surgical staging. It accurately defines the extent of the tumour within bone, in the soft tissues and any involvement of the adjacent joint and neurovascular structures. It is essential to have a least one MR sequence of the whole affected bone to confirm or exclude skip metastases (Fig. 48-15). These are foci of tumour, seen in approximately 5% of cases, arising within the same bone but separate from the main tumour or, on occasion, across the adjacent joint (trans-articular skip metastasis). Static sequences following the intravenous injection of a gadolinium chelate do not contribute to local staging. However, sequential dynamic contrast-enhanced sequences obtained pre- and post-adjuvant chemotherapy can be used to assess tumour response to therapy. FDG-PET has a complimentary role to other imaging in the initial staging of osteosarcoma but has an established role in the evaluation of response to adjuvant chemotherapy and for recurrent disease, both locally and remote. The natural history of osteosarcoma is for haematogenous spread with the production of pulmonary metastases. These are typically peripheral, may be mineralised and, rarely, may result in

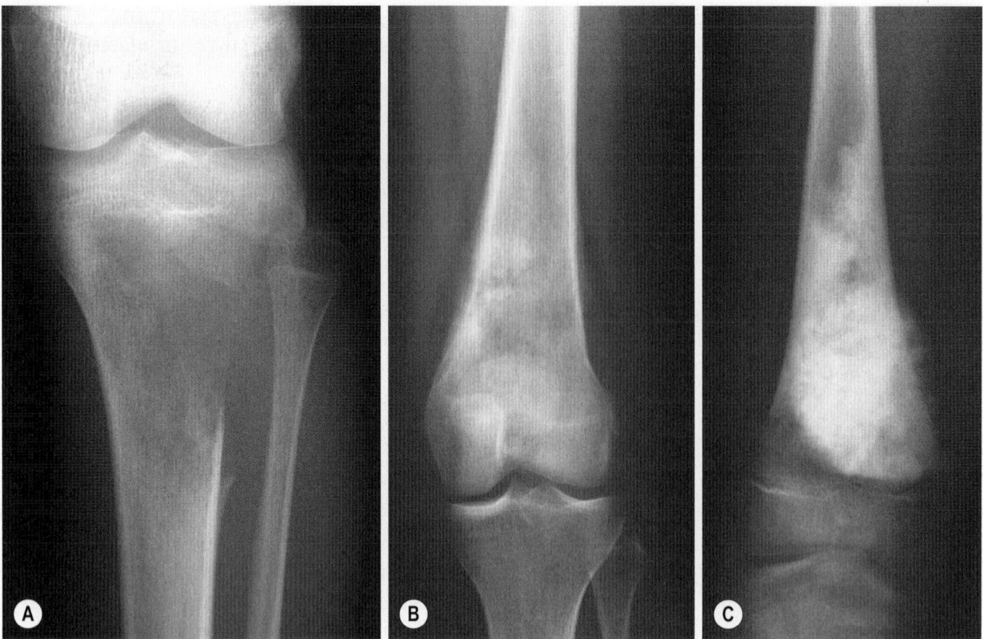

FIGURE 48-14 ■ AP radiographs of three cases of conventional central osteosarcoma arising around the knee: (A) lytic with a Codman angle distally; (B) mixed pattern with lysis and minor malignant osteoid with a lamellar (onion skin) periosteal reaction; and (C) sclerotic with dense amorphous malignant osteoid.

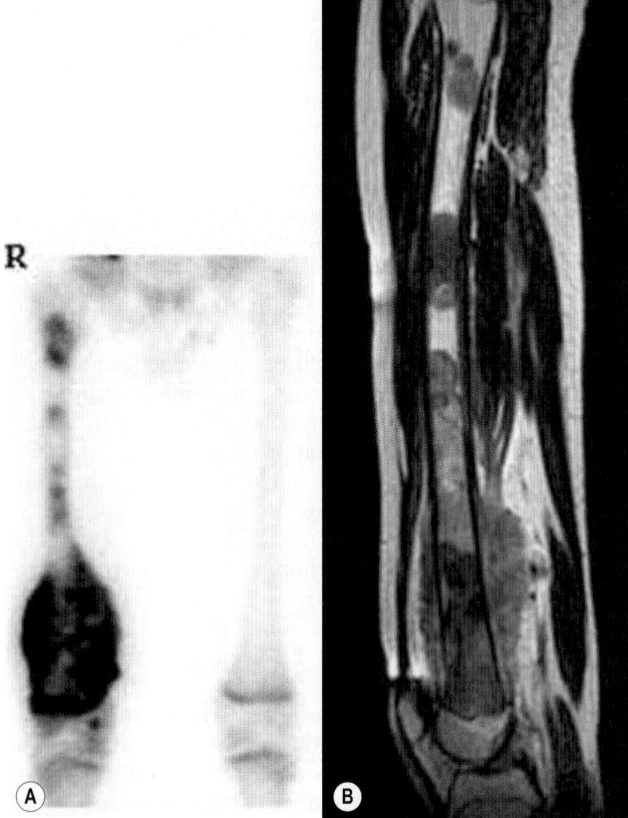

FIGURE 48-15 ■ (A) Bone scintigraphy and (B) sagittal T2-weighted MR images showing a large primary osteosarcoma of the distal femur with multiple proximal skip metastases.

chronic pneumothorax. If sufficiently large, the pulmonary metastases may show increased uptake on bone scintigraphy.

Other Varieties of Central Osteosarcoma. Primary multicentric osteosarcoma is the identification of multiple foci of intramedullary osteosarcoma in the absence of pulmonary metastases. It may be either synchronous or metachronous in presentation. The synchronous type typically consists of mutiple sclerotic metaphyseal lesions developing simultaneously, usually in children or adolescents. In the metachronous type, presentation is with a solitary lytic or sclerotic lesion in a long or flat bone with the development of a second or multiple lesions after a period of greater than 5 months. Some authorities question whether these lesions are truly multiple primaries or an unusual subset of metastatic disease.[21] Suffice to say that the prognosis for the synchronous manifestation is dismally similar to that of the patient presenting with metastatic disease, whereas the metachronous picture can be associated with a better outcome.

Telangiectatic osteosarcoma accounts for approximately 5% of all osteosarcomas and is twice as common in male patients, with a mean age at presentation of 24 years. It is characterised by the formation of multiple blood-filled cavities and hence may be mistaken for an aneurysmal bone cyst (ABC) on both imaging and histology. The femur, tibia and humerus are the most commonly involved bones. Radiographs show a predominantly lytic lesion ± bone expansion.[22] MR imaging reveals multiple fluid–fluid levels (Fig. 48-16) but the identification of solid areas within the tumour on post-contrast-enhanced sequences helps to differentiate telangiectatic osteosarcoma from an ABC.

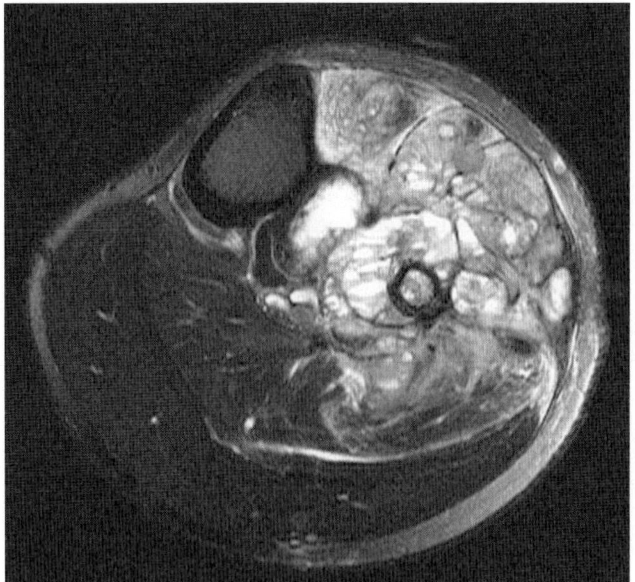

FIGURE 48-16 ■ Axial T2-weighted fat-suppressed image showing a large telangiectatic osteosarcoma arising in the proximal fibula. There are multiple cystic/haemorrhagic areas within the tumour containing fluid–fluid levels.

Small cell osteosarcoma accounts for approximately 1.5% of osteosarcomas. It is a histological variant but tends to show imaging features identical to those of conventional osteosarcoma.

Low-grade central osteosarcoma accounts for approximately 1% of cases of osteosarcoma. As the name implies it is a relatively indolent lesion affecting mainly the femur and tibia. It occurs in a slightly older age group than conventional osteosarcoma, with a mean age at presentation of 34 years. Four radiographic patterns have been described: lytic with coarse trabeculation; predominantly lytic; densely sclerotic; and mixed lytic and sclerotic. The imaging differential diagnosis includes benign fibro-osseous lesions such as fibrous dysplasia.

Surface Osteosarcomas. This designation refers to a group of tumours that arise from the surface of bone and includes parosteal, periosteal and high-grade surface osteosarcoma. All three types account for less than 10% of all osteosarcoma cases.

Parosteal Osteosarcoma. This is the commonest surface osteosarcoma and accounts for approximately 5% of all osteosarcomas. It is a low-grade malignancy, with 60% cases arising on the posterior aspect of the distal femur (Fig. 48-17) and less commonly the proximal humerus and tibia. It occurs at a slightly older age group than conventional osteosarcoma, with most patients affected in the third and fourth decades. The prognosis is excellent, with an over 90% 5-year survival unless there has been dedifferentiation to a high-grade osteosarcoma that occurs in approximately 20% of cases. The characteristic radiographic feature is of a densely sclerotic mass arising on and partially enveloping the posterior distal femoral metaphysis (Fig. 48-17A). Cross-sectional imaging will show that the mass is in part adherent to the underlying cortex with the more peripheral component separated from the cortex by a thin radiolucent line (Fig. 48-17B). Medullary invasion may be seen in approximately 15% of cases. MRI typically shows the main lesion to be of low signal intensity on all sequences due to the sclerotic nature of the tumour. Should foci of intermediate T1- or increased T2-weighted signal intensity be identified at the periphery of the lesion, dedifferentiation should be considered and needle biopsy directed to these potentially higher-grade areas.[23]

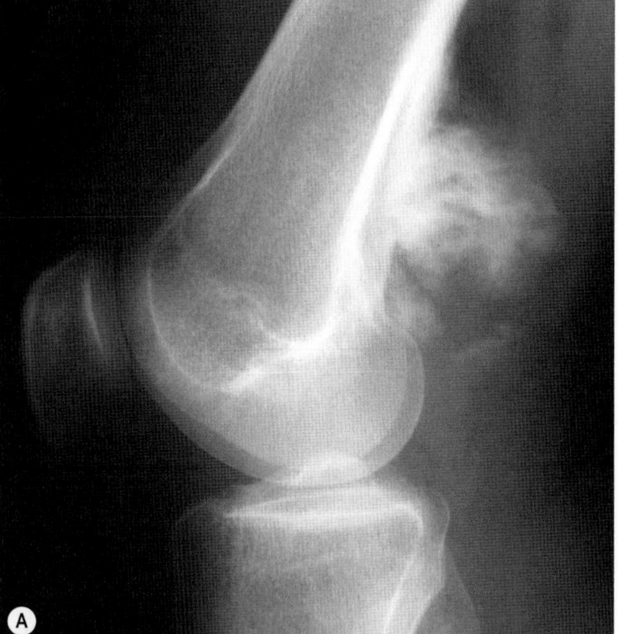

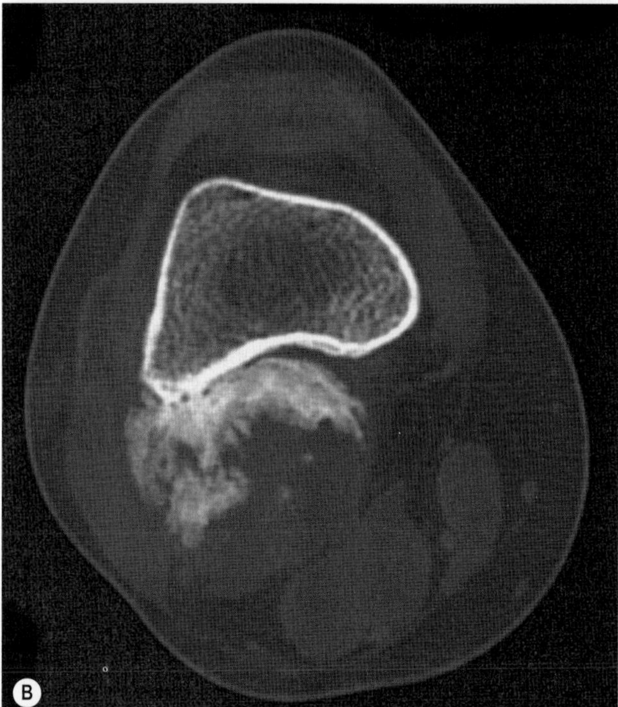

FIGURE 48-17 ■ (A) Lateral radiograph showing a sclerotic parosteal osteosarcoma arising on the posteror surface of the distal femoral metaphysis and (B) CT confirming the malignant osteoid attached in part to the underlying femoral cortex.

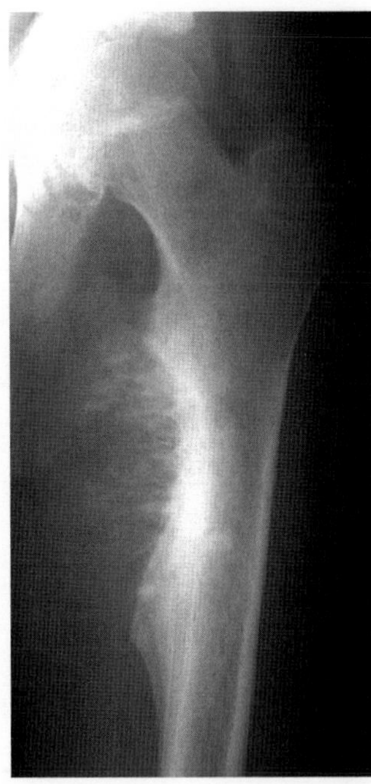

FIGURE 48-18 ■ AP radiograph showing an extensive spiculated periosteal reaction from a periosteal osteosarcoma of the proximal femur.

Periosteal Osteosarcoma. This intermediate-grade sarcoma accounts for less than 2% of all osteosarcomas. Its peak incidence is in the second and third decades with a slight male preponderance. It most commonly arises from the proximal tibial or distal femoral diaphyses. Two radiographic patterns may be seen; a surface lesion with cortical thickening or erosion and a perpendicular ('hair-on-end') periosteal reaction (Fig. 48-18) or a thin peripheral shell simulating a periosteal chondroma.[24] MR imaging may show lobulated hyperintensity on T2-weighted images, reflecting the chondroblastic nature of the tumour. Reactive marrow signal changes may be present but true marrow invasion is rare.

High-Grade Surface Osteosarcoma. This is the rarest of the surface osteosarcomas, accounting for less than 1% of all osteosarcomas. It has the same histological features as conventional central osteosarcoma. The imaging features can be similar to that of periosteal osteosarcoma but more aggressive in that the tumour is usually larger and there is a greater degree of cortical destruction and medullary extension (Fig. 48-19).

Secondary Osteosarcoma. Approximately 5–7% of osteosarcomas are secondary due to malignant transformation in a pre-existing bone lesion. Typical examples are in Paget's disease and following radiotherapy. Rarer examples include medullary infarction, fibrous dysplasia, osteogenesis imperfecta (OI) and chronic osteomyelitis. Care should be taken not to misinterpret hyperplastic callus formation well recognised in OI with malignant osteoid production.

Paget's Sarcoma. Of sarcomas arising in Paget's disease, 50% are osteosarcomas with the remainder spindle cell/pleomorphic sarcomas and uncommonly chondrosarcoma. Many osteosarcomas arising after the age of 50 years are secondary to Paget's disease of bone.[25] There is a rare association between Paget's disease and giant cell tumour of bone that can be multifocal with a predilection for the maxillofacial skeleton. Malignant change to a sarcoma has been reported in 3–14% of patients with Paget's disease but the true prevalence is likely to be under 1% if one takes into account asymptomatic undiagnosed cases in the population. The incidence increases in older patients and the more extensive that Paget's disease is, although it can occur in monostotic disease. There is a decreasing incidence of Paget's disease worldwide and as a consequence the incidence of Paget's sarcoma also appears to be declining.[26] The sex incidence of Paget's sarcoma is similar to that of the primary disease, with men affected twice as often as women. Radiologically, the commonest sites for Paget's sarcoma are the pelvis, femur and humerus (Fig. 48-20). The spine is typically spared. Permeative bone destruction with cortical destruction and evidence of a soft-tissue mass are common features, best shown with CT and MRI (Fig. 48-21). MRI in uncomplicated Paget's disease will tend to show preservation of the medullary fat signal on T1-weighted images. Loss of the fat signal may indicate tumour infiltration as well as other complications such as pseudofracture formation with haemorrhage and oedema.[27] Bone scintigraphy is relatively insensitive to malignant transformation due to the avid, frequently multifocal, uptake of radionuclide in the underlying Paget's disease. Paradoxically, although most sarcomas are osteosarcomas, they may appear as relatively photopenic (cold) on bone scintigraphy (Fig. 48-21B). The prognosis for Paget's sarcoma is extremely poor, with most patients succumbing within a year of diagnosis. This is in part due to the late presentation of the disease, not infrequently already with pulmonary metastases, but also many of the affected patients are of an age that are too frail to undergo prolonged chemotherapy and major surgery. It is important to recognise that other malignancies, such as metastasis, lymphoma and myeloma, may occur in coincidence with Paget's disease, thereby mimicking sarcomatous transformation. Another mimicker of sarcoma is the rare pseudosarcoma, which may also present with a mineralised extraosseous mass.[28] Biopsy is therefore required to make the definitive diagnosis of Paget's sarcoma.

Post-Radiation Sarcoma. Post-radiation sarcoma (PRS), formerly known as radiation-induced sarcoma, refers to bone and soft-tissue sarcomas that develop following previous radiotherapy. They account for 0.5–5% of all sarcomas and the criteria for diagnosis include the following:[29]

1. A history of prior radiation therapy;
2. The development of a neoplasm within the radiation field typically peripheral;
3. A latent period of at least 3–4 years; and
4. Histological proof of a sarcoma, which differs significantly from the originally treated tumour.

The treated tumours most commonly associated with the development of PRS are breast carcinoma, lymphoma, head and neck and gynaecological malignancies. This accounts for the increased incidence in women. The mean age at presentation is in the sixth decade, with a mean latent period before development of PRS of 15

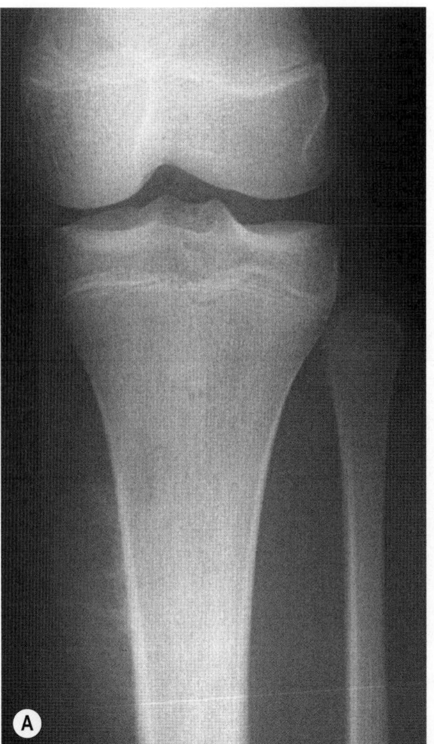

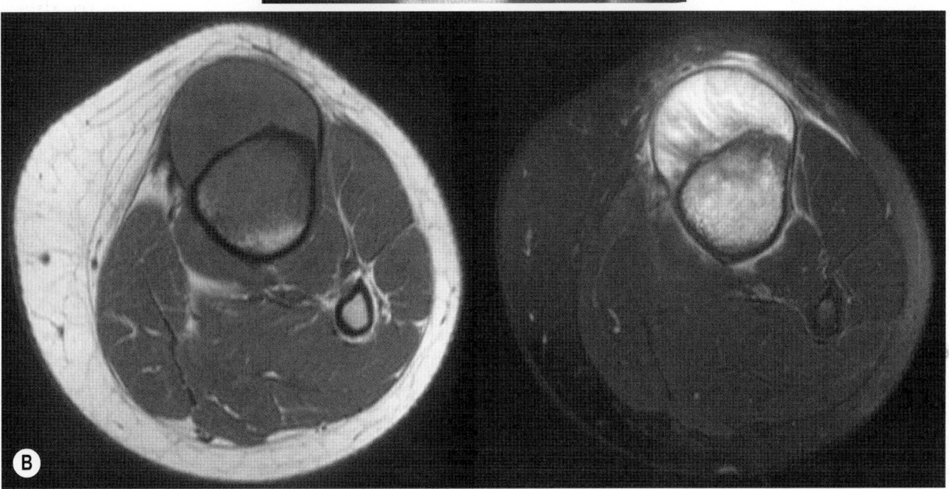

FIGURE 48-19 ■ (A) AP radiograph of a high-grade surface osteosarcoma of the tibia with a spiculated periosteal reaction. (B) Axial T1- and T2-weighted fat-suppressed images showing both the extra and intraosseous components.

years. PRS may be seen in younger individuals, as more paediatric patients undergoing radiotherapy are long-term survivors of their first malignancy. It is considered that a minimum dose of 30 Gy is required to induce a PRS and that the concurrent administration of chemotherapy may increase the risk. The commonest PRS is osteosarcoma, followed by spindle cell sarcoma. The commonest sites are the pelvic and shoulder girdle bones. Typical radiographic features include permeative bone destruction (>80% of cases), soft-tissue mass (>90% of cases) and varying degrees of matrix mineralisation and periosteal reaction (Fig. 48-22).[30] There may be evidence of underlying radiation change including patchy osteopenia, dystrophic calcification and radionecrosis (Fig. 48-23). The MRI appearances of PRS are those of an aggressive tumour destroying bone with soft-tissue extension of intermediate signal intensity on T1-weighted and hyperintense and heterogeneous signal intensity on T2-weighted images. As with Paget's sarcoma, the prognosis for PRS is poor.

FIBROUS ORIGIN

Malignant bone tumours of fibrous origin are classified histologically into those of fibrogenic (e.g. fibrosarcoma) and fibrohistiocytic (e.g. malignant fibrous histiocytoma/ MFH) origin. The nomenclature of fibrous tumours has changed over the years as pathologists have attempted to redefine these tumours. The terms fibrosarcoma and

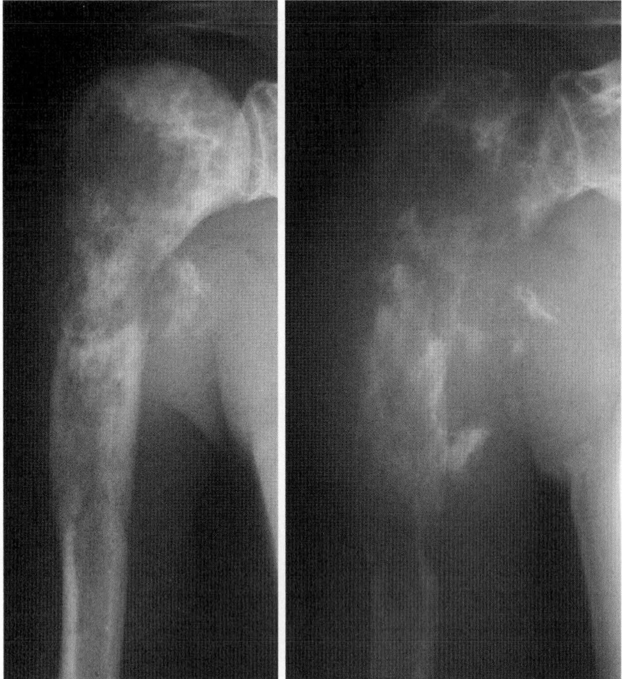

FIGURE 48-20 ■ AP radiographs of the proximal humerus obtained 6 weeks apart showing a rapidly progressive Paget's osteosarcoma.

MFH are less commonly used these days in favour of spindle cell sarcoma and more recently undifferentiated pleomorphic sarcoma (UPS). Because of the considerable overlap of these conditions they are considered as a single entity for the purposes of this chapter. They account for approximately 5% of all malignant bone tumours and occur in adults from 20 to 50 years of age. Up to 20% of cases can present with a pathological fracture. The lesions most commonly affect the long bones (70%), with 50% arising in the lower limb, particularly around the knee. On radiographs the tumours appear aggressive with cortical destruction but little periosteal new bone formation (Fig. 48-24).[31] In the younger age group they can be mistaken for a lytic osteosarcoma; in the third and fourth decades, if subarticular, a giant cell tumour and in the older age group a metastasis. Approximately 25% of cases arise in a pre-existing lesion, notably Paget's disease, post-radiotherapy, bone infarction (Fig. 48-24),[32] dedifferentiated chondrosarcoma, fibrous dysplasia[33] and chronic sinus tracts in osteomyelitis.[34]

MARROW TUMOURS

Malignancies arising from the marrow elements of bone include a group of malignant small round cell tumours comprising Ewing sarcoma, primitive neuroectodermal tumour (PNET), lymphoma, metastatic neuroblastoma and leukaemia, and plasmacytoma/myeloma. The imaging features of lymphoma of bone are covered in Chapter 70 and those of metastatic neuroblastoma, leukaemia and plasmacytoma/myeloma in relevant sections elsewhere.

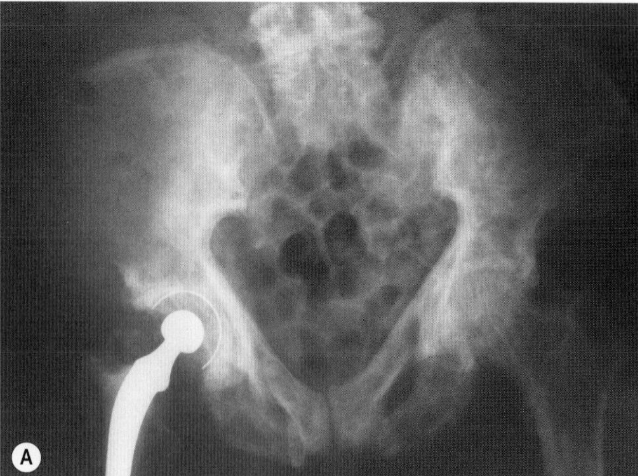

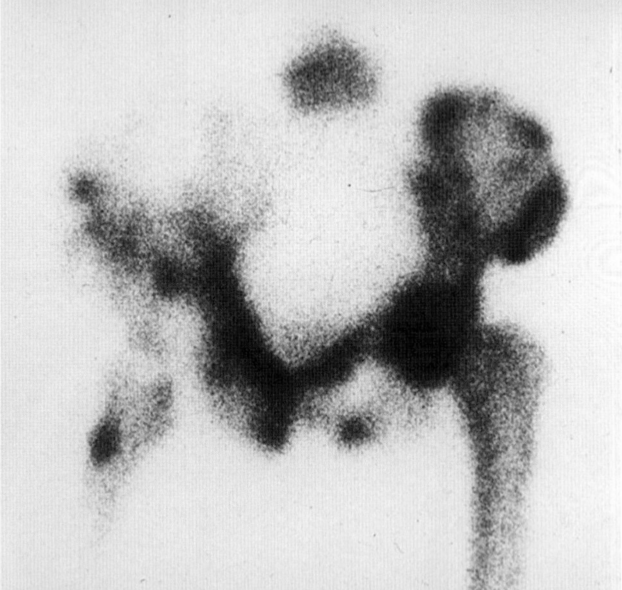

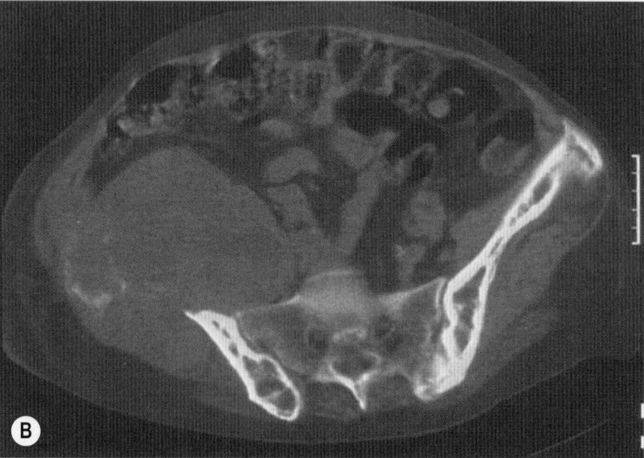

FIGURE 48-21 ■ (A) AP radiograph and (B) frontal image of bone scintigraphy and CT of the pelvis. There is extensive Paget's disease of the pelvis with a large Paget's osteosarcoma destroying the right ilium. The sarcoma appears relatively osteopenic on the scintigraphic image.

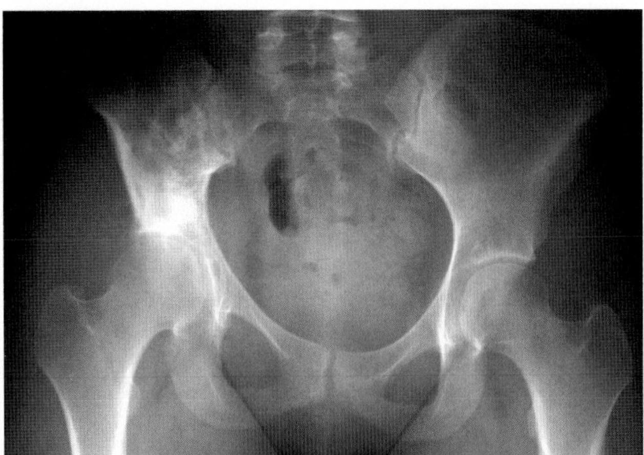

FIGURE 48-22 ■ AP radiograph showing a post-radiation osteosarcoma arising in the right ilium. There is malignant osteoid extending into the soft tissues laterally. The pelvic deformity and mild hypoplasia of the right ilium is secondary to radiotherapy in childhood as part of the treatment for a Wilms' tumour.

Ewing's Sarcoma and Primitive Neuroectodermal Tumour (PNET)

Both are malignant round cell tumours with varying degrees of neuroectodermal differentiation that exhibit similar imaging features and on cytogenetic analysis show specific constant reciprocal translocation between chromosomes 11 and 22. They account for approximately 8% of primary malignant bone tumours, with Ewing's sarcoma the second most common bone sarcoma in children after osteosarcoma. As many as 75% of patients are under the age of 20 years at presentation, most between 5 and 15 years, and 90% are under 30 years. The male-to-female patient ratio is 2 : 1 and 95% occur in Caucasians. Characteristically, presentation is with localised pain and swelling. The presence of systemic symptoms, including pyrexia and an elevated serum ESR, can simulate infection and may indicate disseminated disease. Usually a single bone is involved, but multiple lesions occur at presentation in 10% of cases and commonly later in the disease as Ewing's sarcoma readily metastasises to bone. In contradistinction to other bone sarcomas, most cases show involvement of the diaphyseal (35%) or the metadiaphyseal (60%) regions of a long bone and are typically central/medullary in origin (Fig. 48-25). The bones most commonly affected in order of frequency are

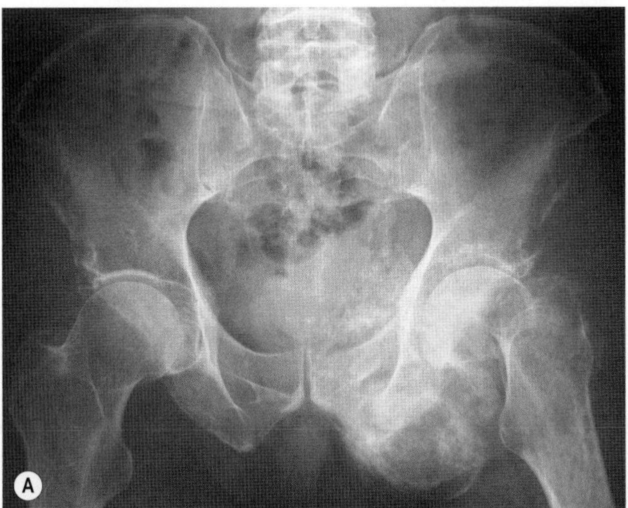

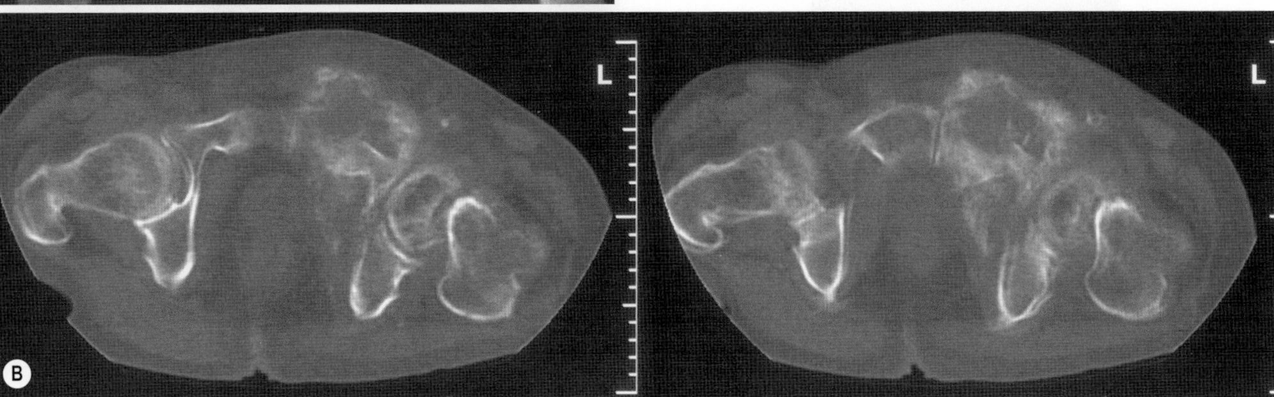

FIGURE 48-23 ■ (A) AP radiograph and (B) CT of the pelvis in a male patient 6 years following surgery and radiotherapy for a rectal carcinoma. There are three pathologies present. A post-radiation osteosarcoma arising from the left pubis, osteonecrosis with an ununited fracture of the femoral neck and a tumour distally in the left femoral neck which could have been a further sarcoma but biopsy proved it to be metastatic.

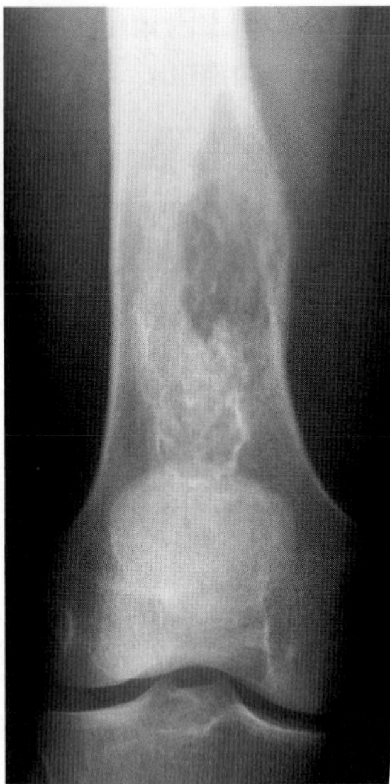

FIGURE 48-24 ■ AP radiograph of the knee showing an undifferentiated pleomorphic sarcoma arising in association with medullary infarction in the distal femur.

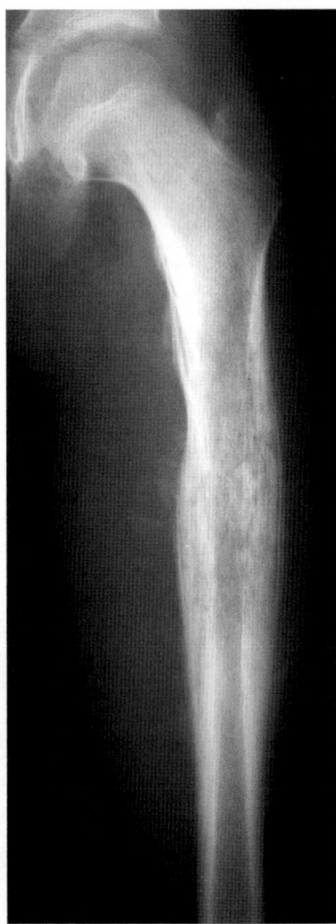

FIGURE 48-25 ■ AP radiograph of an Ewing's sarcoma. Typical features include a central diaphyseal location, permeative bone destruction, a lamellar (onion skin) periosteal reaction with spiculation medially.

the femur and humerus (31%), the pelvic bones (21%—most commonly the ilium) and ribs (<8%). The distal appendicular skeleton, including the hands and feet, is involved in 27% of cases. The Askin tumour is a rare PNET of the chest wall, occurring in children and young adults.[35]

Imaging Features

The radiographic features of Ewing's sarcoma are those of a permeative destructive lesion with a wide zone of transition (Fig. 48-25).[36] The most aggressive lesions may be difficult to identify on radiographs particularly if presentation is early. Soft-tissue extension is evident in 80% of cases. The classic multilamellar ('onion skin') periosteal reaction is uncommon. An interrupted periosteal reaction (Codman angle) is seen at the margins of the tumour in 27% of cases. A vertical 'hair-on-end'/spiculated periosteal reaction is also classic of Ewing's sarcoma seen in 50% of cases but can also be seen in osteosarcoma (Fig. 48-25). Occasionally, Ewing's sarcoma shows a mixed or mainly sclerotic appearance, especially in the flat bones and spine, thereby again mimicking an osteosarcoma (Fig. 48-26). This can be due to a combination of reactive sclerosis and visualisation of a spiculated periosteal reaction end on and is not due to tumour bone as malignant osteoid production is not a feature of this particular tumour. 'Saucerisation' of the outer bone cortex with a soft-tissue mass and eccentric lesions with a relatively small intraosseous component probably represent the rarer periosteal variant of Ewing's sarcoma. The radiographic differential diagnosis can include osteomyelitis, Langerhans cell histiocytosis and stress fracture. MRI accurately defines the medullary infiltration and soft-tissue extension that is of intermediate signal intensity on T1-weighted and intermediate/high signal intensity on T2-weighted and STIR sequences relative to skeletal muscle (Fig. 48-27). Skip metastases

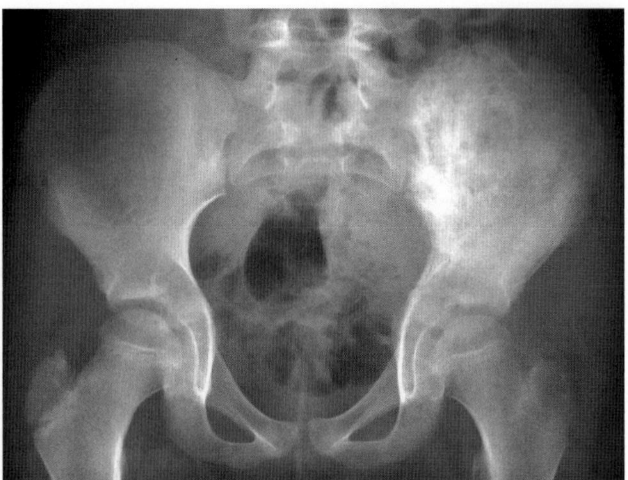

FIGURE 48-26 ■ AP radiograph showing an extensive Ewing's sarcoma of the left ilium. The increased density mimics an osteosarcoma and is due to reactive sclerosis and end-on periosteal new bone formation and not malignant osteoid.

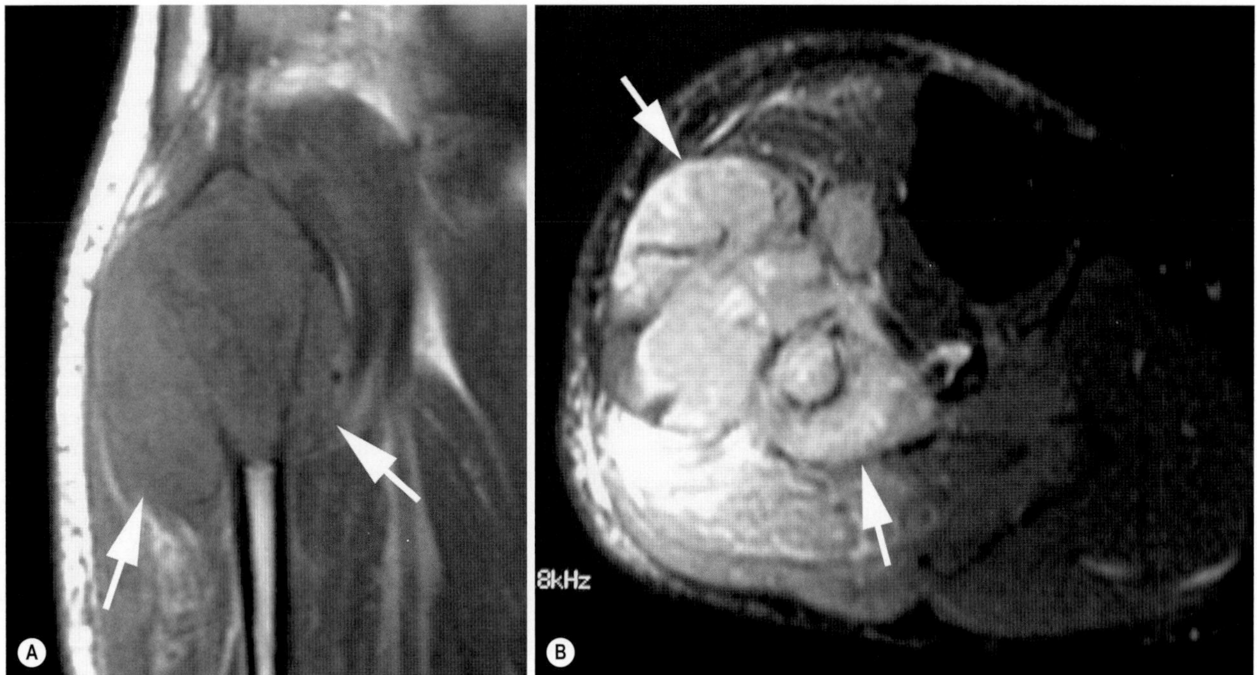

FIGURE 48-27 ■ Ewing sarcoma of the proximal fibula. (A) Coronal T1-weighted spin-echo and (B) axial STIR MR images show a large extraosseous mass (arrows).

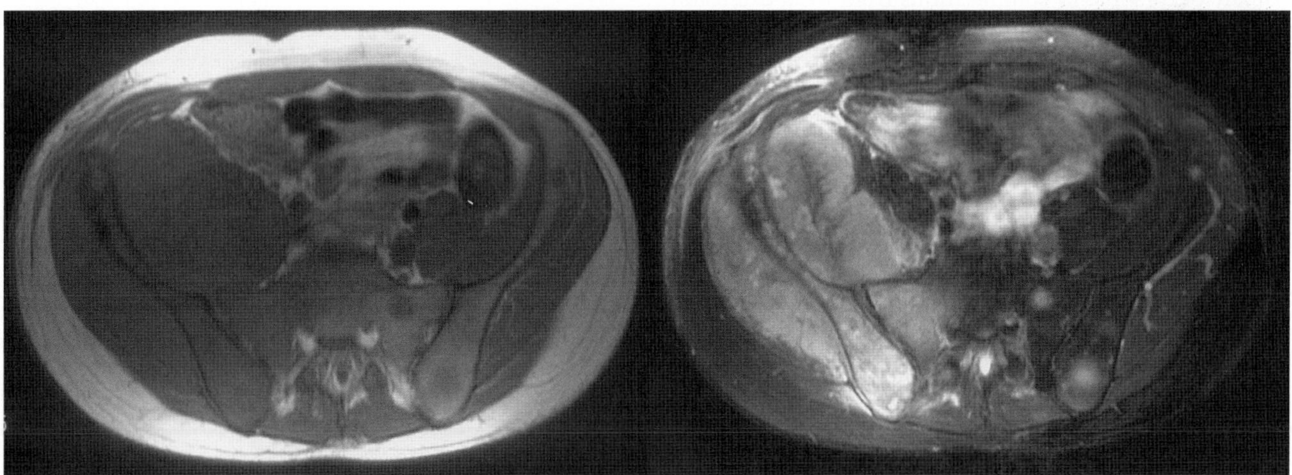

FIGURE 48-28 ■ Axial T1- and T2-weighted fat-suppressed images at initial presentation showing a primary Ewing's sarcoma infiltrating the right ilium with a large intra- and extrapelvic soft-tissue mass. There is also evidence of disseminated disease with foci in the sacrum and left ilium.

(12%) and distant metastases (<20%) in lungs and bone may be identified on initial imaging performed for surgical staging (Fig. 48-28). FDG-PET is more sensitive than bone scintigraphy in the detection of osseous metastases with a performance similar to that of whole-body MRI. FDG-PET may also be used in the assessment of response to adjuvant chemotherapy and detection of recurrence.

NOTOCHORDAL ORIGIN

Chordoma

Chordoma is a low-to-intermediate grade malignant tumour originating from ectopic cellular remnants of the notochord and as such arises from the midline of the axial skeleton. It accounts for 2–4% of all primary malignant bone tumours. Chordoma is the second commonest primary malignancy of the spine and accounts for over 50% of primary sacral tumours. The tumour has a predilection for the sacrococcygeal (50%) and clival (40%) regions, with other areas of the spine rarely involved. They most commonly present between 50 and 70 years of age with men more frequently affected in the older ages, particularly in the sacral region. Chordomas tend to be slow growing and symptoms of pain and related to pressure effects on adjacent structures are often prolonged before the tumour is detected. It is easy to overlook all but the largest of chordomas on radiographs of the pelvis or lumbosacral spine. Large tumours show bone destruction with occasional amorphous calcification. The soft-tissue mass is readily identified on CT or MRI extending anteriorly into the pelvis (Fig. 48-29). The midline origin of the tumour is a useful feature distinguishing it from other sacral tumours such as chondrosarcoma and metastases. The MRI features of intermediate-to-low signal intensity on T1-weighted and high signal on T2-weighted sequences are non-specific. A lobulated hyperintense pattern on T2-weighted images is suggestive of chordoma but can also mimic chondrosarcoma, as does septal enhancement following administration of a gadolinium chelate.[37] Wide excision is the treatment of choice, with radiotherapy reserved for inoperable cases or where wide resection is not possible.[38] Local recurrence, often multifocal, can be seen in up to 40% of cases presumed due to implantation at the time of surgery. Distant metastases are uncommon and death usually occurs due to complications from local extension of the disease. A benign counterpart of chordoma has recently been described, variously termed giant notochordal rest or benign notochord cell tumour.[39] These are benign non-progressive lesions arising at the same sites as chordoma. Whether this condition is a precursor of classic chordoma remains controversial.

FIGURE 48-29 ■ Sacral chordoma shown on axial CT as a predominantly lytic mass with foci of calcification. The mass is shown to have considerable anterior extension into the pelvis.

MISCELLANEOUS TUMOURS

Malignant Vascular Tumours

Primary malignant vascular tumours of bone are rare. The terminology of endothelial tumours is somewhat confusing. Simplistically, there is a spectrum from the low-grade haemangioendothelioma through the extremely rare low-to-intermediate grade haemangiopericytoma to the highly malignant angiosarcoma. The radiographic appearances reflect the biological activity of the tumours from well-defined lytic lesions with no surrounding sclerosis in the low-grade to the permeative bone destruction in the high-grade lesions.[40,41] One important diagnostic feature seen in 25–40% of cases is a multifocal distribution (Fig. 48-30).[42] This is frequently confined to one limb (monomelic) but can be disseminated throughout the skeleton, thereby mimicking metastatic disease.

Adamantinoma

Adamantinoma of long bones is a rare tumour accounting for <0.5% of all primary malignant bone tumours.

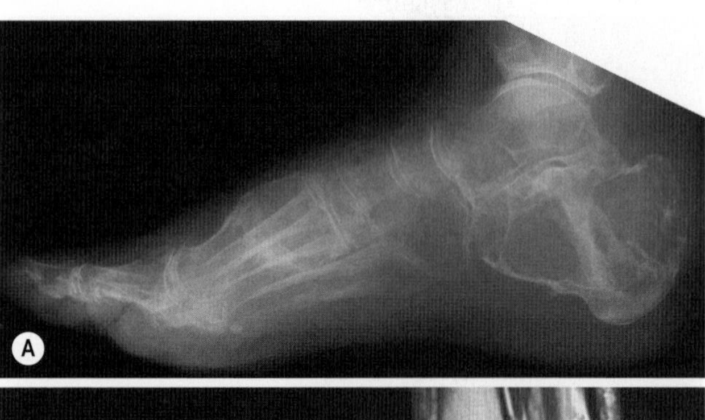

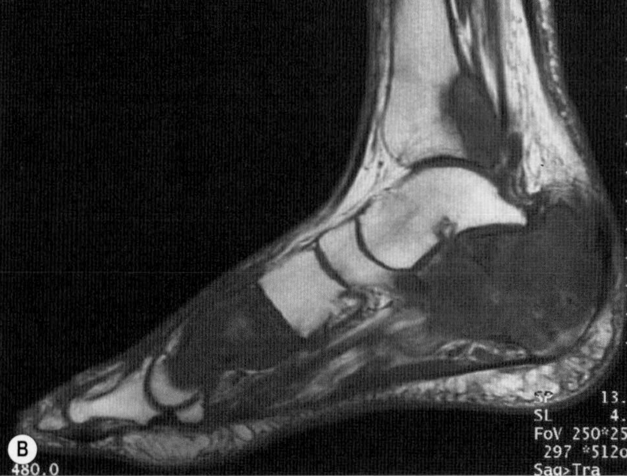

FIGURE 48-30 ■ (A) Lateral radiograph and (B) sagittal T1-weighted image of the foot showing multifocal low-grade haemangioendotheliomas involving the first metatarsal, calcaneus and distal tibia.

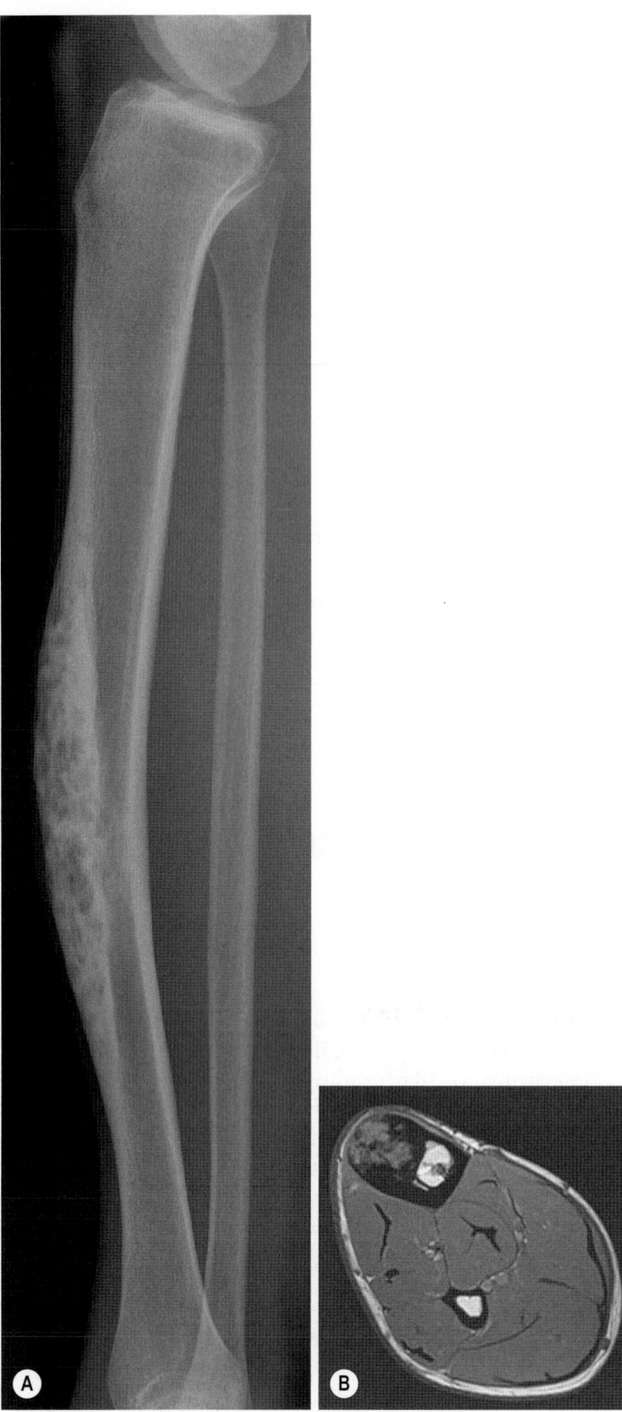

FIGURE 48-31 ■ (A) Lateral radiograph and (B) axial T1-weighted image showing an adamantinoma. Typical features include the anterior, diaphyseal location arising in the tibia.

Although it has some histological resemblance to maxillofacial adamantinoma (ameloblastoma) the two conditions are not related. Most cases in the long bones occur between 10 and 50 years of age, with an average age of 35 years. There is a slight male preponderance but a higher female incidence is found at the younger end of the age range. Patients typically present with local pain and tenderness of several months to several year' duration. Ninety per cent of cases arise in the tibia, mostly in the mid-diaphysis, but almost as commonly towards either meta-diaphysis. The typical radiographic appearances are those of multiple well-defined lucencies with interspersed sclerosis eccentrically originating in the anterior cortex of the tibia (Fig. 48-31). MRI shows marrow extension in 60% of cases, and extraosseous extension and multifocal distribution in 30% cases.[43] It is a locally aggressive tumour with a tendency to recur if incompletely removed. Metastases to the lung have been reported in approximately 10% of cases. The imaging appearances of adamantinoma can be indistinguishable from osteofibrous dysplasia, a benign tumour also with a predilection for the anterior tibial diaphysis. Histological similarities also exist between the two conditions, leading to the concept that osteofibrous dysplasia may be a precursor of adamantinoma. However, longitudinal studies have failed to show progression of osteofibrous dysplasia to adamantinoma. Another suggestion is that the two conditions represent the benign and malignant ends of a spectrum of the same condition.[44]

For a full list of references, please see ExpertConsult.

FURTHER READING

6. Mirels H. Metastatic disease in long bones. A proposed scoring system for diagnosing impending pathological fractures. Clin Orthop Rel Res 1989;249:256–64.
7. Chang ST, Tenforde AS, Grimsrud CD, et al. Atypical femur fractures among breast cancer and multiple myeloma patients receiving intravenous bisphosphonate therapy. Bone 2012;51(3):524–7.
8. WHO. World Health Organisation Classification of Tumours of Soft Tissue and Bone. 4th ed. Lyon: International Agency for Research on Cancer, IARC Press; 2013.
9. Kricun ME. Radiographic evaluation of solitary bone lesions. Orthop Clin North Am 1983;14:39–64.
10. Littrell LA, Wenger DE, Wold LE, et al. Radiographic, CT and MR imaging features of dedifferentiated chondrosarcomas: a retrospective review of 174 de novo cases. Radiographics 2004;24(5): 1397–409.
11. Murphey MD, Walker EA, Wilson AJ, et al. From the archives of the AFIP: imaging of primary chondrosarcoma: radiologic–pathologic correlation. Radiographics 2003;23(5):1245–78.
12. Douis H, Saifuddin A. The imaging of cartilaginous bone tumours. II. Chondrosarcoma. Skeletal Radiol 2012;42(5):611–26.

CHAPTER 49

Soft Tissue Tumours

Paul O'Donnell

CHAPTER OUTLINE

INTRODUCTION

Soft tissue masses are frequently referred for imaging assessment. The exact prevalence and the ratio of benign to malignant are impossible to estimate because:

- Many patients do not seek medical attention for masses that do not appear to be growing and do not impede activities of daily living.
- If medical attention is sought, indolent masses may not be biopsied or excised.
- Formal histological assessment of superficial masses may not be obtained and many are not entered into tumour registries.
- Benign (and some malignant) masses are occasionally excised without imaging.

Soft tissue tumours may be benign, malignant or non-neoplastic and all may present in a similar manner. Benign and non-neoplastic masses are more common, with benign lesions frequently said to occur approximately one hundred times more commonly than malignant.[1] Referrals to hospital will be biased towards clinically suspicious masses and data from tumour centres give a distorted picture. In a study of 358 soft tissue masses referred from primary and secondary care, 95% of cases were benign.[2] In a large study of consultation cases referred to the Armed Forces Institute of Pathology, 68.5% of nearly 40,000 tumours were benign.[3]

The characterisation of soft tissue masses on imaging remains challenging and the histological diagnosis of sarcomas based on imaging, with a few exceptions, is frequently unsuccessful, necessitating biopsy. Benign and non-neoplastic masses may show typical imaging features, but biopsy is often still required to confirm the diagnosis.

IMAGING CHARACTERISATION OF SOFT TISSUE MASSES

Radiographs

Radiographic assessment of a soft tissue tumour has a low diagnostic yield but may still be useful, either alone or as an adjunct to cross-sectional imaging.

The utility of plain radiography has been assessed in 454 soft tissue masses referred to a tumour centre (care is needed in the extrapolation of these results from a referral population to soft tissue tumours in general).[4] There was a positive finding in 62%. The most frequent finding was identification of a mass—most soft tissue tumours show similar density to muscle but a large mass may be seen, as may distortion (but preservation) of adjacent fat planes. In this study, a mass was seen in 31%. When seen on a radiograph, the lesion was more likely to be malignant although in part this depended on the location of the lesion, with visible tumours in the hands and feet more likely to be benign or non-neoplastic and tumours in the thigh, calf and arm more likely to be malignant.

If the mass is large and contains fat in sufficient quantity, its density will be lower than that of adjacent soft tissues. Fat was seen in 7% of the masses: 50% were well-differentiated liposarcomas/atypical lipomatous tumours (see below), with benign fat-containing lesions including lipoma, haemangioma, hibernoma and lipoblastoma.

Foreign bodies may be visualised on radiographs of a mass, as may a surrounding inflammatory reaction. Typically, glass and metal are visible but wood and plastic may not have sufficient density to be seen.

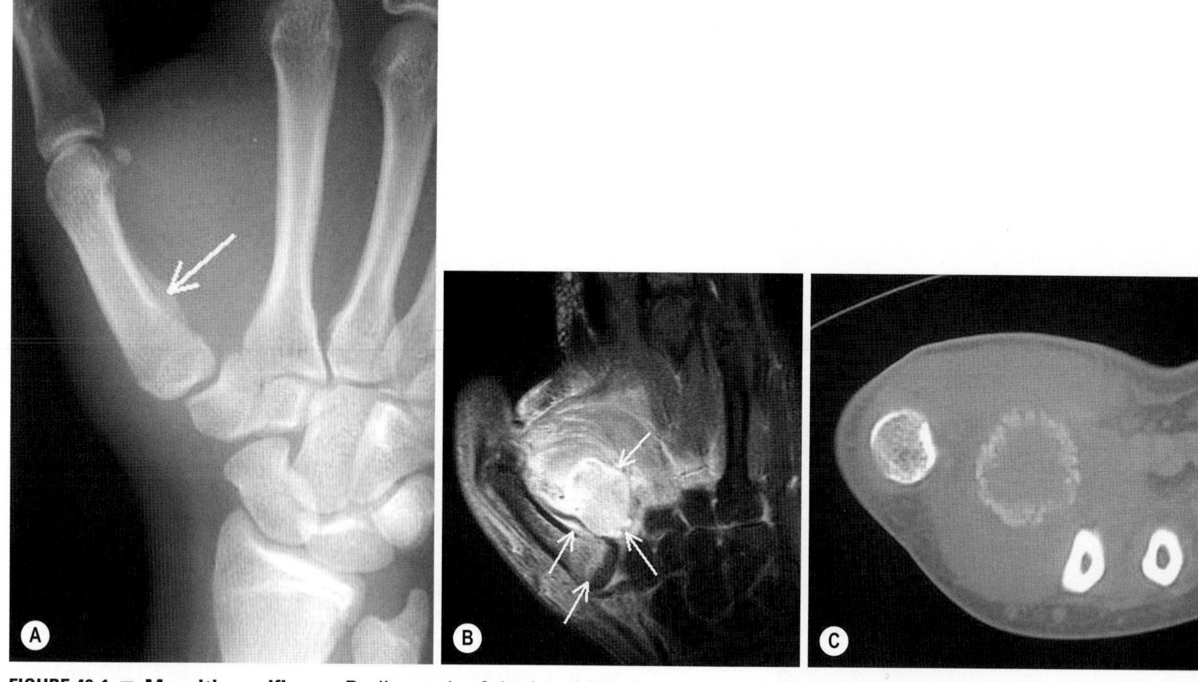

FIGURE 49-1 ■ **Myositis ossificans.** Radiograph of the hand (A) shows a soft tissue mass and periostitis on the palmar aspect of the thumb metacarpal (arrow). Coronal STIR MR image of the hand (B) shows a poorly demarcated hyperintense mass with surrounding soft tissue oedema (arrows). There is also marrow oedema and periosteal reaction in the thumb metacarpal (arrows). Axial CT (C) shows ossification at the periphery of the mass.

Mineralisation was present in 17% of the soft tissue masses in the study. Phleboliths, due to dystrophic mineralisation of thrombus in abnormal vessels, may be seen and are the hallmark of venous malformations. The pattern of calcification may give an indication of the underlying histological nature of the mass. Chondral calcification (for example in soft tissue chondral tumours and synovial chondromatosis) may take the form of punctate foci in comma shapes, rings and arcs, suggesting cartilage. Ossification (for example in myositis ossificans), when mature, forms trabeculae and a cortex, with density at the periphery greater than at the centre. When immature, it forms a rather amorphous, mineralised mass. The pattern of calcification does not always help with the diagnosis. Synovial sarcomas, approximately 30% of which are mineralised, may display chondroid or either type of osteoid matrix.[4]

Abnormality of a bone due to an adjacent soft tissue mass may take several forms. The study by Gartner et al. showed cortical erosion, periosteal reaction, scalloping, intramedullary extension and pathological fracture affecting approximately 14% of subjects,[4] and 39% of these were malignant. Changes were in general non-specific, with benign, non-neoplastic and malignant lesions capable of a wide range of interactions with the adjacent bone. Periosteal reaction was uncommon (4.4%), but 70% of cases showing it were non-malignant.

Computed Tomography (CT)

Evaluation of the soft tissue mass with CT is useful in some cases but, as with radiographs, it is often not tissue specific, as many masses show similar attenuation to muscle. The radiographic features of a soft tissue mass are demonstrated at least as well using CT and it is more sensitive for the identification of small amounts of fat and calcium. As an adjunct to MRI and radiographs, CT is useful for showing the peripheral ossification in myositis ossificans, confirming what may be a difficult MRI diagnosis (Fig. 49-1). CT angiography (and specifically arteriography) is helpful for the preoperative assessment of tumours close to vessels.

Ultrasound (US)

US has been shown to be a useful triage tool for masses referred from primary or secondary care.[2] It can play an important role in confirming a mass is present and not due to a normal anatomical structure or variant (such as an accessory muscle). It can also differentiate solid from cystic lesions. However, once a solid mass has been confirmed, further characterisation with US may be limited, often requiring further assessment with MRI and possible biopsy. As an adjunct to MRI, US can further characterise masses that show fluid signal intensity (cysts and solid myxoid masses), assess vascularity and compressibility (typically of venous malformations (Fig. 49-2)) and allows valuable clinical correlation by the examining radiologist.

Diagnostic features may be present in some lesions and these are more frequently benign or non-neoplastic. Examples include traumatic (muscle/tendon tear, haematoma), infective (abscess, pyomyositis), lipomatous

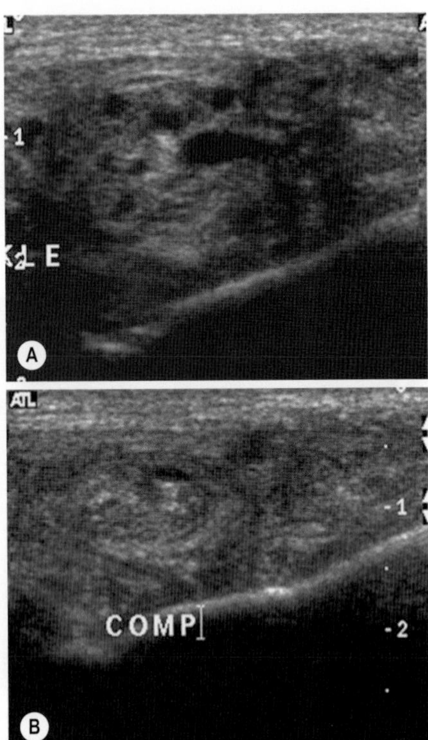

FIGURE 49-2 ■ **Venous malformation.** Ultrasound images without (A) and with (B) compression. A low-reflectivity mass contains tubular structures consistent with vessels, which rarely show blood flow on colour Doppler—occasionally, static or very slowly flowing blood can be seen on grey-scale images. With light probe pressure, the vascular and non-vascular elements are compressed.

(superficial and deep fatty masses—the latter usually need further assessment with MRI), vascular (thrombophlebitis, venous malformation, pseudoaneurysm) and neurogenic (nerve sheath tumours, nerve pseudotumours).

In the differentiation of a malignant from a benign solid mass, the grey-scale appearances are usually non-specific. The assessment of tumour vascularity using colour/power and pulsed Doppler is possible with US and greater success has been claimed. Tumour neovascularity is an important feature of malignancy—tumour vessels are anatomically abnormal, lacking a muscular layer and showing irregular contour. This results in a heterogeneous network of abnormal vessels, often chaotically distributed within the tumour, with abnormal flow characteristics and morphology. A study of benign and malignant masses with high vascularity showed that the pattern of vessels within a mass was of limited value in the distinction of benign and malignant, but that in the presence of an organised pattern, a benign diagnosis was more likely.[5] An organised vascular pattern has been shown in 77% of benign and a disorganised pattern in 80% of malignant soft tissue tumours.[6] The atypical morphology of vessels in malignant masses may result in vessel trifurcations (rather than bifurcations), stenoses, occlusions and an anarchic rather than an hierarchical branching pattern.[7] Identification of any two of these 'major' criteria enabled malignant and benign masses to be distinguished.

Magnetic Resonance Imaging (MRI)

MRI is the technique of choice for local staging of a soft tissue mass, especially if it is in a deep location where US may be less able to assess tumour extent and relations. It is sensitive, can be tissue-specific and allows assessment of most masses, no matter where they are located. Despite this, MRI is often not sufficiently tissue specific to allow confident identification of some deep, solid masses; distinction of myxoid from cystic masses can be difficult without contrast medium and small calcific foci may not be seen. MRI also overlaps with radiography in its ability to identify fat, a foreign body and bone involvement in a soft tissue mass: differentiation of mineralisation and gas may require radiographs or CT, as both show hypointensity on T2-weighted (T2W) images and also on other fluid-sensitive sequences (see below).

Most tumours, and certainly most soft tissue sarcomas, are isointense to muscle on T1-weighted (T1W) images, of intermediate signal intensity on T2 images (similar to fat) and hyperintense on inversion recovery (STIR) or T2W images with fat saturation. As with US, specific diagnoses can sometimes be suggested based on the MRI appearances, more often with benign and non-neoplastic lesions, which may exhibit specific signal characteristics. Examples of MRI signal that allow characterisation and occasionally an MRI diagnosis (in combination with lesion morphology) include T1 hyperintensity, T2 hypointensity and T2 hyperintensity (fluid signal).

Hyperintensity on T1W imaging is commonly due to fat or subacute haemorrhage (methaemoglobin), but may also be due to melanin.

Hypointensity on T2W imaging may be due to calcification, fibrous tissue, chronic haemorrhage (haemosiderin), rapidly flowing blood (for example in an arteriovenous malformation or aneurysm) or gas. A radiograph is useful for excluding calcification as a cause.

Hyperintensity on T2W imaging may be seen in cystic masses, abscesses, myxoid masses (which include intramuscular myxomas, sarcomas and some nerve sheath tumours) and low-flow vascular malformations.

The presence of fluid–fluid levels is a non-specific sign in soft tissue masses: they are rare and equally common in benign and malignant lesions. The presence of haemorrhage is, however, useful—tumour necrosis is often seen in high-grade sarcomas; certain sarcomas (particularly synovial sarcoma) frequently show haemorrhagic foci (in synovial sarcomas up to 47%).

Staging of soft tissue sarcomas is best undertaken with MRI. This requires documentation of the size and local extent of the tumour, including any extracompartmental spread and the relationship of the tumour to adjacent structures such as bones, joints and neurovascular bundles. Initial staging will also usually require a chest radiograph and CT to exclude pulmonary metastases.

WORLD HEALTH ORGANIZATION CLASSIFICATION OF SOFT TISSUE TUMOURS[8]

The most recent version (2002) classified the following types of soft tissue tumours

- Adipocytic
- Fibroblastic/myofibroblastic
- So-called fibrohistiocytic tumours
- Smooth muscle tumours
- Pericytic/perivascular tumours
- Skeletal muscle tumours
- Vascular tumours
- Chondro-osseous tumours
- Tumours of uncertain differentiation

into the categories benign, intermediate and malignant. Several changes were made in this updated classification, including the recognition of two distinct types of intermediate malignancy ('locally aggressive' and 'rarely metastasising') and the reclassification of malignant fibrous histiocytoma, previously considered the commonest type of soft tissue sarcoma, as undifferentiated pleomorphic sarcoma. Many of the changes will be irrelevant to the imaging assessment of a soft tissue mass—the pathological diagnosis is being continually refined, particularly with the evolution of genetic techniques. It should be noted that peripheral nerve and skin tumours, both of which present as soft tissue masses, are considered in separate WHO classifications. Metastases to soft tissue and haematological malignancies, particularly lymphoma, may also present as a soft tissue mass.[9] Imaging is useful in the diagnosis of some of these soft tissue lesions and will be discussed below.

LIPOMATOUS (ADIPOCYTIC) TUMOURS

Lipomatous neoplasms are the most frequent mesenchymal tumours, with subcutaneous lipomas thought to represent up to 50% of all soft tissue tumours[10] and liposarcoma representing the commonest soft tissue sarcoma.[8]

Lipoma

This is a benign adipocytic tumour and the commonest mesenchymal neoplasm in adults. Lipomas typically occur in adults in the fifth to seventh decades with no sex predilection. They are rare in children and may be multiple.[8] Superficial (subcutaneous) tumours are common but lipomas may also occur in deep locations (intramuscular or intermuscular), or even adjacent to bone (parosteal), where they may stimulate a periosteal response. Subcutaneous lipomas are often diagnosed with great accuracy on clinical grounds alone, presenting as small (usually <5 cm), painless, firm, mobile masses.[11] Deep lipomas are often larger, but again usually painless. They cannot be diagnosed clinically and imaging is needed to confirm the diagnosis in deeper lesions. Atypical clinical presentation includes pain due to nerve compression in restricted spaces such as the carpal, tarsal and cubital tunnels.

Lipomas can contain other non-lipomatous elements contributing to a heterogeneous imaging appearance, vessels (angiolipoma), muscle (myolipoma), cartilage (chondrolipoma), bone (osteolipoma—following trauma or ischaemia) or extensive myxoid change (myxolipoma). Fibrous tissue and foci of fat necrosis can also cause a heterogeneous appearance.

Radiographs

Large lipomas are visible as areas of relative lucency (compared with soft tissue) (Fig. 49-3), but small lesions are not visible. Foci of mineralisation (calcification, ossification) are visible in 11%.[11]

Ultrasound

Subcutaneous lipomas are usually elliptical masses, often well-defined, with their long axis orientated parallel to the skin surface (Fig. 49-4). Their reflectivity is variable, while subcutaneous fat is usually low in reflectivity (unless previously inflamed or traumatised); lipomas are relatively reflective, often showing septation orientated along the long axis of the lesion. One study showed 29% had lower reflectivity than surrounding tissues and the

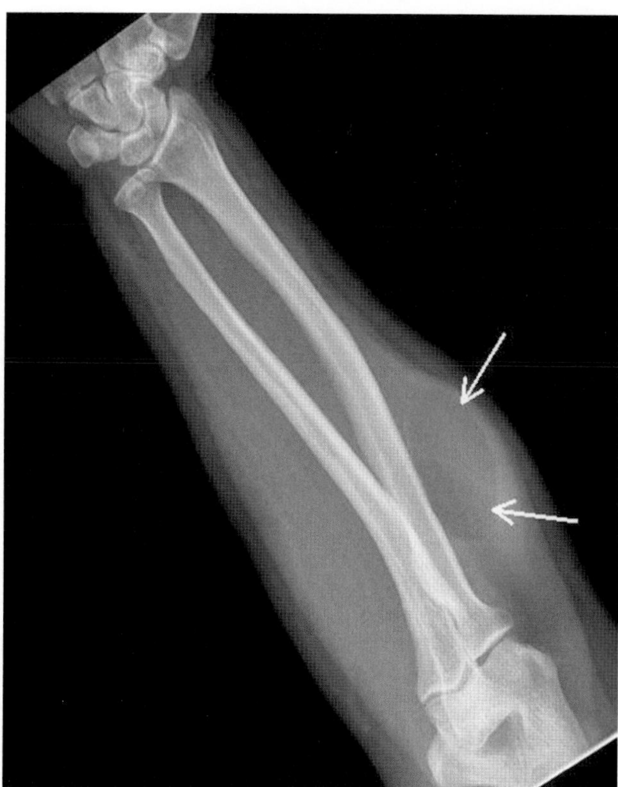

FIGURE 49-3 ■ **Lipoma.** AP radiograph shows an ovoid lucent mass (arrows) projected over the lateral aspect of the forearm.

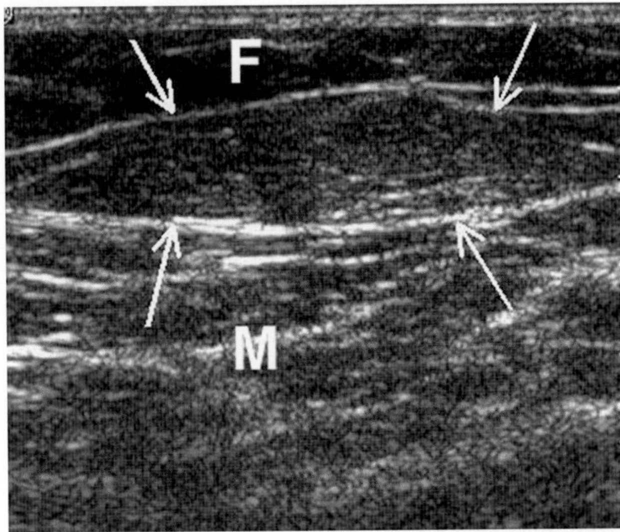

FIGURE 49-4 ■ **Subcutaneous lipoma.** Ultrasound image shows an elliptical mass (arrows), lower in reflectivity than adjacent muscle (M) but more reflective than subcutaneous fat (F). There are thin septations in the long axis of the mass.

remainder was of similar, greater or mixed reflectivity.[12] Light pressure with the ultrasound probe shows the lesions are compressible. They may appear encapsulated although many lipomas appear to blend with the surrounding tissues without evidence of a capsule.

Computed Tomography

This is rarely performed in the case of a subcutaneous lesion, but may show a mass of density similar to that of subcutaneous fat. Non-encapsulated lipomas may be occult. Deeper lesions are more likely to show heterogeneity (non-lipomatous elements, foci of mineralisation).

Magnetic Resonance Imaging

The mass is isointense to subcutaneous fat on T1- and T2W imaging, showing low signal intensity on STIR images and suppression of fat signal on T2W imaging with fat saturation. Fine septa (often immeasurable, typically less than 2 mm) are often seen, but the absence of thick or nodular septa is useful for differentiating a lipoma from a well-differentiated liposarcoma/atypical lipomatous tumour. Fine septa are also less likely to show gadolinium enhancement in benign lesions, which is also useful for differentiation.[13] Focal areas of non-adipose tissue (including fibrosis and necrosis) are not infrequent in benign tumours (particularly deep lesions) and make the distinction from a well-differentiated liposarcoma impossible on imaging alone. Mineralisation (calcification and ossification) may also be seen in benign tumours.

Intramuscular lipomas can be diagnosed with a high degree of confidence; an infiltrative margin and intermingled muscle fibres within and at the periphery of the lesion are features that make it possible to differentiate from other lipomatous tumours[14] (Fig. 49-5).

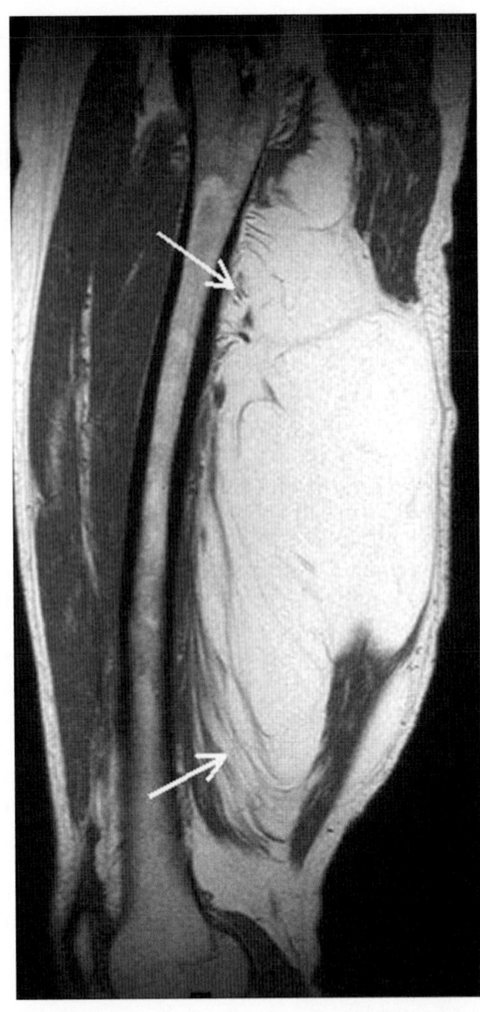

FIGURE 49-5 ■ **Intramuscular lipoma.** Sagittal T1-weighted MR image of the thigh: large, well-differentiated (predominantly fatty) lipomatous mass showing muscle fibres at the periphery (arrows).

Although they may be seen in simple lipomas, the following MRI features are atypical and should suggest the possibility of a well-differentiated liposarcoma:

- incomplete suppression of signal on fat-suppressed sequences
- thick, nodular septa (particularly if they enhance)
- focal non-lipomatous areas.

Other Benign Adipocytic Tumours

Lipoblastoma

Lipoblastoma is a tumour occurring in children—88% of patients are under 3 years old and the median age at onset is 1 year.[15] They usually occur in the extremities and consist of both mature and immature adipocytes (lipoblasts).[8] Lesions in younger patients contain prominent areas of myxoid tissue and MRI appearances may mimic a myxoid liposarcoma. However, they undergo a process of maturation, showing a tendency to develop into lipomas.[16] Imaging reveals a heterogeneous fatty mass on US, CT and MRI, due to myxoid and cystic areas, but, as both lipoma and liposarcoma are rare in young children, the diagnosis can be suggested in the presence of a heterogeneous fat-containing mass in a patient of the correct age.

Hibernoma

Hibernoma is a rare benign tumour composed of brown fat most frequently occurring in the thigh. The tumour appears lipomatous, but usually shows subtly different signal characteristics from those of subcutaneous fat, with hypointensity on T1W imaging and failure to suppress fully on fat-saturated images. Serpentine vessels may be identified within the highly vascular mass, a rare finding in an atypical lipomatous tumour/well-differentiated liposarcoma.[11]

Atypical Lipomatous Tumour/Well-Differentiated Liposarcoma (ALT/WDL)

These lesions are synonymous and classified as intermediate (locally aggressive) malignancies. They account for 40–45% of all liposarcomas and are the commonest subtype of liposarcoma.[8] ALT/WDL are well-differentiated tumours, often predominantly fatty, and show no capacity for metastasis unless dedifferentiation occurs (see below). Although ALT and WDL are identical morphologically and genetically, the term ALT is used for tumours in surgically accessible sites, such as the limbs and trunk, where complete excision is curative. WDL is usually used for tumours in inaccessible sites, such as the mediastinum and retroperitoneum, where complete excision may not be possible and the disease may eventually be fatal following uncontrolled recurrence.

These tumours occur in middle age, most commonly in the sixth decade and there is no sex predilection. They arise in the deep soft tissues of the limbs, retroperitoneum, paratesticular area and mediastinum—rarely they occur subcutaneously.[8] Imaging shows a deep lipomatous mass with varying degrees of heterogeneity. The following features favour a diagnosis of a malignant rather than a benign tumour: lesion size >10 cm, thick, nodular septa, presence of globular or nodular non-adipose areas and fat content less than 75%[17] (Fig. 49-6). Incomplete fat suppression suggests a liposarcoma,[18] while septal enhancement is more likely if the lesion is malignant and may be more important than the thickness of the septa.[13,19] Although on imaging the differentiation of a lipoma in a deep location from ALT/WDL is unreliable, with considerable overlap in the appearances, it is largely irrelevant to initial management. Both are well-differentiated lipomatous neoplasms and would usually be treated by primary excision, with as wide a margin as possible, without prior biopsy.

Other Adipocytic Malignancies

The other major types of liposarcoma are dedifferentiated, myxoid and pleomorphic (pleomorphic liposarcoma is a very rare high-grade tumour). With higher grades of malignancy, fat becomes less conspicuous on MRI, such that there may be no suggestion of an adipocytic tumour in many liposarcomas.

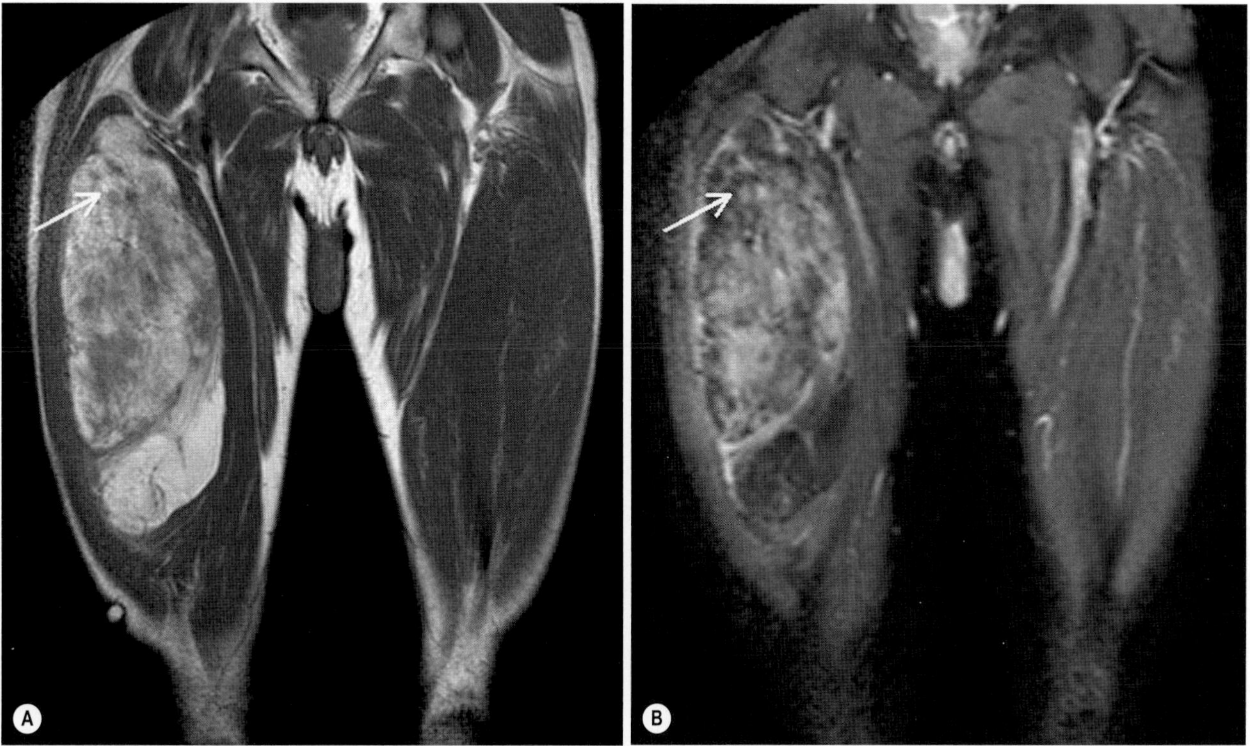

FIGURE 49-6 ■ **Atypical lipomatous tumour/well-differentiated liposarcoma.** Coronal T1 (A) and STIR (B) MR images showing a heterogeneous, partially fatty mass in the right thigh, with extensive areas of non-lipomatous signal, some small nodular foci superiorly (arrows) and thick septation.

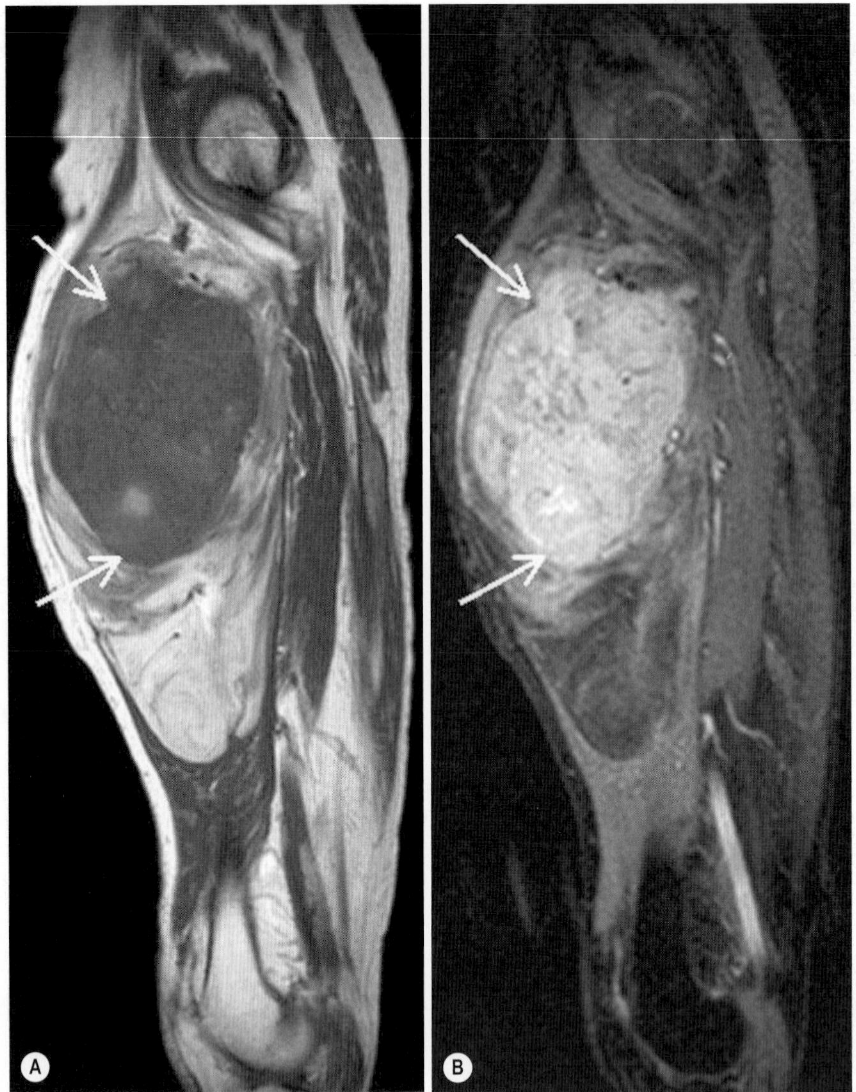

FIGURE 49-7 ■ **Dedifferentiated liposarcoma.** Sagittal T1 (A) and STIR (B) MR images showing a lipomatous mass. At the superior aspect of the mass there is a well-defined non-fatty tumour, corresponding to the dedifferentiated component (arrows).

Dedifferentiated Liposarcoma

Dedifferentiated liposarcoma results from the transition of ALT/WDL to a non-lipogenic sarcoma of variable grade and may occur in the primary tumour (90%) or in a recurrent lesion. The risk of dedifferentiation is greatest in retroperitoneal tumours and occurs in up to 10% of ALT/WDL—this may be time dependent rather than location dependent. It is usually a high-grade tumour, with the dedifferentiated component seen as a discrete non-lipomatous tumour within the fatty mass, reflected in both the histological and radiological appearances (Fig. 49-7). Occasionally, there is a gradual transition from lipomatous to non-lipomatous sarcoma.

Myxoid Liposarcoma

Myxoid liposarcoma is the second most common type of liposarcoma, accounting for approximately 10% of adult soft tissue sarcomas. The tumour consists of a myxoid stroma containing primitive non-lipogenic mesenchymal cells and a variable number of lipoblasts. An imaging diagnosis based on its MRI appearances is frequently possible and dependent on identifying the myxoid component, which resembles fluid, along with a fatty component, usually in the form of thin T1 hyperintense septa (often subtle) (Fig. 49-8). In the most recent WHO classification of soft tissue tumours, round cell liposarcoma, previously considered separately as the cellular, high-grade variant of myxoid liposarcoma, was reclassified as a synonymous lesion.

FIBROBLASTIC/MYOFIBROBLASTIC TUMOURS

Nodular Fasciitis (NF)

This is a fibrous proliferation that forms a rapidly growing mass, usually in the subcutaneous tissues, but is also found in intramuscular and intermuscular (fascial) sites.

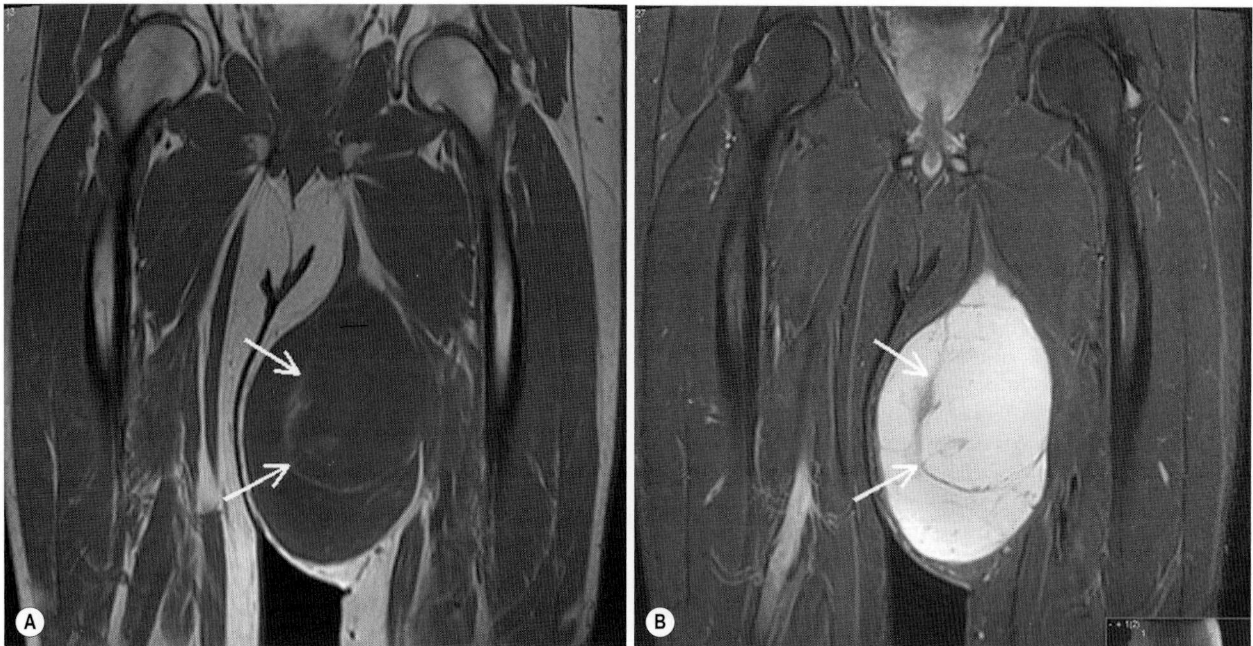

FIGURE 49-8 ■ **Myxoid liposarcoma.** Coronal T1 (A) and STIR (B) MR images showing a large mass at the medial aspect of the thigh with fluid signal characteristics, in keeping with a myxoid tumour, and thin fatty septa (arrows).

Owing to its rapid growth, cellular histology and frequent (although not atypical[8]) mitoses, inappropriately aggressive surgery may be performed. It is said to be the commonest lesion of fibrous origin,[20] occurring in all age groups, but most commonly affecting young adults,[8] with no sex predilection. The most frequent sites of involvement are the upper limb (48%) and trunk (20%),[20] although any site is possible. Imaging shows a mass, which is usually small (< 5 cm in maximum dimension, mean 2.2 cm diameter in one series[20]), and often poorly defined, whose MRI characteristics reflect the histology: the nodule undergoes a process of maturation, with early, cellular lesions containing myxoid tissue (near-fluid signal intensities, but slight T1 hyperintensity compared with muscle), later becoming fibrotic (hypointense on all sequences, including T1). NF has been treated, following confirmatory biopsy, with intralesional steroid injection and surgery, with few recurrences following excision.[21]

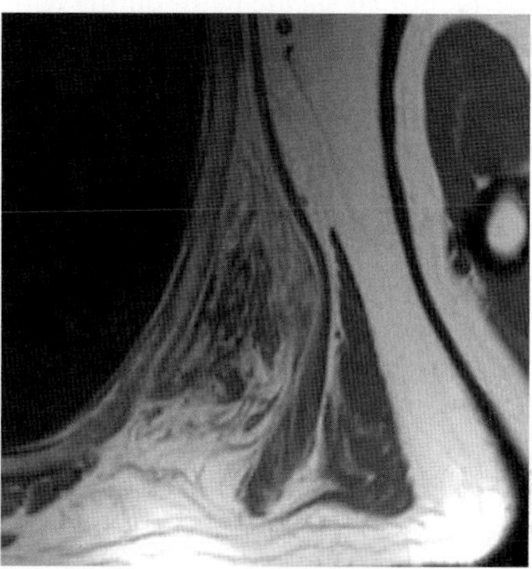

FIGURE 49-9 ■ **Elastofibroma.** Axial T1 image at the inferior aspect of the scapula, showing a soft tissue mass deep to serratus anterior. It consists of fatty (hyperintense) and fibrous (hypointense) striations.

Elastofibroma (EF)

This is a tumour-like lesion (fibroelastic pseudotumour) occurring almost exclusively in elderly patients, consisting of mature adipose tissue entrapped within a fibrous mass, typically found adjacent to the inferior angle of the scapula. When typical in location and appearance on MRI, no biopsy is required and marginal resection suffices. The lesion is common and often bilateral. Over 50% of cases are said to be asymptomatic[22] and it is a frequent postmortem finding.[23] There is a reported prevalence of 2% in subjects >60 years undergoing chest CT for lung disease.[24] EF is thought to arise as a result of friction between the scapula and chest wall, possibly due to manual labour, resulting in collagen degeneration, but familial cases do exist.

Over 99% occur at the typical chest wall location, but other sites, including visceral sites, have been described.[8] US shows non-specific appearances but the mass can be revealed, sometimes fairly dramatically, with shoulder adduction. The appearances on CT and MRI reflect its fibroadipose contents. EF contains alternating striations of fat and fibrous tissue and is typically elliptical, located deep to serratus anterior (Fig. 49-9). The striations parallel the chest wall. Bilateral, symmetrical masses may cause confusion, as the mass may superficially resemble muscle.

Fibromatoses

These are intermediate-grade (locally aggressive) lesions[8] which are further classified as superficial (palmar/plantar) and desmoid-type fibromatosis.

Superficial Fibromatosis

Palmar Fibromatosis (Dupuytren's Disease). Palmar fibromatosis (Dupuytren's disease) is characterised by the development of fibrous nodules and subsequently cord-like bands within subcutaneous tissue, typically located on the ulnar aspect of the palm of the hand. They cause thickening and contraction of the skin and also affect the palmar aponeurosis and flexor tendons, usually of the ring and little fingers. A debilitating flexion deformity may result (Dupuytren's contracture) and it is the severity of the deformity and functional deficit that determines whether surgical resection is needed, although recurrence is frequent. Nodules show low reflectivity on US, but MRI may be more useful as signal characteristics within nodules and cords appear to correlate with cellularity. Cellular lesions (relatively hyperintense to the adjacent tendon on T1- and T2W imaging) are more likely to recur following excision.[25]

Plantar Fibromatosis (Ledderhose Disease). Plantar fibromatosis (Ledderhose disease) is histologically identical to palmar fibromatosis but involves the plantar aspect of the foot where nodules or larger masses arise in the plantar fascia, most often at its medial aspect. Nodules may be small, in which case they are often asymptomatic, and may be identified incidentally during US examination. Larger lesions may cause pain on prolonged standing and walking, and may be multiple. The appearances of a mass arising from the plantar fascia, showing low or intermediate MRI signal intensity, are frequently diagnostic (Fig. 49-10). Treatment is usually conservative, with excision reserved for large, debilitating lesions.[26]

Other Forms. Other forms of superficial fibromatosis include knuckle pads (fibrous masses at the dorsal aspects of the MCP and PIP joints) and Peyronie's (penile) fibromatosis. Superficial lesions in different sites may coexist.

Desmoid-Type Fibromatosis

This encompasses previously used terms such as deep, aggressive or musculoaponeurotic fibromatosis and extra-abdominal desmoid tumour. It is a clonal fibroblastic proliferation occurring in deep soft tissues, typically locally invasive but without the capacity to metastasise.[8] Young adults are most frequently affected, but the lesion may present at any age and in any location. The commoner sites include shoulder, chest wall and back, thigh and head and neck.[8] Abdominal wall and intra-abdominal involvement were previously considered as distinct subtypes.

When a mass occurs in a superficial site, it may appear very firm. Occasionally, this only becomes apparent at the time of needle biopsy, when it may be difficult to puncture the mass due to its consistency. Symptoms arise due to the infiltration or mass effect on adjacent structures, such as joints and nerves; the mass itself is usually painless. US shows a heterogeneous, solid mass which may be in a deep location, mimicking a sarcoma. CT is also usually non-specific, but densely collagenous lesions show higher attenuation, and the poorly defined nature of the mass may be appreciated.[26] The diagnosis may be apparent from MRI, although the appearances are highly variable. The hallmark of desmoid-type fibromatosis is low-signal bands of tissue which represent dense bundles of collagen (Fig. 49-11). Low signal intensity (SI) on

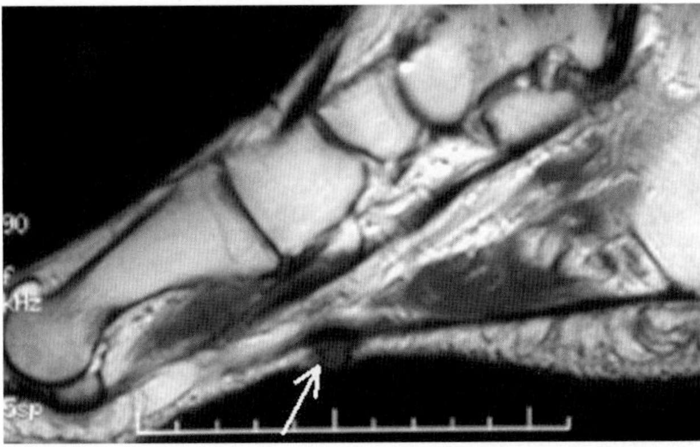

FIGURE 49-10 ■ Plantar fibroma. Sagittal T2 MR image showing a low-signal mass arising from the medial aspect of the plantar fascia (arrow).

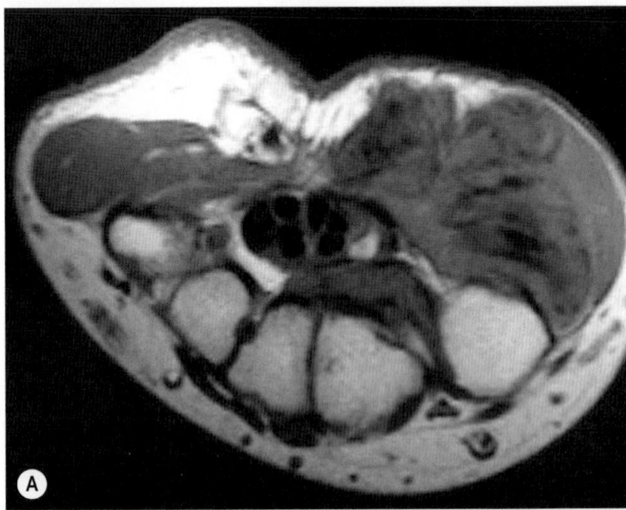

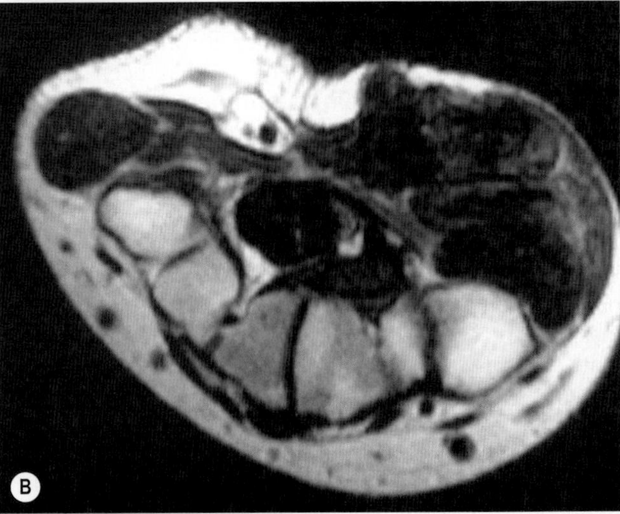

FIGURE 49-11 ■ Desmoid-type fibromatosis. Axial T1 (A) and T2 (B) MR images show a heterogeneous mass in the thenar eminence, which is mildly hyperintense to muscle on T1W imaging and hypointense on T2W imaging. Both sequences show prominent, thick striations of low signal due to bands of dense collagen.

T2W imaging is thought to be due to a combination of high collagen content and low cellularity, with the latter possibly more important, as higher SI areas also show a high collagen content (but greater cellularity).[27] Signal elsewhere in the tumour is typically heterogeneous, but commonly intermediate on both T1- and T2W images.

Intra-abdominal tumours may occur sporadically or in association with Gardner's syndrome (an autosomal dominant condition of adenomatous intestinal polyps, multiple osteomas and desmoid-type fibromatosis).

Fibroma of the Tendon Sheath (FTS)

This typically presents as a painless, fibrous nodule related to flexor tendons, more often in the right hand.[8] The most frequently involved areas are the thumb, index and middle fingers, the palmar aspect of the hand and volar aspect of the wrist (these locations accounting for 80% of cases), but it also occurs in the knee and foot. Triggering of a finger may result, as may pressure symptoms if the lesion arises outside the fingers (for example median nerve pressure from a lesion in the carpal tunnel).[8] The lesion most commonly affects males in the fourth decade. T1- and T2W MRI shows a low-signal nodule or mass related to a tendon, which may have imaging appearances similar to those of giant cell tumour of the tendon sheath (see below), but does not show accentuation of low signal on T2* gradient-echo images ('blooming').

SO-CALLED FIBROHISTIOCYTIC TUMOURS

Pigmented Villonodular Synovitis (PVNS) and Giant Cell Tumour of the Tendon Sheath (GCTTS)

These terms encompass a number of related conditions, arising from the synovium of joints, tendon sheaths and bursae. It should be noted that giant cell tumour of tendon sheath described here is not related to the giant cell tumour of bone. Lesions may present as a localised mass related to a tendon sheath or bursa (GCTTS), as diffuse involvement of a joint or tendon sheath (pigmented villonodular synovitis (PVNS) or tenosynovitis) or as a localised intra-articular mass (localised intra-articular PVNS), most often in the knee.[28] Lesions in the tendon sheath present most commonly as a soft tissue mass.

Localised, mass-like GCTTS is usually painless, but may interfere with tendon function or cause local pressure effects. GCTTS is most often seen in adults with a male : female patient ratio of 2 : 1.[8] Although the lesion may occur at many sites, including the feet, wrists and ankles, most cases (around 85%) occur in the fingers (it is the second most common soft tissue tumour of the hand after ganglia), usually closely related to a tendon sheath (typically flexor). Radiographs are frequently abnormal and may reveal not only the mass but also pressure erosion and cortical destruction (Fig. 49-12); they may also cause bone expansion with intraosseous growth. The lesions may occasionally cause a periosteal reaction and have been reported to show calcification. In one series of hand tumours, 11% of 133 cases showed an abnormality of the adjacent bone.[29]

On US the mass is usually homogeneous and of low reflectivity, showing internal vascularity. Cystic change is not usually seen but there may be posterior acoustic enhancement. The mass may just contact or completely encase the tendon, often extending between tendon and bone, but it does not move with the tendon due to the intervening tendon sheath. Bone erosions may be seen on US. On MRI, haemosiderin contained within the mass may give characteristically low signal intensity on all sequences, especially T2* gradient-echo images. A well-defined mass, showing low-to-intermediate signal on T1- and T2W images and exaggerated low signal on T2*, located on the flexor aspect of the fingers and related to the tendon, is highly suggestive of the diagnosis of GCTTS.

The localised intra-articular form of PVNS is a similar lesion to GCTTS, but is found almost exclusively at the knee and frequently in the infrapatellar (Hoffa's) fat pad.[30] It may also be seen in the suprapatellar pouch and intercondylar notch. Typically, there is a well-defined mass, which shows similar signal intensities on MRI to GCTTS (Fig. 49-13). The lesion may also contain fluid-signal linear foci. As with any predominantly low-signal mass in Hoffa's fat pad (or in any other location), radiographs are useful for excluding mineralisation—soft tissue chondromas also typically occur in this region. Simple excision of the mass is appropriate for typical GCTTS in the hand and localised nodular PVNS. Treatment of diffuse intra-articular PVNS may involve extensive synovectomy, with a much greater chance of recurrence.

Diffuse-Type Pigmented Villonodular Synovitis (Diffuse-Type Giant Cell Tumour)

This term encompasses PVNS, a diffuse synovial proliferation in a joint characterised by recurrent haemarthroses, and similar synovial processes in tendon sheaths (pigmented villonodular tenosynovitis).[8] PVNS presents as a chronic monoarthropathy in a large joint and this condition is further discussed in Chapter 51. Pigmented villonodular tenosynovitis may present as soft tissue swelling along the line of a tendon sheath which will be seen on MRI to contain fluid and synovitis; the latter may show evidence of haemosiderin with low signal intensity on all sequences.

VASCULAR TUMOURS

Haemangioma

The classification of benign vascular lesions is complex and may cause confusion. The International Society for

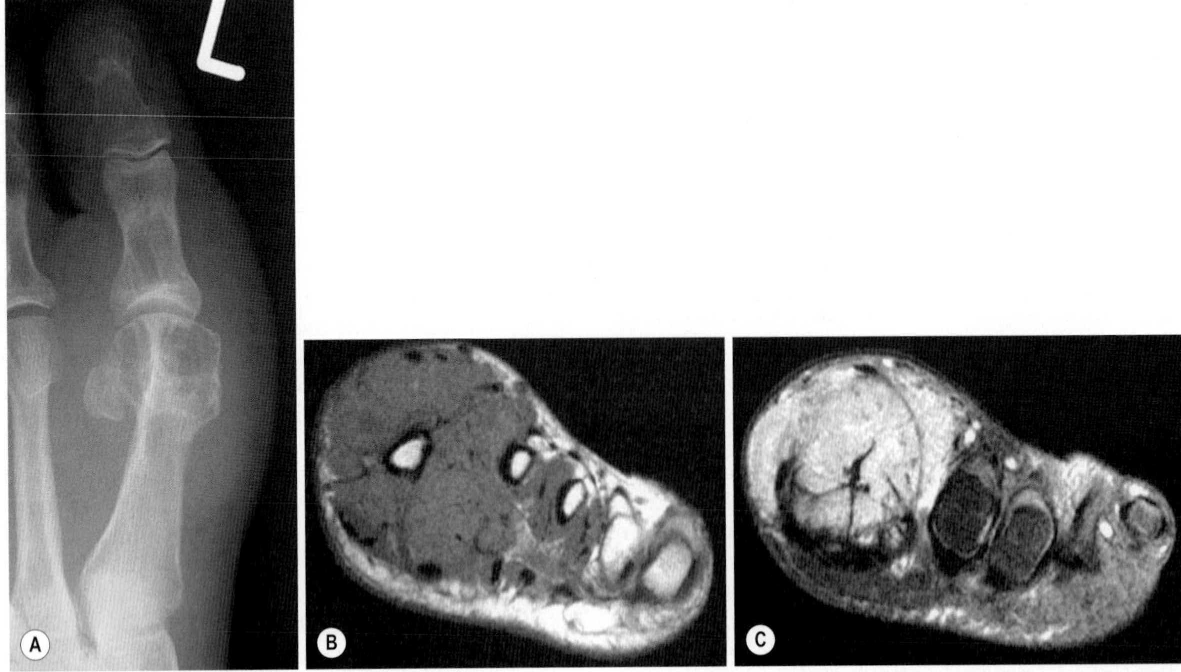

FIGURE 49-12 ■ **Giant cell tumour of the tendon sheath.** (A) Dorsoplantar radiograph shows a large mass in the region of the first metatarsophalangeal joint, with circumferential pressure erosion and lobular lucency in the metatarsal head. Axial T1 (B, slightly proximal) and STIR (C) MR images show a circumferential tumour invading bone at the metatarsal head.

the Study of Vascular Anomalies (ISSVA) differentiates vascular tumours, the most common of which is infantile haemangioma, and vascular malformations. The latter are subclassified into high-flow lesions, containing an arterial component (arteriovenous malformations (AVMs) and arteriovenous fistulas (AVFs)) and low-flow lesions (venous, lymphatic, capillary and mixed (capillary–venous and capillary–lymphatic–venous)).[31]

Haemangiomas are benign vascular tumours of infancy, usually presenting in the first few weeks of life and affecting 2–3% of children.[32] Following an initial period of rapid growth, there is a subsequent slow involution.

Malformations are congenital lesions consisting of dysplastic vascular channels, often unappreciated at birth but which enlarge with the patient and do not regress. High-flow (arteriovenous) malformations may present in childhood or adulthood. Clinical symptoms depend on location and size, but may include pain, tissue overgrowth (rapid growth can occur after minor trauma), bleeding or, with large AVMs, high-output cardiac failure. An abnormality is apparent in the skin, which may be pulsatile, with a palpable thrill and audible bruit.

Many of the lesions referred to as haemangiomas in adults are more accurately described as low-flow, frequently venous, vascular malformations. The WHO classification refers to these lesions as venous haemangiomas.[8] Venous malformations (VMs) account for half to two-thirds of low-flow vascular malformations;[33] lesions are usually purely venous, but may contain capillary or lymphatic elements. They are congenital, but are not always evident at birth. Occasionally, a patch of blue skin discoloration is visible with superficial lesions. With growth of the patient, there is enlargement—fluctuation in size is often reported (depending on enlargement), but there is no significant local warmth of the skin or thrill. The tumour is soft and compressible, exerting no significant mass effect. Eventually, multiple tissue planes and anatomical structures may be affected (skin, fat, muscle, bone). Up to 40% of venous malformations occur in the head and neck, 20% in the trunk and 40% in the extremities.[34]

VMs consist of abnormal venous channels and variable amounts of hamartomatous stroma which contains adipose tissue. The vessels are dysplastic, post-capillary, thin-walled vascular channels which show patchy deficiency of mural smooth muscle—they dilate with time due to repeated stretching, allowing growth and infiltration of adjacent structures.[33] Thrombosis of vessels is frequent and dystrophic calcification within thrombus results in phleboliths. A localised coagulopathy develops within VMs due to consumption of clotting factors, increasing the risk of haemorrhage at surgery or if the lesions are traumatised.[35] Morbidity arises from pain and infiltration of local structures, leading to reduced mobility (muscle involvement and contracture), oedema, ulceration, bleeding and remodelling of the skeleton.[33] As there are no proliferating cellular elements, therapy is targetted at reducing blood flow[34] with techniques including percutaneous sclerotherapy. Imaging is often characteristic.

Radiographs

A lobular mass may be visible, depending on location. The radiographic hallmark of a VM is the phlebolith.

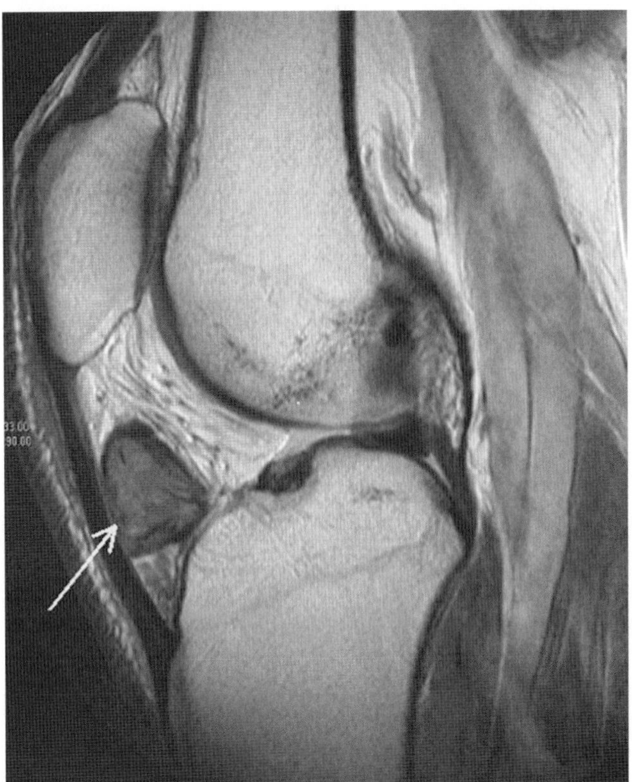

FIGURE 49-13 ■ **Localised intra-articular PVNS.** Sagittal proton density MR image showing a hypointense mass in Hoffa's fat pad (arrow).

These are not always seen, but may be numerous and are seen as a round focus of calcification, often with a lucent centre. Modelling deformity of adjacent bones may be seen (Fig. 49-14).

Ultrasound

Reflectivity is variable on US and the mass may show reflectivity similar to that of adjacent tissues (fat, muscle) and may not be immediately apparent. Low-reflectivity tubular structures suggesting vessels are seen, as are phleboliths. Colour or power Doppler will often show no flow within the mass, but when detected, flow is monophasic and of low velocity. Compressibility with probe pressure is a useful sign on US; the vascular structures and stroma of the mass are easily flattened, reflecting its consistency. Again, this is not a constant feature and depends to an extent on the location, depth and size of the VM, but helps to differentiate it from other soft tissue masses, particularly sarcomas, which in general do not compress (Fig. 49-2).

MRI

VMs show heterogeneous signals, but are generally mildly hyperintense to muscle on T1W imaging and are usually well-defined despite local infiltration. Focal T1 hyperintensity is also frequent, due to small amounts of fat within the lesion and also methaemoglobin (following haemorrhage/thrombosis). Serpigenous channels, which

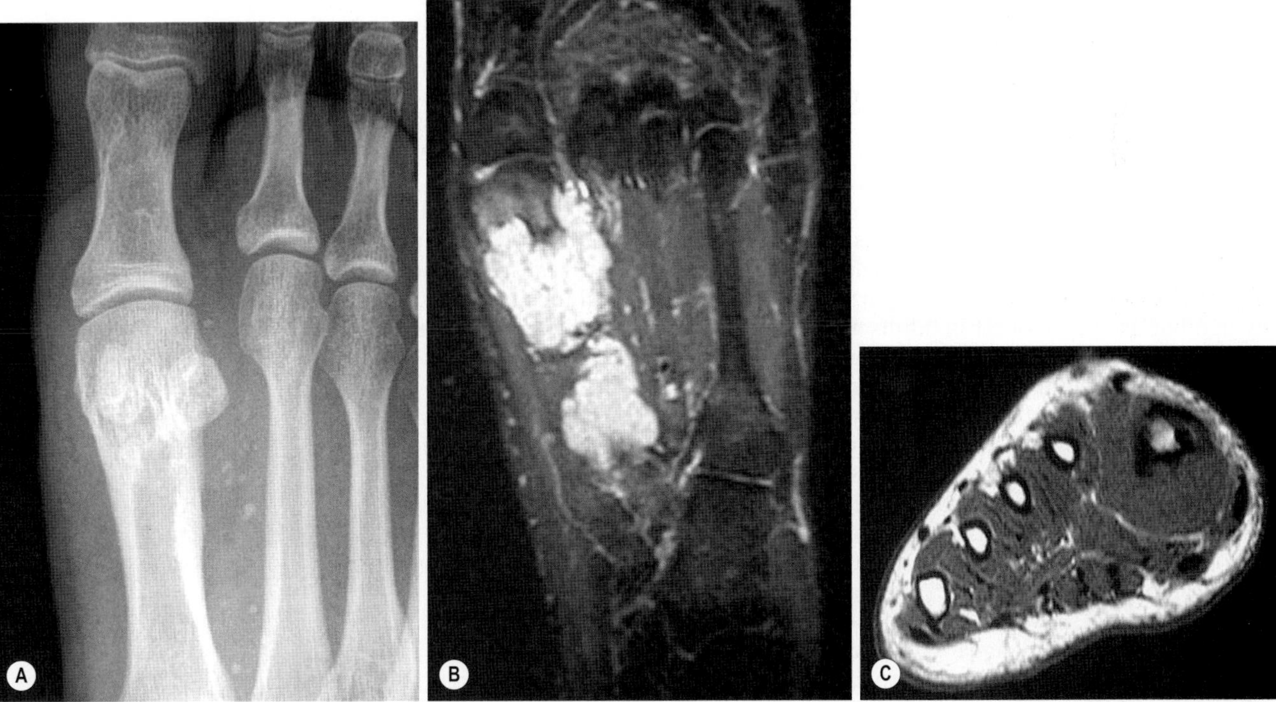

FIGURE 49-14 ■ **Venous malformation.** Dorsoplantar radiograph of the great toe (A) shows soft tissue swelling and phleboliths. Cortical thickening and subtle remodelling of the metatarsal is noted. Axial STIR MR image (B) shows a lobular, hyperintense mass with faint low-signal septation. Coronal T1W imaging (C) shows pressure erosion and cortical thickening of the plantar aspect of the metatarsal by a circumferential mass, which in this case is isointense to muscle.

TABLE 49-1 Syndromes Associated with Vascular Malformations

- Klippel-Trénaunay
- Sturge–Weber
- Maffucci
- Proteus
- Blue rubber bleb naevus

are hyperintense on T2W imaging, are interspersed between the solid, soft tissue matrix. Fluid–fluid levels are common in areas of static blood. Areas of signal void may be due to phleboliths, flowing blood or fibrous septa.[33] Enhancement can be seen on delayed images following intravenous injection of gadolinium contrast medium, but there is no arterial or early venous filling.[34] MRI with gadolinium contrast medium may be useful in differentiating a VM from a lymphatic malformation, the former showing delayed, diffuse enhancement and the latter septal enhancement in the walls of the cystic spaces.[33]

A summary of the features that should be assessed on MRI is:[33]

- classification into high flow (by presence of flow voids and arterial feeding vessels) or low flow;
- description of extent (focal, multifocal or diffuse);
- description of tissue involvement (skin, subcutaneous tissue, muscle, tendon, bone cortex, bone marrow); and
- connection with abnormal vessels (feeding arteries, draining veins).

There are several clinical syndromes associated with vascular malformations (Table 49-1).

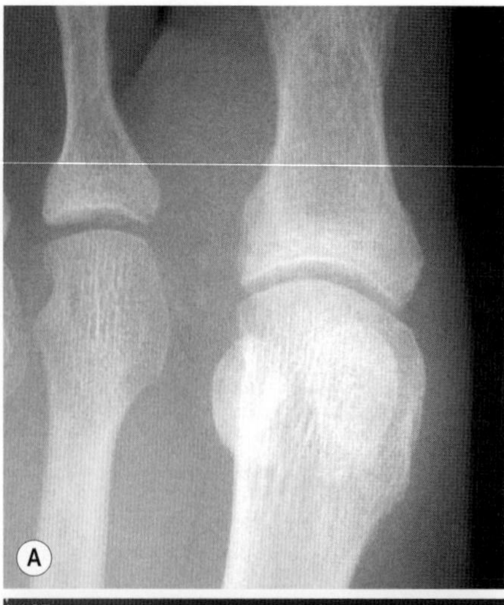

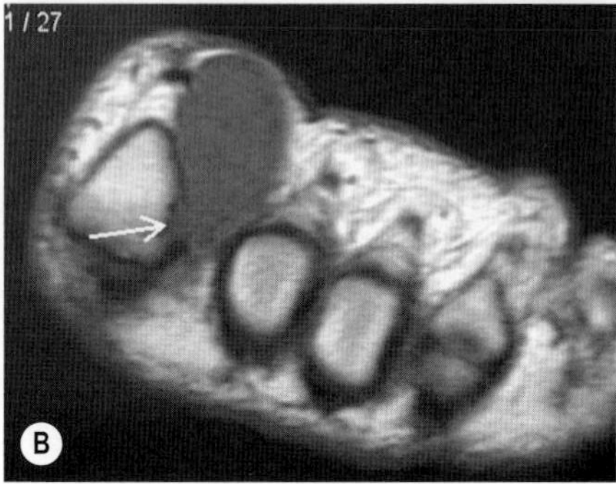

FIGURE 49-15 ■ **Soft tissue chondroma.** A mass between the first and second metatarsal heads contains punctate mineralisation (A). Coronal T1W imaging (B) shows subtle erosion of the lateral aspect of the first metatarsal head (arrow).

CHONDRO-OSSEOUS TUMOURS

Soft Tissue Chondromas

These are benign tumours of hyaline cartilage, occurring outside bone, in extrasynovial locations and not attached to periosteum—other synonyms include extraskeletal chondroma and chondroma of soft parts.[8] They occur at any age but are commonest in adults aged 30–60 years. The commonest location is in the fingers, with 80% occurring in the hands and feet.[36] The masses are usually small (<3 cm diameter), lobular and solitary, and although showing no attachment to periosteum, they may be adherent to tendon sheath or joint capsule; proximity to bone may result in pressure erosion/remodelling[37] (Fig. 49-15). Imaging reflects their cartilaginous nature. Radiographs may show chondral mineralisation (punctate, curvilinear) or rarely ossification[36] and adjacent bone remodelling. MRI shows a lobular chondral mass; hyaline cartilage shows myxoid signal characteristics, with heterogeneous low-signal areas due to calcification. The radiographic differential includes periosteal chondroma (deep to the periosteum), synovial chondromatosis (affecting tendon sheath or arising from an adjacent joint), traumatic and reactive lesions (myositis ossificans, bizarre parosteal osteochondromatous proliferation (BPOP)), tophi and calcification due to connective tissue disorders.[36]

Other benign chondral tumours occurring in soft tissue have been described,[38] including synovial chondromatosis (discussed in Chapter 51) and para-articular (intracapsular) chondroma. The latter represents cartilaginous metaplasia arising from a joint capsule or adjacent connective tissue, most frequently in Hoffa's fat pad, and may present as a mineralised mass. Calcification may progress to ossification, the lesion becoming a para-articular ossifying chondroma[39] or osteochondroma (without connection to bone).

TUMOURS OF UNCERTAIN DIFFERENTIATION

Myxoma

This is a benign soft tissue tumour composed of bland spindle cells in a stroma of abundant myxoid, gelatinous material, classified as a tumour of uncertain differentiation.[8] It is one of a number of myxoid tumours occurring

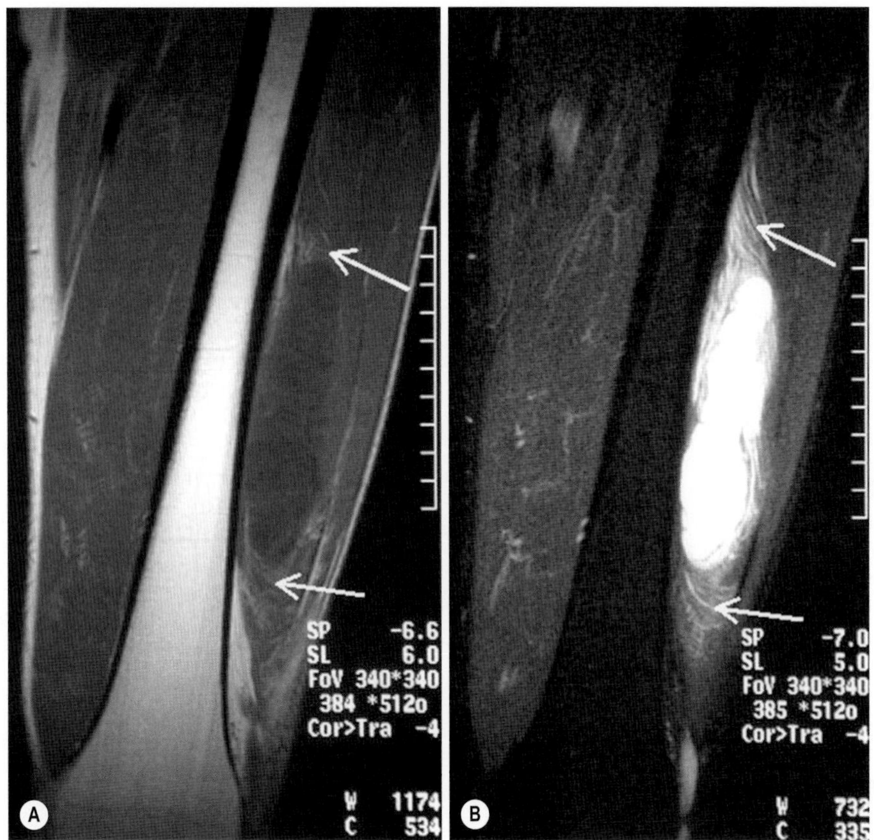

FIGURE 49-16 ■ **Intramuscular myxoma.** Coronal T1 (A) and STIR (B) MR images of the left thigh show an ovoid, poorly defined, heterogeneous mass which is hypointense on T1W imaging and hyperintense on STIR images. A small amount of fat is visible at the poles of the mass (arrows in (A)) and there is adjacent oedema (arrows in (B)).

in soft tissue, all consisting of a background matrix of mucoid material containing a variety of different cell types. While the cell type determines the clinical and biological behaviour, the imaging appearances of these lesions, determined by the myxoid stroma, are broadly similar. Differentiation can also be difficult for the histopathologist.

Most myxomas occur in intramuscular sites, although they may also be intermuscular, subcutaneous or juxta-articular;[40] myxomas also occur outside the musculoskeletal system. Women between the ages of 40 and 70 are most often affected and the most common location for this tumour is the thigh.[40] MRI is the most useful technique for assessment: myxoid tumours often resemble cysts, typically showing low SI on T1W imaging and high SI on T2W and fluid-sensitive sequences. The tumours may be homogeneous, or heterogeneous due to thin fibrous septa and may contain cystic areas; there may be surrounding soft tissue oedema.[40,41] A rind of fat may be seen, most prominently at the poles of the tumour, and this may simulate a 'split-fat sign', typically found in inter- rather than intramuscular tumours (Fig. 49-16). The surrounding fatty and oedematous signal changes reflect the infiltrative nature of the tumour, with fatty changes indicating adjacent muscle atrophy. Following administration of intravenous contrast medium, internal enhancement can confirm that the lesion is not cystic, but occasionally the enhancement is purely peripheral with more prominent enhancement seen in tumours with greater cellularity and reduced myxoid content.[41] US and CT both show non-specific appearances.

The differential diagnosis includes cystic masses, some of which are synovial and para-articular including ganglia, synovial cysts, bursae and seromas. A rare variant of myxoma, the juxta-articular myxoma, can arise adjacent to joints, usually the knee.[42]

Soft Tissue Sarcomas (STSs)

Sarcomas are rare, malignant tumours of mesenchymal origin which account for less than 1% of all primary malignant tumours, but are still three to four times more common than primary bone sarcomas.[43] The greatest incidence is in older patients and in children and adolescents (under 20 years old); soft tissue sarcoma (STS) is very rare, with rhabdomyosarcoma (RMS) most common in younger subjects and non-RMS sarcomas commoner in older children. Many different types of STSs are classified as tumours of uncertain differentiation[8]. The most common STS of late adult life is the *pleomorphic undifferentiated sarcoma* (formerly malignant fibrous histiocytoma), which occurs most commonly in the extremities and retroperitoneum. As its name suggests, this tumour comprises STS which cannot be more precisely categorised.

Most STSs are poorly characterised by imaging. Initial attempts to differentiate benign from malignant soft tissue masses using MRI were unsuccessful and biopsy was recommended in most cases. Signs suspicious of malignancy have traditionally included a deep-seated, large mass with heterogeneous appearances on MRI.[43] More recently, the importance of tumour necrosis (non-enhancing areas, often haemorrhagic) and lesion size (greater than 5 cm at presentation) indicating a high grade lesion have been emphasised[44] (Fig. 49-17). A significant minority of sarcomas is known to arise superficially (in skin and subcutaneous fat). The relevance of lesion depth has been assessed in a referral population of 571 soft tissue tumours and was found to be unrelated to the final diagnosis, while patient age and size ≥5 cm were significant risk factors for malignancy.[45] Although the ability of imaging to reach a histological diagnosis has not advanced, the histopathological approach has been continuously refined using immunohistochemical and genetic techniques. Imaging features may assist in characterisation.

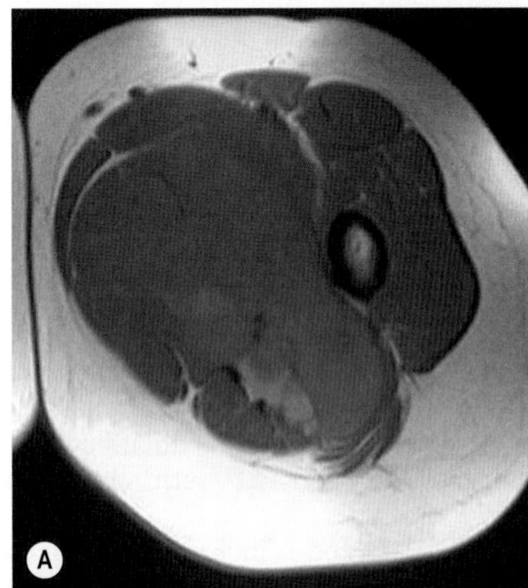

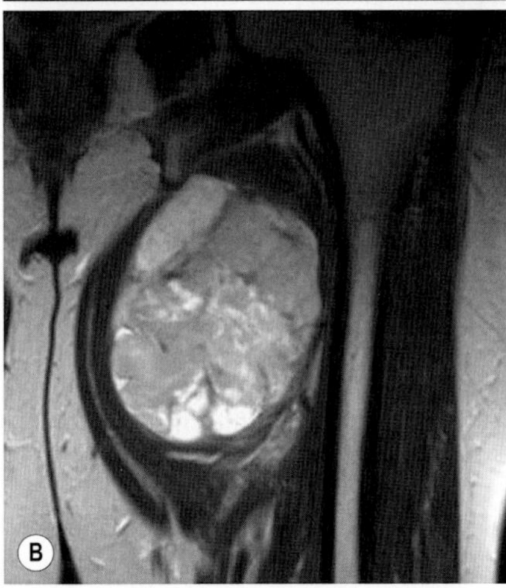

FIGURE 49-17 ■ **High-grade sarcoma.** Axial TW1 (A) and coronal T2W (B) imaging show a large heterogeneous, haemorrhagic mass in the adductor compartment of the left thigh.

Synovial Sarcoma (SS)

Synovial sarcoma accounts for up to 10% of malignant mesenchymal tumours.[46] SS may be found at any age but most patients are aged 15–40 years. It is usually a slow-growing mass located in the extremities, often close to a joint and most commonly in the lower limb. Despite the name, less than 10% are said to be intra-articular. Although it is frequently a large, deep, multilobular and septated mass, it may also be small, homogeneous and slow growing, it is probably for these reasons that it was the malignant tumour most frequently diagnosed as benign using MRI in one study.[47] Imaging findings that may be useful in the diagnosis of SS include calcification (30% of cases) (Fig. 49-18), evidence of haemorrhage (44%), fluid–fluid levels (18%), 'triple signal'—areas of high, low and isointensity compared with fat on T2W imaging (indicating cystic/haemorrhagic elements, fibrous tissue and calcification and solid, non-necrotic tumour) (Fig. 49-19) and bone erosion or invasion (21%).

TUMOURS OF NERVES

Tumours of peripheral nerves are frequent causes of a soft tissue mass. They are classified by the WHO under lesions of the central nervous system, most recently in 2007.[48]

Two broad categories of nerve tumours exist: true neurogenic tumours and pseudotumours involving or arising from nerves. Clinical assessment and imaging are useful in conjunction in determining the nature of nerve lesions.

Benign Nerve Sheath Tumours

Schwannoma (*neurilemmoma*, NL) arises from the Schwann cells surrounding a nerve. They are typically small and slow growing and may arise in peripheral and central locations including sympathetic nerves. Although typically solitary, multiple tumours (schwannomatosis) may occur, either in association with neurofibromatosis type 2 or probably as a separate entity.

Neurofibroma (NF) accounts for slightly greater than 5% of benign soft tissue neoplasms. There are three types, all of which can be seen in neurofibromatosis type 1 (NF1): localised (the commonest type, accounting for >90%), diffuse and plexiform—the latter is one of the defining features of NF1.

- *Localised NF* is usually a slow-growing mass arising from a peripheral nerve, small nerve branch or larger central nerve. Most are solitary and not associated with NF1, but multiple neurofibromas can be found in patients with this condition.

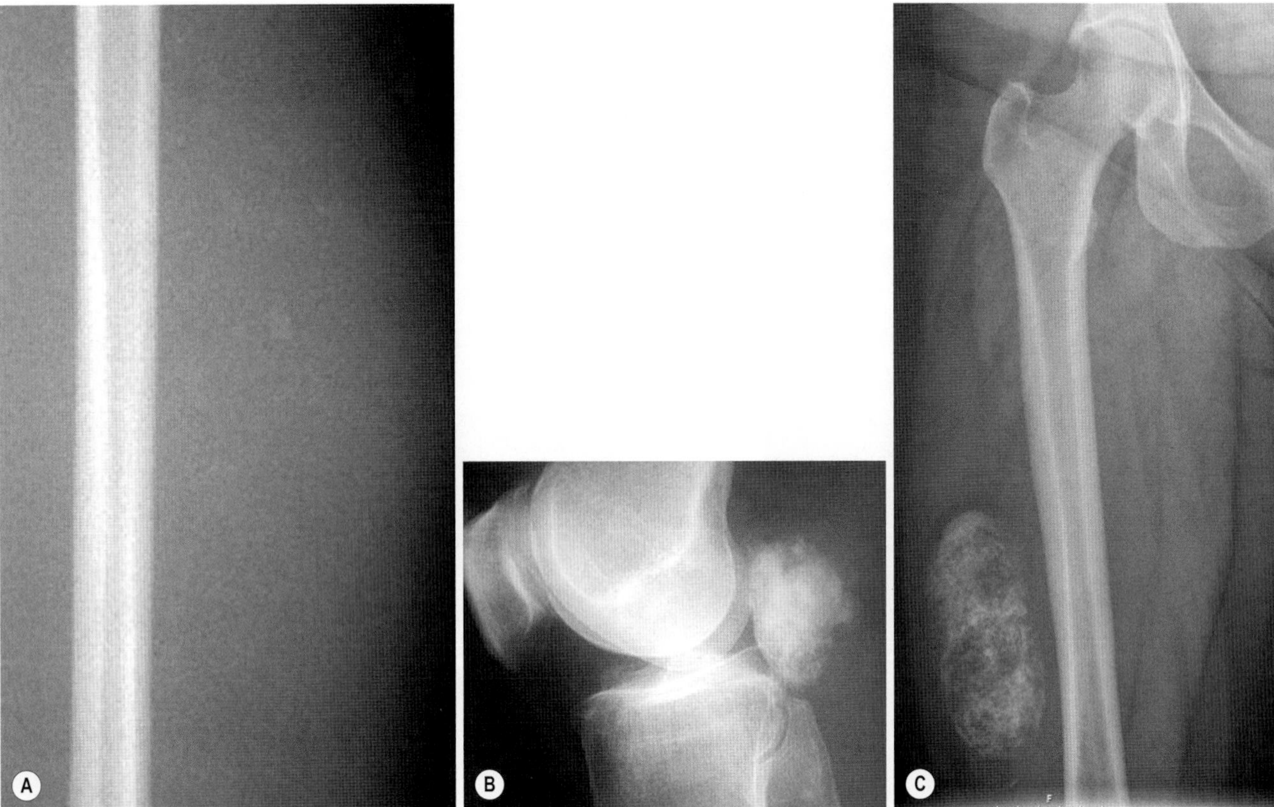

FIGURE 49-18 ■ Patterns of calcification of synovial sarcoma. (A) Faint punctate calcification; (B) heavy ossification; (C) bizarre diffuse mineralisation. There is some evidence to suggest that heavily mineralised or ossified synovial sarcomas have a better prognosis.

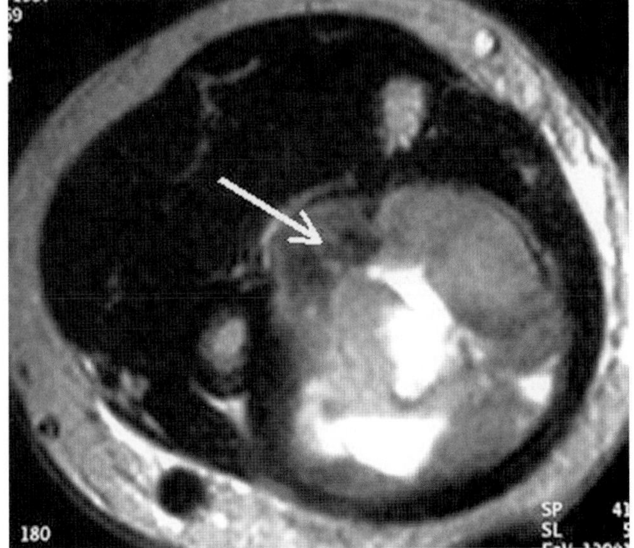

FIGURE 49-19 ■ Synovial sarcoma. T2W imaging shows a triple signal pattern: hyperintense haemorrhage, intermediate-signal solid tumour and low-signal mineralisation (arrow). Fluid–fluid levels are also seen.

- *Diffuse NF* presents as a diffuse area of thickening of the skin and subcutaneous tissues, again it is sporadic but can be associated with NF1 in approximately 10%.[49]
- *Plexiform NF* involves infiltration of a large nerve or plexus, with extension outside the nerve into adjacent tissues, resulting in a lobulated mass, loosely conforming to the morphology of the nerve, described as a 'bag of worms'. There may be associated bone and soft tissue overgrowth (Fig. 49-20).

There are a number of imaging features that suggest a benign nerve sheath tumour:

- *Relationship to a nerve*: The mass may arise in the anatomical location of a nerve, or an adjacent nerve may be visible on imaging studies. However, many arise from small peripheral nerves where no adjacent nerve is visible.
- *Nerve entering/leaving the mass*: Again, the utility of this sign depends on the size of the nerve. If visible, the location of the nerve relative to the mass may be useful in differentiating NLs and NFs. In NLs, the nerve may be eccentrically located relative to the mass, whereas in NF the nerve may enter and leave the mass centrally.
- *Fusiform morphology*.
- *Split-fat sign*: The neurovascular bundle travels in the intermuscular space, surrounded by fat, and an

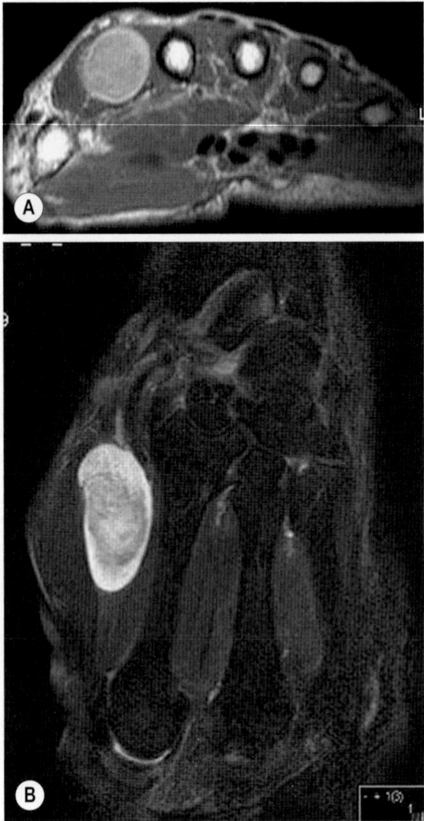

FIGURE 49-20 ■ **Schwannoma.** Axial proton-density (A) and coronal T2W imaging with fat saturation (B) show a well-defined, fusiform mass in the dorsum of the hand, between the thumb and index metacarpals. A fascicular sign is seen in (A) and a target sign in (B).

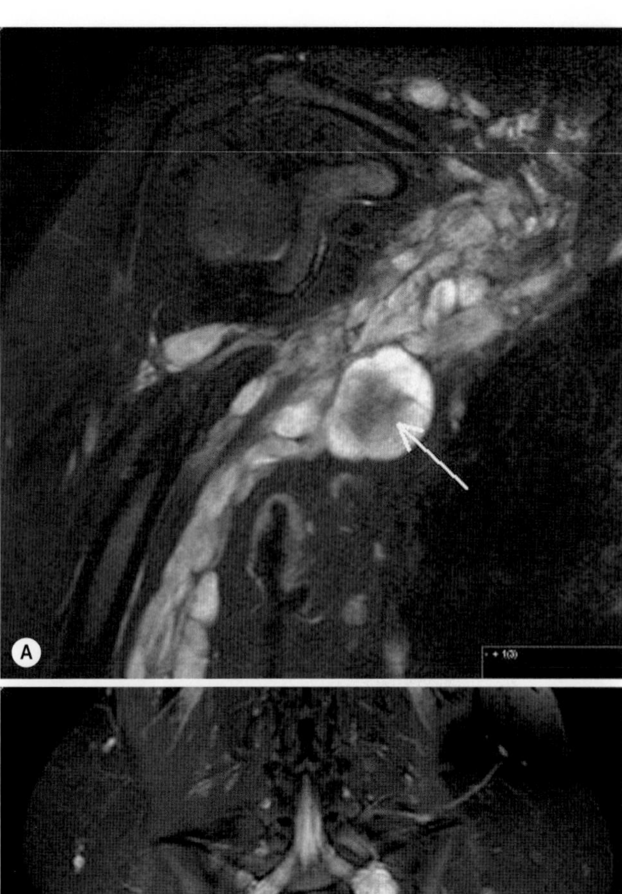

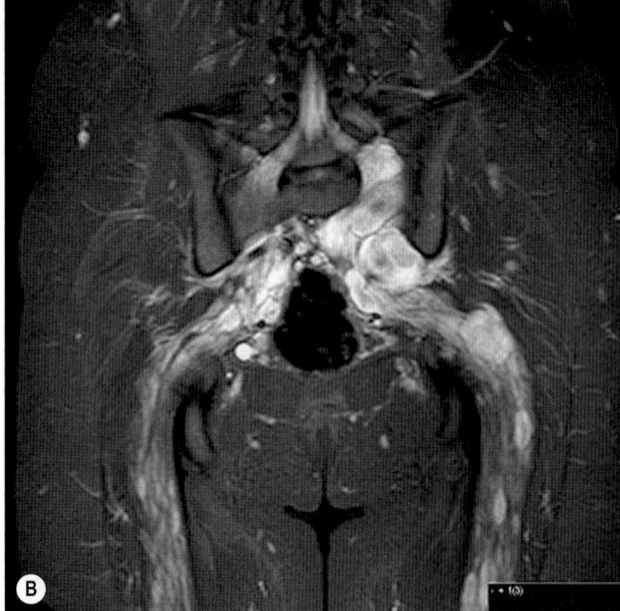

FIGURE 49-21 ■ **Plexiform neurofibromas of the right brachial plexus (A) and sciatic nerves (B).** Coronal STIR images showing marked lobular enlargement of major central nerves in a patient with neurofibromatosis type 1. A target sign is seen in the brachial plexus mass (arrow).

enlarging mass in this region, arising from any component of the neurovascular bundle, may show preservation of the surrounding rim of fat, with displacement of the adjacent muscle.

- *Distal muscle atrophy/denervation*: A variable sign depending on the impact on nerve function.
- *Target sign*: This refers to appearances on T2W imaging and US. On MRI, nerve sheath tumours often show central lower signal (reflecting a more fibrous content) and peripheral hyperintensity (more myxoid content). On US, the central portion shows hyperechogenicity with lower reflectivity in the periphery. This sign is seen most commonly in NFs but may also be seen in NLs (Figs. 49-20 and 49-21) and malignant peripheral nerve sheath tumours.
- *Fascicular sign*: Ring-like areas of hypointensity within the mass on proton-density or T2W imaging, which may correspond to fascicular bundles within the nerve sheath tumour (Fig. 49-21).

Despite the features outlined above, differentiation of NL from NF on US and MRI remains unreliable.

The imaging features of NL which have undergone a process of degeneration ('ancient' change) are often different and may obscure the neurogenic nature of the mass. A heterogeneous mass is usually seen, showing cavitation/cystic change, fluid–fluid levels/haemorrhage and calcification (Fig. 49-22).

Diffuse neurofibroma results in a plaque-like or infiltrative lesion, thickened skin and involvement of the subcutaneous tissues, with marked internal vascularity and enhancement following injection of gadolinium contrast medium.[49]

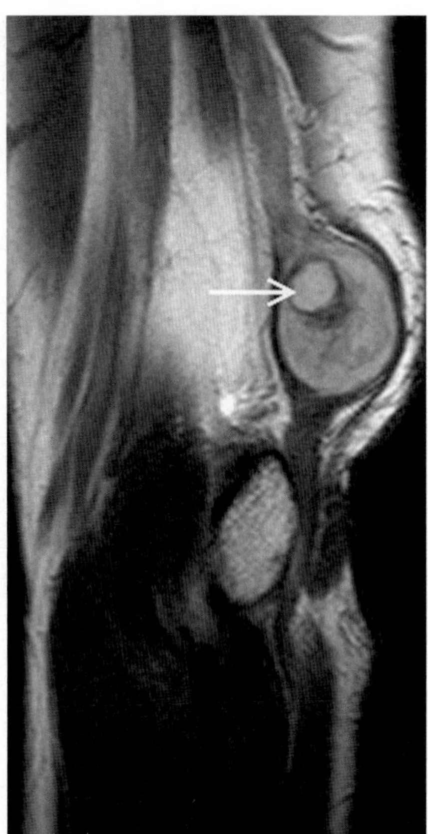

FIGURE 49-22 ■ Ancient schwannoma of the ulnar nerve. Sagittal T2W imaging shows continuity with an eccentric nerve and cyst formation within the tumour (arrow).

Malignant Nerve Tumours

Primary lesions are called malignant peripheral nerve sheath tumours, although several primary non-neurogenic or secondary malignancies may also arise in nerves.

Malignant Peripheral Nerve Sheath Tumours (MPNSTs)

Malignant peripheral nerve sheath tumours account for 5–10% of soft tissue sarcomas. In up to 50% of cases they occur in patients with NF1, affecting 2–5% of subjects with this condition who have an 8–12% lifetime risk of developing this malignancy.[50] MPNSTs in NF1 develop in deep plexiform NFS; the risk of transformation is greater in patients with large central lesions and varies with the precise nature of the genetic defect. In NF1 the tumours tend to be larger (possibly reflecting later presentation) and occur at an earlier age[51] and the prognosis of MPNST in NF1 is significantly worse when compared with that of the general population (5-year survival of 21% compared with 42%).[51]

MPNSTs may show some features of a neurogenic tumour but frequently are non-specific (Fig. 49-23); however, a heterogeneous mass arising from a nerve should raise suspicion, particularly if there is rapid enlargement, neurological deficit and nerve pain.[52] In NF1, there may be development of a mass from a plexiform NF and coincident new pain, change in consistency of the mass and neurological deficit. MRI features include a large, heterogeneous, lobular mass, lacking a target sign, with evidence of haemorrhage (T1 hyperintensity). Enhancement may be peripheral rather than the central enhancement seen in many benign PNSTs.[52] Positron emission tomography has been used to identify areas of malignant transformation within plexiform NFs, with a claimed high sensitivity and specificity.

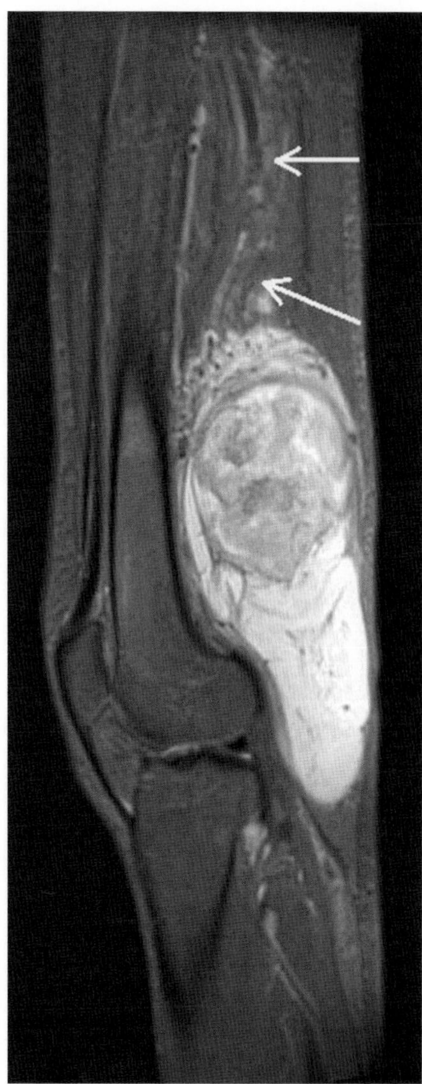

FIGURE 49-23 ■ Malignant peripheral nerve sheath tumour (MPNST). Sagittal STIR MR image: a large, heterogeneous but fusiform mass arises from a grossly enlarged sciatic/tibial nerve (arrows), in keeping with the development of an MPNST from a plexiform neurofibroma.

Tumour-Like Lesions Arising from Nerves (Pseudotumours)

Nerve Sheath Ganglion (Intraneural Ganglion)

As might be expected, imaging shows a lobular area of fluid signal dissecting along a nerve. These lesions present with pain and nerve dysfunction, typically occurring at

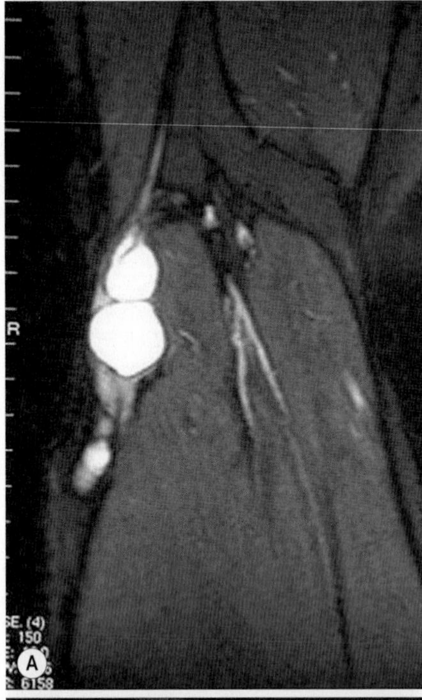

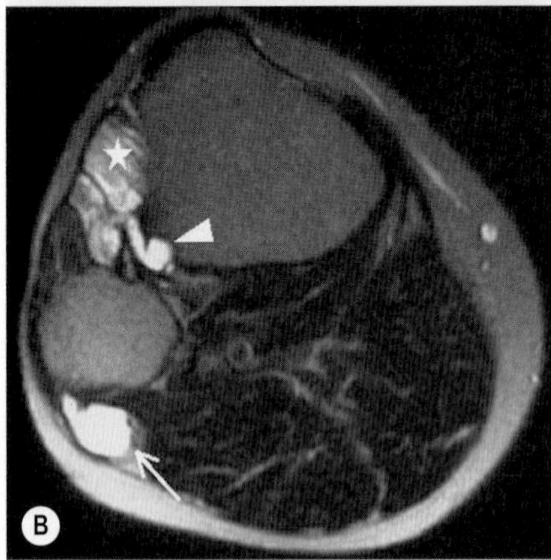

FIGURE 49-24 ■ **Intraneural ganglion.** Coronal STIR (A) and axial T2 with fat saturation (B) MR images of the right knee show a lobular, fluid-signal mass in the common peroneal nerve, compressing the hyperintense nerve (arrow in (B)). Continuation of the ganglion into the articular branch is seen (arrowhead in (B)). There is denervation of the extensor muscles (asterisk in (B)).

the knee (common peroneal nerve, tibial nerve) but have also been described at other locations. Fluid decompresses from a degenerate joint through a capsular defect, dissecting along the epineurium of the articular branch and subsequently into the nerve itself, causing compression of nerve fascicles. In addition to the lobular, elongated, intraneural cystic mass, there may be signs of denervation (Fig. 49-24). Extraneural ganglia may also cause nerve compression but show a different morphology and relationship to the tibiofibular joint[53]—in addition to decompression of the nerve, the degenerate joint may need to be excised to prevent recurrence.

Traumatic Neuroma

Traumatic neuromas usually present with pain, which may be elicited by percussion of the nerve (Tinel's test).

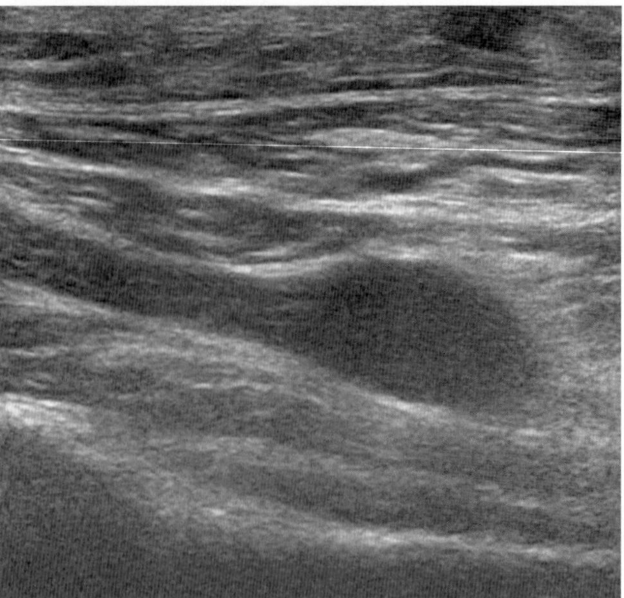

FIGURE 49-25 ■ **Amputation (traumatic) neuroma of the tibial nerve.** Longitudinal ultrasound image showing bulbous mass at the termination of the tibial nerve, which is rather thickened, some years following transtibial amputation.

They are most frequently found in the lower limb after amputation. Within hours of a nerve injury, there is distal degeneration of axons. Attempted repair by macrophages and Schwann cells, if unsuccessful, results in a fusiform (or occasionally laterally located) pseudotumour. Imaging reveals a bulbous mass at the termination of the severed nerve and frequently proximal nerve thickening[54] (Fig. 49-25).

Morton's Neuroma

Morton's neuroma is a common pseudotumour occurring on interdigital nerves in the web space of the forefoot. A small mass develops as a result of perineural fibrosis at the plantar aspect of the web space between the heads of the metatarsals. The lesion is most commonly seen between the third and fourth and, slightly less frequently, the second and third metatarsal heads, usually in middle-aged women. Ultrasound rarely identifies a nerve entering the mass, but does show a well-defined area of low reflectivity in the plantar aspect of the web space, which can be expelled with compression of the forefoot. MRI shows the neuroma best on images coronal to the web space and its low signal intensity reflects its fibrotic nature. T1 images are particularly useful as there is high contrast between the mass and adjacent web space fat.

Lipomatosis of Nerve

Lipomatosis of a nerve was formerly referred to as fibrolipomatous hamartoma or lipofibroma and is classified as an adipocytic soft tissue tumour by the WHO. Involvement of a variety of nerves has been described, but it most frequently affects the median nerve, resulting in a mass and features of neuropathy; and there may be associated macrodactyly. Imaging is characteristic on US and MRI

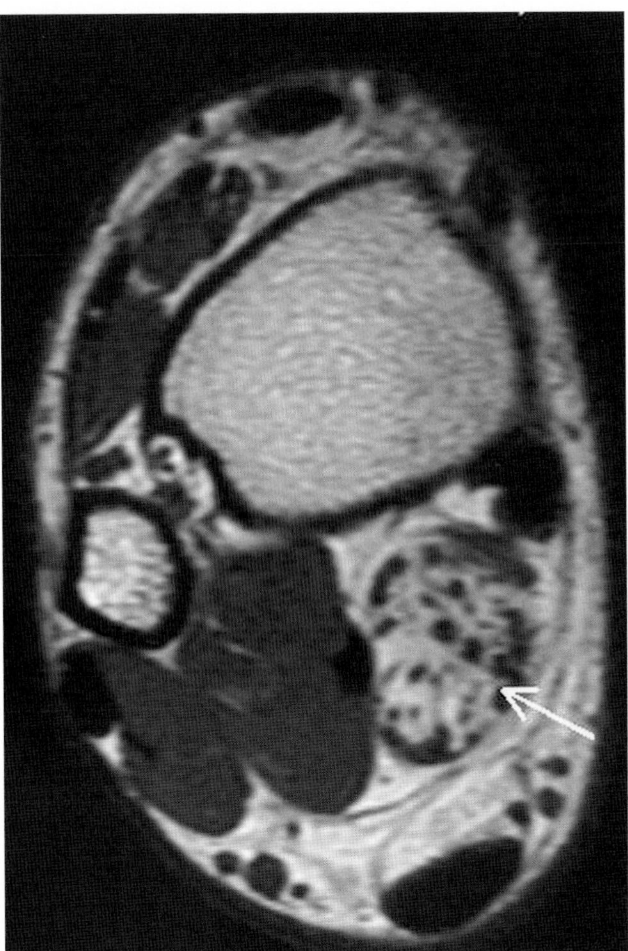

FIGURE 49-26 ■ **Lipomatosis of the tibial nerve.** Axial T1W imaging of the distal right calf shows enlargement of the tibial nerve (arrow). Nerve fibres are thickened and there is intervening hyperintense tissue consistent with fat.

demonstrating thickened nerve fascicles surrounded by adipose tissue within a grossly enlarged nerve (Fig. 49-26).

NON-NEOPLASTIC TUMOUR MIMICS

Many non-neoplastic lesions present as soft tissue masses. In general, imaging can offer a more accurate diagnosis than is often possible for many neoplasms, particularly sarcomas. 'Pseudotumours' are normal variants or non-neoplastic masses that mimic tumours—some examples are given below.

Accessory Muscles

A large number of these exist, but it is the accessory soleus that presents most frequently as a soft tissue mass (Fig. 49-27). The remainder tend to be small and impalpable, but may be identified on cross-sectional imaging examinations. Ultrasound and MRI can be reassuring, showing normal muscle tissue at the site of the mass.

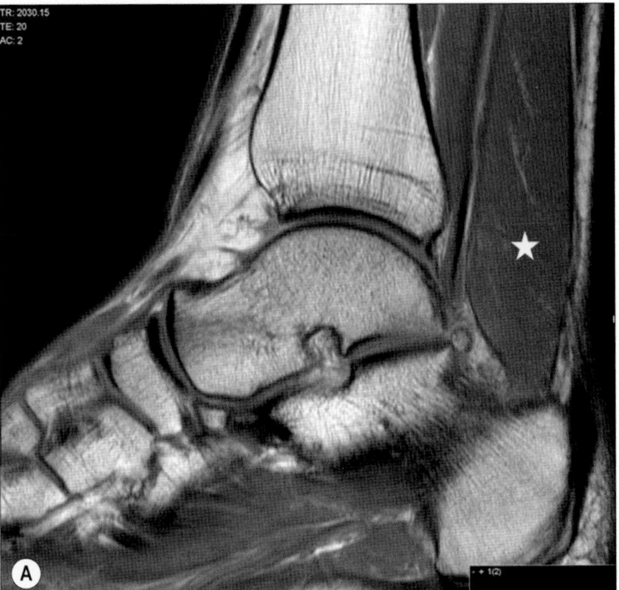

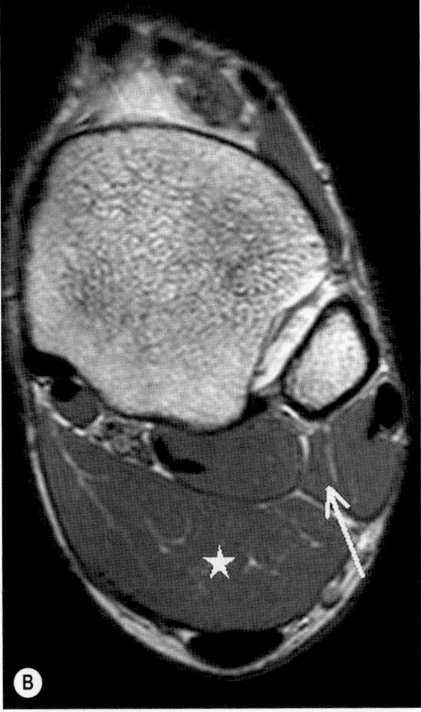

FIGURE 49-27 ■ **Accessory soleus muscle.** Sagittal (A) and axial (B) proton density MR images show the accessory muscle (asterisk) in the posterior calf between the flexor hallucis longus and the tendo Achilles. Another accessory muscle, the peroneus quartus, is also present in this subject (arrow).

Traumatic Lesions

These are frequent causes of a soft tissue mass. They include muscle tears, fascial hernias (Fig. 49-28), haematomas, fat necrosis and aneurysms. The *Morel-Lavallée lesion* is characteristic in site and appearance (Fig. 49-29). It is due to a closed degloving injury, resulting in shearing of the deep subcutaneous fat from the underlying fascia and causes a chronic haematoma, most frequently located over the lateral aspect of the hip and proximal thigh. An

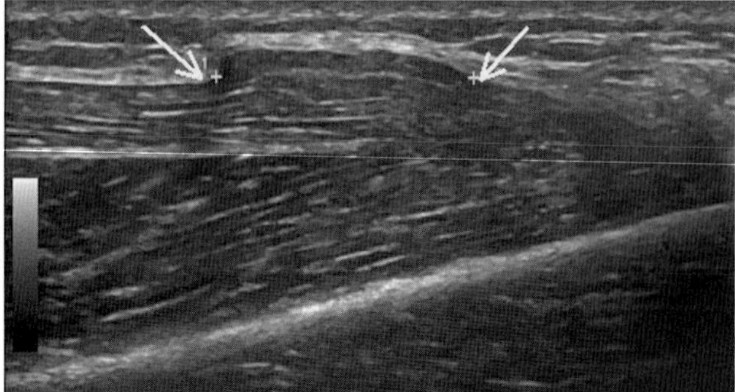

FIGURE 49-28 ■ Muscle fascial hernia. Longitudinal ultrasound image showing herniation of peroneal muscle through a fascial defect (arrows) in the distal lateral calf.

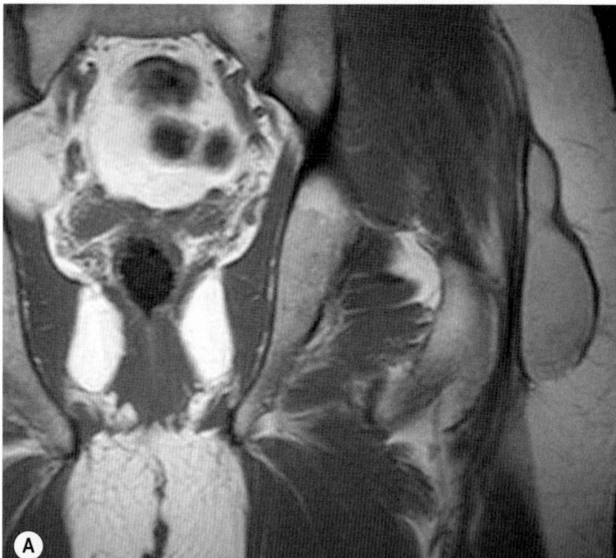

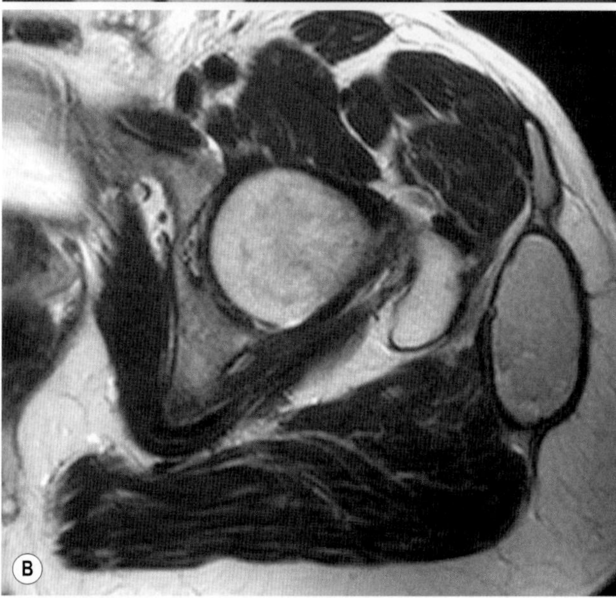

FIGURE 49-29 ■ Morel–Lavallée lesion. Coronal T1 (A) and axial T2W imaging (B). There is an elliptical mass whose appearances suggest chronic haemorrhage (hyperintense on T1W imaging, intermediate SI on T2W imaging with a surrounding rim of low signal), in a characteristic location in the deep subcutaneous fat at the lateral aspect of the hip.

elliptical mass, which frequently shows a low-signal rim and heterogeneous contents in keeping with chronic haemorrhage, is seen on MRI.[55] *Myositis ossificans* is classified by the WHO under fibroblastic/myofibroblastic tumours, but as a localised, self-limiting reactive process.[8] There may be no history of trauma in a significant number, despite representing ossification in the walls of a haematoma following muscle injury. In the early stages, an unmineralised soft tissue mass is apparent and MRI appearances may show extensive oedema around a heterogeneous lesion: careful inspection of the images often shows a characteristic low-signal rim at the margin of the mass and this is diagnostically useful. With time, the mass matures, with progressive peripheral ossification and resolution of pain, but in the early stages, US or CT is useful for identifying subtle mineralisation which may not be visible on radiographs (Fig. 49-1).

Infection/Inflammation

Pyomyositis (infective inflammation before the development of an abscess) causes a diffuse muscle swelling. US may identify a change in reflectivity within the muscle, small microabscesses and surrounding hyperaemia on colour Doppler, whereas on MRI soft tissue abscesses are hyperintense but heterogeneous on T2W imaging with surrounding oedema. Non-infective inflammatory myositis and foreign body reactions may also present as soft tissue masses.

Synovial Disorders

These are frequent causes of a soft tissue mass. Possible lesions include synovial cysts, ganglia, bursae, tenosynovitis. A *popliteal (Baker's) cyst* is one of the most common masses at the knee and often shows characteristic appearances, but it may be complicated by any process that involves the joint, including infection, haemorrhage, inflammatory arthritis and neoplasms.

For a full list of references, please see ExpertConsult.

FURTHER READING

3. Kransdorf M. Malignant soft tissue tumours in a large referral population: distribution of diagnoses by age, sex and location. Am J Roentgenol 1995;164:129–34.
4. Gartner L, Pearce C, Saifuddin A. The role of the plain radiograph in the characterisation of soft tissue masses. Skeletal Radiol 2009;38:549–58.
11. Murphey M, Carroll J, Flemming D, et al. Benign musculoskeletal lipomatous lesions. Radiographics 2004;24:1433–66.
28. Murphey M, Rhee J, Lewis R, et al. Pigmented villonodular synovitis: radiologic-pathologic correlation. Radiographics 2008;28: 1493–518.
31. Enjolras O. Classification and management of the various superficial vascular anomalies: hemangiomas and vascular malformations. J Dermatol 1997;24:701–10.
38. Helpert C, Davies AM, Evans N, et al. Differential diagnosis of tumours and tumour-like lesions of the infrapatellar (Hoffa's) fat pad: pictorial review with an emphasis on MR imaging. European Radiol 2004;14:2337–46.
40. Murphey M, McRae G, Fanburg-Smith J, et al. Imaging of soft-tissue myxoma with emphasis on CT and MR and comparison of radiologic and pathologic findings. Radiology 2002;225:215–24.
45. Datir A, James S, Ali K, et al. MRI of soft-tissue masses: the relationship between lesion size, depth and diagnosis. Clin Radiol 2008;63:373–8.

CHAPTER 50

Metabolic and Endocrine Skeletal Disease

Thomas M. Link • Judith E. Adams

CHAPTER OUTLINE

BONE PHYSIOLOGY AND PATHOPHYSIOLOGY

Though bone appears rigid and inert, it is a highly metabolically active tissue, which is constantly remodelled with osteoblasts building bone and osteoclasts resorbing bone. This dynamic process allows the bone to be an extremely strong tissue that withstands the load-bearing requirements of the skeleton. Bone consists of crystals of hydroxyapatite embedded within an organic matrix, principally consisting of triple helical fibres of Type I collagen. Bones are generally divided into flat and tubular bones. Tubular bones are designed for weight bearing. Flat bones protect internal organs. Anatomically, bone is found in two forms:

- **compact (cortical) bone**, which forms the outer shell of bones,
- **trabecular (cancellous) bone**, which is found mainly in vertebral bodies, the pelvis and the distal regions of long bones.

Bones remodel from birth to maturity, maintaining their basic shape, repairing following fracture and responding to mechanical stresses throughout life. The strength of bone is related not only to its hardness and other physical properties but also to the architectural arrangement of the compact and trabecular bone. The skeleton contains 99% of the total body calcium and therefore plays a vital role in the maintenance of calcium homeostasis.

Bone Cells

Osteoblasts are bone-forming cells, which synthesise and secrete Type I collagen and mucopolysaccharides to form layers of bone matrix (osteoid) which subsequently becomes mineralised. Osteoblasts also synthesise collagenase, prostaglandin E_2 (PGE_2), and bone-associated proteins, osteocalcin and osteonectin. Osteoblasts have receptors for parathyroid hormone, vitamin D, prostaglandin E_2 and glucocorticosteroids.

Osteocytes are derived from the osteoblast and are initially present on the surface of bone but subsequently become encased within bone. Each osteocyte lies within a lacuna and is interconnected to other osteocytes and osteoblasts by cytoplasmic extensions within canaliculi. The osteocyte has a role in maintenance of bone matrix, which is facilitated by the transport of material and fluid via these canaliculi. Osteocytes respond to biomechanical loading, calcitonin and parathyroid hormone, and so play an important role in maintaining constant levels of calcium within the body fluids.

Osteoclasts are multinuclear giant cells that resorb both calcified bone and cartilage and derive from the mononuclear phagocytic cell line of haematopoietic stem cells. Osteoclasts lie on the surface of bone, causing active resorption and forming Howship's lacunae. Osteoclasts in contact with bone develop motile microvilli, which cause the cell to adhere to the bone surface and result in a microenvironment between the osteoclast and the mineralised bone. This brush border of microvilli increases with activation by such factors as prostaglandin, vitamin D and parathyroid hormone. Osteoclasts secrete acid hydrolases and neutral proteases, which degrade the bone matrix following its demineralisation. Figure 50-1 shows the different bone cells and their function in remodelling the bone.

Bone Formation and Turnover

Bone formation (osteoblastic activity) and bone resorption (osteoclastic activity) constitutes bone turnover, a process, which takes place on bone surfaces and continues throughout life (Fig. 50-1). Bone formation and resorption are linked in a consistent sequence under normal circumstances. Precursor bone cells are activated at a particular skeletal site to form osteoclasts, which erode a fairly constant amount of bone. After a period of time the resorption stops and osteoblasts are recruited to fill the eroded space with new bone. This coupling of osteoblastic and osteoclastic activity constitutes the basal

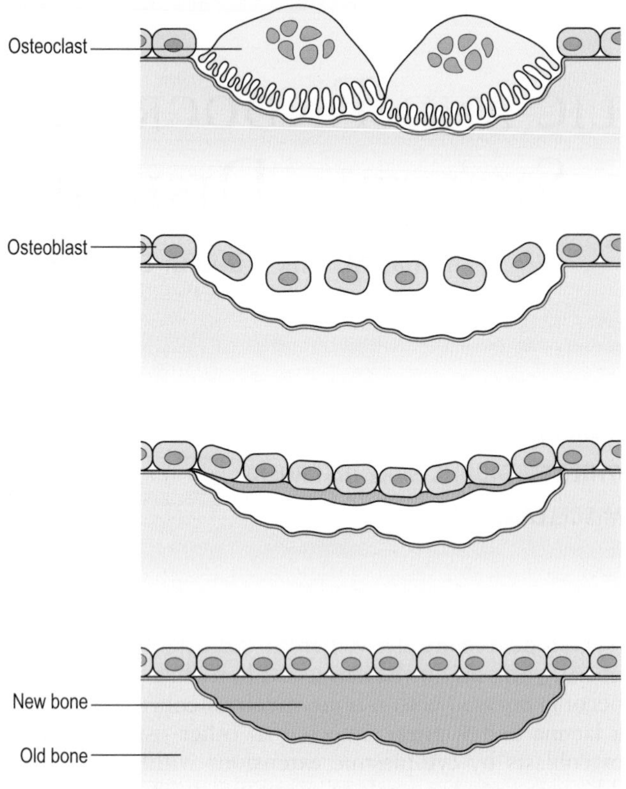

FIGURE 50-1 ■ Bone cells and basal metabolic unit (BMU). Bone turnover continues throughout life so that old bone is replaced by stronger new bone; osteoclasts erode a pit of bone (top) and subsequently osteoblasts are recruited and fill the eroded pit with osteoid, which becomes mineralised. Normally this process is in balance and takes about 3–4 months to complete. If the process becomes uncoupled and erosion is excessive or the pit is incompletely filled with bone, there will be a net loss of bone over time (osteoporosis). Increase in both resorption and formation results in a high turnover state, e.g. Paget's disease.

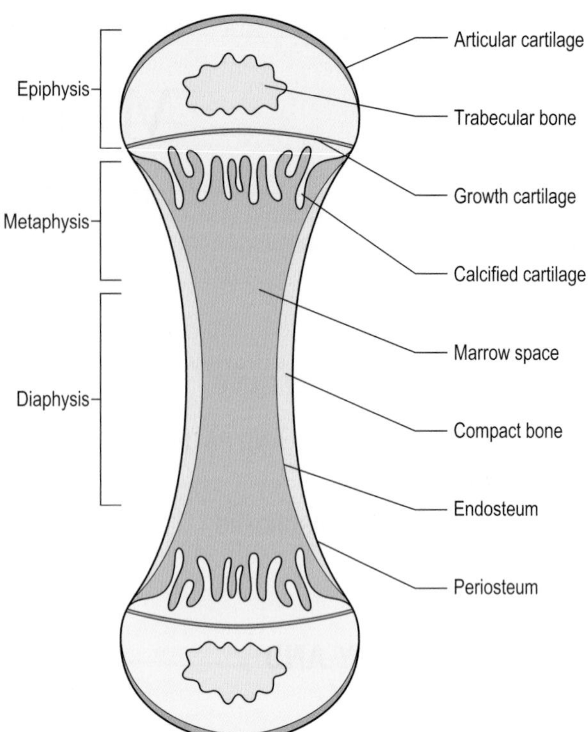

FIGURE 50-2 ■ Tubular bone growth. Tubular bones consist of an outer shell of cortical bone with inner trabecular bone, particularly at the ends of the bones, and haematopoietic marrow. They grow in length by endochondral ossification, which takes place at the physis (growth plate) between the distal epiphysis and the metaphysis.

multicellular unit (BMU) of bone. In healthy young adults the resorptive phase of the turnover cycle lasts about 30 days and the formation phase about 90 days. The length of the turnover cycle increases in later life and the rate of bone turnover is reduced. Uncoupling of the process (excessive osteoclastic resorption or defective osteoblastic function) results in a net loss of bone (**osteoporosis**). If there is both increased bone resorption and formation, this constitutes increased bone turnover. Woven immature, instead of mature lamellar, bone is laid down, as in Paget's disease of bone. Increased activation frequency of resorption units also results in high turnover state (hyperparathyroidism, postmenopausal bone loss). Bisphosphonate therapy reduces the activation of resorption units by inhibiting osteoclasts, and the reversal in the mineral deficit contributes to increase in bone mineral density (BMD).

Defective osteoclastic function prevents normal bone resorption, which is essential to maintain bone health by continuous slow renewal throughout life. Defective osteoclastic function in some diseases (i.e. osteopetrosis) can result in abnormal bone modelling and sclerosis on radiographs; these bone are more brittle and susceptible to fracture. Bone resorption by osteoclasts is a single-stage process in which collagen and mineral are removed together. Bone formation is a two-stage process: osteoblasts lay down osteoid, which subsequently becomes mineralised. Prerequisites for normal mineralisation are vitamin D ($1,25[OH]_2D_3$), normal levels of phosphorus and alkaline phosphatase, adequate intake of calcium and a normal pH. Defects in the mineralisation process will result in rickets or osteomalacia.

Bone Growth and Development

Early in fetal development the framework of the skeleton is in place but without mineralisation. At about 26 weeks of gestation the long bones assume their future shape and proportion. Bones grow in size and change in shape during childhood and adolescence, particularly during the pubertal growth spurt. Skeletal growth occurs primarily by endochondral ossification at the metaphyses and epiphyses (Fig. 50-2). The primary centre of ossification in the tubular bones is in the centre of the cartilaginous template. The secondary, later developing, centres (epiphyses) are located at the ends of the developing bones. In endochondral ossification there is hypertrophy of cartilage cells and glycogen accumulation. Subsequently, these cells undergo degeneration and become calcified (the provisional zone of calcification). The deeper perichondrial cells transform into osteoblasts through a process of intramembranous ossification. These osteoblasts, and vascular tissue, invade the cartilaginous matrix

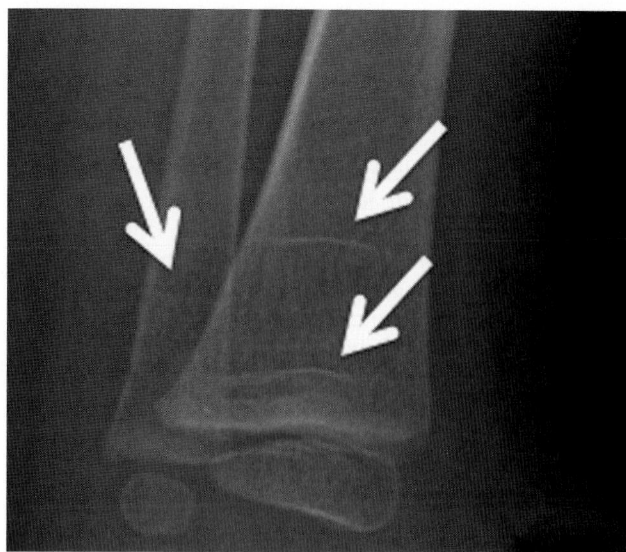

FIGURE 50-3 ■ Growth arrest lines at the distal tibia (arrows). If endochondral ossification ceases for any reason (e.g. period of illness, hypothyroidism), the zone of provisional calcification is left as a thin, horizontal, dense white line when the bone is at that particular stage of development.

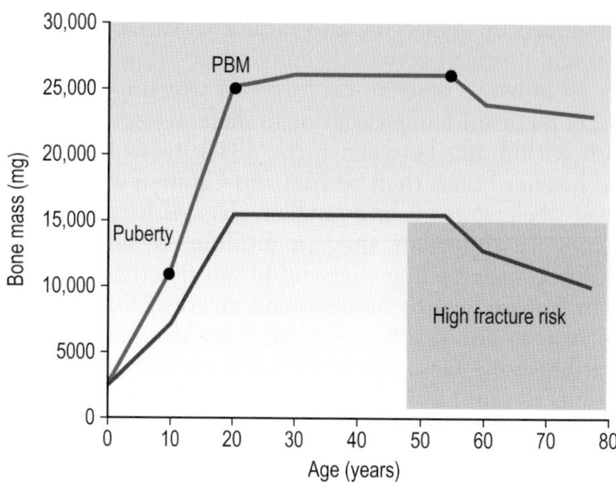

FIGURE 50-4 ■ Bone gain and loss during life. During childhood and adolescence there is accumulation of mineral in the bones which are growing in length and size, particularly at the time of puberty. Bones are larger and heavier in men than in women. Peak bone mass (PBM) is reached in the 20s and remains constant until about 35 years. At the time of the menopause, women lose bone due to oestrogen lack; both men and women lose bone with age. Maximising PBM and minimising bone loss by lifestyle factors such as regular exercise and good nutrition (adequate calcium and vitamin D) and avoiding risk factors (e.g. smoking, excess alcohol consumption) will prevent osteoporosis. Blue line, normal individual; red line, individual failing to achieve potential for skeletal mass. (Adapted from Heaney RP, Abrams S, Dawson-Hughes B, et al. Peak bone mass. Osteoporos Int. 2000;11(12):985–1009.)

and lay down osteoid, which becomes mineralised. Osteoblasts become trapped within the developing bone and transform into osteocytes.

Increase in bone length takes place at the metaphyses of long bones, which adjoin the cartilaginous growth plate. This cartilaginous growth plate remains between the ossification primary and secondary centres until growth ceases and skeletal maturity is reached. The remnant of the cartilage of the epiphyses adjacent to the articular surface becomes the articular cartilage of the adjacent joint. If endochondral ossification ceases for some reason (illness, nutritional deprivation) then the zone of provisional calcification present at that particular stage of skeletal development may remain as a thin white line (Harris growth arrest line) on radiographs (Fig. 50-3).

Bones consist of an outer shell of compact (cortical) bone with a central cavity which contains the marrow space, and 'lace-like' trabecular bone which is prominent in the axial skeleton and at the ends of long bones. Compact cortical bone constitutes about 80% of skeletal mass. Cancellous (trabecular) bone constitutes 20% of total skeletal mass, but contributes importantly to skeletal strength. The bone trabeculae are arranged to resist tensile deforming stresses, either from weight bearing or muscular activity. The number, thickness and distribution of trabeculae are related to biomechanical loading. Trabeculae provide a large surface area on which metabolic processes can take place and have a higher rate of turnover and richer blood supply than compact bone. Around the cortex of the bone is a layer of periosteum and adjacent to the marrow cavity is its endosteal surface. Excessive osteoclastic activity (e.g. in hyperparathyroidism) causes resorption of cortical bone, which may be visible radiologically (cortical 'tunnelling' and erosions) and is indicative of increased bone turnover. Resorption and formation takes place not only within the cortex of bone but also at the periosteal and endosteal surfaces.

As we age, more bone is removed at the endosteal surface than is replaced, resulting in a net loss of bone at this site. This causes the marrow cavity to enlarge and the bony trabeculae to become thinner—some may ultimately disappear. At the periosteal surface, resorption takes place, which is important in maintaining the normal shape of bones as they grow in length. There is a net gain of bone at the periosteal surface throughout life, so that tubular bones progressively increase in width as age advances.

The bones grow during the first two decades of life with a pubertal spurt during adolescence (Fig. 50-4). Skeletal maturity is achieved at an earlier age in girls (16–18 years) than in boys (18–20 years). Some disorders (hypothyroidism, chronic ill health) may retard skeletal development. Skeletal maturation is assessed radiologically from a non-dominant hand radiograph which is then compared with an atlas of hand radiographs of normal American Caucasian boys and girls of different ages[1] or using the Tanner and Whitehouse bone score (TW2) method, which assesses changes in presence, size and shape of certain bones with age.[2]

Following attainment of skeletal maturity, bone is consolidated and peak bone mass is achieved. For cortical bone this is reached at about 35 years of age, and a little earlier for trabecular bone (Fig. 50-4). Although the long bones grow in length at the metaphyses, they are remodelled in shape during development by endosteal resorption and periosteal apposition.

The size and shape of the skeleton and its individual bones are determined by genetic factors, but are influenced by endocrine and local growth factors, nutrition and physical activity. Remodelling allows the skeleton to adjust to mechanical forces to which it is exposed. There is considerable variation in skeletal size and weight, both within and between races. Black races have larger and heavier bones than whites, and Chinese tend to have lower skeletal mass and smaller size. Although genetic factors are important, they are modified by environmental differences such as diet and physical activity.

In mature healthy adults, bone turnover for the whole skeleton is about 2% per year, with maintenance of a constant bone mass. Bone formation is increased during periods of rapid growth and stimulated by physical activity, growth hormone and thyroid hormone. Bone formation is decreased as a consequence of immobilisation, undernutrition, deficiencies of thyroid and growth hormone and glucocorticoid excess. After the attainment of peak bone mass, bone loss, particularly of trabecular bone, is believed to occur from the third decade of life. Bone loss is a phenomenon, which occurs in all races (Fig. 50-4). Generally both men and women lose bone as they grow older, but women lose more than men. Women lose approximately 15–30% of their total bone mass between maturity and the seventh decade, whereas men lose only about half this amount. After the age of 35, women lose bone at an annual rate of approximately 0.75–1.0%, which increases to a rate of 2–3% in the postmenopausal period. This loss affects both cortical and trabecular bone, but the effect on trabecular bone predominates. In contrast, cortical bone is well preserved until the fifth decade of life when there is a linear loss in both sexes, such that men lose about 25% of their cortical bone whilst women lose about 30%. Low bone mineral density may be the result of either low peak bone mass attainment or subsequent accelerated bone loss.

The most common metabolic disorders of bone are: **osteoporosis**, in which there is a deficiency of bone mass leading to insufficiency (low-trauma) fractures; **rickets and osteomalacia**, in which there is a defective mineralisation of bone osteoid due to vitamin D deficiency, hypophosphataemia, lack of alkaline phosphatase or calcium, or severe acidaemia; and **hyperparathyroidism**, in which a tumour or hyperplasia of the parathyroid glands causes increase in parathyroid hormone production and stimulation of osteoclasts. Other metabolic bone disorders include osteogenesis imperfecta, hyperphosphatasia and osteopetrosis. Paget's disease is not strictly a metabolic bone disease, since it can be monostotic or polyostotic and does not involve the entire skeleton, but because it involves increased bone turnover it is often included in this group of disease.

OSTEOPOROSIS

Definition and Epidemiology

Osteoporosis is the most common metabolic bone disease, with increasing significance as the population ages. Fragility fractures due to osteoporosis are one of the most significant challenges to public health worldwide. The elderly represent the fastest-growing age group, and the yearly number of fragility fractures will increase substantially with continued ageing of the population.[3] Approximately 50% of women and 20% of men older than 50 years will have a fragility (insufficiency) fracture in their remaining lifetime in Caucasian populations.[4]

Osteoporosis is defined as a skeletal disorder characterised by compromised bone strength predisposing a person to an increased risk of fracture.[5] Bone strength primarily reflects the integration of bone mineral density (BMD) and bone quality.[5] BMD is expressed as grams of mineral per area or volume, and in any given individual is determined by peak bone mass and amount of bone loss. Bone quality refers to architecture, turnover, damage accumulation (e.g. microfractures), and mineralisation.[5]

Though BMD is only in part responsible for bone strength, dual energy X-ray absorptiometry (DXA) measurements of BMD have been universally adopted as a standard to define osteoporosis in terms of bone densitometry. In 1994 the World Health Organization (WHO)[6] used T-scores to classify and define BMD measurements. A T-score is the standard deviation of the BMD of an individual patient compared to a young, healthy reference population, matched for gender and ethnicity. According to the WHO, normal, osteopenic and osteoporotic BMD are differentiated.

Normal: BMD above (≥) –1 standard deviation (SD) of the young adult reference mean (peak bone mass).

Osteopenia: BMD between (<) –1 and (>) –2.5 SD below that of the young adult reference mean.

Osteoporosis: BMD more than (≤) –2.5 SD below the young adult reference mean.

It should be noted that even in the absence of osteoporotic BMD the *presence of one or more low-impact fragility fractures* is considered as a sign of severe osteoporosis[7] and that not infrequently in these patients the BMD measured with DXA may be in the normal or osteopenic range.

The osteoporosis/osteopenia definition is also applied to older men, but it is not used in men younger than 50, premenopausal women and children or adolescents who have not yet reached peak bone mass. In these patient groups, low bone mass would appropriately be defined as a BMD which is more than 2 standard deviations below the mean BMD matched for age, gender and ethnicity (http://www.iscd.org/visitors/positions/OP-Index.cfm and).[8–10] The WHO definition is *not applicable* to other bone densitometry techniques (quantitative computed tomography, QCT; quantitative ultrasound, QUS) or other anatomical sites (e.g. calcaneus).

Osteoporosis should not be considered as a single disease entity, but rather an end result of many disease processes (Table 50-1). It may result from defective skeletal accretion during bone growth and development. Alternatively, it may result from disease processes in which bone resorption exceeds new bone formation, resulting in a net loss of bone mass and consequent compromise to skeletal strength.

Radiological Features

Osteoporosis is radiographically characterised by decreased radiodensity of bone (Fig. 50-5). However, it

TABLE 50-1 **Main Causes of Osteoporosis**

Primary
Juvenile
Idiopathic of young adults
Postmenopausal
Senile
Secondary
Endocrine
Glucocorticoid excess
Oestrogen/testosterone deficiency
Hyperthyroidism
Hyperparathyroidism
Growth hormone deficiency (childhood onset)
Nutritional
Intestinal malabsorption (e.g. coeliac disease)
Chronic alcoholism
Chronic liver disease
Partial gastrectomy
Vitamin C deficiency (scurvy)
Hereditary
Osteogenesis imperfecta
Homocystinuria
Marfan's syndrome
Ehlers–Danlos syndrome
Haematological
Thalassaemia
Sickle-cell disease
Gaucher's disease
Leukaemia in children
Other
Rheumatoid arthritis
Haemochromatosis

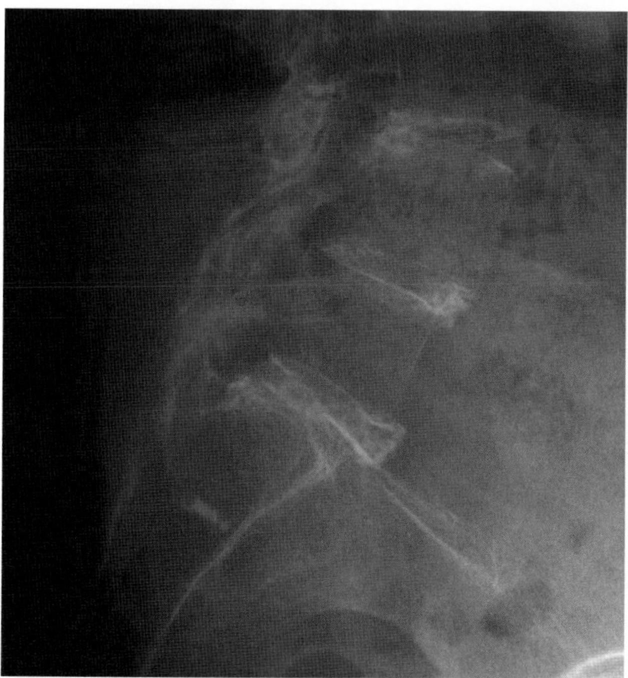

FIGURE 50-5 ■ **Osteopenia.** Lateral radiograph of the lumbar spine showing severe, diffuse osteopenia with degenerative changes of the lumbar spine.

should be noted that radiographs are very limited in assessing the amount of bone loss[11] and only advanced bone loss can be identified. Descriptive terms that have been used to describe reduced bone density in the absence of fragility fractures are 'osteopenia' or 'demineralisation'. The latter is an incorrect term since mineral and collagen are both reduced in osteoporosis. Reduced bone density is often more prominent in areas of the skeleton rich in trabecular bone, particularly in the axial skeleton (vertebrae, pelvis, ribs and sternum). Eventually, changes may also be evident in the bones of the appendicular skeleton. Trabeculae become thin and may disappear completely; they may be sparse, but those that remain may become thickened due to stresses to which the skeleton is exposed (Fig. 50-6). The cortex becomes reduced in width through endosteal bone resorption, and in states of increased bone turnover there will be intracortical tunnelling and porosity.

Osteoporotic bone is less able to withstand the stresses to which the skeleton is exposed compared to normal bone, and this leads to the cardinal clinical feature of low trauma fractures. Such fractures can occur at any skeletal site, but they are most common in sites of the skeleton rich in trabecular bone, particularly the vertebrae, the distal forearm and the proximal femur. These fractures may be associated with considerable pain and deformity. In individuals who suffer hip fractures 20% will die within the next year and 20% will require permanent nursing home care.[4] Even if age-adjusted incidence rates for hip fractures remain stable, the estimated number of hip fractures worldwide will rise from 1.7 million in 1990 to 6.3 million in 2050.[3] It is important to identify patients with osteoporosis and at increased risk of fracture as there are now therapies available (bisphosphonates, selective oestrogen receptor modulators (SERMs), strontium ranelate; teriparatide (parathyroid hormone) and denosumab) which cause relatively small increases in bone mineral density (4–12%) but more importantly reduce future fracture risk by between 40 and 70%.[12,13]

Spine in Osteoporosis

Related to biomechanical forces through the spine, as trabeculae are lost, the process of osteoporosis particularly involves the horizontally orientated secondary trabeculae. The vertical trabeculae actually become more prominent and thickened.[14] This results in a vertical 'striated' appearance to the vertebral body on lateral spinal radiographs and cross-sectional imaging studies. Figure 50-6 shows this pattern in sagittal and coronal reformations of CT images, which was also termed hypertrophic atrophy. This feature is generally seen in several, or all, of the vertebrae when it is related to osteoporosis, which serves to distinguish a similar appearance in a single vertebral body when it is related to haemangioma.

Vertebral fractures are the most common of osteoporotic fractures (Fig. 50-7). The anterior and central mid portion of the vertebrae withstand compression forces less well than the posterior and outer ring elements of the vertebrae, resulting in wedge or end-plate fractures or, less commonly, crush fractures.[15] Vertebral fractures can be graded as mild (20–25% change in shape;

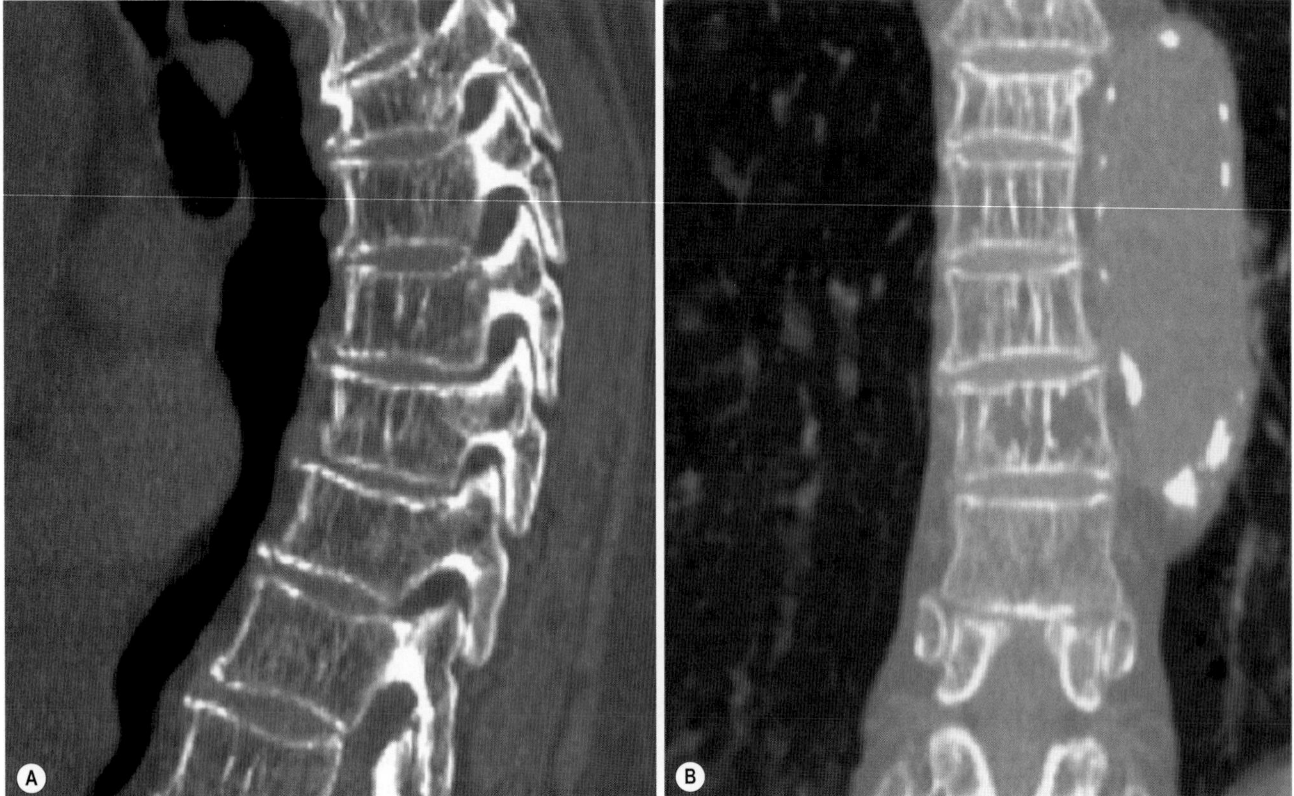

FIGURE 50-6 ■ **Hypertrophic atrophy in osteoporosis.** Sagittal (A) and coronal (B) CT MPRs of the thoracic spine showing diffuse bone loss with prominent vertical trabeculae resulting in a striated appearance.

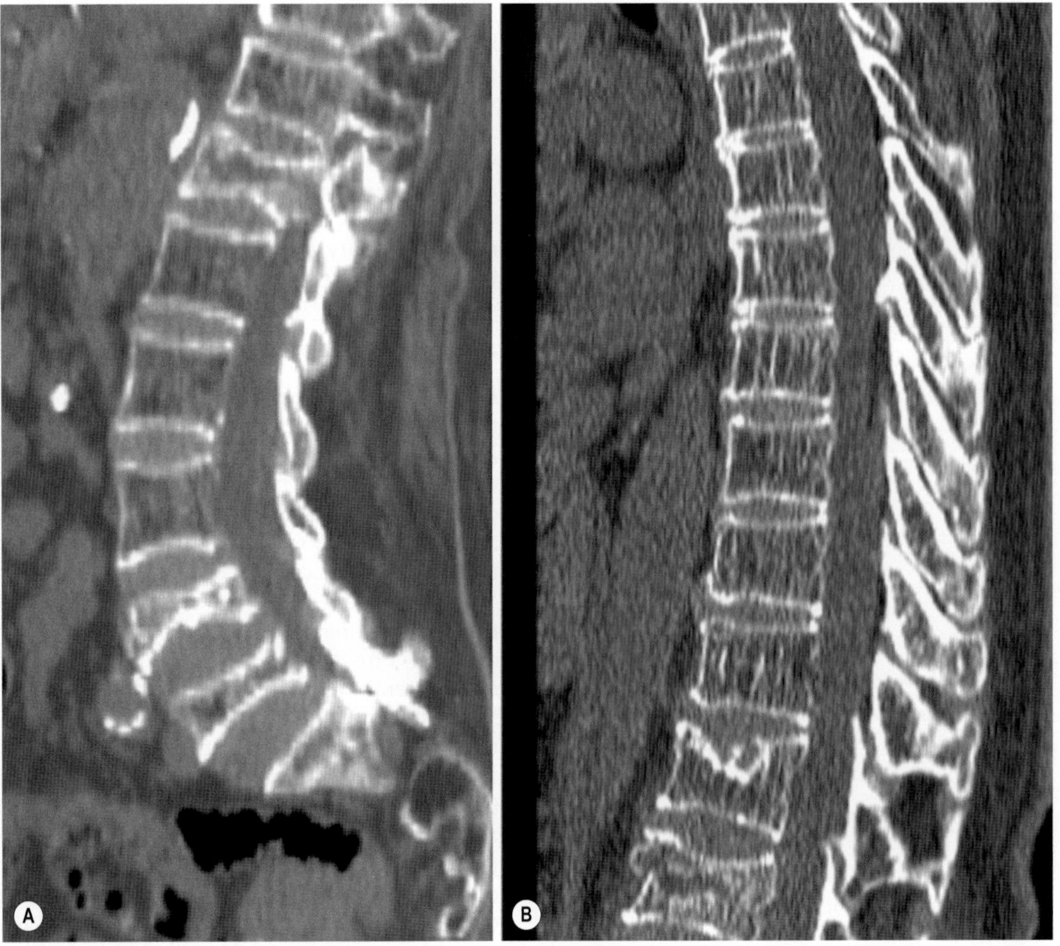

FIGURE 50-7 ■ **Osteoporosis—vertebral osteoporosis and fracture.** Sagittal reconstructions of CT data sets of the thoracolumbar spine showing moderate to severe osteoporotic fractures at T12, L4 and L5 (A) and at the lower thoracic spine with multilevel prominence of the vertical trabeculae and a striated appearance due to loss of the horizontal trabeculae (B).

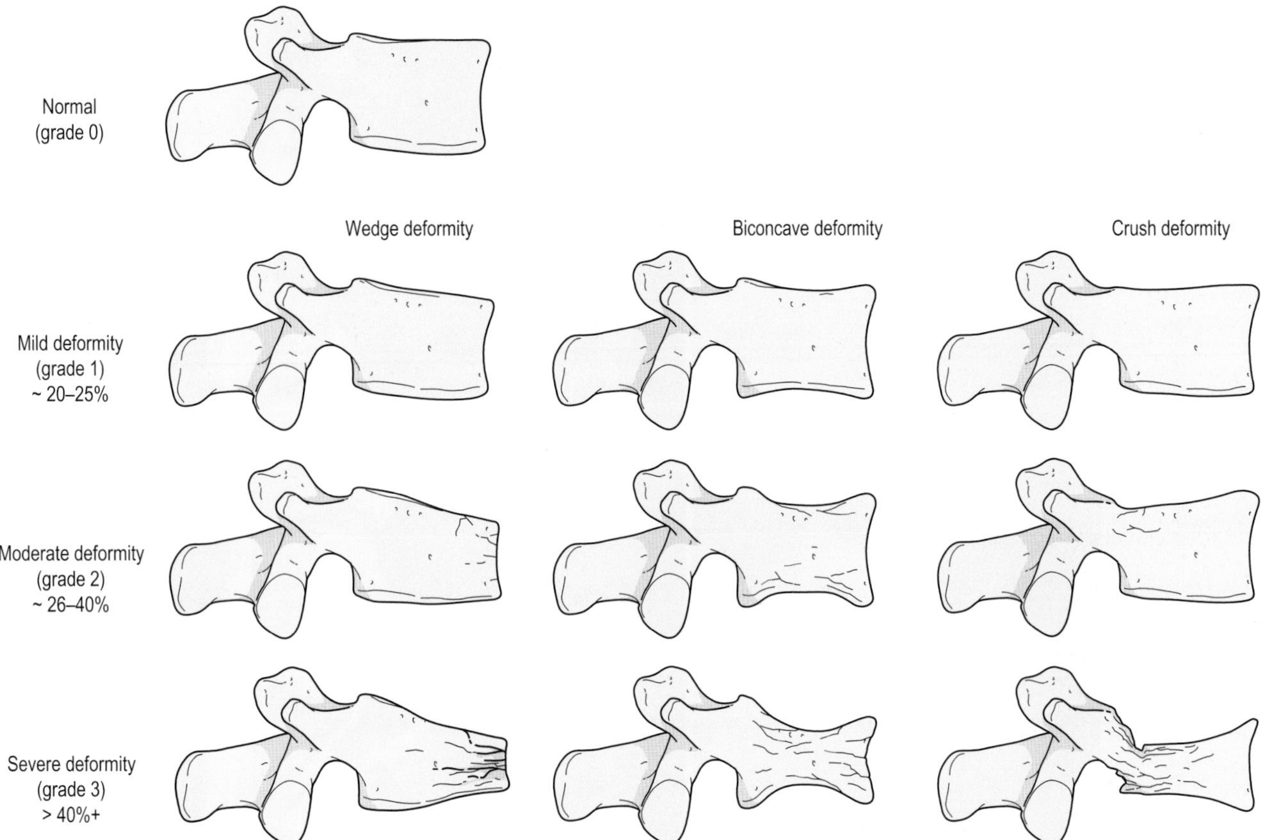

FIGURE 50-8 ■ The semiquantitative method of grading of Genant et al,[16] which is widely used in epidemiology and pharmaceutical studies. Vertebral fractures are strong predictors of future fractures (×5 for vertebral fracture; ×2 for hip fracture). The higher the grade of vertebral fracture, the higher the risk of future fracture.

grade 1), moderate (26–40% change in shape; grade 2) and severe (>40% change in shape; grade 3)[16] (Fig. 50-8). This semi-quantitative grading (SQ) method is the one currently most frequently applied to define the prevalence and incidence of vertebral fractures in epidemiology studies and pharmaceutical trials of the efficacy of new osteoporosis therapies.

The more severe the grade of vertebral fracture, the greater the risk of future fracture. Vertebral fractures are powerful predictors of future fracture (hip ×2; vertebral ×5). If vertebral fractures are present it is therefore extremely important that they are accurately and clearly reported by radiologists as fractures; other terms such as 'deformities', 'collapse', must be avoided. There is evidence that vertebral fractures are being under-reported by radiologists, with the result that patients who should be receiving treatment to reduce their risk of future fractures are not being identified.[17–19] As a consequence, a joint initiative was launched in 2002 between the International Osteoporosis Foundation (IOF) and the European Society of Skeletal Radiology (Osteoporosis Group) to improve the sensitivity and accuracy of reporting of vertebral fractures by radiologists. Vertebral fractures may occur as an acute event related to minor trauma and be accompanied by pain, which generally resolves spontaneously over 6–8 weeks. This resolution of symptoms serves to distinguish osteoporotic vertebral fractures from similar events due to more sinister abnormalities, such as metastases, in which the symptoms are more protracted. However, 30% or more of vertebral fractures may be present in asymptomatic patients. Osteoporotic fractures occur most commonly in the thoracic and thoracolumbar regions and result in progressive loss of height in affected individuals. Osteoporotic fractures are uncommon above T7; if fractures are present above this anatomical region, metastases should be considered. Also if the posterior aspect of the vertebral body is fractured metastases or myeloma should be the first differential diagnosis. Wedging of multiple vertebral bodies in the thoracic spine can lead to increased kyphosis (dowager hump) which, if severe, may result in the ribs abutting on the iliac crests with compromise of respiratory function and reduced quality of life.

Vertebroplasty and Kyphoplasty

Vertebroplasty and kyphoplasty have selected application in patients with osteoporotic vertebral fractures that are persistently painful.[20] The technique is performed mostly by radiologists and orthopaedic surgeons. Vertebroplasty is the injection of cement (methylmethacrylate) into a fractured vertebral body as a means of treating pain. Injection is generally made by passing the introduction needle through the pedicles. Kyphoplasty is the injection of cement into the fractured vertebral body after a balloon has been used to form a cavity and to decompress the

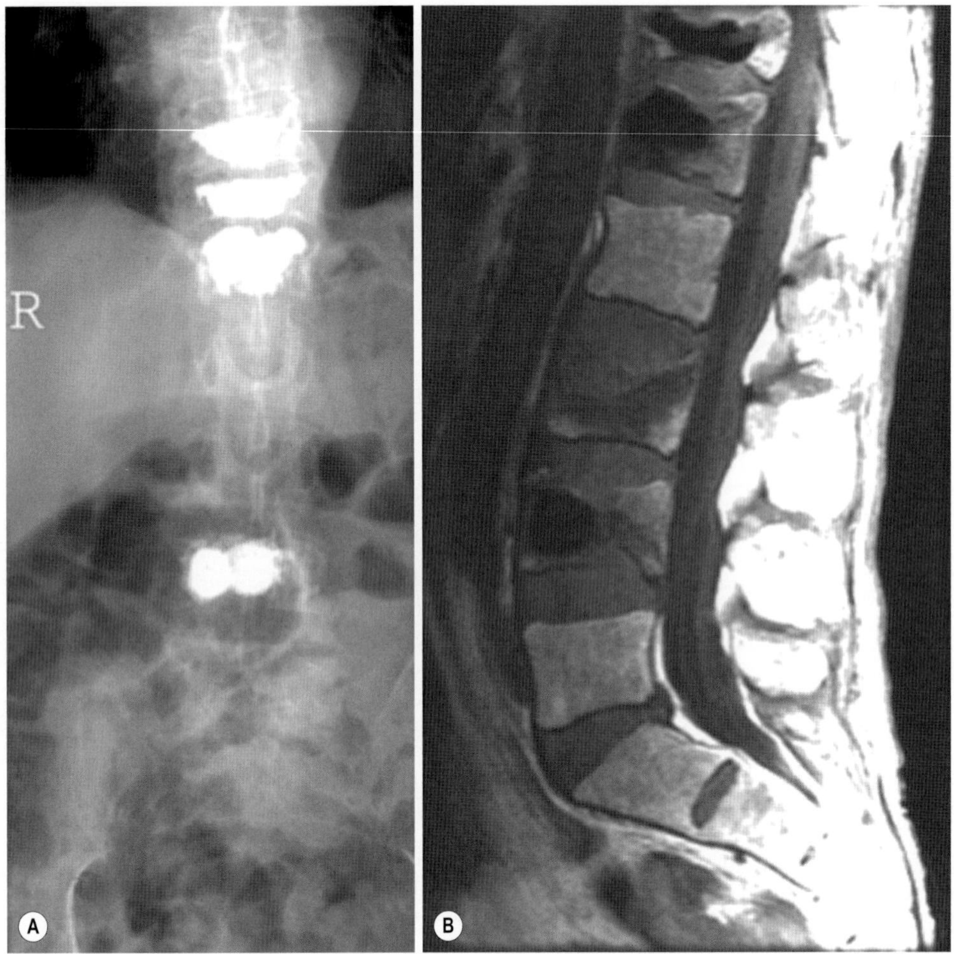

FIGURE 50-9 ■ Osteoporosis—vertebroplasty/kyphoplasty. In selected cases, pain from osteoporotic vertebral fractures which has not responded to conservative (analgesics) and bisphosphonate therapy may be treated by injection of cement (methylmethacrylate) into the vertebral body. The cement is radio-opaque so that it can be visualised during injection, and is seen in the frontal radiograph of the thoracolumbar spine at T11, T12, L1 and L4 (A) and the T1-weighted sagittal MR image at T12, L1 and L4 (B). In kyphoplasty a balloon is introduced through a needle passed through the pedicle and used to increase the height of the vertebral body. A cavity is thus created for the injection of the cement. The cement has rounded configuration in kyphoplasty (seen at L1 and L4) compared to vertebroplasty where the cement is simply injected into the vertebral body (T12).

fracture and correct some of the deformity[21] (Fig. 50-9). Both techniques are intended to relieve pain in patients who have not responded to conservative measures. It has been suggested that vertebroplasty/kyphoplasty should be performed in the first 4–6 weeks after presentation with pain, which requires opiates for pain relief and/or hospital admission.[22] Certainly patients with proven osteoporosis should always be commenced on bone protective/bone enhancing therapy when vertebroplasty is to be performed. Patient selection is crucial to the outcome of the procedure. The pain should arise from vertebral fractures that are temporally related to the onset of symptoms. Magnetic resonance imaging (MRI) with fluid-sensitive sequences and fat suppression can aid the identification of more acute fractures showing bone marrow oedema, typically along the end-plates, in acute and subacute fractures with ongoing bony remodelling.

Two recent trials comparing vertebroplasty with a sham procedure suggested that improvements in pain and pain-related disability associated with osteoporotic compression fractures in patients treated with vertebroplasty were similar to the improvements in a control group.[23,24] Conversely a study published in 2010 concluded that pain relief after vertebroplasty was immediate, sustained for at least a year, and was significantly greater than that achieved with conservative treatment, at an acceptable cost.[25] The chance of successful pain relief by vertebroplasty for osteoporotic fracture is between 70 and 95%.[26] In a previous study kyphoplasty and vertebroplasty demonstrated similar good clinical outcomes during the 12-month follow-up; but kyphoplasty offered a higher degree of spinal deformity correction and resulted in less cement leakage than vertebroplasty.[27]

There are potential risks of vertebroplasty; these may be needle related (pedicle fracture, needle breakage, pneumothorax, haemorrhage, infection), cement related (root compression, cord compression, pulmonary cement emboli), procedure related (pulmonary fat emboli, rib or vertebral fracture), sedation related (respiratory arrest, airway injuries, cardiac arrest) or drug related (allergy). The overall complication rate from reports suggests that symptom-inducing or potentially serious complications occur in approximately 2% of patients treated for osteoporotic fracture.[28]

Most cases are treated under conscious sedation with analgesia, but in some patients general anaesthesia is required. For needle placement, high-quality fluoroscopy in either a biplane or C-arm configuration is recommended. Needles, injector sets and cements are now manufactured specifically for vertebroplasty. Care should be taken to ensure a sterile environment. All patients treated by vertebroplasty or kyphoplasty for osteoporotic compression fractures should be under the care of a clinician with special interest in osteoporosis management and on appropriate medical therapy to reduce future fracture risk.[13]

Osteoporotic Fractures

Fractures that occur in osteoporosis generally heal well with satisfactory callus formation. In some sites the presence of multiple micro-fractures and callus formation can cause osteosclerosis on a radiograph; this must be distinguished from other pathologies such as bone metastases. These insufficiency fractures occur in particular anatomical sites, including the symphysis pubis, the sacrum, pubic rami and calcaneus. Other sites involved are the sternum, supra-acetabular area and elsewhere in the pelvis, femoral neck, humerus and proximal and distal tibia. Some of these fractures may be accompanied by considerable osteolysis, particularly those involving the symphysis pubis. Fragility fractures of the pelvis have been misinterpreted as neoplastic lesions and several previous studies[29–31] focused on the importance of correctly diagnosing sacral fractures to avoid misguiding patient management, which may produce dangerous and costly interventional procedures. Cross-sectional imaging techniques (CT and MR imaging) may help to differentiate insufficiency fractures from other pathologies (Fig. 50-10). On radionuclide bone scintigraphy there is increased uptake in regions of acute insufficiency fractures.

When the sacrum is involved, there is often a characteristic H pattern (Honda sign) of radionuclide uptake. CT and MRI are particularly helpful in defining the fracture lines of insufficiency fractures involving the sacrum (fractures usually occur parallel to the sacroiliac joint) and in the calcaneus. In these sites fractures may not be identified on radiographs because of complex anatomy and overlying structures. MRI is helpful in differentiating vertebral fractures resulting from osteoporosis from those caused by other pathologies (myeloma, metastases). It should be noted that MR is more sensitive than CT in diagnosing pelvic insufficiency fractures.[30]

During the past decade a number of publications focused on osteoporotic insufficiency fractures and demonstrated that findings previously defined as osteonecrosis are actually insufficiency fractures.[29,30,32–35] Previously, the term' spontaneous osteonecrosis of the knee (SONK), was used to describe an osteochondral lesion which was typically observed at the medial femoral condyle but which is now considered to be an insufficiency fracture. Both insufficiency fractures at the medial femoral condyle of the knee and femoral head are frequent findings in older individuals and indicate increased fragility of the skeleton (Fig. 50-11).

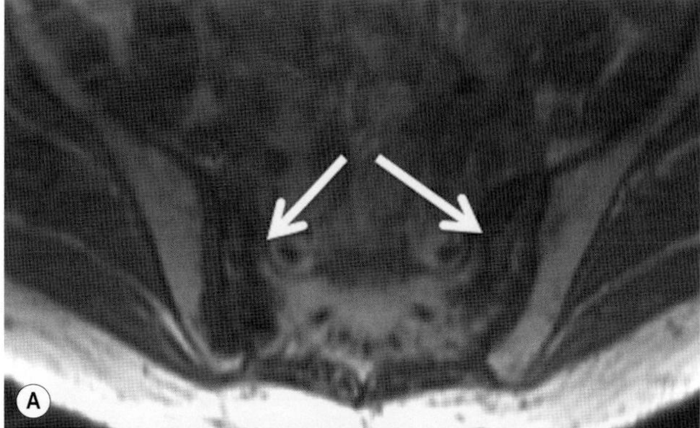

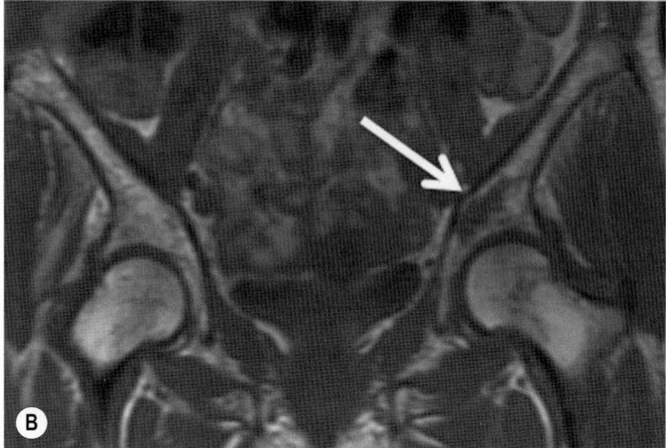

FIGURE 50-10 ■ Pelvic insufficiency fractures. Axial and coronal T1-weighted FSE sequences of the pelvis in a 72-year-old woman with bilateral sacral insufficiency fractures (arrows in A) and a left supra-acetabular fracture (arrow in B). T1-weighted sequences frequently show fracture lines best.

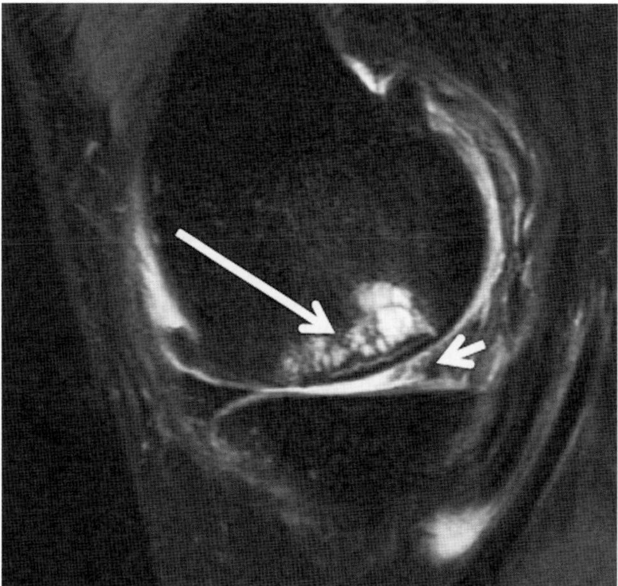

FIGURE 50-11 ■ Medial femoral condyle insufficiency fracture. Sagittal intermediate-weighted fat-saturated MR image of the knee in a 65-year-old man showing a medial femoral condyle insufficiency fracture (long arrow) with meniscal maceration (short arrow).

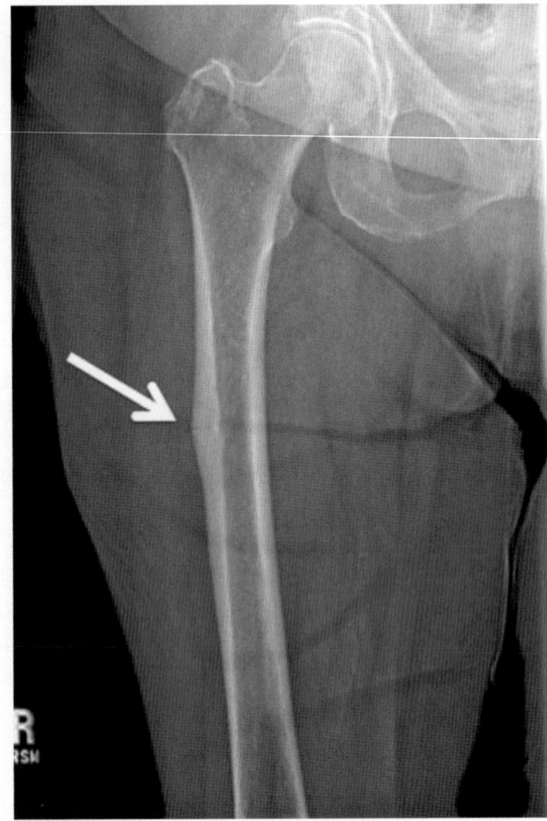

FIGURE 50-12 ■ Atypical proximal femur fracture after bisphosphonate therapy. Radiograph of the right proximal femur showing an atypical, incomplete femoral diaphysis fracture (arrow) after long-term bisphosphonate therapy (arrow).

Recently atypical subtrochanteric and femoral shaft fractures have been reported in older individuals and on long-term bisphosphonate therapy.[36–38] Coexisting factors have been discussed in the aetiology of these fractures such as co-morbidities (e.g. vitamin D deficiency, chronic obstructive airways disease, rheumatoid arthritis, diabetes) and other drugs (e.g. glucocorticoids, proton pump inhibitors).[36–38] The task force of the American Society for Bone and Mineral Research[38] identified a number of major and minor clinical and imaging features of these fractures which include location in the subtrochanteric region and femoral shaft, transverse or short oblique orientation, minimal or no associated trauma, a medial spike when the fracture is complete, absence of comminution, focal cortical thickening and a periosteal reaction of the lateral cortex (Fig. 50-12). There may be prodromal symptoms such as dull or aching pain in the groin or thigh. As these stress fractures may be bilateral in up to 50% of patients and occur anywhere in the femoral shaft, if suspected, imaging should include both femora in their entirety. These fractures are increasingly diagnosed, can occur in bisphosphonate naïve patients and not infrequently only lateral cortical thickening is evident. This may progress to a complete fracture and is therefore a critical finding, which needs to be communicated to the clinician. These incomplete stress fractures are treated with prophylactic internal fixation surgery. The relation of this complication with long-term bisphosphonate therapy has led to consideration of a drug 'holiday' at 5-year review. If the BMD T-score is above −2.5, treatment may be discontinued for two years and then the necessity for recommencement is considered; however, there are no scientific data on which to base such recommendations.

Aetiology

Osteoporosis can be classified as generalised, regional (involving a segment of the skeleton) or localised.

Regional Osteoporosis

This can occur in disuse and reflex sympathetic dystrophy (RSD/regional pain syndrome) following fracture, or related to other pathologies (primary and secondary tumours). Chronic disuse is characterised by a uniform pattern of bone loss; acute immobilisation causes more focal and irregular bone formation and resorption. This results in different patterns of bone loss, which include diffuse osteopenia, linear translucent bands, juxta-articular speckled radiolucent areas and cortical bone resorption.[39] MRI findings in disuse osteopenia are also typical and include accentuation of vertical trabecular lines, presence of subchondral lobules of fat, horizontal trabecular lines, prominence of blood vessels, and dotted and patchy areas of high signal intensity on fluid-sensitive sequences[40] (Fig. 50-13).

RSD/complex regional pain syndrome is a clinical syndrome that can occur in children and adults and may be precipitated by a variety of processes. There is overactivity of the sympathetic nervous system, initially causing pain, soft-tissue swelling and hyperaemia, with excessive bone resorption (probably stimulated by cytokines), which occurs particularly in a peri-articular distribution and may simulate malignant disease. The diagnosis of RSD/complex regional pain syndrome relies on clinical evaluation and radiographs. MRI may provide a differential diagnosis between RSD and other bone pathologies as it demonstrates diffuse signal abnormalities with soft-tissue and bone marrow oedema pattern.[41]

There are also conditions which cause focal or migratory and transient osteoporosis, usually in the region of large joints (hip, knee), the aetiology of which is uncertain. Transient osteoporosis of the hip occurs in younger and middle-aged individuals and middle age, more frequently in men than women. Also, it is typically found in women in the third trimester of pregnancy. There is sudden onset of pain without preceding trauma. Radiographically there is reduction in density of the proximal femur. There may be an underlying abnormality of perfusion of the marrow, which is oedematous. MRI is sensitive in demonstrating bone marrow oedema pattern without focal abnormalities before any radiographic abnormality is evident (Fig. 50-14).[42,43]

Generalised Osteoporosis

There are many causes of osteoporosis, falling into four categories:

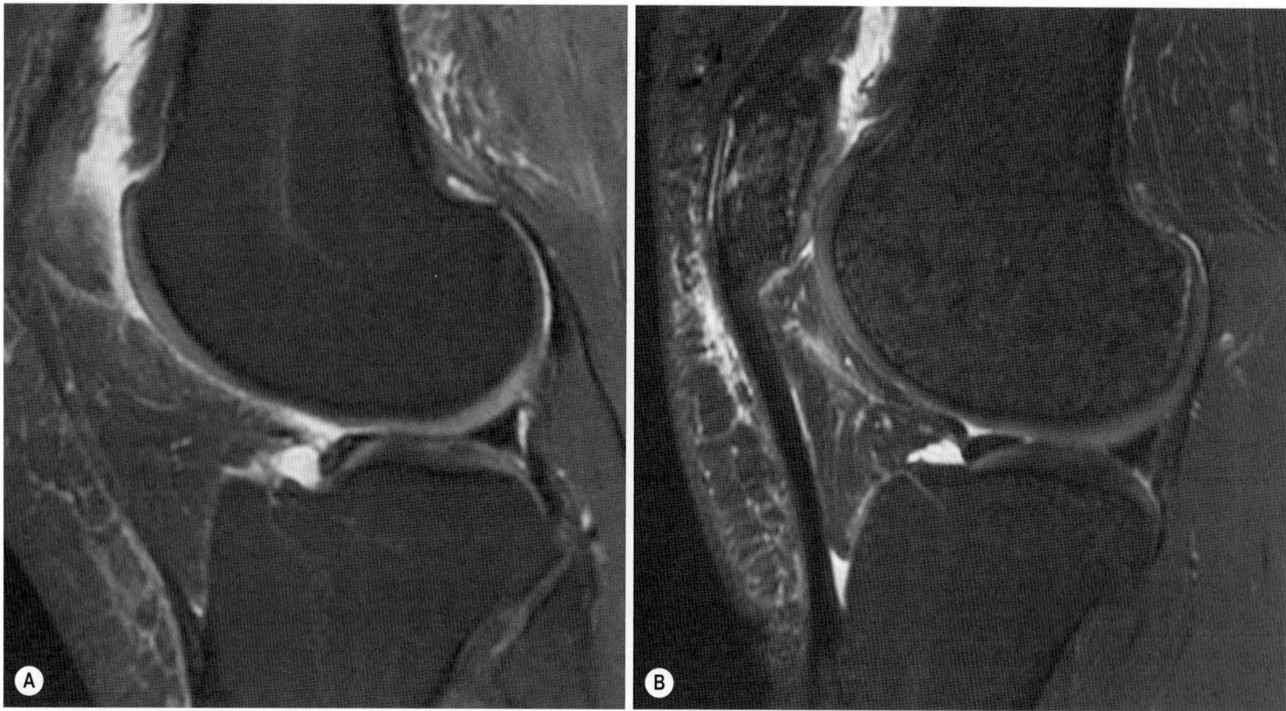

FIGURE 50-13 ■ **Disuse osteopenia.** Sagittal intermediate-weighted fat-saturated MR image of the knee in a 35-year-old man with an ankle fracture showing normal bone marrow signal at the time of the fracture.

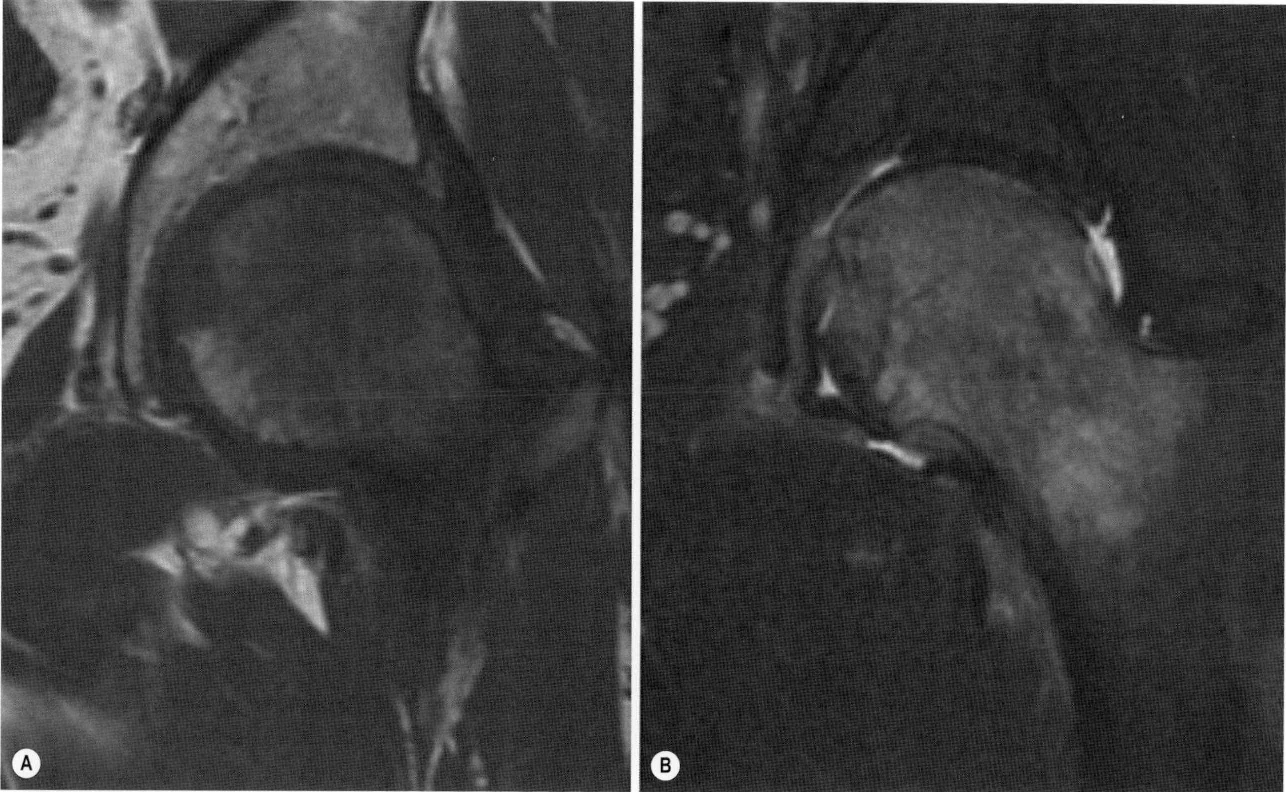

FIGURE 50-14 ■ **Transient osteoporosis of the hip.** Coronal T1-weighted FSE (A) and STIR (B) images of the left hip in a 42-year-old man with transient osteoporosis. Note homogeneous bone marrow oedema pattern without focal linear signal abnormalities, which would suggest a fracture, or deformities as might occur in avascular necrosis of the femoral head with subchondral fracture.

1. Factors which reduce peak adult bone mass
2. Age-related bone loss
3. Bone loss associated with menopause or hypogonadal state
4. Bone loss that is secondary to other medical conditions and drugs (Table 50-1).

Idiopathic Juvenile Osteoporosis (IJO). This self-limiting form of osteoporosis occurs in prepubertal children and must be differentiated from osteogenesis imperfecta and other forms of juvenile osteoporosis. IJO is a rare disorder, first described by Dent and Friedman,[44] and occurs in children aged between 8 and 14 years who have previously been healthy. The disease runs an acute course over a period of 2–4 years, during which there is growth arrest and fractures. There is a wide spectrum of severity, and both cortical and trabecular bone are affected. In the mild form, only one or two vertebral fractures may be present, but in more severe cases fractures involve all the vertebrae and the extremities, particularly the metaphyseal region of the distal tibia. A few affected patients may develop severe kyphoscoliosis, deformities of the extremities, and even die from respiratory failure due to thoracic deformity. The disease is reversible and remits spontaneously. Affected patients may be left with only a mild or moderate kyphosis, short stature and some bone deformity following fractures.[44] Investigations indicate uncoupling of the two components of bone turnover due to both increase in resorption and decrease in formation. The important differential diagnosis in children with vertebral fracture is hypercortisolism and leukaemia. Affected patients do not have the blue sclerae characteristic of osteogenesis imperfecta.

Osteoporosis of Young Adults. This heterogeneous condition occurs equally in young men and women.[45] The disease generally runs a mild course with multiple vertebral fractures occurring over a decade or more, with associated loss in height. Fractures of metatarsals and ribs are also common, and hip fractures may occur. The cause of the condition is uncertain and in some patients it may simply be that inadequate bone mass has been accrued during skeletal growth. Some affected individuals may have a mild variant of osteogenesis imperfecta. Rarely, osteoporosis may present during pregnancy, but whether this is a causal or coincidental association is unknown.

Postmenopausal Osteoporosis. At the time of the menopause, lack of oestrogen will result in some women losing trabecular bone at a rate three times greater than is usual (2–10% per annum). The condition, previously referred to as type I osteoporosis, characteristically becomes clinically evident in women 15–20 years after the menopause. Fractures occur in sites of the skeleton rich in trabecular bone, including the vertebral bodies and distal forearm (Colles' fracture).

Senile Osteoporosis. This condition, previously referred to as type II involutional osteoporosis, occurs in both men and women of 75 years or older and is due to age-related bone loss. This occurs as a consequence of age-related impaired bone formation associated with secondary hyperparathyroidism caused by reduced intestinal calcium absorption due to decreased levels of 1,25$(OH)_2$D production in the elderly.[46] There is reduction in both cortical and trabecular bone. The syndrome manifests mainly as hip fractures and wedge fractures of the vertebrae, but fractures may also occur in the proximal tibia, proximal humerus and pelvis.

Secondary Osteoporosis. A large number of conditions may lead to osteoporosis (Table 50-1). Radiologically these may be indistinguishable from age-related osteoporosis. However, some may have specific and diagnostic radiological features (i.e. subperiosteal erosions of the phalanges in primary hyperparathyroidism). In glucocorticoid excess (endogenous and exogenous), there is reduced bone formation due to a direct effect on the osteoblast, and increased osteoclastic activity, probably mediated through secondary hyperparathyroidism, stimulated by reduced gastrointestinal absorption of calcium. There is also evidence that glucocorticoids induce premature apoptosis of both osteoblasts and osteoclasts. The effect is primarily on trabecular bone. Fractures occur particularly in the vertebral bodies and ribs; the latter may heal with profuse callus formation. Fractures may appear relatively rapidly after starting oral glucocorticoid medication, in particular with high doses and in younger patients (Fig. 50-15).

Osteogenesis Imperfecta

A number of inherited disorders of connective tissue may result in osteoporosis. Osteogenesis imperfecta (OI), or brittle bone disease, results from mutations affecting either the *COL1A1* or *COL1A2* gene of Type I collagen.[47] Although the disease is usually apparent at birth or in childhood, more mild forms of the disease may not become apparent until adulthood, when affected individuals may present with insufficiency fractures and osteopenia (Fig. 50-16). Radiographic features vary according to the type of disease and its severity and include osteopenia and fractures, which may heal with florid callus formation, mimicking osteosarcoma. Bones are thin and over-tubulated (gracile), normal in length or shortened, thickened and deformed by multiple fractures. Intrasutural (Wormian) bones can be identified on skull radiographs. In severe forms of osteogenesis imperfecta the diagnosis may be made before birth by detailed ultrasound in the second trimester. Diagnostic features include cranial enlargement, reduced echogenicity of bone and deformity and shortening of limb bones as a result of intrauterine fractures.

Osteogenesis imperfecta is classified based on distinct characteristics, including blue sclerae, the severity of the disorder and the mode of inheritance (dominant, recessive, sporadic/new mutation).[48] However, accurate classification is difficult because of phenotypic overlap.[47]

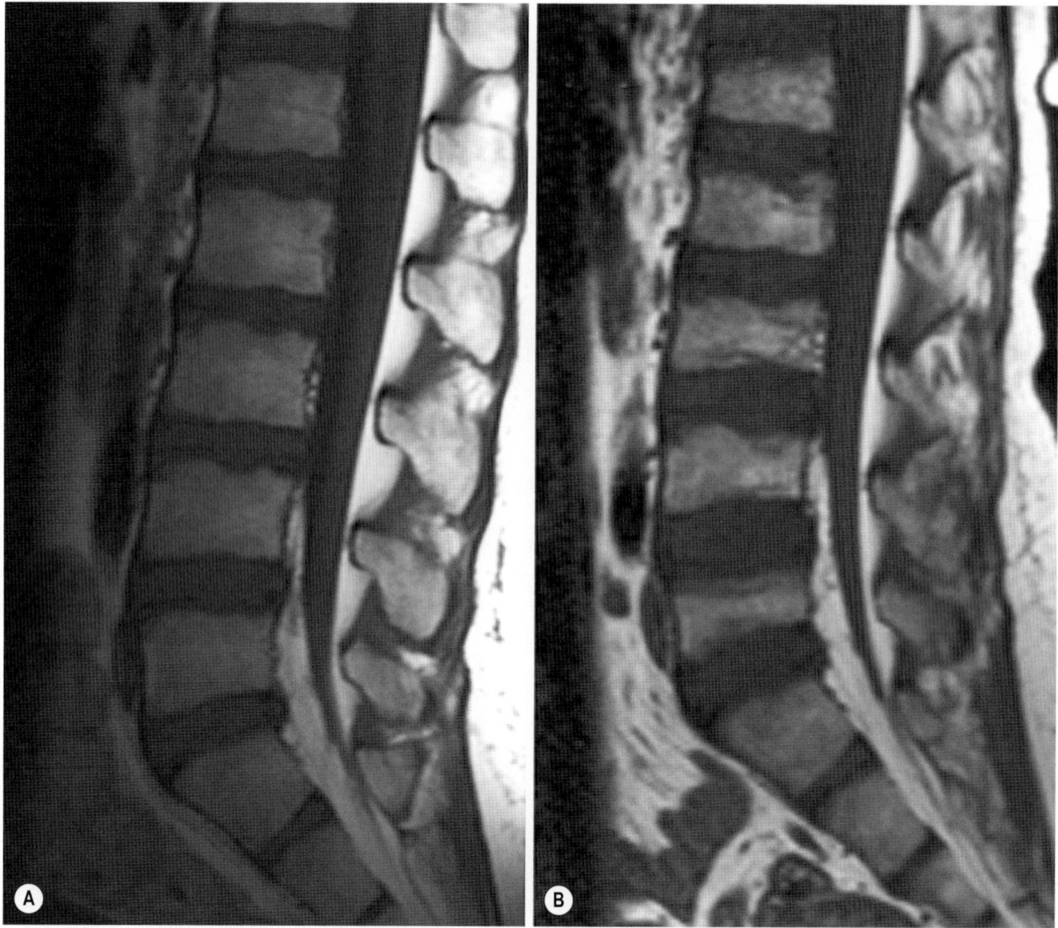

FIGURE 50-15 ■ **Glucocorticoid Induced Vertebral Fractures.** Sagittal T1-weighted MR images of the lumbar spine in an 11-year-old child at the time of glucocorticoid therapy initiation (A) and 3 months later (B) with multiple vertebral fractures having occurred.

Affected subjects who do not have dental involvement are designated as group A. Subjects with dentinogenesis imperfecta are designated as group B.

Type I

This is the mildest and most prevalent form of the disease and may only become apparent in adulthood. There is a history of fractures, generally dating back to childhood. In children the fractures may become radiographically and clinically apparent as the child becomes more active (5+ years), and may take the form of overt fractures or micro-fractures involving the metaphyses. In infancy these features may resemble those found in non-accidental injury.[49] The differential diagnosis can usually be resolved by the presence of associated extraskeletal manifestations of osteogenesis imperfecta (blue sclerae, dentinogenesis imperfecta), or evidence of a family history of the condition. Bone biopsy for diagnosis is rarely required. Affected patients are short in stature, only 10% being of normal height, with joint laxity, blue sclerae and presenile hearing loss. Transmission is by autosomal dominant trait. Radiologically the bones are usually reduced in radiodensity, although some patients may have normal bone density. Bones may be gracile, or modelled normally. Vertebral fractures often occur in the fourth decade and when scoliosis is present, it is mild.

Type II (Lethal Perinatal)

Affected infants are small for dates with deep blue sclerae and shortened and deformed limbs due to multiple fractures. Fractures involve the ribs and death is usually the result of pulmonary insufficiency. Survival is rare beyond the first three months of postnatal life. Other complications include brain and spinal cord injury. Radiologically, multiple fractures are present with a characteristic 'concertina' deformity of the lower limbs. The ribs may appear 'beaded' due to multiple rib fractures, which can occur in utero. The cranial vault is severely under-mineralised and may be distorted by moulding, with Wormian (intrasutural) bones in the occipital and parietal region. Platyspondyly is present. Histology reveals defective endochondral ossification at the metaphyses and epiphyses, which appear disorganised with persistent islands of calcified cartilage and under-mineralised bone. There is defective transformation of woven bone to lamellar bone in both the cortical and trabecular skeletal components. Membranous ossification is also deficient, accounting for the marked calvarial thinning.

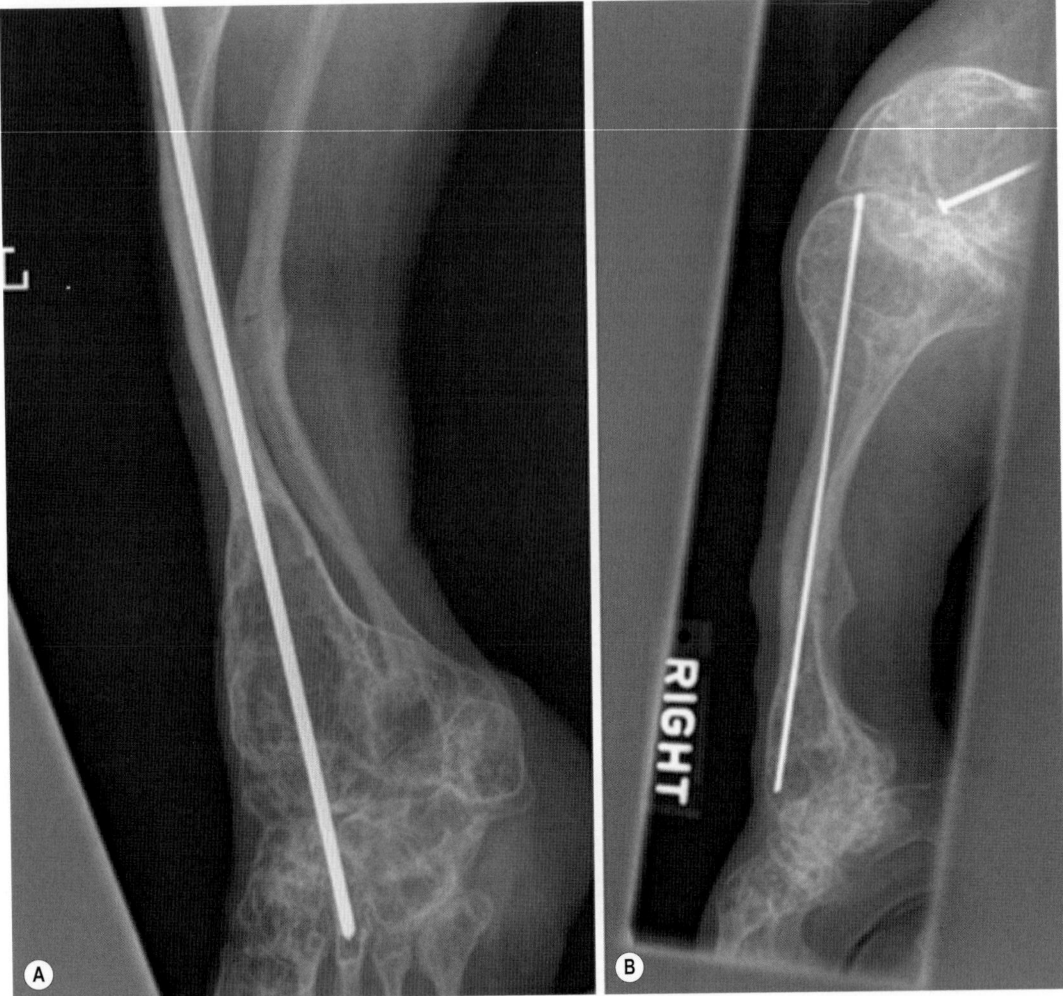

FIGURE 50-16 ■ **Osteogenesis imperfecta.** AP (A) and lateral (B) radiographs of the left distal lower extremity in a 10-year-old child with extensive deformity, incomplete healing fractures and internal fixation with rods. Findings are those of osteogenesis imperfecta, a disorder caused by genetic mutations in Type I collagen resulting in osteoporosis and low-trauma insufficiency fractures (brittle bone disease). The different types vary in clinical presentation and severity.

Type III (Severe Progressive)

This is inherited as an autosomal recessive trait. Fractures are usually present at birth and involve the long bones, clavicles, ribs and cranium, leading to deformity. Although size at birth is normal, growth retardation is evident in the first year of life and many affected patients only reach 0.9–1.2 m (3–4 ft) in height. As growth proceeds, increasing deformity of the calvarium occurs, with associated facial distortion, dental malocclusion and mild prognathism, basilar invagination and progressive hearing loss. Sclerae are blue at birth but this diminishes with age, and sclerae are white in adults. Vertebral fractures occur at an early age and contribute to the progressive and severe kyphoscoliosis, which develops during childhood. Affected patients tend to be wheelchair bound because of the progressive deformities resulting from fractures. Complications include progressive pulmonary insufficiency due to thoracic distortion. Radiologically, the bones may be slender or broad due to recurrent fractures. Epiphyses are abnormal, with expansion and islands of calcified ('popcorn') cartilage. As with other forms of osteogenesis imperfecta, the incidence of fractures declines following puberty.

Type IV (Moderately Severe)

This is inherited as an autosomal dominant trait, can vary in severity and is sometimes confused with either type I or type III OI. There is generally more severe osteopenia and more extensive bone deformity than in type I. The sclerae are blue in children and while this may persist into adulthood, they may also fade to white. Individuals are short in stature with abnormal moulding of the calvarium and basilar invagination in a high proportion of patients. Bones in the axial and appendicular skeleton are osteoporotic and dysplastic, resulting in scoliosis and deformity, particularly of the pelvis. Joint laxity can result in dislocation, particularly of the ankle or knee.

Type V OI resembles type IV disease in terms of frequency of fractures and degree of skeletal deformity. It dominantly inherited or may develop spontaneously and is characterised by development of hypertrophic callus at sites of fractures or surgical intervention. Ossification of the interosseous ligament between radius and ulna may restrict movement in this site.

Quantitative Assessment of the Skeleton

The most important technique to quantify bone mineral density (BMD) is dual energy X-ray absorptiometry (DXA); additional techniques have been used which include quantitative CT, quantitative ultrasound and radiogrammetry. Six-point morphometry is used to quantify change in vertebral shape (deformity) and has an increasing role, with DXA being used to image the whole spine for vertebral fracture assessment (VFA).[50] BMD is the single most important determinant of fracture, accounting for approximately 70% of bone strength. Reduced BMD is a useful predictor of increased fracture risk. The lower the peak bone density, the higher the risk of fracture in later life. Methods of measuring bone density are therefore relevant to the study of skeletal development, the detection of osteopenia and assessment of efficacy of treatment of osteoporosis. Such methods for measuring BMD should be accurate, precise (reproducible), sensitive both to small changes with time and to differences in patient groups (i.e. fracture compared to non-fracture), inexpensive and involve minimal exposure to ionising radiation.

Accuracy expresses how close the measurements made are to the actual BMD measured by chemical analysis. All the quantitative methods available have some inaccuracies caused by variable fat content, either within the marrow of trabecular bone (single energy quantitative computed tomography, QCT) or by the fat content of extra-osseous soft tissue (other photon absorptiometric techniques, DXA). Changes in body composition or marrow fat may introduce errors in the measurement depending upon the technique and measurement site used.

Precision assesses the reproducibility of the measurement technique and is usually expressed as a percentage of coefficient of variation (CV%). A high precision (low CV% in the region of 1%) is essential in longitudinal studies to detect small changes in BMD over reasonable periods of time. Short-term precision principally reflects repositioning errors, whilst long-term precision using calibration phantoms reflects machine instability. Change in BMD is best evaluated by calculating the percentage change; the least significant change from two measures ($p = 0.05$) is given by 2.77 × precision error of the method.[51] As changes in BMD are generally small, an interval of at least 18–24 months should be used between quantitative measures.

Dual Energy X-ray Absorptiometry (DXA)

DXA was introduced in 1987 and is the most widely available bone density technique. It utilises two X-ray beams with differing kVp (30–50 and >70 keV) to enable subtraction of the soft-tissue component allowing measurement of BMD in a given area of bone ('areal' BMD) measured in g/cm^2. This is typically done in the lumbar spine (L1–4), proximal femur (femoral neck and total) and distal radius. Original machines had a pencil beam and coupled detector and acquired data in a rectilinear fashion. Modern systems have a fan beam X-ray source and banks of detectors allowing rapid data acquisition with improved spatial resolution (1 to 0.5 mm). The accuracy of DXA is between 3 and 8%, with precision (CV%) better than 1% in PA spine and total femur, and 1–2% in femoral neck. Radiation dose is low (1–6 μSv for BMD; up to 50 μSv if performed with VFA).[52]

Proximal femur and lumbar spine measurements are performed most frequently. Using an automatic segmentation, which is checked and corrected by the operator, the L1–4 vertebral bodies, femoral neck, intertrochanteric and trochanteric regions are measured. The total femur region of interest is derived from femoral neck, intertrochanteric and trochanteric regions. In addition to areal density values in g/cm^2, DXA provides T- and Z-scores. Z-scores are standard deviations (SD) compared to an age-matched reference population, while T-scores are SD compared to a young adult reference population. Whole-body DXA with regional analysis gives information not only on total and regional BMD but also on body composition (lean muscle mass and fat mass).

In postmenopausal women and men over 50 DXA BMD is used to define osteoporosis (T-score at or below −2.5) and osteopenia (T-score between −1.1 and −2.4).[6] This definition was originally only established for BMD of the proximal femur (neck and total femur regions of interest), but is currently also used for lumbar spine (postero-anterior projection) and distal radius (1/3 radius region of interest) DXA (Fig. 50-17). In premenopausal women, men younger than 50 and children Z-scores are used comparing individual BMD measurements to an appropriate age-matched reference population.[8–10] A Z-score lower than −2 is defined as 'below the expected range for age'. It should be noted that osteoporosis cannot be defined using DXA BMD alone in these populations.

Guidelines for DXA referral vary internationally and were generally performed on a case finding (high fracture risk) strategy, as population screening is not cost-effective. DXA was indicated in women aged 65 and over and in younger and perimenopausal women with risk factors for insufficiency fractures.[9] DXA was also advocated in men 70 years and older and younger men with risk factors for fracture.

Although the T-score of −2.5 was satisfactory as a definition of osteoporosis, it was never appropriate as a level for therapeutic intervention, largely because age is such a strong independent predictor of fracture. In 2008 the WHO introduced the 10-year fracture risk prediction tool (FRAX) which can be accessed at http://www.shef.ac.uk/FRAX/. This tool uses clinical risk factors and the presence of secondary causes of osteoporosis with or without DXA femoral neck BMD to calculate the risk of hip, and other major, osteoporotic fractures.[53,54] With the use of appropriate guidelines,[55,56] which may vary between different nations, FRAX should lead to a more appropriate utilisation of DXA and its results, and more cost-effective intervention strategies.[57]

Individuals being considered for osteoporotic bone protective/bone-enhancing therapy and those already on

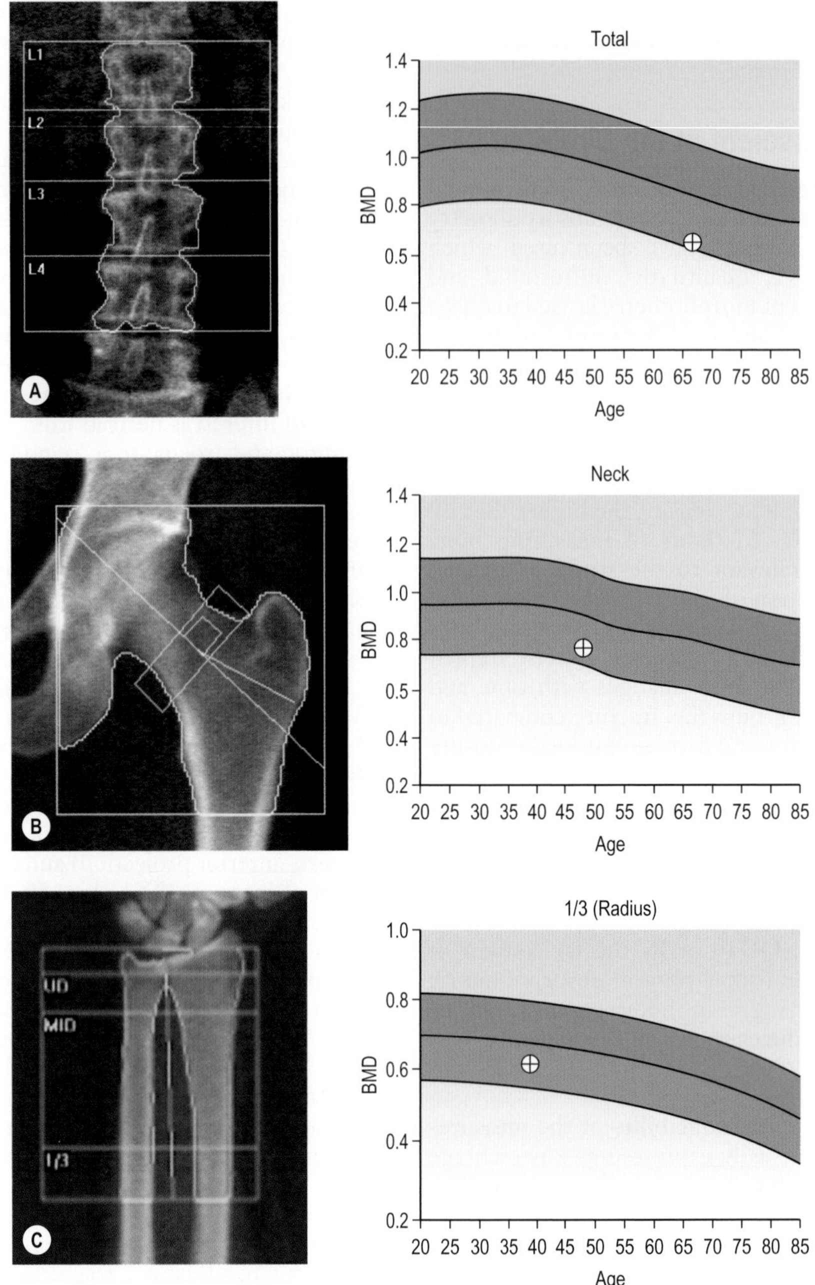

FIGURE 50-17 ■ DXA images of the lumbar spine (A), proximal femur (B) and distal radius (C). DXA provides 'areal' BMD (g/cm^2) and is currently the 'gold standard' method for diagnosis of osteoporosis by bone densitometry in adults (WHO definition T-score –2.5 or below). The blue band shows range of two standard deviations above normal age-matched BMD and the purple band demonstrates range of two standard deviations below the normal age-matched BMD.

therapy should be examined with DXA.[9] Follow-up DXA every 1–2 years is used in clinical practice to verify response to treatment, although measuring serum bone turnover markers will confirm response to bisphosphonate therapy in a shorter period (3–4 months).

DXA has some limitations which need to be considered:

1. It is a 2D image of a 3D bone, which measures density/area (in g/cm^2) of integral (cortical and trabecular) bone and not the volumetric density (in mg/cm^3) as is provided by quantitative CT. Areal BMD is dependent on bone size and will thus overestimate fracture risk in short individuals with small bones, who will have lower areal BMD than normal-sized individuals.
2. Spine and hip DXA are sensitive to artefacts caused by degenerative changes and individuals with significant degenerative disease will have falsely increased areal BMD, which will indicate a lower fracture risk than is actually present. DXA is limited in elderly patients in whom degenerative changes are commonly present (60% in those aged 70 years or more) (Fig. 50-18).
3. All structures overlying the spine such as aortic calcifications, or morphological abnormalities of the vertebrae such as fractures (false elevation of

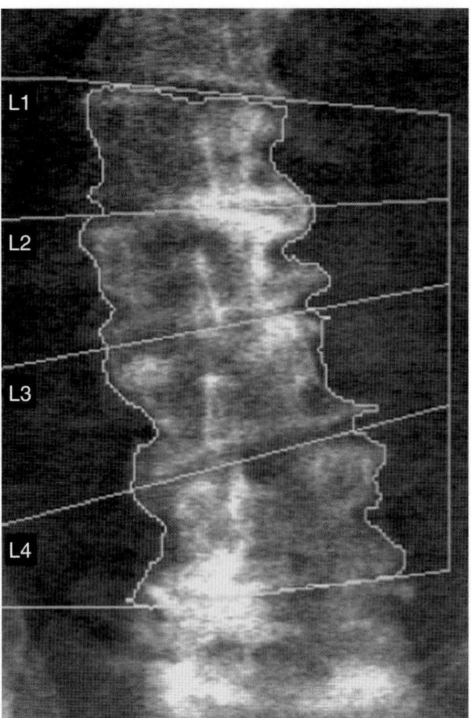

FIGURE 50-18 ■ DXA images of degenerated lumbar spine. DXA image of the lumbar spine demonstrating degenerative changes with sclerosis leading to falsely elevated BMD.

BMD) or laminectomy (false reduction) will affect DXA BMD measurements.

Other causes of falsely high BMD on DXA include vertebral fracture, Paget's disease of bone, sclerotic metastases, vertebral haemangioma, spinal metallic pinning or plating, calcified lymph nodes, residual Myodil and navel rings. Such artefacts require the results from affected individual vertebral bodies to be excluded from analysis, but a minimum of two vertebrae must be available for interpretation.

Treatment with strontium ranelate causes artefactual elevation of BMD, approximately 50% of the increase being due to the high-atomic-number strontium in the bones. DXA can be used for examining peripheral sites: for instance, the distal 1/3 radius is a site consisting predominantly (95%) of cortical bone and measurement here may be helpful in patients with primary or secondary hyperparathyroidism. It can also be used to study regional bone density around a prosthesis following hip arthroplasty.

Quantitative Computed Tomography (QCT)

QCT uniquely allows for the separate estimation of trabecular and cortical BMD and provides a true volumetric density in mg/cm^3. To perform QCT a standard CT unit with a bone equivalent calibration phantom under the patient is used. Density values, measured in Hounsfield units, are transformed into BMD, measured in mg hydroxyapatite/cm^3 using the phantom. Typically, the L1–3 vertebral bodies are measured; either single-slice mid-vertebral 10-mm slice or volumetric MDCT methods can be used to measure BMD (Fig. 50-19); volumetric MDCT techniques are also available to measure proximal femur BMD.

In addition to the true volumetric measurements provided by QCT, the technique has several other important advantages over DXA. QCT can provide separate measures of cortical and trabecular BMD. Trabecular BMD is more sensitive to monitoring changes with disease and therapy, as trabecular bone is more metabolically active than cortical bone.[58] Cross-sectional studies have shown that QCT BMD of the spine allows better discrimination of individuals with and without vertebral fractures.[59,60] QCT is also better suited to examining obese patients as DXA makes assumptions about body composition and so has limitations in measuring BMD in patients with a body mass index over 25 kg/m^2. In such obese patients superimposed soft tissue will falsely elevate measured BMD due to attenuation of the X-ray beams and beam hardening artefact.[61–63]

Limitations of QCT are a higher radiation dose (0.06–2.9 mSv depending on whether lumbar spine or hip is being assessed), although lower doses are utilised for QCT compared with conventional CT[52] and the presence of only a small number of longitudinal studies assessing how QCT predicts fractures. The WHO T-score of −2.5 defining osteoporosis is not applicable to QCT. A T-score threshold of −2.5 for QCT would identify a much higher percentage of apparently osteoporotic subjects and QCT has therefore never been established for clinical use. Currently volumetric QCT techniques are preferred over single-slice techniques[64–67] and in clinical practice absolute measurements of BMD have been defined to characterise fracture risk: 110–80 mg/cm^3 = mild increase in fracture risk; 80–50 mg/cm^3 = moderate increase in fracture risk; and below 50 mg/cm^3 = severe increase in fracture risk. According to the American College of Radiology (ACR) Guidelines for QCT a BMD range of 120–80 mg/cm^3 is defined as osteopenic and values below 80 mg/cm^3 as osteoporotic.[68]

Recommendations for the appropriate use of QCT instead of DXA are (i) very small or large individuals, (ii) older individuals with expected advanced degenerative disease of the lumbar spine or morphological abnormalities and (iii) if high sensitivity to monitor change in BMD is required, such as in patients treated with parathyroid hormone or oral glucocorticoids. A recent study comparing DXA and QCT in older men with diffuse idiopathic skeletal hyperostosis (DISH) demonstrated that QCT was better suited to differentiate men with and without vertebral fractures.[69]

Although QCT is usually applied to the spine and proximal femur, dedicated peripheral QCT units (pQCT) have been developed which allow separate analysis of cortical and trabecular bone in the non-dominant forearm and in other sites of the skeleton, including the tibia. In bone shafts, cortical thickness and cross-sectional bone area can be measured, from which certain biomechanical parameters (stress strain index; moment of inertia) can be extracted. Cross-sectional muscle area and muscle density can also be measured, relevant to studies investigating the interaction of muscle and bone and in sarcopenia.

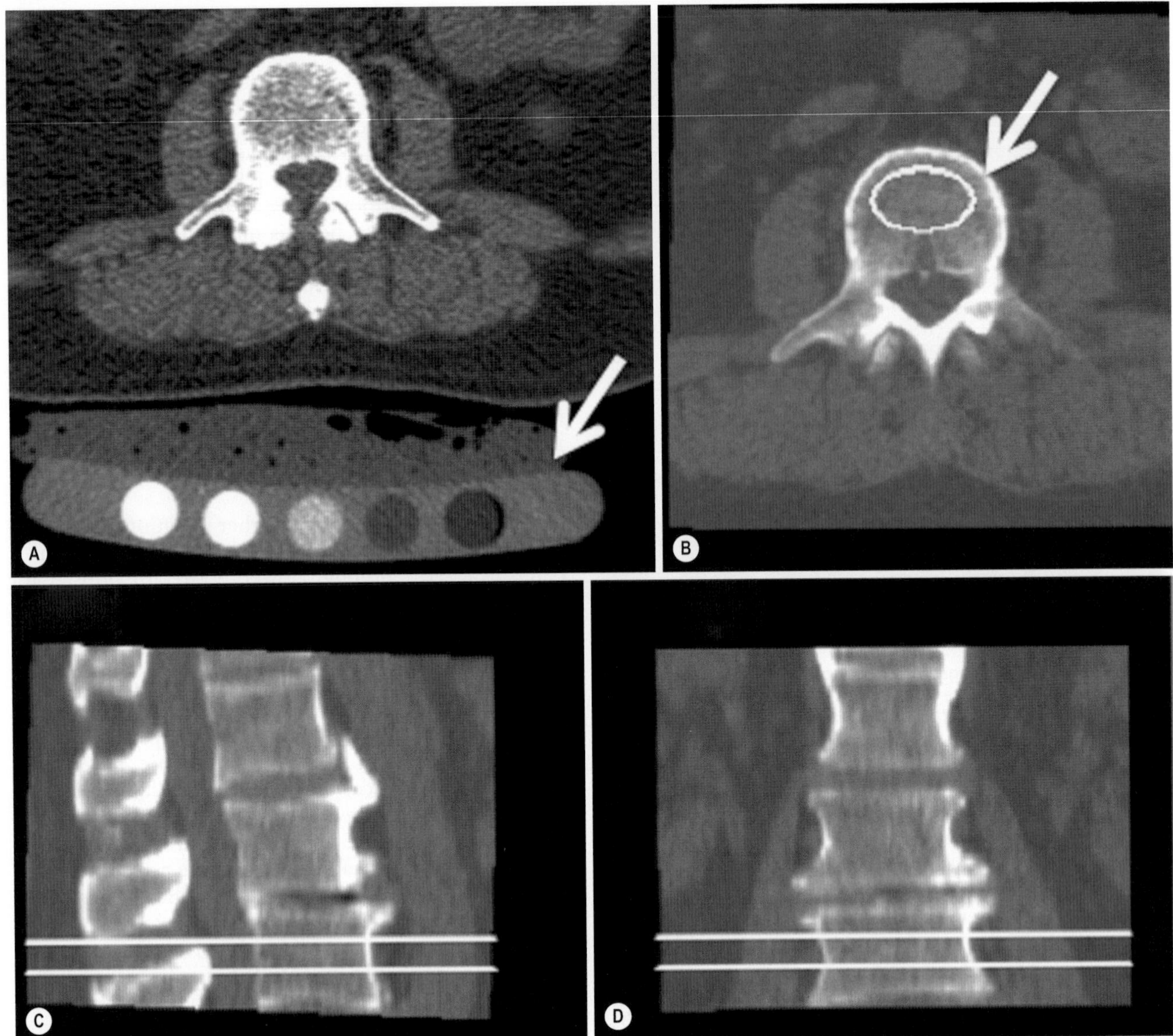

FIGURE 50-19 ■ **Volumetric QCT of the L3 vertebral body.** BMD calibration phantom is shown below patient in (A) (arrow). In (B) the oval-shaped region of interest is depicted (arrow) and (C) and (D) show the volume analysed in the sagittal and coronal images from MDCT acquisition.

Quantitative Ultrasound

Quantitative ultrasound (QUS) is a low-cost technique performed with dedicated devices acquiring data, mostly at the calcaneus. Using a water bath or ultrasound jelly, an emitter and receiver probe are brought in close proximity to the soft tissue surrounding the bone (e.g. calcaneus). The propagation of ultrasound waves through the bone is measured, which is characterised by the velocity of transmission and the amplitude of the ultrasound signal. Velocity is measured as m/s (metre/second) and defined as speed of sound (SoS), which is independent of ultrasound wave attenuation. SoS decreases in osteoporotic bone. In addition, broadband ultrasound attenuation (BUA) is calculated in dB/MHz (decibel/megahertz), which increases in osteoporotic bone. Recent meta-analyses confirmed that both DXA and calcaneal quantitative ultrasonography predicted fractures in an older patient population but that the correlation between the two techniques was low.[70] However, the limitations of QUS are that (i) neither the WHO definition of osteoporosis nor the FRAX 10-year fracture risk calculator are applicable to QUS, (ii) the measures are temperature dependent and (iii) there is no cross-calibration phantom available. Also the method has been applied to a large number of different anatomical sites (fingers, forearm, tibia) without clear recommendations on the preferred site. Consequently, QUS remains largely a research technique.

Radiogrammetry

Radiogrammetry involves cortical thickness measurements on radiographs of various long bones. The bone most frequently used is the second metacarpal of the non-dominant hand, but the method has also been applied to other bones (clavicle, radius, humerus, femur and tibia). In the metacarpal the diameter of the bone in its mid portion (from each periosteal surface) and the medullary width (distance between endosteal surfaces) are measured using callipers.[71,72] A variety of indices have been described, including cortical thickness, metacarpal index and parameters of cortical area. The technique is simple to perform, uses a low radiation dose, and has been widely applied. However, the reproducibility is limited (coefficient of variation (CV) up to 11%). This is because the endosteal surface becomes irregular and more difficult to identify with bone resorption. Now modern computer vision methods (active shape models, ASM) have been applied and improve precision to better than 1% (digital X-ray radiogrammetry, DXR).[73]

Vertebral Morphometry

Over the past decade efforts have been made to standardise the subjective visual assessment of vertebral fracture, and to quantitate alterations in vertebral height and shape. These developments have been stimulated not only by the need for comparable methods to be used in epidemiological studies but also by the fact that the prevalence and incidence of vertebral fractures are used as inclusion criteria and treatment outcome measures in therapeutic trials in which the efficacy of new drugs for the treatment of osteoporosis is being assessed.[50,74]

The technique for spinal radiography should be standardised, with a fixed film focus distance (FFD), and the spine parallel to the radiographic table for the lateral projection. Any scoliosis or tilting of the spine due to poor positioning will cause apparent, but false, biconcavity of the end-plates ('bean-can effect'). Centring is at T7 spinous process for the lateral thoracic spine and L3 spinous process for the lateral lumbar spine projections. Assessments for vertebral fractures are usually made from T4 to L4 on the lateral spinal projections. Vertebral fractures are defined as end-plate, wedge or crush. Changes in shape of the vertebrae (deforming events) are generally defined by the 6-point method, in which the anterior, mid and posterior points of the superior and inferior end-plates of the vertebral body are identified to measure anterior, mid and posterior heights. Vertebral deformity is defined by relating the anterior or mid vertical heights to the posterior height, expressed as a percentage or by specified standard deviations from normal reference data for vertebral size. A vertebral fracture can be defined by grading from 0 (normal) to grade 3 (obvious fracture) in a semiquantitative scheme, which has now largely replaced 6-point morphometry.[16]

The introduction of fan beam technology and improvements in spatial resolution in DXA enabled good-quality (dual and single energy modes) images (postero-anterior and lateral projections) of the thoracic and lumbar spine, from which vertebral fracture assessment (VFA) and morphometric measurements can be made (MXA).[75,76] It may be feasible for this process to be automated by computer techniques.[77] The advantages of VFA over conventional spinal radiography are a lower radiation dose (1/100th),[52] less end-plate distortion since the X-ray beam is parallel to the end-plate at each vertebral level, and the entire spine is visualised on a single image, and BMD measurement can be made on the same equipment.[78]

Other Research Methods

High-resolution multidetector computed tomography (HR-MDCT)[79,80] and high-resolution magnetic resonance imaging (HR-MRI)[81,82] have been used to analyse trabecular bone structure in vivo. One of the most important developments to assess bone architecture over the past 10 years has been the introduction of high-resolution peripheral CT (HR-pQCT)[83–87] (Fig. 50-20). The dedicated in vivo extremity imaging system is

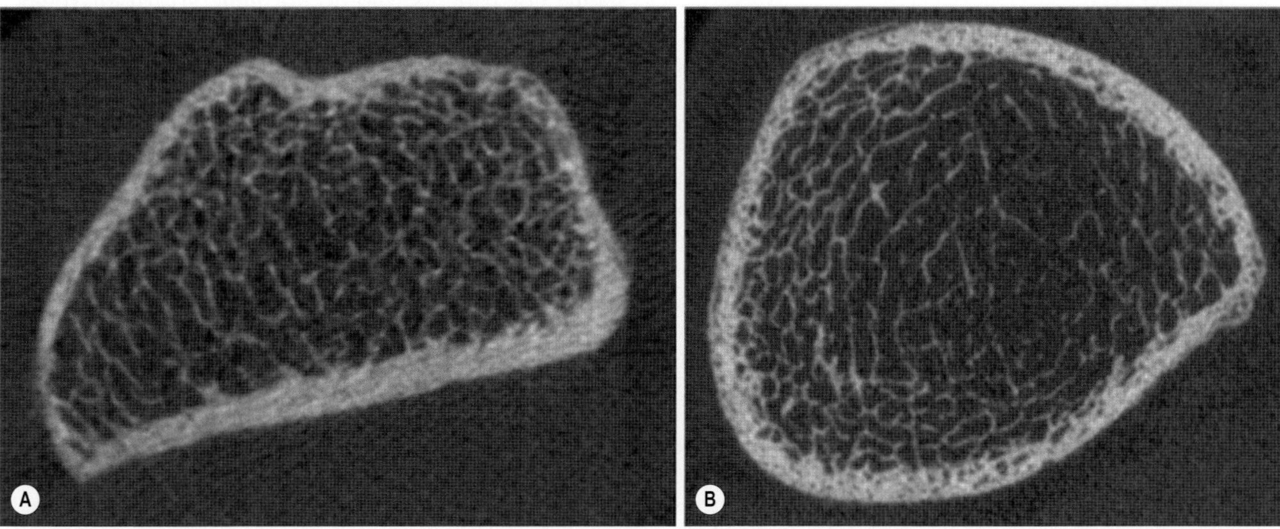

FIGURE 50-20 ■ HR-pQCT images of the distal radius (A) and tibia (B). These high-resolution images demonstrate the trabecular bone structure and the cortical bone architecture, including the cortical porosity. These images can be used to quantify a number of trabecular and cortical structure parameters in addition to biomechanical surrogate markers of bone strength through finite element modelling (FEM).

designed for imaging trabecular and cortical bone architecture and has the advantage of significantly higher signal-to-noise ratio (SNR) and spatial resolution (nominal isotropic voxel dimension of 82 μm) compared to multidetector CT (MDCT) and MRI.[87] In comparison MDCT has a maximum in-plane spatial resolution of 250–300 μm and MRI of 150–200 μm, with slice thicknesses of 0.5–0.7 and 0.3–0.5 mm, respectively. Furthermore, the effective radiation dose is substantially lower compared to whole-body MDCT and does not involve critical, radiosensitive organs (effective dose <3 μSv). The aquisition time for HR-pQCT is long, at approximately 3 min each for the tibia and radius, so motion artefact can be problematic. There are several disadvantages to this technology, most notably that it is limited to peripheral skeletal sites and therefore can provide no direct insight into bone quality in the lumbar spine or proximal femur—common sites for osteoporotic insufficiency fractures.[87]

PARATHYROID DISORDERS

Most parathyroid tumours are functionally active and result in the clinical syndrome of primary hyperparathyroidism. This is the most common endocrine disorder after diabetes and thyroid disease, with an incidence within the population of about 1 in 1000 (0.1%). The incidence is higher in the elderly and is most common in women aged 60 or older. Over the past 50 years the diagnosed prevalence of the condition has increased some tenfold, due principally to the detection by chance of hypercalcaemia in patients, many of whom are asymptomatic.

Hyperparathyroidism

Primary Hyperparathyroidism

The majority (80%) of patients with primary hyperparathyroidism have a single adenoma. Multiple parathyroid adenomas may occur in 4% of cases. Hyperplasia of all glands occurs in 15–20% of patients. Genetic factors are relevant in a proportion of these patients (familial hyperplasia, multiple endocrine neoplasia (MEN) syndromes).

Carcinoma of the parathyroid is an infrequent cause of primary hyperparathyroidism (1%);[88] the malignant tumour is slow growing but locally invasive. Cure may be obtained by adequate surgical excision and there is a 50% or greater 5-year survival rate. Persistent or recurrent disease occurs in more than 50% of patients with parathyroid carcinoma.[88] Surgical resection is also the primary mode of therapy for recurrence since it can offer significant palliation for the metabolic derangement caused by hyperparathyroidism and allows hypercalcaemia to become more medically manageable. However, reoperation is rarely curative and eventual relapse is likely. Chemotherapy and external beam radiation treatments have been generally ineffective in the treatment of parathyroid carcinoma.

Secondary Hyperparathyroidism

Secondary hyperparathyroidism is induced by any condition, or circumstance, which causes the serum calcium to fall. This occurs in vitamin D deficiency, intestinal malabsorption of calcium (e.g. coeliac disease), chronic kidney disease (CKD) (azotaemic osteodystrophy)—through lack of the active metabolite of vitamin D, $1,25(OH)_2D$, and retention of phosphorus. In long-standing secondary hyperparathyroidism an autonomous adenoma may develop in the hyperplastic parathyroid glands, a condition referred to as tertiary hyperparathyroidism. This is usually associated with CKD but it has also been observed in patients with long-standing vitamin D deficiency and osteomalacia from other causes.

Clinical Presentation

Most patients with primary hyperparathyroidism have mild disease and commonly have no symptoms, the diagnosis being made by the finding of asymptomatic hypercalcaemia. The most common clinical presentations, particularly in younger patients, are related to renal stones and nephrocalcinosis (25–35%), high blood pressure (40–60%), acute arthropathy (pseudogout) caused by calcium pyrophosphate dihydrate deposition (chondrocalcinosis), osteoporosis, bone and muscle pain, proximal muscle weakness, peptic ulcer and acute pancreatitis, depression, confusional states and mild non-specific symptoms such as lethargy, arthralgia and difficulties with mental concentration.

Treatment

Surgical removal of the overactive parathyroid tissue in primary hyperparathyroidism is generally recommended.[89] In experienced hands surgical excision is successful in curing the condition in over 90% of patients.[90] The decision to operate, particularly in the elderly and those with asymptomatic disease, requires careful assessment. For patients who do not undergo parathyroidectomy, annual monitoring of serum calcium and creatinine levels and assessment of bone mineral density every 1 or 2 years is recommended, but at present, there is no definitive medical therapy for primary hyperparathyroidism,[90] although a calcimimetic, cinacalcet, which acts through the calcium sensing receptor, has been used in various causes of hypercalcaemia, including primary and secondary hyperparathyroidism.

In secondary hyperparathyroidism treatment should include a combination of dietary phosphorus restriction, phosphate binders, vitamin D sterols, and calcimimetics; parathyroidectomy is effective in suitable candidates refractory to medical therapy.[91]

Radiological Findings

With increased numbers of patients with primary hyperparathyroidism being diagnosed with asymptomatic hypercalcaemia, the majority (95%) of patients will have no radiological abnormalities. In more advanced stages typical radiographic abnormalities are found, that include

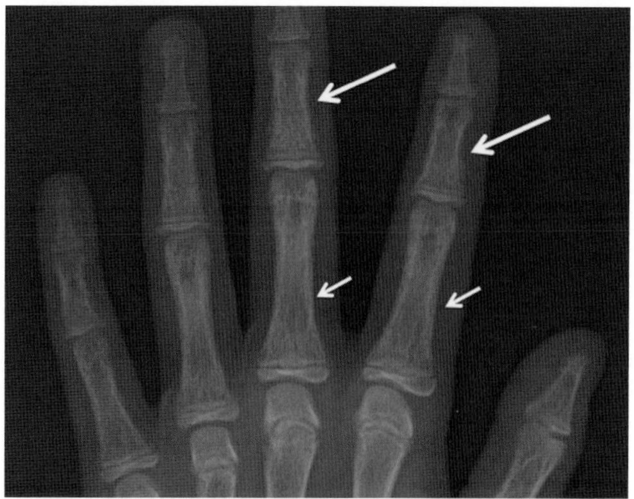

FIGURE 50-21 ■ **Primary hyperparathyroidism.** Radiograph of the left hand demonstrating subperiosteal erosions, particularly in the radial aspect of the middle phalanges of the index and middle fingers (large arrows). Also as a result of increased osteoclastic resorption, cortical 'tunnelling' (areas of resorption within the bone cortex) is evident in the proximal phalanges (small arrows).

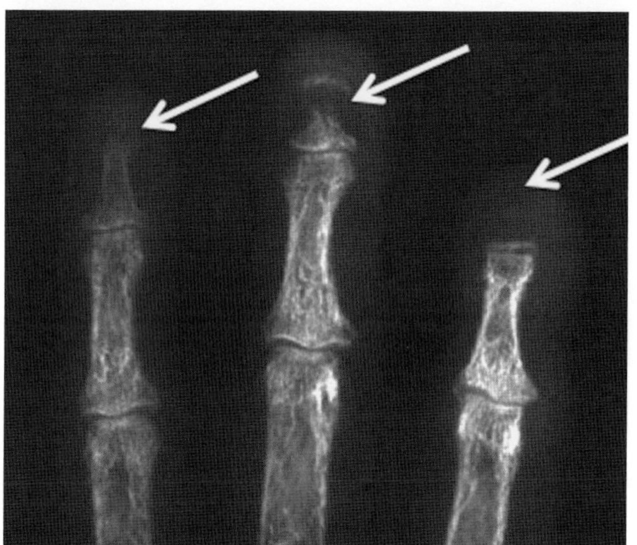

FIGURE 50-22 ■ **Primary hyperparathyroidism.** Radiograph of the left hand showing advanced subperiosteal erosions and acro-osteolysis of the second to fourth digits (arrows).

subperiosteal erosions, chondrocalcinosis, brown tumours and soft-tissue metastatic calcifications, the latter occurring only in secondary hyperparathyroidism associated with CKD in which there is phosphate retention.

Subperiosteal Erosions. Subperiosteal erosion of cortical bone, particularly in the phalanges, is pathognomonic of hyperparathyroidism[92] (Fig. 50-21). The most sensitive site in which to identify this early subperiosteal erosion is along the radial aspects of the middle phalanges of the index and middle fingers. Typically also the tufts of the distal phalanges may be affected. Other sites may be involved, including the distal phalanges (acro-osteolysis) (Fig. 50-22), the outer ends of the clavicle, the

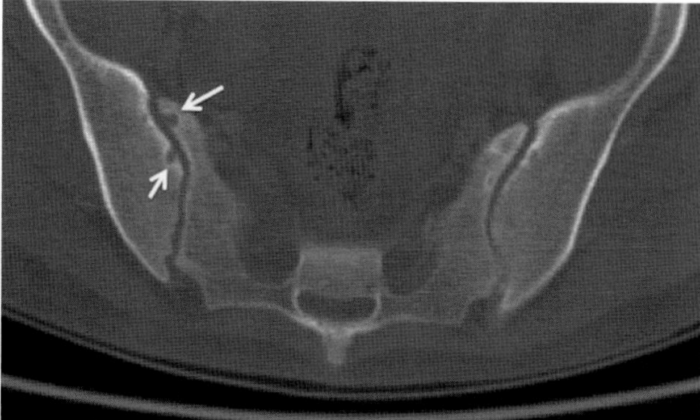

FIGURE 50-23 ■ **Primary hyperparathyroidism.** CT of the sacroiliac joints with subchondral erosions (arrows) mimicking inflammatory sacroiliitis.

symphysis pubis, the sacroiliac joints (Fig. 50-23), the proximal medial cortex of the tibia, the proximal humeral shaft, ribs and femur. However, if no subperiosteal erosions are identified in the phalanges, they are unlikely to be identified radiographically elsewhere in the skeleton. Subperiosteal erosions in sites other than the phalanges indicate more severe and long-standing hyperparathyroidism, such as may be found secondary to CKD. It should be noted that erosions can also affect the joints such as the metacarpophalangeal joints or the sacroiliac joints and, simply based on radiographic findings, differential diagnosis from inflammatory arthropathies, such as rheumatoid arthritis and ankylosing spondylitis, can be challenging.

Intracortical Bone Resorption. This results from increased osteoclastic activity in Haversian canals. Radiographically it causes linear translucencies within the cortex (cortical 'tunnelling') (Fig. 50-21). This feature is not specific for hyperparathyroidism and may be found in other conditions in which bone turnover is increased (e.g. normal childhood, Paget's disease of bone).

Chondrocalcinosis. The deposition of calcium pyrophosphate dihydrate (CPPD) causes articular cartilage and fibrocartilage to become visible on radiographs (Fig. 50-24). Chondrocalcinosis is found in 6–11% of patients with primary hyperparathyroidism.[93] This is most likely to be identified on radiographs of the hand (triangular ligament), the knees (articular cartilage and menisci) and symphysis pubis. Other joints less commonly involved are the shoulder and the hip. Clinically the patients may present with acute pain resembling gout, but on joint aspiration pyrophosphate crystals, rather than urate crystals, are found. However, this is relatively rare and was reported in 25% of patients with CPPD and primary hyperparathyroidism.[93] Affected joints may be asymptomatic, and chondrocalcinosis noted radiographically might bring the diagnosis of hyperparathyroidism to light in an asymptomatic patient. The combination of chondrocalcinosis in the symphysis pubis and nephrocalcinosis on an abdominal radiograph is diagnostic of hyperparathyroidism. Chondrocalcinosis is a feature of primary disease, rather than that secondary to CKD.

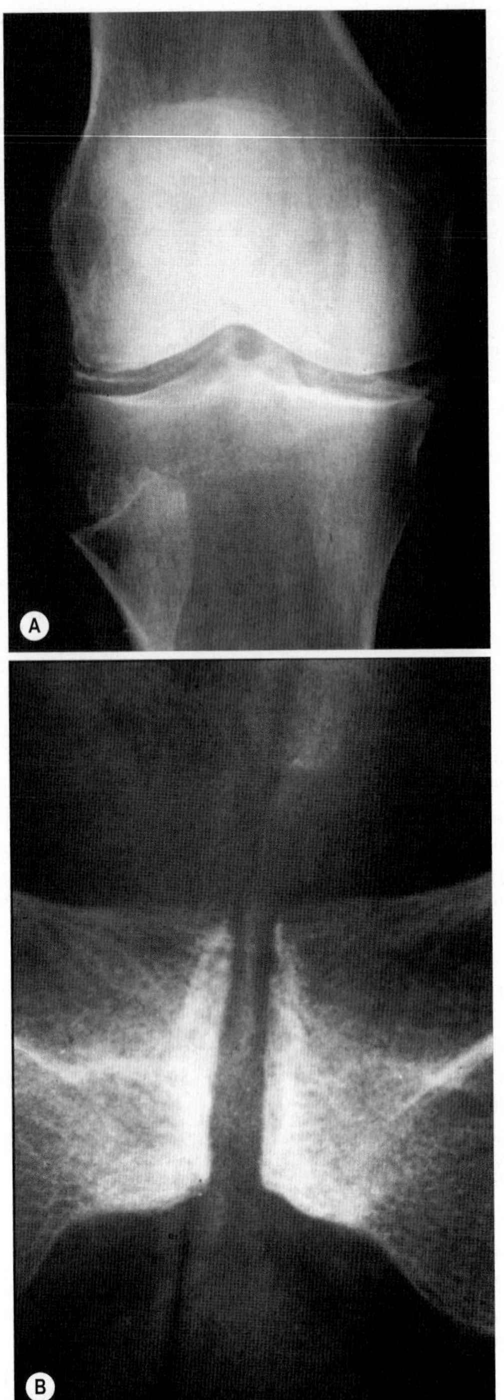

FIGURE 50-24 ■ **Primary hyperparathyroidism.** With chondrocalcinosis (calcification of cartilage) at the knee (A) and the symphysis pubis (B). Other sites where this may be present are the triangular fibrocartilage complex of the wrist and the large joints (hip and shoulder).

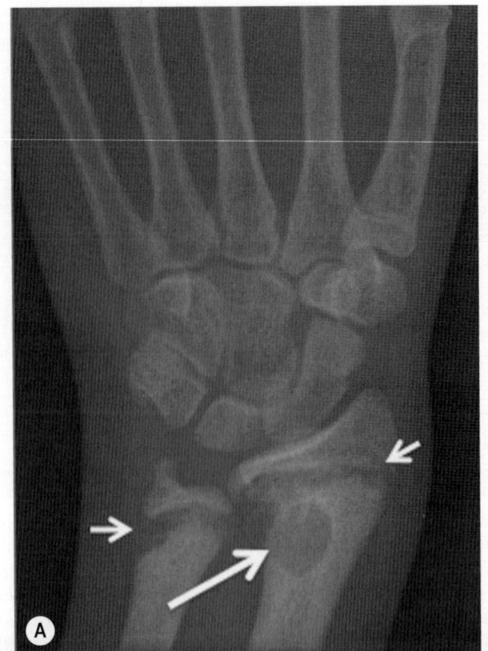

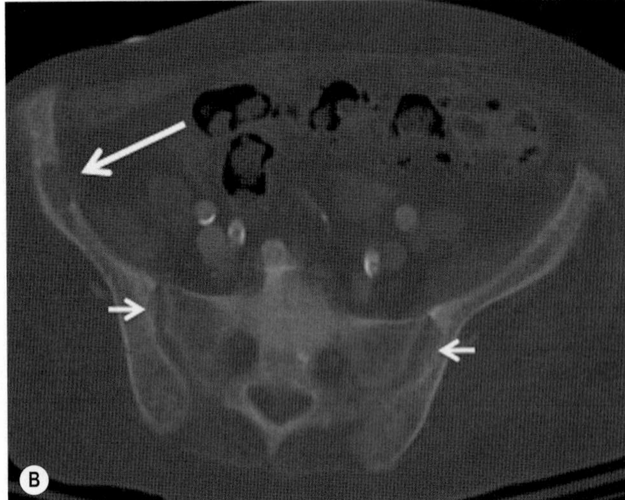

FIGURE 50-25 ■ **Secondary hyperparathyroidism related to chronic kidney disease.** Radiograph of the left hand (A) and CT of the pelvis (B). Brown tumours (osteitis fibrosa cystica) can occur in any site, seen here in the distal radius and the right ilium (arrows). Additionally, resorptive changes are evident at the growth plates and bilateral sacroiliac joints (small arrows).

Brown Tumours (Osteitis Fibrosa Cystica). Brown tumours are cystic lesions within bone in which there has been excessive osteoclastic resorption (Fig. 50-25). Histologically the cavities are filled with fibrous tissue and osteoclasts, with necrosis and haemorrhagic liquefaction. Radiographically, brown tumours appear as low-density, multiloculated cysts that can occur in any skeletal site and may cause expansion of bones. If the clinical history in these patients is not known, brown tumours may be easily interpreted as neoplastic lesions.

Osteosclerosis. Osteosclerosis occurs uncommonly in primary hyperparathyroidism but is a common feature of disease secondary to CKD. In primary disease with normal renal function it results from an exaggerated osteoblastic response following bone resorption. In secondary causes of hyperparathyroidism it results from excessive accumulation of poorly mineralised osteoid, which appears more dense radiographically than normal bone. The increase in bone density affects particularly the axial skeleton. In the vertebral bodies the end-plates

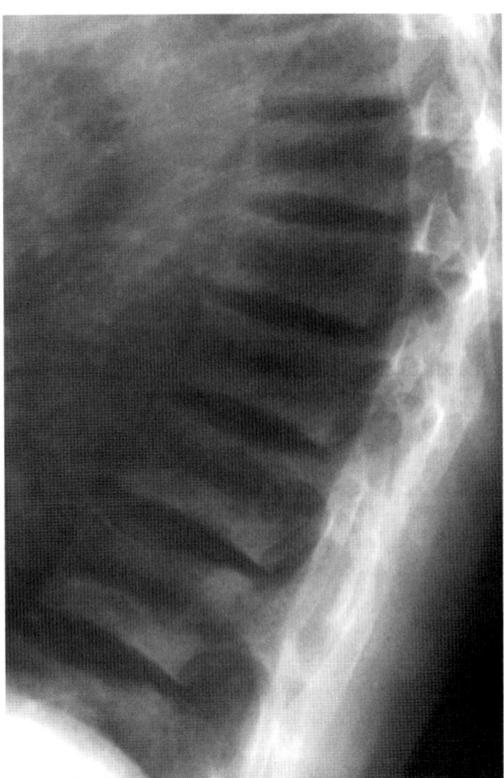

FIGURE 50-26 ■ Secondary hyperparathyroidism. Lateral radiograph of the thoracic spine demonstrating increased sclerosis along the end-plates and increased lucency of the central part, giving a 'rugger jersey' spine appearance. Also note deformity of the vertebral bodies, with loss of height and increased diameter, in addition to wedge-shaped deformities at the upper thoracic spine related to decreased stability and weakness of the abnormal bone.

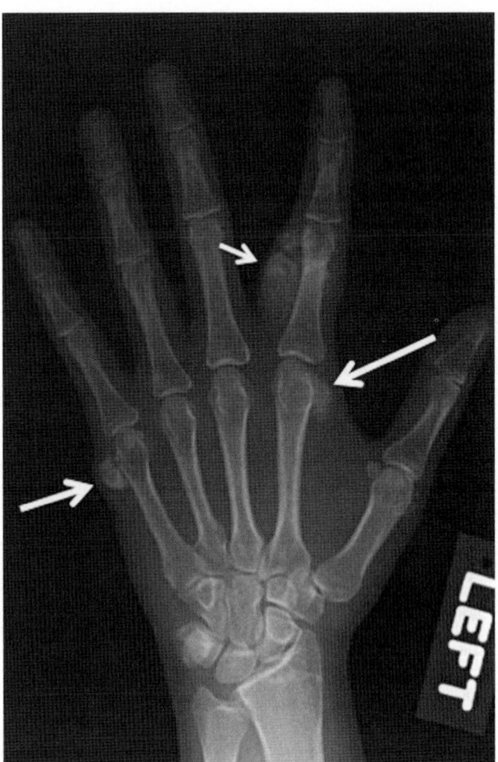

FIGURE 50-27 ■ Secondary hyperparathyroidism related to chronic kidney disease. Phosphate retention leads to increase in the phosphate × calcium product and precipitation of amorphous calcium phosphate in the arteries and soft tissues. AP radiograph of the left hand shows metastatic calcifications around the second and fifth metacarpophalangeal joints (large arrows) and along the second proximal phalanx (small arrow). More typically these calcifications are seen around the large joints.

are preferentially involved, giving bands of dense bones adjacent to the end-plates with a central band of lower normal bone density. These alternating bands of normal and sclerotic bone give a striped pattern described as a 'rugger jersey' spine (Fig. 50-26).

Osteoporosis. With excessive bone resorption, the bones may appear reduced in radiodensity in some patients. This particularly occurs in postmenopausal women and the elderly, in whom bone resorption exceeds new bone formation, with a net reduction in bone mass. This can be confirmed by bone densitometry, which is an integral component in the evaluation of hyperparathyroidism. In primary hyperparathyroidism there is a pattern of skeletal involvement that preferentially affects the cortical, as opposed to the trabecular, bone. BMD measurements made in sites in which cortical bone predominates, e.g. in the distal forearm, may show the most marked reduction.[94] Bone density increases after parathyroidectomy in primary hyperparathyroidism.

Metastatic Calcification. Metastatic calcifications are typically found in secondary hyperparathyroidism; soft-tissue calcification, other than in articular cartilage and fibrocartilage, does not occur in primary hyperparathyroidism unless there is associated reduced glomerular function resulting in phosphate retention. The latter results in an increase in the calcium × phosphate product, and as a consequence amorphous calcium phosphate is precipitated in organs, blood vessels and soft tissues (Fig. 50-27). If there are features of hyperparathyroidism, i.e. subperiosteal erosions and additionally extensive vascular or soft-tissue calcifications, e.g. around joints and in tendons, this implies impaired renal function in association with hyperparathyroidism.

Hypoparathyroidism

Aetiology

Hypoparathyroidism can result from reduced or absent parathyroid hormone production or from end-organ (kidney, bone or both) resistance. This may be the result of the parathyroid glands failing to develop, the glands being damaged or removed, the function of the glands being reduced by altered regulation, or the action of parathyroid hormone (PTH) being impaired. The resulting biochemical abnormality is hypocalcaemia; this can clinically cause neuromuscular symptoms and signs such as tetany and fits.[95] Acquired hypoparathyroidism results from either surgical removal of the parathyroid glands or from autoimmune disorders. Post-surgical hypoparathyroidism is more common and occurs in approximately 13% of patients following thyroid or parathyroid surgery. Idiopathic hypoparathyroidism usually presents during childhood, is more common in girls and is rare in black races. It may be associated with pernicious anaemia and Addison's disease. There may be antibodies to a number of endocrine glands as part of a generalised autoimmune disorder.

Radiological Abnormalities

There may be localised (23%) or generalised (9%) osteosclerosis in affected patients.[96] This particularly affects the skull where the vault is thickened. At an early age of onset, the dentition is hypoplastic. Metastatic calcification may be present in the basal ganglia or in the subcutaneous tissue, particularly around the hips and shoulders (Fig. 50-28). A rare but recognised complication of hypoparathyroidism is an enthesopathy with extraskeletal ossification in a paraspinal distribution and elsewhere.[97] In the spine this skeletal hyperostosis resembles most closely that described by Forestier as 'senile' hyperostosis.[97,98] Differentiating features from ankylosing spondylitis are that there is no erosive arthropathy and the sacroiliac joints appear normal. Clinically the patients may have pain and stiffness in the back with limitation of movement. Extraskeletal ossification may be present around the pelvis, hip and in the interosseous membranes and tendinous insertions elsewhere.

Pseudohypoparathyroidism (PHP)

Pseudohypoparathyroidism describes a group of genetic disorders characterised by hypocalcaemia, hyperphosphataemia, raised PTH and target tissue unresponsiveness to PTH, first described by Albright et al in 1942.[99–101] The condition results from mutations of the *GNAS1* gene.[101] Affected patients are short in stature, have reduced intellect, rounded faces and shortened metacarpals, particularly the fourth and fifth (Fig. 50-29). Metastatic calcification, bowing of long bones and exostoses can occur. Clinical features include tetany, cataracts and nail dystrophy. Some of the clinical and radiological features of PHP may resemble those in other hereditary syndromes, including Turner's syndrome, acrodysostosis, Prader–Willi syndrome, fibrodysplasia ossificans progressiva and multiple hereditary exostosis. In PHP there is end-organ unresponsiveness to PTH since the parathyroid glands are normal and produce PTH. This usually involves unresponsiveness of both bone and kidneys. However, there is a rare variation of PHP in which the kidneys are unresponsive to PTH but the osseous response to the hormone is normal.[102] The condition is referred to as pseudohypohyperparathyroidism, and the histological and radiological features resemble those of azotaemic osteodystrophy.

Radiographic Abnormalities

Abnormalities may not be evident at birth but subsequently patients develop premature epiphyseal fusion,

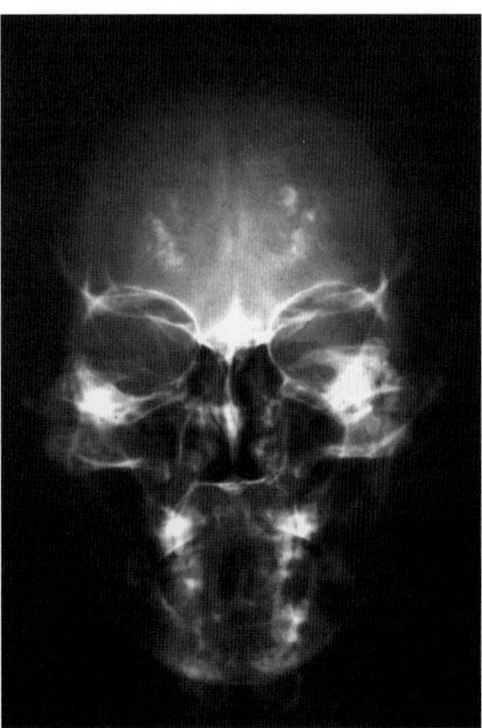

FIGURE 50-28 ■ Hypoparathyroidism. In hypoparathyroidism soft-tissue calcifications are a typical finding, seen in the basal ganglia in this AP radiograph of the skull.

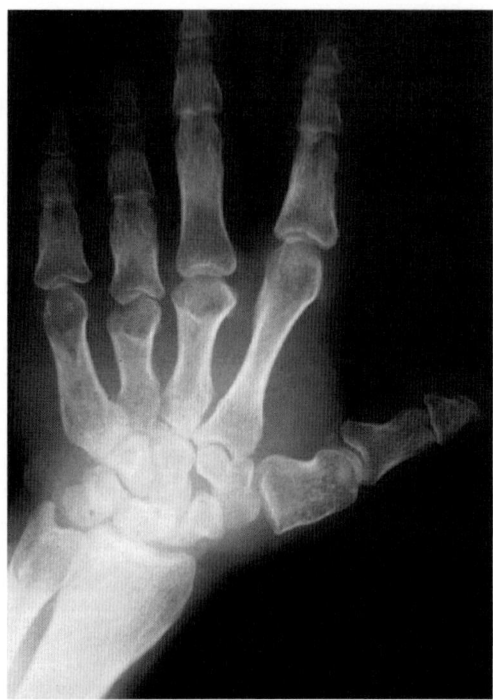

FIGURE 50-29 ■ Pseudo-hypoparathyroidism. In pseudohyperparathyroidism (PHP osteodystrophy of Albright) affected individuals are short in stature, and there are dysplastic features, including shortened metacarpals (brachydactyly), particularly the fourth and fifth, as shown in this AP radiograph of the left hand.

calvarial thickening, bone exostoses and calcification in the basal ganglia and the soft tissue (Fig. 50-28). Metacarpal shortening is present, particularly affecting the fourth and fifth digits (Fig. 50-29). This may result in a positive metacarpal sign; normally a line drawn tangential to the heads of the fourth and fifth metacarpals should not intersect the third metacarpal, but shorting of the fourth metacarpal means that it will. This feature is not specific for PHP and can occur in other congenital (Beckwith–Wiedemann and basal cell naevus syndromes, multiple epiphyseal dysplasia) and acquired (juvenile chronic arthritis, sickle-cell disease with infarction) conditions. Soft-tissue calcification occurs in a plaque-like distribution in the subcutaneous area. Rarely, soft-tissue ossification can occur in a periarticular distribution, usually involving the hands and feet.

Pseudo-Pseudohypoparathyroidism (PPHP)

In these affected individuals the dysplastic and other features are the same as PHP, but there are no associated parathyroid or other biochemical abnormalities. The abnormalities include metacarpal and metatarsal shortening, calvarial thickening and exostoses; soft-tissue calcification and ossification are best identified on radiographs. CT of the brain is more sensitive at identifying basal ganglia calcification than radiographs. BMD may be normal, reduced or increased.

RICKETS AND OSTEOMALACIA

Mineralisation of bone matrix depends on the presence of adequate supplies of 1,25-dihydroxy vitamin D (1,25$(OH)_2$D), calcium, phosphorus and alkaline phosphatase, and on a normal body pH. If there is a deficiency of any of these, or severe systemic acidosis, the mineralisation of bone will be defective. This results in a qualitative abnormality of bone, with a reduction in the mineral-to-osteoid ratio, resulting in rickets in children and osteomalacia in adults. Rickets and osteomalacia are therefore synonymous and represent the same disease process, but manifest in either the growing or the mature skeleton.

In the immature skeleton the radiographic abnormalities predominate at the growing ends of the bones where enchondral ossification is taking place, giving the classic appearance of rickets. At skeletal maturity, when the process of enchondral ossification has ceased, the defective mineralisation of osteoid is evident radiographically as Looser's zones, which are pathognomonic of osteomalacia.[103]

The pro-hormone forms of vitamin D require two hydroxylation stages to form the active metabolite, through which the hormone exerts its physiological action. There are two pro-hormonal forms of 1,25-dihydroxy vitamin D in humans: vitamin D_2 and vitamin D_3. Vitamin D_2 is prepared by irradiation of ergosterol obtained from yeast or fungi, and is used for food supplementation and pharmaceutical preparations. Vitamin D_3 occurs naturally through the interaction of ultraviolet light on 7-dehydrocholesterol in the deep layers of the skin. Vitamin D_2 and D_3 are initially hydroxylated at the 25 position to form 25$(OH)D_2$ and 25$(OH)D_3$, the latter predominating and circulating bound to a specific protein. This hydroxylation occurs predominantly in the liver. A further hydroxylation in the 1 position in the kidney produces 1,25$(OH)_2$D, which is the active form of the hormone.

Vitamin D Deficiency

Deficiency may occur as a consequence of simple nutritional lack (diet, lack of sunlight), malabsorption states (vitamin D is fat soluble and absorbed in the small bowel), chronic liver disease (which affects hydroxylation at the 25 position) and chronic renal disease (in which the active metabolite 1,25$(OH)_2$D is not produced). Consequently, a wide variety of diseases may result in vitamin D deficiency; the radiological features will be similar, being those of rickets or osteomalacia. This similarity of radiological features, but variation in response to treatment, contributed to some of the early confusion. Rickets due to nutritional deprivation was cured by ultraviolet light or physiological doses of vitamin D (400 IU per day), but that associated with chronic renal disease was not, except when very large pharmacological doses (up to 300,000 IU per day) were used. This led to the terms 'refractory rickets' and 'vitamin D resistant rickets' being used for these conditions. Within these terms were included the diseases that cause the clinical and radiological features of rickets, but were related to phosphate, not vitamin D, deficiency, such as X-linked hypophosphataemia, and genetic disorders involving defects in 1α-hydroxylase and the vitamin D receptor.

Genetic Disorders of Vitamin D Metabolism

Prader et al. in 1961 described the condition in which rickets occurred within the first year of life, was characterised by severe hypocalcaemia and dental enamel hypoplasia, and responded to large amounts of vitamin D. The term 'vitamin D dependency' was used for this syndrome. It is now recognised that this disease is due to an inborn error of metabolism in which there is defective hydroxylation of 25(OH)D in the kidney due to defective activity of the renal 25(OH)D 1α-hydroxylase. This results in insufficient synthesis of 1,25$(OH)_2$D. The preferred term for this condition is pseudo vitamin D deficiency rickets (PDDR) and it is inherited as an autosomal recessive trait.[104]

Another inborn error of vitamin D metabolism was described in 1978.[105] Clinically it resembled pseudo vitamin D deficiency rickets but with high circulating concentrations of 1,25$(OH)_2$D. This condition results from a spectrum of mutations which affect the vitamin D receptor (VDR) in target tissues, causing resistance to the action of 1,25$(OH)_2$D (end-organ resistance). Affected patients have complete alopecia.

Oncogenic Osteomalacia

Oncogenic osteomalacia, also termed tumour-induced osteomalacia (TIO), is a rare paraneoplastic syndrome in

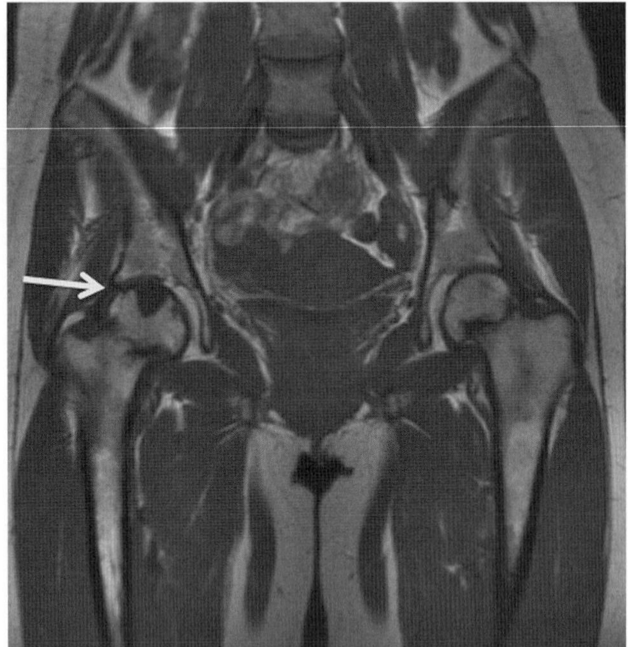

FIGURE 50-30 ■ **Oncogenic osteomalacia.** T1-weighted fast spin-echo coronal MR image of the pelvis showing incomplete bilateral femoral neck fractures and a tumour in the right femoral head (arrow); histologically, this was found to be a mesenchymal tumour which was responsible for oncogenic osteomalacia.

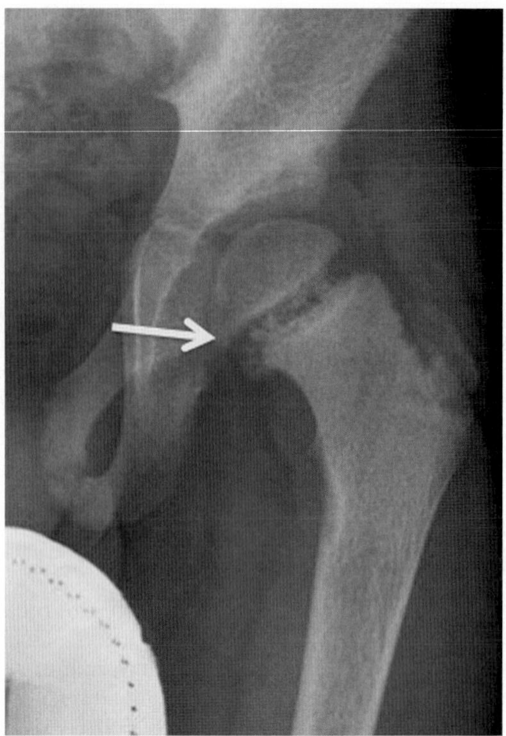

FIGURE 50-31 ■ **Rickets in the immature skeleton.** Evidence of defective mineralisation is evident in sites of endochondral ossification. The growth plate is widened and shows irregular calcification as demonstrated at the hip joint in this AP radiograph of the left hip (arrow).

which patients present with bone pain, fractures, and muscle weakness (Fig. 50-30).[106,107] The cause is a high blood level of the recently identified phosphate and vitamin D-regulating hormone, fibroblast growth factor 23 (FGF23).[108] In oncogenic osteomalacia, FGF23 is secreted by mesenchymal tumours that are usually benign, but are typically very small and difficult to locate. FGF23 acts primarily at the renal tubule and impairs phosphate reabsorption and 1α-hydroxylation of 25(OH)D, leading to hypophosphataemia and low levels of 1,25-dihydroxy vitamin D. Removal of the tumour cures the condition and imaging plays an important role in tumour localisation. A step-wise approach utilising functional imaging (F-18 fluorodeoxyglucose positron emission tomography and octreotide scintigraphy) followed by anatomical imaging (CT and/or MRI), and, if needed, selective venous sampling with measurement of FGF23, is usually successful in locating the tumours.[108]

Radiological Appearances

Rickets. In the immature skeleton the effect of vitamin D deficiency and the consequent defective mineralisation of osteoid is seen principally at the growing ends of bones.[103,109–111] In the early stage there is apparent widening of the growth plate (Fig. 50-31). More severe change produces 'cupping' of the metaphysis, with irregular and poor mineralisation (Fig. 50-32). Some expansion in width of the metaphysis results in the swelling around the ends of the long bones affected. This expansion of the anterior ends of the ribs is referred to as a 'rachitic rosary'. There may be a thin 'ghostlike' rim of mineralisation at

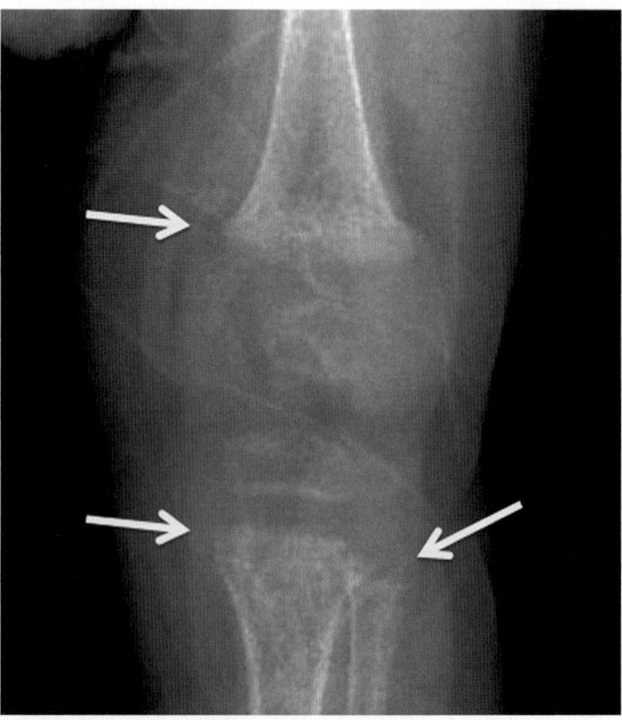

FIGURE 50-32 ■ **Rickets.** Severe osteopenia, widening of the growth plate and cupping of the metaphyses (arrows) in this AP radiograph of the knee.

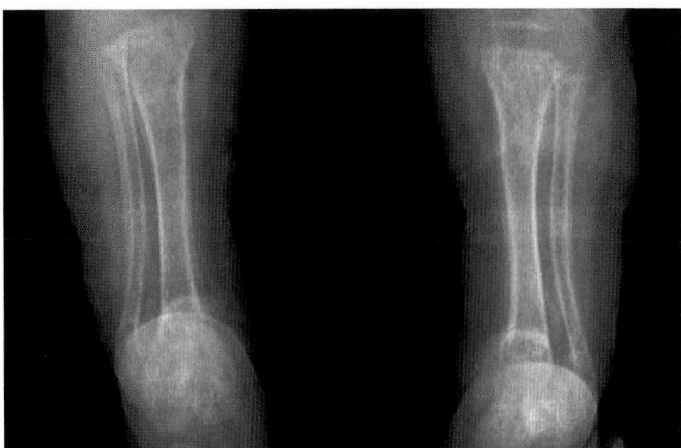

FIGURE 50-33 ■ **Rickets.** Severe osteopenia with medial bowing of bilateral tibia and fibula and cupping of the metaphyses in this AP radiograph of bilateral distal lower extremities.

the periphery of the metaphysis, as this mineralisation occurs by membranous ossification at the periosteum. The margin of the epiphysis appears indistinct as enchondral ossification at this site is also defective. These changes predominate at the sites of bones which are growing most actively, in particular around the knee (Fig. 50-32), the wrist (particularly the ulna), the anterior ends of the middle ribs, the proximal femur (Fig. 50-31) and the distal tibia, and depend on the age of the child. MRI may show abnormalities of the physeal cartilage.[109]

Rachitic bone is soft and bends, and this results in genu valgum or genu varum, deformity of the hips (coxa valga or more commonly coxa vara), deformity of the long bones with bowing (Fig. 50-33), in-drawing of the ribs at the insertion of the diaphragm (Harrison's sulcus) and protrusio acetabuli and triradiate deformity of the pelvis, which can cause problems with subsequent parturition. Involvement of the bones in the thorax and respiratory tract (larynx and trachea) occasionally results in stridor and respiratory distress. In very severe rickets, when little skeletal growth is taking place (i.e. owing to nutritional deprivation or chronic ill health), paradoxically the radiological features of rickets may not be evident at the growth plate. In rickets of prematurity, little abnormality may be present at the metaphysis since no skeletal growth is taking place in the premature infant. However, the bones are osteopenic and prone to fractures. In mild vitamin D deficiency the radiographic features of rickets may only become apparent at puberty during the growth spurt, and the metaphyseal abnormalities predominate at the knee.

With appropriate treatment of vitamin D deficiency, the radiographic features of healing (after 3–4 months) lag behind the improvement in biochemical parameters (after 2 weeks) and clinical symptoms. With treatment, the zone of provisional calcification will mineralise. This mineralised zone is initially separated by translucent osteoid from the shaft of the bone, and may be mistaken for a metaphyseal fracture of child abuse.[112] Reduced bone density and poor definition of epiphyses are helpful distinguishing features for rickets. The section of abnormal bone following healing of rickets may be visible for a period of time, and give some indication as to the age of onset and duration of the period of rickets. Eventually this zone will become indistinguishable from normal bone with remodelling over a period of 3–4 months. The zone of provisional calcification which was present at the onset of the disturbance to enchondral ossification may remain (Harris growth arrest line) as a marker of the age of skeletal maturity at which the rickets occurred. However, this is not specific for rickets and may occur in any condition (e.g. period of ill health, lead poisoning) that inhibits normal enchondral ossification. There will be evidence of retarded growth and development in rickets; this tends to be more marked when the vitamin D deficiency is associated with chronic diseases that reduce calorie intake, general well-being and activity (i.e. malabsorption, chronic renal disease) than with simple nutritional vitamin D deficiency.

Vitamin D deficiency is associated with hypocalcaemia. In an attempt to maintain calcium homeostasis, the parathyroid glands are stimulated to secrete PTH. This results in another important feature of vitamin D deficiency rickets. Evidence of secondary hyperparathyroidism, with increased osteoclastic resorption, is always shown histologically, although not always radiographically.

Metaphyseal chondrodysplasias may mimic rickets and in a variety of inherited bone dysplasias there are metaphyseal abnormalities which may range from mild (Schmid type) to severe (Jansen).[113] Normal serum biochemistry serves to differentiate these dysplasias from other rachitic disorders, which the radiographic abnormalities at the metaphyses may simulate.

Osteomalacia. At skeletal maturity the epiphysis fuses to the metaphysis with obliteration of the growth plate and cessation of longitudinal bone growth. Vitamin D deficiency in the adult skeleton results in osteomalacia, the pathognomonic radiographic feature of which is the Looser's zone[114] (Fig. 50-34). Looser's zones (pseudofractures, Milkman's fractures) are translucent areas in the bone that are composed of unmineralised osteoid. They are typically (but not always) bilateral and symmetrical. Radiographically they appear as radiolucent lines that are perpendicular to the bone cortex, do not usually extend across the entire bone shaft, and characteristically have a slightly sclerotic margin. Looser's zones can occur in any bone but most typically are found in the medial aspect of the femoral neck (Fig. 50-34), the pubic rami, the lateral border of the scapula and the ribs. They may involve the first and second ribs, in which traumatic fractures are uncommon, being usually associated with severe trauma. Other less common sites for Looser's zones are the metatarsals and metacarpals, the base of the acromion and the ilium. They may not always be visible on radiographs; radionuclide bone scintigraphy and MRI may be more sensitive in identifying radiographic occult Looser's zones.

Looser's zones must be differentiated from insufficiency fractures that may occur in osteoporotic bone, particularly in the pubic rami, sacrum and calcaneus. Such insufficiency fractures consist of multiple microfractures in brittle osteoporotic bone and often show florid callus formation, serving to differentiate them from

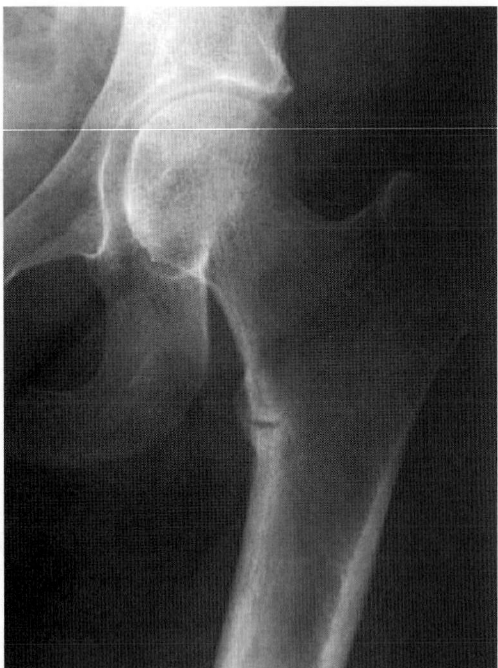

FIGURE 50-34 ■ Osteomalacia. In the mature skeleton following fusion of the growth plates, the pathognomonic radiographic feature is the Looser's zone. These are radiolucent, unmineralised linear areas which are perpendicular to the cortex and which may have a sclerotic margin. They occur most frequently in the medial aspects of the femoral necks (arrow in this AP radiograph of the proximal femur), symphysis pubis, ribs and lateral borders of the scapulae.

Looser's zones.[30,115] Incremental fractures occur in Paget's disease of bone and resemble Looser's zones in appearance, but tend to occur on the convexity of the cortex of the bone involved,[116] rather than medially on the concave side, as in osteomalacia. The other typical features of Paget's disease serve as distinguishing radiological features.[116]

Complete fractures can occur through Looser's zones, but with no evidence of callus formation until the osteomalacia is treated with vitamin D. Then there will be quite florid callus formation around fractures with healing of the fractures and Looser's zones with little residual deformity. As in rickets, osteomalacic bone is soft and bends. This is evident radiographically by protrusio acetabuli, in which the femoral head deforms the acetabular margin so that the normal medial 'teardrop' outline is lost. There may be bowing of the long bones of the legs and a triradiate deformity of the pelvis, particularly if the cause of the vitamin D deficiency has persisted since childhood and has been inadequately treated or untreated.

In osteomalacia, as in rickets, hypocalcaemia acts as stimulus to *secondary hyperparathyroidism*. This may be manifested radiographically as subperiosteal erosion, particularly in the phalanges but other sites (sacroiliac joints, symphysis pubis, proximal tibia, outer ends of the clavicle, skull vault—'pepperpot' skull) may be involved, depending on the intensity of the hyperparathyroidism and how long it has been present. There may also be cortical tunnelling and a hazy trabecular pattern. Generalised osteopenia may occur and vertebral bodies may have biconcave end-plates, due to deformation of the malacic bone by the cartilaginous intervertebral disc ('cod fish' deformity).

Azotaemic Osteodystrophy

The bone disease associated with CKD is complex and multifactorial, and has changed over past decades.[117–119] Whereas originally features of vitamin D deficiency (rickets/osteomalacia) and secondary hyperparathyroidism (erosions, osteosclerosis, brown cysts) (Fig. 50-26) predominated, improvements in management and therapy have resulted in such radiographic features being present in only a minority of patients. Soft-tissue and extensive vascular metastatic calcification (Fig. 50-27) and 'adynamic' bone develop as a complication of disease (phosphate retention) and treatment (phosphate binders). New complications (amyloid deposition, non-infective spondyloarthropathy, osteonecrosis) are now seen in long-term haemodialysis and/or renal transplantation. Radiographs remain the most important imaging technique, but occasionally other imaging and quantitative techniques (CT, MRI, bone densitometry) are relevant to diagnosis and management.

In extreme cases of soft-tissue calcification there may be ischaemic necrosis of the skin, muscle and subcutaneous tissue, referred to as 'calciphylaxis'. This condition can occur in patients with advanced renal disease, in those on regular dialysis, and also those with functioning renal allografts.[120]

Renal Tubular Defects

Glucose, inorganic phosphate and amino acids are absorbed in the proximal renal tubule. Concentration and acidification of urine in exchange for a fixed base occur in the distal renal tubule. Renal tubular disorders may involve either the proximal or the distal tubule, or both. Such disorders result in a spectrum of biochemical disturbances that may result in loss of phosphate, glucose, or amino acids alone, or in combination, with additional defects in urine acidification and concentration. Such defects of tubular function may be inherited and present from birth (Toni– Fanconi syndrome, cystinosis, X-linked hypophosphataemia) or may be acquired later in life (e.g. tubular function being compromised by deposition of copper in Wilson's disease, hereditary tyrosinaemia). Renal tubular dysfunction may also be acquired, with dysfunction being induced by the effects of toxins or therapies (Paraquat, Lysol burns, toluene 'glue sniffing' inhalation, ifosfamide, gentamicin, streptozotocin, valproic acid), deposition of heavy metals or other substances (multiple myeloma, cadmium, lead, mercury), related to immunological disorders (interstitial nephritis, renal transplantation), or with the production of a humoral substance in oncogenic osteomalacia, also termed tumour induced osteomalacia.[108] In these renal tubular-disorders, rickets or osteomalacia can be caused by multiple factors, including hyperphosphaturia, hypophosphataemia and reduced 1α-hydroxylation of 25(OH)D. As the serum calcium is generally normal in these disorders, secondary hyperparathyroidism does not occur.

X-linked Hypophosphataemia (XLH). This genetic disorder is transmitted as an X-linked dominant trait.[121] Sporadic cases also occur through spontaneous mutations. The incidence is approximately 1 in 25,000, and XLH is now the most common cause of genetically induced rickets. The disease is characterised by phosphaturia throughout life, hypophosphataemia, rickets and osteomalacia. Clinically affected individuals may be short in stature, principally due to defective growth in the legs, which are bowed; the trunk is usually normal.[122] Rickets becomes clinically evident at about 6–12 months of age or older. Treatment with phosphate supplements and large pharmacological doses of vitamin D (hence the term 'vitamin D-resistant rickets') can heal the radiological features of rickets and also improve longitudinal growth. The radiological features of XLH are characteristic.[123] There is defective mineralisation of the metaphysis and widening of the growth plate (rickets). The metaphyseal margin tends to be less indistinct than in nutritional rickets and the affected metaphysis is not as wide. Changes are most marked at the knee, wrist, ankle and proximal femur. Healing can be induced with appropriate treatment (phosphate supplements, $1,25(OH)_2D$). The growth plates fuse normally at skeletal maturation. The bones are often short and under-tubulated (shaft wide in relation to bone length) with bowing of the femur and tibia, which may be marked. Following skeletal maturation, Looser's zones appear and persist in patients with XLH (Fig. 50-35A). They tend to be in different sites to those which occur in nutritional osteomalacia, and often affect the outer cortex of the bowed femur, although they also occur along the medial cortex of the shaft. Looser's zones in the ribs and pelvis are rare. Although Looser's zones may heal with appropriate treatment, those that have been present for many years persist radiographically and are presumably filled with fibrous tissue.

Although there is defective mineralisation of osteoid in XLH, the bones are commonly and characteristically increased in radiodensity with a coarse and prominent trabecular pattern. This is a feature of the disease, and is not related to treatment with vitamin D and phosphate supplements, as it is present in those who have not received treatment. This bone sclerosis can involve the petrous bone and structures of the inner ear, and may be responsible for the hydropic cochlea pattern of deafness that these patients may develop in later life.[124] X-linked hypophosphataemia is characterised by an enthesopathy, in which there is inflammation in the junctional area between bone and tendon insertion that heals by ossification at affected sites[125] (Fig. 50-35B). As a result, ectopic bone forms around the pelvis and spine. This may result in complete ankylosis of the spine, resembling ankylosing spondylitis, and clinically limiting mobility. However, the absence of inflammatory arthritis, with normal sacroiliac joints, serves to differentiate XLH from ankylosing spondylitis.

Ossification may occur in the interosseous membrane of the forearm and in the leg between the tibia and the fibula. Separate, small ossicles may be present around the joints of the hands and ossification of tendon insertions in the hands causes 'whiskering' of bone margins.

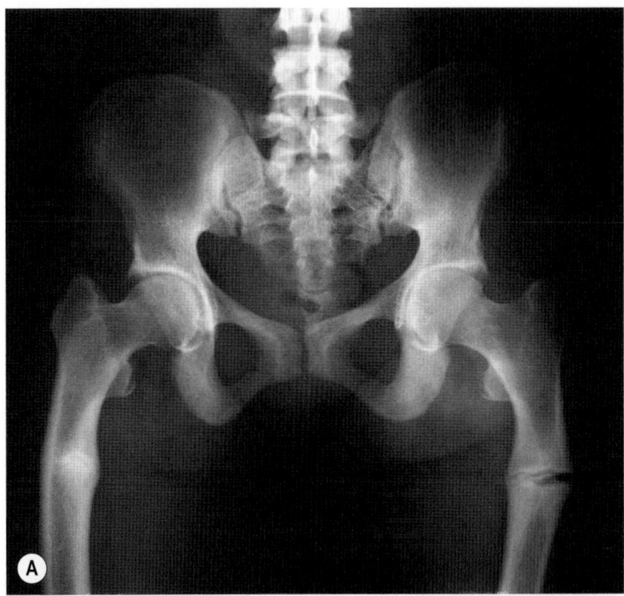

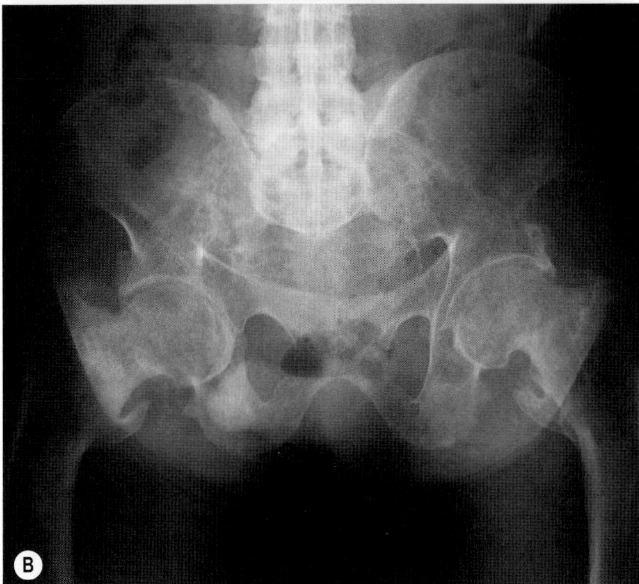

FIGURE 50-35 ■ X-linked hypophosphataemic osteomalacia. This is the most common of the genetic causes of rickets and osteomalacia. The bones may be radiodense with a coarse trabecular pattern. In affected children there will be evidence of rickets. (A) In adults chronic Looser's zones may be present, as in the outer cortex of both femora. (B) There may be evidence of an enthesopathy in older patients with ossification of ligamentous insertion to bone, as present in the pelvis at the psoas insertion to the lesser trochanters. The paraspinal ossification resembles ankylosing spondylitis, but the sacroiliac joints are not eroded, which differentiates the two conditions.

A rare, but recognised, important complication of XLH is spinal cord compression caused by a combination of ossification of the ligamentum flavum, thickening of the laminae and hyperostosis around the apophyseal joints.[126] Ossification of the ligamentum flavum causes the most significant narrowing of the spinal canal and occurs most commonly in the thoracic spine, generally involving two or three adjacent segments. Affected patients may be asymptomatic, even when there is severe spinal canal narrowing. Acute spinal cord compression can be precipitated by quite minor trauma. It is important to be aware of this rare complication of the disease since surgical decompression by laminectomy is curative and is best performed as an elective procedure by an experienced surgeon rather than as an emergency. The extent of intraspinal ossification cannot be predicted by the degree of paraspinal or extraskeletal ossification at other sites. CT is a useful imaging technique for demonstrating the extent of intraspinal ossification.

Extraskeletal ossification is uncommon in patients with XLH before the age of 40 years. The extent to which radiographic abnormalities of rickets and osteomalacia, osteosclerosis, abnormalities of bone modelling and extraskeletal ossification are present varies between affected individuals.[127] In some patients, all the features are present and so are diagnostic of the condition. In others, there may only be minor abnormalities and the diagnosis of X-linked hypophosphataemic rickets may be overlooked.[128]

Other Causes of Rickets and Osteomalacia (Not Related to Vitamin D Deficiency or Hypophosphataemia)

Hypophosphatasia

This rare disorder is generally transmitted as an autosomal recessive trait, but autosomal dominant inheritance has also been reported. The disease is characterised by reduced levels of serum alkaline phosphatase (both bone and liver isoenzymes), with raised levels of phosphoethanolamine in both the blood and the urine. Serum calcium and phosphorus levels are not reduced; in perinatal and infantile disease there can be hypercalciuria and hypercalcaemia attributed to the imbalance between calcium absorption from the gut and defective growth and mineralisation of the skeleton. The latter results in rickets in childhood and osteomalacia in adults. The severity of the condition varies greatly, being diagnosed either in the perinatal period, in infancy or childhood, but in some patients only becoming apparent in adult life.[129] The condition can wax and wane and tends to be more severe in children than when it becomes apparent in later life.

OTHER METABOLIC BONE DISORDERS

A number of congenital and familial disorders can be associated with increased bone density (osteosclerosis) and abnormal bone modelling. These include osteopetrosis, pyknodysostosis, metaphyseal dysplasia (Pyle's disease), craniometaphyseal dysplasia, frontometaphyseal dysplasia, osteodysplasty (Melnick–Needles syndrome), progressive diaphyseal dysplasia (Camurati–Engelmann disease), hereditary multiple diaphyseal sclerosis (Ribbing's disease), craniodiaphyseal dysplasia, endosteal hyperostosis (Worth and Van Buchem types), dysosteosclerosis, tubular stenosis, and oculodento-osseous dysplasia. All are rare and have different natural histories, genetic transmission, complications and radiographic features. Many are dysplasias rather than metabolic bone disorders.

Osteopetrosis

In osteopetrosis there is defective osteoclastic resorption of the primary spongiosa of bone. Osteoclasts in affected bone are usually devoid of the ruffled borders by which osteoclasts adhere to the bone surface and through which their resorptive activity is expressed. In the presence of continued bone formation, there is generalised osteosclerosis and abnormalities of metaphyseal modelling[130,131] (Fig. 50-36). There have been reports of reversal of the osteosclerosis following successful bone marrow transplantation.

Osteopetrosis was first described by Albers-Schönberg in 1904, and is sometimes referred to as marble bone disease, osteosclerosis fragilis generalisata and osteopetrosis generalisata. There are two main clinical forms:

1. The lethal form of osteopetrosis with precocious manifestations and an autosomal recessive transmission.
2. Benign osteopetrosis with late manifestations, inherited by autosomal dominant transmission.

There is also a rarer autosomal recessive (intermediate) form, which presents during childhood with the signs and symptoms of the lethal form but the outcome on life expectancy is not known. The syndrome previously described as osteopetrosis with renal tubular acidosis and cerebral calcification is now recognised as an inborn error of metabolism, carbonic anhydrase II deficiency. Neuronal storage disease with malignant osteopetrosis has been described, as has the rare lethal, transient infantile and postinfectious form of the disorder.

Autosomal Recessive Lethal Type of Osteopetrosis

In affected individuals there is obliteration of the marrow cavity leading to anaemia, thrombocytopenia and recurrent infection. Clinically there is hepatosplenomegaly, hydrocephalus and cranial nerve involvement resulting in blindness and deafness. Radiographically all the bones are dense with lack of corticomedullary differentiation. Modelling of affected bones is abnormal with expansion of the metaphyseal region and under-tubulation of bone. This is most evident in the long bones, particularly the distal femur and proximal humerus. Although the bones are dense, they are brittle, and horizontal pathological fractures are common. The entire skull, particularly the base, is involved and the paranasal and mastoid air cells are poorly developed. Sclerosis of end-plates of the vertebral bodies produces a 'sandwich' appearance. MR imaging may assist in monitoring those with severe disease who undergo marrow transplantation, since success will be indicated by expansion of the marrow cavity. Findings on MR and CT of the brain have been described.

There is an intermediate recessive form of the disease, which is milder than that seen in infants and distinct from the less severe autosomal dominant disease. Affected individuals suffer pathological fracture and anaemia and are of short stature, with hepatomegaly. The radiographic

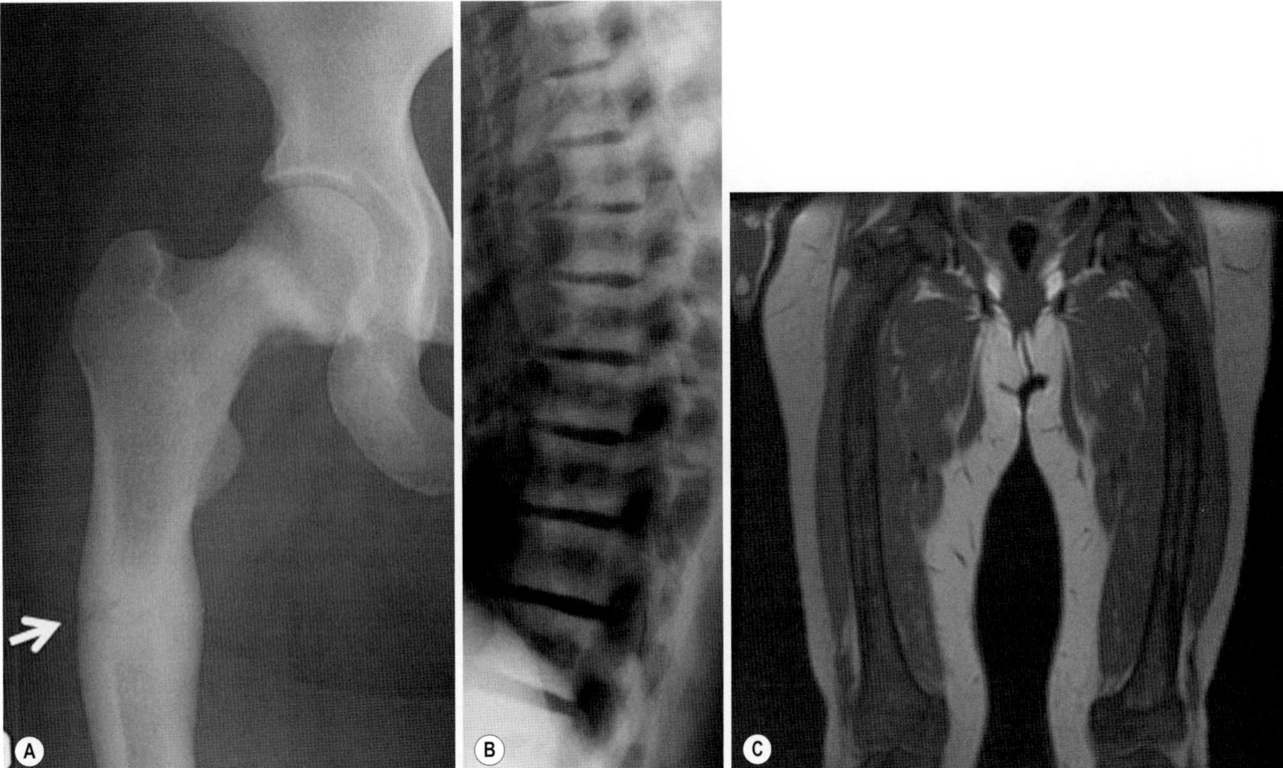

FIGURE 50-36 ■ Osteopetrosis. Osteoclastic function is defective, resulting in dense sclerotic bones which are brittle and prone to fracture. There is evidence of abnormal modelling of the long bones due to the failure of normal osteoclastic periosteal bone resorption which remodels the distal shafts of bones as they grow in length by endochondral ossification. In (A) the AP radiograph of the hip and femur shows increased density of the proximal femur with a remote diaphysis fracture (arrow) and cortical thickening. The lateral thoracic spine radiograph in (B) demonstrates increased sclerosis along the end-plates with a 'sandwich' appearance and the coronal T1-weighted MRI of bilateral femora in (C) shows partial obliteration of the marrow space due extensive sclerosis.

features include diffuse osteosclerosis with involvement of the skull base and facial bones, abnormal bone modelling and a 'bone within a bone' appearance.

Benign, Autosomal Dominant Type of Osteopetrosis (Albers-Schönberg Disease)

This is often asymptomatic, and the diagnosis may come to light either incidentally or through the occurrence of a pathological fracture (Fig. 50-36A). Other presentations include anaemia and facial palsy or deafness from cranial nerve compression. Problems may occur after tooth extraction, and there is an increased incidence of osteomyelitis, particularly of the mandible. Radiographic features are similar to those of the autosomal recessive form of the disease, but are less severe. The bones are diffusely sclerotic, with thickened cortices and defective modelling. There may be alternating sclerotic and radiolucent bands at the ends of diaphyses, a 'bone within a bone' appearance and the vertebral end-plates appear sclerotic (Fig. 50-36B). In 1987, Andersen and Bollerslev classified this form of the disease into two distinct radiological types. In type I fractures are unusual, in contrast to type II in which fractures are common. Transverse bands in the metaphyses are more commonly a feature in type II disease, as is a raised serum acid phosphatase.

Hyperphosphatasia

Hyperphosphatasia is a rare genetic disorder resulting from mutations in osteoprotegerin (OPG), and is characterised by markedly elevated serum alkaline phosphatase levels.[132] Affected children have episodes of fever, bone pain and progressive enlargement of the skull, with bowing of the long bones and associated pathological fractures. Radiographically the features resemble Paget's disease of bone, and it is sometimes referred to as 'juvenile' Paget's disease, osteitis deformans in children or hyperostosis corticalis (Fig. 50-37). There is an increased rate of bone turnover, with woven bone failing to mature into lamellar bone.

Radiographically, this increased rate of bone turnover is evidenced by decreased bone radiodensity with coarsening and disorganisation of the trabecular pattern. In the skull the diploic space is widened and there is patchy sclerosis. The diaphyses of the long bones become expanded with cortical thickening along their concave aspects. The long bones may be bowed, resulting in coxa vara and protrusio acetabulae. The vertebral bodies are reduced in radiodensity, reduced in height with biconcave end-plates. The bowing of the limbs causes affected individuals to be short in height. There is often premature loss of dentition due to resorption of dentine with replacement of the pulp by osteoid.

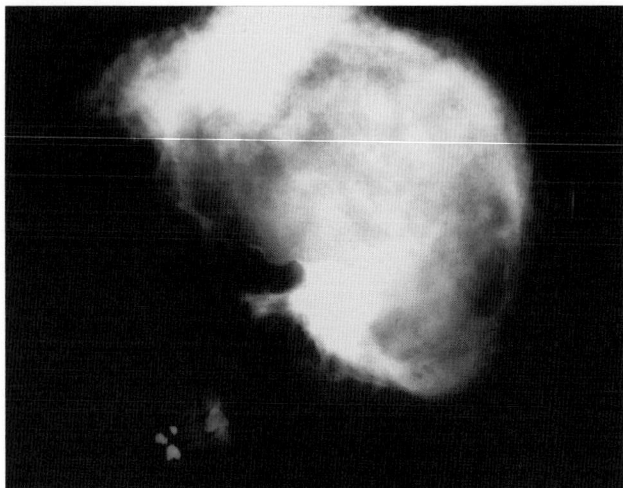

FIGURE 50-37 ■ **Hyperphosphatasia (juvenile Paget's disease).** There is increased bone turnover, resulting in immature woven bone being formed instead of mature lamellar bone. Bones are under-tubulated with a disorganised trabecular pattern, resembling the radiographic features of Paget's disease. In the lateral skull radiograph there is sclerosis, thickening of the skull vault and evidence of bone softening with basilar invagination. Platyspondyly may also be present.

The radiographic features closely resemble those of Paget's disease but are diagnostic as they involve the whole skeleton (as opposed to the monostotic or asymmetrical polyostotic involvement in Paget's disease) and affect children from the age of 2 years. On radionuclide imaging there is generalised increase in uptake, giving a 'super scan' due to excessive osteoblastic activity with absence of evidence of renal uptake.

MISCELLANEOUS

Vitamin D Intoxication

In the past, vitamin D was advocated in the treatment of a variety of conditions, including sarcoidosis, tuberculosis (especially lupus vulgaris), rheumatoid arthritis, hay fever, chilblains and asthma. The treatment had no beneficial effect in these conditions and its use was eventually abandoned. However, this was not before cases of vitamin D intoxication had been described. Vitamin D intoxication has become less common with the introduction of $1,25(OH)_2D$ (calcitriol) and other active metabolites. However, the more recent use of vitamin D to treat cancer, psoriasis and immunological disease may result in a resurgence of interest in vitamin D intoxication. The clinical symptoms include fatigue, malaise, weakness, thirst and polyuria, anorexia, nausea and vomiting due to hypercalcaemia. The latter results in hypercalciuria, nephrocalcinosis, impaired renal function and hypertension. Radiographically, metastatic calcification may be present in tendons, ligaments, fascial planes and arteries, and in the periosteum, resembling periostitis and causing bone sclerosis.

Hypervitaminosis A

Hypervitaminosis A can occur in those who are receiving vitamin A or one of its synthetic derivatives (retinoic acids) for treatment of skin disorders (refractory cystic acne, keratinising dermatoses, psoriasis). The skeletal manifestations include large bone outgrowths from the spine, particularly in the cervical region. In the peripheral skeleton there is evidence of a mild enthesopathy. In affected children there can occur cupping and splaying of the metaphyses, diaphyseal periostitis, particularly in the metatarsals and ulnae, and widening of the cranial sutures.

Fluorosis

Fluorosis results from the long-term ingestion of excessive amounts of fluoride. In some parts of the world fluorosis is endemic (e.g. India). The radiological features that result include osteosclerosis, particularly in the axial skeleton, and an enthesopathy with ossification of ligaments and large spinal osteophytes.[133] The paraspinal ossification may cause compression myelopathy.

Other Endocrine Diseases

Cushing's Disease

Cushing's disease is caused by a basophil pituitary adenoma, usually a micro adenoma (smaller than 10 mm); Cushing's syndrome is caused by a tumour of the adrenal glands (adenoma, carcinoma), ectopic ACTH production by a tumour (e.g. bronchial carcinoma), or iatrogenically by treatment with glucocorticoids. The cardinal skeletal manifestation is osteoporosis, which affects sites rich in trabecular bone (axial skeleton). Low-trauma fractures can occur, and these may heal with exuberant callus formation. Avascular necrosis and bone infarction is also a typical finding.

Thyroid Disease

There may be over- or underactivity of the gland (thyrotoxicosis and myxoedema, respectively). Thyroid disease in adults may be a cause of osteoporosis. Congenital or childhood onset of hypothyroidism (cretinism) results in retarded skeletal maturation, fragmented epiphyses, 'slipper-shaped' vertebrae and Wormian bones in the skull.[134] Thyroid acropachy is the triad of pretibial myxoedema, thyroid eye disease (exophthalmos) and clubbing of the fingers. Radiologically there may be diaphyseal periostitis, predominantly involving the tubular bones of the hand.[135] Patients may be thyrotoxic, euthyroid or hypothyroid.

Acromegaly

Acromegaly is the result of an eosinophilic adenoma of the pituitary gland, usually a macro adenoma (greater than 10 mm in size); if it occurs in children, gigantism results. There is overgrowth of all tissues and organs. The hypertrophied cartilage may initially cause widening of the joints, seen best in the hand radiograph in the metacarpophalangeal (MCP) joints. However, the hypertrophied cartilage is poor in tensile strength and liable to fissures. This results in premature osteoarthritis with relative widening of the joint space (acromegalic arthropathy).[136,137] When the joints in the spine are involved, cord compression can occur. Acromegaly can also result in generalised osteoporosis.

For a full list of references, please see ExpertConsult.

FURTHER READING

7. Kanis JA. Diagnosis of osteoporosis and assessment of fracture risk. Lancet 2002;359(9321):1929–36.
8. Baim S, Binkley N, Bilezikian JP, et al. Official Positions of the International Society for Clinical Densitometry and executive summary of the 2007 ISCD Position Development Conference. J Clin Densitom 2008;11(1):75–91.
17. Delmas PD, van de Langerijt L, Watts NB, et al; IMPACT Study Group. Underdiagnosis of vertebral fractures is a worldwide problem: the IMPACT study. J Bone Miner Res 2005;20(4): 557–63.
30. Cabarrus MC, Ambekar A, Lu Y, Link TM. MRI and CT of insufficiency fractures of the pelvis and the proximal femur. AJR Am J Roentgenol 2008;191(4):995–1001.
38. Shane E, Burr D, Ebeling PR, et al. Atypical subtrochanteric and diaphyseal femoral fractures: report of a task force of the American Society for Bone and Mineral Research. J Bone Miner Res 2010;25(11):2267–94.
52. Damilakis J, Adams JE, Guglielmi G, Link TM. Radiation exposure in X-ray-based imaging techniques used in osteoporosis. Eur Radiol 2011;20(11):2707–14.
74. Link TM, Guglielmi G, van Kuijk C, Adams JE. Radiologic assessment of osteoporotic vertebral fractures: diagnostic and prognostic implications. Eur Radiol 2005;15(8):1521–32.
103. Adams J. Radiology of rickets and osteomalacia. In: Feldman D, Glorieux FH, Pike JW, editors. Vitamin D. 2nd ed. San Diego: Elsevier Academic Press; 2005. p. 967–94.
118. Adams JE. Imaging in metabolic bone disease. Semin Musculoskelet Radiol 2002;6(3):171–2.

CHAPTER 51

Arthritis

Andrew J. Grainger • Philip O'Connor

CHAPTER OUTLINE

IMAGING OF JOINT DISEASE

The imaging of joint disease is complex, with the radiologist required to combine imaging findings and clinical information to accurately characterise arthritis. This chapter details the general principles of the plain radiographic assessment of arthritis and the key features of common arthritic conditions encountered.

Plain Radiographic Interpretation; General Principles

A systematic approach to the review of radiographs for arthritis is required. Important features to identify are:

- Soft-tissue swelling,
- Alteration in joint space,
- Bone changes
  - erosion
  - osteopenia
  - enthesitis.
- Joint alignment.

Finally, the distribution of joint disease provides important information when forming a differential diagnosis.

Soft-Tissue Swelling

Soft-tissue swelling is usually the earliest sign on CR of an inflammatory arthritis, representing synovial hypertrophy, soft-tissue oedema and joint effusion. When seen at the small joints the swelling has a symmetrical spindle shape about the joint. This pattern contrasts with soft-tissue swelling seen in gout, which tends to show a more irregular asymmetrical 'lumpy' appearance. Diffuse swelling of the soft-tissues of a digit is the characteristic finding in the dactylitis seen in hand involvement of the sero-negative inflammatory arthritides (Fig. 51-1). Radiographic soft-tissue abnormality around large joints tends to be limited to the detection of intra-articular effusion or synovitis.

Alteration in Joint Space

Loss of joint space as a result of cartilage destruction is a characteristic feature of many joint diseases. In inflammatory arthritis joint space loss is typically uniform, across the joint. In many joints this is helpful in distinguishing inflammatory arthritis from osteoarthritis (OA), which typically shows non-uniform joint space loss. However, in small joints, both forms of arthritis can show uniform joint space loss (Fig. 51-2).

Preserved joint space in a joint otherwise showing evidence of significant arthropathic change is important and may help with the differential diagnosis. In particular gout and psoriatic arthropathy typically show joint space preservation until late in the disease.

In severe arthritic change bony ankylosis may occur. This is most commonly seen in the sero-negative arthritides and in juvenile arthritis and represents end-stage disease.

Bone Changes

Osteopenia. Periarticular osteopenia is a well-recognised feature of some arthritides but is difficult to reliably identify. It may be more obvious in cases of mono- or pauci-articular joint involvement, where other joints are visible for comparison. An overexposed radiograph can mimic periarticular osteopenia, as can generalised osteoporosis. Often it is easier to identify that there is no evidence of osteopenia, which in itself is a useful observation when forming a differential diagnosis. Sero-negative disease, OA and gout typically preserve or increase bone density (Fig. 51-3).

Erosion. Bone erosion is the hallmark of inflammatory arthritis. Erosions can be described by their relationship to the joint and can be categorised as central, marginal or juxta-articular. Marginal erosions occur at the edge of the joint line involving exposed bone between the edge of the articular cartilage and the joint capsule. They are a classical feature of rheumatoid arthritis (RA). Central erosions occur into bone normally covered by the articular cartilage. They are less common and are typical of inflammatory (erosive) OA. Juxta-articular erosions occur further away from the joint and are characteristic of gout.

Rheumatoid erosions characteristically have no associated bone proliferation when untreated (Fig. 51-4A),

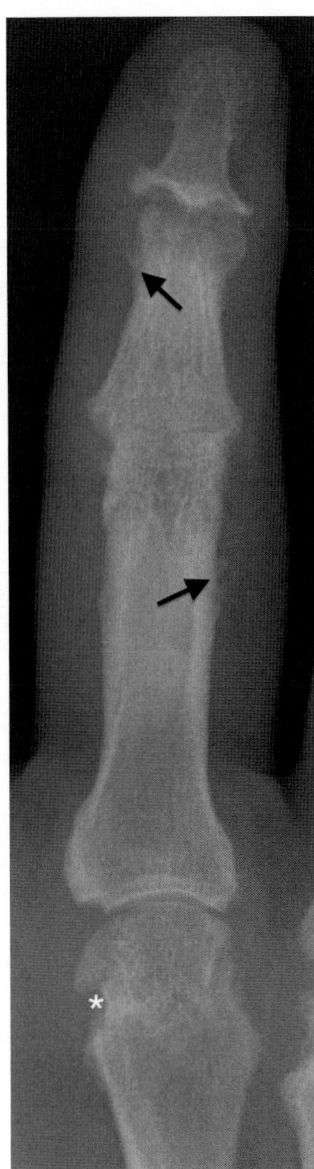

FIGURE 51-1 ■ **Diffuse soft-tissue swelling in the 'sausage' finger of a patient with sero-negative arthritis.** An erosion with bone proliferation (*) and periosteal new bone formation (arrows) is also present.

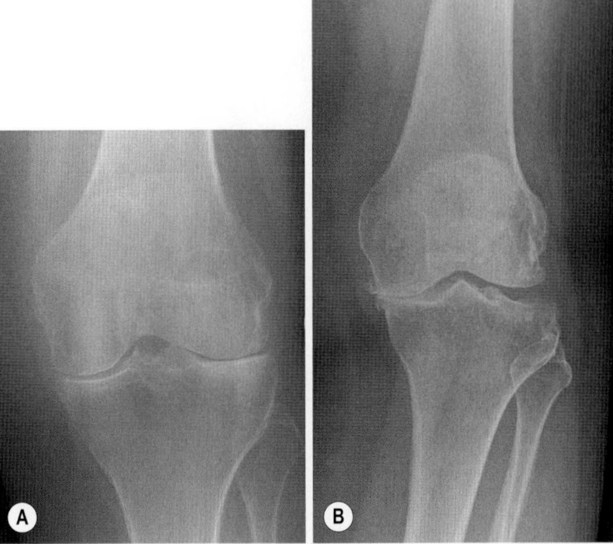

FIGURE 51-2 ■ (A) Rheumatoid arthritis. There is diffuse symmetrical panarticular joint space loss typical for inflammatory arthritis. (B) Osteoarthritis. Joint space loss is confined to the medial compartment; such asymmetrical joint space loss is typical for osteoarthritis. Note also the osteophytes in the medial joint line and subchondral sclerosis in the medial compartment.

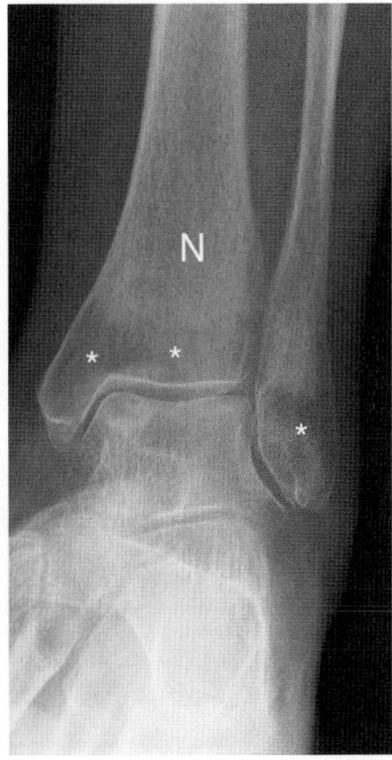

FIGURE 51-3 ■ **AP ankle radiograph demonstrating periarticular osteopenia (*); the distal tibial metaphysis demonstrates normal bone density (N).**

whereas sero-negative erosions typically show proliferative bone formation in or around the erosion (Fig. 51-4B), a useful distinguishing feature. Gout erosions have characteristic overhanging sharply demarcated margins giving them a punched-out appearance (Fig. 51-4C).

Entheseal Disease. Enthesitis is a feature of the sero-negative arthritides. Entheses represent the bony attachment sites of ligaments, tendons or capsule. On radiographs the important bone changes that can be visualised in enthesitis are enthesophyte formation and erosion (Fig. 51-5). Enthesophytes develop at, or immediately adjacent to, the site of an enthesis. They generally have a coarse appearance, with both cortical and medullary bone involved.

Bone Alignment

Joint malalignment is a feature of many arthropathic processes and results from a variety of causes, including tendon or ligament dysfunction and cartilage or bone loss. In most case this represents late changes of arthropathy though joint malalignment can be seen in several conditions without established bone or soft-tissue

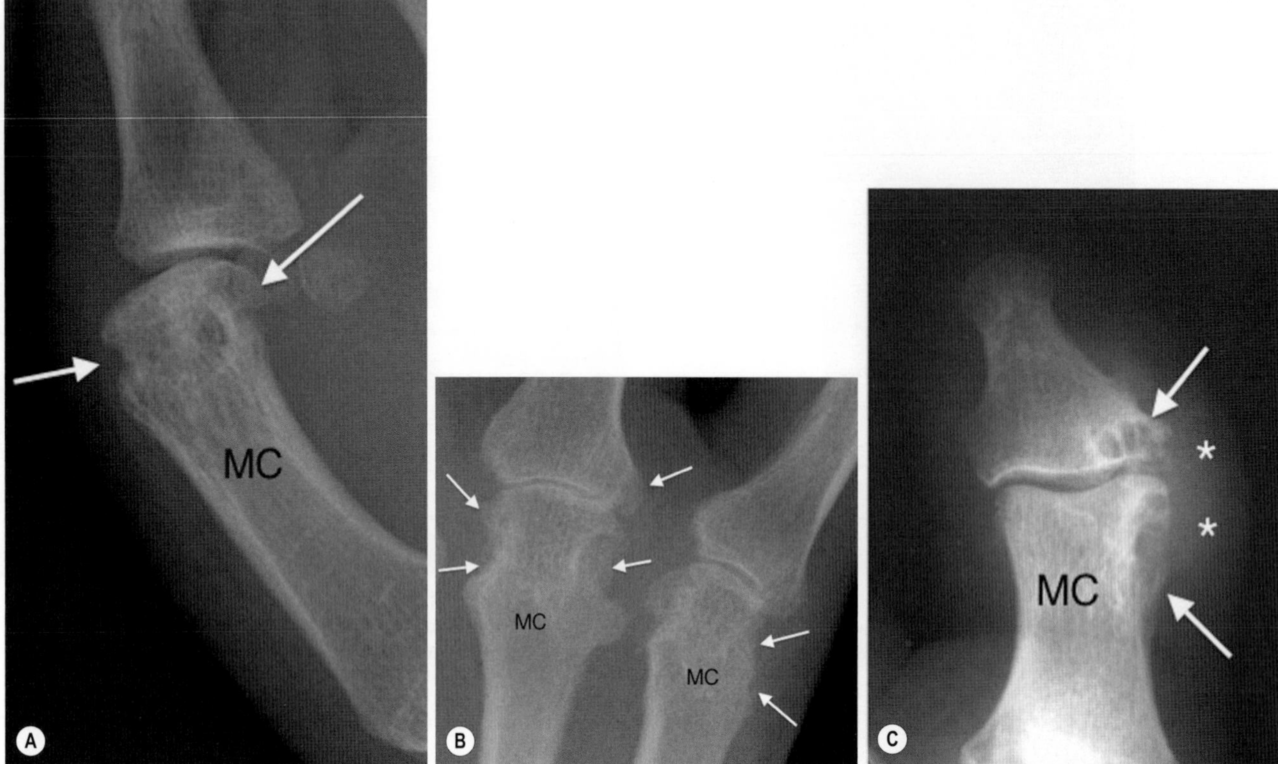

FIGURE 51-4 ■ (A) Rheumatoid arthritis. The metacarpal head (MC) marginal erosions are characteristic of rheumatoid arthritis. There is cortical loss without any associated new bone formation (arrows). (B) Sero-negative arthritis. Again, erosions are seen in the metacarpal head, but in addition to the bone destruction there is associated new bone formation typical for sero-negative arthritis (arrows). (C) Gout. There is asymmetrical dense soft-tissue swelling (*) and well-defined, punched-out periarticular erosion with overhanging margins (arrows).

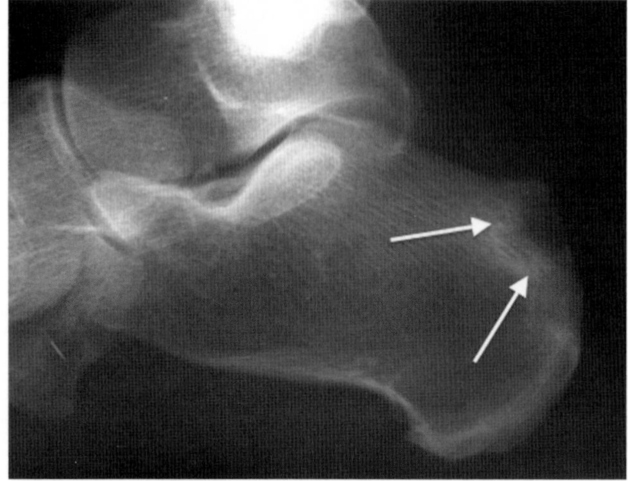

FIGURE 51-5 ■ **Entheseal erosion at the Achilles insertion in sero-negative disease.** There is cortical loss, with reactive new bone formation and sclerosis around the erosion (arrows).

arthropathy. The best known of these is systemic lupus erythematosus (SLE) where subluxations and ulnar deviation of the fingers and toes are seen in patients without bone erosion or cartilage loss (Fig. 51-6).

Distribution of Joint Involvement

An important aid to diagnosis is the distribution of polyarthritic disease when involving the hand and wrist. Symmetrical proximal disease involving the carpal bones and metacarpophalangeal (MCP) joints is typical in rheumatoid arthritis. Distal disease of the interphalangeal joints is characteristic of sero-negative disease and osteoarthritis.

OSTEOARTHRITIS

Osteoarthritis (OA) is a ubiquitous disease and the most common articular disease. It affects the majority of the population at some time and is seen in other vertebrates.

Unsurprisingly, considerable research continues to be centred on understanding the pathogenesis of this condition and developing new ways to treat it. However, it is becoming clear that the disease has a complex aetiology which includes genetic and mechanical factors.[1] Fundamentally, the condition results from an alteration in the normal transmission of forces across a joint. This may occur due to an abnormality in the quality of the tissues at the joint, for instance ligamentous laxity as a result of a connective tissue disorder such as Ehlers–Danlos syndrome, or a change in the biomechanics at the joint such as might arise following trauma. However, it is recognised that there are strong influences on the aetiology of osteoarthritis that occur at a personal level such as genetics, race and ethnicity, diet, obesity, age and gender. It will be appreciated that some of these, such as obesity, will also act to alter joint biomechanics, but in general the understanding of how these and particularly

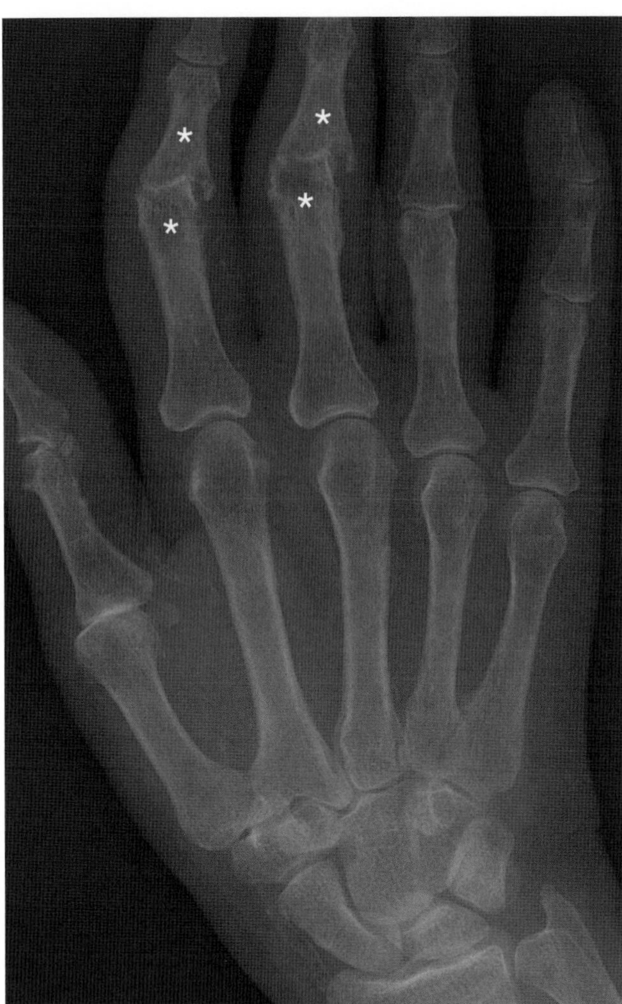

FIGURE 51-6 ■ SLE arthropathy with subluxation and malalignment of the PIP joint of the index and middle finger (*) without erosive change.

genotypes affect the joint structures to bring about osteoarthritis remains unclear and is an important field for research.

The term primary generalised osteoarthritis is used to refer to osteoarthritis occurring without an apparent underlying cause. Secondary osteoarthritis refers to cases where an underlying cause is identified. A wide range of secondary causes exists, but characteristically they tend to result in either altered structure in the constituent parts of the joint, altered loading across the joint or a combination of both (Table 51-1).

Primary Osteoarthritis

Primary osteoarthritis is more common in women than men and has a strong genetic predisposition. It occurs in a typical distribution, characteristically affecting the hands, thumb bases, the hips, knees and first metatarsophalangeal joint in the foot.

Secondary Osteoarthritis

Many conditions, including trauma, may result in secondary osteoarthritis (Table 51-1). In many cases the cause is not identified. Only a single joint may be involved (for instance, when trauma has occurred), or in generalised conditions there may be multiple joint involvement. The radiological findings are identical to those of primary osteoarthritis.

TABLE 51-1 Secondary Causes of Osteoarthritis

Trauma
• Acute
• Chronic repetitive
Systemic metabolic
• Hemochromatosis
• Wilson's disease
• Ochronosis
Endocrine
• Acromegaly
• Hypothyroidism
• Hyperparathyroidism
• Diabetes mellitus
Crystal deposition diseases
• CPPD
• Gout
Other
• Rheumatoid arthritis
• Paget's disease
• Bone/joint dysplasias

Radiographic Findings

Typically, the changes of osteoarthritis seen at the joint represent a combination of destruction and repair, although the balance between these two processes varies.

1. Joint space loss: in common with other arthropathic processes, cartilage thinning is a feature of osteoarthritis, which is seen directly on MRI and identified on conventional radiographs as joint space narrowing. In osteoarthritis, cartilage loss occurs in a more asymmetric distribution across the joint, generally occurring in areas of stress (Figs. 51-2B and 51-7). This results in an uneven pattern of joint space loss, a useful distinguishing feature from other causes of arthropathy.
2. Osteophyte formation: osteophytes are an important diagnostic feature for osteoarthritis, representing the hypertrophic aspect of the disease. They represent new bone formation, generally at the joint margins, although subchondral osteophyte may develop within the joint line itself. They comprise trabeculated bone and may be seen on one or both sides of the joint (Fig. 51-7).
3. Subchondral bone change: the bone deep to the cartilage shows characteristic changes in osteoarthritis. Increased osteoblastic activity brings about sclerosis, while subchondral cysts and bony collapse may also be seen (Figs. 51-7 and 51-8). Cyst formation is thought to be the result of synovial fluid passing into the bone through the damaged cartilage.
4. Loose bodies: as fragments of cartilage and bone are shed into the joint, they may be resorbed but often persist as loose bodies (Fig. 51-8). They may become revascularised and actually grow in situ.

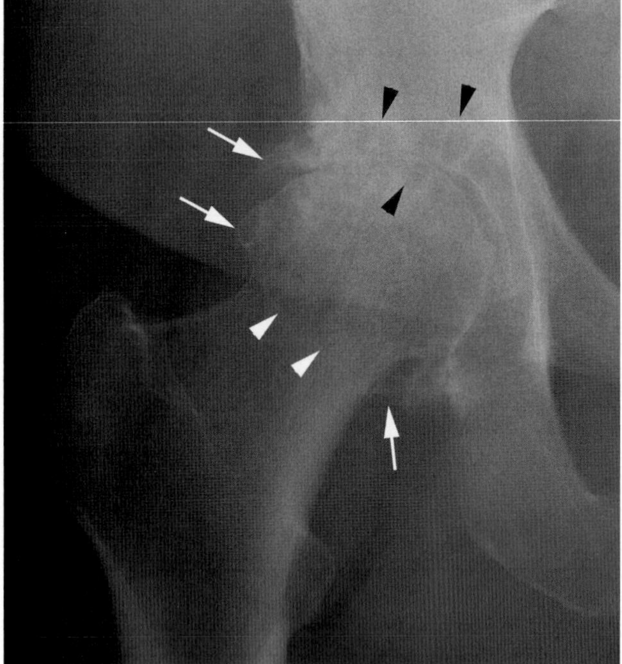

FIGURE 51-7 ■ Severe osteoarthritis of the hip. There is joint space narrowing which has occurred asymmetrically within the joint, in this case affecting the superior joint (the most common pattern of hip involvement). Note also subchondral cyst formation (black arrowheads) and osteophytosis (arrows). The osteophytes form a rim around the femoral head/neck junction and are superimposed over the neck visible as a sclerotic line (white arrowheads), which should not be mistaken for a fracture.

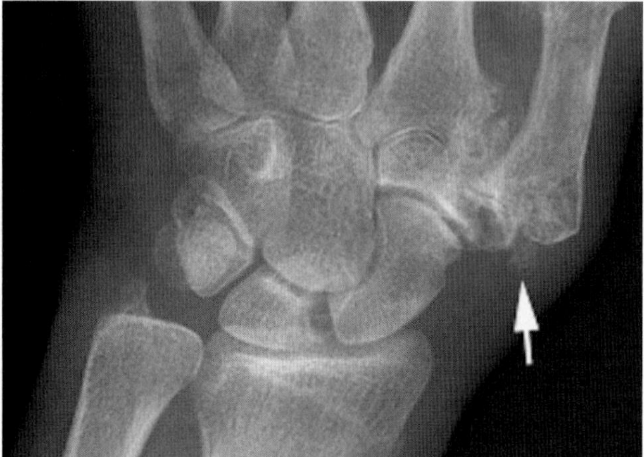

FIGURE 51-8 ■ Severe osteoarthritis affecting the thumb base. There is loss of joint space and subchondral sclerosis along with osteophyte formation affecting the thumb carpometacarpal joint. An osteochondral loose body is present (arrow) and there is joint subluxation. Early involvement of the STT joint is also seen as subchondral sclerosis.

This means it may not be possible to identify the source of a loose body.

5. Joint deformity and subluxation: the diseased joint will commonly show ligamentous laxity, allowing deformity (which may be contributed to by bony collapse and cartilage loss) and subluxation (Fig. 51-8). Further factors leading to deformity relate to reduced proprioception and reduced muscle tone in the elderly.

It has long been recognised that pain experienced by the patient is poorly related to the changes of osteoarthritis seen in a joint on conventional radiographs. One patient may be severely incapacitated, despite only minor changes being evident on the radiograph, while another patient may have very little in the way of symptoms despite radiographically severe changes of osteoarthritis. This has led to investigation of osteoarthritis with more advanced imaging techniques, particularly ultrasound and MRI, in an effort to identify likely pain generators within the osteoarthritic joint. MRI and ultrasound will demonstrate other features such as synovitis, effusion and ligamentous change in addition to the features already described. MRI also demonstrates oedema-like marrow signal in the subchondral bone. Despite this new information, the source of pain in the joint remains unclear, although some evidence suggests that it may be associated with synovitis or bone marrow abnormalities.

Radiographic Changes at Specific Joints

Knee

Osteoarthritis of the knee may show any or all the above features on conventional radiographs. As already noted, joint space loss is usually asymmetrical within a joint in osteoarthritis. The knee demonstrates this observation well as varying degrees of joint space loss are typically seen in the three compartments, often with relative preservation of a compartment despite severe joint space loss elsewhere.[2] The most commonly seen pattern of osteoarthritis involves joint space loss in the medial compartment, often leading to varus deformity (Fig. 51-2B), but on occasion patellofemoral or lateral compartment disease will predominate (Fig. 51-9). Weight-bearing radiographs are more sensitive in identifying joint space loss in the medial and lateral compartments. Semi-flexed views also increase sensitivity to the detection of joint space loss compared to views obtained in extension[3] (Fig. 51-9). 'Skyline' views of the patellofemoral joint are best suited to demonstrate the differential involvement of the medial and lateral facet.

Hip

Again, joint space loss is typically asymmetrical across the joint. The most common pattern involves the superior aspect of the joint with superior migration of the femoral head and narrowing of the superior joint space. As disease progresses, sclerosis and cyst formation may be seen along with flattening of the femoral head (Fig. 51-7). Less commonly, medial joint space loss will predominate (Fig. 51-10). This pattern of joint space loss is more common in women than men. On occasions, central osteophyte forming within the hip joint will displace the femur laterally, giving apparent preservation of joint space. Osteophytes around the femoral head/neck margin will be appreciated as areas of sclerosis on the femoral neck as the anterior and posterior osteophyte overlies the femoral neck. A particular characteristic pattern of

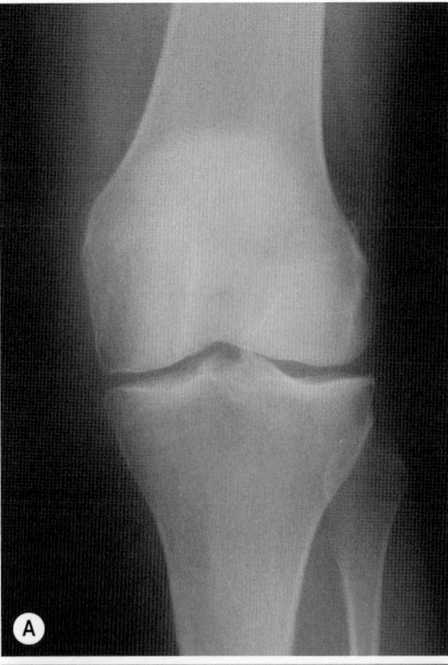

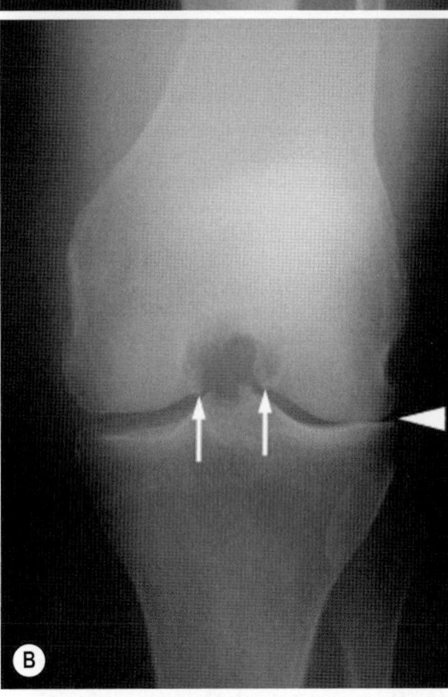

FIGURE 51-9 ■ Knee osteoarthritis showing the effect of weight-bearing on joint space narrowing. (A) Non-weight-bearing radiograph shows some subchondral bone irregularity reflecting the knee osteoarthritis, but the medial and lateral compartment joint spaces look to be relatively well preserved. (B) Radiograph with the patient standing with 30° flexion. Severe loss of lateral compartment joint space is now appreciated (arrowhead). The knee flexion also demonstrates osteophyte in the intercondylar notch (arrows).

osseous hypertrophy is seen along the femoral neck, typically on the medial side, and is known as buttressing.[4] It is appreciated as thickening of the medial femoral neck cortex (Fig. 51-10).

Hands and Wrists

Changes in the hands are characteristically associated with the development of firm nodules, which are generally the result of osteophyte formation or synovial hypertrophy. These are known as Heberden's (distal interphalangeal joint) and Bouchard's (proximal) nodes. The interphalangeal joints (proximal and distal) are typically involved in primary osteoarthritis. However, the pattern of involvement is usually asymmetrical, with different joints on the two hands affected. Metacarpophalangeal joint disease is less frequently seen. At the wrists the disease usually affects the thumb base, involving the thumb carpometacarpal joint and/or the scaphotrapeziotrapezoid (STT) joint (Fig. 51-8).

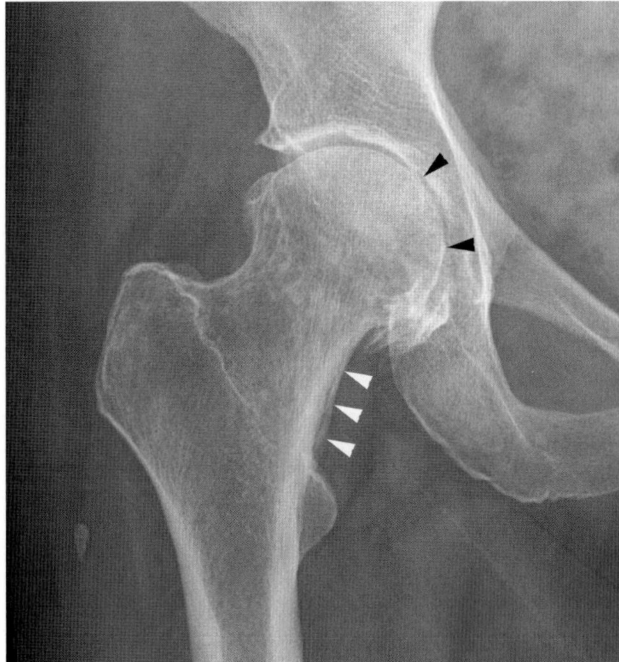

FIGURE 51-10 ■ Severe osteoarthritis of the hip. AP radiograph: In this case joint space loss is in a less common medial distribution (black arrowheads). The study also shows osseous hypertrophy along the medial neck of the femur (buttressing) (white arrowheads). Note also the marginal osteophytes which can also be seen projected over the femoral neck (cf. Fig. 51-7).

Spine

Degenerative changes, representing osteoarthritis of the spine, are also discussed elsewhere. This most commonly occurs in the cervical and lower lumbar spine where degeneration in the intervertebral disc is seen as loss of disc height. Large osteophytes may be seen arising from the vertebral bodies, along with sclerotic change in the vertebral endplates. On occasion, osteophytes will bridge the intervertebral disc space. Typical osteoarthritic change may also be seen in the facet joints where osseous hypertrophy may contribute to spinal stenosis.

Abnormalities of vertebral alignment may also occur as a result of ligamentous laxity and degenerative changes in the disc and facet joints; typically, anterior displacement of the vertebra superior to a degenerative disc is seen with respect to its more caudal neighbour. This can be distinguished from the spondylolisthesis seen in association with pars defects (spondylolysis) because the

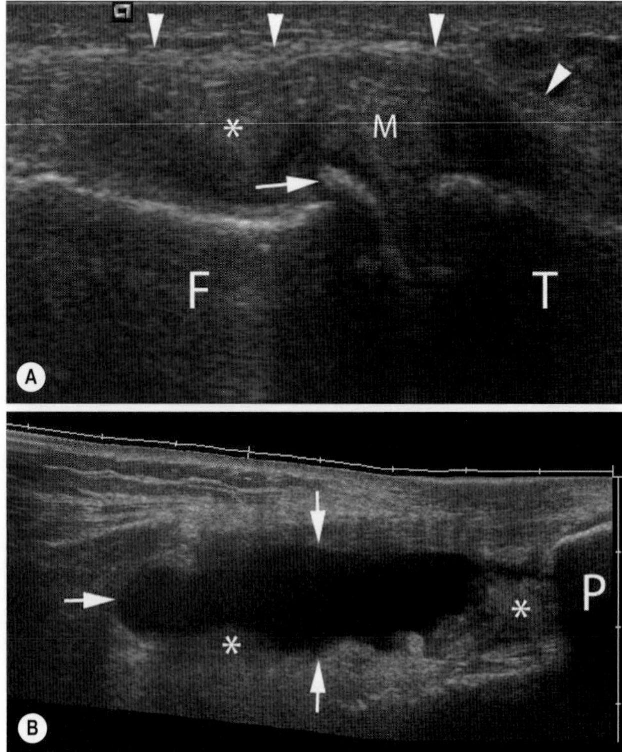

FIGURE 51-11 ■ Knee osteoarthritis. (A) Longitudinal ultrasound image of the medial knee joint. F = femur, T = tibia. There is osteophyte formation (arrow). Note the synovitis (*) surrounded by anechoic joint effusion bulging the overlying medial collateral ligament (arrowheads). The medial meniscus (M) is partially extruded from the joint line. (B) Longitudinal ultrasound image through the suprapatellar pouch. P = patella. There is an anechoic joint effusion distending the pouch (arrows) with synovitis seen along the walls (*).

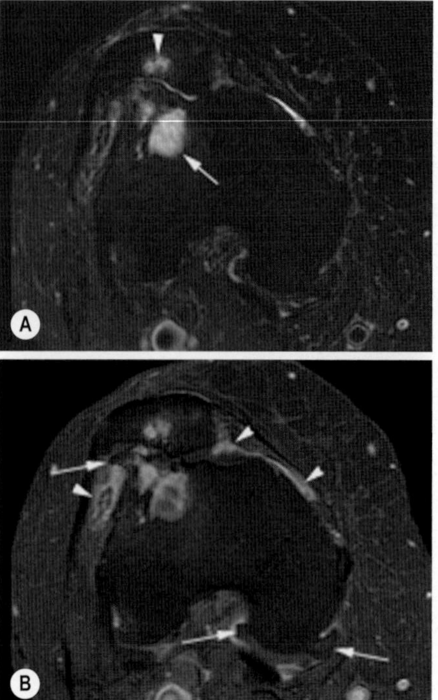

FIGURE 51-12 ■ Patellofemoral osteoarthritis. (A) T2-weighted axial fat-suppressed image. A large subchondral cyst is seen in the trochlea subchondral bone (arrow), along with a subchondral marrow lesion in the patella (arrowhead). The different nature of the two areas of subchondral signal change is difficult to appreciate on the T2-weighted image. (B) T1-weighted axial fat-suppressed image with gadolinium contrast enhancement. The cystic lesion shows enhancement of its periphery with gadolinium contrast with a low signal (cystic) centre. The contrast medium enhances the synovitis (arrowheads). Osteophytes are also appreciated (arrows).

posterior elements of the vertebral body will also slip forward along with the vertebral bodies, as there is no separation of the anterior and posterior spinal elements.

Advanced Imaging

For the most part the advanced imaging of OA remains the preserve of the research environment. However, given the ubiquitous nature of the disease it is not uncommon to identify features of OA on studies undertaken for other purposes or suspected diagnoses.

In recent years it had become recognised that OA is not just a disease of cartilage but affects multiple components of the joint. These include the synovium, ligaments, subchondral bone, articular fibrocartilage (for instance, the menisci in the knee and TFC in the wrist) and the periarticular tendons.

Both MRI and ultrasound readily identify synovitis in OA and this can be marked in osteoarthritis (Figs. 51-11 and 51-12). Osteophytes are also demonstrated by both techniques, ultrasound having been shown to be more sensitive to their detection in the wrist than conventional radiography.[5] While ultrasound is unable to demonstrate the changes in the subchondral bone, MRI will show cystic change and sclerosis but in addition may show oedema-like signal (Fig. 51-12). Research studies suggest this is not due to true oedema within the bone marrow, and thus the term 'bone marrow lesion' is increasingly used in this context.

Erosive (Inflammatory) Osteoarthritis

Erosive osteoarthritis represents a subset of osteoarthritis with more inflammatory and destructive changes. It is usually seen as a polyarthritis classically involving the distal and proximal interphalangeal joints in the hands, although large joint involvement has been described. It is more common in women and has been shown to have a worse outcome than non-erosive OA.[6] While clinical clues may exist as to the inflammatory pattern of disease, the distinction from non-erosive OA is made on the radiographic appearances and the demonstration of erosions. Controversy still exists as to whether this condition represents a separate subgroup of patients with osteoarthritis or represents one end of a spectrum of increasing inflammatory change in osteoarthritis.

The pattern of erosion seen in erosive osteoarthritis is characteristically described as being central in location (occurring in the subchondral bone) and gives rise to the characteristic 'seagull wing' pattern of erosion[7]

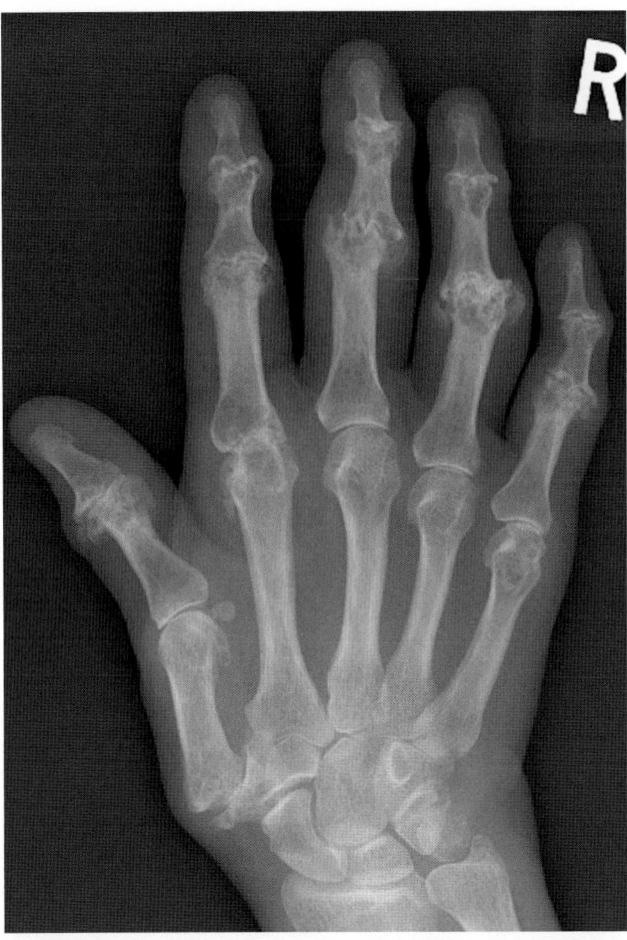

FIGURE 51-13 ■ **Erosive osteoarthritis.** DP radiograph: in addition to the typical osteoarthritis changes seen in multiple joints, including the thumb base carpometacarpal joint, there is erosive change seen at many of the interphalangeal joints. The majority of these are central in location (subchondral) and give rise to the characteristic 'seagull wing' appearance of the distal articular surface (seen for example at the index, middle and ring distal interphalangeal joints).

(Fig. 51-13). Marginal erosions may also be seen but appear to be much less common. Reparative change may occur and can lead to bony ankylosis, not a typical feature of non-erosive OA.[8]

THE INFLAMMATORY ARTHRITIDES

The inflammatory arthritides are characterised by multiple joint involvement with inflammatory change either within the joint, the enthesis or periarticular soft tissues. The management of inflammatory arthritis has changed dramatically in recent years with the advent of powerful biological therapies that, if instigated early, can induce disease remission and prevent the severe joint destruction previously seen. This has led to a greater emphasis on early diagnosis. While CR shows characteristic features of inflammatory arthritis, these represent late findings in the disease process and the use of advanced imaging techniques such as magnetic resonance or ultrasound is becoming more common. These allow early diagnosis and treatment before irreversible joint damage has occurred. Nevertheless, radiography continues to play an important role in the diagnosis and characterisation of inflammatory arthritis and usually forms the initial imaging study.

Rheumatoid Arthritis

Rheumatoid arthritis (RA) is a chronic multisystem autoimmune disorder of unknown aetiology. In Europe it has an incidence of approximately 1%. It is more common in women and is characterised initially by a polyarticular symmetrical synovitis.[9] The later stages of the disease involve joint destruction as a result of bone erosion and cartilage loss. Synovitis is considered to be a strong predictor of bone erosion.[10,11] The hands and wrists are most commonly involved although any synovial joint in the body can be affected. Soft-tissue involvement is seen with the development of tenosynovitis and rheumatoid nodules, which can precede joint changes.

The clinical, and consequently radiological, picture of RA has changed over recent years due to dramatic advances in the way RA is treated. The use of powerful biological agents early in the disease process to arrest joint damage and induce disease remission has resulted in a change in the radiographic assessment of RA, with the detection of early or subtle change increasingly important.[12]

Radiographic Features

The classical plain film appearance of RA is of a symmetrical polyarthritis of the hands and wrists with a proximal distribution typically involving the carpal, MCP and proximal interphalangeal (PIP) joints. Characteristically the distal interphalangeal (DIP) joints are spared, providing an important distinguishing feature from OA and psoriatic arthritis.

The earliest plain film changes are soft-tissue swelling and periarticular osteopenia. At the MCP and PIP joints the soft-tissue swelling is appreciated as spindle-shaped thickening of the soft tissues developing symmetrically about the joint. Periarticular osteopenia can be a difficult radiographic sign to evaluate, particularly when there is symmetrical polyarticular involvement. Joint space loss in RA is usually panarticular, with diffuse joint space loss. Marginal erosions are characteristic of rheumatoid arthritis, and are seen most frequently in the joints of the hands, wrists and feet, erosions being more commonly seen in small joints than large joints. The earliest sites of erosion are typically the radial aspect of the index and middle metacarpal heads and the ulnar aspect of the wrist (Fig. 51-14). Cortical bone loss is first seen as subtle breaks in the bone giving the cortex a 'dot-dash' appearance; subsequently, frank bone erosion is seen (Fig. 51-4A). A form of the disease featuring large cystic areas, typically occurring in active men, has been termed robust rheumatoid and is thought to occur as a result of continued physical activity despite active inflammatory arthropathy.[13]

Ankylosis may occur in the later stages of the disease. Typically this involves the wrist with intercarpal and carpometacarpal fusions.

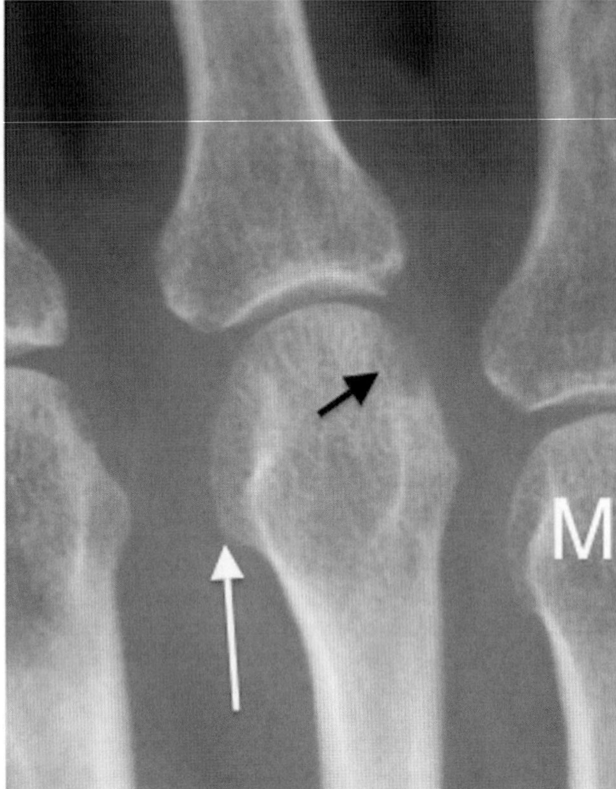

FIGURE 51-14 ■ Rheumatoid arthritis with the earliest feature of erosive change seen along the radial border of this middle metacarpal head. There is localised osteopenia with a 'dot-dash' pattern of deossification (white arrow). Note also the symmetrical soft-tissue swelling and frank erosion of the ulna border (black arrow).

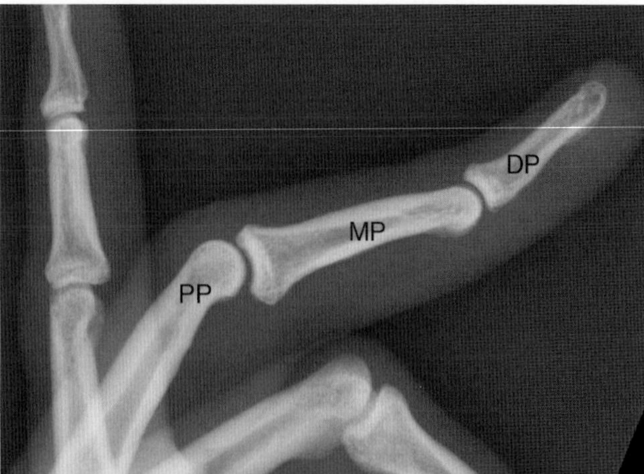

FIGURE 51-15 ■ Boutonnière deformity of the finger with hyperextension of the DIP joint and flexion of the PIP joint. PP, proximal phalanx; MP, middle phalanx; DP, distal phalanx.

Tendon and ligamentous dysfunction along with bone erosion results in deformity and malalignment in the later stages of the disease. Ulnar deviation of the fingers and the radial deviation of the wrist giving a 'zigzag' deformity to the hand is also typical for RA.[14] In the fingers, deformity involving flexion of the PIP joint and extension of the DIP joint (Boutonnière) (Fig. 51-15) or flexion of the DIP joint and extension of the PIP joint (swan neck) are common.

Subcutaneous rheumatoid nodules over the extensor surfaces of joints and in tendons are a common feature of RA seen in around 20% of patients.

Radiographs in Treated Inflammatory Disease

Preservation of bone density may be seen with successfully treated rheumatoid arthritis. In cases where irreversible joint damage has occurred, secondary osteoarthritic change can develop. It is important to recognise this when present, as it can lead to persisting symptoms and inappropriate continuation of biological therapy. The proximal distribution of these secondary osteoarthritic changes and the superimposition of proliferative bone changes on rheumatoid erosions are the key observations in making this diagnosis (Fig. 51-16).

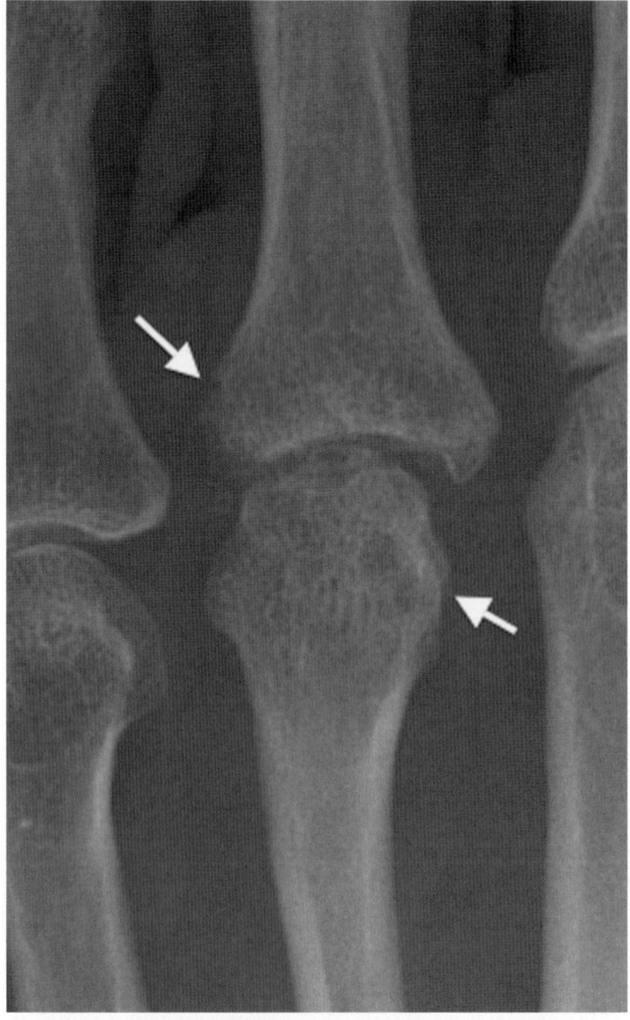

FIGURE 51-16 ■ Rheumatoid arthritis and secondary osteoarthritis. There is rheumatoid erosion and joint space loss with superadded sclerosis and proliferative new bone formation (arrows) indicating the development of secondary OA.

Sero-Negative Arthritis

The sero-negative arthropathies comprise a group of interrelated inflammatory arthritides sharing common features. Chief among these is the characteristic involvement of the entheses with inflammation classically seen at the bony insertions of tendons and ligaments. Other important features are:

- An absence of rheumatoid factors.
- A strong association with the HLA-B27 histocompatibility antigen (although it is important to realise this is not necessary for the development of these diseases, or required for the diagnosis).
- A tendency for axial skeletal involvement (spondyloarthritis).

Four main conditions are considered under this heading: ankylosing spondylitis, psoriatic arthritis, reactive arthritis (formally known as Reiter's disease) and enteropathic spondyloarthritis.

Ankylosing Spondylitis

Ankylosing spondylitis (AS) is a multisystem inflammatory spondyloarthopathy primarily affecting the axial skeleton. It is most common in HLA-B27-positive adolescents and young adults, who present with inflammatory back pain. Sacroiliitis and enthesitis of the axial skeleton is the hallmark of AS. Peripheral joint involvement is seen in up to 30% of patients.[15]

Sacroiliitis. Sacroiliac disease in AS is usually bilateral and symmetrical, with conventional radiographs and CT showing erosive change and subchondral sclerosis progressing if untreated to ankylosis. However, these represent later changes and the earliest feature of sacroiliitis is detected with MRI as subchondral bone marrow oedema. In the past skeletal scintigraphy had a role in the early detection of sacroiliitis but it is generally accepted MRI has greater sensitivity and specificity than CR, scintigraphy and CT (Fig. 51-17).

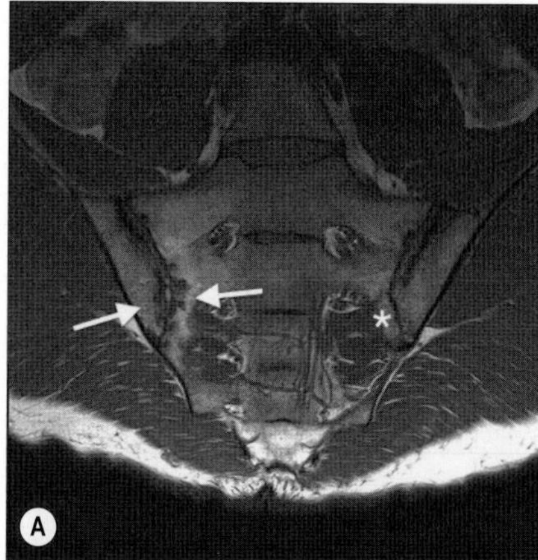

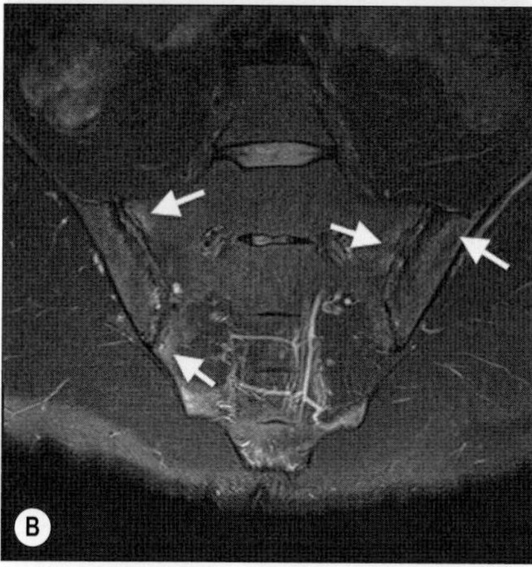

FIGURE 51-17 ■ T1-weighted (A) and T2 fat-supressed (B) coronal MR images of the sacroiliac joints (SIJ) in ankylosing spondylitis. The T1-weighted image readily demonstrates erosion (arrows) in the right SIJ with joint space loss on the left (*), all indicative of damage. Note how poor the T2-weighted image is at demonstrating erosion; however, it shows subchondral oedema (arrows) more reflective of disease activity.

Spinal Disease. Spinal involvement is frequent, with changes seen around the discovertebral unit, costovertebral joints and in the posterior elements of the spine. Occasionally it may precede sacroiliac joint involvement. The changes seen represent enthesitis. Around the discovertebral unit inflammatory change is first seen at the insertion of the peripheral fibres of the annulus fibrosus, Sharpey's fibres. The earliest CR changes of spine disease are seen as sclerosis at these insertion points, identified on the lateral view as sclerotic 'shiny' corners to the vertebral bodies, known as Romanus lesions. Erosive change at these sites is harder to detect radiographically but, along with ossification in the anterior longitudinal ligament, contributes to a characteristic squared appearance to the vertebral bodies (Fig. 51-18).

The MRI equivalent of the Romanus lesions is bone oedema in the corners of vertebral bodies and this will be detected before the sclerosis becomes apparent on CR. Entheseal bone and soft-tissue oedema may also be found on MRI at other sites in the spine before CR changes are found, such as in association with the spinous processes, facet joints and costovertebral joints. With time, erosive change may also become apparent on MRI.

Bone marrow oedema in the corners of vertebrae can also be seen in degenerative disease; AS-related oedema is normally greater in craniocaudal size than transverse diameter and is not usually associated with disc dehydration or loss of disc height.

Proliferative new bone formation occurs later in the disease and can be imaged with CT and radiography. Syndesmophytes, seen initially as thin bone outgrowths, develop typically at the site of Romanus lesions. As is the case with the inflammatory MR changes, they characteristically have a vertical orientation. These are useful features distinguishing them from osteophytes or the more coarse syndesmophytes of psoriatic and reactive arthritis.

If the condition is untreated, progression to fusion is typical, affecting the facet joints as well as the anterior vertebral bodies. The classical spine radiograph is that of the bamboo spine with complete fusion of the vertebral bodies and sacroiliac joints. Fusion between the spinous processes may also be seen. Fusion of the posterior elements of the spine can occur before fusion of the

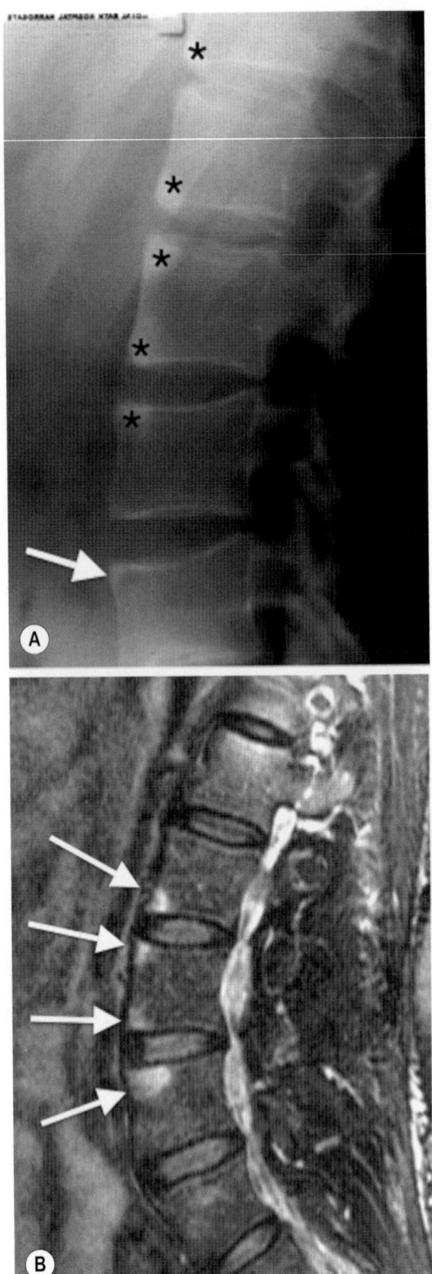

FIGURE 51-18 ■ (A) Ankylosing spondylitis (AS) with sclerosis of the vertebral corners (Romanus lesions). The radiograph shows advanced lesions (*) and an early lesion (arrow). (B) STIR sagittal MR image of a different AS patient with oedema of the vertebral corners (arrows) termed MR Romanus lesions.

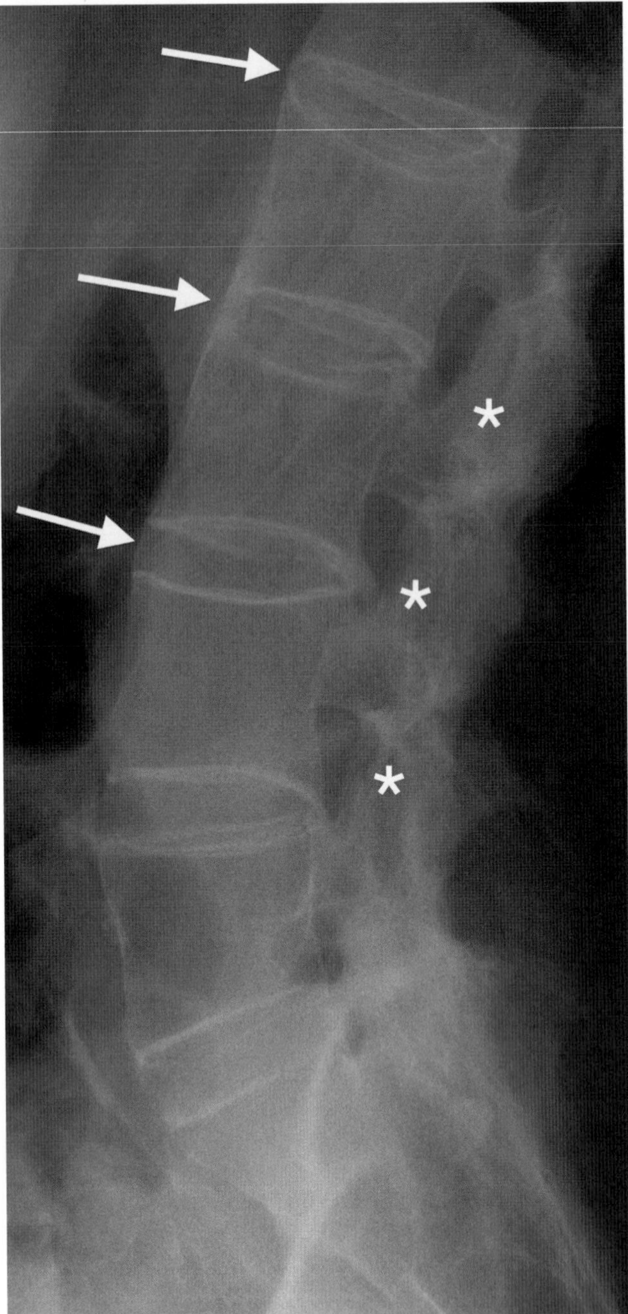

FIGURE 51-19 ■ Ankylosing spondylitis with bamboo spine. Bridging vertical syndesmophytes are seen around the intervertebral discs (arrows). Note no facet joint spaces are visualised, indicating fusion of the posterior joints between L3 and S1 (*).

vertebral bodies and can be difficult to appreciate on plain radiographs (Fig. 51-19).

Spinal fracture is relatively common in AS, despite appearances of sclerosis patients are generally osteopenic and the rigid spine is particularly prone to injury. A transverse fracture through a fused section of spine is highly unstable and is frequently a catastrophic event (Fig. 51-20).

In a largely fused spine, movement may only occur at certain unfused levels. The inflammatory Andersson's lesion may develop where movement occurs and the irregularity and sclerosis present around can be mistaken for infection by the unwary.

Peripheral Joint Involvement. The hip joint is the second most common joint involved after the sacroiliac joint.[16] Patients develop a cuff of entheseal new bone around the femoral head leading to a somewhat flattened appearance to the femoral head that can be misinterpreted as the cam deformity seen in femoroacetabular

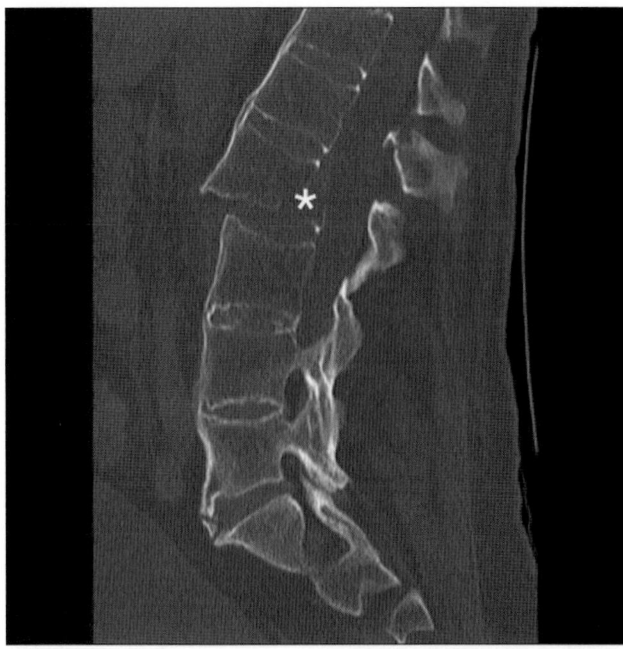

FIGURE 51-20 ■ Spine fracture in ankylosing spondylitis. Sagittal CT reconstruction shows spinal fusion and osteopenia. There is an unstable fracture of the L2 vertebral body (*) with anterior displacement of L2 on L3.

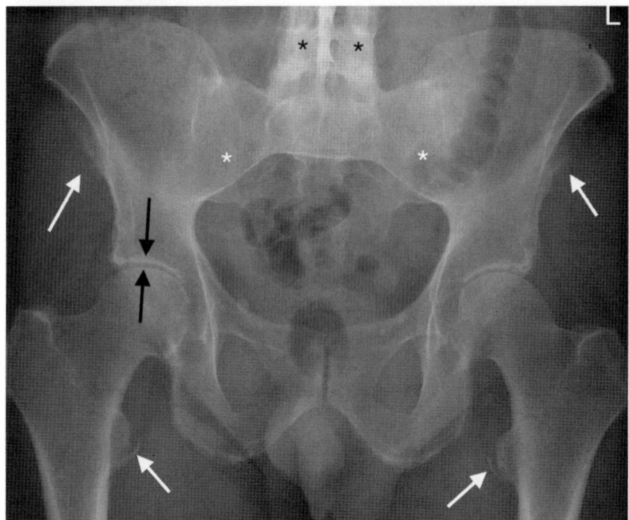

FIGURE 51-21 ■ Patient with ankylosing spondylitis with spinal fusion (black *) and SIJ fusion (white *). There is hip arthropathy with diffuse loss of joint space (black arrows) and flattened configuration of the femoral heads. Widespread entheseal new bone formation is noted around the pelvis (white arrows).

impingement. Joint space loss is diffuse with preservation of bone density. Entheseal new bone is not a prominent feature of AS hip disease per se but is often present in the adjacent hamstring and other pelvic ring entheses (Fig. 51-21).

The shoulder is involved in up to 30% of patients, again showing panarticular joint space loss with preservation of bone density. The entheses of the shoulder are

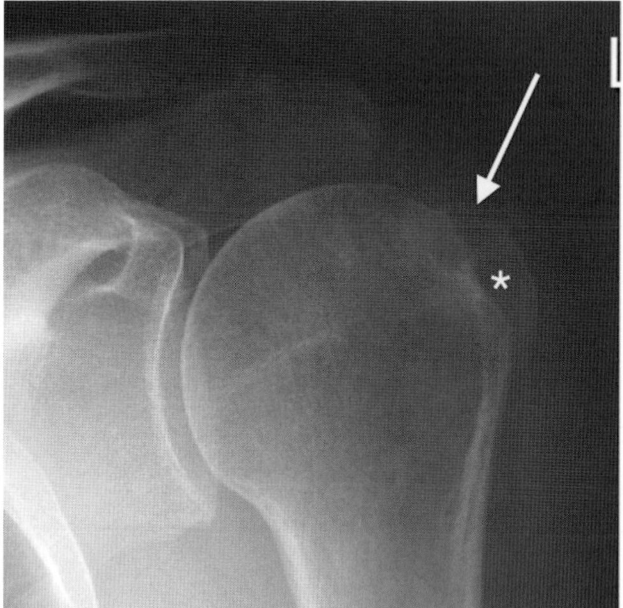

FIGURE 51-22 ■ Patient with ankylosing spondylitis shoulder disease. There is erosion of the rotator cuff insertion on the greater tuberosity (arrow) associated with surrounding proliferative new bone formation (*).

large and readily visualised radiographically. Erosion of the greater tuberosity at the insertion of the rotator cuff with proliferative new bone formation is a common radiographic feature of shoulder disease in AS (Fig. 51-22).

The hands and feet are involved in 15% of patients with AS, who typically present with diffuse swelling of the finger (dactylitis) and characteristic appearances of preserved bone density, proliferative new bone formation entheseal and peripheral joint erosion.

Psoriatic Arthritis

The link between psoriasis and arthritis is complex. Patients with inflammatory arthritis have an increased incidence of psoriasis and vice versa, but there is also an increased incidence of rheumatoid arthritis in psoriatic patients. If sero-positive rheumatoid patients are not included, the link between psoriasis and inflammatory arthritis is strengthened, with 20% of patients with sero-negative inflammatory arthritis having psoriasis.[17]

Five clinical subgroups of psoriatic arthritis (PsA) are recognised:

- Asymmetrical distal interphalangeal arthritis often associated with dactylitis.
- Arthritis mutilans, a severe destructive arthropathy mainly involving the small joints of the hands and feet.
- A pattern of arthritis indistinguishable from RA, which usually has a more benign course.
- Oligoarthritis distributed asymmetrically and involving any synovial joint.
- A pattern of spinal and large joint disease similar to ankylosing spondylitis.

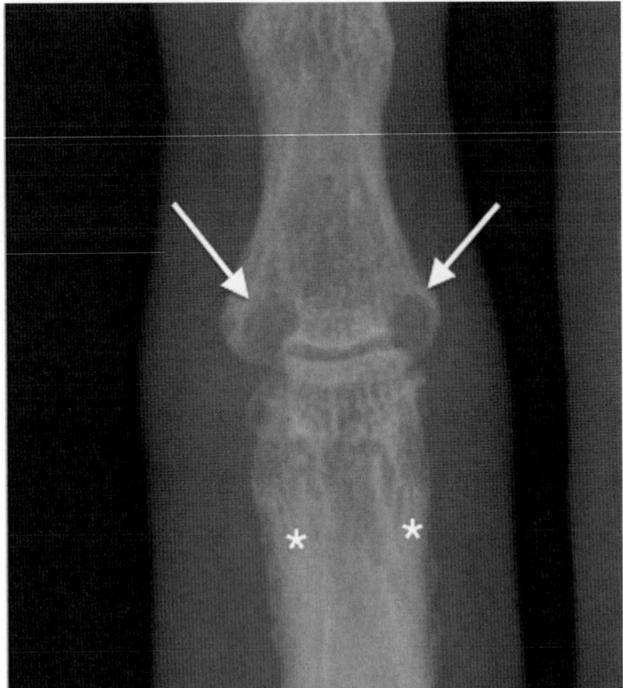

FIGURE 51-23 ■ Psoriatic arthritis. There is erosion of the distal phalanx (arrows) with prominent fluffy enthesophyte formation seen both proximal and distal to the distal interphalangeal joint (*).

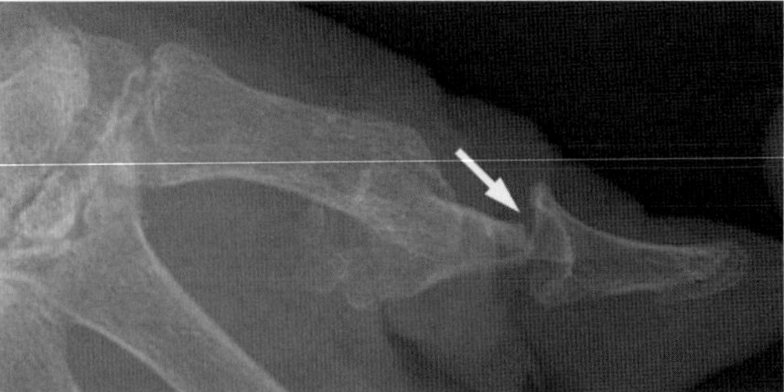

FIGURE 51-24 ■ Psoriatic arthritis. There is a severe deforming arthritis of the thumb and the 'pencil in cup' pattern of erosive change is appreciated at the interphalangeal joint (arrow).

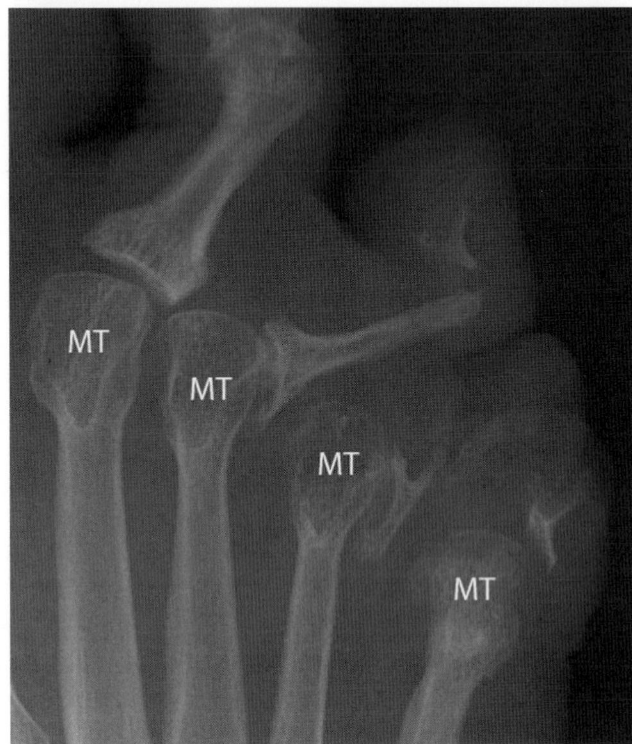

FIGURE 51-25 ■ Psoriatic arthritis. There is arthritis mutilans present with subluxation and erosion of the metacarpophalangeal joints and marked bone loss with a peg-like appearance to the phalanges. MT, metatarsal heads.

The disease classically involves enthesitis and it is suggested that inflammation in the multiple closely related entheseal sites in a digit is the cause of dactylitis.[18] The presence of nail dystrophy among psoriasis sufferers is a significant risk factor for the development of psoriatic arthritis.

Joints of the Hands and Feet. Soft-tissue joint swelling is seen as an early but non-specific radiographic feature of psoriatic arthritis. Global swelling of a digit in the form of dactylitis 'sausage digit' is typical (Fig. 51-1). Periarticular osteopenia is not a feature of psoriatic arthritis and can be useful in distinguishing it from RA. Bone erosion is seen most commonly at the joint margins and shows an entheseal pattern with new bone formation at and adjacent to the erosion site (Fig. 51-23). In the digits, erosions on the distal side of the joint classically merge together to produce a 'pencil-in-cup' appearance considered by some to be pathognomonic of the disease[19] (Fig. 51-24).

Bone loss is not limited to periarticular erosion in psoriatic arthritis and acro-osteolysis (distal tuft resorption) is a well-recognised feature. It can help distinguish psoriatic arthritis from erosive OA. Progressive osteolysis of the terminal phalanges may give them a 'peg-like' appearance, although osteolysis may progress to involve the majority of the phalanx (Fig. 51-25).

Bony ankylosis is a late feature of psoriatic arthritis and commences as a result of fibrous tissue forming within the joint; this can initially give the impression of a widened joint space.

Spinal and Large Joint Disease. Psoriatic spondylitis develops in 20% of patients with peripheral PsA. The clinical presentation is very similar to AS with inflammatory changes developing in the sacroiliac joints and at enthesis sites in the spine. In contrast to AS, psoriatic spondylitis typically shows asymmetrical involvement of sacroiliac joints and spinal syndesmophytes are coarse and more horizontal in orientation. They are also more asymmetrically distributed about the spine (Fig. 51-26). In contrast to AS, costovertebral disease is rare in PsA.

In large joints entheseal disease is less well visualised radiographically. The commonest presentation is one of

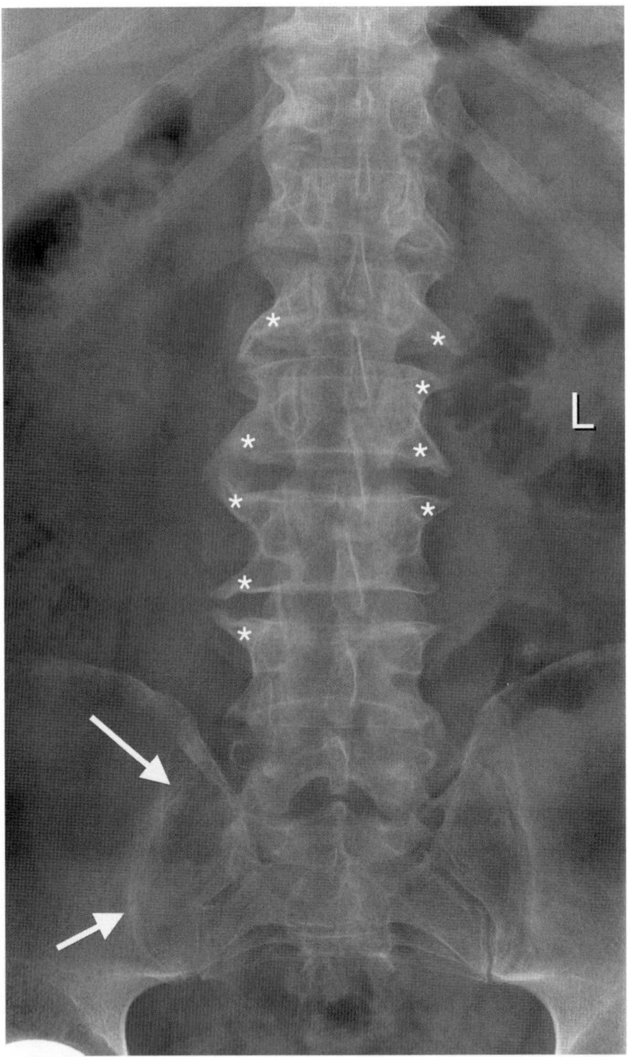

FIGURE 51-26 ■ **Psoriatic arthritis spinal involvement.** There is asymmetric sacroiliitis with loss of joint space (arrows). There are spinal enthesophytes (*), which are more horizontally orientated than those seen in ankylosing spondylitis.

mild large joint oligoarthritis characterised by low-grade diffuse synovitis and recurrent effusions.

Reactive Arthritis

Reactive arthritis is a sterile inflammatory arthritis precipitated by extra-articular infection. It results from a combination of host susceptibility and an environmental trigger and affects a wide variety of joints. It usually occurs 2 to 4 weeks after infection, with gastrointestinal and genitourinary infection the most common triggers. Classically, reactive arthritis involves the small and large joints of the lower limb, with upper limb involvement unusual. As with psoriatic arthritis, joint involvement tends to the asymmetrical. The changes seen in the feet are similar to those seen in psoriatic arthritis, with soft-tissue swelling, joint space narrowing, proliferative marginal erosions and entheseal new bone formation. There may also be sesamoid enlargement as a result of the periostitis. New bone formation at the entheses of the feet is a prominent feature (Fig. 51-27).

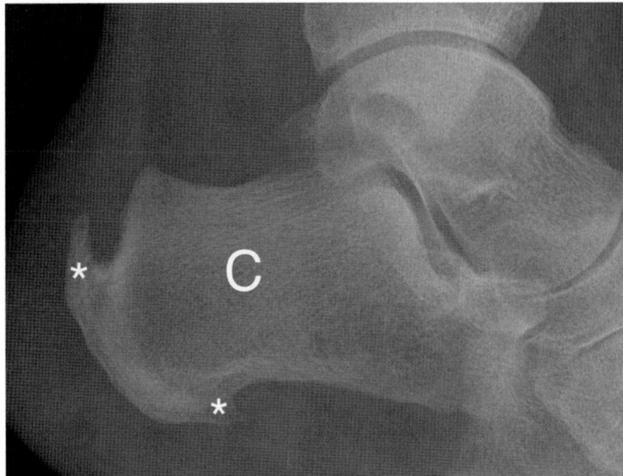

FIGURE 51-27 ■ **Reactive arthritis with prominent new bone formation at the calcaneal entheses (*).** C, calcaneus.

Enteropathy-Associated Arthritis

Arthritis associated with inflammatory bowel disease is very similar to that seen in AS. While axial involvement predominates, 15 to 20% of patients with inflammatory bowel disease exhibit a peripheral arthritis, more frequently seen with Crohn's disease than ulcerative colitis.[20] The sacroiliac involvement is that of relatively asymmetrical involvement with bone oedema progressing to erosion, joint space loss to joint fusion. Peripheral joint involvement commonly involves the wrists, knees, ankles and elbows, with patients presenting with a transient arthritis characterised by effusion and diffuse synovitis. This is frequently asymmetric and occurrences tend to parallel the inflammatory bowel disease activity. The arthritis is characteristically non-destructive and while CR may show soft-tissue swelling and periarticular osteopenia, erosions and joint space loss are unusual.

The Crystal Arthritides

The crystal arthropathies all involve crystal deposition, either in or adjacent to an affected joint. This is a heterogeneous group of diseases resulting in a variety of radiographic findings. Common crystals implicated are monosodium urate (producing gout), calcium pyrophosphate dihydrate and hydroxyapatite.

Gout

Gout is a potentially destructive inflammatory disorder occurring in the setting of hyperuricaemia. Urate crystals are deposited into the soft tissues or joint where they can produce either an acute neutrophil-mediated inflammatory reaction or a more chronic macrophage-mediated response. The variation in response is the result of differing crystal sizes, with larger crystals failing to cause acute inflammatory reactions. Smaller proinflammatory crystals tend to be produced when there are rapid changes in a patient's serum urate levels. Asymptomatic hyperuricaemia is common, occurring in approximately 19%

of individuals in the USA and the UK. Studies show that this hyperuricaemic state can persist for decades, with studies showing only 1 in 8 of patients with urate levels between 7 and 8 mg/dL developing clinical gout over a 14-year period.[21] Factors that increase the likelihood of developing clinical gout are blood urate level > 9 mg/dL and co-morbidities such as renal failure, cardiovascular disease, obesity and diabetes. Gout is much more common in men (95%) than women, men normally developing gout in their fourth to sixth decades with female gout occurring postmenopause. Gout initially presents as an acute intermittent arthritis, but in time may progress to chronic tophaceous gout.

Acute Intermittent Gout. Acute gout presents with severe pain, erythema and swelling in the affected joint, which is usually in the lower limb. In 50% of cases this occurs in the first metatarsophalangeal joint, but the midfoot, ankle and knee are also commonly involved. In imaging terms, the patients have effusion and synovitis in the affected joint. On ultrasound, fine hyperechoic foci may be seen either within the effusion, synovium or on the cartilage surface.[22] These changes can also be seen in the tendon sheaths, especially around the hand and wrist. Frequently, aspiration to exclude infection is required, with microscopy required to confirm or refute the presence of infection and crystals. As the name suggests, the patient is asymptomatic between attacks of acute intermittent gout.

Chronic Tophaceous Gout. When affected joints are no longer pain free between attacks, the patient has developed chronic gouty arthritis. Chronic crystal deposition occurs in both the joints and soft tissues. Joint changes involve effusion, synovitis and erosion, with the small joints of the hands and feet most commonly affected. Large joint disease does occur, with a predilection for the ankle and knee. Crystal deposition within synovium and on the cartilage surface is a prominent feature seen on ultrasound, but also leads to increased effusion and synovitis density on radiographs (Fig. 51-4C). The erosions seen in chronic gout are characteristically periarticular, with a broad base and sharply demarcated overhanging sclerotic margins (Fig. 51-28).

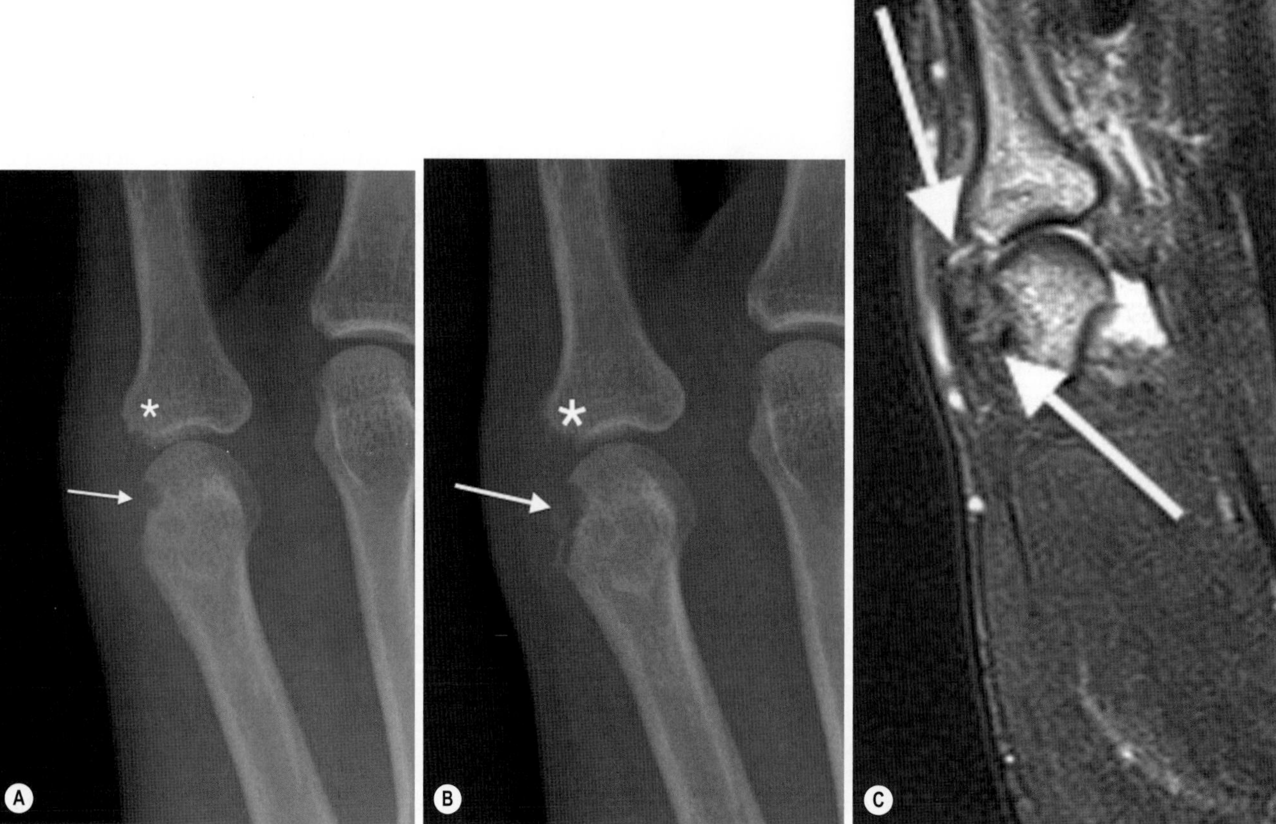

FIGURE 51-28 ■ **Gout.** There is progressive formation of a periarticular gout erosion. (A) There is asymmetrical soft-tissue swelling with cortical loss in the metacarpal head (arrow) and cortical irregularity in the adjacent phalangeal base (*). (B) With time the changes progress to a typical punched-out erosion (arrow) with erosion developing at the phalangeal base (*). (C) Coronal STIR MR. There is asymmetrical soft-tissue thickening, demonstrating characteristic heterogeneous intermediate and low signal (arrows).

Tophi, representing soft-tissue crystal deposition, are a sentinel feature of chronic gout seen as soft-tissue mass lesions occurring most commonly in the hands and wrist (ulnar aspect) and on the extensor surface of the knees and elbows. The asymmetrical soft-tissue swelling is radiographically and sonographically dense due to crystal deposition within deposits (Fig. 51-4C). Tendon crystal deposition is also common in tophaceous gout.

Calcium Pyrophosphate Dihydrate (CPPD) Crystal Deposition Disease

The nomenclature surrounding calcium pyrophosphate deposition disease is confusing and controversial.

- **Chondrocalcinosis**: the presence of cartilage calcification identified radiologically or pathologically. It can be due to a variety or combination of calcium crystals including calcium pyrophosphate dihydrate.
- **CPPD deposition disease**: a specific term indicating a disorder characterised by CPPD crystals in or around joints.
- **Pseudogout**: a clinical condition produced by acute CPPD crystals shedding into joints, resulting in acute attacks of gout-like symptoms. The diagnosis is clinical and cannot be made radiologically.
- **Pyrophosphate arthropathy**: a pattern of joint damage occurring in CPPD deposition disease resembling OA but with some distinct features. Chondrocalcinosis may or may not be present on radiographs demonstrating pyrophosphate arthropathy.

It is important to distinguish between CPPD deposition in cartilage (chondrocalcinosis) or synovium and pyrophosphate arthropathy. Chondrocalcinosis is common in older patients and occurs in association with other conditions such as haemochromatosis, osteoarthritis or Wilson's disease. Pyrophosphate arthropathy has a somewhat variable presentation with an ability to mimic other arthritides.[23] Patients with pyrophosphate arthropathy generally present with an OA-like pattern, although an acute inflammatory component may be seen. Intermittent attacks of pseudogout are said to occur in 10 to 20% of symptomatic patients.[23]

Imaging Findings. Chondrocalcinosis classically occurs in the hyaline and fibrocartilage structures of the knee and wrist but crystal deposition may also occur in virtually any joint. Synovial crystal deposition is also a common feature and is best appreciated radiographically in the suprapatellar pouch of the knee (Fig. 51-29). Chondral pyrophosphate crystals can also be seen on ultrasound examination, having virtually identical features to urate crystals but lying within rather than on the surface of the articular cartilage.[24]

Pyrophosphate Arthropathy. Pyrophosphate arthropathy most commonly shows similar changes to OA with joint space narrowing along with subchondral sclerosis and prominent cyst formation. However, the distribution of these changes is different to primary OA, with a predilection for the patellofemoral compartment in the knee and the radiocarpal compartment in the wrist. Erosion is not a feature of pyrophosphate arthropathy, though remodelling of the femoral aspect of the patellofemoral joint is well recognised (Fig. 51-29). Ligamentous dysfunction resulting in scapholunate and triquetrolunate diastasis is common.

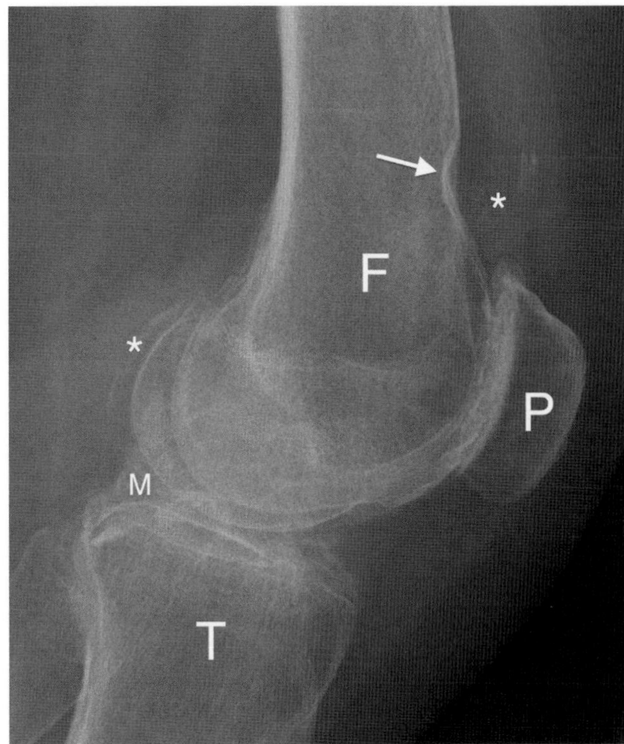

FIGURE 51-29 ■ Pyrophosphate arthropathy with loss of patellofemoral joint space and characteristic remodelling of the distal femoral metaphysis (arrow). There is synovial crystal deposition (*) and meniscal (M) chondrocalcinosis present. P, patella; F, femur; T, tibia.

Calcium Hydroxyapatite Crystal Deposition Disease

Hydroxyapatite (HA) deposition disease is a condition of unknown aetiology, which has both an acute and chronic presentation. Crystal deposition may occur both in the periarticular tissues, most commonly tendons and ligaments, or within the joint itself.[25]

Periarticular HA Deposition Disease. This occurs in both large and small joints. Deposition around large joints is commonest in the hip and shoulder, with small joint involvement most frequently seen in the hands and feet. In the shoulder and hip, HA deposition is within the tendons where is produces an increase in size of the tendon and inflammatory change in the tendon surrounding the deposit. This produces a combination of inflammatory and mechanical symptoms such as secondary external impingement of the shoulder. In small joints HA deposition is usually pericapsular or peritendinous and is associated with acute inflammatory symptoms. HA deposition disease is normally self-limiting, with the vast

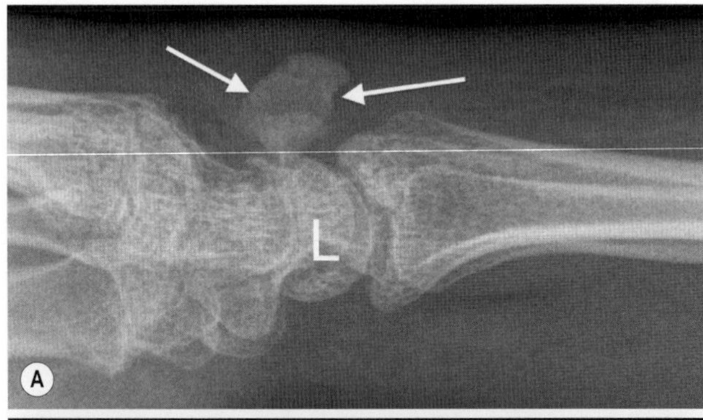

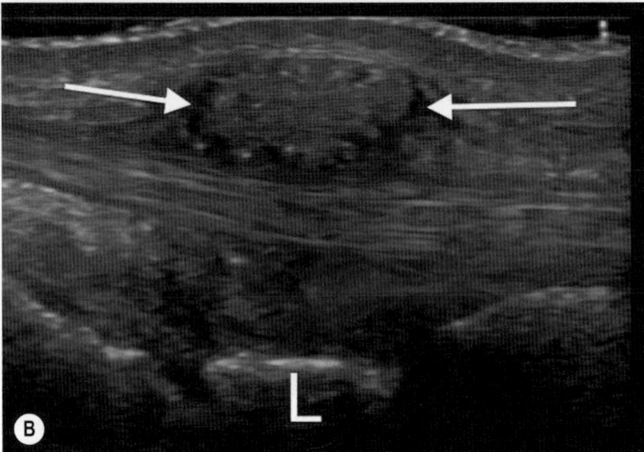

FIGURE 51-30 ■ Hydroxyapatite deposition in the wrist. The lateral wrist radiograph (A) demonstrates a large amorphous calcific deposit (arrows) with no internal architecture typical of an HA deposit. The ultrasound of the same patient (B) shows the deposit has a somewhat heterogeneous echotexture containing bright foci without acoustic shadowing (arrows). L, Lunate.

majority of patients recovering without the need for intervention.

The imaging findings are those of an amorphous calcific deposit, which, unlike soft-tissue ossification, contains no internal structure (Fig. 51-30A). Ultrasonically acute deposits are hyperechoic and cast no acoustic shadow (Fig. 51-30B). As deposits mature, they become denser, leading to acoustic shadowing, and become fragmented. Complications can result for HA deposition, with a small number of patients continuing with persisting symptoms normally as a result of secondary dysfunction and secondary impingement. When deposition occurs in the shoulder or hip close to the enthesis, interosseous extension of the HA deposit can occur which can produce marked intraosseous inflammatory change.

Intra-articular HA Deposition Disease. Intra-articular HA deposition can occur, but the influence this has on the development of arthropathy is poorly understood. The best-described articular condition linked to intra-articular HA deposition is Milwaukee shoulder, characterised by cranial migration of the humeral head as a result of rotator cuff tearing, rapid bone loss in the humeral head with remodelling of the undersurface of the acromion. This has also been termed rotator cuff arthropathy with some authors proposing cuff derangement as the primary aetiological factor with HA deposition a secondary finding.

Connective Tissue Disease

The connective tissue disorders include scleroderma, systemic lupus erythematosus (SLE), dermatomyositis and polymyositis and have certain common features, including arthropathy.

Scleroderma

Systemic sclerosis is commonly associated with joint disease and patients will frequently present with joint pain. CREST syndrome is a common variation of scleroderma seen as the association of *c*alcinosis, *R*aynaud's disease, *oe*sophageal dysmotility, *s*clerodactyly and *t*elangiectasia.

Scleroderma is characterised by excessive deposition of collagen in soft tissues and is associated with fibrosis seen in the skin and internal organs. In the soft tissues flexion contractures and soft-tissue atrophy over the distal phalanges are common findings. However, soft-tissue calcification (calcinosis) is perhaps the most obvious soft-tissue finding of the disease. The calcification is amorphous in appearance and is most commonly seen in the digits, although it may be seen anywhere, including intra-articular locations, characteristically with absence of joint destruction (Fig. 51-31).

Bony resorption is a well-recognised feature of the disease, typically in the tufts of the terminal phalanges, acro-osteolysis. This is much more common in the fingers than the toes. Bony resorption may also be seen at the angle of the mandible, the posterior ribs and diffusely around the wrist.[26] Arthropathy is commonly associated with osteopenia, but joint erosions are uncommon.

Dermatomyositis and Polymyositis

The most common radiographic change of dermatomyositis is the finding of calcification within the subcutaneous soft tissues along muscle or fascial planes (Fig. 51-32). Typically, calcification involves both the skin and skeletal muscles, with the thigh being the most common site of involvement. Joint disease may also occur clinically but radiographs are usually unremarkable or may demonstrate subtle changes such as periarticular osteopenia and soft-tissue swelling. MRI may show other changes within the muscle, which, depending on the stage of the disease, include oedema, fatty infiltration and wasting. Polymyositis has similar radiographic findings but only involves the skeletal muscle.

Systemic Lupus Erythematosus

SLE is a connective tissue disorder predominantly affecting women of childbearing age. Clinical manifestations include systemic malaise and fever, skin rash and articular symptoms. In the later stages of the disease more severe multisystem involvement may be seen.

Articular symptoms are common and have been reported in 76% of patients with this condition.[27] The

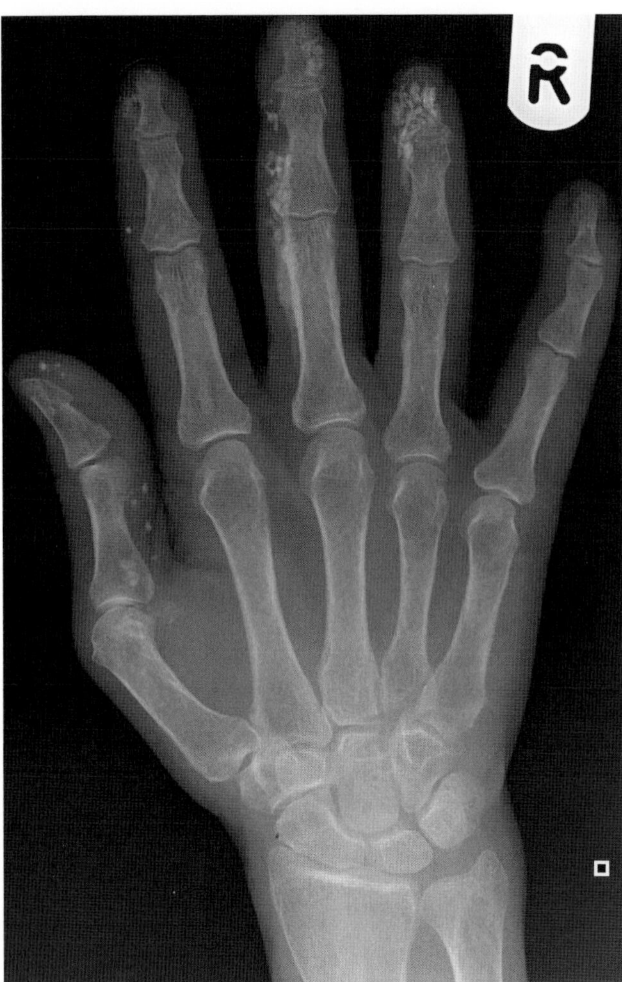

FIGURE 51-31 ■ **Scleroderma (CREST syndrome).** There is extensive soft-tissue calcinosis in the fingers. Soft-tissue atrophy is also evident, particularly over the fingertips.

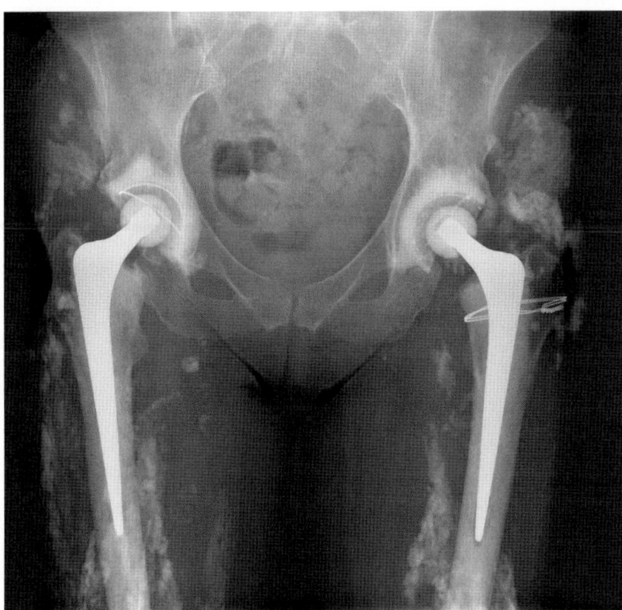

FIGURE 51-32 ■ **Dermatomyositis.** There is extensive soft-tissue calcium deposition. Note how this is associated with the muscle groups and can be seen tracking along these groups and in the associated fascial planes.

hands and wrists are most often affected, although the feet are also sometimes involved. The most frequent finding is synovitis, which will be demonstrated on ultrasound or MRI. Conventional radiographs are often normal, but may show soft-tissue swelling and/or osteopenia.

The most distinctive feature of SLE is a deforming non-erosive arthropathy (Fig. 51-6). This is more frequently seen later in the course of the disease, but may develop as an early feature of the disease.[28,29] In distinction to rheumatoid arthritis, erosions are not typical, having only occasionally been reported.[29] It is suggested that these patients actually represent a group of patients with both SLE and RA.

Deformities are secondary to ligamentous laxity and include ulnar subluxation of the MCP joints and hyperextension at the thumb interphalangeal joint. An important feature of the deformities is their reversibility. This may lead to normal-appearing radiographs despite obvious clinical deformity as the dislocations and subluxations may be reduced by the act of positioning the patient for the radiograph.

Osteonecrosis is a well-recognised feature in SLE and may occur in the femoral head, humeral head, knee and MCP heads. Soft-tissue calcification is a less common radiographic feature in some patients and is usually seen in a periarticular distribution.

Rheumatic Fever (Jaccoud's Arthropathy)

Jaccoud's arthropathy is a rare sequel of rheumatic fever and is initially radiologically indistinguishable from the deforming non-erosive arthropathy of SLE. During an acute attack joint involvement may be manifest as synovitis and effusion, appreciated as soft-tissue swelling on conventional radiographs. With repeated acute attacks, Jaccoud's arthropathy may develop. Late in the disease, erosions, bone projections and contractures may develop as the deformities become irreversible.

Mixed Connective Tissue Disease (MCTD)

Mixed connective tissue disease is recognised as a specific syndrome, which as its name suggests combines overlapping features of the connective tissue diseases and RA. Arthritis is a very common feature of the disease and a wide range of articular and soft-tissue abnormalities may be seen. In the hands these include osteopenia, joint erosions, flexion deformities, ulnar deviation of the phalanges, soft-tissue calcification and atrophy, and resorption of the terminal phalanges. Articular changes are most commonly seen in a proximal distribution similar to that seen in RA, involving PIP and MCP joints and the wrist. Large joint involvement is rare.

Miscellaneous Joint Disease

Diffuse Idiopathic Skeletal Hyperostosis (DISH)

DISH, also known as Forestier's disease, is a common condition found in the late middle-aged/elderly with an unknown aetiology. It is characterised by marked hyperostosis seen at multiple sites, but classically

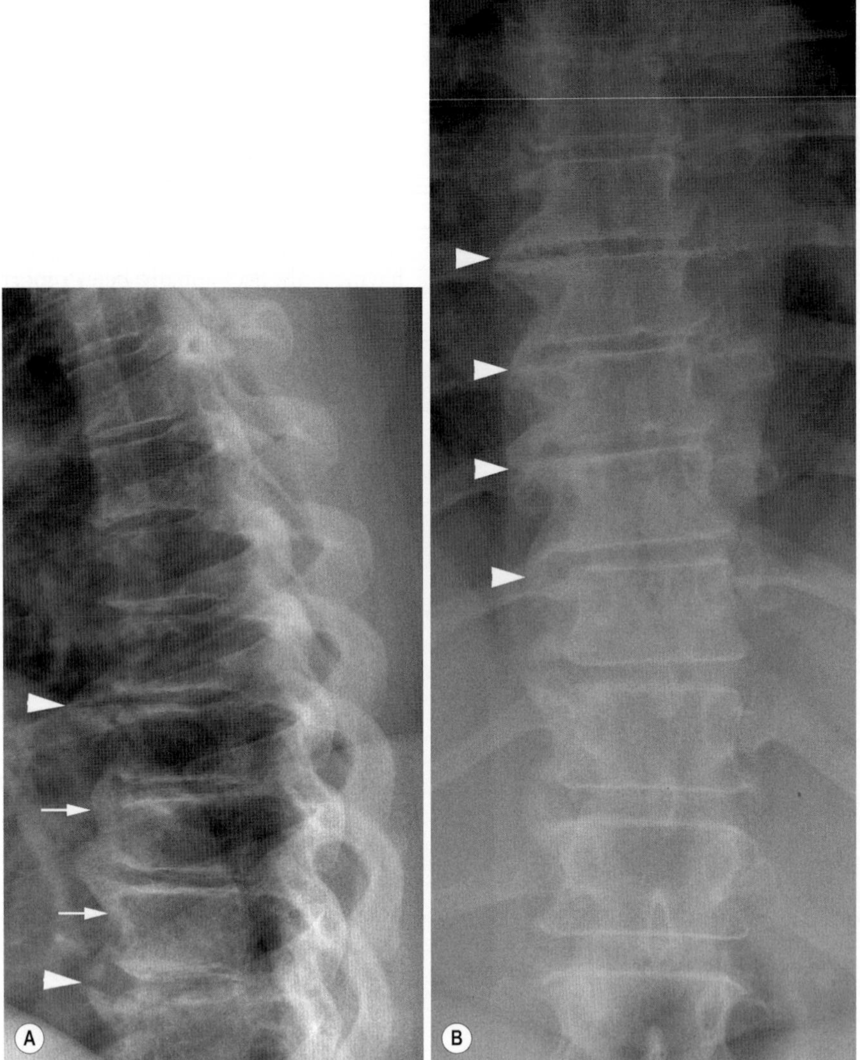

FIGURE 51-33 ■ Diffuse idiopathic skeletal hyperostosis (DISH). (A) Lateral and (B) AP thoracic spine views demonstrate marked bony hyperostosis along the line of the anterior longitudinal ligament (arrows) with large claw-like osteophytes (arrowheads), Note the relative preservation of disc space (in contrast to degenerative disc disease) and characteristic sparing of the left side of the spine shown on the AP view.

involving the spine. Sites of involvement typically occur at enthesis sites where tendons and ligaments attach to bone. Characteristically there is multilevel spinal involvement with flowing ligamentous ossification. Compared with degenerative disc disease, there is relative preservation of disc height. Certain diagnostic criteria are recognised for the diagnosis of spinal DISH and these help in distinguishing it from other causes of diffuse spinal hyperostosis such as ankylosing spondylitis and osteoarthritis.[30] These are:

- the presence of ossification along the anterolateral aspect of at least four contiguous vertebral bodies;
- relative preservation of disc height at the involved levels and absence of other OA features; and
- the absence of facet joint ankylosis or sacroiliac joint erosion or fusion.

The most common site for spinal involvement of DISH is typically T7 to T12, although cervical and lumbar involvement is also frequently seen. Here hyperostosis along the anterolateral aspect of the vertebral bodies is seen, with bridging across the intervertebral disc spaces. A feature of the condition is the tendency to see hyperostosis more commonly along the anterior-right side of the vertebral column (Fig. 51-33). This is thought to be due to inhibition of ossification on the left as a result of aortic pulsation. Compared with the changes seen in spondyloarthritis, the spinal hyperostosis of DISH tends to be more irregular with a wavy surface contour.

DISH is not confined to the spine, with hyperostosis also seen elsewhere in the skeleton, typically associated with the attachments of ligaments to bone. Characteristic sites include enthesis sites about the pelvis, the calcaneus and other tarsal bones, the elbow, hands and the patella.[31]

DISH is fundamentally a radiological diagnosis and generally the symptoms are mild in comparison to the radiographic changes. In addition to stiffness and back discomfort, there may be symptoms of tendinopathy at the enthesis sites and the hyperostosis can cause mechanical symptoms restricting the range of movement at a joint. Hyperostosis in the cervical and upper thoracic spine may give rise to dysphagia. Features resembling DISH may also be seen with retinoid therapy.

Haemophilic Arthropathy

Haemophilia refers to a group of disorders characterised by a tendency to bleed as a result of deficient clotting factors. These disorders may give rise to skeletal manifestations including soft-tissue and intramuscular bleeds. Of the haemophiliac disorders, haemophilia A (factor XIII deficiency) and haemophilia B or Christmas disease (factor IX deficiency) are most frequently associated with bone and joint complications. Both these conditions are X-linked and because of the recessive nature of the gene only manifested in men, although women may act as carriers.

Haemophilic arthropathy arises as a consequence of recurrent bleeds into joints. Most commonly the knees, elbows and ankles are affected. Blood products in the joint lead to an inflammatory response by the synovium and the release of destructive enzymes. The inflamed synovium itself may be a source of haemorrhage, further damaging the joint. Initially, acute haemarthroses may resolve completely with treatment involving administration of the appropriate clotting factor. With recurrent bleeds, complete recovery no longer occurs and restricted joint motion, contractures and muscle atrophy occur. At this stage radiographic changes become evident.

Haemorrhage and synovial inflammation in the joint lead to periarticular hyperaemia and often striking juxta-articular osteoporosis. Before epiphyseal fusion chronic hyperaemia leads to epithelial overgrowth and premature epiphyseal fusion. The synovium of affected joints initially hypertrophies. The ensuing inflammatory cascade leads to bone erosion and cartilage loss (joint space loss), ultimately producing changes of secondary osteoarthritis including subchondral cyst formation and collapse, osteophyte formation and sclerosis. Subchondral cyst formation may be contributed to by intraosseous haemorrhage. In the knee, widening of the intercondylar notch is a well-recognised feature of haemophilic arthritis and widening of the trochlear notch and olecranon fossa may be seen at the elbow (Fig. 51-34). The associated joint effusions and the synovitis may show increased density on conventional radiographs due to the presence of blood products (Fig. 51-34). Ultimately, the synovium undergoes a process of fibrosis and regression.

As with many forms of arthritis the radiographic changes of haemophilic arthritis are relatively late and advanced forms of imaging are becoming commonplace in the management of this condition. Ultrasound readily identifies acute haemarthrosis, although it cannot reliably distinguish between blood and simple effusion or even pus in a joint, so the correct clinical context is required. It will also identify thickened synovium (which may appear hypervascular). A particular use of ultrasound is to distinguish chronically thickened synovium from acute haemorrhage.[32]

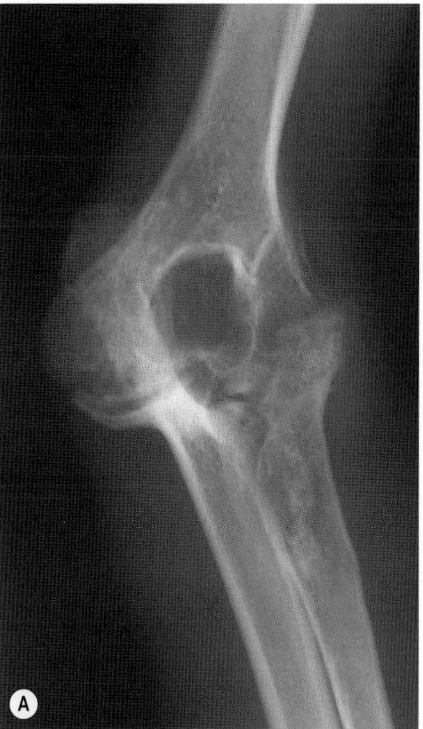

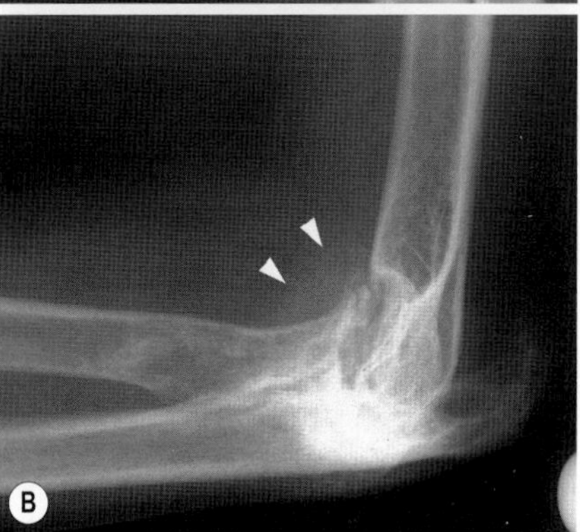

FIGURE 51-34 ■ Chronic haemophilic arthropathy. (A) AP and (B) lateral radiographs of the elbow: there is hypertrophic arthropathy with sclerosis and osteophyte formation. In addition, note the characteristic widening of the trochlea notch and olecranon fossa. On the lateral film, soft-tissue shadowing (arrowheads) representing the hypertrophied synovium is seen and appears dense due to the presence of blood products.

MRI can also assess for the presence of blood in a joint (the signal characteristics will vary depending on the time since the bleed) and for synovial thickening. Fibrosis and haemosiderin in the synovium may give foci of low signal on both T1- and T2-weighted imaging which may show susceptibility artefact on T2* imaging. MRI is also more sensitive than conventional radiographs for the demonstration of bone destruction and cartilage loss (Fig. 51-35).

Other Musculoskeletal Manifestations of Haemophilia. Intramuscular and soft-tissue haemorrhages are frequently seen in patients with haemophilia and may occur spontaneously or following trauma. Commonly involved muscles include the iliopsoas, quadriceps and

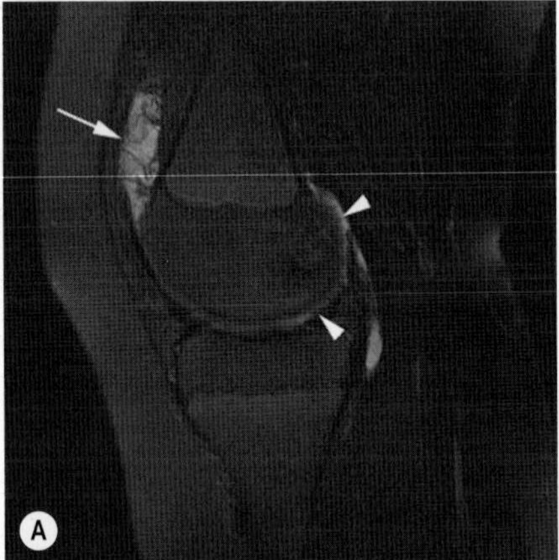

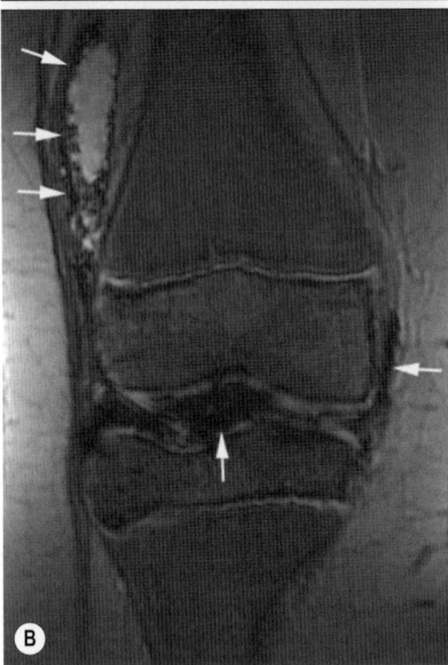

FIGURE 51-35 ■ **Haemophilic arthropathy.** (A) Sagittal fat-suppressed T2-weighted MRI: there is a joint effusion with synovial hypertrophy in the suprapatellar recess which shows low signal on the T2-weighted image (arrows). Cartilage loss is also evident (arrowheads). (B) Coronal T2* gradient-echo MRI: The t2* weighting emphasises the low signal synovium (arrows) which also shows blooming (susceptibility) artefact.

the gastrocnemius.[33] The resulting haematoma can be readily identified on ultrasound, where the early mixed echogenicity becomes progressively anechoic over 3 to 4 days, and MRI, in which case the signal characteristics will depend on the timing of the bleed. Complications of intramuscular haematoma include the development of fibrous tissue leading to contractures and myositis ossificans.[32]

Pseudotumour is a well-recognised complication of both intraosseous and soft-tissue haemorrhage. This is an encapsulated haematoma, which progressively expands. Osseous involvement may result from subperiosteal or intraosseous haemorrhage. The latter results in a well-defined lytic lesion that may be expansile and cause endosteal scalloping. Subperiosteal pseudotumours lead to elevation of the periosteum and pressure effects causing erosion of the underlying cortex. There may be soft-tissue extension and periosteal reaction leading to a differential diagnosis which includes aggressive lesions such as Ewing's sarcoma and infection.[34]

TABLE 51-2 Conditions Associated with Neuropathic Arthropathy

Condition	Prevalence of Arthropathy	Joints Most Commonly Affected
Congenital insensitivity to pain	100%	Ankle, tarsal, knee, hip
Syringomyelia	20–50%	Shoulder, elbow, wrist, cervical spine
Neurosyphilis	5–10%	Knee, hip
Diabetes mellitus	1%	Midfoot, forefoot
Alcohol related	Rare	Foot

Neuropathic Arthropathy

This pattern of arthropathy involves both bony hypertrophic change and destructive change in varying proportions. It is associated with a loss of pain sensation and/or proprioception in the joint and as a result occurs in a number of conditions with neurological sequelae, the joint affected depending on the distribution of neurological disease (Table 51-2).

The radiographic findings associated with a neuropathic joint are similar irrespective of the aetiology and two distinct patterns are recognised, atrophic and hypertrophic neuropathic osteoarthropathy. The most common pattern of involvement is hypertrophic and the findings at an affected joint reflect this, consisting of increased bone density and production of bone debris. Periosteal new bone formation may be seen, as may osteophytes, although these tend to be less well defined than those seen in osteoarthritis. However, alongside these hypertrophic changes, the joint becomes increasingly disorganised with dislocations and bone destruction (Fig. 51-36). Early changes may be difficult to differentiate from osteoarthritis, infection or more rarely tumour. Neuropathic changes are much more commonly seen in the lower limbs than in the upper limbs or spine. Fractures associated with neuropathy are common and may be difficult to diagnose due to surrounding destruction and debris.

The less common atrophic pattern of neuropathic arthropathy usually affects the distal ends of tubular bones and comprises a pattern of osteolysis, which may be mistaken for surgical amputation. This form of the arthropathy generally occurs in non-weight-bearing joints.

Synovial (Osteo)-Chondromatosis

This condition is characterised by the formation of multiple synovial cartilage nodules, which may detach and become free intra-articular bodies. While the condition occurs most frequently in joints, it can occur in any synovial-lined structure so it may also be seen in bursae and tendon sheaths. It is most commonly seen in the knee, hip and elbow and is usually a monoarthritic

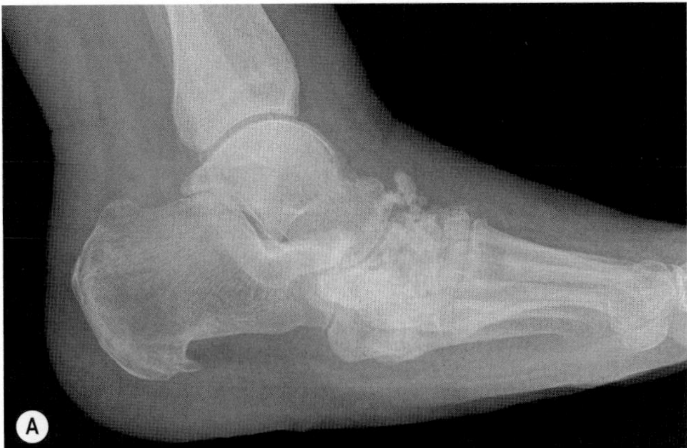

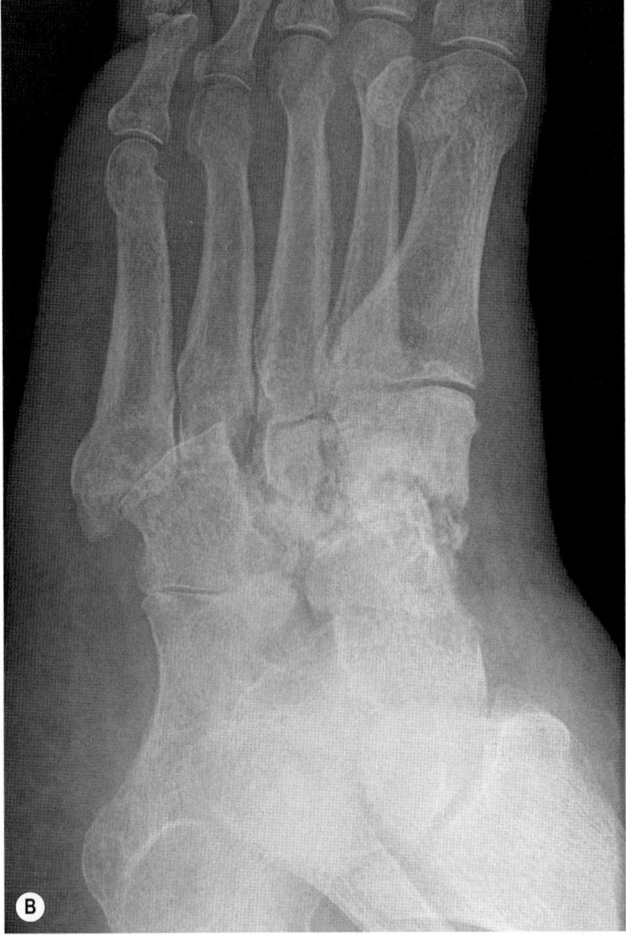

FIGURE 51-36 ■ Neuropathic arthropathy secondary to diabetes mellitus. (A) Lateral and (B) DP oblique views of the foot: there is a hypertrophic arthropathy with sclerosis and osteophyte formation, along with bone destruction and fragmentation and the production of bone debris involving the joints of the midfoot.

process. In the majority of cases the chondral bodies become calcified or ossified and at this stage they are evident on conventional radiographs and the term synovial osteochondromatosis is used (Fig. 51-37). In common with other osteochondral bodies, such as those arising through trauma, even after being shed into the joint space the bodies may continue to grow.

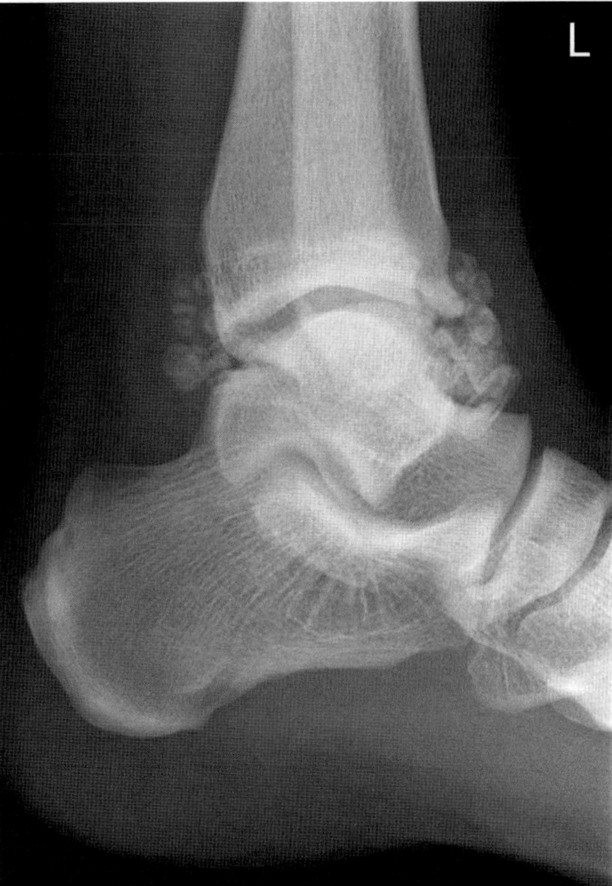

FIGURE 51-37 ■ Synovial osteochondromatosis. Lateral ankle radiograph: there are multiple intra-articular osteochondral bodies in this 42-year-old patient. Note the absence of joint space loss or other features of osteoarthritis.

The condition most frequently occurs in young or middle-aged adults and is described as secondary when seen as a consequence of trauma, degenerative disease or inflammation.

Initially, before calcification of the nodules, radiographs may simply show soft-tissue swelling. At this stage the non-calcified bodies and synovial nodules may be visible on MRI or CT arthrography. As the bodies calcify, they will be seen on all imaging techniques as multiple loose bodies, which may demonstrate trabeculation and may be associated with synovial thickening.

Although the presence of numerous similarly sized ossified bodies, in the absence of joint space narrowing, helps to distinguish synovial osteochondromatosis from loose bodies associated with other arthropathic processes such as OA, it is important to recognise that secondary OA may develop on the background of long-standing synovial osteochondromatosis.

Pigmented Villonodular Synovitis (PVNS)

This uncommon condition results from proliferation of the synovium in joints, bursae or tendons. Most

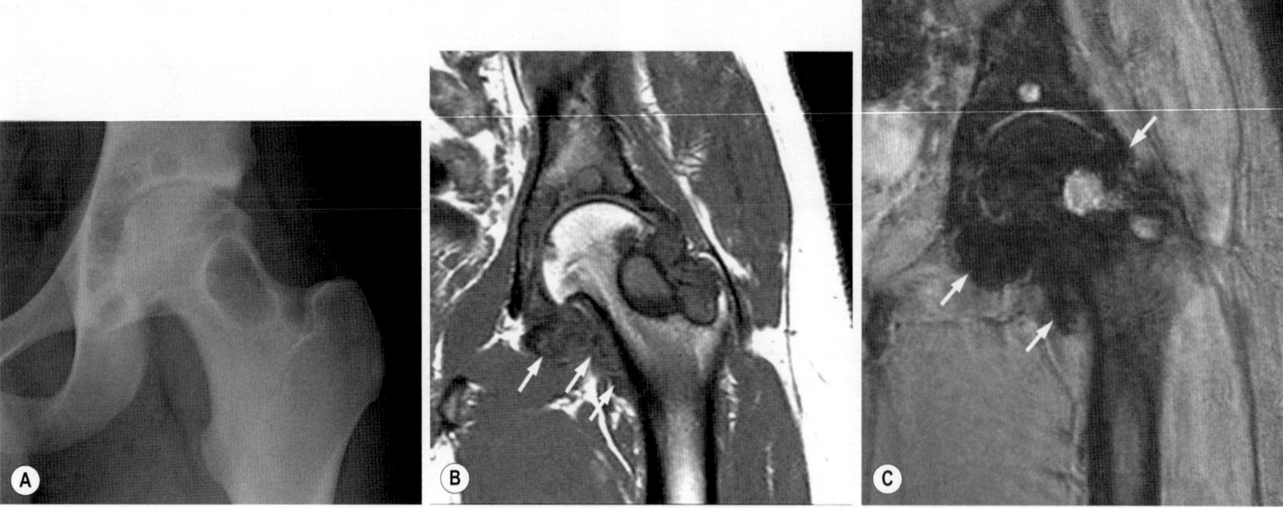

FIGURE 51-38 ■ Pigmented villonodular synovitis (PVNS) of the hip. (A) AP hip radiograph: there is extensive well-defined erosive change involving the acetabular fossa and proximal femur. (B) Coronal T1 MRI shows the extent of the erosive change. Note also the synovial hypertrophy, which shows intermediate to low signal, particularly well seen inferiorly (arrows). (C) Coronal T2* GRE MRI shows the synovitis with characteristic low signal and associated blooming artefact (arrows) due to the presence of haemosiderin.

patients are young adults and present with a chronic monoarthropathy, manifest as intermittent pain and swelling, typically in a large joint. The condition may occur in any joint, but it most commonly affects the knee (around 75%), followed by the hip (15%), with other large joints including the ankle, shoulder and elbow less commonly affected.[35] While the condition typically shows diffuse involvement of the entire synovium, a localised form is recognised, presenting as a synovial nodule most often in the anterior knee.[36]

Radiographs are frequently abnormal and may show features of a joint effusion/soft-tissue swelling. Bone erosion is a relatively common finding and is seen on a background of preserved joint space and reduced bone mineral density (Fig. 51-38). The extent of bone erosion is determined by the capacity of the capsule, with large joints such as the knee showing less frequent erosion than joints with smaller capacity, such as the hip. In the hip, erosion may lead to narrowing of the femoral neck, giving an 'apple-core' configuration.

MRI provides the best clue to the diagnosis due to the presence of haemosiderin in the hypertrophied synovium as a result of recurrent haemarthrosis. Compared with most synovial-based masses, the synovium will frequently shown low signal intensity on both T1- and T2-weighted imaging with accentuation of the abnormality on T2* gradient-echo images which may show blooming artefact in areas of haemosiderin deposition (Fig. 51-38C). Bone erosion, subchondral synovial tissue and 'cysts' are also clearly seen on MRI. Similar appearances (haemosiderotic synovitis) can be seen due to recurrent haemarthrosis in haemophilia and synovial haemangioma (Fig. 51-35).

Articular PVNS is histologically identical to nodular PVNS occurring in tendon sheaths, also known as giant cell tumour of tendon sheath, discussed in Chapter 49.

Lipoma Arborescens

This is a rare intra-articular synovial disorder most commonly seen in the knee. It is a benign condition involving synovial metaplasia, leading to delicate branching fronds of synovium. As the name suggests, the hypertrophied fronds of synovium contain fat, giving characteristic high signal on T1-weighted MRI which is reduced with fat suppression (Fig. 51-39).

Amyloid

Amyloid deposition may occur in synovium and in the surrounding periarticular soft tissues. The radiographic features reflect this with asymmetric soft-tissue masses and well-defined erosions and cysts. An important feature of articular amyloid is the preservation of joint space. The appearances may resemble gout or PVNS. MRI will show deposition of abnormal soft tissue, which is of intermediate to low signal intensity on both T1- and T2-weighted imaging.

Sarcoid

Sarcoidosis is a systemic disease with the potential to involve multiple organs including the lungs and skin. Musculoskeletal involvement is well recognised with joint, bone and muscle involvement described. Most commonly an inflammatory arthralgia is seen (in up to 40% of cases). In the majority of cases radiographs are unremarkable, but soft-tissue swelling and occasionally osteopenia may occasionally be seen.[37] Muscle involvement may be nodular or myopathic, the latter showing non-specific MRI features. Nodular sarcoid infiltration of muscle is evident on MRI and the sarcoid nodules may show a characteristic pattern of signal abnormality,

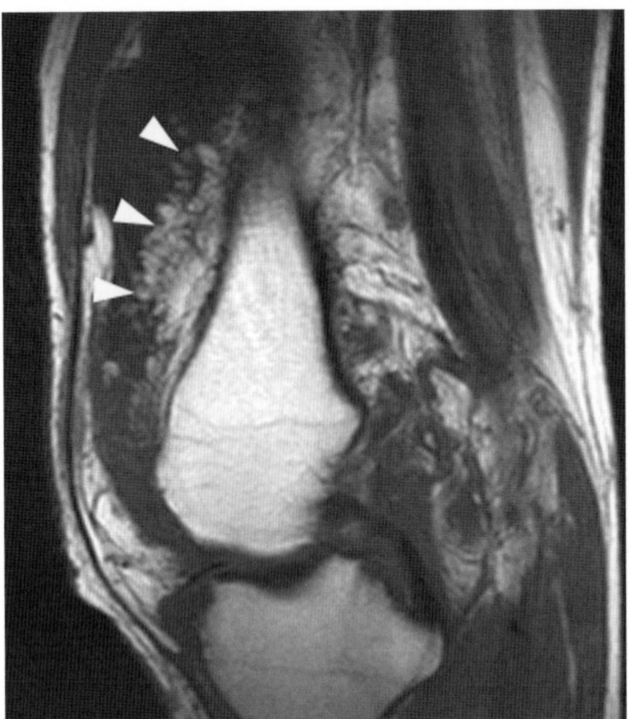

FIGURE 51-39 ■ Lipoma arborescens of the knee. Sagittal T1-weighted MRI: there is frond-like synovial hyperplasia evident in the suprapatellar pouch. This shows the characteristic high T1 (fat) signal of lipoma arborescens.

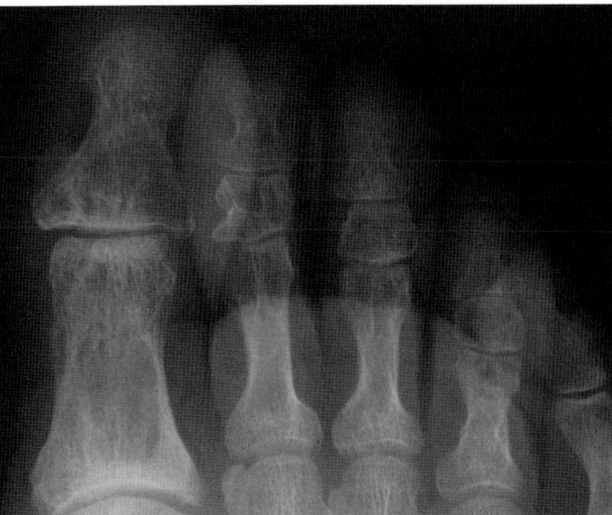

FIGURE 51-40 ■ Osseous sarcoid. DP radiograph of toes: the phalanges show abnormal bone texture with a lace-like pattern resulting from coarsening of the trabeculae. Note also the loss of cortical definition in involved areas.

demonstrating a low signal central zone on all sequences, representing fibrosis and peripheral high signal intensity on T2-weighted imaging.[38]

Bone involvement in sarcoid is seen in between 5 and 10% of patients with the phalanges of the hands and feet characteristically affected.[38] The lesions are frequently asymptomatic and are rarely demonstrated in the absence of skin or pulmonary disease. The most common form of osseous involvement involves coarsening of the trabecular pattern and loss of definition between the cortex and the medulla, giving rise to a lace-like or reticular appearance (Fig. 51-40). Localised cystic lesions may also be seen and may be sharply marginated. A rare form of mutilating sarcoidosis is also recognised.

Hypertrophic Pulmonary Osteoarthropathy (HPOA)

This describes a triad of periosteal new bone formation, finger clubbing and synovitis. It is most commonly seen in patients with pulmonary disease, particularly bronchogenic carcinoma but is recognised to also occur in association with other conditions including inflammatory bowel disease and biliary cirrhosis. If synovitis is the presenting feature, the picture may resemble rheumatoid arthritis. Not all patients will manifest all three components of the condition.

Periosteal new bone formation affects the diaphyses and subsequently the metaphyses of tubular bones, most frequently the radius and ulna, and tibia and fibula (Fig. 51-41). The femora, humeri, metacarpals, metatarsals and phalanges are less commonly involved. If the periostitis is long-standing, the bones have thickened cortices.

The triad of findings is not always associated with an underlying disorder. Primary hypertrophic osteoarthropathy, also known as pachydermoperiostosis, occurs most frequently in men of black African descent. It is associated with thickening of the skin and resulting coarsening of the facies, which may resemble acromegaly, although growth hormone levels are normal.

Multicentric Reticulohistiocytosis

This is a rare disease presenting in adult life most frequently affecting women. The soft tissues are infiltrated by multinucleated histiocytes with the formation of cutaneous nodules associated with erosive arthritis. In some patients the polyarthritis is the presenting feature of the disease, with the cutaneous changes occurring later. The interphalangeal joints of the fingers are most frequently affected, with involvement of the wrists generally occurring before metacarpophalangeal joint involvement. Less commonly, large joint involvement and spinal involvement are seen, although atlantoaxial involvement may be severe and occur early.[39] The erosive arthritis begins in the joint margins and is not associated with osteoporosis. Well-circumscribed erosions are typical, and may closely resemble the appearances of gout and progress to an arthritis mutilans.

Haemochromatosis

Haemochromatosis can be a primary or secondary disorder. Primary haemochromatosis results from a genetic error of metabolism, with increased absorption of iron from the gastrointestinal tract. Secondary haemochromatosis results from increased intake and tissue accumulation of iron from a known cause such as excessive dietary

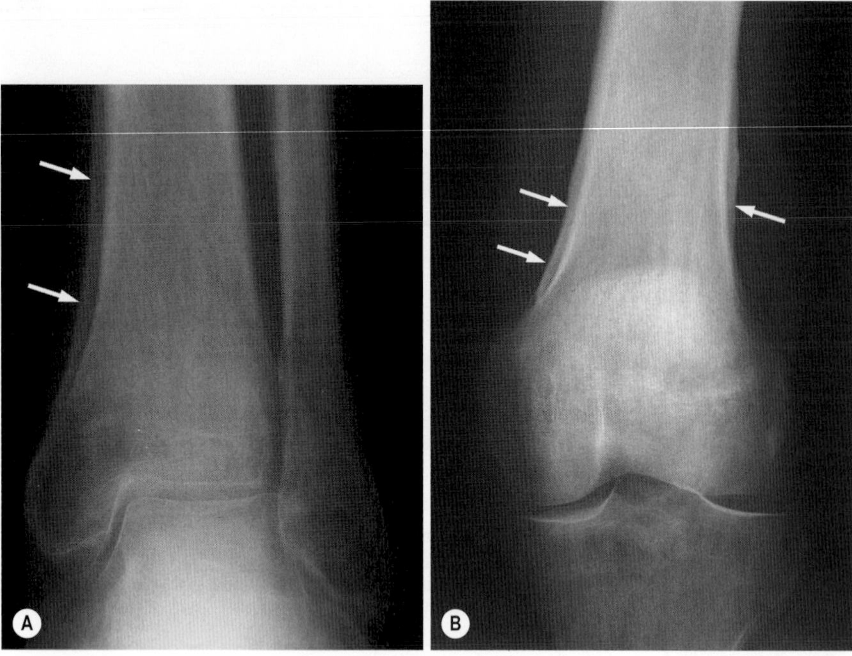

FIGURE 51-41 ■ Hypertrophic pulmonary osteoarthropathy (HPOA) in a patient with a bronchogenic neoplasm. (A) AP radiograph of the distal tibia and fibula showing a lamellar pattern of new bone formation along the medial tibial cortex (arrows). (B) AP radiograph of the distal femur: involvement was severe and relatively unusually there was also femoral involvement.

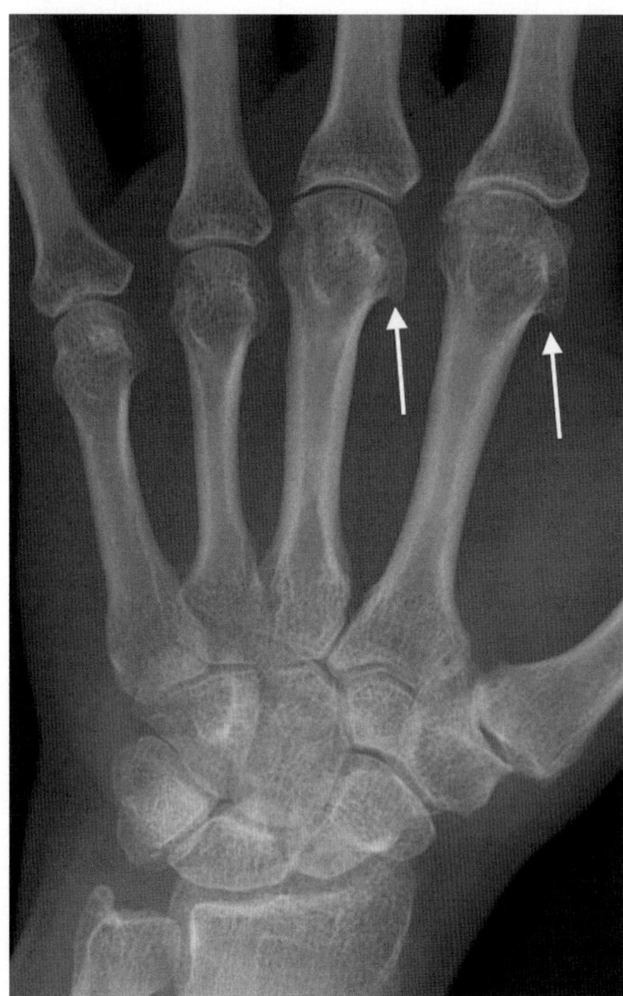

FIGURE 51-42 ■ Patient with haemochromatosis demonstrating classical hook osteophytes arising on the radial aspects of the index and middle finger metacarpal heads (arrows).

intake, cirrhosis, multiple transfusions and refractory anaemia.

Primary haemochromatosis is classically seen in the 40- to 60-year-old male who usually presents with a clinical triad of skin pigmentation, cirrhosis and diabetes, the so-called 'bronze diabetic'. Elevated serum ferritin levels confirm the diagnosis.

Joint disease and chondrocalcinosis are common in haemochromatosis and can be the presenting feature. Appearances resemble OA, but the pattern of joint disease, particularly in the hands, is different, with relative sparing of the interphalangeal joints and predominant involvement of the MCP joints, most frequently those of the index and middle fingers (Fig. 51-42). Another typical feature of the disease is the presence of hook-like osteophytes generally seen on the radial aspect of the metacarpal heads. Chondrocalcinosis is seen in association with the metacarpal changes, usually best appreciated in the wrist. The combination of these findings, although not pathognomonic, should alert the clinician and radiologist to the possibility of haemochromatosis.[23,40]

For a full list of references, please see ExpertConsult.

FURTHER READING

6. Kloppenburg M, Kwok WY. Hand osteoarthritis—a heterogeneous disorder. Nat Rev Rheumatol 2011;8(1):22–31.
12. Villeneuve E, Emery P. Rheumatoid arthritis: what has changed? Skeletal Radiol 2009;38(2):109–12.
18. Benjamin M, McGonagle D. The anatomical basis for disease localisation in seronegative spondyloarthropathy at entheses and related sites. J Anat 2001;199(Pt 5):503–26.
19. Arnett FC. Seronegative spondylarthropathies. Bull Rheum Dis 1987;37(1):1–12.
25. Uri DS, Dalinka MK. Imaging of arthropathies. Crystal disease. Radiol Clin North Am 1996;34(2):359–74, xi.
32. Maclachlan J, Gough-Palmer A, Hargunani R, et al. Haemophilia imaging: a review. Skeletal Radiol 2009;38(10):949–57.

CHAPTER 52

Appendicular and Pelvic Trauma

Nigel Raby • Philip M. Hughes • James Ricketts

CHAPTER OUTLINE

GENERAL CONSIDERATIONS

This chapter will consider skeletal trauma and its consequences. It will be largely confined to appearances on radiographs occasionally supplemented by CT. The soft-tissue aspects of trauma principally imaged with MRI will not be considered in this chapter.

In evaluating any bony injury due to trauma it is essential that two radiographs are obtained, usually at right angles to each other (orthogonal). Many fractures are visible on only one of these radiographs. Inexperienced observers will tend to rely on the anteroposterior (AP) view as this is better understood intuitively. The lateral view, however, will identify at least as many fractures as the AP and may be the only view where the fracture is visible. Time spent becoming familiar with the lateral view will be well rewarded. The old adage 'One view is no view' is particularly relevant when assessing trauma radiographs.

DESCRIBING FRACTURE TYPES

Fractures of bones can be considered to be incomplete or complete. Incomplete fractures are generally confined to injuries in children (Fig. 52-1). There are three types:

1. Plastic bowing injury where the bone is mildly deformed but there is no disruption of the cortex.
2. Torus injury, an impaction fracture with cortical buckling which may be circumferential. There is no true cortical break and the periosteum is intact.
3. Greenstick fracture where there is break of cortex on one side only with buckling of the opposite cortex.

Also seen only in children are fractures related to the epiphyseal growth plate. These have been classified by Salter and Harris into five types (Fig. 52-2).

Complete fractures refer to a fracture which separates one part of bone from the other. The fracture pattern should be described. These fractures can be subdivided by the fracture direction into transverse, oblique, spiral and longitudinal. The presence or absence of angulation, rotation, distraction or shortening with overlap should be stated. The site of the fracture within the bone should be stated. If near a joint, note should be made as to whether the fracture extends to involve the articular surface. This is an important observation as, in general, intra-articular fractures have a poorer prognosis and surgical intervention is more often required.

The term 'comminuted' refers to fractures which have more than two parts of bone at the fracture site, although by convention small bone fragments are often disregarded.

A large triangular bone segment is referred to as a butterfly fragment and a segmental fragment is seen when there is a separate segment of bone between the main fracture components. A compound fracture is one where there is breach of the overlying soft tissue and skin. Although this can sometimes be identified on radiographs it is usually a clinical diagnosis.

It is generally understood that a fracture results in a gap between the bone ends through which the X-ray beam can pass, resulting in a dark or black line on the radiograph. Not so well appreciated is that the presence of a white or sclerotic area of bone is an equally important sign of fracture. In the setting of trauma this finding is due to either impaction or overlap of bone. Both will result in increased bony density. The best-known example

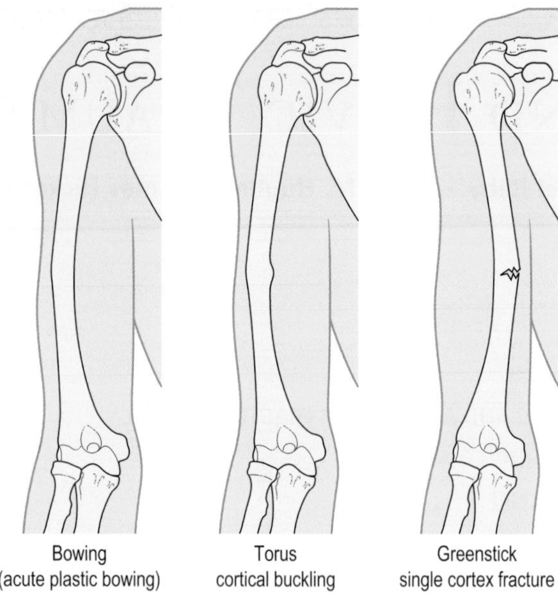

FIGURE 52-1 ■ Children's fractures are often incomplete.

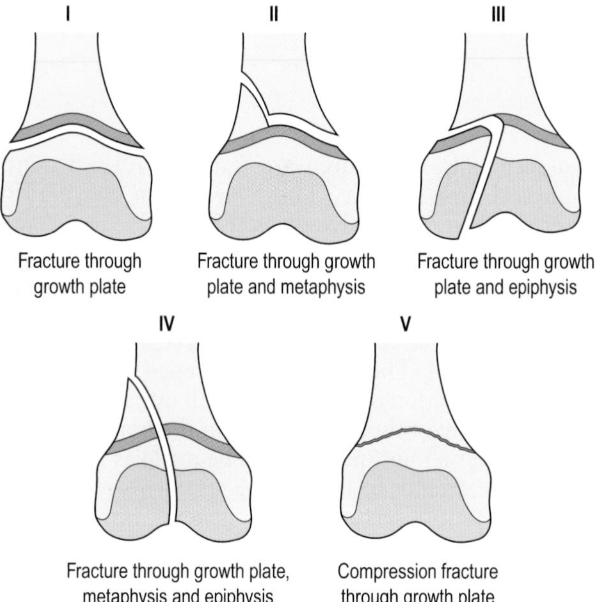

FIGURE 52-2 ■ The Salter–Harris classification of fractures in children involving the growth plate. The numbers refer to the prognosis. Type 1 has the best, type 5 the worst.

of this is an impacted fracture of the femoral neck. However, there are many other situations and sites where this can occur. It is a very useful radiological sign which can help detect subtle fractures. Its value will be demonstrated several times in this chapter.

An avulsion fracture occurs at sites of tendon or ligament attachment when a fragment of bone is pulled off the underlying parent bone as a result of traction from either the muscle tendon kinetic chain or a joint ligament. To describe any injury as an avulsion fracture you must be able to identify the mechanism of injury and state what ligament or tendon attaches to the bone fragment. These should not be referred to as flake or chip fractures unless there is a clear mechanism of a direct impact to the area which would account for the findings; such fractures are rare. Understanding of the above will lead to an appreciation of the severity and significance of the findings. A bone avulsion at the site of tendon attachment occurs due to muscle contraction and will usually be a single-site abnormality (e.g. avulsion of fifth metatarsal base). Ligaments, on the other hand, have no contractile capacity and serve to stabilise joints. For a ligament to avulse a bone fragment there must have been a major distraction or angulation of the joint. This is therefore often associated with other injuries (see discussion of Segond fracture in the section 'The Knee'). A knowledge of major tendon and ligament attachments is essential for correct interpretation of these injuries. The more common examples of this will be described throughout the chapter.

Stress fractures occur when normal bone is subjected to repeated abnormal loading such that microfracturing occurs. Repetition of this loading over a period of time at a rate which exceeds the capacity of reparative processes results in progressive weakening of the bone to the point where a true fracture can occur at the site of stress. A lucent fracture line is, however, often not evident in the early stages of the process. A periosteal reaction and medullary sclerosis may develop at the site of stress and may be the only abnormality on the radiographs. If abnormal loading is continued, a frank fracture will eventually occur. (See examples in the sections 'The Ankle' and 'Foot Injuries'.)

A pathological fracture occurs through an area of abnormally weak bone. The term is usually reserved for fractures occurring at the site of bone involvement by tumour. This may be either primary benign or malignant lesions or secondary malignant deposits. Most commonly pathological fractures occur through the site of a metastatic deposit, including myeloma. Pathological fractures can also occur in weak bone, resulting from osteporosis or metabolic bone disease; these fractures are sometimes referred to as insufficiency fractures.

Dislocation refers to the situation at a joint where the articular surfaces have lost all contact. They may be associated with fractures in addition. Subluxation occurs when the joint surfaces are no longer fully congruous but some articular surface contact is maintained.

THE SHOULDER

The shoulder consists of two separate joints: the glenohumeral and the acromio-clavicular (AC) joint. It is essential that both are carefully evaluated in every patient.

Standard views of the shoulder include an AP radiograph in all cases. A second view is essential but as none are ideal there are local variations. There are three possible additional views: axial, axial oblique and lateral. The authors favour the axial oblique as the patient does not have to move the injured shoulder and it is relatively easy to interpret. Its weakness is that it does not provide a second view of the scapula. A true lateral view can be obtained if a scapular fracture is suspected clinically.

On the AP view it is important to appreciate that the humeral head is an asymmetric structure with more bone

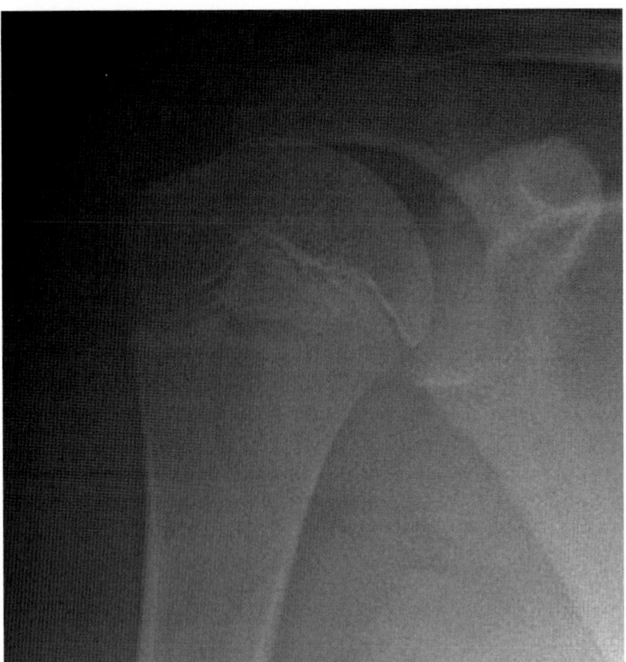

FIGURE 52-3 ■ Anterior dislocation with a large bone fragment which has been sheared off from the posterior aspect of the humeral head.

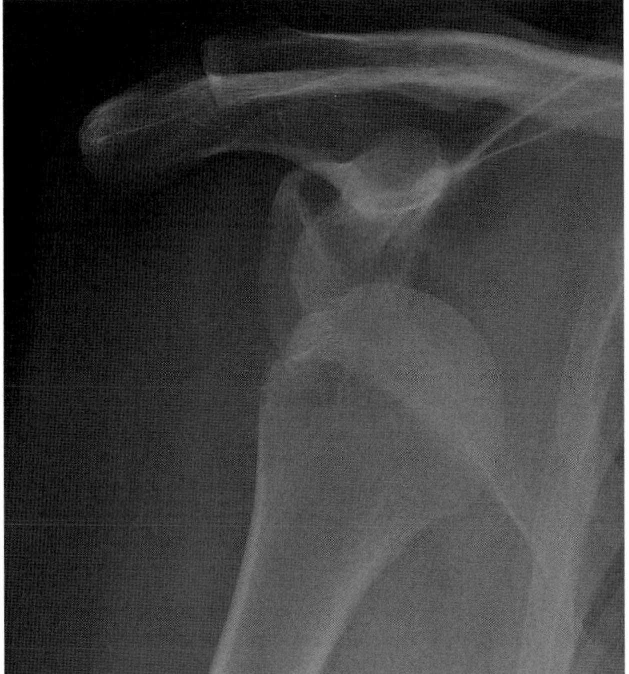

FIGURE 52-4 ■ Anterior dislocation. There is loss of the normal joint congruity. The humeral head lies under the coronoid process.

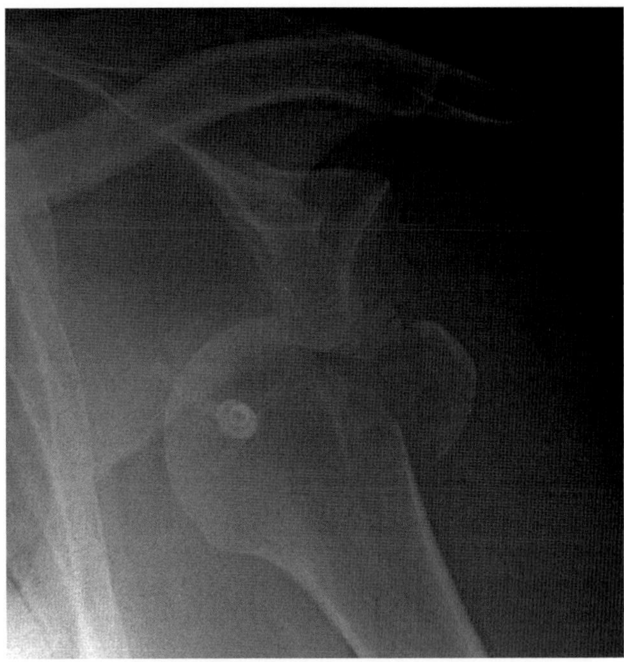

FIGURE 52-5 ■ Adolescent shoulder AP view. The normal epiphyseal plate should not be confused with a fracture. The growth plate lies in an oblique plane with the posterior aspect projected inferior to the anterior aspect.

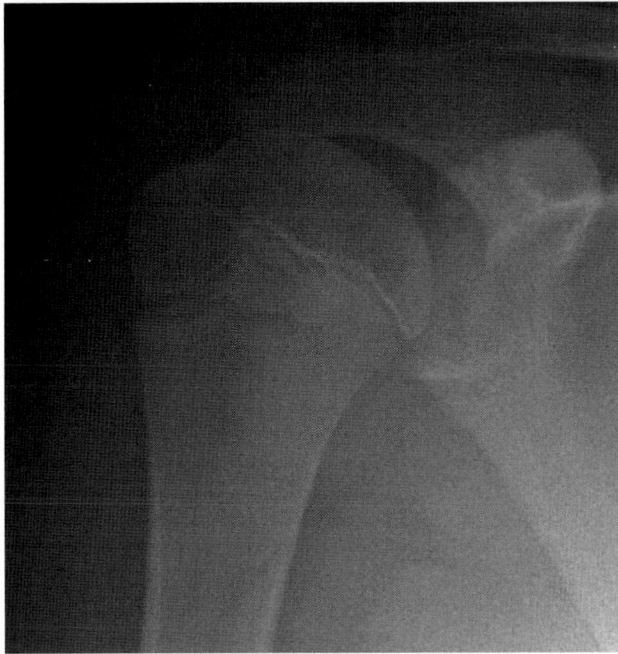

FIGURE 52-6 ■ AP view showing fracture of the inferior glenoid margin known as a Bankart lesion.

lying medial than laterally. The humeral head should be congruent with the glenoid fossa. In the adolescent shoulder the appearance of the unfused epiphysis should not be mistaken for a fracture (Fig. 52-3).

Anterior dislocation is common, accounting for 95% of all dislocations[1] and diagnosis is usually obvious (Fig. 52-4). The humeral head is no longer congruous with the glenoid and is displaced lying in a subcoracoid position.

Anterior dislocations are often associated with fractures, of which there are three types:

1. A fracture of the greater tuberosity sheared off or avulsed as the humerus dislocates (15%) (Fig. 52-5).
2. Fracture of the anteroinferior corner of the glenoid (8%) known as a Bankart lesion (Fig. 52-6). These fractures may be subtle and CT can be used in such cases to clarify the site and extent of the fracture.

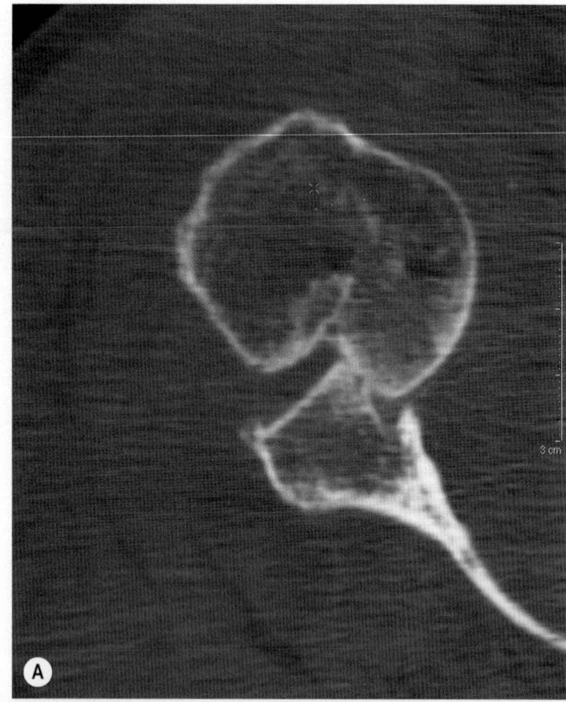

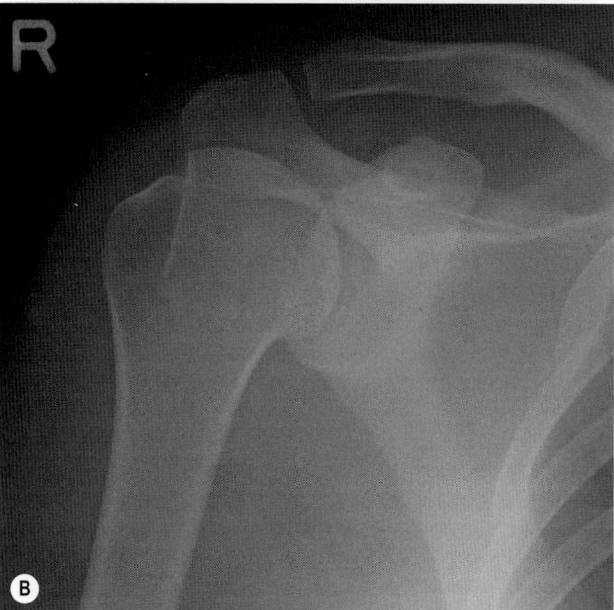

FIGURE 52-7 ■ (A) Anterior dislocation with axial oblique view on CT scan shows the effect of impaction of the glenoid on the humeral head, resulting in a V-shaped bony defect in the humeral head referred to as a Hill–Sachs lesion. (B) The humeral head is now back in joint. Note the defect in the superior contour and the vertical sclerotic line of impacted bone.

3. A V-shaped deformity of the humeral head caused by the impaction of the anterior glenoid rim on the posterosuperior humeral head. This is known as a Hill–Sachs lesion.[2] Once the humeral head is relocated, the signs of a Hill–Sachs lesion are a notch in the superolateral humeral head and a sclerotic vertical line of impacted bone (Fig. 52-7).

Careful search should be made for these fractures in all cases of anterior dislocation.

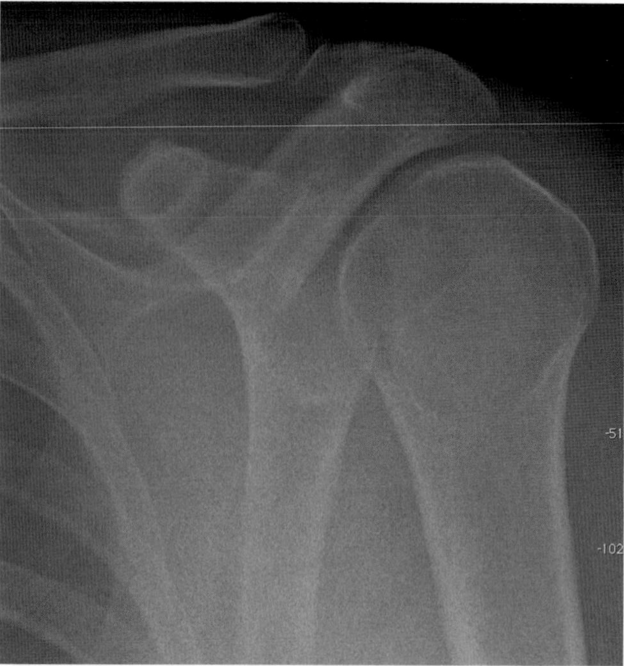

FIGURE 52-8 ■ **Posterior dislocation.** The humeral head has a round symmetrical appearance likened to a light bulb. Posterior dislocation should be suspected but can only be confirmed on the second view.

Posterior dislocation is rare[1] (<5%). The congruity of the humeral head with the glenoid often appears to be maintained on the AP view. The key observation on the AP view is that the normal asymmetrical appearance of the head is replaced by a much more spherical symmetrical appearance referred to as the 'light bulb' sign. Careful scrutiny of the second view is needed to confirm the loss of contact between the humeral head and the glenoid (Fig. 52-8). In many instances the humeral head appears symmetrical but is not dislocated. This is due to the arm being held in internal rotation such as when the arm is in a sling. Thus the second view must be used to determine whether the humeral head is in joint.

Fractures of the humeral head and proximal shaft typically occur following a fall on the outstretched arm. The humeral head is driven into the hard cortical bone of the glenoid. This results in several fracture patterns. Fractures may involve the surgical neck and the greater and lesser tuberosities. This can result in up to four major bone fragments. Comminuted fractures of the humeral head have been classified by Neer depending on the number of major fracture fragments from 1 to 4.[3] In this classification, to qualify as separate bone fragments they must be displaced by 1 cm or angled at 45° or more to the adjacent bone. Based on the above, a multiple part fracture of the humeral head which is undisplaced is classified as a Neer '1 part' fracture.This pattern accounts for the great majority (85%) of such fractures which if they are minimally displaced are not considered as separate fragments. Two-, three- and four-part fractures are seen with fractures involving, respectively, the greater and lesser tuberosities in addition to the surgical neck. Any combination of injuries may occur. Isolated fractures of greater or lesser tuberosity are most often avulsion injuries due, respectively, to the pull of supraspinatous and subscapularis muscles and are comparatively rare outside of the setting of dislocation described above.

Transverse fractures of the humerus involve either the surgical neck or the shaft inferior to this. Medial displacement of the humeral shaft occurs due to pull of pectoralis major muscle.

THE ACROMIO-CLAVICULAR JOINT

Clavicle fractures are very common; as the bone is just under the skin surface, they are easy to detect clinically. Fractures most often involve the middle third (80%). Outer-third fractures occur in 15% of cases. Medial-third fractures are uncommon, accounting for only 5% of cases.[4] The AC joint is held in place by the acromio-clavicular ligament and the two coraco-clavicular (CC) components known as conoid and trapezoid ligaments. Minor disruptions are best detected by looking at the inferior cortex of both the clavicle and the acromion. These should align. If they do not, then there is an AC joint subluxation. The normal distance between the superior surface of the coracoid and the inferior clavicle is no more than 13 mm.

Disruptions are graded from 1 to 3.[5] Grade 1 is sprain of the ligaments only. There is only minor separation, if any, at the AC joint. In grade 2 injuries the AC joint ligaments are torn but the CC ligaments are intact. In a grade 3 the CC ligaments are disrupted. As a result the coraco-clavicular distance may exceed 13 mm (Fig. 52-9). Surgical stabilisation will be required. Detecting the difference between a grade 2 and grade 3 injury may be facilitated if the affected limb is made to weight bear using weights strapped to the wrist to distract the AC joint. More recently direct visualisation of the ligaments by MRI has been suggested.[6]

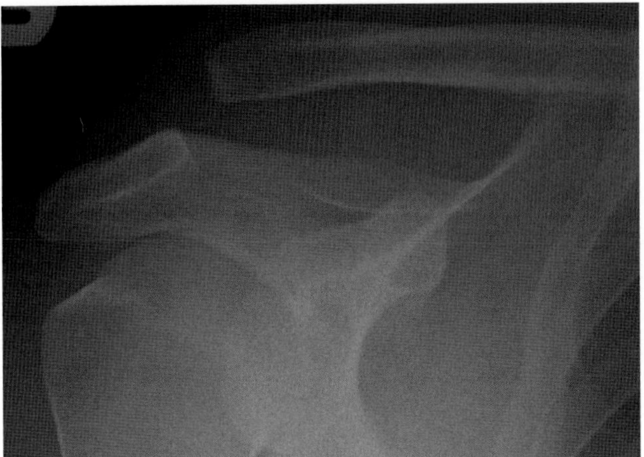

FIGURE 52-9 ■ Grade 3 injury. Distance from coracoid to clavicle is in excess of 13 mm. The coraco-clavicular ligaments will be disrupted and surgical fixation is needed.

THE ELBOW

There are no variations in the standard views of the elbow which are the AP and lateral.

A useful soft-tissue sign in the elbow is the fat pad sign.[7] The normal elbow has small pads of fat closely applied to the distal humerus both anteriorly and posteriorly. These are not normally visible as they lie within the bony fossae of the distal humerus. However, if there is a joint effusion such as may occur following trauma the fluid displaces the fat pads away from the humerus and out of the fossae. These fat pads can then be identified on a lateral radiograph as lucent areas. The anterior fat pad may just be visible normally but if displaced away from the humerus is abnormal. A visible posterior fat pad is always abnormal. The presence of displaced fat pads indicates an effusion[8] and if a fracture is not readily identified further careful inspection of the radiograph is needed to exclude a more subtle fracture which may have been overlooked (Fig. 52-10). In children, a supracondylar fracture is the commonest lesion to be overlooked; in adults, a radial head fracture. Note, however, that the absence of the fat pad sign does not exclude a fracture and effusions are not always caused by trauma.

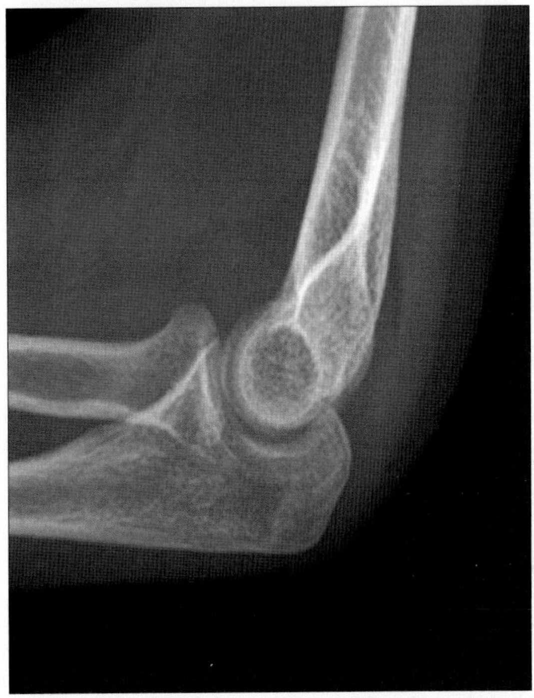

FIGURE 52-10 ■ **Displaced fat pads are visible both anterior and posterior to the humerus.** This indicates that there is a joint effusion. Careful scrutiny of the radiograph is now essential to look for a subtle injury.

Children

Supracondylar fractures are the commonest injury around the elbow in children.[9] Some fractures are grossly displaced with the distal bone fragment displaced posteriorly.The anteriorly displaced humeral shaft often has sharp bone edges which puts the adjacent brachial artery as well as the median and ulnar nerves in jeopardy. However, in 50% they are subtle greenstick-type injuries

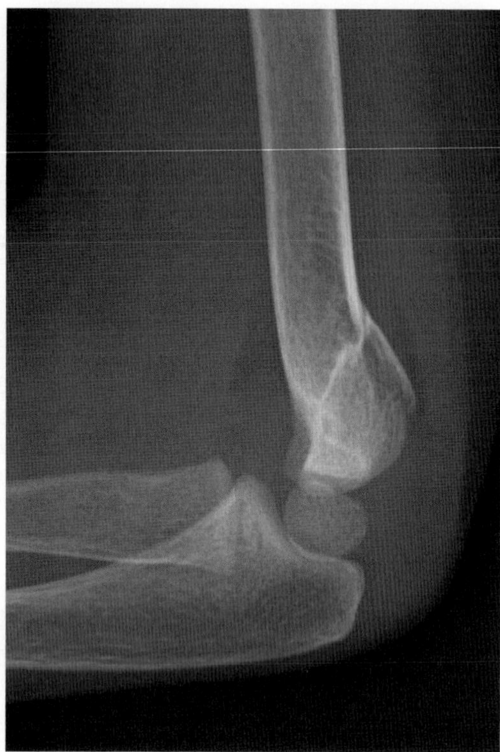

FIGURE 52-11 ■ A subtle supracondylar fracture. This is best identified using the anterior humeral line. A line along the anterior humeral cortex does not pass through the capitellum, which is displaced posterior to the line.

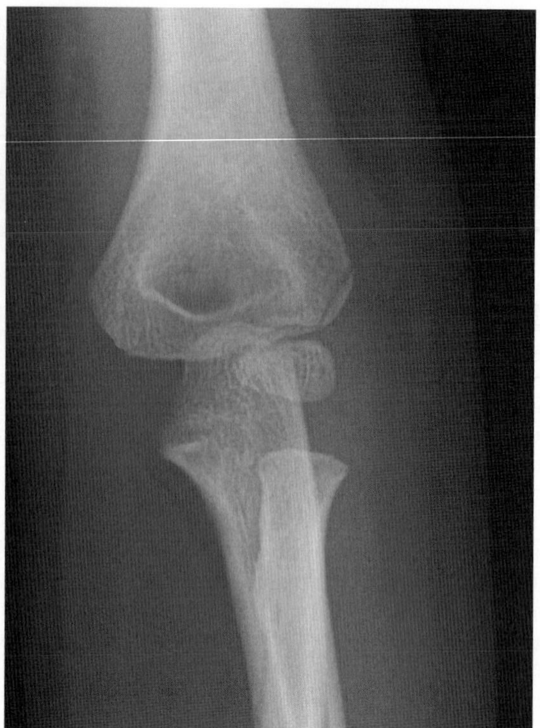

FIGURE 52-12 ■ AP view of child's elbow. A linear lucency is visible at the lateral epicondyle. This represents a fracture and should not be confused with a normal unfused epiphysis. The lateral epiphysis is the last to appear (CRITOL) and as only the capitellum is visible on the radiograph this cannot be the lateral epiphysis and must be a fracture.

(Fig. 52-11). Detection of subtle injuries can be facilitated by using the anterior humeral line.[10] On a lateral radiograph a line drawn down the anterior humeral cortex will pass through the capitellum such that at least one-third of the capitellum lies anterior to the line. If this rule is broken then it is very likely that there is a subtle greenstick or Salter–Harris growth plate injury of the distal humeral, allowing the distal humerus with the attached capitellum to be displaced posteriorly.[11]

The second commonest elbow injury in children is of the lateral condyle.[12] Recognition of these injuries is made difficult by the presence of developing ossification centres in the immature skeleton. There are four in the distal humerus and one each in the radius and ulna. The order of appearance with few exceptions is capitellum, radius, internal epicondyle, trochlea, olecranon, lateral epicondyle—remembered by the mnemonic CRITOL[13] from the first letter of each epiphysis. Knowedge of this order makes it possible to determine whether a bone fragment adjacent to the humerus is a normal ossification centre or represents a fracture. As the lateral epicondyle is the last ossification centre to appear, then if there is a bone fragment adjacent to the lateral aspect of the distal humerus look for the other ossification centres. If it is not possible to identify the five other centres, then the area in question must represent a fracture (Fig. 52-12). It should be noted that although there may only be a small bony component to this injury there will be a large fracture through the growing cartilaginous distal humerus.[14]

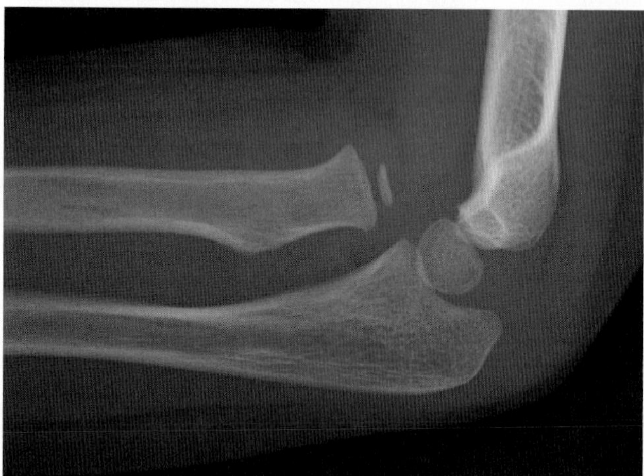

FIGURE 52-13 ■ Lateral adolescent elbow. Fat pads are evident. A line drawn along the proximal radius mid shaft does not pass through the capitellum. The radial head must be dislocated.

Dislocation of the radial head occurs in both children and adults. It may be difficult to appreciate on the AP radiograph but easier on the lateral. A helpful method of detecting these injuries is use of the radio-capitellar line. This line is drawn along the mid shaft of the radius proximal to the tuberosity. It should pass through the capitellum on every view; if not, the radial head is dislocated (Fig. 52-13). This rule is true also in children, although

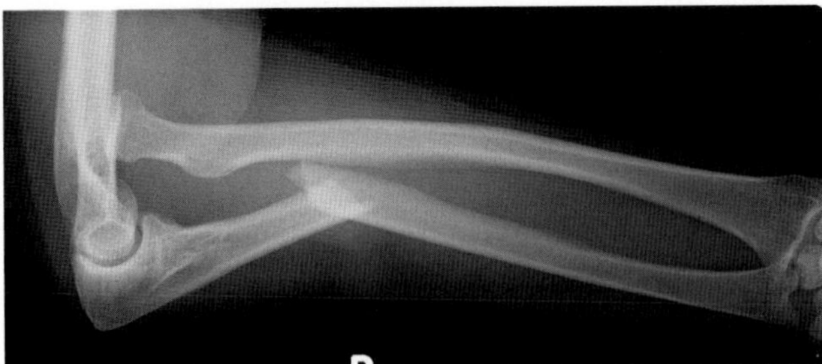

FIGURE 52-14 ■ Radiograph of forearm. There is an obvious fracture of the mid shaft of the ulna with angulation. When this is present there must be an abnormality of the radius. If no fracture is evident, a dislocation of the radial head is almost invariably present, as is the case here. This combination is known as a Monteggia fracture dislocation.

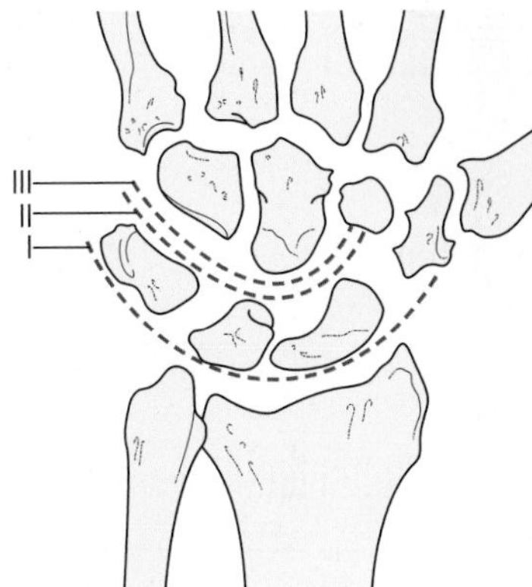

FIGURE 52-15 ■ The carpal arcs.

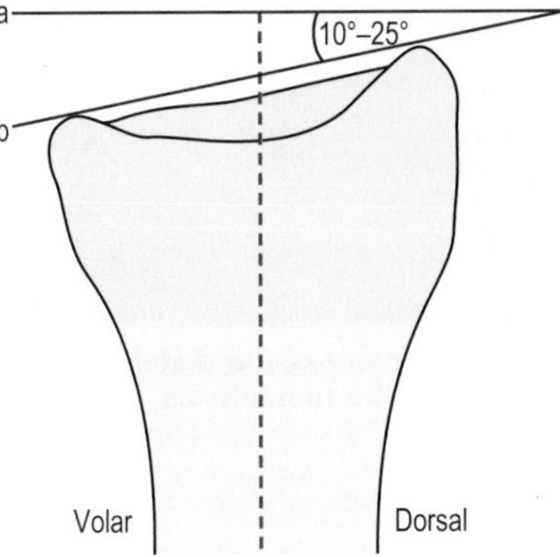

FIGURE 52-16 ■ The normal volar angulation of the distal radius.

care is needed in the very young when the capitellum is small.[15] There is a fracture association which must be recognised. The bones of the forearm are bound strongly at either end by strong ligaments. It is difficult to fracture one of these bones without the other, so fractures of radius and ulna occur commonly together. However, if only one bone appears fractured and, especially if the fracture is angled or overlapped, a covert injury of the other bone is very likely. This typically takes the form of a dislocation of the non-fractured bone. Thus a fracture of the ulnar shaft is often associated with a dislocation of the radial head at the elbow. This is known as a Monteggia fracture dislocation[16,17] (Fig. 52-14). Conversely a radial shaft fracture is associated with a dislocation of the ulna at the wrist. This is known as a Galeazzi fracture dislocation.

Adults

Fractures of the distal humerus in adults rarely cause diagnostic problems. Most fractures are readily apparent. Typically they involve the distal humeral condyles often with inta-articular extension into the elbow joint. Capitellar fractures are uncommon and may be difficult to see on the AP radiograph. The lateral view, however, provides the diagnosis. The displaced capitellum has an appearance like a half moon and is seen lying anterosuperior to the forearm bones. Radial head fractures[18] may involve the radial neck only or may be intra-articular, with disruption of the radial articular surface. The fat pad sign described above is useful in drawing attention to the radial head as a possible site for subtle radial head fracture. The commonest ulnar fracture is of the olecranon.[19] The fracture involves the articular surface with the proximal fracture fragment often displaced due to the unopposed pull of the triceps muscle.

THE WRIST

Standard views for evaluation of the wrist are a postero-antererior (PA) and lateral radiographs. Additional views are required when there is clinical suspicion of a scaphoid fracture.

On an AP radiograph look for the normal uniform spacing of 1–2 mm around each carpal bone and at the carpometacarpal junction. Loss of this spacing should lead to very careful inspection of the abnormal area, as often this will indicate significant carpal or carpometacarpal disruption. One should also observe the arrangement of the carpal bones into three smooth arcs. The first delineates the proximal surface of the proximal row of carpal bones (scaphoid, lunate, triquetral). The second is formed by the distal articular surface of the same bones. The third is along the proximal curvature of the capitate and hamate.[20] These arcs should normally be smooth with no steps or interruption (Fig. 52-15).

On a lateral radiograph the normal distal radius has a volar tilt of approx 10°. This represents the angle between a line drawn along the long axis of the radius and a line drawn from the dorsal to the volar rim of the radius and has a normal range of 2–20° (Fig. 52-16). Alteration of this angle occurs when there is a subtle fracture of the distal radius. Normal relationship of the distal radius and carpal bones is best assessed on the lateral view and this is discussed further in the section on carpal injuries. Displacement of the distal radial epiphysis and disruption of carpal alignment are often only evident on this view. Fractures of the triquetral will usually only be seen on the lateral radiograph. From the above it can be seen that the lateral radiograph is of critical importance in assessing wrist injuries.

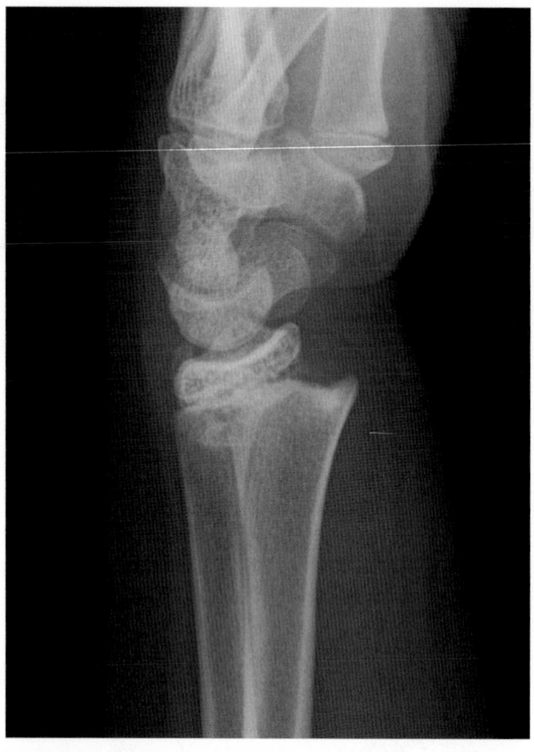

FIGURE 52-17 ■ Displacement of the distal radial epiphysis with a small fragment from the metaphysis. This is a Salter–Harris type 2 fracture.

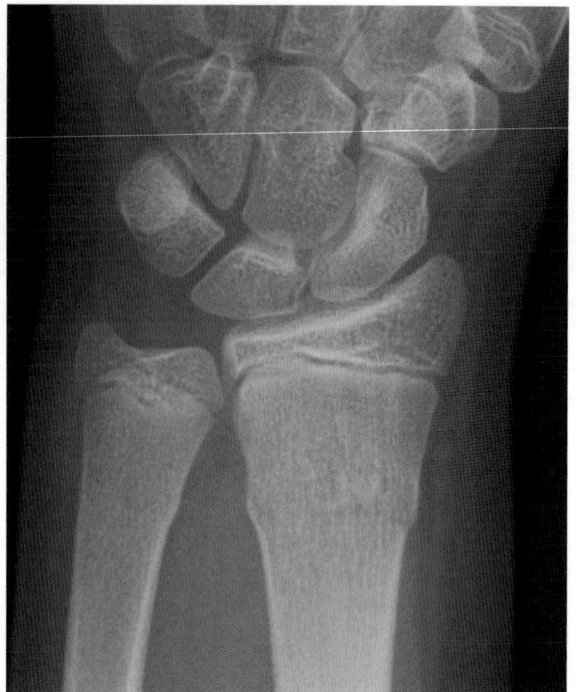

FIGURE 52-18 ■ A buckling of the radial cortex, which indicates a torus injury.

Radius and Ulna

Most commonly, injuries result from a fall on the outstretched wrist. The type of injury sustained is age related.

Children

In young children fractures of the radius proximal to the epiphyseal plate predominate in age group 6–10. These fractures often involve both radius and ulna and may be grossly displaced. After this, until epiphyseal fusion, injuries most commonly involve the epiphyseal plate and are thus Salter–Harris fractures.[9] Typically there is dorsal displacement of the epiphysis with or without an associated fracture fragment from the adjacent metaphysis, resulting in either a Salter–Harris type 1 or 2 injury (Fig. 52-17). Greenstick and buckle or torus fractures of the radius occur only in children (Fig. 52-18).

Adults

Distal radial fracture (Fig. 52-19) is the commonest wrist injury in patients over age of 40.[21] Increasing frequency with age suggests a relationship to osteoporosis. The definition of a Colles' fracture includes the following: (1) fracture of radius within 2 cm of distal radial articular surface but not involving it; (2) dorsal angulation or displacement of distal fragment; and (3) associated fracture of ulnar styloid process. Smith described a variation of the above where the distal radial fragment is displaced and angled volarly and medially. In both of these injuries the articular surface remains intact (Fig. 52-20).

Barton's fracture differs from the above due to involvement of the articular surface of the radius. It is a shearing injury through the articular surface.The term is now often incorrectly ascribed to any intra-articular fracture.

Subtle radial fractures may be detected by observing a minor disruption of the dorsal radius cortex on the lateral radiograph and alteration in the radial angle from the usual 10° volar (Fig. 52-21).

Isolated fracture of the radial styloid process, also known as Hutchinson's or chauffeur's fracture, refers to an intra-articular fracture which runs obliquely across the distal radius from the radial cortex into the joint separating the radial styloid from the parent bone.

Many fractures do not conform exactly with the original descriptions, with combination injuries common. For this reason, rather than using the eponymous names it is better to give a full description of the fracture lines, fragment displacement and angulation and extent of articular involvement.

Carpal Injuries

The scaphoid accounts for at least 60% of all carpal fractures.[21] Typically, when scaphoid injury is suspected, one or two additional radiographic projections are employed with the intention of elongating the scaphoid, projecting it clear of other carpal bones and allowing the X-ray beam to pass through the scaphoid perpendicular

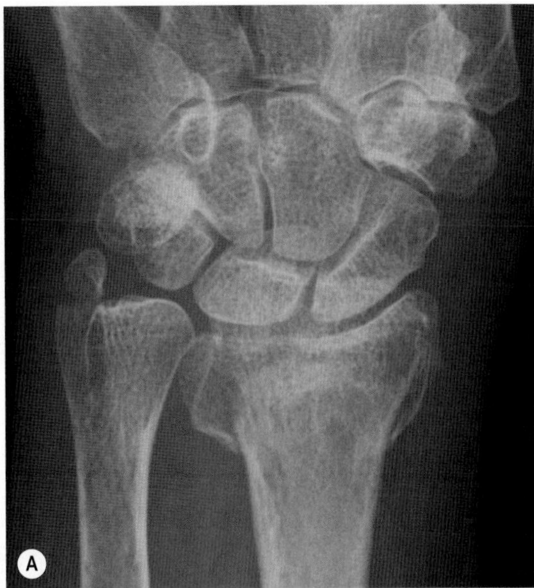

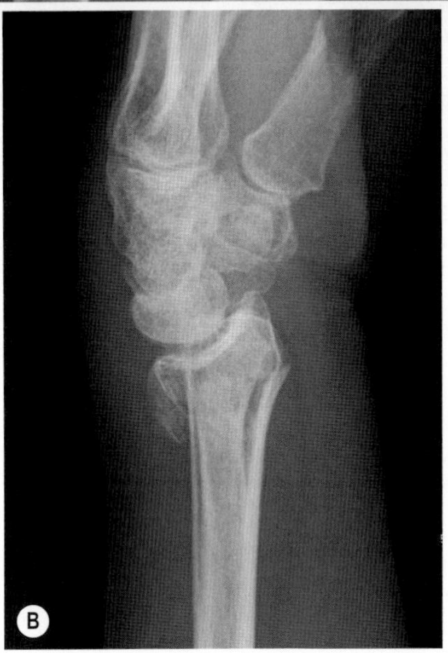

FIGURE 52-19 ■ (A, B) A fracture of the distal radius, which on the lateral is displaced dorsally. There is an associated fracture of the ulnar styloid. There is no intra-articular involvement. This is a Colles' fracture.

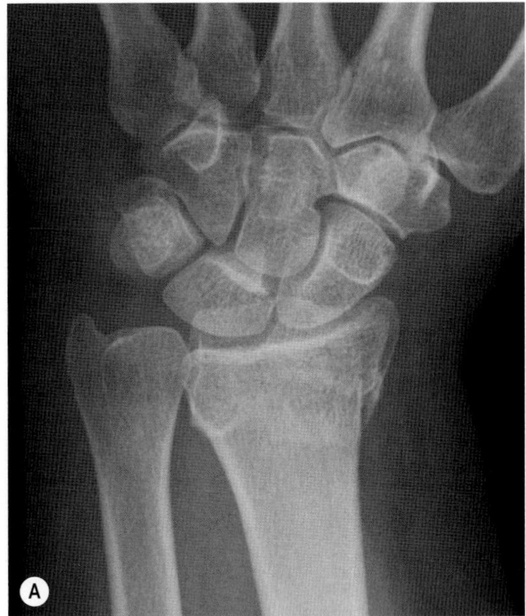

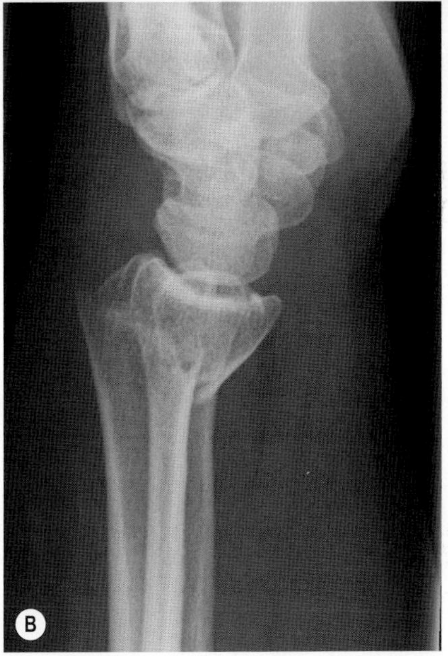

FIGURE 52-20 ■ (A, B) Distal radial fracture with volar displacement and no intra-articular involvement. This is a Smith's type fracture. The appearances on the AP view are virtually identical to a Colles' fracture.

to its long axis. The projections used vary but in the authors' department a second PA view with ulnar deviation plus one with the tube angled at 45° toward the elbow is obtained.

The blood supply of the scaphoid is unusual, with arteries entering distally then passing proximally to supply the rest of the scaphoid. When a fracture occurs through the waist (middle third) of the scaphoid, which is the commonest site (80% of cases), the blood supply to the proximal pole is interrupted. This results in significant risk of avascular necrosis of the proximal pole or non-union of the fracture (Fig. 52-22).

Contrary to common belief, the great majority of fractures are visible on initial radiographs.[22] Nevertheless there are a small number not identified. Accordingly, because of the risk of avascular necrosis and non-union, the patient is managed as if a fracture is present and the wrist is immobilised. The patient is then reviewed at about 10 days when further radiographs are obtained[23,24] in the belief that resorption will occur around a fracture site rendering it visible on delayed radiographs, although this is now questioned. Alternative imaging techniques are now increasingly utilised. Skeletal scintigraphy is sensitive but non-specific. MRI is now the investigation of choice and there is good evidence that this should be undertaken soon after the initial injury[25] (Fig. 52-23).

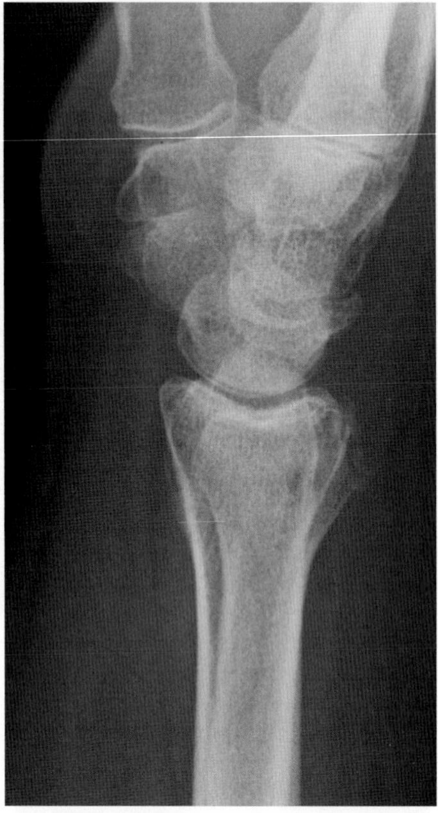

FIGURE 52-21 ■ **Subtle radial fracture.** There is subtle disruption of the posterior radial cortex, indicating an impacted radial fracture. The normal volar tilt of the distal radius is lost.

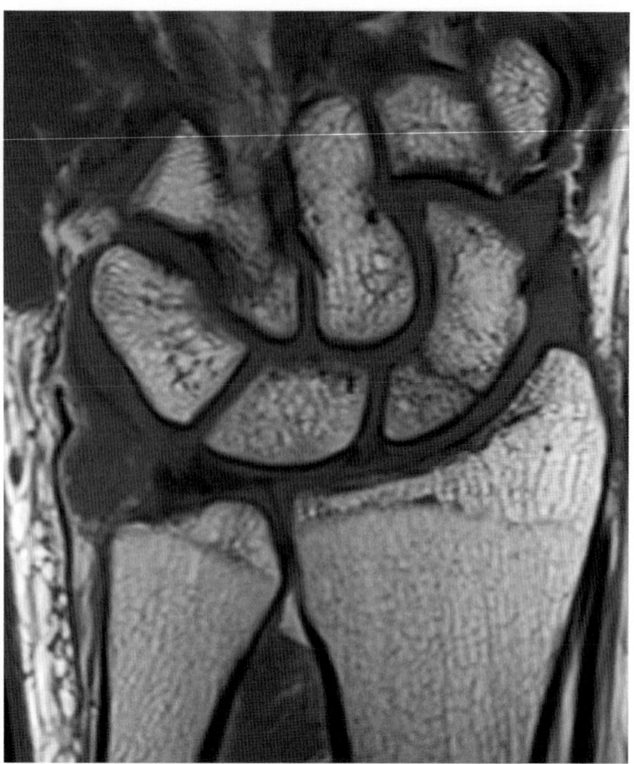

FIGURE 52-23 ■ **MRI of wrist.** There is a fracture through the proximal pole of the scaphoid. No fracture was visible on plain radiographs.

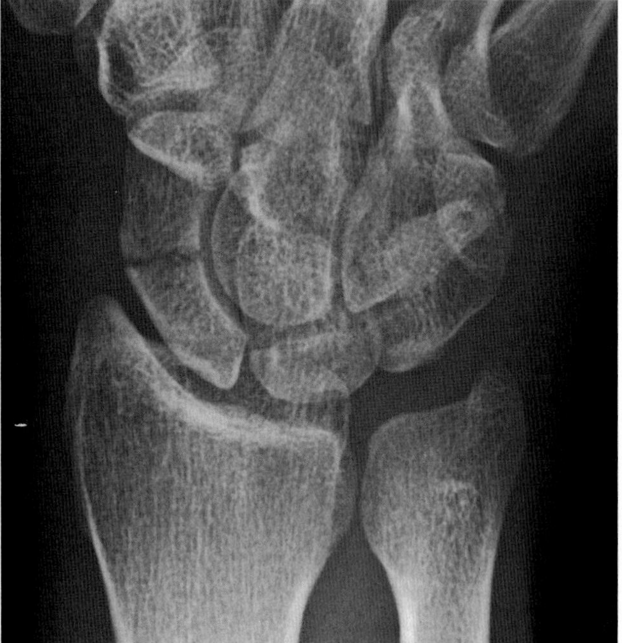

FIGURE 52-22 ■ **Scaphoid fracture.** There is a fracture through the waist of the scaphoid. This is highly likely to interrupt the blood supply to the proximal pole.

TABLE 52-1 Relative Incidence of Carpal Bone Fractures

Scaphoid	68.2%
Triquetrum	18.3%
Trapezium	4.3%
Lunate	3.9%
Capitate	1.9%
Hamate	1.7%
Pisiform	1.3%
Trapezoid	0.4%

After the scaphoid the triquetral is the most commonly injured carpal bone, accounting for 18–20% of injuries[26] (Table 52-1). Typically the fracture is not evident on the PA view but can be seen on the lateral as a bone fragment seen on the dorsal aspect of the wrist (Fig. 52-24). Other carpal bone injuries are all relatively rare, each of the other carpal bone accounting for only 2–3% of injuries. CT or MR has a useful role to play in these injuries, which are often difficult to detect on plain radiography.

Most carpal fractures and dislocations are caused by falling on the outstretched wrist with the wrist forced into an hyperextended position. Carpal dislocations most commonly involve the lunate.[27] On a PA radiograph the lunate normally has a trapezoid appearance. When it is dislocated, it assumes a triangular shape. There is disruption of the normal carpal arcs and the intercarpal

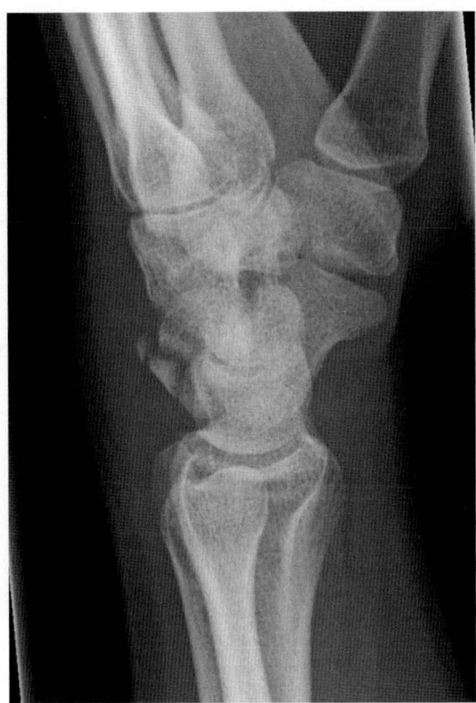

FIGURE 52-24 ■ **Small bone fragments are visible on the dorsum of the wrist.** These indicate a triquetral fracture; there was no abnormality on the AP view.

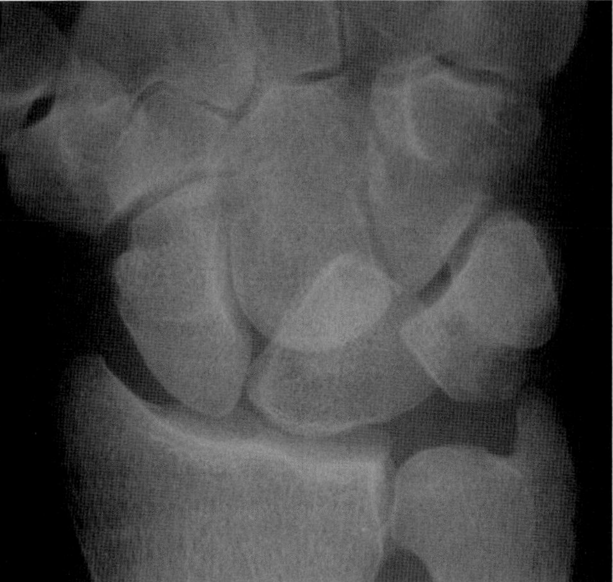

FIGURE 52-25 ■ The lunate has a triangular shape and there is disruption of the carpal arcs with loss of the normal intercarpal spaces.

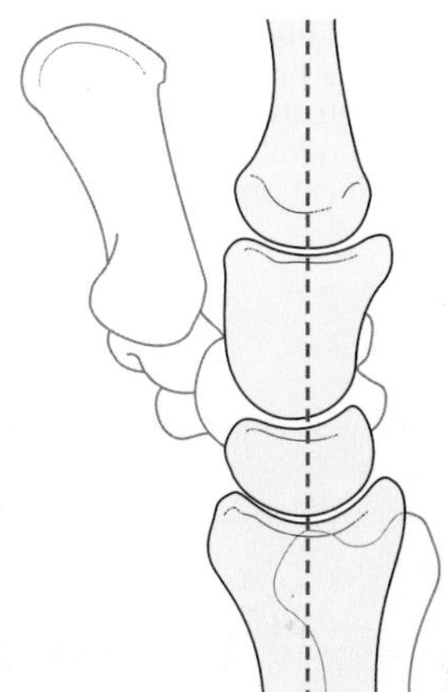

FIGURE 52-26 ■ **Normal alignment of radius, capitate and lunate as seen on a lateral radiograph.**

spaces are lost (Fig. 52-25). It is on the lateral radiograph, however, where the diagnosis is most easily made.[28] On a normal lateral view of the wrist a vertical line drawn through the centre of the lunate should inferiorly pass through the radial articular surface and superiorly should pass through the centre of the capitate (Fig. 52-26). If this rule is broken, a carpal dislocation is certain (Fig. 52-27). Lunate dislocation is most commonly an isolated finding. The lunate will be seen displaced volar to the line. Perilunate dislocation is more common and is often associated with other carpal injuries, most commonly a fracture of the scaphoid. In this injury the lunate remains aligned with the radius but the capitate and the rest of the distal carpal row are displaced in a volar direction (Fig. 52-28).

Scapholunate disassociation is also known as rotatory subluxation of the scaphoid.[29] It is a ligamentous injury occurring with forced wrist extension. On plain radiographs the injury can be identified by noting a widening of the intercarpal distance between scaphoid and lunate; the normal gap is < 2 mm; between 2 and 4 mm suggests possible scapholunate disruption; greater than 4 mm indicates disassociation (Fig. 52-29). This is the so-called 'Terry Thomas' sign named after a 1950s comic with a gap between his front teeth.

Injuries of the Metacarpals and Phalanges

Disruption of the carpometacarpal joint may occur in isolation or may be associated with fracture of either the proximal metacarpal or the adjacent carpal bone.[30] Metacarpal fractures when present aid identification of the injury. These injuries can be detected by observation of the loss of the normal space between the distal carpal row and the base of the metacarpals (Fig. 52-30). Where there is suspicion on the standard radiograph series, a lateral of the hand may add further useful information. A common injury is that of fracture dislocation of the fifth metacarpal and this accounts for 50% of single ray dislocations in the hand.[31]

Transverse and spiral fractures of the metacarpals are common. A punch injury will typically result in a moderately angled fracture of the fifth metacarpal head. Intra-articular fractures of the base of the first metacarpal are known as a Bennett's fracture. The tendon of abductor pollicis longus attaches to the larger fragment, which will tend to displace the fracture unless it is treated with fixation (Fig. 52-31).

Most fractures of the metacarpal and phalanges are apparent on radiographs. There are three fracture types

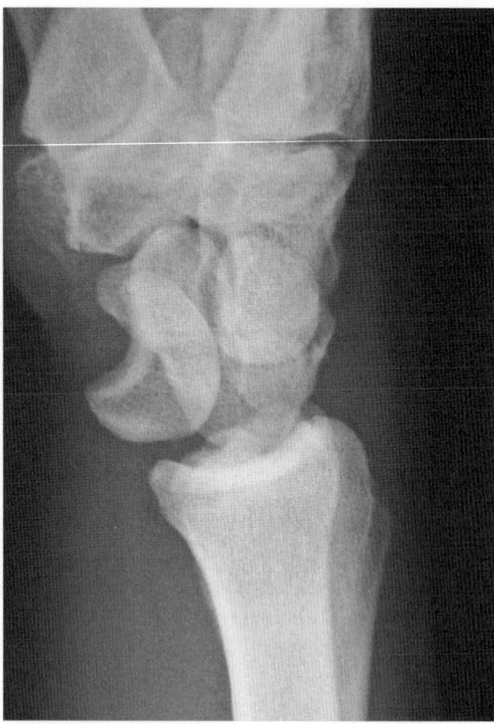

FIGURE 52-27 ■ The lateral view of the carpal injury depicted in Fig. 52-25. The lunate has been displaced volarly. The capitate no longer articulates with the lunate. The radius and capitate are in alignment. The lunate is rotated volarly. These are the features of a lunate dislocation.

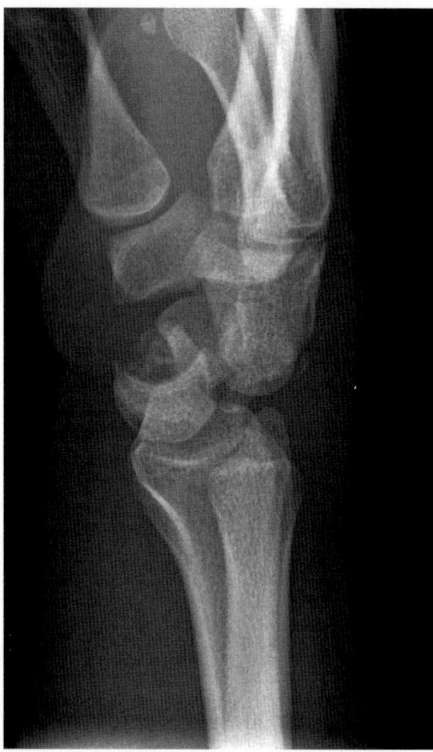

FIGURE 52-28 ■ Perilunate dislocation. Lateral view shows normal alignment of the radius and lunate but the capitate does not articulate with the lunate and lies dorsally. The AP view showed loss of carpal arcs and intercarpal spaces. There were also fractures of the waist of the scaphoid and triquetral. Perilunate dislocation is often associated with additional carpal fractures.

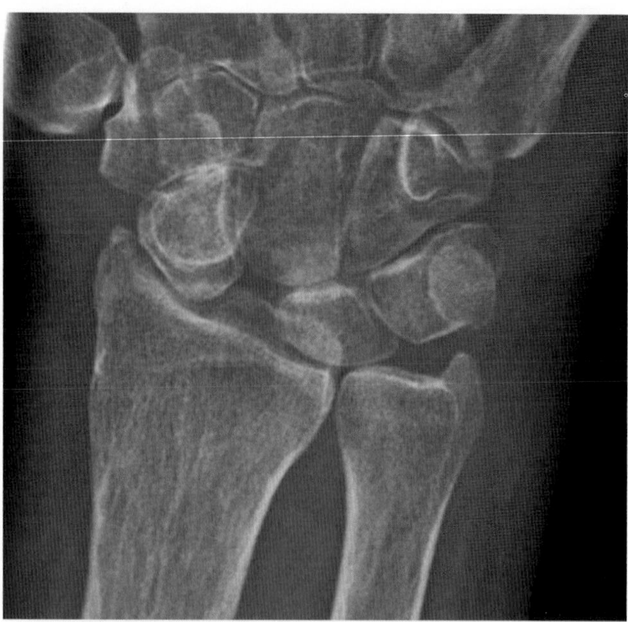

FIGURE 52-29 ■ Widening of the gap between the lunate and the scaphoid, indicating ligament disruption.

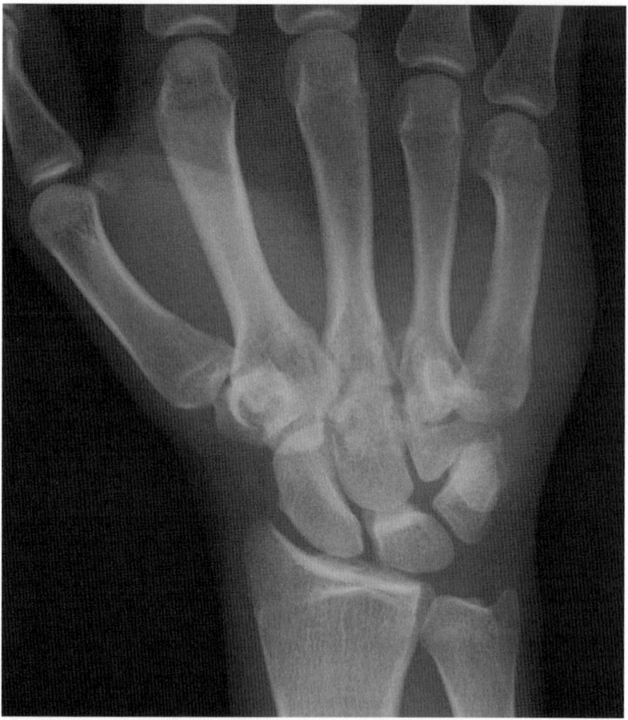

FIGURE 52-30 ■ AP view of wrist. There is loss of the normal spaces between the bases of the fourth and fifth metacarpals and the adjacent hamate. This indicates dislocation at the carpometacarpal junction.

worthy of particular consideration.[32] In all of these the severity and need for surgical intervention are related to the size of the fracture fragment and the extent of articular involvement.

Condylar fractures involve the articular surface of a phalanx, usually distally. These fractures will often require surgical intervention and all should be referred for specialist assessment.

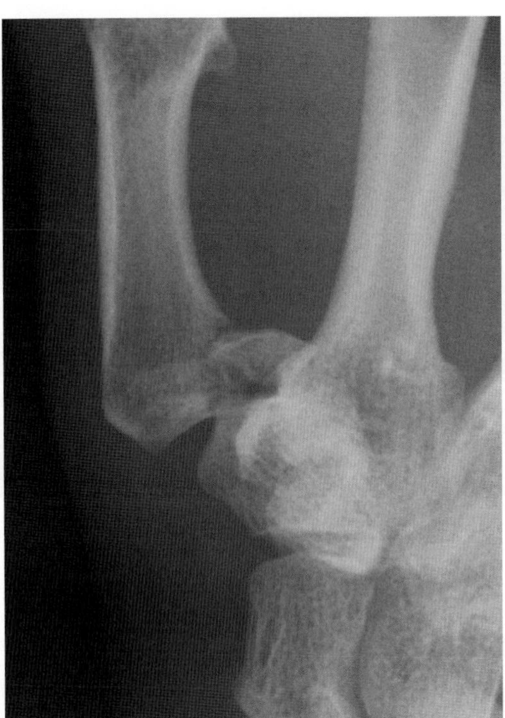

FIGURE 52-31 ■ **Bennett's fracture.** There is an intra-articular fracture of the base of the first metacarpal. The extensor pollicis longus tendon inserts onto the base of the main portion of the metacarpal and will distract and displace the fracture, rendering it unstable. Surgical fixation will be required.

Fractures at the proximal interphalageal joints on the volar aspect are due to avulsions by the volar plate, which is a fibrocartilaginous thickening of the joint capsule.

Articular fractures of the dorsal aspect of the distal phalanges involve the insertion of the extensor tendon, resulting in a mallet finger. A mallet finger deformity is very hard to produce by radiographic positioning alone and patients with a mallet deformity without a fracture frequently have extensor tendon disruption.

Many avulsion injuries of the ulnar collateral ligament of the thumb are soft-tissue ligament injuries only; however, in some cases the ligament avulses a bone fragment from the base of the proximal phalanx (Fig. 52-32). These fractures often occur in skiers, as the thumb is caught in the ski pole straps during a fall, causing hyperextension and twisting, and hence are sometimes referred to as skier's thumb.[33]

PELVIC AND ACETABULAR FRACTURES

Introduction

Fractures of the pelvic ring and acetabulum in young patients are predominantly high-energy injuries and frequently result in visceral injuries which contribute to the associated mortality and morbidity. Recognition of the patterns of pelvic ring injury informs the application of appropriate corrective forces and internal fixation in their treatment. The likelihood of life-threatening pelvic haemorrhage and bladder injury can also be surmised if the severity of the pelvic ring injury is appreciated.

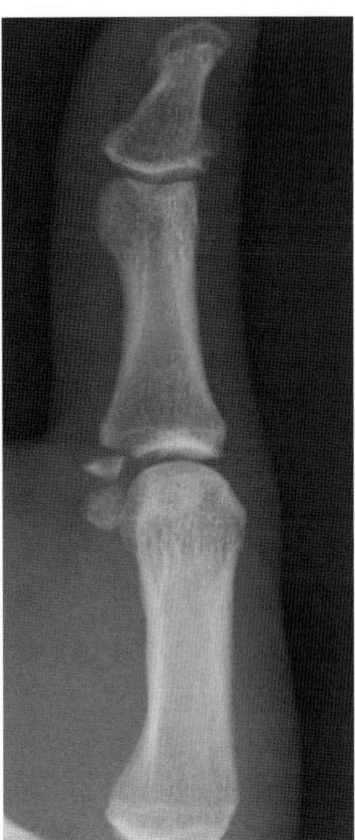

FIGURE 52-32 ■ **AP of thumb.** There is a bone fragment on the ulnar aspect of the base of the proximal phalanx. This indicates an avulsion injury at the insertion of the ulnar collateral ligament. Most of these injuries, however, are ligamentous only, with no bony involvement, and are diagnosed on clinical grounds or with MR.

Acetabular fractures have been classified by Judet and Letournel into five simple and complex types which require an awareness of acetabular anatomy and determine the surgical approach to reduction and fixation. Dependence on standard and oblique (Judet view) radiographs has recently been superseded by computed tomography (CT), with reconstructions that require a practical knowledge by the reporting radiologist. A number of CT features are important in separating fractures that require operative intervention from those that can be managed conservatively.

Avulsion injuries commonly occur in athletes, and affect the apophyseal regions in patients with an immature skeleton. Stress or repetitive injuries can also occur at the tendon insertions but are increasingly seen in the pelvic ring, acetabulum and sacrum as a result of increased sporting activity and more widespread diagnostic application of MRI. Older patients are also prone to pelvic ring injuries in the form of insufficiency fractures consequent upon underlying osteoporosis. This is particularly prevalent following pelvic irradiation.

Pelvic Ring Fractures

Anatomy

The pelvic ring constitutes the sacrum and the two innominate bones which are formed by the fusion of the ilium, ischium and pubic bones. The sacrum and innominate bones are stabilised by ligaments which are important to our understanding of pelvic injury as instability can occur in the absence of fracture as a result of ligamentous disruption. Posteriorly the sacroiliac joints are stabilised by the anterior and posterior sacroiliac ligaments, the latter being amongst the body's strongest ligaments. In the central pelvis the sacrospinous and sacroischial ligaments restrain external rotation of the innominate bones and anteriorly the superior symphyseal ligaments prevent diastasis of the symphysis. The weakest part of the pelvic ring is the anterior pelvis; hence, nearly all injuries disrupt the pubic rami or symphysis initially. Posterior pelvic disruption only occurs after the symphysis is disputed or the rami fractured.

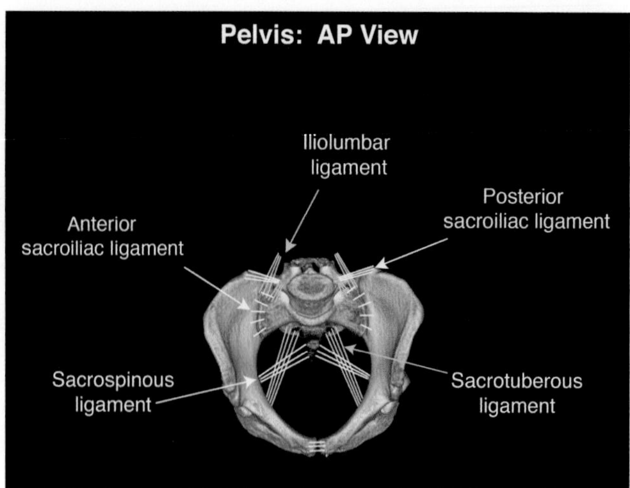

FIGURE 52-33 ■ **Diagramatic representation of the pelvic ring, identifying the primary pelvic ligaments.**

Classification

Previous descriptions of pelvic injury have been eponymous (Malgaine fracture), encompassed presumed mechanism of injury (straddle fracture), or described the fracture appearance (open book), but these descriptions are not systematic and have been replaced with a classification borne out of the increased understanding of such injuries through the experience gained in American trauma centres.

Pennal first recognised the correlation between specific forces applied to the pelvis and patterns of fracture.[34] Subsequently, Tile in 1984 reported the increased risk of haemorrhage with the more severe injuries[35] and finally in 1986 Young and Burgess refined the classification by describing the progression of failure that occurs with particular forces.[36] They described three main patterns of fracture resulting from anterior-posterior compression (APC), lateral compression (LC) and vertical shear (VS) forces. A fourth group with hybrid appearances was described as complex (Fig. 52-33).

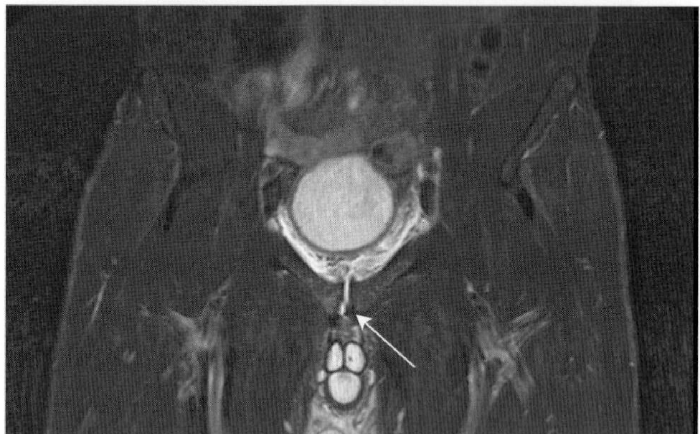

FIGURE 52-34 ■ AP type 1 pelvic ring injury, demonstrating symphyseal diastasis (arrow) and disruption of the symphyseal ligaments.

Anterior Compression Injuries. These injuries commonly occur during head-on collision when forces are applied in the AP plane. The least severe AP pattern of injury, the AP type 1 injury, comprises symphyseal diastasis (<2.5 cm) (Fig. 52-34) and vertical pubic rami fractures. The vertical pattern distinguishes the AP pattern from the oblique/communicated pattern in LC injuries. No significant ligament injury is encountered in AP type 1 injuries, because the pelvis is essentially stable.

AP type 2 injuries demonstrate progressive widening of the symphysis (>2.5 cm) or fracture lines consequent upon disruption of the sacroiliac, sacrotuberous and anterior sacroiliac ligaments. The posterior sacroiliac ligaments are intact. This pattern was previously referred to as the 'open-book' injury, and is unstable to external rotation forces but stable to internal rotation (Fig. 52-35).

AP type 3 injuries include additional posterior sacroiliac ligament disruption, and are unstable to forces in all directions (Fig. 52-36).

The AP type 2 injuries require a symphyseal plate to restore stability while the AP type 3 injuries require anterior and posterior stabilisation.

Lateral Compression (LC) Injury. This is the commonest pattern of injury, accounting for 57% of pelvic ring fractures. There are three types, LC type 1 injuries being the least severe and comprising characteristic oblique or comminuted pubic rami fractures (Fig. 52-37A) or less commonly symphyseal disruption and overlap. Such fractures are usually stable even if associated with minor compression fractures of the anterior rim of the sacroiliac joint.

LC type 2 injuries result from increased force; after the anterior pelvis fails, the innominate bone internally rotates, pivoting on the anterior margin of the sacroiliac joint, disrupting the posterior sacroiliac ligament (LC type 2a) or fracture the iliac blade (LC type 2b). These injuries are unstable to internal rotation forces.

The most severe form of lateral compression injury is the LC type 3 pattern often referred to as the 'roll-over' injury. The side of impact demonstrates the type 2 pattern but the contralateral hemipelvis is externally rotated in the pattern about to be described for AP injuries (Fig. 52-37B).

Vertical Shear. These injuries result from jumping or a fall from a height where the impact is predominantly

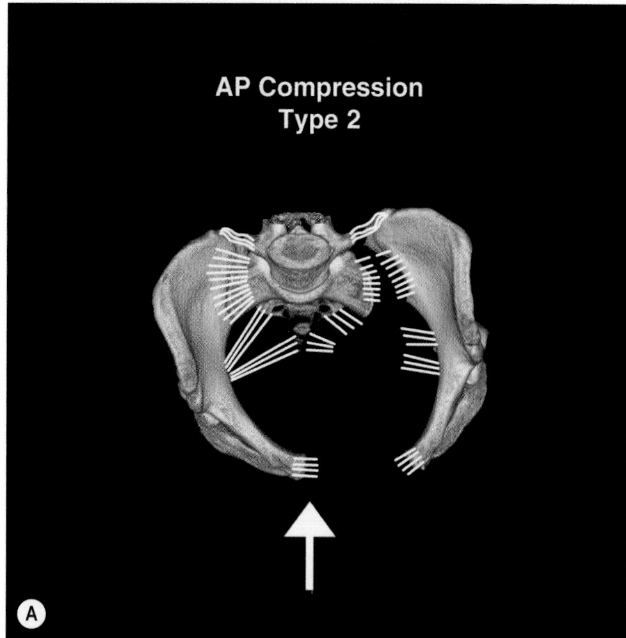

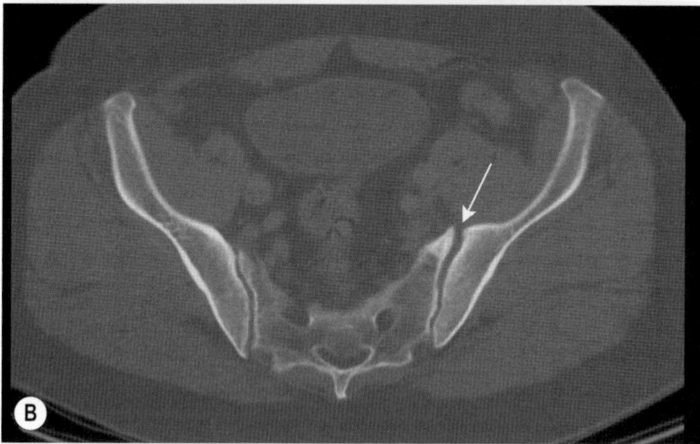

FIGURE 52-35 ■ (A) An AP type 2 pelvic ring injury. Note the disruption of the anterior sacroiliac, sacrospinous and sacrotuberous ligaments. (B) A type 2 pelvic ring injury on axial CT shows a widened anterior joint space in the left sacroiliac joint (arrow); this injury was formerly referred to as an 'open-book' injury.

unilateral. Unlike the AP and LC injuries, the vertical shear injury is of one type, consisting of complete ligamentous disruption, and is associated with multidirectional instability. The pubic rami fractures are vertical, similar to those seen in the AP injuries but the vertical shear injuries demonstrate cephalad displacement on the side of impact (Fig. 52-38).

Complex Injuries. These are uncommon and the majority demonstrate a predominant LC pattern.

Acetabular Fractures

Cross-sectional imaging of acetabular fractures with CT is now standard practice and specialised radiographic views are increasingly an investigation of the past. A good understanding of the three-dimensional anatomy is required to accurately describe and classify these injuries.

Anatomy

The acetabulum comprises a central articular portion which has a cotyloid configuration supported by the arms of an inverted 'Y' created by the anterior and posterior columns. The articular surface has anterior and posterior walls which are identifiable on AP views. The anterior column extends from the superior pubic ramus upward into the iliac blade (Fig. 52-39A), whereas the posterior column is much shorter, running upward from the ischial tuberosity (Fig. 52-39B). The iliopectineal and ilioischial lines define the anterior and posterior columns. The cotyloid articular surface and both columns are connected to the axial skeleton by the sciatic strut or buttress.

Classification

The current classification internationally adopted has an anatomical basis which influences the requirement and

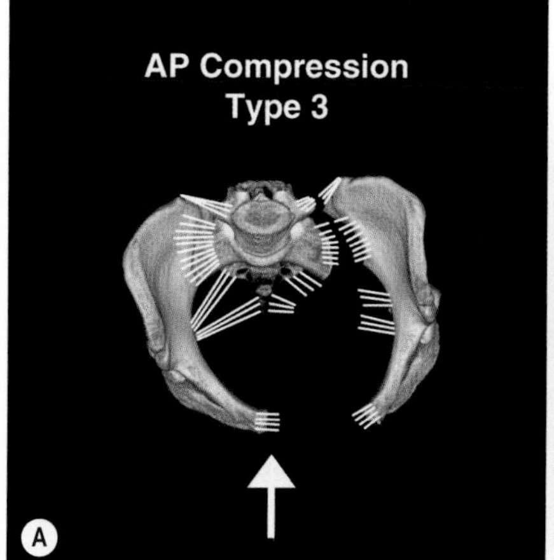

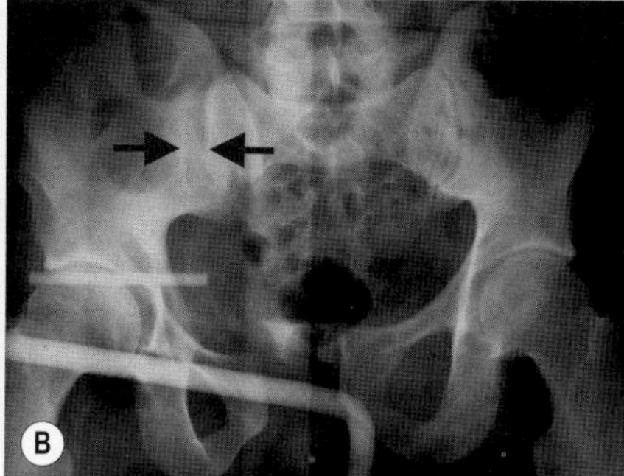

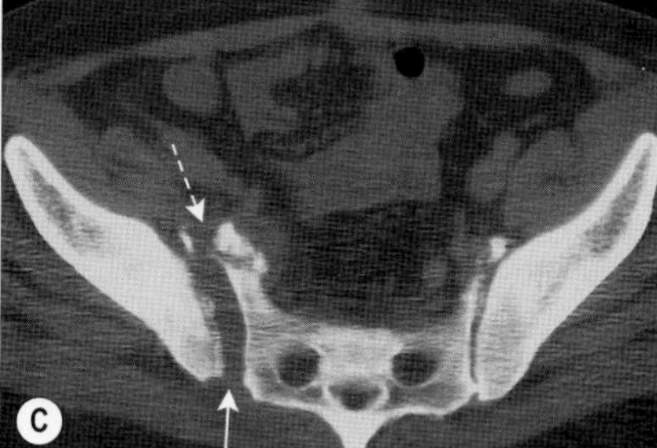

FIGURE 52-36 ■ **AP type 3 pelvic ring injury.** (A) The associated ligamentous disruption: note the disrupted posterior sacroiliac ligament. (B) A widened right sacroiliac joint (arrows): this could represent either an AP type 2 or type 3 based on radiographic appearances; however, the CT in (C) confirms a type 3 injury through the disrupted anterior aspect of the sacroiliac joint (broken arrow) and widened posterior element of the sacroiliac joint resulting from posterior ligament disruption (arrow).

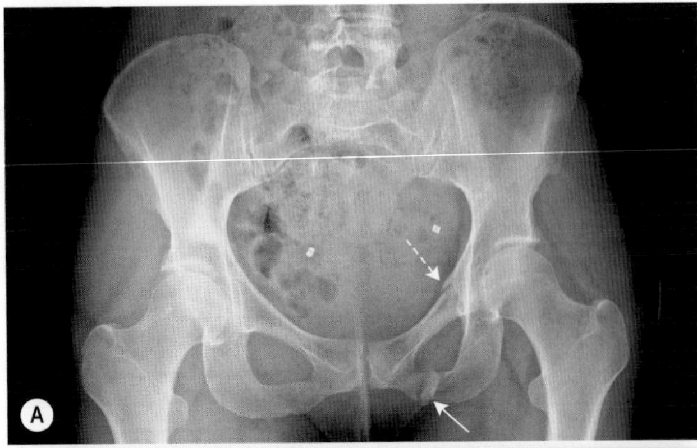

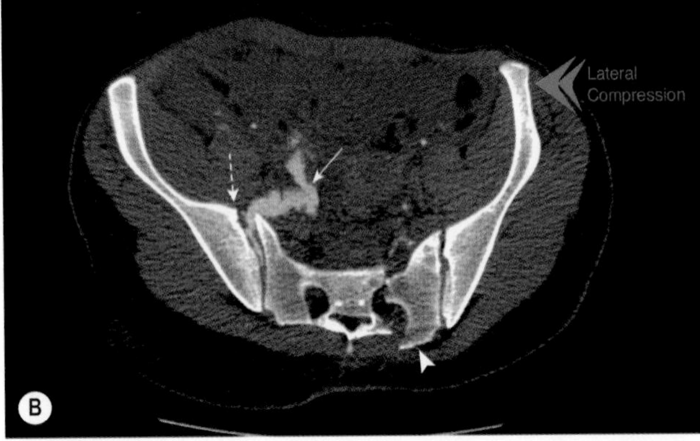

FIGURE 52-37 ■ **Lateral compression injuries.** (A) An LC type 1 injury: the superior pubic ramus fracture has an oblique orientation (broken arrow) and the inferior ramus is a segmental fracture pattern (arrow); no posterior pelvic fractures are evident. (B) A LC type 3 (rollover) injury, lateral compression and internal rotation on the left (arrowhead) and AP type 2 pattern on the right side (broken arrow). Compression fracture of the left sacral ala and active haemorrhage is also demonstrated on this enhanced CT (arrow).

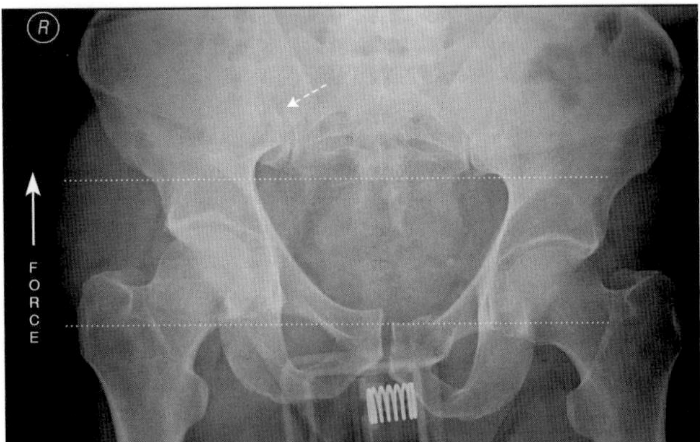

FIGURE 52-38 ■ **Vertical shear injury.** Impact is sustained on the right side, the symphysis and right sacroiliac joint (broken arrow) are disrupted and the right hemipelvis is displaced cephalad.

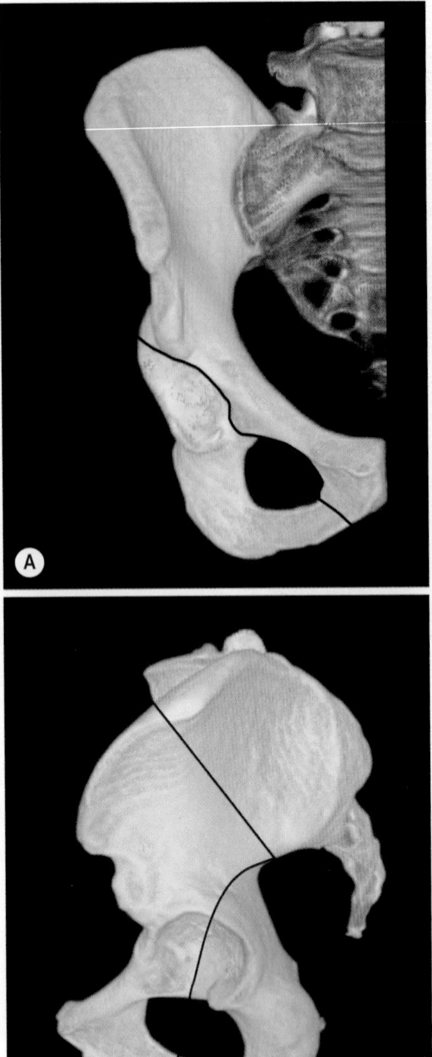

FIGURE 52-39 ■ **Acetabular anatomy.** (A) The anterior (blue) and posterior (yellow) columns coloured on a surface-rendered CT. (B) The columnar anatomy on a surface-rendered lateral projection, anterior column (blue) and posterior column (pink).

approach to surgical repair. The system of classification was first devised in 1964 by Judet[37] and later refined by his colleague Letournel.[38] Five basic or elementary patterns account for the majority of fractures in this classification and comprise, anterior wall, posterior wall, anterior column, posterior column and transverse fractures (Fig. 52-40). Complex patterns represent combinations of the elementary patterns. Common complex injuries include bicolumn, T-shaped and column injuries associated with posterior wall fractures.

Elemetary Patterns

Anterior Wall Fractures. A rare injury is often incorrectly reported when fractures involve the lateral aspect of the superior pubic ramus. These injuries in isolation are rarely displaced, do not involve a major load-bearing surface and are usually managed conservatively.

Posterior Wall Fractures. Posterior wall fractures are amongst the commonest types of acetabular injury and are commonly sustained during head-on collisions when

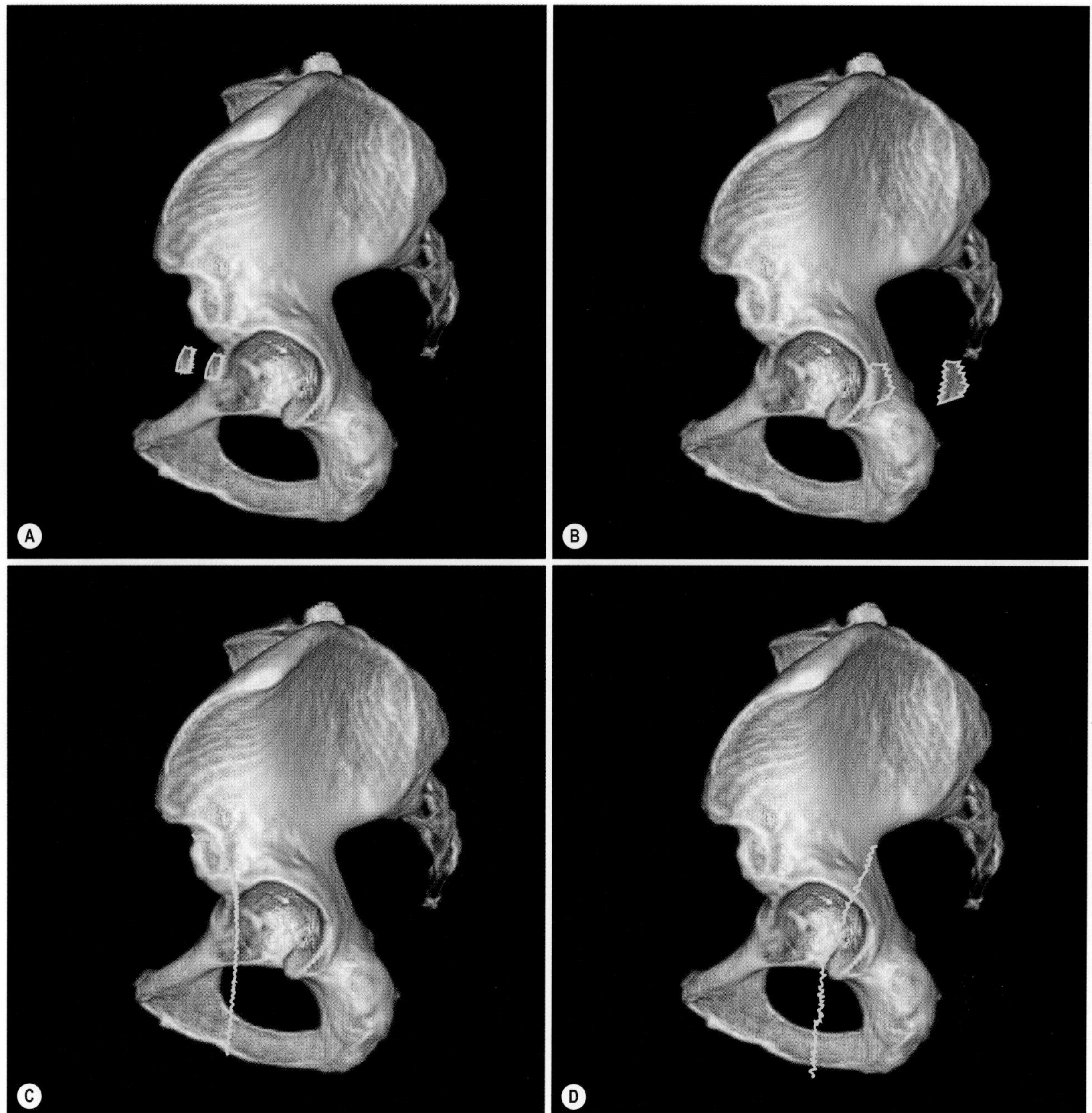

FIGURE 52-40 ■ Elementary patterns of acetabular fractures, Judet and Letournel classification. (A) Anterior wall fracture. (B) Posterior wall fracture. (C) Anterior column injury. (D) Posterior wall fracture.

the force along the femur in a seated individual is directed through the posterior wall, which fractures and the femoral head occasionally dislocates. The posterior wall fracture can be appreciated on the AP view but CT defines its size and displacement with or without impaction, which influences the need to reduce and fix the posterior wall (Fig. 52-41). Fractures accounting for more than 40% of the posterior wall depth will require internal fixation, as will impacted fragments.

Anterior and Posterior Column Fractures. Column fractures have a coronal fracture plane which cleaves the acetabulum into anterior and posterior segments. Both extend through the obturator ring, a prerequisite for a column injury (Fig. 52-42). The anterior column extends anteriorly cephalad to the acetabulum, disrupting the iliopectineal line, whereas the posterior column injury extends posteriorly, disrupting the ilioischial line.

Transverse Fractures. Transverse fractures run across the acetabulum, splitting it into upper and lower halves. The ilioischial and iliopectineal lines are disrupted, but the obturator ring is intact (excluding a column injury; Fig. 52-43).

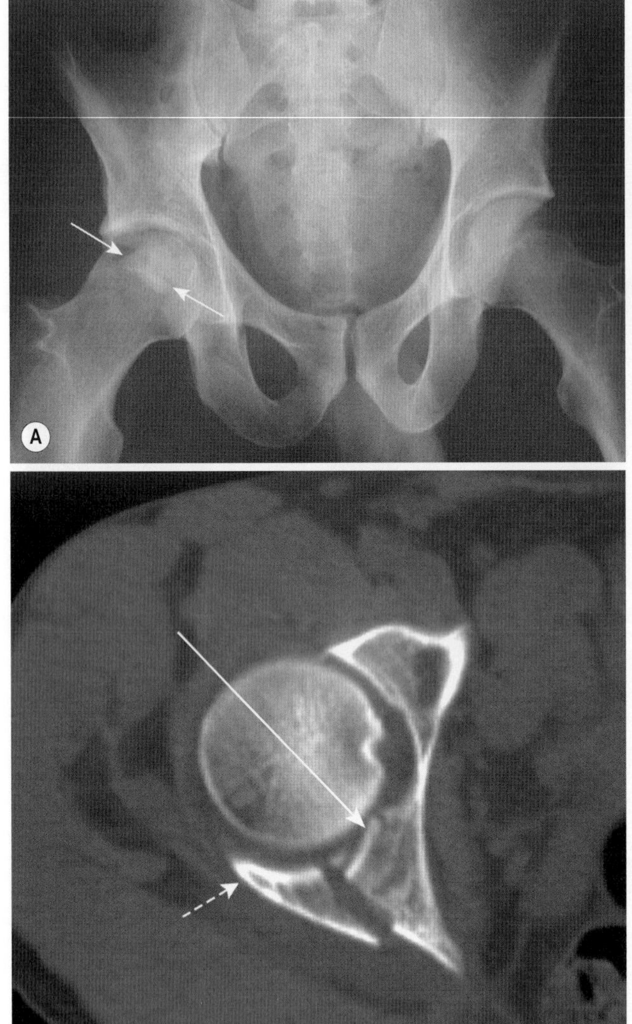

FIGURE 52-41 ■ (A) A posterior wall fracture (arrows). (B) CT of a large posterior wall fracture (broken arrow) (>40%) requiring surgical fixation with an associated impaction fracture (arrow).

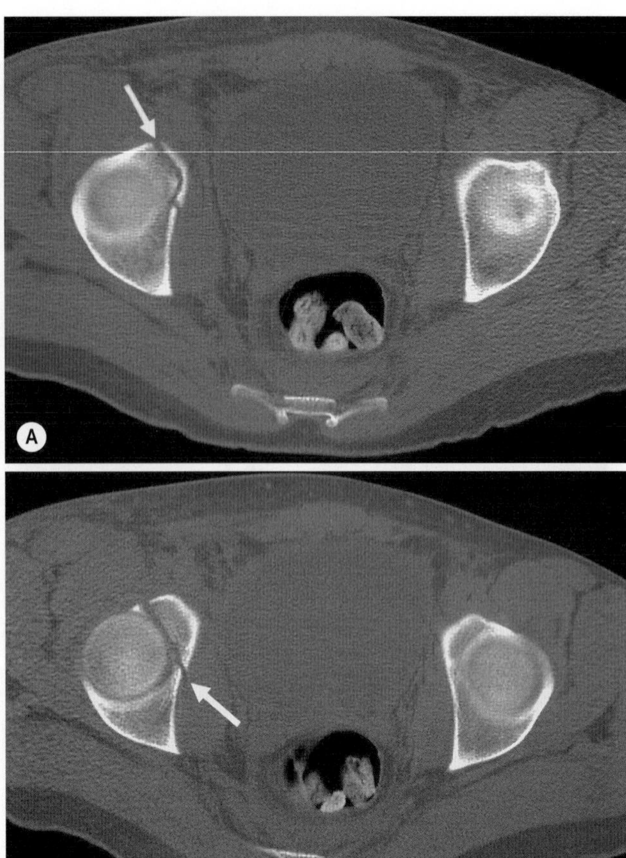

FIGURE 52-42 ■ (A, B) Sequential CT images demonstrating an anterior column fracture, extending from anterosuperior downward, splitting the acetabulum into anterior and posterior segments which then extend down through the rami and thus involve the obturator foramen.

Complex Fractures. The T-shaped and bicolumn are distinguished by the continuity between the acetabular roof and sciatic strut in T-shaped injuries, whereas the bicolumn injuries have no continuity between these structures; the spur sign refers to the disrupted sciatic strut.

Avulsion Injuries

The immature skeleton and unfused apophyses are particularly prone to injury and avulsion. The commonest sites are the anterosuperior iliac spine (sartorius origin), anteroinferior iliac spine (rectus femoris origin) and the ischial tuberosity (hamstring origin; Fig. 52-44).

These injuries may be identified on plain radiographs if a thin sliver of bone is avulsed with the apophysis through the line of provisional calcification. Alternatively, ultrasound or MRI may be requested if the plain radiographs are negative and functional disability is

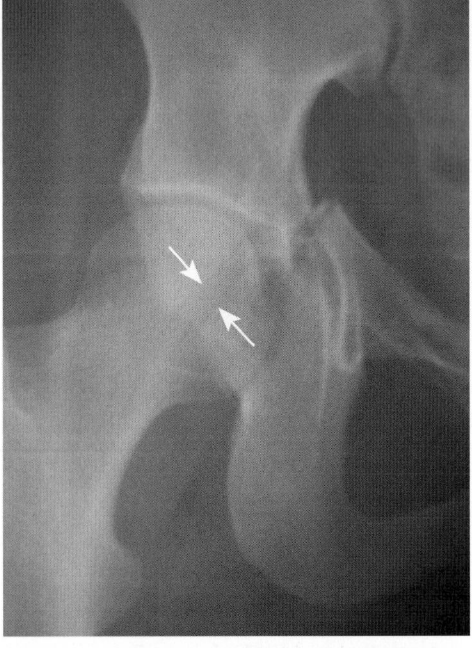

FIGURE 52-43 ■ **A transverse acetabular fracture (arrows) splitting the acetabulum into upper and lower halves.**

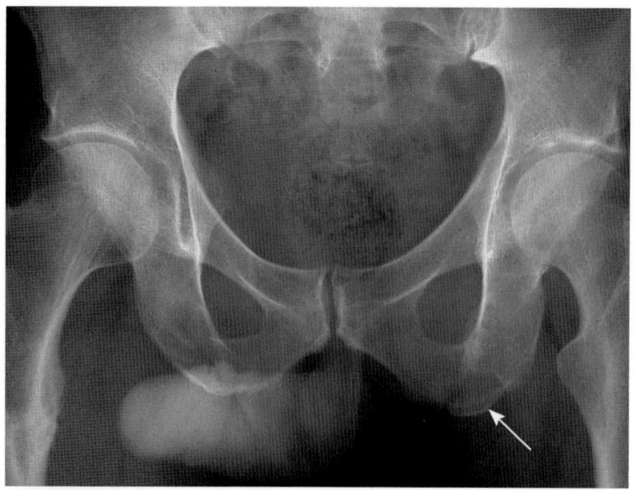

FIGURE 52-44 ■ Hamstring avulsion of the left ischial tuberosity in an adolescent sportsman (arrow).

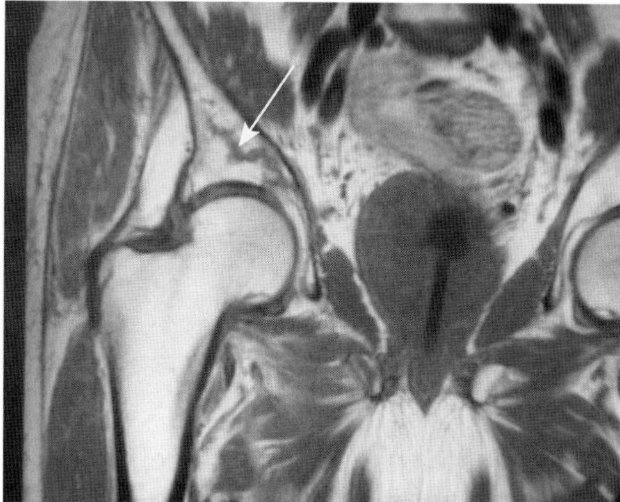

FIGURE 52-45 ■ Incomplete stress fracture (arrow) in the right acetabulum on a T1 spin-echo image, in a 20-year-old Royal Marine.

significant. Surgical repair will be considered for hamstring avulsions.

Insufficiency and Stress Fractures

Stress fractures are sustained through excessive loading, usually but not exclusively during athletic training. The vogue for distance running in particular has precipitated an increase in lower limb stress injuries, including the pelvis. Plain radiographs are usually normal and in these circumstances MRI is the preferred investigation. Stress injuries are usually associated with marrow oedema; this may have a linear orientation and occur anywhere in the pelvic ring (Fig. 52-45). The posterior column of the acetabulum and the sacrum are favoured sites due to their relatively high loading. Sacral fractures or stress reactions often parallel the sacroiliac joint. The fracture line may be identifiable but is often obscured on STIR or fat-saturated sequences and is best demonstrated on T1-SE.

CT, although good at identifying overt fractures, is less capable of identifying stress reactions without a fracture line and does not adequately assess other potential differential diagnoses relating to soft-tissue injury. Nuclear medicine is sensitive at identifying stress injuries but unless the findings are bilateral and symmetric its findings are usually non-specific.

Insufficiency fractures occur when normal loads are applied to a structurally deficient pelvic ring; these fractures are frequently multiple and characteristically are bilateral and relatively symmetric on MRI. This most commonly occurs due to osteoporosis, but other metabolic disorders predisposing to fracture include osteomalacia and parathyroid-related bone disease. Blomlie et al. have also identified insufficiency fractures as occurring in up to 79% of patients receiving radiation therapy for gynaecological malignancy, within 2 years of treatment.[39] The MRI features either resolved or improved within the duration of the study (30 months). MRI is the investigation of choice in elderly patients with pelvic pain where insufficiency fractures are suspected.

Pathological Fractures

Pathological fractures in the pelvis are not uncommon and are most frequently associated with metastatic tumour and myeloma but are also encountered with other disorders, including osteopetrosis and Paget's disease (Fig. 52-46). The diagnosis in metastatic malignancy can be supported by the confirmation of areas of other increased isotope uptake on skeletal scintigraphy. Other processes are also recognised to cause pathological fractures, including osteopetrosis and Paget's disease. Osteolysis associated with fracture can also be encountered in elderly patients following injury to the pubic rami. This process of post-traumatic osteolysis is similar to that recognised in the lateral end of the clavical following injury; it is considered that the absence of load-bearing stress at these sites is a contributory factor. The finding of fractures of the inferior and superior pubic rami is rarely caused by malignancy, helping distinguish tumour from insufficiency fractures. In post-traumatic osteolysis the margins of the fracture appear smooth and well corticated and no bony destruction is seen in the remainder of the pubic ring.

THE HIP

Fracture of the hip is one of the commonest injuries, particularly in elderly patients with osteoporosis. It is the commonest reason for admission to an orthopaedic ward.[40]

The standard view is AP of the pelvis and a lateral of the painful hip. The pelvic radiograph allows comparison of the injured hip with the uninjured side. As these patients will generally be in pain, the lateral radiograph is obtained using the so-called groin lateral projection. This is obtained with a horizontal beam with 20° cephalic angulation centred on the greater trochanter. The opposite thigh is flexed. This does not require any movement by the patient of the painful injured side.

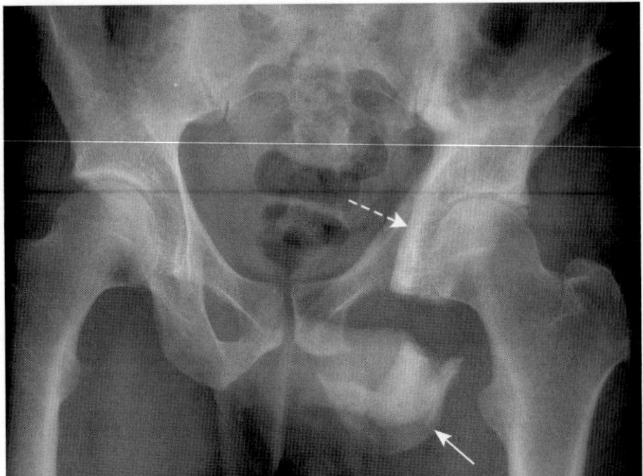

FIGURE 52-46 ■ Pathological fracture through pagetoid left ischial bone (arrow).

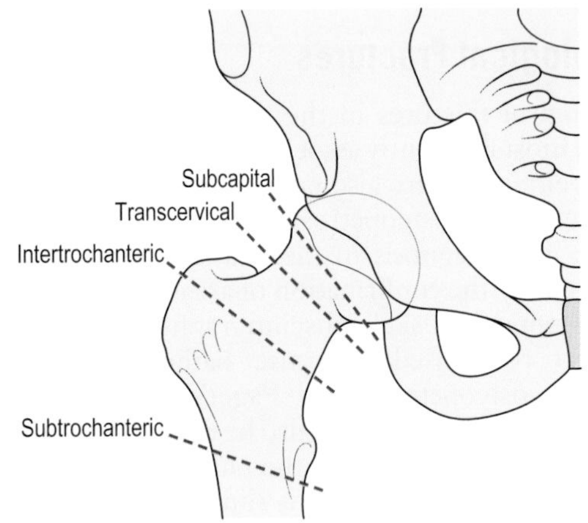

FIGURE 52-47 ■ The sites of proximal femoral fractures.

Fractures are classified by location from subcapital to intertrochanteric (Fig. 52-47). Subcapital and transcervical fractures are intracapsular. The blood supply to the femoral head is derived from recurrent arteries closely applied to the femoral neck. Fractures of the neck and subcapital region interrupt this blood supply, particularly if the fracture is displaced (Fig. 52-48), resulting in avascular necrosis in 15 to 35% of patients. Such fractures are thus treated by hip replacement. Inter- and subtrochanteric fractures are extracapsular and the blood supply is not at risk. These fractures can be treated by plate and dynamic hip screw fixation.

Most fractures are readily apparent but about 15% are difficult to detect. Looking carefully at the trabecular pattern will assist in identifying these: interruption of the trabecular lines indicates a subtle fracture. Impacted undisplaced fractures may be identified by the presence of a sclerotic line and/or interruption of the normal trabecular pattern. Use of the lateral view may be extremely helpful in identifying fractures when there is uncertainty on the AP view (Fig. 52-49).

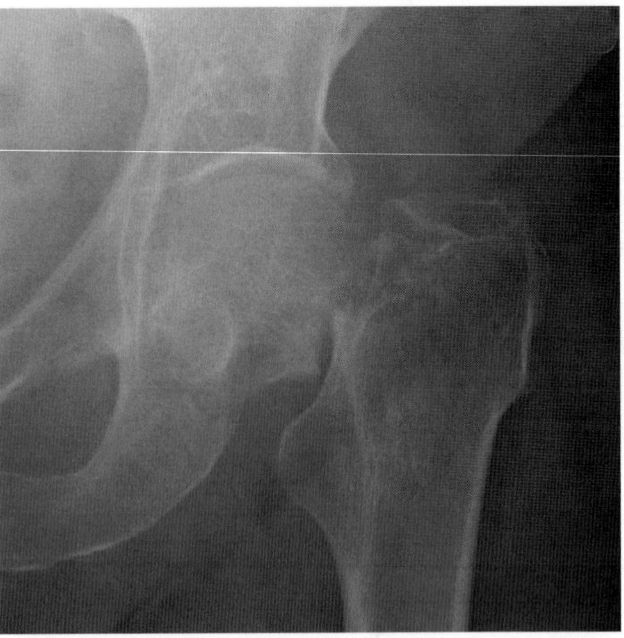

FIGURE 52-48 ■ Displaced subcapital fracture of the femoral neck. The blood supply will almost inevitably be interrupted.

Intertrochanteric fractures, in general, are easier to identify, particularly when severely comminuted (Fig. 52-50), but some fractures may be overlooked when only minimally displaced. Care should be taken when air is trapped in an overlying skin crease. This may mimic a fracture or conversely mask an underlying fracture (Fig. 52-51).

Despite very careful observation, about 1% of fractures are initially occult and cannot be identified on radiographs. If these are not identified and the patient is encouraged to mobilise and weight-bear, then the fracture may become displaced. Because of the risk of subsequent avascular necrosis, great effort must be made to detect these fractures. In the absence of an identifiable fracture on the radiographs, the index of clinical suspicion is used to direct the use of any further investigations. Skeletal scintigraphy can identify occult fractures but may take up to 3 days before it becomes positive; MRI is specific and sensitive and is now the investigation of choice[41,42] (Fig. 52-52).

Hip fractures are often caused by underlying osteoporosis. For this reason, patients under the age of 75 who sustain a hip fracture should be assessed for underlying osteoporosis (usually by DEXA) and treated appropriately.[43]

There are two fractures which may mimic the signs and symptoms of a hip fracture. These are fractures of the pubic rami and greater trochanter. These should be looked for in every patient, but especially when no hip fracture is apparent. If found, they may well account for the patient's symptoms and preclude further investigation for occult fractures. The patient can be advised and managed appropriately.

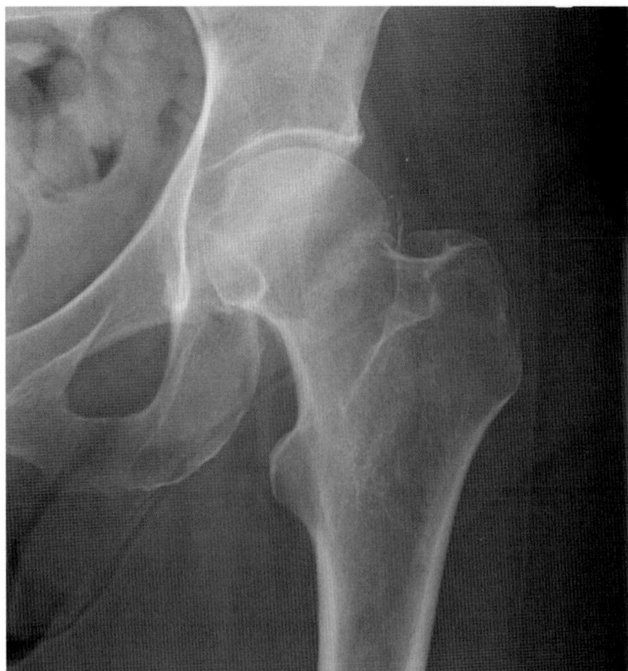

FIGURE 52-49 ■ Subtle interruption of the trabecular lines of the femoral neck. There is ill-defined sclerosis extending across the neck. These signs suggest an impacted fracture.

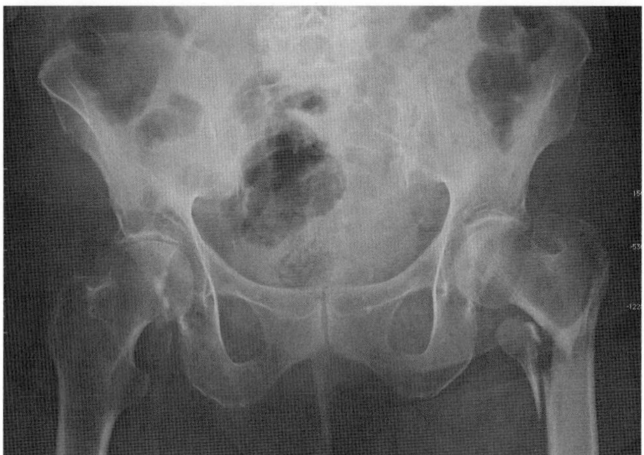

FIGURE 52-50 ■ A comminuted intertrochanteric fracture on the left.

THE KNEE

On the AP radiograph the fibula denotes the lateral side of the knee. The medial and lateral joint spaces are normally equal. The cortices of the tibial plateau both medial and lateral are sharply defined and sclerotic. There is a useful rule of thumb aiding fracture detection. A line dropped perpendicularly from the lateral femoral condyle should meet the margin of the adjacent tibial plateau with (at most) 5 mm of bone lying lateral to the line. If this rule is broken, suspect a lateral tibial plateau fracture.

The lateral view following trauma should be obtained using a horizontal beam: that is with the patient lying flat

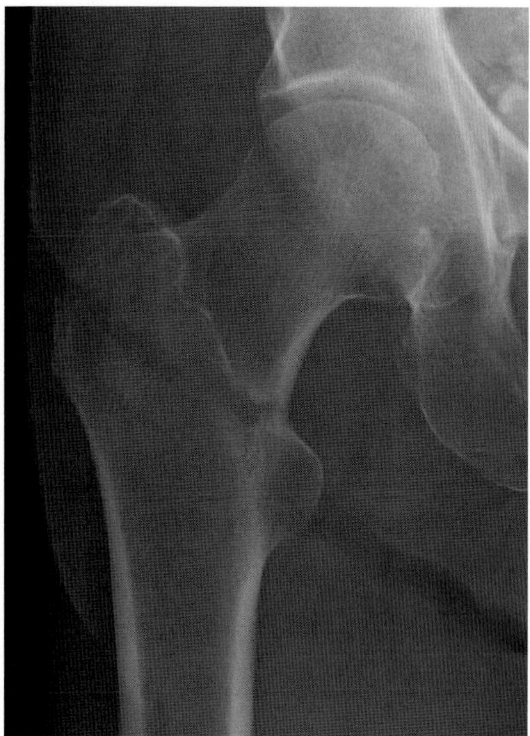

FIGURE 52-51 ■ Air is trapped in the skin crease of the groin, producing a linear lucency traversing the underlying femur. However, on close inspection the lucency crossing the bone is separate from the soft-tissue lucency. Thus this patient has a fracture as well as air in the groin crease.

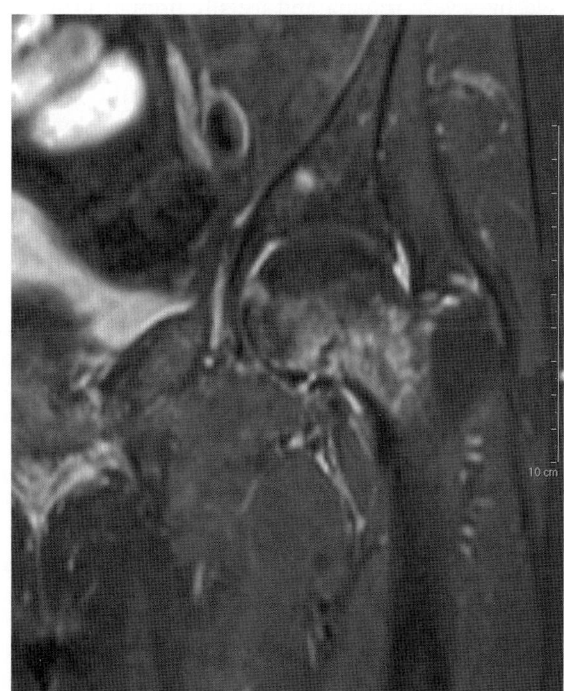

FIGURE 52-52 ■ The AP radiograph of the hip was normal. MRI coronal STIR shows a fracture of the inferior aspect of the femoral neck.

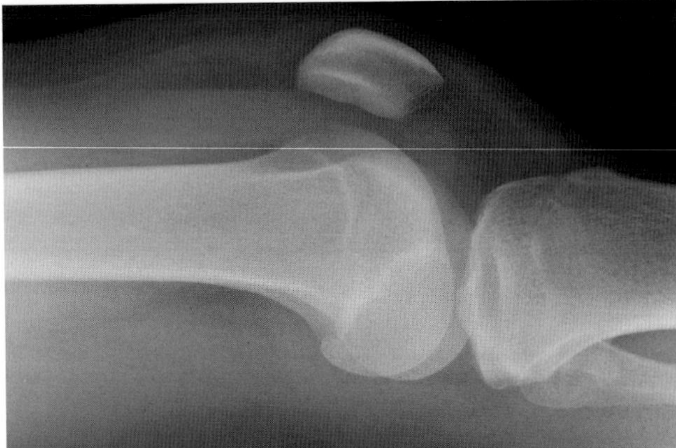

FIGURE 52-53 ■ Horizontal beam lateral radiograph. There is a fluid level evident within the suprapatellar pouch. The dark layer on top represents fluid fat which has layered on top of the much brighter fluid blood. The fluid fat has escaped from the bone marrow, which means there must be a fracture present.

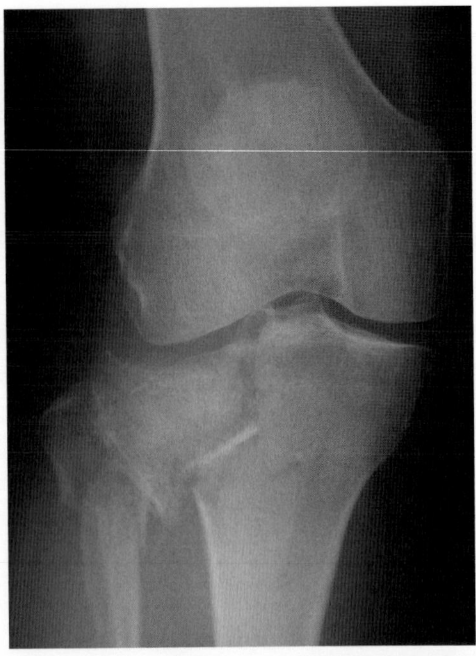

FIGURE 52-54 ■ An obvious fracture of the lateral tibial plateau which has been depressed inferiorly. There is an associated fracture of the fibula.

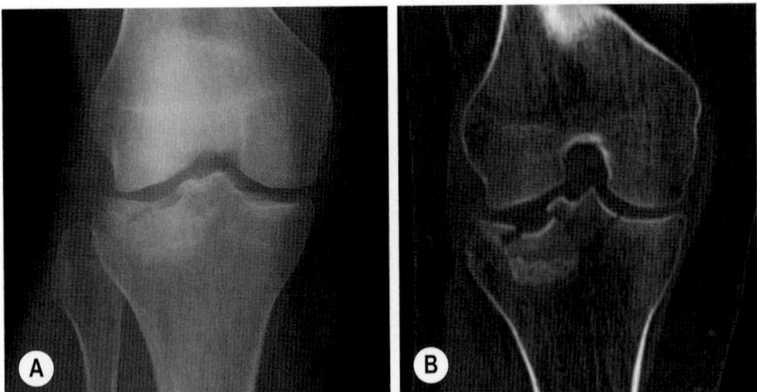

FIGURE 52-55 ■ (A) Area of sclerosis inferior to the lateral plateau indicative of trabecular condensation as a result of a plateau fracture. (B) CT demonstrates the fracture lines and also shows the degree of depression of the fracture. The sclerotic impacted trabeculae correlate with the plain radiographic findings.

and the X-ray beam parallel to the floor. This enables a useful soft-tissue sign to become evident, which is a fluid–fluid level superior to the patella lying within the suprapatellar pouch. It consists of fat layered on blood, known as a lipohaemarthrosis.[44,45] The only fat which is fluid at body temperature is marrow fat. Thus, to be evident on the radiograph there must be a break in a bony cortex, allowing fat to escape into the knee joint; this is usually accompanied by blood. If this sign is present, there must be a fracture and this is almost always visible on the radiograph with careful inspection (Fig. 52-53).

Supracondylar and condylar fractures of the femur are caused by severe trauma and usually present little diagnostic difficulty.

Fractures of the tibial plateau typically occur when the lateral side of the knee is struck, forcing the knee into valgus. The lateral femoral condyle is driven down into the lateral tibial plateau, resulting in fracturing and depression of the plateau. Medial fractures are much less common, accounting for only 10% of such injuries. Most injuries are easily detected (Fig. 52-54). Many now undergo CT, not for diagnosis but to aid surgical planning.[40] The number of fracture fragments and the degree of plateau depression will determine the need for surgery and the type. Depression of the articular surface by more than 10 mm is a key observation in this regard. Tibial plateau depression is measured as the vertical distance between the lowest point on the intact medial plateau and the lowest depressed lateral plateau fracture fragment. More subtle injuries may be detected by use of three observations:

1. Loss of clarity of the normal lateral plateau cortex.
2. Impaction of the subcortical trabeculae resulting in sclerosis (Fig. 52-55).
3. Lateral displacement of the tibial margin beyond a vertical line drawn inferiorly from the lateral femoral condyle. Normally little or no bone lies lateral to such a line (Fig. 52-56).

Small bone fragments around the knee usually signify a significant injury.[47] They should not be dismissed as flakes or chips as many are avulsion injuries by tendons or ligaments.[48] Severe force and distraction of the knee is required to avulse the bony attachments seen on the radiographs. There are two findings of particular significance.

The anterior cruciate ligament (ACL) inserts into the anterior tibial eminence. In adolescents, in particular, this bony attachment is weaker than the ligament. In some instances the ligament is avulsed from this bony attachment, resulting in a bone fragment which is seen within the joint centrally on the AP view and in the anterior half of the joint on the lateral (Fig. 52-57).

The presence of a small bone fragment adjacent to the upper lateral tibia, known as a Segond fracture,[49] is an avulsion injury by the lateral capsular ligament (Fig. 52-58). Its importance is that the mechanism of a forced varus injury that produces this finding results in a very

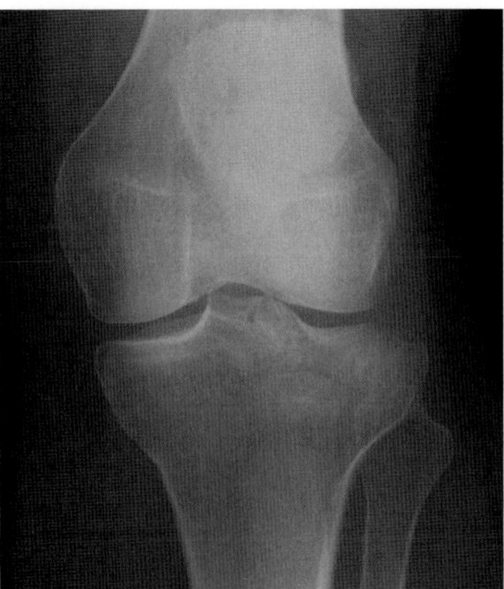

FIGURE 52-56 ■ A lateral plateau fracture with displacement of bone laterally such that a line drawn down the lateral cortex of the femur does not run smoothly onto the lateral margin of the tibia.

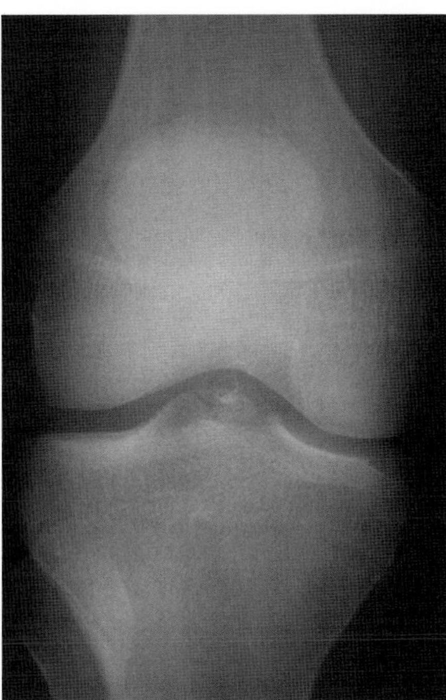

FIGURE 52-57 ■ There are small bone fragments seen centrally in the joint space projected over the tibial spines. Bone fragments in this position are due to avulsion by the anterior cruciate ligament.

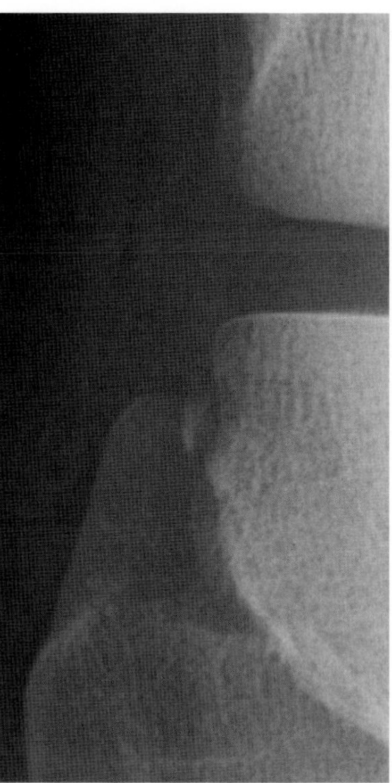

FIGURE 52-58 ■ A very small bone fragment is seen adjacent to the lateral tibia also overlapping the fibula head. This should not be misinterpreted as a minor flake injury. It indicates a high likelihood of injuries of the ACL and medial meniscus.

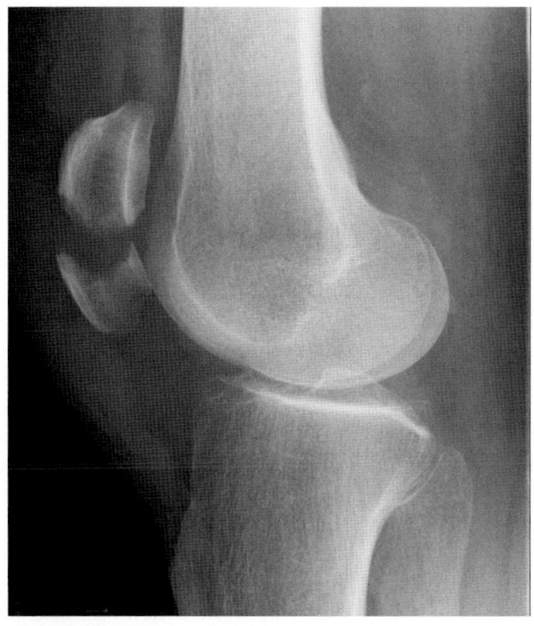

FIGURE 52-59 ■ **Lateral knee.** A horizontal patellar fracture is readily identified.

high incidence of rupture of the ACL and tears of the medial meniscus, both said to be as high as 75–100% of cases.

Patellar fracture is either transverse vertical or stellate (comminuted). Patellar injuries occur either from a direct blow or as a result of contraction of the powerful quadriceps muscles, resulting in a transverse fracture which accounts for 60% of cases. These injuries are readily visible on a lateral view (Fig. 52-59). Vertical fractures are much less common (15%) and are visible on the AP view only with difficulty because of the overlying distal femur. If a patellar injury is suspected clinically and none is seen on conventional radiographs, then an additional radiograph—the skyline (or sunrise) view—should be taken with the knee in flexion; this throws the patella off

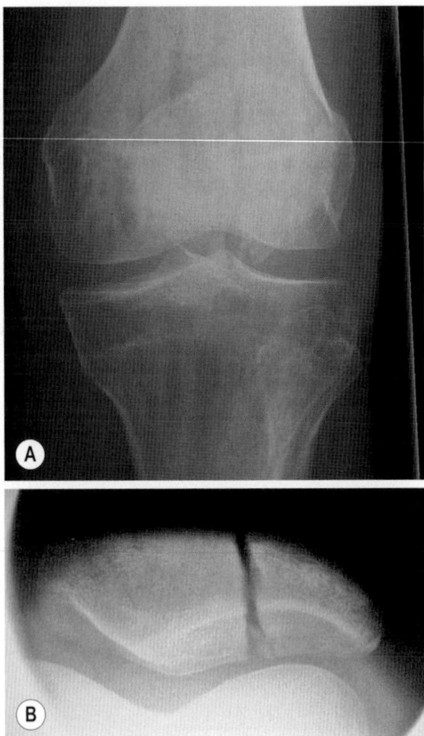

FIGURE 52-60 ■ (A) A vertical patellar fracture is seen with some difficulty. (B) If index of suspicion is high and no fracture is seen, then an additional skyline view will identify such fractures more readily.

the femur and may allow a vertical fracture to be seen (Fig. 52-60). Stellate fractures are usually caused by a direct blow to the patella. They may only be seen on the AP view with difficulty.

Bipartite patella is a normal variant. The bone fragment always occurs in the superior lateral quadrant and has well-defined sclerotic margins (Fig. 52-61). The fragment is usually larger than the defect.

Patellar dislocation is rarely evident as such on plain radiographs. Even when dislocated at the time of injury, this is usually transient and has relocated long before the patient attends the emergency department. The only occasional evidence of the dislocation is when an osteochondral fragment is displaced from the femoral condyle or avulsed from the patella by the medial patellofemoral ligament. These bone fragments may be visible on the radiograph. Again, the skyline view may be helpful in finding these small bone fragments.[50] This is another example of a small bone fragment which signifies a significant injury. It should be distinguished from an ACL avulsion injury described earlier. In the latter, the bone fragment lies centrally in the joint on both views. The former is seen often on one view only and lies away from the joint centre (Fig. 52-62).

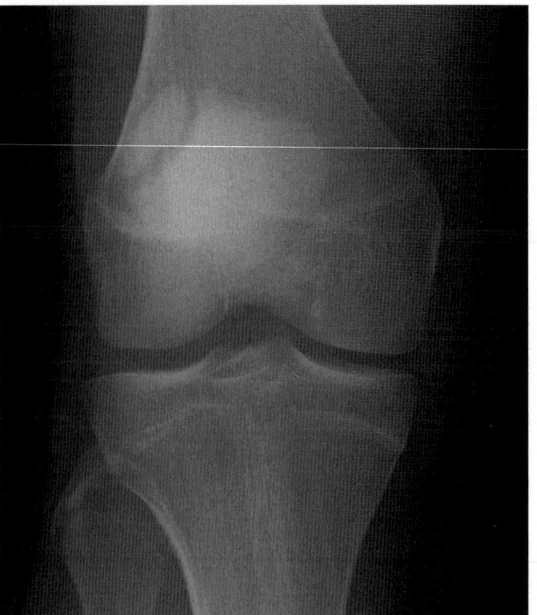

FIGURE 52-61 ■ **Bipartite patella.** The bone fragment seen arising from the superolateral quadrant of the patella is a normal variant, a bipartite patella. It should not be mistaken for a fracture.

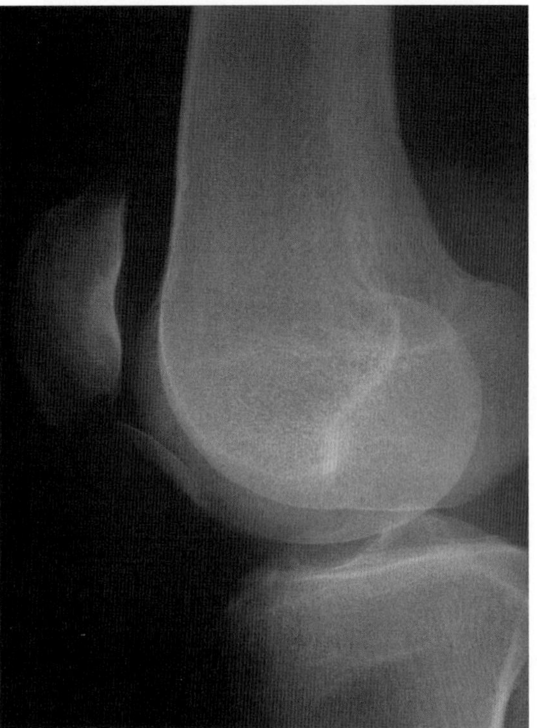

FIGURE 52-62 ■ **There is a curvilinear bone fragment seen in the anterior aspect of the knee.** This is not visible on an AP view. Bone fragments like this are typically found as a result of patellar dislocation, although in the majority of cases there are no radiographic abnormalities.

THE ANKLE

Standard views are an AP mortice view and a lateral. The mortice view is an AP with approximately 10° of internal rotation of the foot, which projects the fibula clear of the talus, making it easier to identify fractures of these structures. The lateral radiograph of the ankle should encompass not only the distal tibia and fibula but also the calcaneus and base of the fifth metatarsal.

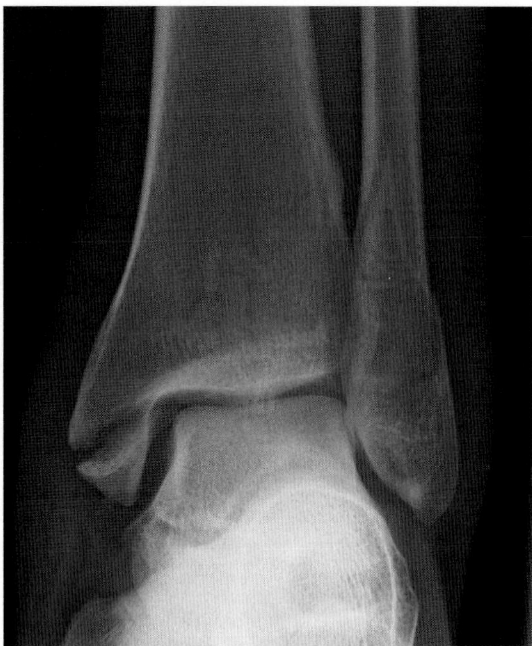

FIGURE 52-63 ■ Fractures of both medial and lateral malleolus. This represents a bimalleolar injury.

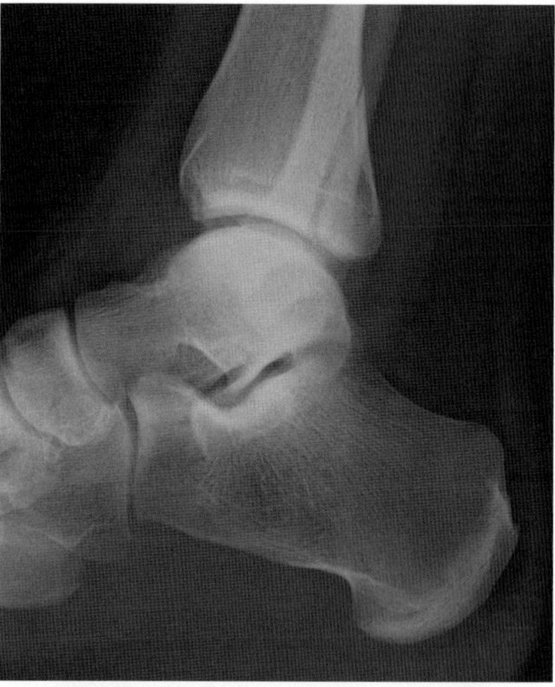

FIGURE 52-64 ■ Fracture of the posterior distal tibial tubercle often referred to (incorrectly) as the posterior malleolus. This is not visible on the AP view. These fractures are often associated with fractures of both medial and lateral malleoli and so would be termed a trimalleolar injury.

The pattern of ankle fractures depends on the position of the foot and the force applied, most often inversion, eversion and rotational injuries. Inversion injuries account for about 80% of these ankle fractures. The fractures involve the malleoli, medial and lateral either singly (unimalleolar) or in combination (bimalleolar; Fig. 52-63). There may also be an associated fracture of the posterior tubercle of the distal tibia, sometimes referred to as the posterior malleolus, resulting in a trimalleolar fracture (Fig. 52-64). Fractures of the distal fibula are often visible only on careful inspection of the lateral view.

A simple commonly used classification of malleolar fractures is the Weber classification.[51] This considers only the position of the fibular fracture in relation to the talar dome. However, the important anatomy is the syndesmosis and associated ligaments of the distal tibia and fibula. The talar dome is merely an anatomical landmark on radiographs, which can be used to try and determine whether a fracture involves the syndesmosis.

Weber A is a fracture of the distal fibula inferior to the talar dome and thus the syndesmosis will be intact (Fig. 52-65). Surgery is not usually required. Weber B fractures at the level of the talar dome may involve the syndesmosis. Surgical treatment is needed in a proportion of these injuries. Weber C fractures are proximal to the talar dome and the syndesmosis is usually disrupted in these cases (Fig. 52-66). These fractures are generally treated with internal fixation. Severity and prognosis of these injuries is also dependent on the number of malleoli involved and the degree of displacement at the fracture sites.

There are more complex comprehensive classification systems for ankle injures but these are beyond the scope of this chapter.

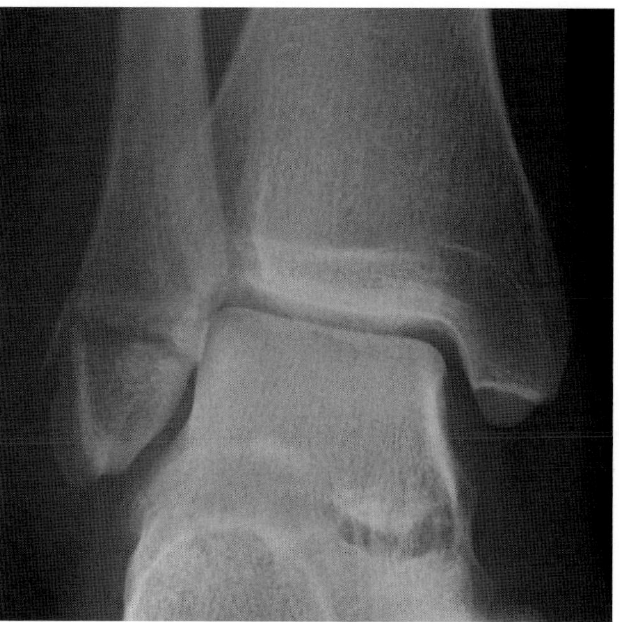

FIGURE 52-65 ■ Fracture of the distal fibula below the level of the talar dome so the syndesmosis is not disrupted. This thus represents a Weber A fracture.

With this type of ankle injury there is also the possibility of an associated high fibular fracture. This should be suspected when there is a medial malleolar fracture or widening of the medial joint space signifying ligament damage. In this circumstance there is a high likelihood

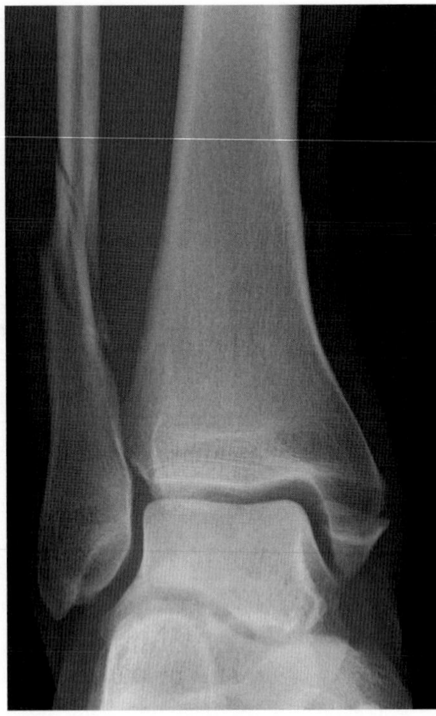

FIGURE 52-66 ■ **The fibular fracture is proximal to the talar dome.** The syndesmosis is usually disrupted in such injuries. Note there is an associated medial malleolar fracture. Therefore this is a bimalleolar Weber C injury.

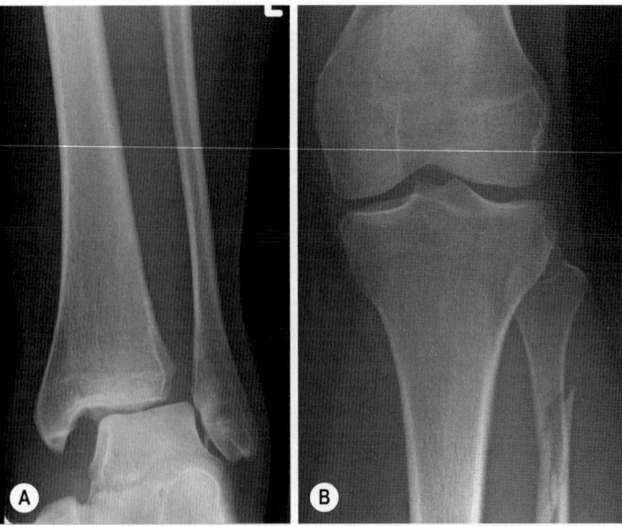

FIGURE 52-67 ■ (A) Widening of the medial joint space of the ankle or, alternatively, lateral talar shift. There must be disruption of the medial ligaments. The syndesmosis is also widened, indicating that it is also disrupted. Such injuries would normally occur in association with fracture of the distal fibula. However, none is evident here. (B) Radiograph higher up the leg, however, reveals a fibular fracture. This high fibular fracture in association with an ankle injury and is known as a Maissonneuve injury.

of a lateral fibular fracture as well. If one is not visible on the ankle radiographs, it is possible that the fibula has fractured but much higher up the leg. Radiographs of this area may then reveal the fracture. This is referred to as a Maissonneuve fracture[52] (Fig. 52-67).

Tillaux fracture describes a fracture of the distal tibia resulting from external rotation. It is an avulsion injury by the anterior inferior tibiofibular ligament. The fracture involves the anterolateral aspect of the tibial articular surface. In juvenile patients with unfused skeletons this will represent a Salter–Harris type 3 injury (Fig. 52-68).

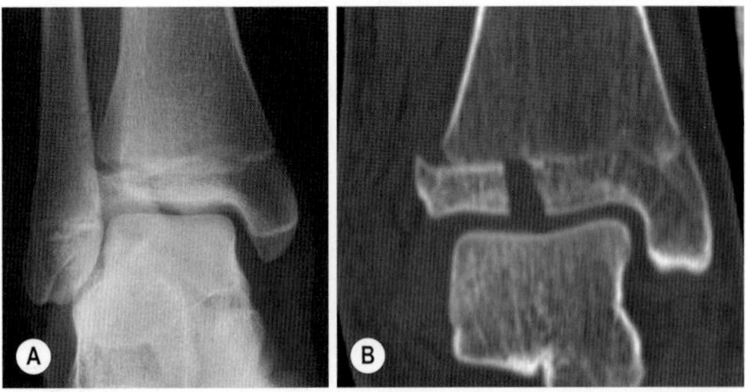

FIGURE 52-68 ■ (A) There is a fracture of the distal lateral tibia running vertically from the articular surface to the epiphyseal plate. (B) Coronal CT reconstruction shows the fracture more clearly and the degree of displacement. This is a Salter–Harris type 3 injury and is known as a Tillaux fracture.

Fractures which disrupt the weight-bearing articular surface of the distal tibia result from a high-energy axial loading. These fractures are generally readily apparent and often associated with comminuted fractures of the tibia and fibula. They are referred to as pilon fractures (Fig. 52-69).

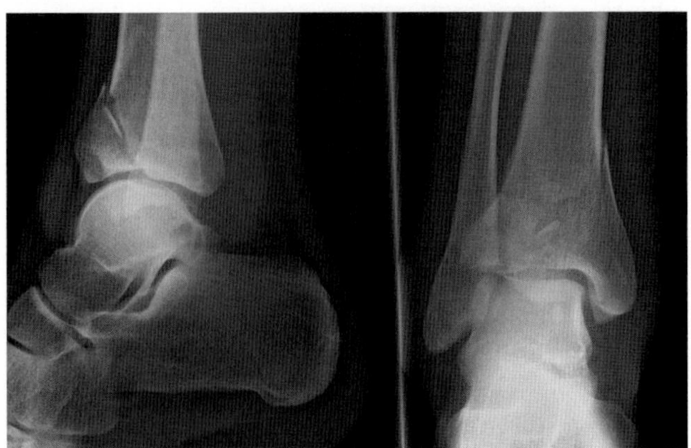

FIGURE 52-69 ■ A complex pilon fracture of the distal tibia which on the lateral view is seen to involve the articular surface with displacement of a large fragment anteriorly. This results from a high-impact injury.

Fractures of the talar dome result from eversion/inversion injuries. The mortice view facilitates their detection when a small bone fragment is separated from the talar articular surface. The cortex of the adjacent talus is irregular, indicating the source of the bone fragment (Fig. 52-70). These fragments may need to be removed if small or fixed if large. If overlooked, continuing pain and early degenerative joint changes are likely.

Calcaneal fractures are caused by a fall from a height on to the heels. They are bilateral in 10% of cases and associated with fracture of the lumbar spine, also in 10%. However, they can also result from a simple inversion

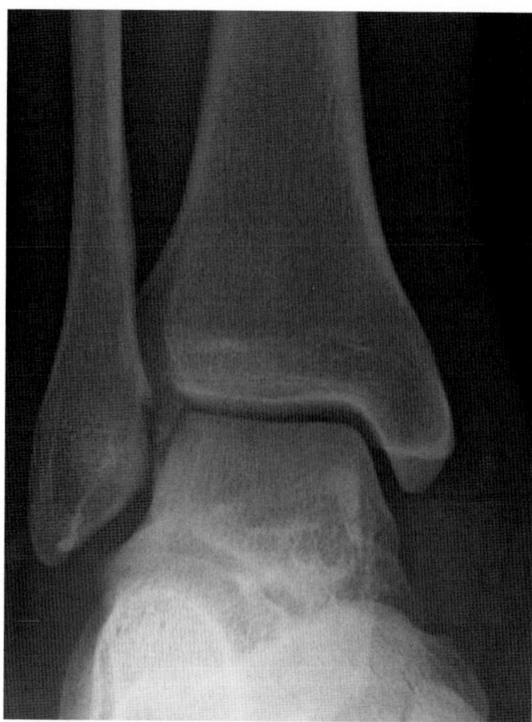

FIGURE 52-70 ■ **A fracture of the talar dome can be seen.** This injury occurs due to an inversion injury and should be carefully looked for. The mortice view facilitates its detection; a standard AP view with overlap of the fibula may make a bone fragment at this point impossible to detect.

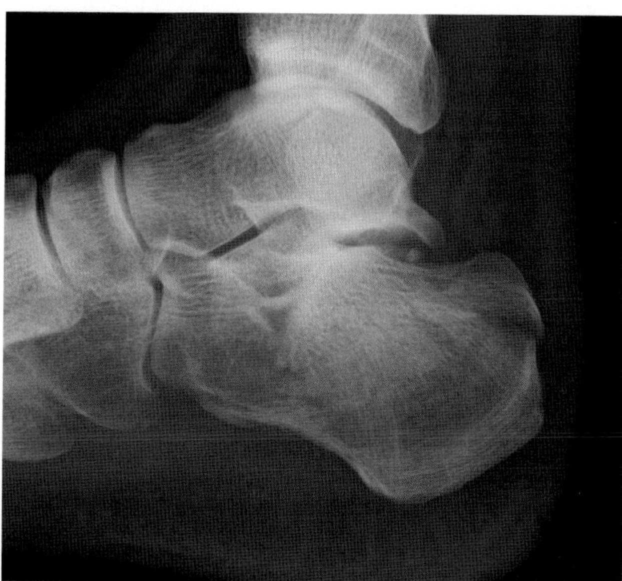

FIGURE 52-71 ■ A tongue-type fracture of the calcaneus with V-shaped fracture line extending from the posterior aspect to the body centrally. There is loss of articular congruity of the subtalar joint.

injury, especially in the osteoporotic patient. Major fractures are easily detected. There are two types of fracture. The tongue type (Fig. 52-71) involves a fracture from the posterior calcaneal cortex extending forwards to the subtalar joint. The second variety is a vertical fracture from

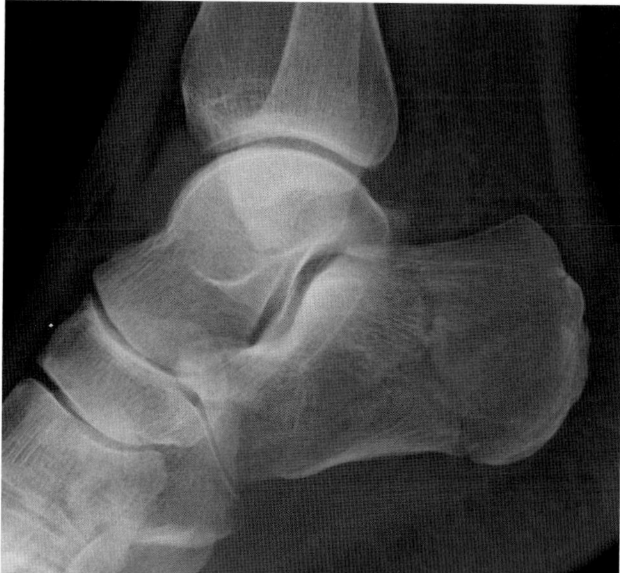

FIGURE 52-72 ■ A vertical fracture line is seen running from superior to inferior, posterior to the subarticular joint. This is therefore an extra-articular injury.

the superior to the inferior calcaneal margin (Fig. 52-72). Both fracture types may occur in the same patient. It is important to determine whether the fracture extends to the articular surface of the subtalar joint.[53] Articular involvement indicates a more severe injury. Whereas the lateral view of the ankle provides a satisfactory view of the calcaneus, an AP view of the ankle does not provide a second view. If calcaneal injury is suspected, a further axial projection radiograph taken at right angles to the lateral is obtained. CT is utilised to aid surgical planning, as these fractures may be very complex.[54]

Some fractures, however, are more subtle. They may be detected by using several observations:

1. Bohler's angle—this is constructed by drawing two lines through the three most superior points on the calcaneus. The first is from the superior aspect of the posterior calcaneus to the highest midpoint, which is the posterior aspect of the articular facet. The second line from this point passes anteriorly and is drawn to the superior tip of the anterior process. These two lines should normally make an angle of 30° (Fig. 52-73). In the presence of a fracture, this angle may be significantly reduced. Note, however, that a normal angle does not exclude a fracture.
2. An abnormal area of sclerosis caused by trabecular impaction signifies an impacted fracture.
3. Loss of the normal congruity of the articulation between the talus and calcaneus at the posterior subtalar joint.

Fractures of the talus most often involve the talar neck: they are uncommon and result from severe force. Fractures of the neck result from severe force driving up into the sole of the foot. It is another bone where the blood

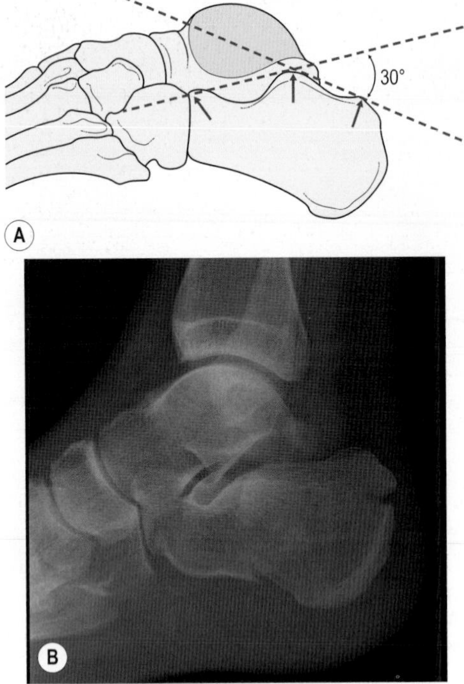

FIGURE 52-73 ■ (A) Line drawing showing how Bohler's angle is constructed and measured. (B) The calcaneus is abnormal with flattening of Bohler's angle as the highest point in the middle is depressed so that joining the three points results in an almost straight line. A posterior fracture is evident.

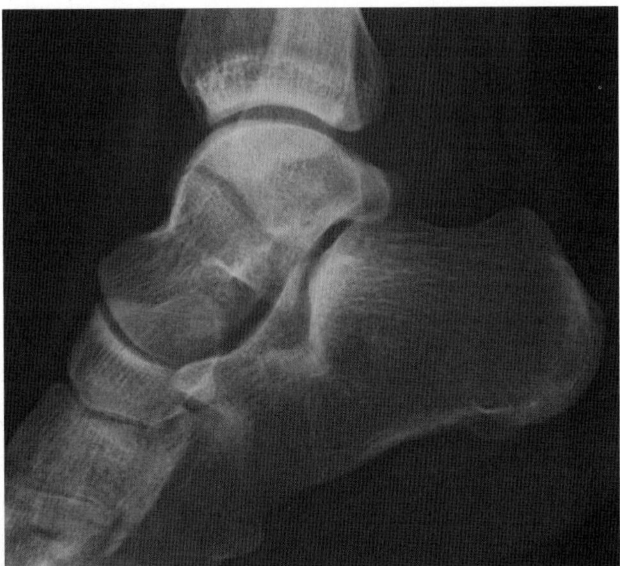

FIGURE 52-74 ■ A lucent line running through the talus indicates a neck fracture which is at risk of developing avascular necrosis caused by interruption of the blood supply.

supply distally may be interrupted by such a fracture with resultant avascular necrosis (Fig. 52-74).

A much more common injury is an avulsion by the joint capsule of a small flake of bone from the dorsum of the talus distally. This injury is of little clinical significance.

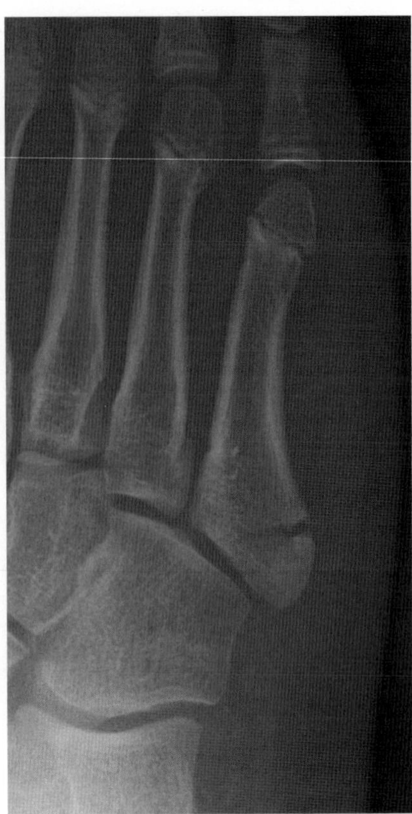

FIGURE 52-75 ■ A fracture of the base of the fifth metatarsal. At this proximal site it is an avulsion injury caused by the pull of the peroneus brevis tendon. These fractures heal well.

FOOT INJURIES

Inversion injury of the ankle may result in a fracture of the foot. It is an avulsion injury caused by the tendon of peroneus brevis muscle which inserts onto the base of the fifth metatarsal.[55] Contraction of the muscle as the ankle inverts may pull off the most proximal portion of the fifth metatarsal. The fracture is easy to see on radiographs of the foot (Fig. 52-75). However, it should also be looked for on ankle X-rays where the lateral radiograph encompasses the base of the fifth metatarsal. This injury should be distinguished from a fracture distal to the articulation between the fourth and fifth metatarsals. This is called a Jones' fracture and has a propensity to heal poorly.[56] It is also caused by inversion of the foot (Fig. 52-76).

In skeletally immature patients there is an unfused apophysis at the base of the fifth metatarsal, which should not be mistaken for a fracture. The apophysis is separated from the metatarsal by a lucency which is longitudinally orientated. Avulsion fractures lie transversely (Fig. 52-77).

Lisfranc injury refers to fractures and dislocations in and around the bases of the metatarsals.[57,58] When there is an associated fracture or the dislocation is severe, the abnormality is readily identified. Most commonly there is a fracture of the base of the second metatarsal with

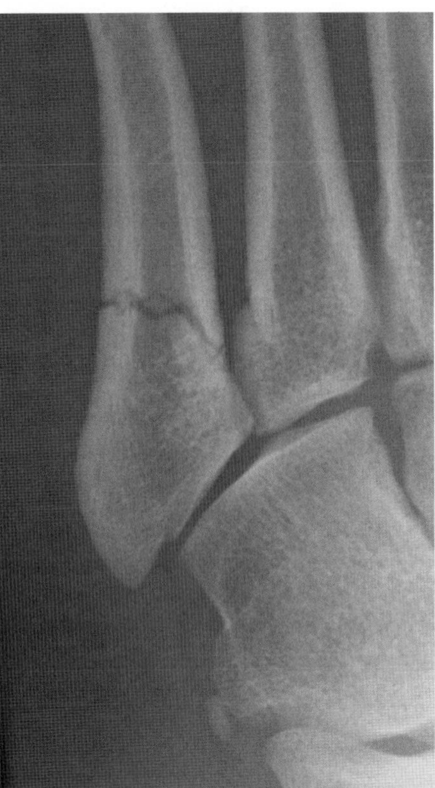

FIGURE 52-76 ■ Fracture of the proximal shaft of the fifth metatarsal. This is known as a Jones' fracture. Fractures at this site have a tendency to heal poorly.

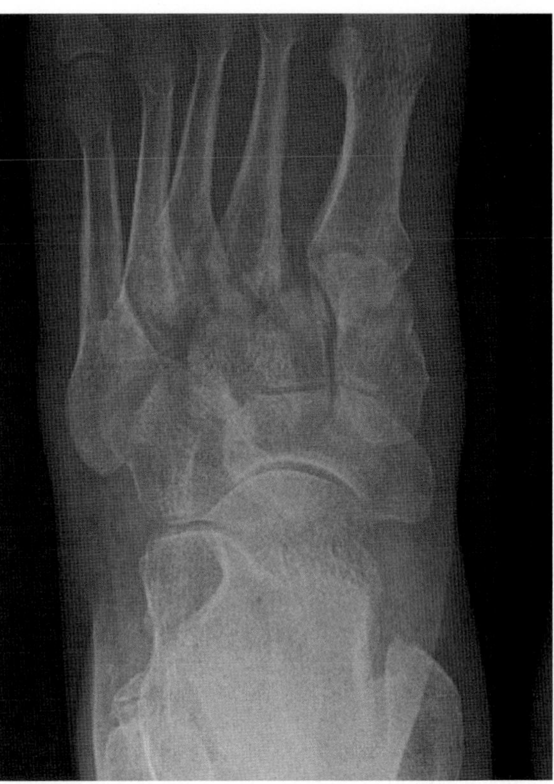

FIGURE 52-78 ■ Lisfranc midfoot injury. The second, third and fourth metatarsals are displaced laterally. There is a fracture at the base of the second metatarsal.

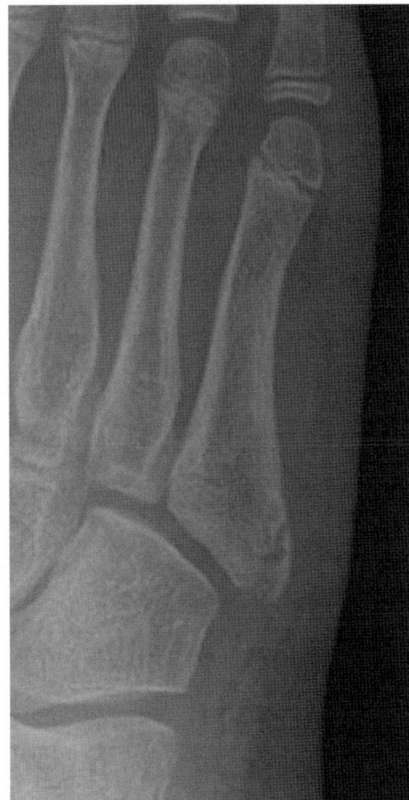

FIGURE 52-77 ■ Immature skeleton. The proximal apophysis of the fifth metatarsal is a normal finding and should not be mistaken for a fracture. Fractures are transverse across the bone shaft; apophyses run longitudinally. Compare with appearances of the fracture in Fig. 52-78.

displacement of the second to fifth metatarsals laterally (Fig. 52-78). More subtle injuries may be identified by observing loss of the normal alignment of the second and third metatarsal bases with their respective cuneiform bones. Normally, a line drawn down the medial cortex of the metatarsal will pass between the medial and intermediate cuneiform on the AP view. On the oblique view a line along the lateral cortex of the metatarsal should pass between middle and lateral cuneiform bones. Some injuries are not visible at all on radiographs and when there is strong index of suspicion clinically, a CT scan may reveal subtle disruptions at this joint.[59]

Stress fractures are caused by repeated low-impact trauma.[60] They are common in the foot, with a predelicition for the shaft of the second metatarsal. Stress fractures are often seen in military recruits from prolonged marching, hence the name of march fracture, but now are more common in those undertaking training for charity distance running events. They are identified radiographically not as a typical lucent line but as an area of periosteal reaction due to increased osteoclastic activity (Fig. 52-79). They are seen most commonly on those undertaking unusual increased activity such as an unaccustomed long distance walking or running.

In patients with a history of inversion injury, Table 52-2 lists injuries that can occur and should be considered when reporting.

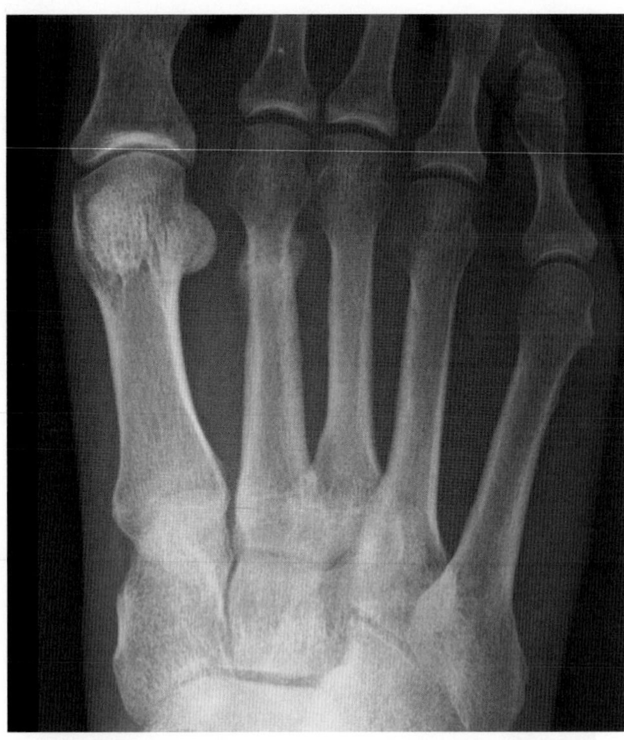

FIGURE 52-79 ■ There is a periosteal reaction around the shaft of the distal second metatarsal. This is the typical appearance of a stress fracture due to unaccustomed exercise. A fracture line will rarely, if ever, become visible.

TABLE 52-2 **Injuries Which May Occur due to Ankle Inversion**

In a patient with a history of inversion injury, consider all of the following:	
Malleolar injuries	Look on lateral carefully for (a) difficult-to-see fibular fractures and (b) post-tibia fractures
High fibular fractures (Maisonneuve)	Medial fractures or talar shift and no fibular fracture visible
Talar dome fractures	
Calcaneal fractures	Look at Bohler's angle Areas of sclerosis Loss of articular congruity
Base of fifth metatarsal	Seen on lateral ankle X-ray

For a full list of references, please see ExpertConsult.

FURTHER READING

Greenspan A. Orthopaedic Imaging: A Practical Approach. 5th ed. Wolters Kluwer/Lippincott Williams & Wilkins; 2011.

Raby N, Berman L, De Lacey G. Accident and Emergency Radiology: A Survival Guide. 2d ed. Elsevier; 2005.

Sarwark J, editor. Essentials of Musculoskeletal Care. 4th ed. American Academy of Orthopaedic Surgeons; 2010.

Solomon S, Warwick D, Nayagam S, editors. Apley's System of Orthopaedics and Fractures. 9th ed. Hodder and Arnold; 2010.

CHAPTER 53

Bone, Joint and Spinal Infection

Balashanmugam Rajashanker • Richard W. Whitehouse

CHAPTER OUTLINE

INTRODUCTION

Bone and joint infections have high rates of morbidity and occasional mortality. A wide range of microbial infections can affect bones and joints, including pyogenic, mycobacterial and fungal organisms. Patients usually present with a high temperature, pain and swelling in the affected bones and/or joints. In younger patients concomitant systemic illness more often occurs. Early diagnosis at acute presentation is important to prevent chronic and recurrent infections, long-term disabilities and treatment failures. Prompt diagnosis is needed particularly in children and also after orthopaedic implant surgeries to prevent the risk of developing serious infections. A multidisciplinary team approach is necessary for effective management of these conditions. Soft-tissue and muscle infections present more acutely and may be potentially life threatening.

It can be difficult to diagnose bone infection early, especially in diabetic patients with pre-existing neuropathic bone and joint changes and in the presence of skin ulceration and cellulitis. A high degree of suspicion and use of appropriate investigations will assist diagnosis. Tuberculous infection of bones and joints pose a particular diagnostic challenge. Septic arthritis is a serious condition, which if untreated leads to destruction of cartilage and adjacent osteomyelitis, with subsequent joint ankylosis and disability. Laboratory tests including white cell count, C-reactive protein, ESR and blood culture are mandatory in the early stages to diagnose these infections. A range of radiological investigations are available currently to enable a prompt diagnosis. It is important that the radiologist is familiar with the clinical spectrum of presentations, appropriate diagnostic tests and the need to perform these without delay to enable prompt management.

EPIDEMIOLOGY

Staphylococcus aureus is the commonest organism causing bone and joint infections in any age group, accounting for up to 80% of cases of osteomyelitis. Gram-negative organisms including *Pseudomonas* and *Enterobacter* are responsible for most of the remaining 20% of cases. Acute infections of prosthetic implants are usually caused by *S. aureus*. Coagulate-negative staphylococci such as *Staphylococcus epidermidis* account for the majority of chronic osteomyelitis associated with orthopaedic implants and account for approximately 90% of pin tract infections. Bacteria adhere to bone matrix and orthopaedic implants via receptors to fibronectin and other receptor proteins. They form a slimy coat and elude the host defence mechanisms by hiding intracellularly and by developing a slow metabolic rate.[1] Osteoarticular *Listeria* infections are rare but do occur in immunocompromised patients and in prosthetic joints.[2] Polymicrobial infection occurs in the majority of osteomyelitidies occurring in the diabetic foot, comprising of mixed Gram-positive and -negative bacteria. Wound swabs are often inaccurate and dominated by contaminants. Cultures from bone biopsy or operative specimens are more reliable in planning appropriate antibiotic treatment.[3] Brodie's abscess, a true small, focal intraosseous collection of pus, is an uncommon manifestation of bone infection, except in East Africa, where reportedly it is a common occurrence.[4] *Staphylococcus aureus* is again the predominant organism cultured in these patients.

Vertebral osteomyelitis usually results from haematogenous seeding or by direct inoculation at the time of spinal surgery. *Staphylococcus aureus* is the commonest microorganism amongst others that include methicillin-resistant *S. aureus* (MRSA), streptococci and *E coli*.[5] As with other orthopaedic implants, coagulase-negative staphylococcal infections are seen after usage of fixation devices.[6]

In children, other than staphylococci, *Haemophilus influenzae* type b, *Streptococcus pneumoniae* and *Streptococcus pyogenes* also occur.[7] One of the significant changes in the epidemiology of bone and joint infections is the increasing incidence of MRSA and the emergence of multidrug resistant (MDR) organisms.[8,9]

Osteomyelitis complicating war injuries is predominantly caused by MDR organisms and include MRSA, Enterobacteriaceae and *Acinetobacter*. There is commonly a history of previous surgical procedures and these conditions usually need further more aggressive management.[10]

Fungal infections of the bone and joints are uncommon and occur predominantly in the immunosuppressed patient. Such infection may resemble tuberculous disease and present as chronic multifocal osteomyelitis or polyarthritis.[11]

CLASSIFICATION

Osteomyelitis can be classified by the type of infection or more commonly by the duration since onset of the illness. Acute osteomyelitis is defined as infection diagnosed within 2 weeks of onset of symptoms whilst subacute osteomyelitis is diagnosed if symptoms exceed 2 weeks' duration. If the infection is diagnosed months after the onset of symptoms, then it is defined as chronic osteomyelitis.[12,13] There are, however, other classifications in the literature, depending on the anatomical areas of bony involvement and on pathogenesis.[14,15]

PAEDIATRIC MUSCULOSKELETAL INFECTIONS

Paediatric, unlike adult, bone infections more commonly occur in healthy bones, without pre-existing trauma, etc. The usual mode of infection is haematogenous, via the arterial blood supply. Acute haematogenous osteomyelitis (AHO) is the most common form of bone infection in children. About 50% of cases occur in children less than 5 years of age and it is twice as common in boys than in girls. Immunocompromised children and children with underlying haematological disorders such as sickle cell disease are more prone to these infections.[16] Infections are commonest in long bones such as the femur, tibia or humerus, with most cases limited to single bone involvement. Less than 10% of cases involve two or more locations,[17] the corollary of which is that multifocal involvement does not exclude acute osteomyelitis (the same is true for septic arthritis).

Pathophysiology

Haematogenous spread is the most common route to bones and joints, though implantation at trauma or surgery and spread from contiguous infection may also occur. Infection usually starts in the metaphysis due to its rich blood supply. From here the infection may spread to the bone cortex and penetrate the loosely attached periosteum, eliciting a periosteal reaction. It may perforate the periosteum and spread to adjacent muscles and soft tissues, forming abscesses. Less commonly, the infection may spread to the epiphyseal plates and joints, causing septic arthritis. In neonates, the metaphyseal capillaries form a connection with the epiphyseal plate, thus increasing the chance of joint infection. In later infancy, these vessels atrophy and there is thickening of the cortex, thus reducing the risk of growth plate involvement and septic arthritis.

Staphylococcus aureus accounts for approximately 60–90% of childhood AHO, followed by group A β-haemolytic streptococci (10%). Other causes include *H. influenzae* and *S. pneumoniae*. *Salmonella* infections were historically common in patients with sickle cell disease but this seemed to reflect the organism prevalence in the population. *Pseudomonas* infections can be seen after puncture wounds of the feet. In neonates, again, *S. aureus* infections predominate, but group B streptococcus and *E. coli* infections are also common.[16,18]

Clinical Features

A few well-recognised clinical presentations of bone and joint infections are seen in children.

Acute osteomyelitis, more common in boys, usually occurs between ages 1 and 10 years. The lower limbs are usually involved. Children usually present with pain and reluctance to use the affected limb. The cardinal signs of acute inflammation, including pain, redness and swelling, may not be present initially, may develop later and may be associated with systemic illness. Often pain is localised and prompt diagnosis and treatment offers a good prognosis.

Chronic osteomyelitis has a more insidious onset over a few weeks and is more difficult to diagnose. There is usually minimal loss of function. Systemic signs are usually absent, but local tenderness may be present. Radiographs are usually helpful as bone changes are usually present by the time medical attention is sought. Chronic osteomyelitis is further discussed under adult infections.

Septic arthritis is also twice as common in boys, with a peak incidence below 3 years of age. Symptoms include pain and swelling around the joint with reluctance to move the limb. Pseudo-paralysis and painful passive movements may be present. There are systemic symptoms and there is rapid progression of symptoms. Diagnosis is more difficult in neonates. The joint is warm and ultrasound can demonstrate a joint effusion. The lower limbs are usually involved, particularly the hip or knee.

Neonatal osteomyelitis and septic arthritis are probably different manifestations of the same condition: 75% of the children are not severely ill and present as failure to thrive. Prognosis is not as good as there is usually a delay in diagnosis.

Disseminated staphylococcal disease presents as a rapidly progressive severe life-threatening illness with virulent bacteraemia and multiorgan involvement, but fortunately is rare.

Investigations and Management

Thorough clinical examination and laboratory investigations are extremely important in diagnosis, before imaging evaluation is performed. Conventional radiography is still one of the most important investigations for diagnosis. The other imaging investigations, ultrasound, CT, MRI and scintigraphic studies are also used. The risk/benefits and costs of these tests, their radiation exposure, requirements for sedation or anaesthesia need to be assessed carefully as investigations are planned.

Plain Radiographs

In acute osteomyelitis, plain radiographs are extremely useful to exclude other lesions such as fractures, Perthes' disease and slipped femoral epiphysis. In septic arthritis the joint space is initially expanded with fluid and may give rise to some asymmetry in the position of the epiphysis, but ultrasound is more reliable to demonstrate fluid in the joint. In subacute osteomyelitis, periosteal reaction, new bone formation and occasionally lucent lesions (Brodie's abscess) in the metaphysical region may be seen. Chronic osteomyelitis shows bone sclerosis, destruction, and periosteal new bone formation.

Ultrasound

Ultrasound has an important role in demonstrating increased joint fluid early in acute septic arthritis and is also used to guide aspiration of the joint effusion for diagnostic and therapeutic purposes (Fig. 53-1). In septic arthritis the cellular debris-laden effusion may be echoic, rendering it less conspicuous. Demonstrating movement of this debris by varying the US probe pressure during the examination may reduce false-negative interpretation. Subperiosteal abscess can be demonstrated as hypoechoic fluid along the bone surface in acute and subacute disease. Soft-tissue abscesses can also be seen as hypoechoic fluid with thick walls that may show increased colour Doppler flow. Direct aspiration under ultrasound guidance and culture and sensitivity of the aspirate is extremely helpful to confirm diagnosis and for further treatment with the appropriate antibiotics. Soft-tissue abnormalities can also be demonstrated with ultrasound, though MRI is more reliable.

Computed Tomography

This investigation is less useful in a paediatric population due to its radiation dose and lack of specific advantages, and MRI is preferred.

Magnetic Resonance Imaging

MRI is the investigation of choice for the diagnosis of acute, subacute and chronic osteomyelitis with high sensitivity and specificity. The characteristic signs of acute osteomyelitis in children include bone marrow oedema, which is seen as low T1 signal in the bone marrow, along with high signal on T2 and STIR images.[19] Abscesses are seen both early and late in disease, as well-defined

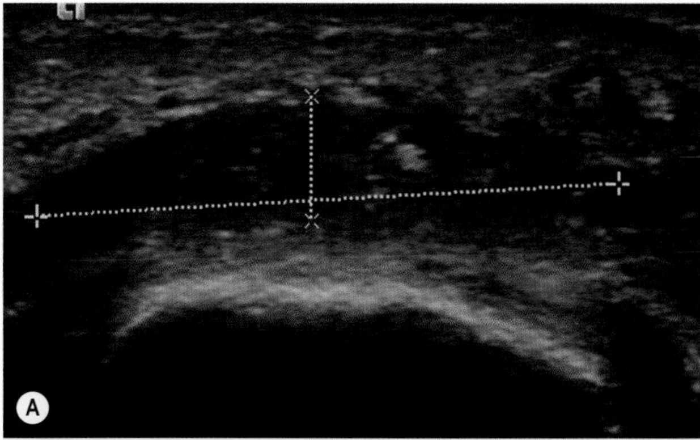

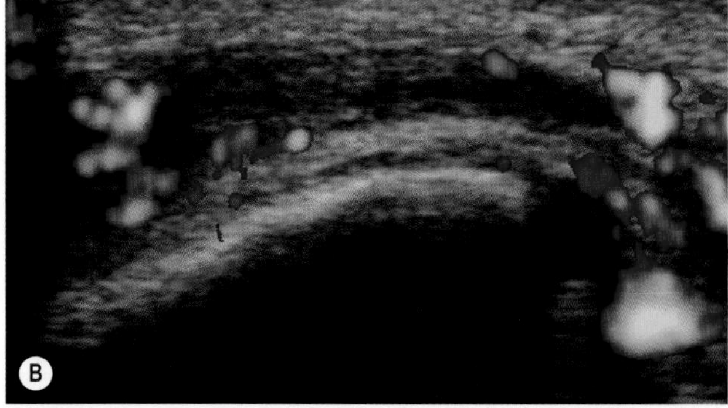

FIGURE 53-1 ■ **Septic arthritis in a child.** (A) Ultrasound of the right knee in a limping 3-year-old child demonstrates the presence of echogenic fluid in the prepatellar bursa. (B) There is increased colour Doppler flow in the surrounding soft tissues and wall of the bursa. The finding of an infected bursa should arouse the possibility of adjacent septic arthritis.

low-signal collections on T1, high signal similar to fluid on T2 images, with enhancing walls on post contrast sequences (Fig. 53-2). This may be seen in the bone, adjacent soft tissues or subperiosteal location due to the loose attachment of the periosteum to the underlying bone in children. Septic arthritis is diagnosed by the presence of a joint effusion, abnormal bone marrow signal localised to either side of the joint or synovial thickening which also shows post contrast enhancement. Physeal involvement is characterised by low T1 and hyperintense T2 signal along the growth plate associated with widening of the growth plate and enhancement on post contrast imaging (Fig. 53-3). Later in the course of the infection, chondrolysis occurs.

Fat-saturated T1-weighted (T1W) images with intravenous contrast medium can increase confidence in the diagnosis of osteomyelitis and also help diagnose complications such as septic arthritis, physeal involvement, intra-osseous, subperiosteal and soft-tissue abscesses. Intravenous gadolinium is most useful to identify non-enhancing abscess collections within a background of soft-tissue and bone marrow oedema and to aid differentiation between granulation tissue and true abscess. It is generally not useful if unenhanced images show no evidence of soft-tissue or bone marrow oedema. The merits of administering intravenous contrast agents should be weighed against its injudicious use in children.[20]

The rim sign is seen in chronic osteomyelitis as a low-signal area of fibrosis surrounding an area of active

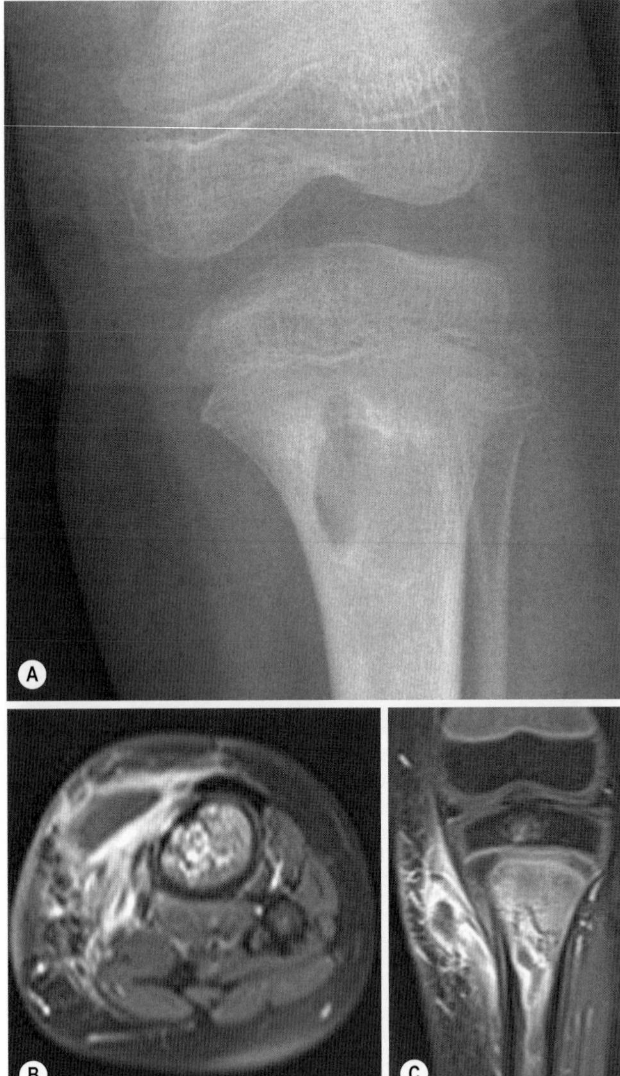

FIGURE 53-2 ■ Osteomyelitis with abscesses in a child. (A) AP radiograph of the left knee showing a lucent metaphyseal lesion of the tibia with surrounding sclerosis. (B) Axial and (C) coronal post-contrast T1-weighted fat-saturated images confirm the presence of a bone abscess, with surrounding oedema of the metaphysis. There is also focal epiphyseal involvement and an abscess in the medial soft tissues.

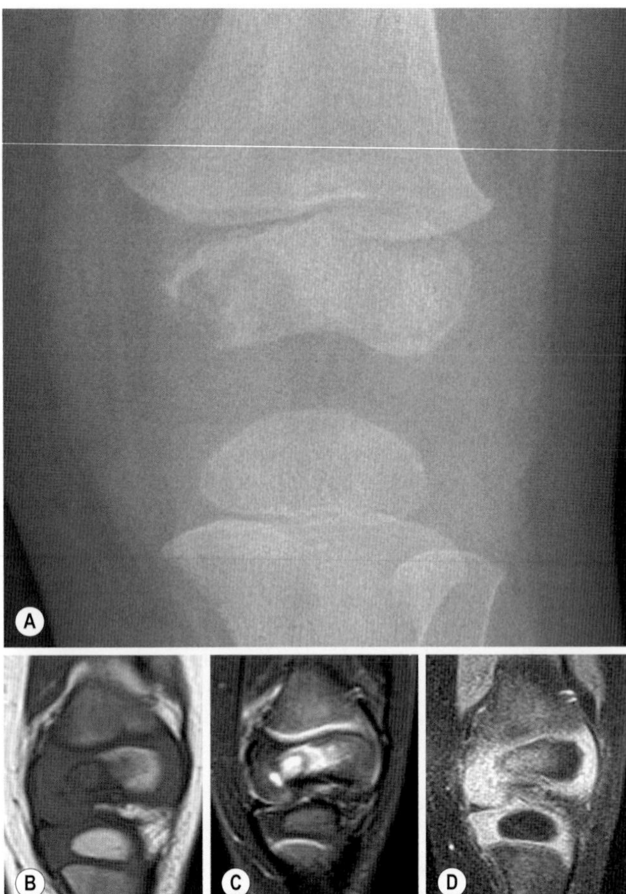

FIGURE 53-3 ■ Osteomyelitis in an 18-month-old child. (A) AP radiograph shows irregularity, erosion and rarefaction of the femoral epiphysis. (B) Coronal T1W image showing low T1 signal at the site of epiphyseal destruction, loss of normal fat signal and destruction of medial aspect of left femoral epiphysis. (C) Coronal STIR image demonstrates high signal in the affected epiphysis. (D) Coronal T1 fat-saturated enhanced image demonstrates abnormal enhancement in the affected medial epiphysis due to active infection.

infection. Active infection has high signal on T2, whereas the rim has low signal on all sequences. There may also be thickening and remodelling of cortex due to chronic infection. Periosteal reaction may not be present at this stage. Bone abscess is seen as fluid signal surrounded by a thick wall that has low signal on T1 and significant enhancement. Abscesses may extend through the cortex into the surrounding soft tissues with the formation of sinuses. There is high T2 signal return from surrounding soft tissues, with loss of normal fat signal on T1 and T2 images (Fig. 53-4).

Post-surgical or interventional procedures cause bone signal changes that can persist for up to 12 months. Hence, whenever possible, MRI should be obtained before any interventions are performed, to avoid the need for additional procedures.[21] Whole-body MRI may be useful to demonstrate multiple sites of involvement.

Nuclear Medicine

In early stages, three-phase ^{99m}Tc-MDP skeletal scintigraphy may be useful for demonstrating increased radioactivity in the affected bone and also for demonstrating multifocal disease. Increased activity may be seen in dynamic perfusion, early blood pool and delayed images. However, such uptake is non-specific and may be seen in other conditions including trauma and tumours. Use of Ga-67 citrate and ^{111}indium-labelled leucocytes will increase the specificity for infection up to 80%.[13]

Chronic Recurrent Multifocal Osteomyelitis (CRMO)

This uncommon form of non-bacterial inflammatory osteomyelitis occurs in children, usually less than 18

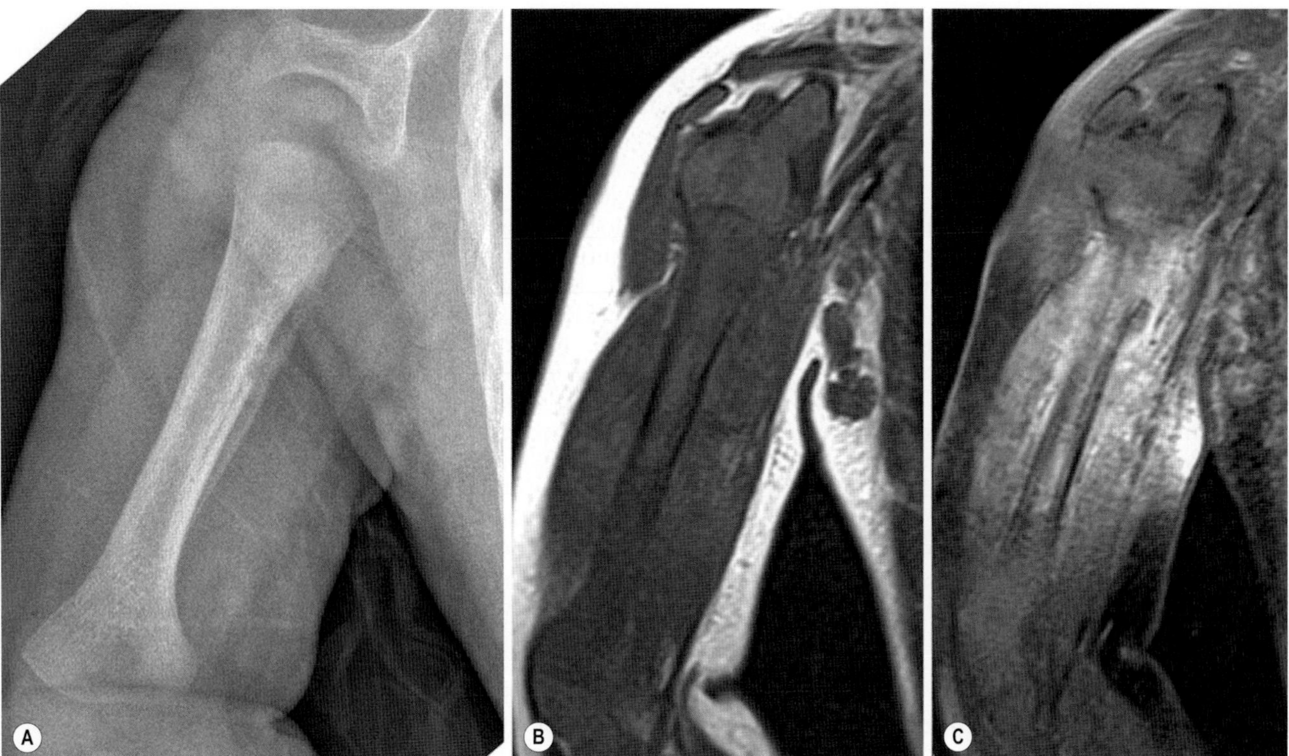

FIGURE 53-4 ■ Osteomyelitis of the humerus in a child. (A) Plain radiograph of a child with humeral osteomyelitis showing abnormal texture of medullary bone, with cortical destruction and periosteal reaction. (B) Coronal T1 and (C) fat-suppressed PD-weighted images show low T1 signal in bone marrow, which is hyperintense on the fat-suppressed PD image. Periosteal reaction, cortical destruction and adjacent soft-tissue oedema (seen as low T1 and high T2 signal abnormality) is also evident.

years of age. The aetiology is not known, but may be related to autoimmune disorders due to its association with inflammatory bowel disease and psoriasis-like skin conditions. A genetic aetiology is also postulated due to an association with mutation of the *LPIN2* gene. It is characterised by recurrent bouts of inflammatory arthritis and features of osteomyelitis which undergo spontaneous remission. It is more common in the lower limbs and may be symmetrical. Metaphyseal lesions occur in approximately 75% of cases. Symptoms are vague and it may present as monoarthritis or polyarthrits. When a single site of disease is present, the term chronic non-bacterial osteomyelitis is used.[22] There may be mild elevation of inflammatory markers but lab diagnosis is generally not helpful. Cultures do not reveal any organisms. Plain radiographs may reveal osteolytic lesions with surrounding sclerosis. Whole-body MRI can be helpful by identifying multiple sites of the disease, some of which may be asymptomatic. Typically MRI reveals periostitis, bone marrow oedema and signs of transphysitis.[23] Many lesions may heal spontaneously, though symptoms may persist for several years. Diagnosis is made by exclusion and from clinical history and typical radiological findings affecting multiple sites and recurrent negative cultures and bone biopsy. Majeed syndrome is an autosomal recessive disorder comprising a triad of CRMO, congenital dyserythropoietic anaemia and inflammatory dermatosis.

SAPHO Syndrome

This is considered as a form of CRMO and occurs in children and young adults, commonest between the second and third decades of life.[23] It is characterised by the presence of synovitis, acne, pustulosis, hyperostosis and osteitis (SAPHO). Skin manifestations and osteoarticular involvement commonly occur. Skin manifestation includes palmoplantar pustulosis and acne. There is bilateral symmetric pain and swelling of the bones and joints. The metaphyses of the tubular bones are commonly affected, though flat bones and axial skeletal sites may also be affected. Biopsy demonstrates acute and chronic inflammatory cells. Relationship to *Propionibacterium acnes* has been postulated but is debatable.[24] Treatment is by non-steroidal anti-inflammatory drugs (NSAIDs) in the first instance but severe cases may need immunosuppressive treatment.

Sclerosing Osteomyelitis of Garré

This is a chronic form of osteomyelitis, usually occurring in children, and commonly affects the mandible. This is considered as a form of CRMO affecting the mandible. Patients present with pain and hard swelling of the mandible. Initial findings include lytic lesions of the mandible associated with sclerosis. With disease progression there is non-suppurative ossifying periostitis with subperiosteal new bone formation and sclerosis.[25] The diagnosis can be made presumptively by radiology, and biopsy reveals features of chronic osteomyelitis, with cultures usually negative.[23]

Necrotising Fasciitis

This is a rapidly progressive life-threatening infection occurring in young children and more common in males. This condition also occurs in adults. Risk factors include immunocompromise, diabetes, intravenous drugs or alcohol abuse and patients with peripheral vascular disease. The condition is polymicrobial in origin, and includes Gram-positive aerobes like group A β-haemolytic streptococcus, *S. aureus*, Gram-negative organisms like *E. coli*, *Pseudomonas aeruginosa* and anaerobes like *Bacteroides*. *Clostridium* infection leads to a gas-producing necrotic infection, gas gangrene, which is rapidly progressive and leads to systemic toxicity and shock. Characteristically, the gas is intramuscular in gas gangrene, giving rise to gas loculi that are elongated and aligned with the muscle fascicles, whilst more globular gas loculi are seen in fasciitis, when a gas-forming organism is present.

The infection involves deep subcutaneous tissues and is associated with a high mortality. Infection causes thrombosis of small blood vessels, leading to necrosis and rapidly involving several facial planes. The condition has been associated with trauma, burns, eczema and varicella infections. The extensive soft-tissue damage leads to multi-organ failure and shock.[26]

Ultrasound can be useful in diagnosing the abnormal muscle echo texture, but MRI is more reliable and is needed to assess the extent of tissue damage and demonstrate the spread of infection along the facial planes. CT may also be useful, but MRI is preferred due to better soft-tissue contrast and lack of radiation. Emergency surgical debridement is needed to stop the progress of this fulminating condition; relevant imaging must therefore be performed immediately.

ADULT MUSCULOSKELETAL INFECTIONS

Spontaneous musculoskeletal infections in adults are less common than in children and are usually due to trauma, previous surgery or underlying immunodeficiency disorders. Trauma and open wounds can result in seeding of bone with microorganisms and to development of osteomyelitis. Whilst haematogenous infection is common in childhood osteomyelitis, in adults, it is mostly responsible for vertebral osteomyelitis. Apart from trauma, infection can also develop in prosthetic implants after surgery. Underlying conditions like diabetes, vascular insufficiency, decubitus ulcers and sinuses can predispose to development of osteomyelitis in adults. Osteomyelitis is classified by the time since onset, as described earlier.[27,28]

Pathogenesis

Healthy adult bone is usually resistant to infection, but when affected can be difficult to treat. The presence of dead bone and implants make it difficult to treat by antimicrobial agents and removal of the debris and the prosthetic implants is necessary to eradicate the infection. The bacteria attach to the bone matrix and orthopaedic implant devices by developing receptors to fibronectin and other structural proteins. They develop a slimy coat and a very slow metabolic rate, hide in intracellular locations and are thus able to elude host defences and antibiotics. The presence of implants also causes cell dysfunction which decreases the ability of polymorphonuclear cells to phagocytise bacteria. Reactions between the bacteria and the host defences cause release of cytokines and consequent osteolysis.[29]

Patients with sickle cell disease are prone to developing enteric bacterial osteomyelitis. In sickle cell disease, there is impaired gut defence due to sickling in the vasculature of gut. This enables the entry of organisms into the bloodstream, and haematogenous spread of infection into the bones. Typically this is *Salmonella* infection but this probably reflects the prevalence of *Salmonella* in countries where sickle cell disease is common.[30]

Clinical Features

Clinical features are variable, but acute infections generally present with pain, swelling and redness of the affected area associated with systemic illness. Joint swelling, reduced mobility and features of overlying cellulitis may be present. In chronic infections, discharging sinuses may be present. Treatment may render chronic osteomyelitis inactive, but reactivation may occur, with recurrence of symptoms (pain, swelling, erythema, fever) and new radiographic features (bone destruction, periosteal reaction). Characteristic radiographic features of chronic osteomyelitis include intraosseous cavities which may contain separated fragments of necrotic bone (a sequestrum) with the surrounding bone becoming thickened and sclerotic (involucrum). The cavity may communicate with the surrounding soft tissue through cloacae in the involucrum, with sinus tracks to soft-tissue abscesses or cutaneous ulcers. Extrusion of sequestra may occur through these sinuses.

Investigations and Management

Laboratory investigations may demonstrate an increased white cell count, elevated C-reactive protein and ESR. In acute infections blood cultures may be positive. Culture of the pus from discharging sinuses is also useful, but generally has a low yield rate for microorganisms. Table 53-1 summarises the main imaging findings in acute, subacute and chronic osteomyelitis.

Plain Radiographs

In acute infections, plain radiographs are useful to exclude other lesions such as fractures or malignancy. Focal abnormalities occur in acute osteomyelitis, usually in the metaphyseal region. These are commonly lytic lesions with a narrow zone of transition but bone sclerosis can also occur. There may be associated soft-tissue abnormalities. In subacute osteomyelitis, periosteal reaction

TABLE 53-1 **Imaging Findings in Osteomyelitis**

	Plain Radiograph	CT	MRI	NM
Acute	Minimal findings Soft-tissue swelling may be seen	Not useful	Bone marrow oedema can occur as early as 24–48 h, seen as low T1, and high T2 signal	May show increased uptake, but takes a few days
Subacute	Lucent or sclerotic lesion, periosteal reaction, soft-tissue swelling	Cortical and marrow abnormalities, including abscess, periosteal reaction, soft-tissue oedema and abscess	Bone marrow changes, cortical abnormalities seen as thickening, bone abscess, periosteal reaction, increased T2 signal in soft tissues, abscess formation. Post-gadolinium T1W sequences outline abscess cavities clearly	Three-phase bone scintigram, ^{111}indium WBC scan and combined studies are useful, especially to assess multifocal involvement. PET-CT generally not used in this context, but may be useful in exceptional circumstances
Chronic	Bone sclerosis, cortical thickening, sequestrum and cloaca, bone destruction, resorption and deformities	Much better than plain radiographs to demonstrate cloaca and sequestrum, periosteal new bone formation and abscess	Better soft-tissue and bone marrow resolution to demonstrate medullary and cortical changes, sequestra and cloaca well demonstrated, useful to outline soft-tissue abscess and sinus tracts	Generally useful if there is a problem with diagnosis. Combined WBC and bone marrow scintigram is useful. May highlight multiple sites of involvement

and cortical thickening also occur. As the disease progresses, bone sclerosis, thickening, resorption and destruction resulting in deformities may occur (Fig. 53-5). Septic arthritis can destroy the joint, resulting in joint fusion and deformities.

Ultrasound

Ultrasound is a simple, non-expensive bedside investigation that can be extremely useful in the acute setting with ease of performing interventions in the same setting. Cellulitis is easily demonstrated as oedema and thickening of the subcutaneous tissues.[31] This creates a cobblestone pattern due to anechoic strands randomly traversing the subcutaneous tissues.

Infective bursitis is demonstrated by the presence of excess fluid in the bursa, wall thickening with increased colour Doppler flow due to inflammatory changes in the affected bursa. Prepatellar and olecranon bursae are the most commonly affected. Fluid aspiration for diagnosis by microscopy and culture under ultrasound guidance also offers therapeutic benefit.

Tenosynovitis shows thickening of the tendon sheath associated with fluid surrounding the tendon itself. There may be non-compressible thickening of the tendon sheath which also demonstrates increased colour Doppler flow due to hyperaemia.[32] It is difficult to differentiate inflammatory tenosynovitis from infection, and aspiration and cytology will confirm the diagnosis (Fig. 53-6).

In the appropriate clinical setting, septic arthritis is confirmed by the presence of fluid in the affected joint and can usually be readily demonstrated by ultrasound, though turbid fluid may be echogenic and more difficult to see. Ultrasound is particularly useful in the hip, where guided diagnostic aspiration can be performed. Early diagnosis can avoid serious consequences, especially in children, where an effusion can be the only sign localising infection to that joint. In the hands, wrists and feet joints, diagnostic aspiration under ultrasound reduces the risk of contamination of other compartments.[26] Thickening of the synovium is seen in septic arthritis associated with lack of compressibility and increased colour Doppler flow due to the presence of inflammation, but can also be seen in other inflammatory and non-inflammatory arthritis.

Abscesses are usually well defined and show hypoechoic or anechoic fluid within, usually with a thick capsule which shows increased Doppler flow. Subperiosteal abscesses can also be demonstrated by ultrasound before a periosteal reaction is evident radiographically, but osteomyelitis generally needs further cross-sectional imaging. Pyomyositis shows abnormal echogenicity in early stages, but in later stages abscess formation is seen (Fig. 53-7). With prosthesis-related infection, ultrasound can be extremely useful to demonstrate fluid collections and diagnostic aspiration can be performed at the same time.

Computed Tomography

High-resolution, multiplanar reconstruction and wide availability result in CT being commonly used in the diagnosis and assessment of osteomyelitis. The main disadvantages of CT are exposure to ionising radiation and limited soft-tissue contrast.

The advantages of CT are that it can demonstrate periosteal reaction, subtle bone erosion, cortical destruction, abscess formation and soft-tissue swelling. CT may also demonstrate thickening of trabeculae and medullary abnormalities. In chronic osteomyelitis CT is better than MRI for the demonstration of cortical destruction and demonstrating the presence of gas (Fig. 53-8). CT is also superior to MRI in the demonstration of sequestra (Fig. 53-9), involucra and cloacae and can guide therapeutic options.[33] Soft-tissue abnormalities can be seen with CT, but MRI is superior for demonstrating these (Fig. 53-10).[34]

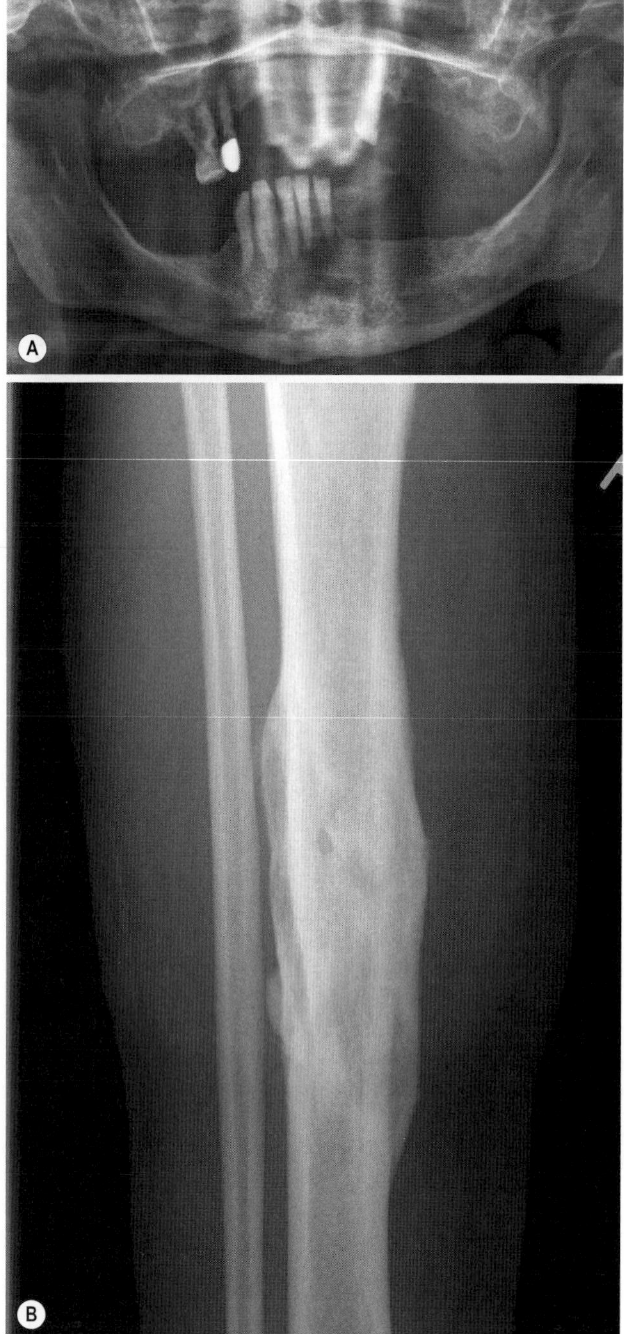

FIGURE 53-5 ■ **Chronic osteomyelitis.** (A) Plain radiograph of the mandible in an elderly patient shows increased bone density and cortical thickening on the left side due to chronic osteomyelitis. There is bone destruction from an associated dental abscess around the roots of the remaining incisors and caries in the remaining right upper molar tooth. (B) Chronic osteomyelitis of the tibia. There is cortical thickening and chronic periosteal new bone formation, forming an involucrum around an indistinct medullary cavity. There is a cloaca.

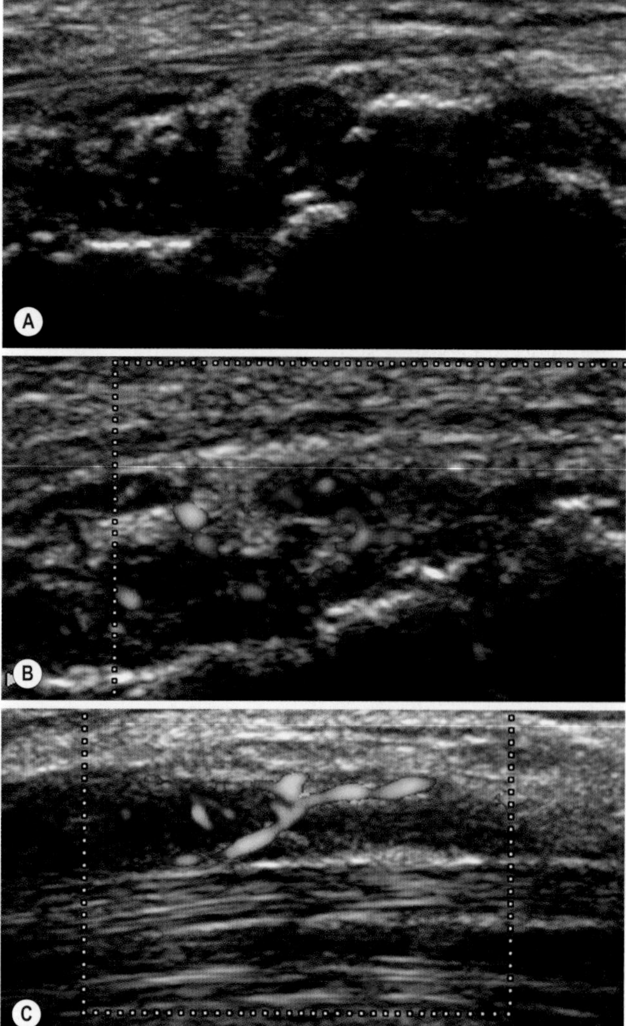

FIGURE 53-6 ■ **Ultrasound extremities.** (A) Ultrasound of the foot shows non-compressible synovial thickening with (B) increased colour Doppler flow over the dorsum of the foot. (C) Tenosynovitis of extensor tendons with synovial thickening and fluid around the extensor tendons of the hand. There is also increased colour Doppler flow suggesting active inflammation. These signs are rather non-specific and are associated with inflammatory conditions, but are also an important early findings in septic arthritis. If clinical symptoms are suspicious, diagnostic aspiration should be performed.

In the spine, CT is much more sensitive in demonstrating trabecular destruction and end-plate erosions than conventional radiography. Paravertebral abscesses may be demonstrated clearly with CT. Vertebral disc space narrowing is not reliably detected on axial images and requires sagittal reconstructions. Spinal canal stenosis and associated fractures of bones can also be clearly demonstrated.[35] In the absence of trauma, the presence of fat/fluid levels in the soft tissues around the bone, especially when associated with spongy bone destruction is an important and specific sign of underlying osteomyelitis.[29]

Periprosthetic infection may be demonstrated by CT. Artefacts due to beam hardening, from high density metallic prosthetic components can be minimised by using an extended CT number scale, a high kVp, acquiring data in thin sections then generating thicker section maximum intensity projection reformations and the use of iterative image reconstruction software designed to suppress metal artefacts.

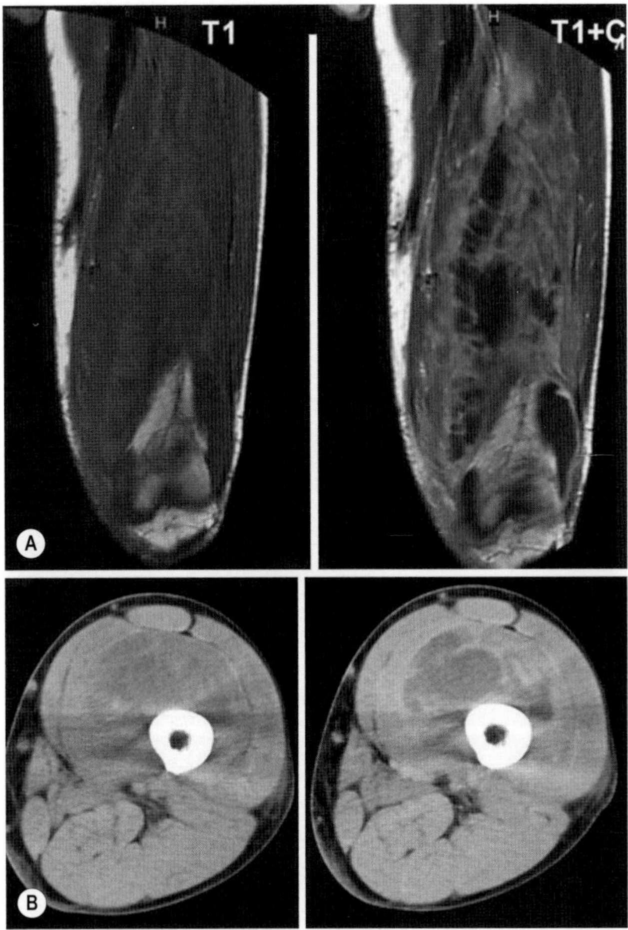

FIGURE 53-7 ■ **Pyomyositis.** (A) Coronal T1 pre- and post-contrast show an extensive intramuscular collection in the vastus intermedius with irregular enhancing walls and septae. (B) Axial CT images before and after intravenous enhancement also demonstrate these features.

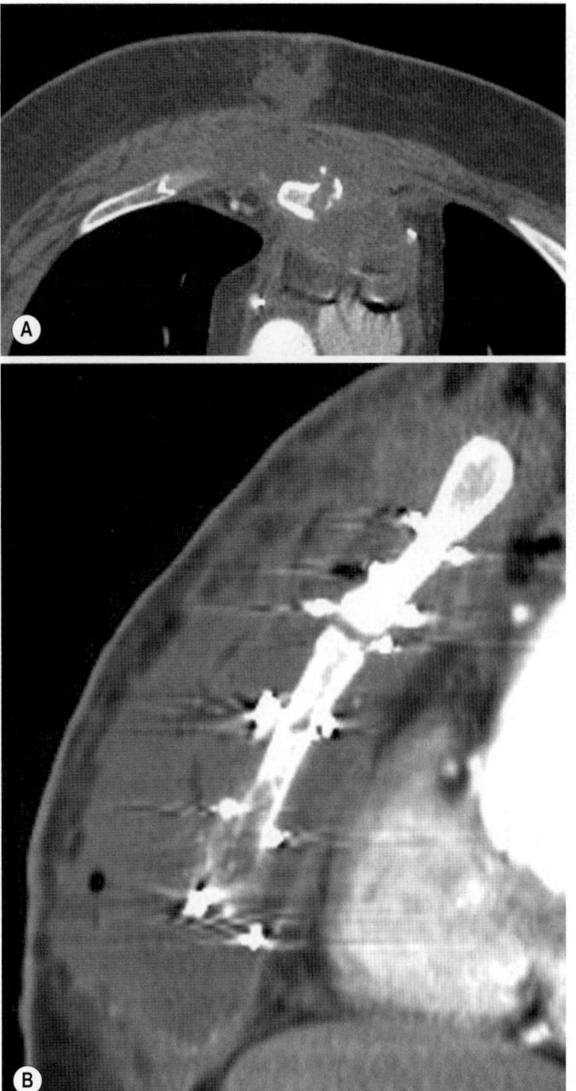

FIGURE 53-8 ■ **Subacute osteomyelitis of the sternum.** (A) Axial CT and (B) sagittal reconstruction through the sternum showing features of osteomyelitis following sternotomy. There is bone destruction and sclerosis along the margins of the sternotomy and a large abscess around the sternum extending to the mediastinum and subcutaneous tissues and containing a gas loculus. Osteomyelitis of the sternum also occurs in intravenous drug abusers.

Magnetic Resonance Imaging

MRI has high accuracy and can be positive as early as 3–5 days after the onset of infection. The good soft-tissue contrast, high diagnostic accuracy and wide availability of MR imaging makes this the investigation of choice in suspected osteomyelitis.

T1- and T2-weighted (T2W) spin-echo (SE) sequences should be obtained in at least two planes: axial and coronal or sagittal. A short tau inversion recovery (STIR) sequence or fat-suppressed T2 sequence is useful to identify the bone marrow oedema and soft-tissue oedema easily. Usual slice thickness is 3–4 mm (Fig. 53-11).[36] Fat-suppressed images can identify ulceration, abscess formation and sinus tracts due to the accentuated fluid signal against a background of suppressed soft-tissue and marrow signals. Gadolinium-enhanced T1-weighted SE images with fat saturation help improve diagnostic confidence, although the overall sensitivity and specificity do not change significantly (Fig. 53-12).[33]

Bone marrow oedema is one of the earliest signs of osteomyelitis. In acute osteomyelitis there is increase in intramedullary water due to oedema, inflammation and ischaemia, resulting in areas returning low T1 signal and increased T2 signal; this is even better appreciated on fat-saturated or STIR images. The marrow oedema is usually ill defined in its early stages. Later on with more localised bone destruction the oedema and signal changes appear well defined.[36]

Bone marrow oedema is more extensive in osteomyelitis than in degenerative or infective arthritis. Cortical disruption may lead to the development of periosteal reaction. Cortical disruption is seen as a break in the normal low signal of the cortical bone. Periostitis shows as thin linear pattern of oedema with enhancement, surrounding the outer cortical margin. Chronic periostitis and periosteal reaction are seen as thickening of low signal of cortical bone in both T1- and T2-weighted images.

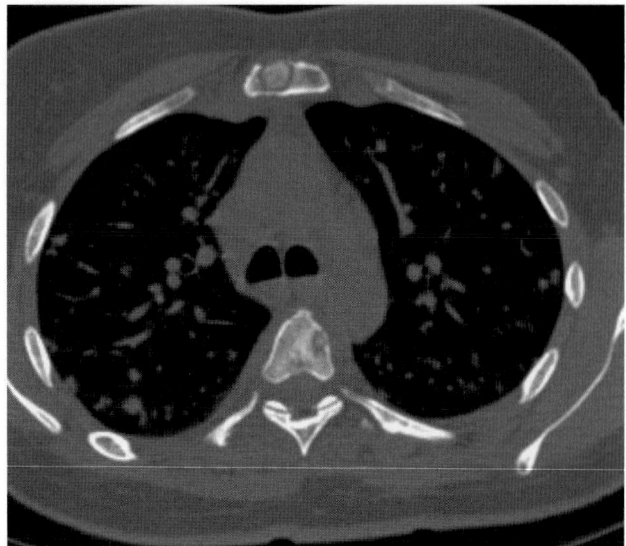

FIGURE 53-9 ■ Chronic osteomyelitis with sequestra. Axial CT thorax demonstrates lytic destructive bone lesions containing central sequestra in the sternum and spine. Pulmonary nodules are also present, due to disseminated TB.

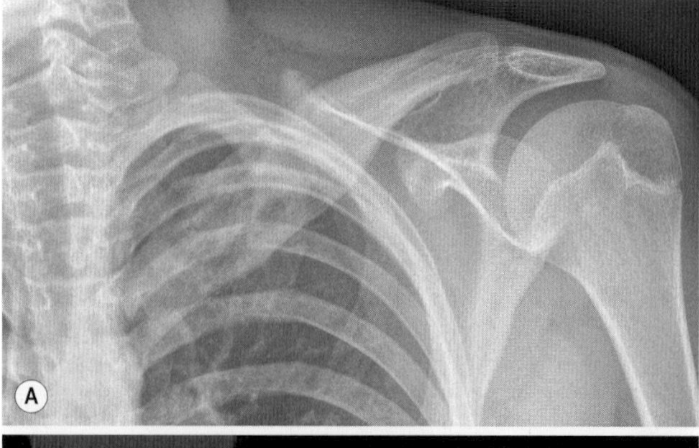

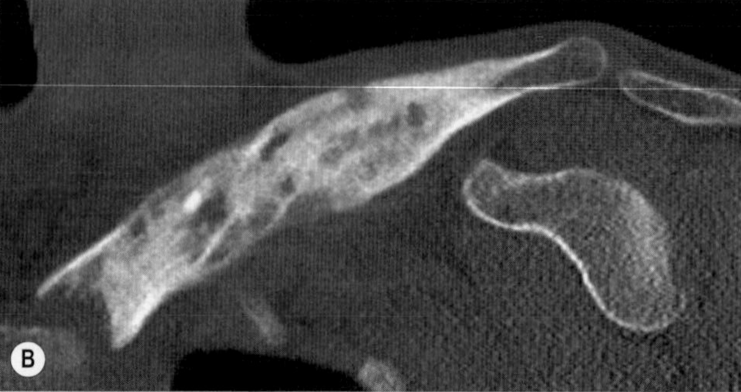

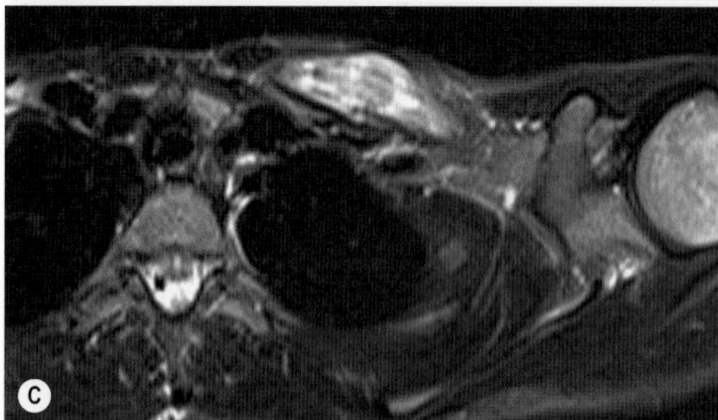

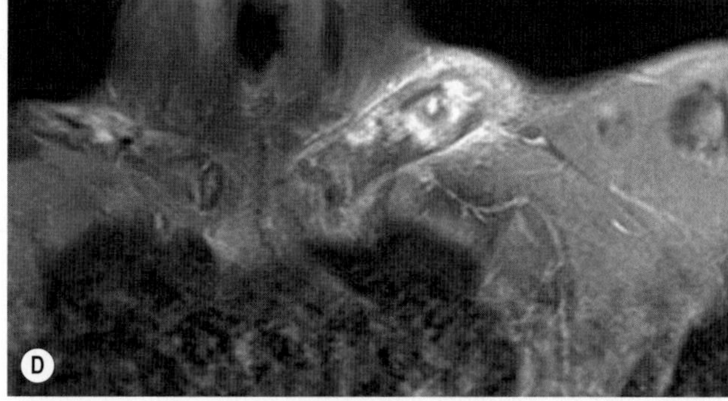

FIGURE 53-10 ■ Chronic osteomyelitis clavicle. (A) Plain radiograph of the left clavicle show features of chronic osteomyelitis. There is sclerosis and diffuse periosteal new bone formation. (B) CT of the clavicle shows diffuse bone sclerosis with multiple cavities and cloaca (arrow). (C, D) MR axial T2W and coronal PD fat-saturated images confirm the above findings. The cloaca is clearly seen in coronal images as a focus of hyperintense signal surrounded by a low signal area (arrow).

In subacute osteomyelitis, an intramedullary abscess (Brodie's abscess) may be seen. The central fluid component has low-to-intermediate T1 signal and hyperintense T2 signal, surrounded by a sclerotic rim which has low T1 and T2 signal (Fig. 53-13).

The MR characteristics of a sequestrum are similar to the bone it is derived from. If it is from cortical bone, it has low signal, with a higher signal if derived from cancellous bone. The exudate in the presence of active infection tends to show a low T1 signal and high T2 signal, which may show enhancement, which is seen to surround the central sequestrum. The involucrum has the signal of normal living bone, but is commonly thickened and sclerotic and may show oedema. A cloaca is seen as a high signal defect in cortical bone at the edge of a cavity. Collections of pus may be seen extending from the cloaca to the subcutaneous tissue (Fig. 53-14).[36]

Soft-tissue oedema is demonstrated as low T1 signal on the background of high signal of the subcutaneous fat and has hyperintense signal compared to normal fat on T2 images. Fat-saturated proton density-weighted images and STIR images can demonstrate the soft-tissue changes more clearly.[37]

MR imaging can be useful in differentiating between acute osteomyelitis and acute bone infarction, especially after intravenous gadolinium contrast agents. Those with osteomyelitis showed a thick, irregular peripheral enhancement around a non-enhancing centre. Medullary infarctions show thin, linear rim enhancement or a long segment of serpiginous central medullary enhancement.[38]

Metal artefact suppression MRI techniques are useful for imaging close to prostheses. These include avoidance of gradient-echo sequences, use of STIR rather than fat suppression, acquiring the images on a high image matrix with a wide bandwidth and repeating sequences with swapped phase and frequency.

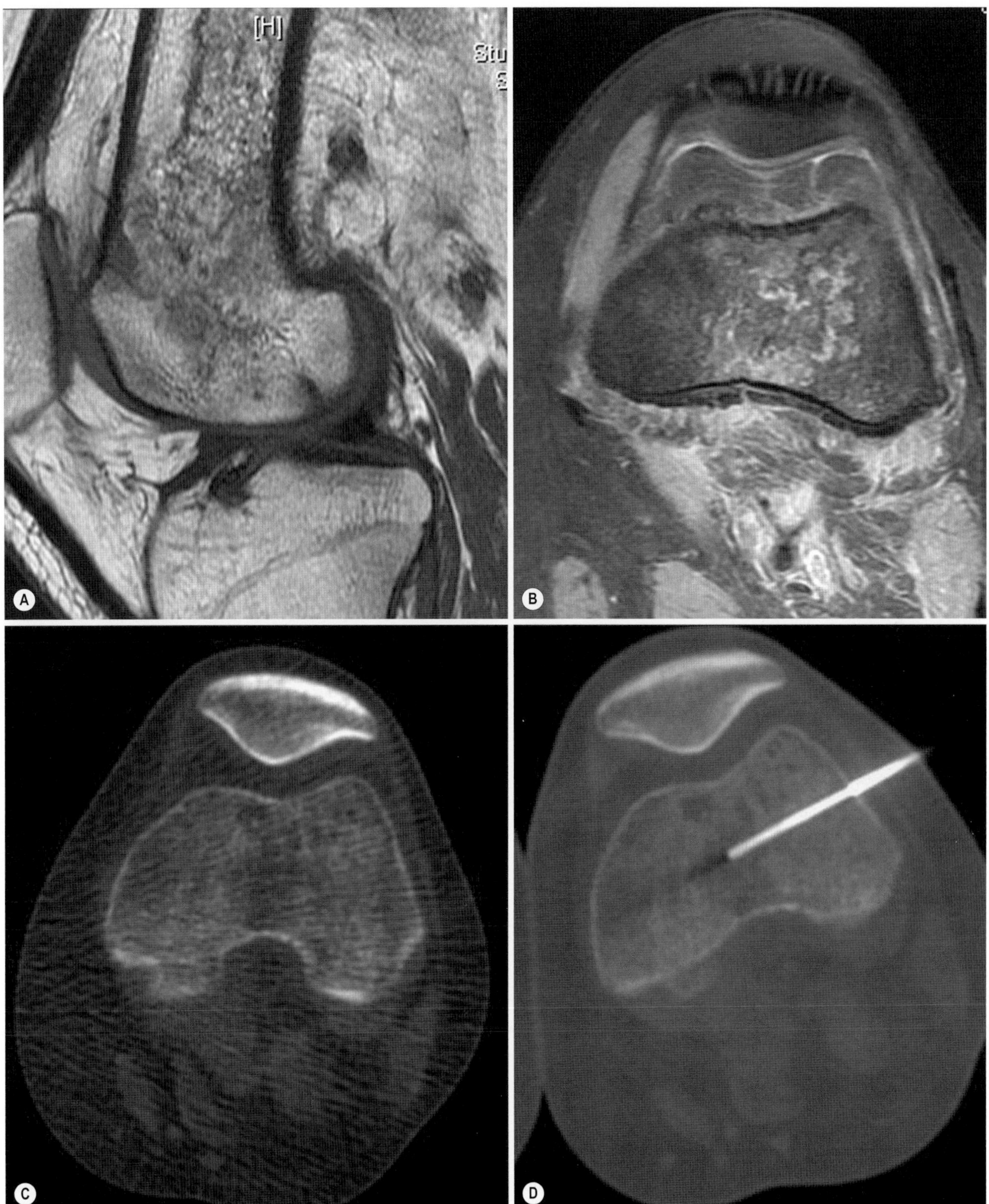

FIGURE 53-11 ■ Osteomyelitis in a young patient with congenital cyanotic heart disease. (A) Sagittal T2 and (B) axial PD STIR images demonstrate abnormal area of the medullary bone in the metaphysis extending into the epiphysis. There is associated soft-tissue oedema seen clearly on the PD images. (C) Axial CT through the epiphyseal region shows patchy trabecular bone lysis. (D) Subsequent biopsy confirmed the diagnosis of osteomyelitis.

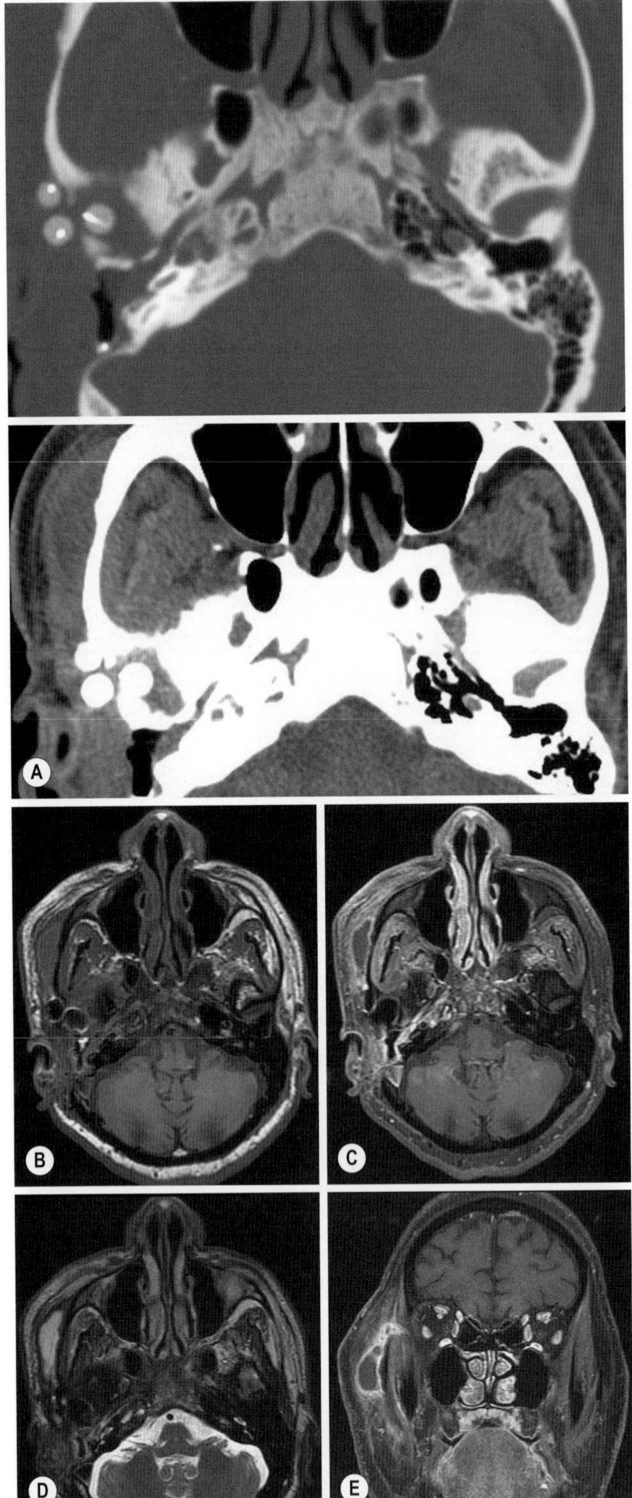

FIGURE 53-12 ■ Osteomyelitis of the zygoma as a complication of middle ear infection. (A) Axial CT image on bone and soft-tissue windows shows soft-tissue filling the right middle ear associated with bone destruction around the temporomandibular joint, antibiotic-impregnated beads within the bone cavity and an abscess around the arch of the zygoma. (B) Axial T1-weighted image, (C) axial fat-suppressed post-enhanced T1-weighted image, (D) axial T2-weighted image and (E) coronal fat-suppressed enhanced T1-weighted image all demonstrate the perizygomatic abscess, evidence of infection in the right middle ear and artefact from the metal wire in the antibiotic beads.

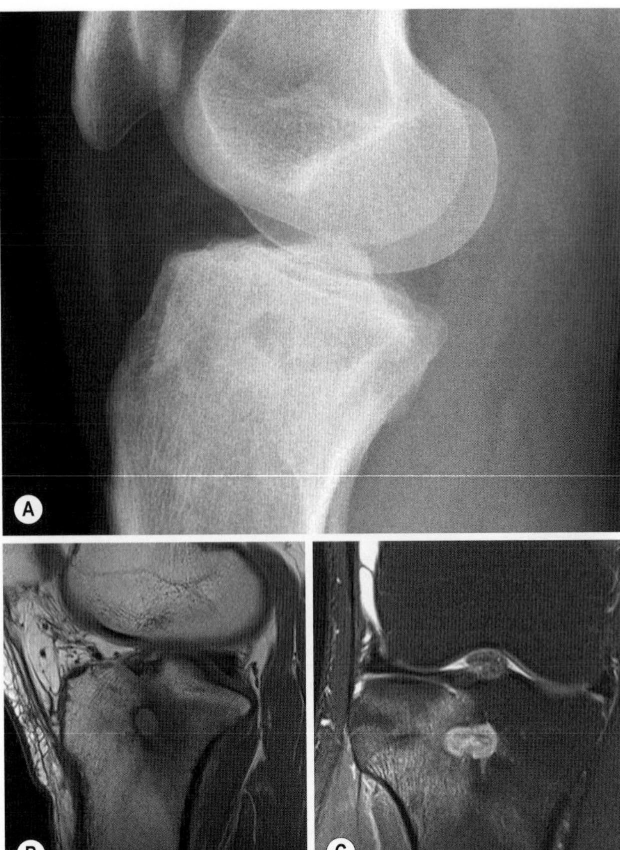

FIGURE 53-13 ■ Brodie's abscess of the tibia. (A) Lateral plain radiograph of the right tibia shows a well-defined lucent lesion with surrounding sclerosis, features of Brodie' s intramedullary bone abscess. (B) Sagittal T1-weighted and (C) coronal PD-weighted with fat suppression show the well-defined Brodie's abscess with surrounding bone oedema.

Nuclear Medicine

Three-phase skeletal scintigraphy is generally useful in the diagnosis of osteomyelitis. However, in the presence of previous trauma, metal devices, neuropathic joints and pre-existing bone conditions, this becomes less reliable and indium and gallium studies play a role. The limiting factor in these investigations is the need for a second investigation such as MRI to confirm the diagnosis due to poor specificity and spatial resolution (Fig. 53-15).

PET-CT has some clear advantages over the conventional. Normal bone cortex has only low FDG uptake and the normal medulla shows slightly increased uptake compared to cortical bone. Hence, in osteomyelitis, increased uptake is a sensitive sign, but it is also positive in trauma, inflammatory diseases, and normal healing processes up to four months after surgery.

Prosthetic joint infection: differentiation between infection and loosening is paramount in the management of these cases, as infection may need removal of the metal prosthesis. FDG may not be accurate here, as hypercellular marrow around a prosthesis secondary to inflammation may show increased uptake both in loosening and infection. Combined ^{111}indium-labelled leucocytes and

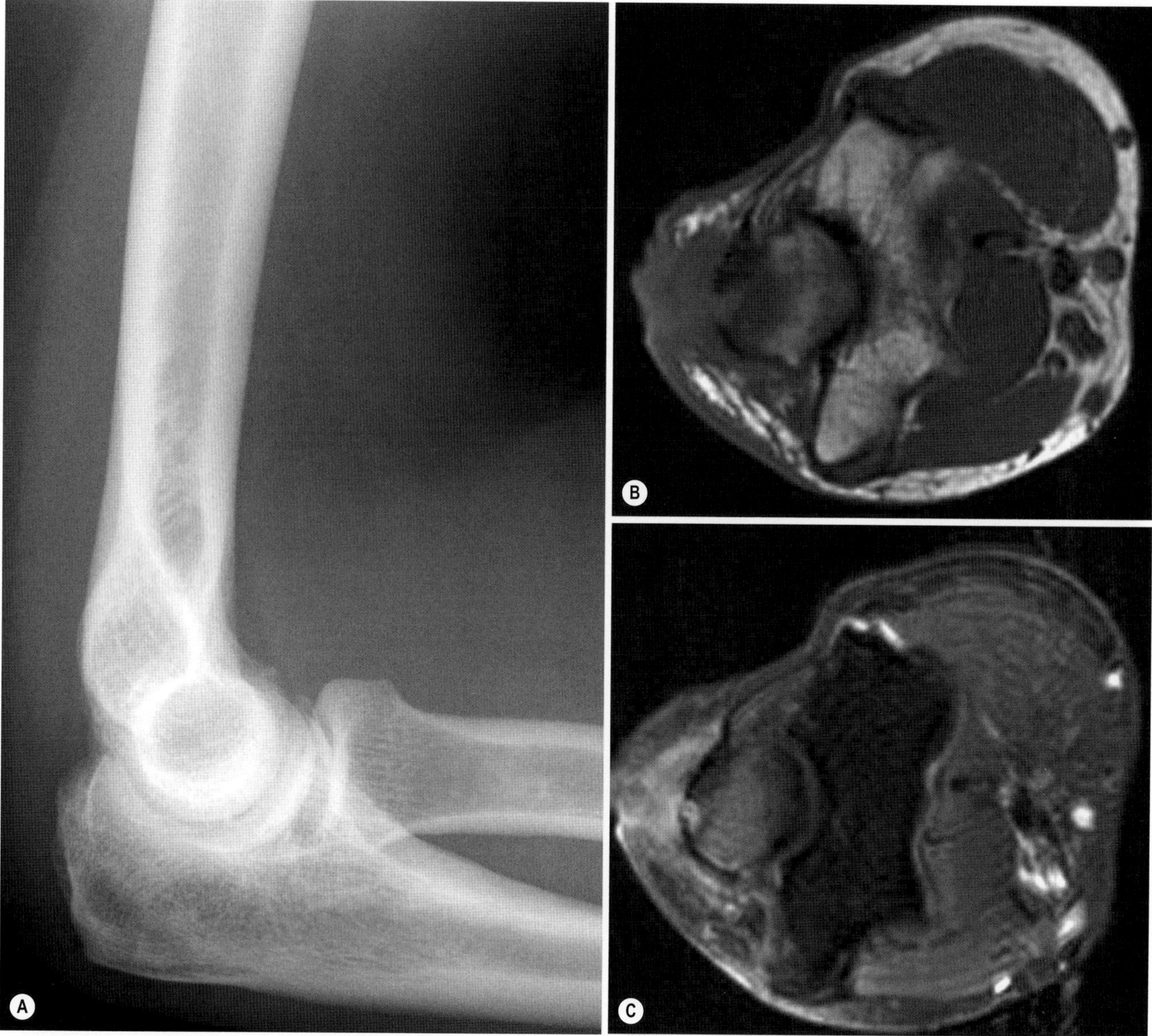

FIGURE 53-14 ■ **Osteomyelitis of the olecranon with a cloaca.** (A) Lateral radiograph of the right elbow shows abnormal bone texture of the olecranon with thinning of the cortex and a focal lytic area due to chronic osteomyelitis. (B) Axial T1-weighted and (C) T1 fat-saturated enhanced images showing abnormal bone marrow signal with low T1 signal which shows enhancement after intravenous contrast medium. There is a well-defined defect in the cortex which represents the cloaca (arrow), with formation of an abscess in the overlying subcutaneous tissue.

^{99m}Tc-sulphur colloids have an accuracy of more than 90% in diagnosing prosthetic infection and are the agents of choice (Figs. 53-16 and 53-17).[39]

Combined skeletal and gallium scintigraphy is the nuclear medicine investigation of choice in diagnosing spinal osteomyelitis and is valuable when there are contraindications for MRI. Gallium SPECT can also be equally useful. However, the procedure requires several patient visits to the department. PET-CT certainly has advantages in this respect and can be useful to diagnose vertebral osteomyelitis and also in localisation of abscesses (Fig. 53-18).

The investigation of choice for diagnosing diabetic foot infections is a labelled leucocyte study with an accuracy of 80%. Combined bone–leucocyte scintigraphy is the investigation of choice in detecting osteomyelitis on the background of neuropathic joints. PET-CT does not appear to have a definitive role in this setting.[40]

Osteomyelitis Secondary to Prosthetic Devices

Infections seen within 3 months of implant surgery are called 'early' and occur due to contamination during surgery or in the early postoperative days. The usual causative organism is *S. aureus*. Subacute infections occur between 3 and 24 months after the implant surgery and are usually caused by virulent coagulase-negative

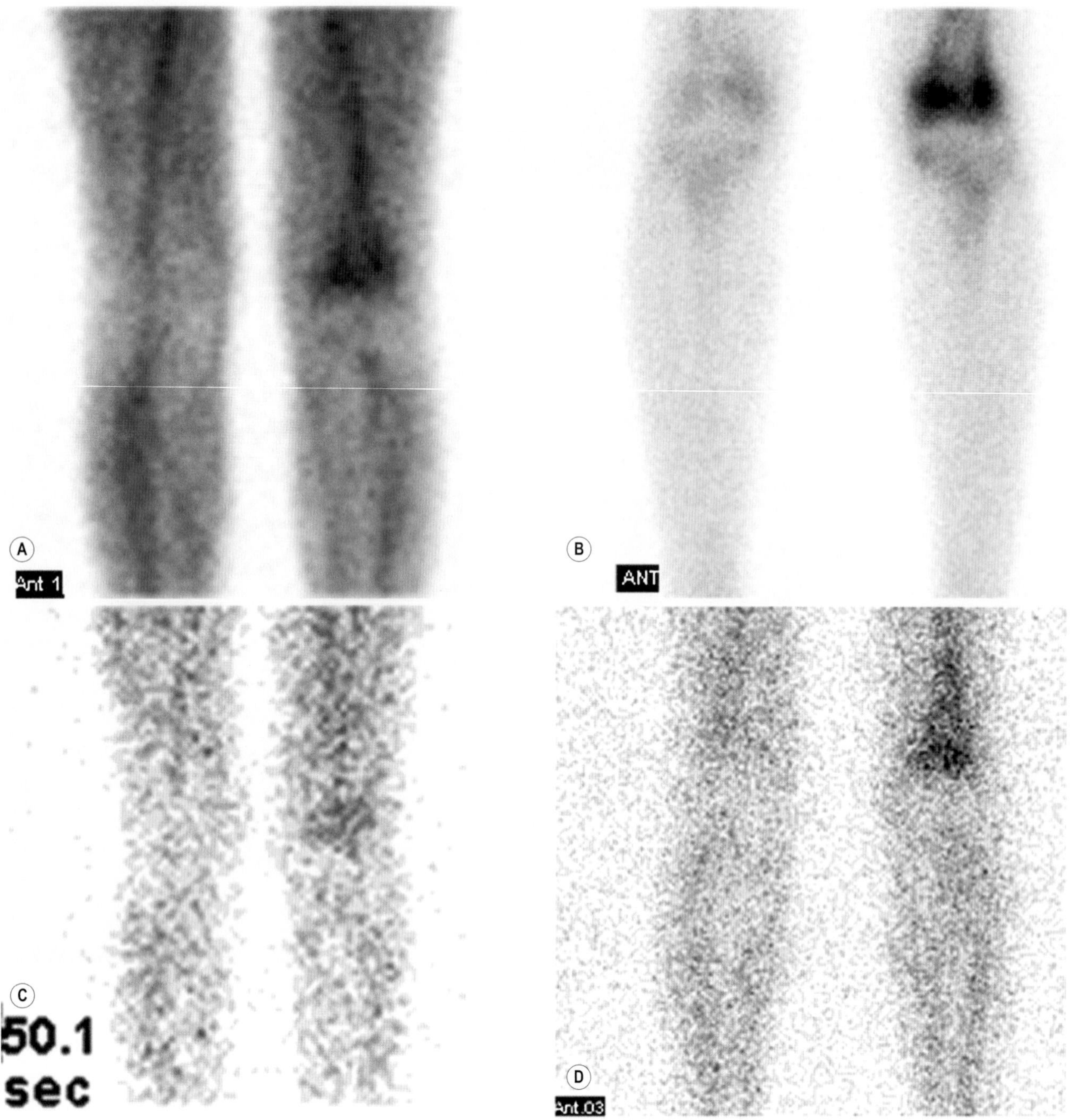

FIGURE 53-15 ■ Osteomyelitis of the left femur: nuclear medicine. (A) Blood pool and (B) delayed ^{99m}Tc bone scintigrams showing increased uptake in the left femoral condyle. (C) First circulation (selected image at 50 s) and (D) 3 days delayed ^{111}In-labelled white cell scintigram showing increased uptake in the same area confirming the presence of osteomyelitis.

staphylococci or *S. epidermidis*. Chronic infections occur after 24 months and are usually due to haematogenous spread of infections from other sources.[8]

Diagnosis of prosthetic infections can be a clinical challenge and may warrant removal of the prosthetic device. Because of the similarities in the imaging appearances of aseptic loosening and prosthetic infection, no single investigation is conclusive. Plain radiography may not be useful in diagnosis but may demonstrate soft-tissue swelling or evidence of loosening. MRI has its limitations due to the presence of artefacts from the metalwork, but sometimes is useful especially after intravenous gadolinium administration to demonstrate bone marrow oedema and fluid collections. Ultrasound is generally the investigation of choice to diagnose fluid collections around the prosthetic device and also to perform diagnostic aspirations for culture and sensitivity. CT with contrast also can demonstrate the presence of deeper collection that is not clearly seen on ultrasound. CT-guided aspirations can also be performed in deeper

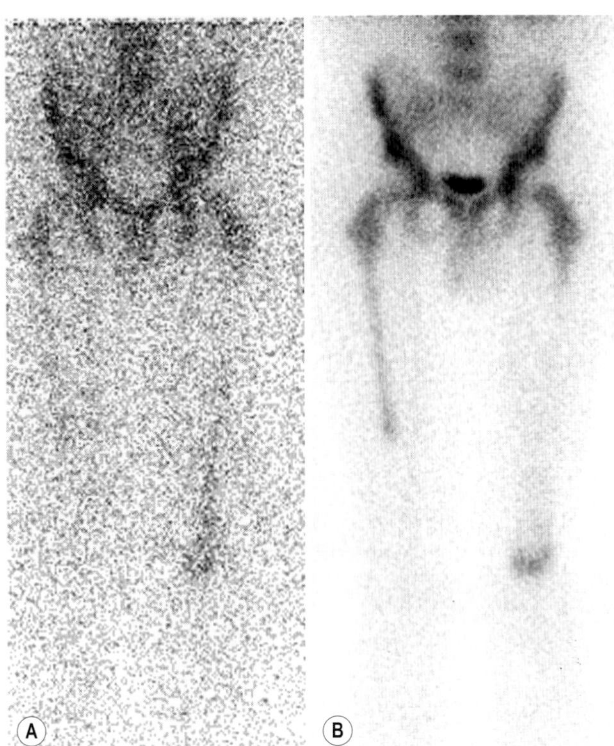

FIGURE 53-16 ■ Osteomyelitis of left femur. Combined ^{111}In and ^{99m}Tc-sulphur colloid bone scintigram. This is currently the gold standard for prosthesis-related bone infection. (A) Sulphur colloid is taken by normal bone marrow of left femur. (B) ^{111}In-labelled white cells accumulate around the site of infection only.

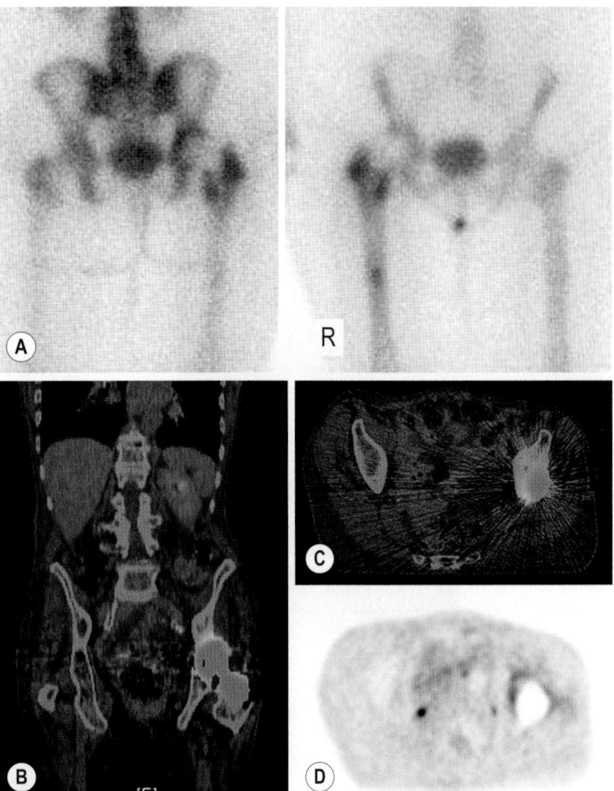

FIGURE 53-17 ■ Prosthesis infection. (A) Anterior and posterior views of a ^{99m}Tc-MDP bone scintigram showing increased uptake around a hip prosthesis. This was proved to be due to infection, though loosening or any other problem around the hip can produce increased uptake. Confirmation with MRI or ultrasound would be necessary. (B) Coronal reformatted fused PET-CT, (C) axial fused PET-CT and (D) axial PET images showing increased uptake around the prosthesis. Again this is non-specific and further evaluation would be warranted to confirm the diagnosis.

collections that cannot be clearly visualised on ultrasound (Fig. 53-19).

Skeletal scintigraphy is widely available and shows increased uptake of tracer around prostheses in the presence of infection. The appearance is generally due to osteolysis and thus can be similar in aseptic loosening. Gallium imaging, the uptake of which is related to inflammation in general, increases the overall accuracy to about 70–80%, but this is still less than satisfactory to separate infection from aseptic loosening.[41,42]

Combined labelled leucocyte and ^{99m}Tc-sulphur colloid imaging is currently the gold standard for imaging of prosthetic infections.[42] Sulphur colloid is taken up in normal marrow whilst labelled leucocytes accumulate at sites of infection as well as bone marrow. Hence if there is activity in the labelled leucocyte images in the suspected area without corresponding activity on sulphur colloid images, then prosthetic infection is confirmed with an accuracy of 95%. There are, however, several limitations including costs, the labour intensive in vitro labelling process, availability, and inconvenience for elderly and unwell patients. ^{111}In-labelled polyclonal immunoglobulin lacks specificity. ^{99m}Tc-sulphur colloid does not consistently differentiate infection from aseptic inflammation.[43]

Anti-granulocyte scintigraphy (AGS) with monoclonal antibodies or antibody fragments labelled with ^{99m}Tc has a reasonably high discriminating ability to identify prosthetic infection with a sensitivity of 83% and specificity of 80%.[44] PET-CT may also play a role in diagnosis of prosthetic infection, but is not widely used for this purpose at the current time and its role is still debatable.[43]

DIABETIC FOOT

Radiology plays an important role in the multidisciplinary approach to management of diabetic foot infections and osteomyelitis. The high risk of amputation in these patients if diagnosis is delayed necessitates the need for prompt and accurate investigation and treatment. The lifetime risk of foot ulceration in diabetic patients is as high as 25% and more than 50% of these become infected, which may need hospitalisation. Osseous involvement occurs in 20–50% of cases.[45,46]

Microangiopathy is the major initiating event in the cascade of foot infection and ulceration in these patients. Microangiopathy reduces the end-organ perfusion reserve despite revascularisation, contributing to development of bone and soft-tissue infections.

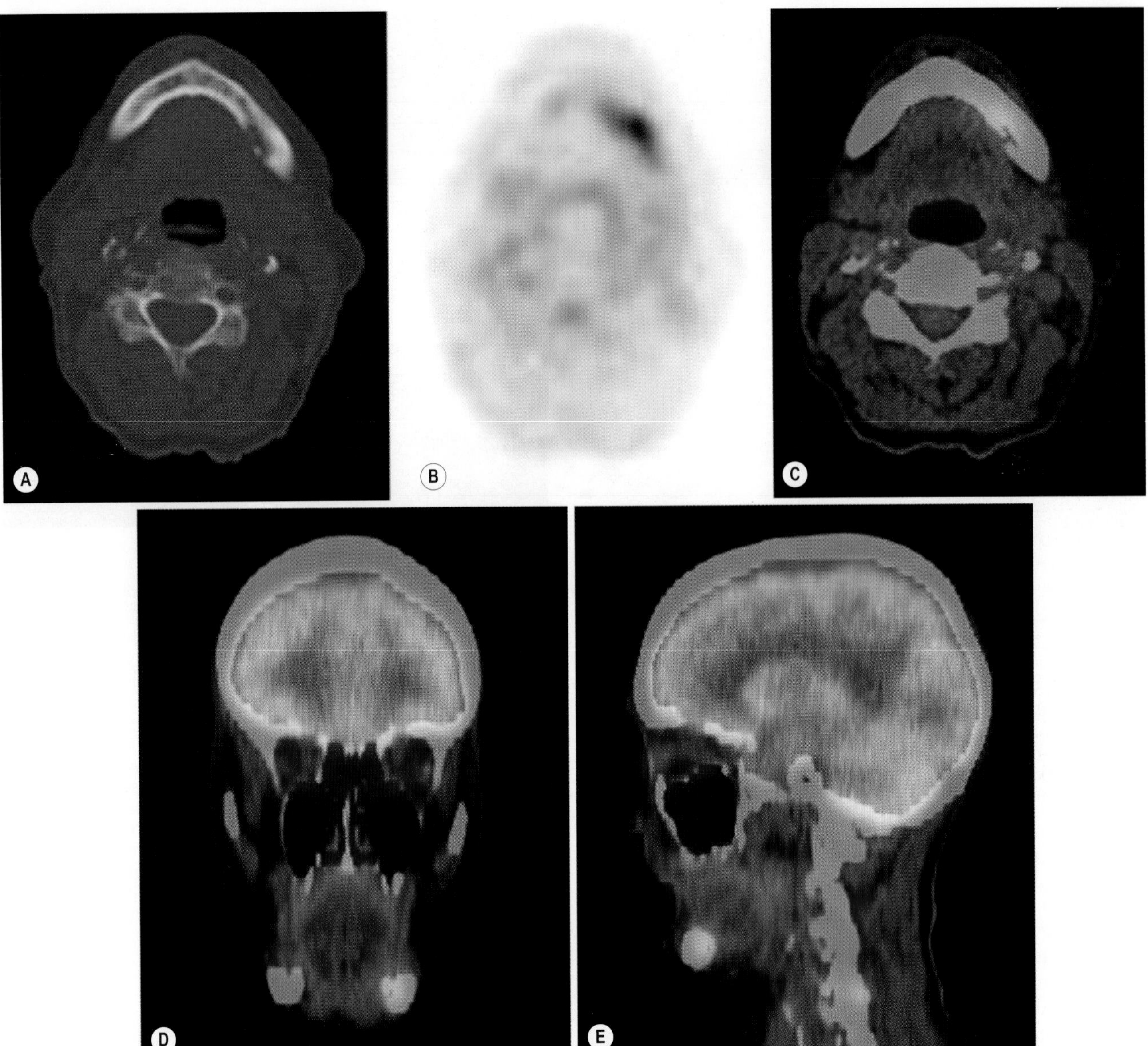

FIGURE 53-18 ■ PET-CT in osteomyelitis. (A) Axial CT through the mandible shows a lytic area with thickening of the adjacent mandible. (B) Axial PET image, and (C) axial, (D) coronal and (E) sagittal PET-CT fusion images show abnormal uptake of tracer in the left mandible, suggesting active infection.

A combination of motor, sensory and autonomic neuropathy contributes to development of foot ulcers, impaired healing and superadded infections.

The cause of foot infection is usually polymicrobial, commonly *S. aureus*, followed by *S. epidermidis*. Extension of soft-tissue infection into the bone causes osteomyelitis.

The clinical presentation of patients with diabetes and a foot complication is extremely important in the diagnostic algorithm. A warm, swollen foot with intact skin is probably an acute Charcot neuroarthropathy, whilst the presence of a cutaneous ulcer that can be probed down to the underlying bone surface is almost 100% diagnostic of underlying osteomyelitis. Imaging tests need to be over 95% sensitive and specific to alter these pre-test likelihoods.

The American College of Radiology introduced appropriateness criteria to select the appropriate imaging investigation(s) which will provide the most help in the management of diabetic osteomyelitis.[47]

Plain Radiography

Plain radiography of the toes, forefoot, foot, ankle or heel (tailored to the suspected site of infection) have Appropriateness Criteria score of 9 (9, most appropriate, to 1, least appropriate) in the diagnosis of osteomyelitis in diabetic foot infections in all forms of clinical presentations (Figs. 53-20 to 53-22). Radiographs have a sensitivity of 60% and specificity of 80% in the diagnosis of acute osteomyelitis in diabetic foot infections.[46]

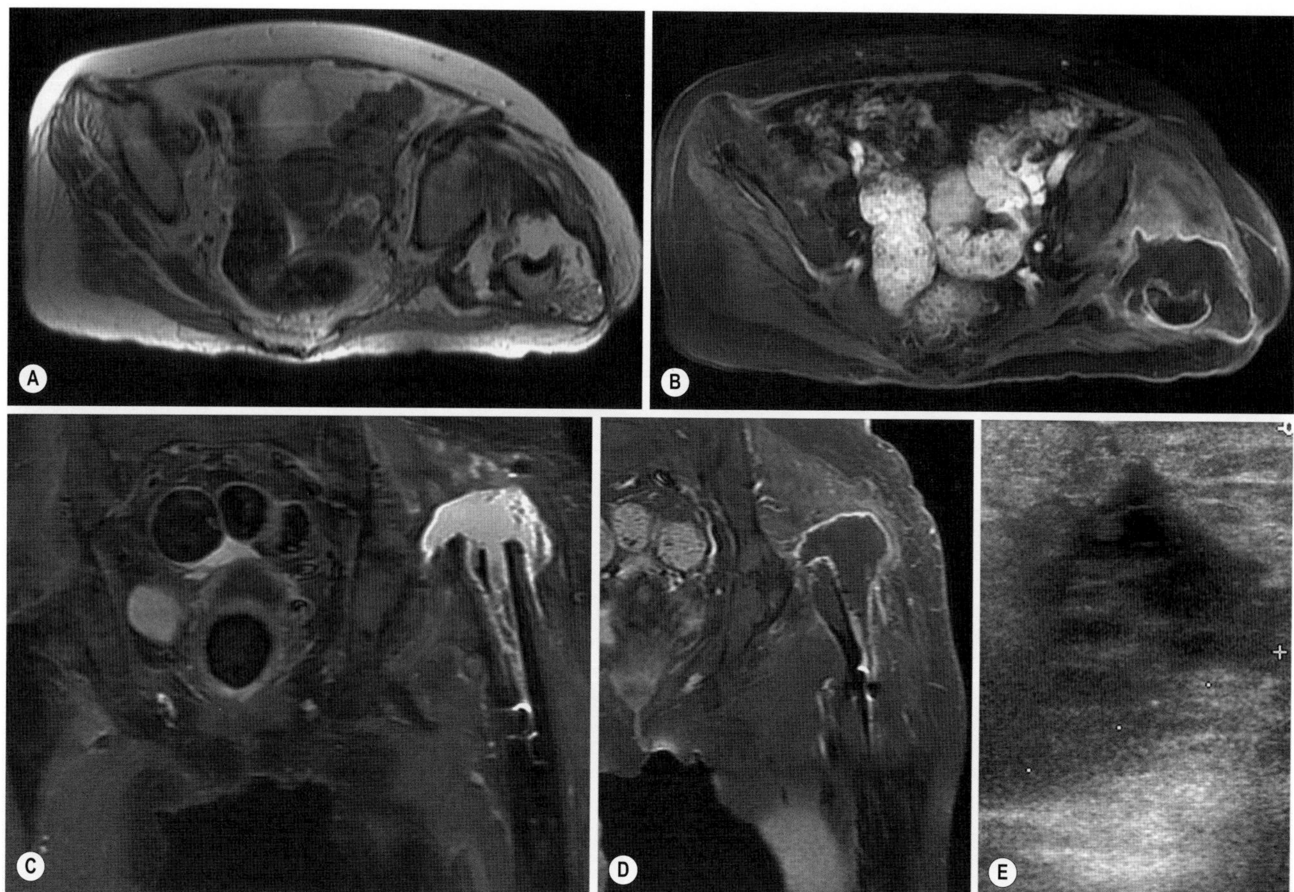

FIGURE 53-19 ■ Girdlestone procedure infection. (A) Axial T2W, (B) axial fat-suppressed post-contrast T1W, (C) coronal STIR and (D) coronal fat-suppressed post-enhanced T1W images through the left hip demonstrate a large abscess in the left hip after removal of a prosthesis. (E) The abscess was localised with ultrasound and aspiration of fluid under ultrasound guidance was performed. Culture of the fluid grew *Listeria monocytogenes.*

The earliest changes include soft-tissue swelling with loss of fat planes, though this is a rather non-specific finding.[48] The classic findings include the triad of *osteolysis, periosteal reaction and bone destruction.* These changes, however, take 10–20 days to be apparent on radiography. The changes may progress to destruction of the cortex, increased bone sclerosis due to sequestrum formation or loss of blood supply with bone necrosis. Bone resorption and auto-amputation occurs in chronic cases. The appearances are often difficult to assess in the presence of associated neuropathic arthropathy. Serial radiography is usually necessary to assess progressive changes. When the diagnosis of osteomyelitis is uncertain, use of MRI with or without contrast or three-phase skeletal scintigram is suggested.

Magnetic Resonance Imaging

After initial radiography, MRI is the investigation of choice in the evaluation of pedal osteomyelitis.[47] Bone marrow and soft-tissue abnormalities are usually demonstrated much earlier compared to plain radiographs. MRI has a sensitivity of 90% and specificity of 82.5% in the diagnosis of osteomyelitis[49] and is superior to ^{99m}Tc bone scanning, plain radiography and white blood cell studies.

High-resolution MRI examines the affected digit or foot with an extremity coil using thin slices (3–4 mm) and a small field of view (8–10 cm). Markers may be helpful for localisation of skin ulceration and clinical sites of swelling, giving increased accuracy of reporting. The patient is usually supine, or the forefoot may be imaged in the prone position with toes in an extremity coil. Imaging in at least two planes is needed for diagnosis and cross-referencing. Axial views are good for the anatomy of tendons and compartments. Sagittal and coronal views help to demonstrate ulcers and sinus tracts, especially when used with fat saturation. A combination of T1 SE, T2 SE or PD Fat Sat and STIR images may be used in different planes. Intravenous contrast medium is often useful. T1 is good for demonstrating the anatomy of bones and tendons. T2/STIR sequences are good for the demonstration of fluid and oedema. Intravenous contrast medium may help to define abscesses and sinuses clearly, but does not have proven value.[50-52]

MR may demonstrate bone marrow oedema, periosteal reaction, cellulitis, joint effusion, sinus tracts, foot ulcerations and callus formation and evidence of gangrene (Fig. 53-22).

Bone marrow oedema is seen as hyperintense signal on T2 imaging, accompanied by corresponding low signal intensity on T1 images. Absence of corresponding

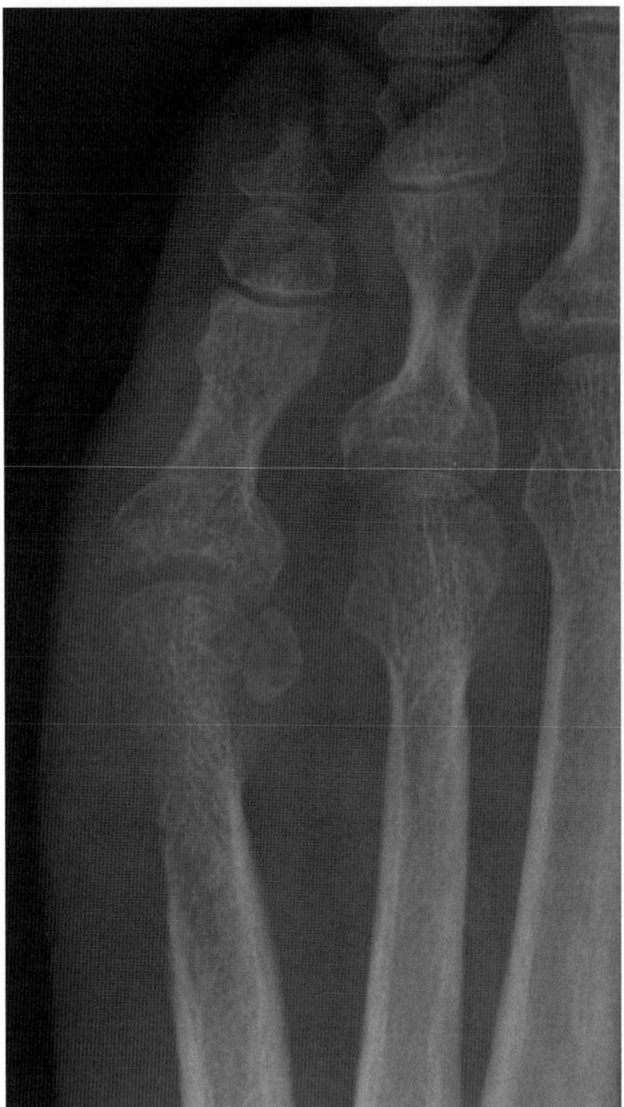

FIGURE 53-20 ■ Diabetic foot osteomyelitis. Cortical bone destruction is evident along the lateral edges of the fifth metatarsal head and base of the adjacent proximal phalanx, with overlying soft-tissue abnormality due to cutaneous ulceration.

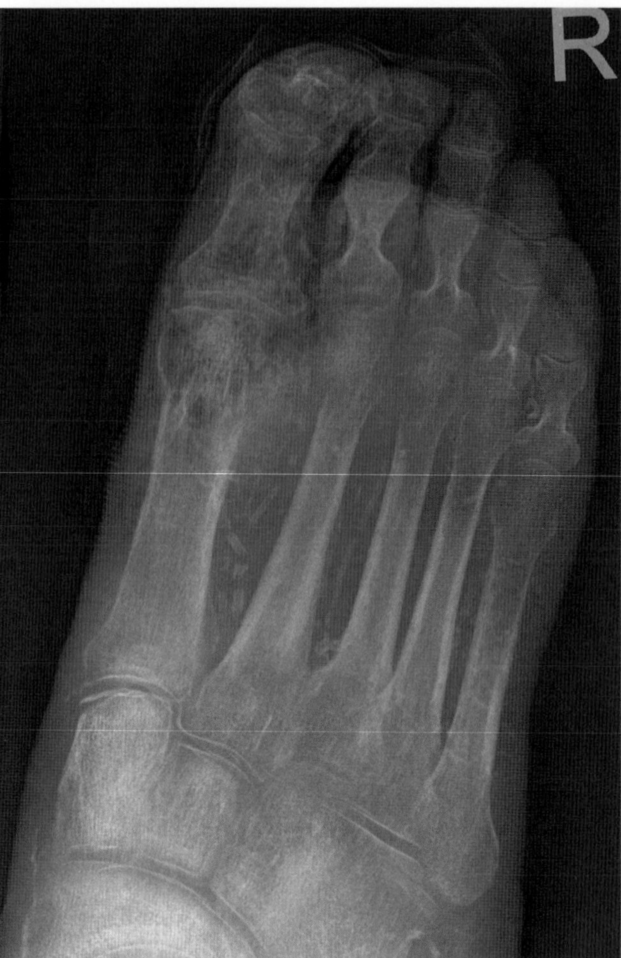

FIGURE 53-21 ■ Diabetic foot complication. Oblique radiograph of the foot shows extensive vascular calcification. There is gas in the soft tissues of the great toe; this more commonly occurs due to air forced in through an open ulcer than a gas-forming organism infection. The loss of soft tissue around the great toe indicates ischaemic mummification of the toe.

low signal changes on T1 images is more likely to represent osteitis than osteomyelitis, even if bone marrow enhancement is present.[53,54] STIR sequences are useful to assess bone marrow oedema, but may overestimate disease by exaggerating high signal against the suppressed signal from normal soft tissues. Periosteal reaction is seen as low signal separated from the cortical bone by high signal fluid collection or oedema; it is usually seen in the metatarsals.[55] Periosteal reaction other than in metatarsals should raise the possibility of infection.

An intraosseous fluid collection is highly indicative of abscess formation. The penumbra sign is also a sign indicative of osteomyelitis; this is an area of intermediate signal on T1 image, surrounding a central low signal area representing the fluid collection. Joint effusion is evidenced by presence of fluid signal in the joint space associated with thickened (and enhancing) synovium.

Skin ulcers are represented as breaches in the skin signal intensity, usually low on T1 and T2 images, and have T2 a hyperintense signal around them caused by oedema. There may be hypertrophy of the edge of the ulcer, which is indurated and has low T2 signal. Sinus tracts are demonstrated as linear fluid containing tracts, hyperintense on T2 images, better seen on fat-saturated T2 or STIR sequences. If the tract is healing or healed, fluid may not be seen and the tract may yield low T2 signal; tract walls will enhance, producing a tramline appearance. Cellulitis is seen as soft-tissue oedema caused by infection and inflammation of the subcutaneous tissue. The normal subcutaneous fat yields high T1 and T2 signal; in cellulitis, low T1 signal and hyperintense T2 signal on fat-saturated sequences are present.[56]

In the diabetic foot it is often difficult to diagnose infections on the background of changes associated with neuropathic joints. This remains the prime diagnostic challenge in imaging of the diabetic foot. Both osteomyelitis and neuropathic osteoarthropathy can demonstrate bone marrow oedema, soft-tissue oedema, joint effusion and enhancement; the conditions often coexist and

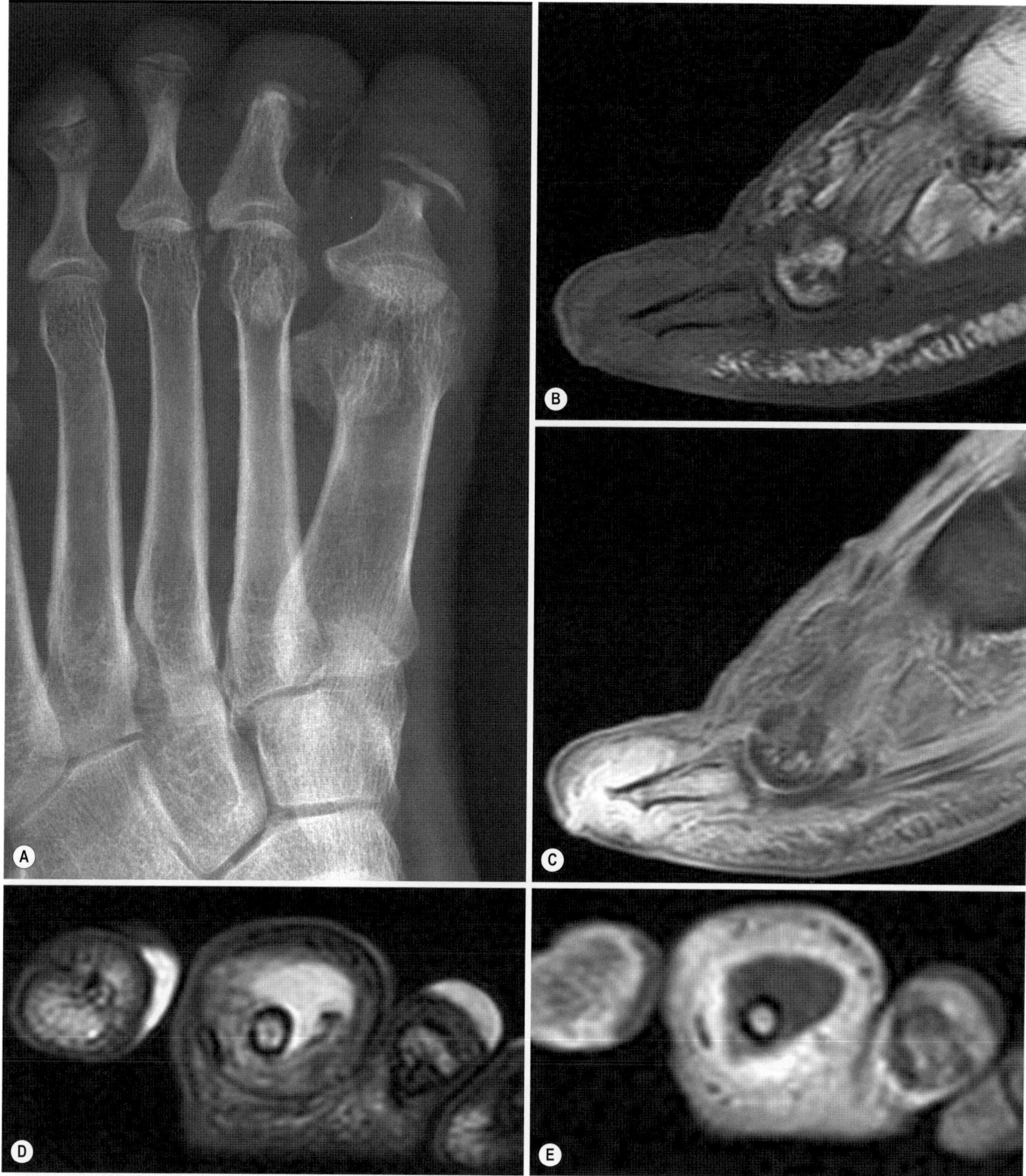

FIGURE 53-22 ■ **Diabetic foot osteomyelitis.** (A) DP radiograph in a diabetic patient showing complete destruction of distal phalanges and most of the middle phalanges of the 2nd–4th toes and the terminal phalanx and bone around the interphalangeal joint of the great toe. This 'sucked candy' appearance can be due to chronic neuropathy, however. (B) Sagittal T1W and (C) sagittal PDW fat-saturated images show the presence of bone marrow oedema, which has low T1 and high T2 signal. There is bone destruction and abscess formation around distal phalanx of the second toe. (D) Coronal PDW fat-saturated and (E) coronal T1 fat-saturated images following intravenous contrast medium demonstrate the extent of abscess formation, confirming active osteomyelitis.

correlation with clinical features is always recommended. There are, however, some features which may help to differentiate between the two and enable one to come to a conclusion of osteomyelitis, in the background of neuropathic joints. Some of these features will be briefly discussed below.

Neuropathic changes include multiple bone involvement, joint deformity, subluxation or dislocation, cortical fragmentation, low signal changes in subchondral bone on both T1 and T2 images, correlating with osteosclerosis on plain radiography. Periosteal new bone is seen exclusively in the metatarsals and phalanges. Neuropathic disease tends to affect intertarsal and tarsometatarsal joints in 60% cases followed by MTP joints in 30%.[57]

Single bone involvement usually favours osteomyelitis. Neuropathy is primarily an articular disease; thus bone marrow oedema may be juxta-articular, centred on subchondral bone, whereas oedema from osteomyelitis may be more diffuse and generally on one side of the joint. However, inflammatory or infective arthritis also tends to produce subchondral distribution of bone oedema. Associated soft-tissue changes, cellulitis, abscess formation and sinus tract suggest infection.

Joint effusion may be present in neuropathic joints with or without infection. However, superadded infection tends to produce thick rim enhancement, whereas neuropathic joint effusion without infection has thin rim enhancement.[56] Bone fragmentation and proliferation, subluxation and dislocations can occur in neuropathic joints with or without infection. Increased erosion occurs after infections, though it is also seen in neuropathic joints without infection.

Intra-articular bodies are more common in neuropathic joints with or without infection. Soft-tissue-related fluid collections are seen more often and are larger near infected joints. Soft-tissue signal abnormalities due to oedema are seen in both entities, but loss of subcutaneous fat signal is seen more with infection. Though ulceration is seen near both infected and non-infected joints, sinus formation is seen only in the presence of underlying osteomyelitis or septic arthritis.

Bone marrow signal abnormalities are seen in both, but intensity and extent of signal abnormalities are greater in the presence of infection. Bone marrow oedema associated with osteomyelitis has low T1, high T2 or STIR signal and shows post-contrast enhancement. Subchondral bone cysts are seen more in neuropathic joints without infection.[56]

Imaging of post-amputation diabetic patients for infection at the amputation margin is also a clinical challenge. The criteria for diagnosis of infection are the same as above after surgery, though it should be borne in mind that signal changes secondary to oedema from surgery should not be mistaken for osteomyelitis. Surprisingly little postoperative oedema is seen after amputation in these patients.[53]

SEPTIC ARTHRITIS

Most septic arthritis results from haematogenous seeding of the synovial membrane.[58] Because synovium lacks a basement membrane infection easily spreads into the joint. Infection can also spread from other source of infections, including endocarditis, sepsis, intravenous drug abuse and inoculation of foreign bodies.

Patients usually present with sudden onset of monoarticular arthritis, associated with systemic symptoms and clinical signs of a joint effusion. Joint effusion may be difficult to detect in shoulders, hips and sacroiliac joints. The knee joint is most commonly affected. Hips, shoulders or ankles are also commonly affected. Sternoclavicular joint infections occur in intravenous drug abusers.[59] In one study, the metatarsophalangeal joint was most commonly affected, followed by small joints of the foot, knee, sacroiliac joints and joints of upper limbs.[60]

Early diagnosis is critical in septic arthritis to avoid disabling outcomes. Delay in diagnosis may lead to development of cartilage and bone destruction due to the release of enzymes by the action of neutrophils, synovial cells and bacteria leading to permanent disability.[61] Before the era of MRI, early imaging findings in septic arthritis were considered non-specific and it was essentially a clinical diagnosis.[62] MRI has improved the diagnostic confidence of septic arthritis and clinical outcome.

Plain radiographs are not diagnostic in early septic arthritis but may reveal signs suggestive of a joint effusion. Subsequent cartilage destruction will result in joint space narrowing, provided the joint is not held open by an effusion. Lysis of the subchondral bone plate, erosions and adjacent bone destruction then occurs (Fig. 53-23). When these latter features are evident the prognosis is poor and diagnosis and urgent management should be achieved before these features have developed. Joint effusion, synovial thickening and increased vascularity can be demonstrated with ultrasound and this is more useful in small and superficial joints. CT may be useful if MRI is contraindicated. CT will reveal joint effusions, and may show bone erosions, bone destruction and synovial enhancement. CT or fluoroscopy may be used for guiding diagnostic aspiration, if ultrasound is difficult.

MRI findings in septic arthritis have now been well established and can occur as early as 24 hours after the onset of infection. MRI is especially useful in deep joints like shoulders and hips where clinical examination is difficult. Gadolinium-enhanced MRI with fat suppression has a sensitivity of 100% and specificity of 77% (Fig. 53-24).[63] There is usually a joint effusion, particularly in the larger joints, which may also be seen in other forms of arthritis. The degree of effusion is not reliable in differentiating between infective and non-infective arthritis. Enhancement of the joint effusion may be present.[60] There may be decrease in the perfusion of the bones. Synovial thickening may be present which is seen as intermediate signal on T2 images. Thickened synovium usually shows significantly more enhancement, compared to normal synovium. Synovial enhancement and joint effusion have the highest correlation with clinical diagnosis of septic arthritis.[60] High-resolution ultrasound may be more useful to demonstrate synovial thickening, especially in smaller joints. Synovial thickening is due to inflammation and vascular proliferation. Synovial outpouring may be present due to increased fluid pressure within the joint.

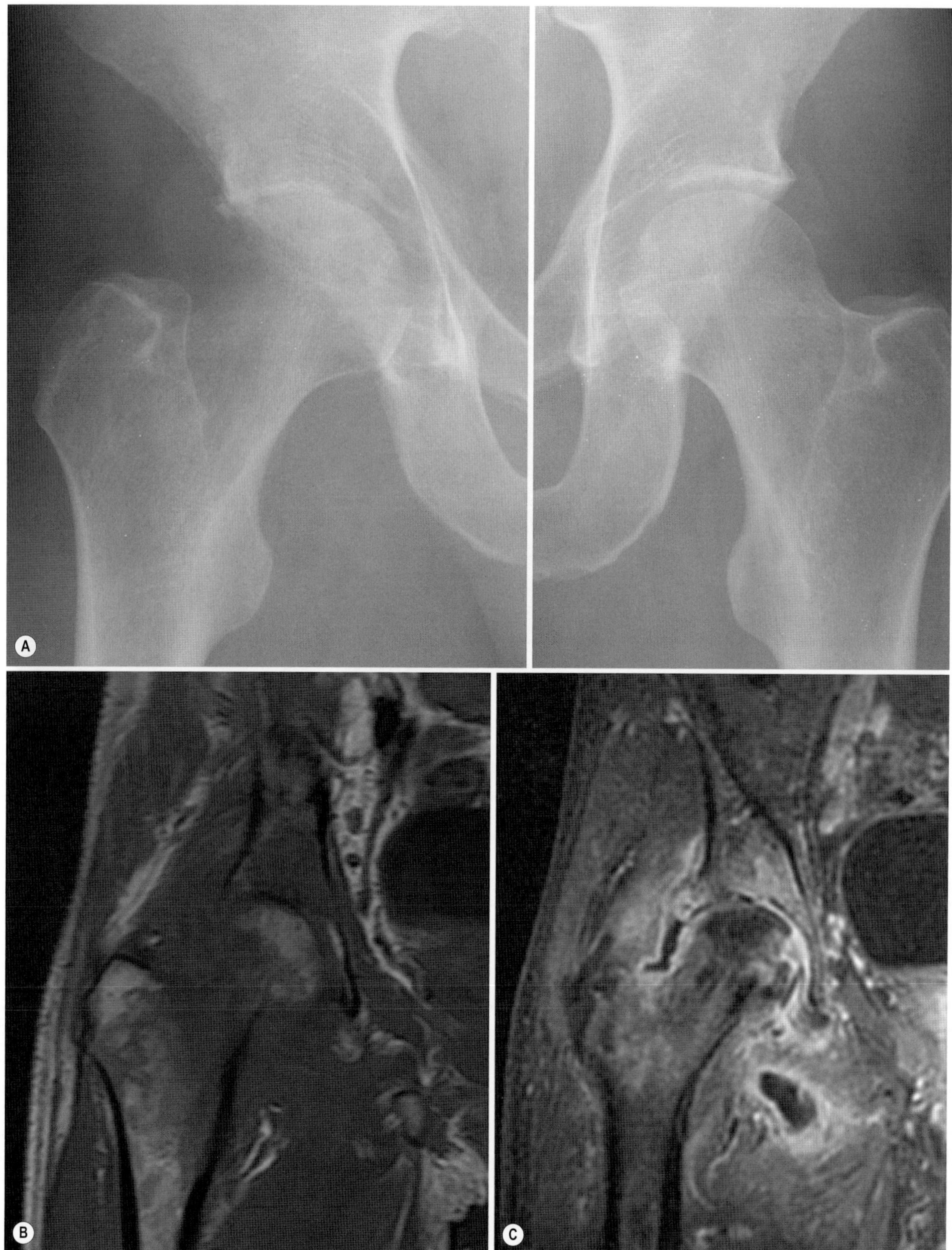

FIGURE 53-23 ■ **Septic arthritis.** Late presentation, three weeks after onset of symptoms in an intravenous drug user. (A) Plain radiograph demonstrates loss of joint space, marked reduction in bone density of the femoral head and partial destruction of the subchondral bone plate in the lateral part of the femoral head. (B) Coronal T1W and (C) enhanced fat-suppressed T1W images show a joint effusion with surrounding enhancement, enhancing bone marrow oedema and an abscess in the adjacent medial soft tissues. Despite immediate surgical arthrotomy and joint washout, the prognosis for this articulation is poor.

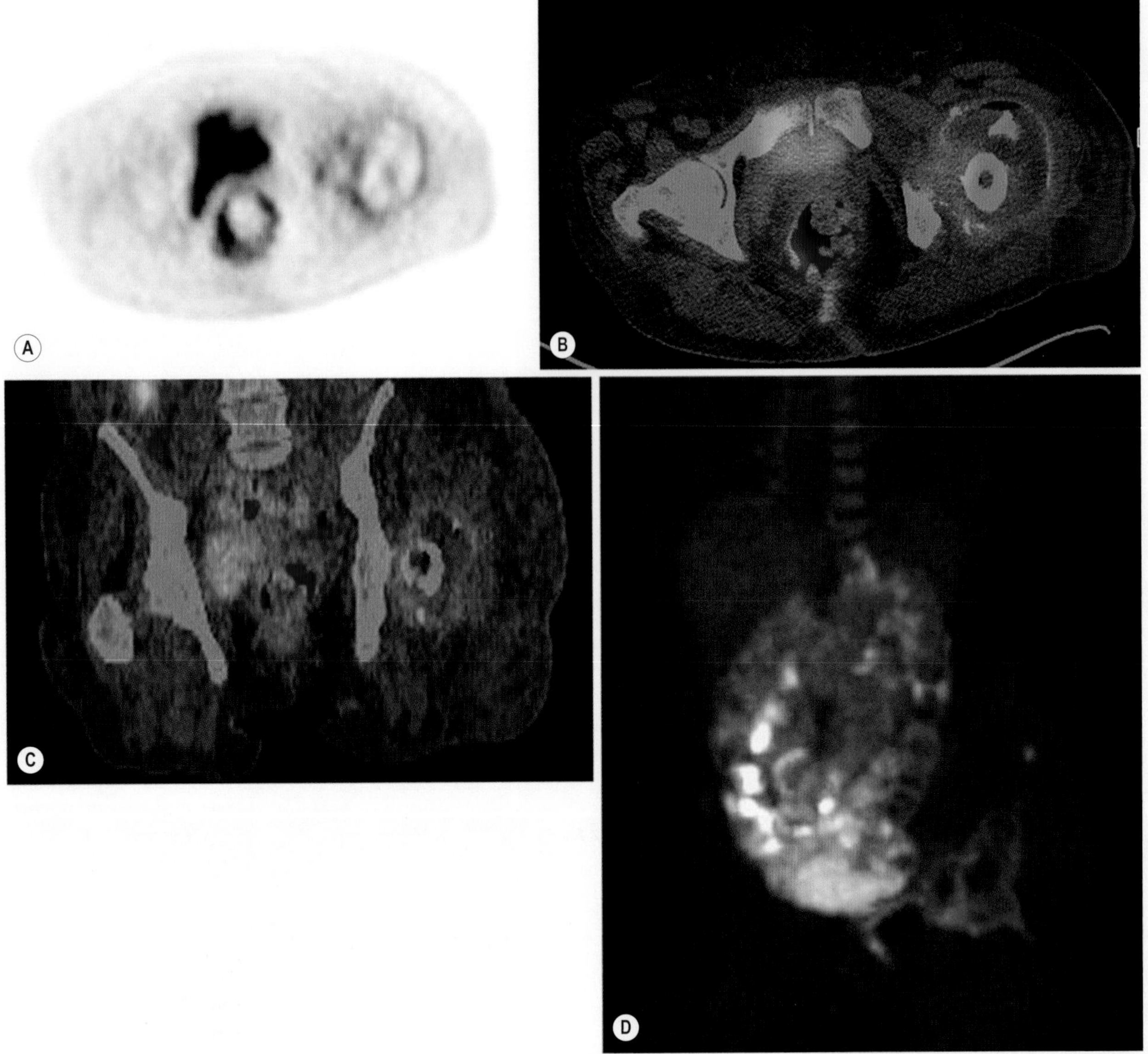

FIGURE 53-24 ■ **Septic arthritis.** (A) Axial PET and (B) axial and (C) coronal fused PET-CT images showing uptake of ^{18}F-FDG along the wall of an abscess cavity surrounding the dislocated proximal left femur after removal of an infected prosthesis. (D) PET MIP image outlines the abscess cavity and sinus tracks.

Septic arthritis progresses to destruction of articular cartilage and then the subchondral bone plate, which can be seen as irregularity of articular cartilage with high signal changes on T2 images with associated bony irregularities and erosions. Bone marrow signal abnormalities may occur due to oedema, and is usually not very extensive. The presence of extensive bone marrow changes, especially low signal on T1 images, should alert one to the possibility of underlying osteomyelitis.[62] Soft-tissue signal abnormalities may also be seen around the affected joints due to inflammation. Cellulitis may develop in muscles, leading to abscess formation in extreme cases.

The diagnosis of septic arthritis is made on the basis of a combination of clinical symptoms and radiology findings. The final diagnosis is made on the presence of positive culture on arthrocentesis, which can be performed under ultrasound, CT or fluoroscopy. Ultrasound is useful for small joints, hips, knees, ankles, paediatric patients and pregnant women. The shoulder, sternoclavicular and sacroiliac joints are more difficult with ultrasound and may require fluoroscopic or CT guidance. If pus is aspirated, as much fluid as possible should be aspirated to achieve decompression.[64] If there is only minimal fluid, saline irrigation of the joint may be performed and the aspirate sent for culture.[65] If culture is negative, a WBC count of more than 50,000/mL is useful to make a diagnosis of septic arthritis.[66] Material for culture should be obtained urgently and antibiotic therapy instigated as soon as possible. Relevant imaging should be performed as soon as possible and should not delay treatment.

MUSCULOSKELETAL TUBERCULOSIS

Tuberculous infections of the bones and joints are common in the developing countries, but are being seen with increasing frequency in developed countries due to increases in immigrant populations and the incidence of HIV, AIDS and other immunosuppressive conditions.

The causative organism is *Mycobacterium tuberculosis*. Haematogenous spread of the bacillus from a primary or reactivated focus in the body, to the bones or vertebrae (see below), is the most common mechanism of bone infection.[67]

Several forms of musculoskeletal tuberculosis are seen, which include tuberculous spondylitis, osteomyelitis, septic arthritis (Fig. 53-25), dactylitis, multifocal bone tuberculosis and soft-tissue infections.[68] Spinal TB is the most common form of tuberculous bone infection and accounts for about 50% of all musculoskeletal infections.[68,69] It is discussed separately in the section on spinal infection.

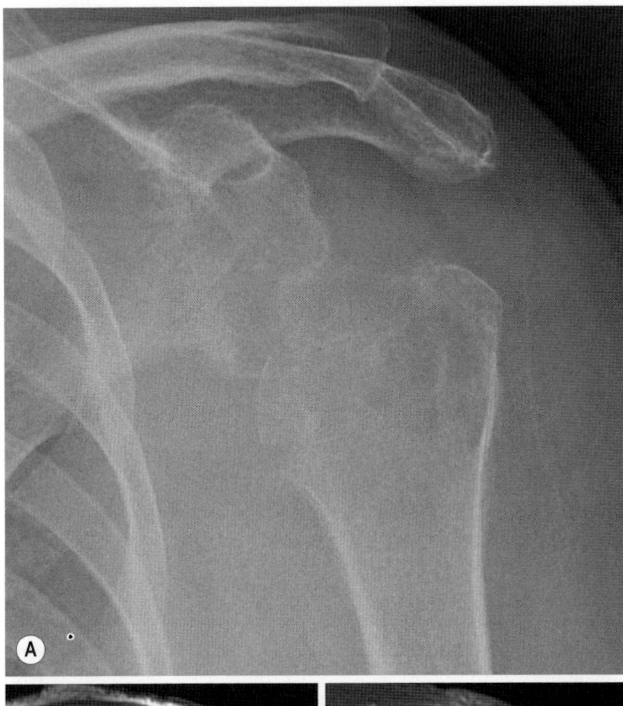

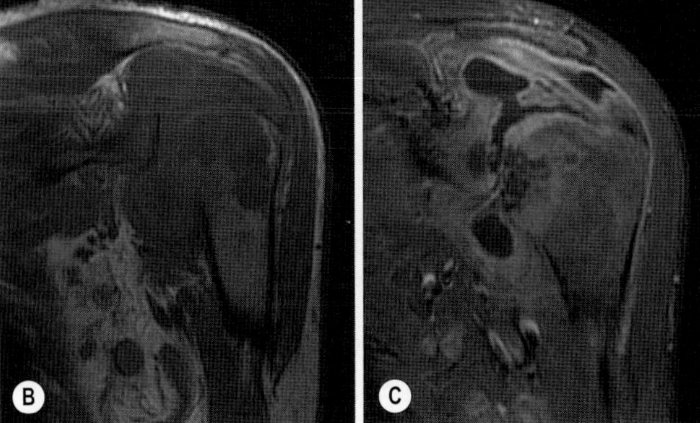

FIGURE 53-25 ■ **Tuberculous arthritis.** (A) Plain radiograph demonstrates extensive bone destruction in the glenoid and humeral head. This appearance in the humeral head has been termed 'caries sicca' (dry rot). (B) MR coronal T1W and (C) coronal enhanced fat-suppressed T1W sequences demonstrate a large joint effusion, extending into the adjacent soft tissues with surrounding enhancing walls and the bone destruction also evident on plain radiograph.

Pathogenesis

Pathologically chronic granulomas develop and are characterised by multinucleated giant cells, lymphocytes and macrophages, with central caeseating necrosis. In the spine this causes rarefaction and destruction of the vertebral end-plates and infection then spreads to adjacent discs.[68] There is late preservation of the intervertebral disc due to a lack of proteolytic enzymes which is somewhat dissimilar to pyogenic spinal infections where disc destruction is an early feature. In long bones, tuberculous arthritis usually starts as a bone infection in the metaphysis, which spreads to the epiphysis and then to the joint. Haematogenous spread is a less common mode of spread in tuberculous arthritis.

In the bones there is rarefaction, trabecular destruction, progressive demineralisation and bone and cartilage destruction. The consequent lytic lesions are well defined, with little surrounding bone regeneration and periosteal reaction. Para osseous abscess formation, called cold abscesses (as they are not warm or tender), may occur. Further extension into the soft tissues leads to sinus formation and skin ulceration.

Investigations (Table 53-2)

Plain Radiography

Plain radiographs are useful in established infection, but in acute infections abnormality is absent or subtle. Small bones may ultimately demonstrate abnormal marrow changes which include lytic lesions with rather thick and well-defined borders. Bony destruction may also be seen in established cases with joint deformities.

Computed Tomography

CT is more sensitive than plain radiographs to demonstrate cortical and trabecular bone destruction, and

TABLE 53-2 **Features Which Aid in Distinguishing Pyogenic from Tuberculous Infection**

Pyogenic Infection	Tuberculous Infection
Clinical symptoms are more acute and severe, with systemic toxicity and raised acute inflammatory markers	Insidious onset, less toxic, present as chronic infections
Subchondral bone marrow oedema prominent	Less prominent
Bone erosions less common	More common
Destruction of articular cartilage more common	Cartilage destruction occurs, but less common
Irregular synovial thickening, that shows avid post-contrast enhancement	Synovial thickening is smooth, and shows enhancement
Surrounding soft-tissue changes are prominent, ill-defined and more extensive	Well-defined inflammation and abscess with little surrounding signal changes, cold abscess
Usually a single site	Multiple sites of involvement common

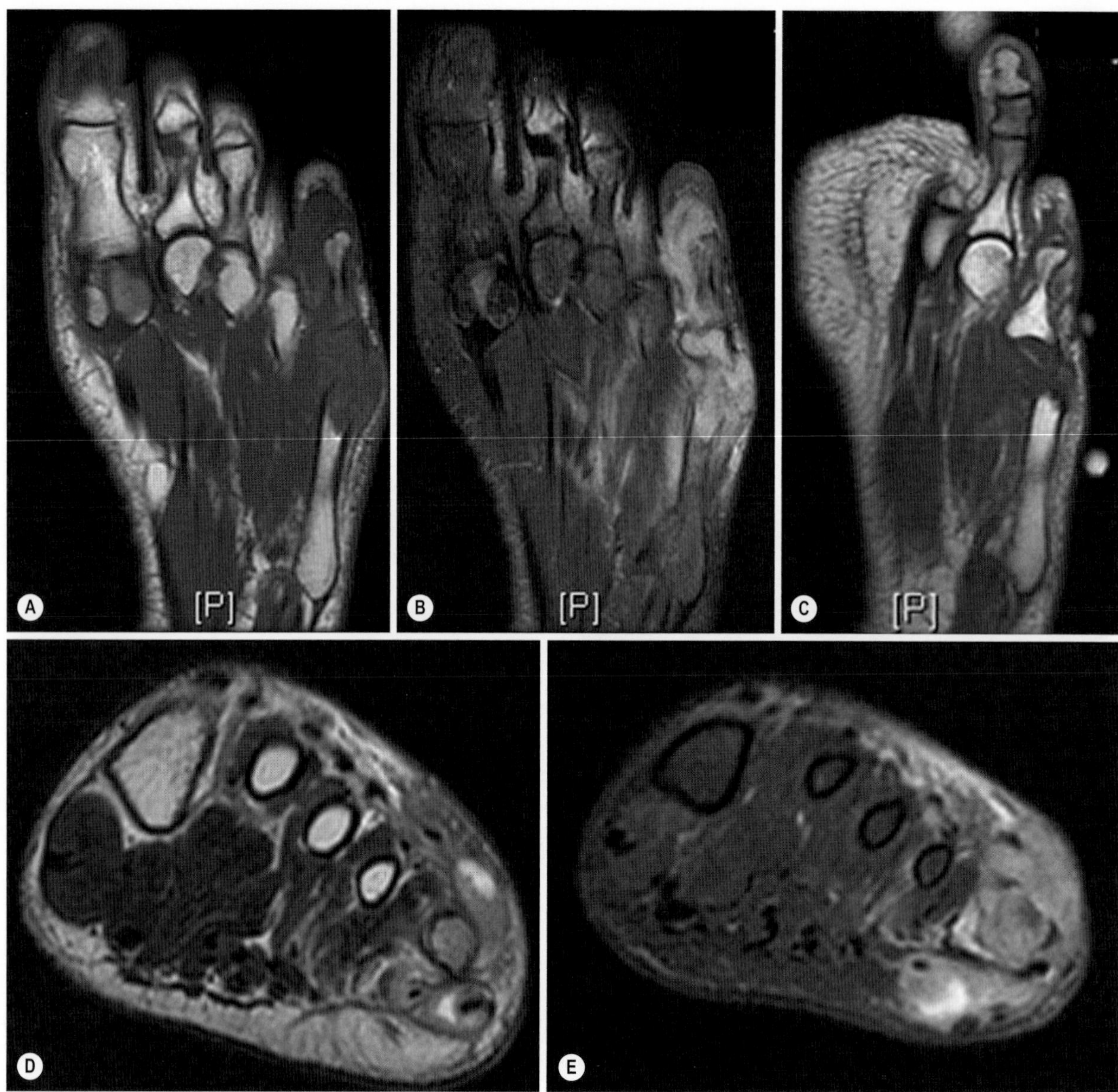

FIGURE 53-26 ■ **Tuberculous arthritis.** (A) Axial T1W, (B) axial PDW with fat suppression, (C) coronal T2 and (D) coronal PDW with fat-suppression images showing tuberculous septic arthritis with destruction of the head of the fifth metacarpal, associated with abscess formation. There is extension of the abscess into the subcutaneous tissues with sinus formation. (E) Axial T1W image, after chemotherapy for TB, showing significant improvement.

periosteal reaction. CT is generally useful for planning guided interventions—drainage of abscesses or planning/guiding bone biopsies.

Magnetic Resonance Imaging

MRI can be useful in distinguishing between tuberculous and pyogenic arthritis, but the features show considerable overlap (Fig. 53-26). Bony erosions are more commonly seen in tuberculous arthritis compared to pyogenic arthritis. Subchondral bone marrow oedema is more prominent in pyogenic arthritis, best seen on T2 images with fat suppression. This may be better seen after gadolinium enhancement. Articular cartilage destruction may be seen in both, but is earlier and more prominent in pyogenic arthritis.[70] Synovial thickening demonstrated as intermediate T2 signal is seen in both conditions. After gadolinium enhancement, synovial changes are more easily analysed and show smooth thickening in tuberculous arthritis compared to irregular thickening in pyogenic arthritis (Fig. 53-27). Surrounding soft-tissue changes are irregular and ill-defined in pyogenic arthritis, while in tuberculous infection tend to be better defined. Abscess cavities in tuberculous infection tend to have smooth and thin walls, with less prominent surrounding inflammation as these are cold abscesses (Fig. 53-28), whereas pyogenic abscesses tend to be more thick walled with pronounced surrounding inflammation.[70,71]

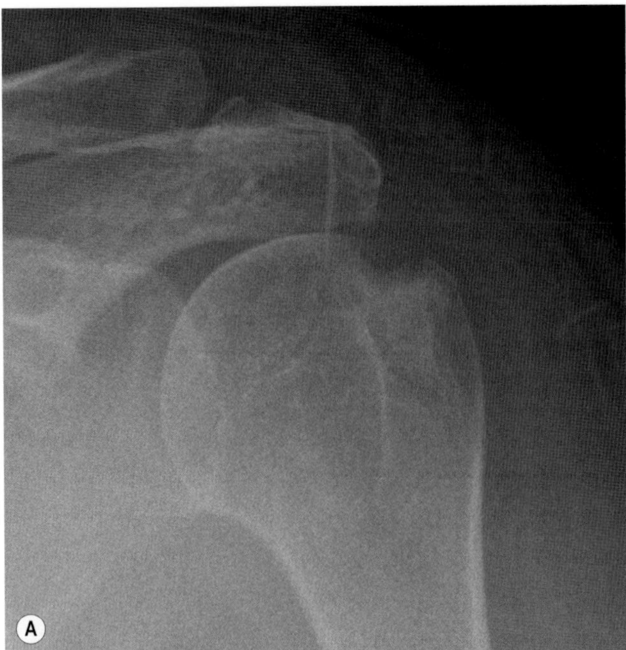

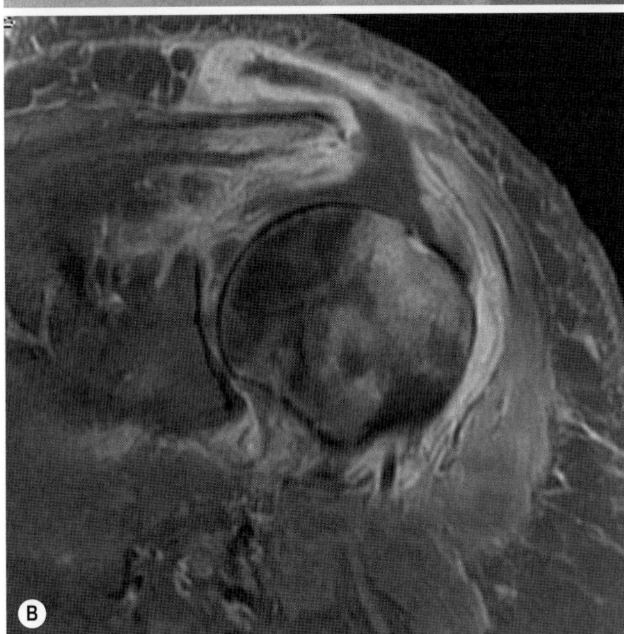

FIGURE 53-27 ■ Pyogenic septic arthritis. (A) Plain radiograph demonstrates a large acute bone erosion at the superior margin of the humeral head articular surface, in a patient with acute sepsis after shoulder arthroscopy. (B) MR coronal-enhanced fat-suppressed T1W image demonstrates marked thickening and enhancement of the synovium, marrow oedema and surrounding soft-tissue enhancement.

UNUSUAL MUSCULOSKELETAL INFECTIONS

Atypical Mycobacterial Musculoskeletal Infections

Atypical mycobacterial infections are also on the rise and are more resistant to treatment than tuberculosis.[72] Musculoskeletal infections occur in approximately 5–10% of atypical mycobacterial infections. Most osseous infections are caused by *Mycobacterium kansasii* and *M. scrofulaceum*, followed by *M. avium-intercellulare* and *M. fortuitum*. The mode of infection may be haematogenous or by direct inoculation from surgical implants or trauma. Patients present with similar symptoms as mycobacterial infections but may be milder and more protracted. Fevers, chills, malaise and weight loss may occur. Early radiographic manifestation includes soft-tissue swelling due to inflammatory changes and regional hyperaemia. General radiographic observations include a tendency for metaphyseal or diaphyseal involvement. Bone resorption, osteolysis with periosteal reaction and bone marrow oedema occur, but take several weeks to be evident radiographically. Multiple sites of involvement, well-defined lytic lesions with marginal sclerosis and osteopenia are less striking than that seen in tuberculosis. In subacute and chronic forms bone abscess, sequestrum, involucrum and cloaca formation occur with the formation of sinus tracts. Spinal involvement, monoarticular arthritis and soft-tissue infections of tenosynovitis, septic bursitis or carpal tunnel syndrome occur and have radiographic changes similar to tuberculous disease.

Hydatid Disease

Infection of bone by the parasitic tapeworm *Echinococcus* is rare, accounting for less than 5% of cases of hydatidosis. Spinal and pelvic sites are commonest. Uni- or multiloculate intraosseous cysts which may expand the bone and extend into adjacent soft tissues are seen but are not specific. Serological tests are positive.

Bone Infections in Sickle Cell Disease

Sickle cell disease is an autosomal recessive condition that occurs as a result of a defect in haemoglobin S, affecting the β-chain. The mild, heterozygous form of the disease is called sickle cell trait, which results in a carrier status, without symptomatic disease. The effect of sickle cell disease is abnormal sickling of red blood cells within the capillaries and blood vessels, which result in vascular occlusion and infarction affecting various organs, called a 'sickling crisis'. Bone infarction can occur, resulting in severe pain. The effect of autosplenectomy due to recurrent splenic infarcts and the presence of bone infarcts predispose these patients to bone infections. Infection is usually caused by *Salmonella* organisms, the source of infection being the gut, followed by staphylococci infections.[73] Long bones and small bones are commonly affected. Radiographic appearances are similar to other forms of osteomyelitis, but a diagnostic challenge can occur due to pre-existing replacement of fatty marrow by red marrow secondary to intramedullary marrow hyperplasia causing abnormal bone marrow signal in the absence of infection. Also aseptic infarction can cause severe bone pain and can cause abnormal signal changes on MRI imaging and be confused with infection. Familiarity with the patterns of MRI appearances of bone infarcts and normal red bone changes is necessary to avoid overdiagnosis of osteomyelitis.

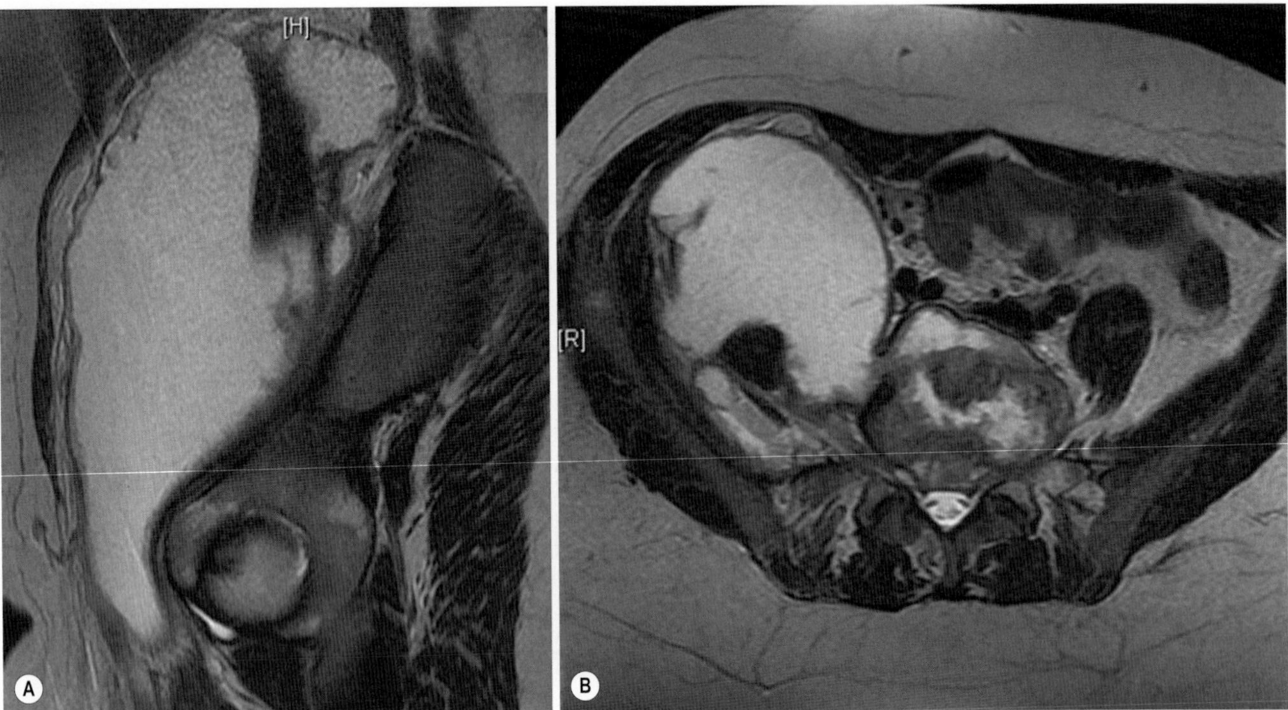

FIGURE 53-28 ■ **Tuberculous 'cold' abscess.** (A) MR sagittal and (B) axial T2W sequences demonstrate a large abscess extending over the surface of the psoas muscle in the pelvis, arising from tuberculous discitis at L4/5.

Bone infarcts typically affect small tubular bones of the hands and feet in children and long bone in adults. Lucency and periosteal reaction occurs in the early stages, which may proceed to sclerosis and bone infarcts and destruction. Avascular necrosis of the epiphyses of the femoral and humeral head is common and can be bilateral.

Blood cultures can be positive in up to 50% of cases and are essential for diagnosing osteomyelitis. Radiographic changes of bone infection are usually subtle in the early stages and may not be evident for up to 10 days after the onset of infection. Osteolysis and periosteal reaction are the initial findings. MRI is the optimal investigation for diagnosing bone infection as it can demonstrate bone marrow changes, abscesses, and periosteal reaction and helps to differentiate from bone infarction and avascular necrosis.[74] Bone infarcts tend to have a serpiginous appearance on MRI and avascular necrosis affects typical sites. Septic arthritis is less common than osteomyelitis. Combined leucocyte-labelled and Tc-sulphur colloid imaging may also help to differentiate between infection and infarction. Early diagnosis and treatment is important in preventing long-term complications in these patients.

Musculoskeletal Fungal Infections

High-risk patients for fungal infections include immunosuppressed HIV-positive patients, organ transplant recipients and patients on chemotherapy and long-term corticosteroids. Travel to endemic areas also increases the risk of infection. Infection occurs through skin inoculation or by the haematogenous route, usually via the lungs. They cause granuloma formation and may show soft-tissue nodules, discharging sinuses, chronic multifocal osteomyelitis and joint infection.[75] Mixed sclerotic and lytic lesions can occur. Synovial thickening and features of chronic granulomatous arthritis are present and resemble osteoarticular tuberculosis.

Aspergillus fumigatus infection occurs via haematogenous spread from invasive pulmonary aspergillosis. The spine is most commonly affected, but infection can occur in other joints. Multifocal osteomyelitis, septic arthritis and discitis can occur. Diagnosis is made by synovial or bone biopsy.

Blastomycosis is endemic in the western United States, and bone infection affects the spine and lower limbs. Radiological features include those of chronic arthritis. Osteolytic lesions resembling bone tumours may occur and need bone biopsy for diagnosis.

Candida osteomyelitis presents as a lytic lesion without significant periosteal reaction, in immunosuppressed patients. Arthritis affects the larger joints.

Cryptococcosis occurs in immunosuppressed patients and may proceed to disseminated infection affecting larger joints, osteolytic lesions in flat bones and avascular necrosis.

Mycetoma tends to cause granulomatous infection of plantar subcutaneous tissue and proceed to cause chronic osteomyelitis, with multiple discharging sinuses. Mixed sclerotic and lytic lesions of bone are seen on radiographs. Chronic infection of the bones and soft tissues of the foot due to fungae or actinomycetes implanted by penetrating injury from thorns was described as 'Madura foot'. The soft-tissue abscesses in this condition characteristically contain multiple small cavities, each with a low

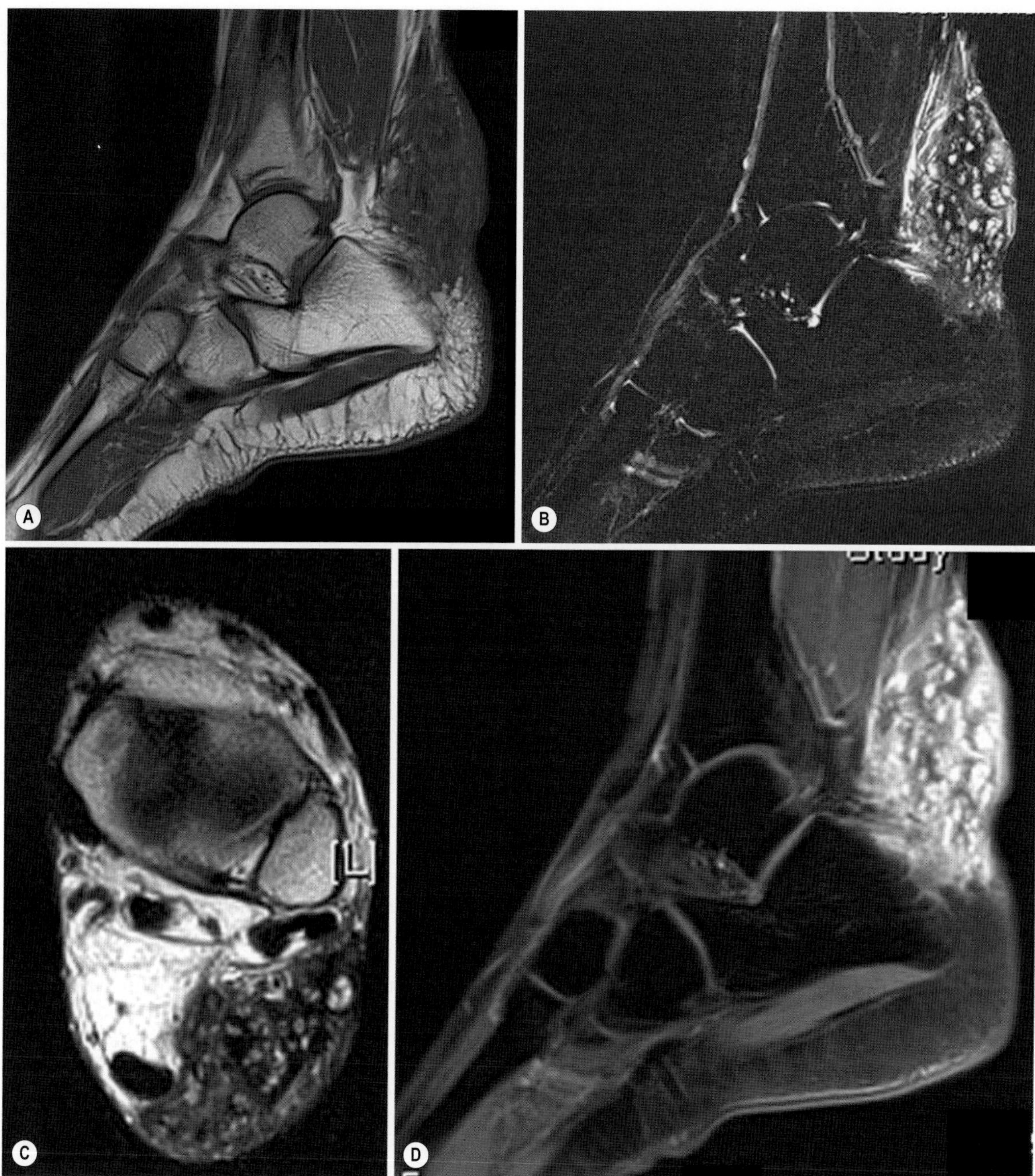

FIGURE 53-29 ■ **Mycetoma of ankle.** (A) Sagittal T1W, (B) STIR, (C) axial T2W and (D) sagittal fat-saturated enhanced T1W images of the ankle. A subcutaneous lesion demonstrating multiple low signal rings with central low signal dots on the T2W image and multiple avid ring enhancements with contrast is seen. The appearances on imaging mimicked a haemangioma, but the 'dot in a ring' appearance is typical of a mycetoma, which was confirmed on biopsy. (Courtesy of Dr R Mehan, Bolton Royal Hospital.)

signal centre on T2W MR imaging (the dot in a ring sign) (Fig. 53-29).

Musculoskeletal Infections in HIV Patients

Bone and joint infections were originally considered relatively rare in patients with HIV infections.[76,77] Infection is usually caused by opportunistic organisms like *Candida*, *Clostridium* and *Mycobacterium avium* complex. However, more recent studies show musculoskeletal infections as a relatively common manifestation in HIV patients.[78] The incidence also increases in IV drug-using HIV-infected patients. Apart from musculoskeletal manifestations of painful articular syndrome and non-infectious arthritis, musculoskeletal infections also occur in HIV patients. These include infectious myositis, septic arthritis, osteomyelitis and tuberculous arthritis.[78] Patients present with fever and arthritic symptoms, commonly affecting knees or ankles. *Staphylococcus aureus*, *Salmonella* and *Penicillium* infections were the commonest seen in these groups.

Radiographic findings include periarticular osteopenia, osteolysis and soft-tissue swellings and share similarities to other forms of osteomyelitis. Outcomes were generally poor in patients with bone infections.

DIFFERENTIAL DIAGNOSIS

Several other disorders may mimic osteomyelitis. *Inflammatory arthritis* may mimic septic arthritis in its early stages and a good clinical history is often the clue to diagnosis. As discussed earlier, both conditions may give rise to joint effusion, synovial thickening and post-contrast enhancement, though symptoms are usually severe with septic arthritis. *Bone infarcts* may mimic osteomyelitis in the acute stages and clinical features and laboratory tests often help in diagnosis. Bone infarcts have serpiginous appearances on MRI imaging, whilst osteomyelitis demonstrates more significant bone marrow oedema and post-contrast enhancement. *Tumours* are an important differential diagnosis in osteomyelitis and share several imaging features, including bone marrow oedema and contrast enhancement. Both lytic and sclerotic lesions with wide zones of transition and cortical destruction can occur with tumours and infection. Biopsy is sometimes needed to confirm the diagnosis and needs liaison with referring clinicians and pathologists. It is axiomatic that biopsy material should always be sent for both histological and microbiological assessment. Acute *diabetic neuropathic joints* are also difficult to differentiate from infection, as discussed earlier in detail. *Degenerative arthritis* can also cause diagnostic difficulties on imaging and clinical symptoms and history is important in management. *Granulomatous diseases* like giant cell tumour or Langerhans cell histiocytosis can also mimic infections of bone. Deposition diseases such as amyloidosis may also cause focal erosive bone lesions similar to infection.

MANAGEMENT

Good clinical history and thorough clinical examination is the most important step in early diagnosis of these infections. Laboratory tests are extremely useful in many instances to highlight the presence of acute infections. Blood cultures should be obtained whenever possible, before the start of treatment with antibiotics, as it helps in choosing the appropriate antibiotics. Culture of pus from sinus tracts, abscess cavities and effusions should also be performed whenever possible to obtain a microbiological diagnosis. It is important to have a multidisciplinary approach to choose appropriate investigations.

Percutaneous biopsy is an alternative to surgery in appropriate circumstances, being cost-effective and less invasive. Percutaneous bone or soft-tissue biopsy may be performed under ultrasonic, fluoroscopic or CT guidance to obtain a definitive diagnosis. This is a relatively safe procedure and extremely useful to confirm the diagnosis as the histological yield from the procedure is high. Abscess cavities and soft-tissue aspirates also require culture and sensitivity, along with cytology and histology, to analyse typical features of certain infections, like caseating necrosis in tuberculosis. Discussion with the referring team is necessary to plan the appropriate route for biopsy, in case the lesion in question turns out to be a malignancy. Departmental protocols should be present to ensure rapid transfer of specimens to the microbiology department in the appropriate transport medium.

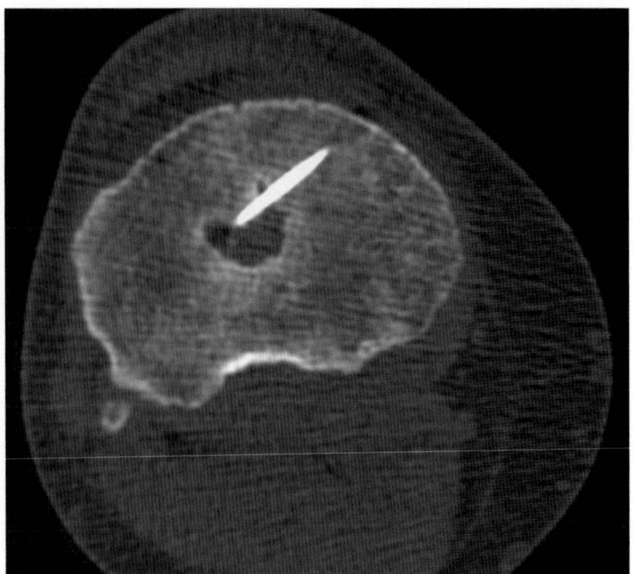

FIGURE 53-30 ■ **CT-guided bone biopsy.** Diagnosis of bone infection is confirmed by bone biopsy. CT remains the most useful tool for planning and guiding biopsy.

Histological examination may reveal changes that are compatible with acute or chronic osteomyelitis. In acute osteomyelitis, there are acute inflammatory cells, neutrophils, congestion and thrombosis of medullary and periosteal blood vessels and necrotic bone. Chronic osteomyelitis shows lack of neutrophils, areas of fibrosis in bones, macrophages, lymphocytes and histiocytes.

Bone biopsy can be usually performed as an outpatient procedure under CT or fluoroscopic guidance (Figs. 53-8 and 53-30). The procedure is performed under local anaesthesia, augmented with nitrous oxide analgesia or conscious sedation if required. The coaxial bone biopsy technique is the one that is commonly used. Once the penetrating cannula is placed on the surface of the lesion, a biopsy needle is inserted and specimen is aspirated.[79] Positive culture rates are usually low and are about 35% for long bones. Cultures from the spine may reveal a higher yield rate, perhaps by sampling the infected disc. Surgical biopsies produce similar yields and thus carry no advantage over percutaneous biopsy. Positive culture rates are very low once antibiotic therapy has been instigated.

Treatment of osteomyelitis and soft-tissue infections needs aggressive antibiotic therapy, surgical debridement and removal of prostheses, depending on the severity of infection. Follow-up is necessary to assess response to treatment and modify treatment accordingly. Septic arthritis requires immediate arthrotomy and joint lavage and optimal antibiotic therapy, adjusted as required by discussion with the microbiologist.

SPINAL INFECTION

Vertebral Osteomyelitis

The incidence of vertebral osteomyelitis is 2.4/100,000 population per annum and tends to increase with increase in age.[80] Vertebral osteomyelitis may be acute, subacute or chronic.

Vertebral osteomyelitis may be pyogenic, tuberculous or rarely fungal, such as *Candida*. Several studies have shown pyogenic infections to be the most common cause, followed by tuberculosis even in TB endemic areas.[81] In some areas brucellosis appears to be the most common.[82]

Pyogenic Vertebral Osteomyelitis

Acute pyogenic vertebral osteomyelitis is usually from haematogenous seeding. Direct extension from adjacent soft-tissue infections and direct inoculation of infection during surgery are also common. The usual causative pathogen is *S. aureus*, but in the presence of spinal implants, coagulase-negative staphylococcal infection also occurs. Low-virulence coagulase-negative staphylococcal infection occurs in prolonged bacteraemia after pacemaker infections.[80] The primary site of infection in acute vertebral osteomyelitis may be urinary tract infections, skin or soft-tissue infections, vascular access sites, septic arthritis or bursitis and endocarditis. There may be underlying disease, including diabetes, coronary artery disease, immunosuppression, cancer or renal failure on dialysis (Fig. 53-31).[80,83]

Pyogenic infection almost always begins in the intervertebral disc. From here, infection spreads into the end-plate and along the longitudinal ligaments. There is ischaemia and necrosis of the disc associated with abscess formation. Contiguous end-plate destruction occurs with extension of the abscess into the paravertebral soft tissues.

Symptoms

Back pain is the commonest clinical presentation and is present in 86% of patients. The lumbar spine is most commonly affected (58%), followed by thoracic (30%) and cervical spine (11%).[83] Vertebral osteomyelitis is complicated by direct seeding in different compartments, including epidural, paravertebral and disc space abscess, with the paravertebral location being the commonest.[84] Systemic signs such as fever may not always be present. Severe sharp pain should alert one to the possibility of epidural abscess. Motor and sensory involvement may occur depending on the degree of spinal cord compression. Neurological complications are particularly common in cervical vertebral infections.

Investigations

Usual inflammatory markers: raised white cell count with neutrophilia. Elevation of the CRP and ESR is invariably present. Blood cultures may be positive in up to 58% of patients. Higher yield rates up to 77% can be obtained from bone biopsy cultures.

Plain Radiographs. Plain radiographs are not very sensitive in acute vertebral osteomyelitis, but are useful in subacute or chronic conditions. Early changes may be seen as minor end-plate irregularities but MRI is much more sensitive. End-plate destruction, paravertebral soft-tissue swelling and kyphoscoliosis are present in established osteomyelitis. In the acute setting, plain radiographs are mandatory to exclude other lesions, such as metastases or fractures.

Computed Tomography. CT is generally only used when there are contraindications to MRI. Enhanced images with multiplanar reformats help to delineate the lesion and demonstrate the extent of any abscess. The main role for CT in vertebral osteomyelitis is to plan and direct the biopsy, thereby confirming the diagnosis and obtaining material for culture (Fig. 53-32).

Magnetic Resonance Imaging. MRI is the investigation of choice for vertebral osteomyelitis and should be promptly arranged, especially in the presence of neurological symptoms and signs, as it also excludes other causes such as intervertebral disc prolapse and malignancy. Motor and sensory symptoms depend on the degree and level of spinal cord or cauda equina involvement.

MRI is extremely sensitive and has 90% accuracy in the diagnosis of acute vertebral osteomyelitis.[85–87] The imaging features are typical for infective discitis and osteomyelitis, and in many instances these entities can be differentiated from tuberculous osteomyelitis. Typically, one disc space and the two adjacent vertebral bodies are involved. The disc usually yields low signal on T1- and increased signal on T2-weighted images associated with loss of the intranuclear cleft. There is destruction of the end-plates of the adjacent vertebrae above and below the disc space. There is adjacent bone marrow oedema and inflammatory tissue. The bone marrow oedema shows as low signal on T1 and high signal on T2 and STIR images, involving the vertebral bodies and end-plates. As the infection proceeds untreated, this may lead to vertebral destruction and collapse. Epidural and/or paraspinal abscess may be noted as high signal fluid collections on T2 images. Intraspinal collections or granulation tissue may cause cord compression. Gadolinium-enhanced T1 images with fat saturation are useful to define the extent and effects of epidural or paravertebral abscess collections (Fig. 53-33). STIR images of the whole spine may be useful to assess multilevel involvement.

In pyogenic osteomyelitis there is usually homogeneous and diffuse enhancement of the vertebral bodies as opposed to the heterogeneous and localised enhancement seen in tuberculous vertebral osteomyelitis. Disc abscess with rim enhancement is more common in pyogenic infections, whilst vertebral intraosseous abscess with rim enhancement occurs more commonly in TB. Paraspinal abscesses are more commonly associated with TB than with pyogenic infections.[87]

Several recent studies have demonstrated the usefulness of diffusion-weighted imaging and apparent diffusion coefficient (ADC) values to differentiate between

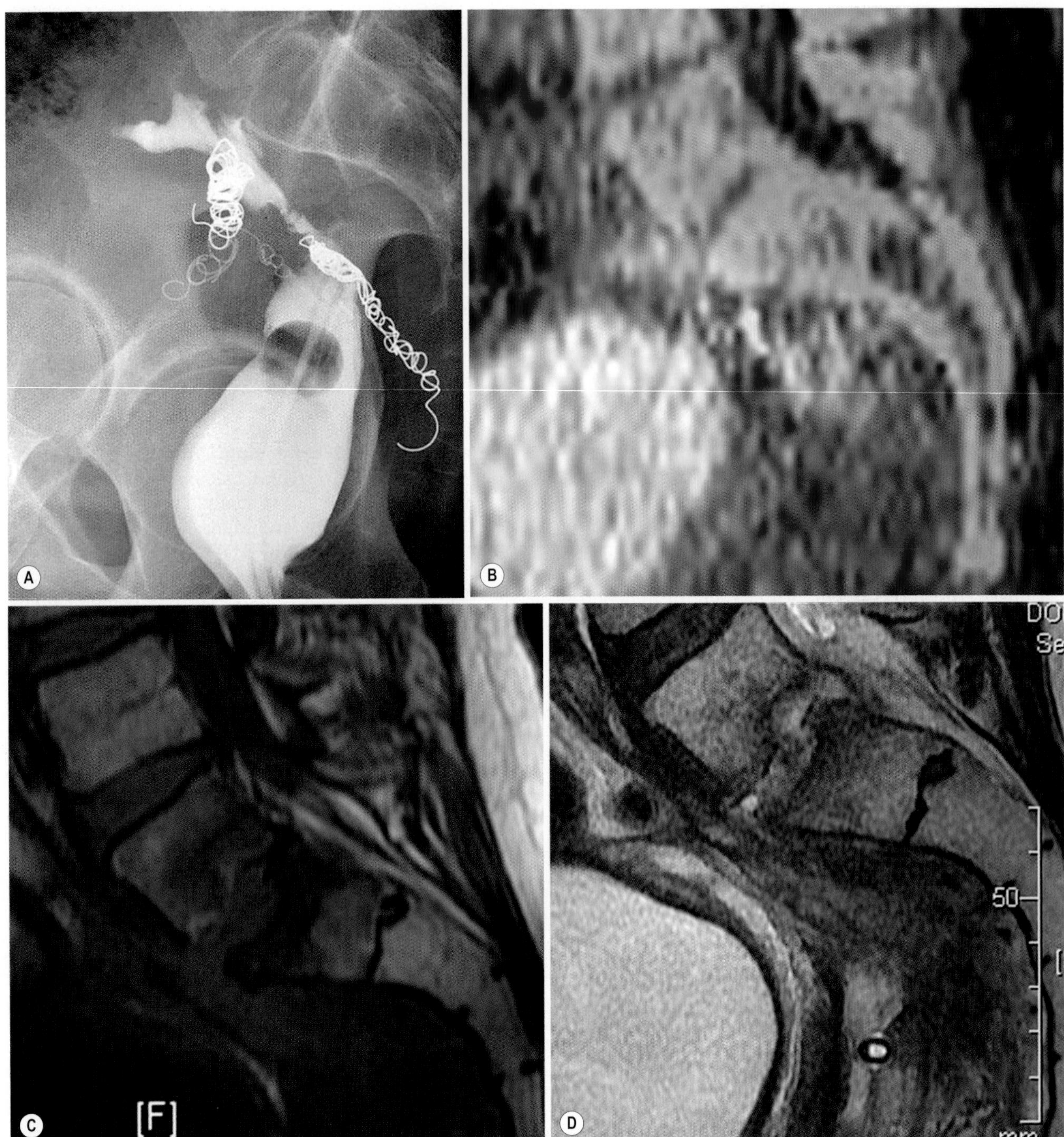

FIGURE 53-31 ■ Pyogenic vertebral osteomyelitis after pelvic sepsis. Patient with a presacral abscess following radiotherapy and AP resection for rectal cancer. (A) Contrast enema showing a sinus track to the prevertebral region at L5/S1. (B) Sagittal fused PET-CT image shows increased uptake of FDG tracer in the presacral region, but not the disc. (C, D) Sagittal T1 and T2 images show the presacral abnormality consistent with granulation tissue extending to the L5/S1 disc, with typical appearances of infective discitis.

infectious and malignant causes of spinal involvement, although results are still somewhat inconsistent.[88,89]

Nuclear Medicine. Skeletal scintigraphy is less important than it was, as most centres rely on MRI. Three-phase ^{99m}Tc bone scintigraphy has about 67% accuracy, but positive results are seen only after a few days. It is also less sensitive to the detection of epidural abscess. ^{111}Indium leucocyte scintigraphy and antileucocyte scintigraphy are more specific, but have sensitivity of around 20%, and hence are not generally useful. Gallium imaging is also a useful adjunct to MRI in the evaluation of spinal infections (Fig. 53-34). Because of limited availability, PET-CT is generally not used in the diagnosis of vertebral osteomyelitis but has been found to be useful in some studies.[90]

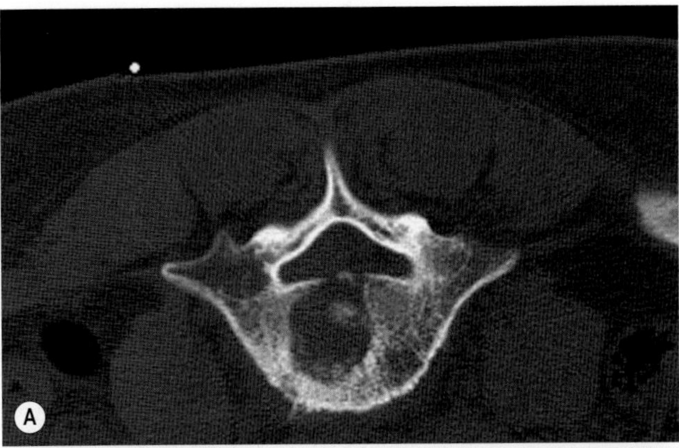

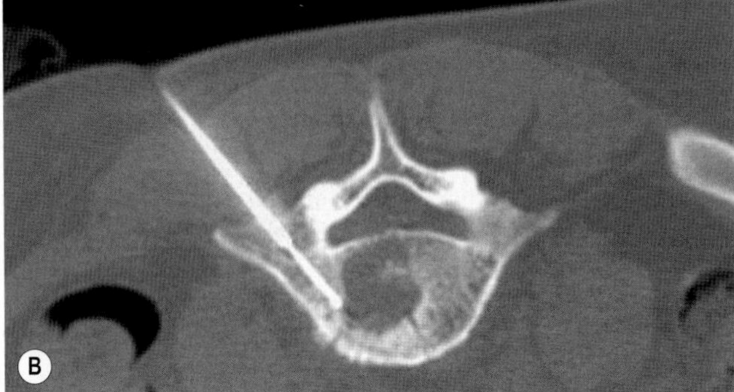

FIGURE 53-32 ■ CT-guided vertebral body biopsy. (A) Preliminary CT with a wire marker on the skin, from which the skin entry site can be measured and marked. (B) CT-guided bone biopsy of the intramedulllary abscess showing needle positioned at the margin of the abscess. Biopsy of the wall for histology, aspiration of the abscess and (if the latter is unsuccessful) gentle instillation and reaspiration of sterile saline for culture is performed.

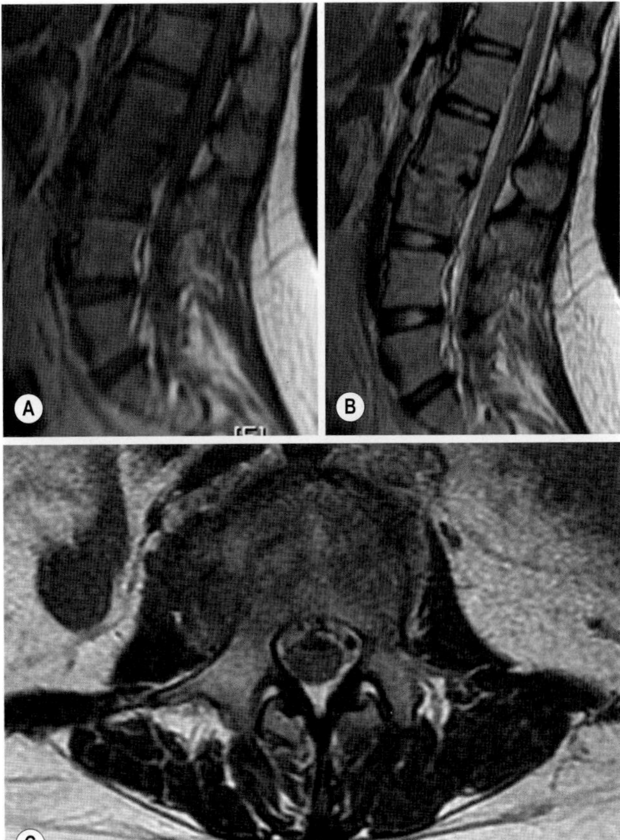

FIGURE 53-33 ■ Bacterial infective discitis. (A, B) Sagittal T1W and T2W images through the spine show involvement of the L2/3 disc with destruction of adjacent end-plates and oedema in the vertebral bodies of L2 and L3. (C) Axial T2W image at the same level shows a paravertebral abscess extending on the right from the involved disc (arrow).

Treatment

Acute vertebral osteomyelitis is usually treated with intravenous antibiotics. Image-guided intervention under CT may be necessary for diagnostic purposes and CT or ultrasound is used for guiding the drainage of abscesses. Surgery is usually required in the presence of implants; in chronic infections due to treatment failure, removal of the implant is generally recommended.

Tuberculous Vertebral Osteomyelitis

Tuberculosis of the spine is still prevalent in developing countries and in TB endemic areas. Poverty, malnutrition and overcrowding predispose to the development of primary tuberculous infection. It is increasingly seen in developed countries in the immigrant population and also increases with the increase in incidence of pulmonary tuberculosis due to immunosuppressive conditions, including HIV infection and AIDS. Tuberculosis of the spine is usually a secondary infection, with spread to the spine occurring by the haematogenous route, usually from primary lung or genital tract infection. Spinal tuberculosis accounts for approximately 50% of all musculoskeletal tuberculous infections.[91,92]

Spinal tuberculosis is most common around the thoracolumbar junction. The incidence decreases on either side of this level but may occur at any level.[92] Infection usually occurs at the anterior ends of vertebral bodies and spreads under the longitudinal ligament to involve contiguous vertebrae. Skip lesions may also occur due to haematogenous spread.

The vertebral body is commonly affected; posterior element involvement is rare but is seen particularly in Asian patients. Three patterns of vertebral body involvement are seen.[92,93]

A paradiscal lesion is the most common form of involvement of spinal tuberculosis. There is involvement of subchondral bone adjacent to an intervertebral disc, with reduction in disc height.

Anterior lesions occur due to spread of infection under the periosteum and anterior longitudinal ligament resulting in loss of blood supply to the vertebral body with development of necrosis and infection. Abscess formation may occur with resultant stripping of the periosteum from the vertebral body, causing scalloping and multiple-level involvements.

Central lesions involve the centre of the vertebral body with loss of height resulting in vertebra plana.

'Gibbus' deformities occur due vertebral body collapse manifesting as acute angulation in the spine. Paraspinal

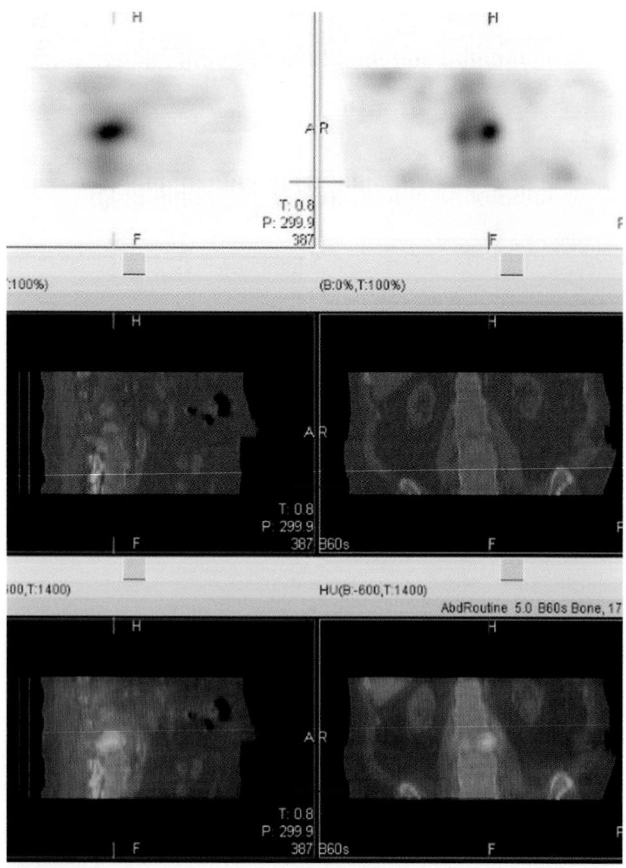

FIGURE 53-34 ■ **Vertebral osteomyelitis: gallium SPECT CT showing vertebral osteomyelitis as hot spots involving the vertebral bodies.** (Courtesy of Dr Ewa Novosinska, Royal Free Hospital, London, UK.)

abscess formation also occurs and typically shows no significant signs of inflammation; hence such abscesses are called cold abscesses (9, 14, and 15).

Table 53-3 summarises features that may help to distinguish pyogenic from tuberculous spinal infection.

Plain Radiographs

In acute infections, plain radiographs may be normal. In subacute infection, bone lucency may be seen in vertebral bodies. End-plate changes and destruction occur with reduction in the intervertebral disc space. Cold abscess formation may cause paraspinal soft-tissue density on AP films. Chronic infection can cause sclerosis of the bone and end-plates, bone destruction with compression fractures and deformities. Gibbus is an acute angulation seen in the spine on lateral views, due to vertebral compression fractures. Other deformities such as kyphosis and scoliosis also occur.

Computed Tomography

The role of CT is usually limited to guiding biopsy but is also useful if there are contraindications, poor patient tolerance or lack of availability of MRI.

Early infection tends to show bone rarefaction and destruction. End-plate changes are more accurately evaluated than on plain radiographs. Sclerosis is seen in advanced disease.

TABLE 53-3 **Differentiation between Pyogenic and Tuberculous Vertebral Osteomyelitis on Imaging**

Pyogenic Spinal Infection	Tuberculosis of Spine
1. Lumbar spine involvement common	More common in thoracic spine
2. Commonly single site with disc space infection and involvement of two adjacent vertebra	Multilevel involvement and skip lesions are common. Spread may occur along anterior longitudinal ligament
3. Disc abscess with end-plate destruction occurs	Intraosseous and paraspinal abscess occurs more frequently
4. Significant surrounding inflammation with diffuse oedema of vertebral bodies	Inflammation is more localised and formation of cold abscess
5. Enhanced images show diffuse vertebral body enhancement, irregular enhancement of thick-walled abscesses	Enhancement of vertebral bodies more localised and show rim enhancement of thin-walled abscess cavities

Sagittal reconstructions of thin-section acquisition shows vertebral body and end-plate changes clearly. Vertebral body collapse and posterior wall retropulsion can be clearly identified even in its early stages. Spinal canal stenosis and cord compression due the bone destruction or soft-tissue inflammatory component can be clearly identified. Intravenous enhancement increases the diagnostic accuracy, outlining the inflammatory granulation tissue and also the thick irregular wall of abscess cavities. Paraspinal cold abscesses are also better seen on CT after intravenous contrast medium. Spinal canal encroachment secondary to vertebral body destruction can be assessed. Multilevel involvement and end-plate changes are also well shown on CT, which is particularly used for planned intervention of spinal tuberculosis. Common indications include drainage of cold abscesses, vertebral body or intervertebral disc biopsy.

Magnetic Resonance Imaging

MRI is the investigation of choice for assessment of tuberculous vertebral osteomyelitis. Usually the affected area of the spine is imaged, but in tuberculous osteomyelitis, it may be be useful to perform imaging of the whole spine to exclude skip lesions. Sagittal T1, T2 and STIR images are obtained with axial T2 images through the involved vertebral bodies (Fig. 53-35).

MRI can also be reliably used to differentiate between tuberculous and pyogenic vertebral osteomyelitis. Patients with tuberculous vertebral osteomyelitis have a significantly higher incidence of a well-defined paraspinal abnormal signal, thin- and smooth-walled abscess cavities, particularly at paraspinal or intraosseous locations, sub-ligamentous spread to three or more vertebral levels and involvement of multiple vertebral bodies. In

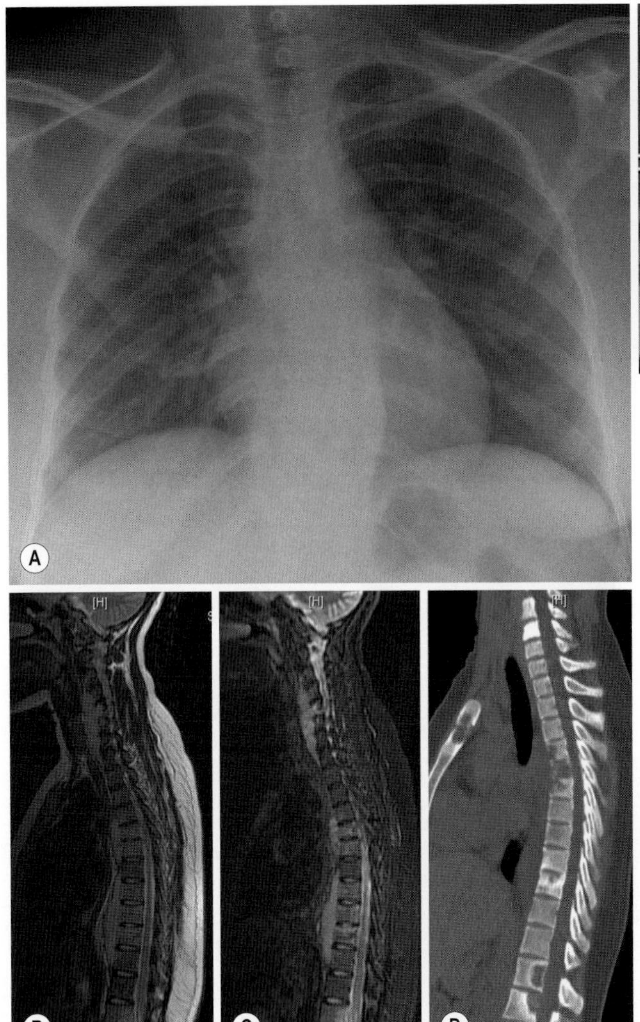

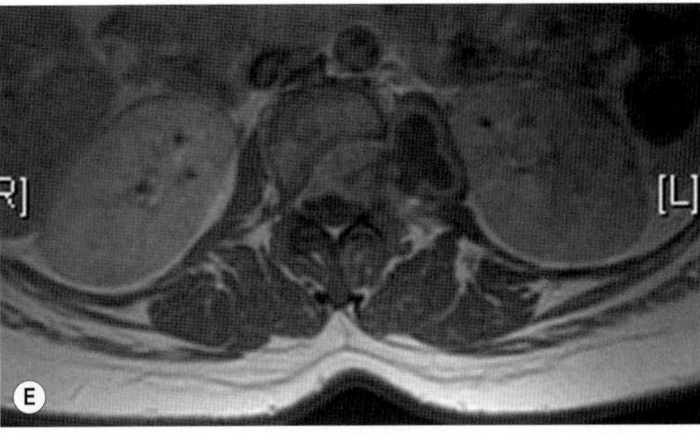

FIGURE 53-35 ■ Multilevel involvement in tuberculous spondylitis. Multilevel involvement is a common presentation in tuberculous vertebral osteomyelitis. This may be caused by spread along the anterior longitudinal ligament. Multilevel haematogenous borne skip lesions also occur. (A) Chest radiograph shows no evidence of underlying pulmonary TB, but there is a mild scoliosis and widened paravertebral soft-tissue planes around the lower thoracic spine. (B, C) Sagittal T2W and STIR images demonstrate multilevel involvement with subligamentous extension at multiple sites. Note the preservation of the intervertebral discs. (D) Sagittal reformatted CT demonstrates lytic lesions at the sites of bone involvement, with surrounding sclerosis. (E) Axial enhanced MRI of lumbar vertebrae shows chronic bone destruction and a large left paraspinal collection which extends laterally to abut the left kidney.

tuberculous spondylitis, there is also an increased incidence of thoracic spine involvement.[94]

Involvement of vertebral bodies and extension to the epidural and paravertebral spaces are commoner than disc space involvement. Bone marrow oedema is seen as low signal on T1 images, but the presence of corresponding high T2 signal may be variable.[95]

In paradiscal lesions, T1 images show low signal with loss of height of disc spaces, with high T2 signal, endplate destruction and paraspinal abscess formation (Fig. 53-36). With anterior lesions there is low T1 and high T2 signals involving the vertebral body, with preservation of disc signal and height. Central lesions involve the centre of the vertebral body and MRI shows abnormal signal of the vertebral body associated with collapse and vertebra plana, classically with preservation of adjacent discs.[96]

Whole-spine fat-suppressed STIR or T2 images are extremely useful to identify high signal bone marrow oedema in vertebral bodies and also high signal in the affected discs, which should be conspicuous against the background of very low signal from adjacent normal vertebrae. Gadolinium-enhanced images are useful for confirmation, revealing enhancement of the bone marrow oedema in affected vertebral bodies. T1 fat-saturated images before and after enhancement are useful to identify abscesses within the vertebral bodies or paravertebral soft tissues. These are typically cold abscesses and hence do not show significant surrounding inflammatory reaction, but there is uniform enhancement of the thin walls (Fig. 53-37). Enhanced images allow accurate assessment of extension and also evaluate the extent of spinal cord compression.[87,92,93]

Though posterior element involvement is not common in tuberculosis of the spine, studies have been published involving only the posterior elements. Posterior element involvement is most common in the thoracic spine, and tends to affect the lamina most commonly, followed by pedicles and articular processes. Spinal cord involvement was seen in many of these patients.[96]

Unusual Spine Infections

Candida albicans is rare but can cause spinal infections.[97] *Aspergillus fumigatus* infections of the spine are extremely rare but occur in immunocompromised people and chronic granulomatous disease. Diagnosis is difficult without microbiology and imaging features are similar to tuberculous disease.[98,99] Treatment is with antifungal

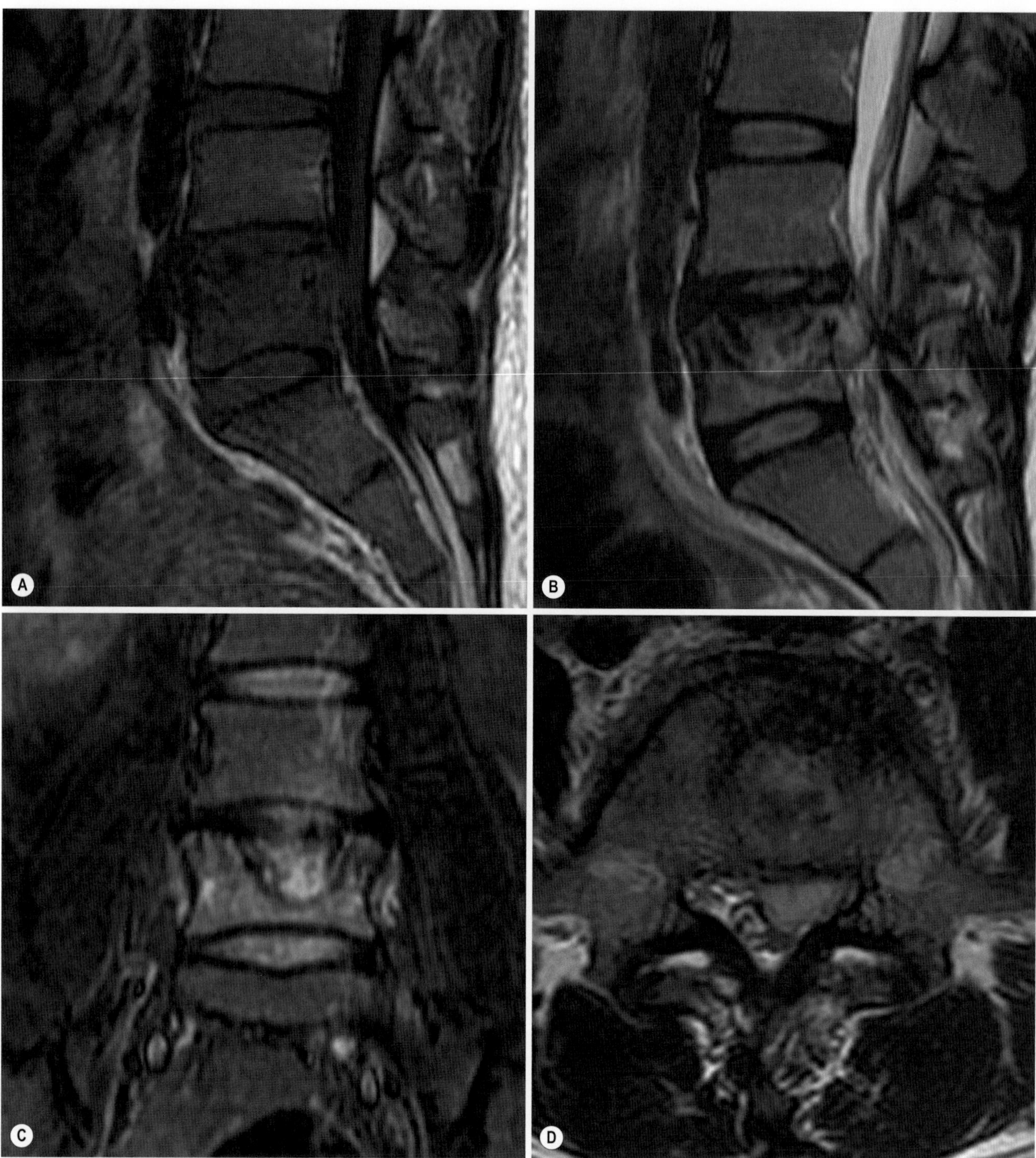

FIGURE 53-36 ■ **Tuberculous vertebral osteomyelitis.** (A, B) Sagittal T1W and T2W images through the spine show discitis of L4/5 vertebra extending to superior end-plate of L5 vertebra, extending to the vertebral body. There is also extension of the abscess into the spinal canal. (C) Axial T2 image at the same level shows the well-defined vertebral body abscess. The abscess component extends into the thecal sac and causes compression of nerve roots on the left. (D) Coronal PD SPIR image shows the well-defined abscess, with relatively little inflammation of surrounding soft tissue, the so-called 'cold abscess'.

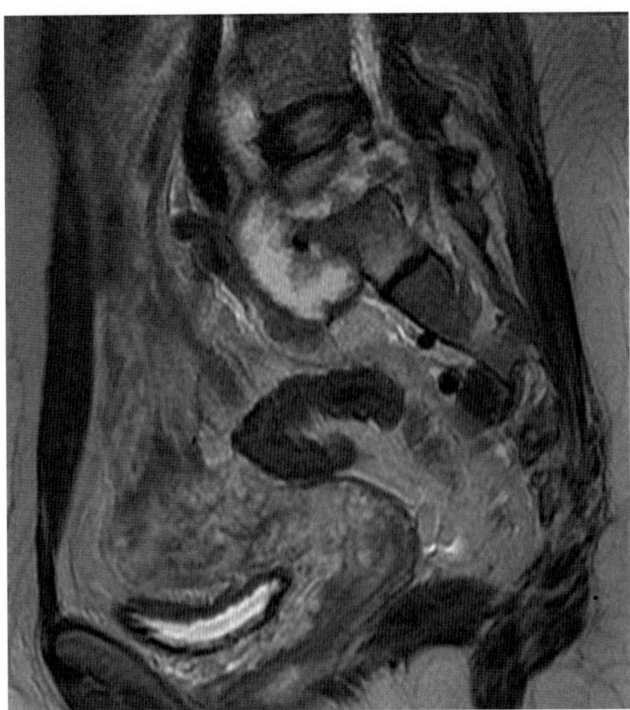

FIGURE 53-37 ■ Tuberculous vertebral abscess presenting as psoas abscess. This young lady was referred for pelvic MRI with a diagnosis of complex ovarian cyst. Pelvic MRI showed this to be psoas abscess extending from spinal TB (see Fig. 53-28). Sagittal T2W image shows the vertebral origin of the psoas abscess. Note the thick, irregular wall to the abscess and the subligamentous spread superiorly, both characteristic of TB.

agents. Atypical *Mycobacterium* infections with *M. intercellulare* and pneumococcal infections have also been reported but are rare.

For a full list of references, please see ExpertConsult.

FURTHER READING

11. Corr PD. Musculoskeletal fungal infections. Semin Musculoskelet Radiol 2011;15:506–10.
23. Khanna G, Sato TS, Ferguson P. Imaging of chronic recurrent multifocal osteomyelitis. Radiographics 2009;29:1159–77.
33. Pineda C, Espinosa R, Pena A. Radiographic imaging in osteomyelitis: the role of plain radiography, computed tomography, ultrasonography, magnetic resonance imaging, and scintigraphy. Semin Plast Surg 2009;23:80–9.
39. Palestro CJ, Love C, Tronco GG, et al. Combined labeled leukocyte and technetium 99m sulfur colloid bone marrow imaging for diagnosing musculoskeletal infection. Radiographics 2006;26: 859–70.
46. Donovan A. Current concepts in imaging diabetic pedal osteomyelitis. Radiol Clin North Am 2008;46:1105–24.
64. Lin HM, Learch TJ, White EA, Gottsegen CJ. Emergency joint aspiration: a guide for radiologists on call. Radiographics 2009;4: 1139–58.
68. De Vuyst D, Vanhoenacker F, Gielen J, et al. Imaging features of musculoskeletal tuberculosis. Eur Radiol 2003;13:1809–19.
79. Wu JS, Gorbachova T, Morrison WB, Haims AH. Imaging-guided bone biopsy for osteomyelitis: are there factors associated with positive or negative cultures? Am J Roentgenol 2007;188: 1529–34.
80. Zimmerli W. Clinical practice. Vertebral osteomyelitis. N Engl J Med 2010;362:1022–9.
83. Mylona E, Samarkos M, Kakalou E, et al. Pyogenic vertebral osteomyelitis: a systematic review of clinical characteristics. Semin Arthritis Rheum 2009;39:10–17.
85. Palestro CJ, Love C, Miller TT. Infections and musculoskeletal conditions: Imaging of musculoskeletal infections. Best Pract Res Clin Rheumatol 2006;20:1197–218.

SECTION E

THE SPINE

Section Editors: Jonathan H. Gillard • H. Rolf Jäger

CHAPTER 54

Imaging Techniques and Anatomy

Thomas Van Thielen • Luc van den Hauwe • Johan W. Van Goethem • Paul M. Parizel

CHAPTER OUTLINE

ANATOMY

Anatomically the spine is organised segmentally, consisting of 7 cervical, 12 thoracic, 5 lumbar, 5 (fused) sacral and 3–5 coccygeal vertebra. Each level, except C1, consists out of the following elements: a vertebral body (corpus vertebrae) anteriorly and a vertebral or neural arch (arcus posterior) posteriorly. Together these two structures enclose the spinal canal.

Functionally the spine can be divided in three so-called columns.[1] The anterior column includes the anterior longitudinal ligament, the anterior annulus fibrosus and the anterior two-thirds of the vertebral body. The middle column comprises the posterior third of the vertebral body, the posterior annulus fibrosus and the posterior longitudinal ligament. The posterior column includes the posterior elements with the pedicles, facet joints, laminae and spinous processes as well as the posterior ligaments.

OSSEOUS ELEMENTS

Vertebral Body

The vertebral bodies have a thin rim of cortical bone and a central framework of mostly vertically orientated trabeculae. This osseous portion contains stores of phosphate and calcium and has a structural support function. Sclerotic bands can be seen in the vertebral body at the site of fusion between two vertebral components. This is typically seen at the neurocentral junction and in the dens axis. In the dens axis there may be remnants of the subdental synchondrosis. These bony structures are optimally evaluated with computed tomography (CT) imaging and to a lesser extent with magnetic resonance imaging (MRI). On CT imaging vascular channels are often visible and in a post-traumatic setting can be mistaken for small fractures.

The centre of the vertebral body is composed of red bone marrow, which is haematopoietically active. Red and yellow bone marrow are not entirely homogeneous and each contain elements of the other. The vertebral marrow is dynamic, changing with age, immune state, oxygenation, coagulation and structural needs.[2] The normal adult distribution of bone marrow is reached by the age of 25. With ageing, the bone marrow assumes a more variable appearance with a reduction in the red cell mass and trabecular bone and increase of the fatty content. These changes appear relatively late in comparison to the changes in the bone marrow in the peripheral skeleton. The distribution of the red bone marrow in a vertebral body is predominantly seen at the metaphyseal equivalents near the endplates and the anterior part of the vertebra.[3] Evaluation of the bone marrow is best done with MRI. In the normal spinal marrow the distribution patterns of fatty and red marrow were categorised into four patterns by Ricci and colleagues[4] (Fig. 54-1). Pattern 1 describes a uniform low signal on T_1–weighted images with high linear signal around the basivertebral vein; this type is most commonly seen in younger patients aged 30 or less. Type 2 is a band-like high T_1 signal limited to the periphery of the vertebral body. Type 3 is characterised by multiple small indistinct (difficult to visualise) high signal intensity foci on T_1-weighted images throughout the vertebral body. These two patterns (types 2 and 3) are seen with increasing age and typically in persons of 40 years and older. Type 4 is a more severe form of type 3 with multiple larger high signal intensity foci (5–15 mm) on T_1 images throughout the vertebral body.

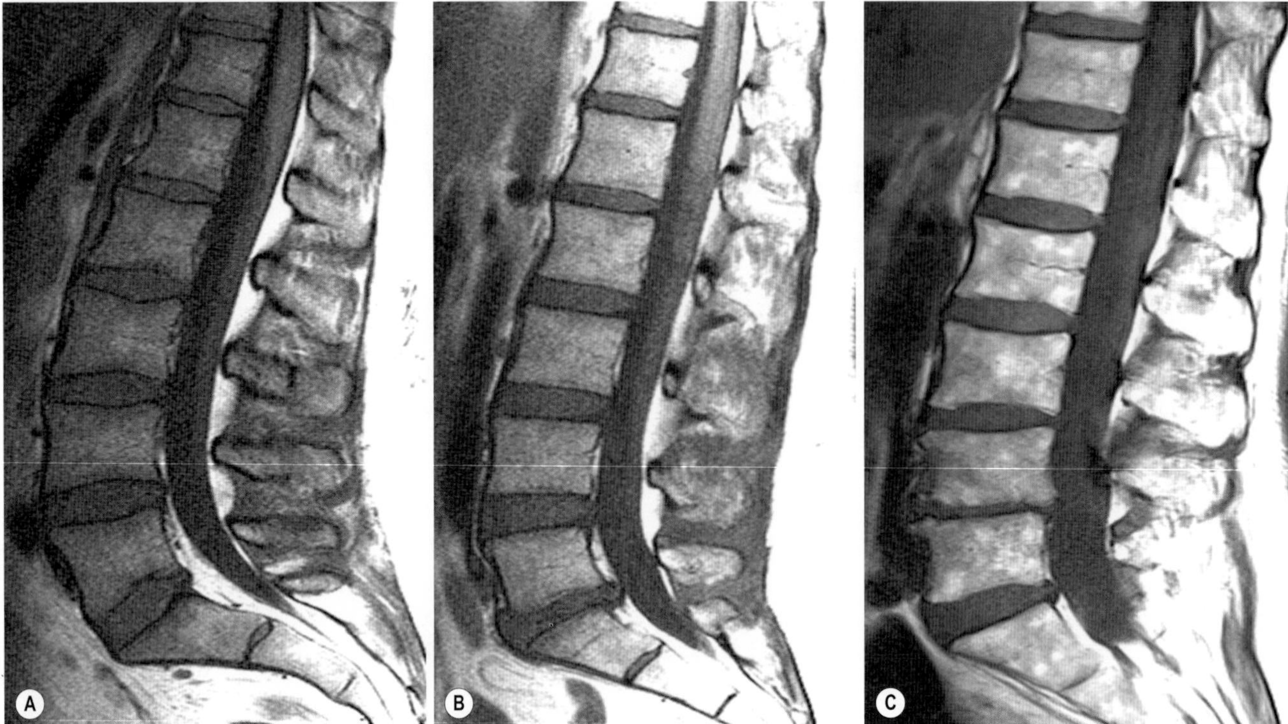

FIGURE 54-1 ■ **Age-related bone marrow changes.** Sagittal T_1-weighted images in a 23 year old (A), 44 year old (B) and 73 year old (C). Normal patterns of bone marrow distribution as described by Ricci and colleagues.[4] (A) Type 1 bone marrow pattern with uniform low signal intensity and a high linear signal around the basivertebral vein. (B) A type 2 pattern with band-like hyperintense signal intensity limited to the periphery and (C) a type 4 marrow pattern in a 73 year old with large hyperintense foci.

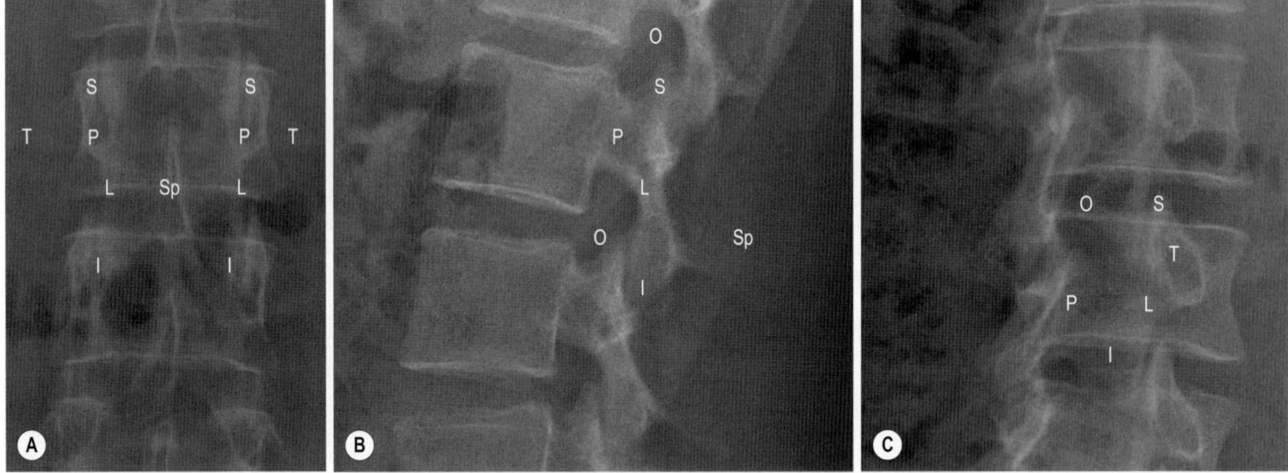

FIGURE 54-2 ■ **Normal imaging anatomy of the spine on plain film radiograph.** Lateral (A), posteroanterior (B) and oblique (C) views. P = pedicle, L = lamina, I = inferior articular process, S = superior articular process, Sp = spinous process, T = transverse process, O = intervertebral foramen.

Neural Arch

The neural arch, also known as posterior arch, forms the bony lateral and posterior border of the spinal canal (Figs. 54-2–54-4). It can be divided into different segments. Between the transverse and spinous process the neural arch is called the lamina. The pedicle is the part situated between the transverse process and the vertebral body. The pedicle of each vertebra is notched at its inferior and superior edge. Together these notches form an opening called the intervertebral foramen. Through this foramen the spinal nerves exit the spinal canal.

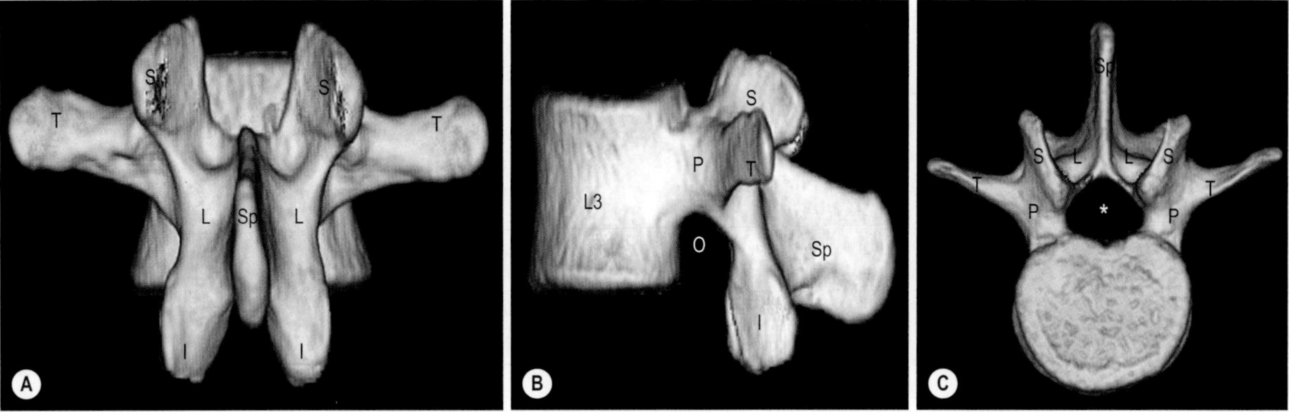

FIGURE 54-3 ■ Normal imaging anatomy of the lumbar spine on CT. 3D reformatted CT images of L3 in posterior (A), lateral (B) and superior (C) views. P = pedicle, L = lamina, I = inferior articular process, S = superior articular process, Sp = spinous process, T = transverse process, O = intervertebral foramen, * = spinal canal.

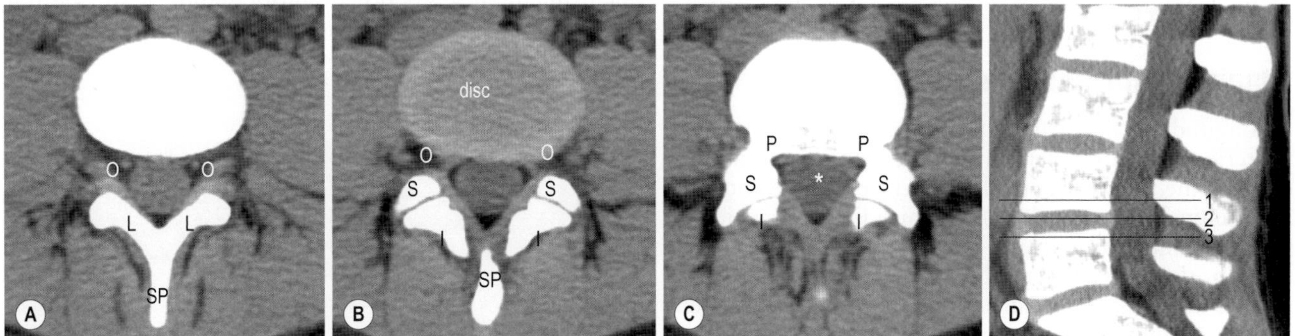

FIGURE 54-4 ■ Normal imaging anatomy of the posterior arch of the lumbar spine on CT. Axial images (A, B, C) at different levels as indicated on the sagittal (D) image. P = pedicle, L = lamina, I = inferior articular process, S = superior articular process, Sp = spinous process, T = transverse process, O = intervertebral foramen, * = spinal canal.

Spinous and Transverse Processes

The spinous process is attached to the most posterior part of the neural arch. The transverse processes arise from the lateral edge of each neural arch (Figs. 54-2–54-4). The spinous as well as the transverse process serve as an important site of attachment for the deep back muscles. As described above, they also divide the neural arch into different anatomical parts.

JOINTS

Facet Joints

The facet joints or the zygapophyseal joints are diarthrodial synovial joints between the inferior and superior articular processes of adjacent neural arches. These articular processes arise from the articular pillars including the bone at the junction between pedicles and the laminae. The superior articular process is located relative anterior to the inferior articular process and faces posteriorly (Figs. 54-2–54-4). In the lumbar spine the joint surface is located in an oblique way at an angle of about 45° between the sagittal and coronal plane. In the thoracic spine the facet joints are almost orientated in the coronal plan.[5]

The inferior facets have a convex shape while the superior articular surface has a concave aspect. In a non-degenerative spine the joint surface is covered with hyaline cartilage, being the thickest in the centre of the joint. In the normal anatomy, as most other joints, the surface of the joints should be smooth and regular with an equal spacing between the two joint surfaces. The distance between the articular processes at the facet joint should be between 2 and 4 mm on plain radiography.[6]

On the posterolateral side, the facet joint is covered with a strong fibrous capsule which is composed of several layers of fibrous tissue and a synovial membrane. On the anterior side of the joint, there is no fibrous capsule. Here, the only border between the spinal canal and the facet joint is formed by the ligamentum flavum and the synovial membrane.[7] The capsule is composed of a superior and inferior recess containing fat pads. These fat pads act as movement-compensating mechanisms and as a lubrication mechanism for the facet joint as they are partially covered with synovial tissue.[5]

Intervertebral Disc—Symphysis

The intervertebral disc consists of the inner nucleus pulposus surrounded by an outer layer, the annulus fibrosus. Embryologically the nucleus pulposus is formed from cells originating from the notochord; in humans these notochordial cells are lost and replaced by chondrocyte-like cells. The nucleus pulposus is macroscopically composed of soft, elastic tissue with a yellow colour.[8] The nucleus pulposus is primarily composed of water, proteoglycans and loose collagen fibres. With normal ageing the water content decreases.

The outer annulus fibrosus is composed of multiple concentric layers of fibrocartilage tissue. The outer layers, also called Sharpey's fibres, continue in the longitudinal ligament and the vertebral bodies. The fibres of each layer are directed in an oblique way (30° angle), forming a meshwork. In this way a very strong flexible structure is formed.

LIGAMENTS

Longitudinal Ligaments

A longitudinal ligament is present at the anterior and posterior part of the vertebral bodies running along the entire spine, providing stability (Fig. 54-5). The anterior longitudinal ligament (ALL) is a thick ligament which is slightly thinner at the level of the vertebral bodies and wider at the intervertebral disc.

The posterior longitudinal ligament (PLL) is situated in the vertebral canal and runs from the dens axis (tectorial membrane) to the sacrum. It is thicker in the thoracic spine and wider in the cervical region compared to the lumbar level. At the level of the vertebral bodies the PLL is separated from the concave posterior wall of the vertebral bodies by the anterior epidural space. This space contains epidural fat, basivertebral veins and the anterior internal vertebral veins.

Ligamentum Flavum

The ligamentum flavum or yellow ligament is a paired structure connecting the spinal laminae forming the posterior wall of the spinal canal (Fig. 54-6). At the lateral side these structures fuse with the capsule of the facet joints, forming a boundary of the intervertebral neuroforamina.[9] The boundary between the two ligamenta flava in the centre is indistinguishable on imaging. The ligamenta flava provide a static elastic force to stimulate the return to a neutral position after flexion or extension. They also limit the flexion motion of the spine and help maintain a smooth posterior lining of the central spinal canal.[10]

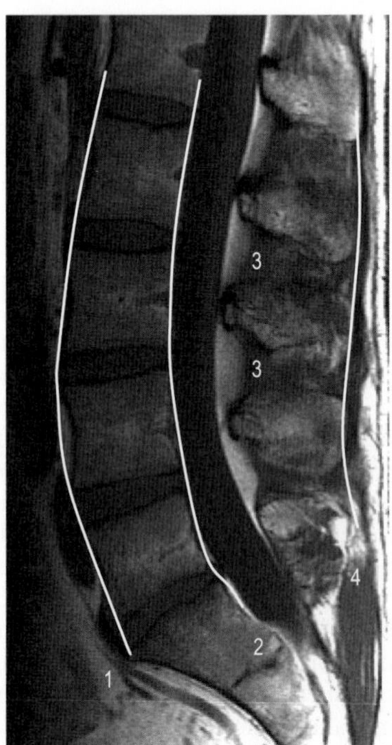

FIGURE 54-5 ■ Normal anatomy of the spinal ligaments. Sagittal T_1-weighted MRI image of the lumbar spine. 1 = anterior longitudinal ligament, 2 = posterior longitudinal ligament, 3 = interspinous ligament, 4 = supraspinous ligament.

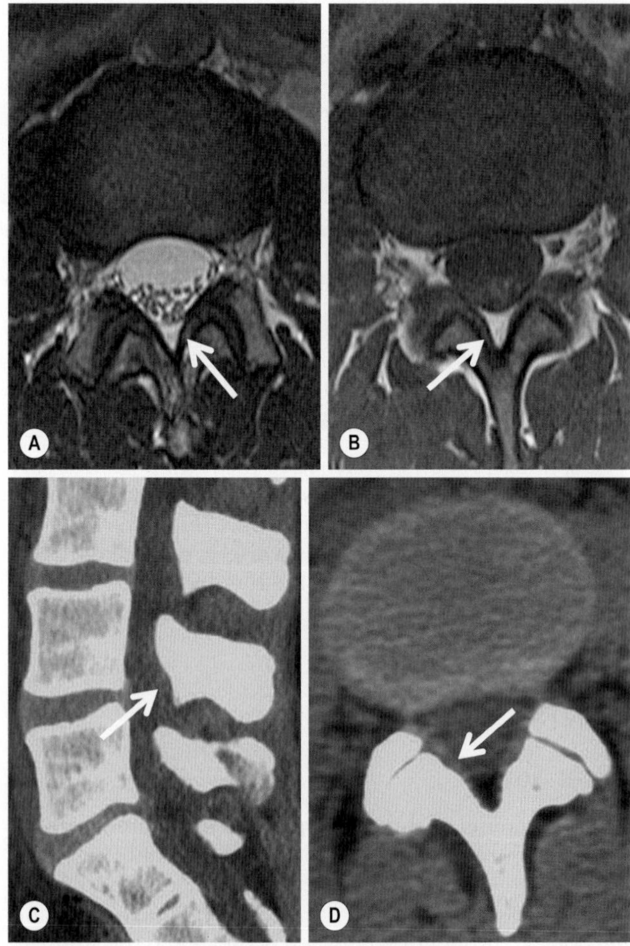

FIGURE 54-6 ■ Ligamentum flavum. Axial T_1-weighted (A) and T_2-weighted (B) images; sagittal (C) and axial (D) reformatted CT images. The ligamentum flavum or yellow ligament (indicated with arrow) is a thin ligament connecting the laminae and forms the posterior wall of the spinal canal.

Interconnecting Ligaments

The posterior elements are heavily reinforced with different ligaments connecting two adjacent vertebra. The supraspinous ligament connects the tips from the spinous processes while the interspinous ligaments connect the base of the adjacent spinous processes (Fig. 54-5). The transverse processes are connected by the intertransverse ligaments. As discussed earlier the laminae of the adjacent vertebra are bound together by the ligamentum flavum.

NEURAL STRUCTURES—SPINAL CORD, SPINAL NERVES, DURA MATER

The shape of the spinal canal varies from oval on the cervical and thoracic level to a triangular shape at the lower lumbar region.[11]

Anteriorly the dura mater is in contact with the posterior longitudinal ligament almost over the length of the whole spine. Laterally the dura mater is in close contact with the medial border of the pedicles. Above and below the pedicles the dura mater is in contact with the epidural fat in continuity with the intervertebral foramina. Posteriorly the dura mater is in contact with the posterior epidural fat separating the dura from the ligamenta flava, the posterior joints and the laminae.

In the kyphotic thoracic regions, the dura can be separated from the posterior elements by a layer of epidural fat of up to 5 mm thick. This fat should not be mistaken for epidural lipomatosis.

The spinal cord and its normal internal structure (grey and white matter) are best evaluated with MR imaging (T_2). It consists of a central butterfly-shaped part which is the grey matter. The measurements of the spinal cord show a wide variation according to the patient.

The conus medullaris is the terminal end of the spinal cord and is in normal anatomy found at the level L1–L2. The spinal cord tapers out into a cone at this level and the nerve roots descend, forming the cauda equina.

The spinal nerves exit the spinal canal through the intervertebral neuroforamina. At the cervical and thoracic level the nerve roots leave the spinal canal horizontally. At the lumbar level the nerve roots first descend in the lateral canal recess before exiting through the neuroforamen.

VASCULAR STRUCTURES

The spinal cord is supplied by three main arteries parallel to the spinal cord: one anterior and two posterior. The blood supply can be divided into three anatomical regions. In the cervicothoracic region the blood is supplied segmentally from arteries originating from the vertebral arteries and the great vessels of the neck (i.e. aorta, carotid and subclavian arteries). The midthoracic region receives most of its blood supply from collateral circulation from superior and inferior arteries and acts as a watershed area. The segmental blood supply is received from small perforants originating from the aorta. The thoracolumbar region is supplied by segmental arteries from the aorta and the iliac arteries. Variably originating from levels Th9 to L2 and in most cases from the left side of the vertebral column, the largest vessel originates from the aorta: the artery of Adamkiewicz.

The venous plexus in the spine is called the Batson plexus. This plexus is unique compared to other plexuses in the body as this venous plexus does not have valves, allowing retrograde flow in the venous network.

CRANIOCERVICAL JUNCTION

The craniocervical junction (CCJ) is the region connecting a spherical (head) and a tubular structure (spine). To stabilise this connection the craniocervical junction is composed of bones, ligaments and muscles.

The bony parts are formed by the occipital bone with a basilar part, squamous part (scale) and the lateral (condylar) part. At the cervical part of the connection, the atlas (C1) consists of an anterior and posterior arch, and two bulky lateral masses. The axis (C2) is formed by a vertebral body, pedicles, foramina transversaria, laminae, spinous process and the dens axis articulating anteriorly with the arcus anterior of the atlas.

The complex organisation of ligaments at the CCJ provides stability but allows a complex range of motion. These ligaments can be divided into the external and internal ligaments. The anterior external ligaments are formed by the ALL running along the anterior side of the vertebral bodies from C2 downward and the anterior atlanto-axial ligament connecting the ALL and the arcus anterior of the atlas. The ligament running between the arcus anterior of the atlas and the os occipitale is the atlanto-occipital ligament. Posteriorly the external ligaments consist of the extension of the ligamenta flava, the posterior atlanto-occipital and the posterior atlanto-axial ligament. The ligamentum nuchae runs from the external occipital protuberance to the spinous process of C7.

The internal ligaments of the CCJ consist anteriorly of a thin apical ligament and thick alar ligaments. The alar ligaments attach the axis to the skull base and run from the lateral aspect of the odontoid process to the anterior part of the foramen magnum. The middle internal ligament (cruciform ligament) is formed by the transverse ligament of C1, the accessory ligaments and the superior and inferior fibres. The transverse ligament is the largest, strongest and thickest craniocervical ligament and maintains stability by locking the anterior part of the odontoid process against the posterior side of the anterior arch of the atlas.[12] It runs posterior to the odontoid process of the dens and attaches bilaterally on the lateral tubercle of C1. The posterior internal ligament is the tectorial membrane. Superiorly this ligament continues as the dura mater; inferiorly the ligament forms the posterior longitudinal ligament.

The function of the muscles in the CCJ is to initiate and maintain movement, and not to limit the movements of this joint. They can be grouped into flexion, extension, abduction, adduction and rotation.

IMAGING TECHNIQUES

Multiple imaging techniques are available to evaluate the spine. The choice of imaging technique depends on the indication (e.g. traumatic or non-traumatic) and on the age of the patient. As MRI has become widely available in most countries it has become the first examination to perform in a non-traumatic setting. Especially in young patients it has the advantage not to use X-rays. In older patients computed tomography can be indicated to evaluate bony degenerative changes. If a contraindication for MRI is present, other imaging techniques (e.g. CT) are indicated.

In post-traumatic imaging CT is the preferred initial imaging technique in blunt spinal trauma patients. CT is also indicated in acute trauma patients when there is no optimal visualisation of the spine on plain film and in patients with unexplained focal pain or neurological deficit with a negative plain film, if unexplained soft-tissue swelling is present or when plain film is abnormal. Plain radiography can be performed in minor injuries. CT offers outstanding information about the bony lesions of the spine and reconstruction in virtually every anatomical plane. A group at the Harborview Medical Center in Seattle, Washington, defined a series of high-risk criteria to decide whether to perform plain radiography or CT imaging as the primary technique when imaging cervical spinal trauma (Table 54-1).[13]

In the evaluation of low back pain (LBP) with or without radiculopathy careful selection of the patients to undergo imaging is indicated to work cost-effectively. Uncomplicated acute (less than 6 weeks) LBP and/or radiculopathy is often self-limiting and imaging is not indicated. Imaging should be considered if any 'red flags' (Table 54-2) are present or if complaints show no improvement after 6 weeks.[14] Plain radiography can be useful in all of the conditions noted in Table 54-2 but can be sufficient if normal in patients with recent significant trauma or osteoporosis or age >70 years. In patients with LBP complicated with red flags, MRI or CT can be justified. MRI is the examination of choice, while CT should be considered in patients with contraindications for MRI or in postoperative patients.

TABLE 54-1 Harborview High-Risk Criteria

If yes to any criteria, high risk for c-spine injury and indication for CT

- Presence of significant head injury
- Presence of focal neurological deficit(s)
- Presence of pelvic or multiple extremity fractures
- Combined impact of accident >50 km/h (>35 mph)
- Death at the scene of the motor vehicle accident
- Accident involved a fall from a height of 3 m or more

TABLE 54-2 'Red Flags' in Low Back Pain

- Trauma, cumulative trauma
- Unexplained weight loss, insidious onset
- Age >50 years with osteoporosis or compression fractures
- Unexplained fever, history of urinary or other infection
- Immunosuppression, diabetes mellitus
- History of cancer
- Intravenous drug use
- Prolonged use of corticosteroids, osteoporosis
- Age >70 years
- Focal neurological deficit(s) with progressive or disabling symptoms, cauda equina syndrome
- Duration longer than 6 weeks
- Prior surgery

PLAIN RADIOGRAPHY

Conventional X-ray imaging is a fast, easy and inexpensive technique which offers a good overview of a large segment of the spine. It is still widely used, but cannot be justified any longer as the definite examination. Plain radiography still has the advantage over CT and MRI for the evaluation of structural malformations and instability with or without dynamic imaging in erect position.

The main disadvantage of plain radiographs is the superimposition of soft tissue and bony structures, making the interpretation difficult. In the lateral view the cervicothoracic junction can be difficult to visualise due to superimposition of the shoulders. To overcome this problem a so-called swimmer's view is made by elevating one arm above the head and letting the other hang down by the side. At the thoracolumbar junction the diaphragm makes it difficult to interpret the lateral view. On the anteroposterior (AP) view superimposition of heart and mediastinum in the thoracic spine and bowel structures in the lumbar spine offer evaluation difficulties.

In a post-traumatic setting, plain radiography can be used to determine the level of the injury to perform a CT of only one specific region. In the cervical spine, studies show that up to 55% of clinically significant fractures can be missed on plain radiography.[15]

In the cervical spine AP and lateral views are the standard views of the cervical spine. To make a good assessment of the spine, a high-quality image with visualisation of the seven cervical vertebral bodies as well as the first thoracic vertebra is necessary (Fig. 54-7). The lateral view is considered the most important view as 90% of pathology can be seen in this image. To evaluate the dens and the atlanto-axial joints an AP 'transbuccal' view is essential (Fig. 54-8). In post-traumatic patients with neck collars, this view can be difficult to perform and if there is any doubt a CT examination should be performed. Oblique views are performed to evaluate the neuroforamina. Two views are taken with the patient turned 45° to either side. The neuroforamen viewed en face is the contralateral side to which the patient has turned the head. The need for these views can be questioned as MRI and especially CT offers a much better evaluation of the (bony) neuroforamina and may demonstrate nerve root compression.

In the thoracic spine, an AP and lateral view is performed. The AP view is used to assess the pedicles (possible metastasis) and the vertebral alignment (scoliosis). When performing the lateral view the convexity of a possible scoliosis should be turned towards the film so the

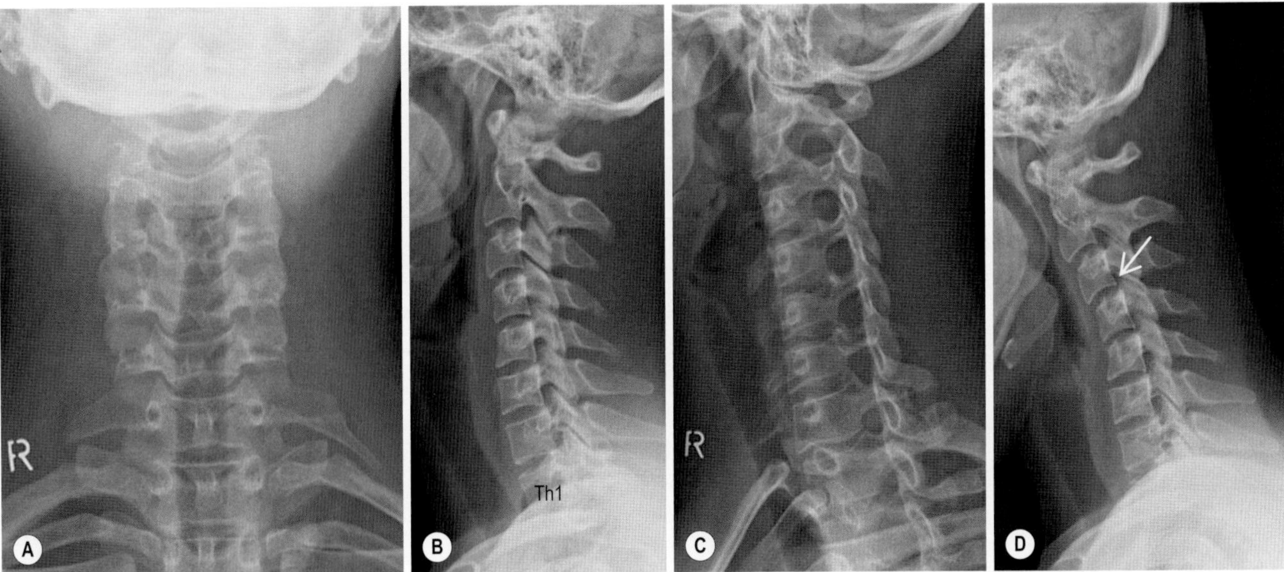

FIGURE 54-7 ■ Normal plain radiography of the cervical spine. AP (A), lateral (B), right oblique (C) and dynamic flexion (D) views of the cervical spine. Decreased cervical lordosis of the cervical spine (B) due to erect positioning of the patient; the upper part of Th1 (Th1) is visualised as it should. In the right oblique (C) there is no obliteration of the left intervertebral neuroforamina. On the dynamic flexion (D) we see a decreased mobility of the lower vertebral segments; the minimal anterolisthesis (arrow) as seen at C3–C4 is normal during flexion.

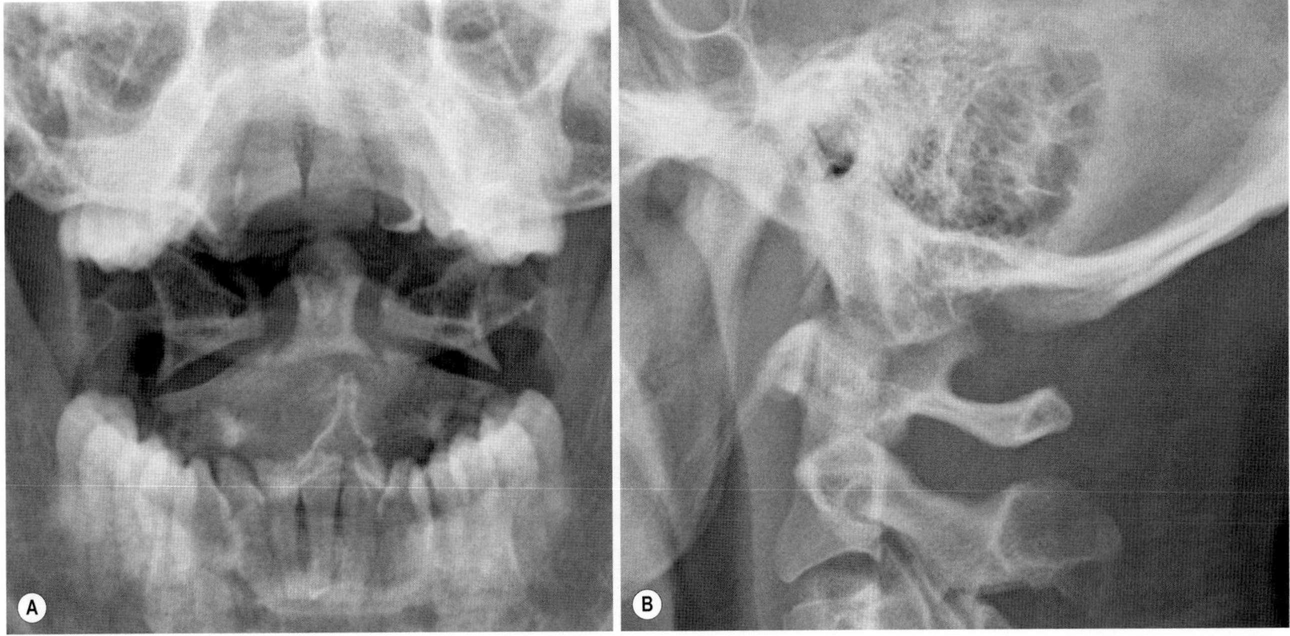

FIGURE 54-8 ■ Plain radiography of the craniocervical junction. AP (A) and lateral (B) views of the craniocervical junction. A complete free projection of the dens should be obtained, although sometimes difficult in post-traumatic patients. In this case the patient's head is turned slightly to the right, causing a discrete asymmetric position of the dens within the atlas. (Note the plumb line between teeth 11 and 21 doesn't project through the centre of the dens.)

divergent X-rays are more parallel to the disc spaces. Autotomography (the patient breaths gently during exposure) is used to blur out the ribs and diaphragm.

In the lumbar spine, the posteroanterior (PA) image of the lumbar spine is taken from posterior to anterior as the divergent X-ray beam will be more parallel to the disc spaces (Fig. 54-9) and to lessen radiation to the organs. When taken from anterior to posterior, flexion of hips and knees will reduce the lumbar lordosis. A spot image of the L5–S1 disc space is made from anterior to posterior with a caudocranial inclination of the tube. The hips and knees are in flexion to reduce the lumbar lordosis. As

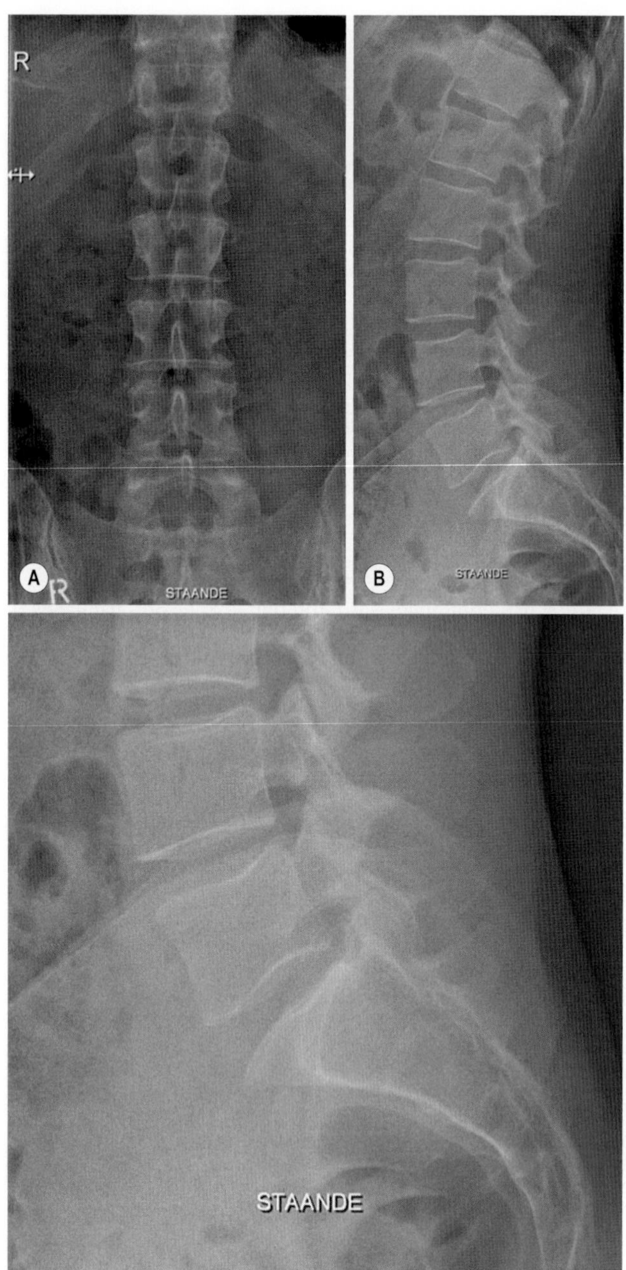

FIGURE 54-9 ■ **Normal plain radiography of the lumbar spine.** PA (A), lateral (B) and lateral spot S1 (C) views. The spot image of L5–S1 is taken anteroposteriorly with the X-ray beam parallel to the intervertebral disc space.

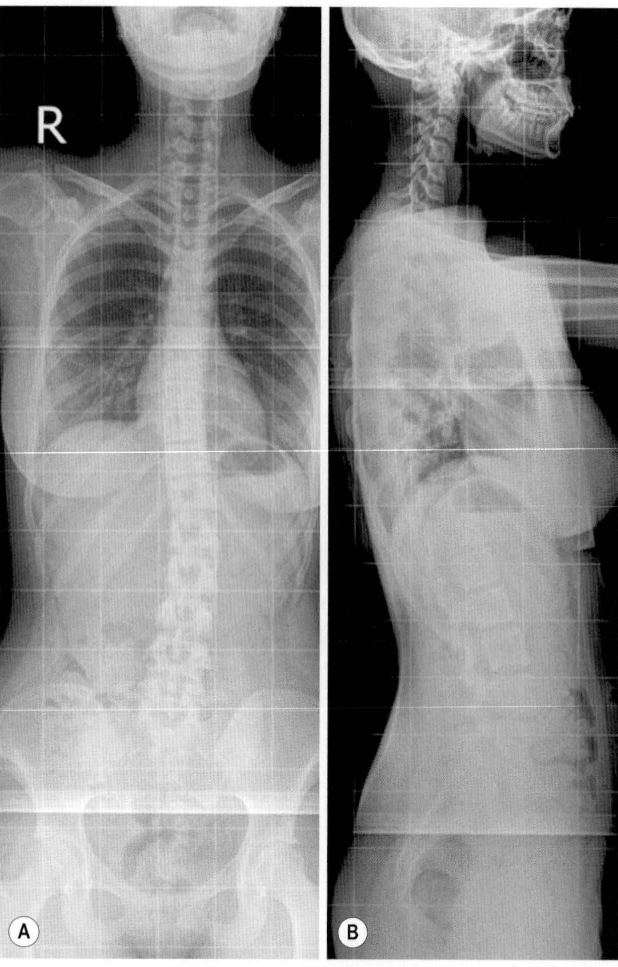

FIGURE 54-10 ■ **Full spine.** AP (A) and lateral (B) views of full spine in erect position. The AP view (A) shows a sinistroconvex scoliosis of the lumbar spine. The plumb line through the centre of C7 projects < 2 cm lateral of the plumb line through the centre of the sacrum, indicating a compensated scoliosis. The lateral view (B) shows a normal thoracic kyphosis and lumbar lordosis.

in the thoracic spine, the convexity of a scoliosis, if present, should be nearer to the radiograph. The PA oblique view is acquired by turning the patient 45°; a torsion of the lumbar spine should be avoided. The oblique view of the lumbar spine is especially useful for evaluating the facet joints and pedicles; this can be used in identification of a spondylolisthesis.

A full-spine AP view is used to evaluate and measure scoliosis and anatomical anomalies of the spine (Fig. 54-10). The lateral view is used to evaluate the thoracic kyphosis and lumbar and cervical lordosis.

Functional (extension/flexion) lateral views can be made to evaluate instability. On these images it is important to look for displacement of the vertebral bodies (anterolisthesis or retrolisthesis) or increased displacement of the vertebral bodies and an increase in distance between the spinous process (Fig. 54-7). In the lumbar spine this is often performed in patients with spondylolisthesis or after surgery to evaluate instability.

MYELOGRAPHY

Myelography and post-myelography computed tomography (Fig. 54-11) for the evaluation of spinal pathology have been largely replaced by MR imaging. MR imaging has the advantage of being non-invasive, painless and without X-ray irradiation and offers multiplanar imaging

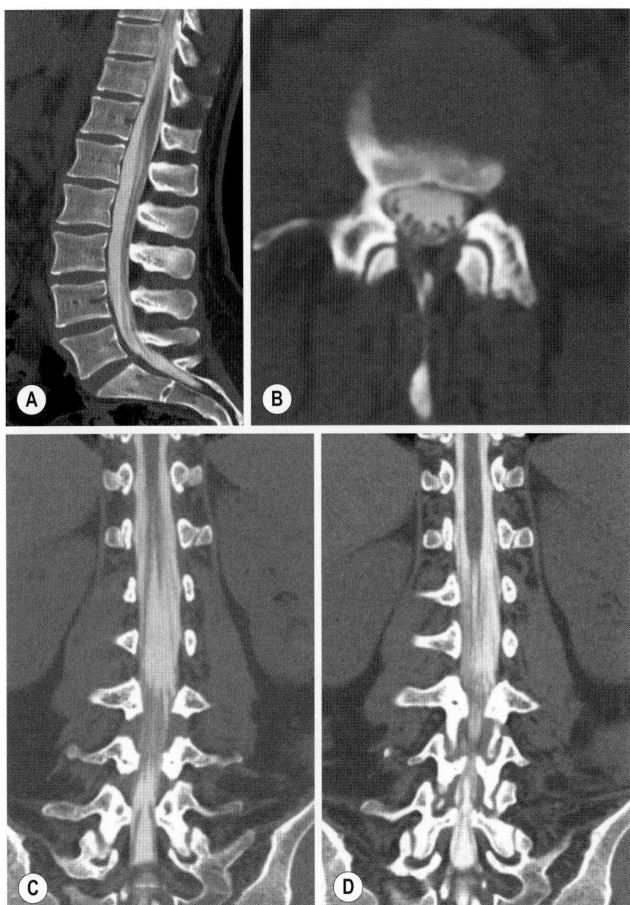

FIGURE 54-11 ■ **Post-myelography CT examination.** Sagittal (A), axial (B) and curved coronal (C, D) reformatted CT images after myelography. Normal imaging study of the spinal canal in a patient with MR-incompatible implants shows the position of the nerve roots of the cauda equina in the spinal canal as well as possible spinal canal stenosis.

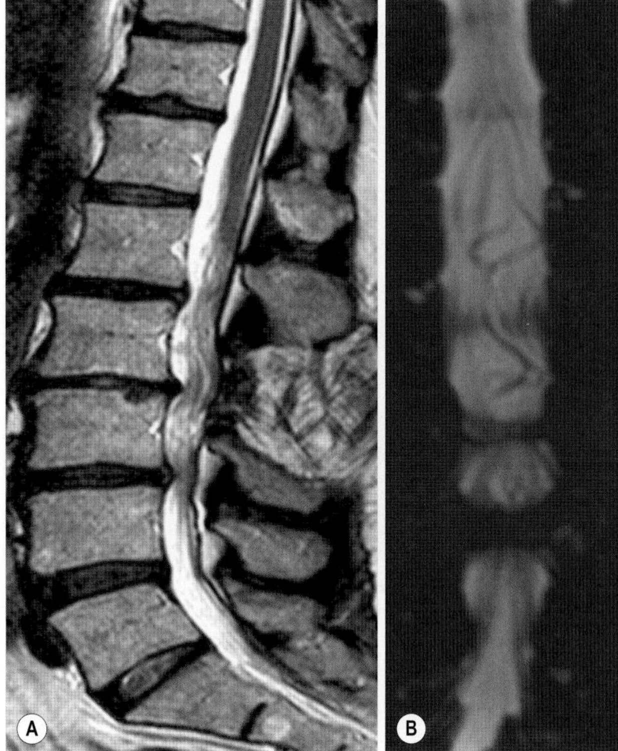

FIGURE 54-12 ■ **MR-myelography.** T_2-weighted (A) and MR myelography (B) images. Postoperative status after laminectomy at L2–L3 for a spinal canal stenosis. Sagittal T_2-weighted image and the myelo-MR show residual redundant nerve roots of the cauda equina proximal to the previous spinal canal stenosis.

possibilities. Therefore an important clinical indication is necessary to perform myelography. Myelographic MR images are obtained without the injection of intrathecal contrast and can be useful for evaluating the spinal canal (Fig. 54-12). The downside is a lower signal-to-noise ratio (SNR) of MR compared to X-ray myelography; thus small lesions can be missed on myelographic MR images.[16]

At this moment only a few indications remain for myelography; contraindications for the patient to undergo MR examinations (e.g. non-compatible pacemaker) are severe claustrophobia or absence of MR imaging. X-ray myelography can be used to dynamically evaluate the spinal canal in patients with spondylolisthesis. Myelography can be used to evaluate processes contacting, impinging or displacing the thecal sac or the nerve roots (e.g. arachnoiditis). Myelography has the advantage over MRI of allowing dynamic and functional evaluation of the cerebrospinal fluid (CSF) and the evaluation of active CSF leakage. Myelography can also be useful in a postoperative spine where artefacts of surgical material may obscure the spinal canal or nerve roots on MRI.[17]

Before starting the examination, patients should be screened. Patients with prior allergic reactions to contrast media should be premedicated. Because intrathecal iodinated contrast medium carries a risk of seizures, medication that provokes seizures should be stopped 48 hours before until 24 hours after the examination. The patients' international normalised ratio (INR) should be normal and ideally less than 1.5 and all woman of childbearing age should be screened for pregnancy.

For myelography a 22- to 26-gauge needle may be used; the smaller the bore, the smaller the risk for CSF leakage after the procedure. Typically a Quincke-type needle with a sharp tip is used for easy penetration of the skin and optimal steering of the needle. A non-ionic contrast agent proved for intrathecal use should be used to reduce neurotoxicity.

The patient is placed in a prone position with the hand above the head and his left knee up providing stability and an oblique view to open the interlaminar spaces. Using fluoroscopy, the level L2–L3 is localised. The region is disinfected and locally anaesthetised. A lumbar puncture is performed and the subarachnoidal location controlled. A test injection with 1–2 mL of contrast medium is performed under fluoroscopy and a 'wisp of smoke' appearance indicates free flow and subarachnoidal placement.

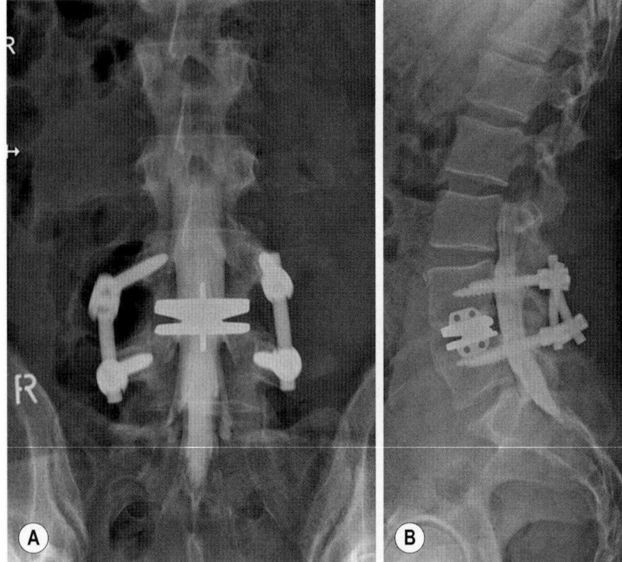

FIGURE 54-13 ■ Plain film myelography. AP (A) and lateral (B) plain film images after myelography in a postoperative patient who had a posterior lumbar intervertebral fusion (PLIF) and disc prosthesis at L4–L5. Myelography shows no spinal canal stenosis.

For lumbar myelography the patient is tilted with the feet down (reverse Trendelenburg) , causing the contrast medium to pool in the thecal sac. AP and oblique views as well as lateral views are performed (Fig. 54-13). The left lateral decubitus is performed as it is easier for the radiologist to position the patient. With the patient in lateral decubitus the table is put flat to take a lateral view of the thoracolumbar junction.[17] The thoracic and cervical myelography is seldom performed and should be done by an experienced radiologist. In most cases a lumbar contrast injection is performed and the table is placed in Trendelenburg position to allow contrast medium to flow to the thoracic and cervical level.

SPINAL ANGIOGRAPHY

Imaging of the vascular structures of the spine is challenging because of the very small vessels, variable and complex anatomy with multiple feeders at different levels. A technique with a high spatial resolution is needed for reliable and accurate visualisation.[18] For this reason digital subtraction angiography (DSA) still remains the gold standard. In clinical practice, however, computed tomographic angiography (CTA) or MR angiography (MRA) can be used to visualise the vascular malformation and the level of vascular feeders. In this way, DSA can be focused on a selection of supplying blood vessels, and examination time, contrast and radiation dose are reduced. A study of 15 patients by Nijenhuis et al. showed that the level of the Adamkiewicz artery can be sufficiently visualised with contrast-enhanced MRA in 14 out of 15 patients, although DSA still offers superior imaging quality.[19] For the evaluation of the spinal arteries on CTA, a high injection rate of 6 mL/s with a high concentration contrast agent is needed to show the spinal cord vessels.[18]

Indications for spinal angiography are suspicion of arteriovenous (AV) malformations, spinal aneurysms, vascular tumours of the spinal cord, meninges or vertebral column (Fig. 54-14). It can also be used for preoperative visualisation of the Adamkiewicz artery in cases of aorta or spinal surgery.[20] On MR imaging, small flow artefacts can simulate a vascular malformation. Thin slices and imaging after gadolinium can be used to differentiate between a flow artefact and a vascular malformation and to avoid spinal DSA.

As spinal DSA is a complex, invasive investigation with risk of morbidity it should only be performed in an experienced centre. Because catheter spinal angiography is an invasive, time-consuming procedure with risk of morbidity and a relative high cost the results of this examination should have a benefit or therapeutical implication for the patient. An intervention with embolisation is also possible when performing spinal angiography.

COMPUTED TOMOGRAPHY

Computed tomography of the spine is the first choice of examination in trauma patients with a high sensitivity in detecting fractures. Although MRI has become more common for the evaluation of the disc space and the spinal canal, CT is still adequate enough to visualise the spinal cord, exclude compression (e.g. haematoma or disc herniation) and is very useful in evaluating the posterior elements and bony changes as facet joint pathology and Baastrup's phenomenon. After surgery, CT can visualise the surgical materials and evaluate possible loosening.

The patient is placed in supine position on the CT table with the neck gently flexed (in non-traumatic patients) to reduce the cervical lordosis. Modern spiral CT allows a fast and continuous acquisition of data to obtain a full data set which makes reconstructions in all anatomical planes as well as 3D reconstruction possible (Fig. 54-15). A digital radiograph, also known as a 'scout' image or 'localiser' (lateral, AP view or both), of the region of interest is performed to make a selection of the volume to be imaged. This scout film can retrospectively be used to localise the level of the acquired data. During examination of the spine it is not necessary to do a breath-hold command.

After the acquisition of the data reconstructions in the sagittal and axial (parallel to the vertebral discs) planes are performed, the slice thickness depends on the region of interest and the indication of the examination. A soft-tissue and bone algorithm is used to enable evaluation of the bone (high resolution of bone structures) and soft tissue. The multislice volume imaging allows reconstructions in virtually every plane as well as curved reconstructions in patients with scoliosis. Three-dimensional volumetric reconstructions can be made to make illustrative images for the clinicians.

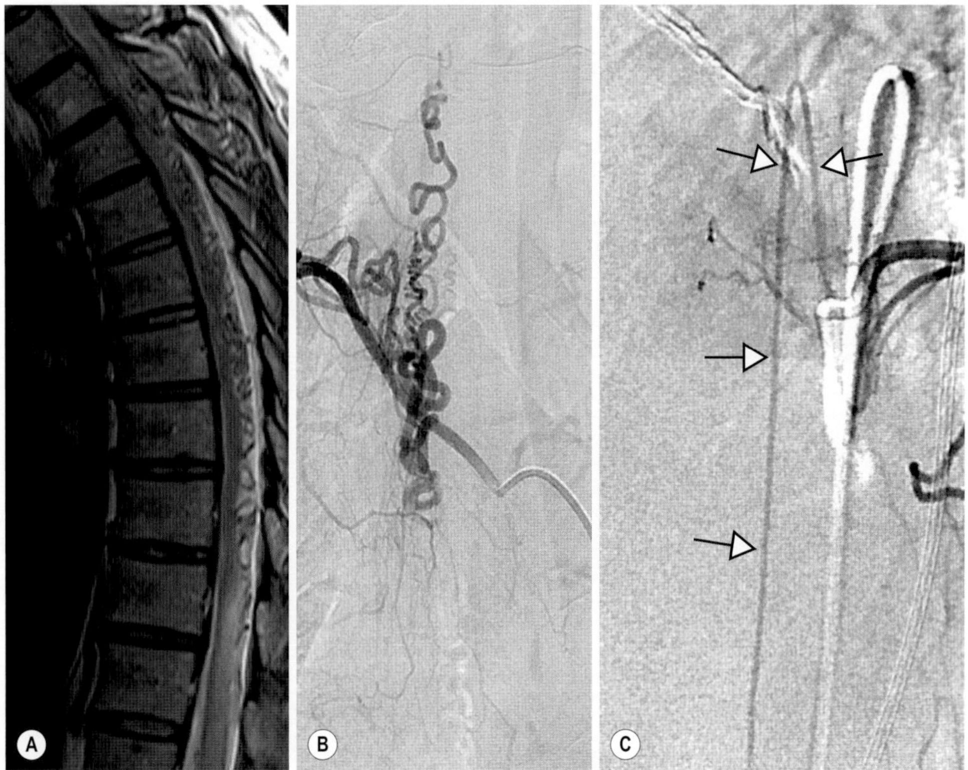

FIGURE 54-14 ■ Sagittal T_2-weighted image (A) of the thoracic spine and selective DSA of the right lumbar artery Th6 (B) and of the left lumbar artery Th8 (C). (A) An AV malformation posterior of the myelum with a high signal intensity in the myelum indicating myelomalacia. (B) The AV malformation selective contrast injection in the right lumbar artery at the level Th6. (C) The Adamkiewicz artery (arrow), with its origin at the left lumbar artery at Th8.

MAGNETIC RESONANCE IMAGING

Magnetic resonance imaging has become the method of choice for imaging of the spine. It is a non-invasive technique and is not associated with radiation exposure. As the signal intensity of CSF, bone, disc, spinal cord and epidural fat are different on most sequences, the contrast resolution can be decreased, which improves the spatial resolution.

The specific parameters of the sequences, the coil type and the reduction of motion artefacts are dependent on the individual manufacturers; the general principles are, however, the same.

The MRI examination starts with acquiring a coronal, low-resolution multislice sequence as a localiser. On these images the most optimal sagittal plane is chosen to make high-resolution images of the spine. A spatial presaturation slab is applied in the cervical spine over the larynx and the carotid artery. In the thoracic spine the same technique is used to reduce artefacts from heart and aorta. The axial images are planned on the high-resolution sagittal images over the regions of interest.

We suggest using sagittal T_1, sagittal T_2, sagittal T_2 with fat suppression (e.g. STIR) and axial T_2 as a routine protocol in MRI of the spine. In the lumbar spine we routinely add axial T_1. According to the clinical information, additional sequences can be added as required.

In the postoperative lumbar spine, again, the routine protocol is used. In addition, sagittal and axial T_1-weighted images after gadolinium (Gd) are acquired.

Spin-Echo T_1-Weighted Imaging

An MR image is called a 'T1-weighted' image when image contrast is based upon difference in longitudinal relaxation time (T_1). T_1 is a time constant specific for each tissue and is characterised by the rate in which the longitudinal magnetisation is restored. T_1 is traditionally produced using spin-echo (SE) sequences with a short repetition time (TR 300–700 ms) and short echo time (TE < 30 ms). If a SE sequence is used with a short TR, spins with a long T_1 relaxation time cannot completely relax and do not contribute to the signal.

In T_1 these tissues (e.g. CSF) are seen as dark structures. Tissues with a short T_1 relaxation time (e.g. fat) conversely have a high signal intensity. T_1-weighted images provide excellent anatomical detail, including bone marrow changes, osseous structures, discs and soft tissue.[21]

Contrast-Enhanced T_1-Weighted Imaging

Contrast agents used in MR imaging contain ions with a high electron spin, causing a shortening of relaxation

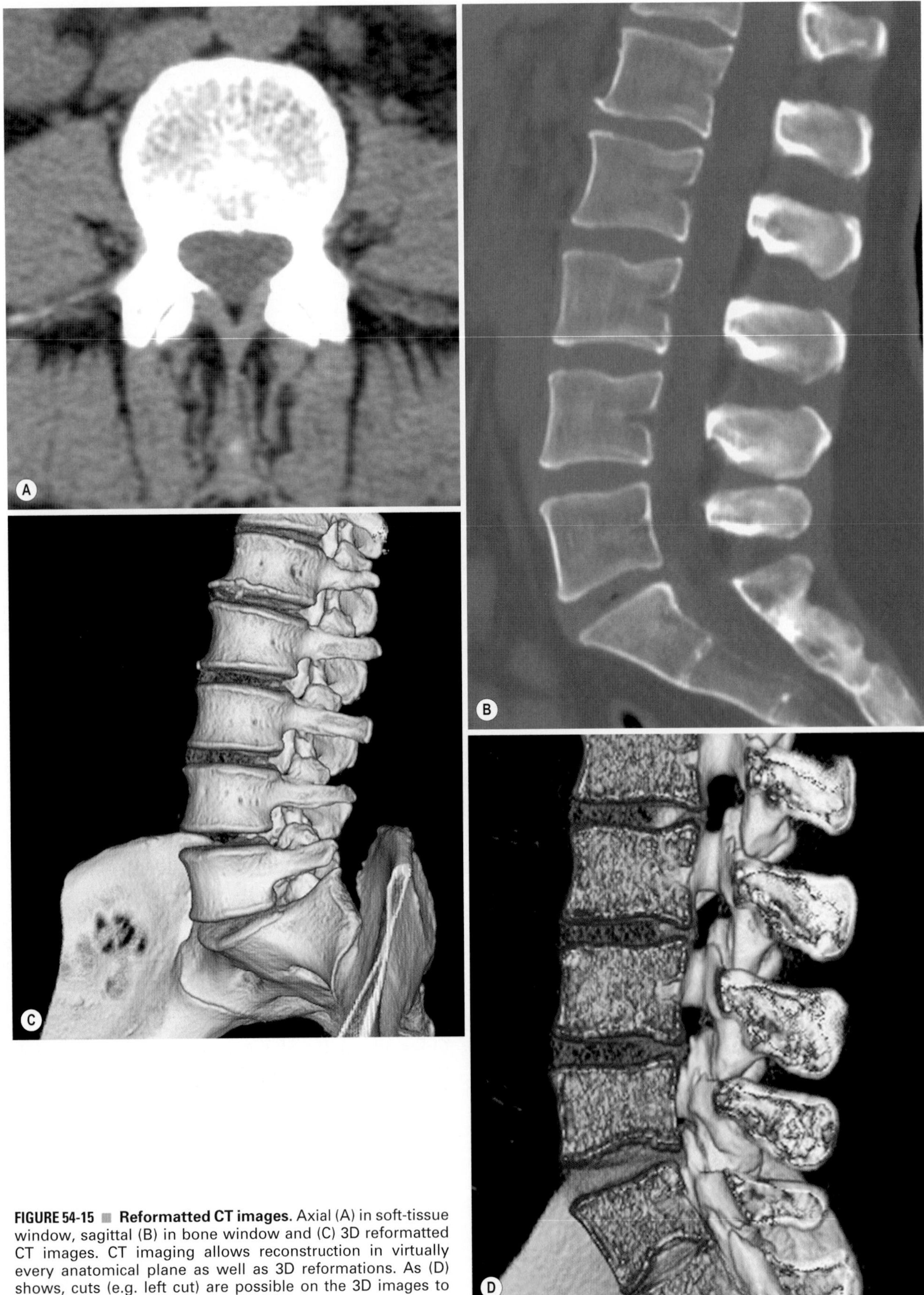

FIGURE 54-15 ■ **Reformatted CT images.** Axial (A) in soft-tissue window, sagittal (B) in bone window and (C) 3D reformatted CT images. CT imaging allows reconstruction in virtually every anatomical plane as well as 3D reformations. As (D) shows, cuts (e.g. left cut) are possible on the 3D images to obtain a 3D view of the spinal canal.

time in adjacent molecules in a magnetic field. The paramagnetic contrast agents for intravenous injection are gadolinium chelates. The standard dose for intravenous injected gadolinium is 0.1 mmol/kg body weight. Gadolinium-based paramagnetic contrast agents are relatively safe and seldom give allergic reactions.[22] Enhancement after injection of paramagnetic contrast agents is seen as an increase in signal intensity and is best seen on T_1. Gadolinium chelates not only shorten T_1 but also T_2. For the evaluation of enhancement it is recommended to perform pre- and post-contrast images over the same region (Fig. 54-16).

The enhancement mechanism is different between intra- and extra-axial lesions. In intra-axial lesions enhancement is caused by disruption of the blood–brain barrier, whereas in extra-axial lesions it is caused by hypervascularity.

Post-contrast imaging can be used to distinguish postoperative fibrosis (scarring) from recurrent disc fragments.[23] In the lumbar spine, fat-suppression techniques before and/or after contrast-enhanced T_1 can further assist in differentiating between enhancing scar tissue and epidural fat and, in rare cases, between postoperative blood and normal epidural fat.[24]

Fat suppression on T_1-weighted images before intravenous injection of gadolinium is of little value because the signal from most pathological lesions, whether inflammatory, neoplastic or infectious, is often low and better visualised against the bright signal intensity of fat. In post-gadolinium T_1-weighted fat suppression can be useful in adults with fatty transformation of the bone marrow. Fat-suppressed images can be particularly useful for evaluating ligamentous structures or lesions involving the paraspinal tissues.[21]

Spin-Echo and Fast Spin-Echo T_2-Weighted Imaging

An MR image is called a 'T_2-weighted' image when image contrast is based upon the difference in transverse relaxation time (T_2 time). In SE sequences, T_2 weighting is achieved by applying a long repetition time (TR 2000–3000 ms) and a long echo time (TE 80–120 ms). T_1 is thus reduced by the long TR while the T_2 contrast is strong due to the long TE. The long TR time imposes a high acquisition time, which is a disadvantage for the conventional SE sequences.

In fast spin-echo (FSE) sequences (also called turbo spin-echo or TSE), multiple phase-encoding steps are acquired per excitation instead of a single step as in conventional SE sequences, causing a reduction in acquiring time.

Imaging characteristics of SE and FSE T_2 are comparable. Fat (including fatty bone marrow), however, is brighter on FSE than on SE sequences; this may mask vertebral metastasis on FSE T_2.

Bright CSF is the hallmark of T_2-weighted images. The spinal cord and nerves have an intermediate signal intensity, causing a maximal contrast between the CSF and neural tissue[21] (Fig. 54-17). T_2-weighted images have a high sensitivity in detecting pathological changes in tissue, especially in which the extracellular matrix has a higher water content.

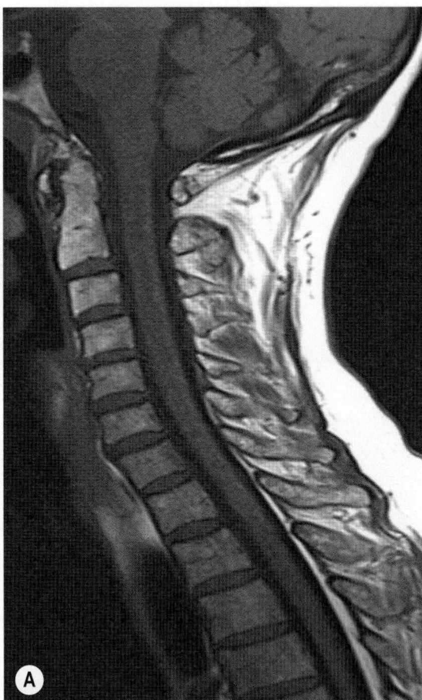

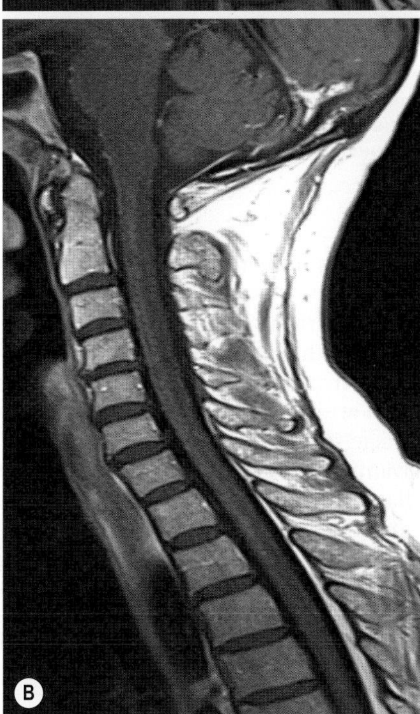

FIGURE 54-16 ■ Sagittal T_1-weighted images before (A) and after (B) injection of gadolinium. The normal enhancement of vascular structures post-contrast indicates the presence of contrast as seen posterior of C2 in and in de venous sinus.

Gradient-Echo Imaging

Gradient-recalled echo (GRE) images appear to be SE or FSE T_2-weighted, as CSF has a high signal intensity; the

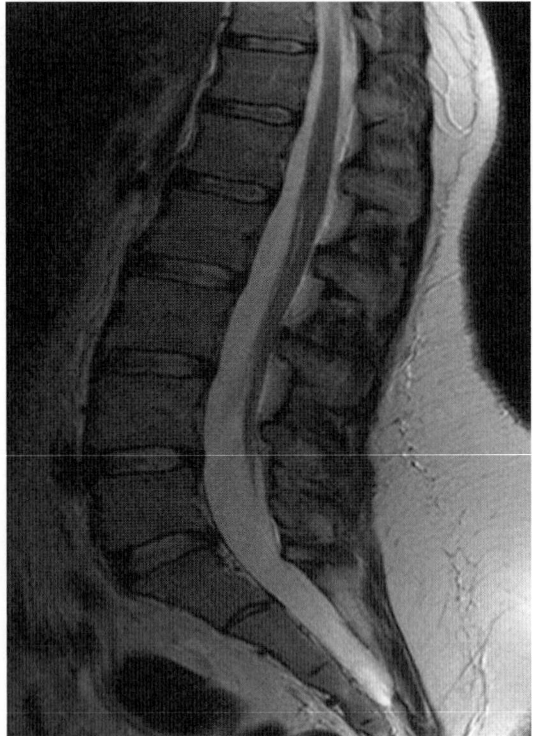

FIGURE 54-17 ■ **T_2-weighted image of the lumbar spine.** Normal sagittal T_2-weighted image of the lumbar spine. On T_2-weighted images there is a maximal contrast between the cerebrospinal fluid and the spinal cord and nerves.

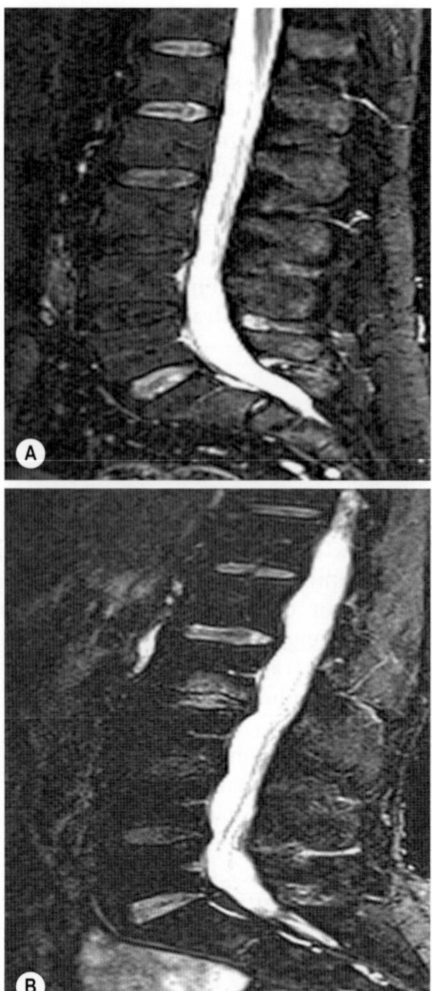

FIGURE 54-18 ■ **Sagittal STIR images** of the lumbar spine in a patient with a normal STIR image (A) with TR 4510 and TE 63. (B) Increased signal intensity on the STIR image (TR 3210, TE 52) in the lower endplate of L2, indicating oedema.

intervertebral discs have a relatively high signal intensity and the vertebrae a low signal. Blood flow creates a high signal intensity on these images.

GRE T_2* has the advantage over conventional SE sequences of offering shorter echo times and, as such, less CSF-pulsation artefacts are especially useful in the cervical and thoracic spine.

A disadvantage of GRE is the low contrast for intramedullary lesions compared with SE or FSE. The signal-to-noise is superior in FSE imaging sequences compared with GRE. GRE images are also more susceptible to local field inhomogeneity of the magnetic field and signal loss is exaggerated in the presence of these inhomogeneities, e.g. metallic implants.

Short Tau Inversion Recovery

Short tau inversion recovery (STIR) has a high sensitivity in detecting musculoskeletal disease because of the synergistic effect of prolonged T_1 and T_2 in abnormal tissue, with improved SNR and fat suppression[25] (Fig. 54-18). This technique is especially favourable in detecting degenerative changes (Modic-changes, facet joint degeneration, spondylolysis, Baastrup) and vertebral metastasis. STIR (and fast-STIR) has also proved to be useful in detecting MS lesions compared with T_2-weighted images.

Because of the longer acquisition time, this technique is more prone to motion artefacts and is not indicated for evaluation of the thoracic spine.[26] STIR images tend to be noisy, but the usefulness is provided by the high SNR.

Diffusion-Weighted Imaging

Diffusion-weighted imaging (DWI) and the calculated apparent diffusion coefficient (ADC) maps are widely used for evaluating many diseases in the brain (Fig. 54-19). In the spine and the vertebral column the research on DWI is much more limited and poses some difficulties, due to the higher magnetic inhomogeneities in and around the spine such as the smaller size, the low SNR and the involuntary motion (respiration and vascular motion). DWI on the spinal cord can be adopted to evaluate spinal cord infarction, active MS lesions, spinal compression and post-traumatic injury. DWI can also be used to detect drop metastasis in children with hypercellular brain tumours.[27] In addition, although still in

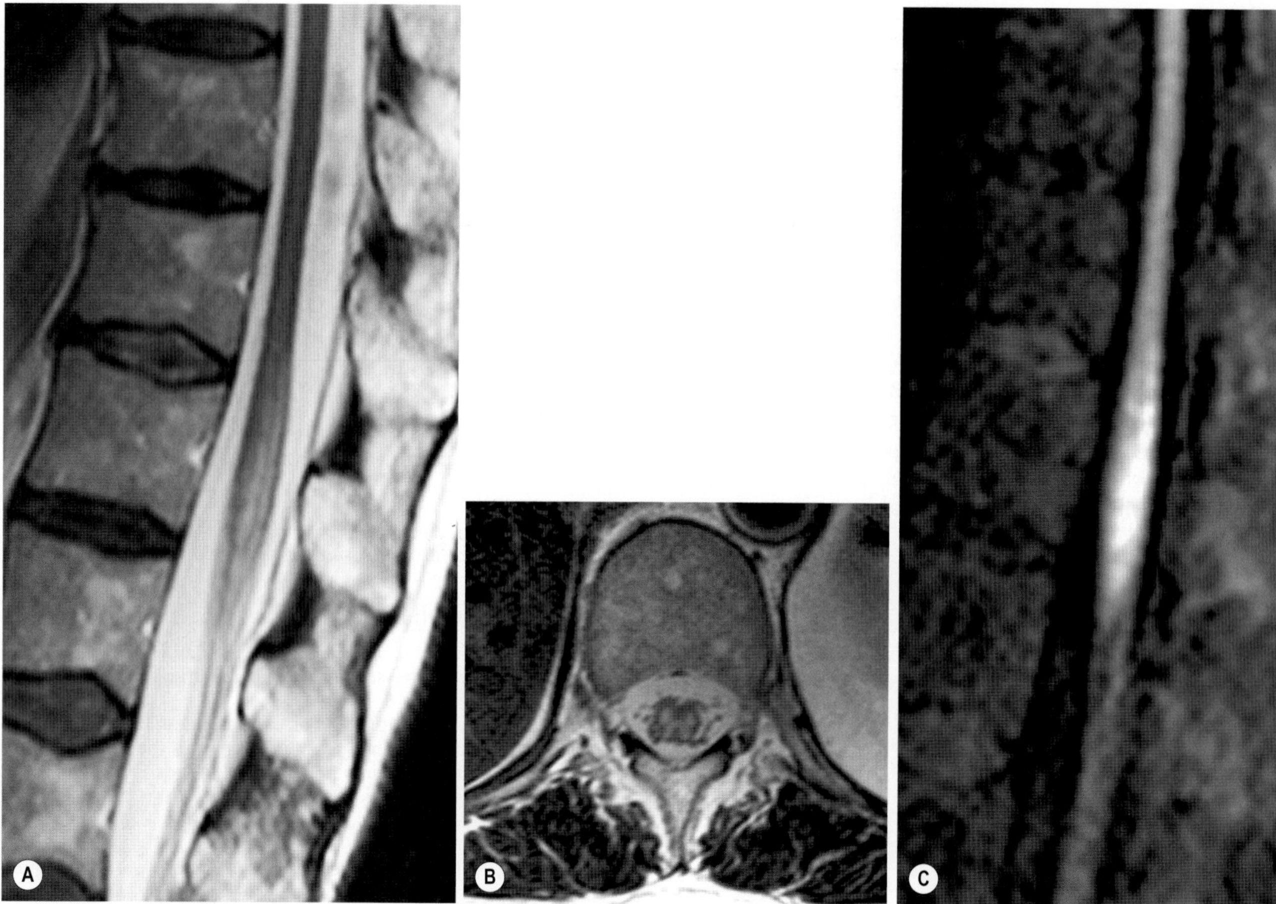

FIGURE 54-19 ■ **Diffusion-weighted imaging: sagittal (A) and axial (B) T_2-weighted and (C) sagittal diffusion-weighted images.** (A) Oedema of the distal and of the spinal cord with hyperintense signal intensity. (B) A hyperintense signal centrally in the grey matter, also known as the 'owl's eye'. The diffusion-weighted image (C) shows diffusion restriction in the distal spinal cord, indicating ischaemia (Images courtesy of Prof. Dr. M. Thurnher, Vienna Austria).

research, diffusion tensor imaging (DTI) can be used to allow characterisation of the structural integrity of the spinal cord.

Fluid-Attenuated Inversion Recovery

The primary goal of fluid-attenuated inversion recovery (FLAIR) sequences is to improve contrast in cases where resolution is less important. FLAIR is a highly T_2-weighted SE sequence with a long inversion recovery time suppressing all the signal from the CSF (black on FLAIR). In the spine this removes the motion artefacts from the CSF.

In FLAIR images most lesions have a high signal intensity; however, cystic lesions and cysts will also appear as black areas (signal voids). In imaging of the lumbar spine on 3 T some studies suggest T_1-weighted FLAIR images to be superior in delineating normal tissue interfaces between soft tissue/CSF-bone or disc/CSF compared with T_1-weighted FSE technique.[28]

Three-Dimensional (3D) Imaging

Volume or 3D imaging is a technique of acquiring thin slices without a reduced SNR or increase in imaging time. GRE and FSE sequences can be used to obtain a 3D data set. When using 3D GRE imaging, a short TR is preferred because of the large number of phase-encoding pulses required. This sequence is vulnerable to motion-induced phase shifts.

An FSE sequence with thin (1–2 mm) slices can be used to cover a segment of the spine. Three-dimensional FSE offers the advantage of reducing flow void artefacts in the CSF.

A 3D data set with thin slices can be used to make reconstructions in multiple imaging planes by using multiplanar reformatting algorithms.

Artefacts

Artefacts are defined as any images (signal or signal loss) that have no anatomical basis but are the result of distorted, additional or suppressed information. Many artefacts are caused by poor choice of technical parameters or defective MRI unit. For example, 3 T compared with 1.5 T MRI gives more artefacts; they are both increased in size as well as in numbers. A good knowledge of normal anatomy and pathology will improve detection of these artefacts.

Susceptibility Artefacts

Magnetic susceptibility artefacts occur at the boundary of two tissues with a large difference in magnetic susceptibility, e.g. the presence of ferromagnetic materials or an air–tissue interface. In the spine this kind of artefact is caused by the presence of metal implants as seen in the postoperative spine and results from a vast difference in magnetic properties between metal implants and human tissue. The sensitivity of the different pulse sequences to these artefacts is echoplanar (EPI) > gradient echo (GRE) > spin echo (SE) > fast spin echo (FSE). Susceptibility artefacts are directly related to field strength.[29] The factors influencing these artefacts are compositions of the material, size and orientation and also the external magnetic field and type of pulse sequence.[30] In order to reduce susceptibility artefacts, GRE sequences should be avoided and, instead, SE or preferably FSE sequences should be used.

Motion Artefacts

These artefacts are caused by discrete movements of the patient. In the cervical spine these artefacts can also be caused by swallowing and in the thoracic spine by cardiac motion.[30] Motion artefacts by swallowing or cardiac movement can be reduced by applying spatial presaturation.

Truncation Artefacts

Truncation artefacts are caused by imperfection in the Fournier transformation. These bright or dark lines are seen parallel to the edges of abrupt intensity changes. These artefacts are more seen on 3-T imaging than in 1.5-T imaging and are a consequence of the improved SNR on 3 T. In the spine these artefacts are especially seen in the interface between spinal cord and CSF, and are a possible cause of overestimation of spinal canal stenosis on MRI. This type of artefact is one of the causes of a band of high or low signal seen near the centre of the spinal cord in mid-sagittal images and is also the source of difficulty for defining the border between the spinal cord and CSF. Their occurrence can be reduced by increasing the spatial resolution (increase matrix size).

Cerebrospinal Fluid Pulsation Artefacts

These artefacts are caused by the pulsatile motion of the cerebrospinal fluid (CSF) caused by to expansion of the CSF during the systolic phase of the cardiac cycle. In the phase-encoding direction this motion can generate linear artefacts parallel to the interface between spinal cord and CSF, producing signal changes in the spinal cord that can be mistaken for intramedullary lesions. Especially in the thoracic spine, areas of turbulent CSF flow related to arachnoidal septa can simulate intradural masses.[31]

For a full list of references, please see ExpertConsult.

FURTHER READING

1. Denis F. The three column spine and its significance in the classification of acute thoracolumbar spinal injuries. Spine 1993;8(8):817–31.
4. Ricci C, Cova M, Kang YS, et al. Normal age-related patterns of cellular and fatty bone marrow distribution in the axial skeleton: MR imaging study. Radiology 1990;177(1):83–8.
5. Grenier N, Kressel HY, Schiebler ML, et al. Normal and degenerative posterior spinal structures: MR imaging. Radiology 1987;165(2):517–25.
12. Tubbs RS, Hallock JD, Radcliff V, et al. Ligaments of the craniocervical junction. J Neurosurg Spine 2011;14(6):697–709.
15. Mathen R, Inaba K, Munera F, et al. Prospective evaluation of multislice computed tomography versus plain radiographic cervical spine clearance in trauma patients. J Trauma 2007;62(6):1427–31.
17. Harreld JH, McMenamy JM, Toomay SM, Chason DP. Myelography: a primer. Curr Prob Diagn Radiol 2011;40(4):149–57.
24. Salgado R, Van Goethem JW, van den Hauwe L, Parizel PM. Imaging of the postoperative spine. Semin Roentgenol 2006;41(4):312–26.
31. Taber KH, Herrick RC, Weathers SW, et al. Pitfalls and artifacts encountered in clinical MR imaging of the spine. Radiographics 1998;18(6):1499–521.

CHAPTER 55

Degenerative Disease of the Spine

Paul M. Parizel • Thomas Van Thielen • Luc van den Hauwe • Johan W. Van Goethem

CHAPTER OUTLINE

INTRODUCTION

The spine is a complex anatomical structure composed of vertebrae, intervertebral discs and ligaments. All of these structures may undergo degenerative and morphological changes with age. The intervertebral discs form the connection between two adjacent intervertebral bodies and have two main functions: allowing movement of the spine and to serve as shock absorbers. Movement at a single level is limited; the combined movement of multiple levels allows a significant range of motion. The cervical and lumbar spine, compared with the thoracic spine, has relative more disc height so the motion in these parts is greater. In the posterior region the facet joints play an important role in the cause of neck and low-back pain. Facet joint syndrome is a range of symptoms that cannot be linked to a single nerve root pattern.

DEGENERATIVE DISC DISEASE

Nomenclature and Classification

Since the first description of a 'ruptured disc' by Mixter and Barr in 1934 with monoradiculopathy,[1] the terminology to grade and report degenerative disease of the spine has been controversial and confusing. Some nomenclature systems are based on description of the observed morphology of the disc contour while others include the pathological, clinical and anatomical features. Cross-sectional imaging is based on other definitions and concepts compared to myelography or discography.[2] In 2001 a new nomenclature was proposed by the Combined Task Forces of the North American Spine Society, the American Society of Spine Radiology and the American Society of Neuroradiology which consists of a classification system for the reporting on imaging studies based on pathology.[3] In this chapter we shall follow the general classification of disc lesions as proposed by the Combined Task Forces. The general classification as proposed by Milette is given in Table 55-1.[4]

TABLE 55-1 **General Classification of Disc Lesions**

- Normal (excluding aging changes)
- Congenital/developmental variant
- Degenerative/traumatic lesion
  - Annular tear
  - Herniation
    - Protrusion/extrusion
    - Intravertebral
  - Degeneration
    - Spondylosis deformans
    - Intervertebral osteochondrosis
- Inflammation/infection
- Neoplasia
- Morphological variant of unknown significance

Age-related Changes in the Intervertebral Disc

The Combined Task Forces reserved the term 'normal' for young discs that are morphologically normal, without

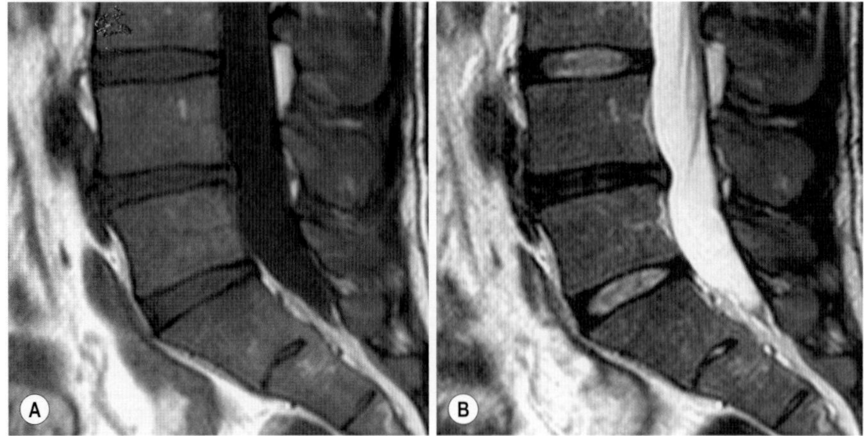

FIGURE 55-1 ■ **'Black disc'.** Sagittal T_1 (A) and T_2 images (B) in a 34-year-old man. Decrease in T_2 signal intensity at the level L4–L5 predisposes the disc to degenerative changes.

signs of disease, trauma or ageing. The normal appearance of an intervertebral disc, however, is age-related due to biochemical and anatomical changes which result in a variable appearance on MRI.[5]

In *infants and young children*, the intervertebral disc is prominent relative to the height of the adjacent vertebral bodies. With increasing age the disc volume decreases. The transition between the nucleus pulposus and the annulus is sharp and becomes less distinct with age.[6]

In *young adults* the disc contour coincides with the margins of the adjacent vertebral endplates. On MR imaging the normal adult disc has a low to intermediate signal on T_1-weighted images and a high signal intensity on T_2-weighted images relative to the bone marrow in the adjacent vertebral bodies.[6] On T_2 the bright nucleus pulposus is indistinguishable from the inner annulus. The normal adult endplates, the outer annulus fibrosus and the ligamentous structures are hypointense on T_1 and T_2. The outer annulus is visualised on T_2 and has a low signal intensity.[7] In young adults diurnal changes in T_2 relaxation are present; these changes disappear after the age of 35 years and are thought to be a normal aspect of ageing.[8]

In the *third decade* the intranuclear cleft appears as a horizontal band of decreased signal intensity on T_2 in the central part of the discs, giving it a bilocular appearance on sagittal images. It resembles a fibrous transformation of the gelatinous matrix of the nucleus pulposus.

In *middle-aged and elderly patients* there is a gradual signal loss of the intervertebral discs on the T_2 images until the disc become hypointense.[9] The loss of signal is best seen on T_2 and correlates to a decrease in water and proteoglycan content and increase in collagen. Though the decrease in T_2 signal of the intervertebral disc is age-related it predisposes to degenerative changes in the discs such as loss in disc height, disc herniation and annular tears (Fig. 55-1). The highest T_2 values are seen near the vertebral endplates and the lower T_2 values are present in the intranuclear cleft and the peripheral annulus fibrosus due to its fibrous nature.

In general in the normal ageing disc the height is preserved, disc margins remain regular and radial annular tears are not a usual consequence of ageing. On the basis of a series of post-contrast MRI studies of the lumbar spine, degeneration and normal ageing have been shown to be two separate processes.[10]

Resnick and Niwayama conclude there are two different processes of degeneration: a first type, which can be considered normal ageing, involves the annulus fibrosus and adjacent ring apophysis (spondylosis deformans) (Fig. 55-2); the second type, called intervertebral osteochondrosis, affects the nucleus pulposus and the vertebral endplates, corresponding to the pathological ageing process.[11]

Anterior and lateral marginal osteophytes are considered as normal ageing while endplate changes and reactive bone marrow are seen as pathological changes. Large amounts of gas in the central disc space seen on X-ray or CT studies are indicative for pathological intervertebral osteochondrosis while small amounts of gas near the apophyseal enthesis should be considered as spondylosis deformans (Fig. 55-3).

Degenerative Disc Disease

The prevalence of degenerative disc disease is linearly related to age. Intervertebral disc degeneration begins early in life.[12] Many other factors (e.g. biomechanical and quality of collagen) are also implicated. Degeneration includes changes involving the endplates (sclerosis, defects, Modic changes and osteophytes) as well as disc changes (fibrosis, annular tears, desiccation, loss of height and mucinous degeneration of the annulus).

The relation between low-back pain and abnormalities in the lumbar spine is controversial as abnormal findings are often seen in asymptomatic patients on plain radiographs, CT studies and MRI studies.[13] Degenerative changes in the disc are already seen in one-third of healthy persons between 21 and 40 years old. The high prevalence of asymptomatic disc degeneration must be taken into account when MRI is used for assessment of spinal symptoms.

Although the validity of disc height as an indication for degenerative disc changes is questionable, the loss of height of the intervertebral space is the earliest sign of

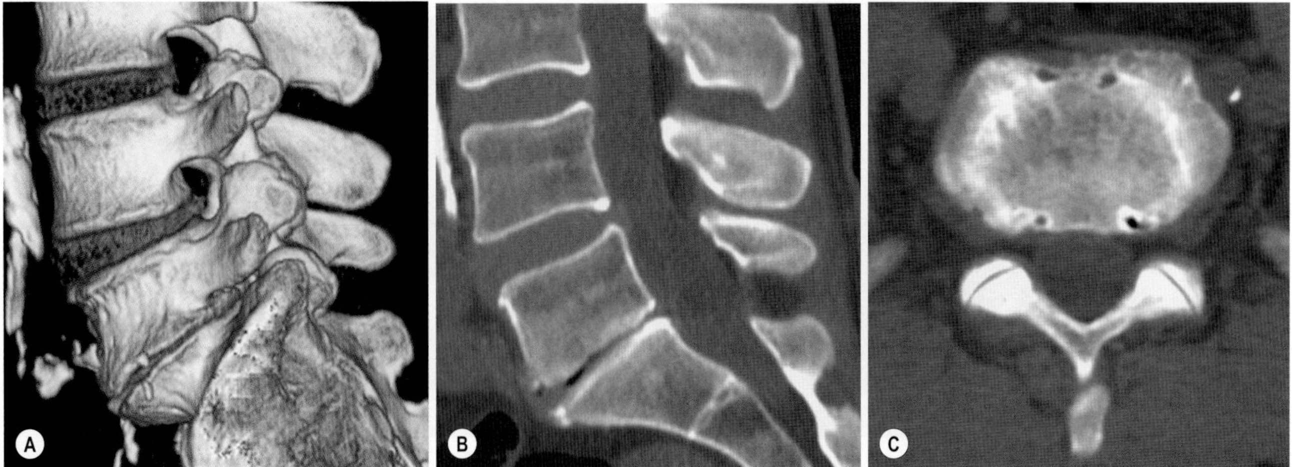

FIGURE 55-2 ■ Spondylosis deformans ('normal ageing') versus intervertebral osteochondrosis ('abnormal ageing') in a 50-year-old woman. Three-dimensional (A), sagittal (B) and axial at L5–S1 (C) reformatted CT images. The L5–S1 intervertebral disc is narrowed with irregular endplates, vacuum phenomenon and concentric protrusion of the disc. At the other levels, mild spondylotic changes are seen at the adjacent ring apophysis, indicating normal ageing.

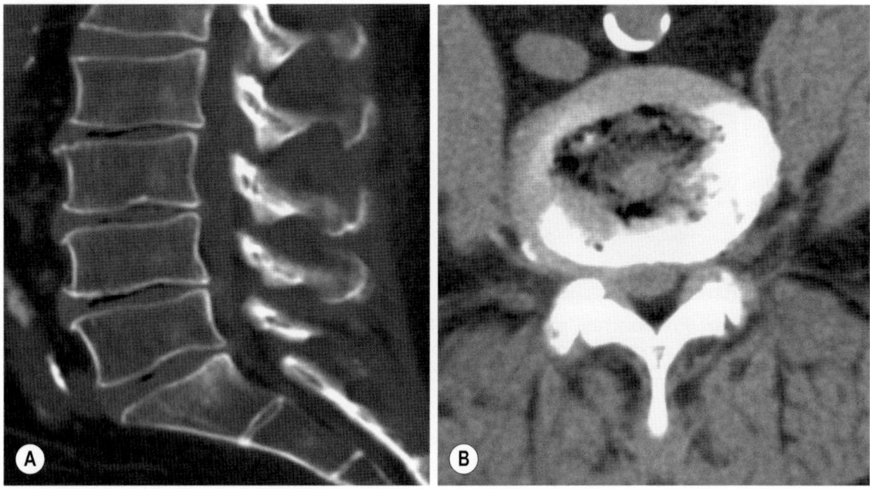

FIGURE 55-3 ■ Vacuum phenomenon in a 56-year-old man. Sagittal (A) and axial (B) CT reformatted images. Intradiscal gas at the levels L2–L3 to L5–S1. This so-called vacuum phenomenon is a sign of advanced degeneration.

disc degeneration on plain radiographs. Loss of disc height has been reported in asymptomatic subjects, indicating there is no direct relationship between clinical symptoms and imaging findings. The position of the patient (lying down or standing) should be taken into account.

Other signs, including sclerosis of the vertebral endplates, osteophytes, vacuum phenomenon and calcification, are more reliable, though they indicate late degenerative changes.

Signal loss on T_2 is an early indicator of intervertebral disc degeneration on MRI.[9] As described earlier, in normal ageing the decrease in signal intensity on T_2 should be uniformly distributed over the different levels. If the signal loss is only seen in one or two levels this should be interpreted as abnormal. This finding is often referred to as 'a black disc', and has been applied to describe discogenic pain syndrome (Fig. 55-1). The degenerative process typically starts at the levels with the highest mechanical stress (motion/weight bearing). In the cervical spine, levels C5–C6 and C6–C7 are most commonly involved and in the lumbar spine the levels L5–S1 and L4–L5.

Annular Tears

With ageing, the intervertebral disc becomes more fibrous and less elastic. The degenerative changes are accelerated when the structural integrity of the posterior annulus fibrosus is damaged by overload. This will eventually lead to formation of fissures in the annulus fibrosus. In the international literature the term 'annular tear' is the most widely used and is also supported by the Combined Task Forces; however, the terminology 'annular fissure' is also used. One should take into account that 'annular tear' does not imply this is caused by trauma.

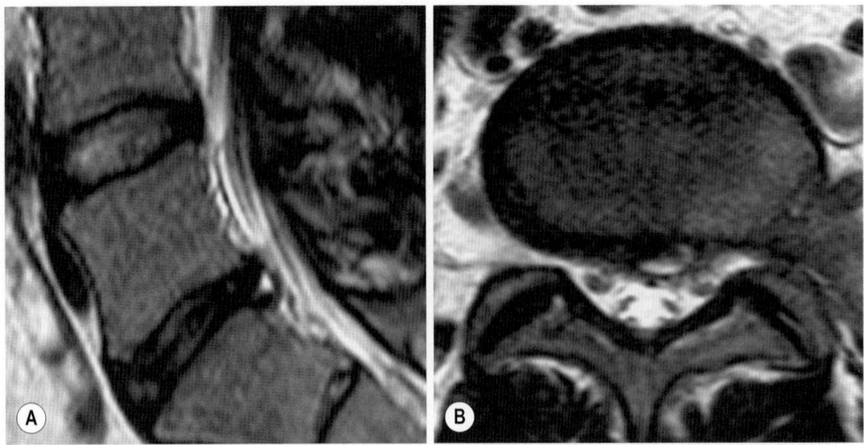

FIGURE 55-4 ■ Radial annular tear. Sagittal (A) and axial (B) T_2-weighted images. The radial tear extends to the outer rim of the annulus fibrosus (A). The axial image (B) shows that, in addition, there is a concentric tear involving the outer circumference of the annulus fibrosus. There is a loss of T_2 signal and decrease in disc height at the level L5–S1.

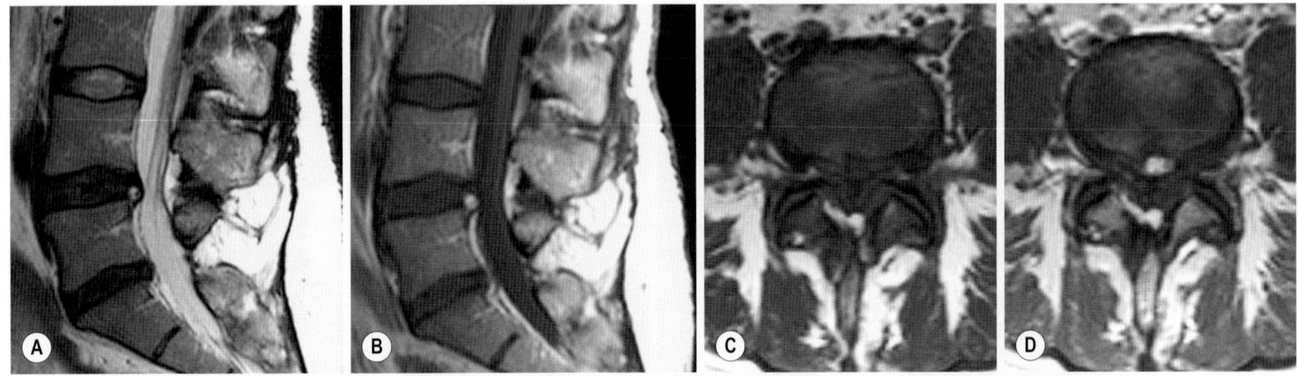

FIGURE 55-5 ■ Enhancing annular tear. Pre-contrast sagittal T_2 (A) and axial (C) T_1 images; post-gadolinium sagittal (B) and axial (D) T_1 images. On the T_2 sagittal image a posterior annular tear and central disc herniation is seen at the level L4–L5. After gadolinium administration, there is a linear area of enhancement in the posterior annulus, indicating a concentric tear.

Annular tears can be divided into concentric, transverse or radial tears:[14]

- *Concentric tears* are circumferential lesions found in the outer layers of the annulus fibrosus. Like onion rings, they represent the splitting between adjacent layers of the lamellae annulus. They are believed to be post-traumatic from torsion overload injuries.
- *Transverse tears* or 'rim lesions' are horizontal ruptures of the Sharpey's fibres near the insertion in the bony ring apophysis. The clinical significance of transverse tears remains unclear, although some authors believe they influence and accelerate degeneration and are associated with discogenic pain.[14] They are believed to be post-traumatic in origin and are often associated with small osteophytes.
- *Radial tears* are annular tears permeating from the deep central part of the disc and extend outwards toward the annulus in either the craniocaudal or the transverse plane (Fig. 55-4). Most of these tears do not reach the pain-sensitive outer layers of the annulus. Radial annular tears are associated with disc degeneration[14] and a complete radial tear is necessary for progressive deterioration of the disc.[15]

The clinical significance of annular tears remains unclear. Some annular tears can cause low-back pain without the presence of modification of the disc contours, also known as discogenic pain.[16] On the other hand, annular tears are often found in asymptomatic patients and can be seen as a part of the ageing process.[17]

On MRI annular tears can be seen as an area of high signal intensity on T_2 or as foci of annular enhancement on gadolinium-enhanced T_1[18] (Fig. 55-5). On T_2 the signal intensity is the same as the adjacent cerebrospinal fluid. Repetitive microtrauma may cause annular tears to enlarge and become inflamed; this can be seen as an area of increased signal intensity. This phenomenon is seen on T_2 and is known as a high intensity zone (HIZ).[19] The HIZ is a combination of radial and concentric annular tears which merge in the periphery of the disc. The presence of a high intensity zone is believed to be related to discogenic pain as it involves the outer, highly innervated layers of the annulus. The value of this sign is, however, limited due to a poor sensitivity and a limited positive predictive value.[20] On T_1 extradural inflammation is seen as a zone of intermediate signal intensity, replacing the fat between the disc and the dural sac; on post-contrast images there is intense enhancement.

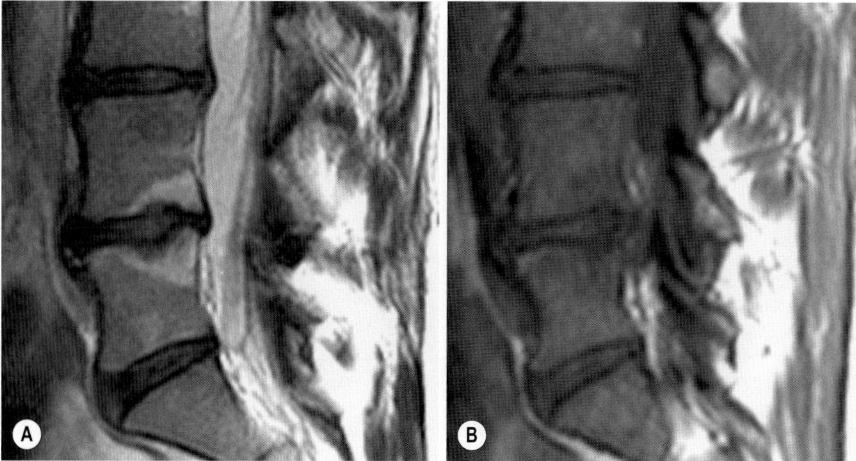

FIGURE 55-6 ■ Intravertebral herniation at L4–L5. Sagittal T_2 (A) and T_1 (B) images. The intravertebral herniations are located in the lower endplate of L4 and the upper endplate of L5. They are surrounded by reactive bone marrow changes, which are hyperintense on the T_2 image and hypointense on the T_1 image (Modic type I changes).

In the cervical spine annular tears, rim lesions and prolapsed disc material are poorly recognised on MRI, even in severely degenerative disc.[21]

In the thoracic spine herniated disc fragments are often associated with abnormal straight or curvilinear densities on CT, also known as the 'nuclear trail sign'. On MRI this finding may also be associated with a comet-tail configuration in the axial plane. This sign indicates advanced disc disruption and degeneration and must be distinguished from an ageing disc that has not failed.

Disc Heriation

Herniation is defined as a displacement of disc material (cartilage, nucleus, fragmented annular tissue and apophyseal bone) beyond the limits of the intervertebral disc space.[3] The definition of the intervertebral disc is the three-dimensional volume defined by the adjacent vertebral endplates and the outer edges of the vertebral ring apophysis, excluding osteophytes. A break in the vertebral endplates or disruption of the annulus fibrosus is thus necessary for disc displacement to occur. Disc herniations through one or both vertebral endplates are called intervertebral herniations. These herniations are also called Schmorl's nodes and are often surrounded by reactive bone marrow changes (Fig. 55-6). One hypothesis is that this type of herniation is caused by a weak spot in the vertebral endplate caused by regression of the nutrient vascular canals leaving a scar.[22] When in young individuals a herniation of the nucleus pulposus through the ring apophysis occurs before bony fusion a small segment of the vertebral rim may become isolated.[23] This is called a limbus vertebra and is most commonly found in the lumbar region and less frequently on the mid-cervical level. They are characterised by a defect in the anterior wall of the vertebra and usually at the anterior superior margin in the lumbar spine and at the anterior inferior margin at cervical level.

A 'bulging' of the disc is defined as a circumferential or generalised disc displacement involving more than 50% of the disc circumference and is not considered as being a disc herniation (Fig. 55-7). The term 'bulging' is not correlated with pathology or aetiology but only refers to the morphological characteristics. A bulging can be physiologically seen on the level L5–S1 and on mid-cervical level, can reflect advanced degenerative changes, can be a pseudo-image caused by partial volume effect, can be associated with bone remodelling or can occur in ligamentous laxity.[3] There are two types of disc bulging: an asymmetrical type, as frequently seen in scoliosis, or the symmetrical type, with equal displacement of the disc in all directions.

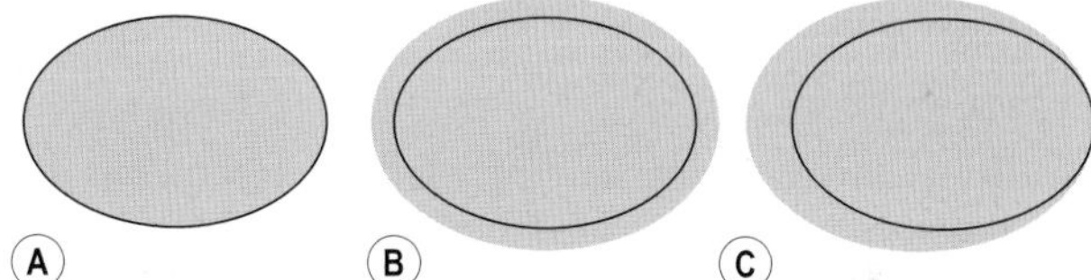

FIGURE 55-7 ■ Bulging disc. Symmetrical and asymmetrical bulging disc on transverse CT or MRI images. Normally the intervertebral disc (grey) does not extend beyond the edges of the ring apophyses (black line) (A). In an asymmetrically bulging disc, the disc tissue extends concentrically beyond the edges of the ring apophyses (50–100% of disc circumference) (B). An asymmetrical bulging disc can be associated with scoliosis. Bulging discs are not considered a form of herniation (C).

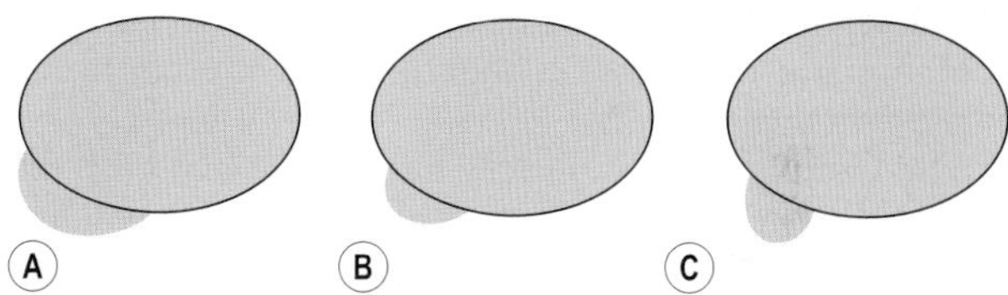

FIGURE 55-8 ■ Disc herniations. Types of disc herniations are seen on transverse CT or MRI images. In protrusions: the base of the herniated disc material is broader than the apex. Protrusions can be broad-based (A) or focal (B). In extrusions (C): the base of the herniation is narrower than the apex (toothpaste sign).

Two types of disc herniations can be differentiated on the basis of the shape of the displaced disc material (Fig. 55-8). A disc herniation is called an 'extruded disc' when

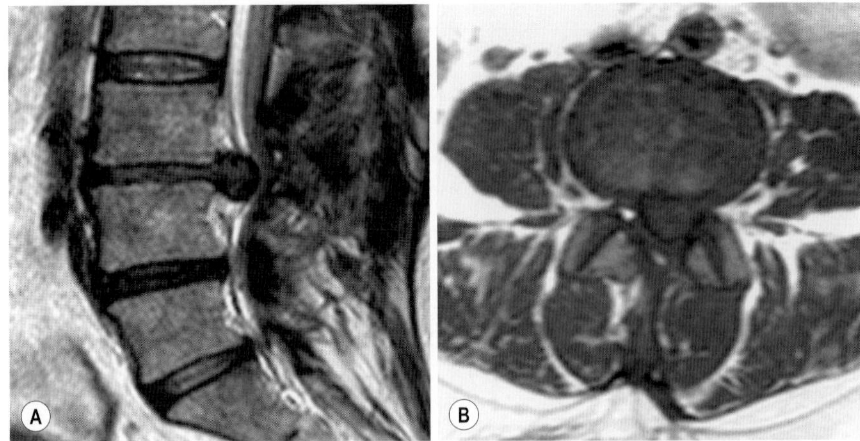

FIGURE 55-9 ■ Massive disc extrusion. Sagittal (A) T2 and axial (B) T1 images. A 45-year-old woman with a massive lumbar disc extrusion at L3–L4 with displacement of the nerve roots and obliteration of the left lateral recess. There is also loss of height of the intervertebral disc L3–L4 and decreased signal intensity of the intervertebral disc at L4–L5, indicating degenerative changes.

the base against the disc is smaller than the diameter of the displaced disc material, measured in the same plane (Fig. 55-9). A 'disc protrusion' is used when the base of the disc is broader than any other diameter of the displaced disc material (Fig. 55-10). A protruded disc can be focal if < 25% of the disc circumference is involved or broad-based when 25–50% of the disc circumference is involved.

When there is no connection between the disc and the displaced disc material, this is called a sequestrated fragment or free fragment and is also described as a disc extrusion (Fig. 55-11). On imaging studies, it is often impossible to determine whether continuity exists. Therefore it is more practical to use the term 'migration', which signifies displacement of disc material away from the site of extrusion regardless of the continuity (Fig. 55-12).

The Combined Task Forces have maintained the distinction between protrusion and extrusion, which is useful because an extrusion is seldom seen in asymptomatic patients.[24] The term 'disc extrusion' is also more acceptable to patients than 'disc herniation'.

A 'contained' herniation refers to the displacement of disc material which is covered by the annulus fibrosus. If this cover is absent, the herniation is 'uncontained'. With discography it is possible to distinguish a contained from an uncontained disc herniation and separate a leaking from a non-leaking disc, depending on the displacement of injected contrast agent. On cross-sectional imaging (CT or MRI) it is often impossible to differentiate contained from uncontained disc extrusions.

Communication with clinicians requires an accurate and simple classification of the disc fragments in the vertical and horizontal direction. The Combined Task Forces have opted for a classification based on anatomic boundaries frequently used by surgeons.[25] In the transverse/axial plane the following zones are used:

- central (posterior midline) (Figs. 55-13 and 55-14)
- paracentral (right/left central) (Fig. 55-15)
- right/left subarticular (lateral recess) (Figs. 55-16 and 55-17)
- right/left foraminal (neural foramen) (Fig. 55-10)
- right/left extraforaminal (outside the neural foramen) (Fig. 55-18)
- anterior zone (anterior and anterolateral).

And in the vertical plane from superiorly to inferiorly:

- pedicle level
- infrapedicle level
- disc level
- suprapedicle level.

Spontaneous Regression of Disc Herniation

Spontaneous regression of a lumbar disc herniation is a common finding, although the underlying mechanism remains unclear. Several hypotheses have been proposed: dehydration or shrinkage of the disc, retraction of the disc in the intervertebral space and resorption due to an inflammatory reaction.[26] Free fragment herniation, herniations with peripheral contrast enhancement on T_1 or high signal intensity on T_2 are predisposing for spontaneous regression[27] (Fig. 55-11). Disc material exposed to the epidural space appears to resolve more quickly than subligamentous disc herniations. While contrast enhancement of the posterior longitudinal ligament indicates an inflammatory response, areas of enhancement in the epidural space below or above the herniated disc indicate venous congestion.[28] Strong contrast enhancement indicates an ongoing absorption process and can be used to evaluate disc reabsorption.

Spontaneous regression of a disc herniation has also been described in the cervical spine and only rarely in the thoracic spine. Median or diffuse soft-tissue herniation in the cervical spine is more likely to regress than focal-type herniations.[29]

Vertebral Endplates and Bone Marrow Changes

With ageing, degenerative changes occur in the vertebral endplates and the vertebral bodies; in 1988 Modic

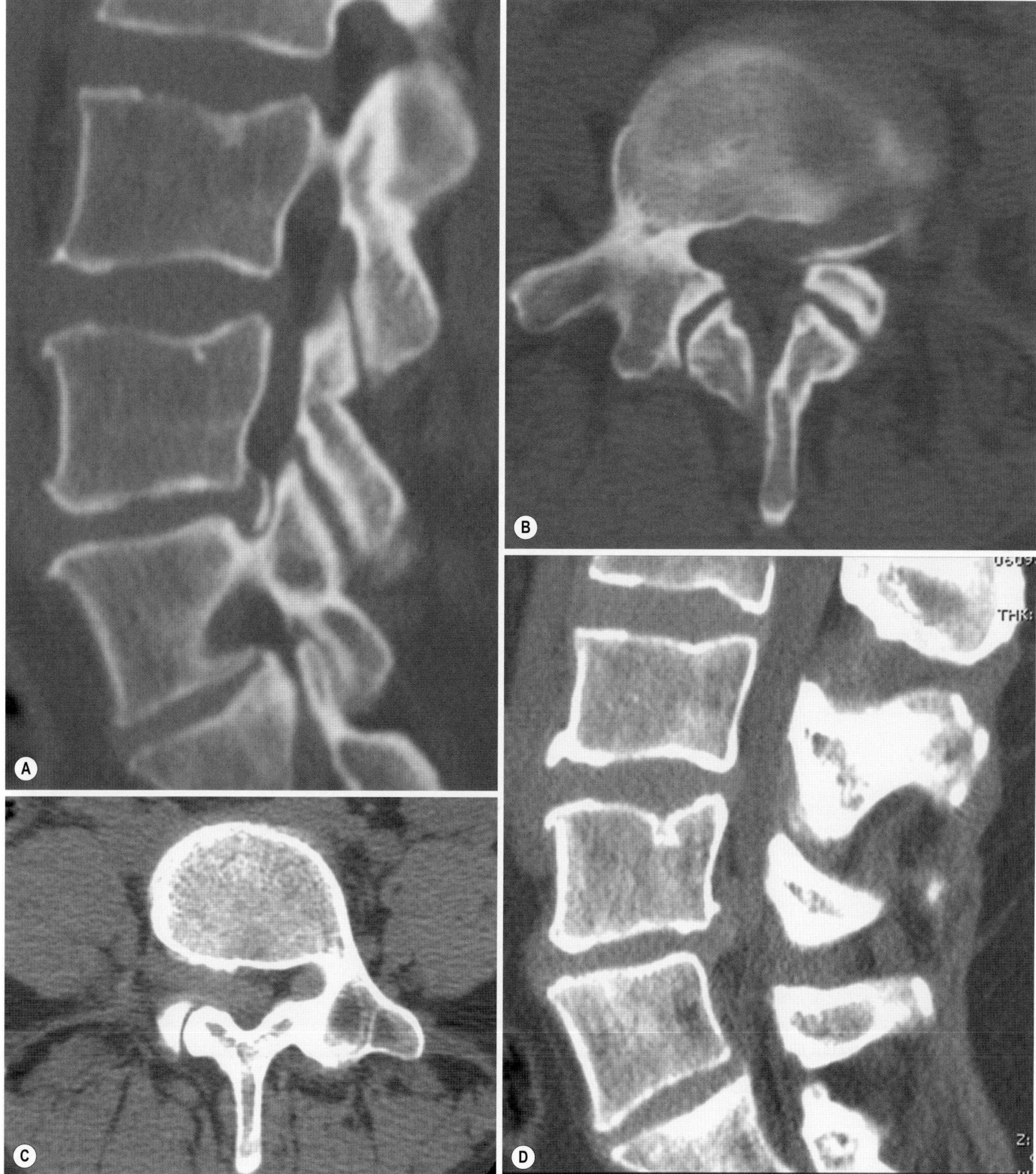

FIGURE 55-10 ■ Foraminal broad-based disc protrusion. Sagittal (A) and axial (B) reformatted CT images in bone window setting; sagittal (C) and axial (D) reformatted CT images in soft-tissue window. (A) and (B) show a broad-based foraminal disc protrusion on the left at L4–L5 with a calcified outer rim. At L5–S1 (C, D) there is a broad-based disc protrusion on the right.

described three degrees of degenerative changes in the endplates and the subchondral bone[30,31] (Table 55-2):

- *Type 1 changes* indicate bone marrow oedema with acute or subacute inflammation. This is seen as a decreased signal intensity on T_1 and increased signal on T_2 (Fig. 55-19).
- *Type 2 changes* indicate replacement of the normal bone by fat and are seen as an increased signal on T_1 and iso- to hyperintense on T_2 (Fig. 55-20). Type 2 changes are the most commonly seen.
- *Type 3 changes* are seldom seen and indicate reactive osteosclerosis, seen as a decreased signal on T_1 and T_2.

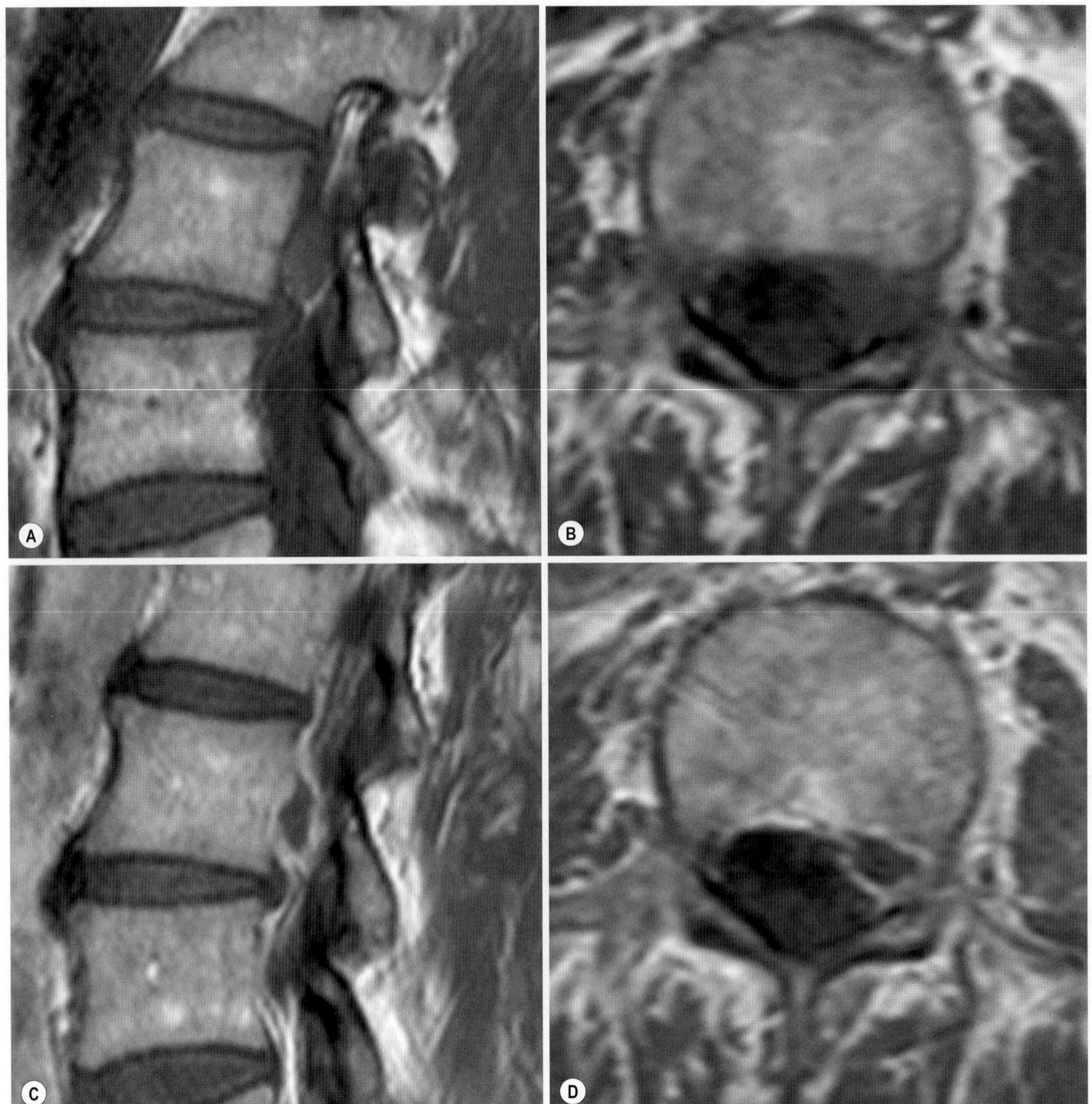

FIGURE 55-11 ■ **Sequestrated disc fragment.** Pre-contrast sagittal (A) and axial (B) T_1 images; post-gadolinium sagittal (C) and axial (D) T_1 images. There is a sequestrated disc fragment posterior to L2. There is a peripheral contrast enhancement on T_1 images post-gadolinium. Peripheral contrast enhancement is associated with a high probability of spontaneous regression.

TABLE 55-2 Signal Intensity Changes in Vertebral Bone Marrow Adjacent to Endplates of Degenerative Discs

Type 1	↓ SI on T_1 ↑ SI on T_2	Inflammatory stage (bone marrow oedema)
Type 2	↑ SI on T_1 ↑ (or ≈) SI on T_2	Fatty stage (local fatty replacement of bone marrow)
Type 3	↓ SI on T_1 ↓ SI on T_2	Reactive osteosclerosis adjacent to the endplates

SI = signal intensity.

Modic changes are commonly seen on MRI in the bone marrow adjacent to the vertebral endplates. Endplate degeneration may affect one or both endplates. If only a part of the endplates is involved, this is most commonly the anterior part.

Modic type 1 changes indicate an acute inflammatory stage; in most cases these changes transform to type 2 changes over a period of 1–2 years, and can be related to a change in patients' symptoms. This evolution is accelerated after osteosynthesis is performed. Modic type 1 changes are often observed in patients with painful lumbar instability.[32] Type 2 and 3 changes are chronic changes and remain unchanged for years.

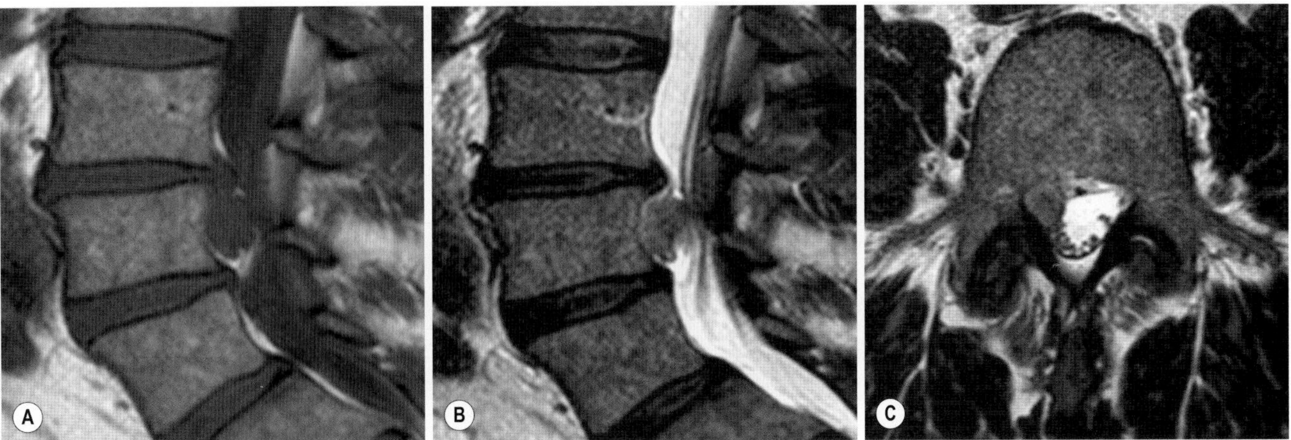

FIGURE 55-12 ■ **Downward migrating disc herniation.** Sagittal T_1 (A), sagittal (B) and axial (C) T_2 images of a 59-year-old man show a large disc fragment descending into the right lateral recess behind the L4 vertebral body. The disc is hypointense on T_2 imaging, indicating a fibrous nature.

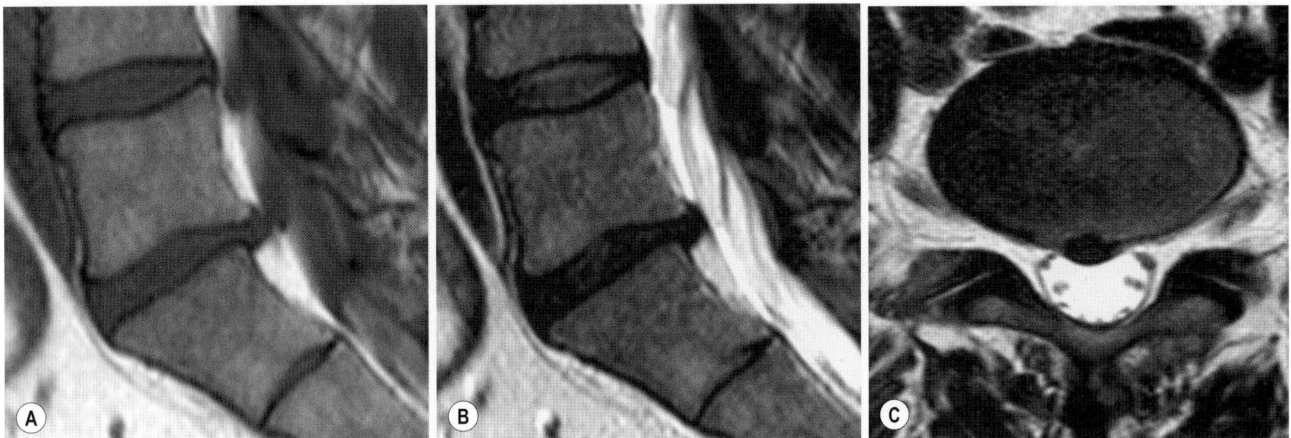

FIGURE 55-13 ■ **Central disc herniation.** Sagittal (A) T_1 image; sagittal (B) and axial (C) T_2 images. Focal central disc herniation at L5–S1 without compression of the nerve roots. The hypointense signal intensity of the disc indicates a fibrous nature.

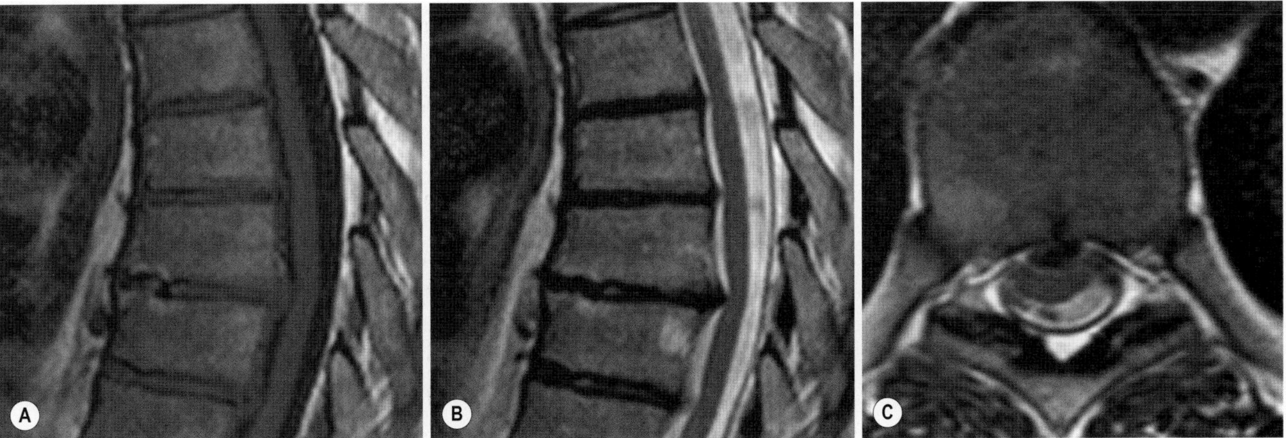

FIGURE 55-14 ■ **Thoracic disc herniation.** Sagittal T_1 (A) image; sagittal (B) and axial (C) T_2 images. Central thoracic disc herniation at the level Th9–Th10. In (C) a small nuclear trail sign is seen.

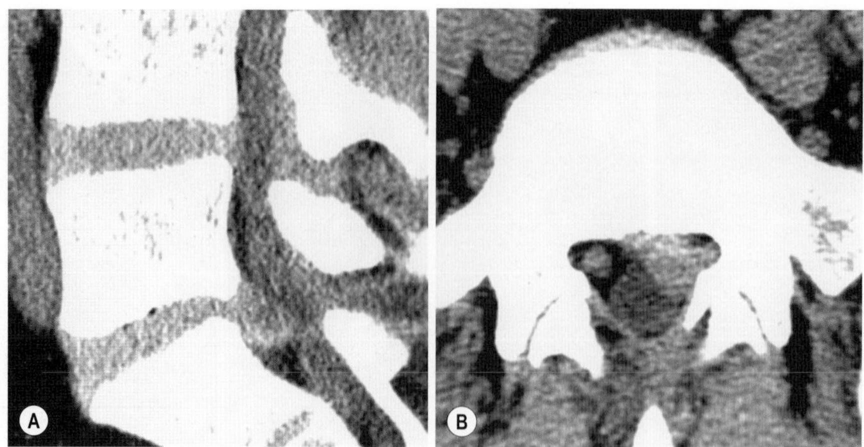

FIGURE 55-15 ■ **Disc extrusion.** Sagittal (A) and axial (B) reformatted CT images show a 42-year-old man with a paracentral disc extrusion on the left side with a descending disc fragment and narrowing of the left lateral recess.

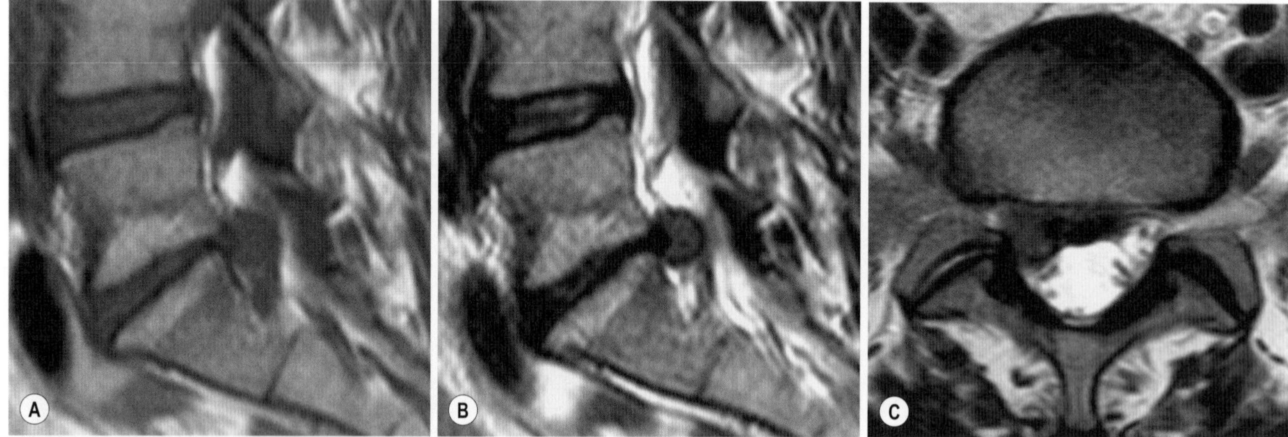

FIGURE 55-16 ■ **Massive lumbar disc extrusion in a 32-year-old woman.** Sagittal T_1 (A) image; sagittal (B) and axial (C) T_2 images. Large subarticular disc extrusion at L5–S1 on the right extending into the right lateral recess. Also note the hyperintense changes in the vertebral endplates at L5–S1 on the T_1 and T_2 images (Modic type 2 changes).

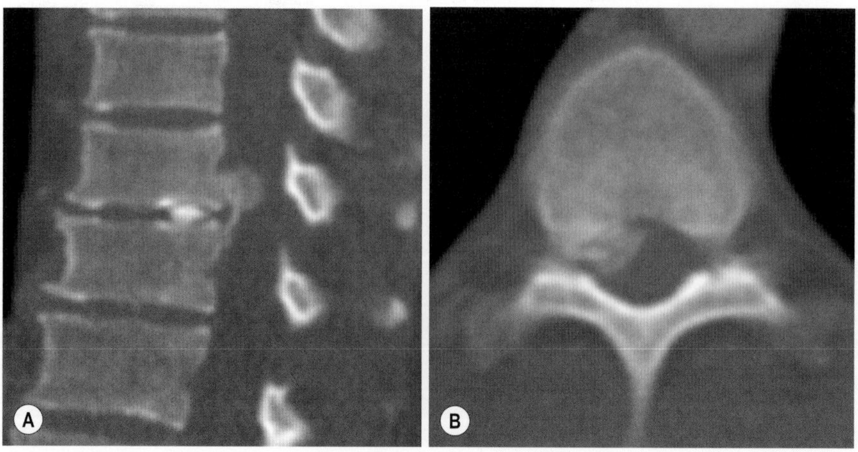

FIGURE 55-17 ■ **Calcified thoracic disc extrusion.** Sagittal (A) and axial (B) reformatted CT images. Calcified ascending disc herniation in the thoracic spine with narrowing of the right lateral recess.

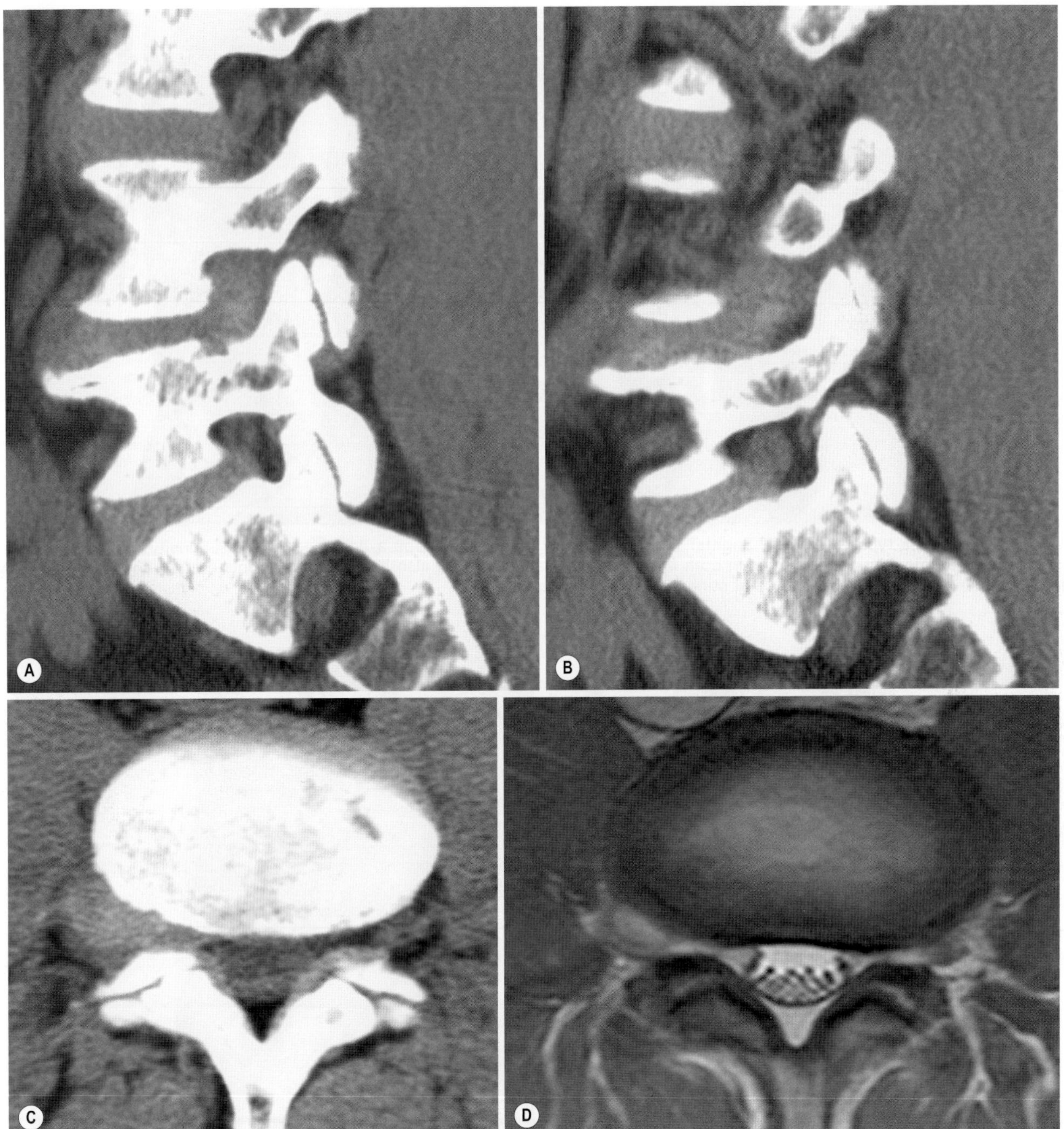

FIGURE 55-18 ■ **Extraforaminal disc herniation.** Sagittal (A, B) and axial (C) reformatted CT images; axial (D) T_2 image. A 52-year-old man with an extraforaminal disc herniation on the right side at level L4–L5 extending into the right neuroforamen causing obliteration of the fat in this neuroforamen.

PATHOLOGY OF THE POSTERIOR ELEMENTS

Facet joint syndrome is defined as a range of symptoms that result in diffuse pain that does not follow a clear nerve root pattern. This is described in the cervical as well as in the lumbar spine. In the past the role of the facet joints as a cause of low-back pain has been underestimated. As the synovial linings and joint capsules of the facet joints are richly innervated, it can be an important source of pain.[33]

As the intervertebral disc and the facet joints work as a three-joint complex, degenerative changes in the disc will change function and anatomy of the posterior elements. On the one hand, facet joint osteoarthritis mostly occurs in the presence of disc degeneration; on the other hand, disc degeneration sometimes occurs without facet joint changes. Therefore, it was suggested that disc degeneration occurs before facet joint

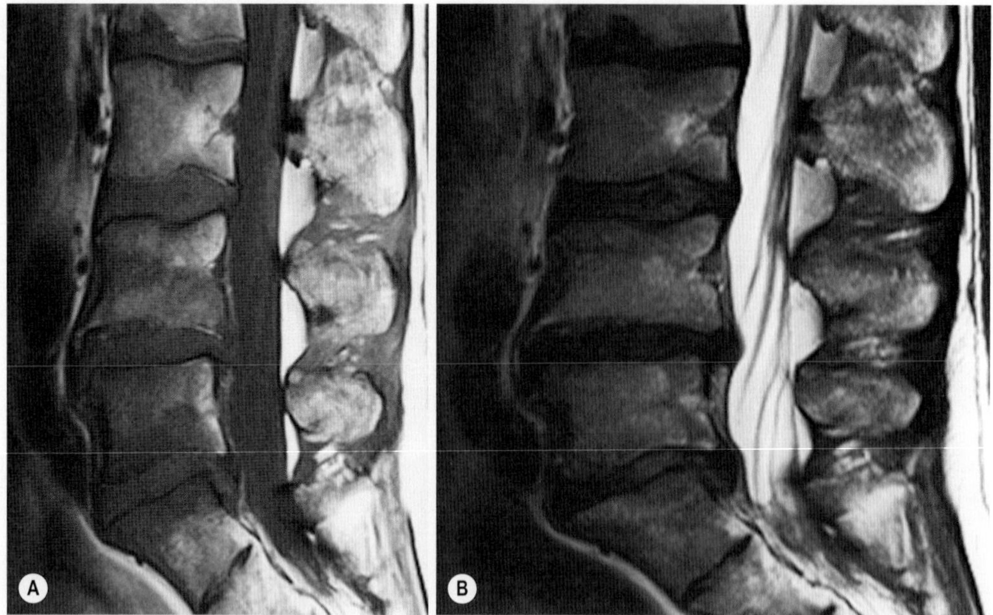

FIGURE 55-19 ■ **Modic type 1 changes.** Sagittal T_1 (A) and T_2 (B) images. There is a decreased signal intensity on T_1 images and increased signal intensity on T_2 images in both endplates at level L5–S1 and also in the upper endplate at L4–L5, indicating bone marrow oedema associated with acute or subacute inflammation.

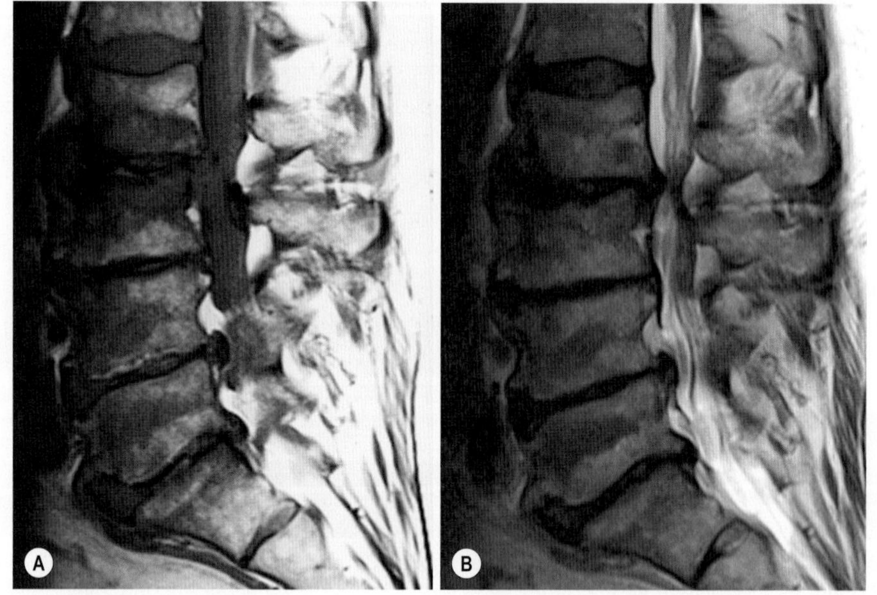

FIGURE 55-20 ■ **Modic type 2 changes.** Sagittal T_1 (A) and T_2 (B) images. There is an increased signal intensity on T_1 and T_2 images at L3–L4, L4–L5 and L5–S1, indicating replacement of normal bone marrow by fat. There are also more acute Modic type I changes at L2–L3.

osteoarthritis, possibly secondary to mechanical changes in the loading of the facet joints.[34] Other factors contributing to facet joint degeneration include weight, lordosis and scoliosis.

A significant association was found between sagittal orientation and osteoarthritis of the lumbar facet joints, even in patients without degenerative spondylolisthesis. Boden et al. observed in a study of asymptomatic patients that more sagittally orientated facet joints at the fourth and fifth lumbar vertebra were associated with herniated discs and spondylolithesis.[35]

Osteoarthritis of the Facet Joints

Degenerative changes of the facet joints are similar to those in peripheral joints and they include osteosclerosis,

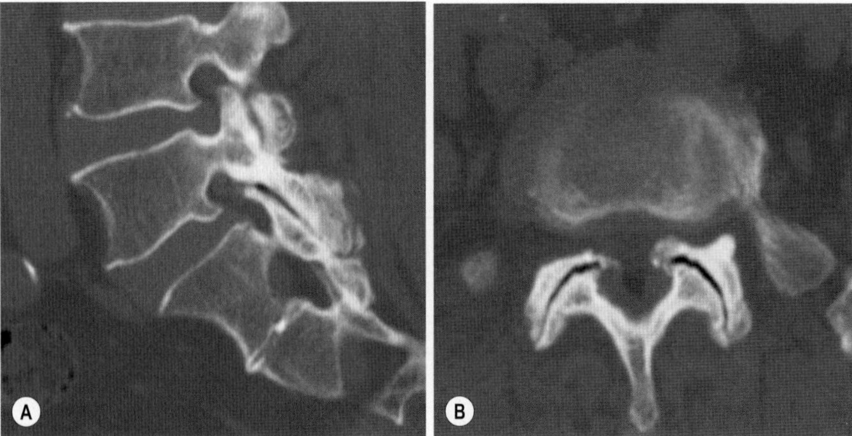

FIGURE 55-21 ■ **Vacuum joint phenomenon in facet joint osteoarthritis.** Sagittal (A) and axial (B) reformatted CT images. Axial CT images show the presence of gas within the L5–S1 facet joints, which may be explained as a result of uneven apposition of the joint surfaces. Associated hypertrophy, juxta-articular calcifications and osteophytes with spinal canal stenosis are present.

thinning of the articular cartilage with erosions and subchondral cyst formation, osteophyte formation, hypertrophy of the articular processes, vacuum joint phenomenon or joint effusion, hypertrophy and/or calcification of the joint capsule and ligamentum flavum.[36] These changes are most commonly found in the lordotic cervical and lumbar segments of the spine.

Hypertrophy is defined as the enlargement of an articular process with normal proportions of its medullary cavity and cortex. This hypertrophy causes distortion of the articular surface, which may cause pain and nerve root compression[36] (Fig. 55-21). Osteophyte formation is an excrescence of bone formation arising from the edges of a joint without a medullary space. Osteophytes protruding ventrally may cause narrowing or stenosis of the lateral canal recesses or the neuroforamina.

Fibrillation and in a later phase fissuring and ulceration of the articular cartilage will develop from the superficial to the deeper layers of the cartilage.[37] In advanced disease the cartilage layers will disappear and subchondral bone sclerosis and cysts will develop. If osteochondral fragments break off the joint surface, these can act as joint mice. Despite the presence of osteophytes and subchondral erosions, the joint space may be preserved. Narrowing of the joint space is frequently observed and may be advanced in patients with facet joint subluxation and erosive osteoarthritis of the facet joint. Widening of the facet joint can be present in severe facet joint degeneration with retrolisthesis due to posterior subluxation.[33]

Weishaupt et al. refined the grading scale of Pathria et al. to grade facet joint osteoarthritis on CT and MRI images[37,38] (Table 55-3, Fig. 55-22).

Standard radiographs including oblique views are a good screening investigation for osteoarthritis of the facet joints although the value is limited.[37,38] The curvature and the double obliquity in the transverse and sagittal plane makes plain film less suited for facet joint imaging as only the portion of the joint parallel to the X-ray beam is visualised. Facet joint narrowing, osteophytes and hyperosthosis may be visualised on standard radiographs as well as spondylolisthesis.

TABLE 55-3 **Criteria for Grading Osteoarthritis of the Facet Joints**

Grade	Criteria
0	Normal facet joint space (2–4 mm width)
1	Narrowing of the facet joint space (< 2 mm) and/or small osteophytes and/or mild hypertrophy of the articular processes
2	Narrowing of the facet joint space and/or moderate osteophytes and/or moderate hypertrophy of the articular processes and/or mild subarticular bone erosions
3	Narrowing of the facet joint space and/or large osteophytes and/or severe hypertrophy of the articular processes and/or severe subarticular bone erosions and/or subchondral cysts

Both CT and MR imaging have a higher contrast and spatial resolution and are better for evaluating more subtle changes as subchondral erosions and cartilage changes. In general there is a moderate to good agreement between CT and MRI findings. It was, however, demonstrated by Weishaupt et al. that CT is superior to MRI in detecting joint space narrowing and subchondral sclerosis.[37]

Associated Soft-Tissue Changes

Soft-tissue changes associated with facet joint degeneration include degenerative cysts (juxtafacet cysts), ligamentum flavum cysts and hypertrophy and/or calcification of the ligamentum flavum.

Degenerative Cysts Arising from the Facet Joints

Degenerative cysts arising from the facet joints are grouped with the ganglion cysts as juxtafacet or juxta-articular cysts. Ganglion cysts have no connection to the joint and have no synovial lining. These synovial cysts are found periarticular and are attached to the joint by a

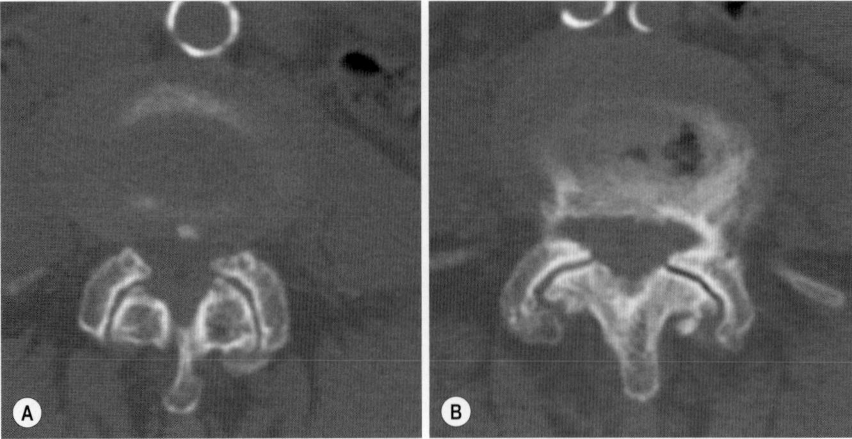

FIGURE 55-22 ■ **Grading facet joint osteoarthritis.** Axial reformatted CT images at L3–L4 (A) and L4–L5 (B). Grade 1 osteoarthritis of the right facet joint L3–L4 (mild hypertrophy) and grade 2 osteoarthritis of the left facet joint (narrowing of the joint space, moderate hypertrophy and osteophytes, subarticular erosion) (A). Grade 3 osteoarthritis of the right facet joint L4–L5 with joint space narrowing, hypertrophy of the articular processes, large osteophytes and subarticular bone erosions can be seen (B).

membrane. The walls are made of loose myxoid connective or fibrocollagenous tissue with a synovial lining and they are filled with yellow or clear mucinous fluid. The consistency of the fluid may vary as haemorrhage and inflammation can be seen.[39]

Juxtafacet cysts are most commonly seen in the lumbar spine and especially at the level L4–L5, which has the most motion in the spine. In the cervical and thoracic spine only a few cases are described. Those in the cervical spine are in half of the cases arising from the cruciate ligament of the atlas.[39] Juxtafacet cysts are increasingly being reported, probably due to the increasing number of MRI examinations performed.[40] Synovial cysts of the facet joints are related to osteoarthritis of the facet joint (Fig. 55-23). The pathogenesis is probably increased motion in the degenerative facet joints. This instability can cause herniation of the synovium through tears in the facet joint capsule.[40] An association between juxtafacet cyst and trauma, chondrocalcinosis, spondylolysis and Baastrup's disease has been reported.

Most juxtafacet cysts arise from the posterior aspect of the facet joint and are situated outside the vertebral canal; anterior cysts into the vertebral canal are four times less frequent.[41]

In the lumbar spine degenerative cysts of the facet joint may cause pain and radicular symptoms by compression of the thecal sac and/or compression of the nerve roots in the lateral recesses. An inflammatory reaction around the juxtafacet cysts may cause sciatica.[40] Depending on the size and location of the cyst, spinal stenosis and/or neurogenic claudication may occur. In the cervical spine facet joint cysts rarely cause radiculopathy.[39]

The natural history of these cysts varies; in a rare case, spontaneous resolution is observed. Haemorrhage is a known complication and causes rapid enlargement, with severe symptoms occurring within months.

In cases of radiculopathy and myelopathy caused by a facet joint cyst, surgery is indicated. Surgical removal is an effective and safe option for treatement. If there is no association with a spinal canal stenosis, a simple excision of the cyst can be performed. In case of associated spondylotic spinal canal stenosis, a removal of the cyst with decompression and laminectomy may be indicated.[39] An alternative and less invasive technique is the percutaneous injection of local anaesthetics and long-acting steroids.

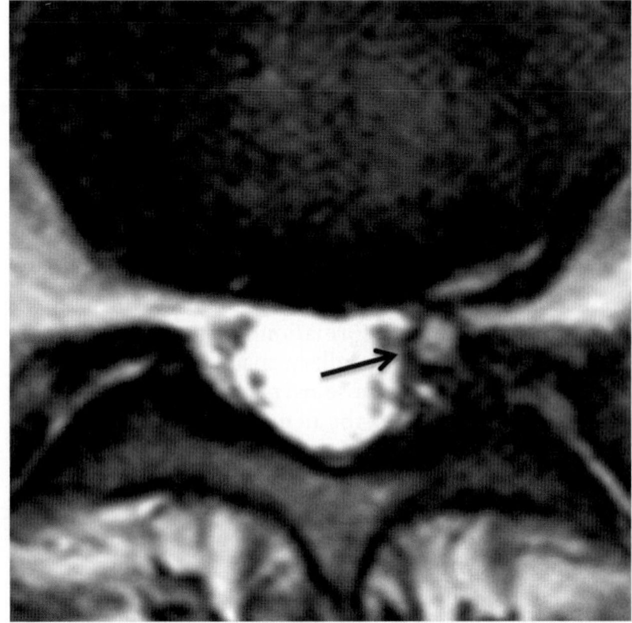

FIGURE 55-23 ■ **Juxtafacet (ganglion) cyst.** Axial T_2 image shows a small cystic lesion (arrow) arising from the anteromedial aspect of the left facet joint L5–S1.

The typical presentation of a synovial cyst is a rounded mass adjacent to the facet joint with low attenuation. This cyst may show egg-shell calcification of the wall and gas inside.[39]

MRI has a high sensitivity and is the imaging technique of choice.[42] Intraspinal synovial cysts are sharply marginated epidural masses near the facet joint. Typical synovial cysts have a hypointense peripheral rim,

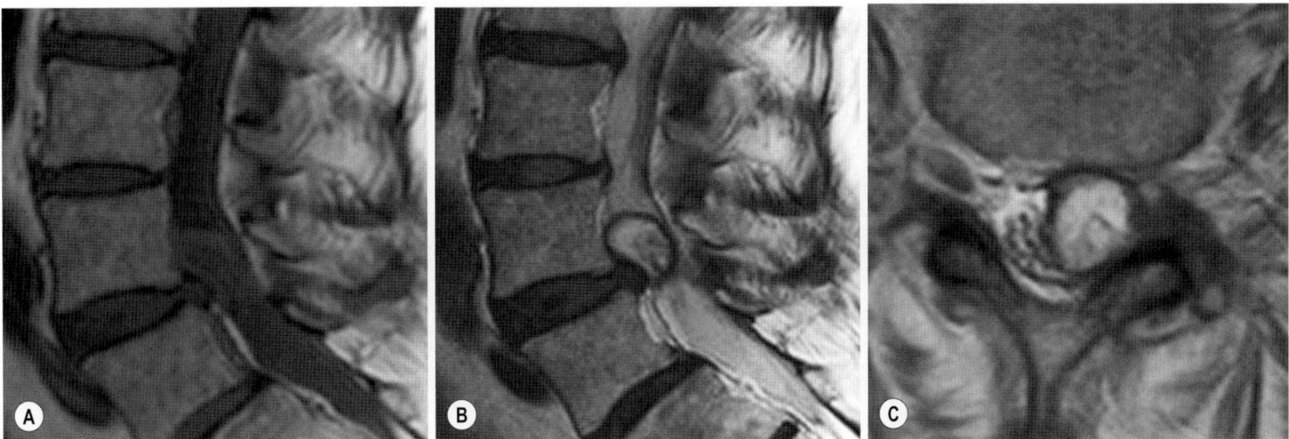

FIGURE 55-24 ■ **Juxtafacet (ganglion) cyst.** Sagittal T_1 (A) image; sagittal (B) and axial (C) T2 images. A large cystic lesion arising from the anteromedial aspect of the left facet joint. The content from the cyst appears mildly hyperintense on T_2 image (B) and is of intermediate signal intensity on T_1 image (A). A low signal intensity rim is observed on the T_2 images (B, C). The cyst causes compression of the thecal sac and obliteration of the left lateral recess is seen.

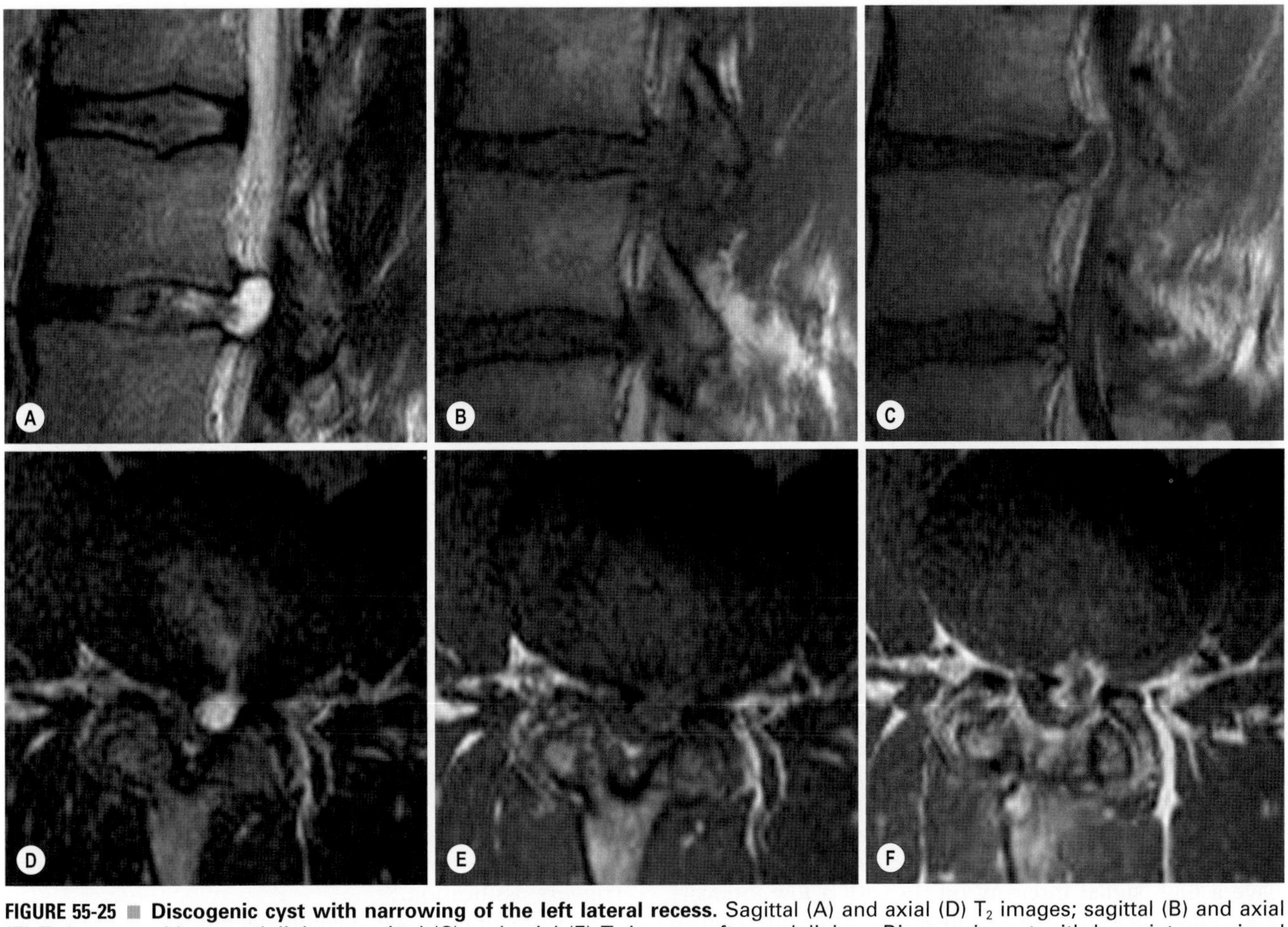

FIGURE 55-25 ■ **Discogenic cyst with narrowing of the left lateral recess.** Sagittal (A) and axial (D) T_2 images; sagittal (B) and axial (E) T_1 images without gadolinium; sagittal (C) and axial (F) T_1 images after gadolinium. Discogenic cyst with hyperintense signal intensity on T_2 images originating from the intervertebral disc L4–L5. This lesion has an intermediate signal intensity on T_1 images and rim enhancement after gadolinium injection. Secondary there is a narrowing of the left lateral recess. Differential diagnosis should be made with a synovial cyst from the facet joints on the basis of its position.

especially on sequences with long TR/TE (Fig. 55-24). This rim enhances after the administration of gadolinium.[43] The signal intensity of a synovial cyst is nearly equal to cerebrospinal fluid on T_1 and on T_2. High signal intensity on T_1 and T_2 indicates subacute blood degradation products.

The differential diagnosis of a mass with this type of signal characteristics in the posterior or lateral spinal canal is broad: juxtafacet cysts, discogenic cysts, cysts of the ligamentum flavum, sequestered disc fragments, infectious cysts or arachnoid cysts and neoplasms (cystic degenerated schwannoma or neurofibroma)[40] (Fig. 55-25).

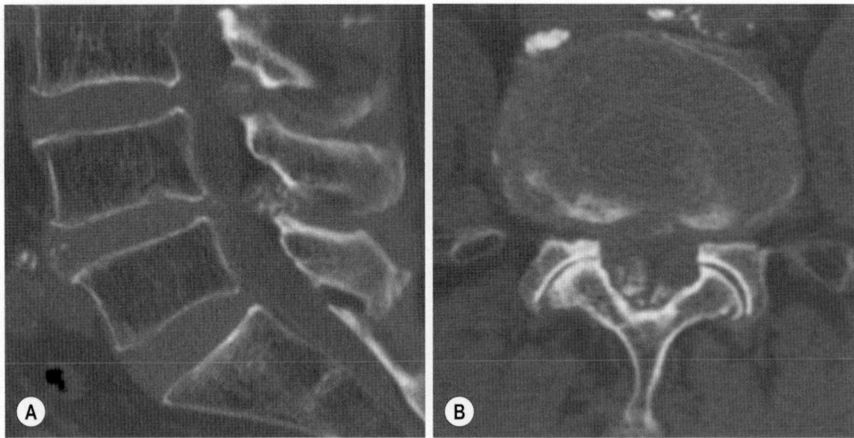

FIGURE 55-26 ■ **Ligamentum flavum hypertrophy and calcification.** Sagittal (A) and axial (B) reformatted CT images. Calcification and hypertrophy of the ligamentum flavum at L4–L5 and in a lesser extend at L3–L4, resulting in a spinal canal stenosis at L4–L5. Calcifications of the ligamentum flavum are also seen in patients with pseudogout. Pseudogout is a crystal-induced arthropathy, which is a debilitating illness in which pain and joint inflammation are caused by the formation of calcium pyrophosphate (CPP) crystals within the joint space. It is sometimes referred to as calcium pyrophosphate disease (CPPD).

Degenerative facet joints are, however, the clue to the most likely diagnosis.

Facet joint arthrography and CT arthrography can be performed if there is any doubt about communication with the adjacent facet joint.

Cysts of the Ligamentum Flavum

Cysts of the ligamentum flavum arise from or are partially embedded in the ligamentum flavum, rather than being close to the facet joints.[40] They are seldom seen and their development may be related to necrosis or myxoid degeneration in a hypertrophied ligamentum flavum.[44] Chronic degenerative changes followed by repeated haemorrhage will form small degenerative cysts; in a later stage these cysts will form one large cyst.[44]

Cyst of the ligamentum flavum are typically located at the level L4–L5, just like juxtafacet cysts. Cysts of the ligamentum flavum have the same imaging characteristics as facet joint cysts. A differentiation may be important, as a simple laminectomy is sufficient for treatment of the ligamentum flavum cysts. On imaging, an extradural, intraspinal mass in close relationship with the ligamentum flavum is seen. On CT imaging, this cyst has a low density compared to the ligamentum flavum. Unlike juxtafacet cysts, no rim calcification has been described.[45] On MR imaging, cysts of the ligamentum flavum are sharply delineated rounded to ovoid cystic masses. They have a high signal intensity on T_2 with a low intensity rim. This rim shows an enhancement after injection of gadolinium.[46]

Ligamentum Flavum Hypertrophy

Symmetrical thickening of the ligamentum flavum is often seen in facet joint arthropathy. It results from facet joint effusion, ligamentous fibrosis, calcification and/or ossification.[47] Degenerative changes are associated with calcifications in the posterior capsule and the ligamentum flavum and the incidence increases with age.[48]

Calcifications of the ligamentum flavum at the insertions are considered normal variants related to traction; calcifications at the periarticular level are thought to be degenerative.[48] Calcifications of the ligament flavum are often seen in patients with diffuse idiopathic skeletal hyperostosis (DISH) and ankylosing spondylitis (Fig. 55-26). They are also observed in patients with metabolic diseases as hypercalcaemia, renal failure, hyperparathyroidism, pseudogout and haemochromatosis.

Calcification of the ligamentum flavum, and especially the posterior longitudinal ligament, is a known cause for radiculopathy and compressive myelopathy in the cervical and thoracic spine (Fig. 55-27). Calcification and/or ossification of the thoracic ligamentum flavum is a rare disease mainly described in the Asian/Japanese literature, and is also known as Japanese disease. Japanese disease mostly affects males younger than 50 years of age. It may cause spinal stenosis with/without myelopathy and/or radiculopathy; the clinical picture consists of progressive myelopathy, resulting in spastic paraparesis.[49] The lower third of the thoracic spine is the most commonly involved, and the cervical spine is only rarely affected. Histopathology of ossification of the ligamentum flavum typically shows mature bone. The ligamentum flavum is progressively replaced by lamellar bone through endochondral ossification. The process starts at the junction between the ligamentum flavum and the joint capsule where a proliferation of cartilaginous tissue triggers ossification.[49]

CT imaging is the imaging technique of choice for evaluating the ossifications. The pathognomonic signs are intense radio-dense lines highlighting the laminae. In most cases these changes are bilaterally present. They usually develop from the medial aspect of the pedicle near the insertion of the ligamentum flavum and progress towards the midline, creating a V-shaped ossification with the anterior concavity situated in the epidural space.[49] Sagittal reconstructions are useful for distinguishing the ossification of the ligamentum flavum from calcifications, which is the only differential diagnosis.

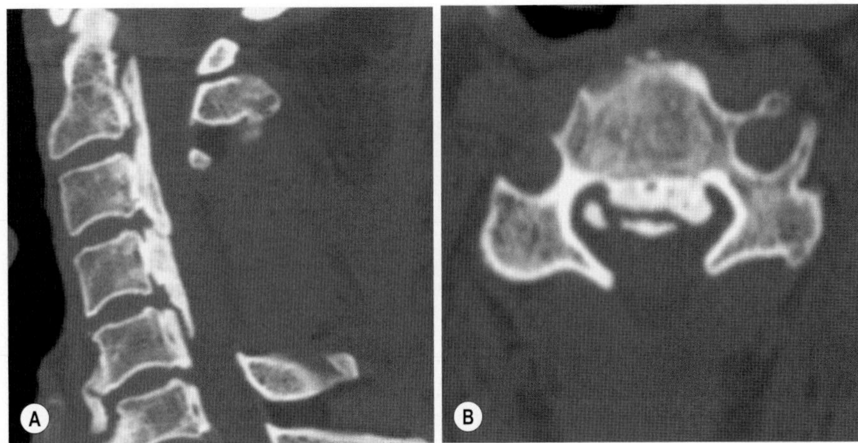

FIGURE 55-27 ■ **Calcification of posterior longitudinal ligament.** Sagittal (A) and axial (B) reformatted CT images show a postoperative condition after posterior laminectomy for a spinal canal stenosis caused by calcifications of the posterior longitudinal ligament from C2 to C5, also known as Japanese disease.

MRI has the advantage of showing changes in the spinal cord as compression of the myelum and myelopathy.

Ossification of the posterior longitudinal ligament is more frequently seen in the cervical spine and less in the thoracic and lumbar spine. Also, thoracic disc herniations may be present in these patients; they also tend to calcify and ossify.[50]

In patients with calcium pyrophosphate dihydrate (CPPD) deposition disease, also known as pseudogout, spinal involvement with calcifications of the ligamentum flavum is rarely seen but may lead to spinal stenosis and spinal cord compression. The lumbar and cervical spine are the most commonly involved. CPPD depositions can also be related to hyperparathyroidism and haemochromatosis.

Degenerative Changes of the Neural Arch

Neural Arch Intervertebral Neoarthrosis

Excessive lumbar lordosis is associated with spine degeneration. Approximation of the adjacent vertebral neural arches may result in abnormal bone contact, resulting in neoarthrosis.[47] Associated remodelling or bony sclerosis of the laminae and pedicles may occur.

Spinous Process Abnormalities and Associated Ligamentous Changes

Baastrup's disease, also known as kissing spine, has been described as a cause of low-back pain (Fig. 55-28). These patients may experience pain caused by irritation of the periosteum or adventitial bursae between abutting spinous processes. It has been described as close approximation and contact of the adjacent spinous processes with enlargement, flattening and reactive sclerosis of the opposing interspinous surfaces.[51] Interspinous bursitis may communicate with the facet joints and can be treated with injection of steroids.

Extension of the synovial cavity to the intraspinal space can result in cyst formation. The cyst can enter the epidural space through the midline cleft of the ligamentum flavum to cause extradural compression.[51] Fatty replacement of the paraspinal musculature is often seen in patients with Baastrup's disease.

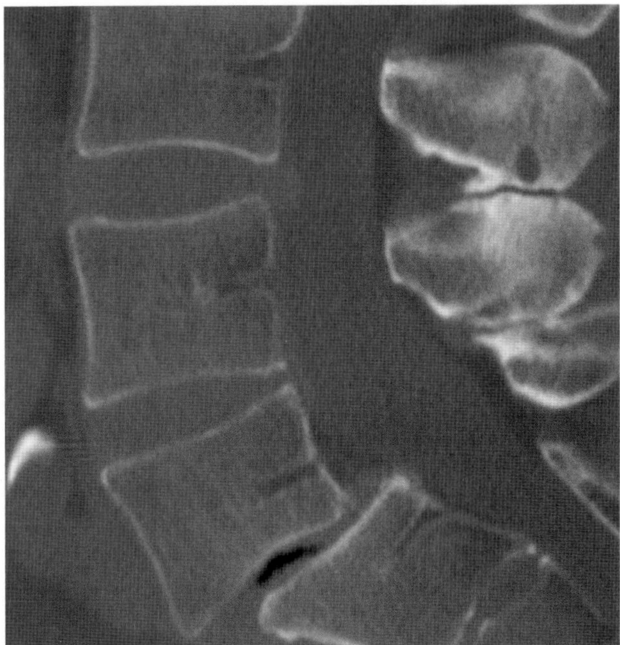

FIGURE 55-28 ■ **Baastrup's phenomenon.** Sagittal reformatted CT image in the midsagittal plane. Grade 2 degenerative spondylolisthesis at the L5–S1 level; malalignment of the spinous processes with anterior slip of the L4 spinous process relative to L5 indicates a type 3 degenerative spondylolisthesis and allows differentiation from isthmic spondylolisthesis. There is collision of the spinous process of adjacent vertebra with progressive interspinous degenerative changes (Baastrup's phenomenon).

Degenerative Spondylolisthesis

A spondylolisthesis, also known as an anterolisthesis, is an anterior displacement of a vertebral body relative to the vertebra below. The reverse, when the vertebral body

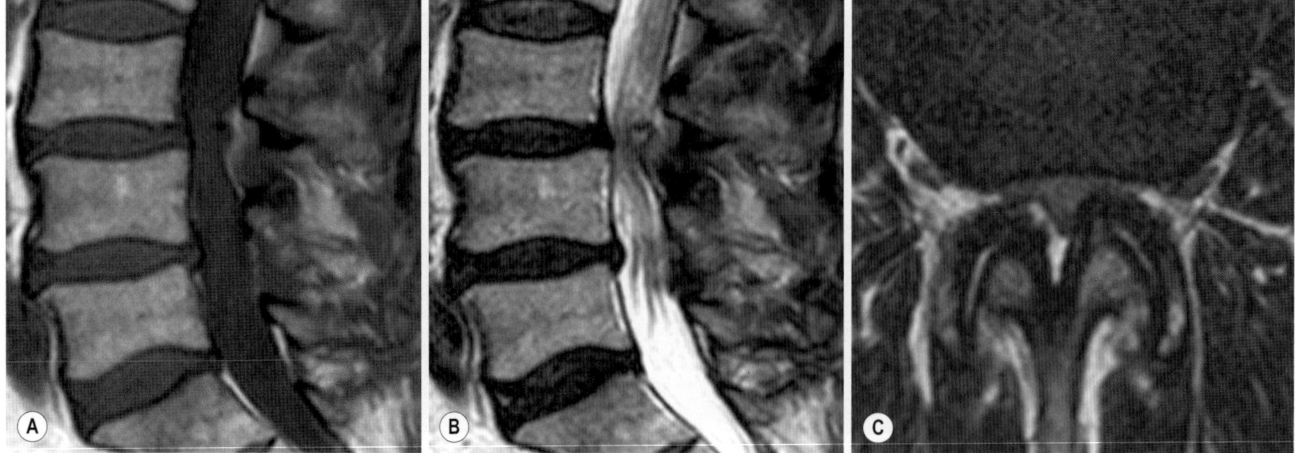

FIGURE 55-29 ■ Spinal canal stenosis L3–L4 with synovial facet joint cyst. Sagittal T_1 (A) and sagittal (B) and axial (C) T_2 images. The axial T_2 image shows an hypertrophic facet joint at L3–L4 with a small synovial cyst at the anteromedial aspect of the left facet joint, resulting in a spinal canal stenosis. Also note the discrete anterolisthesis at L3–L4 caused by facet joint osteoarthritis.

below is displaced anteriorly relative to the superior vertebra, is called a retrolisthesis. Six types of spondylolisthesis can be differentiated: congenital dysplasia of the articular processes, defect of the pars articularis, degenerative changes of the facet joint, fracture of the neural arch, weakening of the neural arch due to bone disorders and excessive removal of bone after spinal decompression. Only the degenerative type will be discussed in this chapter.

The most popular grading method is the Meyerding grading system, which divides the anteroposterior diameter of the superior surface of the lower vertebra into quarters, and grades 1 to 4 are assigned to slips of quarters of the superior vertebral body.

Degenerative spondylolisthesis is the most common cause of lumbar spondylolisthesis above the age of 50. This type of spondylolisthesis is caused by degenerative changes of the facet joints. The grade of slippage is usually limited. A more sagittal orientation of the facet joints is typically observed in these patients.[35] As the neural arch is intact, even small progression in the slip may cause cauda equina syndrome. As facet joint osteoarthrosis is most commonly seen at the level L4–L5, spondylolisthesis is also most common at this level. The incidence increases four times if there is a sacralised L5. Women are four times more affected than men.

Clinical symptoms include low-back pain and leg pain as a result of disc and facet joint degeneration, lateral recess and foraminal stenosis leading to nerve root compression. With progression of the spondylolisthesis the symptoms may change from low-back pain to neurogenic claudication due to central canal stenosis.

On imaging, a lateral plain radiograph shows anterolisthesis with degenerative changes at the facet joint and disc space narrowing. Differentiation with isthmic spondylolisthesis can be made by the malalignment of the spinous processes with anterior slip of the spinous process relative to the one of the vertebral body below[52] (Fig. 55-28).

CT and MRI will show osteoarthritis of the facet joints and associated spondylolisthesis. The sagittal orientation of the facet joints, as well as disc degeneration and/or disc bulging, can be evaluated. Sagittal images may demonstrate narrowing of the intervertebral foramina, the lateral recess and/or the central canal with associated compression of the cauda equine and exiting nerve roots. Anterior slip of the inferior articular process will narrow the inferior aspect of the lateral recess and the intervertebral foramen.[52] Associated thickening of the ligamentum flavum may add to the central canal and lateral recess stenosis.

On MRI, bone marrow changes in the pedicle are a non-specific finding of spondylolisthesis and they are often observed in patients with facet joint osteoarthritis. These bone marrow changes are believed to be a response to abnormal stresses related to abnormal motion and loading caused by degenerative changes in the spinal segment.[53]

DEGENERATIVE SPINAL STENOSIS

Degenerative Spinal Canal Stenosis

A stenosis of the spinal canal is a reduction of the diameters of the spinal canal. The normal size of the spinal canal varies according to the location. Spinal canal stenosis may lead to neurological disorders associated with compression of the nervous structures inside the spinal canal (spinal cord, conus medullaris, cauda equina, nerve roots and meninges).

Acquired spinal canal stenosis is the most common type of spinal stenosis at the cervical and lumbar level, and is less frequent in the thoracic spine (Figs. 55-29 and 55-30).

Degenerative changes of the vertebral bodies and facet joints can be associated with degenerative changes of the ligamentous system (calcification and thickening) and herniated discs.

Posterior and central marginal osteophytes can reduce the spinal canal diameter centrally with possible cord compression. In case of multilevel disease the dural sac can get a 'string of pearls'-like appearance on

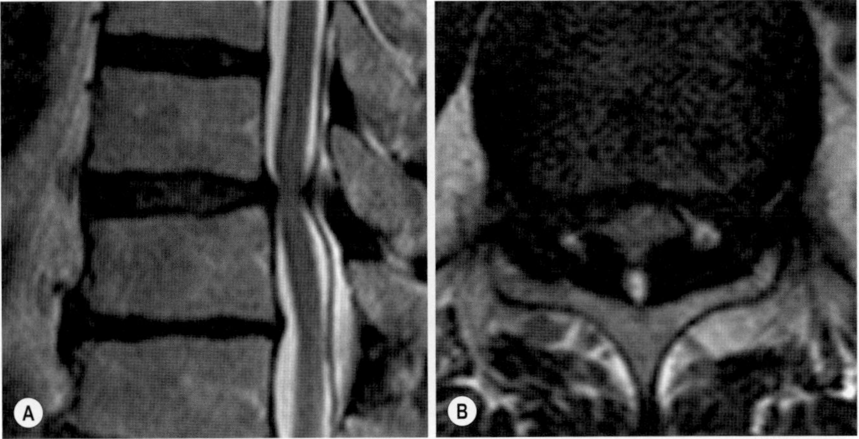

FIGURE 55-30 ■ **Thoracic spinal canal stenosis.** Sagittal (A) and axial (B) T_2 images. There is a lateral stenosis of the spinal canal at a low thoracic level due to hypertrophy of the ligamenta flava (B) and a broad-based disc protrusion.

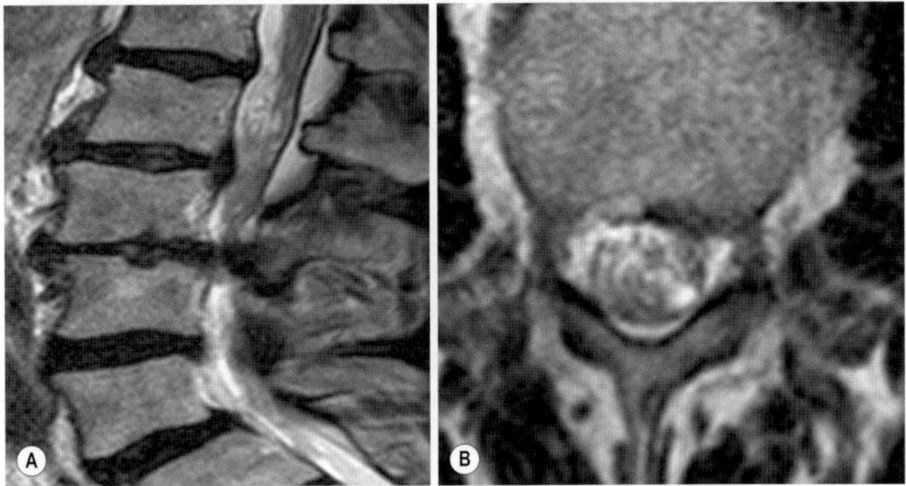

FIGURE 55-31 ■ **Spinal canal stenosis with redundant nerve roots.** Sagittal (A) and axial (B) T2-weighted images. A case of a spinal canal stenosis at L3–L4 as a result of anterolisthesis caused by facet joint osteoarthritis. As seen on the sagittal image (A), it is a case of a concentric spinal canal stenosis with hypertrophy of the ligamenta flava and disc bulging. Proximal of the stenosis there are redundant nerve roots of the cauda equina, as seen on the sagittal (A) and axial images (B).

myelography. A bony protrusion at facet level may cause lateral radicular compression by radicular entrapment in the lateral recess. This phenomenon is more commonly seen at the lumbar level. Disc herniation can also be associated with narrowing of the lateral recess.[54] The compressed nerve root may appear oedematous due to venous congestion and alterations in the blood–nerve barrier.

Posterior and central marginal osteophytosis can lead to the development of a cauda equina syndrome. Compression of the dural sac leads to a reduced space for the nerve roots of the cauda equina. The pressure of the subarachnoidal fluid increases, causing an alteration in the venous drainage, which causes perineural venous congestion and ischaemic damage. Because of its vascular anatomy, the nerve roots of the cauda equina have a higher ischaemic risk if compression is at more than one level. The nerve roots L4, L5 and S1 are predominantly affected. On contrast-enhanced MRI the roots may show enhancement caused by breakdown of the blood–nerve barrier, inflammatory reaction and venous congestion. With high-grade stenosis in the lumbar spine, the nerve roots proximal to the spinal canal stenosis can be elongated, large and tortuous; this phenomenon is called 'redundant nerve roots' (Figs. 55-31 and 55-32).

Osteoarthritis of the facet joints may cause stenosis of the central spinal canal and the lateral or foraminal recesses. This is most commonly seen at the lumbar level. As described earlier in this chapter, hypertrophy and calcification of the posterior ligaments may also cause stenosis of the spinal canal (Fig. 55-33).

Clinical symptoms of a spinal canal stenosis vary with the level of the spinal stenosis. Patients often remain asymptomatic until an acute event happens. The clinical course of the disease can be influenced by age, sex, socioeconomic situation, site and degree of stenosis.[55] Acute or chronic limb pain and paraesthesias are seen in patients with lateral or foraminal radicular compression. Sensory and motor deficits associated with lower limb pain during walking and in upright position are pathognomonic of lumbar canal stenosis. Forward bending and supine position may relieve the symptoms due to an increase size of

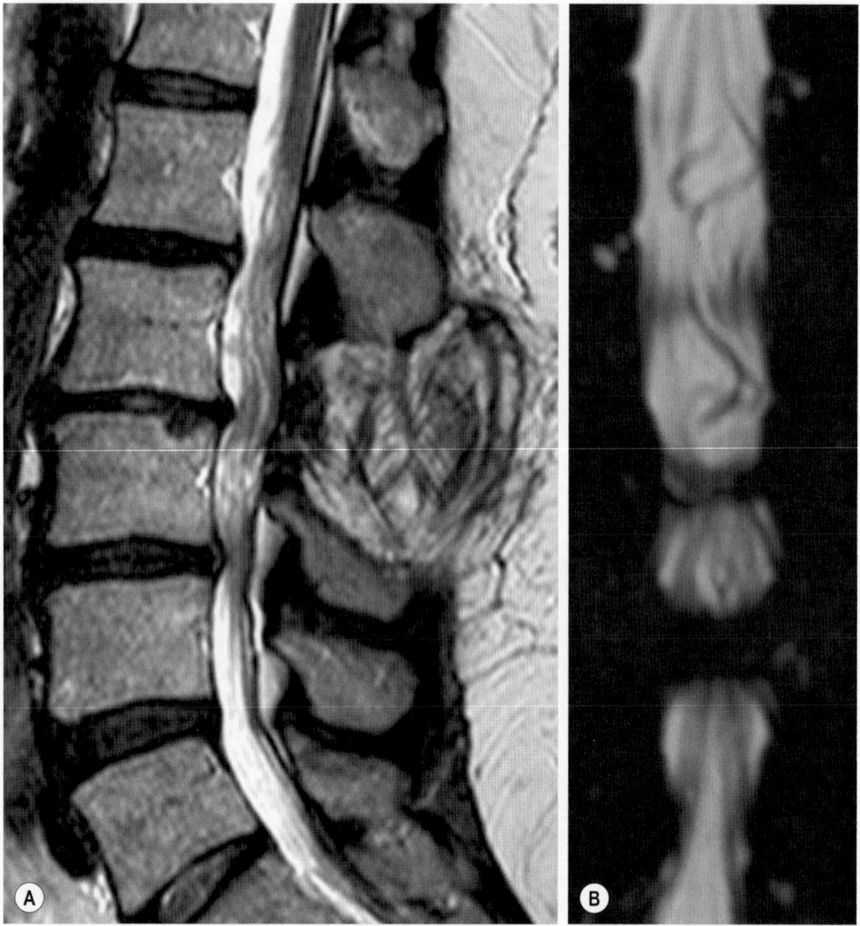

FIGURE 55-32 ■ **Redundant nerve roots.** T_2 (A) and MR myelography (B) images. Postoperative status after laminectomy at L2–L3 for a spinal canal stenosis. Sagittal T_2 image and the MR myelography shows residual redundant nerve roots of the cauda equina proximal to the previous spinal canal stenosis.

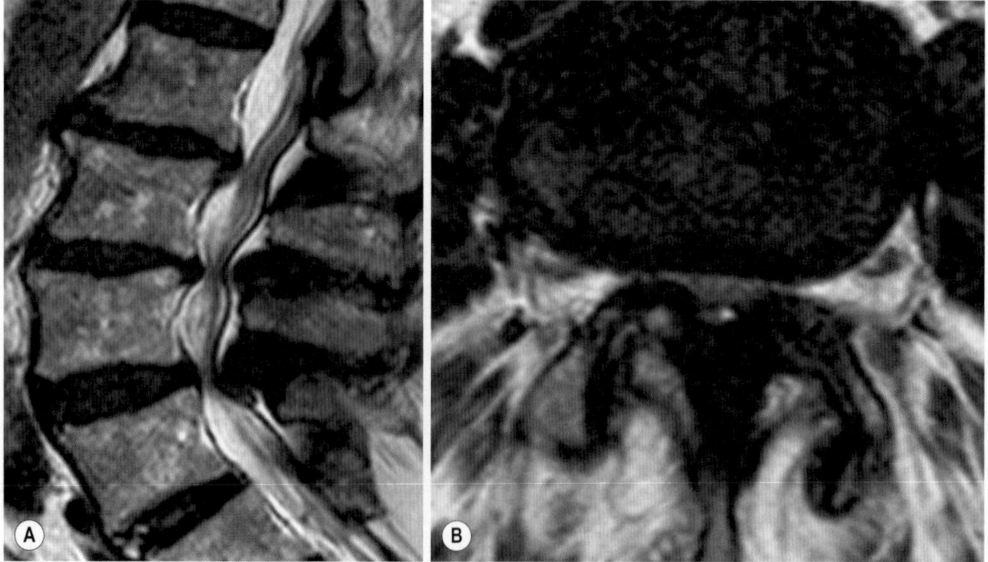

FIGURE 55-33 ■ **Lumbar spinal canal stenosis.** Sagittal (A) and axial at L3–L4 (B) T_2 images. Concentric spinal canal stenosis of the lumbar spine at multiple levels (L3–L4 and L4–L5) caused by hypertrophy of the ligamenta flava, concentric disc bulging and hypertrophic facet joint osteoarthritis.

the spinal canal. Vascular claudication and degenerative changes of knee and hip should be included in the differential diagnosis and need to be ruled out. In patients with lumbar spinal stenosis, a neurogenic bladder caused by mechanic compression of the S2–S4 roots can be present due to their location in the posteromedian area of the spinal canal.

Both CT and MRI imaging are non-invasive techniques which make it possible to evaluate the spinal canal. CT is more useful in evaluation of the bony structures. MR examinations used to be limited to the supine position, which cannot always give a clear answer to some clinical conditions. More recently, standing MR equipment has allowed imaging in a weight-bearing environment.

In the past plain radiographs with myelography have been used to evaluate the spinal canal. At this moment this can still be useful to allow dynamic imaging of the spine.

On imaging, the space available for the cord can be determined to evaluate spinal canal stenosis. At the cervical levels C4–C7 the average anteroposterior diameter is 17 mm and values below 14 mm are considered critical. At the cervical level the diameter of the spinal cord is on average 6.9 mm. It can be useful to assess the perimedullar cerebrospinal fluid (CSF) space compared to the sagittal diameter of the spinal cord. If no perimedullar CSF is present, there is a stenosis.

At the lumbar level a classification of spinal stenosis was suggested by Benoist: severe stenosis (< 10 mm), moderate stenosis (10–12 mm) and mild stenosis (12–14 mm).[55] In MRI imaging a severe stenosis is associated with the absence of epidural fat.

Degenerative Foraminal Stenosis

Facet joint osteoarthritis is an important cause of acquired lumbar spinal stenosis. It can cause a stenosis central, lateral and foraminal. In this section we will focus on the foraminal stenosis; degenerative spinal canal stenosis was discussed in the previous section.

The normal intervertebral foramen has a teardrop-like shape, and its form changes significantly in flexion–extension motions as well as in lateral-bending and axial rotation.[56] Foraminal height ranges between 19 and 21 mm and the superior–inferior sagittal diameter ranges between 7 and 8 mm. Instead of measuring the dimensions Wildermuth et al. introduced a qualitative scoring system.[57]

- Grade 0: normal intervertebral foramina; normal dorsolateral border of the intervertebral disc and normal form at the foraminal epidural fat (oval or inverted pear shape).
- Grade 1: slight foraminal stenosis and deformity of the epidural fat, with the remaining fat still completely surrounding the exiting nerve root.
- Grade 2: marked foraminal stenosis, with epidural fat only partially surrounding the nerve root.
- Grade 3: advanced stenosis with obliteration of the epidural fat.

The foraminal width was found to be related to the dimensions of the spinal canal and pedicle length.[58] Disc narrowing significantly reduces the foraminal height but has only little effect on the sagittal dimensions of the intervertebral foramen. Because of the morphology of the lower lumbar vertebrae, the risk of intervertebral nerve root compression is limited in patients with marked disc degeneration and subluxation of the superior facet joint.[58]

Although lateral recess stenosis may be more common than foraminal stenosis, foraminal stenosis with compression of the spinal nerve within the intervertebral foramen is a distinct feature of lateral spinal stenosis.[59] The emerging and exiting nerve root can be compressed at various levels along its descent. Compression of the nerve may be the result of an enlarged superior articular facet or focal osteophytic spurs. Rostrocaudal subluxation of the facet joints will constrict the upper part of the intervertebral foramen and present an obstacle to the nerve root.[33]

Retrolisthesis and isthmic spondylolisthesis may cause foraminal stenosis, while degenerative spondylolisthesis will rather cause lateral or central stenosis by slipping of the inferior articular processes.[58]

Positional pain differences may be related to position-dependent changes in foraminal size and may therefore only be seen in using positional MRI imaging. This technique may show small changes in forms of neural compromise which are not shown in conventional MR imaging.

For a full list of references, please see ExpertConsult.

FURTHER READING

3. Fardon DF, Milette PC, Combined Task Forces of the North American Spine Society, American Society of Spine Radiology. Nomenclature and classification of lumbar disc pathology. Recommendations of the Combined task Forces of the North American Spine Society, American Society of Spine Radiology, and American Society of Neuroradiology. Spine 2001;26(5):E93–E113.
4. Milette PC. Classification, diagnostic imaging, and imaging characterization of a lumbar herniated disk. Radiol Clin North Am 2000;38(6):1267–92.
17. Boos N, Weissbach S, Rohrbach H, et al. Classification of age-related changes in lumbar intervertebral discs: 2002 Volvo Award in basic science. Spine 2002;27(23):2631–44.
20. Weishaupt D, Zanetti M, Hodler J, et al. Painful lumbar disk derangement: relevance of endplate abnormalities at MR imaging. Radiology 2001;218(2):420–7.
32. Parizel PM, Özsarlak Ö, Van Goethem JWM, et al. The use of magnetic resonance imaging in lumbar instability. In: Szpalski MGR, Gunzburg R, Pope MH, editors. Philadelphia: Lippincott Williams and Wilkins; 1999. pp. 123–38.
37. Weishaupt D, Zanetti M, Boos N, Hodler J. MR imaging and CT in osteoarthritis of the lumbar facet joints. Skeletal Radiol 1999; 28(4):215–19.
40. Apostolaki E, Davies AM, Evans N, Cassar-Pullicino VN. MR imaging of lumbar facet joint synovial cysts. Eur Radiol 2000; 10(4):615–23.
47. Wybier M. Imaging of lumbar degenerative changes involving structures other than disk space. Radiol Clin North Am 2001; 39(1):101–14.
52. Butt S, Saifuddin A. The imaging of lumbar spondylolisthesis. Clin Radiol 2005;60(5):533–46.
55. Benoist M. The natural history of lumbar degenerative spinal stenosis. Joint Bone Spine 2002;69(5):450–7.
57. Wildermuth S, Zanetti M, Duewell S, et al. Lumbar spine: quantitative and qualitative assessment of positional (upright flexion and extension) MR imaging and myelography. Radiology 1998;207(2): 391–8.

CHAPTER 56

SPINAL TUMOURS

Luc van den Hauwe • Johan W. van Goethem • Danielle Balériaux • Arthur M. De Schepper†

CHAPTER OUTLINE

RADIOLOGICAL INVESTIGATIONS IN SPINAL TUMOURS

Computed tomography (CT) and magnetic resonance (MR) imaging are complementary techniques that are needed for evaluation of both the intraosseous extent of the tumour and soft-tissue involvement. MR imaging is the best imaging technique for the evaluation of the epidural space and neural structures.

Plain Film Radiography

Plain film radiography is not the primary imaging technique of choice to image patients with spinal tumours. It is, however, often the first imaging study in the evaluation of patients presenting with back pain. Benign primary bony tumours of the spine are mostly asymptomatic and they are frequently discovered as an incidental finding when plain films are realised on the occasion of a trauma (Fig. 56-1A). Indirect findings that may be associated with intradural spinal tumours are loss of the normal cervical lordosis or torticollis in case of an intramedullary cervical tumour. Scoliosis is almost always present in cases of an extensive spinal cord tumour independent of the histology. These plain film abnormalities are more frequently encountered in children and young adults (58–81%).[1] Indeed, in children, a growing spinal cord tumour (e.g. myxopapillary ependymoma) may expand the bony canal, through pressure erosion, and this enlargement of the spinal canal can be an important feature diagnosed on plain films. Also 'scalloping' of the posterior part of the lower thoracic and upper lumbar vertebrae may be observed in such cases. Intradural extramedullary tumours typically expand into the extradural and paravertebral space. Enlargement of the spinal foramina may be detected on plain films as well as intratumoural calcifications, when present.

Computed Tomography

CT has become the optimal imaging technique for the evaluation of the vertebral bony structures. Multidetector CT (MDCT) allows for rapid and extensive visualisation of the spine and images can be reconstructed in the 3 orthogonal planes. Two-dimensional multiplanar reformatted images are useful in the evaluation of cortical bone destruction and the detection of calcifications (Fig. 56-1B) within the tumour.[2] In case of intradural tumoural pathology, CT may show widening of the bony spinal canal and enlargement of the vertebral neuroforamina. Although CT and MR imaging are diagnostic methods for many cases, CT-guided biopsy may be performed for confirmation, since many bone lesions can have a similar appearance (Fig. 56-2).

Magnetic Resonance Imaging

The imaging technique of choice for the evaluation of spinal tumours is MR imaging (Fig. 56-1C). MR imaging is also very important in the evaluation of lesions of the osseous spine.[3] Protocols may vary slightly between institutions depending on the type of MR system (manufacturer, field strength, etc.), but in general several phased-array coils are used simultaneously to obtain a large field of view.[4] Using advanced parallel acquisition techniques which combine the signals of several coil elements to reconstruct the image, the signal-to-noise ratio is improved along with accelerated acquisition to reduce imaging time. Parallel reconstruction algorithms that reconstruct either the global image from the images produced by each coil, or Fourier plane of the image from the frequency signals of each coil, are used to further improve image quality with better spatial resolution,

†This chapter is respectfully dedicated to the memory of Professor Dr. Arthur M. De Schepper (1937-2013), who died shortly after the typescript of this chapter was completed.

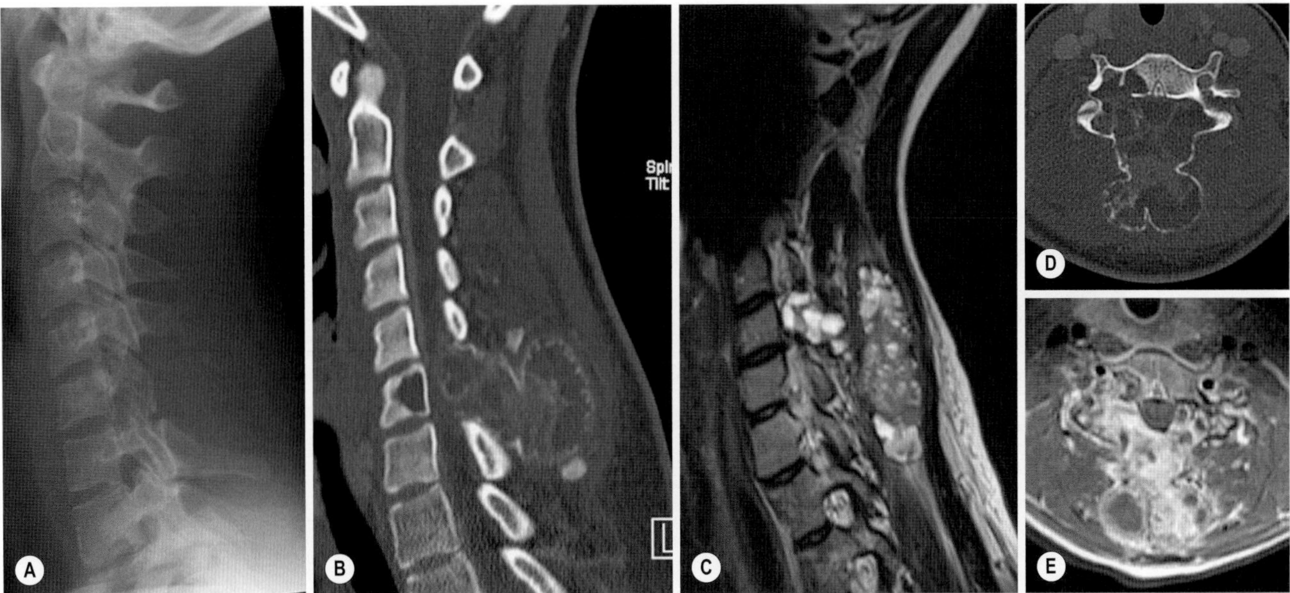

FIGURE 56-1 ■ Comparison of plain film radiography, MDCT and MR imaging in a patient with a giant cell tumour and secondary aneurysmal bone cyst. Plain film (A) shows the absence of the C6 spinous process seemingly replaced by a soft-tissue mass, including some slight calcifications and/or remnants of cortical bone. The full extension of the lesion in the spinal canal, the vertebral body, pedicles and posterior elements becomes evident with the use of MDCT (B and D), and MR imaging (C and E). On these T_2-weighted images, fluid–fluid levels can be observed, which are a hallmark for aneurysmal bone cyst (ABC).

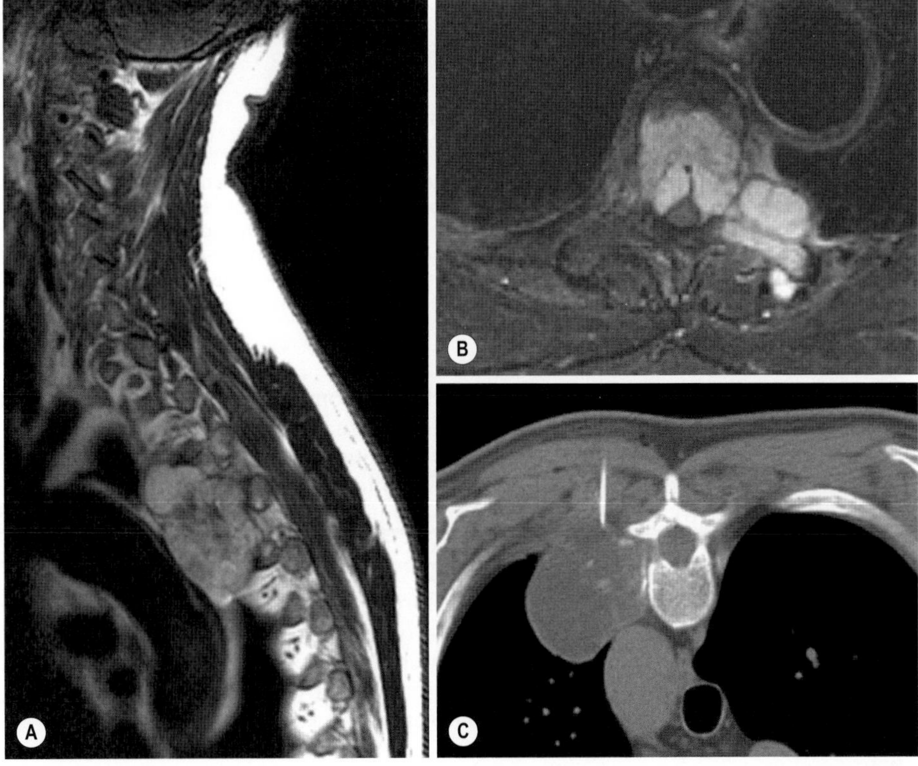

FIGURE 56-2 ■ CT-guided percutaneous biopsy of a vertebral tumour with important paravertebral extension. Sagittal contrast-enhanced T_1 (A) and axial fat-suppressed T_2 (STIR) (B) show the tumour mass extending within the paravertebral soft tissues and anterior epidural space with a typical 'curtain sign'. CT-guided percutaneous biopsy of the large paravertebral mass is performed with the patient in prone position (C). Pathology demonstrated low-grade chondrosarcoma. (Case courtesy of P. Bracke, Brasschaat, Belgium.)

and reduced artefacts.[5] Full-spine and whole-body MR imaging can be performed in this manner. This is important, since it is advantageous to see the whole spine and spinal cord covered in one single examination (Fig. 56-3).

Imaging protocols usually include sagittal and axial T_1 and T_2. T_1 and T_2 offer different and complementary information. T_2 is superior in detecting intramedullary tumours. On the other hand, T_1 is more sensitive than non-fat-suppressed T_2 in detecting bone marrow disease, e.g. vertebral metastases, but short T_1 inversion recovery (STIR) or other fat-suppressed T_2 sequences are also able to increase the detection of certain bone marrow diseases. Suppressing the high signal of CSF in T_2 sequences is

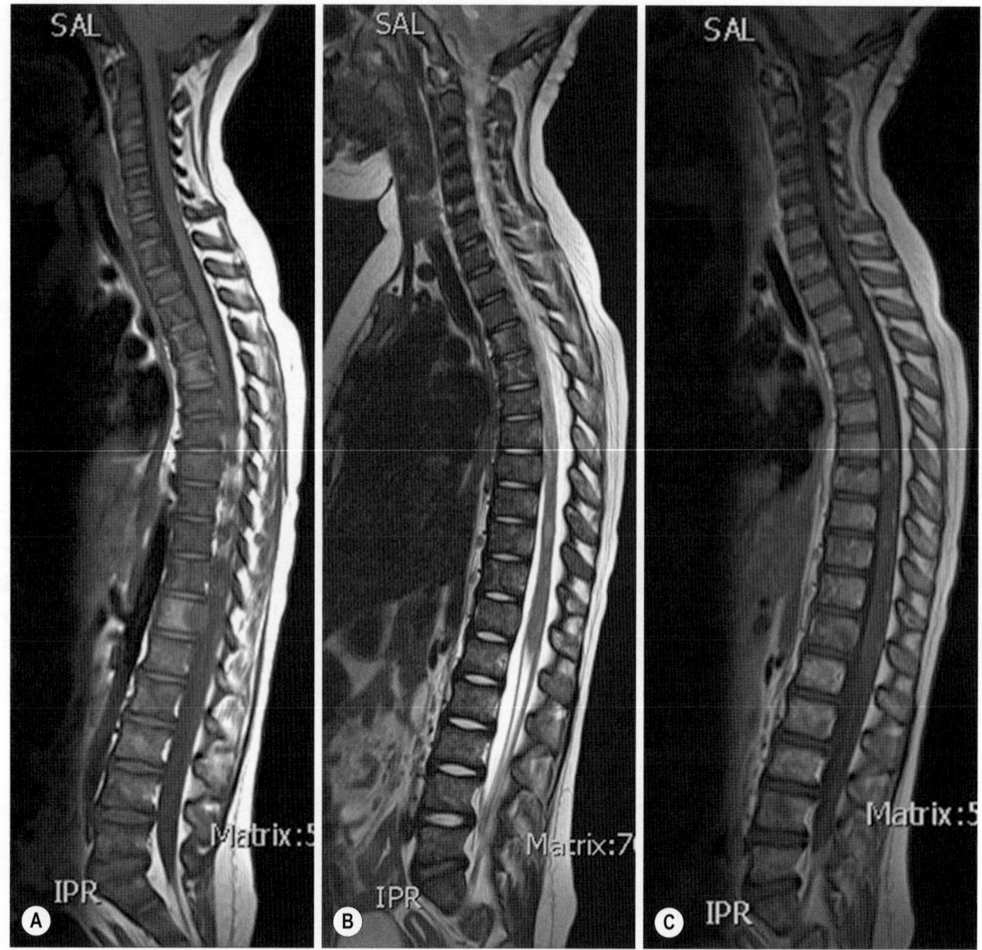

FIGURE 56-3 ■ Full-spine MR imaging in a child with recurrent and metastatic medulloblastoma. Sagittal T_1 (A) shows diffuse heterogeneous signal intensity within the bone marrow of the cervical, thoracic and lumbar vertebrae, indicative of metastatic bone disease. On sagittal T_2 (B), an ill-defined area of high signal intensity within the spinal cord is observed at the Th9–Th10 level with suspicion of more intramedullary lesions more proximally. Sagittal gadolinium-enhanced T_1 (C) not only shows diffuse leptomeningeal enhancement but also confirms the presence of intramedullary metastases and shows enhancement of the vertebral metastases.

very useful in detecting subtle intramedullary lesions. The most common technique to obtain this kind of image is FLAIR (fluid-attenuated inversion recovery), a sequence that nulls out CSF signal. Gradient-echo (GRE) images are useful in order to detect haemorrhagic components often present in spinal cord tumours. In screening for vertebral metastases, an additional sagittal GRE so-called out-of-phase sequence can be used. In the normal adult human, the medullary bone of the vertebral bodies contains approximately equal amounts of water and fat protons. In out-of-phase conditions, the signal of both will cancel out, leaving the vertebrae completely black. In case of vertebral pathology, however, the signal will increase and, as such, vertebral metastases (or other lesions) will clearly stand out.[6] Gadolinium-enhanced sequences, usually performed in the sagittal and axial plane, are used in order to better identify solid enhancing tumour components, and to differentiate tumoural cysts whose borders enhance from associated, so-called reactive, pseudocysts.[7,8] Coronal images may be helpful for the evaluation of paravertebral soft-tissue extension and fat suppression can be used to better demonstrate tumoural enhancement.[2] Some authors recommend contrast-enhanced 3D-GRE T_1 techniques in screening for intradural tumour dissemination.[9] When dealing with extradural tumours, the administration of gadolinium is also useful for biopsy in that it allows differentiation of enhancing viable tumour from areas of non-enhancing necrosis (Fig. 56-2). Moreover, gadolinium-enhanced images better demonstrate epidural extension of the tumour.[2]

Diffusion-Weighted Imaging

Diffusion-weighted imaging (DWI) and diffusion tensor imaging (DTI) have been proven useful in brain tumours. However, these techniques are much more difficult to apply in imaging of the spinal cord. Obtaining spinal cord DWI and DTI has a number of challenges. The spinal cord's small size requires the use of small voxel sizes (higher matrix) for spatial resolution that decreases the signal-to-noise ratio. Images may be degraded because of macroscopic motion related to physiological cerebrospinal fluid pulsations, breathing and swallowing. In

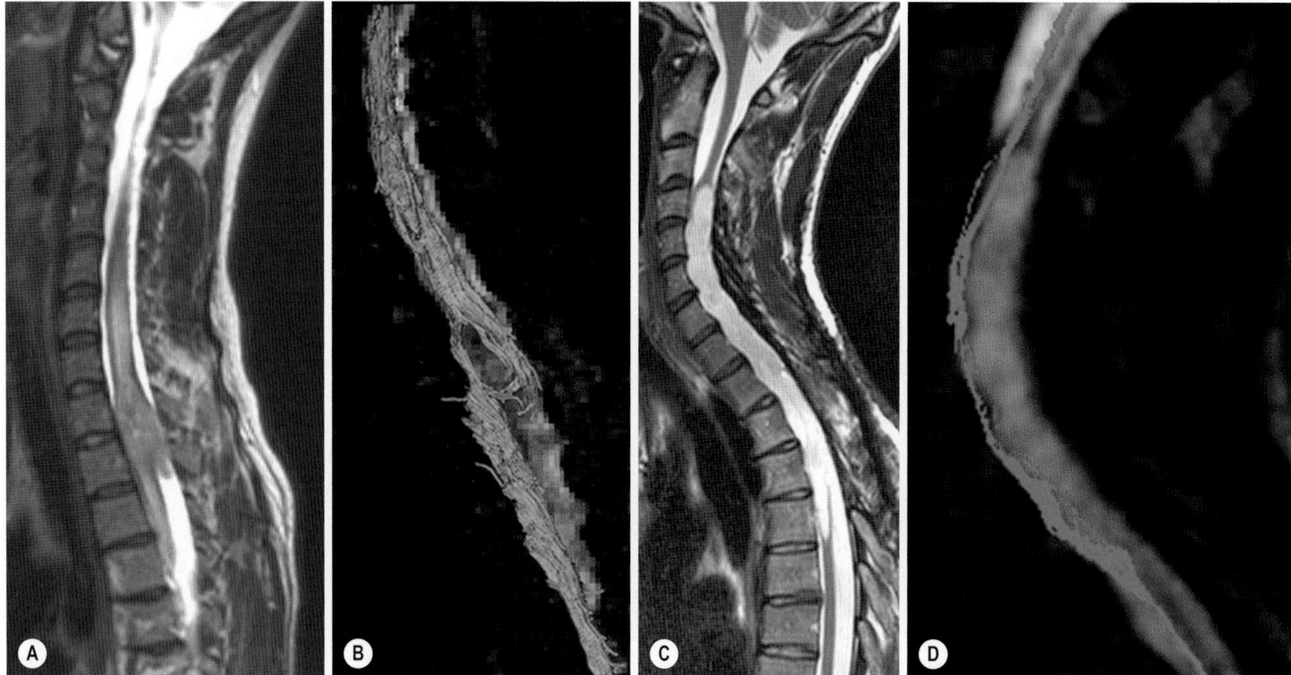

FIGURE 56-4 ■ Value of diffusion tensor imaging (DTI) tractography. Sagittal T_2 (A) and DTI tractography (B) in a patient with spinal cord ependymoma. Peripheral displacement rather than tumoural invasion of the fibres is observed. Sagittal T_2 (C) and DTI tractography (D) in a patient with spinal cord astrocytoma. Fibres are pushed anteriorly by the tumour. (Case (A, B) courtesy of M. Thurnher, Vienna, Austria and W. Van Hecke, Leuven, Belgium.)

addition, local field inhomogeneities reducing the image resolution and the use of echo-planar sequences, typically used in brain imaging, further increases susceptibility effects.[10] Although still under development, fibre tracking based on DTI holds great potential in visualising the fibres within the normal and diseased spinal cord. The effect of a growing spinal cord tumour on the fibre tracts has been demonstrated. If the lesion displaces the fibre tracts rather than infiltrating them it is is suggestive of a well-circumscribed tumour such as ependymoma (Fig. 56-4A, B), which pathologically has a plane of resection between the lesion and the normal spinal cord allowing for a surgical resection compared with a diffusely infiltrating tumour such as fibrillary astrocytoma.[10–13]

Bone Scintigraphy

Bone scintigraphy can be performed when multifocal vertebral lesions with increased radionuclide uptake are suspected. However, bone scintigraphy is limited in its capacity to depict detailed surgical anatomy, particularly compared with CT or MR imaging.[2] Moreover, positive findings may also be attributed to degenerative changes of the spine.

Positron Emission Tomography

Positron emission tomography (PET) has been used extensively to evaluate the grade of malignancy in brain tumours and to differentiate recurrent tumours from radiation necrosis after radiation therapy. In other regions, PET has been used to detect neoplastic lesions such as metastatic ones, and to differentiate neoplastic from non-neoplastic lesions.[14] Only a few reports on the use of PET in patients with intramedullary tumours have been published. Wilmshurst et al. reported the use of both ^{18}F-fluorodeoxyglucose (FDG) and ^{11}C-methionine (MET) and found a correlation with histological malignancy.[15] FDG-PET imaging is also useful in evaluating tumour progression and identifying the most metabolically active components in spinal cord tumours. A prospective study of larger numbers of patients with a wider range of tumour types is required, but this is difficult to achieve given the rarity of spinal cord tumours.[14,15]

CLASSIFICATION OF SPINAL TUMOURS

Spinal tumours may be classified in different ways. The World Health Organisation (WHO) classification of spinal tumours is a universally accepted histological classification. The 2007 WHO classification is based on the consensus of an international Working Group of 25 pathologists and geneticists, as well as contributions from more than 70 international experts overall, and is presented as the standard for the definition of CNS tumours to the clinical oncology and cancer research communities worldwide.[16] The WHO classification of CNS neoplasms is based on the assumption that the tumour type results from the abnormal growth of a specific cell type. The WHO classification also provides a grading system for tumours of each cell type and allows the classification of tumours to guide the choice of therapy and predict prognosis. Based on the grading system, most tumours are of a single defined grade. Although the updated WHO classification does not have a direct impact on the daily practice of the (neuro)radiologist or in the interpretation of images, it is valuable in the communication between clinicians, radiologists and pathologists.[4,16]

Based on their location on imaging findings (MR imaging, and myelography in the past), spinal tumours may be characterised as intramedullary, intradural extramedullary, and extradural spinal tumours.[17] Although this classification is somewhat of an oversimplification, since lesions can reside in several compartments, this approach is very helpful as it narrows the differential diagnosis when a tumour is found in one of these anatomical compartments. Extradural lesions are the most common (60% of all spinal tumours), with the majority of lesions originating from the vertebrae. Metastatic disease is the most frequent extradural tumour, while primary bone tumours are much less frequently observed. Intradural tumours are rare, and the majority are extramedullary (30% of all spinal tumours), with meningiomas, nerve sheath tumours (schwannomas and neurofibromas) and drop metastases being the most frequent ones. Intramedullary tumours are even more uncommon lesions (10% of all spinal tumours). Astrocytomas and ependymomas comprise the majority of the intramedullary tumours.[6]

Intramedullary Tumours

Primary tumours of the spinal cord are 10 to 15 times less common than primary intracranial tumours and overall represent 2 to 4% of all primary tumours of the central nervous system (CNS).[17] They occur with an incidence of 1.1 cases per 100,000 persons. A considerable number of different intramedullary tumours exist; only a few of them are expected to be encountered in a routine practice. The majority of intramedullary tumours are glial tumours; about 90% are ependymomas or astrocytomas. The most frequently encountered neoplasms in adults are ependymoma (40–60%) and astrocytoma. Haemangioblastoma is the third most frequent intramedullary tumour found in adults, but it is rarely seen in children. Astrocytomas are the most common intramedullary tumour in the paediatric age group (60–90% of cases), followed by gangliogliomas. Ependymomas are uncommon in children outside the setting of neurofibromatosis type 2 (NF-2).[18] Astrocytomas and ependymomas are more frequent in the thoracic and the cervical region, respectively, while myxopapillary ependymomas are typically seen in the region of the conus medullaris, filum terminale and cauda equina.[5,6]

MR imaging is the preoperative study of choice to narrow the differential diagnosis and guide surgical resection.[19] Differentiation between ependymomas and astrocytomas before surgery is important for the surgeon because ependymomas of the spinal cord are relatively well circumscribed and they can apparently be completely removed, whereas astrocytomas have a tendency for infiltrating growth that makes complete removal difficult.[20]

Ependymoma

Ependymomas are the most frequent intramedullary tumours in adults; in children these tumours occur sporadically and may be associated with NF-2. Most NF-2-related ependymomas are small intramedullary nodules that may be multiple.[18] The peak incidence for spinal ependymomas is in the fourth and fifth decade, but these tumours also are found in younger patients. Ependymomas arise from the ependymal cells lining the central ependymal canal and, therefore, are frequently located centrally within the cord.[7] This central location explains the more frequently observed sensory symptoms that result from the close proximity to the spinothalamic tracts.[21] Motor deficits only present in the later stage of the disease, thereby delaying the diagnosis. In contrast to sporadic tumours, the majority of NF-2-related spinal tumours are asymptomatic.[22] Intramedullary ependymomas are most often found in the cervical cord and less frequently also the upper thoracic cord. Most ependymomas are low grade (WHO grade 2) with a benign indolent course. The tumours are well demarcated and compress the adjacent cord rather than infiltrating it. Malignant histological subtypes (anaplastic ependymoma; WHO grade 3) rarely occur. There are four histological subtypes of CNS ependymomas: cellular, papillary, clear cell and tanycytic.[6] The cellular form is the most common intramedullary variant.[21] The prognosis for patients with spinal ependymoma depends on the tumour grade, degree of resection and presence or absence of CSF dissemination.[21] In NF-2-patients, these tumours seldom require intervention, even for tumours that expand the cord or have associated cysts. Close surveillance with MR imaging is a reasonable option.[22]

CT may show canal widening, scoliosis and vertebral body scalloping. On MR imaging, ependymomas appear typically as central well-circumscribed iso- or hypointense lesions on T_1 (Fig. 56-5A) and as iso- or hyperintense on T_2 (Fig. 56-5B).[21] Most ependymomas do enhance vividly (Fig. 56-5C) and homogeneously in 91% of the cases. They have usually well-defined borders (Figs. 56-5C, 56-6A), which allows total removal of the tumour in most cases (Fig. 56-6B).[8] Because of their compressive rather than infiltrative nature, a cleavage plane may occasionally be seen on imaging. Diffusion tensor imaging may show how the tumours displace the fibre tracts rather than interrupt them (Figs. 56-4A, B). However, this may also be observed in spinal cord astrocytoma (Figs. 56-4C, D). While astrocytomas usually are very extensive, the mean tumour size of ependymomas is usually three vertebral segments. A so-called 'cap sign' is seen in 20–25% of cases and corresponds to low signal intensity areas seen on T_2 and even better on gradient-echo T_2*, capping at both sides the tumour limits (Fig. 56-6A). Those caps are haemosiderin deposits due to chronic haemorrhage. When present, the cap sign is highly suggestive for the diagnosis of ependymoma.[21] Associated satellite cysts are seen in 60% of the cases, and they may be very large. Delineation of these cysts is easier after gadolinium injection. Syrinx is also a characteristic finding, especially with cervical ependymomas. Spinal cord oedema on either side of the tumour

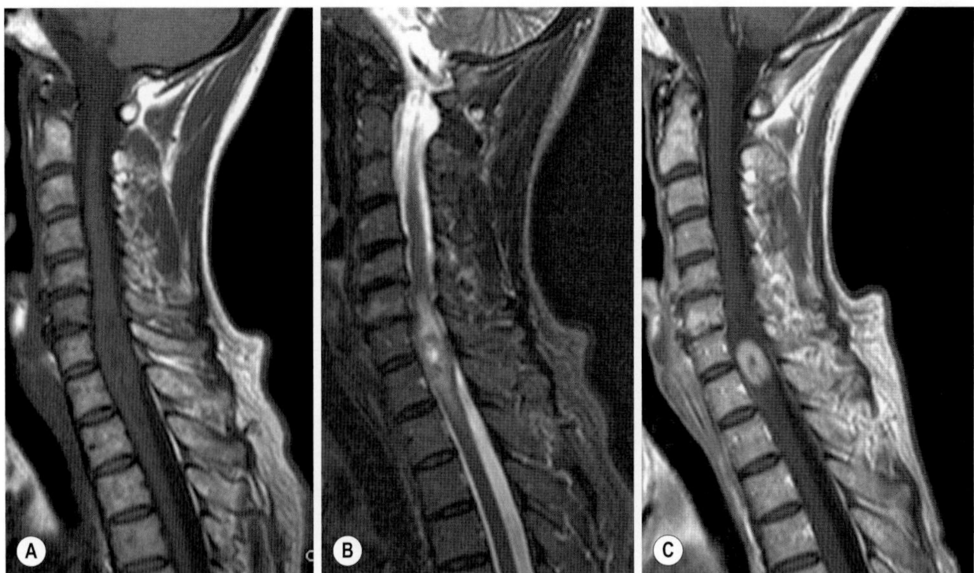

FIGURE 56-5 ■ Spinal cord ependymoma. Sagittal T_1 (A) and T_2 (B) show clearly focal spinal cord enlargement at the cervicothoracic junction. The lesion is iso- to slightly hypointense on T_1, and very heterogeneous on T_2 with areas of low signal intensity within the tumour. There is some associated oedema within the cord. Gd-enhanced T_1 (C) shows focal nodular contrast enhancement centrally within the spinal cord. Straightening of the spine and multilevel degenerative changes of the lower C-spine are observed.

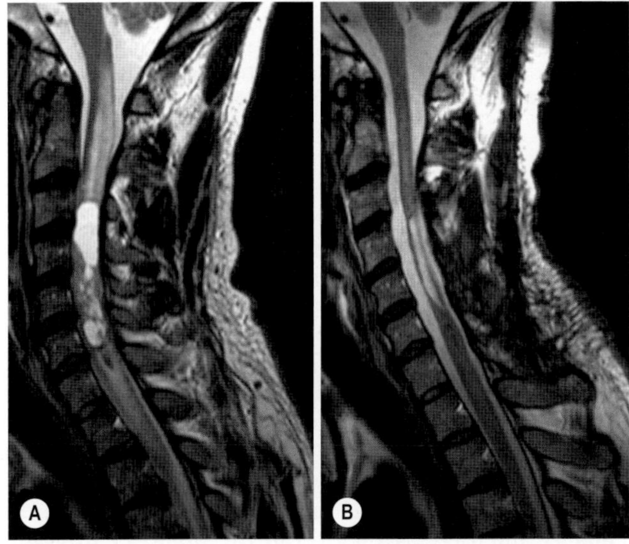

FIGURE 56-6 ■ 'Cap sign' in a grade 2 ependymoma. Preoperative sagittal T_2 (A) shows an expansile lesion arising within the spinal cord at the C3–C7 level. Heterogeneous signal intensity of the tumour with both solid and cystic components. The most typical feature is the bilateral hypointense areas capping the tumour: the 'cap sign' is more frequently encountered in ependymoma. Extensive oedema is observed. Postoperative sagittal T_2 (B) shows complete removal of the tumour.

is variable, but often seen in the large multisegmental tumours.[4]

Myxopapillary Ependymoma

Myxopapillary ependymoma, a WHO grade 1 lesion, is a relatively common spinal intradural neoplasm of the conus medullaris and filum terminale arising from ependymal cells of the filum terminale. It is found predominantly in children and young adults, although it may be observed at older age. There is a slight male preponderance. Patients typical complain of chronic low back pain exacerbating during night. Myxopapillary ependymomas are slow-growing tumours, so they may become very large before the diagnosis is finally made. Associated scalloping of the vertebral body, scoliosis and enlargement of the neural foramina may be observed. Haemorrhage may occur, explaining the sudden worsening of clinical symptoms with occurrence of leg weakness and sphincter disturbances. This greater tendency for haemorrhage may also lead to subarachnoid bleeding and superficial siderosis.

On MR imaging, the lesion is iso- to hyperintense on T_1 (Fig. 56-7A) and hyperintense on T_2 (Fig. 56-7B). The hyperintense signal may be explained by their mucin content. The tumour enhances strongly and is somewhat inhomogeneous after gadolinium injection (Fig. 56-7C). Haemorrhage and cyst formations are common features that contribute to signal inhomogeneity.

The main differential diagnosis is with nerve sheath tumours, such as schwannomas.[18] Although myxopapillary ependymomas are WHO grade 1 lesions, spontaneous and postoperative CSF dissemination along the craniospinal axis as well as dissemination following extradural manipulation of the tumour during spine surgery or following spinal trauma has been reported.[23] In our experience, postoperative radiotherapy is therefore very useful to prevent recurrent disease.

Astrocytoma

Astrocytomas are the most common intramedullary tumours (up to 90%) in children[18] and account for about 30% of intramedullary tumours in adults. The peak incidence for spinal astrocytomas is in the third and fourth decade.[4,6] A slight predominance among males (55%) is

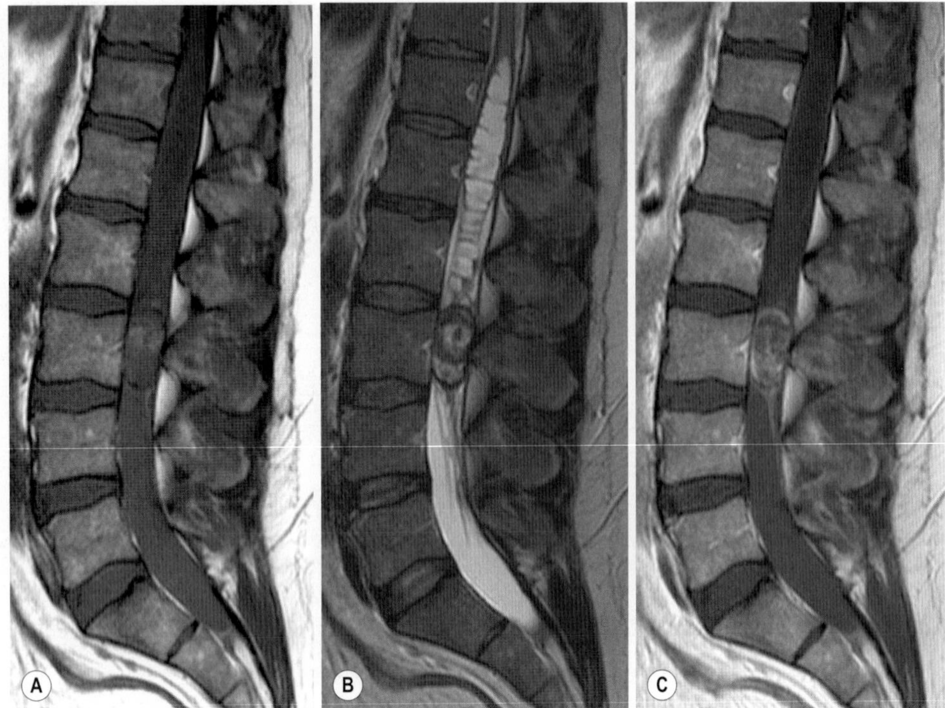

FIGURE 56-7 ■ **Myxopapillary ependymoma.** Sagittal T_1 (A) and T_2 (B) show a well-defined heterogeneous mass at the L3 level. The lesion is slightly hyperintense on T_1, which may be explained by the presence of mucin, but it shows low signal on T_2, and has a low signal intensity rim, suggestive for haemorrhage within the tumour. Inferior to the mass, trapped CSF has high T_1 and T_2 signal, possibly caused by a high protein content. Extensive cyst formation with enlargement of the spinal cord is observed proximal to the tumour with some oedema at the border with the normal cord. Sagittal gadolinium-enhanced T_1 (C) shows enhancement of the tumour mass.

observed in larger series. Histology is the most important prognostic variable. In the paediatric age group, astrocytomas are mostly tumours of low grade (i.e. pilocytic and fibrillary astrocytomas).[19] Pilocytic astrocytomas (WHO grade 1) account for 75% of all intramedullary tumours in the paediatric age group and typically affect children between 1 and 5 years of age, whereas fibrillary astrocytomas (WHO grade 2) account for 7% and tend to occur in older children (around 10 years of age).[18] In adults, the majority (75%) are low-grade (WHO grade 2) fibrillary astrocytomas with 5-year survivorship exceeding 75%. High-grade spinal cord gliomas (WHO grades 3 and 4) are less common and associated with a poor survival. Regardless of WHO grade, spinal cord astrocytomas are infiltrative and associated with poorly characterised boundaries and, consequently, are typically biopsied only since total resection is not possible.[17] The most common site of involvement is the thoracic cord (almost 70%), followed by the cervical cord. They frequently involve a large portion of the spinal cord, spanning multiple vertebral levels in length (Fig. 56-8). Involvement of the entire spinal cord (holocord presentation) is common in children but quite rare in adults.[24] True 'holocord' tumours, however, are rare. In most cases, involvement of the whole length of the spinal cord is caused by extensive spinal cord oedema rather than by a tumour.

Tumours can show areas of necrotic-cystic degeneration (60% of cases), can have a 'cyst with mural nodule' appearance, or can be structurally solid (about 40% of cases). The solid components are iso- to hypointense on T_1 (Fig. 56-9A) and hyperintense on T_2 (Fig. 56-9B), whereas necrotic-cystic components are typically hypointense on T_1 and strongly hyperintense on T_2. The pattern of enhancement is variable and does not define tumour margins.[18] For the most part, low-grade fibrillary astrocytomas do not enhance (Fig. 56-9C), although enhancement may be observed (Fig. 56-8C). Low-grade tumours may evolve over time and become more malignant tumours. Pilocytic astrocytomas, on the other hand, do enhance intensely as they do in the brain. High-grade astrocytomas and glioblastomas tend to be more heterogeneous with necrotic-cystic areas and enhance often in a patchy mode. Intratumoural haemorrhage may be observed and is best seen on gradient-echo T_2*. Associated syringomyelia may occur: the borders of those associated cavities do not enhance after contrast injection (Fig. 56-8C).

Haemangioblastoma

Haemangioblastomas are rare benign (low grade), usually richly vascularised tumours. They represent 2–10% of all spinal tumours and are seen more commonly in adults, with a peak incidence in the fourth decade.[25] Hemangioblastomas can be solitary (80%) or multiple (20%), when associated with von Hippel–Lindau syndrome (VHLs).[26,27] This is an autosomal dominant disease with multiple cerebellar and/or spinal haemangioblastomas (Fig. 56-10),

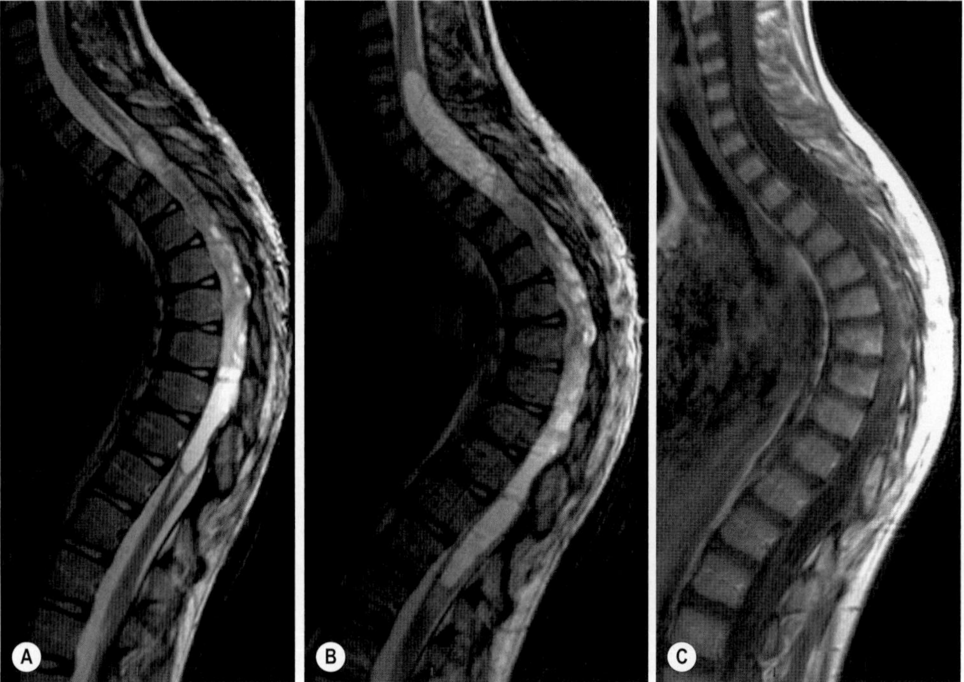

FIGURE 56-8 ■ **Spinal cord astrocytoma.** Follow-up study with sagittal T_2 (A, B) in an 11-year-old girl who had partial resection of the tumour 2 and 3 years before, respectively. Final diagnosis at that time was grade 2 fibrillary astrocytoma. Progressive enlargement of the associated polar cysts proximal and distal to the resected tumour is observed. Also the spinal cord oedema has increased. Sagittal contrast-enhanced T_1 of the most recent follow-up study (C) shows heterogeneous enhancement, not present on the previous examination, which is indicative of progressive disease. Note the hyperkyphosis and scoliosis in this girl, which are frequently indirect signs of intradural spinal tumours in children.

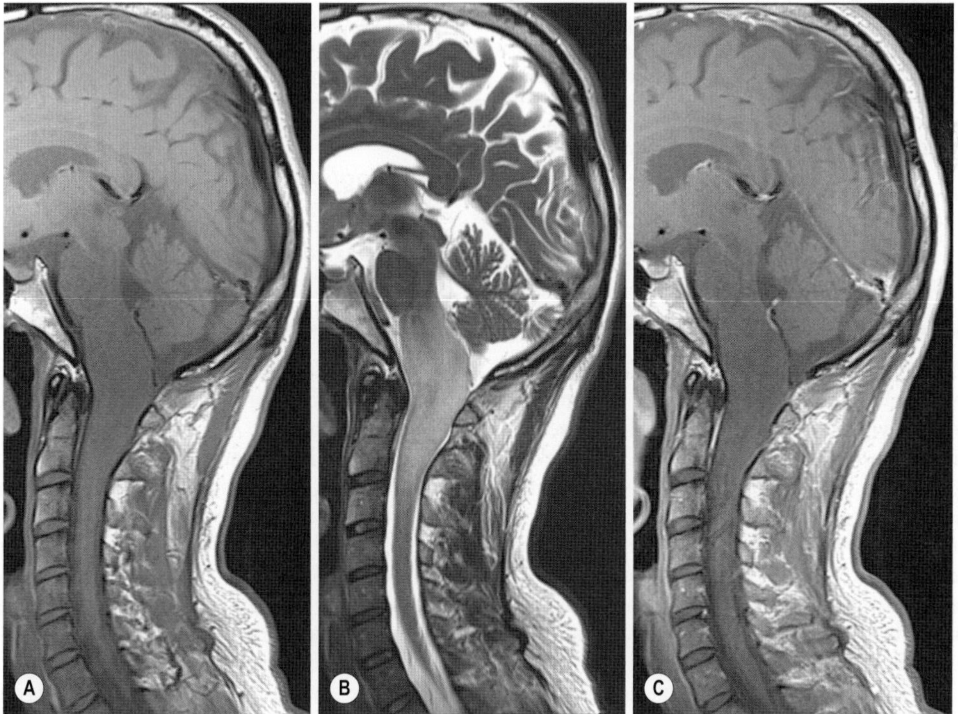

FIGURE 56-9 ■ **Low-grade astrocytoma.** Sagittal T_1 (A) and T_2 (B) show an ill-defined mass with huge swelling of the upper cervical spinal cord and medulla oblongata just extending up to the level of the bulbomedullary junction and even higher in the posterior aspect of the brainstem. Signal characteristics are aspecific, with diffuse low signal intensity on T_1 and high signal intensity on T_2. Sagittal contrast-enhanced T_1 (C) shows no enhancement within the lesion.

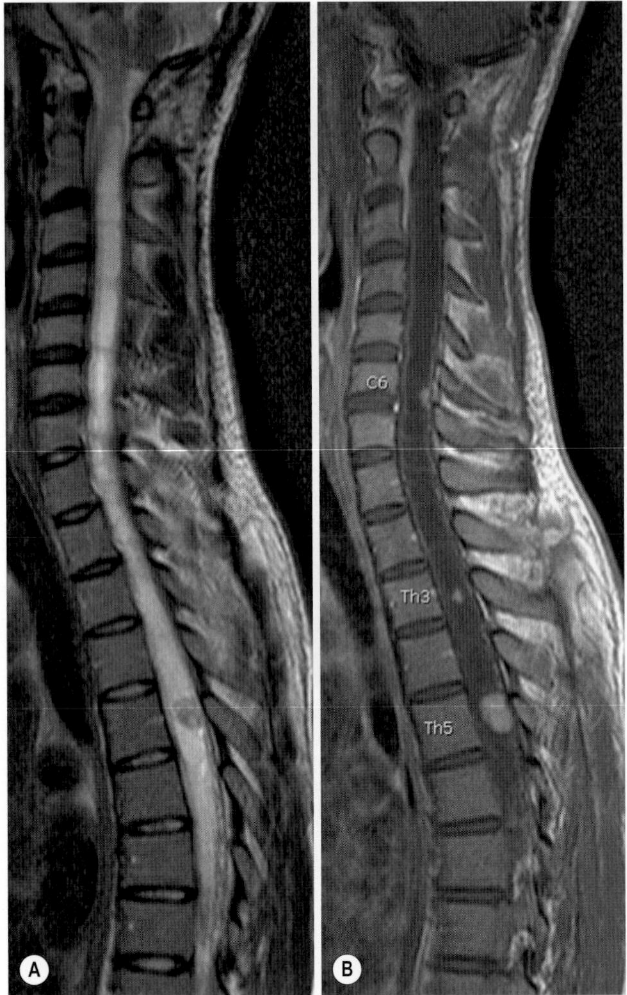

FIGURE 56-10 ■ Multiple spinal cord haemangioblastomas in a patient with von Hippel–Lindau syndrome. Sagittal T_2 (A) shows a diffuse enlarged spinal cord with a slight hypointense nodular lesion at the posterior aspect (subpial) of the spinal cord at the Th5 level. The lesion is surrounded by extensive oedema and multiple associated cysts can be observed proximal to the tumour. Sagittal gadolinium-enhanced T_1 (B) shows strong enhancement within the tumour. Moreover, two smaller additional enhancing nodules at the level of the C6–C7 disc space and Th3 are found. Associated peritumoural cysts show no enhancement.

retinal angiomatosis, renal cell carcinoma and/or phaeochromocytoma in varying degrees.[27] Spinal hemangioblastomas associated with VHLs are usually diagnosed up to 10 years earlier and are associated with less severe neurological symptoms than sporadic lesions. The incidence of spinal haemangioblastomas may be as high as 88% in patients with VHLs,[28] which is much more frequent than previously reported.[29] Therefore, screening spinal MR imaging should be performed in patients with VHLs. Most patients with sporadic disease have a single lesion at the cervical or thoracic level (Fig. 56-11), whereas patients with VHLs have multiple lesions at all spinal levels (Fig. 56-10). Up to one-third of patients with VHLs will develop new lesions every 2 years.[28]

In about 75–85% of cases these are pure intramedullary lesions, but sometimes they may be intradural extramedullary with a variable exophytic component. Pure extradural tumours are very rare.[30] Preoperative evaluation of the precise tumour location is important for total resection and improving the surgical outcome.[30] Haemangioblastomas have two different but rather typical presentations: either a small nodular lesion located in the subpial region and surrounded by extensive intramedullary oedema or a small nodule associated with huge and extensive intramedullary cystic components (Figs. 56-10 and 56-11). The mechanism of this peritumoural cyst formation appears to be the result of an interstitial process that starts with generation of oedema. Vascular endothelial growth factor (VEGF) acting locally in the tumour or hydrodynamic forces, or both, within abnormal tumour vasculature may drive fluid (plasma) extravasation. When these forces overcome the ability of the surrounding tissue to resorb fluid, oedema (with its associated increased interstitial pressure) and subsequent cyst formation occur.[31]

On T_1, the solid tumour nodule is isointense to hypointense relative to the spinal cord; on T_2 it is isointense to slightly hyperintense. A rich vascular network in the tumour, as well as enlarged feeding arteries and dilated draining veins (Figs. 56-11B–D), may best be seen on proton density and T_2. After gadolinium injection, intense and homogeneous enhancement of the subpial nodule is seen.[8] Gadolinium is especially useful in order to pick up small, multiple nodules when associated with large cystic components (Fig. 56-10B). Associated cysts may have signal intensities comparable to CSF, but sometimes a rich protein content results in a higher signal intensity on T_1. Symptomatic small haemangioblastomas have relatively large associated syringes, whereas asymptomatic ones do not.[32] DSA is still performed to identify the feeding arteries to the tumour (Figs. 56-11E, F) and, if possible, to perform preoperative embolisation in order to reduce the bleeding during surgery of those richly vascularised tumours.

Ganglioglioma

Gangliogliomas, being rare tumours in adults (1–2% of all spinal cord tumours),[33] are much more frequently seen in children.[21,34] They represent the second most common intramedullary tumour in the paediatric age group (15% of cases) and mostly affect children between 1 and 5 years of age, as do pilocytic astrocytomas.[18] These tumours are composed of a combination of neoplastic ganglion cells and glial elements. Although they typically are low-grade tumours (WHO grades 1 and 2) with a low potential for malignant degeneration, they have a significant propensity for local recurrence, and the glial element may progress to high grade.[18] Surgical resection is the treatment of choice. After resection, there is a 5-year survival rate of 89%. Their preferential location is in the cervical and upper thoracic cord and may extend to the medulla oblongata through the foramen magnum.[18] Gangliogliomas may extend over more than eight vertebral segments[19] and holocord involvement has been described to be more frequent than in other spinal cord tumours, probably as a result of their slow growth rate.[34] Gangliogliomas are typically eccentrically located (Fig. 56-12).[21]

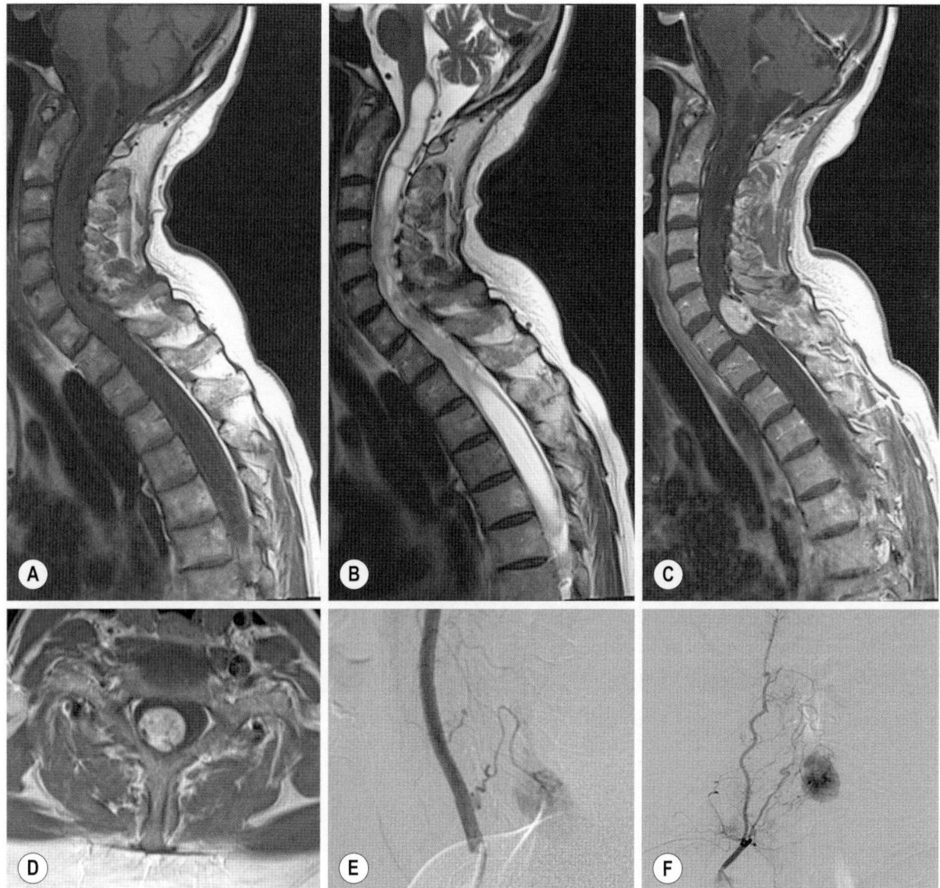

FIGURE 56-11 ■ **Cervical haemangioblastoma.** Sagittal T_1 (A) and T_2 (B) show a diffuse enlargement of the spinal cord. Extensive oedema and multiple cyst formation can be seen extending up to the level of the obex. Sagittal (C) and axial (D) gadolinium-enhanced T_1 show the presence of an intense enhancing tumour at the C7 level. Flow voids can be observed within the enhancing tumour. Enhancement is also visible in dilated veins along the posterior aspect of the spinal cord. DSA (E, F) shows the typical hypervascularisation supplied by enlarged arterial branches arising from the right vertebral and right thyrocervical trunk. (Case courtesy of M. Voormolen, Antwerp, Belgium.)

On imaging, scoliosis and remodelling are common but non-specific findings.[18] Calcification may be seen on CT, but it is much less common than in gangliogliomas that occur intracranially. According to Rossi et al., calcification is probably the single most suggestive feature of gangliogliomas. In the absence of gross calcification, the MR imaging appearance of gangliogliomas is non-specific and does not allow differentiation from astrocytomas.[18] Gangliogliomas have highly variable MR imaging findings. Although propensity for cyst formation has been reported to be common,[19] in other series gangliogliomas were predominantly solid.[18] In a large series of 27 patients with spinal cord gangliogliomas, Patel et al. described several clinical and imaging findings that are characteristic of gangliogliomas: young patient age, long tumour length, tumoural cysts (Fig. 56-12B), absence of oedema, mixed signal intensity on T_1, patchy tumour enhancement (Fig. 56-12C) and cord surface enhancement.[33] They speculated that the mixed signal intensity on T_1 may be caused by the dual cellular population (i.e. neuronal and glial elements) and, in their opinion, this feature was somewhat unique for spinal neoplasms and was uncommonly seen in cord ependymomas or astrocytomas.[33] Perifocal oedema can vary from limited or absent to extensive. Contrast enhancement can be focal or patchy, and it rarely involves the whole tumour mass;[18] absence of enhancement has also been described in a minority of cases.[35]

Less Frequent Intramedullary Tumours

Less frequent tumours include intramedullary metastasis, lymphoma, epidermoid cyst, lipoma, oligodendroglioma, intramedullary schwannoma and teratoma.

Metastasis. Although intramedullary metastases are rare, accounting for only 5% of all intramedullary lesions, their number is growing fast due to the longer survival of many cancer patients (improved chemotherapy, etc.). They are less common than leptomeningeal metastases. The lung and breast are the most common sites of primary malignancies for intramedullary spread.[4] The high sensitivity of MR imaging enables easy detection of intramedullary metastases: however, there are no specific MRI characteristics. Usually, spinal cord metastases are small, nodular, well-defined lesions, surrounded

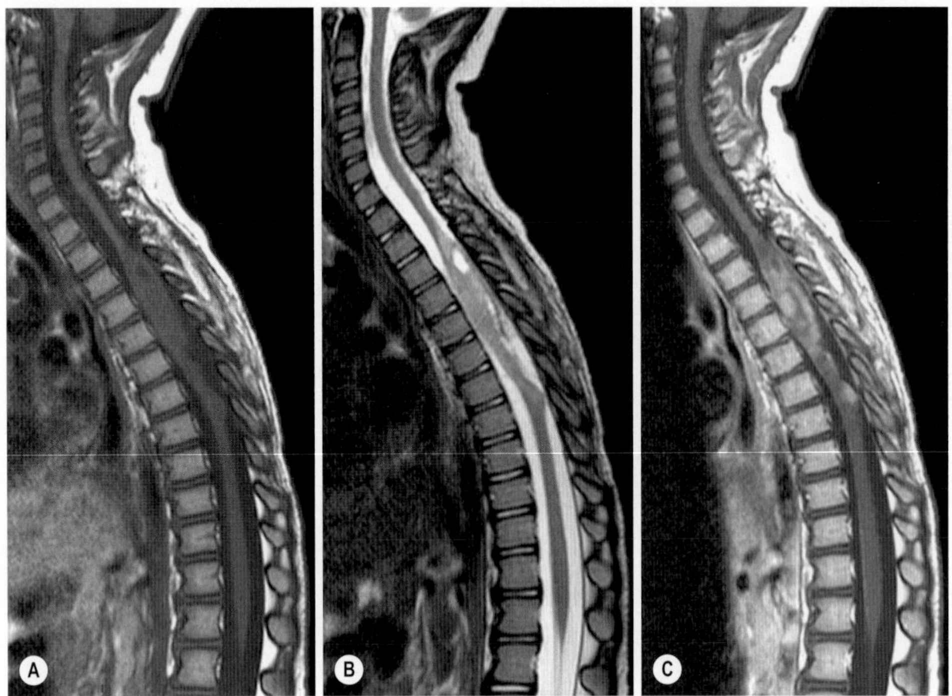

FIGURE 56-12 ■ **Ganglioglioma.** Sagittal T_1 (A) and T_2 (B) show a heterogeneous solid infiltrating tumour in a young child, arising within the thoracic spinal cord, and extending along 5–6 segments. Small intratumoural cysts and discrete peritumoural oedema may be observed on the T_2. Diffuse heterogeneous and patchy enhancement of the tumour is present on sagittal T_1 after gadolinium injection (C). (Case courtesy of A. Rossi, Genoa, Italy.)

by mild to extensive oedema (Fig. 56-13A). The enhancement pattern may be either ring-like or homogeneous and intense (Fig. 56-13B).[36] Recently, two peripheral enhancement features on MR imaging specific for non-CNS-origin spinal cord metastases have been described: a more intense thin rim of peripheral enhancement around an enhancing lesion (rim sign) and an ill-defined flame-shaped region of enhancement at the superior/inferior margins (flame sign).[37] Melanoma metastasis has a more specific appearance, exhibiting a spontaneously hyperintense aspect on T_1 linked to the presence of melanin.

Spinal Cord Tumour Mimics

It may be difficult or impossible to differentiate spinal cord tumours from intramedullary non-neoplastic lesions. In one series of 212 patients undergoing surgery for intramedullary spinal cord 'tumours', Lee et al. reported 4% of non-neoplastic lesions.[38] A variety of lesions may mimic a spinal cord tumour such as vascular cavernous malformations (cavernomas) (Fig. 56-14), tumefactive demyelinating lesions in multiple sclerosis (MS), neuromyelitis optica (NMO) (Fig. 56-15) and acute disseminating encephalomyelitis (ADEM), acute transverse myelitis (ATM), spinal cord contusion and spinal cord infarction. Also, sarcoidosis and vasculitis may mimic a spinal cord tumour. The clinical picture, laboratory findings, electrophysiological testing, and, finally, additional MR imaging of the brain may help to recognise these entities properly, in order to avoid unnecessary biopsy.

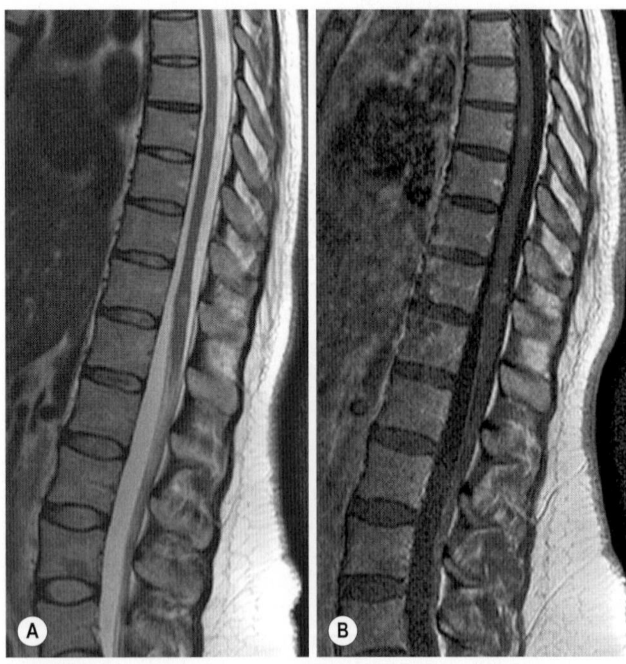

FIGURE 56-13 ■ **Spinal cord metastases.** Sagittal T_2 (A) shows two discrete areas of high signal intensity centrally within the spinal cord at the Th8 and Th11 levels. There is no obvious spinal cord oedema. Sagittal gadolinium-enhanced T_1 (B) shows enhancement of the lesions in this 35-year-old woman with advanced breast carcinoma. MR imaging of the brain, performed at the same time (not shown), demonstrated multiple brain metastases in both cerebral and cerebellar hemispheres.

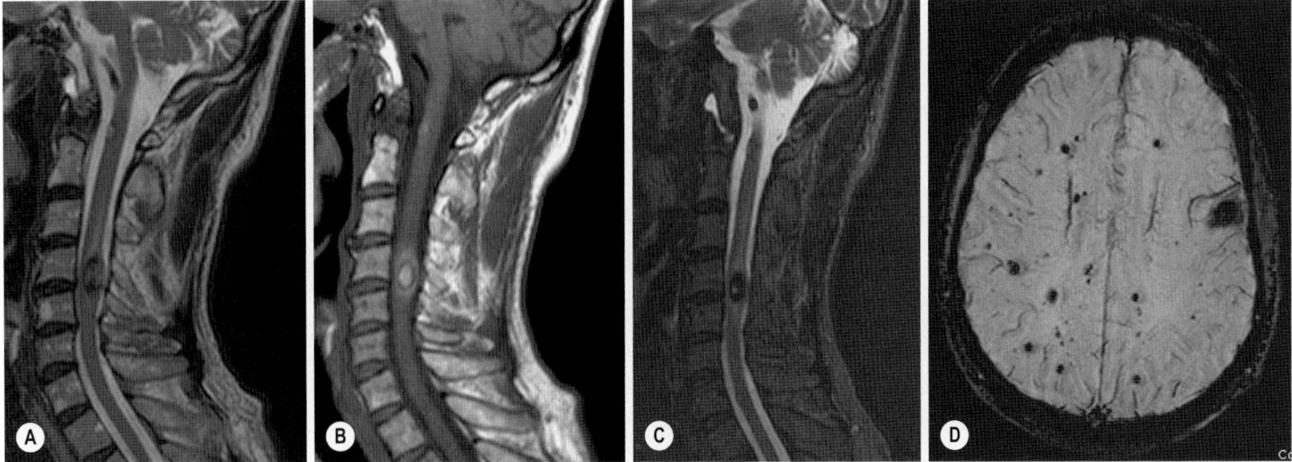

FIGURE 56-14 ■ Multiple cavernomas in a patient with familial cavernomatosis. Sagittal T_2 (A), sagittal T_1 (B) and sagittal GRE T_2* (C). The typical 'mulberry' or 'popcorn' aspect, typical white and black aspect of this C4–C5 lesion. A small, at the C2 level. cavernous malformation, especially on the T_2. This imaging sequence best demonstrates the signs of chronic bleeding within the lesion. There is no perilesional oedema. The lesion is spontaneously partly hyperintense on T_1 and enhances moderately after contrast administration. Axial susceptibility-weighted imaging (SWI) of the brain (D) shows numerous cavernomas.

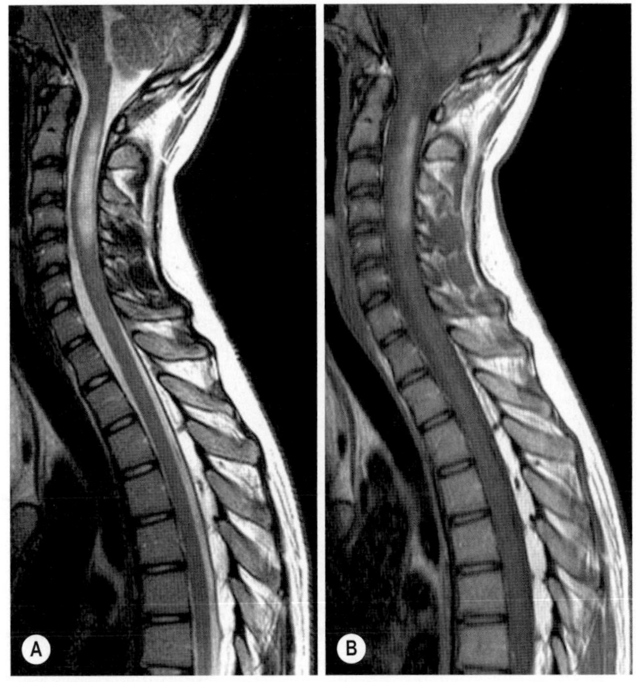

FIGURE 56-15 ■ Neuromyelitis optica. Sagittal T_2 (A) shows an ill-defined area of high signal intensity extending across 3–4 spinal segments; mild enlargement of the spinal cord is noticed. Sagittal gadolinium-enhanced T_1 (B) shows patchy enhancement of the lesion. Knowledge of a clinical history of neuritis optica and normal MR imaging findings of the brain enable the correct diagnosis to be made.

Cavernous Malformation (Cavernoma). Cavernous malformations (also known as cavernous angiomas, or cavernomas) represent 7–10% of all intramedullary tumours. They most commonly involve the thoracic spinal cord segments. These vascular malformations may remain clinically silent for a long period of time before an acute and rapidly progressive neurological deficit occurs due to bleeding. Before the advent of MR imaging, these lesions were extremely difficult to diagnose, especially in the spinal cord, as they usually are small and do not enlarge the spinal cord. Intramedullary cavernous malformations are usually easily recognised thanks to the typical 'black and white' or 'popcorn' appearance due to areas of mixed signal intensity on both T_1 and T_2 or T_2* (Figs. 56-14A–C). Contrast enhancement is variable. As patients with spinal cord cavernomas tend to have multiple other malformations elsewhere in the neuraxis, and also a higher association with familial cavernomatosis, we recommend performing MR imaging of the brain (Fig. 56-14D) whenever the diagnosis of an intramedullary cavernous malformation is suspected.[39]

Intradural Extramedullary Tumours

Intradural extramedullary tumours result in displacement of the cord to the contralateral side and widening of the ipsilateral CSF space. Patients with intradural extramedullary neoplasms frequently present with progressive myelopathy. Weakness is the most common symptom, and diffuse back pain or radicular pain may be present. Most intradural extramedullary tumours are benign. They originate either in a spinal nerve or from the meninges. The differential diagnosis for lesions in this location is limited and can be further narrowed with knowledge of specific imaging characteristics.[40]

Meningiomas and nerve sheath tumours make up for about 90% of all extramedullary intradural tumours. Schwannomas are the most common intradural extramedullary tumours. In the paediatric population, the most common intradural extramedullary neoplasms are leptomeningeal metastases resulting from primary brain tumours.[18,40] Primary tumours in this location are less frequently observed and are mostly schwannomas and neurofibromas in NF-2 and NF-1 patients, respectively.[18]

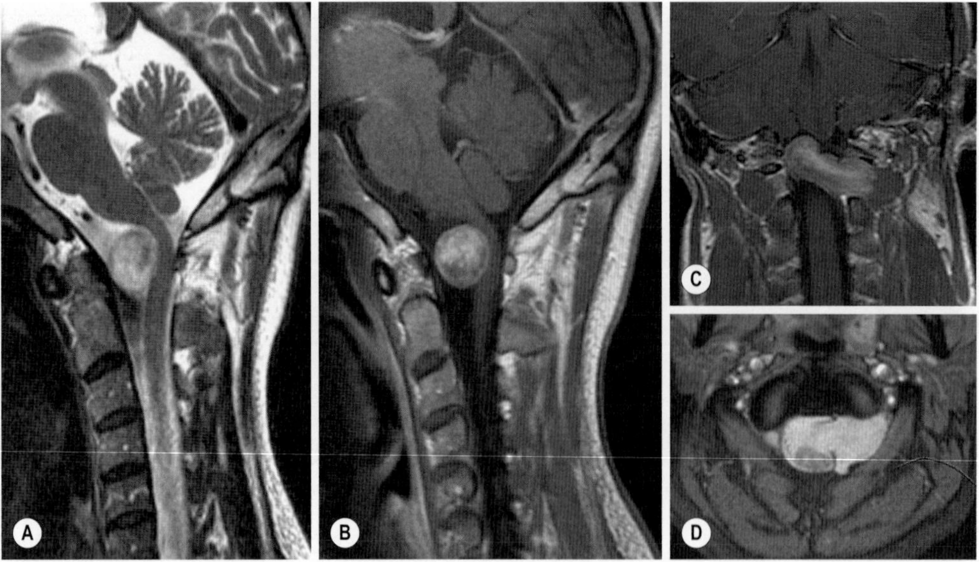

FIGURE 56-16 ■ **Upper cervical neurinoma in a patient with neurofibromatosis type 1.** Sagittal (A) and axial (D) T_2 show a well-delineated mass with high signal intensity. The spinal cord is displaced posteriorly and is compressed by the tumour, which extends through the left C2–C3 neuroforamen. Sagittal (B) and coronal (C) gadolinium-enhanced T_1 show intense contrast enhancement. The axial and coronal planes best show the typical dumbbell aspect of spinal neurinomas involving both the intra- and extradural space, and facilitate discrimination between neurinoma and meningioma (see Fig. 56-20).

Nerve Sheath Tumours: Schwannoma and Neurofibroma

Schwannomas, aka neurinomas or neurilemmomas, are considered benign tumours (WHO grade 1) and represent the most common intradural extramedullary tumours. Schwannomas are usually solitary (Fig. 56-16) and are more commonly seen in adults. Although far less common in children, multiple schwannomas occur in children with NF-2[41] (Fig. 56-17). In these patients the risk of malignant transformation is higher. Typically, schwannomas arise from the dorsal sensory nerve roots.[42] The vast majority (70%) of schwannomas are purely intradural extramedullary tumours, 15% are extradural and 15% have a 'dumbbell' shape involving both the intra- and extradural space (Fig. 56-16). Schwannomas are mostly found at the cervical and lumbar region and less frequently at the thoracic level. On MR imaging, schwannomas are usually well-encapsulated tumours that may have cystic components. They are usually iso-intense to the spinal cord in most cases while some 20% are moderately hypointense on T_1. On T_2, schwannomas are hyperintense (Fig. 56-16A). Calcification and haemorrhage are rare. Contrast enhancement may vary and can be intense and homogeneous or only show faint peripheral enhancement (Figs. 56-16–56-18).[42] Giant schwannomas are typically encountered at the lumbar level and it may be difficult sometimes to discriminate them from myxopapillary ependymoma.[43,44] The distribution of the roots of the cauda equina in the thecal sac on axial imaging may help in distinguishing these tumours: a myxopapillary ependymoma of the filum pushes the roots to the periphery of the thecal sac, whereas a schwannoma of the cauda more often pushes the roots together in an eccentric fashion.[44]

Neurofibromas are not well encapsulated, are ill-defined and often present as multiple tumours. MR imaging usually does not enable differentiation between schwannoma and neurofibroma when the tumour is solitary. In NF-1, multiple plexiform neurofibromas are typically encountered: they are iso-/hyperintense on T_2 and a 'target sign' (hyperintense rim with low/intermediate centre) may be observed. Enhancement is usually mild. Malignant degeneration may occur rarely, mainly in the case of NF-2.

Meningioma

Meningiomas are mainly dural-based intradural tumours. More than 95% of meningiomas are benign tumours (WHO grade 1). They are the second most common intraspinal tumours, occurring most frequently in older patients (peak age in the fifth and sixth decades).[4] Meningiomas are uncommon tumours in the paediatric age group outside the setting of NF-2.[18,40] Overall, 80% of meningiomas are found in the thoracic region, with a female preponderance. In men, however, only half of the meningiomas are in the thoracic region and another 40% are cervical. Meningiomas are mostly located posterolaterally in the thoracic region (Fig. 56-19) and anteriorly in the cervical region (Fig. 56-20).[6] They are usually solitary tumours, but multiple meningiomas, which occur in 2% of affected patients, are most often associated with NF-2.[41] Meningiomas are very slowly growing and major cord compression may be seen with only minor symptoms.

On CT, meningiomas are iso- to hyperattenuating. The hyperattenuation reflects the cellular nature of these lesions, but the presence of calcification also contributes. Hyperostosis may be seen but is not as common as in the

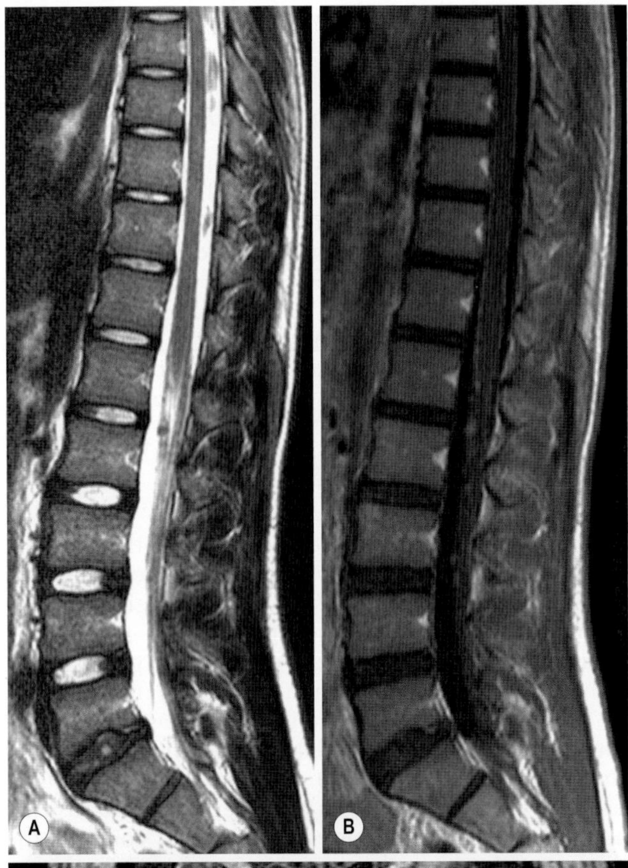

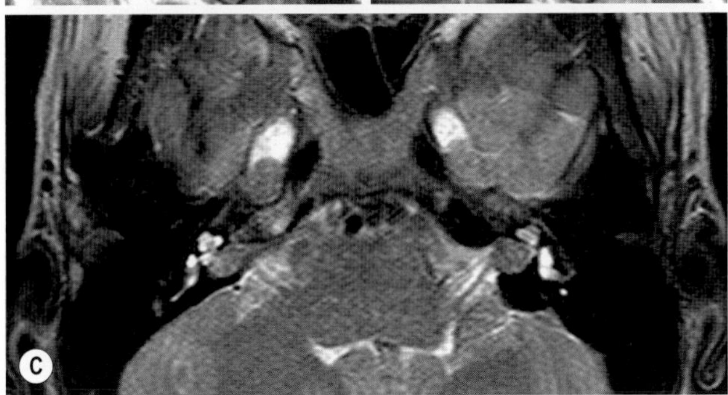

FIGURE 56-17 ■ Multiple schwannomas in a young boy. The MR examination was performed to further characterise a subcutaneous lesion at the L1 level, which was observed clinically. Sagittal T_2 (A) shows some discrete, small nodules attached to the nerve roots of the cauda equina. On sagittal (B) gadolinium-enhanced T_1, many more of these lesions can be observed and show intense contrast enhancement. Axial brain T_2 (C) at the level of the internal auditory canals shows bilateral vestibular nerve schwannomas, pathognomonic for the diagnosis of neurofibromatosis type 2. Bilateral trigeminal nerve schwannomas located within Meckel's cave can be observed.

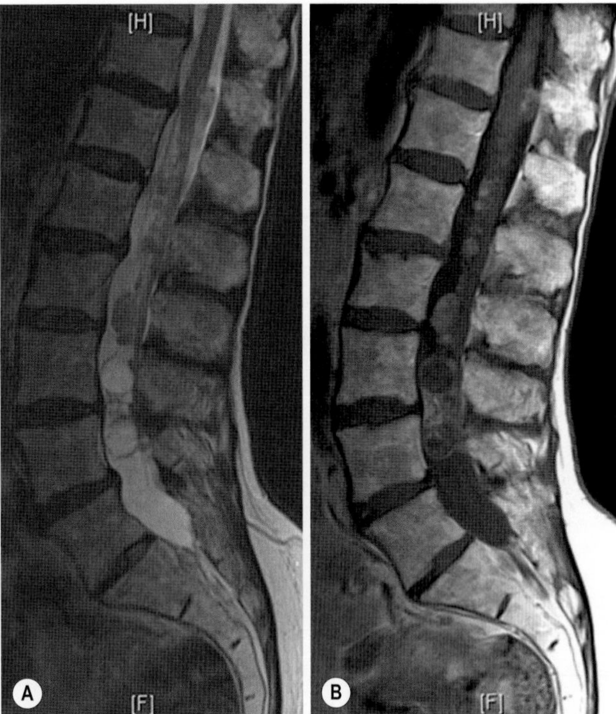

FIGURE 56-18 ■ Multiple neurofibromas in a young woman with neurofibromatosis type 1. Sagittal T_2 (A) and sagittal gadolinium-enhanced T_1 (B) show multiple bulky and nodular tumours arising from spinal nerve roots which are a typically representation of neurofibromatosis type 1. They are iso- to hyperintense on T_2 and show strong homogeneous enhancement. MR imaging of the complete neuraxis is mandatory in the work-up of neurofibromatosis patients.

intracranial forms. This is due, in part, to the more prominent epidural fat within the spine.[40] On MR imaging, meningiomas are iso- to hypointense on T_1 and slightly hyperintense on T_2. There is a strong and homogeneous enhancement with gadolinium (Figs. 56-19B, C and 56-20C, D), except for the calcified areas. Some meningiomas are heavily calcified and dark on all sequences with only little contrast uptake. The classical 'dural tail' may be seen (Figs. 56-19B and 56-20C, D) although this aspect is less frequently and less typically found in the spine compared to the intracranial location.[42] Meningiomas may cause compression and displacement of the spinal cord (Figs. 56-19 and 56-20). Signal changes in the spinal cord secondary to compression can be seen (Fig. 56-21C), but are usually rare.[4]

Metastases

Leptomeningeal metastases are secondary tumours that may arise from a malignant primary neoplasm outside the CNS, such as a breast, lung or other neoplasm (Fig. 56-21), or from the spread of a CNS tumour, i.e. the so-called 'drop metastasis'. Common primary CNS tumours that may spread to the leptomeninges are medulloblastoma (Fig. 56-3), choroid plexus papilloma and carcinoma, ependymoma and high-grade glioma. Leptomeningeal dissemination from CNS neoplasms occurs in younger patients, whereas metastases from lung or breast carcinomas are more frequently observed in older patients.[4] MR imaging is more sensitive than CSF cytology for the detection of subarachnoid spread of primary brain tumours, though CSF cytology may be more sensitive for CSF spread of leukaemias and lymphomas.[45,46] Contrast-enhanced series are the imaging technique of choice to assess for metastasis. Leptomeningeal metastases demonstrate three patterns of enhancement: (1) diffuse contrast enhancement along the pia of the

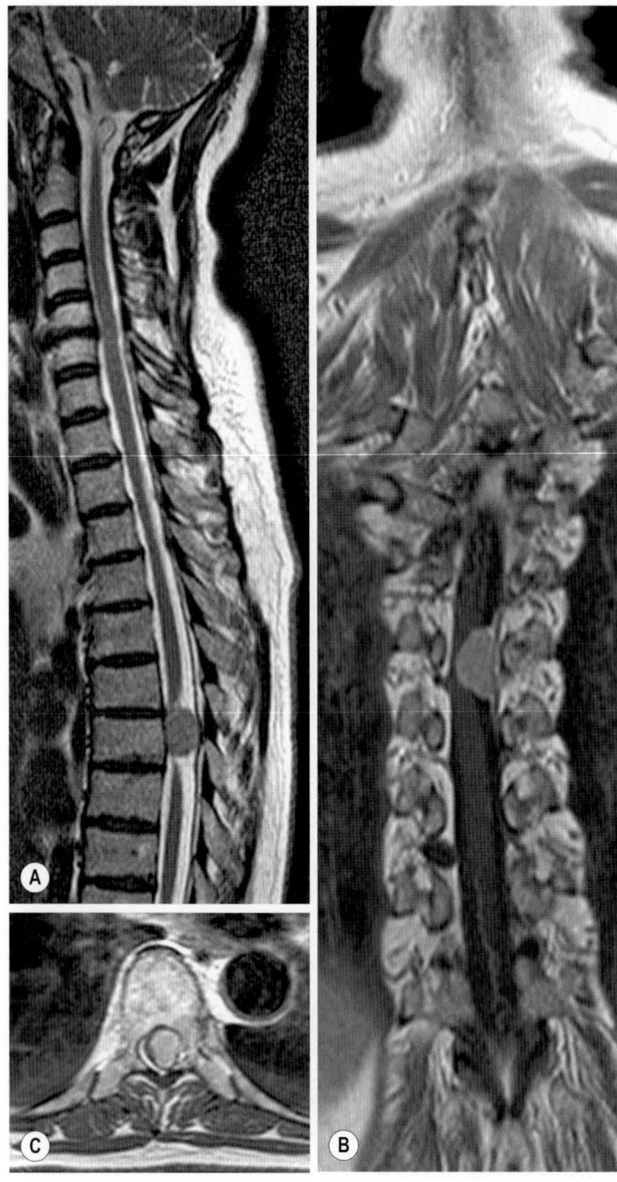

FIGURE 56-19 ■ **Mid-thoracic meningioma.** Sagittal T_2 (A) demonstrates an ovoid intradural extramedullary mass at the Th7 level. The lesion is slightly hyperintense relative to the spinal cord. Coronal (B) and axial (C) gadolinium-enhanced T_1 show avid contrast enhancement. Note the broad attachment to the dura with the presence of a typical dural tail. The tumour causes severe spinal canal narrowing and spinal cord compression and right lateral displacement of the spinal cord.

spinal cord and nerve roots, hence the name 'sugar coating' pattern; (2) multiple small contrast-enhancing nodules in the subarachnoid space (Fig. 56-21B); and (3) as a single contrast-enhancing mass.[4] However, sometimes metastases may not enhance, and careful inspection of T_2 or myelographic sequences is needed (Fig. 56-21C).

Less-Frequent Extramedullary Tumours

Less-frequent intradural, extramedullary tumours include paraganglioma, lipoma, epidermoid and dermoid cysts. In patients with von VHLs, intradural-extramedullary haemangioblastoma[30] and haemangioblastoma arising from the proximal spinal nerve roots[47] have been described (Fig. 56-22).

Intradural Extramedullary Tumour Mimics

The differential diagnosis of intradural extramedullary tumours also include cysts and cyst-like lesions (arachnoid cysts, epidermoid and dermoid cysts, and teratoma, neuroenteric cysts), degenerative lesions (extruded disc fragment, discal cyst, juxtafacet cyst), inflammatory disorders affecting the nerve roots (Guillain–Barré syndrome, arachnoiditis, chronic interstitial demyelinating polyneuropathy (CIDP)) and, finally, infectious and granulomatous disorders (e.g. Lyme disease, sarcoidosis, Wegener's granulomatosis).[4]

Extradural Tumours

Extradural tumours are the most frequently observed spinal tumours; most of them originate from the vertebrae. Two-thirds of all spinal column lesions in children (<18) are benign, but this figure is reversed in adults.[48] Seventy-five per cent of vertebral body lesions are malignant, whereas benign lesions are mostly found in the posterior elements (70%).[48] Metastatic disease, multiple myeloma and lymphoproliferative tumours of the spine (e.g. lymphoma) commonly cause multiple lesions, which, in association with the clinical data, usually allow the diagnosis to be easily made. In contrast, the diagnosis of primary bone tumours must be considered when a solitary lesion is diagnosed.[2] Benign lesions are often asymptomatic and are frequently incidental findings on plain films realised, for example, after trauma. Pain was the most common presenting symptom, affecting 75% of the benign and 95% of the malignant tumours.[49] Extension of the tumour in the anterior epidural space displaces the lateral aspect of the posterior longitudinal ligament. However, this is limited by a strong medial fixation by the medial meningovertebral ligament (ligament of Trolard–Hofmann), giving a bilobular intracanalar aspect in the axial images, which is commonly called 'curtain sign' or 'draped curtain sign'. It may be observed in a variety of spinal tumours (Figs. 56-2, 56-23, 56-25, 56-38, and 56-39), both benign and malignant (Figs. 56-24–56-39), as well in other non-tumoural conditions such as epidural haematoma, epidural and abscesses. Epidural extension of the tumour may cause compression of the spinal cord or cauda equina with (progressive) paraplegia, saddle anaesthesia, urinary retention, incontinence and sexual dysfunction.

A multi-technique approach (CT, MR imaging, bone scintigraphy, PET) is often necessary to define the characteristics and extent of extradural spine neoplasms and bone scintigraphy is useful in detecting multiple lesions and distant metastases.[48] Because of the complex anatomy of the vertebrae, CT is more useful than plain film radiography for evaluating lesion location and analysing bone destruction, sclerosis and/or remodelling.[6] A wide variety of tumours that affect the bony spine may be encountered. It is possible to characterise these lesions based on the age of the patient, multiplicity, level in the spine and location within the vertebra. The differential

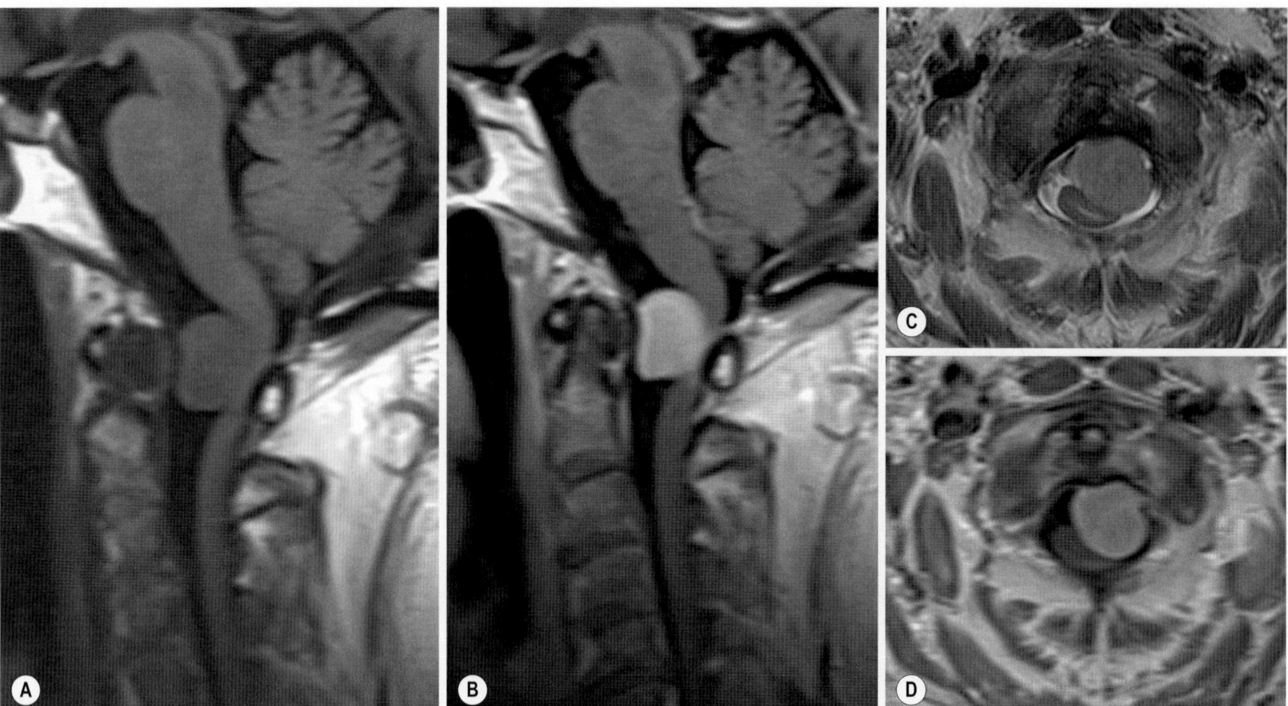

FIGURE 56-20 ■ **Upper cervical meningioma.** Sagittal T_1 (A) and gadolinium-enhanced T_1 (B) show an ovoid intradural extramedullary mass anteriorly in the spinal canal. The lesion is slightly hypointense when compared to the spinal cord and shows intense and homogeneous enhancement. A broad dural attachment can be observed. Compression and posterolateral displacement of the upper cervical cord by the tumour can be seen on the axial T_2 (C) and gadolinium-enhanced T_1 (D). A discrete area of high signal intensity on the axial T_2 can be seen, indicative of spinal cord oedema or compressive myelomalacia.

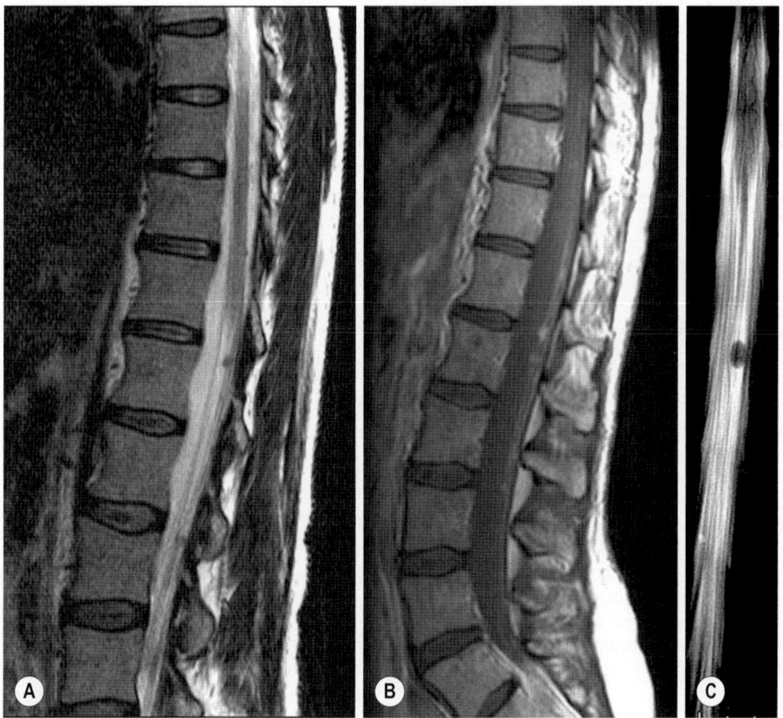

FIGURE 56-21 ■ **Intradural extramedullary metastases in a young woman with aggressive cervical cancer.** Sagittal T_2 (A) and sagittal gadolinium-enhanced T_1 (B) MR myelography (C). Nodular enhancing lesions along the nerve roots of the cauda equina are observed. Without proper clinical information, these lesions are indiscernible from multiple schwannomas as typically encountered in patients with NF-2 (see Fig. 56-17).

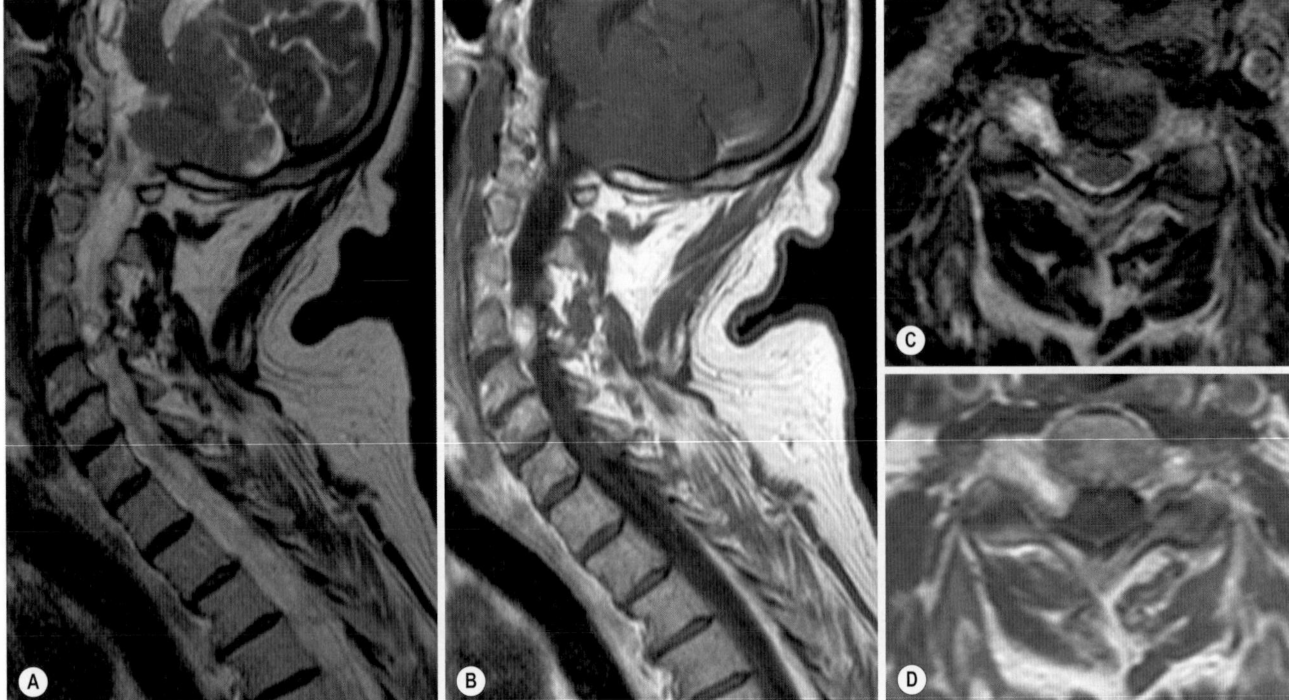

FIGURE 56-22 ■ Haemangioblastoma arising from the right C6 nerve in a patient with VHL syndrome. Sagittal T_2 (A) and contrast-enhanced T_1 (B) show the presence of a mass lesion laterally within the spinal canal. Intense enhancement of the lesion is observed. On axial T_2 (C) and Gd-enhanced T_1 (D), the lesion is arising from the right C6 proximal nerve root and can be classified as a combined intradural–extradural lesion, extending from the spinal canal towards the C5–C6 neuroforamen, which is enlarged.

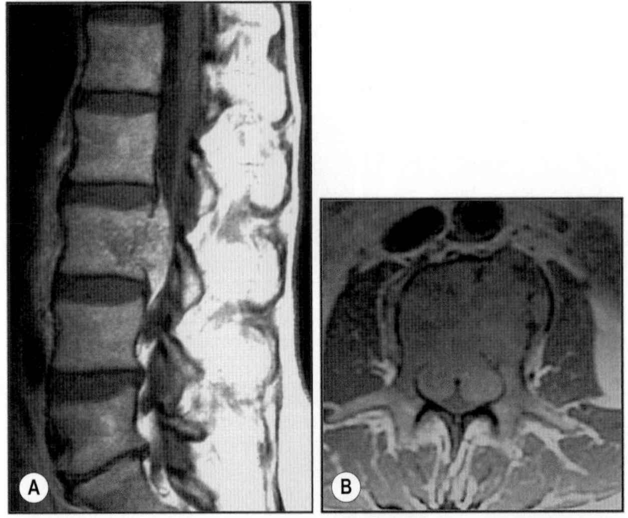

FIGURE 56-23 ■ Curtain sign in a patient with chordoma of L3. Sagittal (A) and axial (B) contrast-enhanced T_1 show a lesion located in the posterior aspect of the vertebral body with destruction of the posterior wall and extension into the anterior epidural space. A 'curtain sign' or 'draped curtain sign' is described whereby the midline is spared because of an intact ventral meningovertebral ligament, running from the anterior wall of the thecal sac to the posterior longitudinal ligament and vertebral endostium. These ligaments are significantly developed at the level of the conus and are known as the sacrodural ligaments of Trolard and Hofmann.

diagnosis can be further narrowed by evaluating the imaging findings, including morphology (border, matrix, expansion, soft-tissue involvement, etc.), density or signal intensity of lesions on CT and MR imaging, as well as pattern of contrast enhancement.[6]

Metastatic Spine Disease

Metastatic disease to the spine is the most frequent spinal tumour. Past or concurrent history of a primary tumour is generally available to suggest this diagnosis, but may need to be ascertained if the history is absent. Osteolytic metastases are most often caused by carcinoma of the lung, breast, thyroid, kidney and colon and (in childhood) neuroblastoma. Osteoblastic metastases are most commonly caused by prostate carcinoma in elderly men and by breast cancer in women. Metastasis to the spine most often involves the thoracic spine (70%), followed by the lumbar (20%) and cervical spine (10%). Multiple spinal levels are affected in about 30% of patients. Most frequently metastasis affects the vertebral body, but all parts of the vertebra may be affected. Vertebral compression fracture and epidural tumour extension are common in metastases.[2,6,48] Spinal metastases usually present as lytic lesions on plain film radiography, but one should keep in mind that metastatic disease is primarily a process of trabecular bone; plain film radiography is a cortical bone imaging technique. There must be 50 to 75% bone destruction for plain film radiographs to identify these lesions. On CT, metastatic disease presents as multiple lytic lesions of different size, with irregular non-sclerotic margins, often with cortical breakthrough

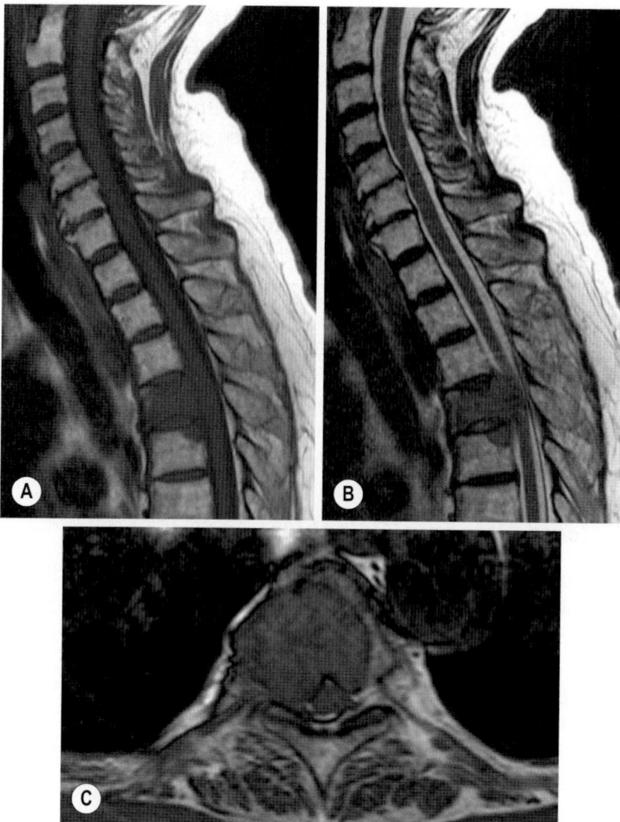

FIGURE 56-24 ■ **MR imaging shows osteoblastic metastatic disease in a woman with breast carcinoma.** Most metastases are hypointense on the sagittal T_1 (A) and when sclerotoc/osteoblastic they are also hypointense on T_2 (B). MRI better delineates the soft tissue extension of the tumour into the paraspinal and epidural soft tissues (C).

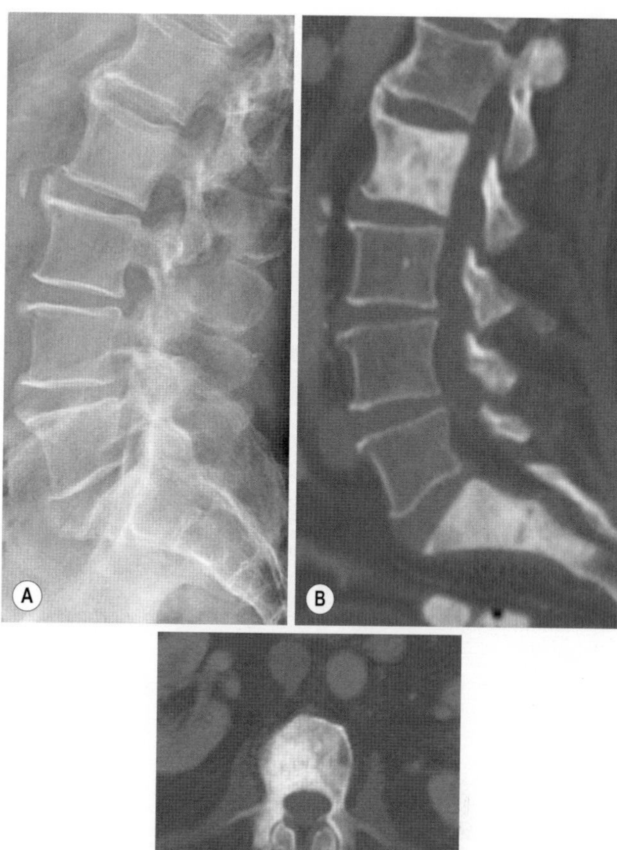

FIGURE 56-25 ■ **Metastatic spine disease in a patient with prostate carcinoma.** Lateral plain film radiography of the lumbar spine (A) shows a slight increased density of the L2 vertebral body. On sagittal (B) and axial (C) CT images, the lesion has the typical aspect of a 'ivory vertebra' due to the bony sclerosis. There is extension of the lesion in the right lateral pedicle. Additional osteoblastic metastases can be observed in S1 and S2.

and paravertebral or epidural extension. Osteoblastic metastases will show increased density and sclerosis and may have the aspect of an 'ivory vertebra' (Fig. 56-24). MR imaging is the preferred imaging technique in the evaluation of patients with suspected spinal metastasis. It allows imaging of the spine in one setting with greater sensitivity than bone imaging and delineates the soft-tissue extension of the tumour into the paraspinal and epidural soft tissues (Fig. 56-25C). On MR imaging most metastases are hypointense on T_1 (Fig. 56-25A). On T_2 they can be either dark (sclerotic) (Fig. 56-25B) or, more frequently, show high signal. Marked enhancement after contrast administration is the rule.

Primary Vertebral Tumours

Primary tumours of the vertebral column make up 10% of all spinal tumours and are rare compared with secondary malignancies. Primary vertebral tumours affect both the adult and the paediatric population and may be benign, locally aggressive, or malignant. Benign primary vertebral tumours include haemangioma, osteoid osteoma and osteoblastoma, aneurysmal bone cyst and eosinophilic granuloma. More locally aggressive primary vertebral tumours include chordoma and giant-cell tumour (GCT), whereas the most frequent malignant tumours are chondrosarcoma, Ewing's sarcoma, multiple myeloma or plasmacytoma, and osteosarcoma.[50] In a review of the Leeds Regional Bone Tumour Registry for primary bone tumours of the spine (1958–2000), chordoma was the most frequent tumour in the cervical and sacral regions, while the most common diagnosis overall was multiple myeloma and plasmacytoma. Osteosarcoma ranked third.[49]

Benign Primary Vertebral Tumours

Vertebral Haemangioma

Vertebral haemangiomas are the most common benign spinal tumours, and the majority of lesions are discovered incidentally on spinal imaging performed for other purposes. In up to 30% of patients multiple lesions are observed. More than half of all vertebral haemangiomas are seen in the thoracic and lumbar spine. Most haemangiomas occur in the vertebral body, but about 10% may extend in the pedicles and even the spinous process may be involved. Two types of vertebral haemangioma exist: benign, asymptomatic lesions (Fig. 56-26), and more

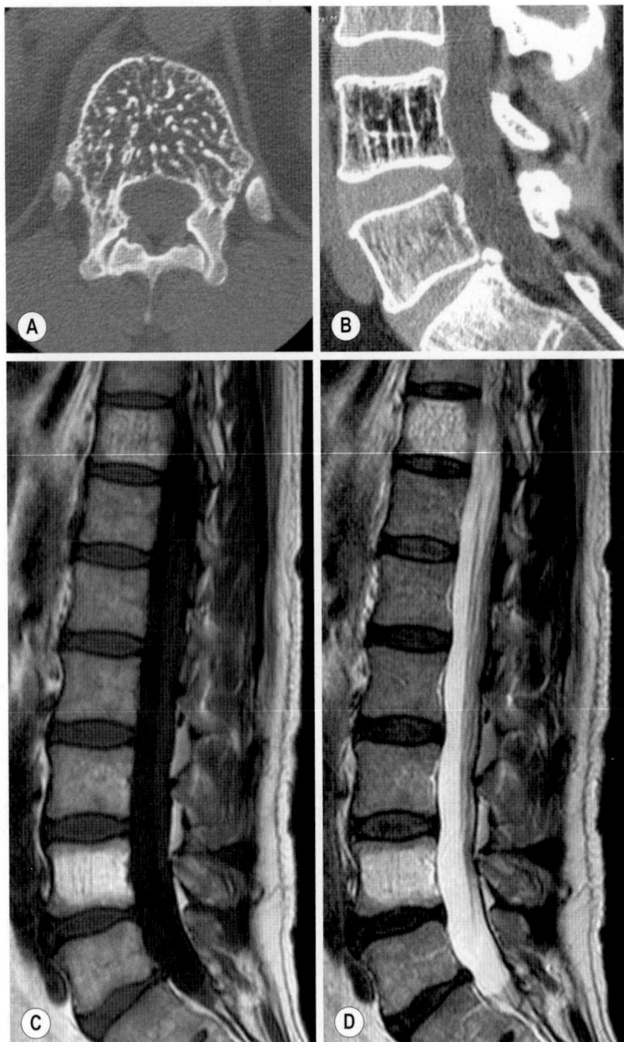

FIGURE 56-26 ■ **Asymptomatic vertebral haemangioma.** Axial CT (A) shows numerous high-attenuation dots within the vertebral bone marrow, simulating the 'polka-dot' pattern on clothing. On a sagittal reformatted image (B) a so-called 'corduroy sign' may be observed: vertically oriented, thickened trabeculations, replacing the normal cancellous bone, surrounded by fatty bone marrow or vascular lacunae. Sagittal T_1 (C) and T_2 (D) MR images show high (fat) signal intensity throughout the Th11 and L4 vertebral body with linear striations of low signal intensity due to thickened trabeculae.

aggressive, symptomatic ones, with compression of the spinal cord (Fig. 56-27).[6] Pregnancy may contribute to the development of aggressive and symptomatic haemangiomas, which is hypothesised to be caused by an increase in blood volume and cardiac output.[51]

The typical radiographic appearance of a haemangioma is characteristic, consisting of parallel linear streaks ('jail bar') in a vertebral body of overall decreased density, or 'honeycomb' pattern which may be also appreciated on sagittal reformatted images (Fig. 56-26B). Transverse CT shows the pattern as multiple dots, also known as 'polka-dot' pattern (Fig. 56-26A), representing a cross-section of reinforced trabeculae.[52] The key features that differentiate haemangiomas from other similar tumours are a hyperintense signal on T_1 (Fig. 56-26C) and T_2 (Fig. 56-26D).[51] The fibroadipose tissue insinuated between the sinusoidal blood channels results in the increased T_1 signal pattern. These lesions will decrease in signal intensity on T_2 with fat saturation and will demonstrate contrast enhancement after gadolinium injection.[48] Low signal intensity on T_1 may indicate a more aggressive lesion with the potential to compress the spinal cord (Fig. 56-27A).[53] Aggressive lesions are characterised by a prominent soft-tissue component that can invade the epidural space and encroach on the spinal cord (Fig. 56-27).[48,54] The radiographic and CT appearances of compressive vertebral haemangiomas can be misleading, with irregular trabeculae and lytic areas; poorly defined, expanded cortex; and soft-tissue expansion.[2] Transarterial embolisation is an effective treatment for painful intraosseous haemangioma and is useful in reducing intraoperative blood loss before decompressive surgery.[55]

Osteoid Osteoma/Osteoblastoma

Osteoid osteomas (OOs) and osteoblastomas are histologically similar benign tumours consisting of osteoblasts that produce osteoid and woven bone.[56] OOs are smaller (less than 1.5 cm), well-contained, self-limited lesions, whereas osteoblastomas are larger (greater than 1.5 cm) and may undergo malignant transformation.[48] The peak incidence for OO is in the second decade. The average age at presentation is 17 years. Men are more affected than women (2–4:1). OO accounts for about 10% of all bone tumours involving the spine.[6] Almost 60% occur in the lumbar spine, 30% in the cervical spine and 10% in the thoracic spine. OO is a lesion of the posterior elements[57] with 50% of lesions arising in the lamina or pedicles and 20% in the articular processes.[48] Localised pain at the site of the lesion—classically worse at night—is the most common clinical presentation.[51] The pain is presumed to be caused by the presence of nerve endings in the nidus that are stimulated by vascular pressure and the production of prostaglandins, which explains the clinical response of these tumours to non-steroidal anti-inflammatory drugs (NSAIDs) such as aspirin.[48] Not infrequently, patients with spinal OO have a painful scoliosis.[6]

Plain film radiography may show a lucent nidus, frequently with small calcifications. Surrounding the nidus is variable bone sclerosis. The complex anatomy of the spine makes the detection and localisation of a radiolucent nidus obscured by reactive sclerosis much more difficult than that of a nidus located in a long bone.[2] Especially when there is extensive bone sclerosis, the nidus is much easier to distinguish on CT.[58] The nidus can be seen on CT as an area of low attenuation with various degrees of surrounding sclerosis (Fig. 56-28).[51] CT is the primary imaging technique used for diagnosis and to guide minimally invasive treatment such as interstitial laser ablation.[59] OOs can also be detected with MR imaging, with the nidus appearing as a hypointense lesion surrounded by marrow oedema on T_2. On T_1, the nidus can have an intermediate signal intensity and areas of signal voids resulting from calcification.[57] Enhancement within the nidus or perinidal marrow can be seen after gadolinium administration and can increase the sensitivity of the imaging study.[57]

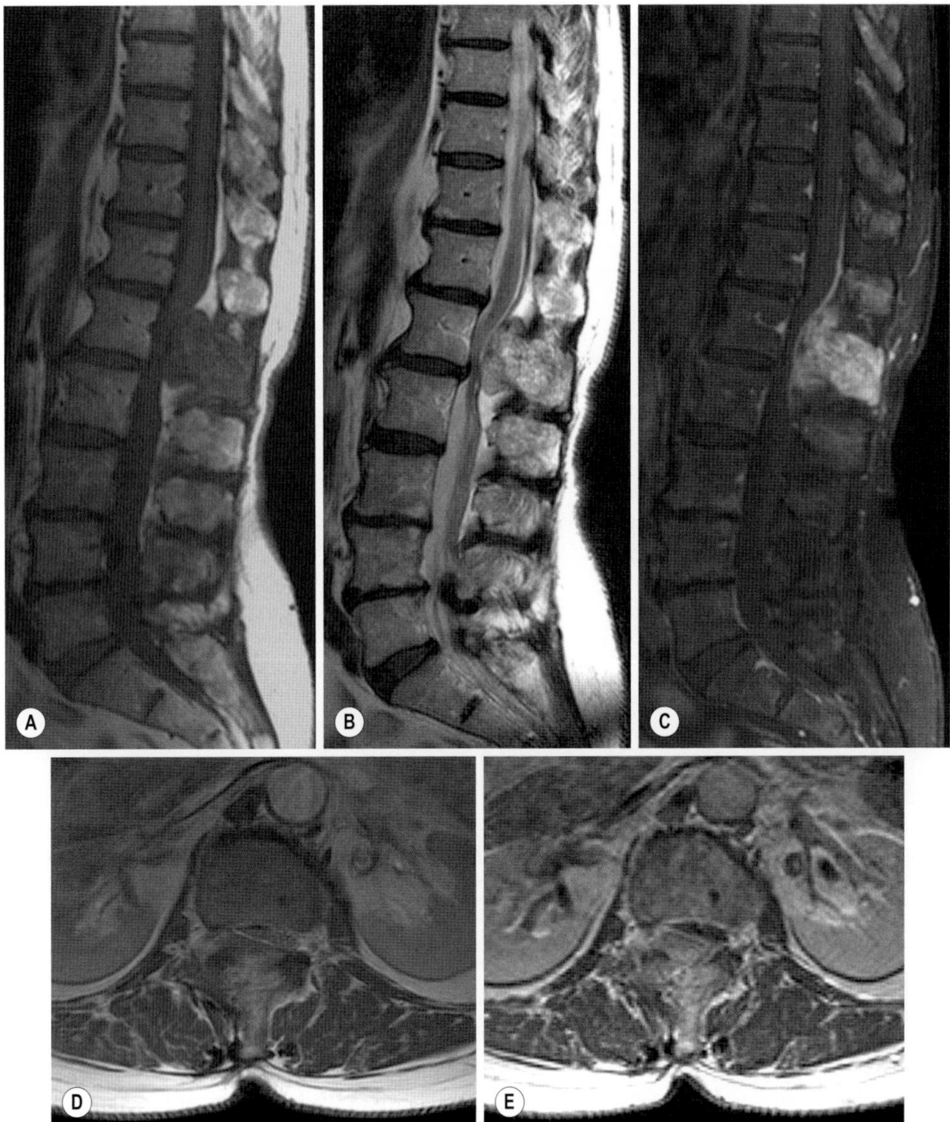

FIGURE 56-27 ■ Aggressive variant of vertebral haemangioma. Expansile lesion involving the posterior elements at the L1 level, leaving the pedicles and vertebral body intact. The lesion has low signal intensity on sagittal T_1 (A). Invasion of the posterior epidural space can be better evaluated on sagittal T_2 (B). Fat-suppressed gadolinium-enhanced T_1 (C) shows strong enhancement of the lesion. Axial T_2 (D) and gadolinium-enhanced T_1 (E) better show the mass effect of the tumour compressing the thecal sac, resulting in spinal stenosis with compression of the cauda equina.

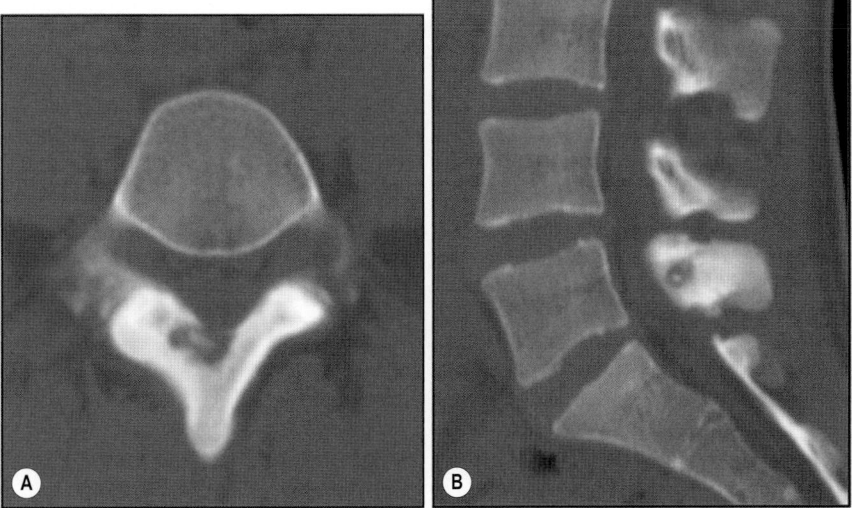

FIGURE 56-28 ■ Osteoid osteoma of the posterior elements. Axial CT image (A) and sagittal reformatted image (B) show a sclerotic bone lesion with a small central lucent nidus and dense calcified centre arising at the junction of the laminae of the L5 vertebra.

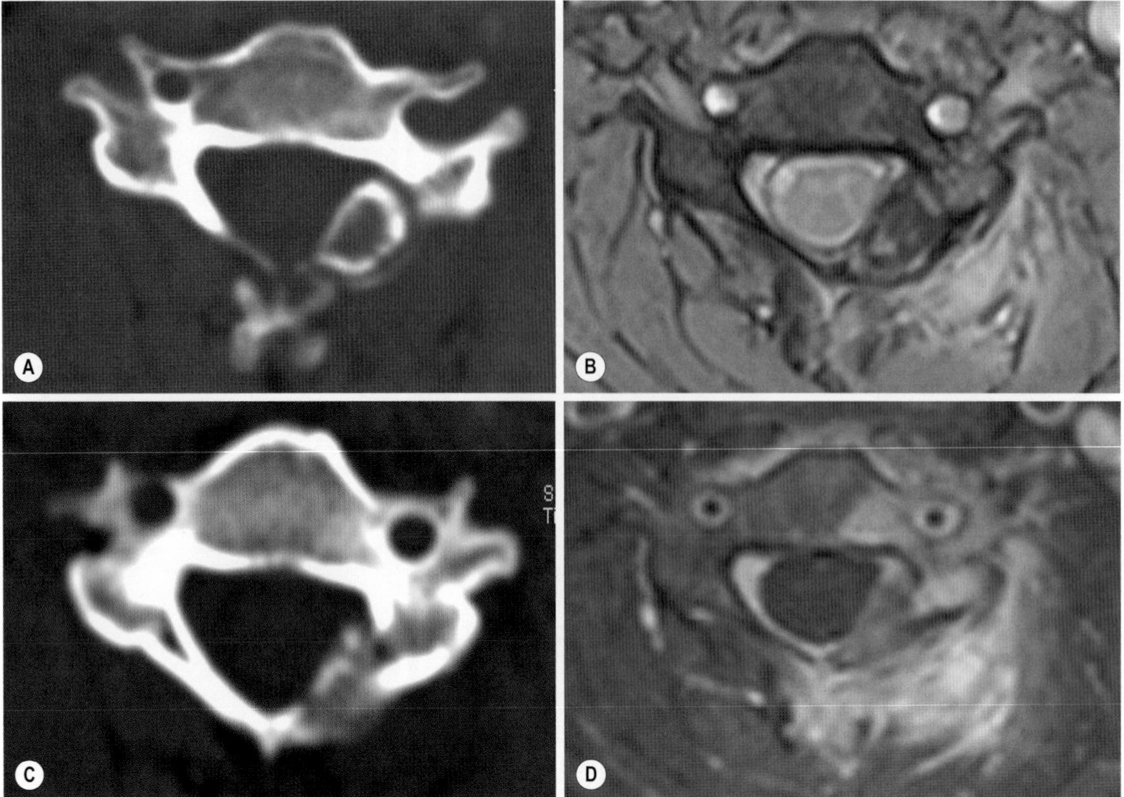

FIGURE 56-29 ■ Osteoblastoma of the vertebral arch. Axial CT images (A, B) demonstrate a partially calcified lesion at the left vertebral lamina. On axial T_1 (C) merely low signal intensity of the calcified lesion's component. Corresponding T_1 after contrast injection (D) shows marked contrast enhancement of the surrounding osseous and soft tissues.

Osteoblastoma

Osteblastomas are related to OOs, and by definition, are larger than 1.5 cm in diameter. They also have the tendency to affect the posterior part of the spine (Fig. 56-29) and present with pain. Osteoblastomas can be more aggressive than OOs and more often require surgical resection. The recurrency rate is about 10%, which is also higher than that seen with OOs.[6] Osteoblastoma has a similar appearance on CT, but displays less reactive sclerosis. The finding of central expansion similar to that of an aneurysmal bone cyst has also been described in spinal osteoblastoma.[51]

Aneurysmal Bone Cyst

Historically, aneurysmal bone cyst (ABC) was considered to be a variant of giant cell tumour (GCT). The microscopic appearances of the two lesions are sometimes strikingly similar, and they are occasionally indistinguishable.[60] Although ABC is classified as a primary bone tumour in many textbooks and scientific papers, Saccomanni states that ABC is a non-neoplastic reactive condition, which is aggressive in its ability to destroy and expand bone. The aetiology of an ABC is uncertain. It may occur in bone as a solitary lesion or can be found in association with other tumours such as GCT (Fig. 56-1) and chondroblastoma.[61] After osteoid osteoma and osteoblastoma, ABC is the third most frequent benign bone tumour.[62] Approximately 20 to 35% of ABC occur in the spine, and ABCs represent 15% of all primary spine tumours.[63]

They afflict predominantly children, with 60% of patients being younger than 20 years.[61] The peak incidence is during the second decade of life, and they are slightly more common in female individuals.[64] They have a predilection for the lumbar spine, followed by equal occurrence in the thoracic and cervical spine. Of aneurysmal bone cysts, 60% occur in the pedicles, laminae and spinous processes;[61] however, the lesions can involve all aspects of the vertebrae, including the vertebral body. Clinical presentation includes pain, neurological deficit, and often scoliosis or kyphosis.[63]

Four radiological stages have been described by Kransdorf et al.: initial, active, stabilisation and healing.[60] In the initial phase, the lesion is characterised by a well-defined area of osteolysis. This is followed by a growth phase, in which the lesion has a purely lytic pattern and sometimes ill-defined margins. Later, during the stabilisation phase, the characteristic soap bubble appearance develops as a result of maturation of the bony shell.[60] The CT appearance of aneurysmal bone cysts is that of a ballooning, multilobulated lytic lesion that resembles a 'soap bubble' with a 'blown-out' appearance (Figs. 56-1B and D).[65] In a series by Hudson, 35% of ABCs showed fluid–fluid levels at CT.[66] Fluid–fluid levels within ABCs are indicative of haemorrhage with sedimentation and are better demonstrated with MR imaging (Fig. 56-30). On T_1, they may have increased signal intensity due to methaemoglobin in either the dependent or non-dependent

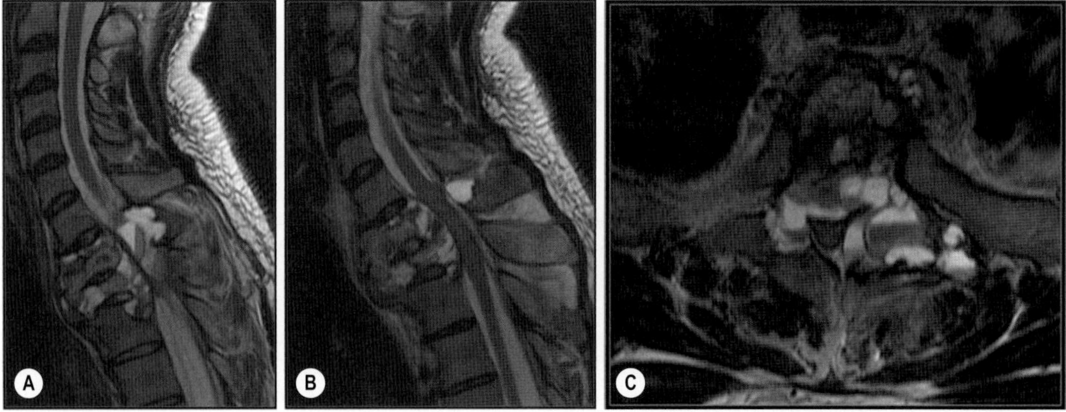

FIGURE 56-30 ■ **Aneurysmal bone cyst.** Sagittal (A, B) and axial (C) T_2 show an expansile process involving several segments of two thoracic vertebrae. Extension toward the spinal canal with spinal cord compression is observed. Presence of multiple fluid–fluid levels proves the haemorrhagic content of the lesions.

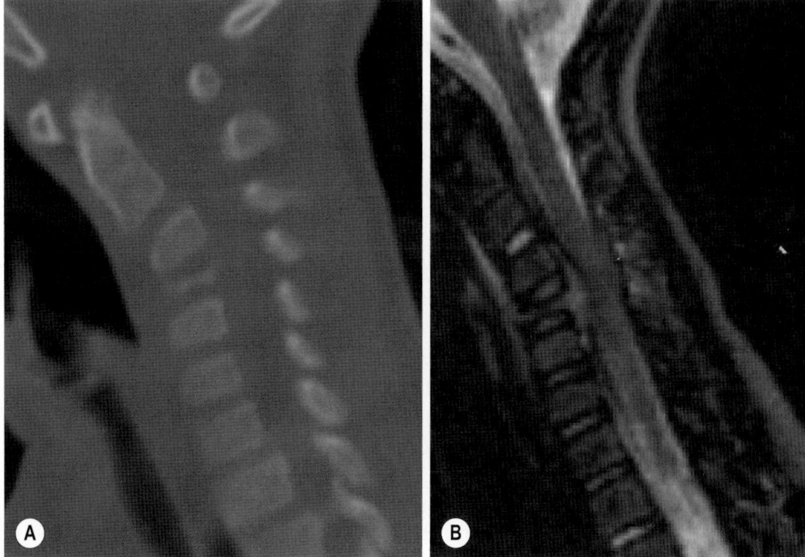

FIGURE 56-31 ■ **Eosinophilic granuloma in a 6-year-old girl with Langerhans cell histiocytosis.** Sagittal CT reformat of the C-spine (A) shows marked C4 vertebral compression ("vertebra plana") with kyphosis. Sagittal T2-weighted imaging (B) demonstrates intact vertebral endplates and adjacent disk spaces. A hyperintense soft tissue mass extending in the prevertebral tissues and anterior epidural space is observed. (Case courtesy of C. Venstermans, Antwerp, Belgium.)

component.[65] This finding is, however, not specific for ABCs, as it is also seen in other bone lesions, which contain areas of haemorrhage or necrosis such as telangiectatic osteosarcoma, GCT and chondroblastoma.[62] The lobulated lesion is surrounded by a hypointense rim on MR imaging corresponding to the intact periosteum or pseudocapsule.[65] The cystic components vary in appearance on T_1 and T_2, which is thought to represent the varying ages of the accumulated haemorrhage products within the cavities. Gadolinium enhancement is seen in up to 96% of lesions (Fig. 56-1E).[51] Peritumoural oedema is best defined on T_2 and STIR.[48] Although CT and MR imaging are diagnostic methods for many cases, it is noted in the literature that biopsy is necessary for confirmation, since many bone lesions can have a similar appearance.[61]

Eosinophilic Granuloma

Eosinophilic granuloma is a rare, benign solitary bone lesion that affects primarily children.[67] The peak incidence for eosinophilic granuloma of the spine is in the first decade. There is a clear male predilection.[6] Eosinophilic granuloma is one of the three clinical presentations of the disorder called Langerhans cell histiocytosis, formerly known as histiocytosis X, which can involve the central nervous system, bone, liver, lungs and lymph nodes. The most frequent sites of skeletal lesions are the skull, femur, mandible, pelvis and spine (least common).[68] In patients with Langerhans cell histiocytosis, the classic presentation of the vertebral lesions is that of vertebra plana, sometimes called 'pancake vertebra' on plain films (Fig. 56-31A).[68] There is a predilection for the thoracic spine, followed by the lumbar and then cervical spine. Vertebral bodies and anterior elements are involved much more commonly than the posterior elements. Lesions may be single or multiple. Eosinophilic granuloma has a highly variable clinical presentation, ranging from non-existent to very painful, sometimes worsening at night and sensitive to salicylate drugs or NSAIDs. The presenting symptoms of cervical eosinophilic granuloma are usually pain and restricted range of motion. In contrast to eosinophilic granuloma of the thoracic spine and lumbar spine, the neurological symptoms are less frequent.

Plain film radiography shows a lytic lesion with sharp borders. It is a classic cause of a single collapsed vertebral body (vertebra plana).[6] Nevertheless, vertebra plana is a rare sign in cervical eosinophilic granuloma.[67] If vertebral collapse is not complete, anterior wedging of the body may be observed. Mild epidural or soft-tissue extension may be seen on CT or MR imaging. Eosinophilic granuloma is isointense on T_1 and hyperintense on T_2. It enhances strongly with gadolinium. There is usually complete preservation of the adjacent discs (Fig. 56-31B). Vertebra plana in children can also occur as a result of a variety of malignant tumours, including Ewing's sarcoma, osteosarcoma and lymphomas. The wide differential diagnoses highlight the necessity for a thorough work-up, usually including an open, CT- or fluoroscopy-guided biopsy.[51,68]

Benign Notochordal Cell Tumours

Benign notochordal cell tumours (BNCTs) are benign tumours arising from embryonic remnants of the notochord, the midline craniocaudal cord of tissue involved in induction of the spine during embryogenesis, which subsequently involutes leaving normal remnants, the nucleus pulposus and abnormal remnants that can persist in adults along the spine.[69] They are found in approximately 20% of autopsy cases.[70] Previously, these tumours have been reported with various nomenclatures including 'ecchordosis physaliphora vertebralis',[71] vertebral intra-osseous chordoma,[72] giant notochordal rest,[72] giant notochordal hamartoma of intraosseous origin[73] and benign chordoma.[74] BNCTs are considered the benign counterpart of chordoma and are now described as a distinct entity, since clinically and histopathologically they lack characteristic features of chordomas and embryonic notochordal remnants.[74,75] However, these lesions may be precursors of chordoma.[74] Some authors hypothesise the existence of a disease continuum from BNCT to incipient and then classic chordoma, as different stages of the same condition.[76] It is conceivable that pre-existing intraosseous BNCTs transform into incipient chordoma (Fig. 56-32) and then extend through the cortex into the surrounding soft tissue. This so-called 'incipient chordoma' has intermediate features between BNCT and chordoma. Histologically, they have the typical features of BNCT, but clinically they tend to behave like aggressive lesions, with osteolysis and extension of the tumour in the adjacent soft tissues.[70] BNCTs should be recognised by radiologists, pathologists and orthopaedic surgeons to prevent unnecessary radical surgery; on the other hand, close follow-up by cross-sectional imaging techniques is necessary to detect incipient lesions early, as they should be treated in the same manner as a classic chordoma.[76]

BNCTs are usually asymptomatic; mild pain is the most common symptom.[74] Most lesions (almost 75%) that are clinically identified arise in the mobile spine, typically the lumbar and cervical regions.[74] A series of seven cases arising from the posterior clivus have been published recently. Radiographic findings may be normal, or may show ill-defined, vague sclerosis within the vertebral body. More rarely, a diffuse prominent sclerosis presenting as ivory vertebra may be seen. Technetium bone scintigraphy show no abnormal uptake. On CT, BNCTs are typically sclerotic, and may replace the entire bone marrow of the vertebral body; cortical disruption or bone destruction are absent.[74] On MRI, BNCTs show a homogeneous low signal intensity on T_1 (Fig. 56-32A) and a homogeneous intermediate-to-high signal intensity on T_2 (Fig. 56-32B).[74] In a retrospective study of 38 patients with histopathological diagnosis of chordomas, Nishiguchi et al. noticed the absence of enhancement on contrast-enhanced series in BNCTs; all chordomas showed some degree of enhancement (Fig. 56-32C).[75] The most important discriminating feature between these two entities is the absence of a soft-tissue component in BNCTs, whereas the presence of a soft-tissue mass should indicate the diagnosis of chordoma.[74]

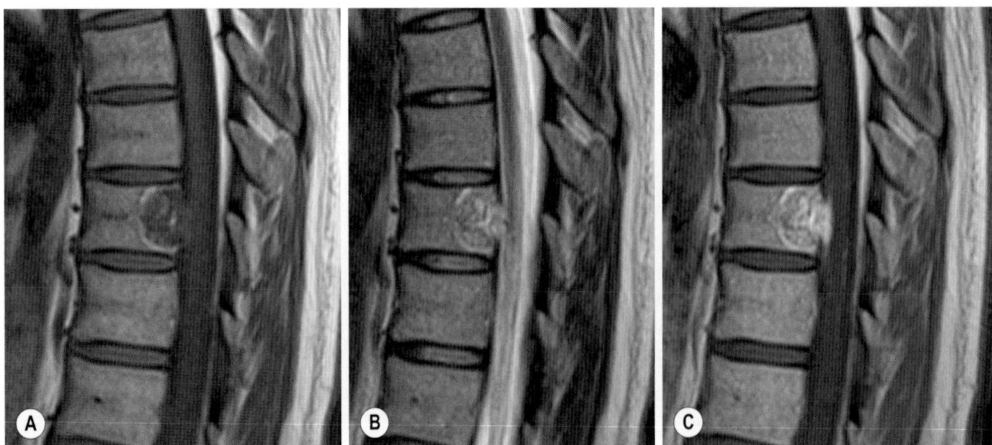

FIGURE 56-32 ■ Follow-up MR examination of a benign notochordal cell tumour (BNCT)-incipient chordoma found initially as an incidental finding in a patient with a motor vehicle accident. Sagittal T_1 (A) shows a geographic, sclerotic hypointense lesion with a discrete hyperintense rim. On sagittal T_2 (B) the lesion is displayed with high signal intensity. The enhancement of the lesion and the extension in the anterior epidural space on the gadolinium-enhanced T_1 (C) suggest transformation of a pre-existing intraosseous BNCT into incipient chordoma.

Locally Aggressive Primary Vertebral Tumours

Chordoma. Chordomas are the most common primary bone tumour of the sacrum and mobile spine.[49] Chordomas are exclusively observed in the spine, with two sites of predilection situated at the two extremities of the spine, the sacrum (50%)[77] (Fig. 56-33) and the skull base (35%).[69] The cervical location is the most commonly involved segment in the mobile spine (Fig. 56-34).[78,79] Chordomas were previously believed to arise from embryonic remnants of the notochord. However, recent studies suggest the possibility that chordomas arise from BNCTs.[70] The peak incidence for chordoma is between 50 and 60 years of age. Men are more affected than women.[80] Chordomas are considered low-grade, slow-growing, locally aggressive lesions.[80,81] Despite the lesion's slow expansion rate, the tumour is often quite large when first discovered, which results in difficulties in the surgical treatment and sometimes leads to a high local recurrence rate and a poor survival rate.[82] Although chordomas are not typically metastatic on presentation, the often late-stage diagnosis of the disease makes distant metastasis more likely. Five per cent of chordomas show metastasis to the lungs, bone, skin and brain at the time of initial presentation, and as high as 65% are metastatic in very advanced disease.[80] Accurate preoperative assessment is important in successful surgical resection with better prognosis.

Chordomas are midline lesions and often appear radiographically as destructive bone lesions, with an epicentre in the vertebral body and a surrounding soft-tissue mass. On CT, an expansive, midline lytic lesion with irregular borders and infiltration of surrounding tissues is observed. Calcification and bone sclerosis are frequently present. Paravertebral and epidural extension of the lesion can be evaluated.[83] Because of the variety of components, most lesions are heterogeneous on MR imaging. The most striking feature of a chordoma is the high signal intensity seen on T_2 (Figs. 56-33B and

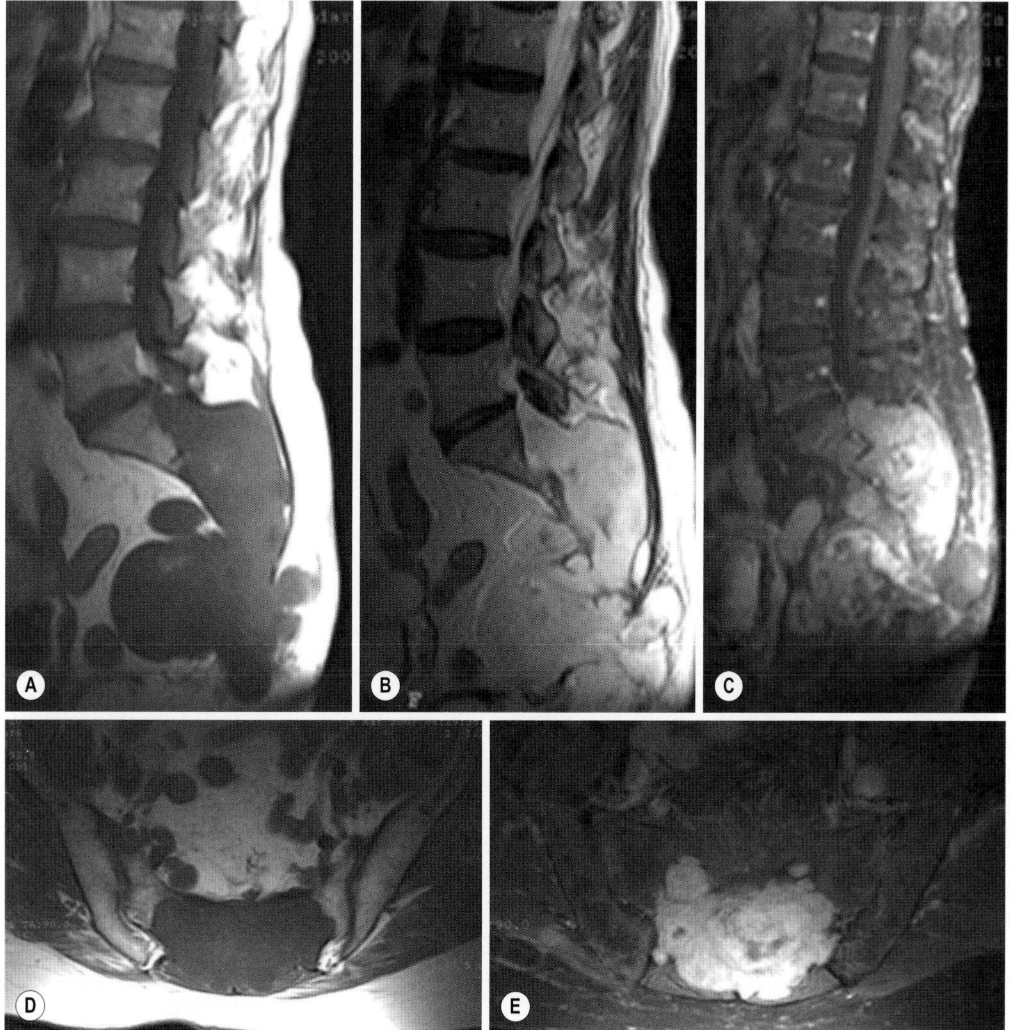

FIGURE 56-33 ■ **Sacrococcygeal chordoma.** A large expansile and multilobulated midline tumour with extensive anterior soft-tissue involvement is found. The tumour looks well-encapsulated, and some internal septations can be seen. The tumour displays rather homogeneous low signal intensity on sagittal T_1 (A) and homogeneous high signal intensity on T_2 (B). Sagittal fat-suppressed contrast-enhanced T_1 (C) reveals heterogeneous enhancement thoughout the mass. Axial T_2 (D) and fat-suppressed contrast-enhanced T_1 (E) show non-involvement of the sacroiliac joints. (Case courtesy of M. Thurnher, Vienna, Austria.)

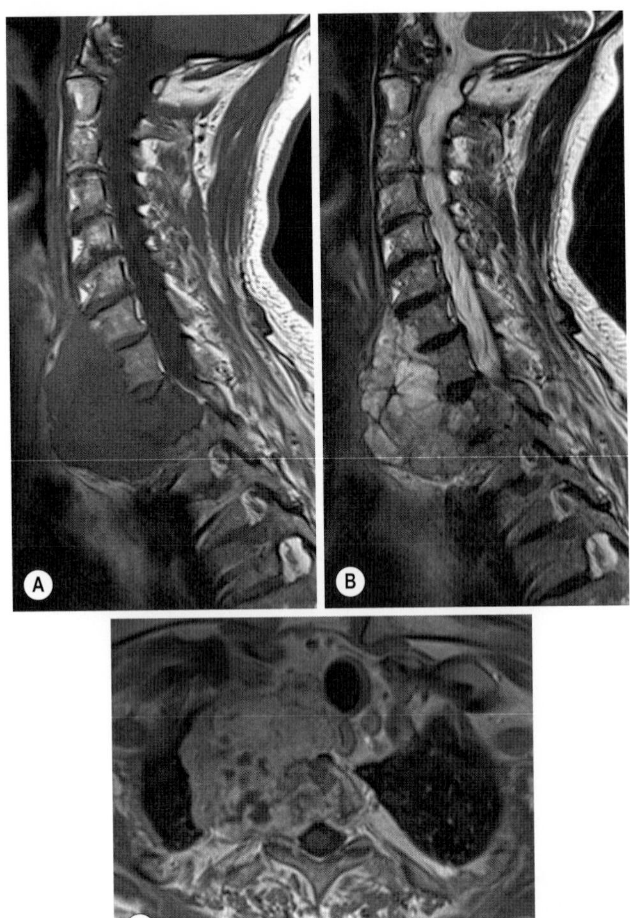

FIGURE 56-34 ■ **Chordoma of the mobile spine.** Sagittal T_1 (A), and sagittal T_2-weighted images and axial T_1 image after Gd injection (C) show a polylobular lesion originating at the body of Th1 and extending anteriorly, invading the anterior aspect of the C6 and C7 vertebral bodies. The lesion is of intermediate signal intensity on T_1 (A) and has mixed, intermediate and high signal intensity on T_2 (B). There is marked, non-homogeneous contrast enhancement of both the osseous and soft-tissue component of the tumour (C).

56-33E). This is due to abundant intra- and extracellular mucin produced by the tumour.[84] Chordomas tend to show hypointense or isointense signal relative to that of muscle on T_1 (Fig. 56-33A). Areas of hyperintensity on T_1 typically represent areas of haemorrhage or high protein content of the myxoid and mucinous collections.[77,84] The presence of haemosiderin in chordomas accounts for the low signal intensity seen with T_2.[84] The pattern of enhancement after gadolinium injection can be variable (Fig. 56-33C), ranging from homogeneous to peripheral septal enhancement.[50] The septal pattern is presumably produced by the presence of chondroid tissues or the degree of the lobules with mucogelatinous contents of these tumours.[84] Chordomas arising in the mobile spine typically show a soft-tissue mass spanning several vertebral segments (Fig. 56-34). Most of the lesions show a so-called 'collar button' appearance on sagittal images. Cervical chordomas display a 'dumbbell' morphology or 'mushroom' appearance without bone involvement and with enlargement of the neuroforamen mimicking a neurogenic tumour.[78] The combination of high signal on T_2 and a lobulated sacral mass that contains areas of haemorrhage and calcification is strongly suggestive of a chordoma.[77]

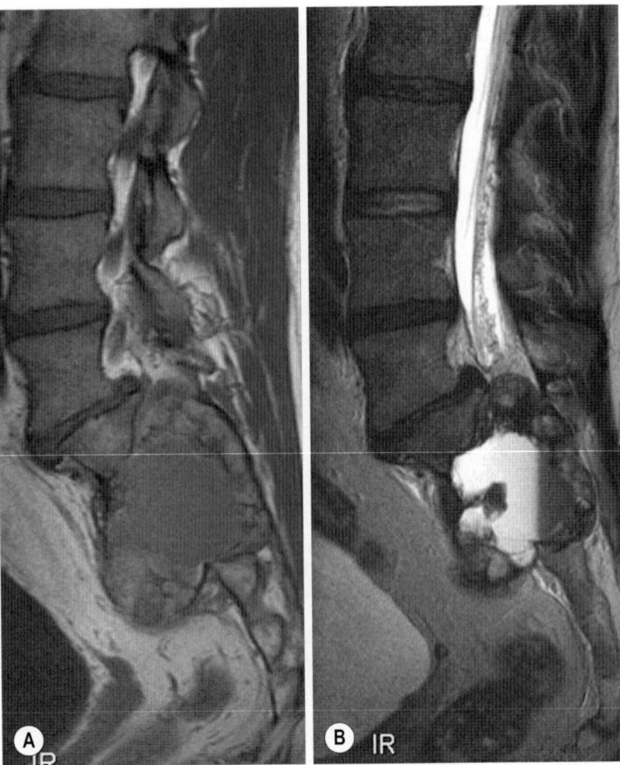

FIGURE 56-35 ■ **Giant cell tumour from the sacrum.** Heterogeneous expansile tumour arising at the S1–S2 level. Low signal intensity components at the periphery of the lesion on both sagittal T_1 (A) and T_2 (B). Large fluid–fluid level with low signal intensity of the dependent part due to sedimentation of blood components on T_2-weighted image.

Giant Cell Tumours. Giant cell tumours (GCTs) involving the spine are rare (7%).[85] They occur in skeletally mature patients in the second to fourth decades of life, more frequently in females.[2] Ten to 15% may have an ABC-like component (Fig. 56-1).[48] Most of these lesions occur in the sacrum, followed in order of decreasing frequency by the thoracic, cervical and lumbar segments of the mobile spine.[85] GCTs are the second most common primary bone tumour of the sacrum (after chordomas), usually located in the upper part of the sacrum and frequently lateralised in a sacral wing (Fig. 56-35).[50] Extension to the iliac wing through the sacroiliac joint is possible.[2] Unlike most benign tumours of the spine, GCTs are found in greater frequency in the vertebral body (55%) but often involve the body and posterior elements (30%).[48] Extraosseous involvement of the soft tissues is seen in 79% of cases.[2] A dramatic increase in lesion size can occasionally be associated with pregnancy and is presumably related to hormonal stimulation.[85]

Plain film radiography demonstrates a well-demarcated lytic and expansile lesion that often crosses the midline in the sacrum and may cross the sacroiliac joints. There is typically a narrow zone of transition.[85] CT better defines the characteristics identified on plain film images and better defines the bone architecture of the lesion. CT demonstrates absence of mineralisation and the lack of a

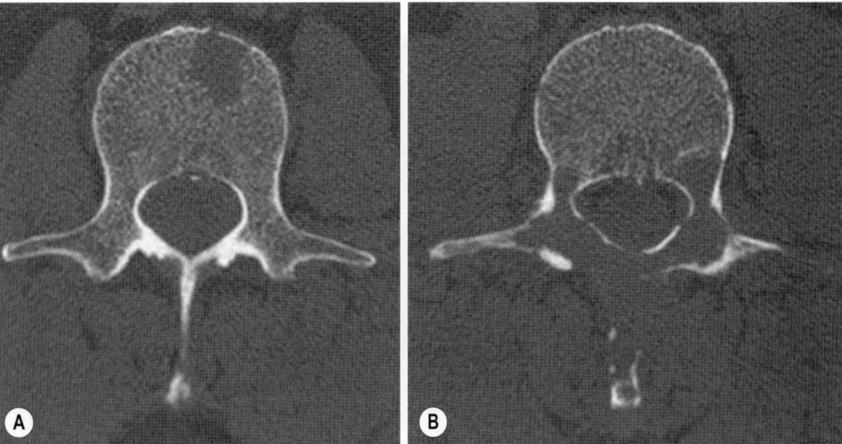

FIGURE 56-36 ■ Multiple myeloma. CT (A, B) shows purely osteolytic lesions in different parts of several vertebrae and in the sacrum.

sclerotic rim at the margins of the tumour. MR imaging characteristics can be helpful in the diagnosis. A low-to-intermediate signal intensity on T_2 (Fig. 56-35B) is often seen within the lesion, which is thought to be secondary to the relative collagen content of fibrous components and haemosiderin within the lesion.[86] The tumour usually has low-to-intermediate signal intensity on T_1 (Fig. 56-35A). These lesions may also demonstrate curvilinear areas of low signal intensity on T_1 and T_2, which may correspond to thickened trabeculae or fibrous septae.[85] Enhancement of the lesion reflects its vascular supply. Cystic areas, foci of haemorrhage, fluid–fluid levels and a peripheral low-signal-intensity pseudocapsule may also be seen.[87,88]

Primary Malignant Vertebral Tumours

In the Leeds Regional Bone Tumour Registry, which focuses on spine tumours, primary malignant tumours of the spine constituted only 4.6% of the cases registered between 1958 and 2000.[49] The most common malignant spine tumours were multiple myeloma and plasmacytoma. The second most common tumour was chordoma. The third most common tumour was osteosarcoma.[89]

Multiple Myeloma and Plasmacytoma

Multiple myeloma and plasmacytoma are the most common malignant vertebral tumours.[49] Multiple myeloma is a disease of infiltrative plasma B cells that can spread to the mobile spine and sacrum. In approximately 5% of patients, the disease may manifest as a solitary plasmacytoma of bone, with a frequent site of presentation being the spine. Two-thirds of these patients have been reported to go on to develop multiple myeloma.[48,89] These lesions occur twice as commonly in men as in women and have peak incidence at approximately 55 years of age. They have a preference for the thoracic spine. The vertebral body is the most common site of involvement because of its rich red marrow content, but the tumour frequently extends to the pedicles (Fig. 56-36B);[87] also epidural extension is a frequent finding. Multiple areas of spinal involvement frequently result in pain and multiple compression fractures with the potential for collapse, spinal instability and neurological deficit from spinal cord compression.

In two-thirds of cases, plain film radiography will show plasmacytoma as a lytic and usually expansile bone lesion with thickened trabeculae and multicystic appearance.[6,87] The tumour preferentially replaces the cancellous bone, whereas the cortical bone is partly preserved or even sclerotic, resulting in a hollow vertebral body or pedicle on CT images (Fig. 56-36). In one-third of cases, the radiographic appearance is less characteristic, with a multicystic 'soap bubble' appearance simulating a haemangioma.[2,87] Plasmacytoma shows low signal intensity on T_1, high signal intensity on T_2 and homogeneous vivid enhancement on post-contrast T_1.[87,90] Curvilinear low-signal-intensity structures extending partially through the vertebral body and resembling sulci seen in the brain, causing a 'mini brain' appearance on axial images, have been described to be typical.[90] These low-signal-intensity structures are likely caused by thickened cortical bone caused by the slow-growing nature of plasmacytoma. This appearance can also be seen on CT. Focal end-plate fractures are well described in patients with plasmacytoma.[91] Involvement of the intervertebral disc and adjacent vertebrae can be used to help differentiate plasmacytoma from metastasis.[2,91]

In patients with multiple myeloma, imaging typically reveals diffuse lytic, 'punched-out' lesions within single or multiple vertebrae (Fig. 56-37). In some cases, there may be no characteristic findings. Diffuse osteoporosis of the vertebral bodies or multiple compression fractures may be observed.[50] Even in advanced stages of this disease, up to 20% of plain films and MR imaging studies may show normal findings. MDCT allows imaging of the entire spine and provides detailed information on osseous involvement in multiple myeloma.[92] Especially in anatomically complex regions such as the pelvis and the thoracic spine, it is superior to plain film radiography. Compared with conventional radiography and MR imaging, MDCT provides more detailed information on the risk of vertebral fractures.[93] For evaluating diffuse bone marrow changes, MR imaging is still the imaging technique of choice. Different signal patterns may be observed, ranging from normal-appearing bone marrow to focal lesions or diffuse bone marrow infiltration. On T_1, a low signal intensity is typically noted (Fig. 56-37A), with marked enhancement after the administration of gadolinium. Lesion conspicuity is increased on T_2 by using fat saturation or STIR techniques (Figs. 56-37B vs

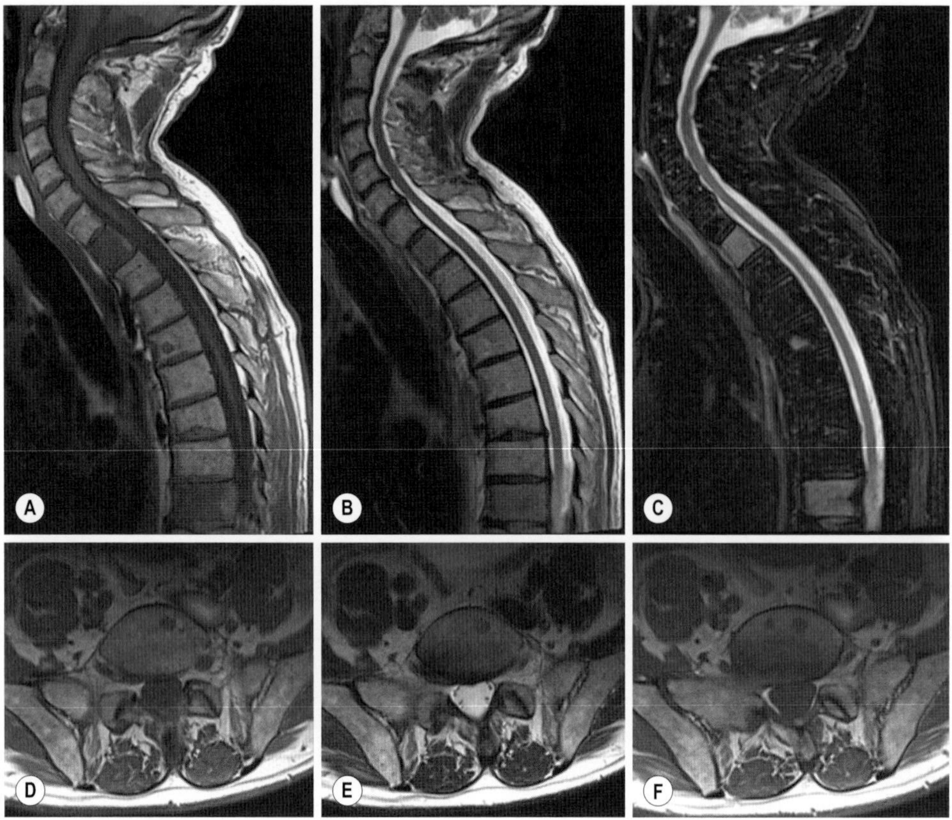

FIGURE 56-37 ■ Multiple myeloma. Sagittal T1 (A), sagittal T2 (B), and sagittal fat-supressed T2 (STIR) (C) and axial T1 (D), axial T2 (E) and axial contrast-enhanced T1-wi (F) reveal lytic, 'punched-out' lesions in the Th4 vertebral body and sacrum. Diffuse bone marrow involvement of Th1 and Th8 vertebral bodies is observed with replacement of the normal fatty bone marrow by low to intermediate signal intensity on T1 and T2. The lesions show marked high signal intensity on STIR.

C). Also T_1 completed after contrast administration should include fat saturation. Focal myeloma lesions in the spine may look similar to metastatic lesions on MR imaging, with pathological fracture, marrow replacement and epidural spread of the tumour.[48]

Chondrosarcoma

The most prevalent types of sarcomas involving the spine are chondrosarcoma, osteosarcoma, and Ewing's sarcoma.[89] Chondrosarcoma is the second most common non-myeloproliferative primary malignant tumour of the spine in adults.[65] Chondrosarcoma is a malignant tumour in which the basic neoplastic tissue is fully developed cartilage without tumour osteoid being directly formed by a sarcomatous stroma. Myxoid changes, calcification or ossification may be present.[89] Chondrosarcomas compose 7 to 12% of all primary spine tumours and account for up to 25% of malignant spine tumours. Men are affected 2 to 4 times more frequently than women; mean age of patients is 45 years. The thoracic and lumbar spine are most frequently affected, with the sacrum being affected only rarely.[94] Chondrosarcoma originates in the vertebral body (15% of cases), posterior elements (40%) or both (45%).[2] Chondrosarcomas of the spine are usually low-grade (either grade 1 or 2) lesions that may arise de novo as primary malignant tumours or as secondary transformations of osteochondromas or Paget's disease.

Although plain films may identify bone destruction and chondroid mineralisation in up to 70% of cases, cross-sectional imaging, including CT and MR imaging in combination, offers the best opportunity to define the tumour matrix and tumour extent (Figs. 56-2 and 56-38).[48] Chondrosarcomas of the spine usually manifest as a large, calcified mass with bone destruction.[95,96] True ossification may be seen, which corresponds to residual osteochondroma in cases of secondary chondrosarcoma.[87] Chondroid matrix mineralisation is better demonstrated with CT (Fig. 56-2C). Calcified matrix is detected as areas of signal void at MR imaging. The non-mineralised portion of the tumour has low attenuation on CT images, low-to-intermediate signal intensity on T_1 (Fig. 56-38A), and very high signal intensity on T_2 due to the high water content of hyaline cartilage (Figs. 56-38B and 56-38D). An enhancement pattern of 'rings and arcs' on gadolinium-enhanced images reflects the lobulated growth pattern of these cartilaginous tumours (Fig. 56-38E).[2]

Ewing's Sarcoma

Although the vertebral column is frequently involved in preterminal metastatic Ewing's sarcoma, primary vertebral Ewing's sarcoma is quite rare, with a reported prevalence of 3.5–15%.[97] Primary vertebral Ewing's sarcoma is usually seen in the second decade of life, with a slight male predilection. Ewing's sarcoma can involve all segments of the spine, with sacral involvement in as many as 50%.[97] The ala is the most frequently affected sacral site (69%); the majority (60%) of lesions in the mobile spine originate in the posterior elements with extension into the vertebral body.[97] Clinical presentation of Ewing's sarcoma is aspecific and includes pain and often neurological deficits.[50]

A permeative appearance that may mimic osteomyelitis is the hallmark of Ewing's tumour of the spine. This characteristic can be demonstrated on plain film

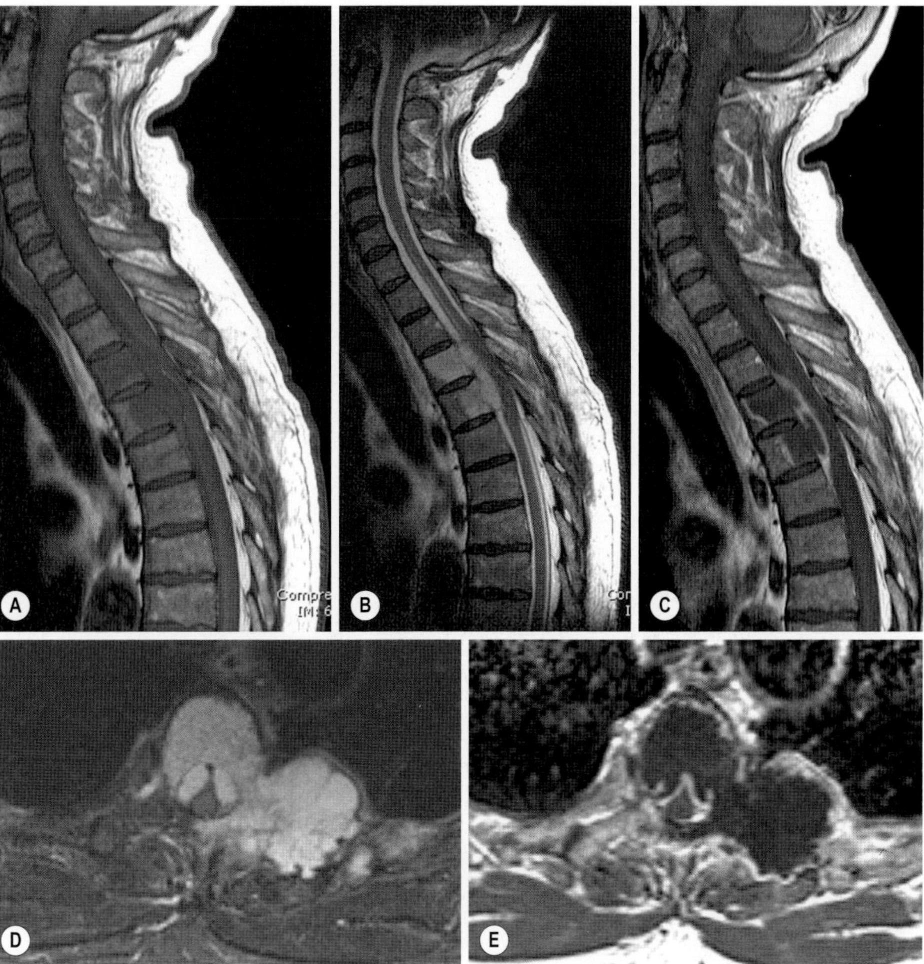

FIGURE 56-38 ■ **Chondrosarcoma.** Sagittal T1 (A), T2 (B) and contrast-enhanced T1 (C) show invasion of the Th3 and Th4 vertebral bodies with low-to-intermediate signal intensity on T1 and very high signal intensity on T2. Extension of the tumour in the anterior epidural space with spinal cord compression is observed. Peripheral irregular enhancement of the tumour. CT-guided percutaneous biopsy of the paravertebral extension of the tumour was performed (Fig. 56.2), and the final diagnosis of low-grade chondrosarcoma was made.

radiography, but CT has greater sensitivity.[98] Vertebra plana may be seen, and two or more adjacent vertebra may be involved. Fifty per cent of tumours have a non-calcified soft-tissue mass.[48] MRI is the imaging study of choice for local tumour staging. The MRI appearance can be extremely variable, depending on matrix formation and the degree of bone and soft-tissue involvement. Most often Ewing's sarcoma is iso- to hyperintense on T_2 (Fig. 56-39A) and isointense on T_1 (Fig. 56-39B and D). Contrast enhancement after gadolinium injection is seen because of the hypercellularity of the tumour (Fig. 56-39C and E).[50] Invasion of the spinal canal is frequent and the paraspinal component is often larger than the intraosseous lesion.[2] FDG-PET/CT is the new standard for initial staging and the detection of recurrence or new metastatic disease.[98] The initial standardised uptake value of the primary tumour has been shown to correlate with tumour aggressiveness.[48]

Osteosarcoma

Osteosarcoma is a high-grade malignant osteoblastic lesion. It is the third most common primary vertebral tumour. Primary vertebral osteosarcoma represents 4% of all osteosarcomas; secondary vertebral osteosarcoma may result from Paget's disease and radiation. Although osteosarcoma, overall, has a peak incidence during the adolescent growth spurt, spinal osteosarcoma tends to occur in an older age group, with a mean age of 38 years.[48] There is no sex- or race-based predilection.[89] Osteosarcoma can be found anywhere in the spine; the thoracic and lumbar segments are involved with equal frequency, followed by the sacrum and the cervical column.[99] In the mobile spine 80% of the lesions are found in the posterior elements with partial vertebral body involvement.[99] Other studies quote a significantly higher percentage of involvement of the vertebral body.[89] Most of the lesions occur at a single spinal segment but 17% involve more than one level. The clinical presentation of osteosarcoma is similar to that of Ewing's sarcoma: patients may present with pain, signs of neurological compression, or a palpable mass.[2] All osteosarcomas, despite their classification as to subtype (osteogenic, chondroblastic, fibroblastic, secondary osteosarcoma), have as their common feature the production of bone (osteoid) by neoplastic osteoblasts.[89]

A multi-technique approach to imaging is vital in defining the presence and extent of spine osteosarcoma. The variable pathological appearance, including osteoid matrix, marked mineralisation, ivory vertebrae, primary lytic pattern and a chondroblastic subtype, leads to a variety of imaging appearances.[99] Plain film radiography may demonstrate cortical destruction, a wide zone of transition, a permeative appearance or bone matrix. CT will better demonstrate these findings (Fig. 56-40) and is the best technique for defining matrix and bone

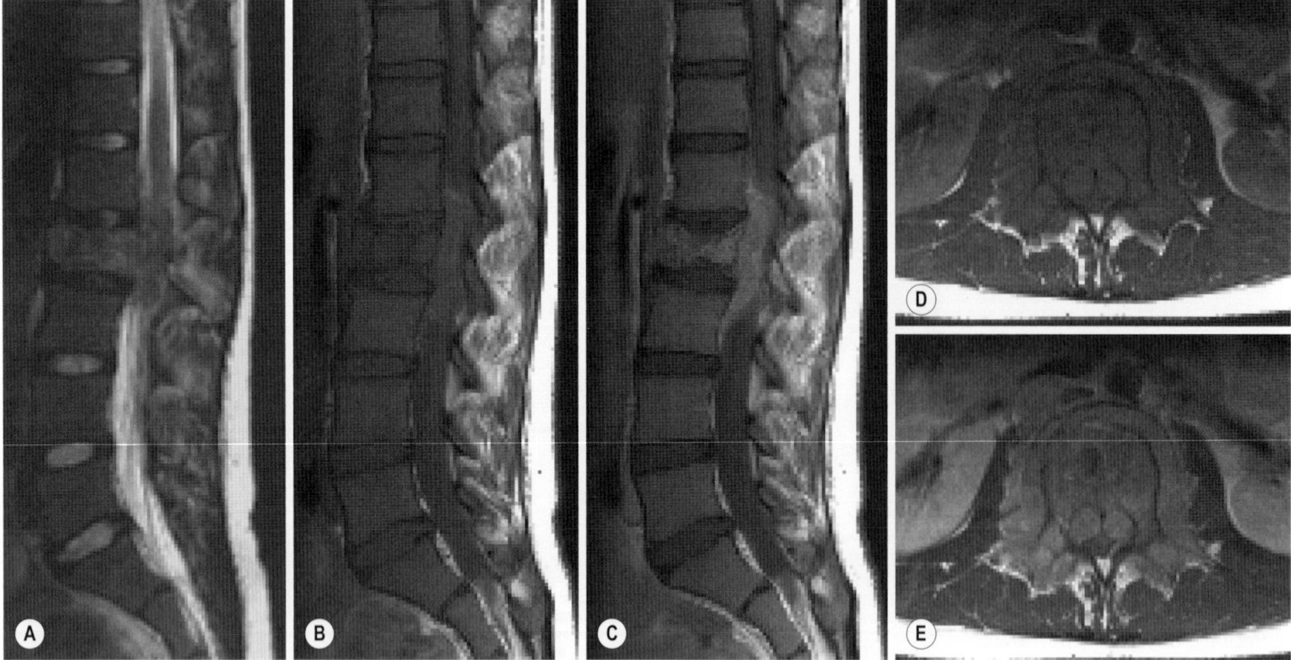

FIGURE 56-39 ■ **Ewing sarcoma of the L2 vertebral body.** The normal signal intensity of the fatty bone marrow is replaced and mild collapse of the vertebral body can be seen on the sagittal images. On the sagittal T2 (A), the lesion has a slight increased signal intensity. On the sagittal and axial T1 (B and D), the tumour is almost isointense and intense gadolinium-enhancement is observed (C and E). Invasion of the spinal canal ('curtain sign') and extension of the tumour in the adjacent paraspinal soft tissues is best demonstrated on the axial images.

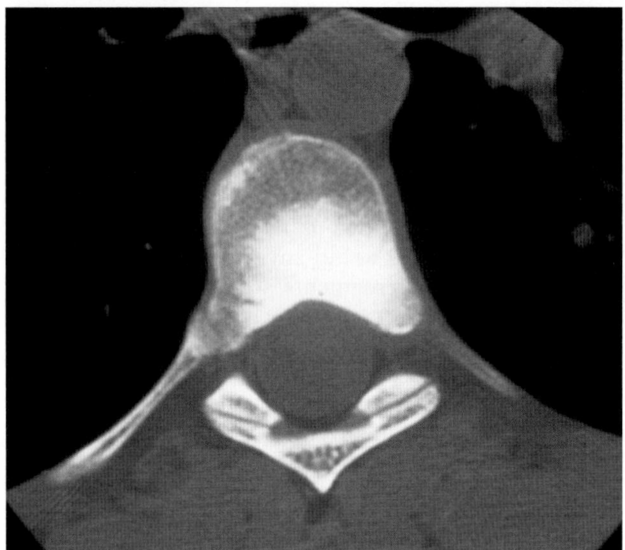

FIGURE 56-40 ■ **Osteosarcoma of the vertebral body.** CT shows a geographic, ill-defined, and non-expansile osteoblastic lesion in the posterior aspect of a thoracic vertebral body.

destruction.[48] Findings on MR imaging are extremely variable, with the signal abnormality based on the pathological subtype of the tumour.[89] Non-mineralised tumours will typically have a low signal on T_1 and high signal on T_2. Densely mineralised tumours, however, may demonstrate decreased signal on both T_1 and T_2. Gadolinium-enhanced images will better show the extension of the tumour in the surrounding soft tissues, particularly the intraspinal extension and the degree of central canal compromise. PET/CT is the current standard of care to stage all patients with bone and soft-tissue sarcomas. PET imaging is also used to monitor treatment response and conduct surveillance for recurrence.[48]

For a full list of references, please see ExpertConsult.

FURTHER READING

2. Rodallec MH, Feydy A, Larousserie F, et al. Diagnostic imaging of solitary tumors of the spine: What to do and say. Radiographics 2008;28(4):1019–41.
4. Abul-Kasim K, Thurnher MM, McKeever P, Sundgren PC. Intradural spinal tumors: current classification and MRI features. Neuroradiology 2008;50(4):301–14.
6. Van Goethem JWM, van den Hauwe L, Özsarlak Ö, et al. Spinal tumors. Eur J Radiol 2004;50(2):159–76.
18. Rossi A, Gandolfo C, Morana G, Tortori-Donati P. Tumors of the spine in children. Neuroimaging Clin N Am 2007;17(1):17–35.
19. Koeller KK, Rosenblum RS, Morrison AL. Neoplasms of the spinal cord and filum terminale: radiologic-pathologic correlation. Radiographics 2000;20(6):1721–49.
21. Smith AB, Soderlund KA, Rushing EJ, Smirniotopolous JG. Radiologic-pathologic correlation of pediatric and adolescent spinal neoplasms: Part 1, Intramedullary spinal neoplasms. Am J Roentgenol 2012;198(1):34–43.
27. Lonser RR, Glenn GM, Walther M, et al. von Hippel-Lindau disease. Lancet 2003;361(9374):2059–67.
40. Soderlund KA, Smith AB, Rushing EJ, Smirniotopolous JG. Radiologic-pathologic correlation of pediatric and adolescent spinal neoplasms: Part 2, Intradural extramedullary spinal neoplasms. Am J Roentgenol 2012;198(1):44–51.
48. Wald JT. Imaging of spine neoplasm. Radiol Clin North Am 2012;50(4):749–76.
65. Murphey MD, Andrews CL, Flemming DJ, et al. From the archives of the AFIP. Primary tumors of the spine: radiologic pathologic correlation. Radiographics 1996;16(5):1131–58.
87. Laredo JD, Quessar el A, Bossard P, Vuillemin-Bodaghi V. Vertebral tumors and pseudotumors. Radiol Clin North Am 2001;39(1): 137–63, vi.

CHAPTER 57

Non-tumoural Spinal Cord Lesions

Farah Alobeidi • Majda M. Thurnher • H. Rolf Jäger

CHAPTER OUTLINE

INFLAMMATORY DISEASE

Multiple Sclerosis

Multiple sclerosis (MS) is a progressive neurodegenerative disorder characterised by multiple inflammatory demyelinating foci called 'plaques'. The spinal cord is commonly involved with changes on autopsy in up to 98% of the cases. One-third of MS patients will have isolated spinal cord involvement. Spinal cord abnormalities in MS include focal lesions, diffuse involvement, axonal loss and spinal cord atrophy. Focal MS lesions appear as oval- or wedge-shaped T_2 hyperintensities located preferentially in the lateral and posterior parts of the spinal cord, which may or may not be swollen. Lesion enhancement is seen less frequently than in the brain, and is commonly subtle (Fig. 57-1). Ring-like or intense nodular enhancement may also occur.

Diffuse signal intensity abnormalities extending over multiple vertebral segments resembling transverse myelitis are seen in primary and secondary progressive MS. Spinal cord atrophy is associated with clinical disability, and is more common in the upper part of the spinal cord.

Tumefactive MS lesions can sometimes present a diagnostic challenge with a clinical presentation and imaging features mimicking tumours. Magnetic resonance imaging (MRI) appearances are classically of large (greater than 2 cm) circumscribed lesions with little mass effect or oedema. They are typically found in the supratentorial white matter but can also involve grey matter and the spinal cord (Fig. 57-2). Approximately half of tumefactive lesions enhance with a typical open ring pattern, with the incomplete portion of the ring on the grey matter side of the lesion (Fig. 57-2). Corticosteroid therapy leads to a dramatic reduction in the size of the lesions.

Acute Disseminated Encephalomyelitis

Acute disseminated encephalomyelitis (ADEM) is an inflammatory demyelinating cental nervous system (CNS) disease of the brain and spinal cord, with a distinct tendency to a perivenous localisation of pathological changes. ADEM develops mostly one or two weeks following a viral disease or prior vaccinations. Cerebrospinal fluid (CSF) analysis shows a high protein level. A high serum titre of IgG specific for myelin oligodendrocyte glycoprotein (MOG) has been described in almost one-half of the studied cases of ADEM.[1]

The spinal cord is involved in 30–40% of the cases. On MR imaging, non-enhancing hyperintense lesions are seen in the spinal cord on long TR sequences (Fig. 57-3). Skip lesions, as well as long segment hyperintensity, may be detected. Complete resolution of abnormalities will usually be seen on follow-up images.

Acute Transverse Myelitis

Acute transverse myelitis (ATM) is an aetiologically heterogeneous syndrome with acute or subacute onset, manifesting as weakness, sensory loss and autonomic dysfunction. It is associated with infectious or systemic autoimmune diseases, but in the majority of cases the aetiology remains unknown (idiopathic). In 2002 diagnostic criteria for idiopathic and disease-associated ATM were proposed by the Transverse Myelitis Consortium Working Group.[2]

The outcome of ATM ranges from full recovery to complete inability to walk or even death from respiratory failure. On MR imaging, intramedullary T_2 high signal intensity with cord swelling will be seen. Enhancement may be present. In comparison with spinal cord involvement in MS where focal lesion do not take more than half of the cross-sectional area of the cord, lesions in TM tend to involve more than two-thirds of the cross-sectional area of the cord (Fig. 57-4).

Depending on the length of the signal abnormality, TM can be divided into longitudinally extensive TM (LETM) when signal abnormalities extend more than two segments and acute partial TM (APTM) when signal abnormalities extend less than two vertebral segments.

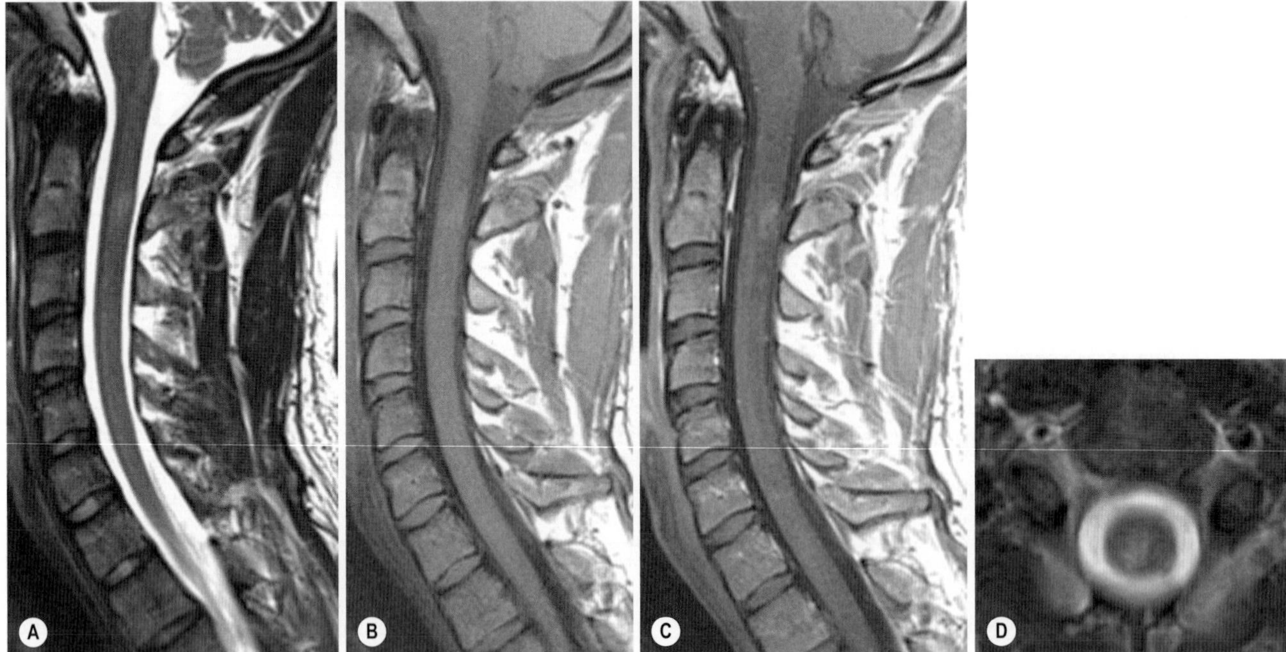

FIGURE 57-1 ■ Multiple sclerosis in a 30-year-old female patient. (A) Sagittal T_2 demonstrates an ill-defined hyperintense lesion in the spinal cord at the level of C2. The lesion is isointense on T_1 (B) and shows subtle enhancement on post-contrast T_1 (C). (D) Axial T_2 shows dorsal location of the demyelinating plaque.

Neuromyelitis Optica

Neuromyelitis optica (NMO) is a severe inflammatory disorder that predominantly affects the optic nerves and the spinal cord. It has a relapsing course in 80% of the cases and females are more commonly affected (9:1). The discovery of aquaporin-4 antibodies in 2004 has substantially changed our understanding of the disease, which was for many years debated and considered as an MS subtype.[3] Antibodies to aquaporin-4 (AQP4-Ab or NMO-IgG) are sensitive and highly specific serum markers of NMO, and will be positive in 60–90% of NMO patients. Patients with NMO present either with optic neuritis (unilateral or bilateral) or with LETM and spinal symptoms.

In optic neuritis MRI shows hyperintensity of the optic nerves with enhancement. Spinal cord involvement manifests itself as intramedullary T_2 hyperintense signal often extending more than three vertebral segments (LETM) with cavitations and patchy enhancement. On follow-up magnetic resonance (MR) defects, atrophy and central cavities, predominately located in the area of the posterior fascicle, have been described.[4] In some cases MRI findings may resemble spinal cord ischaemia with bilateral ventral hyperintensities.[4] Contrary to the common belief that brain lesions are not present in NMO, recent studies reported brain abnormalities in up to 40–60% of NMO patients. Periventricular signal intensity abnormalities (around the third and fourth ventricle, and in the periaqueductal region) can be detected on MRI, corresponding to brain areas with the highest aquaporin concentrations. Extensive lesions in the cerebral hemispheres have also been described.[5] Enhancement on brain MRI is not common (13–36%), with 'cloud-like enhancement', which appears as multiple patches of enhancing lesions being the most common type.[6]

NMO has been associated with other autoimmune diseases, including hypothyroidism, Sjögren's syndrome (SS), systemic lupus erythematosus (SLE), pernicious anaemia, ulcerative colitis, primary sclerosing cholangitis, rheumatoid arthritis, mixed connective tissue disorders and idiopathic thrombocytopenic purpura.

Systemic Lupus Erythematosus

Systemic lupus erythematosus (SLE) is a relapsing and remitting, chronic, multisystem autoimmune disease. Although the frequency of neuropsychiatric lupus has been reported as high as 95%, SLE-related myelitis is rare, with prevalence varying between 1 and 2%. Involvement of the spinal cord in SLE usually occurs during a time of acute exacerbation and is occasionally the first manifestation of SLE in an undiagnosed patient.

SLE myelitis manifests mostly as transverse myelopathy. The pathophysiological mechanism of TM in SLE is uncertain, although vasculitis and arterial thrombosis resulting in ischaemic cord necrosis have been suggested. Studies have suggested a higher incidence of antiphospholipid and NMO-IgG antibodies in those with SLE myelitis than in the general SLE population and this has contributed to our understanding of the disease process.[7]

The mid-thoracic cord is most commonly affected, resulting in a sensory level and frequently in paraplegia, which may be complete. Cervical myelopathy and cauda equina involvement, on the other hand, often cause only partial motor and sensory loss. MRI demonstrates T_2

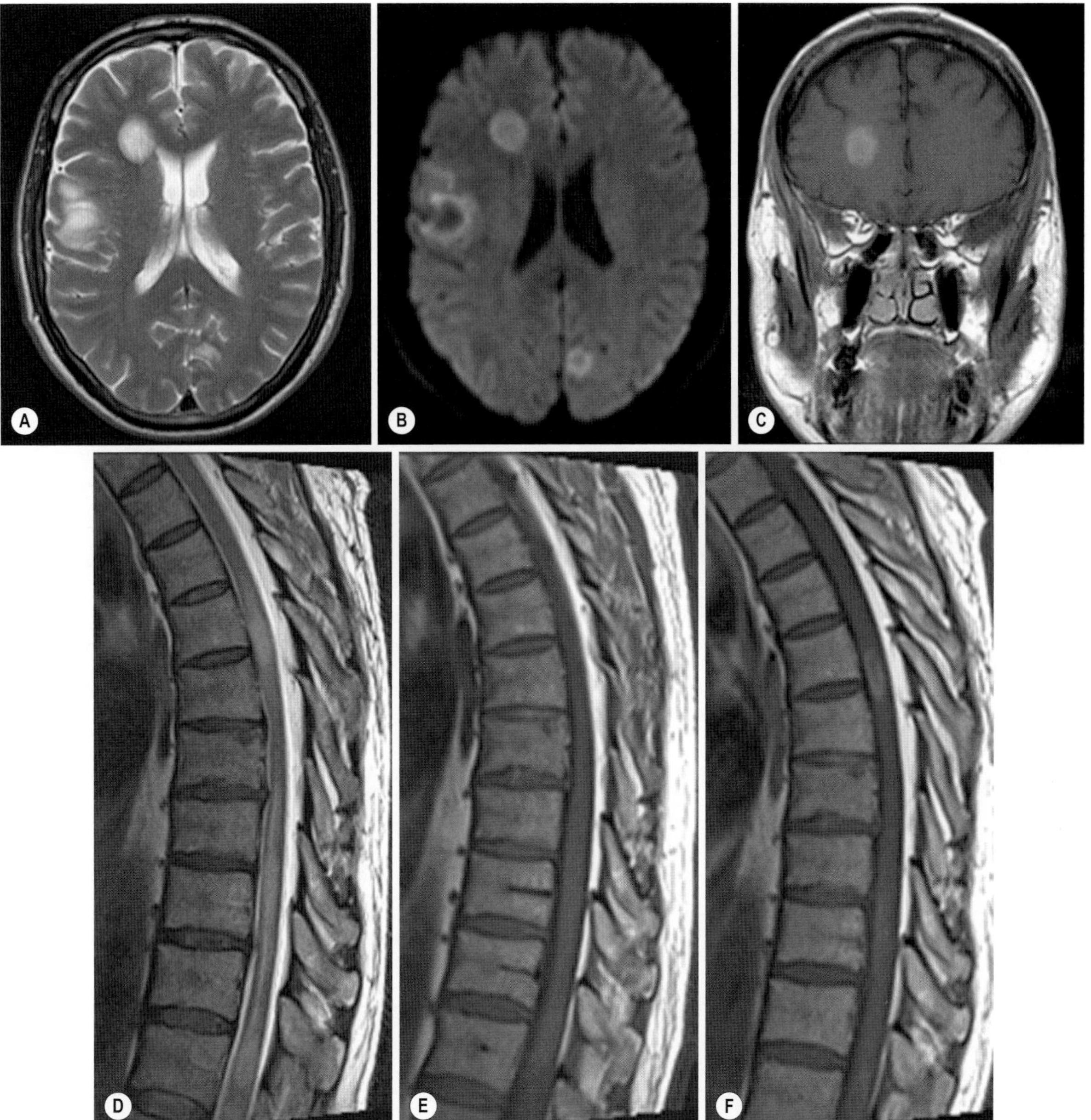

FIGURE 57-2 ■ **Tumefactive MS.** (A) Axial T_2 demonstrating multiple hyperintense lesions within the right frontal and left occipital lobes. The lesions are relatively well defined with little mass effect. Other lesions were also present (not shown). (B) DWI shows a rim of restricted diffusion in the larger lesion; the ring is incomplete laterally, which is a typical finding in tumefactive MS lesions. (C) Coronal post-contrast T_1 demonstrating enhancement of the right frontal lobe lesion. (D) Sagittal T_2 of the thoracic spine demonstrating multiple T_2 hyperintense lesions, the caudal of which extends over several segments. The lesions are not clearly seen on (E) sagittal T_1, but demonstrate ring-like enhancement post-contrast administration on (F) sagittal T_1 post contrast.

hyperintensity and oedema, frequently with spinal cord expansion. Lesions may demonstrate patchy enhancement during the acute phase (Fig. 57-5). Improvement or resolution of these findings correlates with clinical improvement. Indeed, some patients may have a normal MRI if they have already received treatment.

Sarcoidosis

Sarcoidosis is a systemic condition of unknown aetiology characterised histologically by non-caseating granulomatosis. Although CNS sarcoidosis is found in approximately 25% of cases on post-mortem examination, symptomatic involvement in life is uncommon. Clinical presentation depends on the site of involvement and is often non-specific.

Spinal involvement may be osseous, discal, meningeal or involve the cord itself. The most common spinal cord manifestation is leptomeningeal enhancement. This is best seen on sagittal contrast-enhanced T_1 images as thin linear or nodular enhancement, which frequently extends along the surface of the nerve roots. Dural

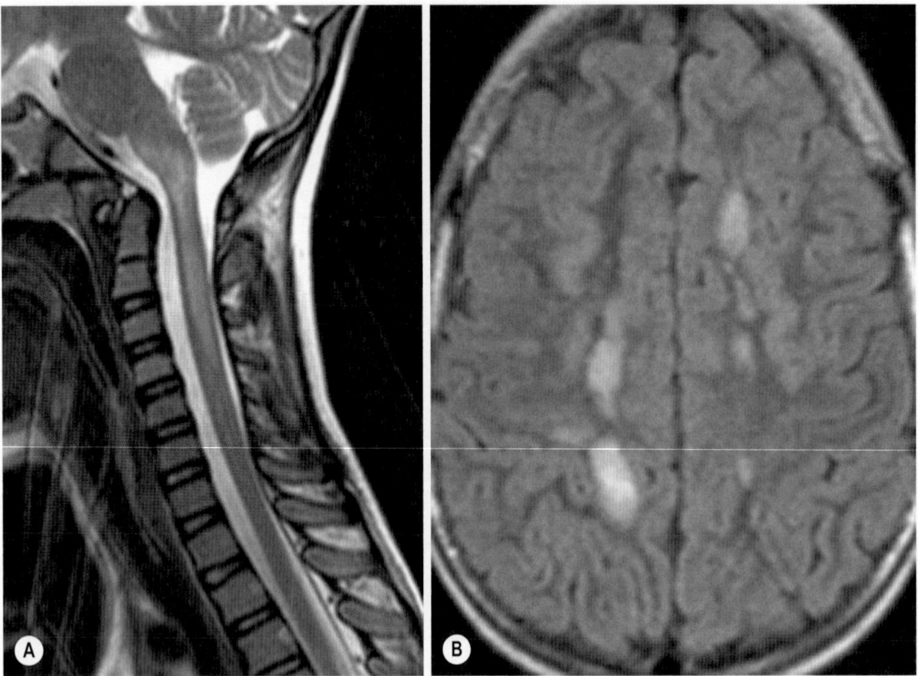

FIGURE 57-3 ■ Acute disseminated encephalomyelitis (ADEM) with brain and spinal cord involvement in a child with acute onset of symptoms following viral infection. (A) Sagittal T_2 of the cervical spine shows homogeneous high-signal-intensity abnormality in the cervical spinal cord and medulla oblongata. On post-contrast T_1 no enhancement is observed (not shown). (B) On an axial FLAIR MR image of the brain, multiple hyperintense white matter lesions are detected.

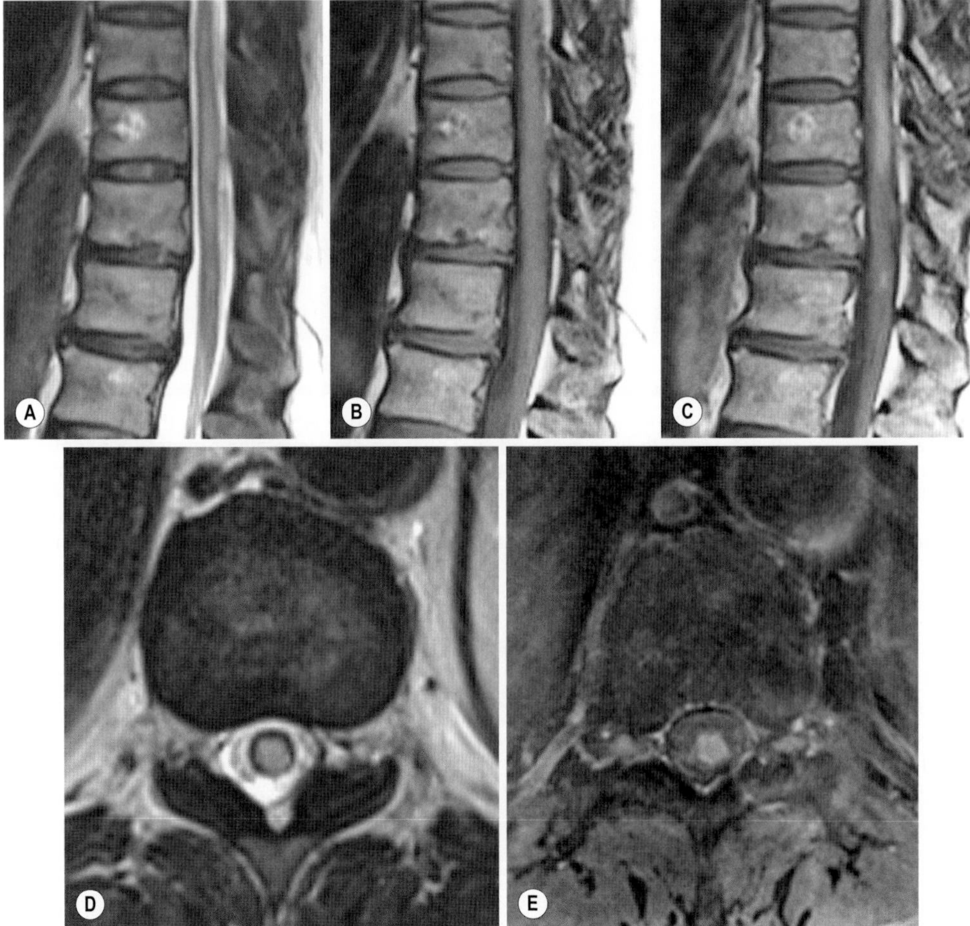

FIGURE 57-4 ■ Acute transverse myelitis (ATM). (A) Sagittal T_2 showing diffuse hyperintensity extending over several segments. Sagittal T_1 pre four (B) and post four (C) contrast showing enhancement of the lesion. Axial T_2 (D) and axial post-contrast T_1 (E) demonstrate that the lesion occupies more than two-thirds of the spinal cord cross-section.

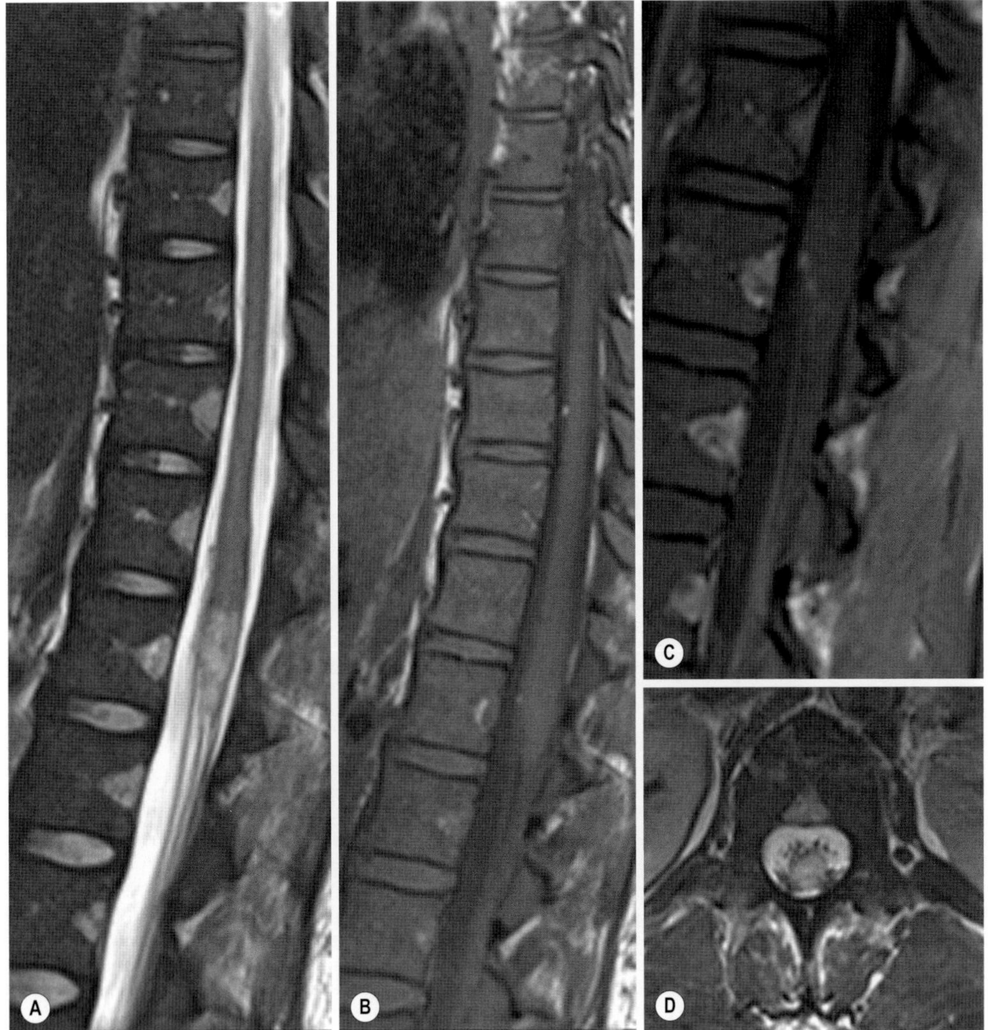

FIGURE 57-5 ■ **Systemic lupus erythematosus.** (A) Sagittal T_2 and (B) sagittal T_1 of the thoracolumbar spine demonstrating a lesion within the conus medullaris. A smaller, similar-appearing lesion was present in the same patient in the cervical spine (not shown). (C) Magnified post-contrast sagittal T_1 sagittal show faint enhancement of the lesion. (D) On axial T_2 the lesion occupies most of the transverse section of the conus medullaris.

involvement is more nodular in appearance, often with enhancing dural-based mass-like lesions that may mimic meningiomas.

Intramedullary spinal lesions are uncommon and frequently associated with severe neurological deficit. MRI demonstrates an enhancing mass that is hyperintense on T_2 sequences with associated fusiform enlargement of the spinal cord. These findings are, however, non-specific and can mimic intramedullary tumours, TM, MS and fungal infections. When the cauda equina is involved there is enhancement and clumping of the nerve roots.

The diagnosis of CNS sarcoidosis can represent a challenge on spinal cord imaging alone and is supported by the presence of typical appearances of brain sarcoidosis, such as involvement of the hypothalamic–pituitary axis, leptomeningeal enhancement or dural masses, as well as other diagnostic tests, such as elevated serum ACE levels.

DEMYELINATING POLYNEUROPATHIES

Although not strictly diseases of the spinal cord, demyelinating polyneuropathies merit a brief mention here as they can affect the cauda equina and other intradural nerves, leading to abnormal findings on an MRI of the spine.

Guillain–Barré Syndrome

Guillain–Barré is an acute immune-mediated polyneuropathy. Affected individuals have a typical areflexia and ascending paralysis type of symmetrical weakness, with or without sensory loss, that starts in the feet and hands and progressively moves up the limbs to the trunk over a few days. The trigger is frequently a viral illness with the production of antibodies that cross-react with myelin in the peripheral nervous system.[8] Approximately 80%

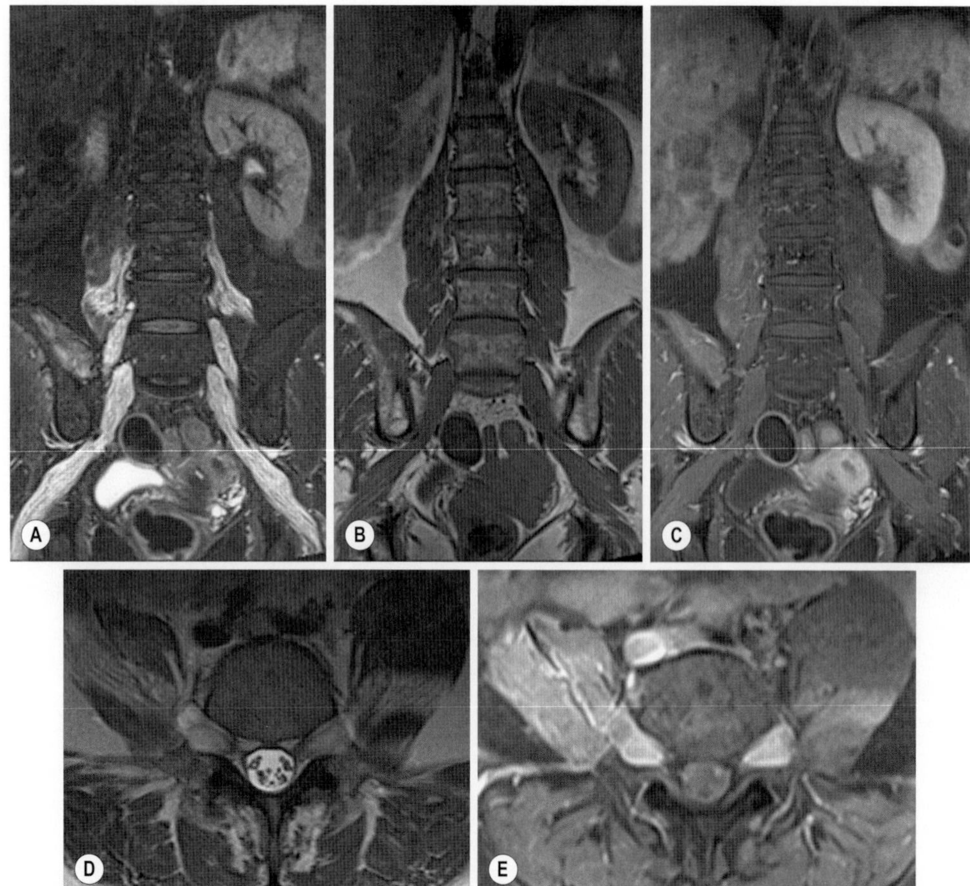

FIGURE 57-6 ■ Chronic inflammatory demyelinating polyneuropathy (CIDP). Coronal (A) fat-suppressed (FS) T_2 demonstrating grossly enlarged T_2 hyperintense nerves. (B) Pre-contrast T_1 and (C) FS post-contrast T_1 show diffusion enhancement of the nerves. Note that there is asymmetry of the psoas and pelvic muscles with atrophy, T_2 hyperintensity and enhancement typical for acute denervation. (D) Axial T_2 at level of L4 and (E) axial post-contrast FS T_1 confirm T_2 hyperintensity and enhancement of both the intradural and extradural nerves as well as the asymmetry and enhancement of the psoas muscles.

make complete or near-complete recovery over a few weeks from onset, with approximately 10% developing persistent symptoms that may have a relapsing and remitting course. In approximately 10% of cases, it can be life threatening if the respiratory muscles are affected.

Diagnosis is usually clinical and supplemented by nerve conduction studies and CSF examination. MRI demonstrates nerve thickening and enhancement, which is non-specific and is seen in other inflammatory disorders but is a useful diagnostic adjunct.

Chronic Inflammatory Demyelinating Polyneuropathy (CIDP)

This is an immune-mediated chronically progressive or relapsing symmetric sensorimotor disorder. It can be considered the chronic equivalent of acute inflammatory demyelinating polyneuropathy, the most common form of Guillain–Barré syndrome. In contrast to Guillain–Barré syndrome, CIDP has an insidious onset and evolves in either a slowly progressive or a relapsing manner. Preceding infection is infrequent. As with Guillain–Barré syndrome, the mainstay of treatment is immunosuppressive or immunomodulatory intervention. MRI findings are similar, with enhancing thickened nerve roots. Acute and subacute muscle denervation is demonstrated by hyperintensity within the affected muscle on fluid-sensitive sequences, such as T_2-weighted or STIR images. In chronic denervation, muscle atrophy and fatty infiltration demonstrate high signal changes on T_1-weighted sequences in association with volume loss. CIDP may therefore show both these changes depending on the stage of imaging (Fig. 57-6).

VASCULAR DISEASES

Spinal Dural Arteriovenous Fistula (SDAVF)

Over 80% of spinal arteriovenous malformations represent SDAVFs located in the spinal dural mater, usually close to a root sleeve.[9] Such fistulae are most commonly located in the thoracolumbar region but can occur at any

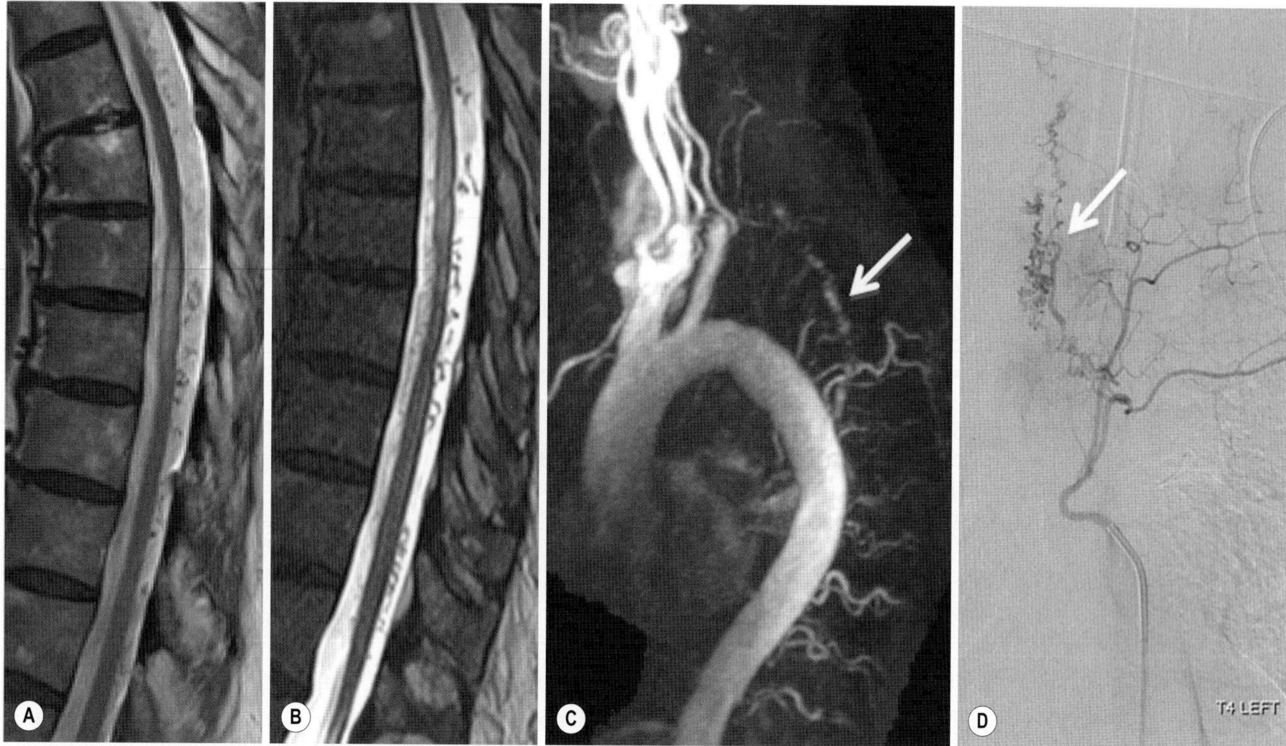

FIGURE 57-7 ■ **Spinal dural arteriovenous fistula (SDAVF).** (A) Sagittal T_2 demonstrating intrinsic T_2 cord hyperintensity in keeping with spinal cord oedema. Serpiginous flow voids of the dilated perimedullary veins are more prominent on the dorsal surface and appear more conspicuous on (B) the CISS sequence. (C) Sagittal reconstruction of TWIST sequence at the level of the thoracic aorta suggests presence of a fistula in the upper thoracic cord (arrow). A SDAVF was confirmed by DSA (D) following selective catheterisation of left supreme intercostal trunk which demonstrated the fistulous point (arrow).

level, though in the cervical spine only around the foramen magnum except in extremely rare cases. The fistula is usually supplied by one or two branches of a nearby radiculomeningeal artery and shunts often via a single vein into intradural radicular veins. The increase in spinal venous pressure results in slow venous drainage and stagnation because radicular veins and intramedullary veins share a common venous outflow. This results in the clinical findings of progressive myelopathy. SDAVFs are more common in middle-aged to elderly men and the typical presentation is of a slowly progressive gait disturbance, difficulty climbing stairs and paraesthesia. Bowel and bladder incontinence, erectile dysfunction and urinary retention are often seen late in the course of the disease but may be the presenting feature.

Diagnosis is often made by radiologists, based on typical MRI imaging features that guide definitive diagnosis by spinal DSA. T_2 sequences show an ill-defined central intramedullary hyperintensity extending over multiple levels with associated cord expansion. There may be a hypointense rim, most likely due to deoxygenated blood within dilated capillary vessels surrounding the congested oedema.[10] Engorged perimedullary veins can be seen as flow voids, which are more pronounced on the dorsal surface compared to the ventral surface. Although these are readily depicted on standard T_2 sequences, they become much more conspicuous on heavily T_2-weighted sequences (constructive interference in steady state (CISS), fast imaging employing steady-state acquisition (FIESTA) or 3D turbo spin-echo (3D TSE)) (Fig. 57-7). There may be diffuse post-contrast enhancement of the spinal cord, reflecting breakdown of the blood–brain barrier. The coiled perimedullary veins are easily depicted following contrast enhancement. It should be noted that normal pial veins can be prominent at the level of the lumbar enlargement of the spinal cord and that the distribution of abnormally enlarged veins is a poor guide to the location of a dural fistula. The site of the fistula can, however, be sometimes shown by dynamic contrast-enhanced magnetic resonance angiography (MRA). Multiplanar reformats of 4D dynamic MRA sequences, such as time-resolved angiography with interleaved stochastic trajectories (TWIST), can show non-invasively the site of the SDAVF in cases where the diagnosis is uncertain and can guide digital subtraction angiography (DSA), helping to avoid unnecessary superselective injections of all possible arterial feeders (Fig. 57-7).[11]

These lesions are an absolute indication for DSA. When searching for a dural fistula, imaging should be slow, say one frame rate every 2 s due to delayed venous return. A large number of arteries may have to be injected before the lesion is found. The study should not be regarded as negative unless: (A) all the spinal arteries from the foramen magnum to the coccyx have been opacified adequately, or (B) the veins thought to be abnormal have been opacified and shown to drain normally.[12] If a lesion is found, adjacent levels should also be injected and the major radiculomedullary arteries supplying the region must be identified.

Treatment aims to stop disease progression, with prognosis dependent on the symptoms and stage of disease pre-treatment. Embolisation of arteries supplying a dural fistula may be feasible, provided the vessel to be embolised can also be shown *not* to supply the spinal cord. The aim of treatment is to exclude the shunting zone (i.e. the most distal part of the artery together with the most proximal part of the draining vein).[13] Of course this is not always possible and a more proximal occlusion will lead to a transient improvement of symptoms, although fistula recurrence is high in these cases. Early surgical intervention should be considered for incomplete embolisations, as delay of secondary intervention is associated with a poor outcome.[14]

Spinal Arteriovenous Malformations (SAVMs)

In contrast to SDAVFs, spinal arteriovenous malformations (AVMs) are fed by spinal arteries, either radiculomedullary and/or radiculopial, located in an intra- or perimedullary location, respectively. There are two distinct subtypes: (A) glomerular AVMs (also known as plexiform or nidus type), the most common, contain a cluster or nidus of abnormal vessels between the feeding artery and draining vein and (B) fistulous AVMs (also known as AVM of the perimedullary fistula type or intradural AV fistula) which are direct AV shunts commonly located superficially on the cord.[15] Drainage is via spinal cord veins or perimedullary veins. In contrast to SDAVFs, these lesions are more prone to haemorrhage, a useful discriminating feature on MRI. Depending on the AVM location, haemorrhage may be intramedullary or subarachnoid. Lesions can also cause symptoms via venous congestion in a pathophysiology mechanism similar to SDAVF.

The dilated intra- and/or perimedullary veins are demonstrated on MRI as serpiginous flow voids on T_2 sequences, which enhance post-contrast administration. If there is venous congestion, oedema is present, seen as ill-defined intramedullary T_2 hyperintensity with cord expansion. If haemorrhage is present, various intramedullary signal intensities are seen, depending on the age of the blood. A subarachnoid haemorrhage may be present. There may also be an intranidal aneurysm (Fig. 57-8).

Embolisation of AVMs can sometimes be therapeutic but frequently it is palliative or 'targeted' to eliminate false aneurysms or to reduce hypertension or as a precursor to surgical treatment.

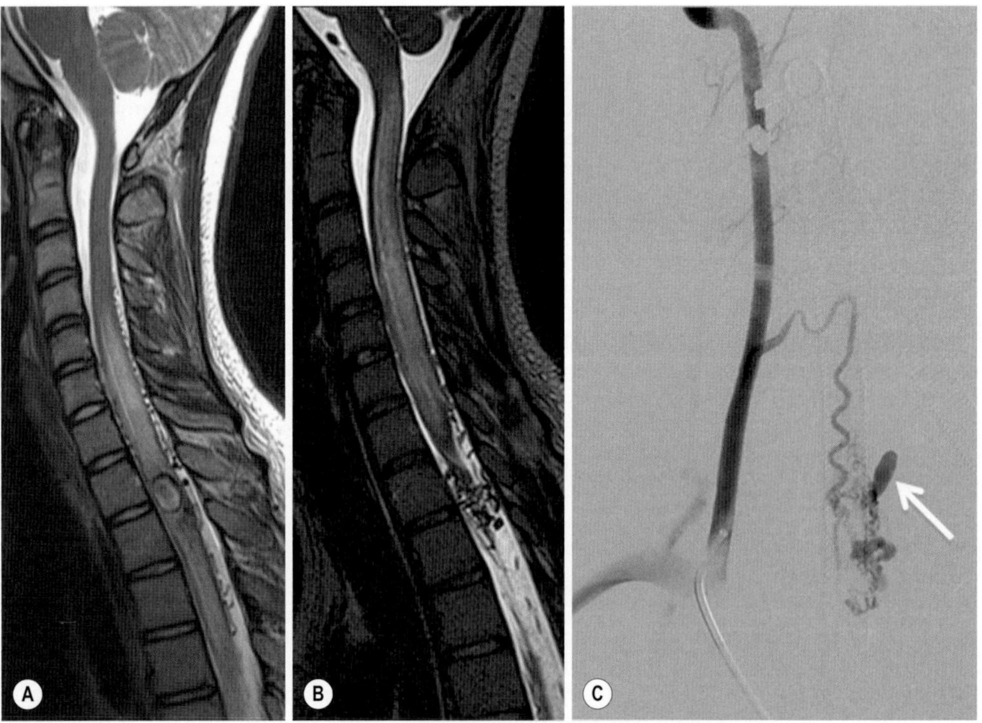

FIGURE 57-8 ■ **Spinal arteriovenous malformation (SAVM).** (A) Sagittal T_2 MRI demonstrating an intramedullary lesion at $T_1/_2$ with a hypointense rim in keeping with haemosiderosis. Note the cord expansion and associated cord oedema. Note also the serpiginous flow voids, which are more prominent on the dorsal surface of the cord. These are much more conspicuous on heavily weighted T_2 sequences such as (B) CISS sequence, right parasagittal slice. (C) Selective catheterisation of the right vertebral artery on DSA confirms the presence of an arteriovenous malformation. Note the intranidal aneurysm (arrow).

TABLE 57-1 **Summary of Spinal Vascular Malformations and Fistulas**

Type	Angio-architecture	Age (years)	Typical Clinical Presentation	Haemorrhage	Notes
Dural	Fistula	40–70	Progressive myelopathy	Rare	Male predominance, rarely cervical
Perimedullary (type I) (micro)	Fistula	30–70	Progressive myelopathy	Rare	Clinical and MR findings mimic SDAVF
Perimedullary (type II) (micro)	Fistula	20–40	Acute neurological deficit	Common	Commonly at conus
Perimedullary (type III) (macro)	Fistula	2–30	Acute neurological deficit	Common	Associated with Oslu–Weber–Rendu
Intramedullary	Nidus	10–40	Acute neurological deficit	Common	Flow-related aneurysms
Extradural	Fistula	Any	Asymptomatic to progressive myelopathy	Rare	Symptoms due to venous drainage pattern
Complex	Fistula	5–20	Acute or progressive neurological deficits	Common	Partial treatment often best pattern

A summary of SDAVFs and spinal AVMs, together with other types of vascular malformations and fistulas, is shown in Table 57-1.[16]

Spinal Cord Cavernous Malformation (SCCM)

Cavernous malformations (also known as cavernomas, cavernous angiomas and cavernous haemangiomas) are vascular malformations composed of sinusoidal-type vessels in immediate apposition to each other without any normal intervening parenchyma. In contrast to the brain where they are relatively common, SCCMs are more rare. They can be extradural, intradural-extramedullary or most commonly, intramedullary. Four clinical presentation subtypes have been described:[17] (A) discrete episodes of neurological deterioration separated by variable time intervals (hours or days) during which various degrees of recovery are made; (B) slowly progressive myelopathy; (C) acute neurological deficit with rapid decline; and (D) acute neurological deficit with gradual decline over weeks or months. Small repeated haemorrhages have been suggested as the underlying pathophysiological mechanism for episodes of repeated acute neurological deficit.

MRI appearances are characteristic with heterogeneous lesions on both T_1- and T_2-weighted sequences displaying typical 'popcorn' appearances, due to blood products of different ages. Due to haemosiderin staining, there is a T_2 low-intensity rim and hypointense 'blooming' on gradient-echo sequences. There may be minimal contrast enhancement, cord expansion or oedema (Fig. 57-9).

Symptomatic SCCM should be surgically removed at an early stage to avoid recurrence or rebleeding.[17]

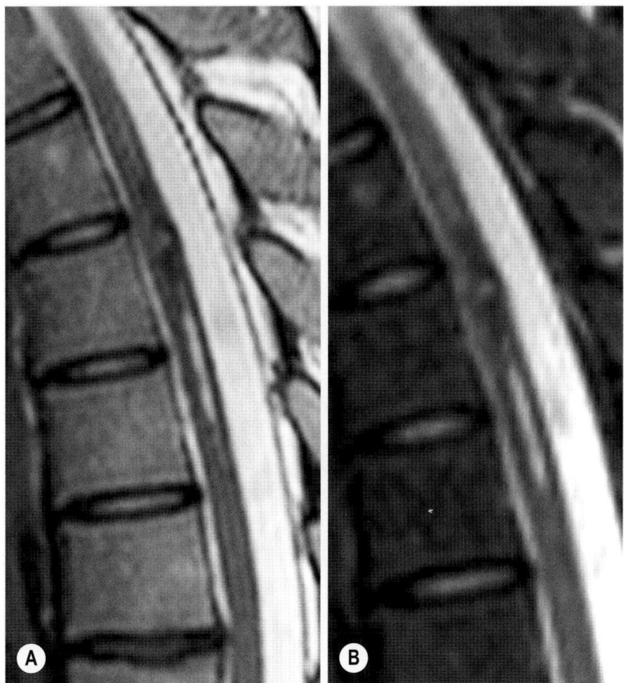

FIGURE 57-9 ■ Spinal cord cavernous malformation (SCCM). (A) Sagittal T_2 and (B) with fat suppression demonstrating intramedullary lesion with heterogeneous signal intensity and T_2 hypointense rim in keeping with blood products. Note the associated intrinsic cord T_2 hyperintensity, which extends for several segments above and below the lesion.

Spinal Cord Infarction

In contrast to its cranial counterpart, spinal cord infarction is rare due to its rich anastomotic blood supply. Complication following aortic aneurysm repair and aortic dissection are the most common causes of spinal cord infarction, although frequently no definite case is identified. Clinical presentation is acute, evolving over minutes, in contrast to other myelopathies and spinal cord lesions. The neurological deficit is frequently bilateral and accompanied by pain, with symptoms dependent on the level of involvement. Spinal cord infarcts are more often located in the thoracolumbar cord than the cervical cord and are frequently located

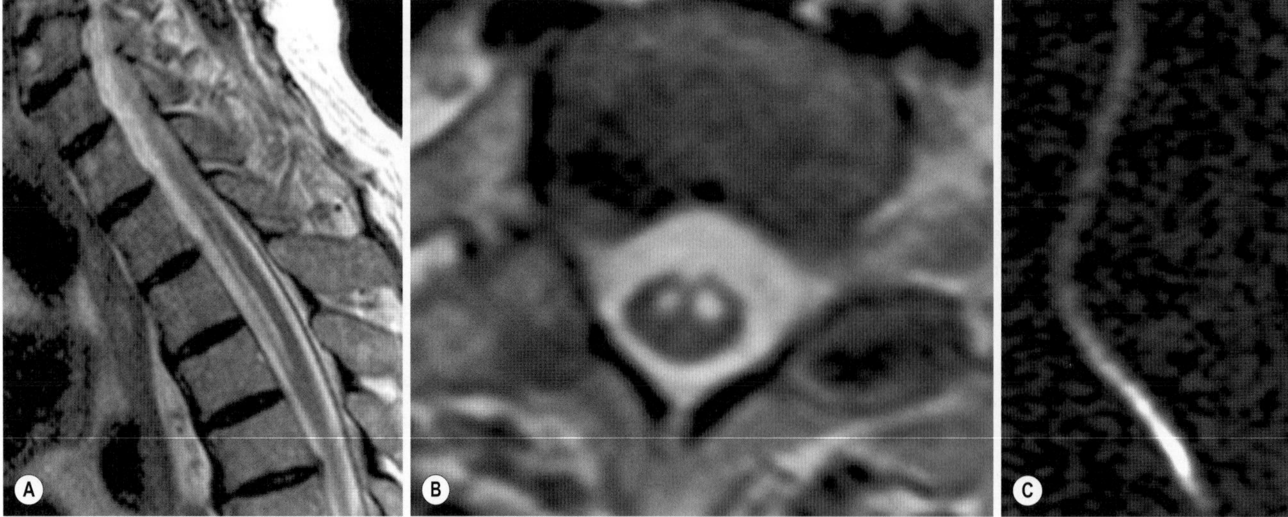

FIGURE 57-10 ■ Acute spinal cord ischaemia with acute onset of symptoms in a male patient following aortic repair. (A) On sagittal T_2 of the cervicothoracic spine linear hyperintensity is shown in the ventral part of the spinal cord extending over three vertebral segments. (B) Axial T_2 demonstrates 'snake's eyes' appearance, indicating involvement of the ventral grey matter of the spinal cord. (C) Sagittal trace DWI demonstrates high signal consistent with restricted diffusion.

in the central and anterior territories of the anterior spinal artery. This results in a classical sensory pattern loss of superficial pain and temperature discrimination, with relative preservation of light touch, vibration and position sense. Weakness and sensory loss for all techniques are found at the segmental levels of the spinal cord infarct.

In acute cases, MRI demonstrates high T_2 signal intensity in the central aspect of the cord; this may result in an 'owl's eyes' or 'snake's eyes' appearance on axial imaging through the lesion due to involvement on the anterior part of the grey matter. There will be some enhancement on post-contrast imaging due to breakdown of the blood–brain barrier. Diffusion-weighted imaging (DWI) is particularly sensitive to acute ischaemic change and should be performed in suspected cases of acute infarcts, which will appear as areas of restricted diffusion (Fig. 57-10).

Spinal Cord Vasculitis

Vasculitis of the spinal cord can be primary or idiopathic, known as primary angitis of the CNS, or secondary to a wide range of immune-mediated and inflammatory conditions such as SLE, Sjögren's and Behçet's disease to name a few.

MRI demonstrates multiple T_2 hyperintense focal intramedullary lesions. On axial images, these are frequently located in the dorsal and lateral aspects of the cord, resembling MS plaques. In the acute phase the lesions enhance following contrast administration and similar lesions can also be shown in the brain (Fig. 57-11). Follow-up MRI studies will show regression of the enhancement of some/all of the lesions.

Imaging findings are non-specific, with a wide differential diagnosis including MS, ADEM, sarcoidosis, infections and metastases, which have been discussed elsewhere in this and other chapters. A diagnosis of spinal vasculitis should only be made after clinical correlation, a review of the brain imaging and results of other diagnostic tests.

SPINAL CORD INFECTION

Spinal cord infection can be bacterial, viral, fungal or parasitic in origin.

Bacterial spinal cord abscess is a rare entity, with epidural abscess being far more common. In most described cases of *Staphylococcus aureus* abscesses, meningitis and epidural abscess were simultaneously present. Bacterial spinal cord abscesses have been described in intravenous drug abusers, in the setting of an intracardiac right-to-left shunt, following lumbar punction, and also in otherwise healthy individuals. On MRI, bacterial intramedullary abscesses will have ring-like or peripheral enhancement, high-signal-intensity centre and marked spinal cord oedema.

Tuberculous spinal cord abscess is a rare form of spinal tuberculosis, compared to extradural collections in tuberculous spondylodiscitis. The lesions exhibit low signal intensity on T_1 and high signal on T_2 with peripheral enhancement of the capsule. In cases of tuberculous myelitis T_2 hyperintensity in the spinal cord with or without enhancement will be observed (Fig. 57-12). Intramedullary tuberculoma is rare and the thoracic cord is the most common location. The MRI appearance is characterised by hypointense ring enhancement, with or without

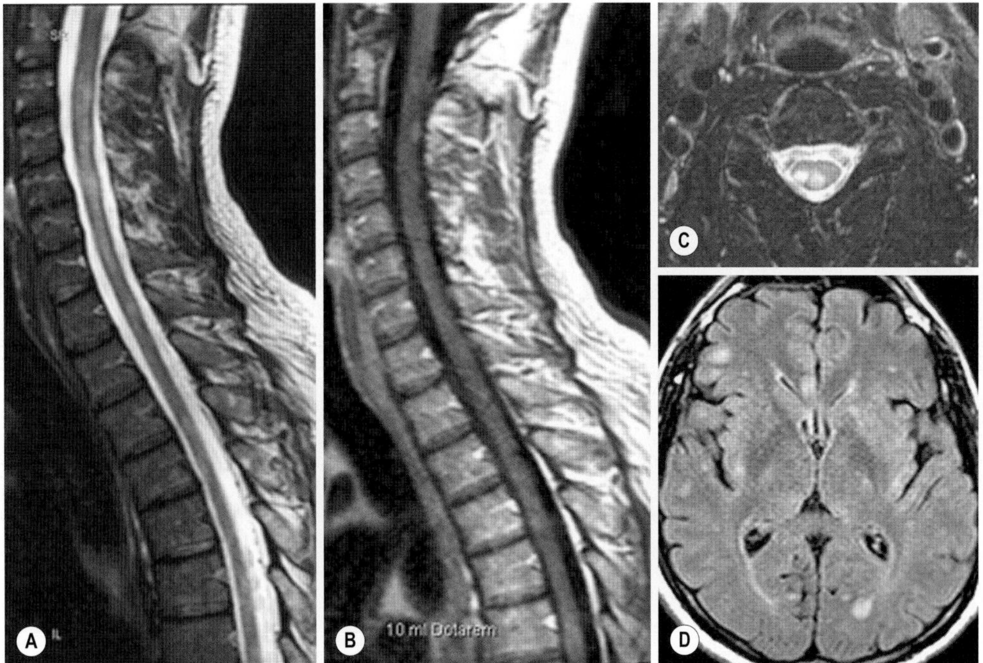

FIGURE 57-11 ■ **Vasculitis with brain and spinal cord involvement.** (A) The sagittal STIR images show multiple focal hyperintense lesions. (B) Only one of these lesions (at the level of C3) shows a subtle enhancement on post-contrast T_1. (C) Axial fat-suppressed T_2 confirms that the lesions are located in the dorsal and lateral parts of the spinal cord, resembling MS lesions. (D) Multiple focal lesions are seen on an axial FLAIR image of the brain.

central hyperintensity on T_2 images and hypo- to isointense rings on T_1 images.

Viral myelitis seen in immunocompromised individuals is mostly due to cytomegalovirus (CMV) infection, and is a common complication after solid organ transplantations. Imaging findings are non-specific with intramedullary T_2 hyperintensity (Fig. 57-13). Varicella-zoster virus (VZV) may also cause myelitis with similar imaging appearances and can occur in immunocompetent as well as immunocompromised individuals.

Fungal spinal cord infections are due to *Aspergillus* or *Candida* species and are mostly seen in immunocompromised patients.

Parasitic myelitis is rare, and has been described in toxoplasmosis and cysticercosis. Patients with toxoplasmic myelitis almost always have cerebral involvement. On MRI, enhancing intramedullary lesions with extensive cord oedema will be seen. Although spinal cord toxoplasmosis is uncommon, in AIDS patients presenting with evolving myelopathy and enhancing lesions in brain and/or spinal cord toxoplasmic myelitis should be considered.

In intramedullary cysticercosis the appearance on MRI depends on the stage. In the early vesicular stage there is a well-defined T_2 hyperintense cyst in the spinal cord. On T_1 the cyst will have low signal intensity with high-signal-intensity scolex. In a later stage (colloidal stage) the thickened cyst capsule shows high signal on T_1 and low signal on T_2. The cyst content appears hyperintense on T_1 and scolex becomes invisible. Peripheral enhancement is seen in cyst degeneration.

DEVELOPMENTAL AND CYST-LIKE LESIONS

The commonest congenital malformation found in adults involves the caudal part of the neural tube. A useful descriptive term is lipomyelomeningodysplasia, which emphasises the various elements. Other conditions result in a dorsal dermal sinus that runs from a skin dimple to the spinal canal, some terminating in intraspinal dermoids or epidermoids. The neuroenteric canal or adhesion may persist, or form at other levels such as the upper cervical region, resulting in neuroenteric cysts along the connection between the foregut and spinal canal; a persistent cutaneous communication results in a dorsal enteric fistula. Aberrant neuro-endodermal adhesions are probably also the origin of diastematomyelia. Finally, excessive retrogressive differentiation can lead to various degrees of sacral and sacrolumbar dysgenesis, often referred to as the caudal regression syndromes.

Intramedullary Lipoma

This consists of a mass of adipose tissue located mainly between the posterior columns of the spinal cord. A tongue-like extension along the central canal is often found, in keeping with its embryogenesis. The overlying dura mater is usually intact and the lipoma entirely intradural; however, there may be a dural defect to which spinal cord and lipoma become adherent. Such

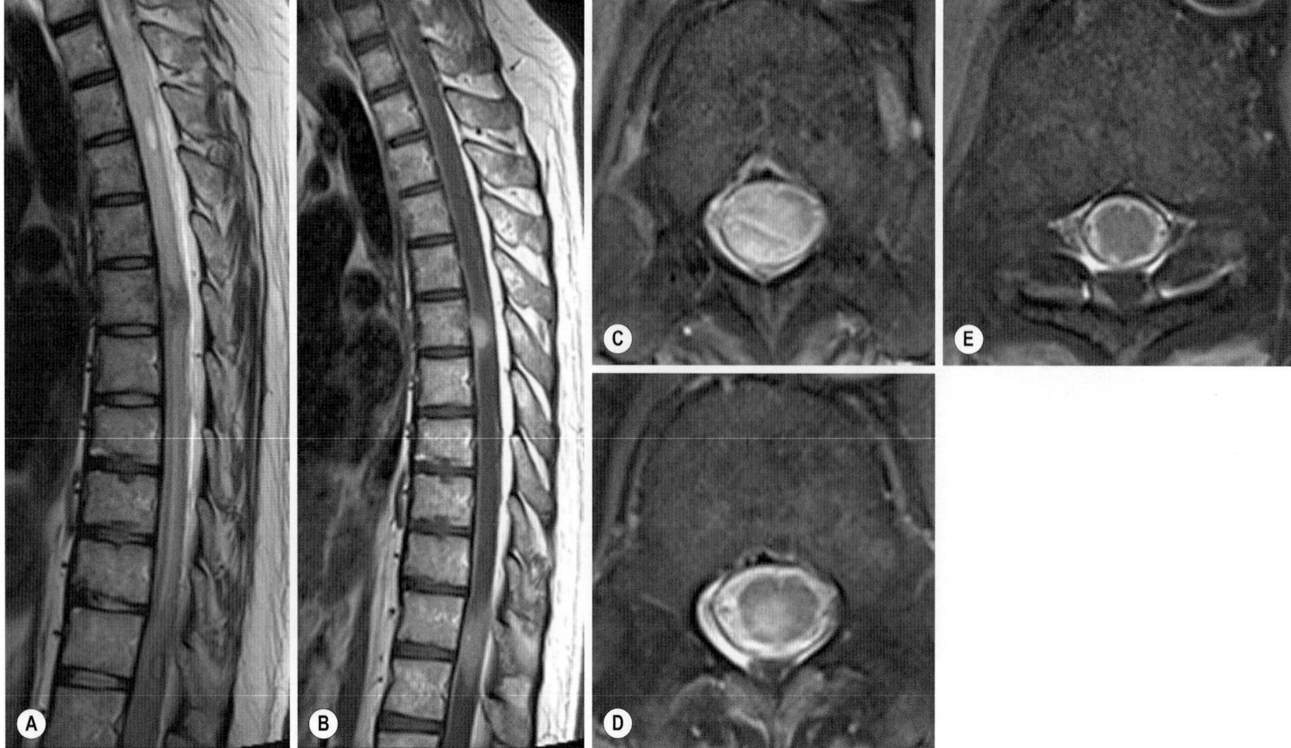

FIGURE 57-12 ■ Spinal TB in male recently moved from India. (A) Sagittal T_2 of the thoracic spine demonstrating multiple intramedullary lesions, of different signal intensities and associated widespread T_2 hyperintensity. These findings are in keeping with TB granulomata and associated spinal cord oedema. The most inferior lesion on this image has a T_2 hypointense rim suggestive of haemorrhage. (B) Following contrast enhancement, some of the lesions enhance. Note also the extensive leptomeningeal enhancement, particularly along the ventral aspect. There is also patchy intramedullary enhancement at the cervicothoracic junction. (C–E) A series of axial contrast-enhanced T_1 through the lower thoracic cord demonstrate cord expansion and enhancement of the intramedullary lesion as well as of the surrounding leptomeninges and CSF space, which appears bright, mimicking a T_2 sequence.

lesions occur most often near the thoracocervical or craniovertebral junction. CT and MRI demonstrate the fatty nature of the tumour. They may be associated with other conditions such as diastomatomyelia (Fig. 57-14). Non-fatty elements may also be present, resulting in a heterogeneous appearance.

Lipomyelomeningodysplasias

These represent a spectrum of abnormalities ranging from an abnormally low location of the conus medullaris with minimal or even absent lipoma, to massive lipomatous formations involving all elements of the spinal and adjacent subcutaneous tissues. The abnormality may not be apparent clinically, hence the term occult spinal dysraphism. Unlike myelocele, Chiari malformation is present in only 6%. Patients frequently present in adult life, sometimes only with back pain and minimal neurological signs.

MR is the optimal investigation, although ultrasound (US) has been advocated in children. MR demonstrates all aspects of the abnormalities including the origin of nerve roots and associated lesions such as cysts in the spinal cord. In over 80%, the spinal cord terminates at or below the level of the third lumbar vertebra, and is usually tethered to the dorsal aspect of the dura, where it fuses with the fatty tumour. Nerve roots issuing from an apparently thickened filum terminale indicate that it contains significant nervous tissue and therefore should not be divided surgically.

Diastematomyelia

The spinal cord is split into two usually unequal hemicords, each with a central canal and anterior spinal artery, but giving rise to only ipsilateral spinal roots. Any level can be involved, including the filum terminale and medulla oblongata, but most are thoracic.[18] The cleavage usually extends over several segments and only rarely do the hemicords not reunite caudally. The hemicords are enclosed in a common dural tube in 50% of cases, usually in the cervical region, but in the remainder each is enclosed in its own dural tube, with a bony or cartillagenous spur arising from malformed lamina often lying between them. Abnormal traction may be exerted by such a spur at the point of reunion of the hemicords. Clinical abnormalities are often absent, but in some symptomatic cases progression apparently was halted by excision of tethering spurs. MRI shows the abnormality well (Fig. 57-14).

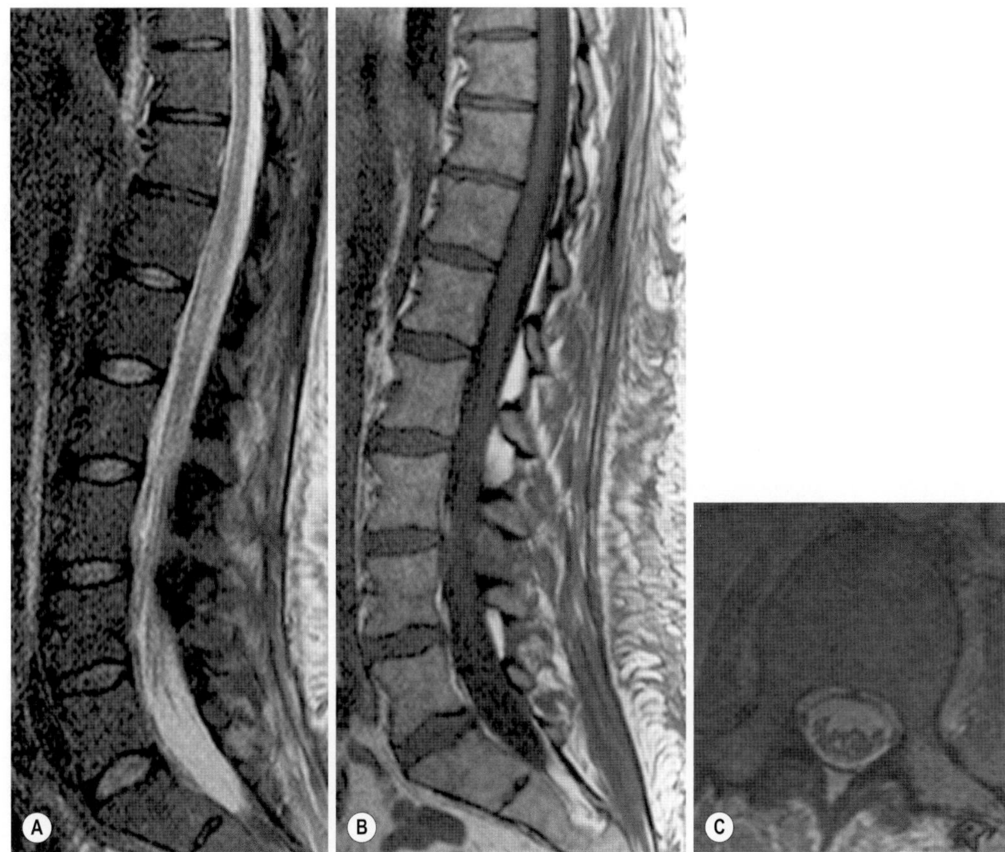

FIGURE 57-13 ■ Cytomegalovirus (CMV) myelitis in an immunocompromised patient after heart transplantation. (A) On sagittal STIR images subtle high signal intensity is detected in the conus medullaris. (B) On sagittal post-contrast T_1 images only subtle enhancement and clumping of cauda equina was detected on (C) axial T_2. In the CSF analysis PCR was positive for CMV.

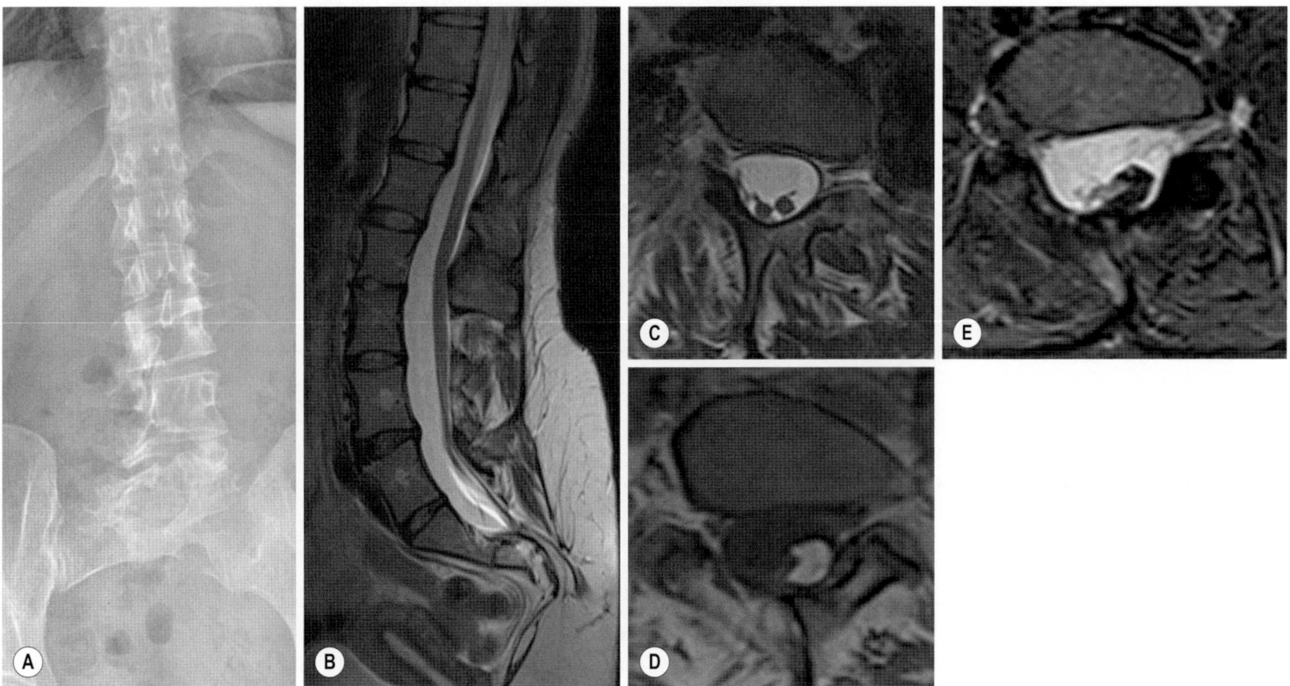

FIGURE 57-14 ■ Diastematomyelia. (A) AP thoracolumbar radiograph demonstrating deformity of L4 and L5 vertebrae and the sacrum with absence of the coccyx. There is a mild lumbar scoliosis concave to the right. (B) Sagittal T_1 of the lumbar spine demonstrating an ill-defined low-lying conus at the L4–L5 level. The nerve roots are tethered caudally and herniate through a bony defect in the posterior elements. There is agenesis of the lower sacrum and of the coccyx. (C) Axial T_2 through the lower thoracic spine clearly demonstrates the split cord. (D) Axial T_1 through the lower dural sac demonstrates an intradural extramedullary left-sided high-signal-intensity lesion. This suppresses on (E) fat-suppressed axial T_2 at the same level. The appearances are in keeping with a lipoma.

Neuroenteric and Other Developmental Cysts

Intraspinal neuroenteric cysts are intradural, usually unilocular cysts lined by gastrointestinal or bronchial epithelium that occur in either the cervical (often near the craniovertebral junction) or lower thoracic regions.[19] They compress the spinal cord (usually the anterior aspect) and may invaginate into its substance; occasionally the spinal cord is split into two halves as in diastematomyelia. Plain radiography may show focal expansion of the spinal canal, and thoracic lesions in particular may be associated with butterfly or hemivertebrae (Fig. 57-15). On MRI the cyst contents may yield a slightly higher

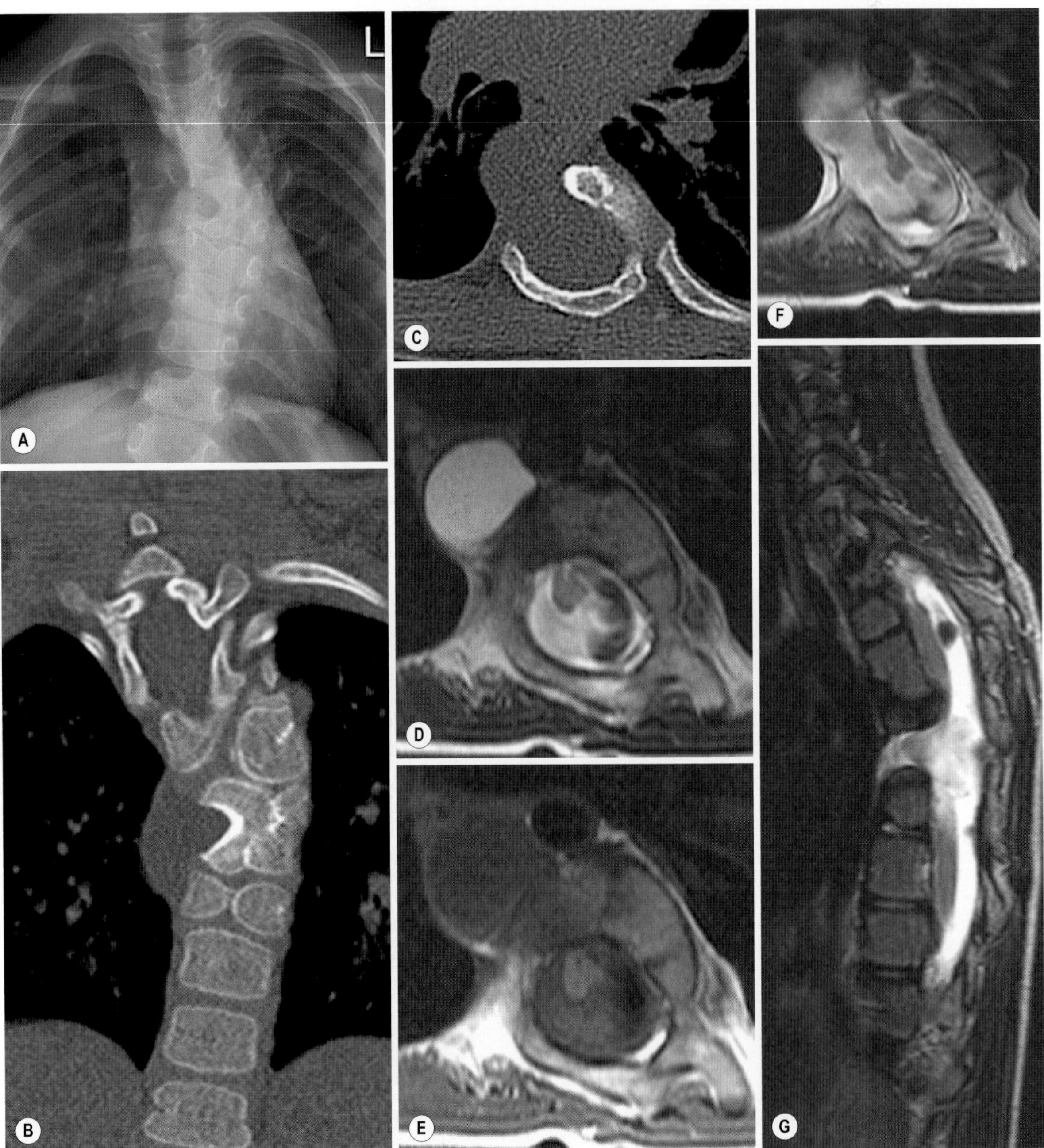

FIGURE 57-15 ■ **Neuroenteric cyst.** (A) Chest radiograph and (B) coronal multiplanar reformat of CT thorax in same patient. There is a complex segmentation anomaly within the mid-thoracic region associated with kyphoscoliosis, consisting of congenital fusion and butterfly vertebrae. There is an associated right paraspinal mass. (C) Axial CT through the lesion shows that it is in direct continuation with the spinal canal through a large ventral bony defect. (D) Axial T_2 and (E) axial T_1 at the level of the lesion demonstrating that the lesion is cystic. (F) Axial T_2 through the bony defect demonstrates the direct continuity of the cyst with the spinal canal. The appearances are in keeping with a neuroenteric cyst. The thoracic cord is also seen to extend through the bony defect. The neural tissue is seen to lie to the left of the neuroenteric cyst. (G) Sagittal T_2 in the right paramidline demonstrating the direct communication with the spinal canal.

signal than cerebrospinal fluid, on T_1 as well as T_2 sequences, but are clearly demarcated from cord substance. Communication with the spinal canal is clearly demonstrated by both CT and MRI (Fig. 57-15).

Dermoid and epidermoid cysts are rounded intradural and sometimes intramedullary lesions. Imaging may demonstrate fat within them and calcification. They may be associated with other forms of dysraphism, and in about 20% a dorsal dermal sinus can be traced running obliquely downwards from the lesion to a skin dimple on the lower back, which may also be a source of intradural sepsis.[20]

Ependymal cysts usually occur with other types of dysraphism. They represent little more than focal dilatations of the central canal of the spinal cord, usually appearing as a swelling near the lumbar enlargement.

Chiari Malformations

These represent a group of abnormalities characterised by dislocation of the hindbrain into the spinal canal. Chiari described four types, but his types III and IV are rare and the Chiari II is seen mainly in the paediatric practice. The Chiari I lesion is not really a malformation at all: it may be acquired in conditions associated with raised intracranial pressure (tumours, venous hypertension), lowered intraspinal pressure (lumbo-peritoneal shunts) and conditions that diminish the volumes of the posterior fossa (craniosynostosis, basilar invagination). It may develop in the first 3 years of life[21] in the absence of any cause other than probable slower growth of the posterior fossa relative to the hindbrain during this period when both are growing most rapidly.

Chiari Type I Lesion (Cerebellar Ectopia)

This is defined as descent of otherwise normal cerebellar hemispheres below the foramen magnum, usually involving the tonsils. However, in about 50% of cases, the medulla oblongata shows elongation of the segment between the pontomedullary junction and dorsal column nuclei with the obex of the fourth ventricle coming to lie in the cervical canal, where it may or may not be overlain by the cerebellar tonsils.

Elongation is sufficient to produce a kink on the posterior surface of the medulla oblongata in about 15%, where the tail of the fourth ventricle rolls down over the upper one or more segments of the spinal cord. The prevalence of Chiari type I lesion in the normal population has been considerably overestimated on MRI, and is probably under 1%.[22]

Chiari Type II Malformations

In these malformations the cerebellum is dysplastic. The inferior vermis is everted rather than inverted so that the nodulus becomes the most inferior part of the cerebellum and the fourth ventricle is reduced to a coronal cleft. The cerebellar herniation then consists mainly of inferior vermis. The medulla oblongata is invariably elongated, usually enough to become kinked. Hydrocephalus and dysplasia of the cerebral hemispheres, cranial vaults and meninges are frequent. A meningomyelocele is present in 98% or more of cases, and may play an important role in embryogenesis.

These hindbrain abnormalities may be associated with compression and progressive degeneration in parts of the brainstem, cerebellum and upper spinal cord. In Chiari type I malformations, symptoms commonly do not appear until adult life and about 50% of symptomatic cases are associated with syringomyelia. Syringomylia occurs most commonly when the cerebellar tonsils lie between the neural arches of C1 and C2, whereas cerebellar syndromes predominate when the tonsils lie lower than the neural arch of C2.[23]

In up to 15% of type I lesions, occipitalisation of the atlas and basilar invagination are present.

MRI is by far the best way to demonstrate hindbrain abnormalities, which are present in over 5% of symptomatic cases (Fig. 57-16). However, descent of the cerebellum through the foramen magnum of up to 3 mm is present in up to 20% of normal subjects on mid-sagittal MRI sections due to the shape of the foramen magnum and partial volume effects with the more laterally placed biventral lobules, and MRI in the coronal plane is more reliable (Fig. 57-16).[22]

Meningoceles

Varying degrees of dural ectasia usually accompany the spinal dysraphisms. Both generalised and focal dural ectasia may occur in systemic disorders such as neurofibromatosis, Ehlers–Danlos and Marfan's syndromes. It may occur in erosive arthropathies, especially ankylosing spondylitis,[24] where focal ectasia sometimes forms pockets or saccules invaginating into the walls of the spinal canal, including the vertebral bodies and neural arches. Such lesions also occur idiopathically.

Anterior Sacral Meningocele

This lesion consists of a unilocular, complex lobular or even multilocular presacral cystic mass, containing CSF, which communicates with the intraspinal subarachnoid space.

There is a large usually eccentric anterior defect in the lower part of the sacrum, and the sacral canal is expanded. Varying degrees of sacral and coccygeal agenesis may be associated. On plain radiographs, the eccentric anterior sacral defect gives the remaining part of the sacrum a pathognomonic scimitar appearance. The pelvic mass may be shown by US, CT or MRI, the latter invariably demonstrating communications with the sacral canal (Fig. 57-17).

Occult intrasacral meningocele is a variant of this condition. The sacral canal is expanded by a meningocele that lies below the normal level of termination of the thecal sac. There is no anterior sacral defect and no intrapelvic extension.

Lateral Thoracic Meningocele

This lesion commonly presents as a paravertebral mass on chest radiography. It is commonly solitary and usually is found on the right; 70–85% of lesions are associated with neurofibromatosis. There is typically an angular

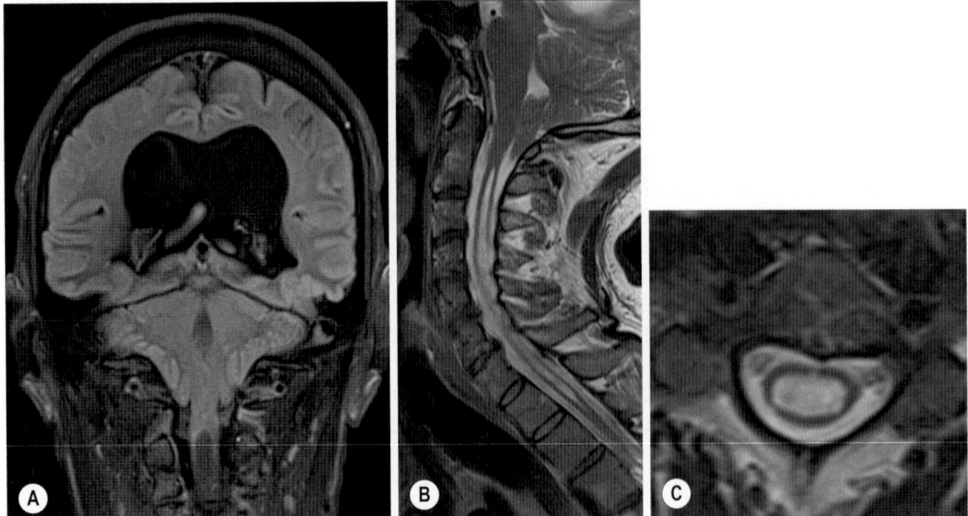

FIGURE 57-16 ■ **Chiari I malformation.** (A) Coronal FLAIR demonstrating bitonsilar herniation. Note the secondary hydrocephalus. (B) Sagittal T_2 demonstrating the Chiari malformation and an associated extensive cervical syrinx cavity. (C) Axial T_2 showing syrinx cavity of CSF density.

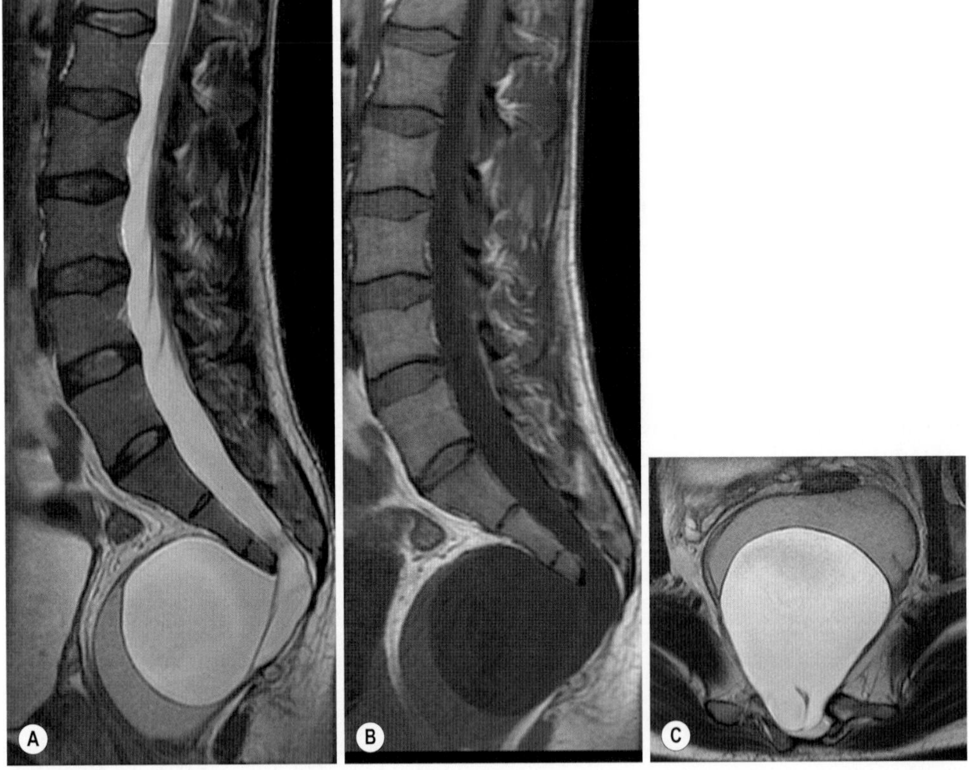

FIGURE 57-17 ■ **Anterior sacral meningocele.** (A) Sagittal T_2, (B) sagittal T_1 and (C) axial T_2 of the lumbar spine demonstrating a large presacral cystic mass that is in direct continuation with the vertebral canal through an anterior vertebral defect. Note the agenesis of the coccyx and the lower sacrum.

kyphoscoliosis towards the side of the meningocele, and pressure erosion of the margins of the relevant intervertebral foramen is evident.

Anterior Thoracic Meningocele with Ventral Herniation of Spinal Cord

This is an increasingly recognised condition very occasionally providing explanation for an otherwise unexplained chronic thoracic myelopathy in adults.[25] It is most readily recognised on mid-sagittal MRI of the thoracic spine, where the spinal cord is displaced anteriorly in contact with a vertebral body at or very near an intervertebral disc, commonly at about T6. The meningocele may not be easy to show on axial images. Appearances are often misinterpreted as an intradural arachnoid cyst displacing the spinal cord anteriorly, from which the condition needs to be distinguished.

Intraspinal Arachnoid Cyst

Extradural arachnoid cysts arise from defects in the dura mater, either congenital or inflammatory (e.g. ankylosing spondylitis); intradural arachnoid cysts arise from arachnoidal duplications or spinal arachnoiditis. Symptoms of pain or neurological disability may arise when the spinal cord or cauda equina is compressed, bearing in mind that size and intracystic pressure may vary considerably. Occasionally, the spinal cord or roots herniate through a dural defect and become entrapped. Plain radiographs may show expansion of the spinal canal when the cyst is extradural. MRI shows these lesions well (Fig. 57-18). Signal from fluid in the cyst, and often from the subarachnoid space below it, is usually higher than from CSF elsewhere due to reduced mobility. Effects on the spinal cord, namely compression and rarely myelomalacia or syringomyelia, are shown. Small herniations of neural tissue through the dural defects may require thin imaging sections and high-resolution imaging techniques to show them. Aspiration and drainage of arachnoid cysts compressing the spinal cord may be accompanied by immediate and dramatic improvement in clinical condition.[26]

Care must be exercised not to overdiagnose intradural arachnoid cysts in the thoracic region. The retromedullary subarachnoid space in the thoracic spine is commonly wide, and partly loculated by usually incomplete septae; the spinal cord usually is closely applied to the anterior margin of the bony canal and may have a flattened appearance over an exaggerated kyphosis.

Perineural arachnoid cysts (Tarlov cysts) occur commonly in the sacrum, especially on the second sacral root. They can be large, multiple and are often associated with eccentric pressure erosion of the sacral canal and are well shown by MRI. Clinical significance, even of large cysts, is doubtful.[27]

Syringomyelia

The term 'syringomyelia' describes conditions in which there is a cavity within the spinal cord, lined mainly by glial tissue and containing fluid that is similar or identical

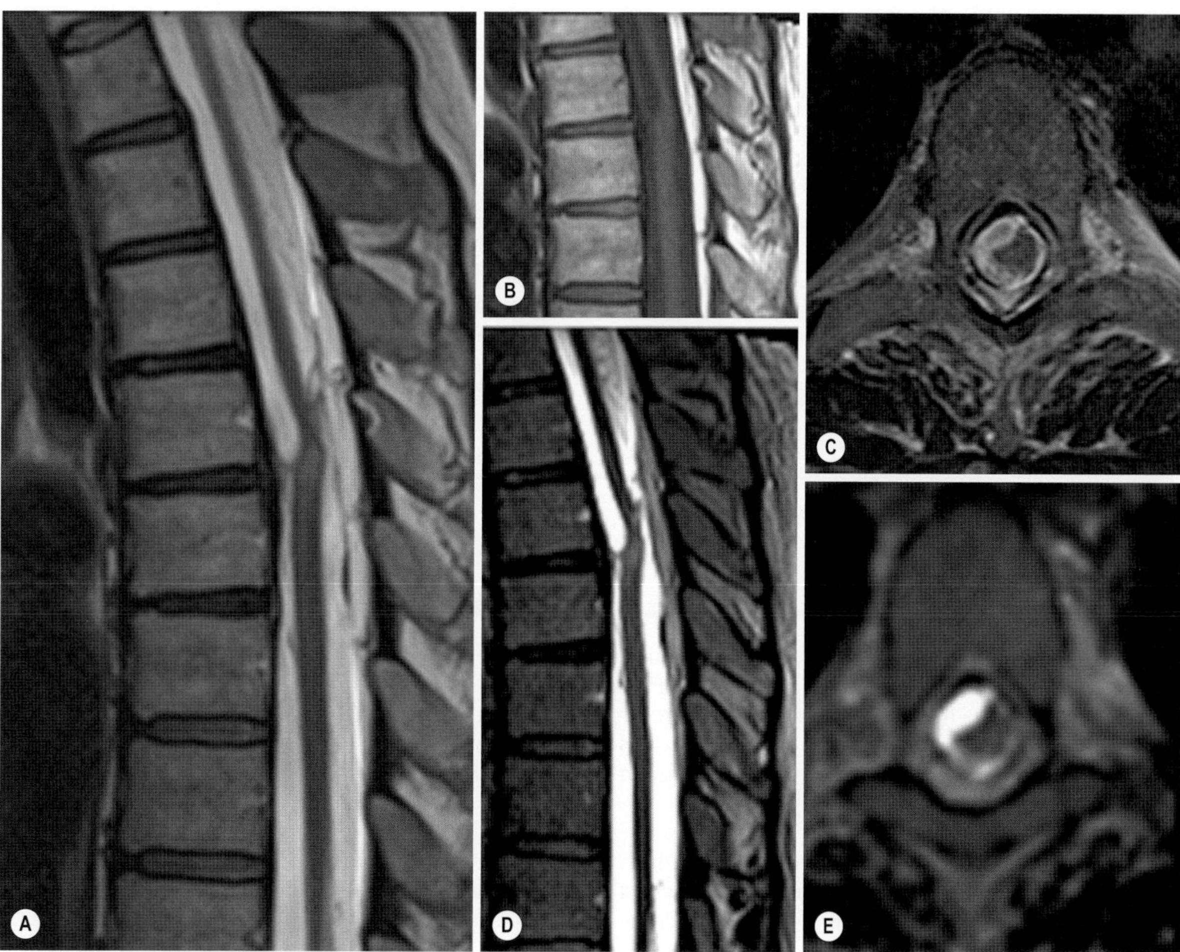

FIGURE 57-18 ■ Intraspinal arachnoid cyst. (A) Sagittal T_2, (B) sagittal T_1 and (C) axial T_2 of the thoracic spine demonstrating an abnormal appearance to the mid-thoracic cord, which is moulded and displaced to the left by a right anterior intradural extramedullary lesion of CSF signal intensity. There is focal volume loss and subtle intrinsic signal change within the cord at this level in keeping with focal myelomalacia from compression. The conventional T_2 (A and C) images demonstrate CSF flow-related artefact in the lesion (focal areas of signal drop). This artefact is not present on (D) sagittal CISS and (E) axial CISS images, which demonstrate the lesion more clearly.

with CSF. It is associated with a number of distinct pathological processes, including cerebellar ectopia and trauma.[28] Whatever the cause, the cavity seems capable of propagating, probably due to hydrodynamic forces, into normal cord tissue. Usually it involves many segments or the whole spinal cord, but sometimes smaller isolated cavities are found confined to only a few spinal segments, often referred to as fusiform syrinx. The cervical cord is involved most often, although occasionally only the thoracic cord. Only about 10% of cysts extend cranial to C2, where they split into two or deviate to right or left in a plane ventral to the floor of the fourth ventricle. Small cavities usually involve the bases of the posterior columns, and commonly the central cord canal for part of their extent; larger cavities are associated with more extensive loss of cord substance. Double cavities are sometimes present and individual cavities may be multilocular. The spinal cord is enlarged in about 80% of cases, normal in size in 10% and diffusely atrophic in 10%. The size of the spinal cord may vary in response to posture and respiration. Size variation usually is not associated with changes in clinical state, nor does the severity of clinical disability relate to the size of the cyst and remaining cord substance.[29]

Between 70 and 90% of cases of syringomyelia are associated with cerebellar ectopia, the cerebellar tonsils usually lying at the level of C1 or between C1 and C2 (Fig. 57-16).[23] It is postulated that intermittent obstruction of the outlets of the fourth ventricle and of CSF flow across the foramen magnum, combined with a patent communication between the fourth ventricle and the central canal of the spinal cord, together produce secondary degeneration of cord substance by causing intermittent distension of the central canal but alternative hypotheses exist.[30] The term syringohydromyelia is often used for this type of cord cavitation.

Other causes of cavitation of the spinal cord can result in appearances indistinguishable from syringohydromyelia. These include intramedullary tumours, spinal cord trauma and inflammatory processes discussed earlier in this chapter, which can result in colliquative necrosis (myelomalacia), which may organise into cavities that propagate into normal cord substance. Finally in about 10–20% of patients with spinal cord cavities, no cause or association can be found.

Syringomyelia and its cause are well demonstrated by MRI, which shows a well-circumscribed cavity of a similar signal to CSF on T_1 and T_2 sequences (Fig. 57-16). Pulsatile cysts may show flow-related signal changes.[31] Dynamic MRI, using phase-contrast techniques, has been used to study CSF movement, especially at foramen magnum level.[32]

A moderate correlation is found between the presence and location of the cavity on MRI and clinical features, but *not* between clinical severity and size of the syrinx relative to remaining cord substance, *or* with its degree of distension.[33–35] MRI is good for monitoring the mechanical success of operative strategies,[36] of which three are in current use, the third being new and controversial, deriving from an alternative theory of causation: (A) foramen magnum decompression; (B) syringo-subarachnoid, peritoneal or pleural shunting; and (C) lumbo-peritoneal shunting.[37,38] All seem equally effective in obtaining, and generally maintaining, collapse of the syrinx in 70–80% of cases. Unfortunately, however, clinical outcome and extension of cord cavitation on interval images seem to bear no relation to whether the cavity remains collapsed.[36]

NEURODEGENERATIVE AND METABOLIC DISEASES

Motor Neuron Disease (MND)

This condition comprises a group of progressive neurodegenerative diseases affecting the upper and lower motor neurons of the brain and spinal cord. They can be classified according to the type of motor neuron it affects. In amyotrophic lateral sclerosis (ALS) both upper and lower neurons are affected at two or more levels; progressive muscular atrophy (PMA) involves only the lower motor neurons, whilst primary lateral sclerosis (PLS) involves only upper motor neurons. Rarely, the disease is restricted to the bulbar muscles, secondary to disease affecting the motor nuclei in the medulla, when it is termed progressive bulbar palsy (PBP).

ALS, also known as Lou Gehrig disease, is the most common of the motor neurodegenerative diseases and almost all cases evolve to this. Most cases are sporadic, with only approximately 5–10% being familial, inherited in an autosomal dominant pattern.[39] Most commonly the presentation is a mixed pattern of hand weakness and atrophy of the intrinsic hand muscles, together with hyperreflexia and ataxia reflecting lower and upper motor neuron involvement, respectively. Limb fasciculations are common. With disease progression comes weakness and atrophy of the lower limb, dysarthria, dysphagia and tongue fasciculations. Prognosis is poor, with death from respiratory failure.

MRI plays a role in excluding other diagnoses, such as MS or radiculopathy, but can be normal. Positive MRI findings are of symmetrical T_2 hyperintensity in the lateral columns, best appreciated on axial imaging,[40] correlating well with histopathological findings affecting primarily the lateral corticospinal tracts.

Spinal Muscular Atrophy (SMA)

This is a large group of genetically associated autosomal recessive neuromuscular disorders, characterised by loss of the spinal lower motor neurons in the anterior horns with no sensory or pyramidal tract involvement. The genetic defects associated with SMA types I–III are localised on chromosome 5q11.2-13.3.[41] The international SMA consortium meeting recognises four distinct subtypes based on age of onset: (A) type I, acute infantile form; (B) type II, chronic infantile or intermediate form; (C) type III, juvenile form; and (D) type IV, adult form.[42] MRI may reveal focal atrophy of the cervical cord with an associated small area of T_2 hyperintensity. These findings are non-specific and associated with focal myelomalacia from other causes, for example following trauma.

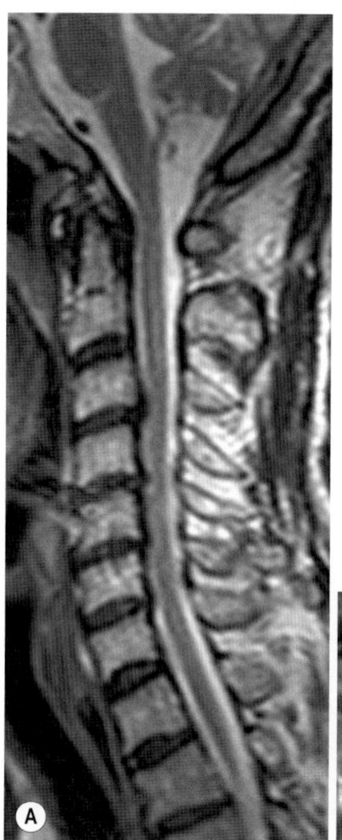
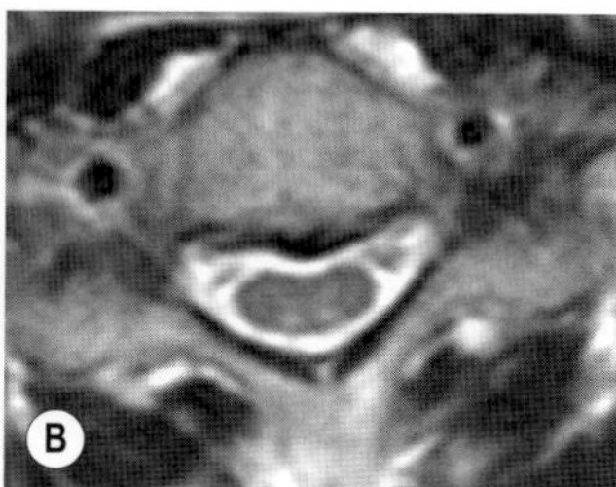

FIGURE 57-19 ■ **Subacute combined degeneration of the spinal cord (SCD) in a 60-year-old man after gastrectomy.** (A) Sagittal T_2 showing linear high signal intensity in the cervical spinal cord extending over two segments, without associated cord swelling. (B) Typical bilateral dorsal hyperintensities are demonstrated on axial T_2.

Spinocerebellar Ataxia

This term encompasses a large group of progressive inherited neurodegenerative disorders characterised by ataxia and poor coordination of hand, speech and eye movements which are progressive. They are classified by mode of inheritance and the causative gene. The most common of the autosomal dominant group is spinocerebellar degeneration, itself consisting of different subtypes. Friedreich's ataxia is the commonest of the autosomal recessive forms.

Friedreich's Ataxia (FRDA)

This is the most common inherited ataxia. It is caused by mutations in the frataxin gene, causing loss of large primary neurons in the dorsal root ganglia, sensory fibres in peripheral nerves, degeneration of the posterior and lateral columns of the spinal cord and atrophy of the cerebellar dentate nucleus. It presents with progressive limb and gait ataxia, dysarthria, loss of position and vibration senses and areflexia.

MRI of the spine demonstrates thinning of the cervical spinal cord, particularly in the anterior posterior dimension. There is also frequently intramedullary T_2 hyperintensity, which is symmetrical within the posterior or lateral columns of the spinal cord.[43]

Subacute Combined Degeneration of the Spinal Cord (SCD)

This is a progressive myelopathy presenting with sensory symptoms in the context of dietary deficiency of vitamin B_{12} or co-proteins. Vitamin B_{12} deficiency can be due to malabsorption syndromes, previous gastrectomy, pernicious anemia and dietary deficiencies (e.g. in strict vegetarians). The lateral and dorsal spinal cord columns are affected, and improvement is often only partial after treatment. A typical MR imaging finding is a linear hyperintensity on sagittal T_2 located bilateral dorsally in the cord (Fig. 57-19) that regresses on treatment. Lesions, which are most often seen between C2 and C5, may enhance after IV contrast medium. However, MRI may also remain negative.[44]

For a full list of references, please see ExpertConsult.

FURTHER READING

Agosta F, Filippi M. MRI of spinal cord in multiple sclerosis. J Neuroimaging 2007;17(Suppl 1):46S–9S.

Borchers AT, Gershwin ME. Transverse myelitis. Autoimmun Rev 2012;11:231–48.

Bot JC, Barkhof F. Spinal-cord MRI in multiple sclerosis: conventional and nonconventional MR techniques. Neuroimaging Clin N Am 2009;19:81–99.

Lycklama G, Thompson A, Filippi M, et al. Spinal-cord MRI in multiple sclerosis. Lancet Neurol 2003;2:555–62.

McKeon A, Lennon VA, Lotze T, et al. CNS aquaporin-4 autoimmunity in children. Neurology 2008;71:93–100.

Pavone P, Pettoello-Mantovano M, Le Pira A, et al. Acute disseminated encephalomyelitis: a long-term prospective study and meta-analysis. Neuropediatrics 2010;41:246–55.

Pittock SJ, Lennon VA, Krecke K, et al. Brain abnormalities in neuromyelitis optica. Arch Neurol 2006;63:390–6.

Sellner J, Lüthi N, Bühler R, et al. Acute partial transverse myelitis: risk factors for conversion to multiple sclerosis. Eur J Neurol 2008;15:398–405.

Thomas T, Branson HM, Verhey LH, et al. Demographic, clinical, and magnetic resonance imaging (MRI) features of transverse myelitis in children. J Child Neurol 2011;27(1):11–21.

Wender M. Acute disseminated encephalomyelitis. J Neuroimmunol 2011;231:92–9.

Weinshenker BG, Wingerchuk DM. Neuromyelitis optica: clinical syndrome and the NMO-IgG autoantibody marker. Curr Top Microbiol Immunol 2008;318:343–56.

Wingerchuk DM, Lennon VA, Pittock SJ, et al. Revised diagnostic criteria for neuromyelitis optica. Neurology 2006;66:1485–9.

CHAPTER 58

Postoperative Spine

Tomasz Matys • Nasim Sheikh-Bahaei • Jonathan H. Gillard

CHAPTER OUTLINE

INTRODUCTION

Imaging plays an important role in the assessment of the postoperative spine. The main objectives of imaging are to evaluate the alignment of the spinal column, the position of implants and the status of fusion or fracture healing, and to demonstrate potential complications in case of persistent or new postoperative symptoms.[1,2] Postsurgical appearances may be complex, and knowledge of indications for surgery, type of the procedure, hardware and biomaterials used and pertinent clinical information is essential to avoid misinterpretation.[3] In this chapter we discuss principles of spinal surgery and briefly review its potential complications with emphasis on these most often encountered in radiological practice.

PRINCIPLES OF SPINAL SURGERY

The goals of spinal surgery can be broadly categorised into three main groups:

1. Decompression of neural structures, for example by removal of herniated disc material, widening of a stenosed spinal canal, or removal of a displaced fracture fragment.
2. Stabilisation of the spinal column in order to reduce pain caused by motion segments, ensure stability after a fracture or resection of spinal elements, prevent progression of deformity, or reduce its degree.
3. Excision of spinal tumours.

In order to achieve decompression, several surgical techniques are employed, usually in combination.[1,4] Removal of intervertebral disc material is performed by discectomy or minimally invasive microdiscectomy; access to herniated disc may require removal of the margins of the lamina (laminotomy), unilateral laminar resection (hemilaminectomy) and resection of the ligamentum flavum (flavectomy). Techniques used in spinal canal decompression include laminoplasty (osteotomy of one lamina with contralateral partial osteotomy to allow formation of a unilateral gap), bilateral laminectomy with the removal of the posterior elements and deroofing of the spinal canal and/or facetectomy (excision of a part or entire facet joint). Neural foraminal decompression is achieved by foraminotomy. More extensive techniques used in the management of traumatic fractures and primary or metastatic spinal tumours include resection of one or both pedicles (pediculectomy), vertebral body (corpectomy) or entire vertebra (vertebrectomy).

Stabilisation can be the primary goal of surgery, or can be performed in combination with decompressive or excision procedures that impair spine stability. In the majority of cases, a stabilisation procedure consists of instrumentation and bone grafting. Types of fixation devices used include translaminar or facet screws, and transpedicular screws in conjunction with rods, plates, hooks, wires or clamps.[1] It is important to realise that metalwork, although usually left in place indefinitely, is only relied upon for temporary support until uninterrupted osseous union is achieved. Bone fusion can be promoted by a variety of graft materials.[5] Autologous bone grafts are most often harvested from the iliac crest, another part of the spine, or for purely cortical bone, from the tibia or fibula. Ground-up (morselised) cancellous bone chips are used to promote osteogenesis (Fig. 58-1A), while cortical bone is used for structural support (Figs. 58-1B, C). Allograft bone substitutes are obtained from the tissue bank and include femoral rings, fibular struts and bone chips that can be used on their own or to supplement allografts. Synthetic graft substitutes include recombinant bone morphogenetic protein (BMP), demineralised bone matrix (DBX) and ceramics

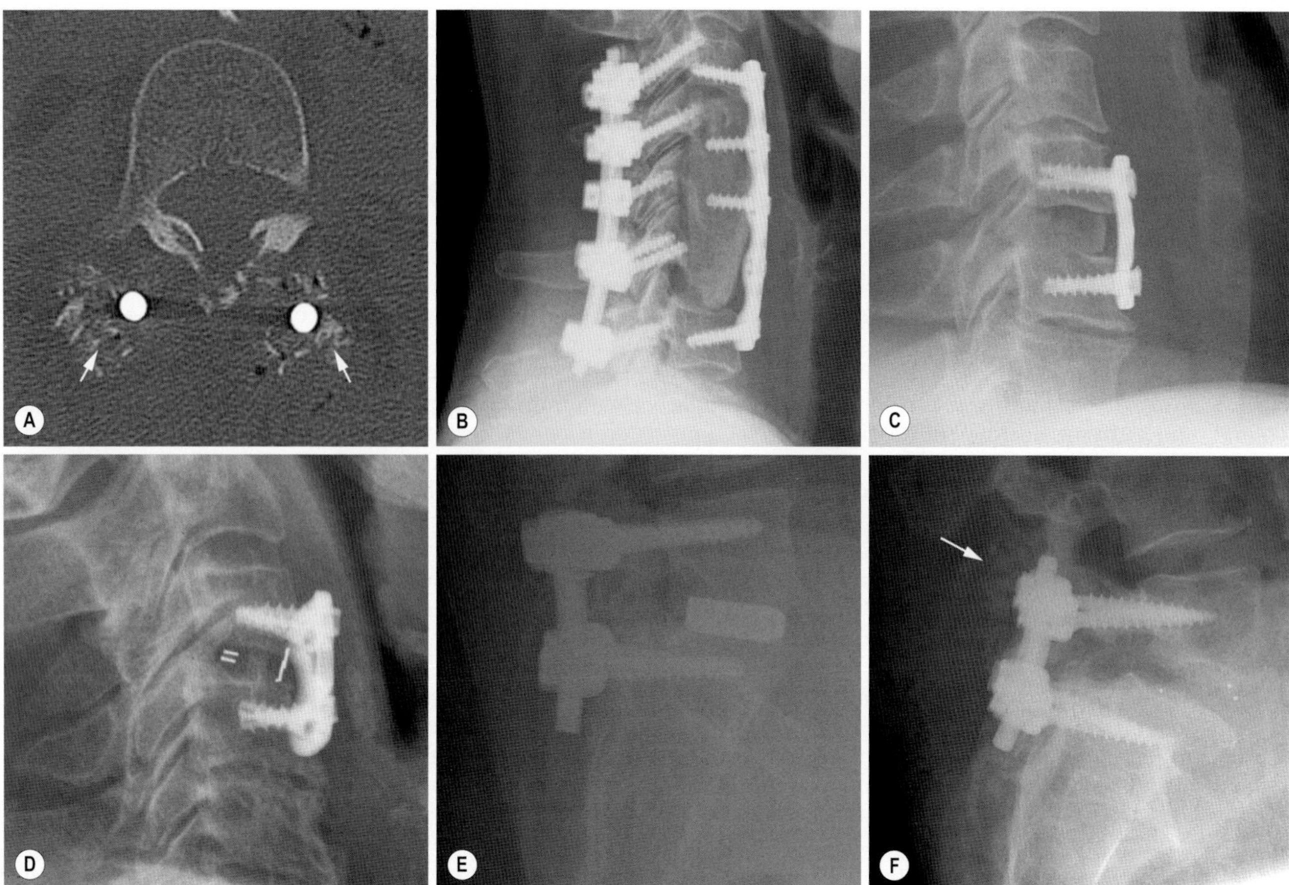

FIGURE 58-1 ■ (A) Axial CT image showing morselised bone chips (arrows) in a patient with lumbar fixation. (B) Lateral radiograph of the cervical spine showing autologous bone graft from iliac crest used for structural support in a patient with C4–C6 corpectomies for chordoma treatment. Note anterior plate and posterior fixation with pedicular screws and rods spanning C3–C7 levels. (C) Interbody cortical autologous bone graft in a patient after anterior cervical discectomy and fusion (ACDF). (D) Synthetic radiolucent interbody cage used in ACDF; note radiopaque cage markers in the intervertebral space. (E) Lateral radiograph of the lumbar spine in a patient after posterior lumbar interbody fusion (PLIF) with radiopaque cage. (F) Patient with transforaminal lumbar interbody fusion (TFLI) using radiolucent cage; radiopaque cage markers are visible as dots in the intervertebral space. Also note bone chips posterior to the fixation hardware (arrow).

(tricalcium phosphate, hydroxyapatite or calcium sulphate), available in a variety of forms and consistencies. Increasingly, synthetic cages[6] manufactured from metal (titanium or tantalum) or non-metallic radiolucent material such as carbon composite polymers, polyetheretherketone (PEEK) or bioabsorbable polylactic acid (PLA) are used instead of cortical bone for structural support in vertebral interbody fusion procedures (Figs. 58-1D–F). Such implants provide immediate load-bearing capacity while fusion occurs in their core packed with autologous cancellous bone, allograft or synthetic bone substitute.

Spinal surgery can be performed from anterior, posterior or combined approaches. An anterior approach is primarily used in the cervical spine for procedures such as anterior cervical discectomy and fusion (ACDF), and anterior instrumentation for corpectomy, peg fracture fixation with anterior screws, cervical foraminotomy and disc replacement. The traditional open anterior approach in the lumbar spine has been more difficult, but with increasing use of minimally invasive surgery (MIS)[7] and endoscopic surgical techniques this route is now more frequently used, for example for anterior lumbar interbody fusion (ALIF). A posterior approach is used in discectomy, foraminotomy, spinal canal decompression, various types of fixation using pedicle, translaminar or transfacet screws, and insertion of interspinous spacers, as well as posterior lumbar interbody fusion (PLIF) and transforaminal lumbar interbody fusion (TLIF). Anterior and posterior approaches can be combined in '360° fusion' procedures in which anterior interbody fusion is accompanied by posterior stabilisation with translaminar or pedicle screws, and facet joint or intertransversal fixation. Scoliosis correction surgery may require an anterior or posterior approach, depending on individual anatomical considerations and involved spinal segment.[1,2,7]

IMAGING TECHNIQUES IN POSTOPERATIVE SPINE

Plain radiographs are commonly used in routine follow-up of the instrumented spine to assess hardware migration, loosening or breakage. Radiography is inexpensive, is quick to perform and is the only technique allowing imaging with the patient in an upright position. Anteroposterior and lateral projections can be supplemented with dynamic flexion and extension views to assess motion at the fusion site and adjacent segments suggestive of pseudoarthrosis and instability. Serial radiographs may be helpful in demonstrating subtle changes in implant positioning.

More precise evaluation of implant position, alignment and integrity and fusion status is provided by CT. As the majority of implants are made of titanium, which has lower radiographic density than steel, beam hardening artefacts are generally minimal. The amount of artefact is further reduced by using helical acquisition (which also enables multiplanar reformats), high tube voltage and current, narrow collimation, thin sections and low pitch. Reconstruction with smooth or standard kernel may be preferable as bone kernel algorithm can accentuate artefacts. Average intensity projection (AIP) may be helpful in assessing hardware integrity.[8] In non-implant-related complications and non-instrumented spine, CT has been largely superseded by MRI, but may still play a role in patients with claustrophobia or contraindications to entering the magnet.

MRI is the technique of choice in non-hardware-related complications due to its ability to image soft tissue and neural structures, and conspicuity of contrast enhancement. It may demonstrate early complications such as haemorrhage, infection or dural leaks, and helps differentiate causes of persistent or recurrent symptoms.[3,9] Protocols vary depending on institutional experience, especially with regards to routine use of fat suppression and gadolinium contrast medium—while some authors advocate a contrast-enhanced T1 sequence in all postoperative patients,[3] other institutions rely on unenhanced T2-weighted images for routine assessment.[10] Early postoperative appearances can be difficult to interpret and misleading due to signal changes in intervertebral disc, endplates and epidural soft tissues that may mimic the appearances of disc herniation and lead to false impression of residual disc material. Bone removal can be difficult to assess on T2-weighted images, and T1-weighted sections are better suited for this purpose.[3,9] The presence of spinal implants is not a contraindication to MRI. Susceptibility artefacts from metallic implants are less problematic at lower field strengths and can be minimised by avoiding gradient-echo sequences, using fast spin-echo techniques, high receiver bandwidth, small voxel size, short TE and anterior-to-posterior frequency-encoding direction.[11]

INTRAOPERATIVE AND PERIOPERATIVE COMPLICATIONS

Intra- and perioperative complications can be related to injury of structures and organs during approach to the surgical site, or to surgical technique including hardware misplacement. For example, an anterior approach to the cervical spine puts at risk the recurrent laryngeal nerve, with transient or permanent palsy due to excessive retraction or transection. Injury to vertebral artery is a rare but potentially catastrophic event. The most dreaded complication is the spinal cord injury; direct iatrogenic trauma is uncommon, but spinal cord function may be impaired by patient positioning or intraoperative hypotension, especially if there is a pre-existing cord compression or contusion. Paraspinal visceral structures that are at risk of injury during approach or by screws of excessive length or aberrant course include trachea, oesophagus, lung, pleura, thoracic duct, aorta and great vessels, heart, ureter, peritoneum and bowel.[1,7] Imaging in cases of damage to these structures should be tailored to the clinical scenario and specific organ and injury pattern.

Hardware-related complications in the perioperative period are mostly related to misplaced transpedicular screws. CT is the best technique for demonstrating screw placement, which should be wholly contained within the respective pedicles and covered by cortical bone from all sides (Figs. 58-2A, B); the screw tip should approach, but not breach, the anterior cortex of the vertebral body. Misplaced screws (Figs. 58-2C, D) may impinge on the spinal canal or neural foramen, threatening the spinal cord, cauda equina or exiting nerve roots. The reported rate of misplacement is high and may exceed 40%;[1] however, clinically significant impingement or injury of neural structures is less common. The incidence of radiculopathy is reported at 7% and the nerve root is most at risk of injury or irritation if the medial or inferior border of the pedicle is violated. The need for screw removal or revision is dictated by neurological symptoms, taking into account the degree of misplacement.

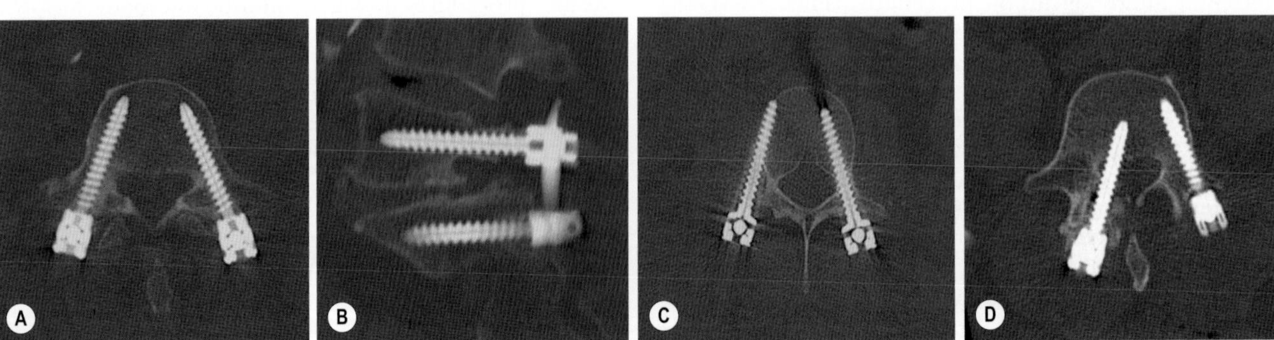

FIGURE 58-2 ■ Axial CT image (A) and sagittal oblique reformat (B) demonstrating satisfactory placement of transpedicular screws. (C) Misplaced right screw coursing laterally to the pedicle. (D) Misplaced right screw coursing medially to the pedicle through the lateral recess.

EARLY COMPLICATIONS

Early complications of spinal surgery include haemorrhage, cerebrospinal fluid (CSF) leak and infection.[1,7,9]

Postoperative haemorrhage is uncommon (less than 1% of patients) and usually occurs in the immediate postoperative period. In the cervical spine, expanding neck wound haematoma can lead to airway compression and is a surgical emergency;[12] the role of imaging is limited as the diagnosis is usually clinical and urgent wound exploration should be performed without delay. Symptoms of spinal cord or cauda equina compression in the early postoperative period are suspicious for epidural haematoma.[1] Small amounts of asymptomatic epidural haemorrhage are present in most procedures involving the spinal canal, but symptomatic haematoma requiring evacuation occurs in less than 0.5% of patients on average, being the highest in the thoracic spine at 4.5%.[13] MRI is the technique of choice for identifying the extent of haemorrhage and compression of neural structures. Findings include an epidural mass with T1 signal dependent on age of the haematoma (iso- or hypointense in acute haemorrhage, hyperintense in chronic haematoma) and heterogeneously hyperintense on T2-weighted sequences, with no contrast enhancement (Fig. 58-3).

CSF leak is an equally uncommon complication of spinal surgery, occurring as a result of unrecognised or improperly repaired dural breach. Extravasation of CSF into surrounding tissues leads to formation of a pseudomeningocele. CSF can also egress through the surgical wound or drain track, resulting in a cutaneous CSF fistula. MRI is an investigation of choice as it readily demonstrates fluid signal intensity collections in the paraspinal soft tissues related to the thecal sac; communication with the thecal sac can sometimes be visualised. There is no enhancement, or thin peripheral enhancement only (Fig. 58-4). Pseudomeningocele needs to be

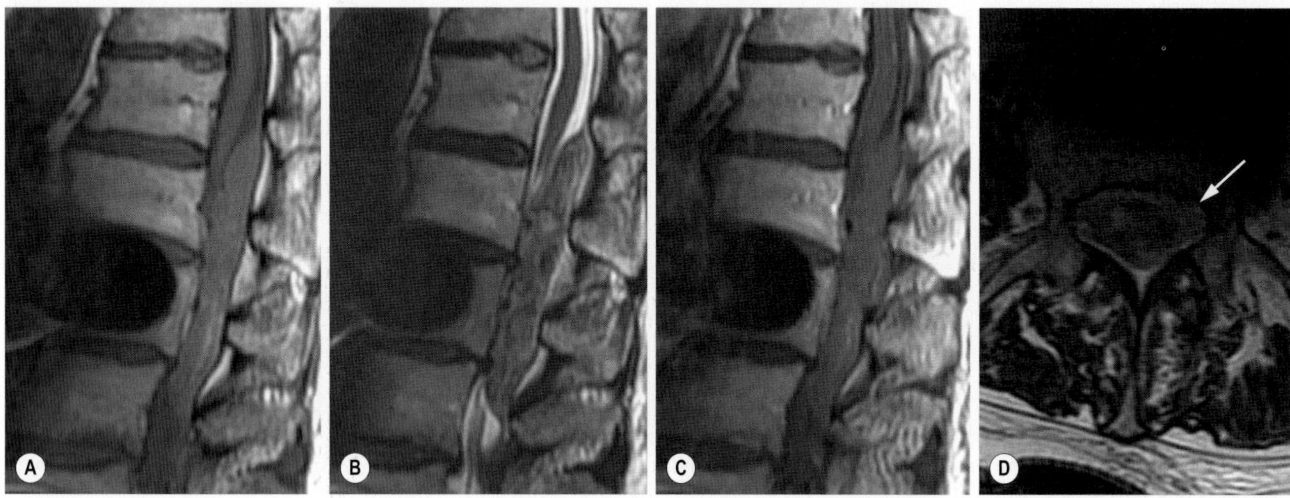

FIGURE 58-3 ■ Epidural haematoma. Sagittal MRI images demonstrate epidural mass slightly hyperintense to spinal cord on T1-weighted images (A) and of heterogeneous signal on T2 sequence (B), with no enhancement following gadolinium administration (C). Roots of cauda equina are displaced anteriorly and to the left (arrow) and compressed (D).

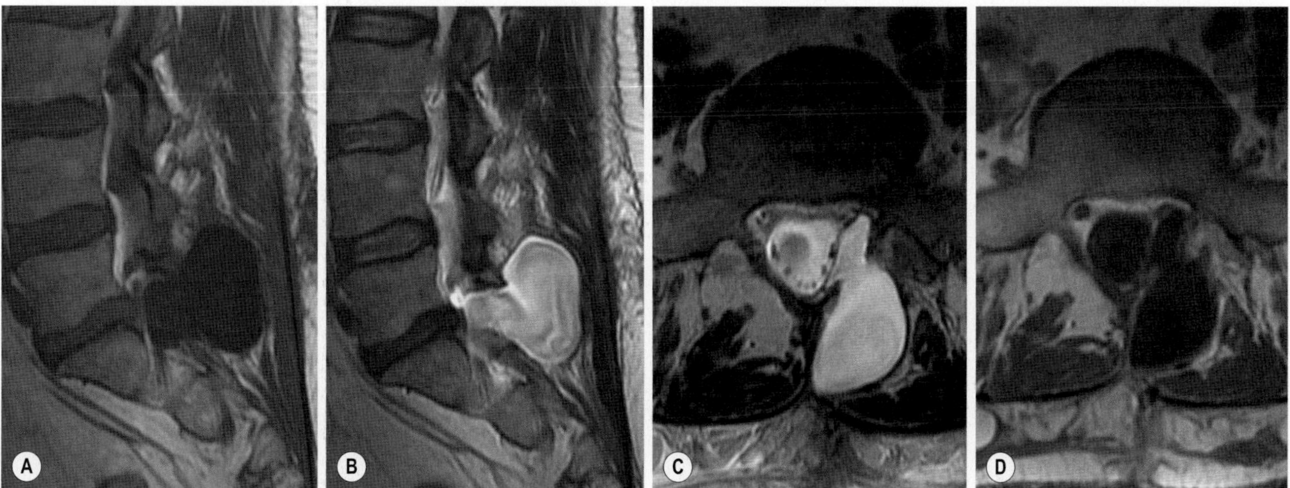

FIGURE 58-4 ■ Pseudomeningocele in a patient after left S1 nerve root decompression procedure. Sagittal T1-weighted (A) and T2-weighted (B) images demonstrate fluid intensity collection in the posterior paraspinal soft tissues. Axial T2 image (C) shows fluid collection related to the extradural part of S1 nerve root and extending through flavectomy defect to the left of the spinous process. Post-contrast T1 image (D) shows lack of enhancement.

differentiated from true meningocele with expansion of the dura through the surgical spinal canal defect, postoperative haematoma and abscess. A CT myelogram can be helpful in localising the exact site of extravasation and outlining the fistulous track. Pseudomeningocele may be associated with signs of intracranial hypotension (CSF leakage syndrome) such as dural thickening and enhancement, 'sagging' midbrain, tonsillar herniation, venous distension, pituitary gland enlargement and subdural haematomas or hygromas.[2]

Postoperative infections complicate 0.2–3% of spinal procedures and include a spectrum of wound infections, discitis, vertebral osteomyelitis, and epidural abscess, which can occur in isolation or combined. Most cases are caused by direct staphylococcal infection and should be suspected in all patients with persistent back pain occurring weeks to months after surgery. The white cell count often remains within normal limits but erythrocyte sedimentation ratio and C-reactive protein levels are elevated. In infection limited to the surgical wound there are no intervertebral disc or vertebral body signal changes (Fig. 58-5). Features of intervertebral disc involvement on MRI include loss of disc height, T1 hypointensity with T2 hyperintensity, and contrast enhancement of the intervertebral disc space; similar signal changes and enhancement in adjacent endplates indicate extension of disc infection and vertebral osteomyelitis (Fig. 58-6). An associated paraspinal abscess appears as enhancing soft tissue with areas of fluid intensity; thick enhancing rim and surrounding oedema can also be seen. The diagnosis of spondylodiscitis in the early postoperative period may be difficult as intervertebral space and endplate changes

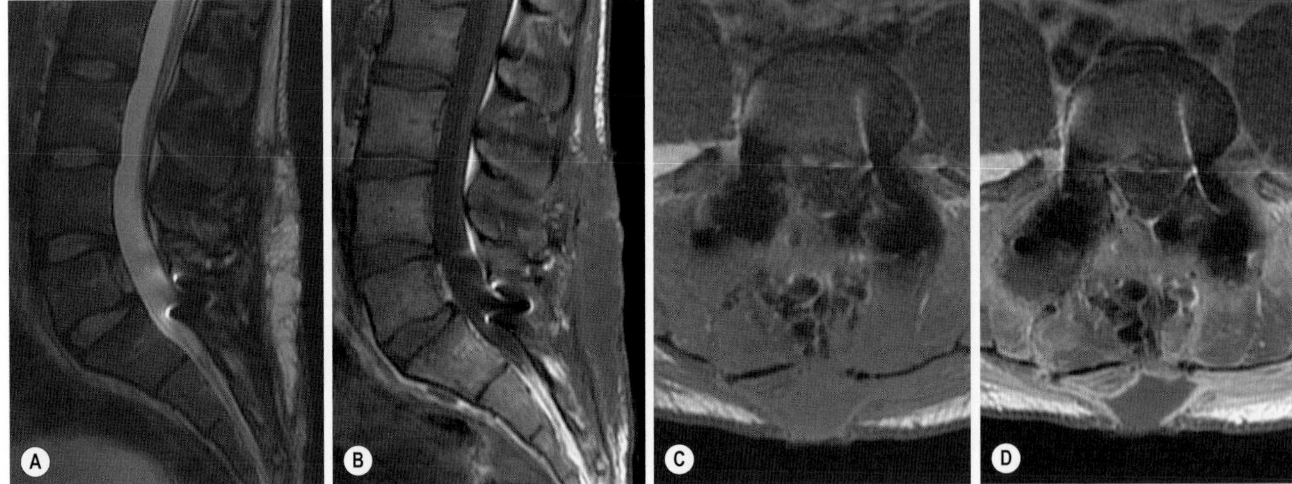

FIGURE 58-5 ■ Wound infection in a patient with posterior lumbar fixation. Sagittal T1 (A) and T2 (B) images demonstrate complex mass in the posterior paraspinal and subcutaneous soft tissues. Axial T1-weighted images before (C) and after administration of gadolinium (D) demonstrate avid ring enhancement around fluid collection in subcutaneous soft tissues close to the skin surface, and diffuse enhancement in the paraspinal soft tissues. Note normal signal intensity in intervertebral discs and vertebral bodies.

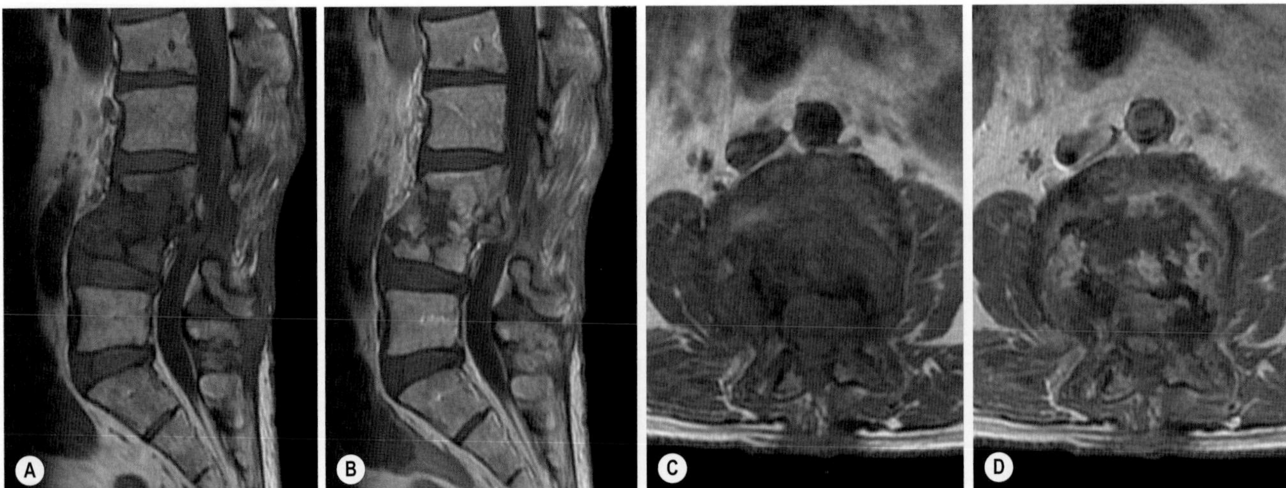

FIGURE 58-6 ■ Discitis and vertebral osteomyelitis in a patient after microdiscectomy. Sagittal (A, B) and axial (C, D) T1-weighted images obtained before (left) and after (right) administration of gadolinium demonstrate destruction of the L3/4 intervertebral disc and collapse of adjacent vertebral bodies with hypointense marrow. There is contrast enhancement of the remaining intervertebral disc, adjacent vertebrae and paraspinal soft tissues.

are seen in the normal postoperative spine; a combination of imaging features (such as coexistence of intervertebral space enhancement, peridiscal signal changes and enhancing paraspinal mass) may be helpful.[3,14] Clinical correlation is crucial, and diagnosis may require percutaneous disc biopsy; this should be performed with a cutting needle, as aspiration leads to high proportion of false-negative results. The most serious form of postoperative infection requiring emergency surgical decompression or percutaneous drainage is spinal epidural abscess.[15] It can accompany spondylodiscitis or occur in isolation, and should be suspected when the patient demonstrates the triad of localised axial back pain, fever and progressive neurological deficit, ultimately leading to paraparesis. MRI demonstrates T1 hypointense, T2/STIR hyperintense epidural collection. The presence of contrast enhancement helps differentiate spinal epidural abscess from epidural haematoma, which otherwise can have similar appearances.

LATE COMPLICATIONS

Late complications of spinal surgery include delayed hardware failure and displacement leading to pseudoarthrosis and instability, as well as adjacent segment disease. A specific clinical entity termed 'failed back surgery syndrome' refers specifically to patients who have undergone lumbar spine surgery for degenerative disease (discectomy, foraminal stenosis or instability) and continue to experience symptoms due to a number of potential causes detailed below.

As mentioned earlier, hardware is used in spinal surgery to provide temporary support only and is destined to fail if the osseous fusion does not occur. In most cases hardware failure is, therefore, a manifestation of a lack of bony fusion and development of pseudoarthrosis. Factors that increase the risk of fusion failure include old age, smoking, diabetes, obesity, poor bone quality (e.g. in osteoporosis) and multilevel instrumentation. On plain radiographs pseudoarthrosis should be suspected if there is resorption of the bone graft, progressive misalignment, more than 4 mm translation or more than 10° of angular motion between adjacent vertebrae on flexion and extension views.[1,2] Features of pseudoarthrosis on cross-sectional imaging include a line between the bone and graft material that is lucent on CT, and a low T1 signal on MRI. Hardware failure such as fractured or extruded screws, fractured plates and rods and misplacement or subsistence of interbody cages can be evident on plain radiographs (Figs. 58-7A, B). CT allows more precise assessment of implants (Fig. 58-7C), and MRI may be helpful in evaluating compression of neural structures (Fig. 58-7D). On CT, the screws should be scrutinised for the presence of peri-implant lucency indicative of loosening; this is usually obvious in advanced cases (Fig. 58-7E), but early changes may be more subtle (Fig. 58-7F).

Adjacent segment disease is an accelerated occurrence of degenerative disc and facet changes at the level above and below the level of fusion due to altered spine dynamics. Imaging findings include typical degenerative changes such as loss of disc height, disc herniation, endplate signal alterations and facet joint hypertrophy. The most important differential diagnosis is discitis and vertebral osteomyelitis, which, however, are likely to involve the site of surgery or fusion rather than the adjacent levels.

Failed Back Surgery Syndrome

Failed back surgery syndrome (FBSS) is a clinical entity defined as significant persistent back pain following surgical intervention with or without radiating pain and/or various degrees of functional incapacity.[16] Despite advances in technology and techniques, the number of patients suffering from FBSS has increased in recent years with increasing rate of spinal surgery.[17] The incidence of FBSS following lumbosacral spine surgery is reported to be between 10 and 40% in different studies.[9,18]

The aetiologies for FBSS can be classified in three main categories: preoperative, intraoperative and postoperative. The main preoperative risk factors are psychosocial influences, for example depression, anxiety or hypochondriasis.[19,20] Revision or repeated surgery is another preoperative risk factor, with the success rate decreasing to nearly half after second surgery and declining even further after subsequent operations.[21–23] Intraoperative causes of FBSS include poor technique, inadequate or overaggressive decompression and operation on the incorrect level. Overaggressive decompression may lead to spinal instability, which is seen in up to 14% of cases with FBSS. The incidence of incorrect operation level is widely variable in different studies, ranging from 0.03 to 3.3%,[24,25] and is increased in the presence of unusual patient characteristics such as morbid obesity, physical deformity or congenital variations. Emergency surgery, involvement of multiple surgeons or multiple procedures in a single surgical visit[26] and limited exposure in microscopic techniques[17] also increase the risk.

Postoperative causes for FBSS are those in which neuroimaging plays an important role. Residual or recurrent disc herniations are common following spinal surgery and can present with persistent or recurrent pain. Recurrent disease is seen in 7–12% cases of FBSS.[2] In the first few days after surgery it is difficult to differentiate the residual disc herniation from inflammatory tissue and debris. In the following weeks the inflammatory process and mass effect subside and avidly enhancing granulation tissue forms. After several months the granulation tissue reorganises to form epidural fibrosis, which demonstrates diffuse but weaker enhancement.[9] Differentiation between epidural scar and disc material is one of the most important and challenging aspects of postoperative spine imaging. Both disc material and epidural fibrosis are hypo- to isointense on T1-weighted and iso- to hyperintense on T2-weighted sequences, and gadolinium-enhanced T1-weighted images are crucial in their differentiation. Contrast-enhanced MRI has an accuracy of 96–100% for differentiating between fibrosis and disc material.[4] Recurrent or residual disc material does not enhance, or there is mild enhancement around the disc (Fig. 58-8). It is important to remember that contrast medium will penetrate the disc with time and the central part may show enhancement if imaging is delayed. It is

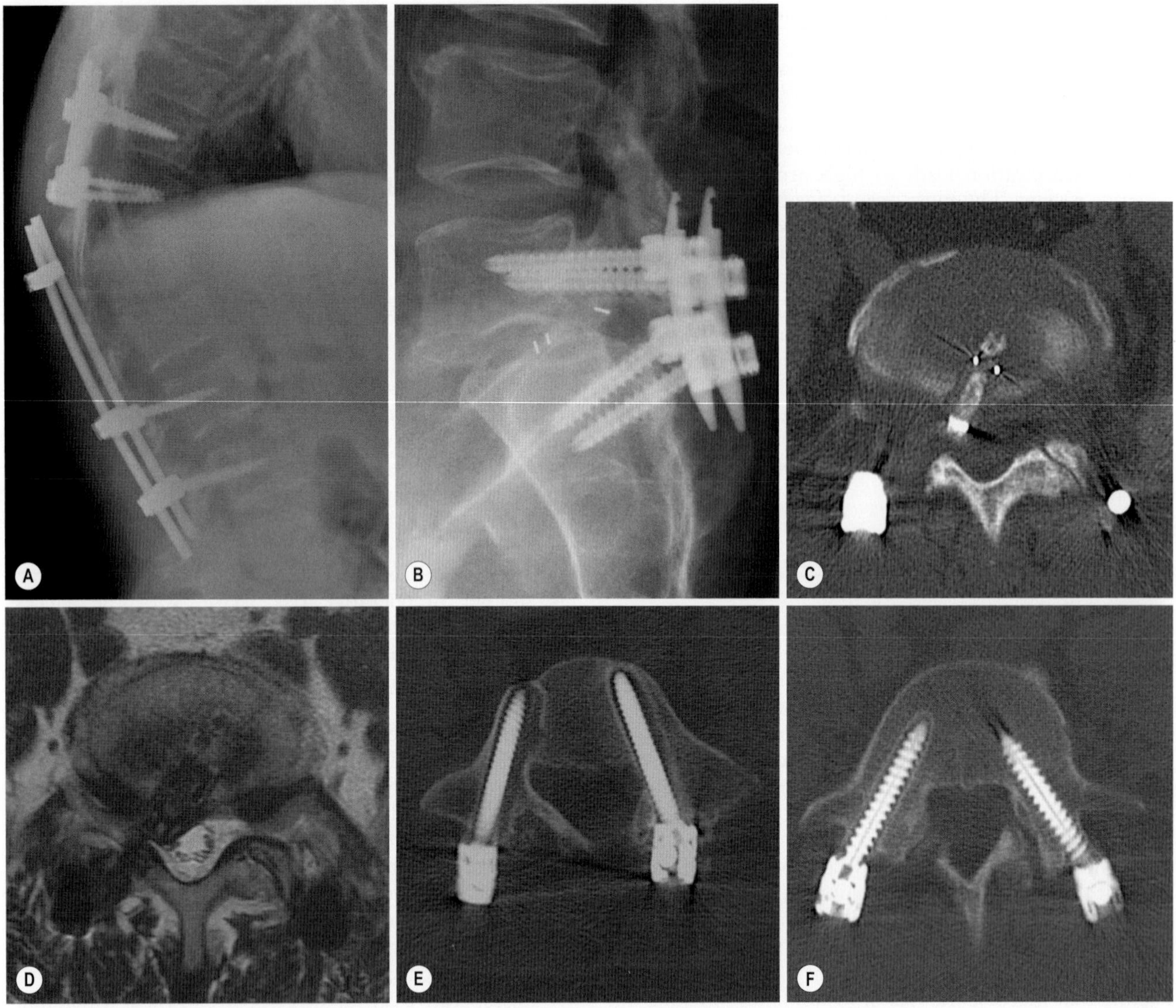

FIGURE 58-7 ■ Examples of late hardware failure. (A) Fractured rods in a patient with posterior thoracolumbar fixation of a burst fracture. (B) Posterior cage migration in a patient with transforaminal lumbar interbody fusion (TLIF); note that posterior radiopaque marker of the interbody cage lies within the spinal canal. (C) CT in the same patient allows better visualisation of the misplaced cage, and (D) axial T2-weighted MRI image demonstrates compression of the descending right S1 nerve root in the lateral recess by the misplaced cage. (E, F) Examples of various degree of peri-implant lucency indicating screws loosening; compare with normal left screw in (F).

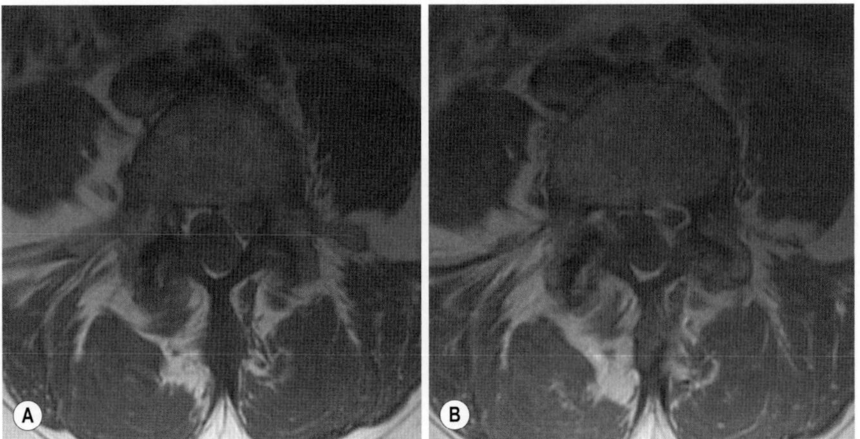

FIGURE 58-8 ■ Example of a recurrent disc herniation. (A) Unenhanced T1-weighted axial image demonstrates epidural lesion abutting the left anterior aspect of the thecal sac. (B) Gadolinium-enhanced image demonstrates peripheral enhancement, but the centre of the lesion remains of low signal.

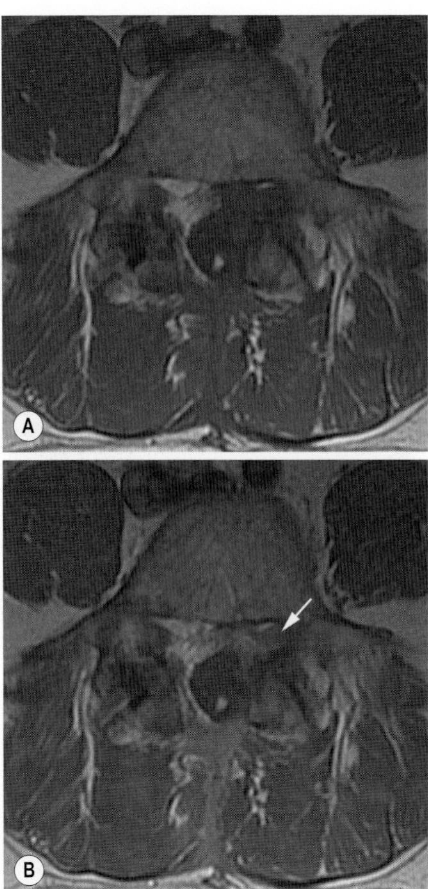

FIGURE 58-9 ■ Example of epidural fibrosis. (A) Unenhanced T1-weighted axial image demonstrates epidural lesion adjacent to the left anterior aspect of the theca. (B) Gadolinium-enhanced image demonstrates avid enhancement of the scar that extends along the left aspect of the thecal sac and is in continuity with postoperative scar tissue in the midline. Exiting nerve root (arrow) is surrounded by the enhancing tissue.

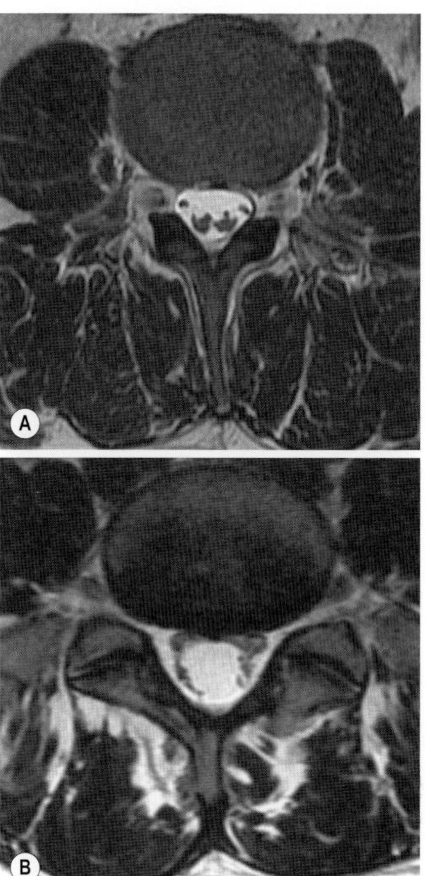

FIGURE 58-10 ■ Sterile arachnoiditis in patients following lumbar surgery. Axial T2-weighted images demonstrate clumping of nerve roots (A) and 'empty sac' sign (B) with nerve roots adherent to the periphery of the theca and absent in their usual dependent location.

therefore crucial that post-gadolinium images are obtained immediately after contrast injection. Herniated disc usually has smooth margins, lies anterolateral in the epidural space and tends to displace or compress the nerve roots and theca. On the other hand, epidural fibrotic tissue enhances early and uniformly, has irregular configuration with minimal mass effect and can occupy anterior-to-posterior aspects of the epidural space. It can also encase and retract the theca and nerve roots rather than displace them (Fig. 58-9). As epidural fibrosis is an inevitable finding following any surgery involving manipulation of the epidural space, it may be considered a normal postoperative change in the absence of significant theca deformity or tethering of nerve roots. Therefore, it is important to remember that symptoms may not be caused by the presence of epidural scar tissue, and that there is no correlation between severity of symptoms and the amount of scarring. Different studies have shown that epidural fibrosis can be responsible or contribute to pain in 20–36% of FBSS patients.[27,28] There are different theories regarding how epidural fibrosis causes persistent pain, including limitation of movement and inflammation,[29] hypoxic damage to the nerve[30] or disturbance in CSF flow, resulting in nerve hypersensitivity.[31]

Sterile arachnoiditis is another postoperative cause of FBSS which has been reported in 6–16% of cases following spinal surgery.[4] The MRI features of arachnoiditis include 'clumping' of nerve roots and 'empty' theca caused by peripherally distributed nerve roots and their adhesion to the theca (Fig. 58-10), as well as an intrathecal soft-tissue 'mass' with a broad dural base representing a large group of matted nerve roots.

Nerve root enhancement on MRI is frequently seen in the early postoperative period, when it may reflect transient inflammation.[9] Enhancement present after 6 months should, however, be considered a pathological feature,[32] and suggests ongoing radiculitis as the cause of pain.[9] In asymptomatic patients nerve root enhancement is only rarely seen beyond this time point. In contrast, almost two-thirds of symptomatic patients demonstrate nerve root enhancement that strongly correlates with clinical symptoms, especially when combined with nerve thickening and displacement.[32]

Stenosis involving the central or juxta-articular portion of the spinal canal or neural foramen is an important cause of persistent or recurrent pain reported in 25 to

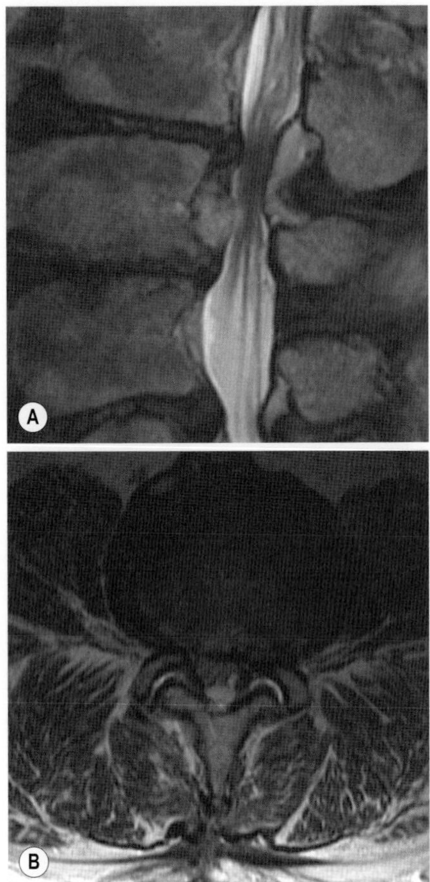

FIGURE 58-11 ■ **Moderate spinal canal stenosis demonstrated on sagittal (A) and axial (B) T2-weighted images.**

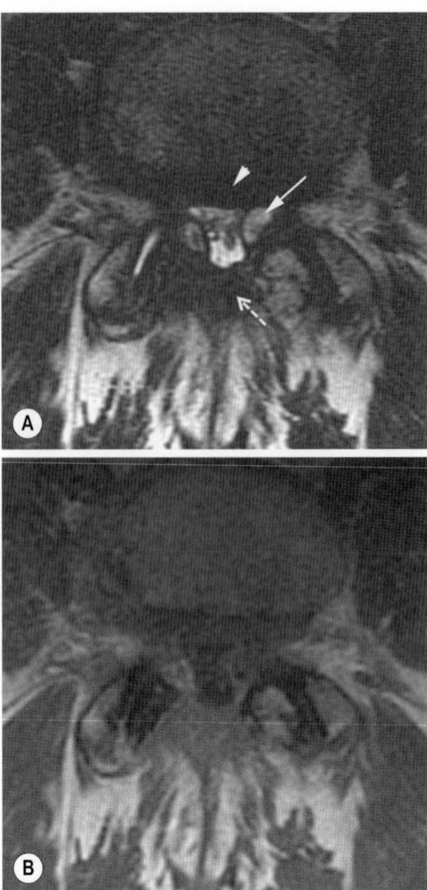

FIGURE 58-12 ■ Axial T2-weighted (A) and contrast-enhanced T1-weighted images (B) demonstrate a small synovial cyst (arrow) related to the left facet joint. Also note recurrent disc (arrowhead) and enhancing scar (dashed arrow) posteriorly. There is mild spinal canal stenosis.

29% of patients with FBSS.[33] Stenosis can be a consequence of accelerated degenerative changes after an operation. Loss of intervertebral disc height after discectomy is another cause. The best diagnostic clue on imaging is a trefoil appearance of the spinal canal on axial, and an hourglass appearance on sagittal imaging (Fig. 58-11). A sagittal diameter of the spinal canal less than 10 mm is considered absolute spinal canal stenosis.[2]

Postoperative synovial cysts (Fig. 58-12) are an uncommon cause of FBSS reported in 1% of cases. They are secondary to alteration of the facet joint biomechanics following surgery, with removal of ligamentum flavum as a potential predisposing factor. The important diagnostic clue is continuity of the cyst with the facet joint and the usual presence of fluid signal.[4]

IMAGE-GUIDED PERCUTANEOUS CEMENT BONE AUGMENTATION

Percutaneous cement bone augmentation interventions include vertebroplasty and kyphoplasty. The main indication for these procedures is pain associated with osteoporotic vertebral fractures refractory to medical therapy.[34,35] They may also be used in treatment of pathological vertebral fractures associated with lytic metastases and multiple myeloma, as well as traumatic fractures. The treatment of asymptomatic vertebral compression fractures and prophylactic intervention in non-fractured vertebrae remain a matter of debate. It should be noted that effectiveness of vertebroplasty in relieving pain and improvement of function in patients with osteoporotic compression fractures has recently been in question in view of results of controlled randomised clinical trials showing no clinical benefit of the procedure,[36,37] or only modest reduction in pain with no difference in functional outcomes.[38] While the future role of cement bone augmentation remains to be established, differences between the techniques used and potential complications deserve a brief mention.

In vertebroplasty there is intraosseous injection of bone cement (usually PMMA; polymethylmethacrylate) into the vertebral body using a needle introduced via transpedicular approach under fluoroscopic guidance (Fig. 58-13A, B); extrapedicular or posterolateral approach can also be used. Partial restoration of vertebral height is sometimes accomplished, but is not a primary goal of the procedure. In kyphoplasty, before cement injection, inflatable tamps (balloons) are introduced into the vertebral body. Expanding tamps crush the trabeculae and create a cavity into which cement is instilled; some height

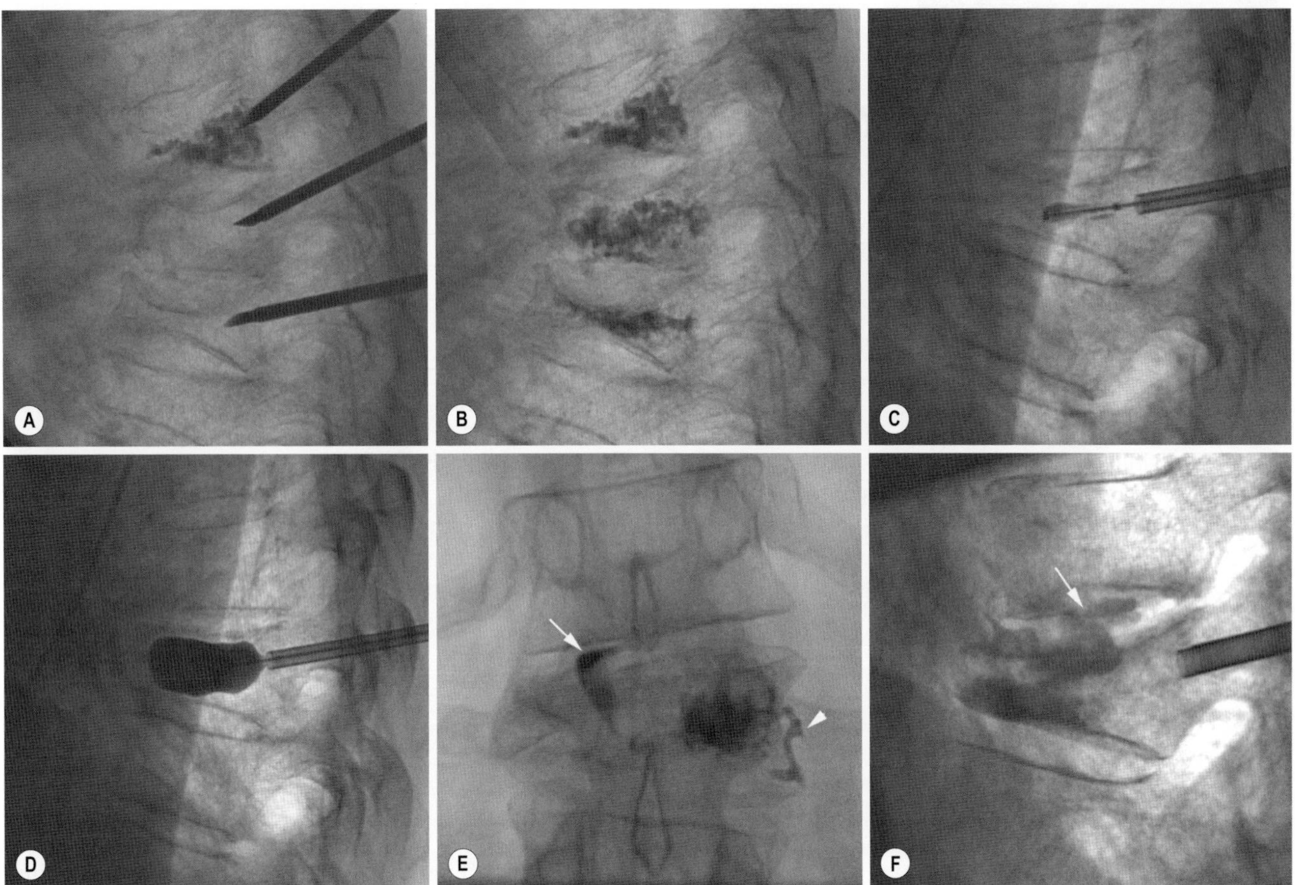

FIGURE 58-13 ■ Fluoroscopic images obtained during cement bone augmentation procedures. (A) Vertebroplasty on three adjacent levels showing transpedicular needles in situ and cement being injected at the most superior level. (B) Final effect of the vertebroplasty shown in (A). (C) Inflation of the balloon inside the vertebral body during kyphoplasty. Note partial reduction of the fracture (D) with some restoration of vertebral body height. (E, F) Extravasation of cement into the intervertebral space (arrows) increases risk of adjacent vertebral fracture post procedure. There is minor extravasation into a paravertebral vein (arrowhead in E).

restoration is more likely to be achieved (Figs. 58-13C, D). Variation of kyphoplasty aimed to maintain the degree of height restoration between the tamp deflation and cement injection involves deployment of balloon-mounted stents inside the vertebral body (stentoplasty).[39] The main potential complication of vertebroplasty is leakage of cement outside of the vertebral body, with extravasation into paravertebral veins (Fig. 58-13E); large extravasation with penetration of cement into systemic venous circulation may result in cement pulmonary emboli. Epidural or neural foraminal extravasation may lead to compression of neural structures requiring surgical decompression. Cement extravasation into the intervertebral space (Fig. 58-13F) has been shown to increase the risk of fractures of adjacent vertebrae post procedure.[35,40] Cement extravasation is less likely to happen in case of kyphoplasty thanks to lower viscosity of cement, which is instilled into a preformed cavity under lower pressure.[35] Other complications associated with needle placement include injury to epidural venous plexus, nerve roots or spinal cord.

For a full list of references, please see ExpertConsult.

FURTHER READING

1. Benzel EC. Spine Surgery: Techniques, Complication Avoidance, and Management. 2nd ed. Philadelphia: Churchill Livingstone; 2005.
2. Ross JS. Specialty Imaging. Postoperative Spine. Philadelphia: Wolters Kluwer, Lippincott Williams & Wilkins; 2012.
3. Salgado R, Van Goethem JW, van den Hauwe L, Parizel PM. Imaging of the postoperative spine. Semin Roentgenol 2006;41: 312–26.
4. Ginat TD, Murtagh R, Westesson P-eA. Imaging of postoperative spine. In: Atlas of Postsurgical Neuroradiology: Imaging of the Brain, Spine, Head, and Neck. 1st ed. Berlin: Springer; 2012.
8. Douglas-Akinwande AC, Buckwalter KA, Rydberg J, et al. Multichannel CT: evaluating the spine in postoperative patients with orthopedic hardware. Radiographics 2006;26(Suppl 1):S97–110.
9. Van Goethem JW, Parizel PM, Jinkins JR. Review article: MRI of the postoperative lumbar spine. Neuroradiology 2002;44:723–39.

CHAPTER 59

SPINAL TRAUMA

James J. Rankine

CHAPTER OUTLINE

CLINICAL ASPECTS

The cervical spine and thoracolumbar junction are the most common sites of spinal trauma. Specifically, the most common sites for fractures and dislocations are the lower cervical spine (C4–7), the thoracolumbar junction (T10–L2) and the craniocervical junction (C1–2). These mobile areas, particularly the cervical spine, can be injured with relatively little force. Patients with cervical trauma may present as 'walking wounded' to the accident and emergency departments with no other injuries and so despite the increasing use of CT as a first-line investigation, many patients with cervical trauma continue to be initially investigated with conventional radiographs. Approximately 15% of spinal fractures occur at more than one level and are non-contiguous, so the clinician must carefully assess the whole spine.[1]

In contrast to the cervical and lumbar spine, the thoracic spine is a relatively rigid structure, restricted in mobility by the thoracic cage. The thoracic spine, ribs and sternum constitute a bony ring and in common with fractures of bony rings elsewhere in the body, the ring often fractures at more than one point. A displaced fracture of the sternum should raise clinical suspicions of a fracture of the thoracic spine. Since greater forces are usually required to cause a thoracic spine fracture, associated vascular injury should be considered. For these reasons thoracic and lumbar trauma is most appropriately imaged as part of a polytrauma CT with intravenous contrast medium.

Patients with osteoporosis may sustain thoracic axial load compressive fractures with little or no history of injury and are often initially assessed by conventional radiographs. The lack of force involved in the injury should not imply to the clinician that these are fractures that always run a benign course. The compressed vertebral body can develop avascular necrosis, leading to delayed post-traumatic collapse and spinal deformity, termed Kummell's disease.[2] It is important that these patients are followed up clinically, and where appropriate their osteoporosis is pharmacologically treated.

Conventional radiographs cannot exclude injury in any part of the spine. While CT is sensitive to bony injury, it cannot exclude ligamentous disruption. This is particularly important in cervical trauma where the spine can be rendered unstable due to ligamentous disruption without any bony injury. The removal of spinal immobilisation in the light of negative conventional radiographs, or CT, should be performed in a controlled manner under senior supervision. Any clinical concerns, which are principally the degree of pain on gentle movement or the development of any neurological signs or symptoms, warrants an MRI examination, regardless of the findings on CT or conventional radiographs. It is important that the clinician managing a patient with spinal trauma is aware of the limitations of conventional radiographs and CT.

Patients with spinal injury should have regular neurological observations performed. Any clinical deterioration in the neurology warrants an urgent assessment by MRI to investigate the possibility of an epidural haematoma, which can be surgically drained. Urgent surgical intervention cannot correct any neurological dysfunction sustained at the time of injury, but can prevent worsening neurological damage from an expanding epidural haematoma compressing the spinal cord.

IMAGING TECHNIQUES AND EVALUATION

CERVICAL SPINE

Conventional Radiographs

A full conventional radiographic examination of the cervical spine as a minimum includes a lateral view, anteroposterior (AP) view and an AP odontoid peg view. The lateral view should include the cervical–thoracic junction, and if not then a 'swimmer's' view is performed where the arm adjacent to the radiographic plate is elevated and the beam is centred above the shoulder further from the plate and angled 15° in a cephalad direction. A full conventional radiographic examination is most appropriate in injury isolated to the cervical spine, with relatively low forces and where removal of immobilisation and clinical reassessment would be considered with negative findings. In many other situations, especially in the context of polytrauma, it is more appropriate to proceed directly to CT without conventional radiographs. Many institutions continue to perform a lateral radiograph as part of the initial assessment of the patient in the resuscitation room. Of the conventional radiographic projections, the lateral is the single most useful but with such rapid access to CT now available in most institutions the value of performing any conventional radiographs is debatable. The lateral radiograph no longer constitutes part of the primary survey in the ATLS guidelines[3] but cervical immobilisation must continue until the spine can be radiologically and clinically cleared.

Despite the diminishing role of conventional radiographs they remain a common means of initially assessing many patients and, since the principles of interpreting the radiographs also apply to the interpretation of the sagittal and coronal reformats produced by a CT examination, it remains an important skill.

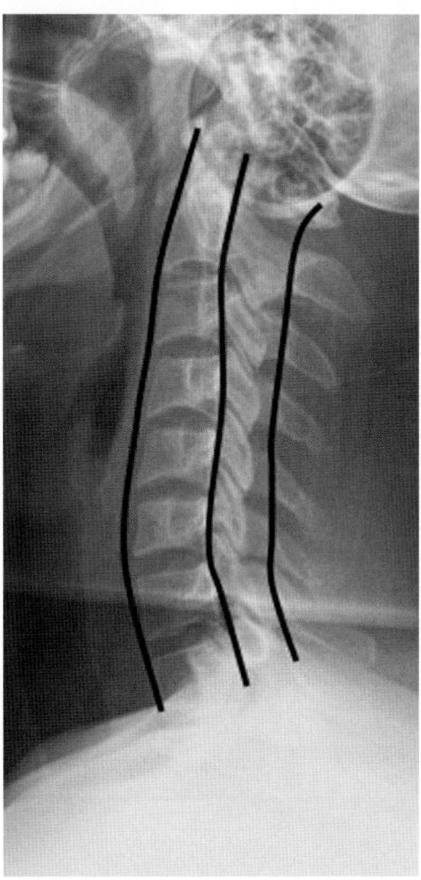

FIGURE 59-1 ■ Alignment on the lateral cervical spine radiograph is assessed by visually assessing the smooth contour of the spinal lines.

Alignment is assessed by visually assessing the spinal lines on the lateral radiograph (Fig. 59-1). They should all appear smooth and without interruption. The anterior spinal line passes along anterior borders of the vertebral bodies and the anterior aspect of the odontoid peg. The distance between the anterior arch of C1 and the odontoid peg should not exceed 3 mm in adults and 5 mm in children. The posterior spinal line passes along the posterior borders of the vertebral bodies. The junction of the laminae with the spinous processes forms the spinolaminar line. The lamina of C2 is normally up to 2 mm posterior to the spinolaminar line. The facet joint line marks the posterior aspect of the facet joints and in a true lateral projection the facet joints on each side are superimposed, giving a single line. The distance between this line and the spinolaminar line should be the same at all levels. The appearance of a double facet joint line at a particular level is evidence of an abnormality of rotation at that level which is usually caused by a fracture dislocation of the facet joints (Fig. 59-2). The appearance of a double facet joint line is termed the 'bow tie' sign.

Slight anterior subluxation of C2 on C3 is a common normal appearance in children. In this situation the malalignment causes disruption of the anterior spinal line and the spinolaminar line (Fig. 59-3). This distinguishes it from the Hangman's fracture, where the anterior spinal line is disrupted but the spinolaminar line is not, since the posterior elements are no longer connected to the vertebral body (see later).

Malalignment can occur with angulation of the spine in the absence of anterior subluxation. The distance between the spinous processes should be roughly equal at all levels, taking into account the normal downward slope of the C7 spinous process A kyphotic angulation of the spine associated with widening of the gap between two spinous processes implies rupture of the posterior ligamentous structures at that level (Fig. 59-4).

Noting the central position of the spinous processes assesses alignment on the AP radiograph. The spinous processes of the cervical spine may appear bifid (the spinous process separates into two portions). This is a normal anatomical finding at many levels and in this situation the central point of the posterior elements is the point midway between the two tubercles of the spinous process (which may be unequal in size).

When assessing the AP through mouth odontoid peg view, normal alignment is demonstrated by noting that the lateral margins of the C1–C2 facet joints are

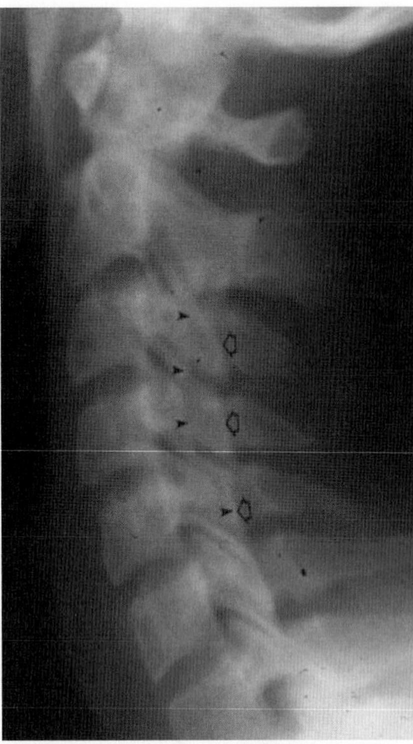

FIGURE 59-2 ■ Unilateral facet joint dislocation. The appearance of a double facet joint line, termed the bow tie sign (arrowheads and block arrows), on the lateral cervical radiograph is evidence of rotation of the spine.

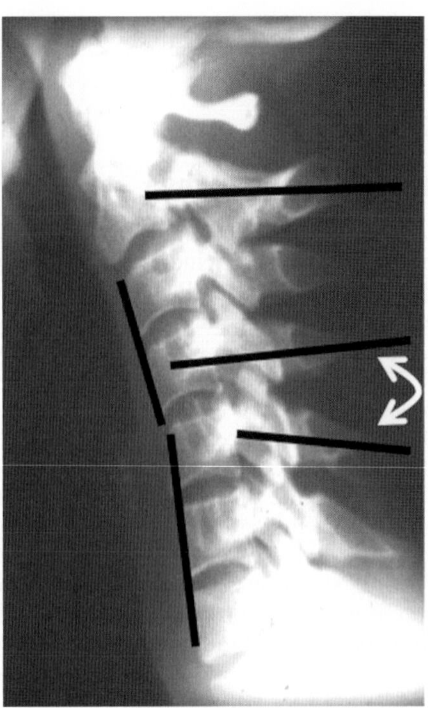

FIGURE 59-4 ■ Posterior ligamentous disruption. There is angulation of the anterior spinal line at C4–C5. The posterior lines mark the position of the spinous processes with fanning between the C4 and C5 spinous processes.

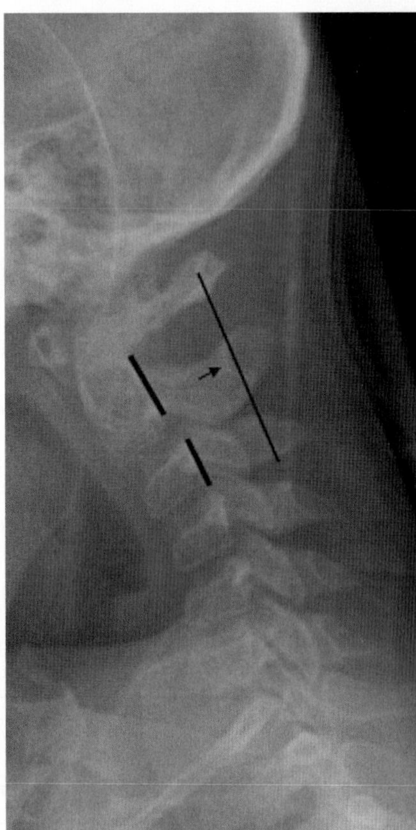

FIGURE 59-3 ■ Physiological subluxation of C2 on C3 in a 6-year-old child. There is disruption of the anterior and spinolaminar lines. The spinolaminar line of C2 (arrow) lies anterior to the spinolaminar line joining C1 and C3.

symmetrically aligned with no overlap. On the lateral view the integrity of Harris' ring should be examined at the base of the odontoid peg. This ring does not represent a distinct anatomical structure but is a composite shadow that includes the C2 body (Fig. 59-5).

The bones are assessed for fractures, cortical disruption and separate bony fragments. A well-corticated round opacity situated at the site of the anterior longitudinal ligament should not be mistaken for an avulsion. The lack of cortical disruption of the adjacent vertebral body and the absence of soft-tissue swelling are indicators of this normal finding, which is thought to represent a remnant of an ununited secondary vertebral ossification centre.

Soft-tissue swelling is assessed on the lateral radiograph. Superior to the level of the larynx the distance between the anterior aspect of the vertebral bodies and the posterior aspect of the air in the oropharynx should be no greater than one-third of the AP diameter of a vertebral body width. Inferior to the level of the larynx (usually C3 or C4 and frequently seen due to calcification in the laryngeal cartilage) it should be no greater than the AP diameter of the vertebral body. Intubation distorts the soft tissues behind the oropharynx, making the interpretation of soft-tissue swelling unreliable in intubated patients.

Lateral flexion and extension radiographs have traditionally been used to assess stability of the spine. Movement of the acutely injured spine in the presence of ligamentous disruption can cause neurological injury so there is no role for flexion and extension radiographs in the acutely injured spine. The stability of the spine and the presence of ligamentous disruption should be assessed by MRI. There remains a role for flexion and extension radiographs in the assessment of delayed instability, but this is likely to be some months after the acute event and should only take place after appropriate imaging and treatment of the acutely injured spine.

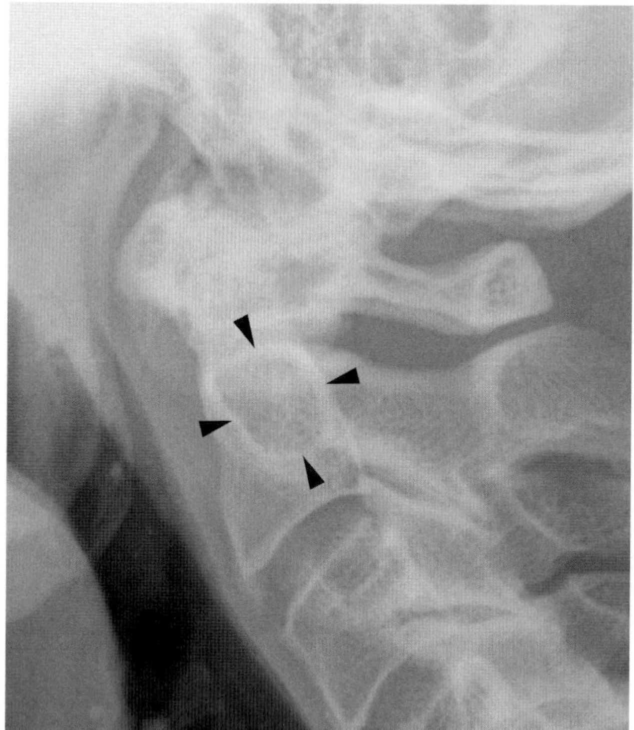

FIGURE 59-5 ■ Harris' ring. The normal lateral cervical spine film shows an an apparent ring at the base of the odontoid peg (arrowheads). This does not correspond to a single anatomical structure but is a composite shadow which includes the C2 vertebral body.

CT

CT of the cervical spine should include the spine from the cranio-cervical junction to the level of the third thoracic vertebral body. The precise imaging parameters will depend on the CT system being used, but an appropriately thin slice thickness should be selected to allow good-quality coronal and sagittal reformats. The alignment and soft-tissue swelling is assessed on these reformats using the same basic principles as the interpretation of the conventional radiograph. The axial sections are particularly useful for diagnosing bone fractures.

The presence of malalignment and soft-tissue swelling will often give an indication of ligamentous disruption in the absence of any bony injury but this is not always the case. If there is continued clinical concern following a normal CT, then MRI is warranted as CT cannot exclude a purely ligamentous disruption.

MRI

MRI of the cervical spine is best performed with the standard head and neck coils for the particular system being used to allow the best resolution with a small field of view. As there are frequently fractures at multiple levels the whole of the spine should be imaged in the sagittal plane. Axial sections can be planned from the sagittal slices and targeted at areas of abnormality. The principles of the sequences used and the image interpretation apply equally to the cervical spine and thoracolumbar spine.

The sagittal sequences should include T1- and T2-weighted fat-saturated sequences. A short tau inversion recovery (STIR) sequence can be used as an alternative to the T2-weighted fat-saturated sequence since it is a robust sequence that provides reliable fat suppression. Bone and soft-tissue injury is more clearly demonstrated with fat-saturated sequences and injuries can be missed on standard turbo spin echo T2-weighted sequences (Fig. 59-6).

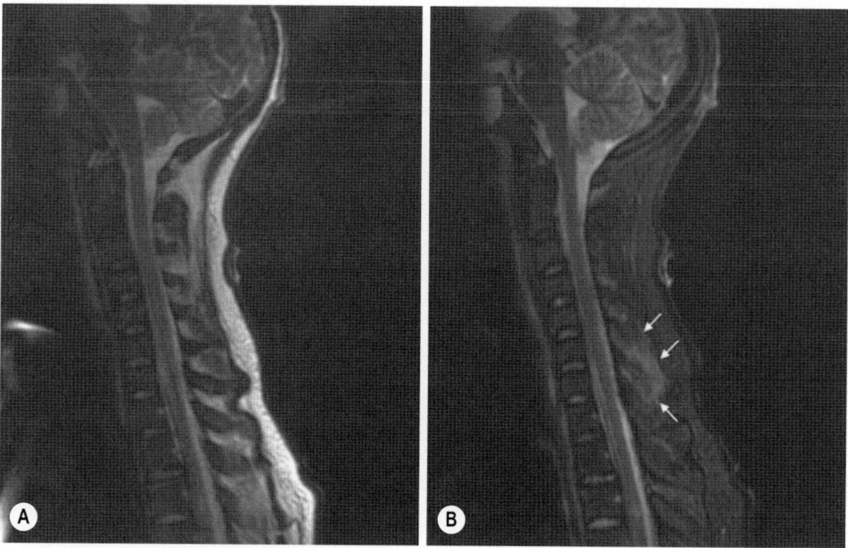

FIGURE 59-6 ■ (A) Sagittal T2-weighted and (B) STIR MRI. There is a fracture of the posterior elements of C5, which is demonstrated by oedematous change on the STIR sequence (arrows) but not seen on the T2-weighted sequence.

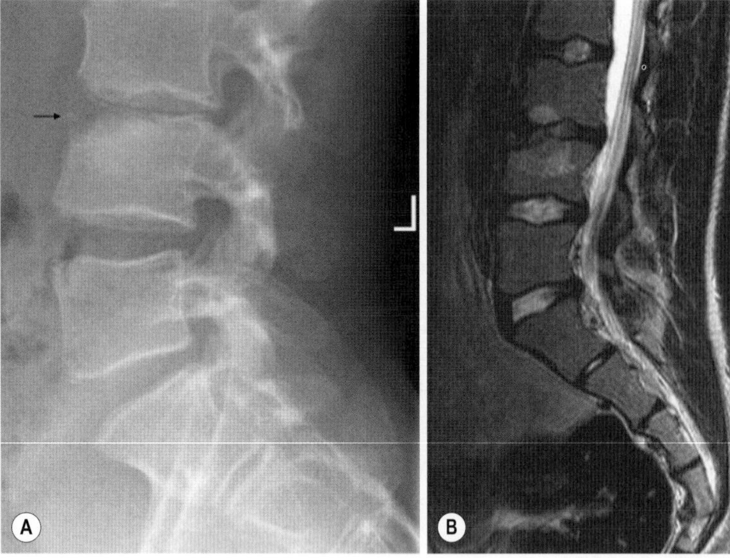

FIGURE 59-7 ■ Limbus vertebrae. (A) Conventional radiograph and (B) sagittal T2-weighted fat-saturated MRI in a 14-year-old male. The antero-superior endplate of L4 is depressed with a separate bone fragment (arrow). The MRI demonstrates that the intervertebral disc has prolapsed anteriorly, separating the bone fragment from the vertebral body. There is associated bone oedema, indicating this is a relatively recent occurrence.

Gradient echo sequences may be used when assessing neurological injury since these better demonstrate haemorrhage, an important prognostic indicator for poor neurological recovery.

THORACOLUMBAR SPINE

Conventional Radiographs

The conventional radiographic examination of the thoracic and lumbar spine includes AP and lateral views. The upper thoracic spine is particularly difficult to image on the lateral view due to the substantial overlying bone and soft tissues of the shoulders. CT, as part of a polytrauma CT protocol, most appropriately images the thoracic spine, as greater forces are required to cause a fracture of the relatively rigid thoracic cage. Conventional radiographs of the thoracic spine are rightly becoming a rare investigation.

Soft-tissue swelling due to a paravertebral haematoma is best demonstrated on the AP view of the thoracic spine where it causes focal widening of the mediastinum. Alignment is assessed on both the AP and lateral views. There should be an equal distance between the spinous processes and on the AP view the spinous process should be central with a symmetrical appearance of the pedicles and vertebral body.

The greater degree of mobility of the spine at the thoracolumbar junction renders this area particularly prone to injury and it is a relatively easy area to demonstrate with conventional radiographs due to the even quantity of overlying soft tissue. Patients with osteoporosis can sustain vertebral body compression fractures with fairly minimal forces. Often the challenge in interpreting the conventional radiograph is in determining what is an acute injury and what is old. Acute fractures tend to have sharp cortical margins and lucent fracture lines, whereas old injuries have smooth cortical margins and sclerosis. Ultimately, clinical correlation and, if necessary, MRI are a more reliable indicator of the age of a fracture than conventional radiographs.

A limbus vertebrae is a common developmental abnormality that should not be confused with an acute injury (Fig. 59-7). In the lumbar spine it most commonly affects the superior endplate of L4. These usually occur during adolescence before the endplates develop their full structural integrity. The intervertebral disc can prolapse anteriorly, lifting off the ring apophysis, typically occurring without any history of injury. The typical site and well-corticated appearance of the bone fragment are clues that this is not an acute injury.

CT

CT of the thoracic and lumbar spine should be performed as part of a polytrauma CT protocol that includes an intravenous contrast agent for the assessment of vascular injury. The precise imaging parameters will depend on the particular CT system but the axial imaging should allow sagittal and coronal reformats of sufficient diagnostic quality. The sagittal reformats of the thoracic spine should include the sternum since this is part of the bony ring of the thoracic cage and the integrity of the sternum is important in the stability of a thoracic fracture.

Because of the relatively rigid nature of the thoracic spine, injury usually involves bony fractures. CT is therefore very useful for diagnosing or excluding a thoracic spine injury. The thoracolumbar junction, on the other hand, is a relatively mobile structure and behaves more like the cervical spine in that purely ligamentous injury can occur without bony fractures. The presence of epidural fat within the spinal canal adjacent to the ligamentum flavum provides a natural soft-tissue contrast for assessing the posterior ligaments, an anatomical feature which is not present in the cervical spine (see later). However, ultimately, MRI remains the gold standard for assessing purely ligamentous injury.

SPECIFIC INJURY PATTERNS

CERVICAL SPINE

Atlanto-Occipital Dissociation

Dissociation between the cranium and cervical spine is an unusual injury since it is usually incompatible with life. It more commonly occurs in children. A simple assessment of normal cranial–cervical alignment is provided by tracing a line down the clivus that should extend onto the tip of the odontoid process. With cranio-cervical dislocation this line will fall anterior or posterior to the tip of the odontoid peg (Fig. 59-8).

C1 Injuries

Rotatory Subluxation

Fixed rotatory subluxation occurs most frequently in children and typically occurs following a respiratory illness in the absence of trauma. The hallmark feature is fixed rotation between C1 and C2. An inadequately positioned CT performed with the head rotated to one side can mimic a rotatory subluxation since the function of the C1–C2 joint is to allow rotation of the head relative to the spine. Re-positioning the head and reimaging will correct the rotation, whereas in fixed rotatory subluxation the rotation between C1 and C2 persists when the patient rotates the head to either side. With this pattern of malalignment there is usually no history of trauma and when diagnosed in the context of acute trauma it is most frequently a case of misdiagnosis due to inadequate positioning at the time of CT rather than true rotatory subluxation and the first step should be to review the positioning of the patient and if necessary repeat the examination.

FIGURE 59-8 ■ Atlanto-occipital dissociation. (A) A line drawn down the clivus passes onto the anterior aspect of the odontoid peg (dashed line). (B) Sagittal STIR sequence. The apical ligament (arrow), which is the superior extension of the posterior longitudinal ligament, is stripped off the clivus. The cranium is anteriorly subluxed relative to the cervical spine. There is oedema (arrowhead) related to the posterior ligamentous disruption.

Jefferson Fracture

Fractures of the C1 ring, in common with fractures of bony rings elsewhere in the body, usually fracture at more than one site. A Jefferson fracture describes a fracture involving the anterior and posterior ring due to an axial force transmitted through the occipital condyles onto the atlas. The disruption of the anterior and posterior ring results in malalignment of the C1–C2 facet joints. The diagnosis can be made on conventional radiograph open mouth peg views, where overhanging of the lateral mass of C1 will be seen relative to the margins of C2 (Fig. 59-9A). However, CT will best demonstrate the site and any associated soft-tissue mass (Fig. 59-9B). On the open mouth peg view, simple asymmetry of the spaces between the odontoid peg and lateral masses is not diagnostic of this fracture pattern. Incomplete ossification of the posterior arch of C1 is a common normal variant that should not be confused with a fracture.

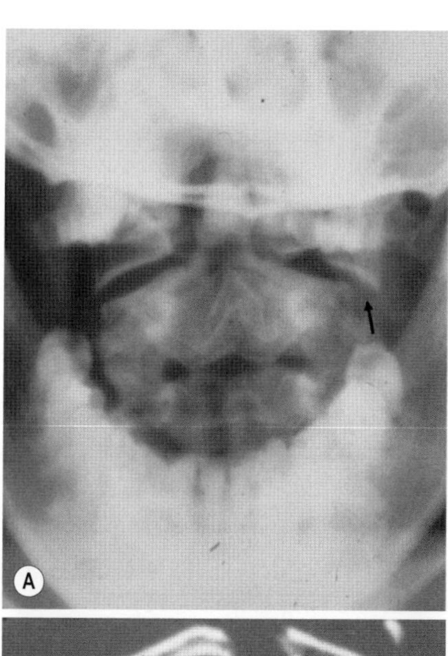

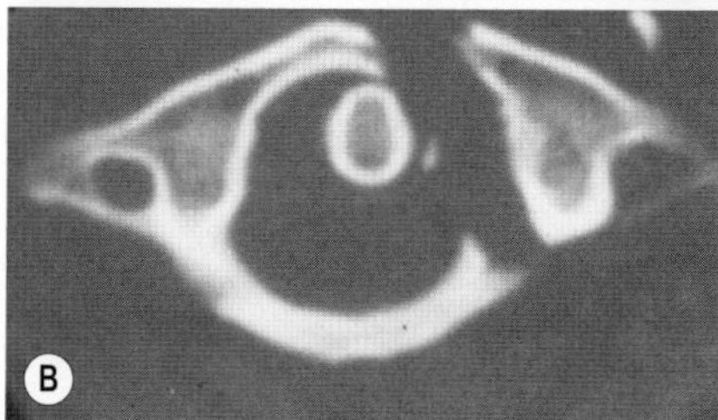

FIGURE 59-9 ■ Jefferson fracture. (A) Open mouth odontoid peg view. There is overhanging of the C1–C2 facet joint on the left (arrow)—compare with the right. (B) Axial CT demonstrates anterior and posterior ring fractures.

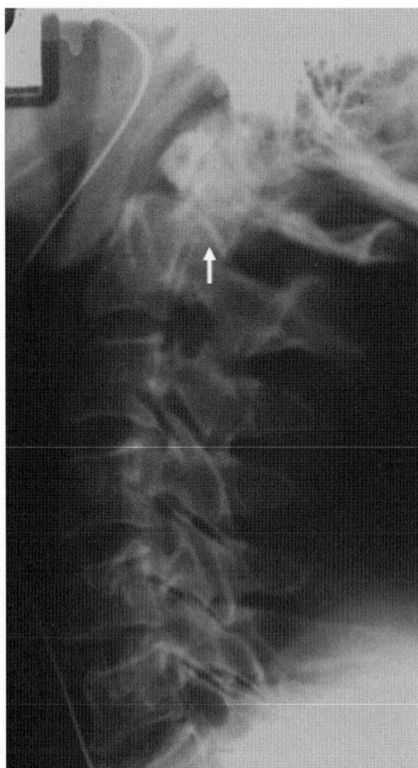

FIGURE 59-10 ■ Fracture of the base of the odontoid peg with posterior displacement (arrow). The anterior spinal line runs up the anterior aspect of the arch of C1 and not the odontoid peg.

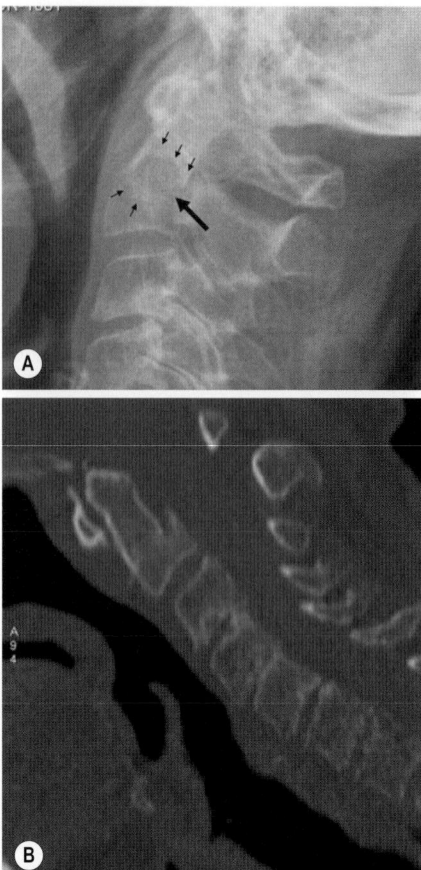

FIGURE 59-11 ■ Undisplaced type III odontoid peg fracture. (A) Harris' ring (arrows) is disrupted posteriorly (large arrow)—compare with Fig. 59-5. (B) CT Sagittal reformat showing the fracture is minimally displaced.

C2 Injuries

Odontoid Fractures

Fracture of the odontoid peg is a relatively common injury. The classic diagnostic feature is displacement of the anterior C1 arch relative to C2 (Fig. 59-10). Displacement is usually posterior though the fracture can displace anteriorly. With an undisplaced fracture the only diagnostic clue may be soft-tissue swelling anterior to the upper cervical spine.

The fracture either occurs through the base of the odontoid peg (type II fracture) or extends into the body of C2 (type III). A type III fracture has a better prognosis for bony union since there is a greater vascular supply in the vertebral body than in the peg. The diagnosis of an undisplaced type III fracture can be difficult but is aided by examining Harris' ring (see Fig. 59-5).[4] A type III fracture extends into the body of C2 and can be seen as a disruption of the ring (Fig. 59-11).

A type I fracture describes an avulsion of the tip of the odontoid peg, a controversial condition that is never encountered in clinical practice in acute trauma. An os odontoideum is a well-corticated ossification centre above a rudimentary peg which is not a feature of acute injury though some consider it the sequela of a type I injury.

Hangman's Fracture

A hangman's fracture is a traumatic spondylolisthesis of C2 where a fracture occurs through both pedicles, separating the posterior elements from the vertebral body (Fig. 59-12). The C2 vertebral body subluxes anteriorly relative to C3 but the posterior elements remain normally aligned. Because the spinal canal effectively widens in AP diameter at the level of slip there is often little or no neurological injury despite sometimes marked spondylolisthesis.

Hyperflexion Injuries

Flexion forces to the spine can cause rupture of the posterior elements, resulting in kyphotic angulation and anterior displacement. Typically there may be little in the way of anterior soft-tissue swelling since all the soft-tissue injury occurs posteriorly. If no associated bony injury occurs, then the diagnosis rests on demonstrating the abnormality of alignment (see Fig. 59-4).

There may be a fracture of the anterior aspect of the vertebral body, the flexion teardrop fracture. The bony fragment is typically relatively large and elongated in the cranio-caudal direction of the spine, which distinguishes it from the hyperextension tear drop, which is usually a small fragment. Since significant spinal displacement is required at the time of injury to cause such a compression fracture there is a strong association with severe neurological injury.

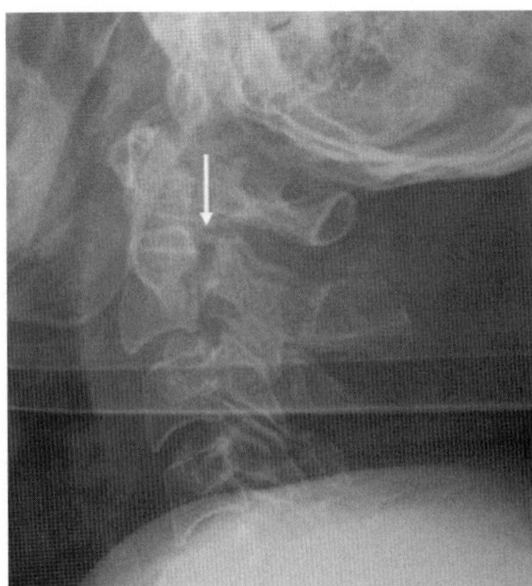

FIGURE 59-12 ■ **Hangman's fracture.** There is a fracture between the pedicles and body of C2 (arrow). There is slight anterior subluxation of C2 on C3 but the spinolaminar line of C2 remains behind the spinolaminar line of C1 and C3 (compare with physiological subluxation depicted in Fig. 59-3).

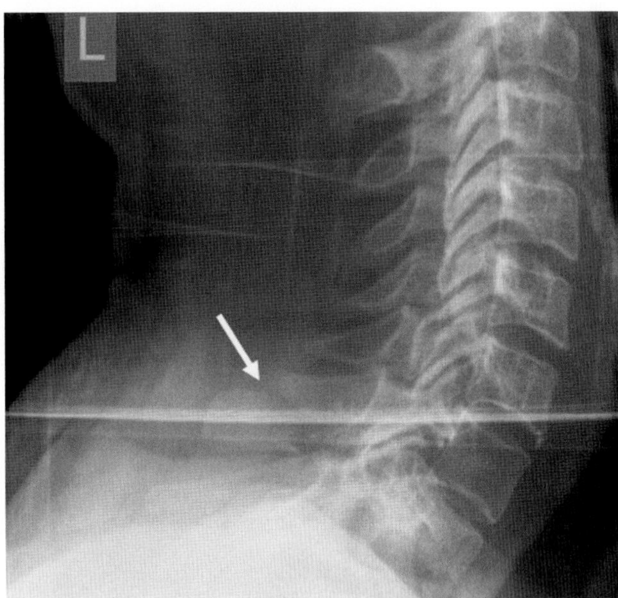

FIGURE 59-14 ■ **Clay-shoveler's fracture.** There is a fracture of the spinous process of C7 (arrow), which does not extend to the spinolaminar line.

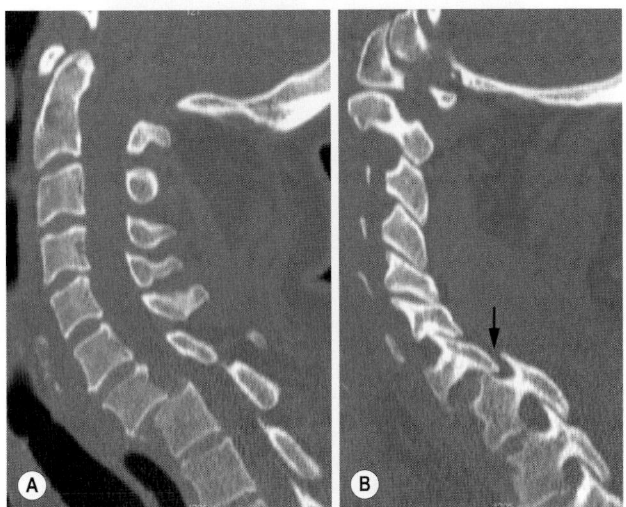

FIGURE 59-13 ■ **Bilateral facet joint dislocation.** (A) Sagittal CT reformat. There is greater than 50% forward slip of C7 on T1. (B) Parasagittal reformat through the facet joint demonstrates that the joints are 'locked' in a dislocated position (arrow).

Bilateral subuxation of the facet joints can occur with little in the way of bony injury. The facet joints can lock in a displaced position, the so-called perched facet joints (Fig. 59-13). The displacement of the spine can be 50% or greater of the vertebral body width.

A hyperflexion force with resistance of the posterior paraspinal muscles can produce a 'clay-shoveler's' fracture (Fig. 59-14). This is a fracture of the lower cervical or upper thoracic spinous process and is one of the few cervical fractures that can be considered stable. The fracture should not extend across the spinolaminar line as this suggests injury to the posterior ligaments and hence instability.

Hyperflexion Rotation Injury

A rotational force applied along with flexion can result in a unilateral dislocation of a facet joint. The key conventional radiographic feature is the demonstration of a rotational abnormality at a single level (see Fig. 59-2). Malalignment in the sagittal plane may be very minimal so the abnormality of rotation is a key diagnostic feature. CT demonstrates the 'reverse hamburger' sign on the axial sections through the facet dislocation (Fig. 59-15). The use of CT in this injury has demonstrated that a dislocation of the facet joint is frequently associated with a fracture of the joint and that these are not usually purely ligamentous injuries as previously thought.

Hyperextension Injuries

Extension force to the spine can result in rupture of the anterior longitudinal ligament and posterior displacement and angulation. There is typically soft-tissue swelling anterior to the spine at the site of the ligamentous disruption and since the malalignment may be very subtle the presence of this soft-tissue swelling is a key sign. There may be an associated hyperextension teardrop fracture, which is usually a small fragment (Fig. 59-16).

Neurological abnormality implies that a hyperextension dislocation occurred at the time of injury though the spine may be relatively normally aligned subsequently. This is the usual mechanism of injury when a patient has clinical signs of neurological damage in the presence of relatively normal conventional radiographs and CT imaging. The term *spinal cord injuries without radiological abnormality* (SCIWORA) has been applied in the past to this situation, a condition more commonly seen in children. However, any patient with neurological abnormality following acute trauma warrants an MRI which

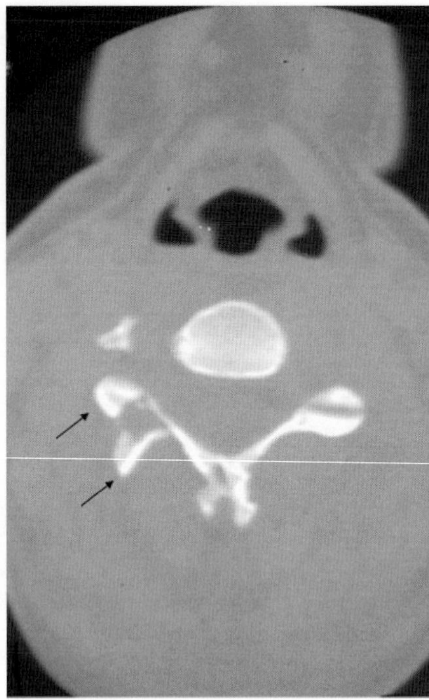

FIGURE 59-15 ■ Unilateral facet joint dislocation. The left facet joint has a 'hamburger' appearance. The right facet joint is dislocated and fractured, giving the appearances of the 'reverse hamburger' sign (arrows).

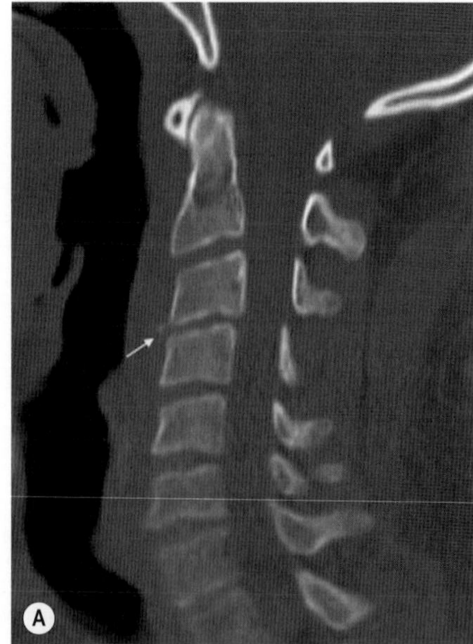

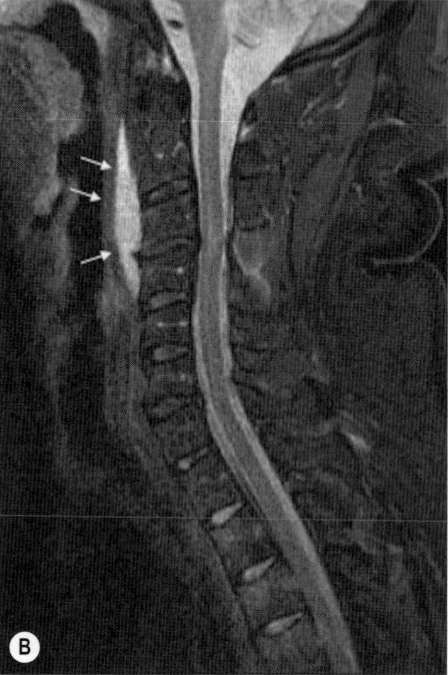

FIGURE 59-16 ■ Hyperextension injury. (A) Sagittal CT reformat. There is a small hyperextension teardrop fracture (arrow). There is slight malalignment at C3–C4 with retrolisthesis. (B) Sagittal STIR MRI. There is a large amount of anterior soft-tissue swelling (arrows). There is evidence of cord injury with cord oedema.

will demonstrate the soft-tissue injuries, so the term SCIWORA is probably an anachronism.

THORACIC AND LUMBAR SPINE

Classification Systems

Classifying a spinal fracture provides an important tool for the radiologist in communicating with the treating surgeon. For the surgeon it provides a guide to the management, the most crucial decision being the need for surgical internal fixation versus conservative treatment. Ideally a classification system would identify those injuries which are unstable: that is liable to continuing deformity or neurological injury under normal physiological loads. Denis described a three-column concept of the spine, the middle column involving the posterior aspect of the vertebral body and posterior longitudinal ligament, the anterior column the structures anterior to this and the posterior column the structures posterior.[5] Traditional teaching has been that any injury that involves two of the three columns is unstable but this is a gross simplification. One of the commonest thoracic and lumbar injuries is the burst fracture that according to Denis' concept involves the anterior and middle columns and is therefore unstable, yet many burst fractures are stable and treated non-operatively. Conversely, apparently minor endplate fractures in the presence of osteoporosis can progress to avascular necrosis and delayed vertebral collapse and deformity. The purely anatomical disruption of the spine is only one factor in determining the management of the patient, but it is important for the radiologist to accurately identify the extent of the bony and ligamentous disruption.

More recent classification systems have been described to take into account the anatomical information available on MRI. Oner et al.[6] described a classification system that categorised all the possible relevant structures seen on MRI, which included the endplate, the disc and the ligamentous structures. The AO classification system[7] provides a comprehensive system for describing the mechanism and anatomical disruption of the spine. The problem for the reporting radiologist in these systems lies in their complexity: the AO system has 22 different categories.

The system described in this chapter is necessarily simplistic and based on the Denis classification that has a mechanistic and anatomical approach. The importance in pattern recognition is in identifying those situations in which the degree of ligamentous disruption is likely to be greater than initially apparent on conventional radiographs or CT. MRI can then be performed in these cases, allowing a more accurate description of the anatomical disruption.

Flexion Compression and Flexion Distraction Injuries

The flexion compression fracture results in loss of height of the anterior aspect of the vertebral body but the posterior ligamentous structures are intact. The flexion distraction injury ruptures the posterior bony and/or ligamentous structures by distraction and causes a variable degree of compression of the anterior column (Fig. 59-17). The posterior ligamentous structures that are ruptured include the posterior longitudinal ligament, the ligamentum flavum, the interspinous ligament and the supraspinous ligament. Often the posterior distraction will occur through the posterior bony elements, the so-called bony Chance fracture, named after the British radiologist who first described the injury.[8] These are relatively easy to identify since the bony injury can be seen on conventional radiographs and is easily demonstrable by CT. The fracture may occur through one vertebra, passing through the pedicles and spinous process at a single level. In this pure bony Chance fracture the posterior ligaments remain intact and while these fractures are usually surgically fixed there is a good prognosis since bony injury heals better than ligamentous disruption. The fracture may pass through the pars interarticularis and involve the posterior ligaments of the adjacent level, usually the level above. This is an important observation since it will determine the extent of surgical fixation. With the advent of CT multislice technology, allowing reformats of high quality, it is becoming apparent that CT can define the posterior ligamentous structures. The presence of epidural fat adjacent to the ligamentum flavum provides a natural anatomical contrast to the density of the ligament. The intact ligament should have a smooth contour, whereas irregularity implies a rupture. With rupture of the ligament, haemorrhage occurs into the epidural fat, giving a 'dirty fat' sign (Fig. 59-18). However, ultimately, MRI remains the most accurate means of demonstrating ligamentous disruption

If the flexion distraction injury involves the posterior ligamentous structures without posterior bony injury this is referred to as a soft-tissue Chance injury (Fig. 59-17B). Without bony injury present these can provide a diagnostic challenge on conventional radiographs and CT, as they can be confused with the simple flexion compression

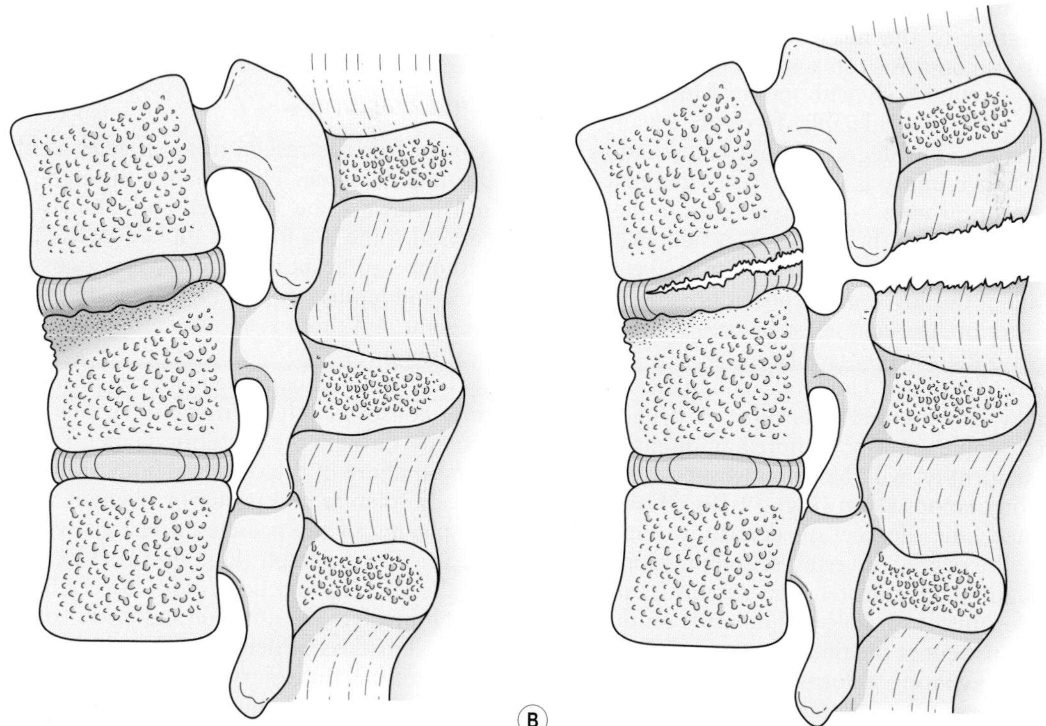

FIGURE 59-17 ■ **Flexion compression and flexion distraction injuries.** (A) Flexion compression fracture. There is loss of height of the anterior aspect of the vertebral body. The posterior ligaments are intact. (B) Flexion distraction injury. There is rupture of the posterior ligaments and only slight compression of the anterior vertebral body. The illustration shows disruption at the level of the intervertebral disc without posterior bony fracture, a 'soft-tissue Chance' injury. However, the fracture may pass through the bone elements of the posterior arch (bony Chance fracture).

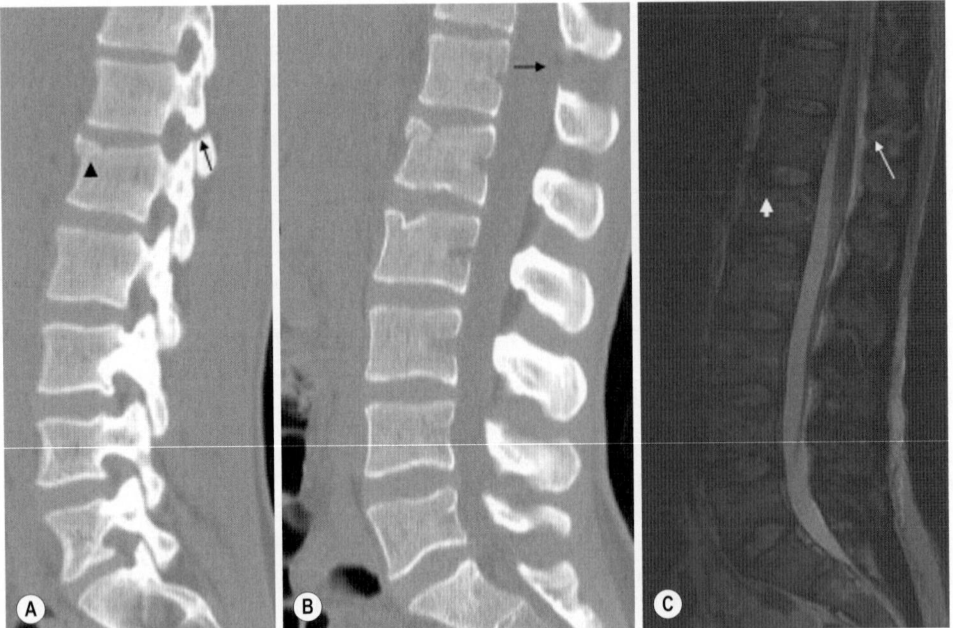

FIGURE 59-18 ■ **Flexion distraction injury with bony and ligamentous involvement.** (A) There is anterior compression of the vertebral body (arrowhead) and a fracture through the pars interarticularis (arrow). (B) The distraction injury extends through the interspinous ligament of the level above. There is a 'dirty fat' sign with loss of the normal epidural fat (arrow). (C) Sagittal T2-weighted MRI; there is compression of the anterior aspect of the vertebral body (arrowhead) and interspinous ligament disruption of the level above (arrow) with disruption of the ligamentum flavum and high signal passing through the interspinous ligament.

injury with intact posterior ligaments. The diagnostic clues begin before the imaging, with the degree of clinical suspicion relating to the mechanism of injury. Elderly patients with osteoporosis can sustain compression fractures of the vertebral body with minimal force, whereas it usually requires considerable force to fracture the young adult spine. The degree of bony compression in a soft-tissue Chance injury is usually fairly minimal since the flexion occurs around a fulcrum anterior to the spine: for instance, in a lap seat belt injury. Considerable vertebral body collapse is more suggestive of an axial compressive injury and if this involves the posterior vertebral wall then the posterior ligamentous structures will be intact since this is a burst fracture (see later).

The main diagnostic clue to a soft-tissue Chance injury is a kyphotic spinal deformity. A kyphosis can occur with a simple anterior compression injury but the degree of deformity will be commensurate with the degree of bony compression (Fig. 59-19). With a soft-tissue Chance, the degree of deformity cannot be explained by the degree of vertebral compression, which is usually slight. Unfortunately the demonstration of a kyphotic deformity is variable and depends on the positioning of the patient at the time of imaging (Fig. 59-20). The lack of a kyphotic deformity cannot therefore be used as evidence of intact posterior ligaments.

In addition to carefully reviewing the lateral films for evidence of a suspected Chance injury, evidence of bone or soft-tissue injury to the posterior elements may be evident on the AP film, which should also be carefully reviewed. Fracture through the pedicles or spinous processes and/or widening of the gap between adjacent spinous processes (which should normally be equidistant) are important features of Chance injuries (Fig. 59-21).

Burst Fractures

A burst fracture results from an axial compressive force through the spine. This is one of the commonest thoracic and lumbar spine fractures and can also occur in the cervical spine if a force is applied to the top of the head without significant neck flexion or extension. In the thoracic and lumbar spine a typical mechanism is a fall from a height and there is an association with bilateral calcaneal fractures.

The vertebral body, pedicles and posterior bony structures constitute a bony ring so that there is commonly a fracture through the posterior elements in addition to the burst fracture of the vertebral body. This combination of a body fracture and posterior element fracture can lead to splaying of the pedicles, a feature which can be seen on an AP radiograph (Fig. 59-22). The hallmark feature on the lateral projection is loss of vertebral body height, which involves the anterior and posterior vertebral body walls. This loss of height of the posterior vertebral wall distinguishes this injury from a flexion compression and flexion distraction injury in which the posterior wall is intact. Compression of the posterior vertebral wall in the context of other typical features of a burst fracture effectively excludes disruption of the posterior ligaments since the posterior structures have been compressed and not distracted (Fig. 59-23).

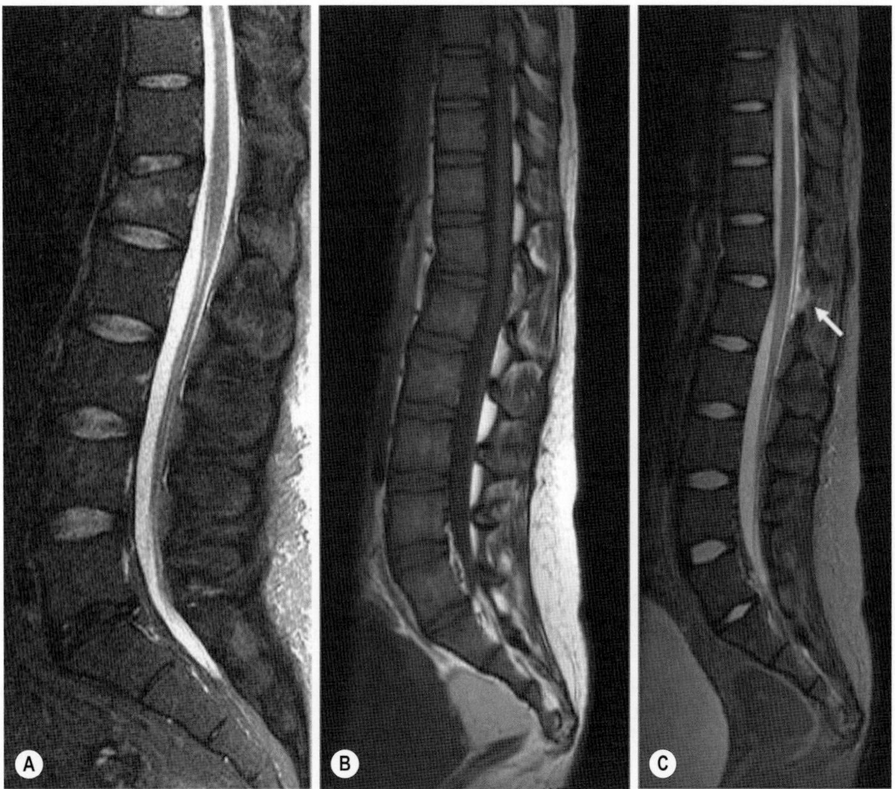

FIGURE 59-19 ■ Comparing the kyphosis in flexion compression and flexion distraction injuries. (A) Flexion compression injury, sagittal STIR MRI. There is a moderate degree of anterior compression of the vertebral body but only minimal kyphosis. The posterior ligaments are intact. (B) Sagittal T1-weighted and (C) sagittal STIR MRI. Flexion distraction, soft-tissue Chance injury. Kyphosis in the absence of any vertebral body compression. There is disruption of the posterior ligaments (arrow).

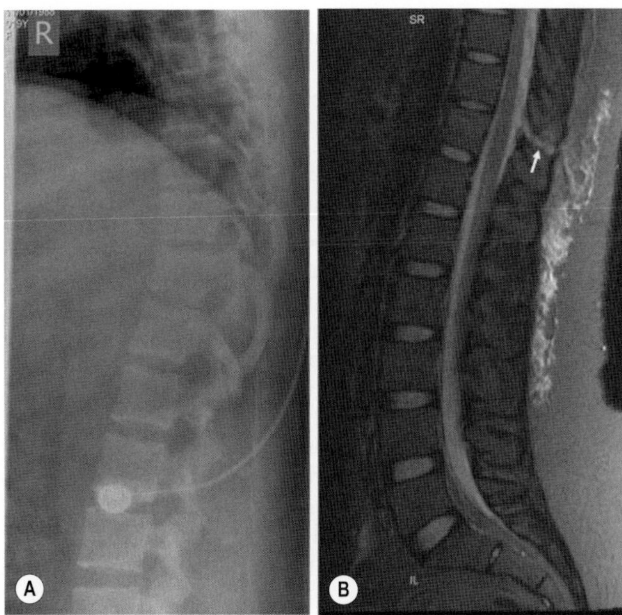

FIGURE 59-20 ■ Soft-tissue Chance injury. (A) Lateral radiograph shows a kyphotic deformity. (B) Same patient, sagittal STIR MRI. With the patient lying supine in the MRI unit there is no spinal deformity despite an interspinous ligament disruption (arrow).

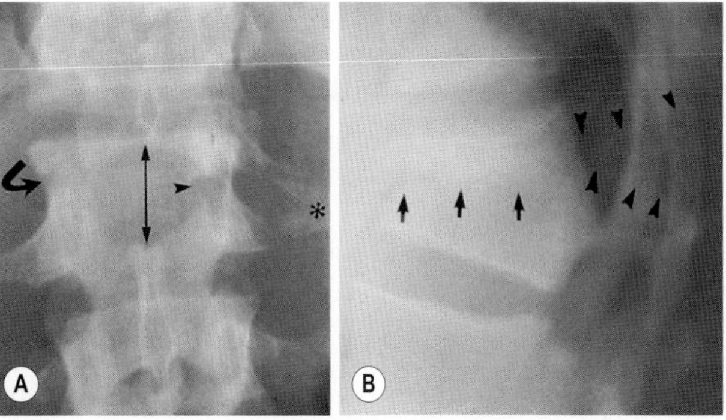

FIGURE 59-21 ■ Bony Chance fracture of L1. The AP projection (A) shows a comminuted fracture of the left transverse process (*), transverse fracture of the left pedicle (arrowhead), separation of the T12 and L1 spinous processes (double arrow) and a fracture of the right superolateral cortex of L1 (curved arrow). In the lateral projection (B) the arrowheads indicate a distraction transverse fracture of the spinous process and laminae and the arrows indicate the horizontal fracture of the body with anterior wedging.

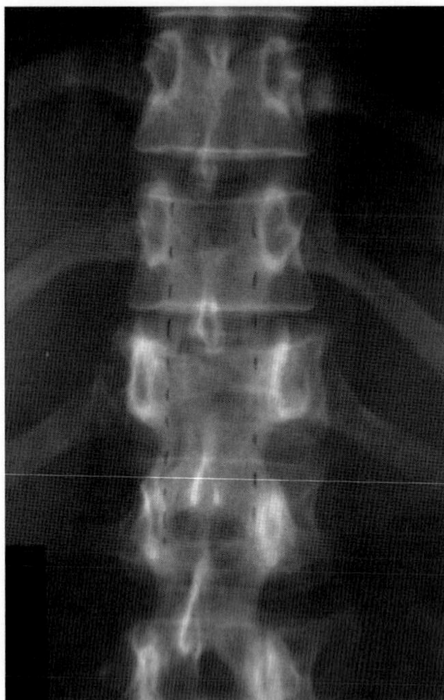

FIGURE 59-22 ■ **AP radiograph of a burst fracture.** The pedicle of the fractured vertebra lies outside a line joining the inner aspects of the pedicles of the level above and below (dotted line).

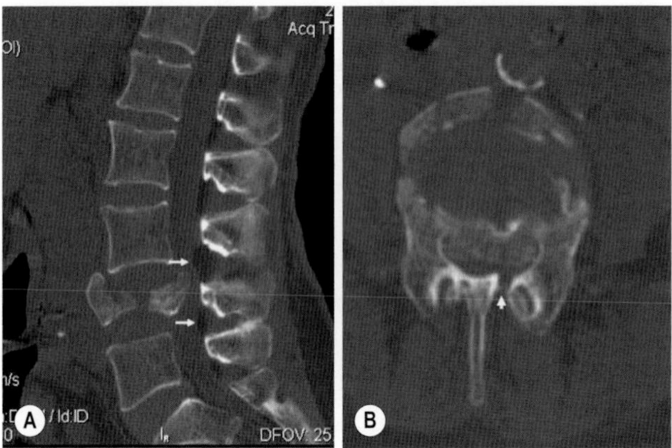

FIGURE 59-23 ■ **(A) sagittal and (B) axial CT of a pincer burst fracture.** There is loss of height of the vertebral body affecting the anterior and posterior walls. The presence of normal epidural fat (absence of the 'dirty fat' sign)(arrows) is evidence of intact ligaments. Note the ligamentum flavum buckles into the spinal canal. There is a fracture of the lamina (arrowhead).

There may be a mild kyphotic deformity if the anterior vertebral body collapses more than the posterior wall. A fragment from the anterior vertebral body wall may separate, resulting in a 'pincer burst' fracture. A progressive kyphotic deformity can develop in this situation if the fragment fails to unite with the rest of the vertebral body. For this reason pincer fractures are usually surgically fixed.

Lateral asymmetrical collapse of the vertebral body may lead to a lateral plane deformity (lateral angulation or curvature) evident on the AP projection and CT coronal reformats. Whilst there is frequently a degree of angulation deformity at the fracture site there is no step in the alignment without a spondylolisthesis on the lateral or sagittal projections and no lateral step on the AP or coronal views. This distinguishes a burst fracture from a fracture dislocation, which may have fractures of the anterior and posterior vertebral body walls but also has complete ligamentous disruption including all the posterior ligaments, a highly unstable injury.

The axial CT section through a burst fracture shows the typical appearance of encroachment of the posterior vertebral wall into the spinal canal and burst fractures are strongly associated with neurological injury (Fig. 59-23B). Wilcox et al. performed high-speed video filming and pressure monitoring at the moment of burst fracture in an animal model.[9] They demonstrated that all the neurological injury occurs at the moment of the burst fracture and the resting state of the fragment in the canal has no bearing on subsequent neurological injury. This resting position of the fragment is the appearance demonstrated on CT and, whilst the size of the fragment in the canal may seem alarming, surgeons no longer routinely surgically remove these fragments, given it has no bearing on the neurological outcome.[10] If, following neurological improvement, the patient subsequently develops signs of canal stenosis, this can be addressed later, after the acute event.

The CT appearances of a burst fracture are so characteristic that the role of MRI is principally in demonstrating the associated neurological injury. Since there is frequently a fracture of the bony posterior elements, oedematous change will frequently be seen in the interspinous ligament adjacent to the fractured lamina. This should not be confused with a rupture of the ligament. The ligamentum flavum frequently appears buckled, a result of loss of height of the vertebral body, but no defect will be seen in the ligament.

Fracture Dislocation

A combination of flexion and rotation can result in a fracture dislocation in the thoracic and lumbar spine. These are high force injuries, which are frequently associated with severe neurological injury and often cord transection. There will be varying degrees of bony disruption, but the full width of the spine is always involved, with complete ligamentous disruption, making these the most unstable of injuries.

The key diagnostic feature is a step in the alignment in either the sagittal or coronal profile, frequently both (Fig. 59-24). Any step in alignment within the thoracic spine implies a fracture dislocation since a step in alignment is not encountered in other conditions. In the lumbar spine a spondylolisthesis is frequently encountered due to degenerative disease at L4–L5 and spondylolysis at L5–S1. A step in the lateral plane can be seen in association with a degenerative lumbar scoliosis but these conditions have typical features and, in the absence of other features of injury, should not cause any diagnostic confusion.

An MRI should always be performed in these injuries to investigate the neurological injury and as a preoperative plan. Fragments of bone, disc or haematoma within the canal can worsen the neurological injury if realignment of the spine causes these to exert a greater pressure effect on the cord. In the case of cord transection with complete neurological paralysis, this will not be a consideration although the spine is frequently still surgically stabilised to aid the patient's rehabilitation.

THE RIGID SPINE

The patient presenting with a fracture through an otherwise fused spine presents specific problems in their diagnosis and management. The commonest causes of spinal fusion are ankylosing spondylitis (AS) and diffuse idiopathic skeletal hyperostosis (DISH). The lack of a motion segment in the fused spine gives it the biomechanical properties of a long bone. When a fracture occurs through the fused spine it always occurs through the full width of the spine and is highly unstable. The presence of osteoporosis in a fused spine, coupled with the biomechanical properties of an extended lever arm, can result in a fracture with a minimal history of trauma. The clinician must be aware of the possibility of a highly unstable fracture in a patient with new onset of symptoms in the fused spine, even in the absence of any history of trauma. In treating these fractures extensive surgical fixation is required to overcome the biomechanics of an extended lever arm, similar to the principles of long bone fixation.

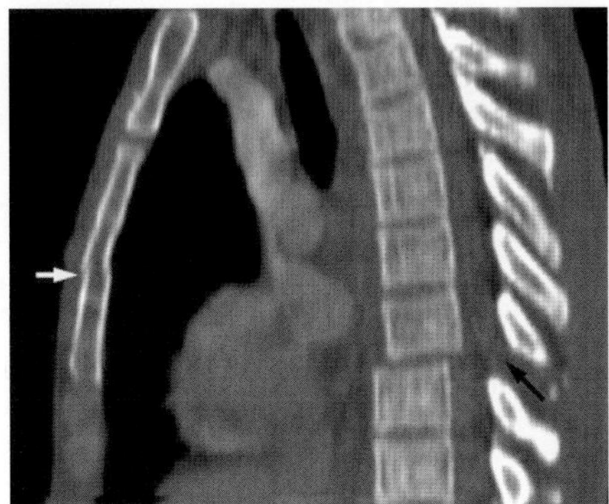

FIGURE 59-24 ■ **Fracture dislocation of the thoracic spine.** There is a step in the alignment and disruption across the spine with complete disruption of the posterior ligaments (note the 'epidural dirty fat' sign); there is an associated fracture of the sternum (arrow).

The fracture through the fused spine usually runs in the transverse plane. If the fracture is undisplaced and the bones are osteoporotic the fracture line may be very indistinct and require high-quality coronal and sagittal CT imaging. The presence of gas within the fused spine is an indicator of motion and hence fracture (Fig. 59-25). This is the result of vacuum phenomenon, the same process found in the vertebral disc at a motion segment.

There is an increased chance of fracture at more than one level in the fused spine and the whole of the spine should be imaged, just as one would do with a long bone. MRI provides a reliable means of imaging the whole spine but this is not always possible in the severely kyphotic spine of a patient with AS who may not fit into the bore of an enclosed magnet.

NEUROLOGICAL INJURY

Spinal Cord

MRI provides an important prognostic indicator for neurological recovery following spinal cord injury. The

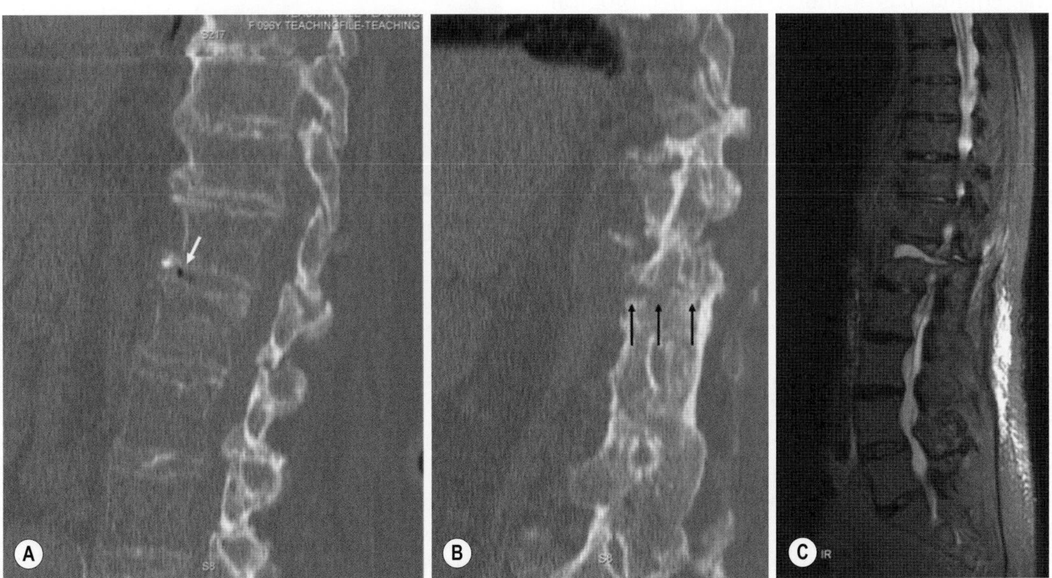

FIGURE 59-25 ■ **Fracture through the ankylosed spine in a patient with ankylosing spondylitis.** (A) The presence of vacuum phenomenon is evidence of spinal movement (arrow). (B) Sagittal CT through the facet joints. There is a faint fracture line (arrows) through the fused facet joints. (C) Sagittal STIR MRI demonstrates a fracture through the full width of the spine. The fracture through the vertebral body is difficult to define on CT, as the bone is very osteoporotic.

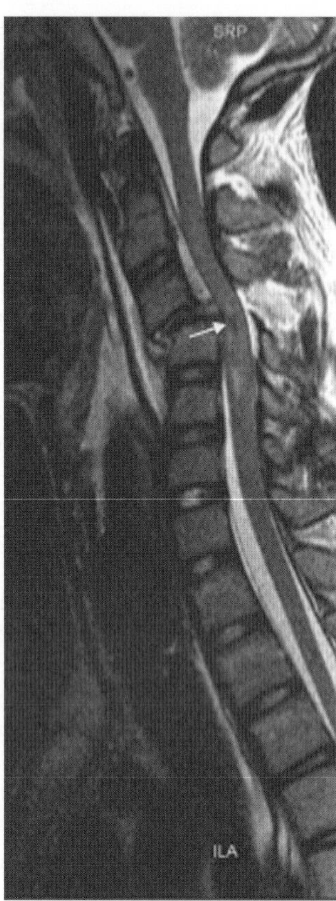

FIGURE 59-26 ■ **Sagittal T2-weighted MRI.** Low signal within the cord (arrow) is evidence of a cord haematoma. High signal inferior to this is cord oedema.

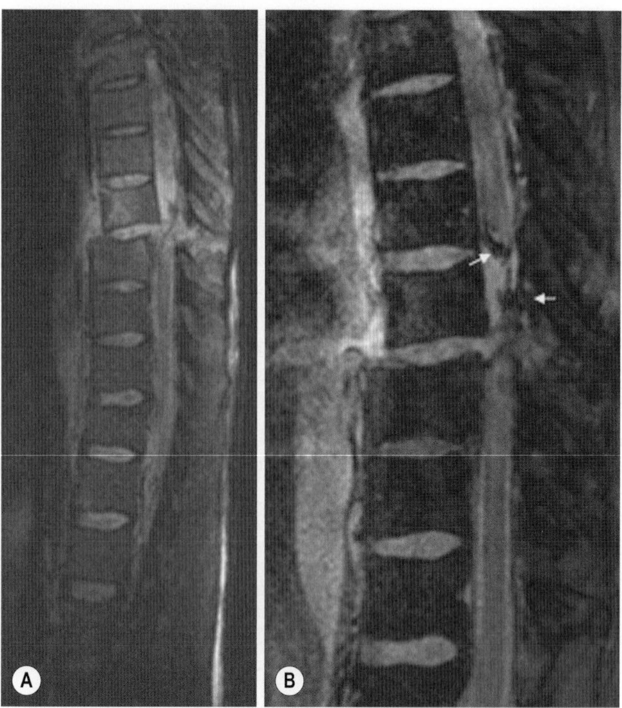

FIGURE 59-27 ■ **Fracture dislocation with cord transection.** (A) Sagittal STIR MRI and (B) gradient echo. The presence of blood is more clearly seen on the gradient echo sequence (arrows), which lies within the gap at the site of the cord transection.

position of a burst fracture either above or below the level of the conus is important prognostically as trauma to the cauda equina has a much better neurological outcome than spinal cord injury. Mild cord oedema has a good prognosis for neurological improvement, whereas cord haemorrhage is a poor prognostic indicator and cord transection clearly has the worst prognosis. Haematomas within the cord less than 4 mm in diameter have a better neurological outcome than larger haemorrhages.[11]

In the acute setting haemorrhage within the cord will appear hypointense on T2-weighted turbo spin echo imaging due to the presence of deoxyhaemoglobin (Fig. 59-26). At a variable time after this, which may be up to 10 days, this becomes hyperintense due to the presence of methaemoglobin. The zone of hyperintensity begins at the periphery of the collection. None of these appearances will usually be confused with the uniform appearances of cord oedema, but gradient echo sequences can be used since these are more sensitive to the presence of haemorrhage (Fig. 59-27).

Delayed worsening of neurology after a spinal cord injury may be due to the development of a spinal cord syrinx (Fig. 59-28). Progressive enlargement of a syrinx can compromise the residual neurological function and surgical drainage of the syrinx may be required.

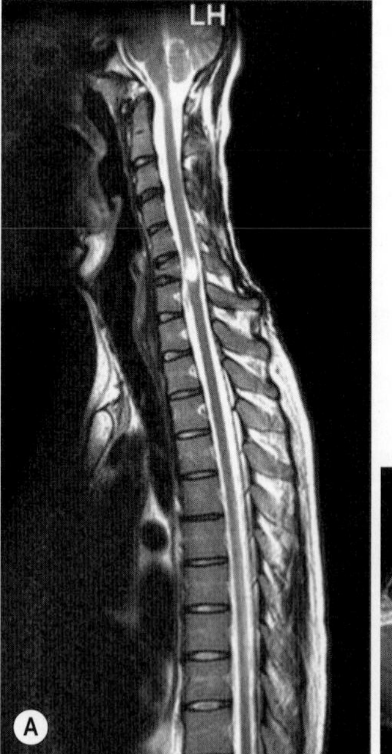

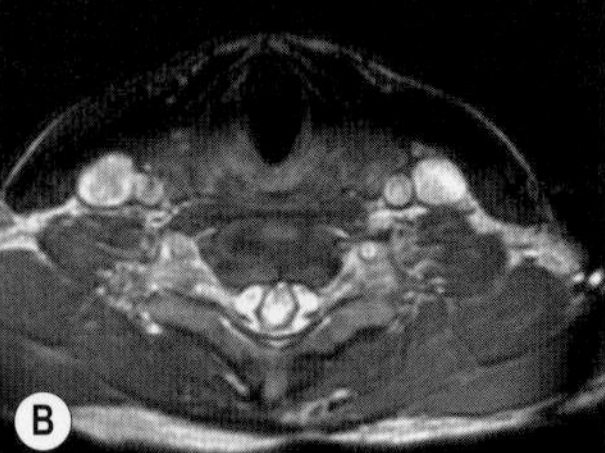

FIGURE 59-28 ■ **Delayed post-traumatic spinal cord syrinx.** T2-weighted MRI sagittal (A) and axial (B). A syrinx has developed at the site of previous spinal cord injury.

Brachial Plexus Injury

Nerve roots in the cervical spine can be avulsed from the cord, resulting in a brachial plexus injury. Whilst these commonly occur with an associated spinal injury in the

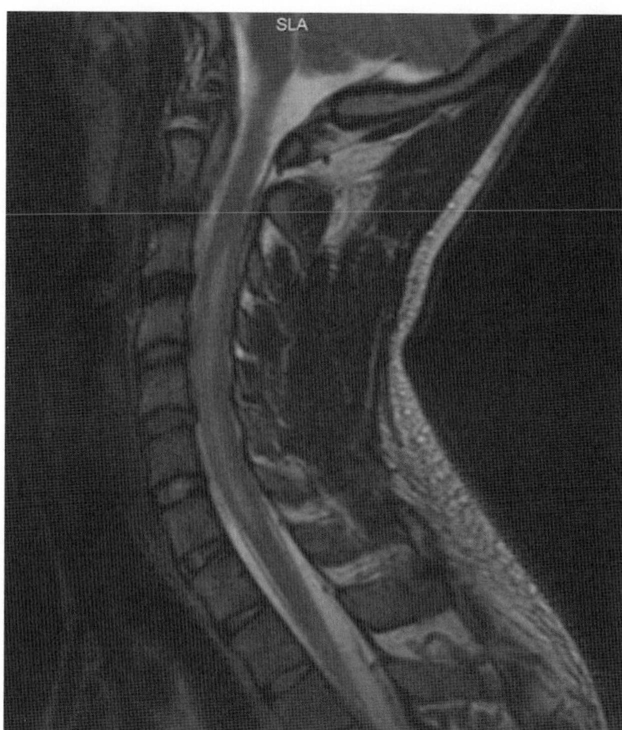

FIGURE 59-29 ■ **Sagittal T2-weighted MRI.** There is diffuse cord oedema due to nerve root avulsions at multiple levels.

polytrauma patient, the mechanism is one of a closed traction force applied to the shoulder and transmitted to the cord via the brachial plexus. Brachial plexus avulsion may be accompanied by diffuse spinal cord oedema, which should not be mistaken for the direct cord injury associated with a cervical spinal fracture (Fig. 59-29).

The lowest four cervical spinal nerves, C5–C8 and the first thoracic nerve T1 form the brachial plexus. Seventy-five per cent of cases of clinical brachial plexus injury involve avulsion of the roots from the cord[12] with 25 per cent confined to the distal brachial plexus.

MRI has largely replaced CT myelography in the diagnosis of nerve root avulsions with heavily T2-weighted 3D 'myelography' sequences, allowing the optimum slice orientation to demonstrate the intradural nerve roots. A complete nerve root avulsion is usually accompanied by a dural tear, resulting in a traumatic meningocele (Fig. 59-30). The demonstration of intact nerve roots in a patient with clinical brachial plexus injury suggests that the injury has occurred more distally within the brachial plexus, usually in the infraclavicular region.

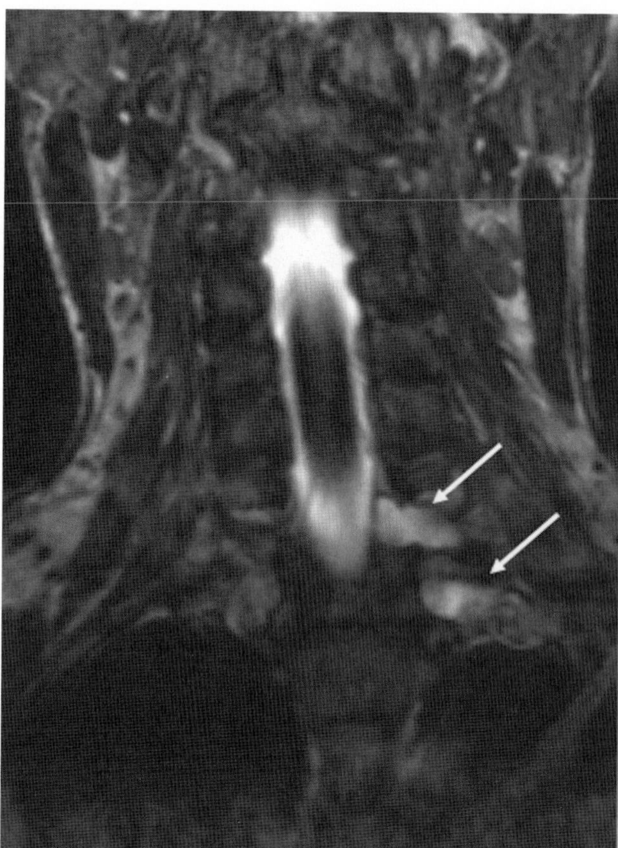

FIGURE 59-30 ■ **Coronal T2-weighted MRI 'myelogram' sequence.** Brachial plexus avulsion at C8 and T1 on the left with traumatic meningoceles (arrows).

For a full list of references, please see ExpertConsult.

FURTHER READING

6. Oner FC, van Gils AP, Dhert WJ, Verbout AJ. MRI findings of thoracolumbar spine fractures: a categorisation based on MRI examinations of 100 fractures. Skeletal Radiol 1999;28:433–43.
7. Magerl F, Aebi M, Gertzbein SD, et al. A comprehensive classification of thoracic and lumbar injuries. Eur Spine J 1994;3:184–201.
8. Chance GQ. Note on a type of flexion fracture of the spine. Br J Radiol 1948;21:452–3.
9. Wilcox RK, Boerger TO, Allen DJ, et al. A dynamic study of thoracolumbar burst fractures. J Bone Joint Surg Am 2003;85:2184–9.
10. Boerger TO, Limb D, Dickson RA. Does 'canal clearance' affect neurological outcome after thoracolumbar burst fractures? J Bone Joint Surg Br 2000;82:629–35.
11. Boldin C, Raith J, Fankhauser F, et al. Predicting neurologic recovery in cervical spinal cord injury with postoperative MR imaging. Spine 2006;31:554–9.
12. Chuang DC. Management of traumatic brachial plexus injuries in adults. Hand Clin 1999;15:737–55.

SECTION **F**

NEUROIMAGING

Section Editors: H. Rolf Jäger • Jonathan H. Gillard

CHAPTER 60

Overview of Anatomy, Pathology and Techniques; Aspects Related to Trauma

Joti Jonathan Bhattacharya • Kirsten Forbes • Peter Zampakis • David J. Bowden • John M. Stevens

CHAPTER OUTLINE

OVERVIEW OF ANATOMY, PATHOLOGY AND TECHNIQUES

Modern imaging techniques depict the brain in ever more exquisite detail in all three orthogonal planes. Since neuroradiology forms an important part of radiology training and a substantial part of most radiologists' daily work, familiarity with some of the intricacies of neuroanatomy becomes increasingly important; radiology remains in large part applied anatomy. The brain, at the macroscopic level, is a largely symmetric structure aiding the identification of abnormalities. Here we offer an overview of brain and vascular anatomy as shown on current imaging techniques, beginning with a brief summary of brain development. Imaging techniques for the brain and vasculature are then reviewed.

ANATOMY OF THE BRAIN AND VASCULAR SYSTEM

Embryology

The brain derives from the rostral end of the embryonic neural tube, formed of neural ectoderm. The initially fairly uniform neural tube develops three swellings, the primordial cerebral vesicles (prosencephalic, mesencephalic and rhombencephalic), which subsequently give rise to five vesicles.[1] At this stage it remains one cell thick, with a pseudostratified epithelium containing the neural stem cells. The cavity of the neural tube represents the future cerebral ventricles and the central canal of the spinal cord, ending anteriorly at the membrane of the lamina terminalis. Thus the anterior wall of the third ventricle (lamina terminalis) represents the rostral end of the neural tube (Fig. 60-1).

Bulges appearing on either side of the prosencephalic vesicle represent the developing telencephalic vesicles and, subsequently, cerebral hemispheres, and their opening, the future interventricular foramen (of Monro). With growth, the wall of the neural tube thickens and nutrition, which was initially by simple diffusion from the amniotic fluid to the neural plate, and after closure of the tube by diffusion from the surrounding primordial vascular plexus, is no longer sufficient. a depression appears in the roof of the developing third ventricle and adjacent cerebral hemispheres, invaginating a layer of ependyma and vascular pia mater, to form the choroid plexus (Fig. 60-2).

Thus the original function of the choroid plexus appears to be oxygenation and nutrition of the deep portions of the brain.[2] Subsequently, penetrating vessels grow into the brain substance. With growth of the cerebral hemispheres, neuronal proliferation occurs in the periventricular zone, followed by migration of neurons along radially oriented glial cells to reach the pallial surface of the brain. This results in formation of the cerebral cortex, with its characteristic lamination. Over most of the hemispheric surface a six-layer neuronal structure can be identified: the isocortex (neocortex). Paul Broca traced the isocortex to its medial edge (Latin: *limbus*), thus identifying a medial limbic lobe (the hippocampus and associated structures) which was found to have a simpler three-layer structure, the allocortex. An intermediate band of cortex between the isocortex and allocortex can be discerned, termed the mesocortex. Other

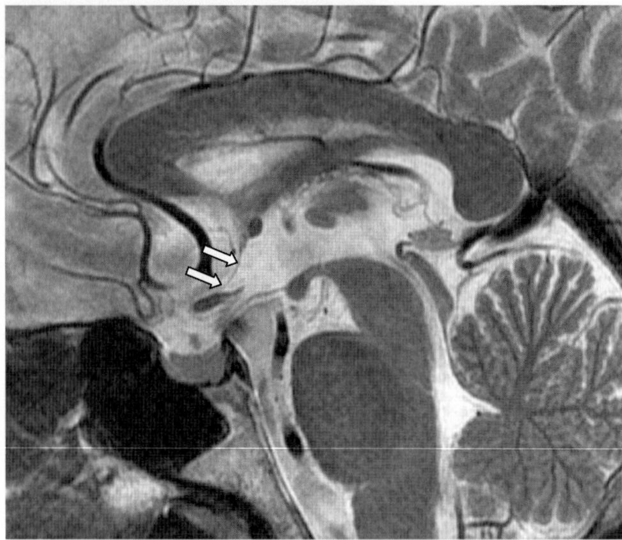

FIGURE 60-1 ■ Midline sagittal T2 MR image through the third ventricle. The thin membrane of the lamina terminalis (white arrows) corresponds to the anterior end of the embryonic neural tube.

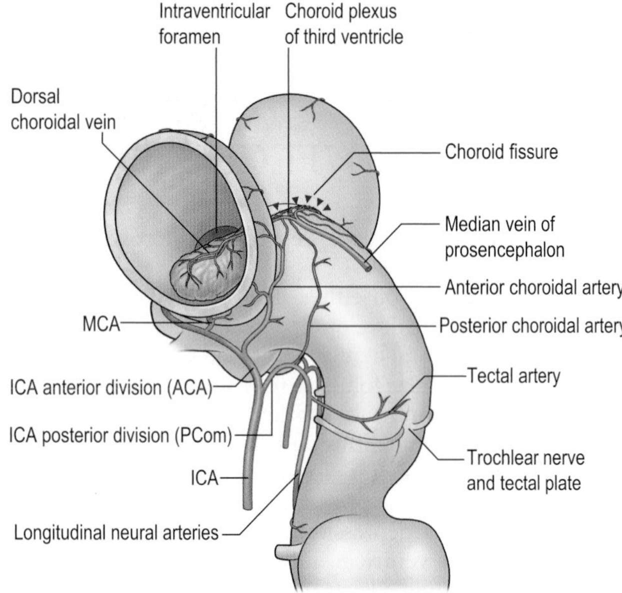

FIGURE 60-2 ■ Schematic of early embryo. The bulging telencephalic vesicles (here cut open to reveal the choroid plexus and interventricular foramen) represent the future cerebral hemispheres. Choroid fissure has appeared in the roof of the future third ventricle, forming the choroid plexus, which is proportionately much larger than in the adult. The choroid plexus is drained by the median prosencephalic vein, a forerunner of the vein of Galen.

terminologies (archicortex, paliocortex, archipallium, etc.) are obsolete and better avoided. The developing cerebral hemispheres are initially separate, with the first crossing fibres developing in the lamina terminalis to form the anterior commissure. Superior to this, formation of the corpus callosum begins, progressing posteriorly. The surface of the hemispheres from an initially smooth (lissencephalic) appearance becomes progressively convoluted. The mesenchymal soft tissues overlying the brain, deriving mainly from the neural crest, differentiate into skull, dura mater and enveloping the brain the vascular meninx primitiva. Cavitation within the meninx primitiva separates the pia mater from arachnoid mater, producing the subarachnoid space, and modification of the primordial vascular plexus produces the surface vessels of the brain.

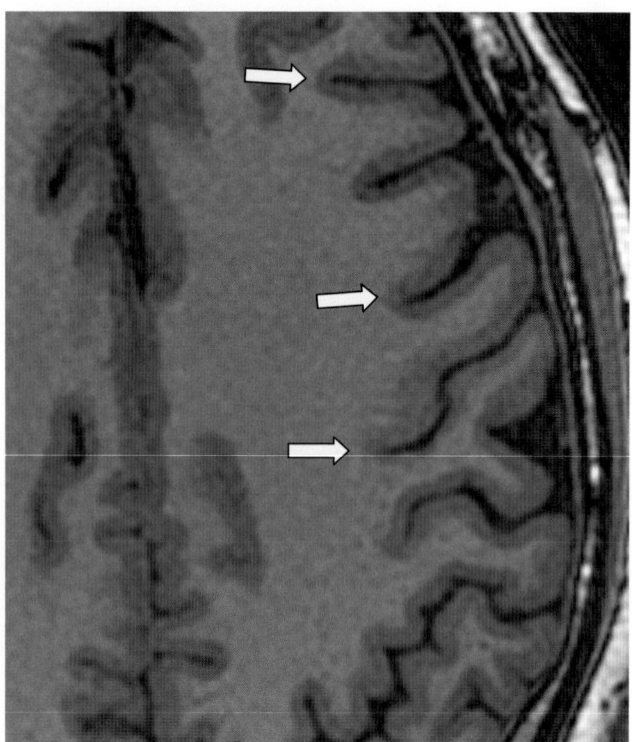

FIGURE 60-3 ■ T2 MR image demonstrates cortical thickness. Note that cortex is thicker over surface and sides of gyri, and thinnest in the depths of the sulci (arrows).

Cerebral Cortex, Lobar Anatomy and Deep Grey Matter Structures

If we consider neuroradiology begins with the first radiograph of a skull taken in 1895,[3] we could imagine the disappointment of those pioneers as they realised that the brain was invisible to the 'new radiation'. Indeed most of the history of neuroradiology has involved the quest for an image of the brain. This was achieved with the first CT images in 1972. The cerebral hemispheres can now be examined in superlative detail by MRI at 1.5 and 3 T, and high-field systems are offering the beginnings of MR microscopy, to probe details of the cerebral cortex.

The cerebral cortex itself consists of arrays of neurons (estimated to number 100 billion, each one communicating synaptically with many adjacent neurons in a system of astonishing complexity) which on Nissl staining appear to be arranged in layers.[4,5] The cortex varies from 2 to 5 mm in thickness. Cortical thickness, though not its internal structure, is readily apparent on standard T1 IR and T2 sequences (Fig. 60-3).

Isocortex, as described above, has six layers, allocortex has three, with mesocortex in between, all layers being numbered from superficial to deep. Probably, equal numbers of glial cells are present in the cortex, interacting metabolically with neurons and synapses as well as with the rich network of cortical capillaries. Precise

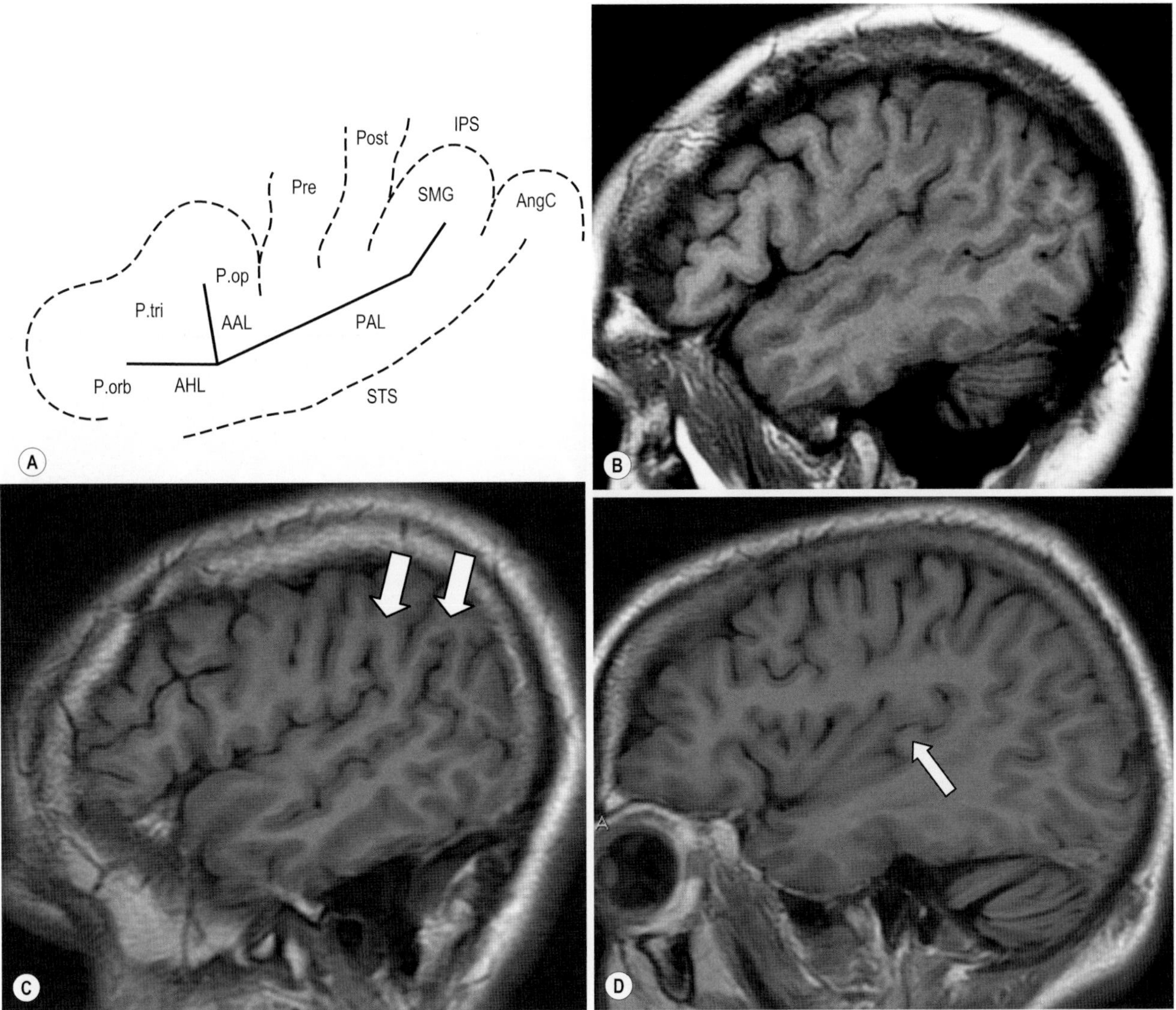

FIGURE 60-4 ■ Sulcal and gyral relationships of the lateral hemisphere. Schematic and sagittal MR images. (A) Schematic showing Sylvian fissure in bold. Adjacent sulci of frontal, parietal and temporal lobes represented by dashed lines. Note that the anterior ascending and horizontal limbs of the Sylvian fissure divide the M-shaped inferior frontal gyrus, below the inferior frontal sulcus, into three parts. Broca's area (motor speech) classically occupies the pars opercularis. Wernicke's area (receptive speech) is usually centred on the supramarginal gyrus. (B) The M-shape of the inferior frontal gyrus is well defined in this image. Low signal change in the supramarginal gyrus is evident in this patient with receptive dysphasia and an infarct of Wernicke's area. (C) The inverted horseshoe-shaped supramarginal and angular gyri are well shown in this image (arrows). (D) More medial parasagittal image demonstrates the triangular-shaped insular cortex. Note the consistent bulge of Heschl's gyrus (primary auditory cortex) arising from the superior surface of the temporal lobe (arrow). Abbreviations: PAL, posterior ascending limb; AAL, anterior ascending limb; AHL, anterior horizontal limb; P.op, pars opercularis; P.tri, pars triangularis; P.orb, pars orbitalis; Pre, precentral gyrus; Post, postcentral gyrus; IPS, intraparietal sulcus; SMG, supramarginal gyrus; AngG, angular gyrus; STS, superior temporal sulcus.

functions of glial cells are not clear-cut, but they are certainly not mere supporting cells.[6] The surface of the cortex is formed by a continuous layer of superficial astrocyte foot processes with associated basement membrane forming the glia limitans to which is applied the pia mater, with a potential subpial space intervening.

The cortical mantle over the surface of each hemisphere is folded into a series of elevated gyri separated by sulcal clefts. These form the basis of the separation into the lobes of the brain, which were originally named for the overlying skull bones. Gratiolet (in 1854) adopted this schema, adding precise boundaries which became widely adopted.[7] The lobar terminology represents a convenient though arbitrary system (which has varied over time and between authors) and is largely devoid of ontogenic significance. Six lobes in each hemisphere are often described: frontal, parietal, occipital, temporal, insula and limbic. With familiarity, patterns emerge from the initially bewildering array of brain convolutions allowing quite accurate identification of the major subdivisions.[8,9] The interhemispheric fissure and Sylvian (or lateral) fissure (Fig. 60-4) are immediately obvious.

The central sulcus is the other main landmark of the hemisphere separating the precentral gyrus (motor) from the postcentral gyrus (sensory) and can usually be confidently identified on axial and sagittal images (Fig. 60-5). From these landmarks other sulci and gyri can be sequentially identified.[8,10,11]

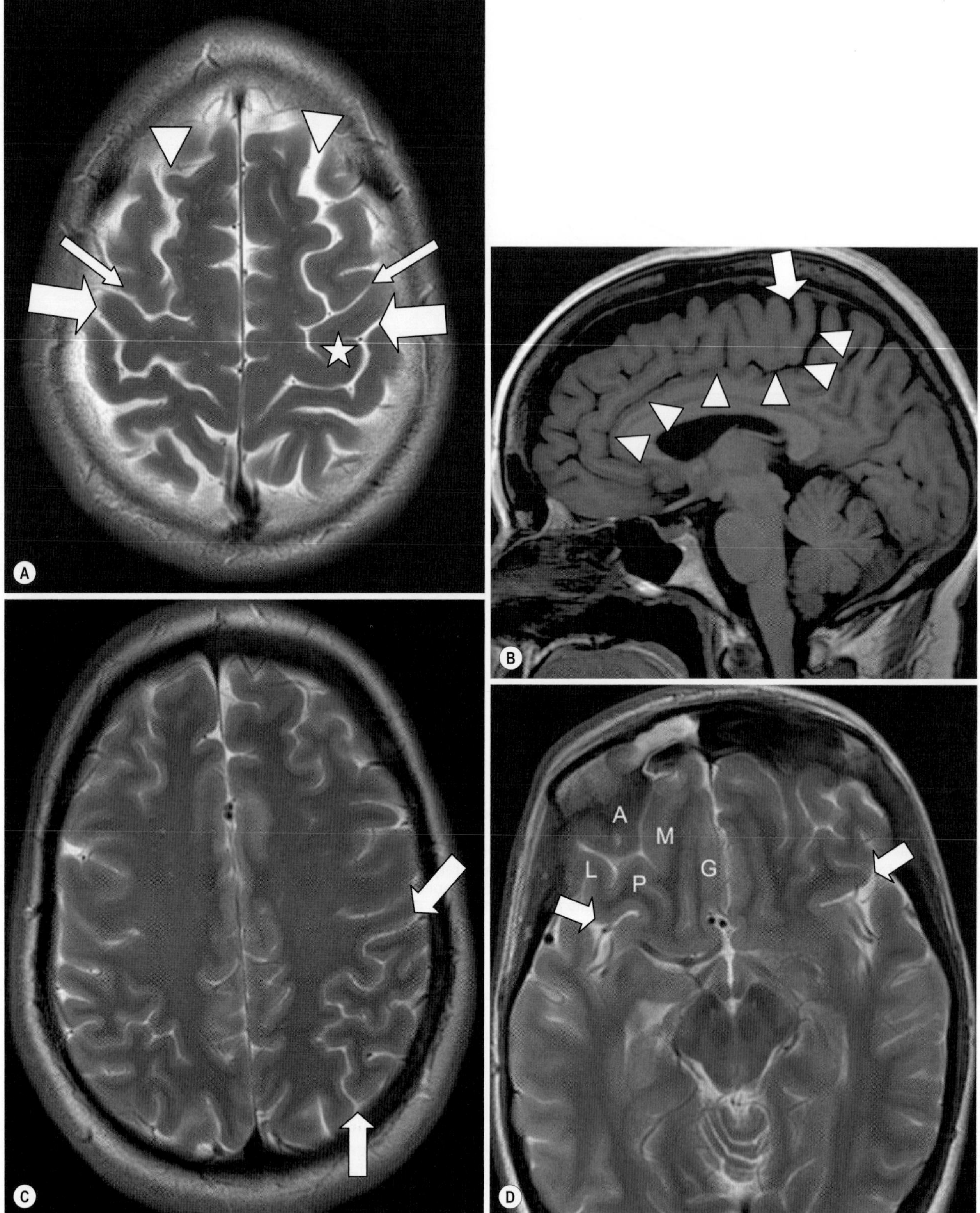

FIGURE 60-5 ■ (A) Axial T2 MR image near vertex. The superior frontal sulcus (arrowheads) is readily identified on most brains between the superior and middle frontal gyri. It typically meets the precentral sulcus (small arrows) almost at a right angle. Posterior to this lies the central sulcus. The bulge in the precentral gyrus (star) represents the hand motor area. (B) Sagittal T1 image. Paralleling the corpus callosum, the cingulate sulcus (arrowheads) as it approaches the splenium turns towards the brain surface. This extension, the pars marginalis of the cingulate sulcus, lies immediately posterior to the central sulcus (large arrow). (C) On axial images, the intraparietal sulcus (arrows) separates the superior parietal lobule (medially) from the inferior parietal lobule (laterally). Anteriorly, it merges with the postcentral sulcus. (D) More caudally, the frontobasal sulci are demonstrated. Note the H-shaped orbital sulci separating the anterior (A), posterior (P), medial (M) and lateral (L) orbital gyri. Gyrus rectus (G) is separated from the medial orbital gyrus by the olfactory sulcus. Arrows indicate the Sylvian fissure.

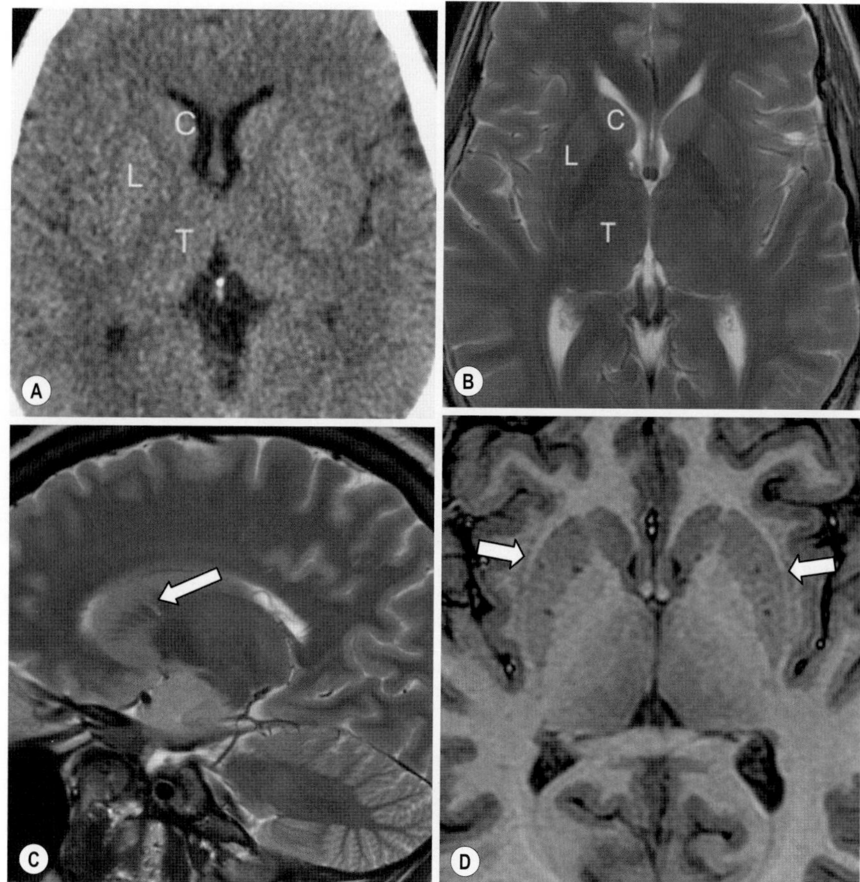

FIGURE 60-6 ■ (A, B) Standard axial CT and T2 MRI images through the basal ganglia and internal capsule. The caudate (C) and lentiform nuclei (L) and the thalami (T) are well demonstrated by CT and MRI together with the intervening V-shape of the internal capsule. (C) Parasagittal T2 image through the basal ganglia. Note the striated appearance of the grey matter bridges crossing the internal capsule, linking the caudate and lentiform nuclei (arrow). (D) T1 axial image shows the thin grey matter layer of the claustrum between the lentiform nucleus and the insula cortex, separating the white matter of the external capsule medially from the extreme capsule laterally.

The deep grey matter structures principally comprise the basal ganglia, amygdala and thalamus and are well demonstrated by CT and MRI (Fig. 60-6). The basal ganglia are part of the extrapyramidal system including the caudate nucleus, globus pallidus, putamen, nucleus accumbens and substantia nigra. The globus pallidus and caudate are linked across the intervening internal capsule by a series of grey matter bridges giving a striated appearance, the origin of the term corpus striatum for this region.

Beneath the internal capsule, these nuclei are linked by the nucleus accumbens. Physiological punctate calcification of the basal ganglia is commonly seen with ageing on CT images after the age of about 30 years.[12,13] Iron deposition is also encountered in the basal ganglia, increasing with age from the second decade (Fig. 60-7).[14] Similarly, calcification in the pineal gland is seen in about 40% of subjects by the age of 20 years (Fig. 60-8).[15]

The thalami are paired large nuclear masses forming most of the lateral walls of the third ventricle, above and behind the hypothalamus. They often are in contact across the ventricle at the massa intermedia. The posterior border, or pulvinar, bulges convexly into the quadrigeminal cistern and overlies the medial (visual) and lateral (olfactory) geniculate bodies.

White Matter Centre

The anatomy of the white matter of the brain has generally received little attention in the imaging literature, which is surprising given the ubiquity of white matter diseases. The medullary core of the brain is formed of bundles of axons, supporting glial cells and penetrating blood vessels. Its whitish colour derives from the fatty myelin sheaths contributed by oligodendrocytes (in the periphery myelin sheaths are formed by Schwann cells). The lipid content accounts for the low density of white matter on CT images and for the characteristic high signal on T1 and low signal on T2 MRI sequences. The white matter is less metabolically active than grey matter and consequently receives a much smaller proportion of the brain's blood supply. On axial anatomic or imaging sections the white matter core presents an oval aspect, Vieussens (eighteenth century) terming the component in each hemisphere, the centrum semiovale (Fig. 60-9).[16] Long after Schwann (1839) established the cell theory, anatomists considered the white matter to be an amorphous continuum, which paradoxically, in imaging terms it has remained until recently. Tractography with MRI diffusion tensor imaging (DTI) can now reveal white matter bundles and their pathways in the living brain. Some of the larger tracts are apparent even on standard sequences. It is conventional in neuroradiology to describe lesions as lying in the subcortical (U-fibres immediately below the cortex), deep (white matter core) or periventricular (thin band of white matter adjacent to the ependyma) white matter.

Axons entering or leaving the cortex can be classified into several types (Fig. 60-9). Thus subcortical U-fibres link one gyrus locally to adjacent gyri with a U-shaped band deep to the sixth layer of the cortex.

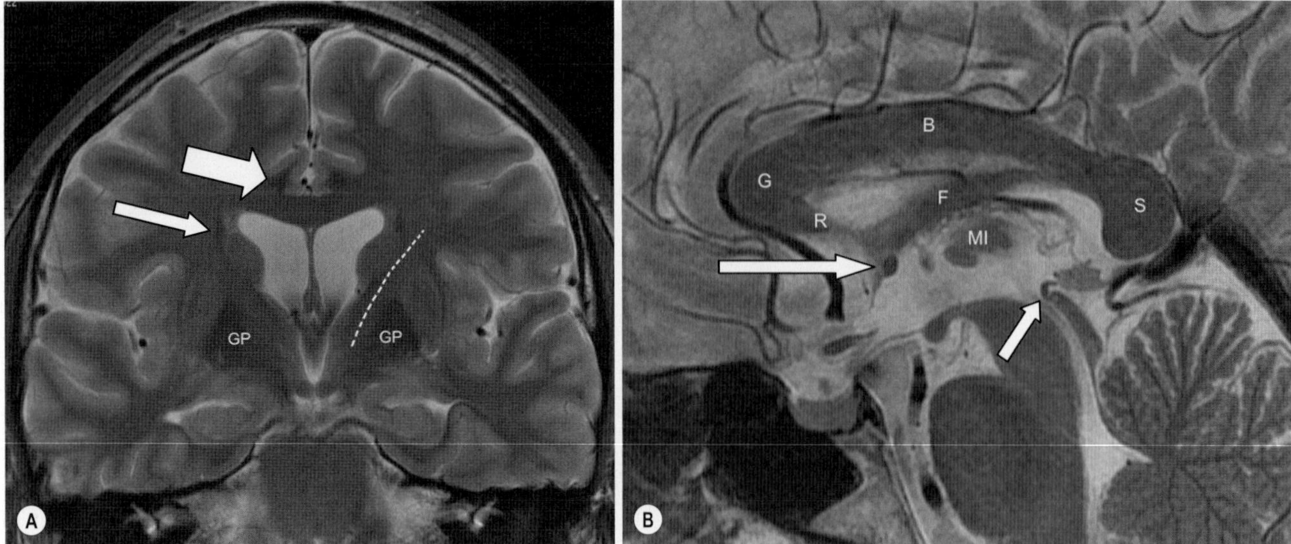

FIGURE 60-7 ■ (A) Coronal T2 MR image. Low signal bundles of the cingulum (arrow) within the cingulate gyrus and the superior longitudinal fasciculus (thin arrow). The internal capsules are well seen (dotted line) between the caudate and lentiform nuclei. Note low signal of iron deposition in the globus pallidus (GP) and the flow voids of CSF passing through the foramen of Monro. (B) Sagittal T2 MR image. The corpus callosum genu (G), rostrum (R), body (B) and splenium (S) are shown. Note the anterior commissure (long arrow) and posterior commissure (short arrow) forming the posterior border of the cerebral aqueduct. Also shown are the fornix (F) and the massa intermedia (MI), or thalamic adhesion, within the third ventricle.

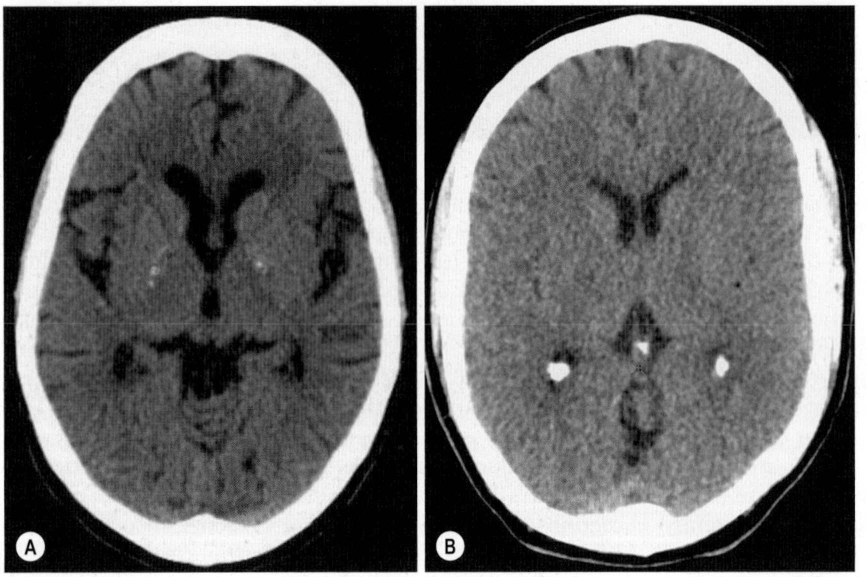

FIGURE 60-8 ■ **Axial CT images.** (A) Normal age-related calcification of the globus pallidus on each side. (B) Midline calcification of the pineal gland. Note the paired internal cerebral veins immediately anterior to the pineal calcification. Typical calcification is also present in the choroid plexuses in the trigones bilaterally.

Ascending/descending tracts carry sensory information to the thalamus and cortex, or project motor fibres via the internal capsule to traverse the brainstem. For example, the corona radiata and internal capsule bearing the descending corticospinal tract, corticocerebellar tracts traverse the cerebellar peduncles and the ascending spinothalamic tracts.

Association tracts link cortical areas in different lobes of the same hemisphere. The most prominent are the superior longitudinal fasciculus (SLF I, II and III) running in the white matter of the parietal lobe linking parieto-occipital and frontal lobes, the arcuate fasciculus, the extreme capsule, the fronto-occipital fasciculus (running with the subcallosal bundle of Muratoff, the combination being visible on standard T2 sequences MRI), the uncinate fasciculus linking anterior and mesial temporal structures with the frontobasal region, and the cingulum bundle, also visible on standard MRI (Fig. 60-7).

Commissural tracts are crossing fibres linking corresponding regions of opposite hemispheres, the largest of these being the corpus callosum, a mammalian innovation only absent in marsupials and monotremes. This dense bundle of fibres containing up to 190 million axons has a rostrum, genu, body and splenium. Anteriorly, its fibres fan out into the forceps minor and posteriorly from the larger splenium into the forceps major. Consisting of densely packed axons with relatively low metabolic requirements, it is less susceptible to ischaemic disease but is a typical site of demyelination, particularly on its ventricular surface. It also provides a common route of

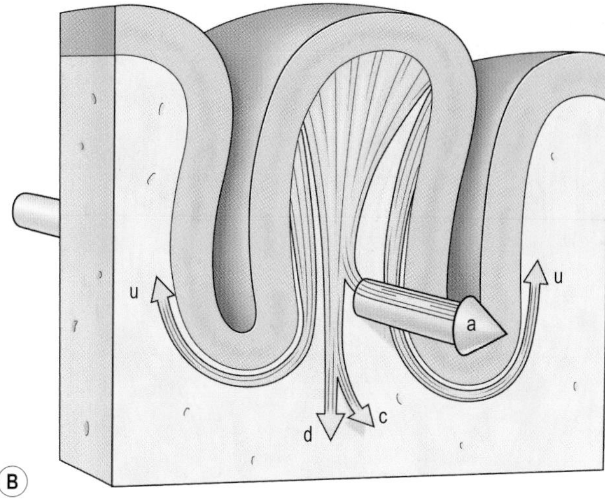

FIGURE 60-9 ■ (A) Axial T2 MRI demonstrates the white matter core of the cerebral hemispheres, the centrum semiovale (CS). (B) Schematic demonstrating the several types of white matter tract: subcortical U-fibres (u), ascending/descending tracts (d), association tracts (a) and commissural tracts (c).

spread for aggressive neoplasms (butterfly glioma). The anterior commissure (AC), a dense bundle of axons, runs in the anterior wall of the third ventricle and is well demonstrated on sagittal and axial sections. The posterior commissure (PC), although more difficult to visualise directly on sagittal images, can be readily pinpointed since it is located at the point where the cerebral aqueduct opens into the third ventricle. The AC–PC line is a basic imaging plane for stereotaxic procedures and is thus easily drawn on sagittal images. There are several other smaller commissures, including the fornix (or hippocampal) commissure and the habenular commissure.

Limbic System, Hypothalamus and Pituitary Gland

Following the isocortical mantel over the hemisphere to its medial edges, the structures of the limbic system are encountered. These include the amygdala, hippocampus, parahippocampal gyrus, cingulate gyrus, subcallosal gyri and associated structures.

Limbic structures are associated with memory processing, emotional responses, fight-or-flight responses, aggression and sexual response: in summary, with activities contributing to preservation of the individual and the continuation of the species. These structures are demonstrated in detail by coronal and sagittal MRI. The limbic system is often rather misleadingly described as a phylogenetically ancient part of the brain: the hippocampus is unequivocally a mammalian innovation while the isocortex itself has equally ancient antecedents.

The core limbic structures are located in the medial temporal lobe readily amenable to high-resolution MRI.

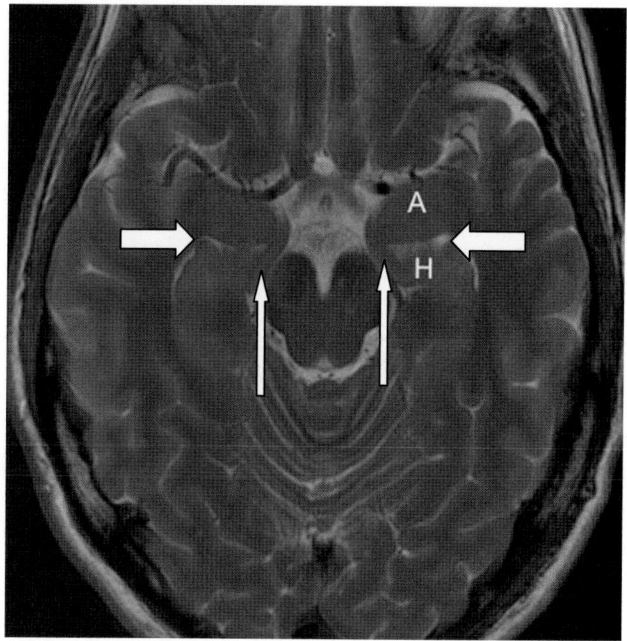

FIGURE 60-10 ■ **Axial T2 MR image of mesial temporal structures.** The uncal recess of the temporal horn of the lateral ventricle turns medially, separating the amygdala (A) from the hippocampal head (H). The uncus lies medially (thin arrows).

The amydala is the most anterior structure, separated from the hippocampal head by the uncal recess of the temporal horn (Fig. 60-10). The medial lying uncus (hook) has anterior amygdaloid and posterior hippocampal components.

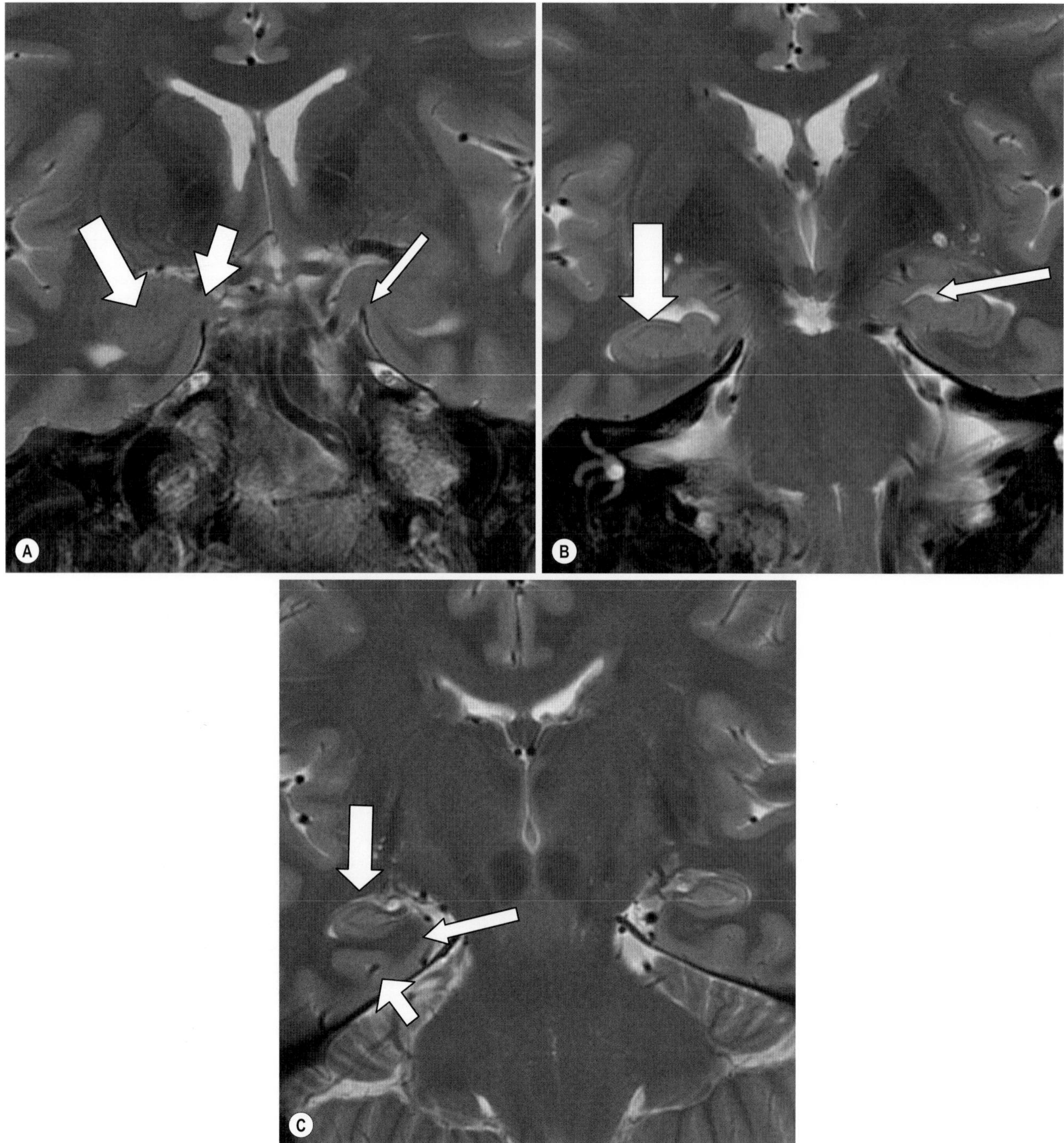

FIGURE 60-11 ■ Coronal T2 MR images from anterior to posterior, demonstrating the main limbic structures of the mesial temporal lobe. Compare with the structures on the schematic picture. (A) Amygdala (large arrow), uncus (short arrow), free margin of tentorium cerebelli (thin arrow). (B) Hippocampal head (large arrow), uncal recess of temporal horn separating posterior aspect of amygdala superiorly from hippocampal head inferiorly. (C) Body of hippocampus (large arrow), parahippocampal gyrus (long arrow), collateral sulcus (short arrow). (D) Schematic illustration of hippocampal structures.

The hippocampal head, body and tail are well shown on coronal imaging, along with the parahippocampal gyrus (Fig. 60-11).

The white matter connections of the hippocampus via the fibria-fornix system are visualised on coronal and sagittal images. A thinned layer of hippocampal tissue, the indusium griseum, extends over the corpus callosum but is not visible on standard imaging.

The hypothalamus forms the floor of the third ventricle and its side walls anteriorly following an oblique line inferiorly from the foramen of Monro to the midbrain aqueduct. It consists of a group of nuclei serving a number of autonomic, appetite-related and regulatory functions for the body as well as controlling and producing hormonal output from the pituitary gland. The hypothalamus is intimately linked to other limbic structures and might be considered the output for the limbic system.

The pituitary infundibulum (or pituitary stalk), a hollow conical structure, extends inferiorly from the hypothalamus to the pituitary gland. The pituitary

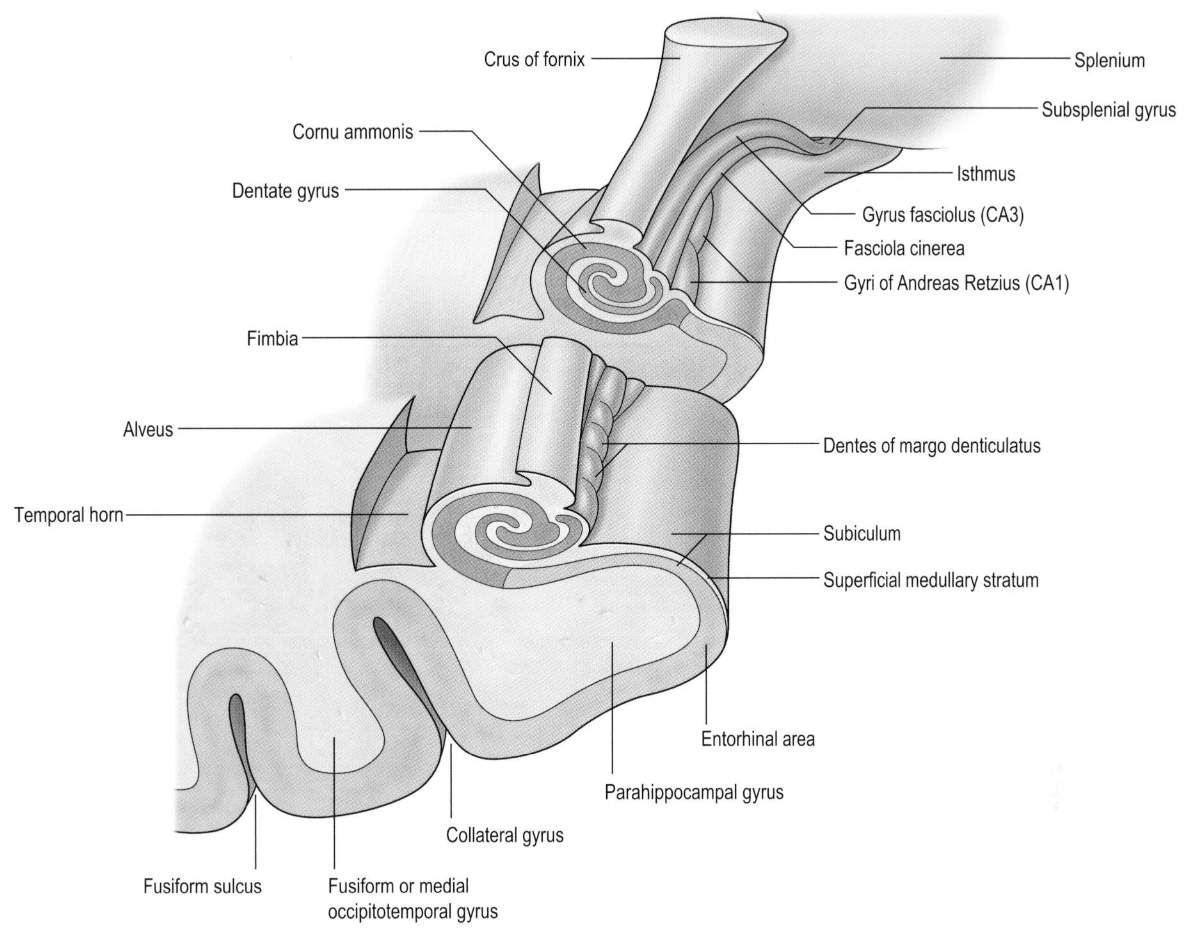

FIGURE 60-11, Continued

gland varies considerably in size, with sometimes only a thin rim of glandular tissue visible at the floor of the pituitary fossa. In young females, the gland may fill the fossa with a convex upper border. Anterior and posterior lobes can be distinguished on MRI, the posterior lobe often returning a high signal on T1-weighted images due to neurosecretory granules in the neurohypophysis. Both gland and stalk show strong contrast enhancement.

Ventricular System and Subarachnoid Space

The ventricular system, filled with cerebrospinal fluid, is the mature derivative of the cavity of the neural tube. Thus, the telencephalon contains the lateral ventricles; the diencephalon, the third ventricle; the midbrain, the cerebral aquaduct and the brainstem, the fourth venrticle (Fig. 60-12). The ventricles are lined by modified glial cells constituting the ependyma.

The lateral ventricles are divided into frontal horn, body, occipital (posterior) and temporal horns. The junction of the body, occipital and temporal horn is known as the trigone indented posteromedially by the calcar avis, the impression of the deep calcarine fissure. The sites of the original outpouchings of the telencephalic vesicles form the interventricular foramina of Monro linking the lateral ventricles with the anterosuperior aspect of the third ventricle. The third ventricle is a midline, slit-like cavity bordered laterally by the bulky grey matter of the thalami that frequently make contact with each other centrally as the massa intermedia. Antero-inferiorly and inferiorly lies the hypothalamus. A number of important structures are identified in the walls of the third ventricle on sagittal midline MRI slices (Figs. 60-7 and 60-13).

From the posteroinferior aspect of the third ventricle, the cerebral aqueduct (of Silvius) traverses the midbrain emerging into the rhomboid-shaped fourth ventricle (Fig. 60-14). The floor of the fourth ventricle is formed by the pons and medulla oblongata and it is roofed by the cerebellum, with its tented apex, the fastigium. There are two lateral apertures, the foramina of Luschka and a single posterior one, the foramen of Magendie allowing efflux of cerebrospinal fluid (CSF) into the subarachnoid space. At the inferior aspect of the fourth ventricle the embryonic continuation of the neural tube cavity into the central canal of the spinal cord is commonly obliterated in the adult.

As described above, the cavity of the ventricular system is invaginated, from the choroid fissure by the choroid plexus, a vascular membrane with pial and ependymal layers. Anterior and posterior choroidal arteries enter this membrane. Choroid plexus is present in both lateral ventricles and extends through the interventricular foramina into the third ventricle forming the roof. In the fourth ventricle the choroid plexus extends laterally into both foramina of Luschka, often projecting into the

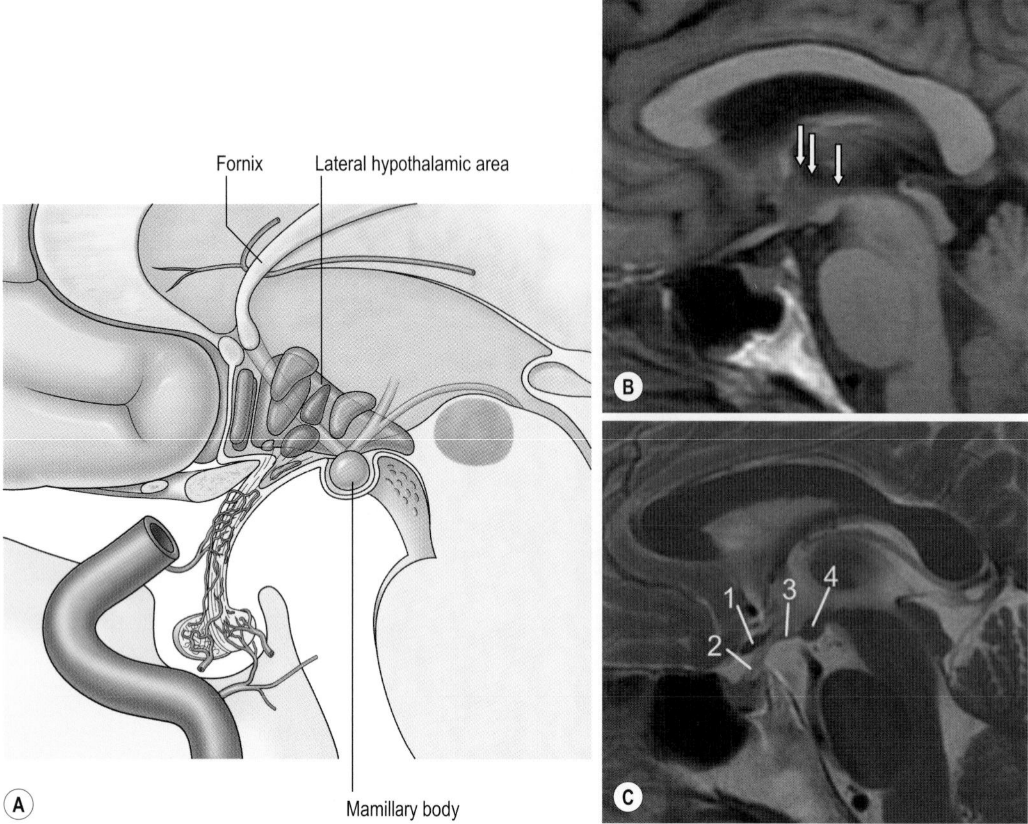

FIGURE 60-12 ■ (A) Schematic diagram depicting the nuclei of the hypothalamus in the lateral wall and floor of the third ventricle. Preoptic nuclei in red. Paraventricular and anterior nuclei in yellow. Medial and infundibular nuclei in blue. Posterior nucleus and mamillary body in orange. Blood supply to the pituitary gland is also shown with the superior and inferior hypophyseal arteries arising from the internal carotid artery. (B) Sagittal T1 image. Hypothalamic border (hypothalamic sulcus) is well seen in this example (arrows). (C) Sagittal T2 image demonstrates the structures in the floor of the third ventricle: Optic chiasm (1), pituitary infundibulum (2), tuber cinereum (3) and mamillary bodies (4).

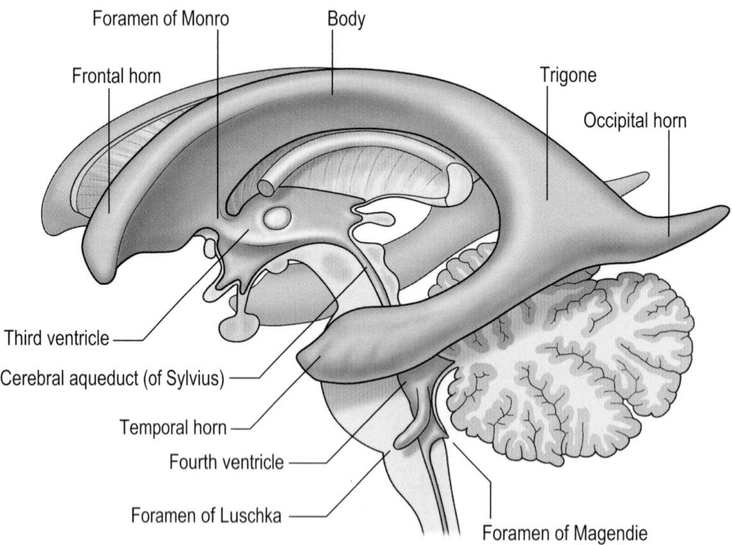

FIGURE 60-13 ■ **Schematic illustration of the components of the ventricular system.** Note the two anterior recesses (chiasmatic and infundibular) and the two posterior recesses (pineal and suprapineal) of the third ventricle.

subarachnoid space. Fourth ventricular choroid plexus is supplied by branches of the posterior inferior cerebellar artery.

CSF flows from the fourth ventricular foramina into the subarachnoid space (Fig. 60-15). Over the superior convexity of the brain, the subarachnoid space is thin. At the base conversely, because of irregularity of the inferior surface of the brain and skull, the spaces become widened in places which are known as subarachnoid cisterns, named for adjacent structures.

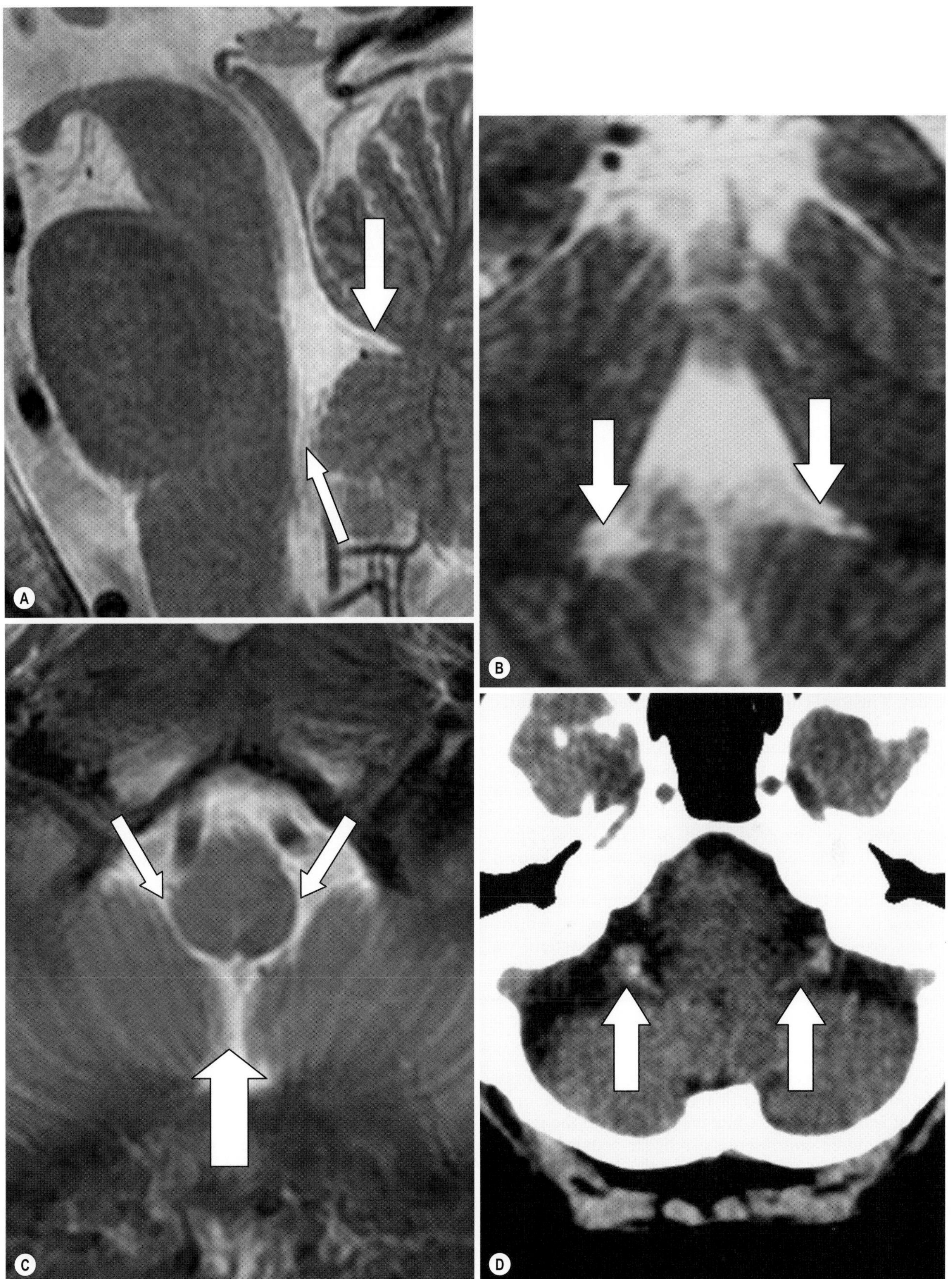

FIGURE 60-14 ■ (A) Sagittal T2 MR image. Flow void of CSF within the aqueduct is present. The tented apex of the fourth ventricle, the fastigium (large arrow) and the foramen of Magendie (small arrow) are well shown. (B) The rhomboid shape of the fourth ventricle is apparent in coronal images. The lateral recesses (arrows) funnel into the foramina of Luschka. (C) Axial MR image through the caudal fourth ventricle demonstrate the foramen of Magendie (large arrow) and foramina of Luschka (small arrows). (D) Axial CT. Tufts of choroid plexus typically project through the foramina of Luschka into the subarachnoid space and may be calcified (arrows).

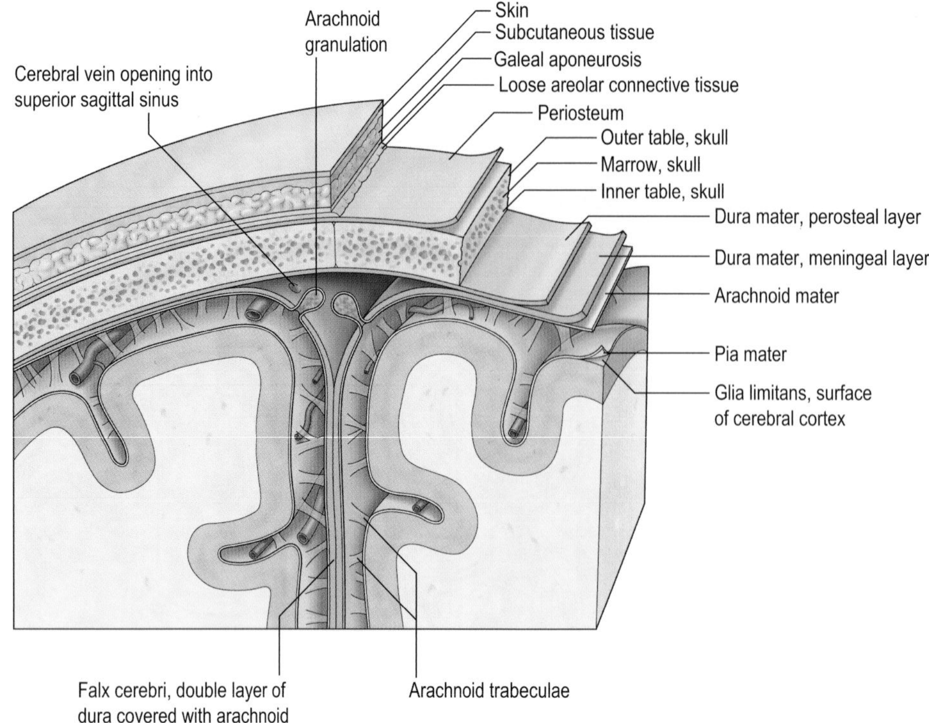

FIGURE 60-15 ■ Schematic showing the relationship of the subarachnoid space to the surrounding meninges.

CSF is produced in part from the choroid plexuses, and in part from transudation of fluid from brain capillaries into the ventricles at a rate of approximately 500 mL per day. The total volume of CSF in the ventricles, intracranial and spinal subarachnoid space is about 150 mL. Thus, total CSF volume is turned over several times a day. Previous concepts that the majority of CSF is reabsorbed into the dural venous sinuses at the arachnoid granulations no longer appear tenable.[17,18] Whether the granulations are involved at all in CSF reabsorption remains debatable and their major functions are unknown in adults as well as infants in whom they are not fully formed. The major routes of CSF reabsorption appear to be along the cranial nerve linings, large vessel adventitia and the cribriform plate into the lymphatic system, via the spinal, especially lumbar, epidural space as well as directly back into the capillaries and venules of the brain.

Cerebellum

The cerebellum occupies the bulk of the posterior fossa, lying posterior to the fourth ventricle and brainstem to which it is linked by the white matter tracts of the paired superior, middle and inferior cerebellar peduncles. It is separated from the occipital lobes by the dural fold of the tentorium cerebelli. The cerebellum displays much finer folding than the cerebral hemispheres, the folds being termed folia. There are two cerebellar hemispheres joined by a midline portion, the cerebellar vermis, which is divided into a number of lobules readily identified on sagittal MRI (Fig. 60-16). Cerebellar cortex overlies the cerebellar white matter. Within the white matter on each side are the cluster of paired deep cerebellar nuclei, the largest of which are the two dentate nuclei. The principal functions of the cerebellum involve the coordination of skilled voluntary movements and muscle tone, each cerebellar hemisphere serving this function for the same side of the body.

Brainstem

The brainstem is usually considered to include the midbrain, pons and medulla oblongata and extends from the posterior commissure at the opening into the third ventricle to the pyramidal decussation at the cervicomedullary junction. This may be divided into the hindbrain or rhombencephalon, comprising the medulla oblongata and pons (as well as the cerebellum which develops from them) and the mesencephalon or midbrain.

The midbrain (Fig. 60-17) consists of the anteriorly lying cerebral peduncles containing the descending and ascending tracts. These are separated by the grey matter nuclei of the substantia nigra from the midbrain tegmentum. The tegmentum extends posteriorly to the cerebral aqueduct (of Silvius). Posterior to the aqueduct lies the tectal (or quadrigeminal) plate with its superior and inferior colliculi. Cranial nerve IV arises here also, the only cranial nerve to arise from the dorsal surface of the brainstem. Grey matter structures within the midbrain include the substantia nigra and red nuclei, readily identified on MRI, as well as the upper cranial nerve nuclei. The medial forebrain bundle bringing limbic fibres from the septal area and hypothalamus ends in the reticular formation, a loose array of neurons, part of the limbic midbrain.

The pons (Fig. 60-17) comprises a bulbous convexity anteriorly, the basis pontis, containing masses of transversely oriented fibres which enter the large middle cerebellar peduncles on each side. Amongst these fibres are the dispersed bundles of the corticospinal tracts which

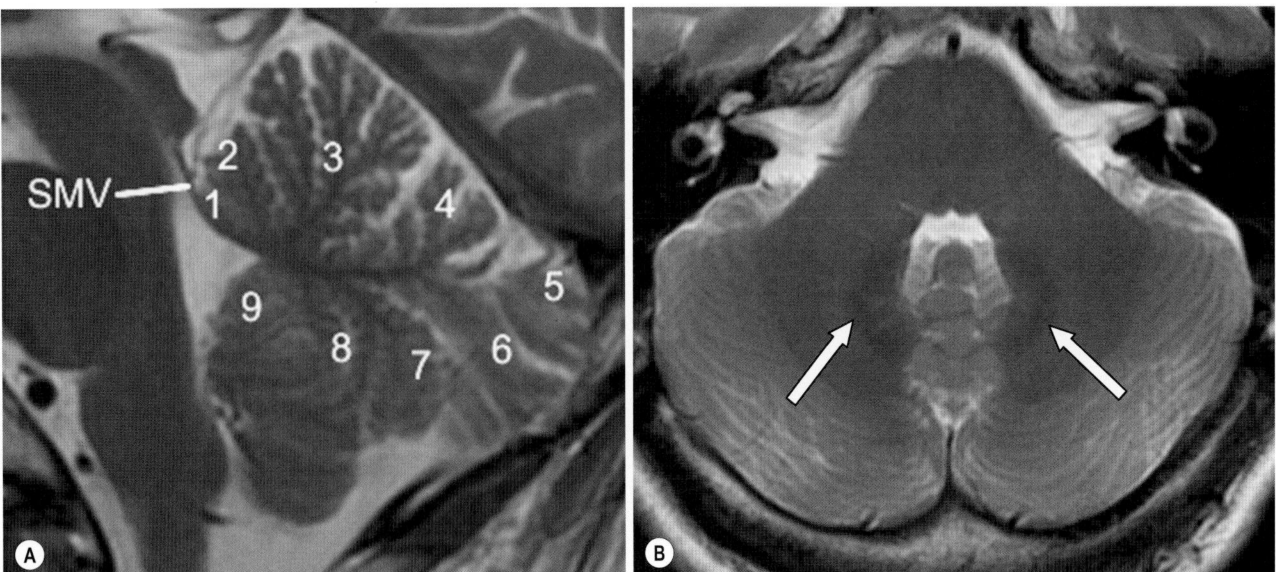

FIGURE 60-16 ■ T2 MR images. (A) Sagittal image of cerebellum. Lobules of vermis are demonstrated: lingula (1), central (2), culmen (3), declive (4), folium (5), tuber (6), pyramid (7), uvule (8) and nodule (9). The roof of the fourth ventricle is formed by the superior medullary velum (SMV). (B) Axial image at level of pons and internal auditory meatus. Iron deposition in the dentate nuclei gives low signal change (arrows).

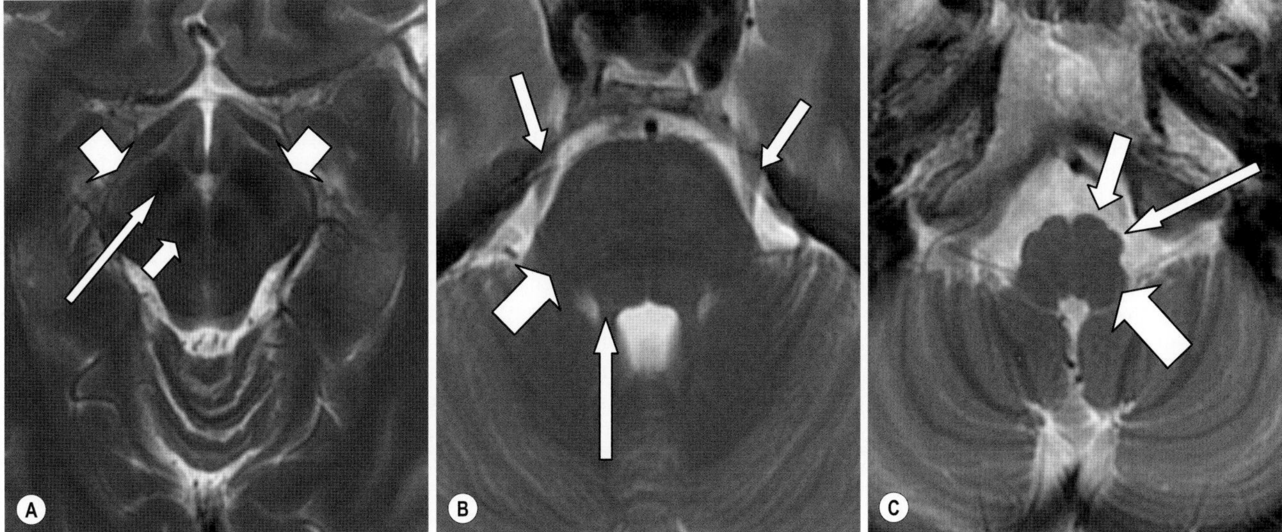

FIGURE 60-17 ■ Axial T2 MR images through brainstem. (A) Midbrain. Note the low signal indicating iron accumulation in the red nuclei (short arrow) and substantia nigra (long arrow). The cerebral peduncles contain the ascending and descending tracts from the cerebral hemispheres (broad arrows). (B) Pons. The trigeminal nerves can be seen running anteriorly into Meckel's cave (short arrows). The superior (long arrow) and middle cerebellar peduncles (broad arrow) are separated by CSF in the inferior extension of the ambient cistern. (C) Medulla oblongata. On each side three bulges are visible in the contour of the medulla: the pyramids (short arrow), olives (long arrow) and the inferior cerebellar peduncle (broad arrow).

separate as they leave the midbrain and reform as they enter the pyramids of the medulla. The posterior part of the pons, the pontine tegmentum, forms the floor of the upper part of the fourth ventricle, and contains cranial nerve nuclei (V, VI, VII, VIII).

The medulla oblongata (Fig. 60-17) consists of an inferior closed portion, with its central canal extending into the spinal cord, and a superior open portion related to the inferior portion of the fourth ventricle. The closed part of the medulla extends from the C1 spinal roots to the obex at the lower margin of the fourth ventricle. The ventral surface of the medulla is marked by two bulges on each side: medially lie the pyramids and laterally, the olives. The medulla transmits ascending sensory tracts posteriorly and descending motor tracts anteriorly both of which cross the midline, or decussate within the closed medulla (sensory decussation lying slightly higher). The lower cranial nerve nuclei lie within the medulla but are not visible with imaging. In cross-section the medulla oblongata is, however, well demonstrated on MRI.

Cerebral Vasculature

The internal carotid arteries (ICA) supply the anterior cerebral circulation while the vertebral forming the

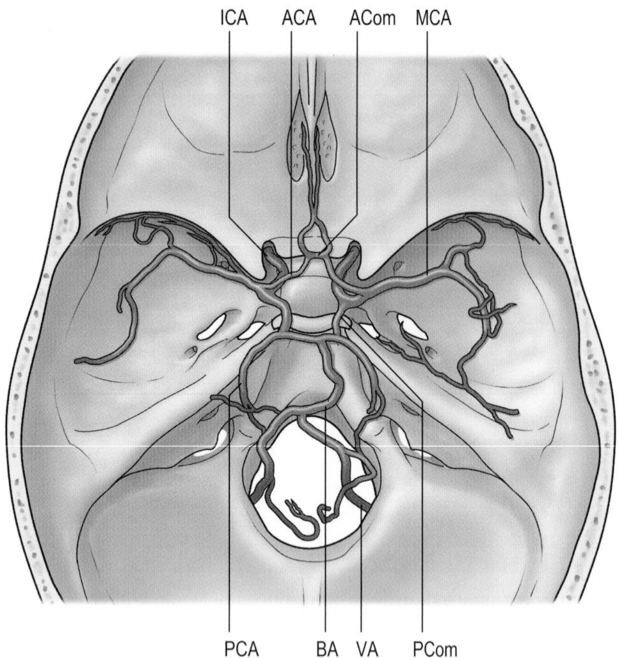

FIGURE 60-18 ■ CTA of a relatively symmetrical and complete circle of Willis. Anterior cerebral artery (ACA), anterior communicating artery (ACom), internal carotid artery (ICA), middle cerebral artery (MCA), posterior communicating artery (PCom), posterior cerebral artery (PCA), basilar artery (BA), vertebral artery (VA).

basilar artery supply the posterior circulation (Fig. 60-18), the two meeting at the circle of Willis. The external carotid arteries (ECA) supply most extracranial head and neck structures (except the orbits) and make an important contribution to the supply of the meninges. There are numerous anastomoses between the external carotid arteries and the anterior and posterior circulation.

The aortic arch gives rise to three main branches, brachiocephalic, left common carotid and left subclavian arteries. The common carotid arteries run within the carotid sheath, lateral to the vertebral column, and bifurcate usually at the fourth cervical vertebrae into external and internal carotid arteries.

Anterior Circulation

The internal carotid artery can be divided into a number of segments C1–C5. The cavernous segment (Fig. 60-19) gives branches to dura, pituitary gland and cranial nerves before its first major branch, the ophthalmic artery.[19] The tentorial and inferior hypophyseal vessels may arise as a meningohypophyseal trunk. The inferolateral trunk supplies adjacent cranial nerves and anastomoses with the ECA. After leaving the cavernous sinus, it pierces the dura and enters the subarachnoid space at the level of the anterior clinoid process (Fig. 60-20). The posterior communicating artery is of very variable size, sometimes occurring as a fetal-type posterior cerebral artery. The anterior choroidal artery supplies the posterior limb of internal capsule, cerebral peduncle and optic tract, medial temporal lobe and choroid plexus. The supraclinoid segment of the ICA divides into the anterior (ACA) and middle cerebral arteries (MCA).

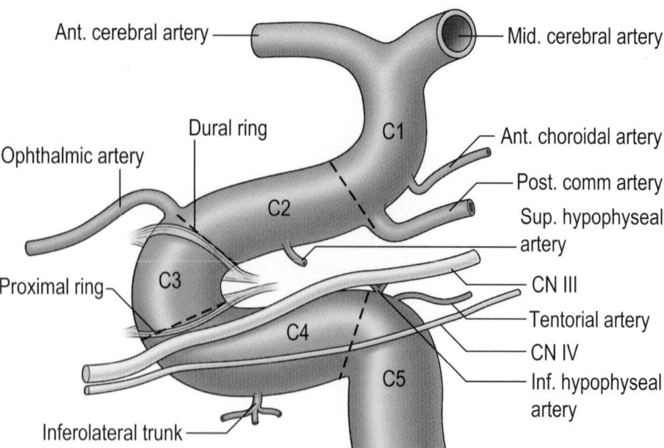

FIGURE 60-19 ■ Schematic illustration of the carotid syphon. The emergence of the ICA from the petrous bone into the cavernous sinus is shown inferiorly (not labelled) and the dural rings where it exits the cavernous sinus are shown proximal to the ophthalmic artery. The close relationship of the cranial nerves to the artery is indicated (CN V and VI are not shown). The segments of the ICA are numbered. Small branches of the ICA are shown and the close relationship of the origins of the posterior communicating and anterior choroidal arteries are apparent.

The anterior cerebral artery[20,21] is divided into three anatomical segments: horizontal or precommunicating segment (A1), vertical or postcommunicating segment (A2) and distal ACA including cortical branches (A3). The A1 segment is joined to the contralateral A1 segment by the anterior communicating artery. The A1 segment gives rise to perforating branches, the medial lenticulostriate arteries. The recurrent artery of Heubner is the largest of the perforating branches doubling back on the parent artery, arising from the A1 or A2 segment. One or other A1 segment may be hypoplastic, or the A2 segments may fuse to give a midline azygous anterior cerebral artery. Cortical branches of the ACA supply the medial aspect of the cerebral hemisphere.

The middle cerebral artery[22] is divided into four anatomical segments: horizontal segment (M1), insular segment (M2), opercular segment (M3) and cortical branches (M4 segments). Medial and lateral lenticulostriate arteries are perforating branches that arise from the M1 segment supplying the basal ganglia and capsular regions. The M1 segment divides as a bifurcation or trifurcation. Cortical branches supply the lateral surface of the cerebral hemispheres.

Posterior Circulation

The vertebral arteries usually arise as the first branches of the subclavian arteries (V1), then entering the foramen transversarium of the sixth cervical vertebra. They run upwards through each vertebra (V2) before arching around the anterior arch and behind the lateral mass of the atlas (V3) to pierce the dura mater and enter the subarachnoid space at the level of the foramen magnum (V4), fusing with their fellow in front of the lower pons, to form the basilar artery (Fig. 60-21). The left vertebral artery is commonly larger. The vertebral arteries give muscular branches, which anastomose with the ascending pharyngeal and occipital arteries, posterior meningeal

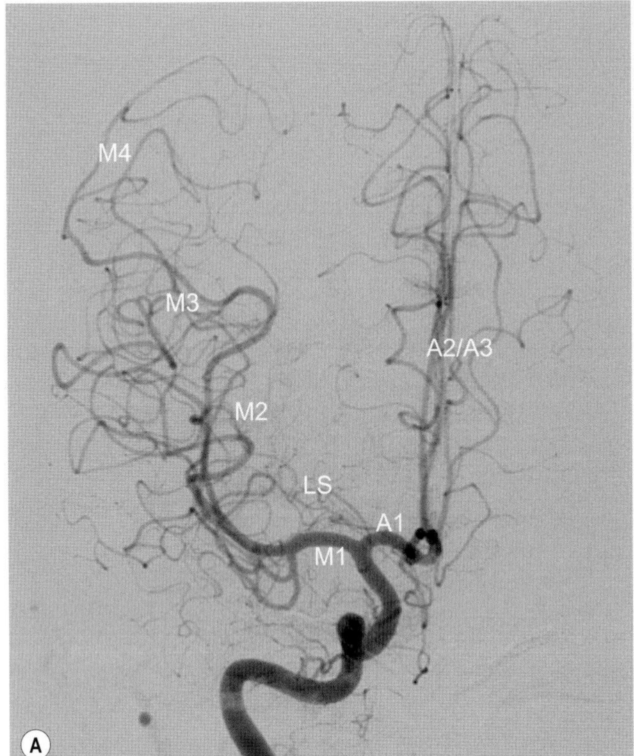

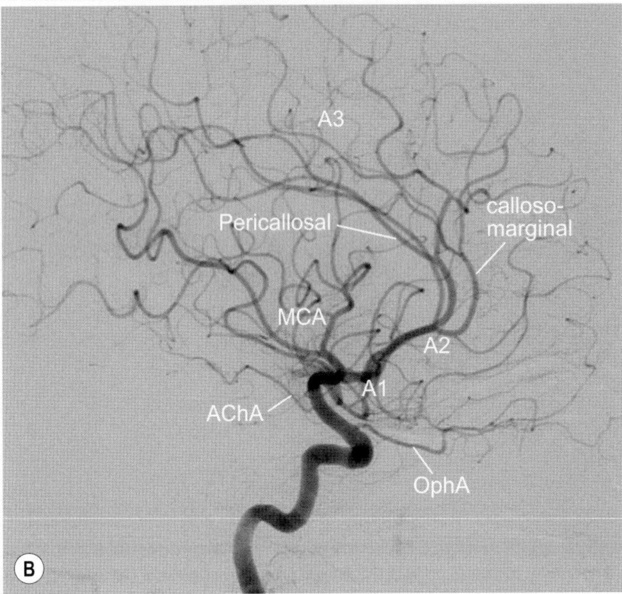

FIGURE 60-20 ■ Digital subtraction angiography (DSA) of the ICA. (A) AP view. (B) Lateral view. Segments of the MCA (M1–4), and ACA (A1–3) are visible. Anterior choroidal artery (AChA), ophthalmic artery (OphA), lenticulostriate arteries (LS).

branches, as well as supplying the cervical spinal cord. After entering the cranial cavity, each vertebral artery gives off a posterior inferior cerebellar artery (PICA) supplying the brainstem, inferior cerebellar hemisphere, vermis and the choroid plexus.

The basilar artery runs superiorly on the anterior surface of the pons giving off anterior inferior cerebellar (AICA), superior cerebellar (SCA) and posterior cerebral arteries on both sides as well as perforating branches. It terminates just above the tip of the dorsum sellae.[23]

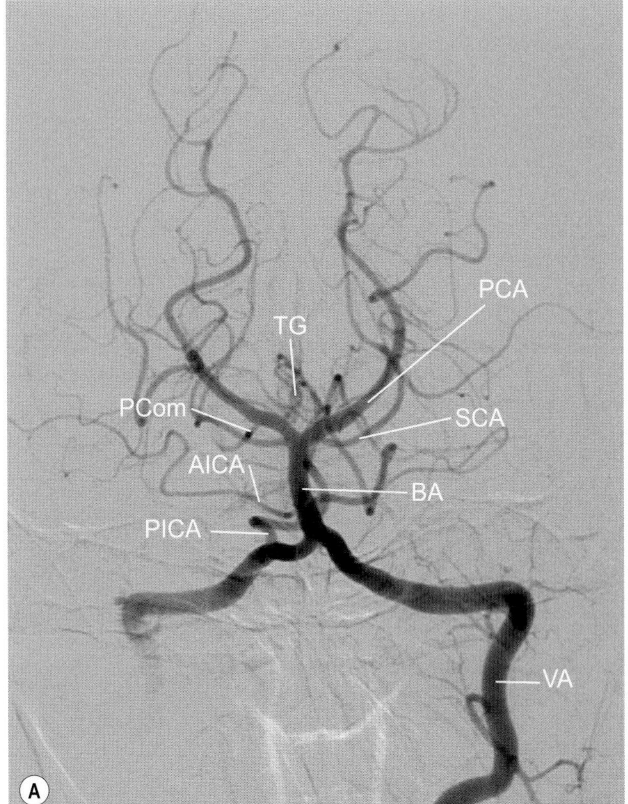

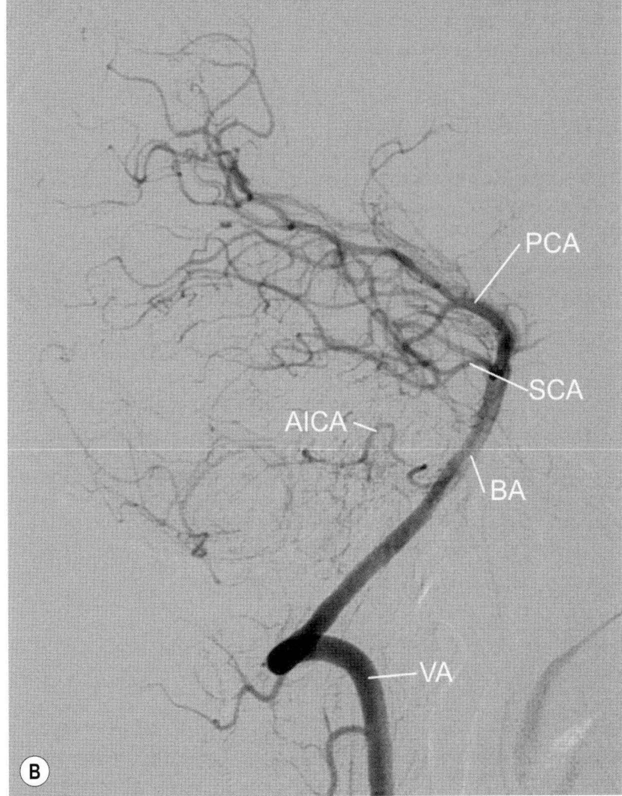

FIGURE 60-21 ■ DSA of the vertebrobasilar circulation. (A) AP and (B) lateral views. vertebral artery (VA), basilar artery (BA), posterior inferior cerebellar artery (PICA), anterior inferior cerebellar artery (AICA), superior cerebellar artery (SCA), posterior cerebral artery (PCA), posterior communicating artery (PCom), thalamogeniculate (TG) perforating arteries.

The AICAs enter the cerebellopontine angle, and supply the surrounding structures; their branches include the internal auditory arteries, to the nerves in the internal auditory meatus. The cerebellar branches anastomose with those of the PICA. The SCAs arise several millimetres below the posterior cerebral arteries from which they are separated by the tentorium cerebelli. They pass around the brainstem to fan out over the superior surface of the cerebellar hemispheres.

The posterior cerebral arteries are the terminal branches of the basilar artery, each of which has four segments. P1 (precommunicating) segment joins the posterior communicating artery to become the P2 (ambient) segment and then P3 (quadrigeminal) segment. The P4 segment is the terminal segment, and includes the occipital and inferior temporal branches. There is reciprocity in calibre of the precommunicating (P1) segments of the posterior cerebral arteries and the posterior communicating arteries: at one extreme is the so-called fetal origin of the posterior cerebral artery. Here, the P1 segments may be hypoplastic and even invisible on vertebral angiography. The posterior communicating arteries and P1 segments give off the thalamoperforating arteries and thalamogeniculate arteries, which enter the posterior perforated substance. Posterior choroidal arteries, medial and lateral arise from the P2 segment. Cortical branches arise from the P2 segment (anterior and posterior temporal arteries) and from the P4 segment, supplying a considerable portion of the inferior surface of the temporal lobe and the medial surface of the occipital lobe, including the visual cortex.

External Carotid Artery

The major branches of the external carotid artery are shown in Fig. 60-22; in general they are named simply for their territory of supply.

Anastomotic Pathways

There are three main categories of collateral supply to the brain: extracranial–intracranial anastomoses, the circle of Willis and leptomeningeal collaterals. The extracranial—intracranial collaterals are actual or potential anastomotic connections between branches of the external carotid artery and the internal carotid or vertebral arteries. These play a role in chronic cerebrovascular occlusive disease and their knowledge is of vital importance for interventional endovascular procedures.[24]

The circle of Willis[25] plays a critical role as a collateral supply in acute and chronic cerebrovascular occlusive disease. The circle of Willis is well demonstrated with axial projections of MR or CT angiograms. A complete circle of Willis is only found in about 40% of people and various segments of the circle may be sufficiently small or absent to be ineffective as a collateral channel. Common variations include absence or hypoplasia of one of the A1 segments and of one or both posterior communicating arteries. The fetal origin of the posterior cerebral artery from the internal carotid artery occurs in 20–30%.

There are other developmental connections between the anterior (carotid) and posterior (vertebrobasilar) circulation that may persist into adult life, the commonest, the trigeminal artery found in less than 1% of normal people (Fig. 60-23). The so-called otic artery is most likely fictitious.[26]

Leptomeningeal (pial) collaterals are end-to-end anastomoses between distal branches of the intracerebral arteries that can provide collateral flow across vascular watershed zones. These are highly variable and are of

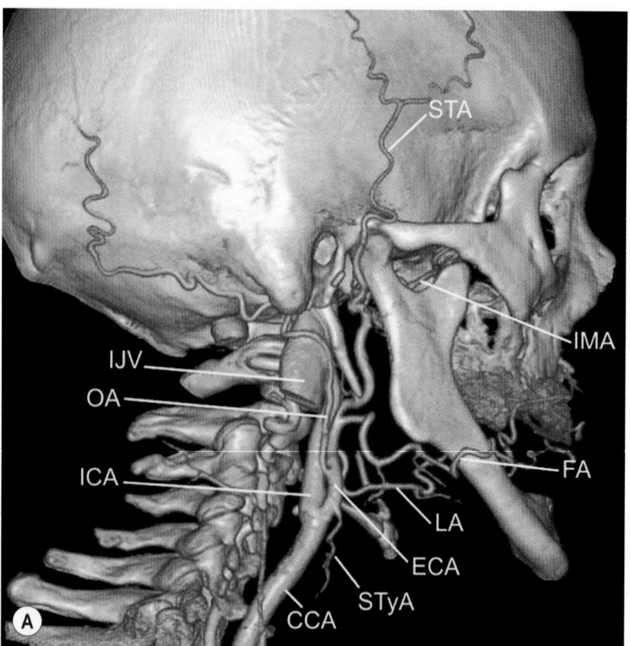

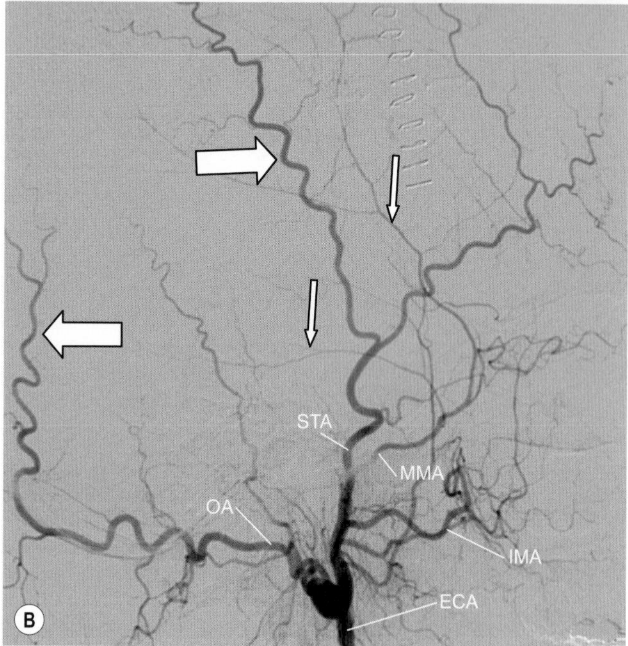

FIGURE 60-22 ■ (A) CTA image of external carotid arteries. Common carotid artery (CCA), internal carotid artery (ICA), external carotid artery (ECA), superficial thyroid artery (STyA), lingual artery (LA), facial artery (FA), occipital artery (OA), internal maxillary artery (IMA), superficial temporal artery (STA). The ascending pharyngeal artery arises at the CCA bifurcation following the course of the ICA but is not visible on this study. Internal jugular vein (IJV). (B) DSA of external carotid artery. The middle meningeal artery (MMA) is the first branch of the IMA. Note that the scalp branches have a 'corkscrewing' course (large arrows) readily distinguished from the meningeal branches, which have a much straighter course (small arrows).

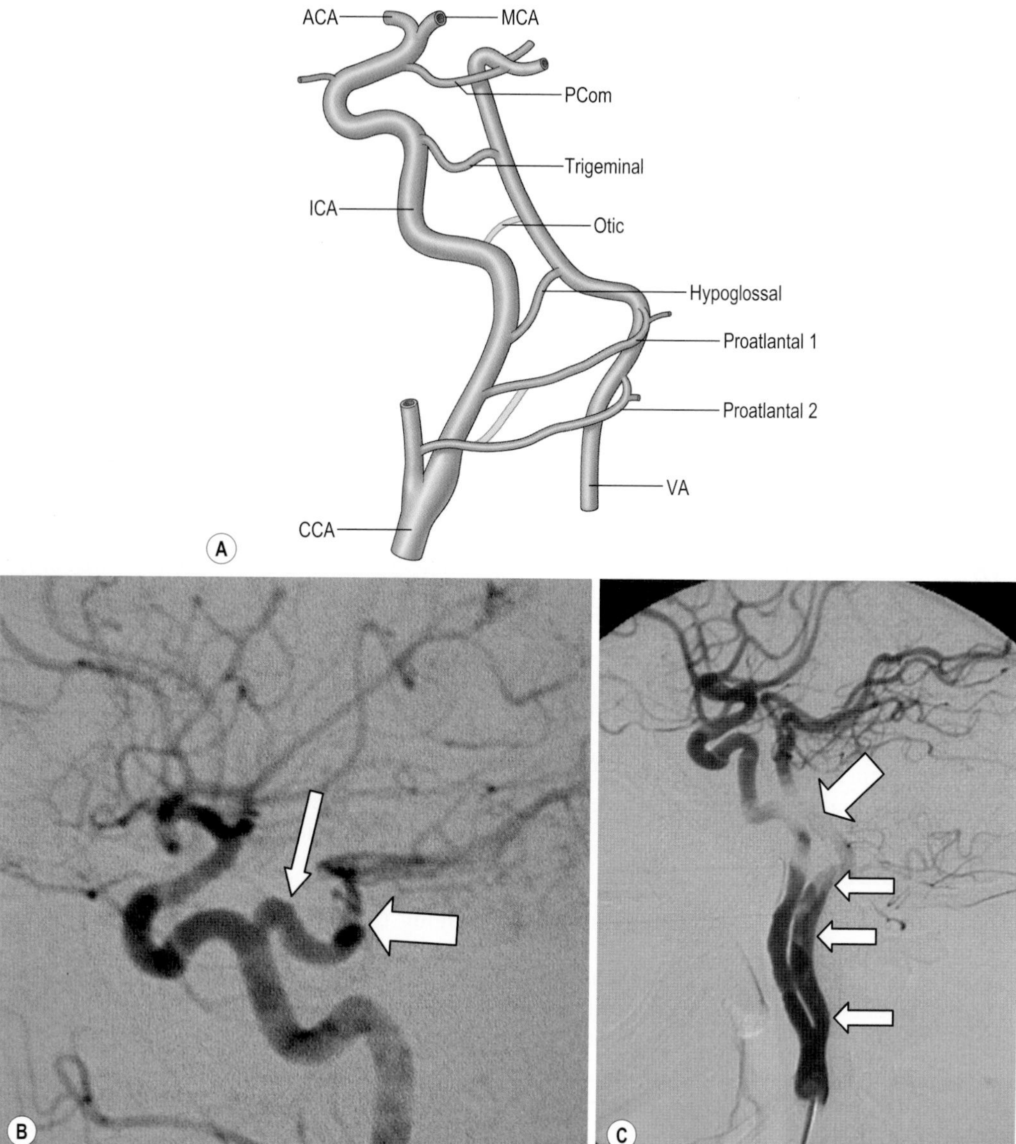

FIGURE 60-23 ■ (A) Schematic diagram showing the series of embryonic anastomoses between the anterior and posterior circulation which form and regress until the final one, the posterior communicating artery, is established. (B) DSA: the persistent trigeminal artery (small arrow) is most frequently encountered. (C) DSA: the persistent hypoglossal artery (small arrows) is extremely rare, arising from the ICA and traversing the hypoglossal canal to reach the basilar artery. Broad arrows in (A) and (B) indicate the basilar artery.

great importance in acute occlusion of intracerebral vessels.

Intracranial Veins

The dural sinuses run within the major dural septa: the superior sagittal sinus between the layers of the upper part of the falx cerebri and the inferior sagittal sinus in the lower border of the falx, running backwards to join the great vein of Galen.[27] The straight sinus is formed by the confluence of the vein of Galen and inferior sagittal sinus and runs downwards towards the torcular herophili. The transverse (or lateral) sinuses are often asymmetric in size; the right is usually the dominant one. They become the sigmoid sinuses as they turn downward to discharge into the internal jugular veins, which run in the lateral portion (the pars vascularis) of the jugular foramina.

The superior petrosal sinuses extend from the cavernous sinus to the sigmoid sinuses. The inferior petrosal sinuses connect the cavernous sinus to the jugular.

Cerebral veins consist of two groups: the deep, subependymal veins and the superficial cortical veins. The former are rather constant, while the latter are extremely variable. In the angiographic series, the cortical veins fill before the deep ones. The deep and superficial groups are in fact joined by fine medullary veins.

The septal veins course directly posteriorly on the septum pellucidum, to join the thalamostriate veins. They meet at the foramina of Monro, forming the venous angle, from which the internal cerebral veins run posteriorly on the roof of the third ventricle, near the midline. The confluence of internal cerebral and basal veins of Rosenthal gives rise to the midline great vein of Galen, which enters the straight sinus.

Most superficial cortical veins drain upwards and medially to the superior sagittal sinus. Veins in the inferior frontoparietal and temporal regions drain to the superficial middle cerebral vein, thence to the sphenoparietal sinus and cavernous sinus. Inferior parietal, posterior temporal and occipital veins drain directly to the transverse sinuses. Two large cortical veins running posterosuperiorly across the parietal lobe to the superior sagittal sinus and posteroinferiorly over the temporal lobe to the transverse sinus are the superior and inferior anastomotic veins (of Trolard and Labbé, respectively); it is uncommon for both to be well developed.

The anatomy of the posterior fossa veins is very variable. There are three principal drainage pathways: the vein of Galen, the superior petrosal sinus and direct tributaries into the transverse and straight sinuses.

TECHNIQUES FOR IMAGING THE BRAIN AND CEREBRAL VASCULATURE

Computed Tomography

In the acute neurological setting, speed and ready availability of computed tomography (CT) have led to it being the common first-line imaging choice. Recent advances in CT have positively impacted neuroimaging, offering lower dose and faster and higher resolution imaging.

Indications, Risks and Benefits

The radiologist should have a good understanding of the specific indications, risks and benefits of CT, as well as those of alternative imaging techniques.[28] There is a wide range of indications for CT of the brain, used either as a primary technique of investigation or as a secondary technique when MRI is unavailable, contraindicated or unsuccessful (Table 60-1).[29]

In the acute setting, CT offers rapid detection of surgically treatable conditions, such as haemorrhage, hydrocephalus, extra-axial collection or mass lesions, allowing quick treatment decisions. Acute head trauma is one of most frequent primary indications, with CT replacing skull radiography, allowing rapid detection of potentially life-threatening primary and secondary findings of intracranial trauma.[30,31] The speed and ease of CT is integral to its utility in acute stroke, allowing exclusion of intracranial haemorrhage, detection of early ischaemic changes and rapid progression to thrombolysis. The addition of CT angiography and perfusion allows assessment of vascular patency and changes in cerebral perfusion.[32] Computed tomography offers a first-line assessment of intracranial haemorrhage: when combined with CT angiography, most causative intracranial aneurysms and many vascular malformations can be identified.[33]

Beyond the brain, CT offers exquisite assessment of bone and is widely used to detect and characterise bony lesions or fractures of the calvarium, skull base or spine. Brain and cervical spine imaging can be easily combined, allowing detection of the third of patients with moderate to severe head injuries who also have cervical spine trauma.

As CT uses ionising radiation, it requires medical justification of the investigation and radiation dose, using low-dose techniques where possible to adhere to the ALARA (as low as reasonably achievable) principle. Imaging alternatives, commonly magnetic resonance imaging (MRI), should always be considered, especially where radiation dose is of higher concern, such as children.[34] Further, MRI may provide more detailed information on the underlying pathological process and therefore may be a more appropriate investigation.

TABLE 60-1 **Indications for CT of the Brain**

Primary Indications	Secondary Indications (when MRI Is unavailable or contraindicated, or if radiologist deems CT to be appropriate)
Acute head trauma	Diplopia
Suspected acute intracranial haemorrhage	Cranial nerve dysfunction
Vascular occlusive disease or vasculitis (including use of CT angiography and/or venography)	Seizures
Aneurysm evaluation	Apnoea
Detection or evaluation of calcification	Syncope
Immediate postoperative evaluation following surgical treatment of tumour, intracranial haemorrhage, or haemorrhagic lesions	Ataxia
Treated or untreated vascular lesions	Suspicion of neurodegenerative disease
Suspected shunt malfunctions, or shunt revisions	Developmental delay
Mental status change	Neuroendocrine dysfunction
Increased intracranial pressure	Encephalitis
Headache	Drug toxicity
Acute neurological deficits	Cortical dysplasia, and migration anomalies or other morphological brain abnormalities
Suspected intracranial infection	
Suspected hydrocephalus	
Congenital lesions (such as, but not limited to, craniosynostosis, macrocephaly and microcephaly)	
Evaluating psychiatric disorders	
Brain herniation	
Suspected mass or tumour	

However, MRI examination times are much longer and availability may still necessitate CT in the first instance.

Technique and Protocols

There continue to be rapid advances in CT technology, which have major implications for neuroimaging techniques and protocols. Knowledge of current technology and upcoming changes are vital for the practising radiologist.

Spiral CT has revolutionised CT and offers major advances for neuroimaging. Rapid, continuous imaging of the area of interest, by use of slip-ring technology, enables acquisition of a volume data set. Improvements in hardware, most notably, multidetector configuration, and software, have both improved speed, and spatial resolution in the *z*-axis, enabling the acquisition of isotropic data. The ability to cover whole organs in one tube rotation offers major advantages for assessment of both cerebral vasculature and perfusion.[35]

Data can be resampled according to need, and edited (e.g. skull removal), allowing the radiologist to highlight relevant data and optimise interpretation. Multiplanar reformatting (MPR) of data is useful in many situations in both brain and spine. Sagittal images provide good visualisation of the midline structures such as the craniocervical junction and pituitary fossa (Fig. 60-24), while coronal images improve assessment of structures in the axial plane, e.g. the superior aspects of the brain, floor of the middle cranial fossa. Slice thickness can be manipulated according to need and streak artefacts can be reduced from the skull, allowing better visualisation of the posterior fossa and sellar regions.

While volume rendering (VR) and multiple intensity projection (MIP) have particular utility for neurovascular imaging, VR can also be helpful for depicting complex fractures of calvarium, skull base or spine, allowing assessment of integrity and alignment. Single slice techniques, however, still offer an equivalent assessment of the brain in the axial plane and have the advantage that the gantry can be angled to avoid irradiation of the globes.[36]

Intravenous contrast is most commonly administered to further evaluate a known pathology with blood–brain barrier breakdown, such as tumour or abscess, or a suspected pathology within an area of observed abnormality: for example, vasogenic oedema. The addition of intrathecal contrast provides exquisite myelographic images, allowing detailed assessment of intracranial subarachnoid spaces: for example, in CSF leak (Fig. 60-25). For the spine, CT myelography offers an alternative to MRI in assessment of spinal cord or nerve root compression.

Viewing the Images

Ionising radiation produced by CT is absorbed to varying degrees by the body, reflecting the linear attenuation coefficient and electron density. Thus, a grey scale of variable densities (Hounsfield units) is produced, ranging from −1000 for air to +1000 for bone/calcification, with water as 0.

Contrast between structures is maximised by limiting the grey-scale spectrum to a central window level and width that focuses on the likely densities within. This narrows the viewing spectrum to benefit the grey-scale capabilities of the human eye, which are considerably less than a CT imaging device. For the brain, a window level set in the range of 35–50 and width of 70–150 provides a good baseline setting. Assessment using specific bone window settings, with a higher window level and width, e.g. 80–500/600–2000, is key not only for trauma patients but also for all patients and should be performed to detect bone lesions. A bony reconstruction algorithm and filter can enhance fine bony detail (Fig. 60-26). Variable window width and centre level settings are also helpful to accentuate contrast differences between oedematous and normal brain, for example in detection of acute stroke,[37] while letting structures outside the set window level be distinguished such as haemorrhage and calcification.

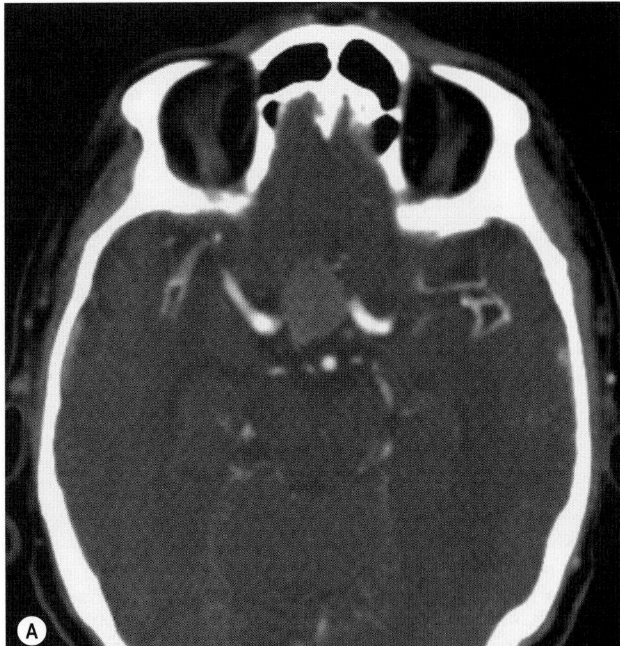

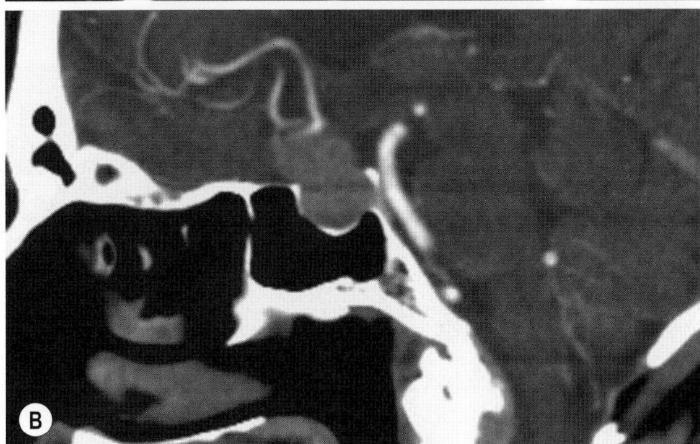

FIGURE 60-24 ■ (A) A 60-year-old man, with reducing vision. Spiral CT (dual bolus contrast) reveals an enhancing suprasellar mass. (B) Sagittal reformat provides a good assessment of midline structures and confirms this as a mixed sellar/suprasellar mass lesion. It was confirmed pathologically as a pituitary macroadenoma.

Slice thickness should be optimised according to personal preference and need. Thicker slices offer less noise,

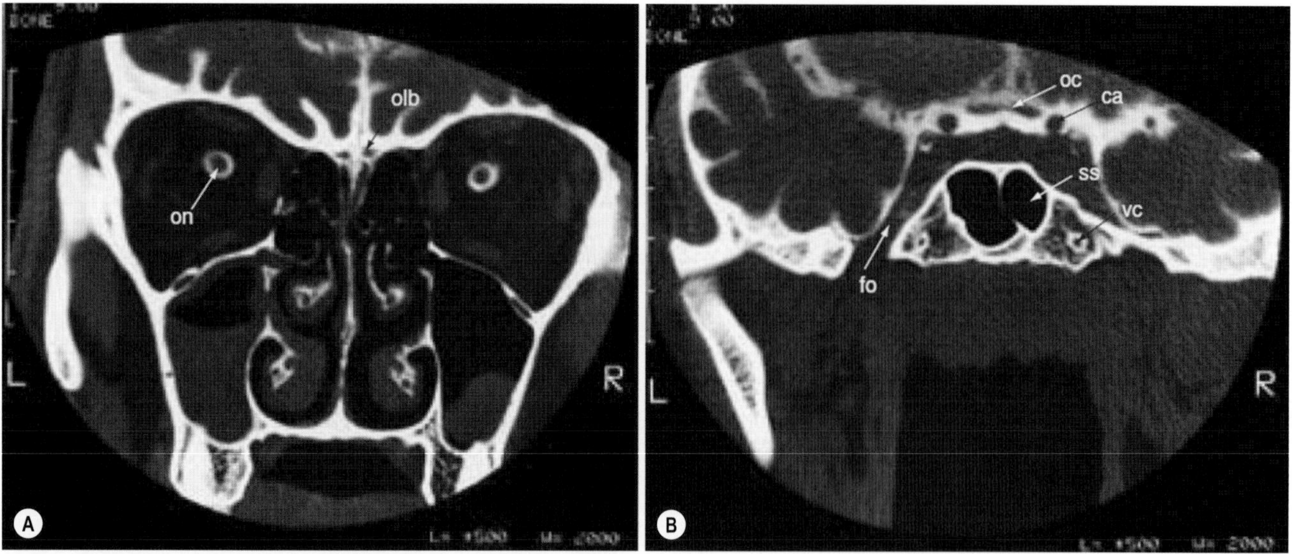

FIGURE 60-25 ■ Thin-section (1.5 mm) CT slices at the (A) level of the olfactory grooves and (B) foramen ovale. The intrathecal contrast outlines the subarachnoid space and extends into the optic nerve sheaths, outlining the optic nerves. ca = carotid artery, fo = foramen ovale, oc = optic chiasm, olb = olfactory bulb, on = optic nerve, ss = sphenoid sinus, vc = vidian canal.

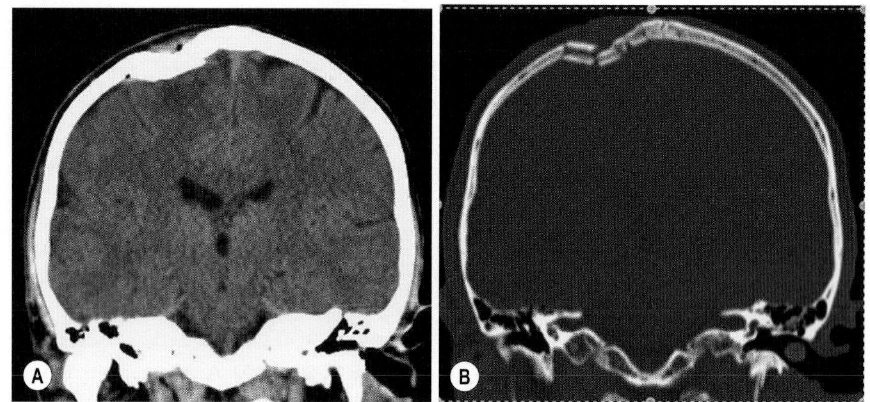

FIGURE 60-26 ■ (A) A 20-year-old man following blunt trauma. Coronal reformat of spiral CT, viewed on soft-tissue windows (window centre 35, width 70), shows a depressed right posterior skull fracture, with underlying parenchymal oedema. (B) Assessment of the comminuted fragments and displacement is optimised by use of a high-resolution bone algorithm and filter (window centre 800, width 2000).

while thinner slices reduce partial volume and artefacts, e.g. posterior fossa. Further viewing possibilities are also available where iterative data reconstructive techniques are used. This reconstructive technique reduces noise, and ultimately dose, producing a smoother appearance.[38] It can be blended with back-projection techniques, to produce best subjective viewing conditions (Fig. 60-27).

Magnetic Resonance Imaging

MRI is a key diagnostic technique for imaging of the neuraxis, allowing detailed assessment of the anatomy and pathological findings of the brain and spine.

Indications, Risks and Benefits

The choice of cross-sectional neuroimaging technique is dependent on a number of factors, including the clinical status of the patient, the speed of examination required and the suspected pathology. Some of the indications for MR of the brain are listed in Table 60-2.[39]

The full extent of involvement and the underlying pathological process are commonly easier to define using MRI. The superior soft-tissue contrast of MRI ensures that many pathological findings are detected earlier than CT. In many cases, this is due to the high inherent sensitivity of MRI to water, which is increased at an early stage in many parenchymal lesions. MRI also offers a high contrast for other compositions, such as fat and subacute haemorrhage, which show T1 shortening (Fig. 60-28). The technique can be used for follow-up of parenchymal haematoma, to confirm expected evolution and help exclude underlying tumour or vascular malformation.[40]

When clinical symptomatology points to the posterior fossa, MRI should be performed whenever possible. Both

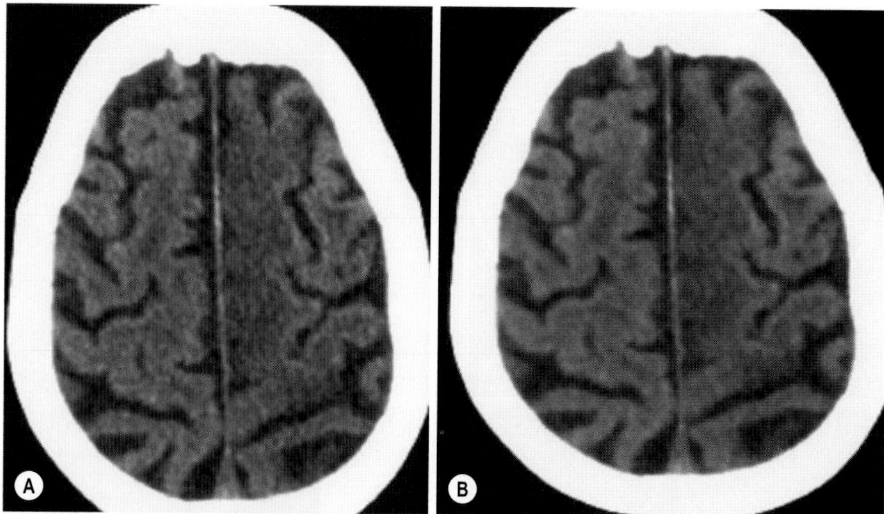

FIGURE 60-27 ■ A 67-year-old woman with anterior cerebral artery infarct. (A) Reduced-dose CT brain, reformatted using filtered back projection, shows a slightly noisy appearance. Low attenuation with sulcal effacement of the left paramedian frontal lobe present, in keeping with anterior cerebral infarction. (B) Same examination reconstructed by iterative reconstruction reduces image noise and has a much smoother appearance.

TABLE 60-2 **Indications for MRI of the Brain**

Primary Indications	Extended Indications
Seizures Cranial nerve dysfunction Diplopia Ataxia Acute and chronic neurological deficits Suspicion of neurodegenerative disease Primary and secondary neoplasm Aneurysm Cortical dysplasia and other morphological brain abnormalities Vasculitis Encephalitis Brain maturation Headache Mental status change Hydrocephalus Ischaemic disease and infarction Suspected pituitary dysfunction Inflammation or infection of the brain or meninges, or their complications Postoperative evaluation Demyelination and dysmyelination disorders Vascular malformations Arterial or venous/dural sinus abnormalities Suspicion of non-accidental trauma	Suspicion of acute intracranial haemorrhage or evaluation of chronic haemorrhage Neuroendocrine dysfunction Functional imaging Brain mapping Blood flow and brain perfusion study Image guidance for intervention or treatment planning Spectroscopy (including evaluation of brain tumour, infectious processes, brain development and/or degeneration, and ischaemic conditions) Volumetry Morphometry Tractography Post-traumatic conditions

brainstem and cerebellum are best depicted on MR, without the streak artefacts from the skull base that are common on CT. Further, MRI should be used as the primary investigation for assessment of spinal disease, including symptoms of spinal cord dysfunction or neural compression. It provides best assessment of the soft tissues of the spine, including the intervertebral discs, as well as valuable information on bone integrity, alignment and marrow composition. For patients in whom MR is not suitable, CT offers an alternative.

A safe MR examination necessitates that patients are interviewed and screened prior to the examination to exclude individuals who may be at risk or have contraindication to exposure to the MRI environment: for example, ferrometallic clips. Patients suffering from anxiety or claustrophobia may require sedation or anaesthesia. The examination is significantly longer than CT and is dependent on sequences used, which can be problematic for some patients. Under certain clinical conditions, very rapid acquisitions such as echo-planar imaging

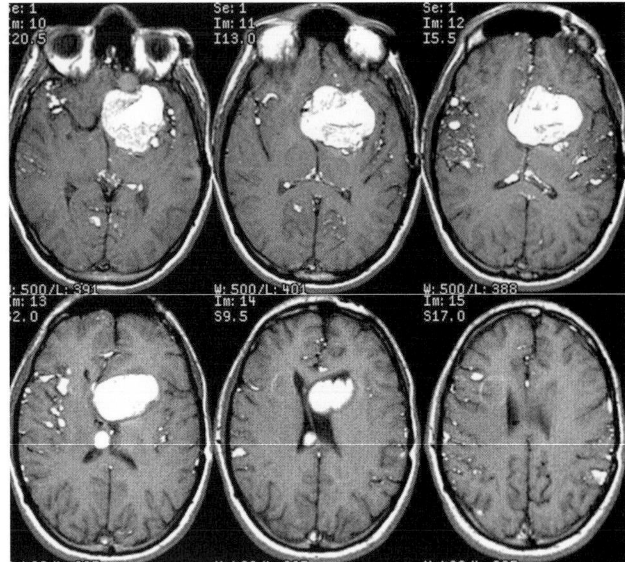

FIGURE 60-28 ■ A 25-year-old male patient with headaches. Axial T1-weighted MR images (unenhanced) reveal a T1 hyperintense mass lying to the left of the midline, with scattered globules of T1 hyperintensity within the subarachnoid spaces and ventricular system. Findings are in keeping with a ruptured dermoid, with spread of fat within cerebrospinal fluid.

or single-shot fast spin-echo imaging can be performed, although this necessitates lower-resolution techniques. Motion correction can be extremely helpful, particularly in the moving or confused patient (Fig. 60-29).[41]

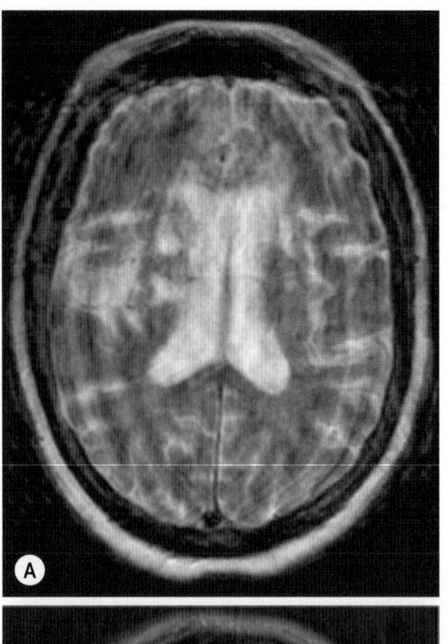

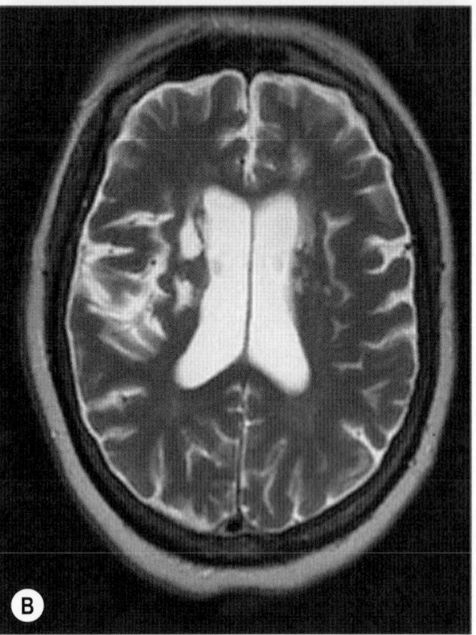

FIGURE 60-29 ■ A 78-year-old woman with multifocal chronic deep white matter infarcts. (A) Axial T2-weighted FSE MR image acquired using conventional sequence is severely degraded by motion artefact. (B) Axial T2-weighted FSE acquired with motion correction (PROPELLER) during the same examination shows correction of any patient motion and marked improvement in image quality.

Technique and Protocols

Most imaging of the neuraxis is performed using superconducting magnets of 1.5 T or higher. Use of 3 T MRI is becoming more widespread for structural and functional imaging, offering the advantage of either shorter imaging times, or higher resolution, which can offer benefit in subtle pathologies.[42] There are significant advantages of higher-field imaging for more specialised sequences, including MR angiography, MR spectroscopy and functional MRI, due to inherent higher signal to noise. Ultra-high magnetic fields, up to 7 T, will likely become more available in the future, offering further advantages in these areas.[43]

Advances in coil technology have lead to widespread use of multichannel coils, speeding up imaging time by use of parallel imaging. Combined coils, such as brain and spine, have now become commonplace, removing the necessity to change coil during an examination of the brain and spine.

A wide variety of pulse sequences are available for MR imaging of the neuraxis, constantly evolving with advancing techniques. The exact protocol used depends on both the clinical question and the available hard and software. Most imaging examinations of the brain or spine use a multi-contrast approach, incorporating at least both T1-weighted and T2-weighted imaging, which can be acquired using a number of different techniques. T2-weighted FLAIR sequences are commonly added, due to their high sensitivity to lesion detection, with particular utility in cortical and periventricular regions, where suppression of cerebrospinal fluid enhances lesion detection.

Images should be optimised using variable image parameters, including TE, TR, flip angle. Slice thickness, spatial resolution, signal-to-noise ratio, acquisition time and contrast are all interrelated and should be carefully controlled. A maximum slice thickness of 5 mm with a 2.5-mm gap should be used in the brain, but thinner slices often offer benefit and, when obtained with a 3D technique, offer the option of multiplanar reconstruction. Such T1 volume studies are commonplace, but there is now increasing availability of volume T2-weighted sequences. T2*-weighted imaging, using a gradient-echo sequence, or susceptibility-weighted imaging (SWI), is

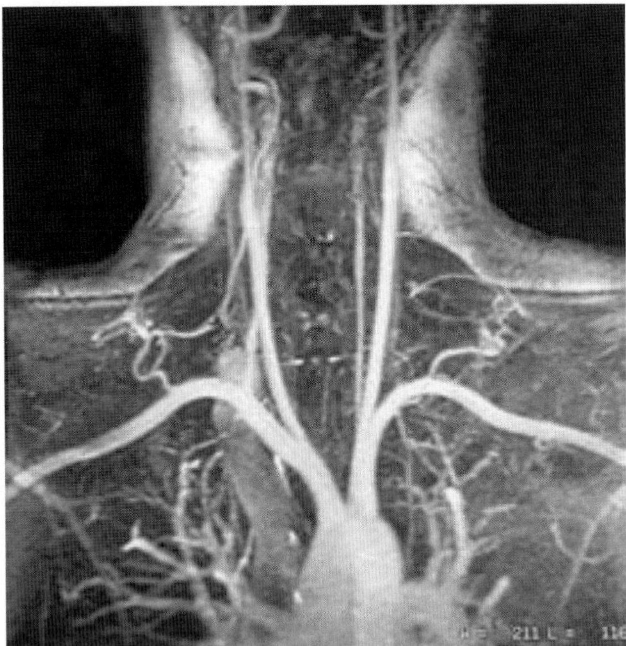

FIGURE 60-30 ■ Contrast-enhanced MRA of aortic arch. A 3D gradient-echo sequence has been acquired during the first pass of an intravenously injected gadolinium bolus. It shows the origins of the great vessels.

important for detection of acute or chronic haemorrhage or calcification and has a significant impact on the detection of cerebral microhaemorrhages, the clinical importance of which is being increasingly recognised.[44]

Intravenous administration of gadolinium can be used to assess the integrity of the blood–brain barrier. Care should be made with the choice of agent, especially where patients have renal dysfunction, in order to limit the risk of nephrogenic systemic fibrosis.[45]

Contrast medium administration is useful in a wide range of indications: for example, in the assessment of tumours or infection. It can be useful to detect acute demyelinating plaques, where enhancement is indicative of improved response disease-modifying treatments.[46] MR angiography or venography of the neurovascular circulation can be performed using intravenous contrast, either targeted to a specific vascular phase or using a time-resolved technique, to assess the vasculature (Fig. 60-30). Alternatively, unenhanced techniques, commonly time-of-flight or phase contrast can be used.

Diffusion-Weighted Imaging

Diffusion-weighted imaging is key to include as part of an acute stroke protocol for detection of cytotoxic oedema, but also has a wider utility: for example, in encephalitis, abscess, brain tumours and metabolic conditions.[47] This technique exploits the presence of random motion (Brownian motion) of water molecules to produce image contrast.[48] A pair of diffusion sensitising gradients around the 180 refocusing RF pulse of a T2-weighted sequence assess whether molecular motion has occurred. Mobile molecules acquire phase shifts, which prevent their complete rephasing and result in signal loss, proportional to the degree of motion. The degree of phase shift and signal loss depends also on the strength and duration of the diffusion sensitising gradient, which is expressed by the '*b*-value': 1000 s mm^{-2} is commonly used in stroke imaging. The apparent diffusion coefficient (ADC) can be calculated and provides a quantitative assessment of water movement in tissue.

A further feature of diffusion in the brain is its directional dependence, or anisotropy. This is particularly prominent in compacted white matter tracts, and least evident in grey matter. DTI explores anisotropy in a variety of directions on a pixel-by-pixel basis. This technique has utility in assessment of white matter structure and lesions thereof, such as diffuse axonal injury.[49]

MR Perfusion Imaging

Perfusion imaging can be performed for a variety of indications, such as stroke or tumour. T2*-weighted techniques exploit the magnetic susceptibility effects within the brain tissue during the first pass of an intravenously injected gadolinium-based contrast agent, causing a transient signal drop on temporal imaging.[50] The sequential changes in signal intensity, plotted as a time–signal intensity curve, allow generation of the relative cerebral blood volume (rCBV), proportional to the area under the curve. Other measurements that can be derived are time to peak and mean transit time (MTT) of the gadolinium bolus. Using tracer kinetics, the relative cerebral blood flow can be estimated by dividing the rCBV by the MTT.

The technique, however, at present is only semiquantitative and cannot provide absolute values. An emerging non-contrast technique, arterial spin labelling, does not require exogenous contrast medium and has the advantage of providing absolute values of perfusion parameters.[51] Alternatively, T1-weighted perfusion imaging can assess accumulation and distribution of gadolinium. Pharmacokinetic modelling can be used to gain data on contrast leakage, including permeability, which can provide useful functional information: for example, in neuro-oncology.[52]

Magnetic Resonance Spectroscopy

Magnetic resonance spectroscopy (MRS) allows investigation of biochemical changes in brain pathologies, by detection of metabolites on ^{1}H-MRS peaks.[53] A change in the resonance intensity of these marker compounds may reflect loss or damage to a specific cell type. The acquisition of long echo time data allows the detection of *N*-acetylaspartate (NAA), creatine (Cr/PCr) and choline (Cho) in normal brain, and lactate in areas of abnormality. The methyl resonance of NAA produces a large sharp peak at 2.01 ppm and acts as a neuronal marker, as it is almost exclusively found in neurons in the human brain. The creatine peak (3.03 ppm) arises from both phosphocreatine- and creatine-containing substances in the cell and choline (3.22 ppm) is thought to arise from choline-containing substances in the cell membrane. The acquisition of short echo time data detects further resonances from additional metabolites, such as *myo*-inositol, glutamate and glutamine.

Current clinical uses in neuroimaging include assessment of brain tumours, stroke, metabolic conditions and demyelination.

Functional MRI

Functional MRI (fMRI) can be used to study cortical activation. It measures a tiny increase in signal intensity on T2*-weighted acquisitions in the relevant cortex during neuronal activation.[54] During cortical activation there is an increase in rCBF and thus an increase in oxygen delivery to the activated brain, which exceeds the local oxygen metabolic requirement. There is a net increase in oxyhaemoglobin concentration in the venules and veins in the vicinity of the activated brain, which results in a tiny increase in MR signal, the so-called *b*lood *o*xygenation *l*evel-*d*ependent or, BOLD effect. The magnitude of this MR signal change is tiny and quantitative comparison must be made between the MR signal during the resting state and the activation state during multiple repetitions in order to detect activation.

Although fMRI is being increasingly used for brain mapping, it does have clinical applications, such as identification of eloquent cortex, prior to surgery in patients with structural lesions.[55]

Nuclear Medicine

Single-Photon Emission Computed Tomography

Single-photon emission computed tomography (SPECT) images are formed from detection of gamma rays emitted during radionuclide decay. Gamma rays or photons are detected by a gamma camera, which, if rotated about the patient's head, allows reconstruction of tomographic slices of distribution of activity in that part of the patient.

Clinical applications of SPECT include dementia, cerebrovascular disease, epilepsy, encephalitis and head injury.[56] Radionuclide imaging of the brain requires radiopharmaceuticals that cross the blood–brain barrier. SPECT may be used to produce images of rCBF using a variety of radiopharmaceuticals: e.g. ^{99m}Tc-hexamethylpropyleneamine oxime (HMPAO) (Fig. 60-31). SPECT can also be used to image uptake at neurotransmitter receptors using various radiopharmaceuticals, usually labelled with ^{123}I. Many different SPECT radiopharmaceuticals are taken up into intracranial tumours: for example, ^{201}Tl.

SPECT is available in most nuclear medicine departments, is relatively inexpensive and has good patient acceptability, although it has inherently poorer resolution than PET.

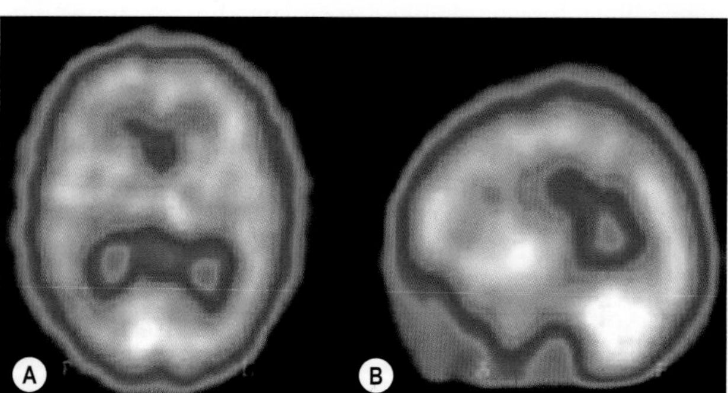

FIGURE 60-31 ■ **SPECT.** Normal ^{99m}Tc-HMPAO SPECT of the brain, axial (A) and sagittal (B) images.

Positron Emission Tomography

Positron emission tomography (PET), like SPECT, produces tomographic images.[56] Positron-emitting radioisotopes decay by emission of positrons, which combine with an adjacent electron in an annihilation reaction with the emission of two high-energy gamma rays in opposing directions. Detection of these simultaneously emitted photons allows calculation of their site of origin and, therefore, a map of radiopharmaceutical distribution in the patient. PET can be used to study different physiological processes in the brain.

A cyclotron is required to generate positron-emitting isotopes that can be made from a variety of biologically interesting compounds. Physiological parameters can be derived: for example, cerebral glucose uptake, using[1,8] fluorodeoxyglucose (FDG); oxygen metabolism, using $^{15}O_2$ or ^{11}CO; and rCBF, using $H_2{}^{15}O$. A number of radiopharmaceuticals are available for PET receptor imaging. FDG, [^{11}C]-methionine and [^{18}F]-α-methyltyrosine are used for tumour imaging.

The disadvantages of PET compared with SPECT are its limited availability and high cost due to the necessity of a cyclotron close to the PET unit.

VASCULAR IMAGING TECHNIQUES

Imaging techniques for the assessment of intra- and extracranial vessels have evolved over recent decades with traditional digital subtraction angiography (DSA) no longer the universal reference standard. Following introduction of new CT and MR applications, the role of DSA is increasingly restricted to the endovascular treatment of diseases as well as for the diagnosis of certain pathological conditions such as small dural or pial AV fistulas or head and neck pathologies. This section discusses the techniques of vascular imaging (invasive and non-invasive). Doppler ultrasound is covered elsewhere.

Conventional Catheter Digital Subtraction Angiography

General principles and basic arteriographic techniques are described elsewhere. Most diagnostic cerebral angiography is performed under local anaesthesia. Using the standard Seldinger technique, the transfemoral route is almost exclusively used for catheterisation of the cerebral vessels. There has been a move towards using 4Fr catheters, often with multipurpose or vertebral curves, with Sidewinder curves reserved for difficult access.

A complete diagnostic study may involve catheterisation of six vessels. Internal and external carotid runs are necessary to exclude or verify the presence of dural or pial AV fistulas. And separate catheterisation of the two vertebral arteries may be needed. Angiographic runs usually start with the internal carotid artery. Contrast medium can be injected manually or by pump injector. For 3D DSA, an automatic pump injection (20 mL of contrast medium at a rate of 5 mL s^{-1}) is needed for smaller-calibre 4Fr catheters.

A biplane angiography unit is of major advantage in neuroangiography. It allows simultaneous acquisition of two projections (such as AP and lateral or two oblique views) during a single injection, reducing the number of contrast medium injections.

Routine cerebral angiography is carried out with a frame rate of two or three images per second, while for the investigation of teriovenous malformations (AVMs) a frame rate of six images per second is usually preferred. Flat detector (FD)-equipped angiography machines have become the norm for neuroangiographic imaging. With this equipment, it is possible to obtain not only high-quality 3D vascular volumes (3D rotational angiography) but also CT-like images (FD-CT) of brain parenchyma that allow detection of intraparenchymal and subarachnoid haemorrhages. This technological breakthrough also allows for removal of the bony structures and offers high-resolution 3D images of the cerebral vessels. As a result, planning of endovascular treatment of aneurysms or AVMs is much easier, even in difficult anatomical locations, such as the carotid siphon[57] (Fig. 60-32). The ability to obtain CT images of the brain also reduces the need to transfer patients from the angiography suite to a CT facility, should complications occur.

Nowadays, the indications for diagnostic DSA have been dramatically reduced. In departments where CTA is routinely used, cerebral angiography is used to resolve discrepancies between two non-invasive methods and as an integral part of endovascular interventional procedures.

DSA is still required in most patients with subarachnoid haemorrhage and negative CTA, in order to exclude a small dural or pial fistula. In cases of intraparenchymal haematoma, DSA is part of the diagnostic work-up, in order to exclude or to reveal the presence and angioarchitecure of a brain AVM. DSA is now less commonly required in carotid artery disease to confirm a significant stenosis suspected on non-invasive imaging, or to reveal intracranial haemodynamic changes, due to severe stenosis. Preoperative angiography is sometimes performed in glomus jugulare tumours and meningiomas to assess tumour vascularity, and is frequently combined with preoperative embolisation in very vascular tumours.

The principal modern use of intra-arterial angiography is related to therapeutic interventions, such as brain aneurysm or AVM embolisation, or in the context of intra-arterial treatment of acute stroke.[58] Follow-up DSA after aneurysm and AVM treatment remains widely used. Ongoing improvements in magnetic resonance angiography (MRA) technology are likely to further reduce indications for DSA, but patients with non-MRI compatible implants will continue to need catheter angiography.

There are very few absolute contraindications to cerebral angiography. A well-documented history of untoward reactions to contrast media is probably the most important contraindication. Severe renal failure is a relative contraindication, because haemodialysis can follow the DSA. Treatment with anticoagulant drugs does not contraindicate arteriography, provided the prothrombin level is within the normal therapeutic range.

Local and general complications of arteriography are discussed elsewhere. Specific risks of catheterisation of the aortic arch or cervical arteries include cerebral thromboembolism and damage to the arteries by the catheter or guidewire, which include spasm, thrombosis and dissection. Older patients with severe atherosclerotic disease should be treated with extreme caution, during catheterisation, because of the higher possibility of thromboembolic complications.[59] Reported risks of cerebral angiography in studies published over the past 15 years are reported to vary from 0.3 to 1.5%.[60,61]

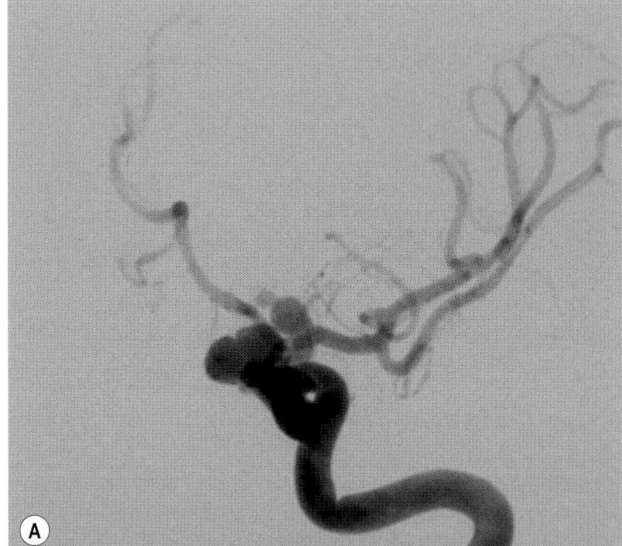

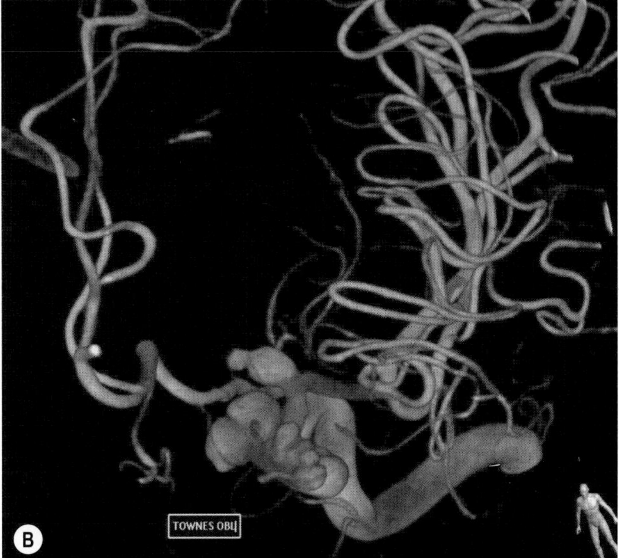

FIGURE 60-32 ■ (A) Standard 2D DSA image showing multiple aneurysms of the carotid syphon and ICA termination. (B) A 3D image can be rotated into any projection to display the aneurysms more clearly, assisting in planning the endovascular approach.

Computed Tomography Angiography (CTA)

Selective imaging of blood vessels with CT has become possible with the introduction of helical CT systems. Over the past decade, the use of multidetector CT angiography has revolutionised the demonstration of intra- and extracranial vessels. Even more recently, dual-energy CT has increased diagnostic capabilities of tomography.[62]

Modern multidetector CT units are able to cover an area from the aortic arch up to the circle of Willis or the entire intracranial circulation from the skull base to the vertex with a single data acquisition. Timing of data acquisition in relation to the administration of contrast medium is critical for maximum arterial opacification. All modern CT systems provide an automated bolus detection system. This is more satisfactory because it adjusts for individual variations in circulation time.

For the cervical arteries, the reference axial image for the smart prep should be at the level of aortic arch, while for the intracranial angiogram, it may be placed at a level cranial to the carotid bifurcation (C4-C5 vertebrae). Typical volumes of 100–120 mL of contrast medium are given at a rate of 3–4 mL s^{-1}.

The quality of CT angiograms depends heavily on postprocessing of the image data. Separation of vessels running close to bone (near the skull base and cranial vault) may be difficult. These difficulties can be at least partially resolved by using thick-section multiplanar reformats (which can be angled in such a way to exclude bone) and by interactive viewing of the source data. With newer technology of dual-energy systems, accurate highlighting of bone structures on CTA data sets is very easy. The highlighted pixels can be removed by a single click, removing the bony structures. The dual-energy approach reliably isolates even complex vasculature, for example, at the base of the skull where CTAs are difficult to interpret,[63] and plaque characterisation in carotid stenosis is more reliable.

In neurovascular angiography, the immediate availability and fast examination time in MDCT have proven highly beneficial in the non-invasive investigation of supra-aortic extracranial and intracranial vessels for the vast majority of pathologies. In most centres where MDCT is available, CTA is the first and often the only examination needed for diagnosis. In the setting of possible thrombectomy, in acute stroke, CTA is usual in the diagnostic algorithm.[64]

Studies have shown that CTA is an excellent tool for the detection of intracranial aneurysms in cases of subarachnoidal haemorrhage. CTA has been used successfully for the evaluation of carotid artery stenosis, cervical artery dissection and intracranial vascular stenosis.[65–67] It has also been suggested that it could be the only diagnostic test in patients with perimesencephalic subarachnoid haemorrhage, although this remains controversial.[68]

CTA is also used to examine the cerebral venous system (CT venography) for suspected superficial or deep cerebral venous system thrombosis.

CTA has certain advantages over MRA: it can be used in claustrophobic patients and patients with cardiac pacemakers, or other implants that preclude MR data acquisition. It is also quicker and more easily performed than MRA. Its disadvantages are the use of ionising radiation and iodinated contrast media.

Magnetic Resonance Angiography

The basic principles of MRI are discussed elsewhere. MRA relies on inflow of unsaturated spin (time-of-flight (TOF) MRA) or the accumulation of phase shifts proportional to the flow velocity (phase contrast MRA). MRA may be used in conjunction with gadolinium-based contrast media (contrast-enhanced (CE) MRA). Both TOF and phase contrast techniques can be performed with a 2D or 3D data acquisition.

MRA is useful for the evaluation of extracranial atherosclerotic disease, as well as for the detection of intracranial arterial or venous pathology. For the cervical vessel disease, a systematic review and meta-analysis showed that MRA is highly accurate for the diagnosis of high-grade ICA stenoses and occlusion with both TOF and CE techniques, CE MRA is highly accurate for distinguishing occlusions from high-grade stenoses, whereas both CE MRA and especially TOF MRA appear to be poor diagnostic tools for moderate ICA stenosis.[69] For imaging of the intracerebral vessels, 3D TOF MRA is the technique of choice, with a single-slab 3D TOF acquisition being adequate for imaging the circle of Willis. Data are usually displayed as maximum intensity projections, but inspection of the source data should always be performed to resolve difficult cases, to confirm the suspicion of an artefact or to clarify possible false-positive results.

Over recent years major advances in MRA techniques allowed for the measurement of arterial blood flow in various cerebrovascular conditions (quantitative MRA (QMRA)), detection of aneurysms (3D TOF MRA), assessment of intracranial stenosis and, to a limited extent, AVMs.

MRA is, however, still usually not the first-choice examination in everyday practice, especially for the evaluation of SAH or intracerebral hematomas. It is, however, widely used for the follow-up of aneurysms after endovascular treatment (Fig. 60-33).

Phase contrast MRA is based on the detection of phase shifts generated by a flow-encoding gradient. Although generally inferior to 3D MRA, it is more sensitive for detection of slow flow (with the appropriate velocity encoding) and can therefore be used for imaging cerebral veins. It does not suffer from T1-contamination artefact and it can provide information about the direction of blood flow.

The administration of a gadolinium-based contrast medium has been shown to have some benefit in conjunction with intracranial 3D TOF MRA for conditions such as AVMs and intracranial stenosis, while, more recently, contrast-enhanced, time-resolved 4D MRA has shown promising results for the pretreatment assessment of AVMs.[70]

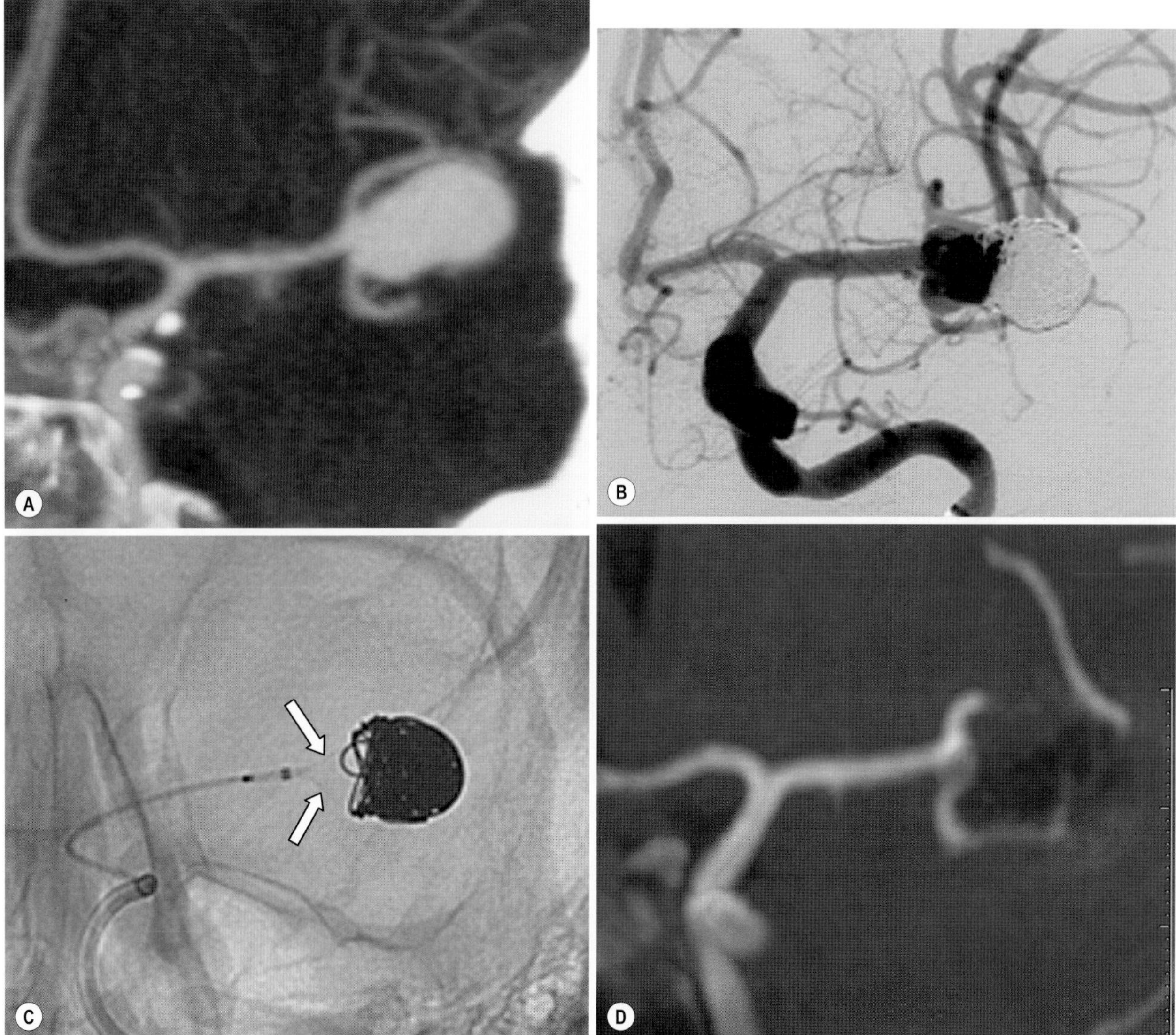

FIGURE 60-33 ■ **Patient with ruptured left MCA aneurysm.** (A) CTA shows wide-neck aneurysm. (B) Initially treated by coiling. Loose packing at aneurysm neck led to compaction and refilling of the aneurysm. (C) Re-treatment with intrasaccular flow diverter (WEB device) (arrows). (D) A 6-month follow-up MRA shows complete occlusion of aneurysm, and demonstrates the normal convexity of the recess of the WEB device.

TRAUMA TO THE SKULL AND BRAIN

HEAD INJURY

Head injuries are either open (penetrating) or closed (non-penetrating), the latter being by far the more common in civilian practice. The main indication for imaging is suspected intracranial haemorrhage where prompt neurosurgical evacuation may modify outcome. Because it shows haemorrhage particularly well, CT generally is recommended in preference to MRI for this purpose. Furthermore CT is more widely available on a 24-h basis and is easier to perform following major trauma. Thus there are clear recommendations from the Royal College of Radiologists[71] and the National Institute of Clinical Excellence (NICE)[72,73] about the indications for and appropriate timing of CT following trauma. During the subsequent clinical course, imaging may be required to assess neurological deterioration or other complications, or perhaps failure to improve, and later to make a final assessment of overall damage for long-term prognosis. For many of these less acute indications, MRI may be preferred. Despite the numerous published guidelines for imaging of the head and cervical spine in trauma, they are only guidelines and many individual brain injury units have their own variations. The principles behind these, however, are simply the application of common sense on a case-by-case basis.

Skull Fractures

Detection of fractures of the cranial vault by plain radiography of the skull is now appreciated to be less useful in assessing the probability of intracranial haemorrhage

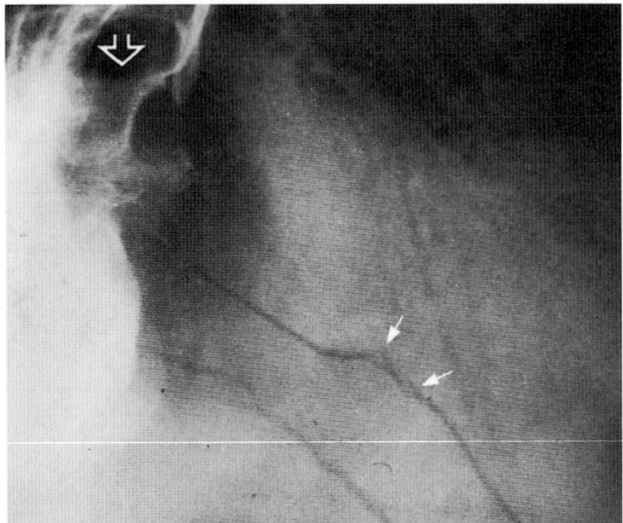

FIGURE 60-34 ■ Bilateral vault fracture, with fluid level in sphenoid sinus (open arrow). Two fracture lines are seen; the more anterior (upper on this radiograph) is better defined and is therefore on the side nearer the radiographic plate. Apparent islands of bone within (small arrows) are typical of an acute fracture. This radiograph has been obtained with the patient in the supine brow up position.

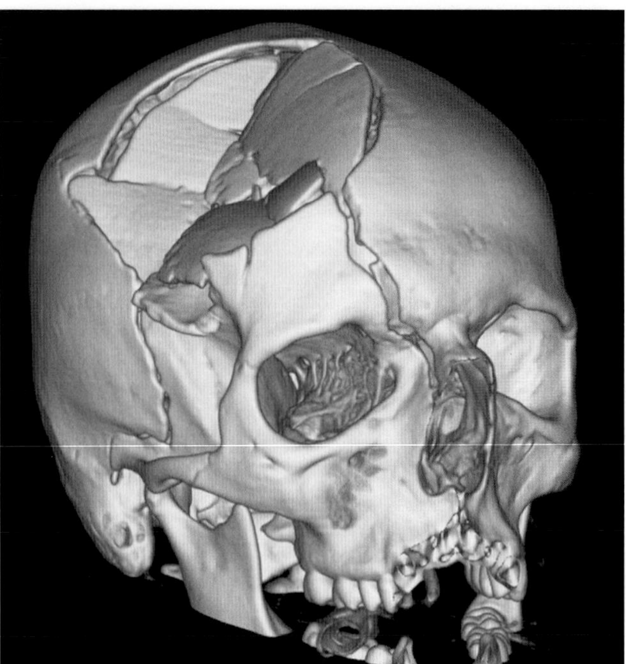

FIGURE 60-35 ■ **Stellate comminuted depressed fracture produced by a direct blow.** CT volume rendered image.

than had been previously suggested. Clinical assessment appears to be a better guide and this, in turn, guides the need for CT. Thus the role of skull radiography has greatly diminished. In any event simple linear fractures are often of little consequence in themselves. Like fractures elsewhere, these may be simple or comminuted. They sometimes branch, and must be distinguished from vascular markings (Fig. 60-34), including the groove in the squamous temporal bone caused by a deep temporal artery.[74] Acute fractures are usually straighter, more angulated, more radiolucent and do not have corticated margins. A fracture passing through a sinus or air cell is effectively compound, and of much greater potential significance than a simple fracture. A compound fracture is one in which the cranial cavity is in real or potential communication with the exterior. Depressed fractures (Fig. 60-35) are usually comminuted and often compound; bone fragments embedded in brain substance often are removed or relocated to reduce the risk of post-traumatic epilepsy. Acuteness of the fracture may be determined by demonstrating overlying scalp swelling on CT. Fractures of the skull base are important because of bleeding or leakage of CSF; air and fluid within the sphenoid sinus may indicate that the leptomeninges have been torn. CT is extremely helpful in assessing fractures of the skull base, including the petrous bone, where it may also reveal ossicular dislocation, a treatable cause of traumatic hearing loss. Growing fractures (leptomeningeal cysts) usually occur after severe head injuries early in life.[74] The dura mater underlying a linear fracture is torn, often with laceration of the underlying brain. Exposure of the remodelling bone to pulsation of the CSF results in progressive widening of the fracture line over weeks or months.

Traumatic Haemorrhage

Trauma may cause bleeding into the scalp, between the cranial vault and the dura mater (extradural—but also termed epidural), between the dura and arachnoid mater (subdural), or into the subarachnoid space, brain or ventricular system. The aim of imaging in the acute stage is to identify patients with intracranial bleeding requiring surgery; they represent less than 1% of patients with well-documented head injury. CT is the imaging procedure of choice, rather than MRI, as haematomas are about the most readily recognisable abnormality on plain CT.

Extradural Haemorrhage

The **acute extradural (or epidural) haematoma** is a relatively stereotyped lesion (Figs. 60-36 and 60-37). Because the dura mater tends to adhere to the skull, the haematoma is seen on CT sections as a biconvex dense area immediately beneath the skull vault, convex towards both the brain and the vault. The temporoparietal convexity is the most common site, in which lesions are easily detected on axial sections. The haematoma often lies beneath a fracture of the squamous part of the temporal bone. They tend not to cross cranial sutures. Areas of low density within them may indicate continuing bleeding (Fig. 60-37), and add further urgency to the assessment. Frontal, vertical and posterior cranial fossa collections (Fig. 60-38) can be difficult to diagnose; coronal images may be required. Even then, shallow extradural haematomas may be overlooked, especially when adjacent to contused or haemorrhagic brain. Wide-window CT images may help distinguish the intermediate density of the clot from bone and underlying brain. The underlying brain is displaced, but often appears intrinsically normal. MRI can be helpful on occasions (Fig. 60-39).

Subdural Haemorrhage

Subdural bleeding is often, but not always, associated with damage to the brain, and arises from rupture of veins

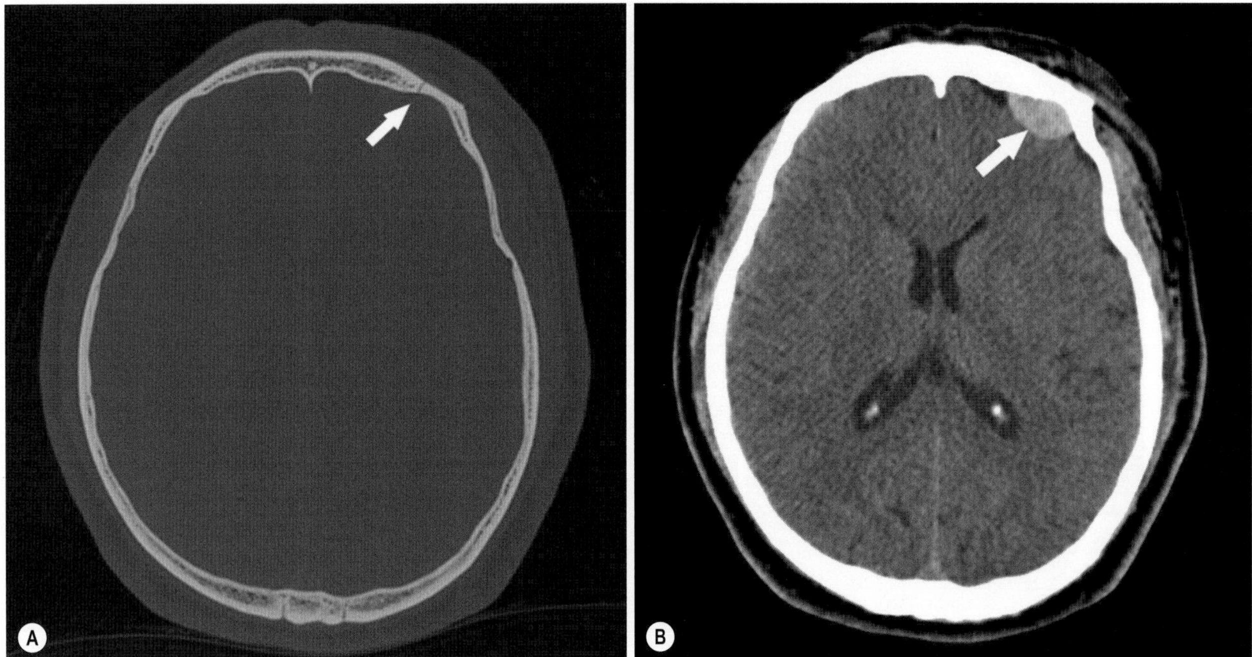

FIGURE 60-36 ■ (A, B) CT: axial 'brain and bone windows' from equivalent levels demonstrate an undisplaced fracture of the left frontal bone (A, arrow), with a small extradural haematoma overlying the adjacent frontal lobe (B, arrow). Soft-tissue contusion overlying the fracture site is also noted.

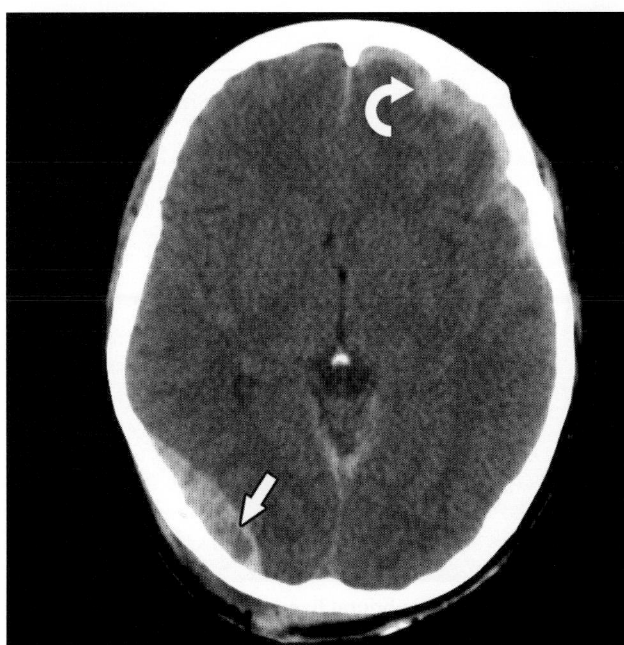

FIGURE 60-37 ■ **Trauma.** CT: a biconvex extradural haematoma overlies the right parieto-occipital region. Note the central low attenuation (arrow) within the haematoma, indicative of active haemorrhage. A crescent of fresh subdural blood is also seen overlying the left frontal and temporal lobes (curved arrow).

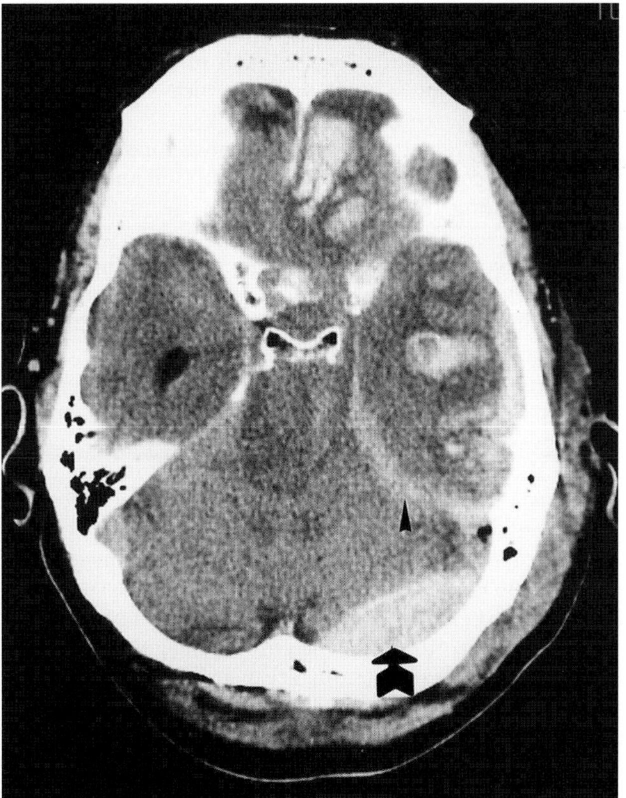

FIGURE 60-38 ■ **Trauma.** CT: A biconvex density of blood over the left cerebellar hemisphere indicates an extradural haematoma (thick arrow). A crescent of fresh subdural blood spreads over the left temporal lobe and tracks along the tentorium in a comma-shaped fashion (arrowhead); this feature differentiates it from an extradural. Typical sites of haemorrhagic contusions are also seen; gyrus recti and temporal lobe.

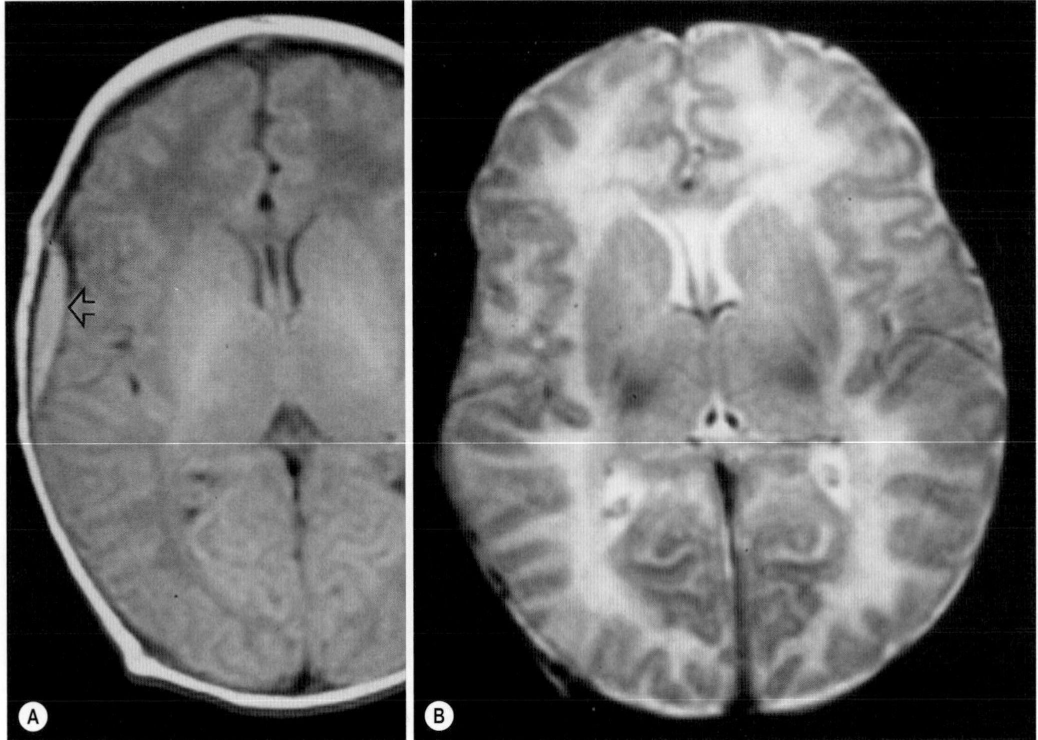

FIGURE 60-39 ■ **Acute extradural haematoma.** MRI in a neonate with traumatic delivery. (A) Axial T_1-weighted image (750/16). Slightly hyperintense epidural collection (arrow) in the right temporal region. (B) Axial T_2-weighted image (3000/120), epidural collection is hypointense and is invisible except for deformation of the underlying cortex. This is the MR signature of deoxyhaemoglobin.

which cross the subdural space; vault fractures are much less commonly present in patients with subdural haematomas than extradural bleeds.

Subdural haematomas are seen most commonly over the cerebral convexities, under the temporal and occipital lobes, or along the falx cerebri. They lie in the virtual space between the dura and arachnoid maters and may be extensive. This is because the blood within them, while under less pressure, is less restricted and tends to spread out over the surface of the brain; bleeding may even extend over an entire cerebral hemisphere. They may follow minor head injuries, and sometimes seem to develop spontaneously, especially in the elderly and in patients with haematological abnormalities. In such situations they are often diagnosed during the investigation of persistent headache, or perhaps transient but repetitive focal neurological deficits. Large ones requiring operative evacuation are usually associated with a reduced conscious state of the patient.

On axial CT and MRI, the cerebral surface typically is concave (Fig. 60-40), but on coronal images may appear more convex. Acute lesions are usually hyperdense on CT, but mixed density is also common. They become progressively less dense over time, and typically end up of similar density to CSF within a few weeks or months. During this evolution there is often a period when the attenuation of the haematoma is similar to that of cerebral tissue; the resulting 'isodense subdural' haemotoma[75] can be difficult to identify (Fig. 60-41) and is a well-recognised pitfall on CT which continues to cause problems.[76] MRI is better at making this diagnosis when these

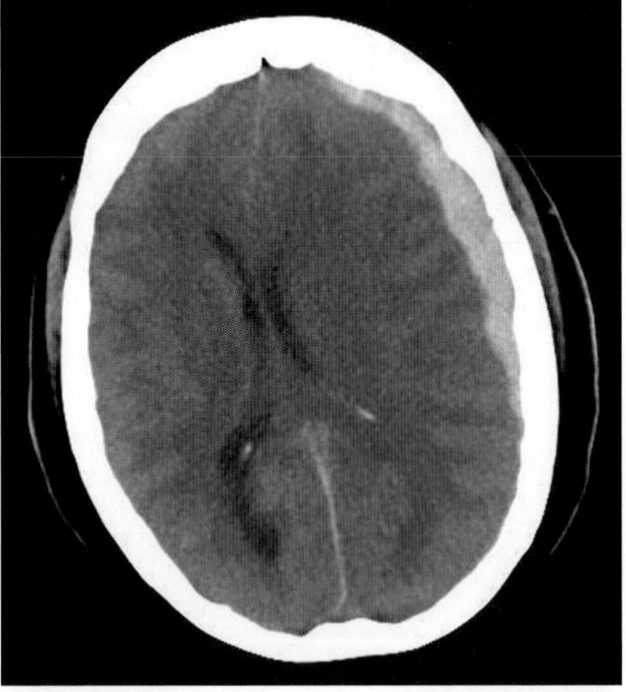

FIGURE 60-40 ■ **Acute subdural haematoma.** CT: Heterogeneous density of irregular shape occupies extra-axial space overlying the left cerebral convexity. There is quite severe mass effect exhibited by effacement of convexity sulci, narrowing of the left-sided ventricular system and midline shift. (Courtesy of Dr Dan Scoffings.)

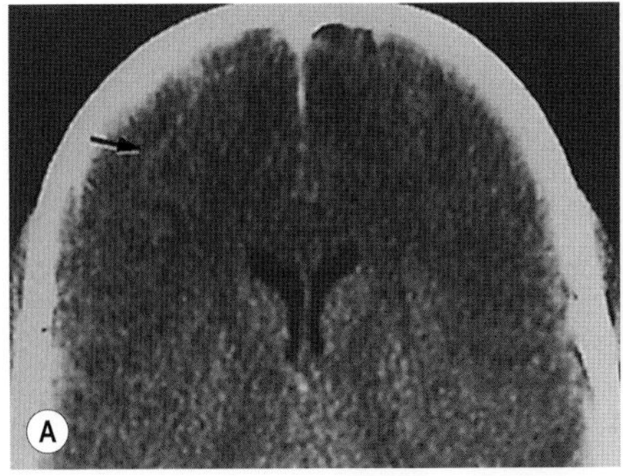

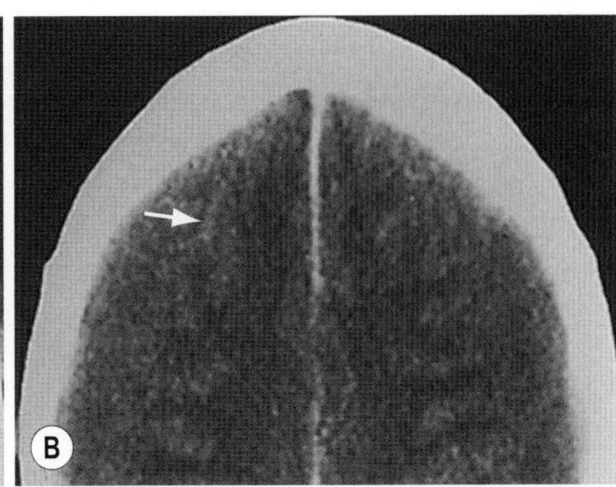

FIGURE 60-41 ■ Bilateral isodense subdural haematomas on contrast-enhanced CT. The ventricles (A) are slit-like and displaced medially, giving a 'rabbit's ears' appearance. A higher section (B) indicates that the normal grey–white interface lies too near the midline; the cortex appears abnormally thick. On close inspection, both sections show cortical vessels (arrows) displaced away from the cranial vault.

lesions are of some long-standing. Most resolve spontaneously with time, but some persist, sometimes for years. Occasionally these lesions enlarge progressively at a variable, but usually slow, rate and eventually may require evacuation. The high morbidity of these lesions, particularly in the aged, is due in large part to the associated swelling, contusion or laceration of the underlying brain. It is often evident that midline displacement is greater than would be accounted for by the mass of the haematoma alone. Dilatation of the contralateral ventricle is a bad prognostic sign.

The interhemispheric subdural haematoma extends along the falx cerebri and may spread onto the tentorium, giving a characteristic comma shape on axial CT sections (see Fig. 60-38).

Coronal CT sections may be useful in distinguishing supra- and infra-tentorial bleeding. Sub- or extradural collections low in the posterior cranial fossa, which may be life-threatening, may be overlooked, and the presence of unexplained hydrocephalus after acute head injury should prompt thorough examination of that region (see Fig. 60-42).

The CT attenuation of the blood in a subacute subdural haematoma slowly decreases: as a rule of thumb, it remains denser than the brain for 1 week, and is less dense after 3 weeks (Fig. 60-43). There is thus an interim period of up to 2 weeks when it may be 'isodense' with brain (see Fig. 60-41). Not all isodense haematomas are subacute: an acute bleed can be isodense in a very anaemic patient, and if there is continued leakage of venous blood, a chronic haematoma may not be of low density. Indirect signs may then be crucial: midline shift, with compression of the ipsilateral ventricle; contralateral ventricular enlargement; effacement of cerebral sulci; and medial displacement of the junction between the white and grey matter ('buckling'). Some of these signs may be absent if there are bilateral collections; the frontal horns may then lie closer together than normal, giving a 'rabbit's ear' configuration (see Fig. 60-41). Intravenous contrast medium, by highlighting the vessels on the surface of the brain, may remove any doubts about the extracerebral location of the lesion. The increasing use of MRI for nonacute problems should help overcome this diagnostic problem in the future.

Chronic subdural collections are usually biconvex. Their density is less than that of brain, approaching that of CSF. Fluid–fluid levels may be seen between denser blood elements in the more dependent portions and

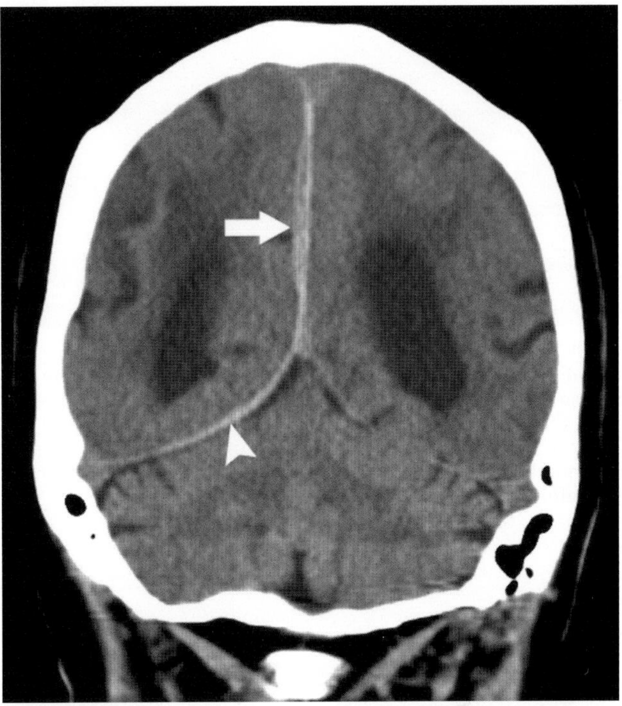

FIGURE 60-42 ■ CT: Coronal reformatted image demonstrates a subtle parafalcine subdural haematoma (arrow) with layering over the tentorium cerebelli (arrowhead). Reformatted coronal images are useful for identifying the latter, which may be difficult to identify on axial images.

serous fluid above, particularly if haemorrhage has been repeated. The membrane on their deep surface frequently shows contrast enhancement.

PRIMARY CEREBRAL DAMAGE IN CLOSED HEAD INJURY

This is commonly associated with intracerebral haemorrhage, usually small and multifocal. An important feature is that the haemorrhages tend to enlarge and become more conspicuous over the initial few days after injury. Primary cerebral damage may be described as either superficial or deep. Interestingly, these patterns of injury usually are mutually exclusive. Deep damage generally is considered to occur more commonly in high speed accidents and to have a worse prognosis, but exceptions are encountered quite frequently, and as in all forms of head

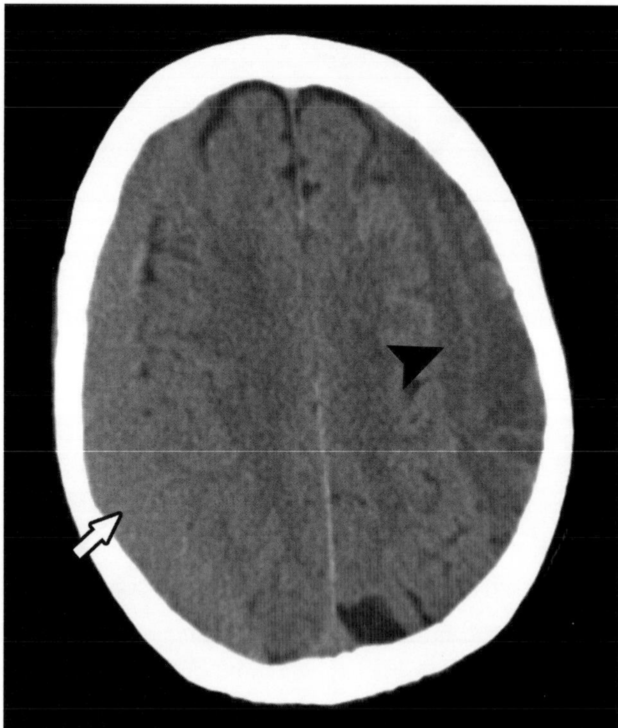

FIGURE 60-43 ■ Bilateral subacute haematomas. CT: The subdural haematoma overlying the right cerebral convexity is isodense to brain parenchyma (arrow), and results in mass effect with effacement of the adjacent cortical sulci. The subdural collection overlying the left convexity (arrowhead) is of lower attenuation than brain parenchyma but denser than CSF, and is therefore older than that on the right side.

injury, prognosis must be guarded in the initial few months following the injury.

Superficial Primary Cerebral Damage

This consists of cerebral contusions (see Fig. 60-38) and cortical lacerations. The underlying white matter also usually is damaged to a variable extent. The lesions usually are quite extensive, and typically involve the inferior parts of the frontal lobes and the anterior parts of the temporal lobes, but they can be found elsewhere. The mechanism is rotation of the brain with respect to the skull, especially the sphenoid ridges and the anterior cranial fossa. The term contrecoup contusion often is used because commonly this type of cerebral damage lies diametrically opposite the site of impact, as defined by skull fracture or scalp haematoma (Fig. 60-44). However, the cause is rotation, not linear acceleration of the brain. On CT, contusion appears as superficial low density areas with mild to moderate mass effect, which tends to increase a little in the initial days and subsequently contracts into a region of focal atrophy and sometimes cavitation. Multiple, usually small hyperdense haemorrhages are often present within the low density areas in the early stages. On MRI, they appear as mixed signal lesions, later contracting to regions of persistent mainly cortical cerebral damage. MRI is not much more sensitive in assessing the extent of contusions than CT.

Deep Primary Cerebral Damage

This pattern of injury is considerably less common. The mechanism here is differential rates of rotational acceleration within brain substance itself, producing shearing forces which damage axons and microvasculature. The injury is microscopic and may not be detected at all by

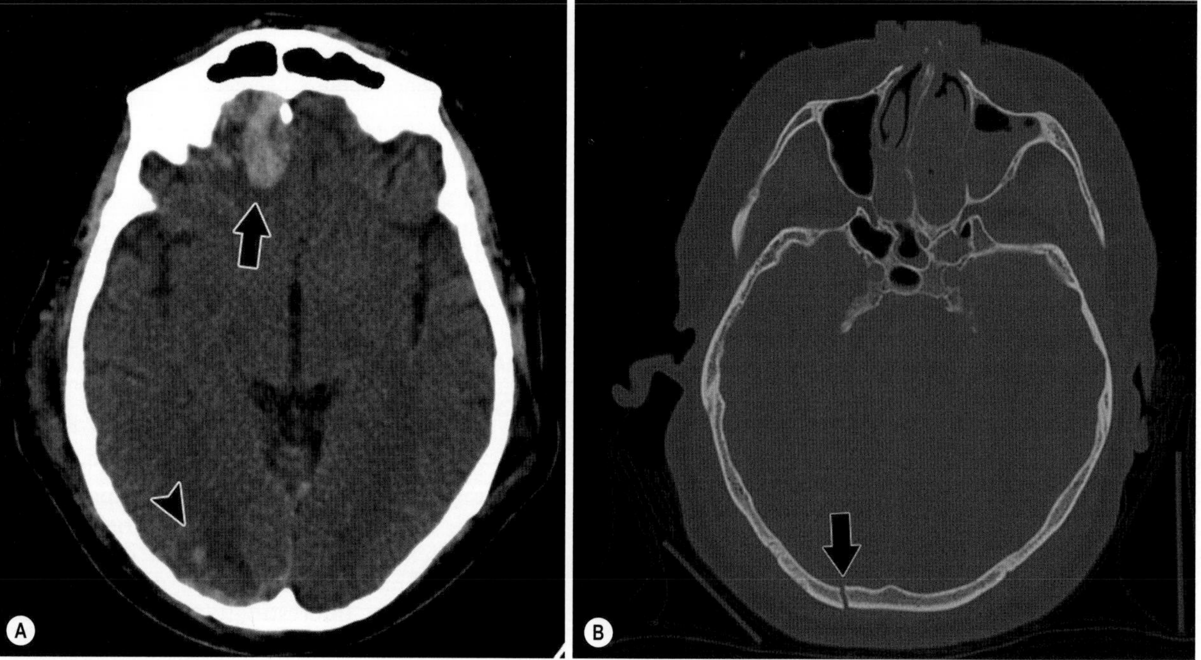

FIGURE 60-44 ■ Contrecoup injury. (A) Haemorrhagic 'contrecoup' contusion is demonstrated within the anterior right frontal lobe (arrow). A 'coup' contusion of the occipital lobe resulting from the direct impact is also seen (arrowhead), adjacent to a fracture of the right occipital bone (B, arrow).

CT or MRI, unless diffuse atrophy subsequently develops in the brain. Its presence is most often recognised on imaging by the presence of so-called marker lesions. These probably represent small areas of microvascular damage with haemorrhage or infarction, but they are a reliable guide to the presence of diffuse axonal injury, though not to its extent. They are small multifocal lesions, and tend to occur in more or less characteristic sites: high parasagittal cerebral white matter, corona radiata, posterior corpus collosum and subcortical white matter almost anywhere. They usually are not visible on CT unless haemorrhagic; many more may be on MRI, whether haemorrhagic or not. Susceptibility-weighted MRI (T_2 'star' acquisitions) often shows still more lesions, even long after the event, as small dark patches of haemosiderin (Fig. 60-45). Characteristically the surrounding brain appears normal. Quantitative diffusion tensor imaging has been considered to demonstrate the axonal damage in a few reported cases, but only when it has been exceptionally severe.

When the vascular component of the shearing injury is severe there may be larger haemorrhages in the basal ganglia and elsewhere, a pattern sometimes termed diffuse axonal injury of the brain.

Primary Brainstem Injuries

These usually only occur with deep cerebral damage. The most common is a haemorrhagic lesion in the dorsolateral midbrain. Another is the pontomedullary rent, usually not compatible with life and therefore rarely seen on imaging.

OTHER TYPES OF INTRACRANIAL HAEMORRHAGE AFTER CLOSED HEAD INJURY

Subarachnoid Haemorrhage

Head injury is probably the most common cause overall of subarachnoid haemorrhage. It commonly accompanies superficial cerebral damage, but may be minor and inconspicuous and is usually not recognised radiologically or clinically.

Intraventricular Haemorrhage

When isolated, intraventricular haemorrhage usually seems to be the result of tears in the attachments of the septum pellucidum to the corpus callosum.

Isolated Large Intracerebral Haemorrhage

Although rare, intracerebral haemorrhage is encountered from time to time and is often a source of diagnostic confusion. Cerebral angiography may show a false aneurysm.

SECONDARY CEREBRAL DAMAGE WITH CLOSED HEAD INJURY

This results mainly from the effects of raised intracranial pressure, local pressure cones and fluctuations in systemic

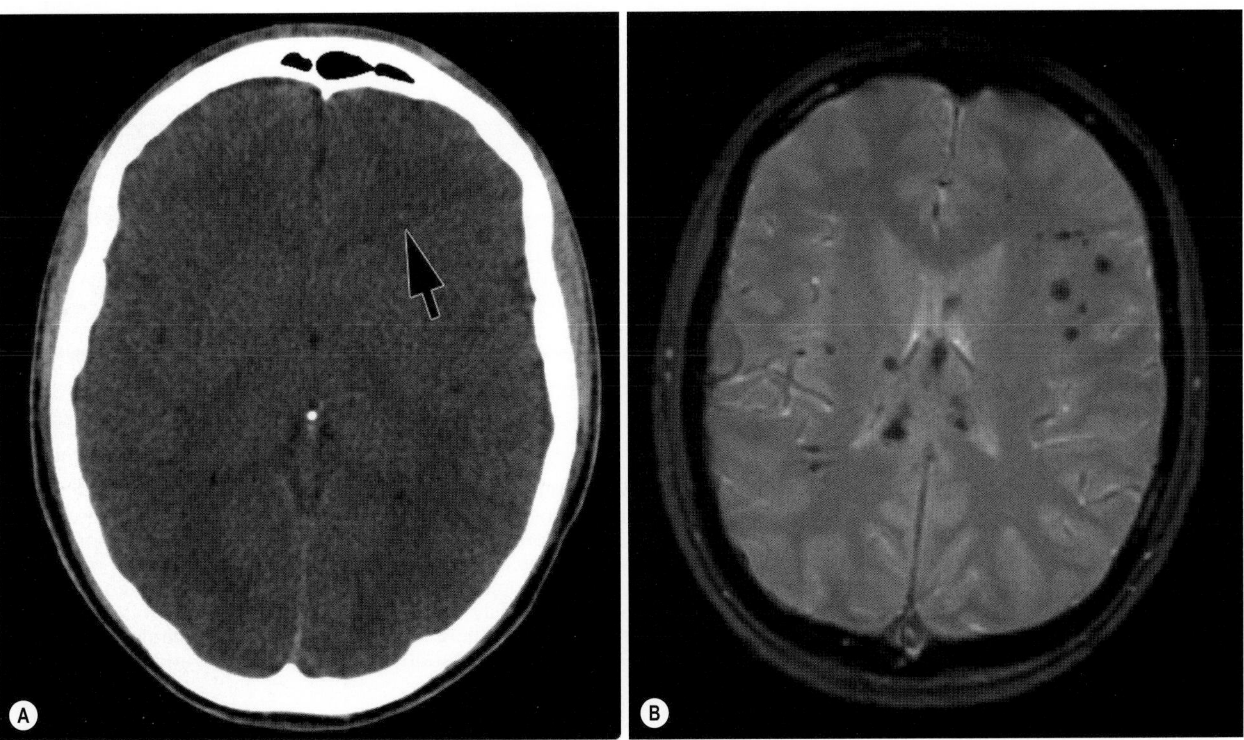

FIGURE 60-45 ■ **Diffuse axonal injury.** On unenhanced CT imaging (A) a subtle focus of high attenuation is present at the grey–white matter interface (arrow). (B) Axial T_2*-weighted MR image (660/25) at the equivalent level demonstrates numerous further foci of haemorrhage not seen on CT, manifesting as multiple hypointense punctate foci within the subcortical and deep white matter of both hemispheres and within the corpus callosum.

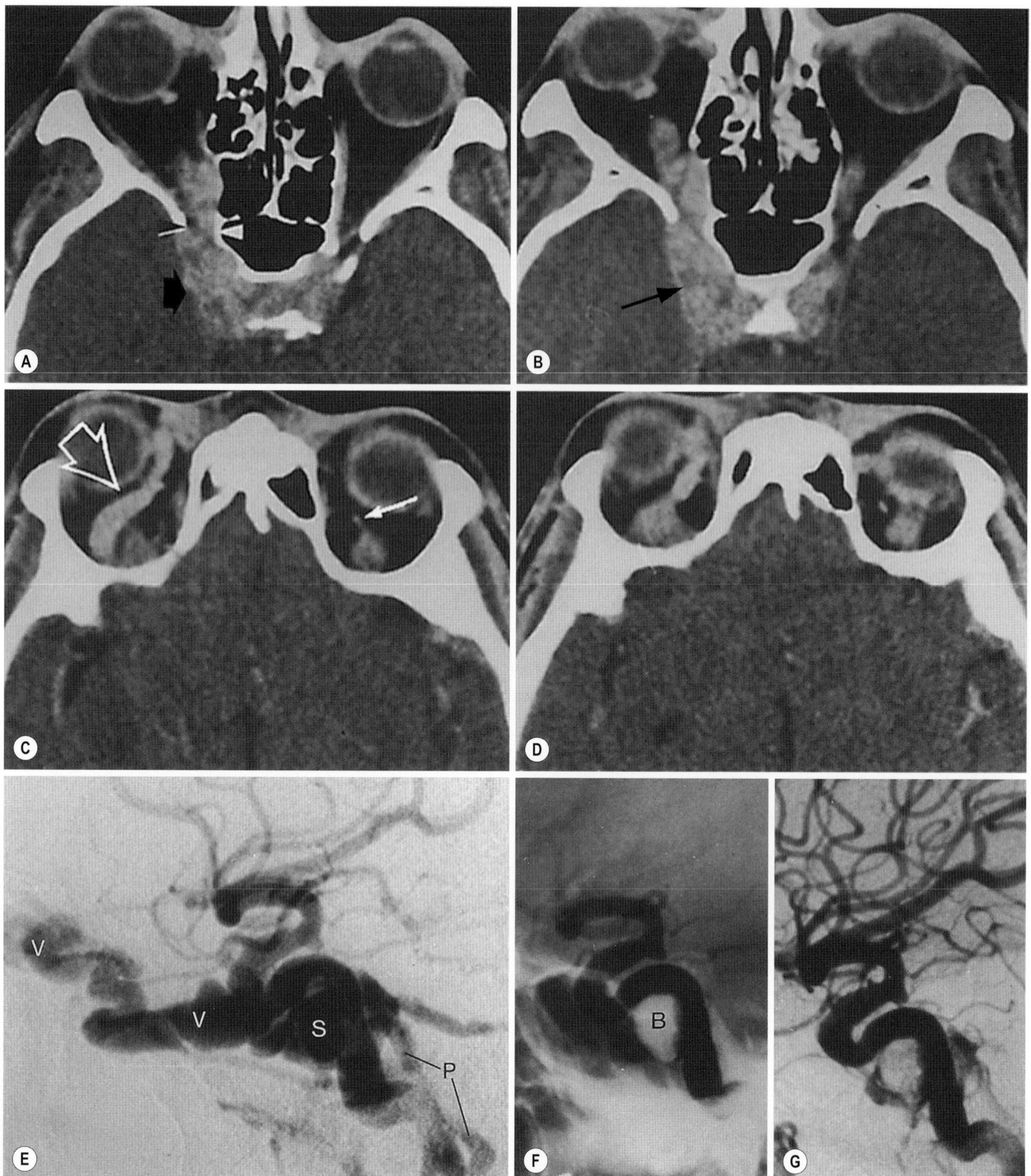

FIGURE 60-46 ■ **Post-traumatic caroticocavernous fistula.** (A–D) Axial contrast-enhanced CT: the right cavernous sinus (A, arrow) is enlarged, and a large enhancing mass runs forwards into the orbit through a widened superior orbital fissure (A, arrowheads). A sigmoid structure (C, open arrow) in the upper part of the right orbit represents the greatly dilated superior ophthalmic vein (cf. normal left side in C, small white arrow). Some of the extraocular muscles are thicker than on the left, and there is marked right proptosis. (E) Intra-arterial DSA, lateral projection, arterial phase, following injection into the right internal carotid artery. Contrast medium floods into the cavernous sinus (S), and drains anteriorly into a grossly dilated superior ophthalmic vein (V); there is also shunting posteriorly and via the inferior petrosal sinus (P). Intracranial arterial filling is poor. (F, G) After therapeutic detachment of a balloon (B) in the cavernous sinus (F, lateral projection), shunting particularly anteriorly, is greatly reduced, and intracranial filling much improved (G).

blood pressure and blood oxygen saturation. A common serious problem in the initial 2 or 3 d after a major head injury is diffuse cerebral swelling due to an increase in the cerebral blood volume, appropriately referred to as hyperaemic brain swelling, and less appropriately as brain oedema. It is a potent cause of raised intracranial pressure in this period and may trigger drastic neurosurgical decompression by wide craniectomies. The appearance of brain substance on CT and MRI is not affected, so it is not directly recognisable by imaging alone.

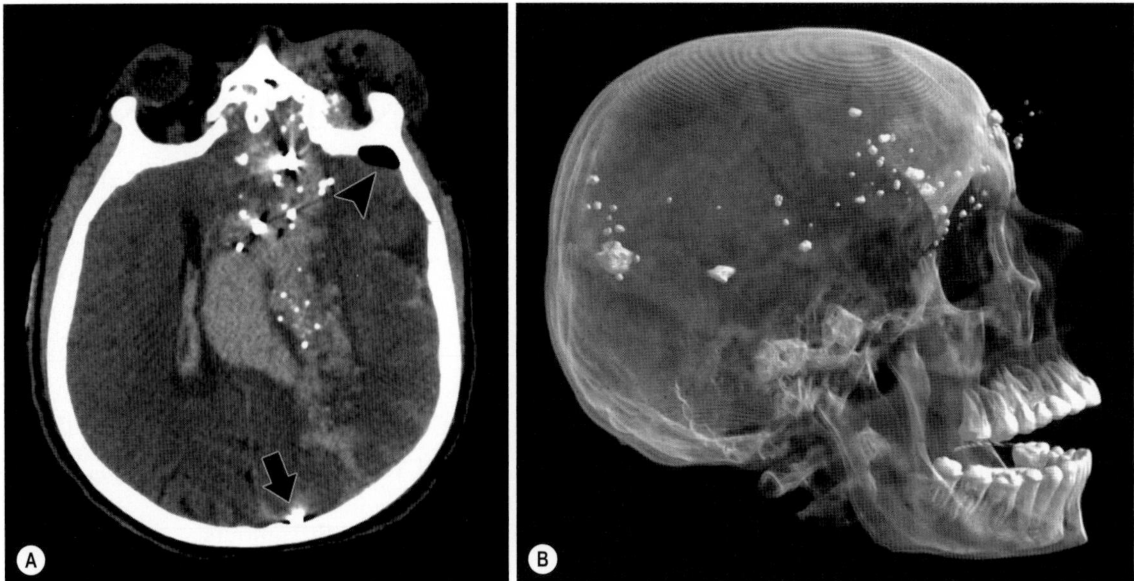

FIGURE 60-47 ■ **Gunshot injury.** (A) Axial CT: The site of projectile penetration is through the left frontal sinus and has resulted in extensive intraparenchymal haematoma with extension into the lateral ventricles, in addition to pneumocephalus (arrowhead). Multiple metallic density projectile fragments lie along the projectile tract, the larger fragments resulting in streak artefact. Note the large fragment adjacent to the occipital bone, with no exit site (arrow). (B) A partially transparent volume-rendered image is useful for identifying the relative position of the numerous projectile fragments.

Secondary cerebral damage consists of infarctions and brainstem haemorrhage. Infarcts most commonly occur in the cortical distributions of one or both posterior cerebral arteries, and haemorrhages are most often found in the ventral mid-brain and upper ponds. Both probably, but certainly the latter, are due to pressure cones across the tentorial incisura.

OTHER COMPLICATIONS WITH CLOSED HEAD INJURIES

Hydrocephalus requiring shunting is an uncommon complication and generally is of a communicating type.

CSF fistulae are associated with skull base fractures and may present with otorrhoea or rhinorhhoea. Most heal within 10 d or so, but a small number may persist or become intermittent, and eventually require surgical repair. Detailed imaging may be necessary to identify the site of the leak.[77] CSF leaks are associated with intracranial air, which may be extradural if the meninges are intact, or if they are torn, subarachnoid or intraventricular. These are often referred to as aerocoeles or pneumocephalus.

Cranial nerve palsies are usually associated with skull base fractures and are immediate and permanent. Delayed cranial nerve palsies also may occur in the absence of fracture and may be reversible. Virtually any nerve or branch that traverses the skull base can be involved.

An arteriovenous fistula may be an immediate or a delayed complication (Fig. 60-46). The most common occurs between the internal carotid artery and the cavernous sinus,[78] and is termed a direct carotid cavernous fistula. These usually are torrential, and may require urgent endovascular treatment to preserve vision, sometimes at a time when the overall outcome is in the balance. Alternatively they may be chronic and the patient may present with an alarming engorged exophthalmos.

Penetrating Head Injuries

Although uncommon, such injuries are increasing in frequency in civilian practice. Appearances on imaging vary with the penetrating agent and the trajectory of the cerebral penetration. Intracerebral haemorrhage usually dominates the appearances on imaging (Fig. 60-47). Direct vascular injury is more common than in closed head injury, resulting in larger haemorrhages and more frequent false aneurysms.

For a full list of references, please see ExpertConsult.

FURTHER READING

2. Lasjaunias P, Berenstein A, ter Brugge K. Surgical Neuroangiography. 2nd ed. vol 1 Clinical Vascular Anatomy and Variations. Berlin: Springer-Verlag; 2001. pp. 480–96.
5. Nieuwenhuys R, Voogd J, van Huijzen C. The Human Central Nervous System. 4th ed. Berlin: Springer-Verlag; 2008. pp. 491–510.
43. van der Kolk AG, Hendrikse J, Luijten PR. Ultrahigh-field magnetic resonance imaging: the clinical potential for anatomy, pathogenesis, diagnosis, and treatment planning in brain disease. Neuroimaging Clin N Am 2012;22:343–62, xii.
47. da Cruz LCH Jr, editor. Clinical Applications of Diffusion Imaging of the Brain. London: Elsevier; 2011.
54. Stroman PW. Essentials of Functional MRI. Boca Rotan, FL: CRC Press; 2011.

CHAPTER 61

Benign and Malignant Intracranial Tumours in Adults

Ruchi Kabra • Caroline Micallef • H. Rolf Jäger

CHAPTER OUTLINE

RADIOLOGICAL INVESTIGATIONS IN INTRACRANIAL TUMOURS

Plain radiographic findings in brain tumours are of historical interest and may show signs of raised intracranial pressure (such as erosion of the lamina dura of the dorsum sellae, or a 'J-shaped' sella), tumour calcification or enlargement of middle meningeal artery grooves in meningiomas.

Magnetic resonance imaging (MRI) is the preferred investigation for patients with suspected intracranial tumours. It provides a better soft-tissue differentiation and tumour delineation than CT and advanced MR imaging techniques, such as diffusion-weighted (DWI) and perfusion-weighted (PWI) imaging and MR spectroscopy (MRS), allow the assessment of physiological and metabolic processes.

Intra-arterial angiography for brain tumours is now mostly performed in conjunction with preoperative or palliative tumour embolisations.

COMPUTED TOMOGRAPHY

Most clinically symptomatic brain tumours are detectable on CT, by virtue of mass effect and/or altered attenuation. Intra-axial tumours are usually of low attenuation on non-enhanced CT images. Primary intracranial lymphoma is usually iso- to slightly hyperdense to the brain parenchyma. High attenuation areas within a tumour indicate tumour calcification or recent intratumoural haemorrhage. Tumours frequently exhibiting these two features are listed in Table 61-1.

Bone-window settings can reveal bone erosion or hyperostosis, associated with extra-axial tumours.

Contrast enhancement improves the visualisation of strongly enhancing mass lesions such as meningiomas, schwannomas, metastases and certain types of glial tumours.

CT perfusion has emerged as a technique to assess the relative cerebral blood volume (rCBV) and permeability changes in brain tumours.[1] The newer 320-detector row CT system provides full brain coverage.[2] CT perfusion has the advantage of a direct relationship between the CT attenuation coefficient and contrast material concentration in tissue.

MAGNETIC RESONANCE IMAGING

Structural MRI

The MRI protocol for structural tumour imaging should include T2-weighted, fluid-attenuated recovery

TABLE 61-1 **Commonly Calcified and Haemorrhagic Lesions**

Commonly Calcified Lesions	Commonly Haemorrhagic Lesions
Oligodendrogliomas (90%)	GBM (grade 4 glioma)
Choroid plexus tumours	Oligodendroglioma
Ependymoma	Metastases
Central neurocytoma	– Melanoma
Meningioma	– Lung
Craniopharyngioma	– Breast
Teratoma	
Chordoma	

(FLAIR) sequence and T1-weighted images before and after injection of a gadolinium-based contrast medium.

Most tumours appear hypointense on T1 and hyperintense on T2 and FLAIR images. The latter provide a particularly good contrast between normal brain tissue and glial tumours and show signal loss in cystic tumour components.[3] Highly cellular tumours such as lymphomas and primitive neuroectodermal tumours have decreased water content and therefore appear relatively hypointense on T2 images. Intratumoural haemorrhage or calcification is also hypointense on T2 images and becomes more conspicuous on T2* or susceptibility-weighted images (SWI) where magnetic susceptibility effects are stronger. Hyperintensities on T1 images can be due to haemorrhage, calcification, melanin (in metastatic melanomas) or fat.

Enhancement with gadolinium is seen in vascular extra-axial tumours such as meningiomas, and in intra-axial tumours which disrupt the blood–brain barrier. This is generally a feature of high-grade intra-axial tumours, but can also be present in certain low-grade tumours, such as pilocytic astrocytomas and WHO grade II oligodendrogliomas. The visibility of contrast enhancement on MR can be improved by doubling or tripling the gadolinium dose,[4] or by using high relaxivity gadolinium compounds.[5] Post-contrast FLAIR sequences are useful to assess leptomeningeal disease.

MR images may be acquired in an intraoperative setting where an MR imaging facility is available in an operating theatre environment. With tumours, in particular, images may be acquired during surgery, thus guiding the extent of lesion resection in near real time while preserving eloquent regions of the brain.

Advanced Physiological and Molecular Imaging Methods

DWI, PWI, MRS, functional MRI (fMRI) and positron emission tomography (PET) provide additional information about brain tumours which can be useful in specific clinical settings.

MR Perfusion Imaging

There are three main methods of PWI:

1. Dynamic susceptibility-weighted contrast-enhanced (DSC) imaging exploits the susceptibility effects of gadolinium, which, because of its paramagnetic properties, causes a transient signal loss on T2*-weighted images during the passage of a gadolinium bolus.
2. Dynamic contrast-enhanced (DCE) imaging measures the increase of signal intensity on a series of T1-weighted images following gadolinium administration.
3. Arterial spin labelling (ASL) uses magnetically labelled blood as endogenous tracer to assess blood flow and does not require an injection of a contrast medium.

DSC is currently the most widely used perfusion technique in brain tumours. rCBV measurements derived from DSC correlate closely with angiographic and histological markers of tumour vascularity and the expression of vascular endothelial growth factor (VGEF).[6] It provides an indirect measure of tumour neovascularity and high-grade glial tumours tend to have higher rCBV values than low-grade tumours.[7] Leakiness of contrast agent into the extravascular space due to disruption of the blood–brain barrier can lead to inaccuracies of the rCBV calculations in DSC PWI, especially in high-grade tumours. Several mathematical models have been developed to correct for this problem which can also be minimised by administering an extra gadolinium dose prior to DSC PWI ('preloading dose').[8]

In DCE PWI, T1-weighted images are acquired beyond the duration of the first pass of the gadolinium bolus, typically for about 5 min. The shape of the time–signal intensity curve is influenced by tissue perfusion, vascular permeability and the extravascular-extracellular space. Several mathematical models can be used to quantify contrast leakage into the extravascular space as a measure of microvascular permeability. The most frequently used parameter is the transfer coefficient K^{trans} which is influenced by endothelial permeability, vascular surface area and flow. DCE images can also be analysed using a model-free approach by looking at the slope of the time–signal intensity curve.[9]

ASL uses labelling of endogenous hydrogen to measure cerebral blood flow (rCBF).[10] As hydrogen is freely diffusible and crosses the blood–brain barrier immediately, it is not possible to measure tissue blood volume in the same way as with DSC PWI where the tracer (gadolinium) stays (or is assumed to stay) predominantly in the intravascular compartment. Studies of brain tumours have demonstrated, however, a good correlation between rCBF measurements obtained with ASL and rCBV measurements derived from DSC PWI[11] and the clinical use of ASL techniques in neuro-oncology is likely to increase.

MR Diffusion Imaging

DWI measures Brownian motion of water molecules within tissue. The apparent diffusion coefficient (ADC)

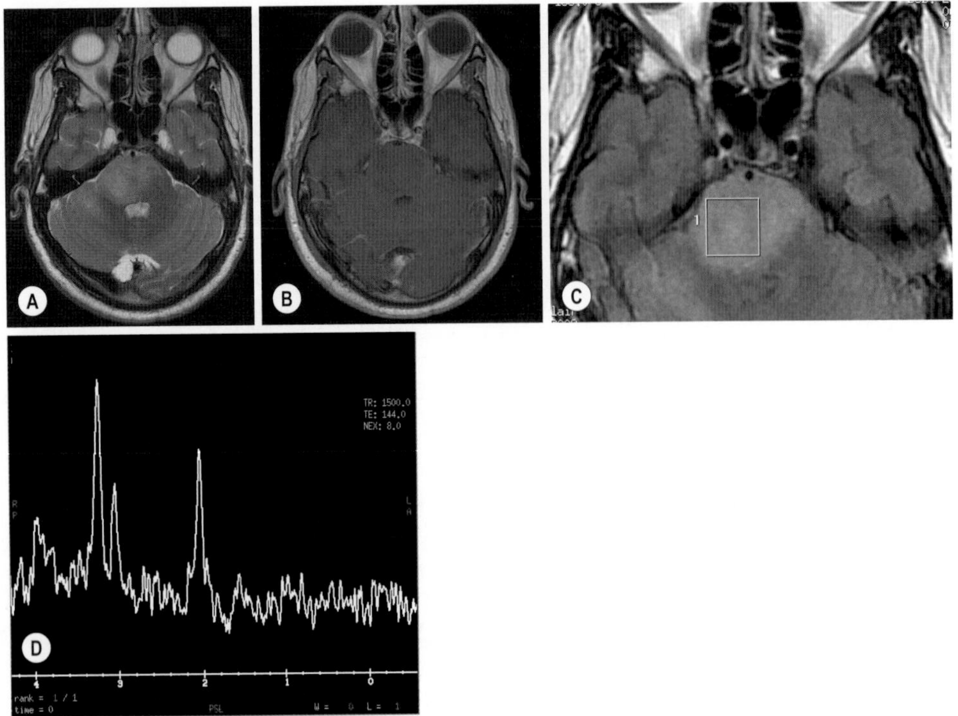

FIGURE 61-1 ■ Proton magnetic resonance spectroscopy. Single voxel magnetic resonance spectroscopy. Diffusely infiltrative brain stem glioma which is hyperintense on T2WI (A) and hypointense on contrast-enhanced T1WI (B). A magnified FLAIR image (C) demonstrates placement of the spectroscopy voxel within the tumour. The spectrum (D) demonstrates that the choline peak (3.22 ppm) is elevated and much higher than the creatine peak (3.03 ppm) and the *N*-acetylaspartate peak (2.01 ppm). (CHO = choline, PCr/Cr = creatine, NAA = *N*-acetylaspartate)

describes the overall water diffusibility in tissue and is an indicator of disruption of tissue microstructure, cellular density and matrix composition in tumours. ADC measurements correlate inversely with the histological cell count of gliomas[12] and positively with the presence of hydrophilic substances in the tumour matrix.[13]

There is increasing evidence that DWI using multiple (low and high) *b* values is helpful in brain tumours.[14]

Diffusion tensor imaging (DTI) provides additional information about the direction of water diffusion.[15] The tendency of water to move in some directions more than others is called anisotropy and can be quantified using parameters such as fractional anisotropy (FA). Compact white matter tracts show normally a high degree of anisotropy that can be lost if they are infiltrated by tumour cells which destroy the ultrastructural boundaries formed by myelin sheaths.

Post-processing of DTI allows the depiction of important white matter tracts and their connections (tractography), which can be displayed in direction-encoded colour images. Tractography is useful in the preoperative assessment of brain tumours and helps to differentiate between displacement and infiltration of white matter tracts.[16]

MR Spectroscopy

MRS analyses the biochemistry of a brain tumour and provides semiquantitative information about major metabolites.[17,18] A common pattern in brain tumours is a decrease in *N*-acetylaspartate (NAA), a neuron-specific marker, and creatine (Cr), and an increase in choline (Cho), lactate (Lac) and lipids (L) (Fig. 61-1). The concentration of Cho is a reflection of the turnover of cell membranes (due to accelerated synthesis and destruction) and is more elevated in regions with a high neoplastic activity. Lactate (Lac) is the end product of non-oxidative glycolysis and a marker of hypoxia in tumour tissue. This is of interest, as tumour hypoxia is now recognised as a major promoter of tumour angiogenesis and invasion. Lac is probably associated with viable but hypoxic tissue, whereas mobile lipids is thought to reflect tissue necrosis with breakdown of cell membranes.

The choice of echo time (TE) is an important technical consideration for performing MRS. It can be short (20–40 ms), intermediate (135–144 ms) or long (270–288 ms). MRS with a short TE has the advantage of demonstrating additional metabolites which may improve tumour characterisation, such as *myo*-inositol, glutamate/glutamine (Glx) and lipids, but is hampered by baseline distortion and artefactual NAA peaks. Intermediate echo times have a better defined baseline and quantification of NAA and Cho is more accurate and reproducible. Long echo times lead to a decrease of signal to noise.

MRS is presently a sensitive but not very specific technique. Single voxel spectroscopy provides good-quality spectra but is prone to sampling errors. Chemical shift imaging (CSI) is technically more demanding but provides 2D or 3D spectra and larger area coverage. With 3T MRI systems it is now possible to obtain a 16 × 16 × 16 array of spectra with a voxel size of 1 cm^3 in 5–10 min.[19]

fMRI

Blood oxygen level-dependent (BOLD) imaging detects changes in regional cerebral blood flow during various forms of brain activity. Paradigms using motor tasks, language and speech productions and memory are able to show activation of relevant cortical areas. The main use of fMRI in tumour imaging is the preoperative localisation of eloquent cortical regions which may have been displaced, distorted or compressed by the tumour[18] and identifying any evidence of functional reorganisation. This can improve the safety of surgery and allow for a more radical resection. The BOLD effect is an **indirect** measure of neuronal activity that may be influenced by numerous physiological factors as well as the MR relaxation properties of soft tissue such that activation within a tumour may reflect angiogenesis rather than eloquent function and susceptibility effects from blood products, for instance, may mask areas of brain activation. Other important caveats include the inability of discriminating between indispensable and expandable brain regions and accurate assessment of the distance between a lesion and an area of functional activity. To this effect, other non-BOLD techniques such as arterial spin labelling (ASL) are being developed and may reduce these pitfalls in the futures.

When possible an indicated fMRI should be combined with MR tractrography in order to minimise intra-operative injury to white matter tracts connected to eloquent cortical areas (Fig. 61-2).

Positron-Emission Tomography (PET)

The most widely used PET tracer in oncological imaging is fluorodeoxyglucose [^{18}F] (FDG), which provides a measure of glucose metabolism that correlates closely with the proliferative activity of tumours. Its limitation in neuro-oncoly is the high physiological baseline glucose metabolism of the brain., which may result in a poor lesion to background contrast. New PET radiopharmaceuticals, for brain tumour imaging[20] include amino acid analogues such as [^{11}C]methionine (MET) and [^{18}F]fluoroethyl-L-tyrosine (FET), nucleoside analogues such as [^{18}F]fluorothymidine (FLT) and hypoxia markers such as [^{18}F]fluoromisonidazole (F-MISO). Radioactively labelled choline, [^{11}C]choline (CHO) or [^{18}F]choline, can be used to assess membrane cell turnover and 68Ga-DOTATOC shows a high uptake in meningiomas.[21]

PET imaging is currently mostly used in combination with computed tomography (PET/CT), but the availability of PET/MRI systems is likely to increase in future, allowing simultaneous acquisition and registration of high-resolution MR sequences and molecular information from PET.

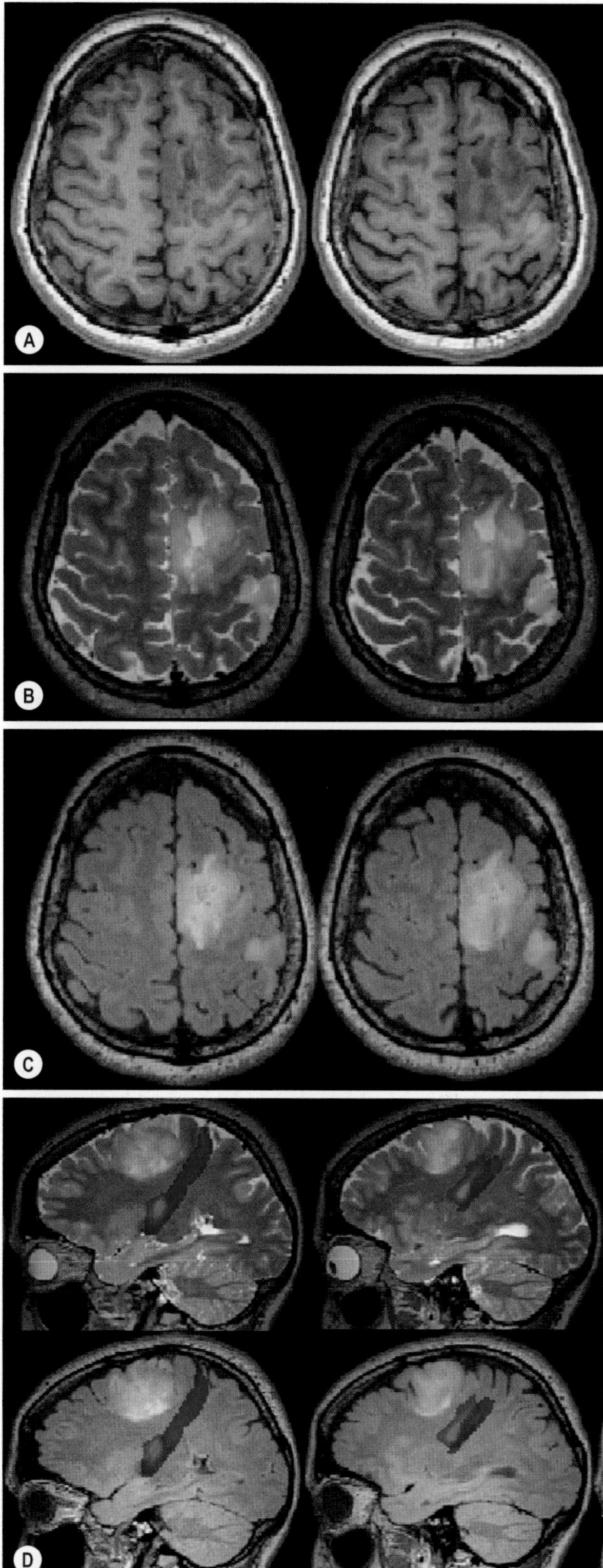

FIGURE 61-2 ■ fMRI in a patient with a frontal low-grade glioma. The fMRI of right-hand movement shows activation in the left pre- and post-central gyri, posterolateral to the tumour which appears hypointense on TW1 (A), and hyperintense on T2WI (B) and FLAIR images (C). Sagittal images of DTI (D) show non-invaded corticospinal tracts posterior to the tumour (right hand in red and, right foot in blue).

CLASSIFICATION OF INTRACRANIAL TUMOURS

There are several ways of classifying brain tumours: primary versus secondary intra-axial (arising from the brain parenchyma) versus extra-axial (arising from tissues covering the brian, such as the dura), and various regional classifications (supratentorial, infratentorial, intraventricular, pineal region and sellar region tumours).

The World Health Organisation (WHO) classification of intracranial tumours is a universally accepted histological classification of brain tumours. It was extensively revised in 1993 with the incorporation of immunohistochemistry into diagnostic pathology and updated in 2000, when genetic profiles were added, stratifying neoplasms by their overall biological potential.[22,23] The latest revision is from 2007 with the introduction of eight new entities and three new variants to the previous classification.[24] The WHO classification no longer relies on standard pathological features alone but includes information from immunochemistry and molecular tumour profiling. An outline of this classification is given in Table 61-2.

Intra-axial tumours, which conform largely to the tissue types 1, 4, 5 and 9, will be discussed first, followed by extra-axial tumours corresponding to the tissue types 2, 3, 6, 7 and 8.

TABLE 61-2 **Abbreviated WHO Classification of Brain Tumours**

1	**Tumours of Neuroepithelial Tissue**
1.1	Astrocytic tumours
1.2	Oligodendroglial tumours
1.3	Oligoastrocytic tumours
1.4	Ependymal tumours
1.5	Choroid plexus tumours
1.6	Other neuroepithelial tumours
1.7	Neuronal and mixed neuronal-glial tumours
1.8	Pineal region tumours
1.9	Embryonal tumours
2	**Tumours of Cranial and Paraspinal Nerves**
2.1	Schwannoma
2.2	Neurofibroma
3	**Tumours of the Meninges**
3.1	Meningioma
3.2	Mesenchymal tumours
3.3	Haemangioblastoma
4	**Lymphoma and Haematopoietic Tumours**
5	**Germ Cell Tumours**
5.1	Germinoma
5.2	Teratoma
5.3	Choriocarcinoma
5.4	Other germ cell tumours
6	**Cysts and Tumour-Like Conditions**
6.1	Rathke's cleft cyst
6.2	Epidermoid cyst
6.3	Dermoid cyst
6.4	Colloid cyst
7	**Tumours of the Sellar Region**
7.1	Pituitary adenoma
7.2	Craniopharyngioma
7.3	Others
8	**Local Extension from Regional Tumours**
9	**Metastases**

INTRA-AXIAL TUMOURS

NEUROEPITHELIAL TUMOURS

Neuroepithelial tumours account for 50–60% of all primary brain tumours and represent a broad spectrum of neoplasms arising from or sharing morphological properties of neuroepithelial cells. They include glial neoplasms, choroid plexus tumours, tumours with predominant neuronal phenotype (ganglioglioma, dysembryoplastic neuroepithelial tumour and neurocytoma), pineal tumours and embryonal tumours (neuroectodermal tumours, medulloblastoma).

Gliomas

Gliomas are the commonest neuroepithelial tumours and may originate from astrocytic or oligodendrocytic cell lines. Assessment of the DNA profile and gene expression in tumours plays an increasing role in the characterisation of gliomas and has prognostic implications.[25]

Presently the most relevant molecular and gene abnormalities are isocitrate dehydrogenase (IDH1 or IDH2) mutation, 1p and 19q chromosomal translocation, methylation status of the DNA repair gene 0-6-methylguanine-DNA-methyltransferase (MGMT) and overexpression of the epidermal growth factor receptor (EGFR).

Astrocytic Tumours

Astrocytomas account for approximately 75% of glial neoplasms and range from the benign pilocytic astrocytomas (WHO grade I) to glioblastoma (WHO grade IV), the most malignant astrocytic tumour, and show a distinct age distribution: pilocytic astrocytomas (WHO grade 1) occur mainly in children and young adults; infiltrative low-grade astrocytomas (WHO grade II) are most frequent in the third decade of life; anaplastic astrocytomas (WHO grade III) have a peak incidence around 40 years; and glioblastoma (WHO grade IV) usually occurs after 40 years.

Pilocytic astrocytomas are non-invasive, well-circumscribed, potentially resectable neoplasms which are classified as WHO grade I. They have a low proliferative potential, do not show any IDH mutations and have a predilection for the posterior fossa (Fig. 61-3) and optic nerve/chiasm in children and young adults. Cerebral pilocytic astrocytomas are much less common and usually seen in an older age group (Fig. 61-4). Pilocytic astrocytomas have usually a cystic component and show enhancement, which can be nodular or ring-like. Infratentorial pilocytic astrocytomas in adults are frequently mistaken for haemangioblastomas, which have a similar appearance and represent the commonest primary intra-axial tumour below the tentorium cerebelli in adults, associated in about 20% with von Hippel–Lindau disease. There is evidence that DSC perfusion imaging may help distinguish between the two, as haemangioblastomas have a considerably higher rCBV than pilocytic astrocytomas.[26]

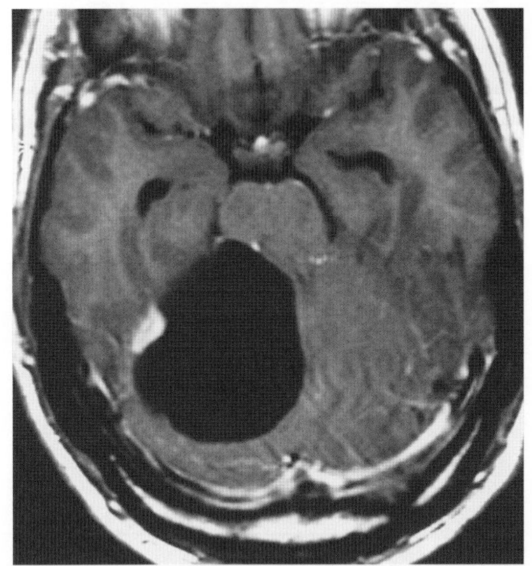

FIGURE 61-3 ■ Cerebellar pilocytic astrocytoma. Axial T1W post-gadolinium MRI. There is a cystic lesion in the cerebellum with a small, enhancing mural nodule but otherwise non-enhancing cyst wall. The fourth ventricle is compressed, causing hydrocephalus (note enlargement of the temporal horns). The differential diagnosis of this lesion is a cerebellar haemangioblastoma.

Diffuse astrocytomas (WHO grade II) are infiltrating low-grade tumours which occur typically in the cerebral hemispheres of young adults, involving cortex and white matter with less well-defined borders than pilocytic astrocytomas. WHO grade II astrocytomas have a low mitotic activity but show a propensity to progress to a higher histological grade, usually within 3–10 years. They frequently show IDH1 and IDH2 mutations, which have a favourable impact on overall survival.[27] WHO grade II astrocytomas appear iso- or hypodense on CT and show areas of calcification in up to 20%. MRI is better in defining the extent of the low-grade gliomas (Fig. 61-5). They are hyperintense on T2 images and FLAIR images and hypo/isointense on T1 images and show no contrast enhancement as opposed to pilocytic (WHO grade I) and anaplastic (WHO grade III) astrocytomas.

Anaplastic astrocytomas (WHO grade III) are high-grade gliomas with an increased mitotic activity and raised immunohistochemical proliferation indices. The majority of anaplastic astrocytomas show contrast enhancement but up to a third may be non-enhancing.[28] Infiltration of the peritumoural tissues is more extensive than in grade II lesions.[29,30]

Pleomorphic xanthoastrocytoma (PXA) is a rare, relatively benign low-grade tumour arising near the surface of the brain, with a predilection for the temporal lobe, and presents usually with epilepsy in children and young adults. The tumour is usually well circumscribed, may enhance strongly and has a cystic component in over 50%. Despite its fat content, it is T1 hypointense and T2 hyperintense on MRI. It can occasionally transform to a more aggressive anaplastic WHO grade III tumour.

Glioblastoma (WHO grade IV) has the worst prognosis but is unfortunately also the commonest primary intracranial neoplasm in adults,[31] showing poorly differentiated, often highly pleomorphic glial tumour cells with florid microvascular proliferation and necrosis. About 90% of glioblastomas arise de novo (primary glioblastoma) and 10% are from malignant transformation of

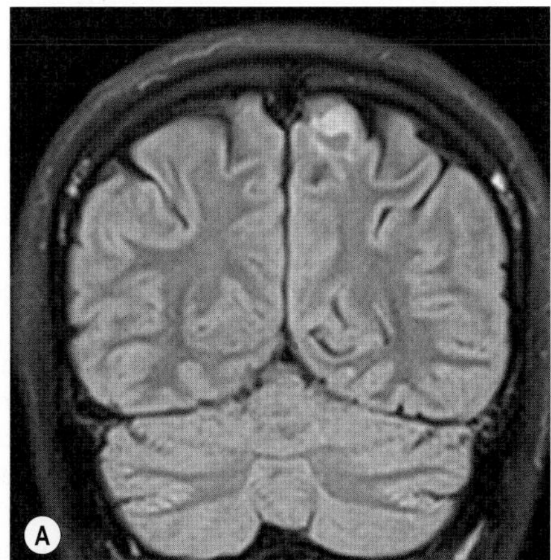

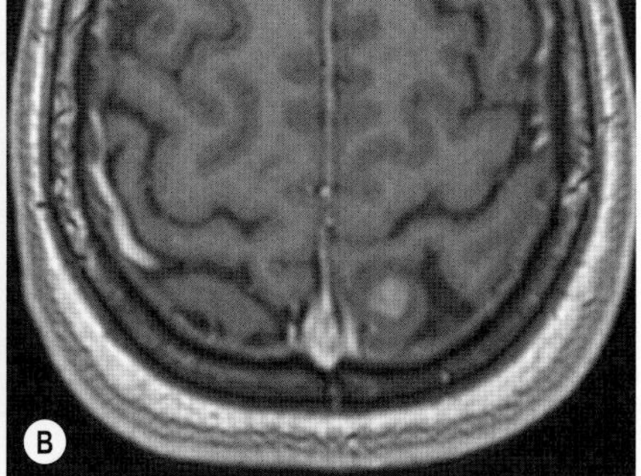

FIGURE 61-4 ■ Cerebral pilocytic astrocytoma in a young adult female patient presenting with epilepsy. FLAIR image (A) shows a well-defined, partially solid (hyperintense) and partially cystic (hypointense) lesion involving the left parietal cortex. The contrast-enhanced T1WI (B) shows uniform enhancement of the solid component.

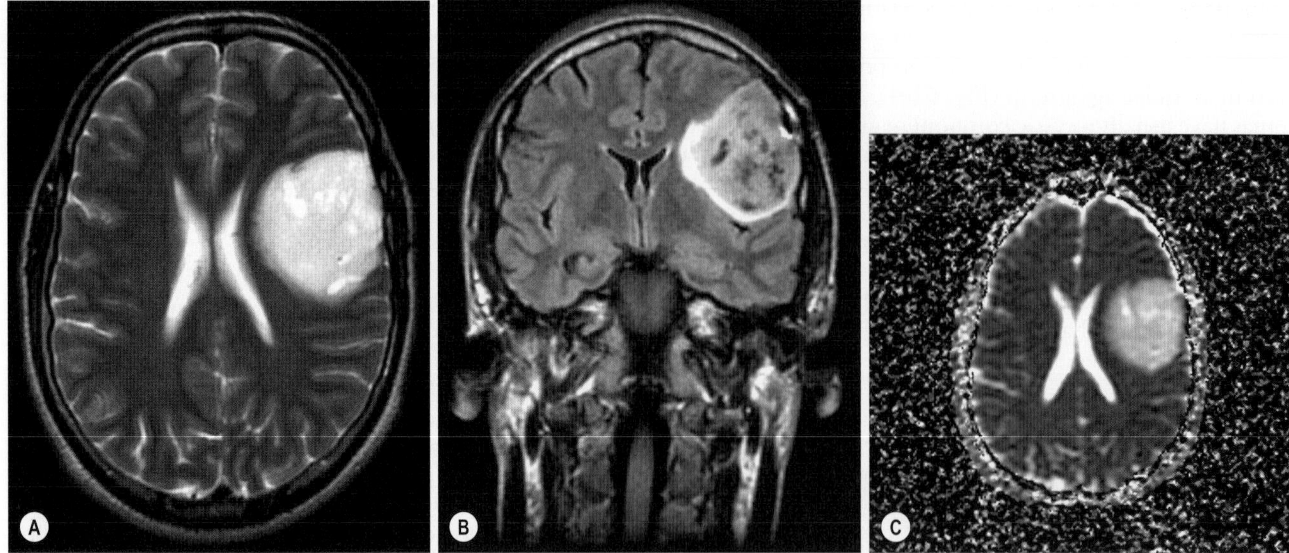

FIGURE 61-5 ■ Low-grade glioma (WHO grade II astrocytoma). Axial T2W (A), FLAIR (B) images showing a left frontal hyperintense mass lesion with well-defined borders and small cystic areas. On the ADC map (C) the glioma is easily identified as an area of increased diffusivity compared to normal brain parenchyma.

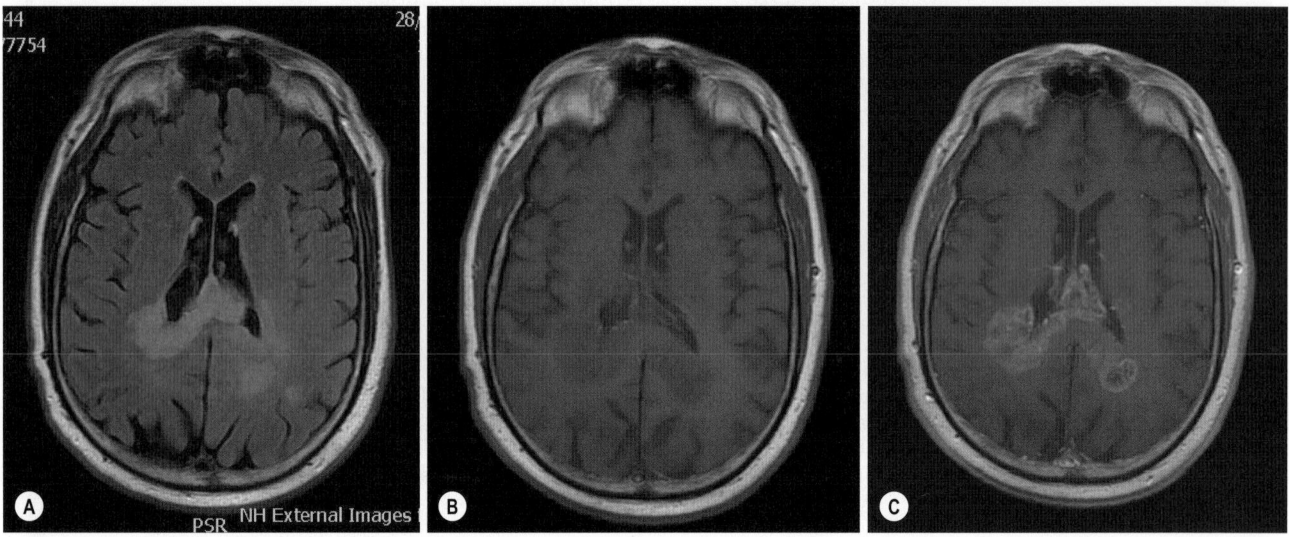

FIGURE 61-6 ■ Glioblastoma. A 55-year-old patient with a 'butterfly' glioblastoma. The tumour appears hyperintense on FLAIR images (A) and infiltrates and thickens the splenium of the corpus callosum and surrounds the trigones of both lateral ventricles. On the pre-contrast T1WI images (B) the glioblastoma appears hypointense and the post-contrast T1WI (C) shows widespread inhomogeneous enhancement of the tumour.

lower-grade astrocytomas (secondary glioblastoma). The two groups have different genetic characteristics: primary glioblastomas, which occurs in a slightly older age group, show EGFR overexpression and secondary glioblastomas show IDH mutations like the lower-grade gliomas from which they arise. Methylation of the DNA repair gene MGMT is associated with a better response to temozolomide and better prognosis in glioblastomas.

The MRI appearances of glioblastomas are heterogeneous, showing a mixture of solid tumour portions, central necrosis and surrounding oedema. The solid portion is usually T1 hypo and T2/FLAIR hyperintense but to a lesser degree than the areas of central necrosis and surrounding oedema, which have signal intensities similar to CSF on T2 images. The oedema is usually infiltrated by strands of tumour cells, which cannot be detected on standard MR images. The solid portion of the glioblastomas may show complete or partial or enhancement with contrast (Fig. 61-6). The extent of enhancement of the solid tumour seems to correspond to different molecular profiles and appears to have an influence on patient survival.[32,33]

The standard treatment for glioblastoma (GBM) consists of surgery (with a variable extent of resection depending on tumour location and the patient's clinical status), followed by a combination of radiotherapy and chemotherapy with temozolomide. Second-line treatment includes anti-angiogenesis drugs and other experimental drugs. The assessment of tumour response and progression in GBM had traditionally been based on measurements of enhancing tumour portions known as Macdonald criteria.[34] With the advent of combined chemoradiation as standard therapy and antiangiogentic drugs as second-line treatment, new phenomena such a pseudoprogression and pseudoresponse have to be taken into account and have made an assessment solely based on assessment of enhancing tumour portion unreliable.[35,36] The Response Assessment in Neuro-Oncology (RANO) Working Group has therefore published recommendations for updated response criteria for high-grade gliomas.[37]

Pseudoprogression is due to an inflammatory reaction, which results in a temporary increase of contrast enhancement and oedema, usually within 12 weeks of chemoradiation, and subsides subsequently without additional treatment (Fig. 61-7). Pseudoprogression is more frequently observed in patients with methylation of the DNA repair gene MGMT, and is associated with a better prognosis (longer overall survival). There are certain histological similarities between the inflammatory response in pseudoprogression and classical radiation necrosis

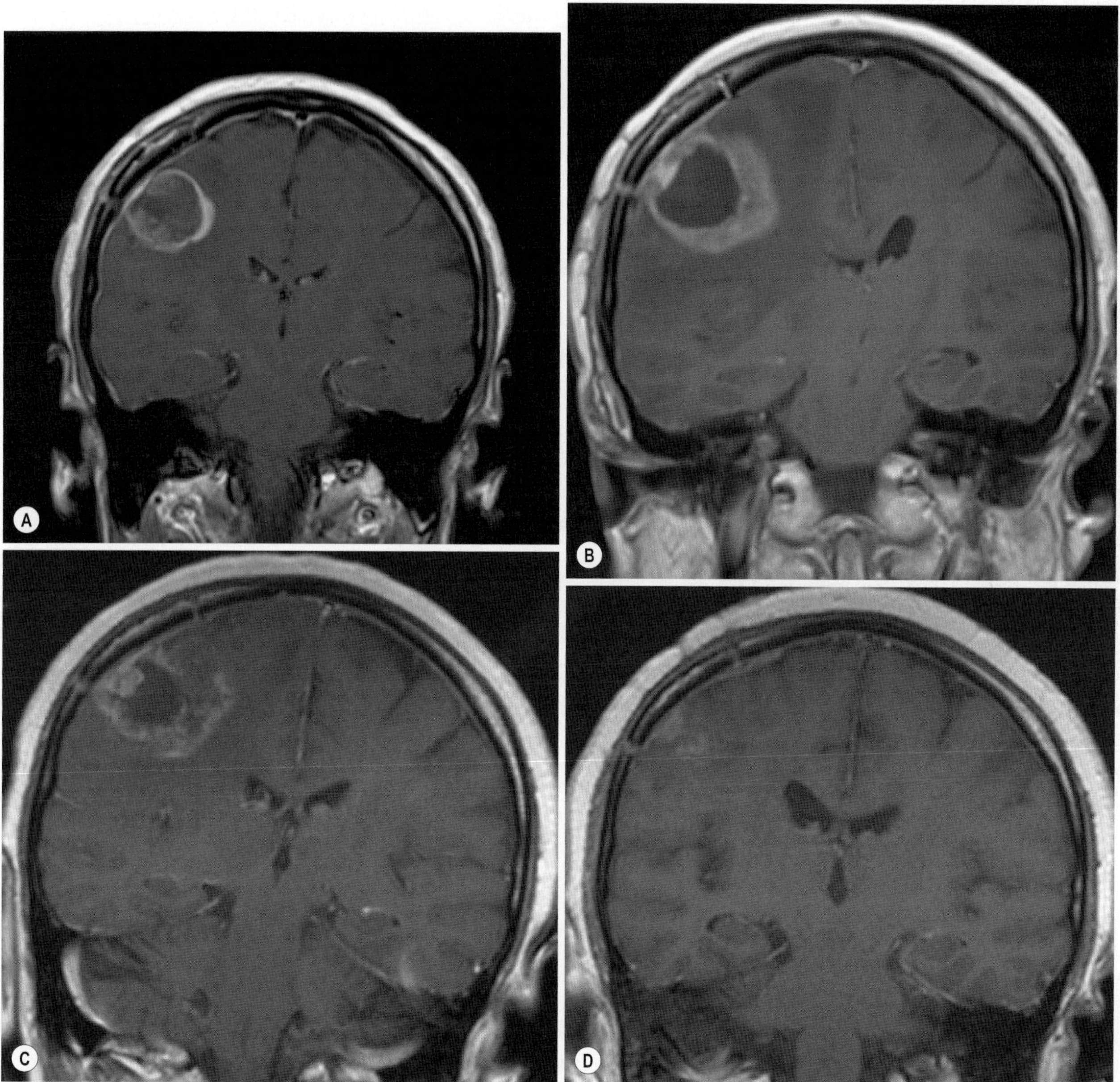

FIGURE 61-7 ■ **Pseudoprogression.** Series of contrast-enhanced T1WI in a patient with glioblastoma before (A) and at 6 weeks (B), 16 weeks (C) and 6 months (D) after treatment with temozolomide and radiotherapy. The baseline images (A) show an irregular ring-enhancing mass lesion. Six weeks following combined chemoradiation (B) there is an increase of enhancement and associated oedema. Both the enhancement and oedema decrease subsequently (C, D) without altering the treatment, leaving a small amount of residual enhancement at the site of the tumour after 6 months (D). The time course of these appearances is typical for 'pseudoprogression', an inflammatory response to chemoradiation associated with a favourable outcome.

which is a delayed complication of radiation treatment occurring 6–12 months after treatment. Advanced MR imaging such as DSC and DCE perfusion imaging shows promise in differentiating theses two conditions from true tumour progression.

Pseudoresponse is characterised by a decrease of enhancement and oedema following the administration of antiangiogenic drugs without improved survival.[37,38] In pseudoresponse the tumour progresses by infiltrative patterns without neoangiogenesis, resulting in an increase of non-enhancing T2/FLAIR hyperintense tumour portions (Fig. 61-8).

Antiangiogenic treatment can also be associated with non-enhancing areas of markedly decreased ADC, which appears to correspond to an atypical gelatinous necrotic tissue rather than tumour and are associated with improved outcome.[39]

Oligodendrogliomas account for 10–15% of all gliomas and occur predominantly in adults. They are diffusely infiltrating neoplasms, which are found almost exclusively in the cerebral hemispheres, most commonly in the frontal lobes, and typically involving subcortical white matter and cortex (Fig. 61-9). The WHO classification distinguishes between WHO grade II (well-differentiated low-grade) and WHO grade III (anaplastic high-grade) oligodendrogliomas. The former are slowly-growing tumours with rounded homogeneous nuclei; the latter have increased tumour cell density, mitotic activity,

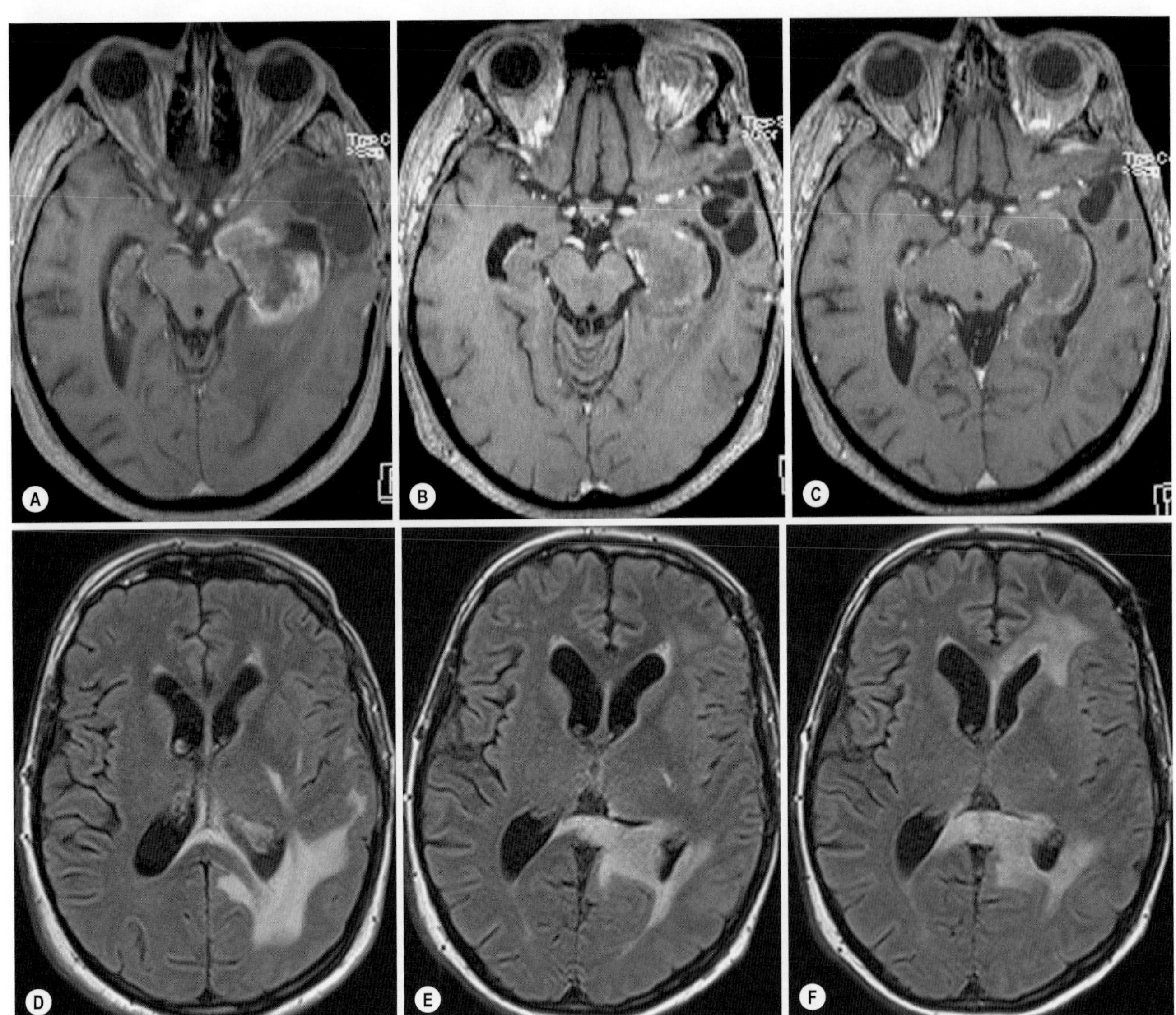

FIGURE 61-8 ■ Pseudoresponse. Series of contrast-enhanced T1WI (A–C) and FLAIR images (D–F) in a patient with glioblastoma receiving anti-VGEF therapy as second-line treatment. The baseline images show an enhancing tumour component in the left temporal lobe and a non-enhancing FLAIR hyperintense component in the left peritrigonal region extending into the splenium of the corpus callosum (D). Six weeks after anti-angiogenesis treatment there is marked decrease of enhancement (B) and some resolution of oedema in the left peritrigonal region (E); there is, however, thickening and increased signal intensity of the splenium of the corpus callosum consistent with increasing amount of tumour infiltration. Sixteen weeks post-treatment the enhancement remains minimal (C) but there has been a further increase in the non-enhancing infiltrative tumour in the splenium of the corpus callosum and also around the frontal horn of the left lateral ventricle (F). These appearances are typical for 'pseudoresponse'.

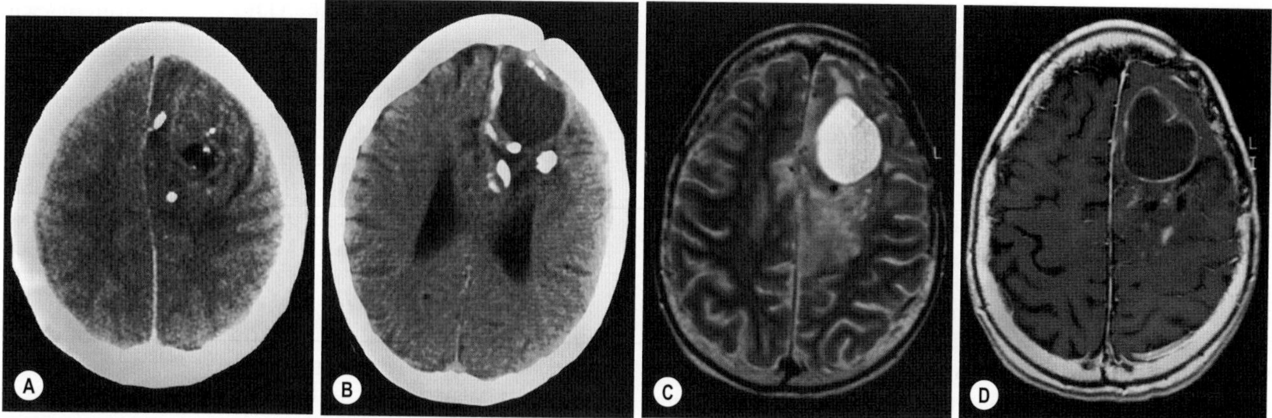

FIGURE 61-9 ■ WHO grade II oligodendroglioma. CT after IV contrast medium (A) shows a large left frontal tumour that involves the cortex. It is predominantly solid with irregular enhancement, but there are also cysts and coarse calcification. Follow-up after 2 years with CT (B), T2W MRI (C) and T1W post-contrast MRI (D) shows more extensive cyst formation and calcification than on the first image. The calcification is much less apparent on MRI and appears as non-specific low signal areas. Posterior infiltration of the tumour is, however, best seen on MRI (C). Note that the patient had undergone a left frontal craniotomy after the first CT.

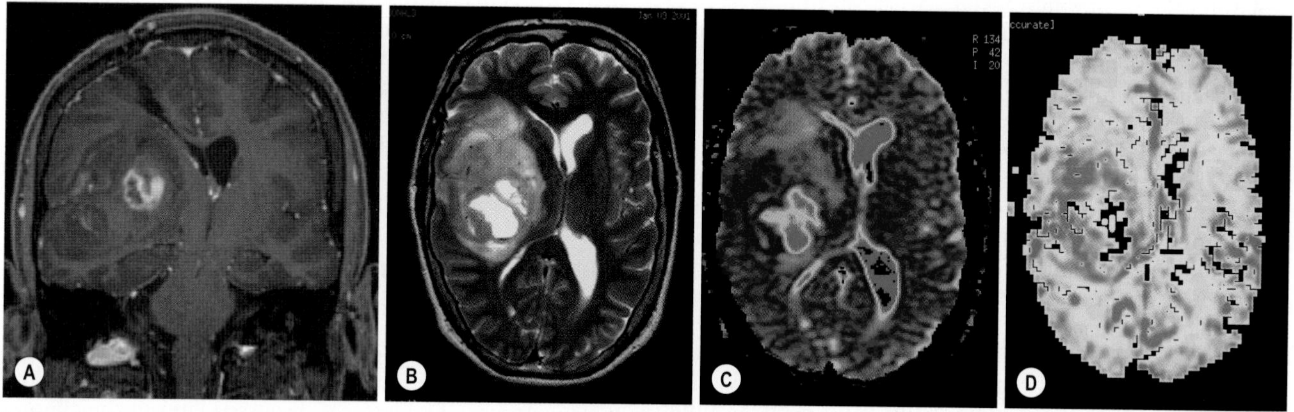

FIGURE 61-10 ■ Grade III oligodendroglioma. Post-contrast T1WI (A), T2WI (B), ADC map of diffusion-weighted MRI (C) and rCBV of perfusion-weighted MRI (D) of a WHO grade III oligodendroglioma. There is patchy enhancement within the tumour (A). The T2WI (B) show a central hyperintense cystic area surrounded by more hypointense solid tumour components which have a decreased ADC corresponding to the dark blue areas in (C) and increased rCBV, corresponding to the dark red areas in (D).

microvascular proliferation and necrosis. Both low- and high-grade oligodendral tumours express proangiogenic mitogens and may contain regions of increased vascular density with finely branching capillaries that have a 'chicken wire' appearance. This contributes to their appearance on contrast-enhanced MRI and MRP. Up to 90% of oligodendrogliomas contain visible calcification on CT, which can be central, peripheral or ribbon-like (Fig. 61-9).[40] On MRI, intratumoural calcification appears typically T2 hypo- and T1 hyperintense and causes marked signal loss on T2* or SWI images. Intratumoural haemorrhage, which occurs uncommonly in oligodendrogliomas, may have a similar appearance. Contrast enhancement is variable and often heterogeneous. Unlike in astrocytomas, contrast enhancement is not a reliable indicator of tumour grade it oligodendrogliomas: it occurs in about 20% of WHO grade II tumours and in over 70% of WHO grade III oligodendrogliomas.[41] Low-grade oligodendrogliomas may also have an elevated rCBV on PWI.[42]

Allelic loss on the chromosomes 1p and 19q is present in 80% of oligodendrogliomas and is associated with better response to chemotherapy. Oligodendrogliomas with 1p/19q loss appear to have a significantly higher rCBV than those with intact 1p and 19q[43] (Fig. 61-10). Conventional MR images may provide a further clue to the oligodendroglioma genotype: tumours with intact 1p/19q show more homogeneous signal on T1- and T2-weighted (T1W, T2W) images and have sharper borders than the tumours with chromosome deletions.[44,45]

MRS of low-grade tumours with oligodendral elements shows increased levels of *myo*-inositol/glycine as well as glutamine and glutamate.[17]

The Role of Advanced Physiological MR Imaging in Glial Tumours

The use of PWI, DWI and MRS as an adjunct to structural imaging can improve the prediction of the histological tumour type and grade, tumour infiltration of surrounding tissue, treatment response and patient survival. These techniques are also helpful for differentiating treatment-related complications from tumour progression. Low-grade (WHO grade II) oligodendrogliomas tend to have higher rCBV values and lower ADC values than WHO grade II astrocytomas.[46] This can be explained by increased vascular density and higher cellular density in low-grade oligodendrogliomas and differences in tumour matrix composition.

Several studies have shown the use of PWI to distinguish low-grade from high-grade glial tumours. The formation of new blood vessel (angiogenesis) represents an important aspect of tumour progression and growth in glial tumours, and is reflected in the much higher rCBV values of WHO grade III and IV tumours compared to WHO grade II tumours. PWI significantly increases the sensitivity and positive predictive value of conventional MR imaging in glioma grading with a sensitivity of 95% for distinguishing low-grade from high-grade gliomas when an rCBV threshold of 1.75 is used.[47]

Combining minimum ADC with maximum rCBV measurements further improves the accuracy of glioma grading, particularly the distinction between WHO grade II and III tumours.[48] For oligodendrogliomas ADC values were better than rCBV values in distinguishing between WHO grade II and III tumours.[41]

DWI appears also useful to identify the MGMT promotor methylation status in glioblastomas. Tumours with methylated MGMT, which have a better prognosis, demonstrated a significantly higher minimum ADC.[49]

In MRS, glial tumours are characterised by an increase in Cho and decrease in NAA, which can be expressed in a choline to NAA index (CNI). Low-grade tumours have generally a lower CNI than high-grade tumours; WHO grade IV tumours show additionally an increase in lipid and lactate as markers of hypoxia and necrosis.[19]

Infiltration of peritumoural regions in gliomas can also be assessed with physiology-based MR techniques.[16,19] The peritumoural regions of high-grade gliomas show a more marked decrease in ADC, fractional anisotropy and NAA and increase in CBV compared to low-grade tumours. This is a reflection of the more invasive nature of these tumours, which destroy ultrastructural boundaries with a consequent decrease in ADC and FA; and replace normal brain tissue, resulting in a drop of NAA. Metastases, on the other hand, are surrounded by 'pure' vasogenic oedema, which contains no infiltrating tumour cells. The peritumoural regions in metastases show therefore no increase in rCBV or decrease in FA.

Physiological and molecular MR imaging have also a role in predicting patient survival and treatment response.

Measurements on baseline rCBV in gliomas are strongly predictive of patient outcome[50] and have proved to be a better predictor of time to progression than histological grading.[51] Diffusion tensor imaging can be used to grade the invasiveness of glioblastoma, which correlates with progression-free survival.[52]

Response to radiation and/or chemotherapy may be evident on PWI, DWI and MRS before any significant tumour volume changes occur.[19] Indicators of a good response to therapy are an early decrease of rCBV and an early increase of ADC.[53,54] Treatment with antiangiogenic agents usually results in a rapid decrease of permeability (K^{trans}) and rCBV.

Treatment complications can also be assessed with PWI, DWI and MRS. The role of these methods in distinguishing radiation necrosis from tumour recurrence is well established,[9,55,56] and there is increasing evidence that these techniques are also helpful in the diagnosis of pseudoprogression.[36,57,58]

Radiation necrosis is a late complication of radiotherapy or gamma knife surgery, and can present as an enhancing mass lesion, difficult to distinguish from recurrent tumour on conventional imaging.[56] FDG-PET, PWI and DWI may help to distinguish between radiation necrosis and tumour recurrence (Fig. 61-11).[56,59] In radiation necrosis the enhancing lesion has a low glucose metabolism (FDG uptake) and low rCBV, both of which tend to be high in tumour recurrence. On DCE perfusion imaging, recurrent tumours show a much higher maximum slope of enhancement than radiation necrosis.[9] ADC measurements of the enhancing components in recurrent tumour are significantly lower than in radiation necrosis, mirroring the higher cellular density in recurrent neoplasms.

In addition to the above indications, PWI, DWI and MRS may in future be increasingly used in the context of stereotactic tumour biopsies and help to direct tissue sampling towards areas with maximal angiogenesis, cellular density and metabolic activity.

Tumours of Predominantly Neuronal Cell Origin

These include gangliocytomas, gangliogliomas, dysembryoplastic neuroepithelial tumours (DNET) and central neurocytomas. The latter is discussed later in the chapter in the section 'Intraventricular Tumours'.

Gangliogliomas and Gangliocytomas

These are slow-growing tumours with a low malignant potential, which occur preferentially in young adults and in the temporal lobe presenting with epilepsy. Gangliogliomas contain a mixture of neural and glial elements with neoplastic large ganglion cells; gangliocytomas have only neuronal elements. CT and MRI show peripherally located mixed solid/cystic lesions which commonly calcify. Enhancement can be variable and is often peripheral (Fig. 61-12).

Dysembryoplastic neuroepithelial tumours (DNETs) are highly polymorphic tumours that arise during embryogenesis. They are preferentially located in the supratentorial cortex and frequently manifest through intractable complex partial seizures. DNETs appear variable on imaging but are usually hypodense on CT and T1 hypointense and T2 hyperintense on MRI (Fig. 61-13). Small intratumoural cysts may be present and cause a 'bubbly' appearance. Calcification is seen in about 25% and they enhance in 20–40% of cases. Thinning of the overlying bone is present in approximately half of the cases, reflecting the extremely slow growth of these tumours which allows bone remodelling to occur.[60]

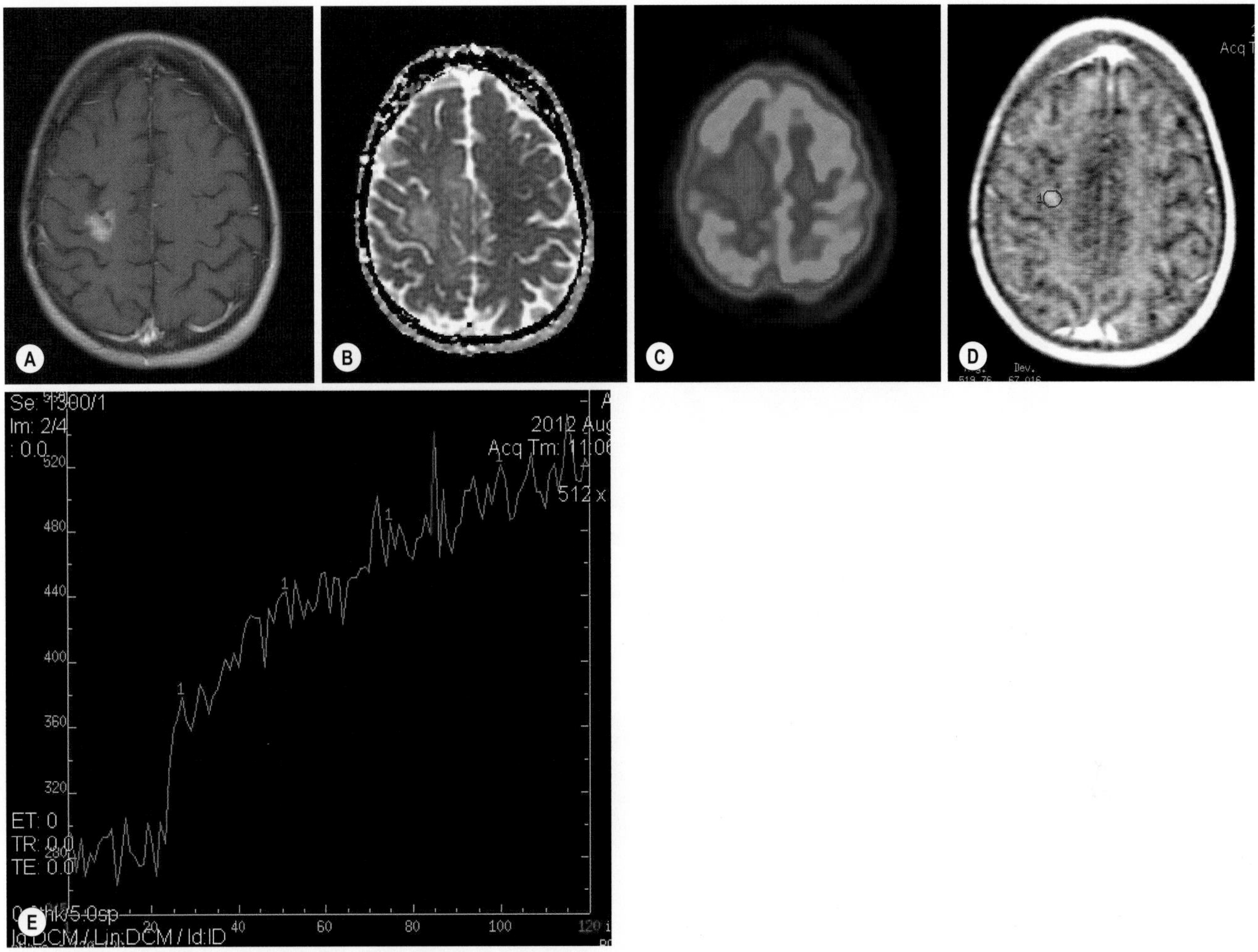

FIGURE 61-11 ■ **Radiation necrosis.** Contrast-enhanced T1WI (A), ADC map (B), FDG-PET (C) and DCE perfusion imaging (D, E) in a patient with radiation necrosis following radiotherapy for a high-grade glioma. On the contrast-enhanced T1WI (A) there is an enhancing area which is indistinguishable from tumour recurrence. The corresponding region shows an increased ADC (B) and decreased glucose metabolism on the FDG-PET (C). A ROI placed over this area on DCE perfusion images (D) demonstrates a slow rise of signal intensity without washout (E). All the findings in (B–E) are typical for radiation necrosis and not for tumour recurrence.

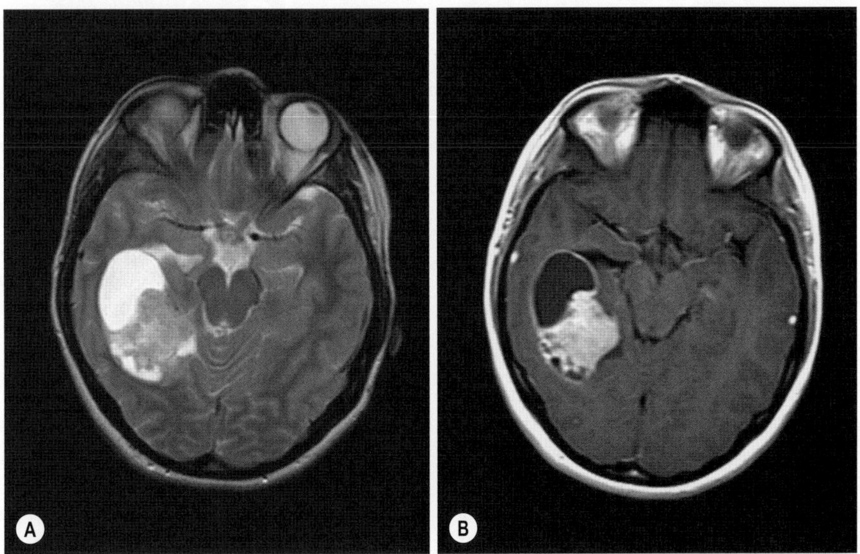

FIGURE 61-12 ■ **Ganglioglioma (WHO grade I).** T2WI (A) and post-contrast T1WI (B) of a WHO grade I ganglioglioma showing a well-defined, non-infiltrating tumour with a cystic component anteriorly and markedly enhancing solid component posteriorly. There is also enhancement of the cyst wall.

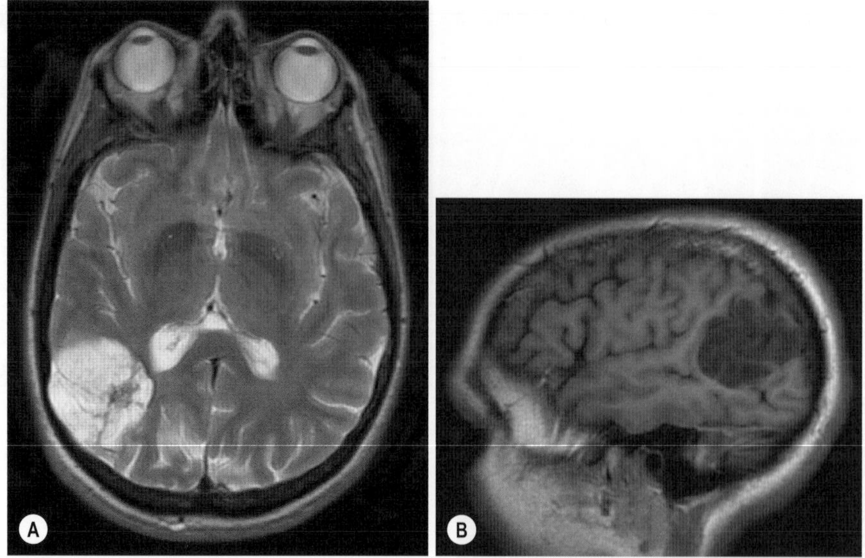

FIGURE 61-13 ■ **Dysembryoplastic neuroepithelial tumour (DNET).** An axial T2WI (A) and a sagittal T1WI (B) showing a T1-hypointesne and T2-hyperintense cortically based tumour with a 'bubbly' appearance. Thinning and remodelling of the overlying bone is also demonstrated.

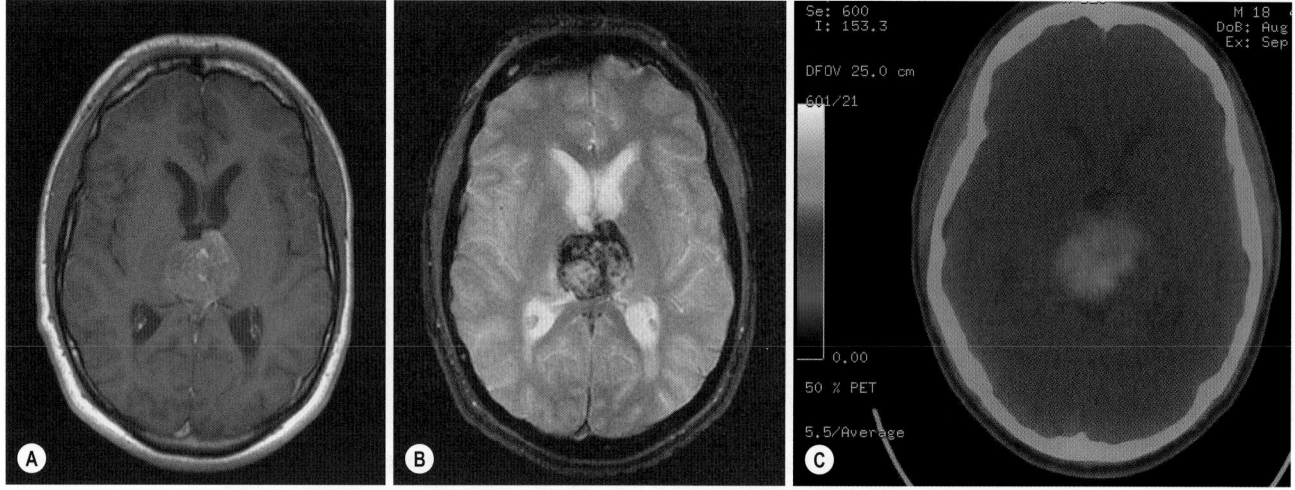

FIGURE 61-14 ■ **Pineal tumour.** Pineal germ cell tumour in an 18-year-old male patient presenting with Parinaud's syndrome. Contrast-enhanced T1WI (A) shows an enhancing pineal region tumour compressing the third ventricle, which contains areas of susceptibility artefact (signal dropout) on T2*WI (B) and avid tracer uptake on a choline PET (C).

Pineal Region Tumours

Pineal region tumours account for approximately 1% of intracranial tumours in adults, whereas they represent 10% of all paediatric brain tumours. They present either with obstructive hydrocephalus secondary to aqueduct compression or with problems with eye movements and accommodation, caused by compression of the underlying tectal plate. More than half of all pineal region tumours are of germ cell origin (germinoma, teratoma, yolk sac tumours and choriocarcinoma).[61] The diagnosis of a germ cell tumour is often made by the presence of marker proteins (such as α-fetoprotein or chorionic gonadotrophin) in the cerebrospinal fluid.

Germinomas account for the majority of pineal region tumours and occur primarily in young men. They are usually rounded, and often iso- or hyperdense on CT and grey matter isointense on standard MRI. They show marked, homogeneous contrast enhancement and virtually never calcify. They tend to displace physiological calcification within the pineal gland. Germinomas may be multifocal (the second commonest site being the hypothalamic region associated with diabetes insipidus which usually occurs only late in suprasellar astrocytomas) or show diffuse subependymal and subarachnoid spread, best appreciated on contrast-enhanced T1 images.[62] They show restricted diffusion on DWI due to dense cellularity with high choline and reduced NAA and MRS.

Teratomas appear more lobulated and inhomogeneous on CT and MRI, reflecting fat content and calcification. The margins of these tumours are often irregular and enhancement is usually inhomogeneous (Fig. 61-14).

The remaining pineal region tumours are mainly of pineal cell (pineoblastomas, pineocytomas) or glial origin (astrocytomas). Pineocytomas are largely histologically benign tumours, usually occurring in young adults, that lack specific imaging features although they tend to enhance and, by contrast with germinomas, contain physiological pineal calcification centrally within the mass. Pineoblastomas occur in children and belong to the group of primitive neuroectodermal tumours (PNETs). They behave like cerebellar medulloblastomas, with frequent seeding via the CSF. They tend to be of low signal intensity on T2 images and can appear bright on DWI. Benign pineal cysts are common and must be differentiated from pineal tumours. They are smooth and well defined and can exhibit rim enhancement. Their signal on T1, proton density-weighted and FLAIR images may be higher than CSF due to their protein content. They do not, however, cause hydrocephalus or a midbrain syndrome.

Embryonal Neuroepithelial Neoplasms

The revised WHO classification (2007) lists the following embryonal neuroepithelial neoplasms: medulloblastomas and its variants, primitive neuroectodermal tumour (PNET) and atypical teratoid/rhabdoid tumour (ATRT). Medulloblastomas are the commonest posterior fossa tumour in children and arise classically from the super medullary velum at the roof of the fourth ventricle (Fig. 61-15). Gene expression profiling has identified for distinct molecular subgroups of medulloblastomas with different clinical outcomes. PNETs are extracerebellar and have a poorer prognosis than medulloblastomas, as have ATRTs, which occur nearly always in children below 5 years of age.

Imaging features of the embryonal neuroepithelial neoplasms reflect their high cellular density and they appear hyperdense on CT, hyperintense on DWI and of intermediate-to-low density on T2 images.

They enhance with IV contrast medium and have a propensity for dissemination in the subarachnoid space with leptomeningeal deposits. Staging of these tumours requires therefore a contrast–enhanced MRI of the entire neuroaxis.[30]

LYMPHOMAS

Lymphoma of the CNS can be primary (PCNSL) or secondary in patients with systemic lymphoma. Secondary CNS lymphoma is more common and occurs usually with non-Hodgkin's lymphomas, Hodgkin's lymphomas having a very low risk of CNS involvement.

Immunocompromised patients have an increased risk of developing PCNSL, but the incidence in the HIV-infected population has markedly decreased since the widespread introduction of antiretroviral therapy. In contradistinction, there has been an increased incidence of PCNSL in the immunocompetent population.

Primary CNS lymphoma (PCNSL) invariably involves the brain parenchyma, whereas secondary CNS lymphoma affects the leptomeninges in two-thirds and the brain parenchyma in one-third of cases.[63]

PCNSL appears as a single (less frequently multiple) lobulated enhancing mass, often abutting an ependymal or meningeal surface Enhancement is usually uniform in immunocompetent patients and irregular or ring-like in immunocompromised patients. The high cellular density and nucleus-to-cytoplasm ratio make PCNSL appear hyperdense on CT (Fig. 61-16) and hypointense on T2 images. The ADC of PCNSL is lower than in gliomas[64] or toxoplasmosis,[65] which is an important differential diagnosis in immunocompromised patients. PCNSL grows in an angiocentric fashion around existing blood vessels without extensive new vessel formation. PCNSL show findings on PWI which differentiates them from high-grade gliomas. They tend to have a much lower rCBV than high-grade gliomas and characteristically show a high percentage signal recovery, overshooting the baseline on the time–signal intensity curves of DSC studies.[66]

A characteristic clinical feature of PCNSL is a rapid resolution of the tumour following administration of steroids and/or radiotherapy

Secondary CNS lymphoma can cause enhancement of the leptomeninges, subependyma, dura, cranial nerves and superficial cerebral lesions.[63] Lymphoma has a high glucose metabolism on FDG-PET, which can be more apparent than contrast enhancement (Fig. 61-17).

METASTASES

The primary neoplasms that most commonly metastasise to the brain are carcinoma of the lung, breast and malignant melanoma. Generally, metastases appear as multiple rounded lesions with a tendency to seed peripherally in the cerebral substance, at the grey/white matter junction. They can, however, occur anywhere in the cerebrum, brainstem or cerebellum, and can also spread to the meninges. Metastases are characterised by oedema in the surrounding white matter which is often disproportionate to the size of the tumour itself. On T2 images, the neoplastic nodule may blend with the surrounding oedema, giving a picture of widespread vasogenic oedema and obscuring the diagnosis. Most metastases enhance strongly with IV contrast medium, either uniformly, or ring-like if the metastasis has outgrown its blood supply. Most metastases from lung and breast are similar in density to normal brain parenchyma on CT, but some types are spontaneously dense, particularly deposits from malignant melanoma.[67]

Haemorrhage occurs in about 10% of metastases, resulting in high signal on T1 images and high or low signal on T2 images. Similar signal characteristics can also occur in non-haemorrhagic metastases from melanoma, due to the paramagnetic properties of melanin (Fig. 61-18). Small metastases and those that are not

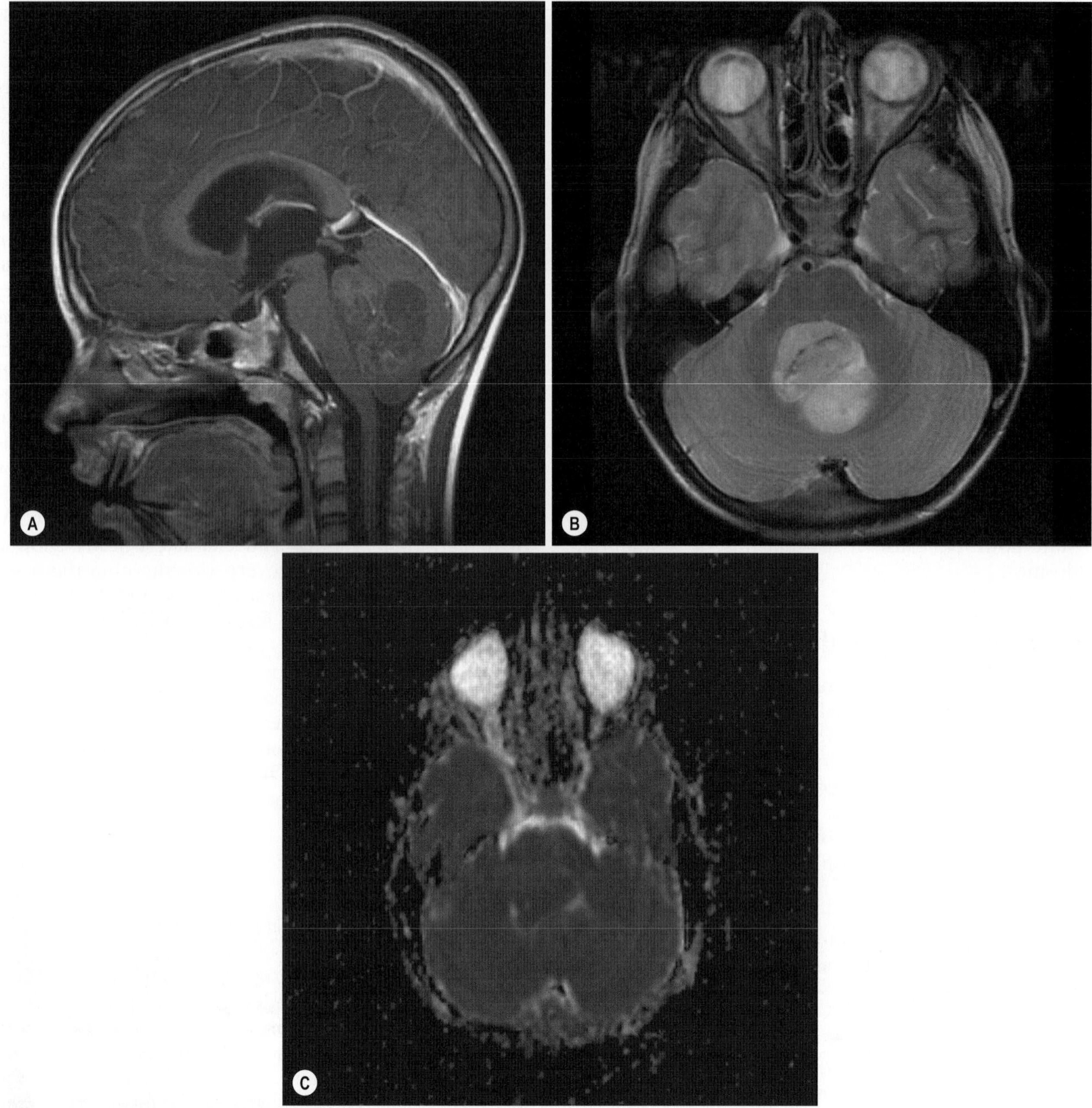

FIGURE 61-15 ■ Medulloblastoma. Sagittal gadolinium-enhanced T1W (A), axial T2W images (B) and ADC map (C) demonstrate a heterogeneously enhancing mass posterior to the fourth ventricle, which is obliterated. The increased cellularity of this tumour is reflected by its relative hypointensity on the ADC map. (Courtesy of Dr R. Gunny.)

made conspicuous by surrounding oedema are often only detected on contrast-enhanced studies. Increasing the contrast dose or relaxivity of gadolinium compounds can improve the sensitivity for detection of metastases on MRI.[5]

Advanced MR imaging methods can also contribute towards the diagnosis and differential diagnosis of metastases. DWI may help to predict the histology of metastases. Well-differentiated adenocarcinoma metastases are hypointense on trace-weighted DWI, whereas small cell and neuroendocrine metastases are hyperintense, due to their higher cellularity.[68,69] On standard MRI it may occasionally be difficult to distinguish a single metastasis from a glioma. PWI and MRS of the peritumoural rather than intratumoural region were shown to be useful in differentiating the two, as mentioned above.

DWI is helpful to differentiate cystic metastasis from cerebral abscesses (Fig. 61-19).[69] The latter contain more viscous fluid and pus and show a more marked restriction of water diffusion than necrotic tumours. Abscesses appear therefore bright on trace-weighted DWI and dark on ADC maps (Fig. 61-20).

INTRAVENTRICULAR TUMOURS

Approximately a tenth of all primary intra-axial brain tumours involve the ventricular system. The precise anatomical location of the tumour within the ventricles often provides an important clue to the nature of the lesion. Common intraventricular tumours and cysts and their sites of predilection are summarised in Table 61-3. Intraventricular tumours arising from neuroepithelial tissue (ependymomas, central neurocytoma and choroid plexus tumours) are discussed first.

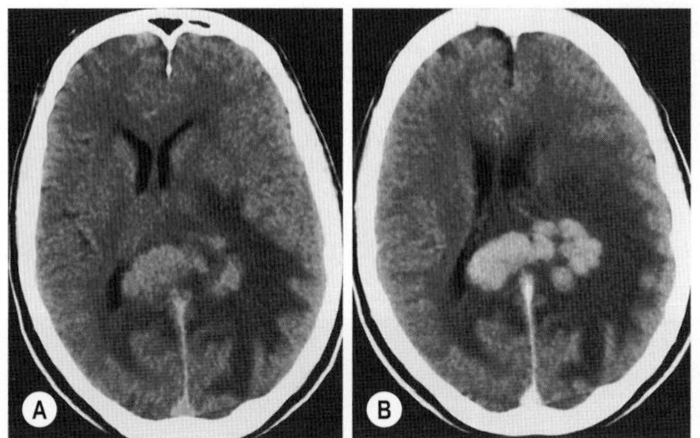

FIGURE 61-16 ■ **Primary cerebral lymphoma.** CT before (A) and after IV contrast medium (B). An irregular mass that is hyperdense to grey matter expands the splenium of the corpus callosum and extends into the left hemisphere. It is surrounded by extensive white matter oedema and enhances avidly with contrast.

Ependymoma

Ependymomas arise from neoplastic transformation of the ependyma and account for about 5% of adult primary brain tumours, being twice as frequent in children. Ependymomas are usually intraventricular, although extraventricular rests of ependymal cells may give rise to hemisphere tumours. Supratentorial tumours occur in young adults and fourth ventricular ependymomas (Fig. 61-21), which frequently extend through the foramina of Magendie and Luschka, and have two age peaks, at 5 and 35 years of age. They are well-demarcated lobulated mass lesions which show calcification on CT in over 50% and are of mixed signal intensity on MRI (predominantly hyperintense on T2 and iso- to hypointense on T1 images). MRI may demonstrate small cysts but calcification is less conspicuous than on CT. Enhancement is mild to moderate and often heterogeneous.

TABLE 61-3 **Intraventricular Lesions**

Tumour	Typical Site
Colloid cyst	Foramen of Monro/third ventricle
Meningioma	Trigone of lateral ventricle
Choroid	Fourth ventricle
Ependymoma	Lateral ventricle (more common in children) and fourth ventricle
Neurocytoma	Lateral ventricles (involving septum pellucidum)
Metastases	Lateral ventricles, ependyma and choroid plexus

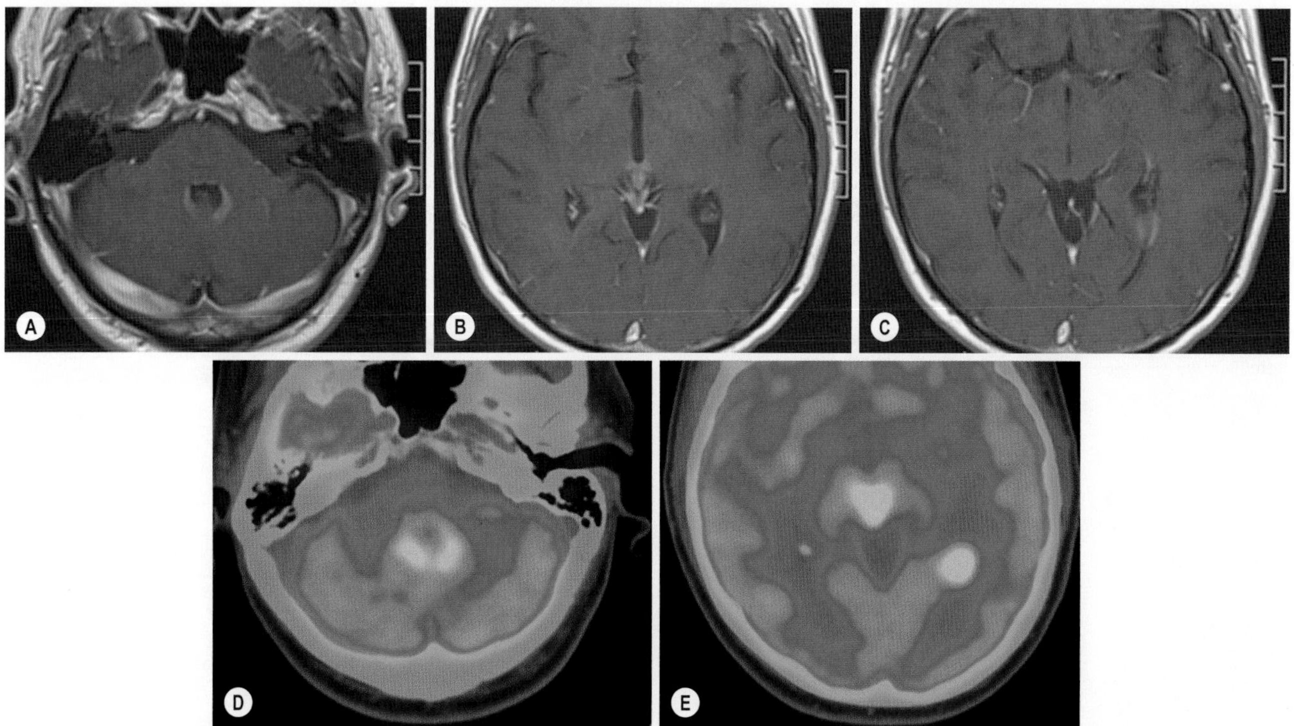

FIGURE 61-17 ■ **Secondary cerebral lymphoma.** Contrast-enhanced T1WI (A–C) and FDG-PET/CT (D, E) in a patient with secondary CNS (B-cell) lymphoma showing focal thickening and enhancement of the ependyma lining the fourth ventricle (A), the third ventricle posteriorly and left occipital horn (B) and atrium of the left lateral ventricle (C). These lesions are more conspicuous on the FDG-PET which show avid tracer uptake (D, E).

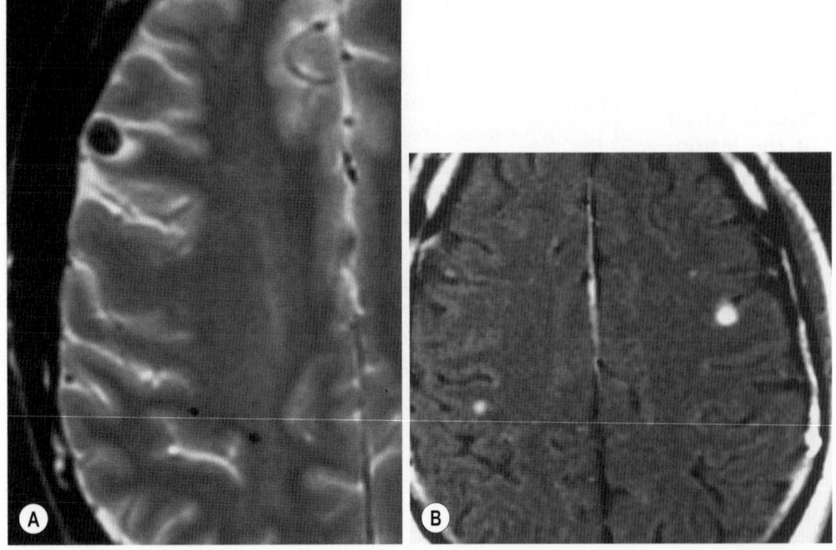

FIGURE 61-18 ■ Metastases. (A) Melanoma (MRI): axial T2W (2000/80). There are at least three foci of signal hypointensity in the right hemisphere, the largest in the right posterior frontal cortex and the others deeper in the subcortical parietal region. This T2 shortening is attributable to melanin. (B) Axial post-contrast T1W with magnetisation transfer (650/16). At a slightly different level, this post-contrast study discloses at least four rounded hyperintense metastatic deposits, all in the cortex or subcortical regions.

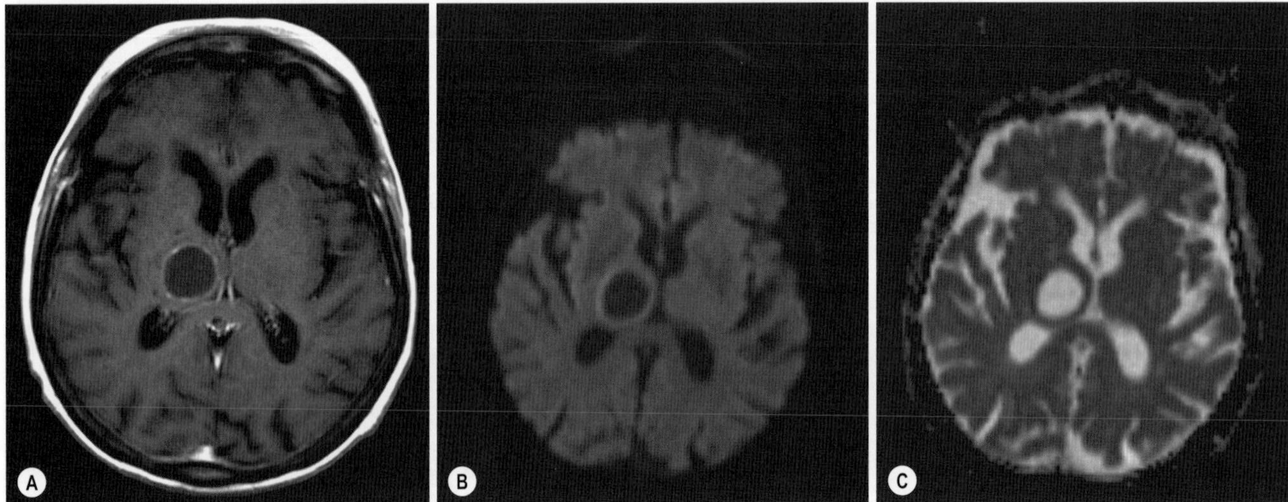

FIGURE 61-19 ■ Cystic metastasis from CA breast. Axial T1W post-contrast image (A) demonstrates a peripherally enhancing, centrally necrotic lesion in the right thalamus. The lesion appears dark on the trace-weighted DW image (B) and bright on the ADC map (C), which is consistent with a relatively unrestricted diffusion in the centre of the mass.

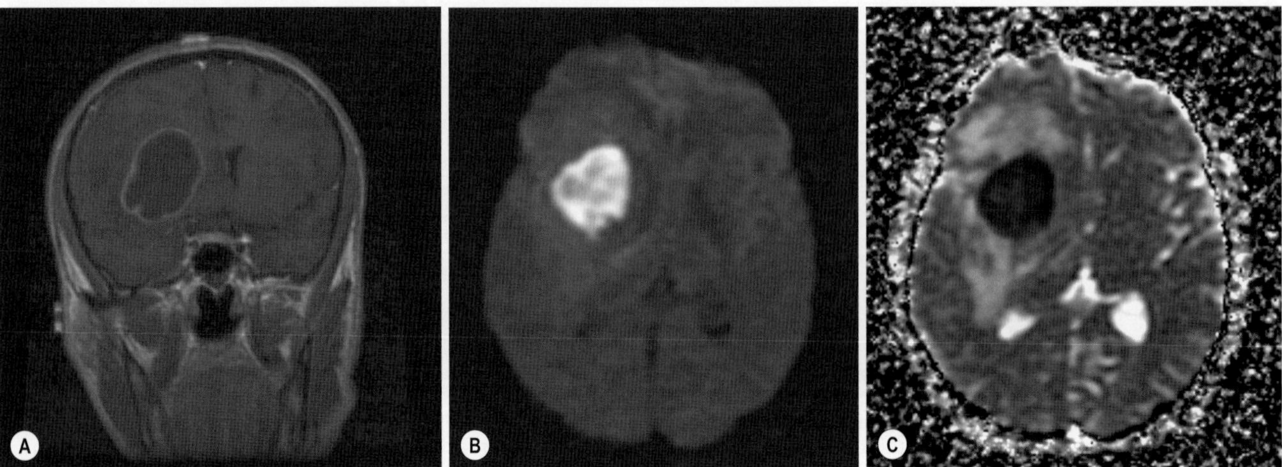

FIGURE 61-20 ■ Brain abscess.

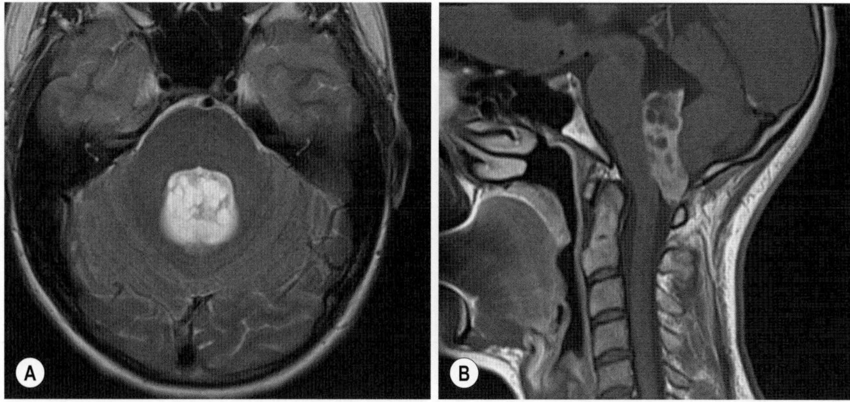

FIGURE 61-21 ■ Ependymoma of the fourth ventricle. (A) The axial T2WI demonstrates a relatively well-circumscribed hyperintense partially solid and cystic mass expanding the fourth ventricle. (B) Sagittal post-contrast T1WI shows a heterogeneously enhancing mass expanding the inferior part of the fourth ventricle and extending through the foramen of Magendie. There is dilatation of the ventricular system in keeping with obstructive hydrocephalus.

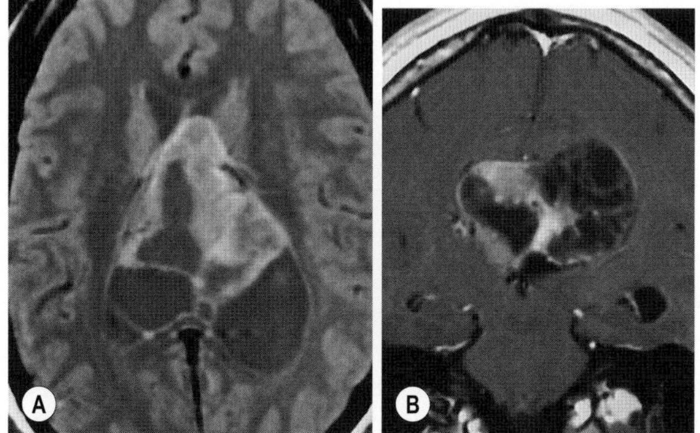

FIGURE 61-22 ■ Central neurocytoma. Axial proton density (A) and coronal T1W post-gadolinium (B) MRI. A partly cystic, multi-septated, enhancing mass, which is related to the septum pellucidum, fills the bodies of both lateral ventricles and causes hydrocephalus with dilatation of the left temporal horn.

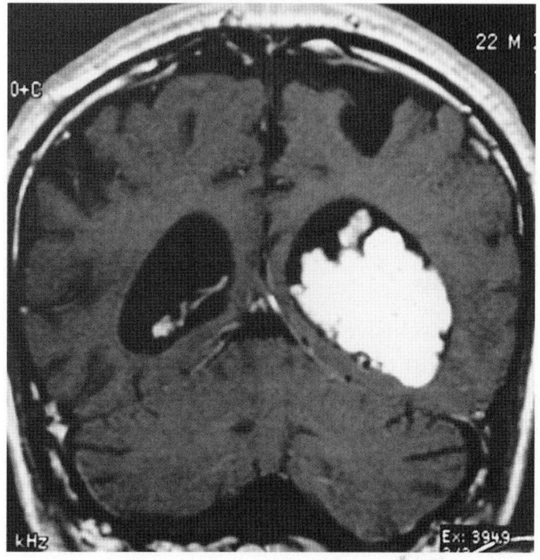

FIGURE 61-23 ■ Choroid plexus papilloma. Coronal T1W post-gadolinium MRI. There is a lobulated, strongly enhancing tumour in the trigone of the left lateral ventricle. Both lateral ventricles are dilated due to hydrocephalus associated with this tumour.

Central Neurocytoma

Central neurocytomas are slow-growing intraventricular tumours of purely neuronal origin.[70] They may rarely arise outside the ventricular system. Before the advent of immunohistological methods they were frequently misdiagnosed as subependymal oligodendrogliomas. These relatively benign tumours occur predominantly in the second and third decades of life, and represent probably the commonest lateral ventricular masses in this age group. They typically arise from the septum pellucidum and occupy the frontal horns and bodies of the lateral ventricles, and sometimes extend through the foramen of Monro. CT frequently shows calcification and small cysts. MRI shows a heterogeneously enhancing mixed-signal intensity mass containing septated cysts, susceptibility artefact from calcification and grey-matter-isointense nodules (Fig. 61-22). Obstructive hydrocephalus is common.

Choroid Plexus Tumours

Choroid plexus papillomas are WHO grade I tumours and much more common than the more aggressive atypical choroid papillomas (WHO grade II), which show a higher mitotic count, or choroid plexus carcinomas (WHO grade III). The location and incidence of choroid plexus papillomas vary with age. They are relatively more common in childhood (3% of primary brain tumours), presenting as a 'cauliflower-like' mass in the trigone of the lateral ventricle (Fig. 61-23). In adults, papillomas are less common, and occur predominantly in the fourth ventricle. CT shows an iso- to hyperdense mass with punctate calcification and homogeneous enhancement. On MRI the papillomas appear as lobulated, intraventricular masses of heterogeneous, predominantly intermediate signal intensity on both T1 and T2 images, with intense contrast enhancement. Angiography, which is rarely indicated, shows a highly vascular mass supplied predominantly by the anterior and posterior choroidal arteries. Choroid plexus

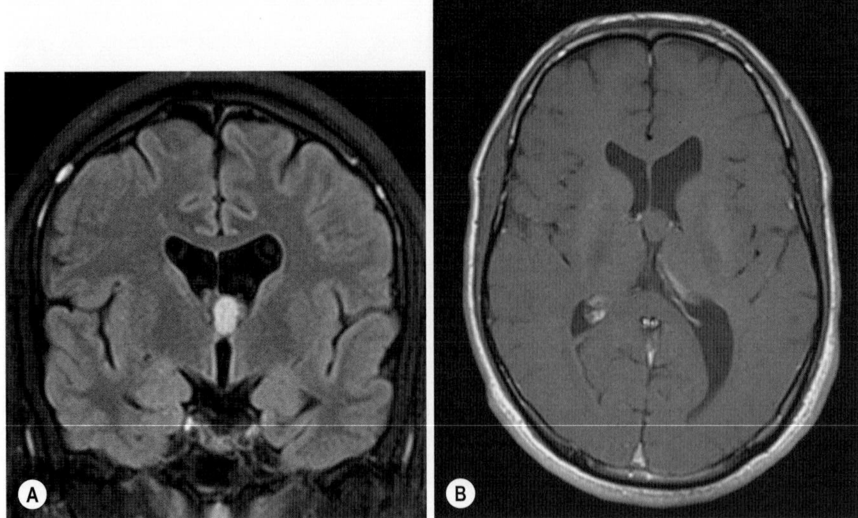

FIGURE 61-24 ■ **Colloid cyst.** FLAIR image (A) shows a well-circumscribed mass at the foramen on Monro, which is homogeneously hyperintense due to proteinaceous cyst content. It does not enhance and appears isointense on post-contrast T1WI (B). There is mild dilation of the left lateral ventricle.

carcinomas are rare, highly malignant tumours that invade the adjacent brain parenchyma to a greater degree than papillomas.

Colloid Cyst

This occurs exclusively at the paraphysis, which lies in the posterior lip of the foramen of Monro, between the third and lateral ventricles. They tend to cause hydrocephalus, by intermittently or continuously obstructing the outflow of cerebrospinal fluid from the lateral ventricles and are smooth, spherical lesions, which are characteristically hyperdense on unenhanced CT imaging. Their MR appearance varies depending on the cyst content (calcium, cholesterol, haemosiderin); some can have similar a signal to CSF, but most are of high signal on T2 and T1 FLAIR images (Fig. 61-24).

Meningioma

This is the commonest cause of a mass in the trigone of the lateral ventricle after the first decade of life. The CT and MRI appearances are similar to those of extraventricular meningiomas (see below): a well-defined, globular lesion which is usually hyperdense on CT and may give similar signal to cerebral cortex on T1 and T2 images. They usually show marked contrast enhancement on CT and MRI.

EXTRA-AXIAL TUMOURS

Primary extra-axial neoplasms arise from the meningothelial arachnoidal cells (meningiomas), mesenchymal pericytes (haemangiopericytoma) or cranial nerves (schwannomas, neurofibromas) and include developmental cysts or tumour-like lesions (epidermoid and dermoid cysts). Metastatic involvement of the meninges and tumours in specific regions (around the sella turcica and skull base) are discussed separately. Overall, meningiomas represent the commonest non-glial intracranial neoplasm, accounting for approximately 20% of all primary intracranial tumours. Multiple meningiomas and cranial nerve tumours are found in neurofibromatosis type 2. Extra-axial lesions occur much more frequently in adults than in children and account for the majority of primary infratentorial tumours in adults, with three lesions sharing a predilection for the cerebellopontine region: vestibular schwannoma, meningioma and epidermoid cysts.

When analysing an extra-axial lesion, it is important to pay attention to associated bone changes: meningiomas tend to induce a hyperostotic bone reaction, whereas epidermoid cysts and schwannomas tend to cause bone thinning resulting in enlargement of, for example, the middle cranial fossa or internal auditory meatus. Other features distinguishing extra- from intra-axial mass lesions are 'buckling' and medial displacement of the grey–white matter interface, a CSF cleft separating the base of the mass from adjacent brain, and a broad base along a dural or calvarial surface.[71]

MENINGIOMAS

Meningiomas originate from arachnoid cell rests, related to arachnoid granulations of the dura mater, and may assume a spherical, well-circumscribed shape or be flat, infiltrating ('en plaque') lesions.[72]

There are several histological types of meningioma, including meningothelial, fibrous/fibroblastic, transitional and psammomatous tumours. The WHO

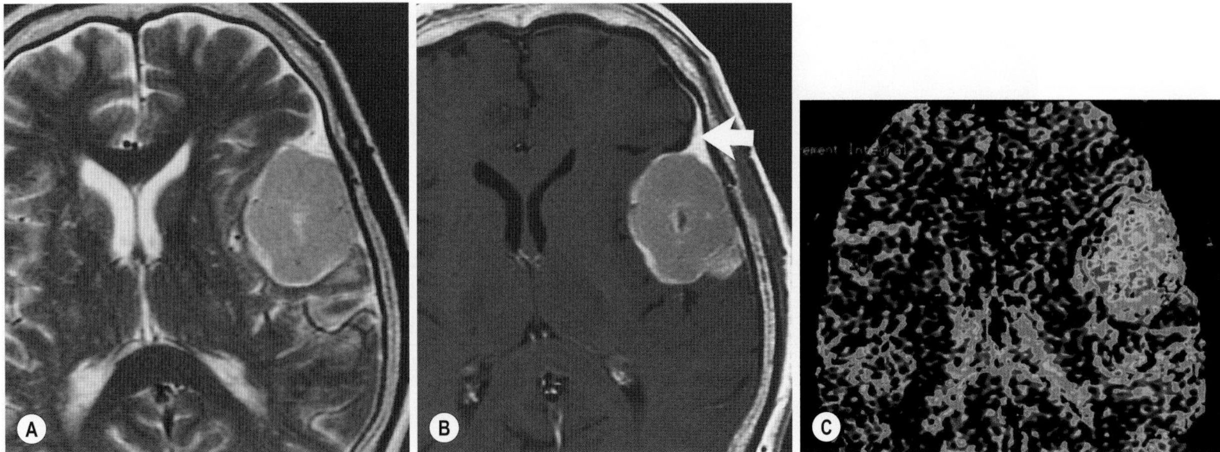

FIGURE 61-25 ■ Meningioma with perfusion-weighted imaging. Axial T2W (A), gadolinium-enhanced T1W (B) and perfusion-weighted (C) MRI. A grey matter isointense mass deeply indents the left cerebral convexity (A). Its broad dural base, the surrounding displaced cerebral sulci and the small pial vessel between the tumour and the brain surface (arrowhead) are all features of an extra-axial lesion. The tumour enhances and there is a 'dural tail' (arrow) (B), which is a frequent radiological finding in meningioma, but is not pathognomonic (see Fig. 61-30). Perfusion-weighted MRI (C): a colour map of the relative cerebral blood volume (rCBV) shows increased blood volume of the tumour compared with normal cortex and white matter, confirming its highly vascular nature.

classification for brain tumours distinguishes three types of meningiomas.[24]

The majority of meningiomas are typical (WHO grade I) meningiomas and have a good prognosis, with a low recurrence rate following surgical resection. Diagnosis of a grade II (atypical) meningioma is based on evidence of a high mitotic index, various patterns of disordered growth or brain invasion (although this is not formally a pathological criterion, it corresponds prognostically to WHO grade II). Grade III (anaplastic) meningiomas demonstrate excessive mitotic activity and have a sarcoma-, carcinoma- or melanoma-like appearance under light microscopy.[73]

Of meningiomas, 90% are supratentorial, arising, in decreasing order of frequency, from the parasagittal region, cerebral convexities, sphenoid ridge and olfactory groove. Infratentorial meningiomas are most frequently located on the posterior surface of the petrous bones and clivus and can mimic vestibular schwannomas. Bone sclerosis is in favour of meningioma and enlargement of the internal auditory meatus is much more common in schwannomas.

Many meningiomas are incidentally discovered on CT or MRI performed for other indications. CT is well suited to demonstrate effects on adjacent bone such as hyperostosis associated with benign meningiomas or bone destruction associated with atypical meningiomas. Sixty per cent of meningiomas are spontaneously hyperdense and up to 20% contain calcification[74] and enhancement is usually intense and uniform.

On MRI, meningiomas appear frequently isointense to cerebral cortex on both T1 and T2 images and may be difficult to detect without IV contrast medium. Meningiomas can have 'capping cysts' of similar MRI signal intensity to CSF. As on CT, meningiomas enhance vividly and homogeneously, except for the uncommon cystic and very densely calcified tumours, which may produce foci of low signal within the mass. There may also be a linear, contrast-enhancing 'dural tail' extending from the tumour along the dura mater. The 'dural tail' sign, once thought to be pathognomonic for meningioma (Fig. 61-25), can also be seen with other tumours such as schwannoma or metastasis.

Vasogenic oedema is not infrequently associated with meningiomas. The extent of the vasogenic oedema does not correlate with the size of the meningioma and, as with metastases, even small lesions can cause quite extensive oedema. The presence of intra-axial oedema, however, is thought to correspond to an increased likelihood of recurrence.[75]

Meningiomas abutting the superior sagittal or transverse sinuses can compress or invade these venous structures. The distinction between compression and occlusion is important for preoperative planning, and can be made by MRA or CTA.

Physiological MR imaging methods may also of help in the diagnosis and prognostication of meningiomas using non-invasive methods.

MRS may show an alanine peak, which is characteristic for a meningioma but is seen in less than 50% of cases. However, no MRS data have been clinically correlated to patient outcomes.[76]

DWI has been used to investigate the differences between typical and atypical meningiomas with conflicting results. A decrease in ADC values of benign meningiomas at follow-up was thought to raise suspicion of transformation to a higher grade[77] following initial reports of significantly lower ADC values in non-typical meningiomas.[78] However, a more recent study did not show any significant correlation between ADC values and meningioma histology.[79]

Meningiomas have usually a markedly elevated rCBV on PWI, which can be used to differentiate them from dural metastases, which tend to have a lower rCBV.

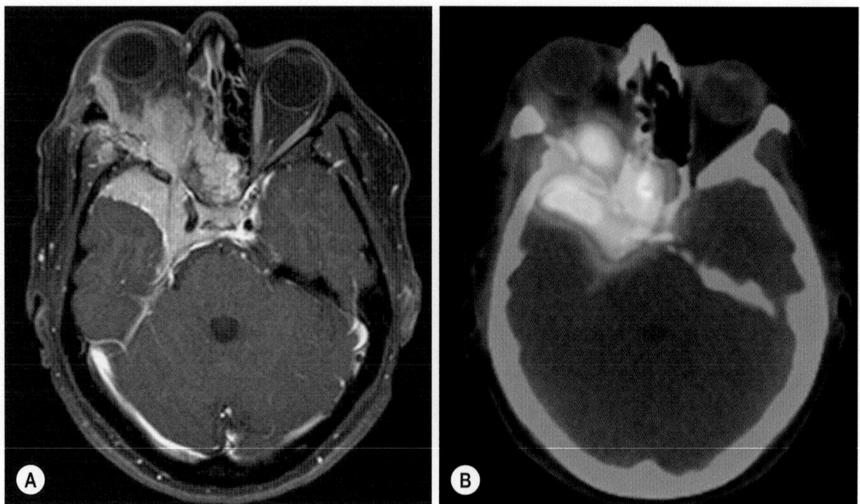

FIGURE 61-26 ■ Meningioma. Post-contrast T1W1 (A) demonstrates an avidly enhancing extra-axial mass centred on the right planum sphenoidale and extending to the petrous apex, cavernous sinus, orbital apex and also involving the right optic nerve sheath and intraconal structures, as well as the sphenoid and ethmoid sinuses. On PET imaging (B) there is avid ^{68}Ga-DOTATOC uptake, which is a somatostatin analogue, due to the high density of somatostatin receptors in meningiomas.

Furthermore, the CBV of peritumoural odema has been found to be higher when surrounding malignant meningiomas[80] (Fig 61-25).

On PET imaging meningiomas show a high uptake of ^{68}Ga-DOTATOC (Fig. 61-26), which can be useful for differentiating meningiomas from other similarly looking tumours and to distinguish residual/recurrent tumour from postoperative enhancement or to improve radiotherapy planning in skull base meningiomas.[21]

Angiography is now mostly performed in the context of preoperative embolisation to minimise intraoperative blood loss. The cardinal angiographic findings are supplied from meningeal vessels and a dense, homogeneous, persistent blush. Parasitisation of cortical vessels by tumours over the cerebral convexity or of branches of the ophthalmic artery by subfrontal masses is not rare.

With preoperative embolisation now being frequently performed, it is important to be aware of the post-embolisation MRI appearances of meningiomas which typically include a decrease in enhancement and reduced perfusion of the devascularised segment of the meningiomas.[81]

Haemangiopericytomas enter into the differential diagnosis for meningiomas. Features suggestive of a haemangiopericytoma rather than meningioma are a lobulated (rather than spherical) dural-based mass, absence of calcification and hyperostosis and multiple areas of flow void on MRI, reflecting the high vascularity of these tumours.[82]

CRANIAL NERVE SHEATH TUMOURS

Cranial nerve sheath tumours, originating from cranial nerves, account for 6–8% of primary intracranial tumours. Most are benign neoplasms arising from Schwann cells ('schwannomas') of the nerve sheaths. Schwannomas arise eccentrically from the sheath and compress the parent nerve rather than invading it. All cranial nerves except I (olfactory) and II (optic), which are white matter tracts of the cerebrum, have nerve sheaths, but schwannomas usually grow on the sensory nerves, most frequently from the superior vestibular division of the vestibulocochlear nerve (often inaccurately called 'acoustic neuroma') and, with decreasing frequency, from the trigeminal, glossopharyngeal and lower cranial nerves. Pure motor cranial nerves rarely form schwannomas. Multiple cranial nerve schwannomas are found in neurofibromatosis type 2 and bilateral vestibular schwannomas are pathognomonic of this condition. Neurofibromas are benign tumours, composed of fibroblasts, reticulin and a mucoid matrix in addition to Schwann cells. Cranial nerve tumours are T1 iso/hypointense and T2 hyperintense, and larger lesions often contain areas of cystic degeneration. Cranial nerve tumours almost invariably show marked enhancement with IV contrast, which is solid in two-thirds and ring-like or heterogeneous in one-third of cases.

Vestibular schwannomas account for over 80% of cerebellopontine lesions. They smoothly erode the posterior edge of the porus acusticus, widening the internal auditory meatus (IAM) and often present as an oval component within the cerebellopontine angle cistern, giving rise to the 'ice-cream cone' appearance.[83] CT has been largely replaced by MRI for imaging tumours of the cerebellopontine angle with a sensitivity approaching 100% and a very high specificity.[84] Thin-section T2 imaging with sequences such as CISS/DRIVE/C-FIESTA resolve the 7th and 8th nerves in detail (Fig. 61-27). Tumours as small as 4 mm causing focal nerve thickening can be detected, and MRI is often used for screening patients with asymmetrical sensorineural hearing loss.[85] If the findings are equivocal, gadolinium-enhanced images refute or confirm the suspicion of a tumour.

T2* W or SWI images demonstrate microhaemorrhages in most vestibular schwannomas, which is a useful differentiating feature from meningiomas.[86]

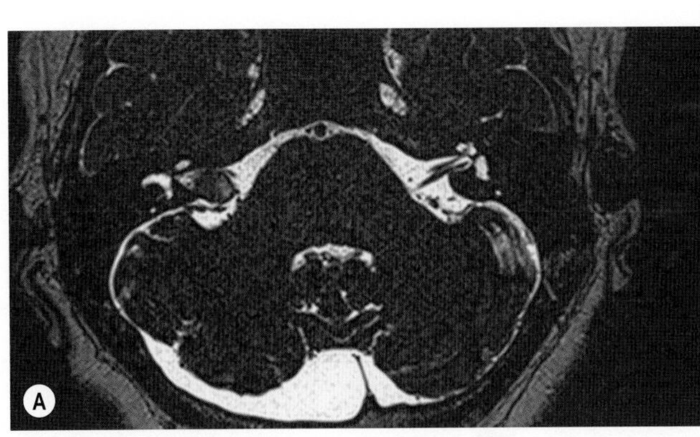
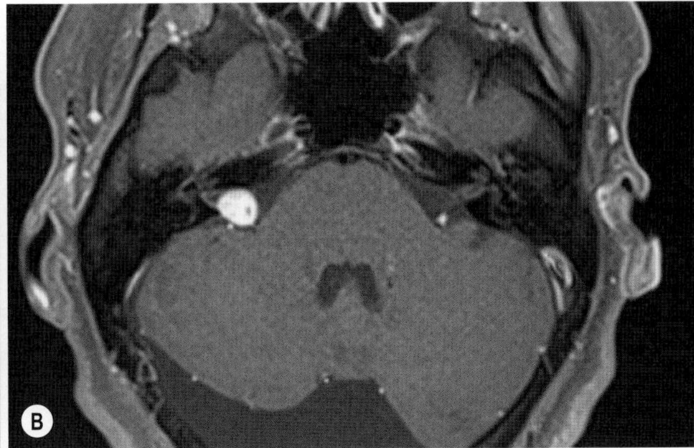

FIGURE 61-27 ■ Vestibular schwannoma. (A) Thin-section T2W CISS imaging shows a vestibular schwannoma with a small cystic component medially, expanding the right internal auditory meatus. (B) Post-contrast T1WI demonstrates marked enhancement of the tumour.

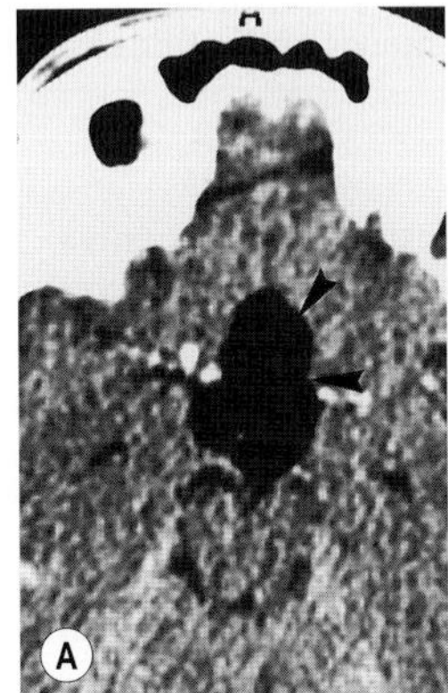
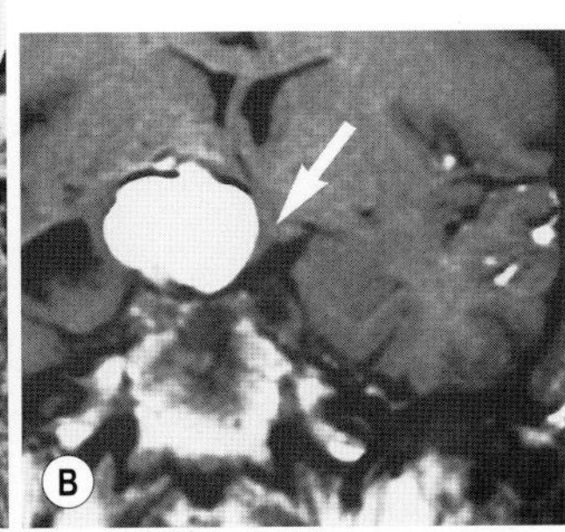

FIGURE 61-28 ■ Suprasellar dermoid tumours. CT (A). There is a midline, fat density tumour (arrowheads) occupying the suprasellar region. (B) Coronal T1W MRI of a different patient with a ruptured dermoid tumour. There is a lobulated high signal mass in the chiasmatic cistern, compressing and displacing the optic chiasm to the left (arrow). Fat globules, which have spilled into the subarachnoid space, are seen as high signal foci in the left Sylvian fissure. The patient has had previous surgery via a right temporal approach, causing right temporal atrophy and enlargement of the right temporal horn.

Vestibular schwannomas appear usually isointense to normal brain parenchyma on DWI, and have raised ADC values. Meningiomas can have similar appearances on DWI[87] but PWI demonstrates significantly lower rCBV measurements in vestibular schwannomas than in meningiomas.[88]

EPIDERMOID AND DERMOID TUMOURS

Epidermoid and dermoid cysts, or 'pearly tumours',[89] result from inclusion of ectodermal epithelial tissue or cutaneous ectoderm, respectively, during the closure of the neural tube.

Intracranial dermoids account for 0.04 to 0.6% of all intracranial tumours and are usually located along the midline. Dermoids contain all skin elements, including fat, and appear therefore of very low density on CT and of high signal intensity on T1 images (Fig. 61-28). They may rupture and release their contents into the subarachnoid space, which is demonstrated as fatty globules within the basal cisterns or ventricles. Dermoid cysts often remain asymptomatic, but can present with aseptic meningitis in the event of rupture.[90]

Epidermoid cysts represent approximately 0.2 to 1.8% of all intracranial tumours and can be central (chiasmatic and quadrigeminal plate cisterns) or eccentric (cerebellopontine angle, middle cranial fossa, Sylvian fissure). Although present at birth, these lesions grow slowly by accumulating desquamated epithelium and conform to the shape of the portion of the subarachnoid space they occupy, sometimes invaginating into the brain parenchyma. On CT, epidermoid cysts generally appear as well-circumscribed, lobulated, non-enhancing, homogeneously hypodense lesions (of similar density to CSF). There is typically no surrounding oedema.[91] On MRI, epidermoid cysts have a signal intensity close to that of CSF on T1, T2 and FLAIR images which can make them difficult to distinguish from other cystic lesions[92] such as arachnoid cysts (Fig. 61-29). The latter often have better defined margins and cause bone thinning. DWI is the most helpful MRI sequence for making the diagnosis of epidermoid tumours. They appear bright on DWI, as opposed to arachnoid cysts, which appear dark, like CSF.

MENINGEAL METASTASES

Meningeal metastases may involve the pachymeninges (dura mater), leptomeninges (arachnoid and pia mater) or both. Contrast-enhanced MRI is much more sensitive than contrast-enhanced CT for detection of metastatic meningeal involvement. Carcinomatosis of the dura mater, common in carcinoma of the breast, manifests itself as focal curvilinear or diffuse contrast enhancement closely applied to the inner table of the skull, which does not follow the convolutions of the gyri. Focal segmental lesions may be difficult to distinguish from en plaque meningioma (Fig. 61-30). Leptomeningeal carcinomatosis produces linear or finely nodular contrast enhancement of the surface of the brain, extending into the sulci and following the convolutions of the brain. It may be

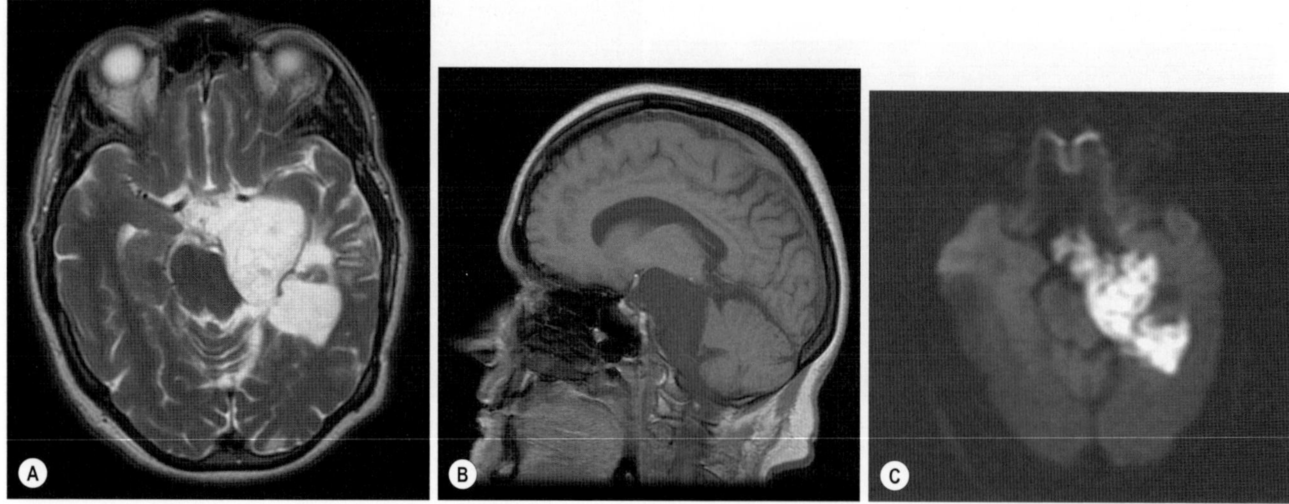

FIGURE 61-29 ■ **Epidermoid tumour.** Axial T2W image (A) and sagittal gadolinium-enhanced T1W image (B) show a large non-enhancing lesion of similar signal intensity to CSF, which occupies the chiasmatic and ambient cisterns, and distorts the medial aspect of the left temporal lobe. On the trace-weighted DW image (C), the lesion appears markedly hyperintense, indicating restricted diffusion.

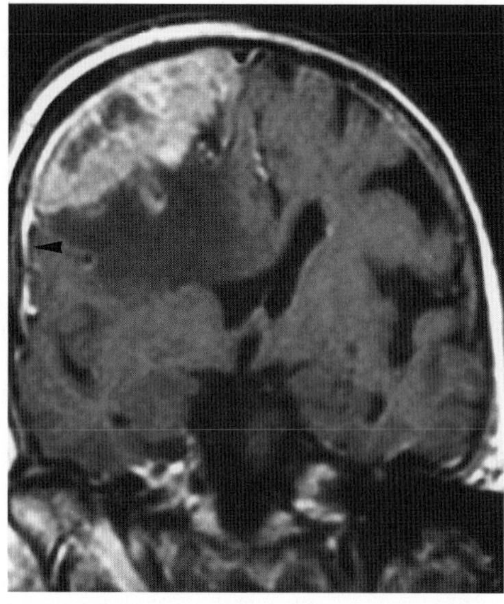

FIGURE 61-30 ■ **Dural metastasis from carcinoma of the breast.** Coronal T1W post-contrast MRI. There is a heterogeneously enhancing mass with an irregular surface that arises from the dura over the right cerebral convexity. It displaces the underlying brain and causes considerable low signal oedema within it. There is a 'dural tail' extending away from the tumour (arrowhead).

indistinguishable from infective meningitis or sarcoidosis. Leptomeningeal disease is commonly seen in leukaemia, lymphoma and breast or lung cancer.

SKULL BASE TUMOURS

Tumours of the skull base include a large pathological spectrum, such as metastases, myeloma/plasmacytoma, meningioma, caudally extending pituitary adenomas, direct extension of nasopharyngeal malignancies as well as tumours and inflammatory lesions arising in the paranasal sinuses. Two specific lesions of the central and posterior skull base are discussed below: chordomas and glomus jugulare tumours.

Chordomas

Chordomas originate from malignant transformation of notochordal cells and their most frequent location in the skull base is the spheno-occipital synchrondrosis of the clivus, followed by the basiocciput and petrous apex: tumours away from the midline are considerably less common. Chordomas are locally invasive and uncommonly metastasise. They present usually with pain and lower cranial nerve palsies. Both MRI and CT are usually performed to assess intracranial chordomas.[93] Bone destruction and calcification are well demonstrated on CT with bone window settings and the tumour is hyperattenuating in relation to the adjacent neural axis. MRI demonstrates a mass which is of intermediate-to-low signal intensity on T1 images and of very high signal intensity on T2 images, frequently containing septae of low signal which gives a characteristic 'soap-bubble' appearance[83] (Fig. 61-31). The solid components show variable, but often marked, contrast enhancement. Fat-suppressed T1W spin-echo sequences are particularly helpful for demonstrating the extent of the tumour and distinguishing pathological enhancement from the high signal of adjacent clival fat. Partial encasement or displacement of the intracranial vessels is common but arterial narrowing or stenoses are rare. Both MR and CT angiography can readily assess the relationship of the tumour to the surrounding vessels and hence aid in surgical planning.

The differential diagnosis includes chondrosarcoma, metastasis and nasopharyngeal carcinoma.

Glomus Jugulare Tumours

Glomus jugulare tumours (chemodectomas) arise from paraganglion cells, the precursors of the chemo- and

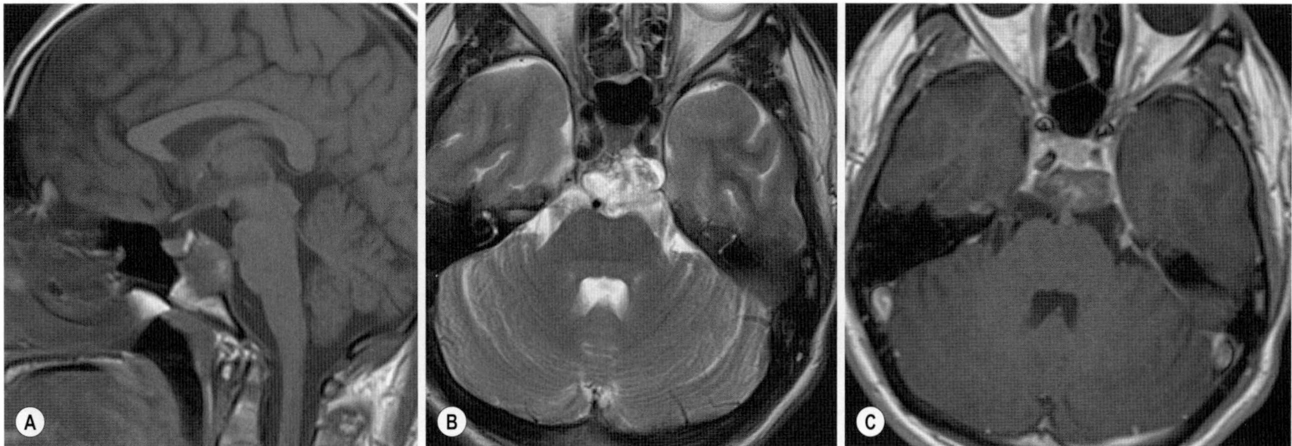

FIGURE 61-31 ■ **Chordoma.** Sagittal T1W image (A) shows a mass arising from the clivus. The mass has partially replaced the normal hyperintense bone marrow and destroyed the cortex posteriorly. On axial T2WI (B) the mass is predominantly hyperintense with with septae of low signal, giving a 'soap-bubble' appearance. Contrast-enhanced T1WI (C) shows patchy enhancement of the tumour.

baroreceptors of great vessels. The most common site is the jugular bulb and their presentation is with pulsatile tinnitus, deafness, vertigo and lower cranial nerve palsies. The tumour causes enlargement of the pars vasorum of the jugular foramen, and any associated bone destruction is well demonstrated on CT (Fig. 61-32). Glomus jugulare tumours enhance intensely on CT and MRI due to their extreme vascularity. On MRI, they appear hyperintense on T2 images and tend to contain areas of flow void corresponding to dilated vessels. These tumours frequently obstruct the internal jugular vein, which may show signal changes indicative of thrombosis.[94]

PITUITARY REGION TUMOURS

Imaging of the pituitary gland and sellar/parasellar region requires high-resolution images, as the pituitary gland is of small volume and in close proximity to many important structures.[95] The differential diagnosis for sellar and parasellar masses is large and, in addition to pituitary tumours, non-neoplastic lesions such as arachnoid cysts or giant aneurysms (Fig. 61-33) must be considered.

Pituitary Adenomas

Pituitary adenomas are the most common neoplasms in the sellar region and comprise 10 to 15% of all intracranial neoplasms. They are classified as microadenomas (diameter < 1 cm) and macroadenomas (> 1 cm) and become symptomatic either because of their endocrine activity (microadenomas and functioning macroadenomas) or by the mass effect they exert (non-functioning macroadenomas) on adjacent structures such as the optic nerves and chiasm, which leads to visual symptoms.

Non-functioning microadenomas are not uncommon and can be found incidentally on MRI studies performed for other reasons.

MRI is the investigation of choice for the detection of microadenomas. Two methods are typically employed, sometimes in conjunction. The first is a standard spin-echo (SE) T1 pre- and post-contrast imaging in the coronal and sagittal plane using a high-resolution technique (3-mm thin slices with small intervals). Fat-saturated T1 images should be performed after administration of IV contrast medium to eliminate high signal from fat in the clivus and clinoid processes, which could be mistaken for enhancement. The second method utilises the different potential enhancement characteristics of adenomas versus normal pituitary tissue by performing dynamic pituitary MRI, which involves the acquisition of a series of rapid images with a time interval of approximately 10–15 s following contrast.[96] A newer imaging technique employs spoiled gradient recalled (SPGR) acquisition in the steady state sequence which gives 1-mm-thin sections and excellent soft-tissue contrast. However, it has the disadvantage of a lower signal-to-noise ratio than SE sequences.[97]

Functioning microadenomas can produce prolactin (prolactinomas), ACTH (in Cushing's disease) or growth hormone (eosinophilic microadenomas). Prolactinomas are the most common functioning microadenomas and tend to arise laterally within the anterior lobe of the pituitary gland. They may depress the floor of the sella turcica or expand one side of the gland, causing a subtle upwardly convex bulge and contralateral displacement of the infundibulum. Microadenomas are best shown on contrast-enhanced images and usually enhance later and/or to a lesser degree than normal pituitary tissue (Fig. 61-34).

The primary treatment of prolactin-secreting microadenomas is medical and the role of imaging in cases of hyperprolactinaemia is therefore mainly to exclude a macroadenoma. Precise localisation of the microadenoma is, however, important in ACTH and thyroid-stimulating hormone (TSH)-producing adenomas, which are treated surgically. In cases where MRI is inconclusive, inferior petrosal and/or cavernous sinus venous sampling may be necessary to lateralise an adenoma in pituitary-driven Cushing's disease. Sensitivity and specificity of more than

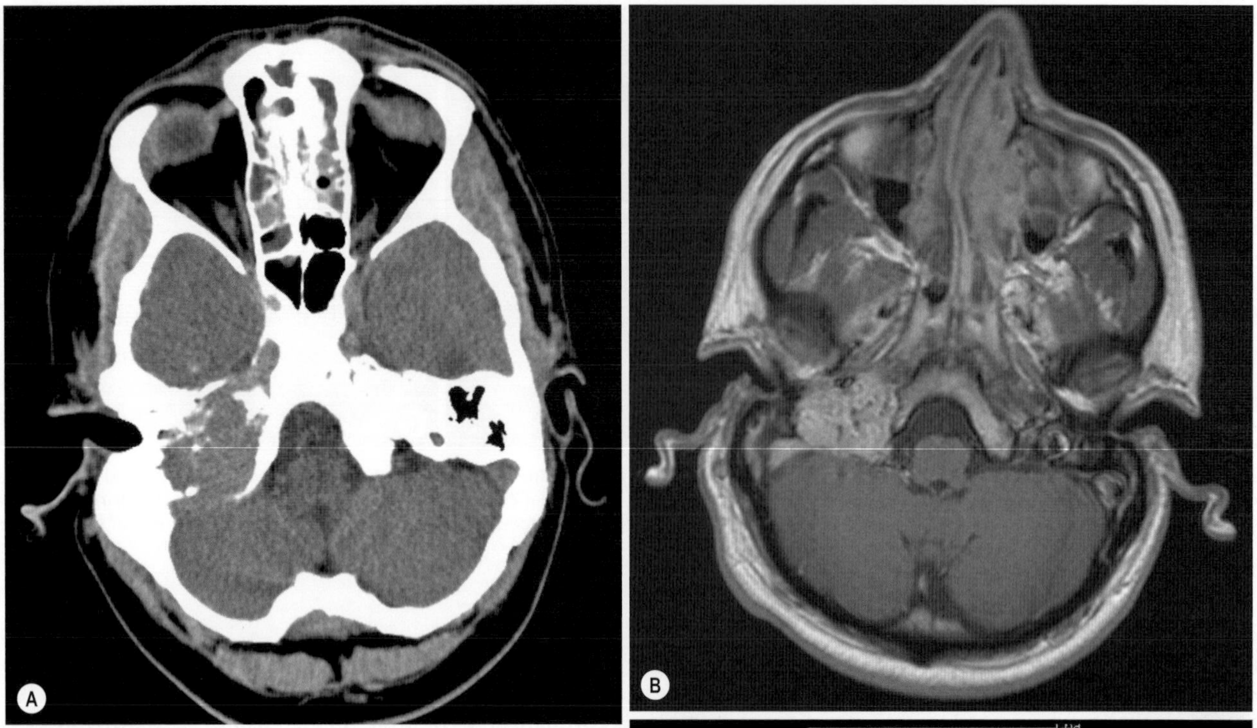

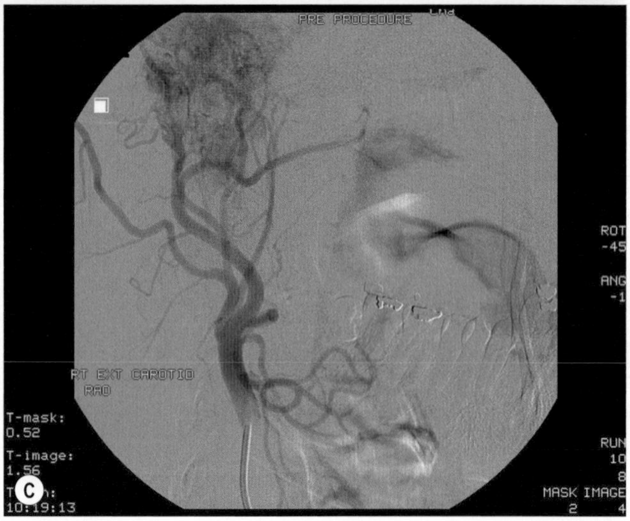

FIGURE 61-32 ■ **Glomus jugulare tumour.** An axial CT (A) demonstrates expansion of the right jugular foramen and bone destruction in the adjacent petrous bone by a mass that is markedly enhancing on an axial T1W post-contrast image (B). The mass contains areas of flow voids, corresponding to the dilated tumour vessels seen on the right external carotid artery angiogram (C). (Courtesy of Dr. M. Adams.)

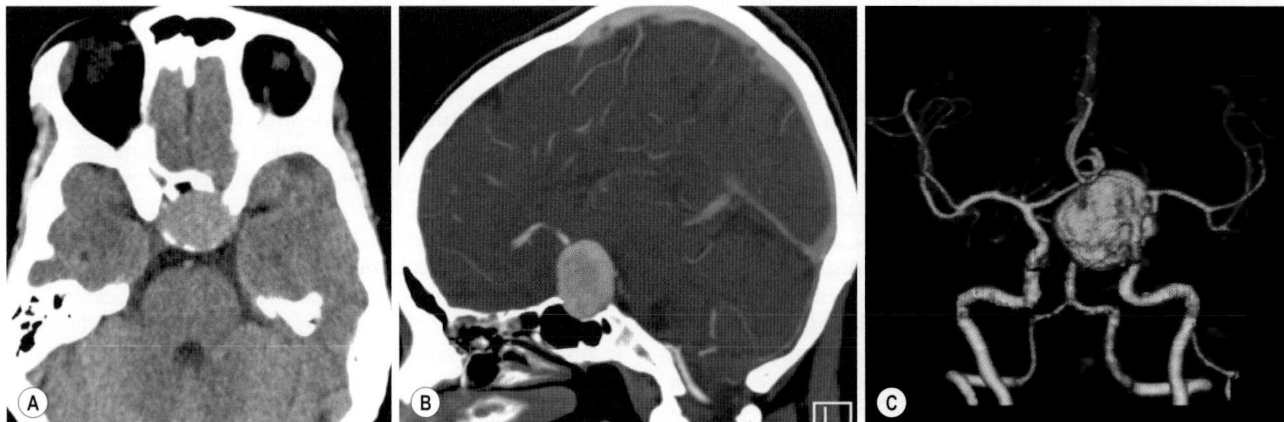

FIGURE 61-33 ■ **Aneurysm.** Axial-unenhanced CT (A) shows a homogeneous, intermediate-density mass expanding the sella turcica. Sagittal MPR images of the CTA angiogram (B) demonstrate this lesion to be highly vascular (B) and volume-rendered reconstructions (C) of the CTA confirm a left cavernous ICA aneurysm. A 'do not biopsy' lesion!

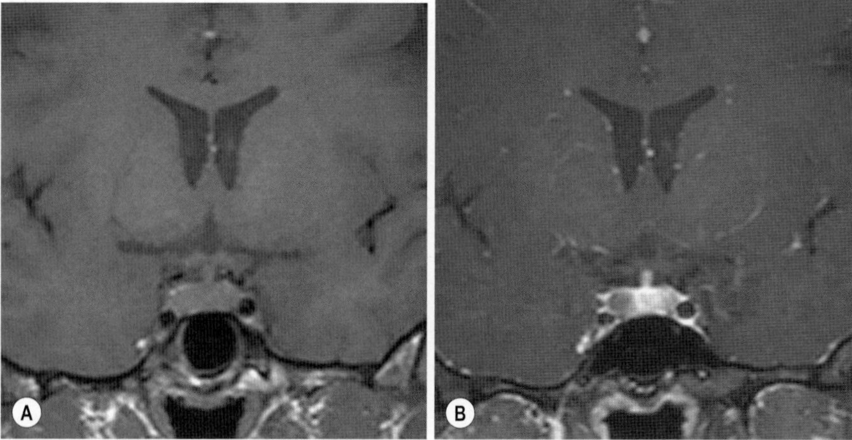

FIGURE 61-34 ■ **Pituitary microadenoma.** Pre-contrast T1WI (A) demonstrates asymmetrical enlargement of the anterior lobe of the pituitary gland on the right. Post-contrast T1WI (B) shows a right-sided microadenoma (<10 mm) abutting the cavernous sinus. It enhances to a much lesser degree than normal pituitary tissue, which makes it easily discernible.

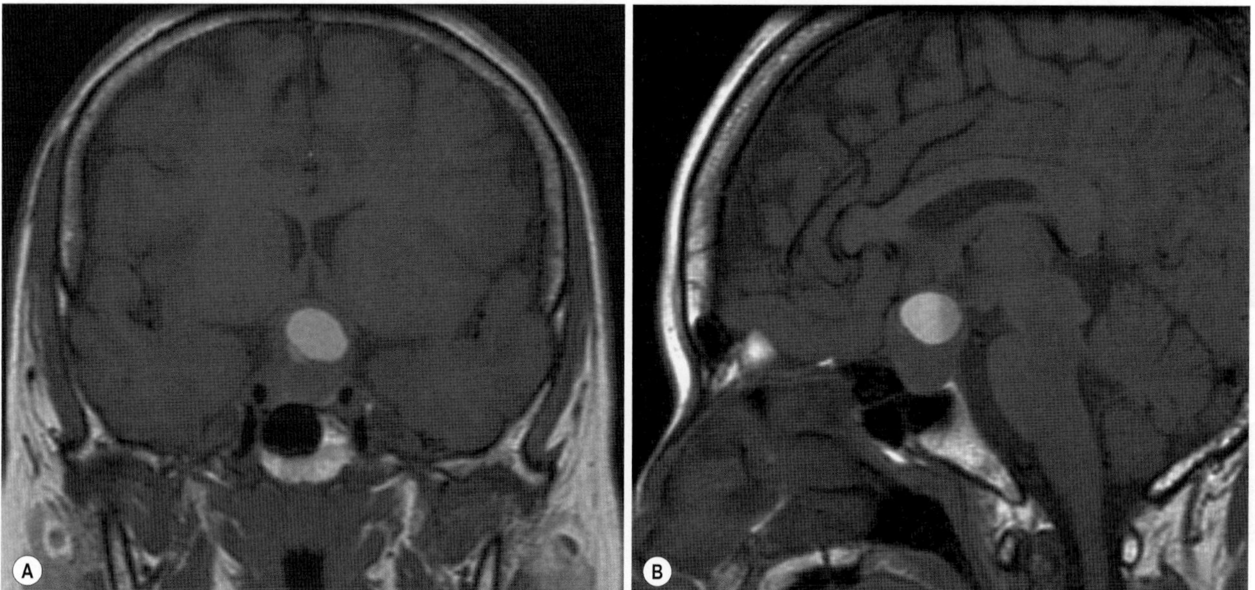

FIGURE 61-35 ■ **Pituitary apoplexy due to haemorrhage into a pituitary macroadenoma.** Coronal (A) and sagittal (B) T1W images demonstrate a hyperintense area at the superior aspect of the tumour that contains a fluid level and is consistent with a recent intratumoural haemorrhage. The optic chiasm is stretched across the apex of the mass.

90% is reported in detection of these lesions, but lesion localisation is not as high when compared with MRI.[98] Eosinophilic microadenomas can cause enlargement of the sella along with other features of acromegaly.

Macroadenomas balloon the pituitary fossa and can have a suprasellar component or extend inferiorly into the sphenoid sinus and clivus. Suprasellar extension leads first to elevation, then to compression of the optic chiasm and intracranial optic nerves, and large tumours may compress brain parenchyma, often in the region of the hypothalamus. Most macroadenomas are isointense with brain parenchyma on unenhanced T1W images and hyperdense on CT. Administration of IV contrast may show uniform or heterogeneous enhancement and facilitates the detection of cavernous sinus invasion, which is often a poor prognostic sign.[99] Enhancement and thickening of the dura (forming a 'dural tail') is frequently seen with large macroadenomas and is a helpful sign of an aggressive lesion, believed to be caused by venous congestion due to compression or invasion of the adjacent cavernous sinus.[100] Macroademomas may contain cystic or haemorrhagic components. Acute haemorrhage into a pituitary macroademona can lead to rapid expansion of the gland, resulting in acute compression of the optic chiasm (pituitary apoplexy). Haemorrhage appears hyperintense on non-enhanced T1W images and, in the acute stage, hyperdense on CT (Fig. 61-35).

Craniopharyngiomas

Craniopharyngiomas are suprasellar tumours which occur most frequently in childhood, but may arise in adult life, and have a second peak of incidence at about the 6th decade. Symptoms are due to compression of the optic chiasm or to raised ICP secondary to obstruction of the foramen of Monro.

They arise from epithelial remnants of Rathke's pouch, from which the anterior pituitary develops, and can be cystic, solid or mixed cystic/solid (Fig. 61-36). Craniopharyngiomas tend not to expand the pituitary fossa unless they become very large which is a differentiating feature from pituitary macroadenomas.

The two main pathological subtypes are the adamantinomatous and squamous-papillary varieties, which vary in age at presentation, tumour location and imaging characteristics.[92] The adamantinomatous type, more common in children, is more likely to have large T1 hyperintense cystic components, whereas the squamous-papillary type, more frequent in adults, is more likely to be predominantly solid and associated cysts return low signal on T1W images, similar to CSF.

The solid components of craniopharyngiomas show intense contrast enhancement and may be partially calcified.

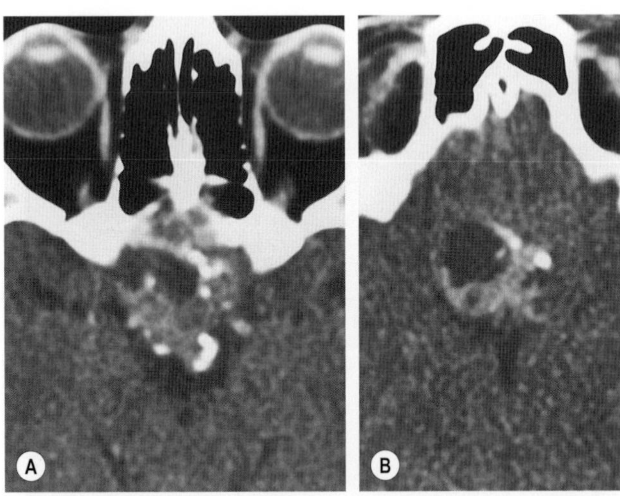

FIGURE 61-36 ■ **Craniopharyngioma.** CT following IV contrast medium. There is a partly calcified, partly cystic lesion in the suprasellar region. There is inhomogeneous enhancement of the solid tumour components.

Rathke's Cleft Cysts

Symptomatic Rathke's cleft cysts are less common than craniopharyngiomas and usually lie within the pituitary gland, but can also be found adjacent to the infundibulum, above the sella. On MRI, they appear frequently as T1 hyperintense cysts, reflecting the proteinaceous nature of the cyst fluid, but may also exhibit similar signal characteristics to CSF. In contradistinction to craniopharyngiomas, Rathke's cysts usually demonstrate thin and uniform walls which infrequently enhance following IV contrast.[101]

Other Sellar Region Tumours

Parasellar meningiomas can arise from the dura mater of the cavernous sinus or the tuberculum, dorsum or diaphragma sellae. Clinical presentation is with cranial nerve palsies or visual symptoms. Parasellar meningiomas are strongly enhancing masses which expand the cavernous sinus and frequently encase and narrow the cavernous portion of the internal carotid arteries. Suprasellar meningiomas often show a forward extension along the dura mater of the anterior cranial fossa and are associated with dilatation ('blistering') of the sphenoid sinus. Intracranial extension of optic nerve sheath meningiomas characteristically involves the planum sphenoidale.

Optic nerve gliomas are astrocytic tumours that occur in childhood and may involve the optic nerves, optic chiasm and optic tracts (Fig. 61-37). These tumours can be associated with NF1 but chiasmic tumours are more frequently seen in patients who do not have NF1.[102]

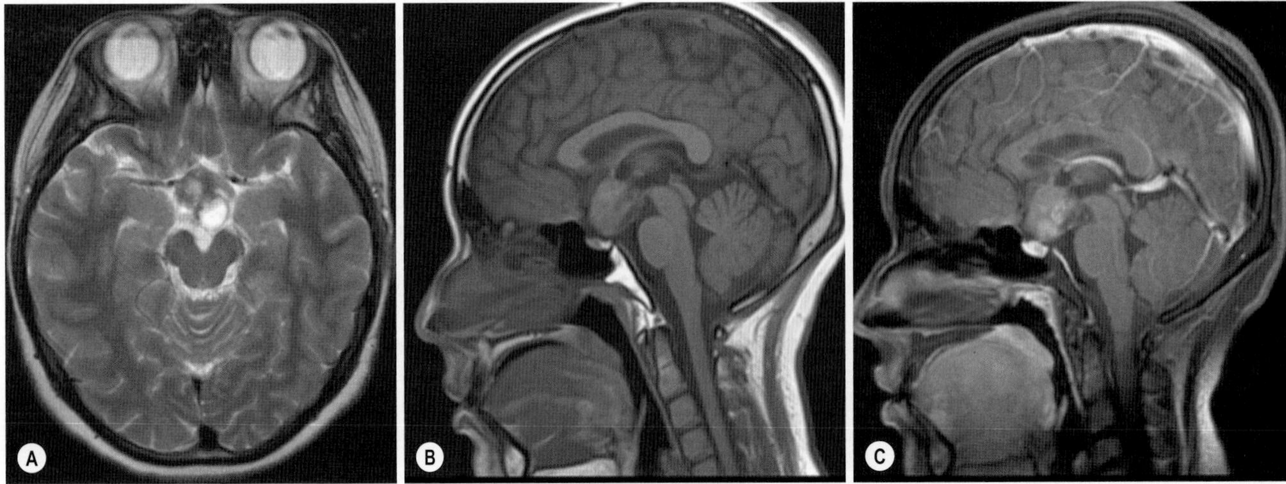

FIGURE 61-37 ■ **Intracranial optic nerve glioma.** T2WI (A), non-enhanced T1WI (B) and post-contrast T1WI (C) in a patient with an optic nerve glioma showing a mass centred on the optic chiasm with a cystic component posteriorly and solid T2 isointense (A) and T1 isointense (B) components that show heterogeneous enhancement (C). A normal enhancing pituitary gland is seen inferior to the mass (C).

Metastases, particularly from breast carcinoma, can cause thickening of the pituitary stalk and can present with diabetes insipidus. Similar appearances may be seen in histiocytosis and sarcoidosis.

For a full list of references, please see ExpertConsult.

FURTHER READING

5. Essig M, Anzalone N, Combs SE, et al. MR imaging of neoplastic central nervous system lesions: review and recommendations for current practice. Am J Neuroradiol 2012;33(5):803–17.
24. Louis DN, Ohgaki H, Wiestler OD, et al. The 2007 WHO classification of tumours of the central nervous system. Acta Neuropathol 2007;114(2):97–109. Erratum: Acta Neuropathol 114(5):547.
29. Wilms G, Demaerel P, Sunaert S. Intra-axial brain tumours. Eur Radiol 2005;15:468–84.
30. Young RJ, Knopp EA. Brain MRI: tumor evaluation. J Magn Reson Imaging 2006;24:709–24.
40. Ricci P. Imaging of adult brain tumors. Neuroimaging Clin N Am 1999;9:651–69.
63. Haldorsen IS, Espeland A, Larsson EM. Central nervous system lymphoma: characteristic findings on traditional and advanced imaging. Am J Neuroradiol 2011;32(6):984–92.
72. Drevelegas A. Extra-axial brain tumors. Eur Radiol 2005;15: 453–67.
83. Bonneville F, Savatovsky J, Chiras J. Imaging of cerebellopontine angle lesions: an update. Part 1: enhancing extra-axial lesions. Eur Radiol 2007;17(10):2472–82.
95. Rennert J, Doerfler A. Imaging of sellar and parasellar lesions. Clin Neurol Neurosurg 2007;109(2):111–24.

CHAPTER 62

Neurovascular Diseases

Amrish Mehta • Brynmor P. Jones

CHAPTER OUTLINE

STROKE

Stroke is the third leading cause of death in Western populations and is the largest single cause of adult disability. It has a tremendous medical, social and economic impact. Over 130,000 cases develop in the UK every year. The annual cost to the NHS, UK families, businesses and public sector exceeds £7 billion.[1]

'Stroke' is an imprecise term used to describe the sudden onset of a persistent neurological deficit caused by partial or complete blockage (ischaemic stroke) or rupture of a cerebral blood vessel (haemorrhage). Ischaemic stroke, which constitutes the great majority of cases (~ 85%),[2] will be discussed in this section. An account of intracranial haemorrhage will follow in the next section.

A transient ischaemic attack (TIA) by definition resolves within 24 h. This includes amaurosis fugax, a transient loss of vision in one eye. The risk of stroke following a TIA is higher than previously thought, maybe up to 8% in the first week and 12% within a month,[3] and even more in those awaiting endarterectomy for a symptomatic carotid stenosis.[4] Indeed, up to 44% of clinical TIAs have recently been shown to actually represent small completed brain infarcts on imaging,[5] and in this situation, the risk of a persistent neurological deficit from a subsequent event is further increased.[6]

Whilst still essential for the exclusion of non-ischaemic causes of the fixed deficit and to identify surgical remedial lesions, imaging is now pivotal in modern acute stroke management and the strategies to recanalise the occluded artery.

Pathophysiology

Normal cerebral blood flow (CBF) is 50–55 mL/100 g brain tissue/min. Cerebral autoregulation responds to a fall in cerebral perfusion pressure (CPP) with vasodilatation and recruitment of collateral vessels, thus increasing cerebral blood volume (CBV) and reducing resistance, in order to maintain CBF. The average time a blood cell remains with a particular volume of tissue rises due to vasodilatation and collateral flow, resulting in a prolonged mean transit time (MTT) and thereby allowing improved oxygen delivery. After the vessels are fully dilated the autoregulatory system cannot properly respond to any further reduction in CPP and therefore CBF starts to decline. Oxygen extraction goes up to compensate, but once this is maximal any further fall in CBF causes cellular dysfunction. The loss of normal neuronal electrical function occurs when CBF falls to 15–20 mL/100 g/min. This may, however, be reversible, depending on the severity and duration of the ischaemia, such that irreversible infarction is likely to occur within minutes if the CBF <10, but moderate ischaemia (10–20) may be reversible for a few hours. At levels of CBF <10, hypoxaemia leads to failure of the ATP-driven cell integrity systems (glutamate, NMDA, Na^+/K^+), resulting in cell depolarisation and influx of Na^+ and water. Cellular swelling and cell death occurs (cytotoxic oedema). In time, structural breakdown of the blood–brain barrier occurs due to ischaemic damage to capillary endothelium. Leakage of intravascular fluid and protein into the extracellular space and later net influx of water to the infarcted area cause vasogenic oedema.[7–9] It is important to note that CBV generally remains preserved in infarction, unless there is a profound reduction in CPP, where it has been postulated that microvascular collapse due to inability of the vessels to remain patent may eventually result in a reduction in CBV.[10]

Following recanalisation of the occluded vessel, either spontaneously (33% within 48 h)[11] or following treatment, the ischaemic region becomes reperfused. This will occur with both viable and non-viable tissue.[12] Indeed, a state of 'post-ischaemic hyperperfusion' ensues where persistently vasodilated vessels result in an elevated CBV.[13] CBF is also elevated.

The Penumbra Model

Following a thromboembolic cerebral arterial occlusion, the decline in regional CBF in the affected brain parenchyma is not uniform. The accepted model, validated in animals and humans, is centred upon an infarct core with very low CBF and cell depolarisation. A peripheral zone—the penumbra—has moderately diminished CBF, resulting in loss of electrical function but preserved cell integrity. The duration of ischaemia in the penumbra is critical, and strategies to recanalise the vessel and restore normal CBF are likely to convey the greatest benefit here. Failure or, more crucially, a delay in achieving this, however, may lead to progression to infarction, especially as this tissue is poorly autoregulated and more vulnerable. Surrounding the penumbra is a zone of benign oligaemia. Here CBF is only mildly impaired and tissue is likely to survive.

Stroke Classification

The most commonly used classification system of ischaemic stroke (TOAST)[14] discriminates between large vessel thromboembolic, cardioembolic, small vessel and 'other' aetiologies. Precise allocation into these subtypes is sometimes difficult and strokes are not infrequently undetermined. A few points to consider are:

- Deep white matter infarcts are typically small vessel in nature but can result from emboli originating from large vessel atheroma or from a cardiac source.
- Middle cerebral artery (MCA) territory infarcts can arise from emboli from the heart or carotid artery, or from in situ thrombosis in the middle cerebral artery.
- Small peripheral infarcts in a vascular territory are usually embolic but the source is not always clear (i.e. cardiac vs carotid vs MCA) (Fig. 62-1).
- Peripheral infarcts involving multiple vascular territories must be from a proximal source and most likely the heart.
- The basilar artery supplies the posterior cerebral arteries (PCAs) unless the posterior communicating artery(s) is/are large, in which case emboli from the carotid circulation may enter their territory. Brainstem infarcts are commonly result from occlusion of short perforating vessels. A combination of infratentorial, thalamic and occipital infarcts suggests an occlusion of distal basilar artery, or 'top of the basilar' syndrome (Fig. 62-2).[15]

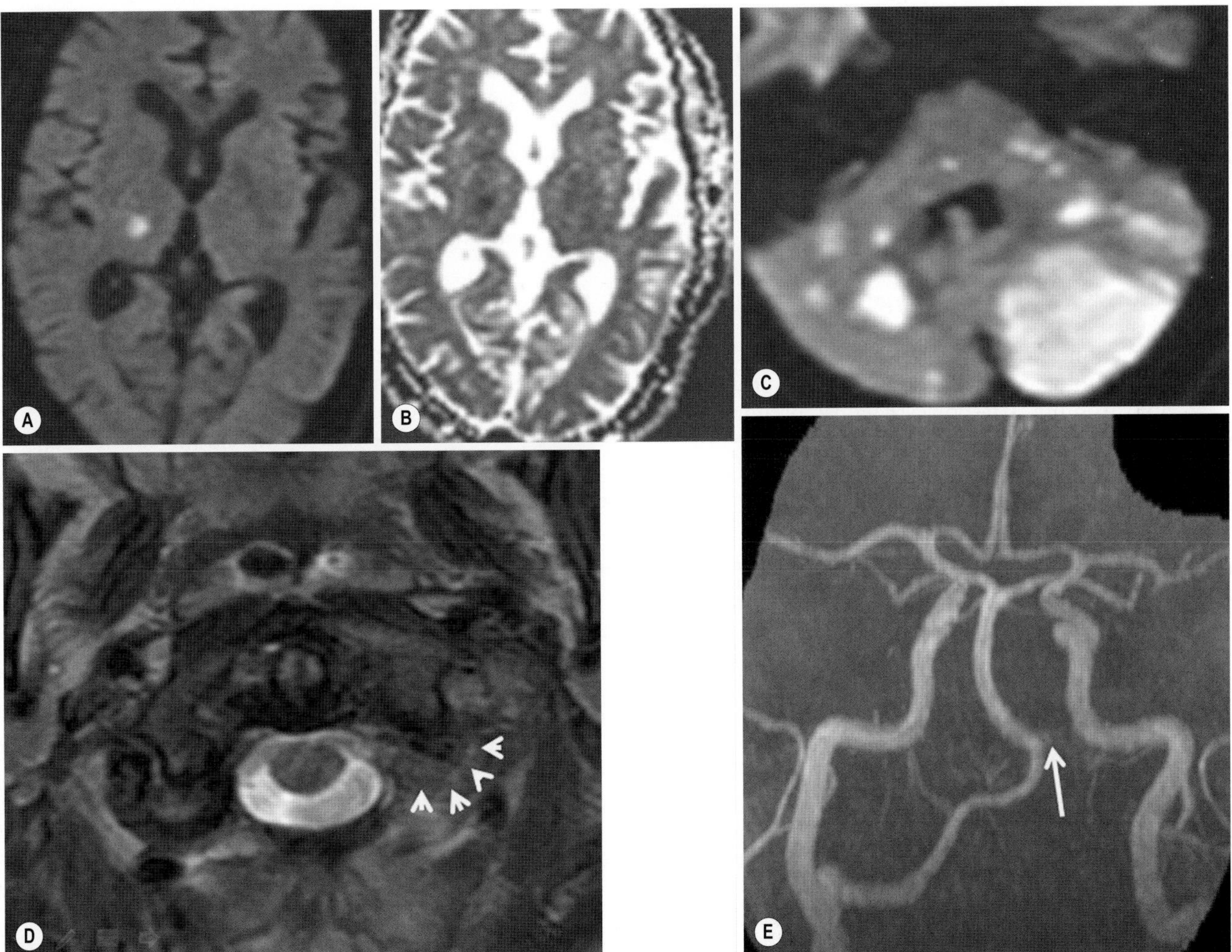

FIGURE 62-1 ■ There are multiple embolic posterior circulation infarcts in the right thalamus (hyperintense on DWI, A, and hypointense on ADC, B), and both cerebellar hemispheres (C). Note the absence of the normal flow-related signal void in the left vertebral artery at the skull base (D, white arrowheads) and absence of flow in the left vertebral artery on the TOF MRA (E, white arrow).

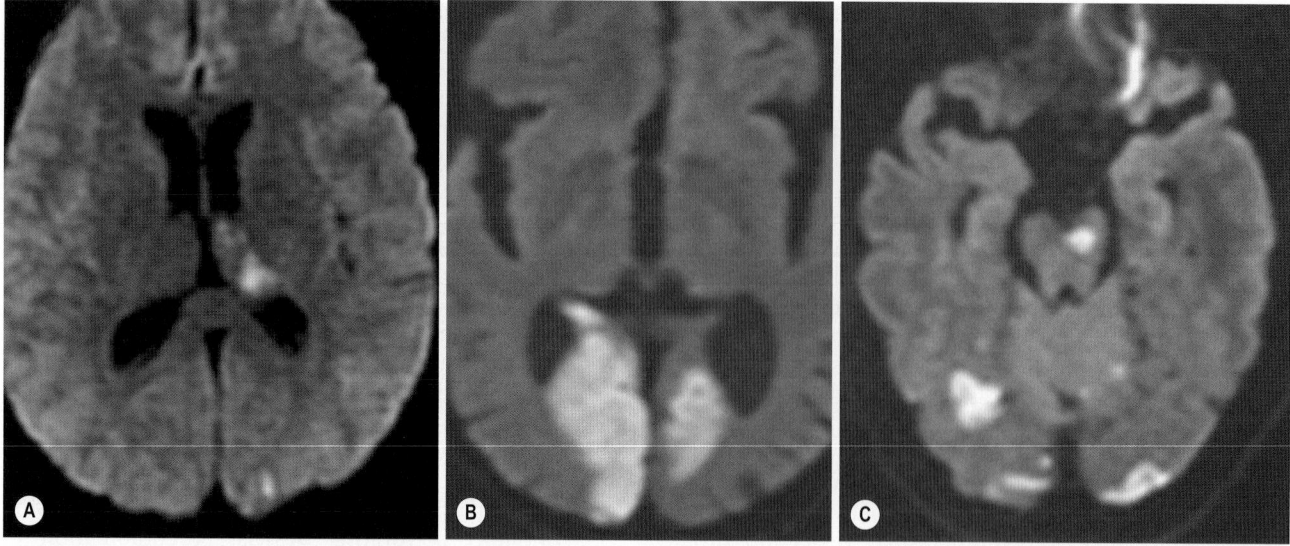

FIGURE 62-2 ■ **Basilar tip syndrome.** Multiple bilateral acute PCA territory infarcts depicted by hyperintensity on DWI are demonstrated in the left thalamus (A), both occipital lobes (B) consistent with impairment of flow at the basilar tip. In a different patient (C), there are multiple acute embolic infarcts in the posterior cerebral and superior cerebellar artery territories.

Causes

Large Vessel Thromboembolic Stroke (40%)

- Most commonly due to thrombus at the site of atherosclerotic plaque or embolisation more distally (artery-to-artery).
- Sites: carotid bifurcation > intracranial internal carotid artery (ICA) > proximal MCA (> anterior cerebral artery (ACA)); vertebral artery origins > distal vertebral (VA) > basilar artery.
- Also vasculopathy (e.g. large vessel vasculitis, dysplasia such as fibromuscular dysplasia (FMD)), dissection.
- Haematological causes: deficiency of protein C/S/ antithrombin III; polycythaemia; pregnancy, oral contraceptives; paraneoplasia.

Cardioembolic Stroke (15–30%)

- Intracardiac thrombus: myocardial infarct, enlarged left atrial appendage, aneurysm, arrhythmia (especially paroxysmal atrial fibrillation (AF)); valvular disease—endocarditis, prosthetic valves, inadequate anticoagulation; right-to-left shunts.
- Cardiac tumours.

Small Vessel or Lacunar Stroke (15–30%)

- Small infarcts (<1.5 cm) in deep perforator territories; typically
  - Lenticulostriate perforators from M1 segment of MCA with infarcts in the lentiform nuclei, internal capsules and corona radiate.
  - Thalamic branches from posterior choroidal perforators from basilar tip, proximal PCAs and posterior communicating arteries cause infarcts in the thalami and posterior internal capsules.
  - Perforators from the basilar artery and its major branches resulting in brainstem infarcts.
- Small vessel pathology: hypertension/diabetes, etc. = ischaemic microangiopathy.
- Also vasculitis/ drugs/ radiation.
- Rarely Susac's syndrome/intravascular lymphoma/CADASIL (cerebral autosomal dominant arteriopathy with subcortical infarcts and leucoencephalopathy).

Borderzone Infarction

Also known as watershed ischaemia, this occurs at the boundaries of the major vessel territories—superficially between the leptomeningeal collaterals of the MCA and ACA which also extend into the corona radiata deep to the superior frontal sulcus, and those of the MCA and PCA. In the deep white matter of the inferior corona radiata and external capsules lies the deep borderzone between the cortical branches and deep M1 perforators of the MCA (Fig. 62-3).

Postulated mechanisms include local (e.g. carotid stenosis) and global (e.g. cardiac insufficiency) hypoperfusion, but embolic infarcts at these sites can also occur.

Borderzone ischaemia in the posterior fossa is uncommon but usually occurs between the superior cerebellar artery (SCA) and posterior inferior cerebellar artery (PICA) territories, and occasionally between the SCA, PICA and anterior inferior cerebellar artery (AICA) territories.

Global Hypoxic–Ischaemic Injury

Inadequate oxygen supply to the entire brain can be the consequence of severe hypotension or impaired blood oxygenation. Global hypoperfusion can result in watershed infarcts as described above, but profound hypoxia

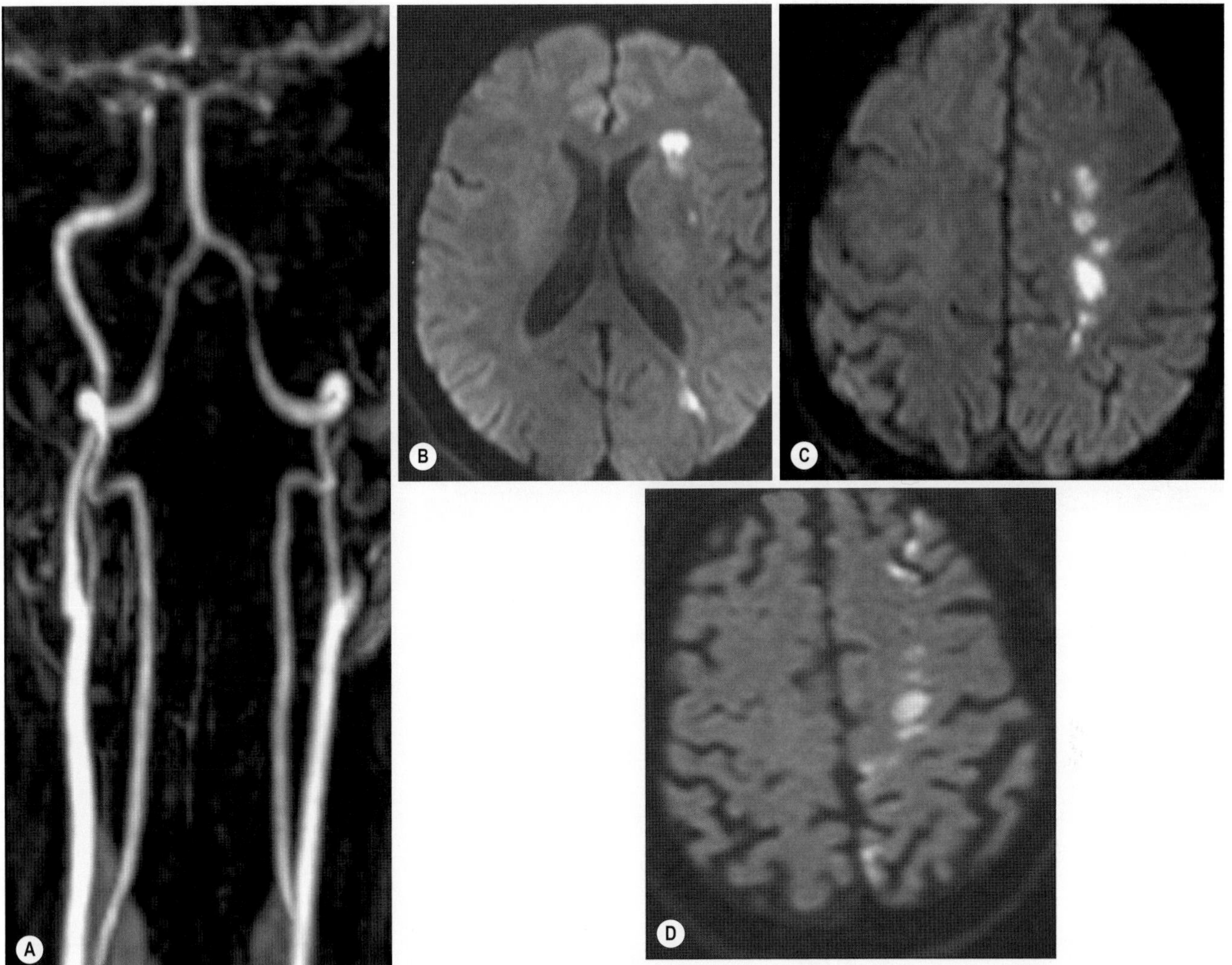

FIGURE 62-3 ■ **Borderzone ischaemia.** There is severe impairment of flow or occlusion in the left ICA from just after its origin (A). This is associated with acute infarcts on DWI in a typical distribution in the left frontal and parietal lobes (B–D), between the MCA and ACA, and MCA and PCA territories. These are presumed to be secondary to hypoperfusion in the left ICA territory. A linear distribution deep to the superior frontal sulcus is very suggestive of ACA–MCA borderzone ischaemia (C, D).

can also cause symmetric ischaemia in the basal ganglia, thalami and hippocampal formations. Anoxia due to defective blood oxygenation such as in carbon monoxide poisoning tends to cause infarcts in sensitive regions, typically, as in this case within the globus pallidus (Fig. 62-4).

Imaging Strategies and Goals in Acute Stroke

Standard Imaging

Brain imaging must be incorporated into the management paradigm of acute stroke. Currently, the only licensed therapy for vessel recanalisation in the acute period involves the administration of intravenous thrombolytic agents—mainly tissue plasminogen activator (tPA). This was derived from key studies (NINDS, ECASS-3 and SITS-MOST)[16–18] which demonstrated significant improvements in the degree of disability at 3 months in patients with ischaemic stroke treated with iv tPA provided they were within 4.5 h of onset, had sustained infarcts of less than one-third of the MCA territory and were less than 80 years old. Traditionally, imaging has been directed at these criteria, employing non-enhanced cranial computed tomography (NECT). Within the past 3 years in the UK following government-initiated restructuring of metropolitan stroke services and considerable investment, thrombolysis rates have risen dramatically from <1% to around 15% in most major hyperacute stroke units (HASUs)—with improvements in outcomes already becoming apparent.[19] In most of these centres, NECT continues to form the mainstay of acute stroke imaging.

Objectives of NECT in Acute Stroke

- To exclude haemorrhage and allow administration of aspirin therapy[20]
- To exclude an alternative cause of the fixed neurological deficit. Around 30% of patients presenting with a stroke-like episode have a non-vascular cause[21]

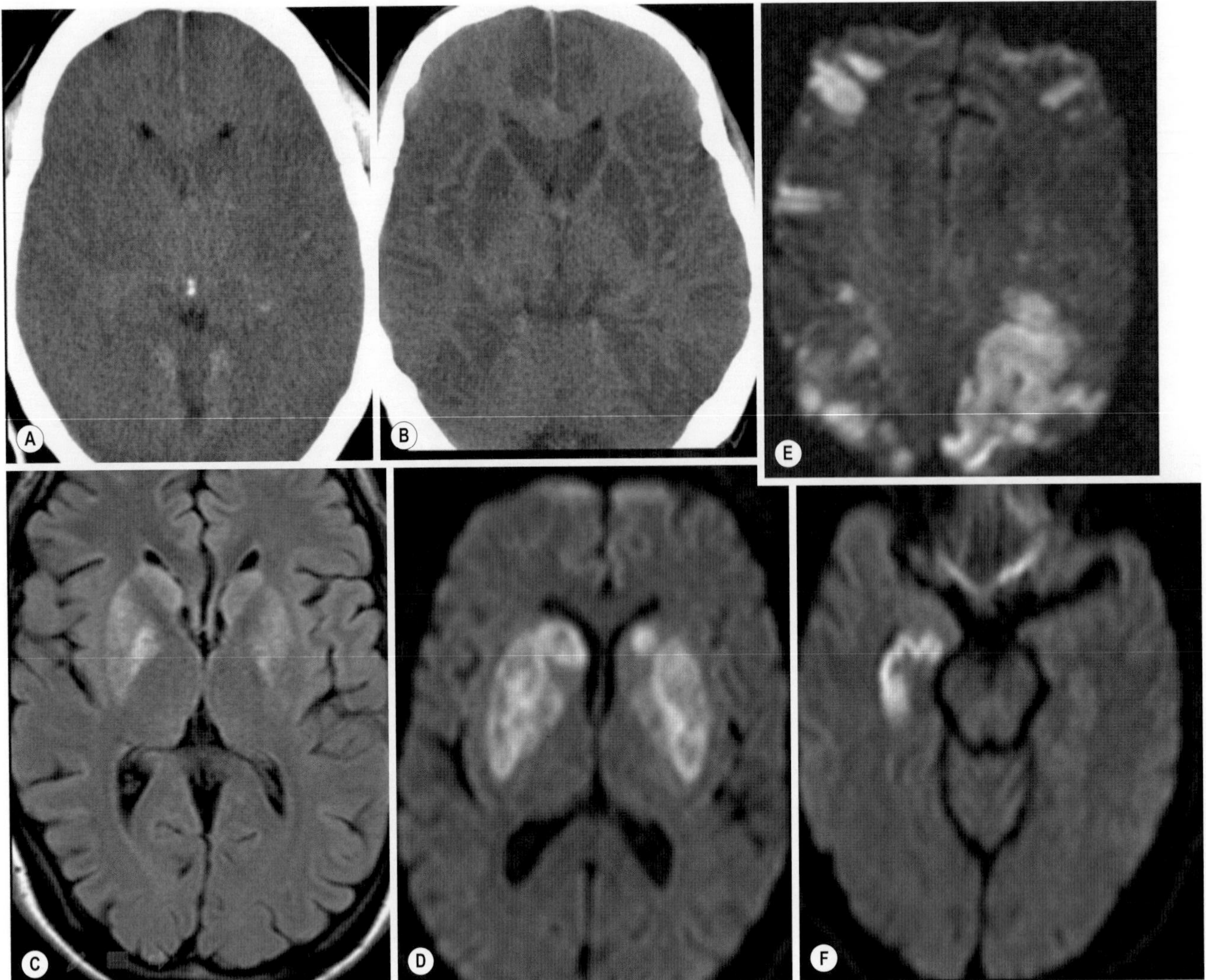

FIGURE 62-4 ■ Global hypoxic—ischaemic insult. The cranial imaging manifestations of global hypoperfusion or hypo-oxygenation typically vary according to their severity and age of the patient. In adults, the most common patterns are shown. On plain CT, bilateral symmetric grey matter hypodensity involving the basal ganglia, thalami and cerebral cortex is typical, acutely with cerebral swelling (A). When profound, the normal grey–white matter relationship is reversed (B). Signal change and restricted diffusion is demonstrated in the affected areas on MRI. Again, this is bilateral and symmetric. The basal ganglia are involved on FLAIR (C) and DWI (D), whilst the frontal and parietal lobes are infarcted in (E). Note that the hippocampal formations are also sensitive to global insults (F).

- To exclude infarcts > 1/3 MCA territory
- To establish that the infarct corroborates the clinical timeline and does not obviously appear subacute
- In cases of suspected posterior circulation stroke, to attempt to identify an obviously thrombosed basilar artery

Hyperacute Infarct Imaging Signs

A dense artery is the earliest detectable change on computed tomography (CT). As it is caused by fresh thrombus occluding the vessel it can be seen at the onset of the ictus. Thrombus may rapidly disperse, so this sign is not always present. When found in the proximal MCA or terminal ICA, it correlates with large infarcts and very poor outcomes[22] although it has a better prognosis if limited to an MCA branch within the sylvian fissure (the sylvian fissure 'dot' sign) (Fig. 62-5).[23] MCA calcification can mimic this sign but is often bilateral. The basilar artery may also appear dense in the case of posterior circulation infarcts, particularly the 'top of basilar' syndrome. The early parenchymal signs on CT are reduced grey matter density and brain swelling, manifest as effacement of sulci (Fig. 62-6). These changes are traditionally thought to reflect cytotoxic oedema, which reduces the Hounsfield number of grey matter so it is indistinguishable from adjacent white matter. In early MCA infarcts this causes a reduction in clarity of the margins of the lentiform nucleus and cortex, particularly in the insula. Hypodensity on early CT examinations affecting more than 50% of the MCA territory is associated with a high mortality rate,[24] and intravenous thrombolysis is contraindicated when more than one-third of the MCA territory is involved. However, infarct size evaluation is notoriously difficult in the acute

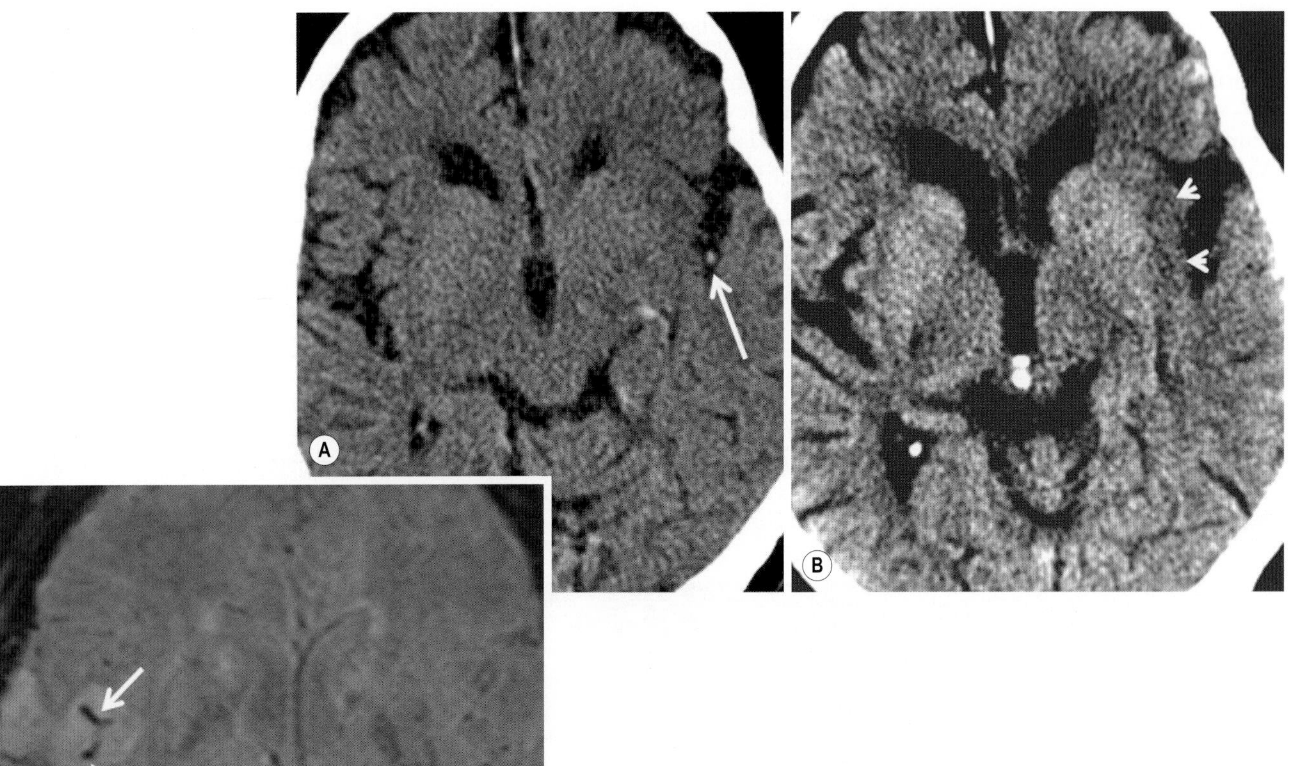

FIGURE 62-5 ■ **Sylvian 'dot' sign.** (A) There is thrombus within an M2 division of the left MCA—shown as a hyperdense dot in the left sylvian fissure (white arrow). This caused by an acute left MCA territory infarct involving the left insula with loss of conspicuity of the cortex. This is made more conspicuous by adjusting the window settings to W = 35, L = 35: the 'stroke' window (B, white arrowheads). Thrombus within a right M2 branch of a different patient is shown here as marked linear hypointensity ('blooming') on the SWI sequence (C, white arrows). This is caused by exaggerated sensitivity to susceptibility artefact afforded by SWI—in this case from deoxyhaemoglobin in acute thrombus.

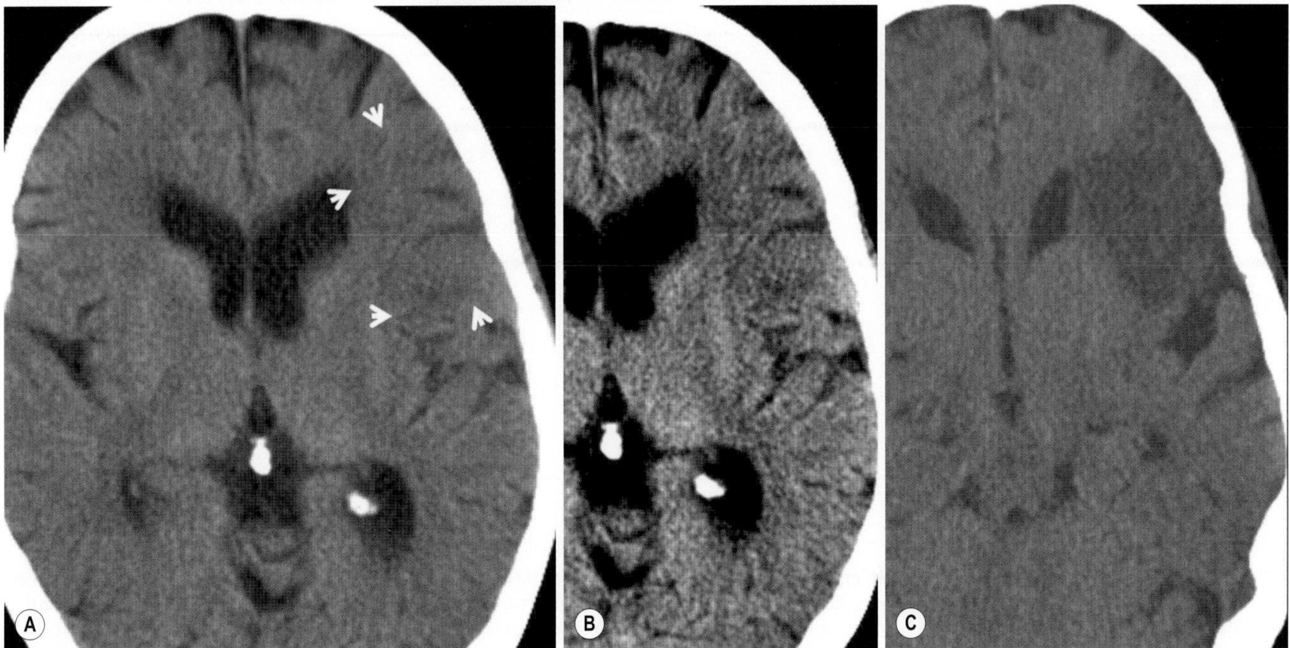

FIGURE 62-6 ■ **Evolution of infarct on CT.** In the hyperacute phase, there is subtle parenchymal swelling with sulcal effacement, and very mild cortical low attenuation with loss of grey–white matter differentiation (A, white arrowheads). This is more conspicuous when window settings are adjusted to 35/35 (B). Subacutely, there is well-demarcated and conspicuous wedge-shaped parenchymal low attenuation, with sulcal effacement (C).

phase, due to the lack of convincing parenchymal changes in 50–60% of NECT within 2 h. The sensitivity of CT for infarcts has been reported to be only 30% at 3 h[25] and 60% at 24 h. These difficulties have led to the development of the Alberta Stroke Program Early CT Score (ASPECTS).[26] ASPECTS can be used to predict outcome and risk of post-thrombolysis haemorrhage. It correlates well with diffusion weighted imaging (DWI) findings at presentation[27] and facilitates more accurate interpretation of emergency CT by nonexperts.[28] Even in patients not suitable for thrombolysis it seems intuitive that a methodical approach such as ASPECTS is likely to increase accuracy and reliability of CT interpretation, at least for supratentorial events (Fig. 62-7). The sensitivity to subtle grey matter low attenuation is enhanced using the 'stroke window' setting when reviewing images (window width = 35/window level = 35).

ASPECTS Infarct Size Scoring System

- Two NECT axial slices are examined (a, level of basal ganglia and internal capsule; b, bodies of the lateral ventricles)
- Ten regions are identified (four deep and six cortical)
- Starting with a score of 10, 1 point is deducted for each of these areas that is involved.
- If the score is <7, the infarct is considered >1/3 of an MCA territory

The key advantages of NECT are that it is very rapid, accessible, simple and safe. Speed is essential as the therapeutic window is closing all the time.

On magnetic resonance imaging (MRI), thrombus may cause loss of a normal arterial flow void. However, arterial high signal may be seen in a patent vessel on

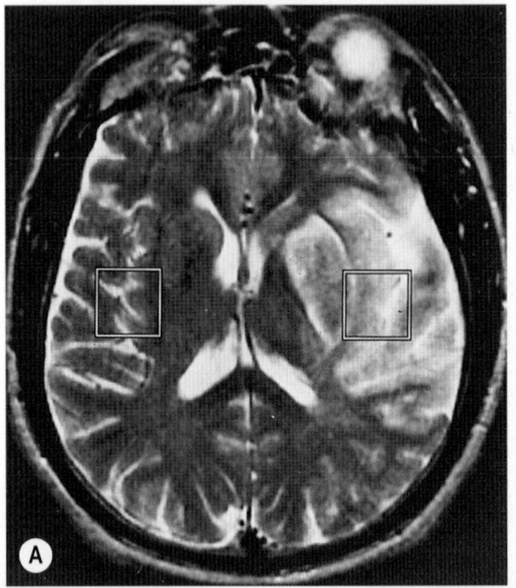

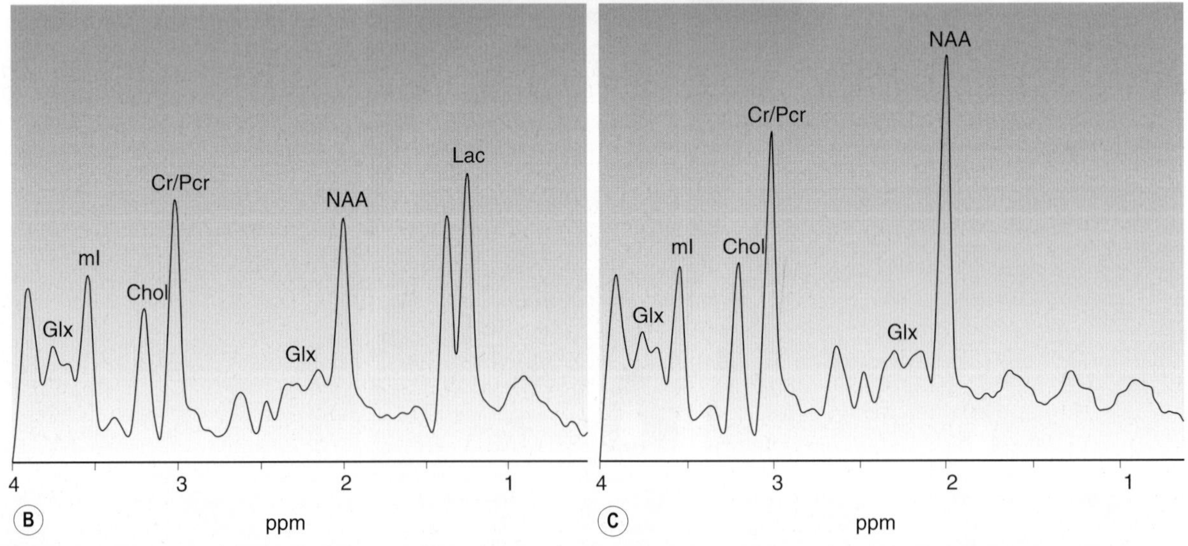

FIGURE 62-7 ■ **ASPECTS for early ischaemic change on CT.** A = anterior circulation; P = posterior circulation; C = caudate; L = lentiform; IC = internal capsule; I = insular ribbon; M1 = anterior middle cerebral artery (MCA) cortex; M2 = MCA cortex lateral to insular ribbon; M3 = posterior MCA cortex; M4, M5 and M6 are anterior, lateral and posterior MCA territories immediately superior to M1, M2 and M3, rostral to basal ganglia. Subcortical structures are alotted three points (C, L and IC), MCA cortex is alotted seven points (insular cortex, M1, M2, M3, M4, M5 and M6). A point is lost for each area that shows early ischaemic change (low density or swelling). The range of scores is 0–10, representing an infarct of the entire territory and normal findings, respectively. (From Barber P A, Demchuk A M, Zhang J et al 2000 Validity and reliability of a quantitative computed tomography score in predicting outcome of hyperacute stroke before thrombolytic therapy. Lancet 355:1670–1674 with permission from Elsevier.)

fluid-attenuated inversion recovery (FLAIR) MRI due to altered flow, a useful qualitative sign of reduced perfusion when the parenchyma usually still appears normal.[29] Intravascular enhancement due to sluggish flow in affected vessels—probably veins—may be seen on contrast-enhanced CT and MRI acutely.[30] Parenchymal MRI changes include cortical swelling and T1/T2 prolongation, more obvious on T2 sequences, particularly FLAIR. Parenchymal hyperintensity is often absent or very subtle in infarcts prior to 3 h,[31,32] suggesting that early parenchymal low density on CT may be due to abnormal perfusion (reduced CBV) rather than oedema.[33] Furthermore, brain swelling on CT without accompanying low density does not always progress to infarction. Such cases may also be due to abnormal perfusion, but a compensatory increase in CBV rather than a reduction.[34] Thus, whilst it is generally accepted that swelling with obvious low density on CT is an indication of infarction, perhaps subtle low density or swelling without low density are sometimes signs of compromised perfusion that may be reversible, particularly the latter. Diffusion-weighted imaging (DWI) has a pre-eminent role in acute stroke imaging due to its extremely high sensitivity and specificity,[35] with parenchymal hyperintensity as early as 5 min following the onset of infarction. DWI should be interpreted in conjunction with an apparent diffusion coefficient (ADC) map, which is derived from the DWI data and in the clinical environment is displayed as a grey scale 'image' for ease of use. 'Restricted diffusion' in acute infarcts returns high signal on DWI and appears dark on the ADC map (Figs. 62-8 and 62-9). Whilst DWI hyperintense areas (with appropriate ADC hypointensity) are considered to and almost always do represent areas of irreversible ischaemia, recently investigators have reported that following early recanalisation with either intravenous agents or mechanical embolectomy, DWI-positive areas may not progress to infarction. This phenomenon does not occur commonly and the proportion of the overall insult which appears to reverse is relatively small. Moreover, the effect is reduced in tissue with more profoundly reduced ADC. Nevertheless it does suggest that DWI-defined early ischemic injury physiologically represents the combination of irreversible ischemic core and a small potentially reversible surrounding area (Fig. 62-10).[36–38]

Whilst NECT has a much higher sensitivity than spin-echo MRI for the detection of acute haemorrhage, T2*-weighted gradient-echo imaging (GRE) has equivalent or superior sensitivity compared with CT.[39–41] The sensitivity for detection of deoxygenated haemoglobin—the key moiety in acute haemorrhage—is further enhanced with the susceptibility-weighted imaging (SWI) sequence.[42]

Advanced Imaging

The availability of neuroradiological expertise, multislice CT technology and improved access to MRI in some, typically neuroscience, units allows the delivery of advanced imaging techniques. These include 'penumbral imaging' which attempts to establish the relationship of the irreversible core infarct with any potentially salvageable but ischaemic penumbra; angiographic imaging to identify the site of vascular compromise and additional techniques such as permeability imaging and SWI. In the setting of hyperacute stroke, the challenge is to deliver this information rapidly.

Objectives of Penumbral Imaging

- To more accurately delineate the size of the core infarct
- To establish whether a penumbra of salvageable tissue is present

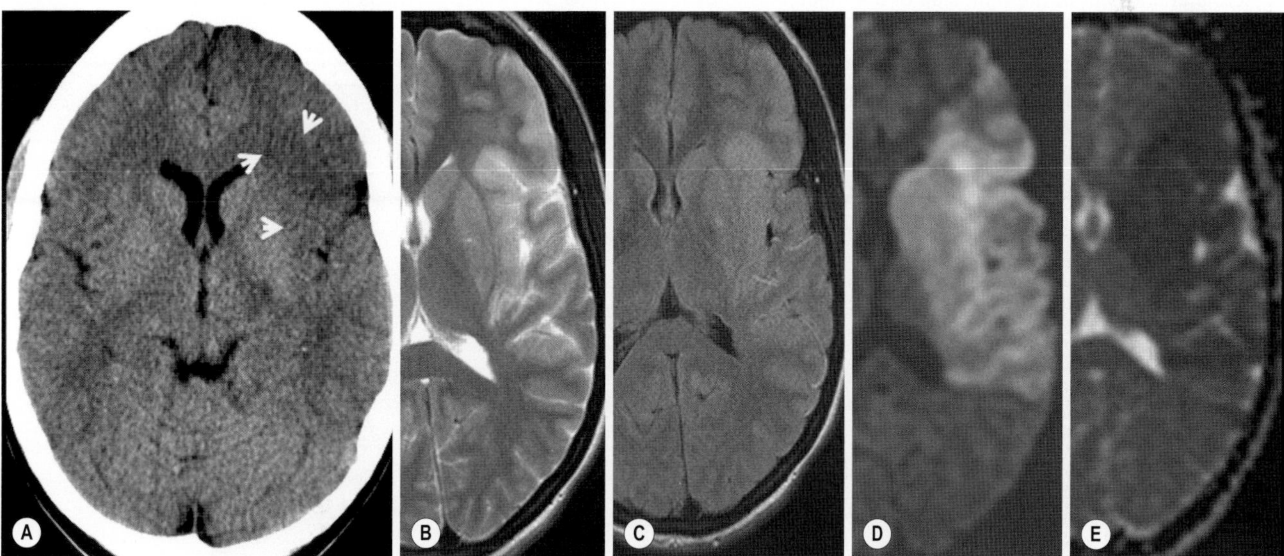

FIGURE 62-8 ■ An acute left MCA territory infarct presenting 7 h after onset is visible on CT (A) as low attenuation in the left frontal operculum and left insula. At this stage, not only is the infarct shown as T2 hyperintensity and gyral swelling but also more extensive involvement of the left MCA territory is identified on T2-weighted and FLAIR imaging (B, C). However, the full extent of involvement—including the basal ganglia—is only clearly demonstrated on DWI (D) as hyperintensity and on the corresponding ADC map (E) as hypointensity.

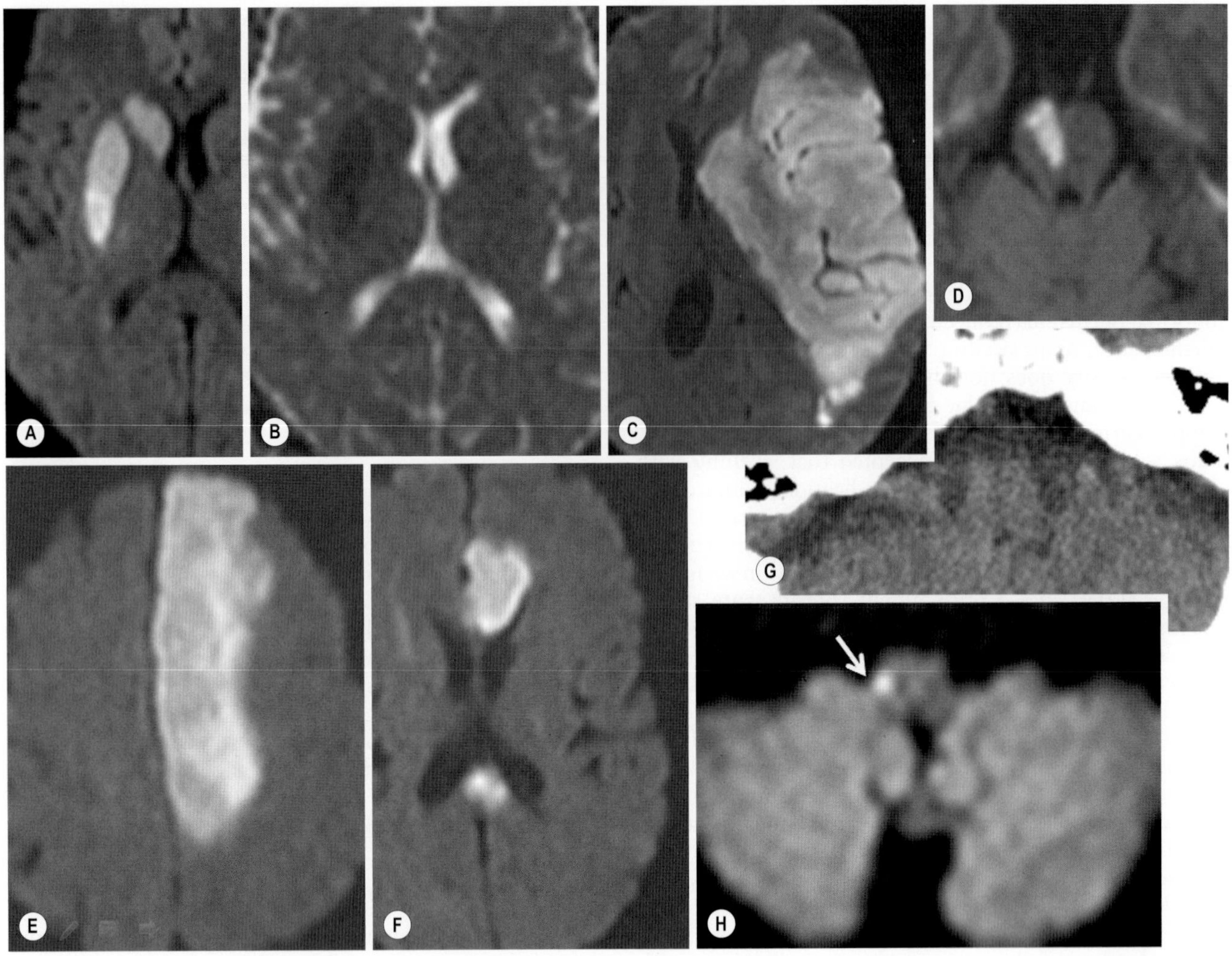

FIGURE 62-9 ■ **Acute territorial infarcts on DWI.** Acute right-sided striatal infarct with hyperintensity on DWI (A) and hypointensity on ADC (B). Other acute infarcts involving the entire left MCA (C) and left ACA (E, F) territories. Note the involvement of the left side of the genu and splenium of the corpus callosum in (F). However, the splenium is often supplied by the PCA. (D) A typical perforator infarct in the pons involving the anteromedial aspect of the basis pontis. A small right PICA territory infarct involving the posterolateral aspect of the right side of the medulla is shown on DWI (G, white arrow), but is inconspicuous on CT (H).

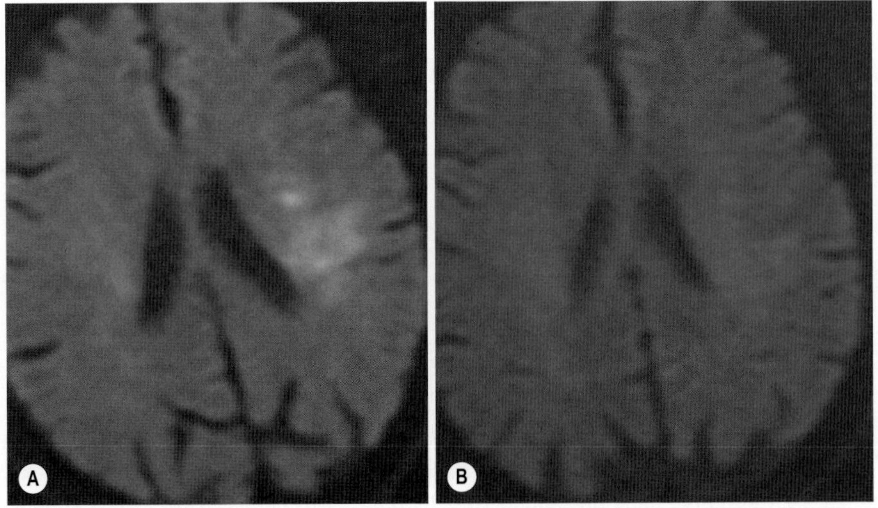

FIGURE 62-10 ■ **DWI reversibility.** This patient presented with right hemiparesis at 4 h post onset. Initial DWI at presentation (A) showed a modest area of restricted diffusion consistent with a small core infarct. However, on the subsequent MRI performed at 24 h post iv thrombolysis (B), there has been some resolution of the DWI abnormality, rather than progression to an established infarct.

- To evaluate the size and severity of ischaemia of the penumbra

The following should be considered in this analysis:

- Large core infarcts have a poorer outcome, regardless of penumbra size or severity. Specifically, core volumes greater than 70 mL are associated with adverse outcomes regardless of recanalisation therapy.[43]
- Core infarcts with small penumbra are described as 'matched' defects and carry reduced reperfusion benefit. However, some units proceed with thrombolysis in this situation because of the possibility of partial reversibility of the DWI-positive volume.
- Large areas of salvageable tissue, known as 'mismatch,' are likely to benefit most from recanalisation therapy.[44–46]
- Areas of mildly ischaemic penumbra may reperfuse spontaneously—known as 'benign oligaemia'.
- Appropriate patient selection using penumbral imaging may extend the therapeutic time window beyond 4.5 h.[47–49]

Perfusion Imaging. In the context of stroke, perfusion imaging with CT (CTP) and perfusion weighted MRI (PWI) is most often performed using a first-pass intravenous contrast technique. In PWI, this is achieved using dynamic susceptibility contrast enhancement (DSE-MRI), which relies on the long-range susceptibility effects of gadolinium resulting in a reduction in signal intensity as it transits through brain tissue. By mathematical deconvolution of the time-density (CT) or time-negative signal intensity (MRI) curves which are generated, 3 parameters are usually studied:

- relative cerebral blood volume (rCBV)—essentially the area under the curve
- relative cerebral blood flow (rCBF)—related to the gradient of the curve at contrast arrival
- mean transit time (MTT)—calculated from the Central Volume Principle: MTT = CBV/CBF

These are typically depicted as colour maps. However, there is considerable debate in the literature as to which of the parameters is the most reliable surrogate marker of core and of penumbra. Earlier studies employed first-generation perfusion scanning protocols with shorter acquisition times of 40–50 s which resulted in potential underestimation of both CBV and MTT due to failure to image the whole of the time–density or time signal–intensity curves, Furthermore, standard post-processing algorithms with no correction for the delay in contrast arrival—such as due to a stenosis or haemodynamic instability—exposed the interpretation to underestimation of CBF and overestimation of MTT.[50–54] Whilst new protocols allow for longer acquisition times (60–70 s), and many of the latest-generation post-processing platforms now correct for delay, there is still considerable variability and lack of standardisation in the parameters generated from scanning machines and platforms (or even different versions of the same platform) from different vendors.[55–59] This is particularly true with CT perfusion. Recent reports suggest that newer techniques do allow more accurate and reliable characterisation of the core and penumbra on imaging.[60–62] These are given in Table 62-1.

TABLE 62-1 Thresholds for Determining Infarct Core and Penumbra With CT and MR Perfusion Imaging

	CTP	PWI-MRI
Infarct core	Thresholded CBF (nominally better than CBV)	DWI
Ischaemic penumbra	Thresholded MTT (probably better than CBF)	Thresholded MTT and CBF

As alluded to earlier, the size of the infarct core is the single most important imaging parameter in determining whether recanalisation therapy would be appropriate. Whilst fluorodeoxyglucose (FDG) positron emission tomography (PET) is considered the most accurate, it is clearly not the most practical for clinical use. In descending order, DWI, thresholded CT-CBF, CT-CBV (both from CT perfusion) and CTA-source data are more sensitive and precise than NECT.[63] Unfortunately, for CT perfusion, the threshold at which the CBF should be set to establish the core varies between platforms but is generally 70–85% reduction compared with the normal contralateral side.[61] It remains unclear as to why perfusion imaging derived CBV approximates to the DWI-defined core, when experimentally, CBV rarely falls in an infarct. Additionally, a volume of tissue which has infarcted but then becomes rapidly reperfused may become masked and appear normal on CBV.[64]

Delay-corrected MTT is considered the most reliable biomarker of the penumbra in CT perfusion when appropriately thresholded, at 150% relative to the contralateral normal side.[62] This threshold discriminates between the genuinely 'at-risk' tissue and the region of benign oligaemia. Simultaneous evaluation of CBF should corroborate this as CBF will generally be preserved or only mildly reduced in benign oligaemia, but more significantly diminished in at-risk tissue (Fig. 62-11).

T_{max} is an additional parameter generated by perfusion imaging—at the time of the CBF calculation—and has been used as a penumbra biomarker.[48]

Mismatch is usually accepted as the volume of penumbra, being at least 20% larger than the core.

Angiographic Imaging. Improvements in endovascular device design and the availability of fast, non-invasive angiographic techniques to rapidly identify the site of the occluded vessel are driving a revolution towards intra-arterial thrombolysis and probably, more effectively, endovascular mechanical embolectomy in acute stroke treatment. In comparison with iv tPA therapy, these strategies are not only more successful in recanalising occluded cerebral vessels[65–67] but also are likely to deliver more favourable outcomes in the treatment of strokes from occluded major vessels such as the distal ICA and proximal MCA, and may well prolong the therapeutic window significantly beyond 4.5 h in selected patients. Furthermore, endovascular procedures to recanalise an occluded basilar artery are considered appropriate even up to 18 h. In addition, mechanical embolectomy can be employed when there is a contraindication to tPA, most notably anticoagulant therapy and recent surgery.

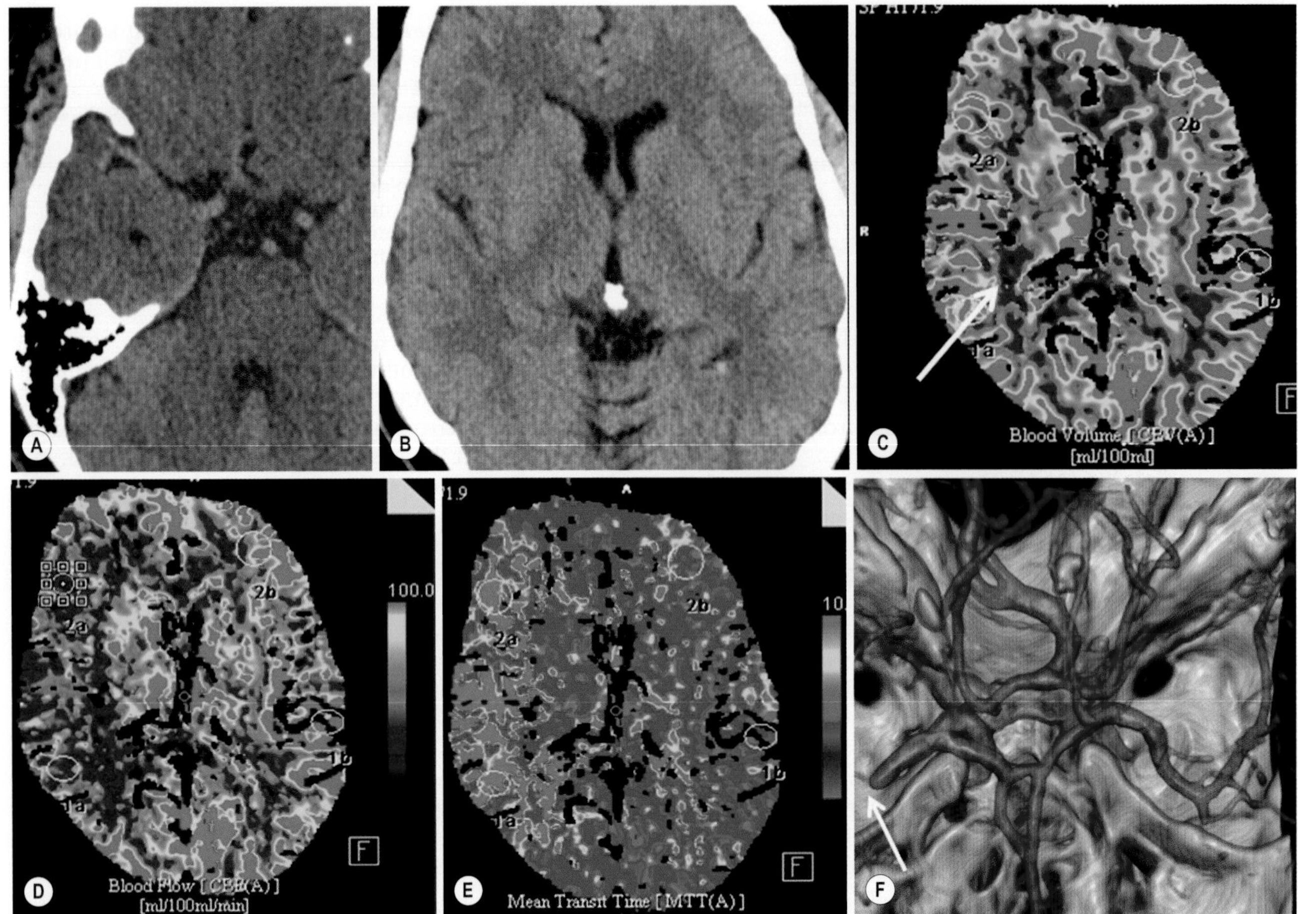

FIGURE 62-11 ■ Ischaemic penumbra on CT perfusion. (A, B) Within 2 h of left-sided hemiparesis, the non-contrast enhanced CT was normal. Note that there is no vessel hyperdensity. (C) However, there is a small area of reduced CBV in the right temporo-occipital white matter (white arrow), indicating only a very small 'core' of irreversibly infarcted tissue. (D, E) The CBF and MTT perfusion maps demonstrate a large volume of ischaemic but potentially salvageable tissue, with prolonged transit times (warm colours, E) and reduced cerebral blood flow (cold colours, D). (F) Volume-rendered image from a CT angiogram shows occlusion of the M1 segment of the right middle cerebral artery (white arrow).

In the US, the MERCI™ device has been approved for use up to 8 h post onset.[66] Current technology primarily involves a stent-clot retriever device.

However, procedure-related complication rates are high and there is a paucity of Level 1 data demonstrating a clear overall benefit. Indeed, only one randomised controlled trial has been conducted, evaluating intra-arterial therapy—in this case intra-arterial thrombolysis. This did demonstrate a significant improvement in outcomes compared with intravenous heparin.[68] In several non-randomised control trial open label trials, functional outcomes were poorer than with iv tPA. Longer times to recanalisation (relating to anaesthesia, endovascular access and device deployment) and the selection bias of more severe strokes likely account for much of this.[69]

Nevertheless these techniques are set to become a more common therapeutic option for strokes where the thrombus is in the distal ICA or proximal MCA, or in the basilar artery.[70] Therefore, initial angiographic imaging to identify an appropriate endovascular target is a necessity. As shown above, this can be most effectively achieved using CT, as part of a multimodal examination also delivering penumbral information with CT perfusion. However, data sets are large (typically >200 slices from the aortic arch to the circle of Willis) and reviewing these can take time. By contrast, interpretation of the maximum intensity projection (MIP) images of an MRA is rapid (Figs. 62-12–62-14).

Useful information regarding the extracranial neck arteries is also provided with CT angiography (CTA) or magnetic resonance angiography (MRA). In particular, possible embolic sources in the aortic arch and carotid bifurcation are well demonstrated, as are alternative aetiologies such as vessel dissection.

When acquired correctly (i.e. with saline chase following the iv contrast injection), the thin-slice CT angiographic images of the head (known as the CTA-source data) approximate to relative cerebral blood volume maps. When reviewed on a 35 window width/35 window level setting ('stroke window'), low density on the CTA-source data depicts the infarct core and correlates well with CBV maps from perfusion CT.[63]

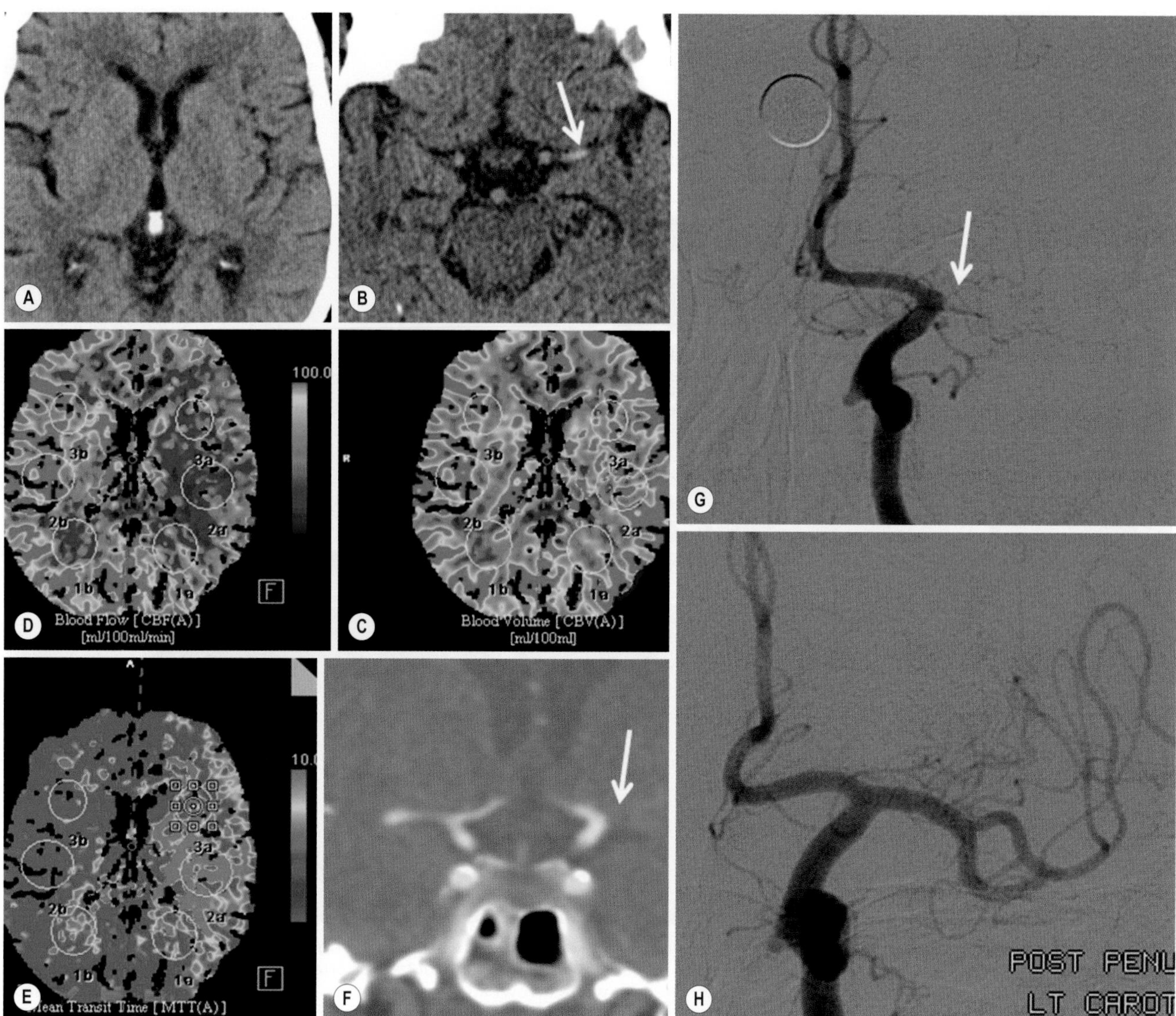

FIGURE 62-12 ■ Mechanical thrombectomy to recanalise an occluded left MCA following identification of a large penumbra using CTP. Within 90 min of the onset of severe right hemiparesis and receptive aphasia, the plain CT showed a hyperdense left M1 segment (B, white arrow) but no parenchymal changes (A). There is also no evidence of a core infarct on the CBV maps (C) but there is significant mismatch with a large penumbra on both CBF (D) and MTT (E) maps. CT angiography confirms occlusion of the left MCA from its origin (F, white arrow), as does the digital subtraction catheter angiogram performed prior to endovascular intervention (G). Following a single pass with a stent clot-retriever device, there has been complete recanalisation of the left MCA (H).

Assessment of Collateral Flow. The importance of perfusion to ischaemic brain tissue via an alternate route is becoming increasingly recognised. This 'collateral' flow—chiefly via leptomeningeal vessels—if adequate is likely to sustain ischaemic tissue for hours or even days after a vessel occlusion. In these areas, CBF and CBV are likely to be preserved whilst the MTT is prolonged. Improved collateral supply is associated with milder deficits, smaller final infarcts and improved outcomes after major vessel occlusions.[71] Imaging the collateral supply is challenging and a number of studies have employed a variety of techniques, from catheter angiography[72] to CTA,[73] MRA[74] and transcranial Doppler ultrasound.[75] CTA is likely to be the most accessible method, as part of the multimodal approach to acute stroke imaging.

Additional Advanced Imaging Techniques. Perfusion imaging, including PET, is also used for elective assessment of haemodynamic reserve and stroke risk. For example, perfusion may be normal at rest despite a significant carotid stenosis but show reduced blood flow following acetazolamide challenge, which is the reverse of normal.[76,77] Single-photon emission computed tomography (SPECT) with ^{99m}Tc-HMPAO will show a perfusion defect as soon as vascular occlusion occurs, although care must be taken in interpretation of HMPAO SPECT studies 10 days or more after the onset of stroke due to hyperfixation of the radiopharmaceutical in infarcted tissue.[78] Quantification of the degree of ischaemia using HMPAO SPECT will predict risk of intracranial haemorrhage following intra-arterial thrombolysis[79]

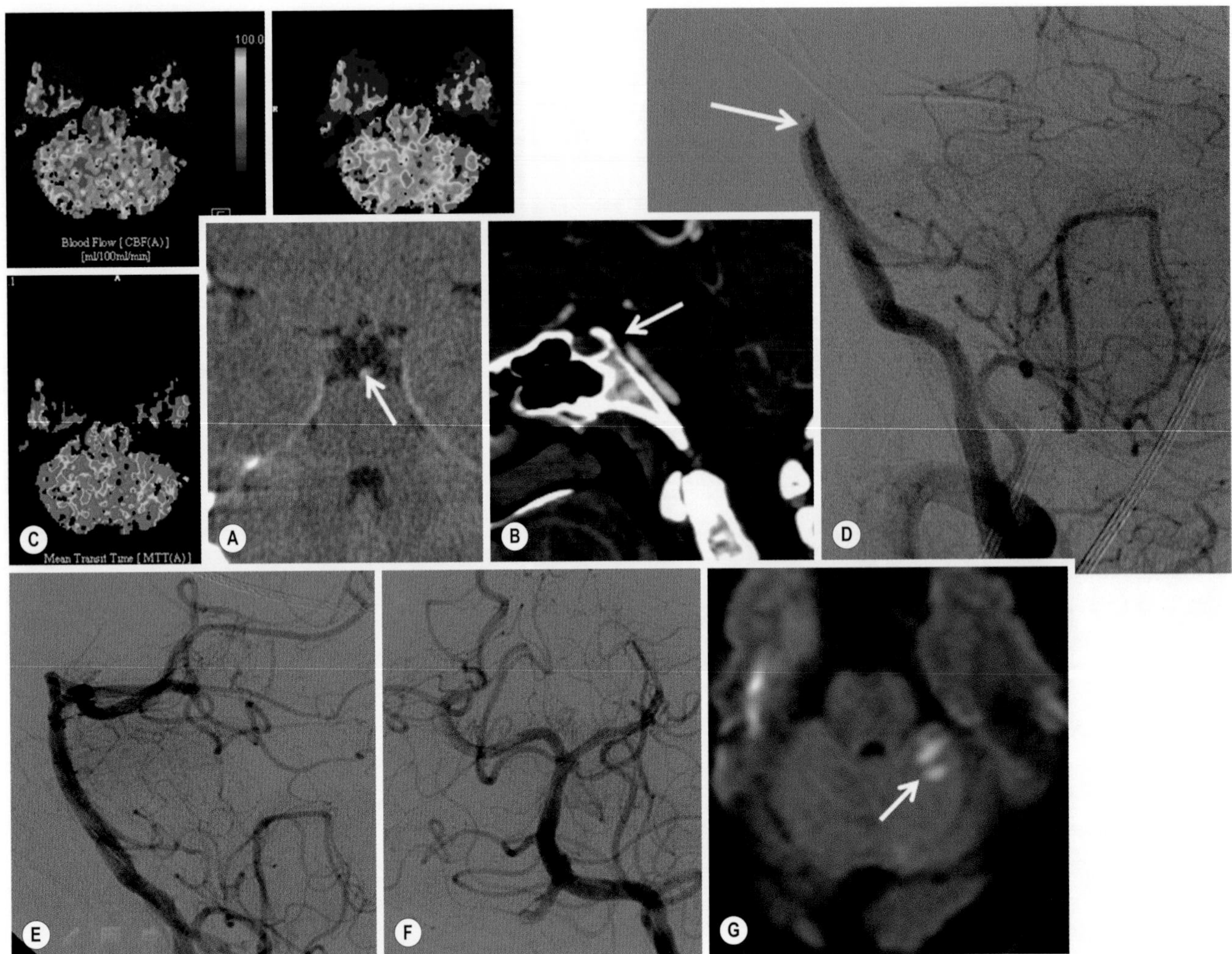

FIGURE 62-13 ■ **Basilar artery thrombectomy.** A young woman presenting with a stuttering progressive reduction in consciousness, a complex ophthalmoplegia and nystagmus was shown to have a hyperdense distal basilar artery on plain CT (A, white arrow). CT angiography confirmed occlusion of the distal basilar artery (B, white arrow) and hypoperfusion was present in the superior aspects of both cerebellar hemispheres on CTP (C, warm colours on MTT). Mechanical thrombectomy, deploying a thrombo-aspirator device, was performed, resulting in complete recanalisation of the basilar artery, shown on digital subtraction angiography following left vertebral artery injection (E and F, compared with D), with total clinical recovery. An MRI performed at 24 h shows only a small infarct in the left superior cerebellar hemisphere (G, white arrow).

but there is currently no practical use for isotope studies in the acute setting.

In addition to the increased sensitivity for acute haemorrhage, SWI also depicts the acutely thrombosed segment of a major intracranial vessel as a prominent, markedly hypointense, expanded, serpiginous structure due to the exaggerated 'blooming' effect.[42] Furthermore, early studies suggest that the ischaemic but potentially salvageable brain tissue may be shown on SWI as tissue with prominent hypointense parenchymal and pial vessels due to engorgement of veins with deoxygenated blood (Figs. 62-15C and 62-15E).[80]

Permeability imaging, which provides imaging biomarkers of the integrity of the blood–brain barrier, can be performed using longer-acquisition CT perfusion or dynamic contrast-enhanced perfusion MRI (DCE-MRI), which is also a first-pass contrast-enhanced perfusion study but evaluates the T1 effects of contrast passage, as opposed to the T2* (susceptibility) effects of DSE described earlier. There is some evidence that increased permeability in infarcted/ischaemic brain tissue is predictive of subsequent haemorrhage following recanalisation therapy in both animal and human experiments.[81–87]

CT or MRI? Penumbral imaging can be achieved effectively on both CT and MR platforms, using perfusion techniques. Despite the superior characterisation of the acute infarct with DWI, whole brain coverage with PWI, rapid visual assessment of vessel occlusion on MRA and at least comparable ability (to NECT) of GRE T2* or SWI to identify acute haemorrhage (Fig. 62-15), multimodal CT appears to have maintained its foothold in most UK neuroscience units. This is largely due to the near-whole head coverage of perfusion CT in machines with 128 slices or more, the rapid acquisition times, much greater access, the reliability of CT angiography (to be discussed later) and rapid more often automated post-processing. Logistical issues regarding immediate access

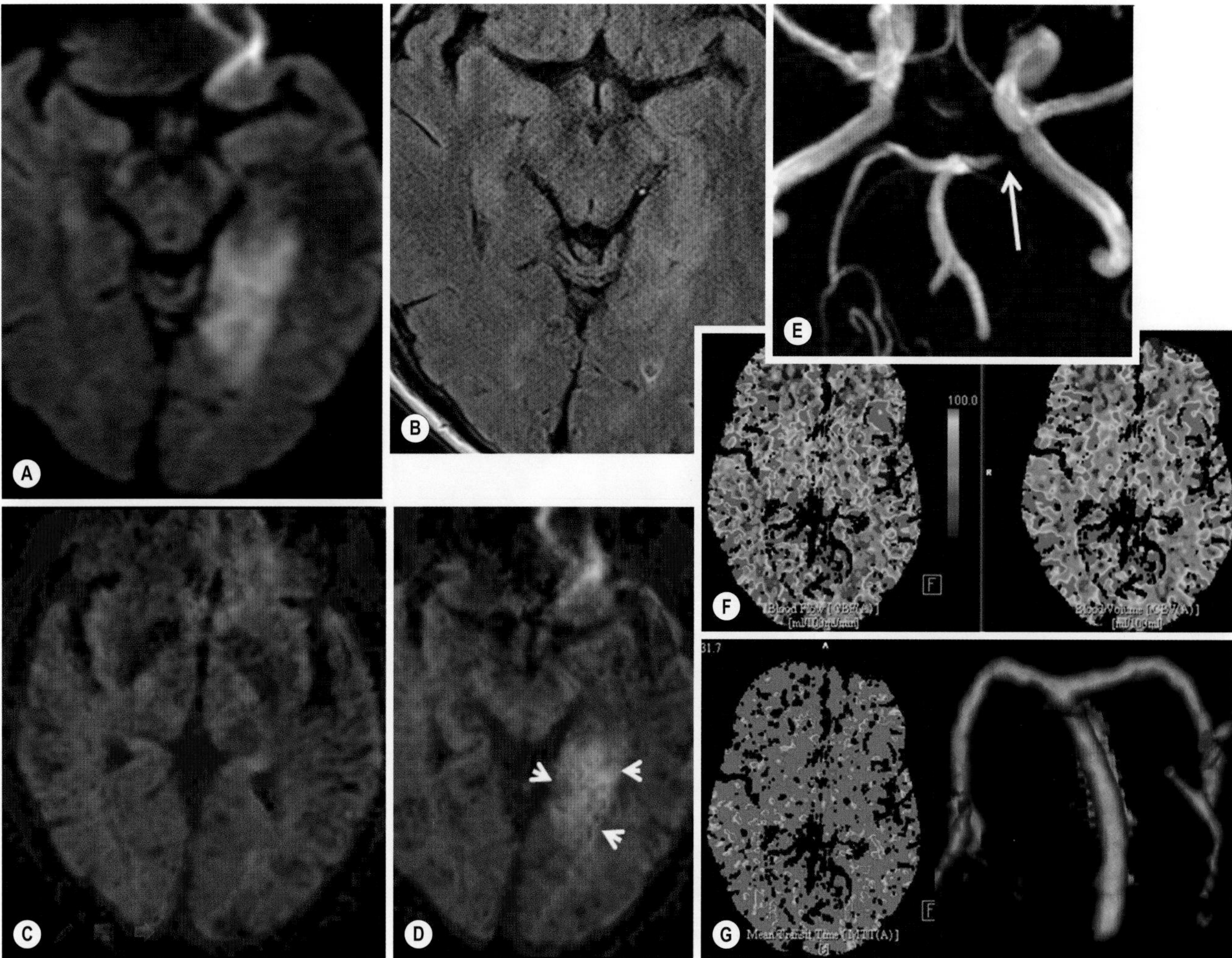

FIGURE 62-14 ■ Recanalisation of the left PCA with intravenous thrombolysis in a patient who woke up with a right hemiparesis and visual disturbance. (A) DWI MRI demonstrates hyperintensity consistent with an acute infarct in the left PCA territory but which is only minimally hyperintense on the FLAIR sequence (B), indicating onset within the last 4.5 h. MRI perfusion fused with DWI shows a significant penumbra with elevated MTT depicted in red against the acute infarct in white (C and D, white arrowheads). The time-of-flight MRA shows severe impairment of flow in the left PCA (E, white arrow), which recanalises completely following iv thrombolysis on CT angiography (G) with restoration of the normal perfusion parameters on CT perfusion (F).

to MRI, prolonged imaging times (not just acquisition, but safety and patient transfers) and post-processing has hampered the role of MRI—particularly evident in the poor recruitment to MRI-based multicentre stroke trials.

CT perfusion techniques also appear to afford more quantitative capability than standard dynamic susceptibility MR perfusion imaging. This permits the utilisation of thresholds for cerebral blood flow and mean transit time to attempt to identify at-risk tissue as discussed earlier. However, there is variability between CT machines, processing platforms and software versions, which precludes the application of this uniformly.

Arterial spin labelling MR perfusion (ASL) provides an assessment of cerebral blood flow without the need for a contrast injection.[88] It is less sensitive to susceptibility and motion effects but is affected by delay phenomena (as with contrast). It is currently a specialised technique, beginning its translation from research environments into clinical practice (Table 62-2).

TABLE 62-2 **Multimodal Stroke Imaging Platforms**

	CT	MRI
Multimodal technique	NECT + CTA + CTP	DWI + PWI + SWI + FLAIR + T1W + CEMRA
Times		
Acquisition	3–5 min	11–13 min
Total imaging time	8–12 min	20–40 min
Post-processing	5 min	5–10 min
Total	13–17 min	25–50 min

NECT = non-contrast-enhanced CT; CTA = CT angiography; CTP = CT perfusion; DWI = diffusion-weighted imaging; PWI = perfusion-weighted MRI; SWI = susceptibility-weighted imaging (for acute haemorrhage); CEMRA = contrast-enhanced MRA.

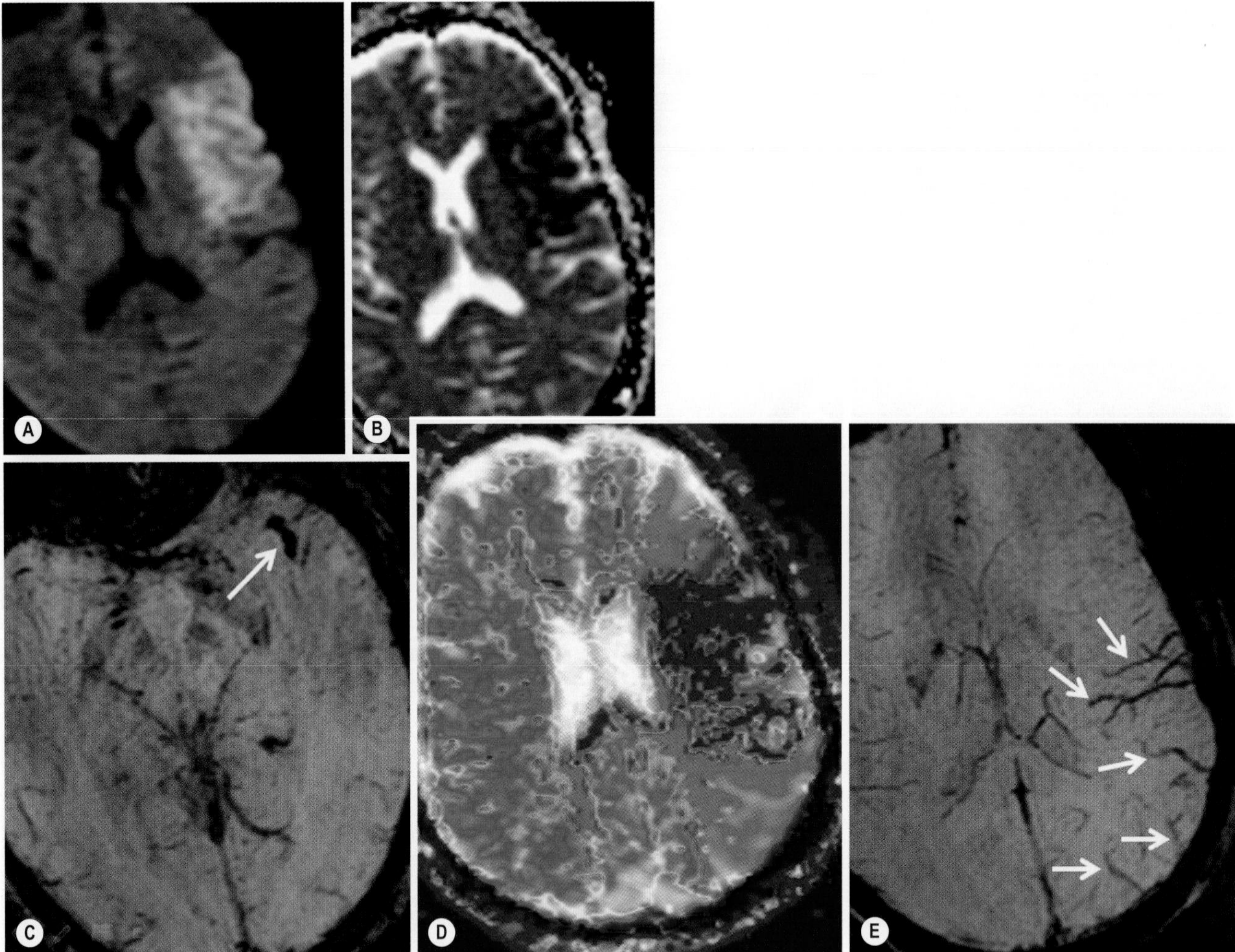

FIGURE 62-15 ■ Acute stroke MRI imaging. This patient presented at 5 h following the onset of right hemiparesis and dysphasia. There is an acute left MCA territory infarct represented by parenchymal hyperintensity on DWI (A) and hypointensity on ADC (B). There is a short segment of profound linear hypointensity ('blooming') in the proximal left M2 on SWI (C, white arrow) consistent with intraluminal thrombus. MRI perfusion fused with DWI (D) reveals a significant mismatch with a large area of ischaemic penumbra (red area) in relation to the core infarct (blue area). Prominent hypointense vessels on SWI are also shown in the ischaemic territory beyond the core infarct and may represent the penumbra (E, white arrows). Despite this, this patient was not thrombolysed due to the size of the core infarct and time of presentation.

Multimodal CT can therefore be more easily incorporated into the management of acute stroke patients without substantial detriment to the therapeutic opportunity.

The main clinical application of penumbral imaging in hyperacute stroke is for the assessment of suitability for thrombolytic therapy in:

- Cases presenting 3–6 hours after onset.
- Cases with an unclear time of onset, for example 'wake-up' strokes. That is, where the onset was whilst the patient was asleep and no precise time of onset is known. FLAIR imaging can also be helpful here. The degree of mismatch between the DWI and FLAIR hyperintensity may allow assessment of the volume of infarcted tissue within 6 hours of onset. Tissue infarcted for less than 3 hours is likely to be negative or only very subtly abnormal on FLAIR, whilst tissue infarcted for more than 4.5 h is most likely to be hyperintense on FLAIR (Fig. 62-16).[31,32]
- Clinically severe strokes to determine whether the deficits can be accounted for by a large area of reversible ischaemia (potential benefit with therapy) or a substantial core infarct, where the risk of post-thrombolysis haemorrhage is significantly higher.
- And when considering mechanical thrombectomy as a rescue therapy when iv treatment has failed.

Subacute and Chronic Infarct Imaging Signs

In the **subacute phase** there is structural breakdown and blood–brain barrier disruption. Fluid leaks into the extracellular space, causing well-demarcated low attenuation on CT and T2 hyperintensity on MRI that involves both grey and white matter in large infarcts. The severity and duration of brain swelling depends on infarct size. It usually increases during the first week, persists during the second week and then regresses. Other diagnoses such as tumour or infection should be considered if there is

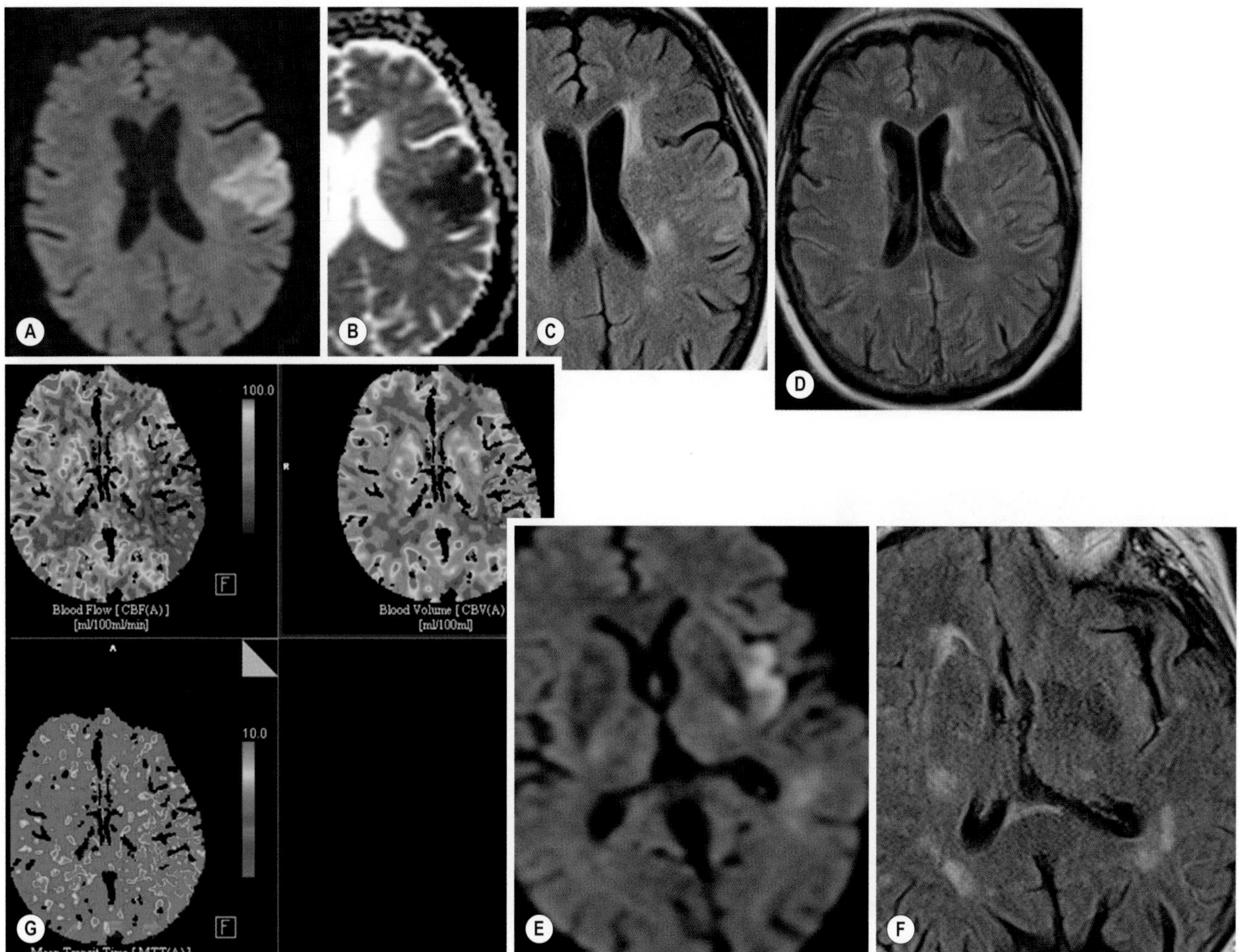

FIGURE 62-16 ■ Wake-up strokes. (A–D) This patient presented with a right hemiparesis having woken from sleep. Whilst there is an acute infarct depicted by hyperintensity on the DWI (A) and hypointensity on the ADC map (B), there is also clear cortical hyperintensity in this area on the FLAIR sequence (C). This suggests that the onset was very likely to be longer than 3 h previously and closer to 6 h. MRI perfusion did not demonstrate a significant penumbra, with no CBF deficit (D). This patient was not treated with recanalisation therapy. (E–G) By contrast, this patient who also awoke with symptoms of a left MCA territory infarct, was treated with iv thrombolysis. DWI MRI showed a small core infarct in the left insula (E), which was only minimally hyperintense on FLAIR (F), and therefore considered to be within 4.5 h of inctus. CT perfusion demonstrated mismatch with a moderately large area of potentially reversible ischaemia in the left temporoparietal region (G).

extensive white matter oedema without cortical involvement or prolonged brain swelling.

Contrast enhancement on CT and MR due to blood–brain barrier disruption is common in the subacute stage; indeed on MRI it occurs in almost all cases by the end of the first week[89] and persists for several months. The pattern is variable and therefore not always specific; however, gyriform enhancement, if present, is most characteristic of a cortical infarct (Fig. 62-17F). Lack of enhancement of large cortical lesions on MRI suggests alternative diagnoses such as low-grade glioma.

Haemorrhagic transformation due to secondary bleeding into reperfused ischaemic tissue occurs during the first 2 weeks. It is shown in up to 80% of infarcts on MRI,[90] appearing hyperintense on T1 and hypointense on T2 images, and particularly GRE and SWI images (Fig. 62-18). It is often seen in the basal ganglia and cortex, where it can assume a gyriform pattern. The occurrence and severity of haemorrhagic transformation correlates with the size of the infarct and degree of contrast enhancement in the early stage[91] and its risk is also increased with cardioembolic infarcts, and in the setting of diabetes and thrombolysis treatment. It is worth noting that gyriform cortical T1 shortening (hyperintensity) in the subacute and indeed chronic phases more often represents cortical laminar necrosis—due to the migration and congregation of lipid-laden macrophages—than haemorrhagic transformation. Furthermore, this effect is also observed following other cortical insults such as encephalitis.

Chronically, encephalomalacia and volume loss develop, causing enlargement of adjacent sulci and ventricles. The density on CT and signal intensity on MRI, including FLAIR, approaches that of CSF (Fig. 62-17). Occasionally, and mostly in children, this enecephalomalacia may be cystic in nature, acquiring paradoxical mass effect. Wallerian degeneration is sometimes visible as faint T2 hyperintensity in the ipsilateral corticospinal

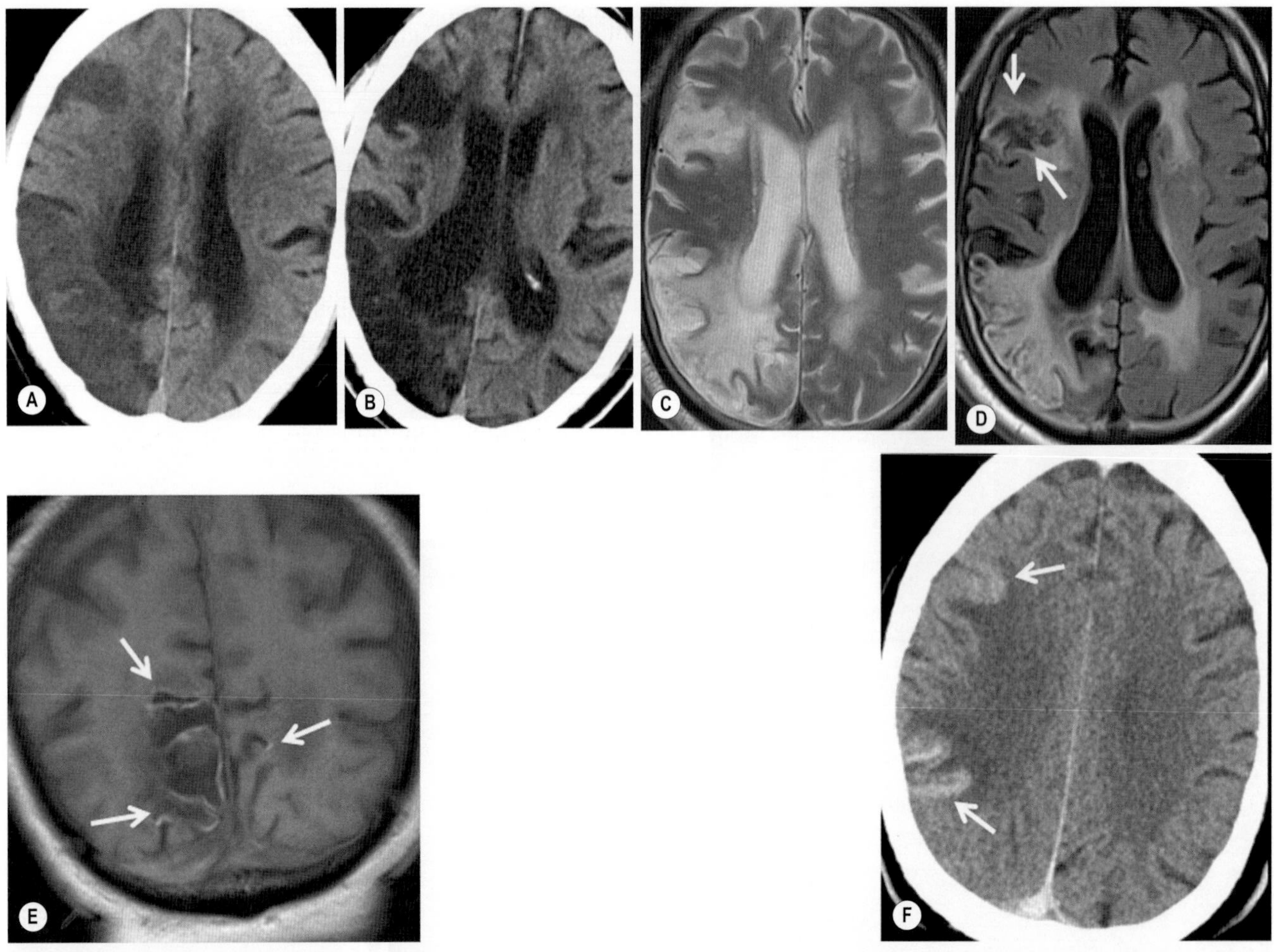

FIGURE 62-17 ■ **Subacute and mature infarcts.** On CT, there is a progressive reduction in attenuation (lower density) with infarct maturation accompanied by increased lesion delineation and volume loss as evidenced by sulcal prominence and ex-vacuo dilatation of the ventricles (A, B). A similar process is depicted on MRI with increased T2 (and FLAIR) hyperintensity (C, D) until the tissue reaches the signal intensity of fluid. At this stage, the infarcted tissue is hypointense on FLAIR with a hyperintense margin of gliosis (D, white arrows). Gyriform cortical T1 hyperintensity in the infarcted tissue develops in the subacute phase, and is known as cortical laminar necrosis (E, white arrows). Gyriform enhancement occurs early in cortical ischaemia due to breakdown of the blood–brain barrier, and may persist for several months (F, white arrows).

tract with related asymmetrical brainstem atrophy. With large middle cerebellar artery infarcts, contralateral cerebellar volume loss is also occasionally observed. Rarely, dystrophic calcification occurs in the very late phase.

On DWI, normalisation of the DWI and ADC signal occurs within 5–10 days ('pseudonormalisation') during which small infarcts can be masked. Larger lesions will still be obvious on structural images. Prolonged restriction of diffusion in small white matter infarcts lasting several weeks has been reported, the explanation for which is not entirely clear.[92] Beyond this period, loss of structural integrity results in increased water mobility and the imaging appearance reverses to low signal on DWI and bright on the ADC map.[93,94] This state is described as 'free diffusion' (Fig. 62-19). In mature infarcts, tissue with very long T2 relaxation times (markedly T2 hyperintense) may appear as high signal on DWI due to T2 effects dominating the signal—the so-called 'T2 shine through' effect. Such areas are easily distinguished from genuinely acutely infarcted tissue as they will also be hyperintense on the ADC map. Another potential pitfall of DWI is acute haemorrhage, which can return a high signal resembling an infarct. However, there is often also a low signal margin produced by susceptibility effects.[95] Analysis of other sequences should indicate the correct diagnosis.

On perfusion imaging, CBV in the infarcted region increases in the early subacute stage[96] due primarily to collateral supply.

Atheromatous Extracranial Vascular Disease

Atheroma can occur at vessel origins (including vertebral arteries), at the carotid bifurcation, and in the distal course of internal carotid or vertebral arteries. The carotid bifurcation is the commonest site and represents a significant source of emboli. Thirty per cent of transient ischaemic attacks progress to cerebral infarction, of which 20% are within the first month, and the majority within the initial few days. Such stenoses are also a cause of hypoperfusion strokes if haemodynamically significant.

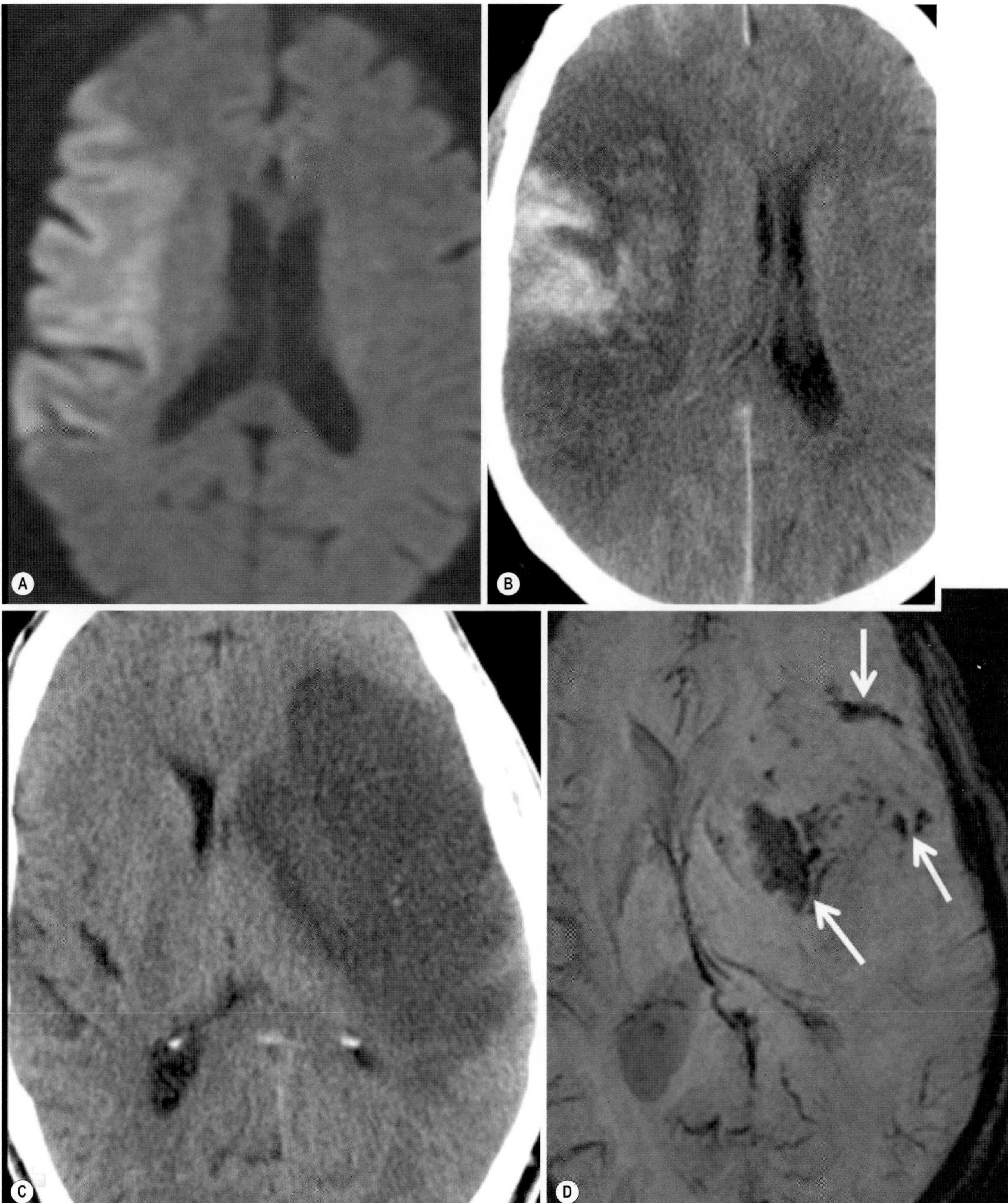

FIGURE 62-18 ■ **Haemorrhagic transformation.** Haemorrhage within an infarct is more common in large infarcts and in those involving the basal ganglia, and following efforts to recanalise occluded major vessels. (A) The DWI of this patient demonstrated a large right MCA territory infarct. Sixty hours after symptom onset, the patient clinically deteriorated. A CT examination revealed a moderate area of acute haemorrhage (hyperdensity) within the infarct, with ipsilateral mass effect and midline shift (B). In (C), a large left MCA territory infarct is complicated by haemorrhagic transformation. Although only subtly hyperdense in the basal ganglia on CT (C), the exquisite sensitivity of SWI to markedly hypointense blood products detects their presence easily (D, white arrows).

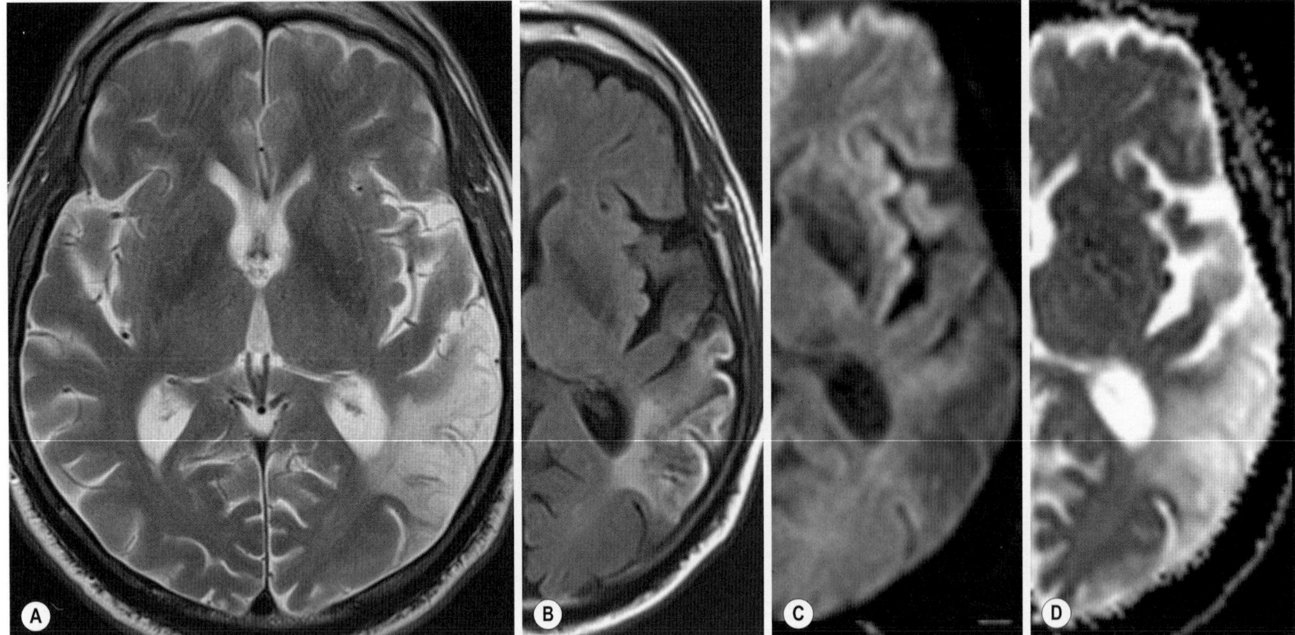

FIGURE 62-19 ■ MR imaging of a patient 6 months after a left MCA territory infarct reveals marked T2 hyperintensity on T2-weighted imaging (A)—which nulls centrally on FLAIR (B)—and free diffusion on DWI (hypointensity on DWI (C) and hyperintensity on ADC (D)). This is associated with local volume loss.

The North American Symptomatic Carotid Endarterectomy Trial (NASCET)[97] and the European Carotid Surgery Trial (ESCT)[98] found that patients with symptomatic 70–99% stenosis of the internal carotid artery benefited from endarterectomy surgery. Stenosis measurements in these trials were performed on conventional catheter angiograms, using slightly different methods, which are illustrated in Fig. 62-20. Surgery also reduces the risk of stroke in asymptomatic carotid stenosis of 70% or more as measured by ultrasound.[99] Symptomatic 50–69% stenoses may be a suitable target for intervention but in both cases the benefits are smaller and the advantages of surgery could more easily be outweighed by poor patient selection or excess morbidity from surgery (or angiography).[100] Carotid intervention should not be considered for a stenosis of less than 50% regardless of symptoms. More recently, the Asymptomatic Carotid Stenosis Trial (ACST) demonstrated that endarterectomy confers a reduction in stroke risk amongst patients younger than 75 years old, with greater than 70% stenosis of the internal carotid artery provided that the operative risk was not higher than in the trial itself.[101,102]

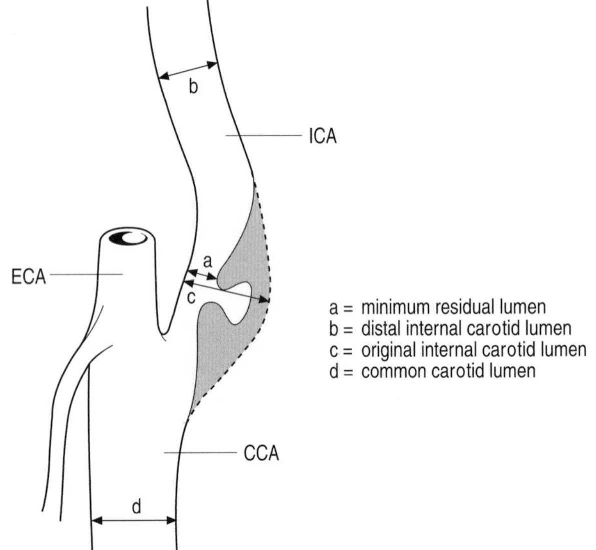

FIGURE 62-20 ■ Different ways of measuring percentage of carotid artery stenosis (adapted from 86): (A) NASCET method = [1 − (*a*/*b*)] × 100; (B) ESCT method = [1 − (*a*/*c*)] × 100; common carotid method = [1 − (*a*/*d*)] × 100.

Imaging Options for Carotid Stenosis

Conventional digital subtraction catheter angiography (DSA) is invasive, potentially hazardous,[103] expensive, and not widely available. Most carotid imaging is now performed with Doppler ultrasound, CTA, MRA performed without exogenous contrast injection such as 2- or 3-dimensional time-of-flight (TOF) methods, or contrast-enhanced MRA (CEMRA) performed dynamically after an intravenous bolus of gadolinium-based contrast.[104] These non-invasive techniques are now very widely available, although access for patients with TIA varies among hospitals,[105] and DSA is no longer in routine use. In both a systematic review of the world literature and individual patient data meta-analysis performed recently in 2009,[106,107] sensitivities and specificities of these techniques were as follows: 70 to 99% stenosis, sensitivity: ultrasound (US), 0.89; CTA, 0.76; MRA, 0.88; CEMRA, 0.94; specificity: US, 0.84; CTA, 0.94; MRA, 0.84; CEMRA, 0.93. Fewer data were available for milder stenoses but accuracy was poorer. Hence, it is widely accepted

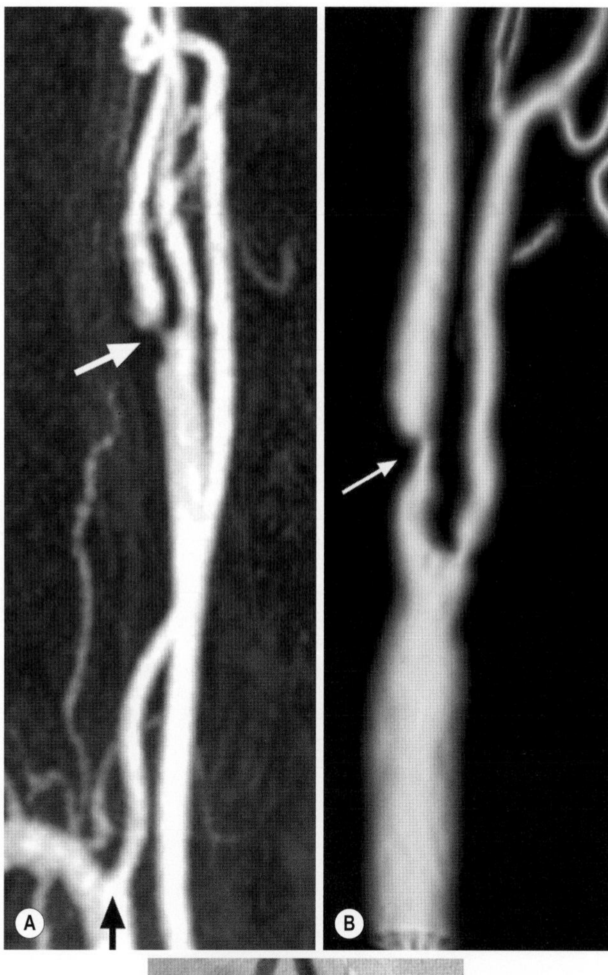

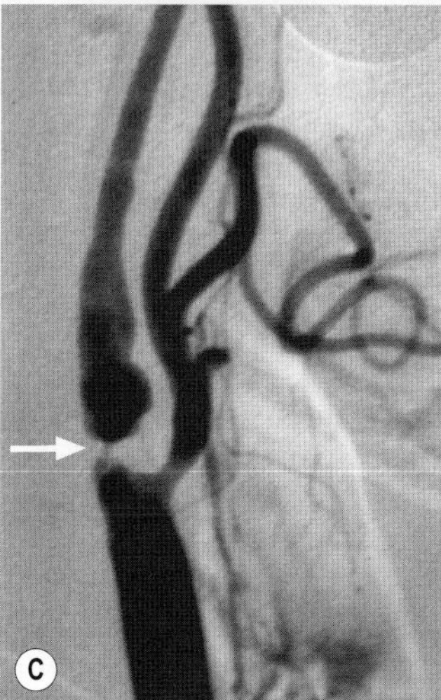

FIGURE 62-21 ■ **Carotid bifurcation atheroma.** Examples of internal carotid artery stenoses (white arrows) from different patients on (A) CEMRA MIP, (B) CTA volume rendering and (C) DSA. Note the right vertebral artery origin is clearly demonstrated (A, black arrow).

that CEMRA is the most accurate method of carotid stenosis evaluation (Fig. 62-21). However, it should be pointed out that in the experience of the authors, CTA performed on 128-multidetector CT is at least as accurate as CEMRA. Indeed, this is supported by the data from very recent case series.

Vessel Plaque Imaging. Ultrasound and MRI techniques are able to identify high-risk plaques with a high risk of rupture and distal embolism.[108,109] Isotope imaging with FDG-PET and ^{11}C-PK11195 detect intraplaque inflammation which is thought to be involved in emboli formation.[110,111]

Imaging Signs

Doppler ultrasound (USS) demonstrates plaque location, extent and morphology. Hyperechoic lesions, typically with acoustic shadowing, represent plaque calcification whilst hypoechoic plaque indicates an increased risk of stroke. Doppler flow velocity and characteristics correlate well with the degree of vascular stenosis but cannot reliably distinguish between complete occlusion and 'trickle' flow. USS may also underestimate the degree of narrowing due to fresh or free-floating thrombus.

A narrowed vessel flow void on MRI indicates stenosis whilst an absent flow void usually indicates occlusion, especially if there is intraluminal high signal. However, this appearance can also represent severely impaired flow distal to a tight stenosis.

There is good correlation between a normal time-of-flight MRA and absence of disease (high specificity). It is, however, rather prone to overestimation of the degree of stenosis. Also, as the technique is heavily flow dependent, turbulence, a reduction in flow and a genuine stenosis can all generate an apparent vessel narrowing. A 'flow-gap' does not differentiate occlusion from very slow flow. Whilst many of the flow-dependent artefacts are significantly reduced by the luminal CEMRA, they are not eliminated. As stated earlier, this technique gives better plaque morphological and extent assessment. However, the ICA distal to a severe stenosis can appear spuriously narrow.

CT angiography (CTA) is a luminal contrast technique and does not suffer from flow-dependent artefacts. It has a very high specificity and, with newer-generation MDCT, affords an excellent assessment of a stenosis. Juxtaluminal hypodensity indicates large fatty plaque and free-floating thrombus—at particular risk of embolism—are well characterised. Furthermore, arterial and slightly delayed phases can usually discriminate between occlusion and trickle-flow defines tandem lesions. Accurate stenosis assessment can be difficult in segments of heavy calcification—not an uncommon problem.

CEMRA and CTA both allow a full assessment of the arterial tree from the aortic arch to the circle of Willis and beyond.

Non-Atheromatous Extracranial Vascular Narrowing

Causes of non-atheromatous extracranial vascular narrowing include arterial dissection, fibromuscular dysplasia (FMD), extrinsic compression (for example, from nasopharyngeal tumours and soft-tissue infection), radiation vasculopathy (with intimal fibrosis and accelerated atherosclerosis) and catheter spasm.

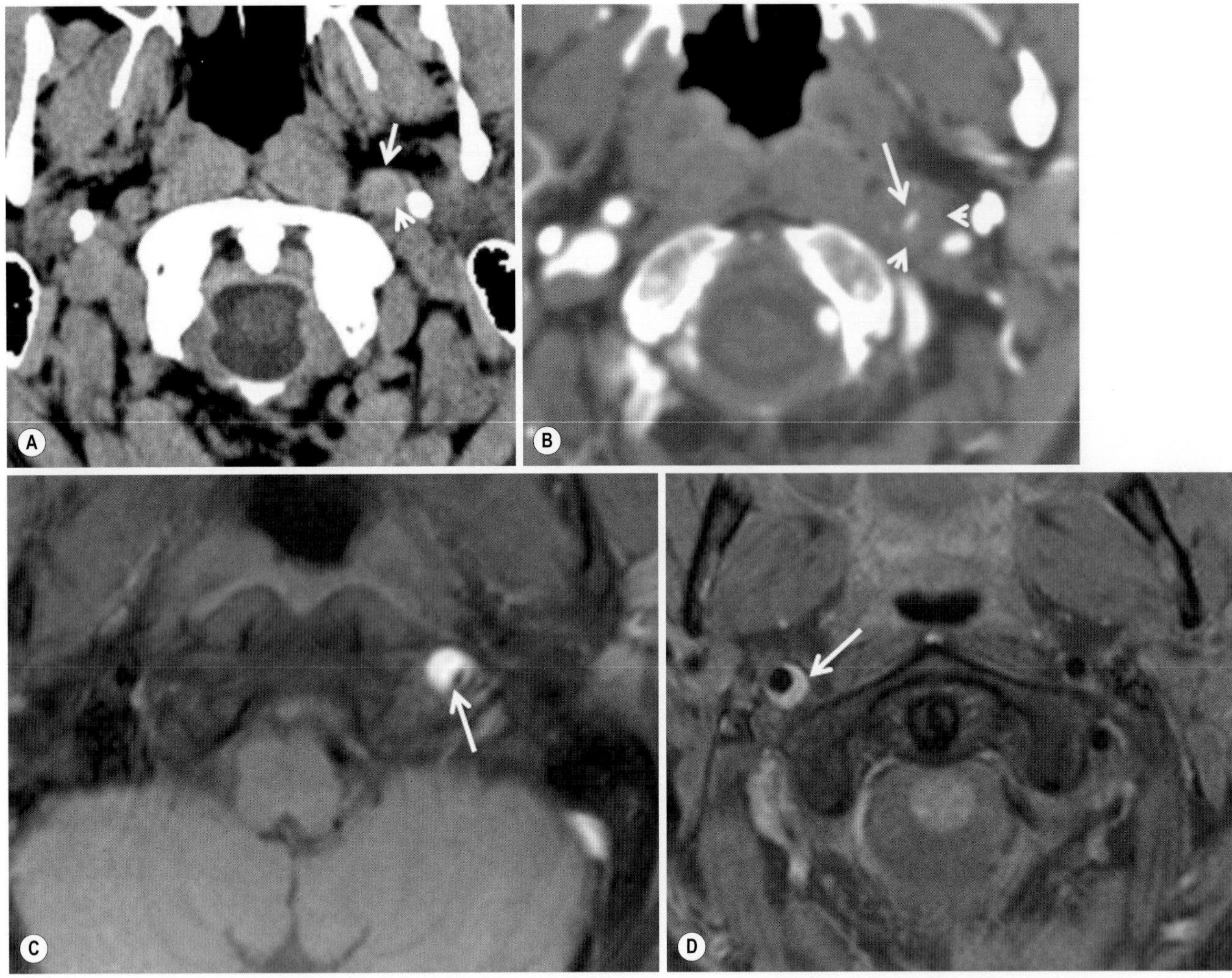

FIGURE 62-22 ■ **Carotid artery dissection.** A patient presented with neck pain and left-sided Horner's syndrome. Plain non-contrast-enhanced CT at the skull base demonstrated an expanded and heterogenous ICA (A, white arrow) with impression of crescentic hyperdensity (white arrowhead). CT angiography revealed a very narrow-calibre lumen (B, white arrow) within an expanded non-enhancing vessel (white arrowheads). Subsequent fat-saturated T1-weighted MRI shows the hyperintense intramural haemorrhage expanding the left ICA and surrounding the narrowed lumen (C, white arrow), and in another patient with a right ICA dissection (D, white arrow).

Arterial Dissection

Dissection of the cervical arteries is an important cause of stroke, particularly in younger patients, in whom it accounts for 20% of acute ischaemic strokes. Dissection of the internal carotid artery is most common, occurring proximally after the bulb and at the skull base. The vertebral artery is susceptible because of its bony canal and in children due to the arcuate foramen posterior to the lateral mass of C1. Whilst arterial dissection can occur spontaneously, cervical trauma, underlying vasculopathy such as fibromuscular dysplasia and connective tissue disorders such as Ehlers–Danlos syndrome, can precipitate the injury. The risk is also increased amongst patients with migraine, hypertension and in the setting of ilicit drug use.

Carotid artery dissection can occasionally be diagnosed on the routine NECT and axial MRI of the skull base, where an expanded vessel with crescentic hyperdensity on CT, or 'fried egg' appearance on MRI, can be observed. The latter arises from a true lumen with variable patency (ranging from normal flow void to abnormal signal due to occlusion or slow flow) with a surrounding cresecent of intramural haemorrhage in the false lumen. The conspicuity of the T1 hyperintense intramural clot is enhanced on T1 fat-saturated images (Fig. 62-22). Angiographic images typically demonstrate a smooth, tapered reduction of the luminal calibre often with luminal irregularity. The intraluminal flap may also be visible, as may pseudoaneurysmal dilatation. Although DSA classically shows differential opacification and contrast washout in the true and false lumens if they are both patent, most of these features can be shown on MRA or CTA and the diagnosis can usually be made without recourse to DSA. The diagnosis of a vertebral artery dissection is usually more difficult. T1 fat-saturated images are less rewarding in their demonstration of the intramural haematoma due to the signal emanating from the plexus of veins that typically surround the vertebral arteries in their cervical course. Careful scrutiny of the CTA axial images for vessel irregularity, the intimal flap, overall vessel expansion and the possibility of coexisting dissecting aneurysms is warranted.

Fibromuscular Dysplasia (FMD)

FMD occurs predominantly in middle-aged women and most often affects the cervical ICA (75%). The vertebral (12%) and external carotid arteries may also be involved. Disease is bilateral in 60% of cases. Angiographic images, almost always with non-invasive techniques, demonstrate alternating luminal narrowing and dilatation, the resulting appearance often described as a 'string of beads' (Fig. 62-23). This 'corrugation' typically affects the mid ICA, usually 2 cm distal to bulb. Uni- or multifocal tubular stenoses are less common, and where observed, the degree of stenosis is usually modest (less than 40%). FMD can occasionally be observed intracranially and is associated with aneurysms.

Intracranial Vascular Disease

Ischaemic Microangiopathy

There are a number of causes of small vessel disease in the brain (see Table 62-3). By far the most common is ischaemic microangiopathy, the risk factors for which are age, hypertension, diabetes mellitus, hyperlipidaemia and smoking.[112] More than 95% of those over 65 years of age have white matter lesions on MRI, but these are usually limited in extent.[113] Arterioles of the long penetrating arteries become occluded, the outcome probably depending on vessel size. Occlusion of a larger perforating vessel causes a lacunar infarct; blockage of smaller arterioles results in ischaemic demyelination and gliosis. Although highly variable in distribution, it predominantly affects the periventricular and deep cerebral white matter, basal ganglia, thalami and the ventral pons. CT shows white

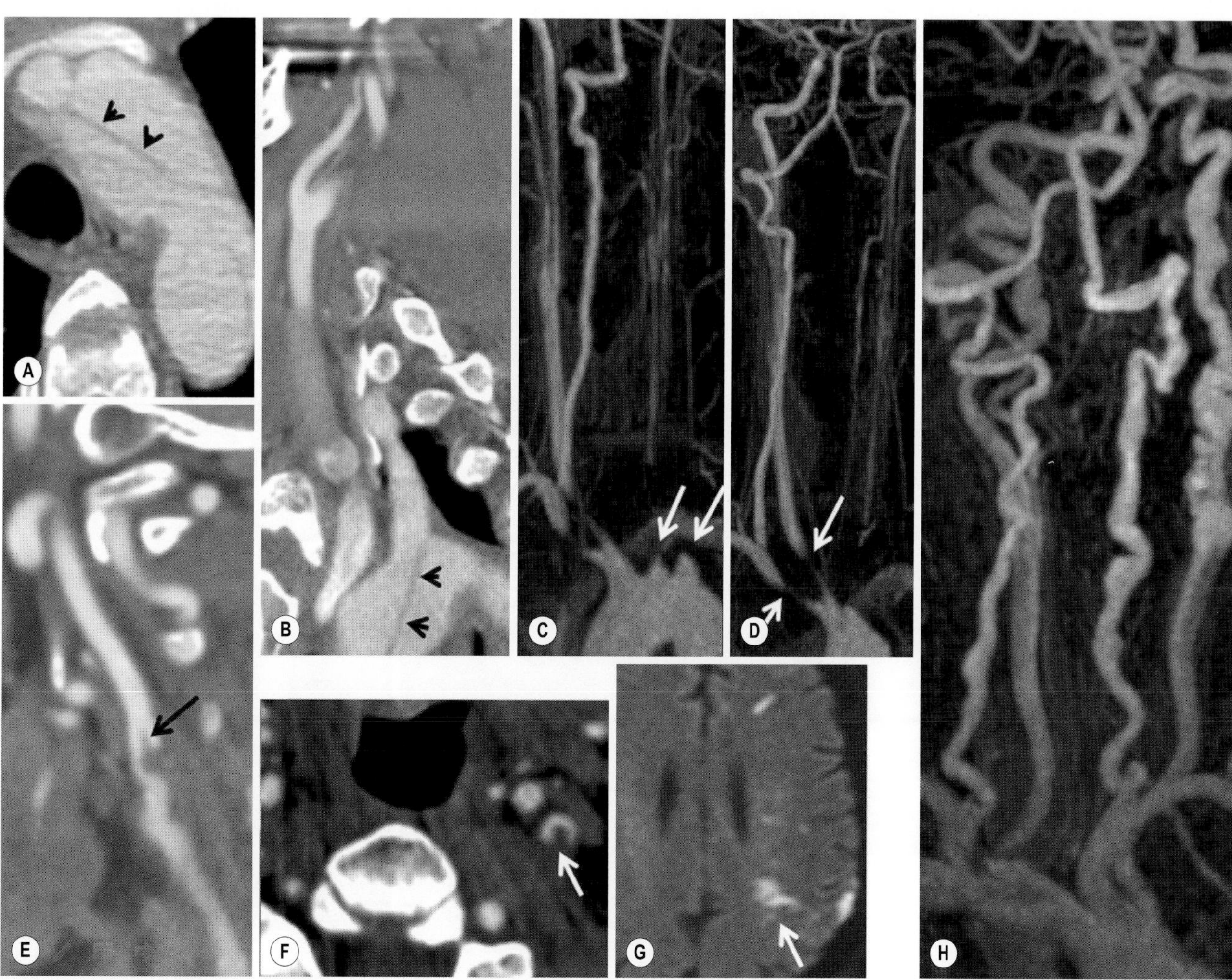

FIGURE 62-23 ■ **Extracranial arterial abnormalities.** An aortic arch dissection extends to involve the origin of the left CCA (A, B). The initimal flap is clearly visible (black arrowheads). Takayasu's arteritis (C, D). This large vessel vasculitis typically affects the great vessel origins, most commonly beginning with the left subclavian artery. In this case, there is occlusion of the left subclavian and common carotid arteries (C, white arrows) with severe stenosis of the right subclavian and common carotid arteries (D, white arrows). Free-floating thrombus (E–G). Low-density atherosclerotic plaque arising from the intima of the vessel wall projects into the lumen of the left internal carotid artery origin (E, black arrow; F, white arrow) and d is associated with small acute embolic infarcts in the left middle cerebral artery territory (G; white arrow) on DWI. Fibromuscular dysplasia. A contrast-enhanced MRA (H) of a 47-year-old female patient reveals extensive 'beading' of the left CCA, left ICA and left vertebral artery, and to a lesser extent right ICA in the neck. This pattern of alternating luminal dilatation and mild narrowings is typical.

matter hypodensities ('leukoariosis') but MRI, particularly FLAIR, is much more sensitive.

Whilst distinguishing an acute infarct from a background of established disease on CT is extremely challenging, DWI will easily identify its site. New infarcts develop every few months in small vessel disease and are clinically silent unless they arise in eloquent areas, although they will be shown on fortuitously timed DWI.[114] It is important to realise that these white matter changes are non-specific and similar appearances may be encountered in other microangiopathic diseases such as vasculitis,[115] and occasionally inflammatory processes affecting the CNS.

TABLE 62-3 Causes

Common	Uncommon	Rare
Ischaemic microangiopathy	Drug-related hypertension/ vasculopathy	Moya moya
Vasospasm (SAH)	Sickle cell disease	Intravascular lymphoma
	Radiation vasculopathy	Intracranial dissection
	Intracranial atheroma	Intracranial FMD
	Vasculitis	CADASIL
	Amyloid angiopathy	Susac's syndrome
		Neurocutaneous syndromes

Acutely, lacunar infarcts are often rounded with a hazy outline and may fluctuate in size in the subacute phase—most often enlarging. When mature, however, they become sharply delineated, shrink in size—typically less than 1.5 cm diameter—and cavity-like. The gliotic hyperintense rim of a mature lacune on FLAIR differentiates it from a perivascular space.

Ischaemic microangiopathic disease is often associated with microhaemorrhages in the deep nuclei and scattered more peripherally.[116] These are depicted as small foci of susceptibility artefact on T2* GRE and SWI (microbleeds are not visible on CT) (Figs. 62-24 and 62-25). They are also present in around 6% of asymptomatic

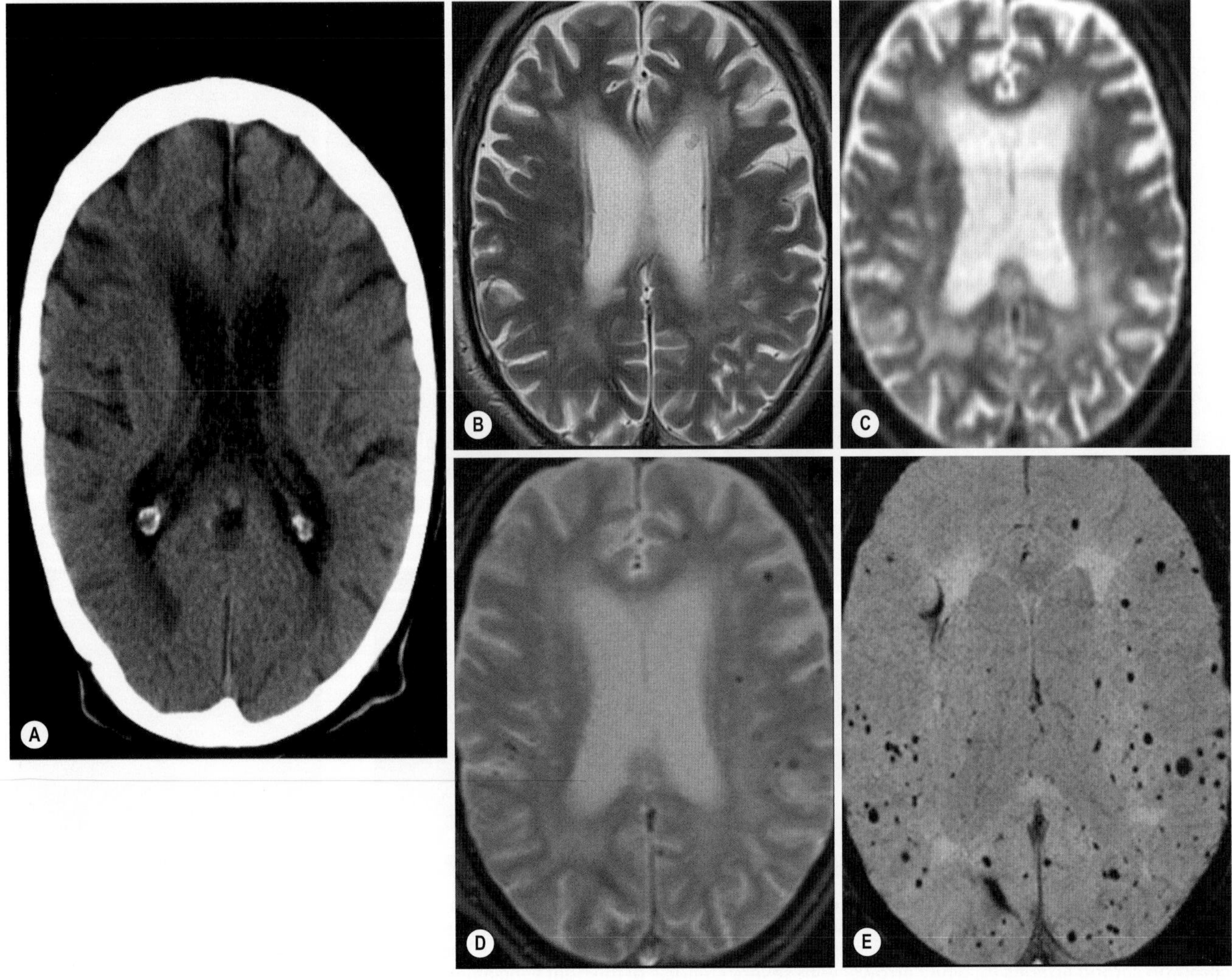

FIGURE 62-24 ■ Sensitivity to haemosiderin deposition. No microhaemorrhages are apparent in the brain parenchyma on plain CT in this patient with amyloid angiopathy (A). There is progressively increasing sensitivity to their presence from a standard T2-weighted spin-echo sequence (B), through the b = zero diffusion-weighted acquisition (C), gradient-echo T2* sequence (D) and, finally, susceptibility-weighted imaging (E), which affords exquisite detection of microhaemorrhages by demonstrating multiple foci of susceptibility artefact depicted as marked hypointensity.

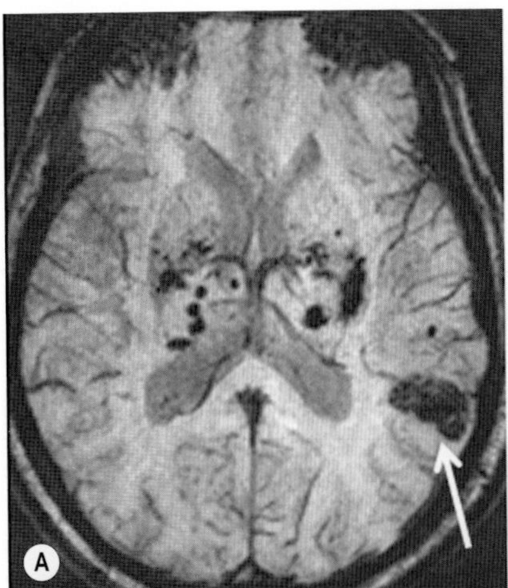

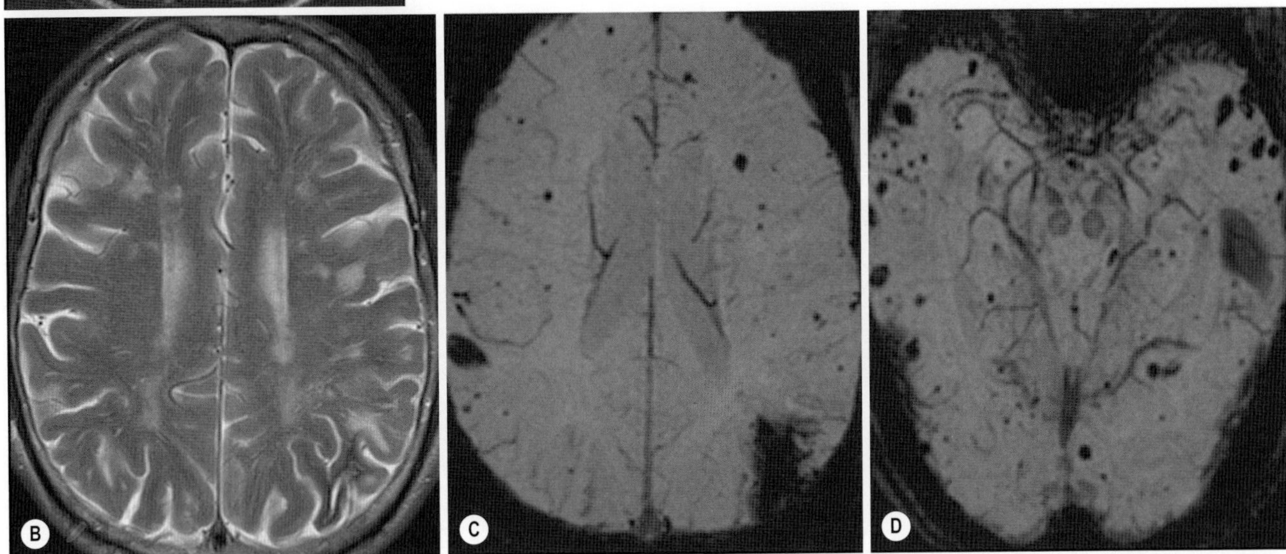

FIGURE 62-25 ■ Distribution of microhaemorrhages. Multiple hypertensive microhaemorrhages are shown in the deep grey nuclei in this patient with severe microangiopathic ischaemic disease (A), whilst the distribution of microhaemorrhages is typically more peripheral and lobar in a patient with amyloid angiopathy (B–D). Again, the SWI acquistion (C, D) far exceeds the routine T2-weighted sequence (B) in the sensitivity to such lesions. Note, however, the presence of a previous lobar haemorrhage (A, white arrow).

older people, associated with age, hypertension and radiological extent of small vessel disease.[117] They are a marker of vascular fragility in hypertensive small vessel disease, their distribution mirroring symptomatic haemorrhages. There is some evidence that they present an increased risk for parenchymal haemorrhage in antiplatelet therapy.[118] However, this and the impact of anticoagulation are still under investigation. Similarly, it is not clear whether they increase the risk of post-thrombolysis haemorrhage.[119,120]

Moya Moya

Moya moya is the literal Japanese term for 'puff of smoke', describing the angiographic appearance of abnormal, dilated and irregular collateral vessels that develop secondary to progressive occlusion of the supraclinoid internal carotid arteries. Moya moya represents an idiopathic arteriopathy, which, although primarily involving the supraclinoid ICAs, often progresses to the proximal anterior and middle cerebral arteries, and occasionally the posterior circulation (typically the basilar tip). It is mainly seen in patients from Japan and the Pacific Rim. In advanced cases there may be extensive dural, leptomeningeal and pial collateral circulation. The characteristic vascular changes can also be shown on MRA or CTA and MRI may show associated infarcts. The latter are usually in the borderzones (Fig. 62-26). A moya moya-like pattern may be found in other conditions such as sickle cell disease, Down's syndrome, previous radiotherapy or tuberculous meningitis and Type 1 neurofibromatosis.[80]

Vasculitis

This heterogeneous group of inflammatory diseases mainly affects smaller parenchymal and leptomeningeal vessels. Conditions that cause cerebral vasculitis, other than primary (isolated) angiitis of the central nervous system, include infection, cocaine ingestion and autoimmune diseases such as systemic lupus erythematosus, polyarteritis nodosa, giant cell arteritis and Sjögren's syndrome, sarcoidosis and Wegener's disease.

Appearances on MRI are typically non-specific. White matter hyperintensities with a subcortical distribution are more common and there may be foci of haemorrhage, leptomeningeal enhancement and occasionally infarcts. Medium vessel disease is rare, arising secondarily due to disease of the vasa vasorum. Involved areas may resemble territorial strokes but do not evolve appropriately.

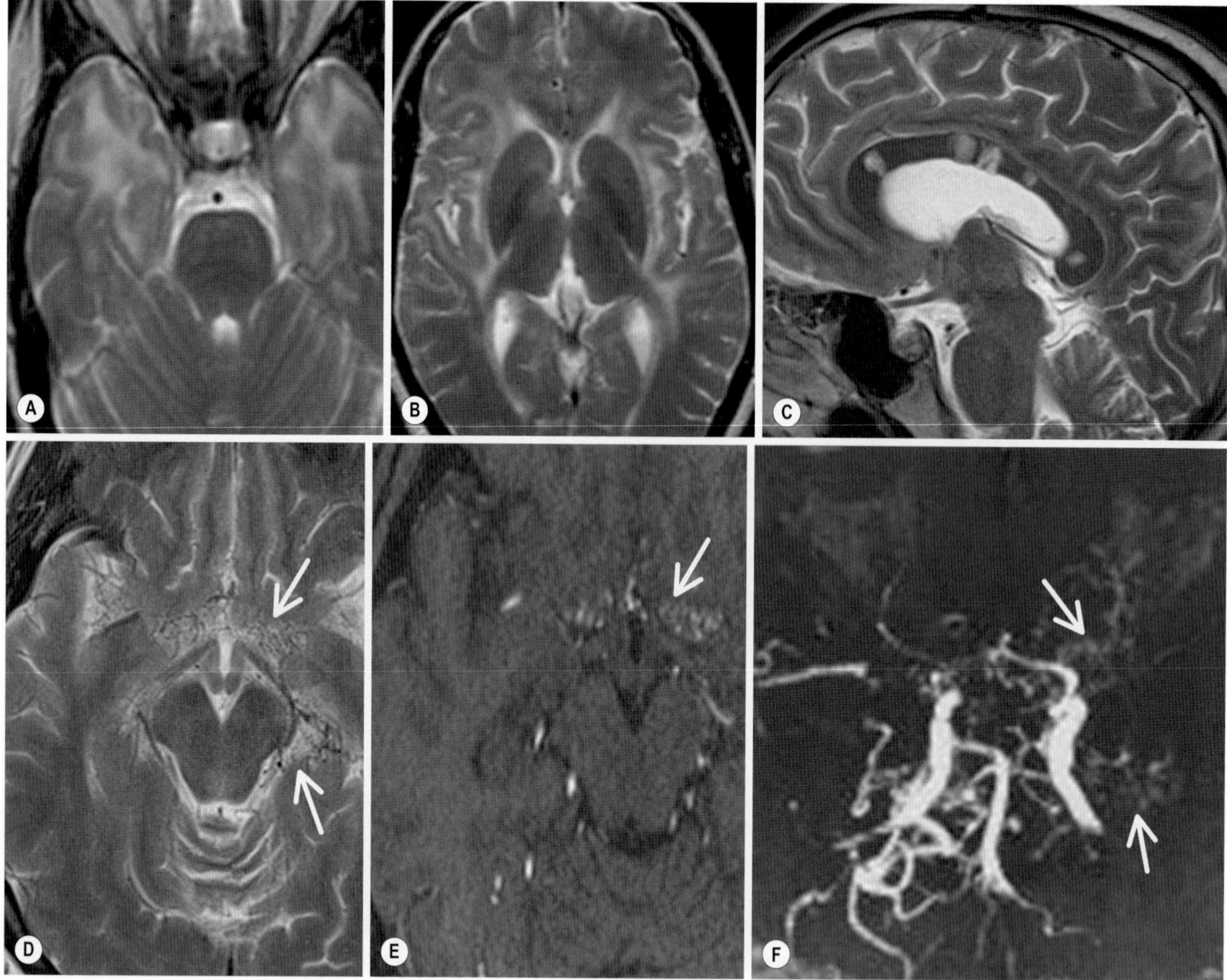

FIGURE 62-26 ■ CADASIL (A, B). Extensive confluent white matter signal abnormality typically involving the anterior temporal lobes and subinsular regions. Basal ganglia involvement and microhaemorrhage are also often noted. Susac's syndrome (C). Small multifocal, often rounded lesions in the corpus callosum in a patient presenting with headache, encephalopathy, retinal branch occlusions and hearing loss. Moya moya syndrome (D–F). There is absence of the normal flow void on the T2-weighted spine-echo image (D) and flow signal on the time-of-flight MRA (axial raw data E, maximum intensity projection F) within both terminal ICAs, middle cerebral arteries, right ACA and left PCA due to the terminal occlusive vasculopathy. In an attempt to compensate, a myriad of fine abnormal collateral vessels have developed in the anterior perforated substance and left choroidal fissure (white arrows).

DSA catheter angiography is superior to MRA and CTA, particularly for smaller, more peripheral vessels. Angiographic signs suggesting a vasculitis include stenoses, occlusion, thromboses or arterial beading, although they are not specific. Aneurysms are also observed. However, angiography is frequently negative and it should not be regarded as the gold standard investigation; a brain or meningeal biopsy is often necessary to make a firm diagnosis.

Cerebral Venous Thrombosis (CVT)

Cerebral venous thrombosis is an easily overlooked diagnosis that should always be considered in the presence of headache, seizures or encephalopathy. Thrombus forms in dural sinuses and/or superficial cortical veins/or extending to internal cerebral veins from straight sinus leading to venous hypertension and haemorrhage. Venousinfarction ensues if anticoagulation is not implemented early.

Cerebral, osseous or air cell infection, local trauma, dehydration, pregnancy, the oral contraceptive pill, smoking and vasculitis (especially Behçet's disease) are not uncommon precipitants but in their absence a thrombophilia screen will be necessary.

Imaging signs pertain both to the thrombosed cortical vein or dural sinus and the 'upstream' parenchyma. An acutely thrombosed sinus, or less commonly superficial cortical vein, typically appears hyperdense and expanded on NECT, and as a hypodense centre within an enhancing periphery in post-contrast CT examinations, especially on CT venography. This is the so-called 'delta' sign. On most MRI sequences, there will loss of the normal flow void, and the thrombosed vessel may be hyperintense on both T1- and T2-weighted imaging. Rarely, very acute thrombus can appear hypointense on T2 and be mistaken for a flow void, and slow flow can result in loss of the flow void, mimicking thrombosis. Loss of flow signal and/or irregularity and severe narrowing indicate thrombus on MR venography. This is a phase contrast angiographic technique where a low-velocity encoding optimises depiction of venous flow. In practice, however, recanalisation versus a hypoplastic sinus versus slow flow can often be difficult to differentiate with MRI and MRV alone. In the authors' opinion, detailed assessment of the NECT and structural MRI images is usually most helpful. SWI can be particularly useful in CVT. In addition to the exaggerated hypointensity and expansion of the thrombosed vein or sinus (described as 'blooming'), multiple prominent serpiginous veins may be observed in the venous territory indicating venous congestion.[121] As mentioned earlier, this sequence is also very sensitive to acute haemorrhage. Phase images generated as part of the SWI sequence may also enable identification of an occluded cortical vein,[122] being hypointense compared with normally patent veins.

The imaging appearance of the parenchymal lesions depends on whether there is venous hypertension or infarction or secondary haemorrhage. Disproportionate parenchymal swelling and oedema (MRI, high T2/FLAIR signal; CT, low density) with early fragmented haemorrhage is typical. The distribution of parenchymal lesions is important: bilateral (although sometimes asymmetric) involvement of the thalami and to a lesser extent basal ganglia is typical in internal cerebral vein and/or straight sinus thrombosis; the posterolateral aspects of the temporal lobe and/or inferior parietal lobule are commonly involved in thrombosis of the vein of Labbé and/or lateral venous sinus; cortical and subcortical lesions, often bilateral but asymmetric, are frequent in superior sagittal sinus occlusion (Figs. 62-27 and 62-28).

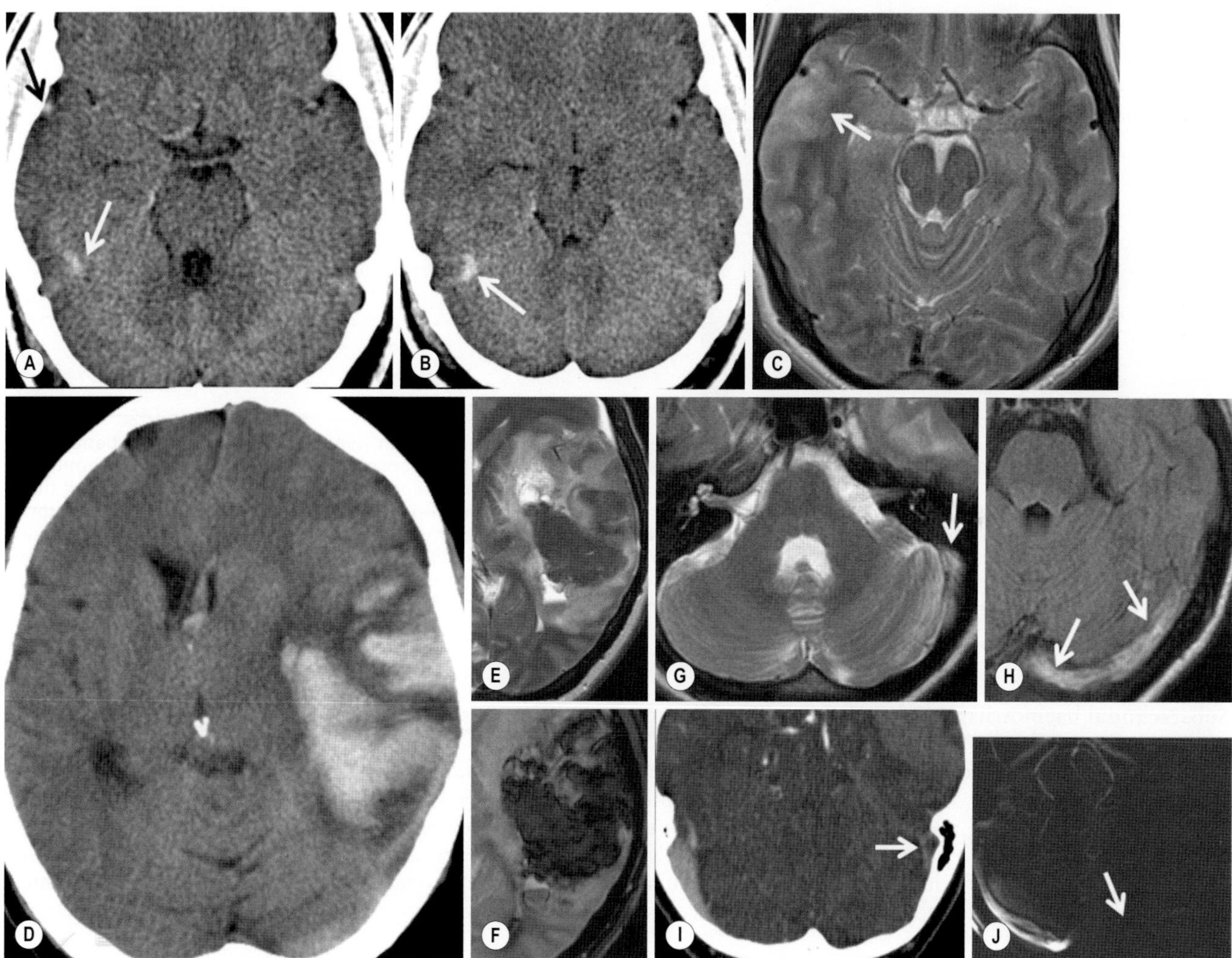

FIGURE 62-27 ■ Cerebral venous thrombosis. (A–C) This young male patient presented with headache and seizures. Serpiginous hyperdensity on CT within a vessel on the surface of the right temporal lobe (A, black arrow) and approaching the right lateral venous sinus (A, B, white arrows) is consistent with the 'string sign' of cortical venous thrombosis—in this case, involving the right vein of Labbé. There is a small area of early venous ischaemia in the anterolateral aspect of the right temporal lobe on T2-weighted MRI (C, white arrow). Lateral venous thrombosis. (D–J) A large acute parenchymal haemorrhage in the left frontal and temporal lobes was discovered on plain CT (D) in this patient who presented with seizures and encephalopathy. Hypointensity on the T2-weighted MRI (E) and SWI (F) are consistent with acute blood products. There is a considerable degree of surrounding parenchymal oedema shown as high signal intensity on T2W. A causative left lateral sinus thrombosis is identified on T2W (G, white arrow) and FLAIR (H, white arrows) with loss of the normal related signal void and confirmed by a filling defect within the left lateral sinus on the CT venogram (I, white arrow; compare with right lateral sinus) and absence of flow-related signal in this sinus on MR venography (J, white arrow).

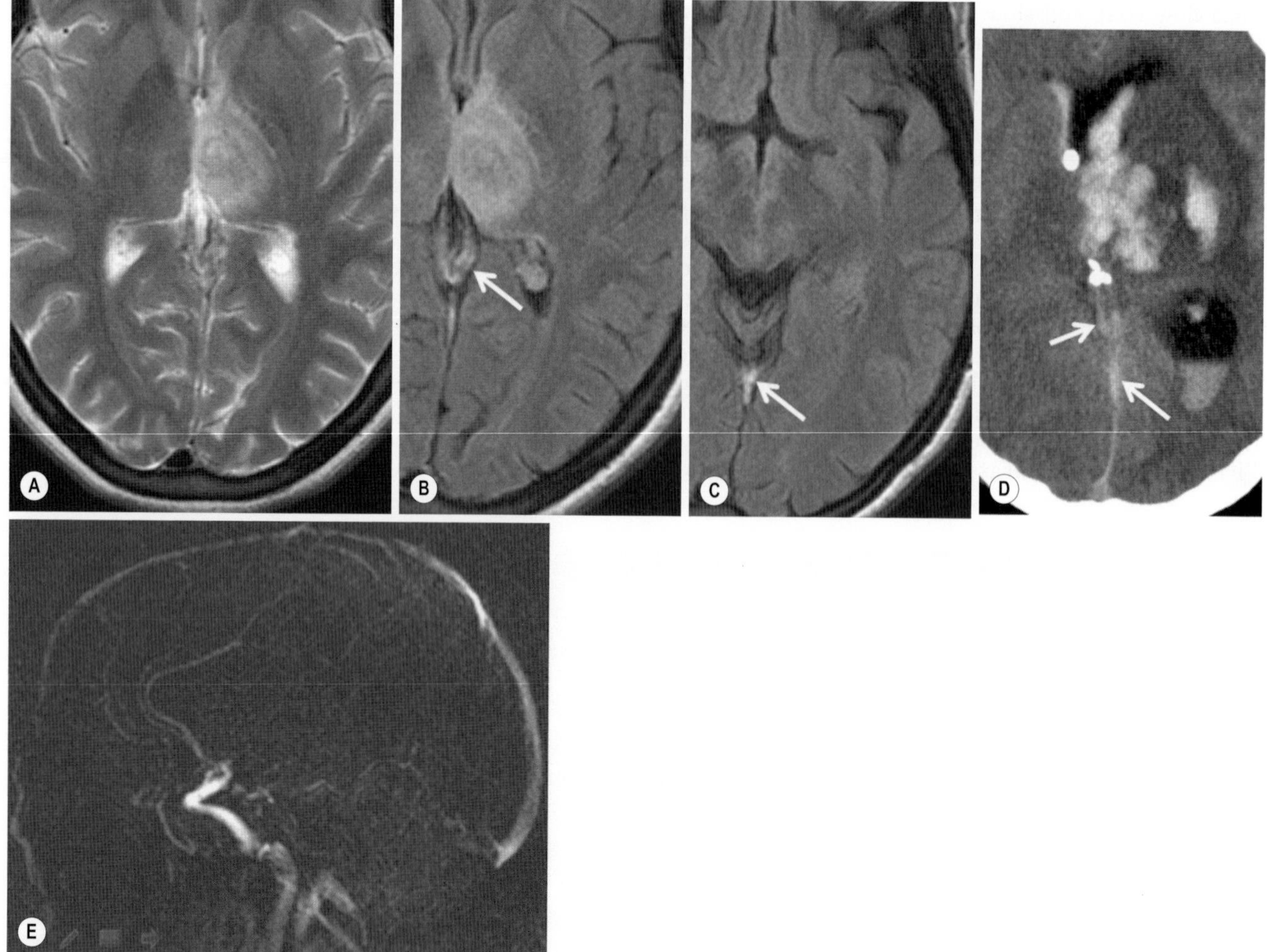

FIGURE 62-28 ■ Deep venous thrombosis. (A–E) This young female patient presented with headache and right-sided hemiparesis whilst playing in a prolonged hockey competition in summer, followed by reduced consciousness. The initial MRI examination (A, C) demonstrates signal abnormality and swelling consistent with venous hypertension, oedema and ischaemia in the left thalamus. There is abnormal signal within and expansion of the left internal cerebral vein and straight sinus on FLAIR (B, C, white arrows) in keeping with thrombus. The MR venogram does not show any flow in the deep venous system (E). A clinical deterioration is accompanied by haemorrhage and venous infarction in the left thalamus (D), with additional involvement of the left lentiform nucleus and right thalamus. Intraventricular haemorrhage and hydrocephalus has developed. There is persistent hyperdensity within both internal cerebral veins and the proximal straight sinus (D, white arrows).

Subarachnoid haemorrhage is also often observed in this setting.

Overall, CVT is a difficult diagnosis to make and often requires more than one investigation. Scrutiny of the initial NECT is usually rewarding. CT venography is optimal for major dural venous sinus thrombosis, whilst MRI/V is more likely to identify subtle parenchymal lesions and thrombosis of the internal cerebral veins, straight sinus and cortical veins. On MRI, assessment of all of the major venous structures on all sequences is important as individual sequences can be misleading. Although, DSA catheter angiography is now rarely required, it most accurately defines the extent of disease and most reliably demonstrates recanalisation. Most commonly, it is utilised as a prelude to endovascular therapy if there is clinical deterioration despite medical management.

NON-TRAUMATIC INTRACRANIAL HAEMORRHAGE

Intracranial haemorrhage can be traumatic or spontaneous (non-traumatic) and is usually described in relation to the anatomical compartment in which it occurs.

SUBARACHNOID HAEMORRHAGE (SAH)

The incidence of SAH has remained stable over the last 30-40 years and is quoted at 9 per 100,000 person-years.[123]

Classically, SAH presents with a sudden-onset severe headache. In almost half of patients a period of unresponsiveness occurs, with 30% patients developing a focal neurological deficit. Severe acute-onset headaches are not uncommon. The majority will be innocuous and it should be noted that with this isolated symptom only 10% of patients will have had a subarachnoid haemorrhage.[124] However, with mortality rates approaching 50% and a post ictus dependency rate of 30%,[125] SAH and subsequently acute severe-onset headaches cannot be taken lightly.

Spontaneous SAH is most commonly due to a vascular abnormality, with a ruptured aneurysm accounting for approximately 80% (Table 62-4).

TABLE 62-4 **Causes of Subarachnoid Haemorrhage**

- Aneurysm (80%)
- Non-aneurysmal perimesencephalic (10%)
- Traumatic

Rare Causes

- Arteriovenous malformations
- Dural venous sinus or cortical vein thrombosis
- Intracranial dissection
- Drug abuse—cocaine
- Pseudoaneurysms—vaso-occlusive disorders with flow aneurysm on collateral vessels. Mycotic aneurysms
- Reversible cerebrovascular vasoconstrictive syndrome

In 10% no structural or vascular abnormality is demonstrated. This most frequently occurs when the subarachnoid blood is confined to the perimesencephalic area of the basal cisterns and is termed 'non-aneurysmal perimesenchephalic SAH'. These patients (who by definition have a negative catheter angiogram) have a very good long-term prognosis.[126] The risk of further bleeding is thought to be no higher than that in the general population. Variations in venous anatomy found with this pattern of SAH suggest a venous origin.[127] Rarer causes of SAH such as vascular malformations, venous thrombosis and drug abuse account for a much smaller proportion of cases.

Initial Investigation of Acute SAH

NECT is positive for SAH in 98% within 12 h of ictus onset[128] but this falls to less than 75% by the third day.[129] Acute SAH causes increased density of the cerebrospinal fluid (CSF) spaces on CT (assuming sufficient elevation of the CSF haematocrit). Most aneurysms are located on or close to the circle of Willis and blood is therefore seen in the basal cisterns, although the entire intracranial subarachnoid space may be opacified and intraventricular blood is common. In some cases the distribution of the surrounding blood may indicate the aneurysm location (Fig. 62-29).

A lumbar puncture should be performed when there is a strong clinical suspicion of SAH but a negative CT. Ideally this should take place at least 6 h, and ideally 12 h, following the ictus. This enables red blood cell lysis to

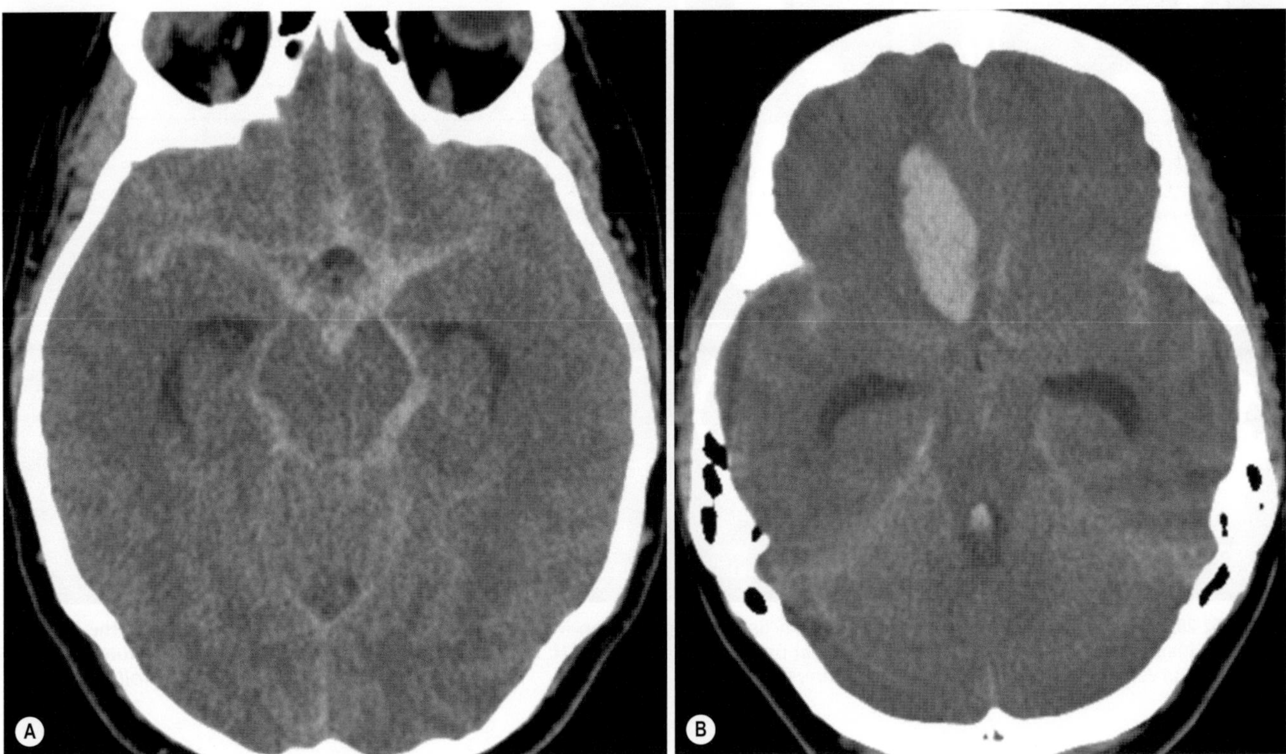

FIGURE 62-29 ■ **Distributions of acute SAH.** (A) Diffuse SAH within basal cisterns. (B) SAH with a focal parenchymal haematoma in the right inferior temporal lobe. This is very suggestive of an anterior communicating complex aneurysm—note the temporal horn dilatation in keeping with hydrocephalus.

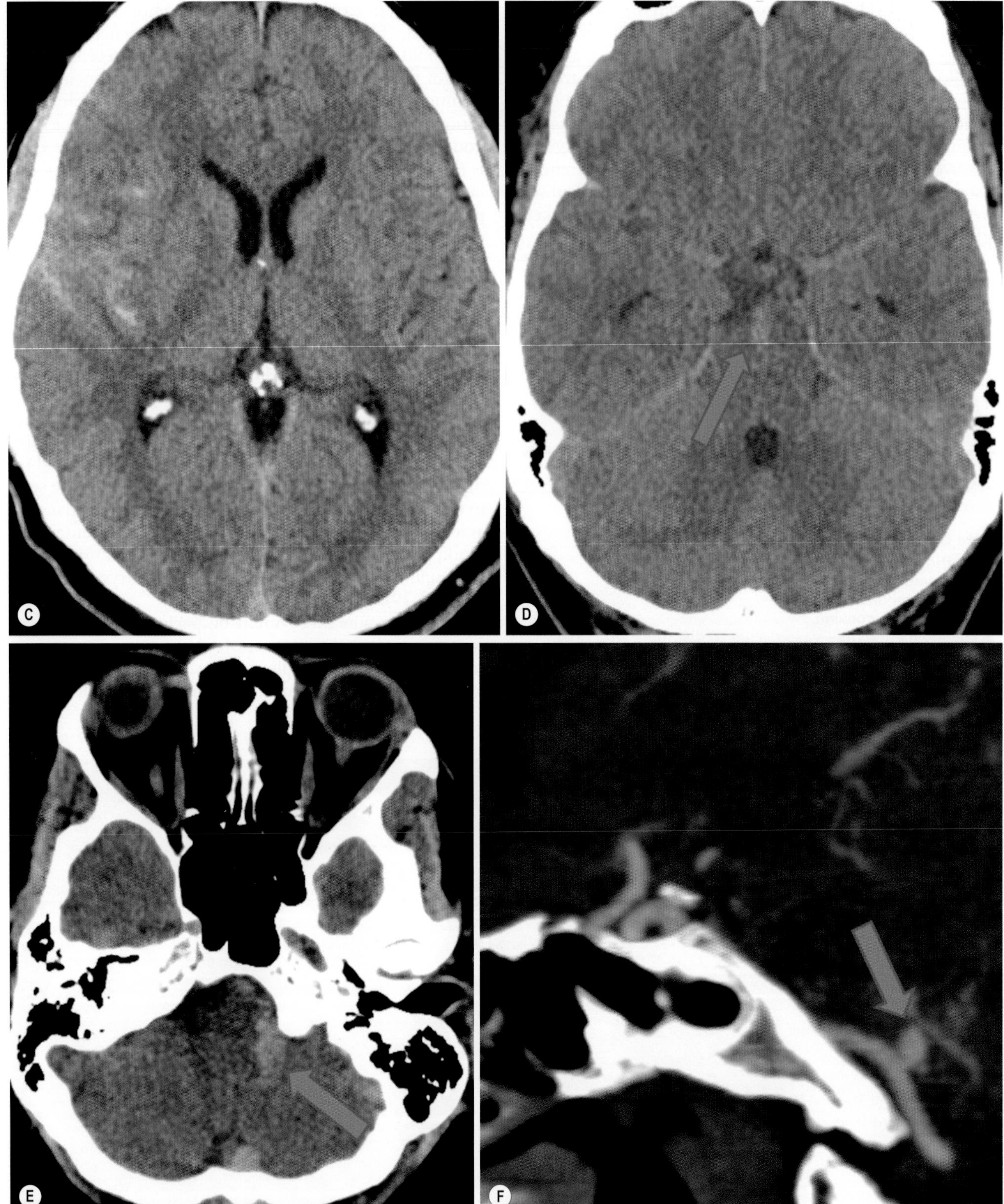

FIGURE 62-29, Continued ■ (C) SAH in the right sylvian fissure suggests an MCA anuerysm. (D) Small amount of SAH in the interpeduncular fossa—in keeping with a non-aneurysmal perimesencephalic SAH. (E) SAH adjacent to left side of the brainstem suggests a PICA aneurysm. (F) CTA confirms a PICA aneurysm. *Continued on following page*

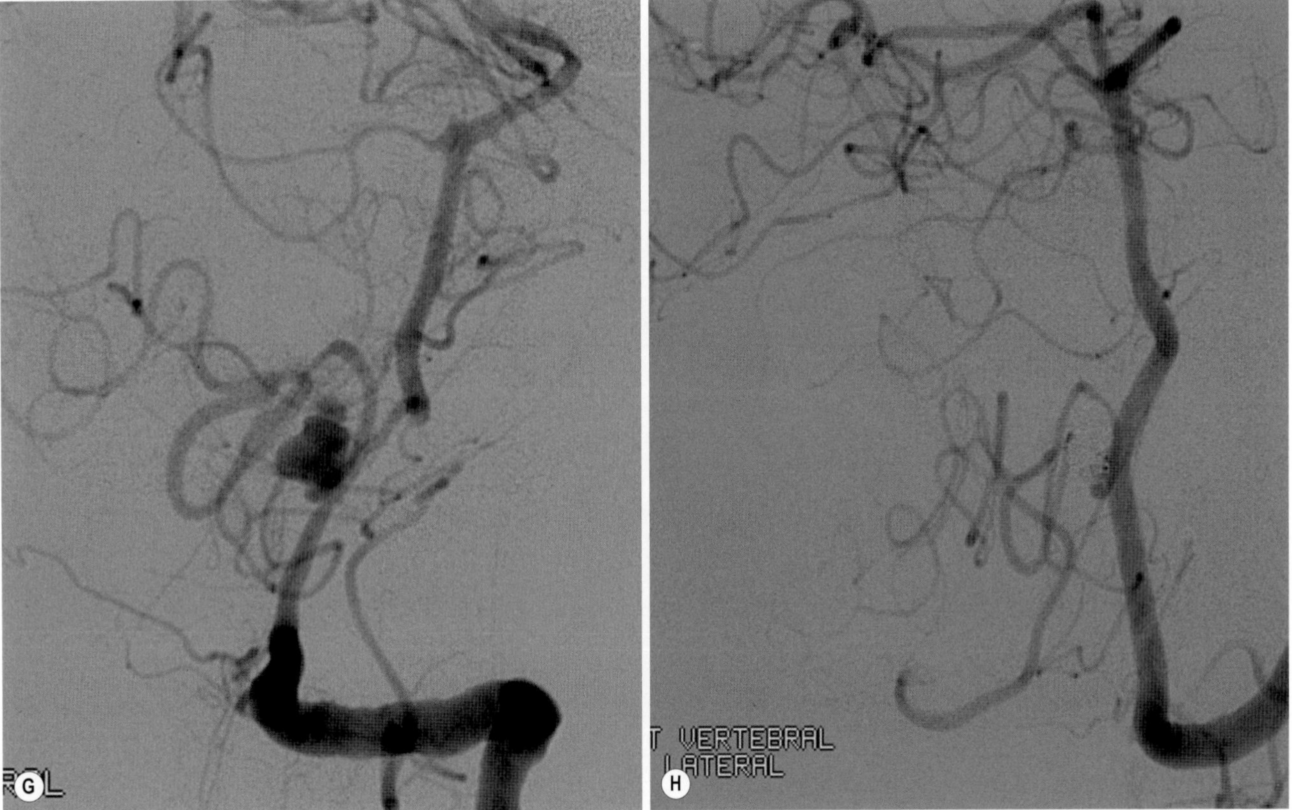

FIGURE 62-29, Continued ■ (G) DSA demonstrates the same PICA aneurysm. (H) Aneurysm is excluded from the circulation by endovascular insertion of platinum coils.

occur and thus blood degredation products such as bilirubin can be detected.[130,131]

Spin-echo MRI sequences are unreliable in SAH but by using a T2* gradient-echo or FLAIR sequence, sensitivities of 94–100% and 81–87% can be achieved in the acute (less than 4 days) and subacute (more than 4 days) periods, respectively.[132] The susceptibility effects of paramagnetic iron cause low signal on gradient-echo sequences; on FLAIR the CSF appears high signal due to the presence of increased protein. FLAIR may remain positive for up to 45 days after a haemorrhage,[133] at a time when the blood has long since become invisible on CT. However, FLAIR imaging is less sensitive at low CSF red blood cell concentrations following normal CT.[134]

Abnormal signal within the sulcal spaces on FLAIR sequences is not specific for SAH. Supplemental inspired oxygen,[135] leptomeningeal vascular engorgement and contrast medium leakage into the subarachnoid space after an acute infarct[136] can all cause the CSF to return high signal on FLAIR. CSF flow and pulsation artefact within the basal cisterns and at the foramen magnum is a common cause of artefactual abnormal signal which is commonly encountered in daily practice.

In the subacute period, CT and MRI will demonstrate a number of the complications associated with acute SAH. Of these, communicating hydrocephalus and ischaemia secondary to vasospasm are the most important. It is very common to see mild dilatation of the ventricles, particularly the temporal horns, at diagnosis. Indeed it may be a useful clue to the diagnosis if the presence of blood is not obvious. It usually resolves over several days, but may progress and necessitate CSF diversion. Vasospasm usually occurs between 4 and 11 days after the haemorrhage and is a significant cause of morbidity during this period.[137] It is more likely if the initial CT shows a large amount of subarachnoid blood.

MRI in chronic repeated SAH may show evidence of superficial siderosis with haemosiderin staining of the leptomeninges, particularly around the midbrain and in the posterior fossa. Such patients often present with symptoms related to the lower cranial nerves, ataxia or gradual cognitive decline. Location of an occult bleeding site is often not possible in these cases. The haemosiderin staining is often best appreciated on T2* GRE or SWI imaging (Fig. 62-30C).

Aneurysmal SAH

Aetiologically, cerebral aneurysms account for the majority of acute SAH cases. Aneurysms may be saccular, fusiform, or dissecting.[138] Fusiform aneurysms can be regarded as an extreme form of focal ectasia in hypertensive arteriosclerotic disease. Intracranial aneurysms can also develop following an arterial dissection or following direct vessel wall infection.

The majority are saccular aneurysms, which are usually round or lobulated and arise from arterial bifurcations, predominantly in the circle of Willis. Giant aneurysms, by definition, measure over 25 mm in diameter and account for approximately 5% of all cerebral aneurysms. They

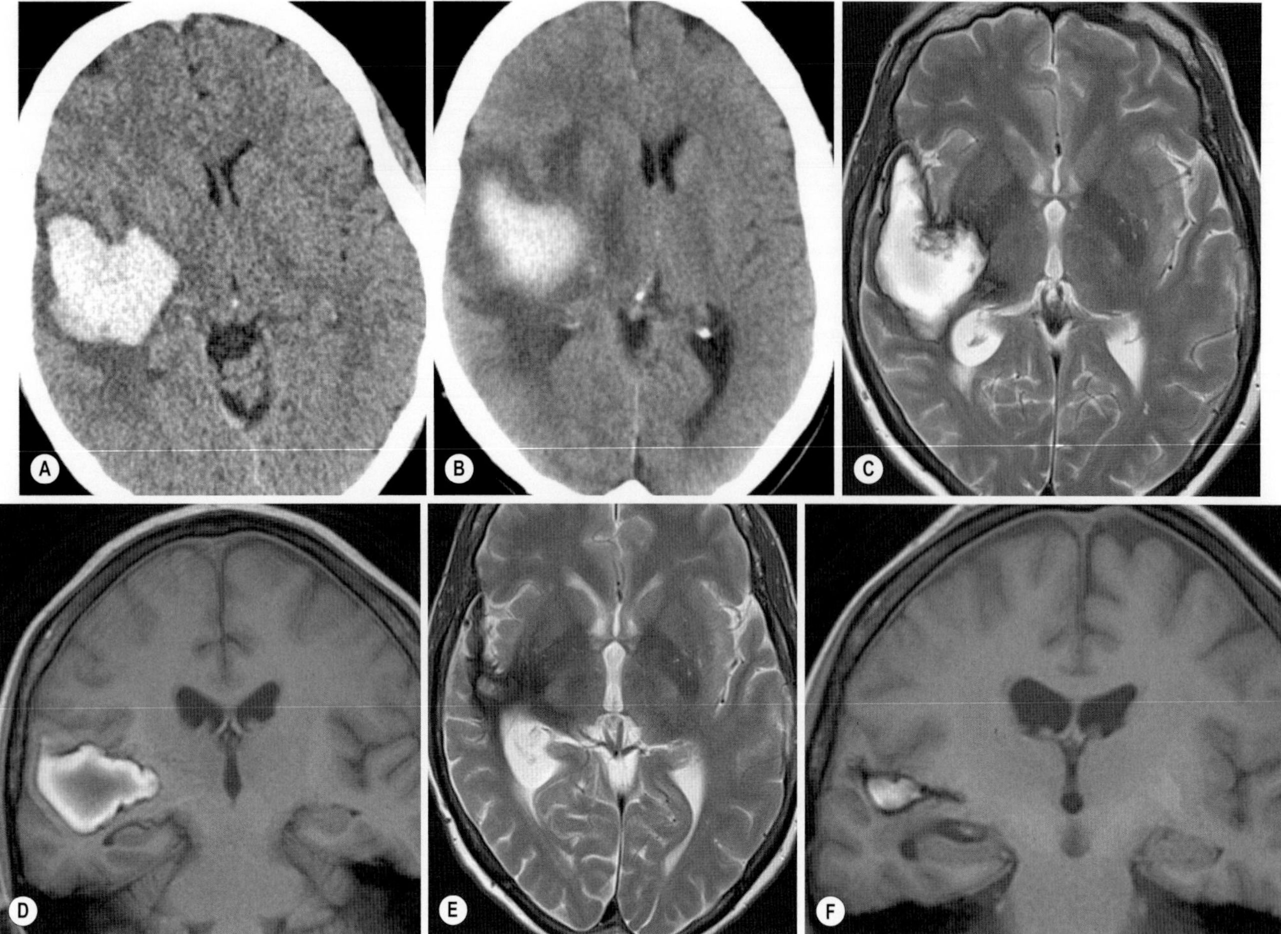

FIGURE 62-30 ■ Evolution of intraparenchymal haemorrhage. (A) Acute primary haematoma on CT. Note the homogeneous appearance with only a small peripheral rim of hypodensity. (B) Two weeks later the haematoma is less hyperdense but there is more surrounding oedema. (C, D) MRI at 1 month. The haematoma remains prominant but the surrounding oedema has resolved. There is a peripheral haemosiderin rim. There is T1 shortening (D) predominantly in the periphery. (E, F) At 5 months there has been shrinkage of the haematoma cavity which still shows residual T1 shortening (F). There is adjacent parenchymal haemosiderin staining with local loss of volume evidenced by the enlarged trigone of the right lateral ventricle.

often contain layers of organised thrombus. Aneurysms tend to present with SAH or mass effect on adjacent structures, most commonly a posterior communicating artery aneurysm resulting in extrinsic compression upon the cisternal segment of the third cranial nerve. Around 90% of intracranial aneurysms arise from the carotid circulation, the remaining 10% from vertebral or basilar arteries.[138] The anterior and posterior communicating arteries give rise to approximately one-third each of all intracranial aneurysms, with another 20% from middle cerebral arteries and 5% from the basilar termination. The remainder arises from other vessel origins and bifurcations. It should be remembered that 20% of aneurysms are multiple.

Aneurysmal SAH will often diffuse quickly throughout the CSF spaces giving little clue to its site of origin. More focal cisternal or parenchymal haematomas can be helpful in localising the source of the haemorrhage. A clot in the septum pellucidum, possibly extending into one or other frontal lobe, is virtually diagnostic of an aneurysm of the anterior communicating artery. Aneurysms of the distal anterior cerebral artery related to pericallosal branches are less common. Aneurysms of the MCA bleed into the sylvian fissure, sometimes with a clot in the temporal lobe. Aneurysms of the posterior communicating artery (which arise from the internal carotid artery at the origin of this vessel) are a frequent cause of SAH but can also present with an isolated third nerve palsy due to pulsatile pressure on the nerve.

Aneurysms of the posterior circulation are commonly located at the basilar artery termination and if they rupture blood may be seen in the interpeduncular fossa, brainstem or thalami; prognosis is frequently poor. The second commonest site in the posterior circulation is at the origin of one of the posterior inferior cerebellar arteries. They often haemorrhage into the ventricular system via the fourth ventricle and the haematoma localises around the craniocervical junction and the spinal subarachnoid space.

Larger aneurysms are shown on standard structural CT and MRI. On CT they appear as rounded enhancing lesions. Giant aneurysms have an enhancing lumen and a wall of variable thickness that often contains laminated thrombus and may be calcified. On spin-echo MRI sequences a patent aneurysm appears as an area of flow void. Areas of increased signal intensity within the aneurysm may represent mural thrombus or turbulent, slow flow.

Surrounding white matter oedema suggests a mycotic aneurysm, particularly if very extensive. Mycotic aneurysms are caused by septic emboli and tend to occur peripherally, typically on the branches of the MCA. They commonly present with haemorrhage, usually with a peripheral intraparenchymal clot, which, while not specific, is highly suggestive of such a lesion in a patient with known septicaemia or bacterial endocarditis.

Angiography in Acute SAH

The investigation of acute SAH requires expedient evaluation of the intracranial arterial circulation.

Digital subtraction catheter angiography (DSA) remains the gold standard for the imaging of intracranial aneurysms and vascular malformations. Its high spatial and temporal resolution allows accurate characterisation of the smallest aneurysms and enables endovascular treatment or surgical planning. Three-dimensional angiography rotational angiography (3D DSA) has further improved accuracy as it helps to resolve aneurysms which may be obscured by overlying vessels.[139–141] It reduces the need for multiple angiographic runs and provides high-resolution 3D images of the cerebral vessels that show the relationship of an aneurysm to adjacent vessels. Manipulation at the workstation permits the image to be rotated and viewed from any angle. This technique, however, is invasive, with an approximately 0.5–2% complication rate.[142,143] It is costly, requires specialist operator skills and equipment and is largely confined to neurosciences centres.

The last decade has seen dramatic advances in non-invasive imaging of aneurysms. Modern multidetector CT scanners with sophisticated post-processing computer software now provide fast, non-invasive intracranial angiographic data which approaches the sensitivity of catheter angiography. Results of several systematic reviews and meta-analysis show that CT angiography has a very high diagnostic value for the detection of intracranial aneurysms, particularly those of 3 mm[144–146] and over in size. Smaller aneurysms, particularly at the skull base, can be difficult to resolve. However, recent publications on multidetector scanners (320 detector rows) often using bone subtraction algorithms showed equivalent sensitivity and specificities with 3D DSA.[147–150]

Given its availability, speed and accuracy, CTA is the standard initial investigation of choice for investigating SAH in the acute setting. It takes only a few minutes to prepare the patient and plan the examination and on a multidetector CT system the whole head is imaged in less than 10 s. This is ideal in patients with SAH, who are often restless and unwell. It provides rapid diagnosis and enables endovascular and surgical treatment planning. This may negate the need for diagnostic catheter angiography prior to treatment, although catheter angiography is still required when the treatment strategy is not clear.

It is essential to methodically review source images on a workstation, in addition to multiplanar reformats and 3D surface renderings. Particular care should be taken close to the skull base, where adjacent bone may reduce the conspicuity of small aneurysms. CTA images can be degraded by vasospasm or inadequate opacification if the images are not acquired during the arterial phase of contrast enhancement. It is apparent on visual inspection when this is the case. The images can be rotated in multiple planes (like in 3D DSA), allowing for accurate evaluation of the anatomy of an aneurysm and its neck. However, the greatest benefit of CTA is its ease of use. It seems superficially attractive to consider devolving CTA to the general hospital environment. However, accurate interpretation requires experience in neurovascular radiology and CTA is part of the overall care of SAH patients, which is currently delivered in a neuroscience environment.

Practice varies in patients with a negative CTA following acute SAH. There is a body of opinion that a single technically adequate CTA is sufficient following a classical perimesencephalic SAH.[151] Some institutions now rely solely on CTA for all diagnostic imaging in SAH. However, in most centres it remains routine practice to confirm a negative CTA result with DSA. It is also used if for any reason aneurysm anatomy is not adequately displayed on CTA. Other vascular causes of SAH such as small vascular malformations are also more accurately assessed with this method.

CT angiography should be performed as soon as possible following SAH since the aneurysm re-bleed rate is greatest during the first 48 h and vasospasm can adversely affect the quality of angiograms performed several days after the haemorrhage. If a negative angiogram is marred by vasospasm, a repeat study is indicated.

Aneurysms can be treated by surgical clipping or endovascular coiling. The latter is performed via a microcatheter placed in the aneurysm sac through which a number of electrically detachable platinum coils with or without a gel coating are deployed (Figs. 62-31 and 62-32). The coiling may be assisted by the use of a catheter-mounted balloon or insertion of a stent across the aneurysm neck to prevent the coil ball prolapsing into the parent vessel. A multicentre randomised comparison of surgical clipping and endovascular coiling showed superior outcomes at 1 year for coiling over clipping (death or dependency 23.5 vs 30.9%; absolute risk reduction 7.4%). This difference was maintained at 7 years with a lower risk of epilepsy but more episodes of re-bleeding in the coiled group.[152] There is still a role for surgical clipping if the anatomy of the aneurysm is unfavourable for endovascular treatment.

Imaging of Incidental Intracranial Aneurysms

Increasingly, saccular aneurysms are discovered incidentally on scans for other indications and this represents a management problem. A large-scale study, International Study of Unruptured Intracranial Aneurysms (ISUIA) suggests that the annual risk of haemorrhage from

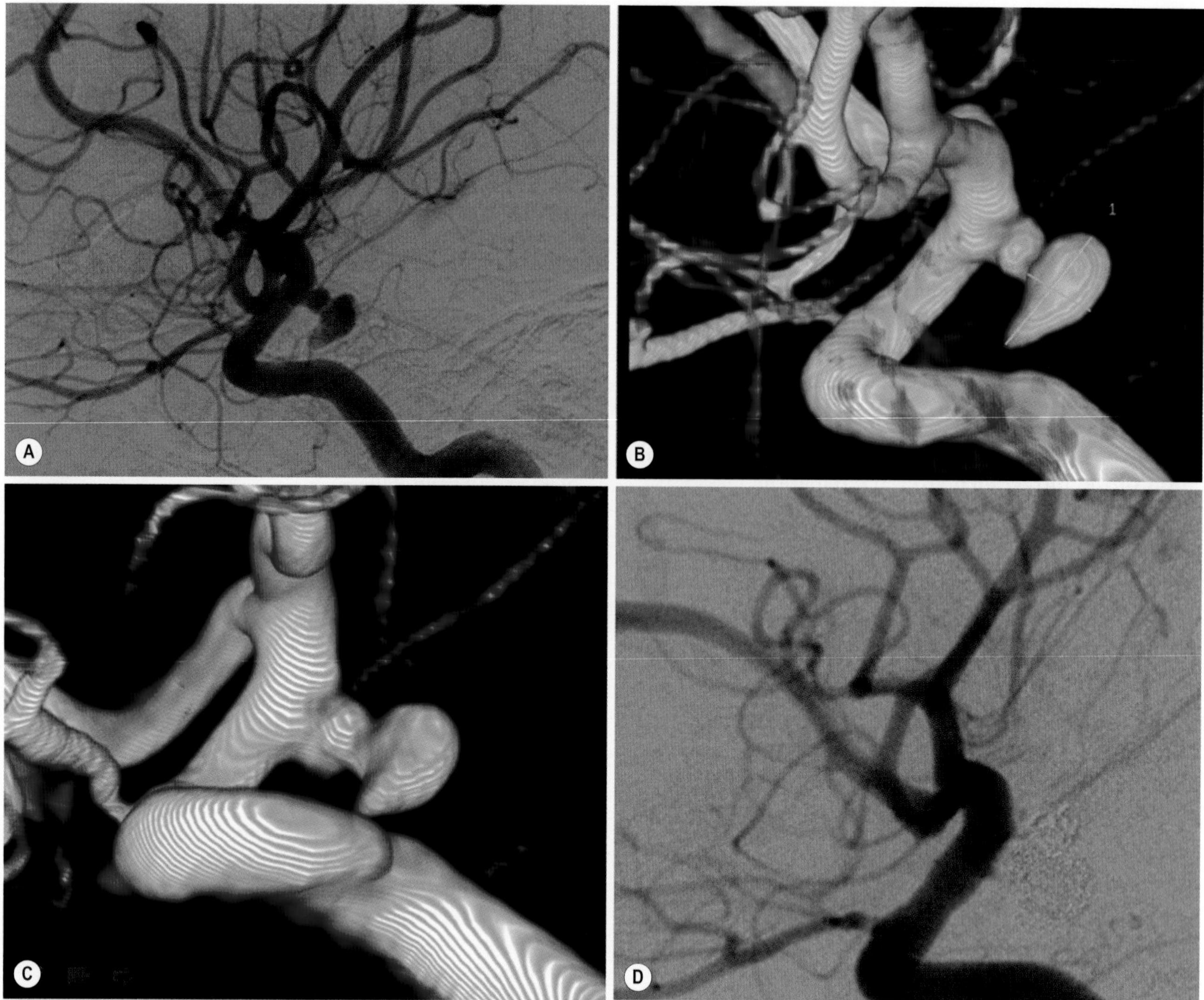

FIGURE 62-31 ■ A 37-year-old female patient presents with an acute-onset painful right third nerve palsy with pupil involvement. CT angiography demonstrated the presence of a lobulated posterior communicating artery (Pcomm) aneurysm. (A) The Pcomm aneurysm is demonstrated at DSA. (B, C) The size and position of the aneurysm neck is further appreciated with the volume-rendered images from the 3D rotational DSA. (D) After endovascular coiling, the aneurysm is completely excluded from the circulation.

small incidental aneurysms is substantially lower than previously thought and the risks of elective intervention higher.[153,154] Current data indicate that there is no benefit from treating aneurysms of the anterior circulation that are 7 mm or less in diameter, regardless of the patient's age, if there is no prior history of SAH. The difference between the risks of haemorrhage and treatment may favour intervention for larger or posterior circulation aneurysms (including posterior communicating aneurysms) depending on aneurysm size and remaining life expectancy.[154]

With no ionising radiation, MRA is considered to be the preferred method of imaging for intracranial aneurysms in the non-acute setting. These include screening of patients with two first-degree relatives who have suffered subarachnoid haemorrhage or those with connective tissue disorders who are at higher risk of aneurysm formation. It is also the preferred method of investigation for follow-up of incidental aneurysms and increasingly in follow-up assessment of endovascularly treated aneurysms.[155–157] Three-dimensional TOF MRA is the most widely accepted technique because it provides good spatial resolution and is relatively insensitive to signal dropout from turbulent flow. Resolution is further improved at higher field strengths and a number of studies have shown accurate detection of aneurysms down to the size of 1 mm,[158–160] although aneurysms less than 3 mm and those at the carotid siphon are those most easily missed. Like CTA, MRA images can be easily manipulated on the work station. Recent SAH may cause image degradation on TOF MRA due to T1 shortening from haemorrhage. Giant aneurysms are rarely visualised in their full extent on 3D TOF MRA because of slow and turbulent flow in their fundus. The lumen is properly opacified on CTA, which also shows mural thrombus and the aneurysm wall.

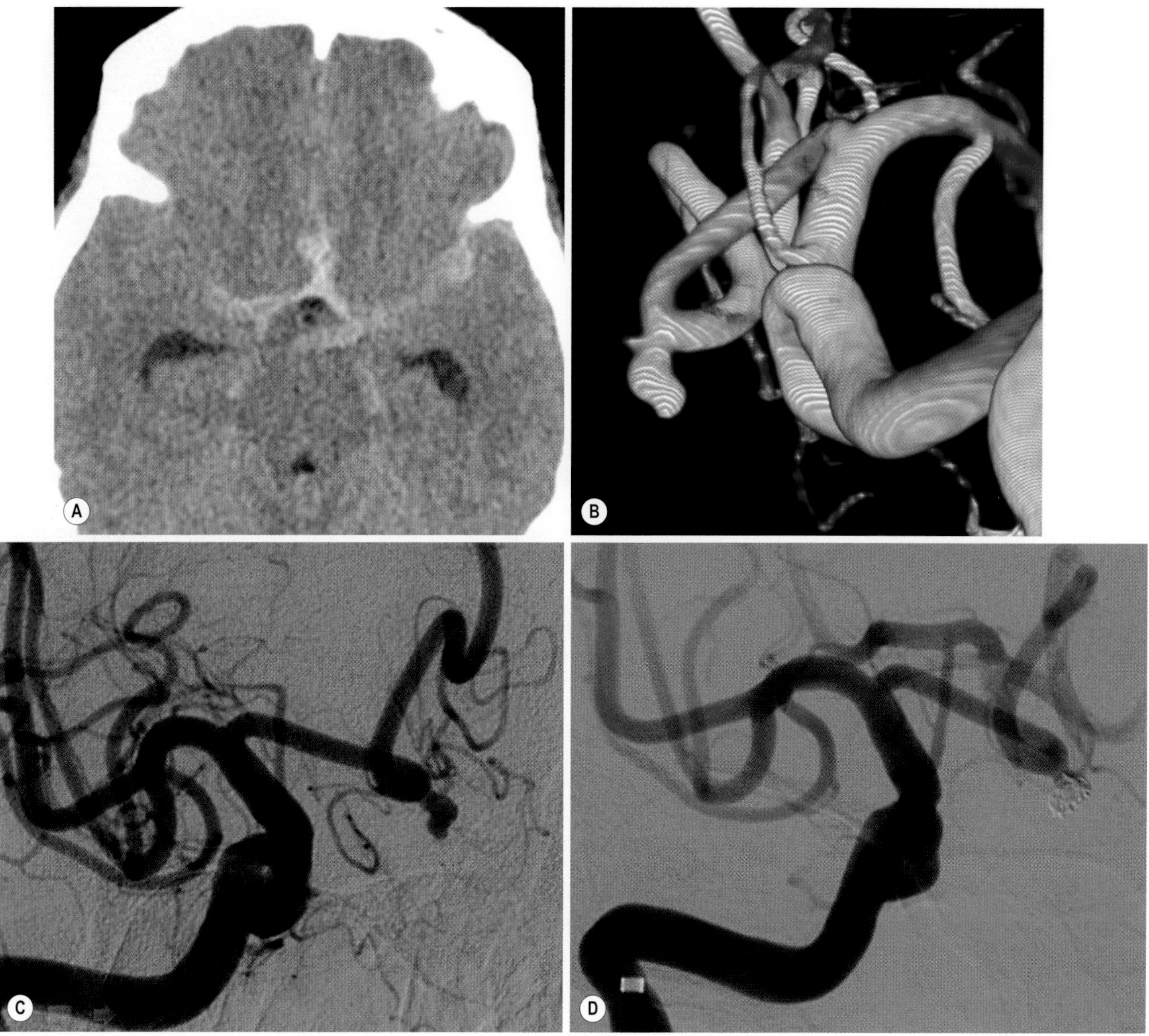

FIGURE 62-32 ■ A 50-year-old presents with an acute-onset headache. (A) NCECT demonstrates acute subarachnoid blood. (B, C) 3D DSA characterises the lobulated anterior communicating artery aneurysm prior to endovascular coiling where it is completely excluded from the circulation (D).

INTRACEREBRAL HAEMORRHAGE

Non-traumatic intracerebral haemorrhage accounts for 10–15% of all strokes. It has a higher mortality rate than other types of stroke, with less than 40% of patients surviving the first year. Primary haemorrhage occurs most commonly in the elderly from the rupture of small perforating vessels damaged by atherosclerotic hypertensive change or amyloid angiopathy. This accounts for up to 80% of spontaneous parenchymal haemorrhage. The preferential sites of hypertensive haemorrhage are the striato-capsular/thalamo-capsular regions, pons and cerebellum.[161–164] Larger hypertensive bleeds in the basal ganglia can extend into the ventricles or subarachnoid spaces. Peripheral or lobar haemorrhages in the elderly are suggestive of amyloid angiopathy, particularly if they are multifocal.[165] Both pathologies are often accompanied by a background of microbleeds.[166] These are best identified on T2* gradient-echo or susceptibility-weighted imaging. Hypertensive microbleeds tend to have a central predominance, whereas those associated with amyloid angiopathy are most often peripheral (Fig. 62-30).

Secondary haemorrhage can be due to a coagulopathy (usually on a background of hypertensive or amyloid angiopathy), underlying vascular malformation, haemorrhagic transformation of arterial and venous infarction (Fig. 62-33) and tumour. 'Recreational' drugs such as cocaine and ecstasy[167] and vasculitis are other rare but important causes.

Intracranial haemorrhage caused by aneurysms is usually associated with SAH, but very occasionally a ruptured aneurysm can cause an apparently isolated intracerebral clot (particularly if the surrounding subarachnoid space has been 'sealed off' by preceding SAH). This should be considered whenever a parenchymal haematoma extends to involve the sylvian fissure or basal cistern.

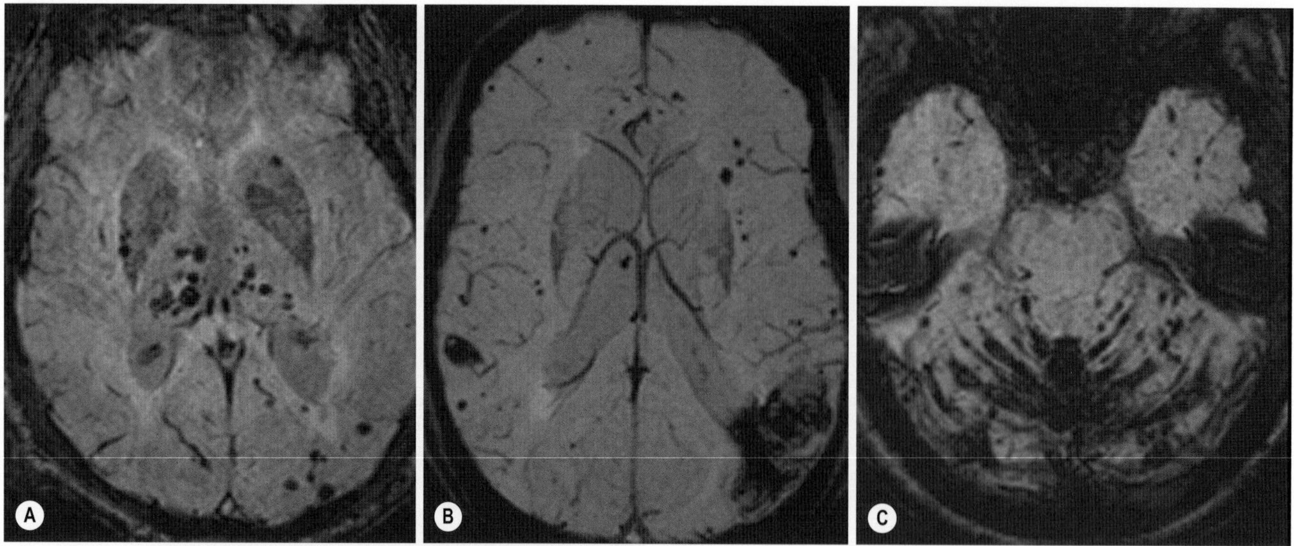

FIGURE 62-33 ■ SWI images demonstrate (A) cerebral microhaemorrhages related to hypertension. Note the predominantly ganglionic distribution. (B) Small lobar haemorrhages and predominantly peripheral microhaemorrhages in a patient with amyloid angiopathy. (C) Extensive haemosiderin staining over the cerebellar folia in a patient with siderosis of unknown aetiology.

TABLE 62-5 **Temporal MR Characteristics of Parenchymal Haematomas**[169]

Time	Stage	Biochemical form	SI on T1-weighted image	SI on T2-weighted image
Immediately to several hours	Hyperacute	Oxyhaemoglobin in RBC	↔	↑
1 to 3 days	Acute	Deoxyhaemoglobin in RBC	↔ ↓	↓↓
3 to 7 days	Early subacute	Methaemoglobin in RBC	↑↑	↓↓
1 to several weeks	Subacute to chronic	Extracellular methaemoglobin	↑↑	↑↑
Weeks to indefinitely	Remote	Ferritin and haemosiderin	↓	↓↓

SI = Signal intensity relative to grey matter.

Appearance on CT and MRI

Acute parenchymal haemorrhage is reliably detected on CT, appearing as increased density. Calcified or highly proteinaceous material and contrast enhancement of tumours can reach a similar density to fresh blood clot, but the clinical context or correlation with unenhanced images should prevent confusion. Hyperacute, unclotted blood will appear less dense, which may cause a blood–fluid level to be visible. This appearance is most commonly due to haemorrhage from coagulopathies (usually anticoagulant medication). Very rarely in severely anaemic patients with a haematocrit level below 20% haematomas can be isodense to the surrounding brain.[168] Deep or extensive haemorrhage may extend into the ventricles, forming a haematoma, or a blood–fluid level in the occipital horns, which are dependent with the patient supine.

Typically an acute primary parenchymal haematoma is homogeneous with only a fine rim of surrounding low density. Extensive oedema at presentation suggests an underlying abnormality. Features favouring a neoplastic haemorrhage are a more complex structure, extensive surrounding vasogenic oedema and enhancing areas not immediately adjacent to the blood clot. In some cases the diagnosis can only be made after follow-up studies.

Over the course of several days, an untreated haematoma becomes less dense, from the periphery towards the centre, and therefore appears smaller, although the surrounding oedema usually increases. The time of ictus is important, as small haemorrhages can look identical to infarcts on CT by 8–9 days, which clearly has important treatment ramifications. MRI will help to distinguish between the two. Vasogenic oedema may develop in the surrounding white matter and should contrast medium be given at this stage, it usually produces a halo of enhancement. After several weeks, the blood products become hypodense and are eventually absorbed to leave a focal, often slit-like, cavity or area of atrophy.

The MRI appearance of intracerebral haemorrhage changes over time as red cells break down and degrade, ultimately taken up by macrophages as haemosiderin.[169] These physiological phenomena result in a relatively characteristic temporal pattern of MRI appearances on T1 and T2 spin-echo sequences (Table 62-5).[169]

Factors such as protein and water content, fibrin formation and clot retraction can alter the sequence and timing of changes in appearance on MRI (Fig. 62-34).

Gradient-echo and more recently susceptibility-weighted imaging[170,171] is much more sensitive to the magnetic field inhomogeneities induced by blood degradation products than spin-echo sequences. This applies to both acute and old haemorrhage (deoxyhaemoglobin and haemosiderin, respectively).

Angiography in Intracerebral Haemorrhage

The indications for angiography in intraparenchymal haemorrhage are determined by clinical factors as much as imaging appearance. It is unlikely a treatable vascular abnormality will be found in a basal ganglia bleed in an elderly hypertensive patient, whereas a haemorrhage in the same location in a young, normotensive patient warrants further investigation with angiography to exclude an arteriovenous malformation (AVM). It is also noteworthy that some 'recreational' drugs are associated with aneurysm formation and rupture, so angiography is often appropriate in such patients.[167]

The timing of angiography depends on the size and mass effect of the haematoma. CTA is used in the emergency setting for the detection of ruptured AVMs and aneurysms as it is much easier and quicker to perform in very sick patients. It allows the neurosurgeons to assess the location and extent of the vascular abnormality and to plan their surgical approach prior to evacuation of the haematoma. In a stable patient not requiring urgent haematoma evacuation it is usually preferable to defer angiography until the haematoma has resolved because smaller vascular lesions can be compressed by an acute haematoma and not be apparent angiographically. It is not yet established that a small arteriovenous fistula or malformation can be reliably excluded using CTA/MRA, so DSA is still preferred for elective investigation of such patients. Dynamic contrast-enhanced CTA and MRA studies which are time resolved are demonstrating good results in comparative studies with catheter angiography in patients with vascular malformations.[172–174]

ARTERIOVENOUS MALFORMATIONS

Intracranial vascular malformations can be classified according to the presence or otherwise of arteriovenous shunting.[175] The former comprises cerebral (or subpial) AVMs and dural fistulae; the latter includes developmental venous anomalies (DVAs), cavernous angiomas ('cavernomas') and capillary telangiectasias. DSA is still the method of choice for the investigation of cerebral AVMs and dural fistulae. Cavernous angiomas and telangiectasias are angiographically occult or 'cryptic' vascular malformations which tend to have characteristic appearances on MRI.

Cerebral (subpial) AVMs are probably congenital anomalies consisting of direct arteriovenous shunts without a normal intervening capillary bed. Some are essentially fistulous—direct shunting from an artery to a vein; others have a plexiform nidus or a combination of the two. They lie within the brain substance or cerebral sulci and are supplied by branches of the internal carotid artery or vertebrobasilar system, sometimes recruiting additional supply from meningeal arteries. Cerebral haemorrhage is the commonest clinical presentation, others being epilepsy, headache or focal neurological deficit.

They are usually detectable on CT or MRI as serpiginous areas of high density (with marked contrast enhancement) or mixed signal, respectively. CT may show calcification and the MR signal comprises areas of flow void and high signal, which may represent thrombosis or flow-related enhancement. There may be haemorrhage at different stages of evolution. AVMs may be surrounded by areas of ischaemic damage that are low attenuation on CT and hyperintense on T2-weighted MRI. Dilated feeding arteries and early opacification of draining veins indicating shunting are the angiographic hallmarks of these lesions (Fig. 62-35).

Dural arteriovenous fistulae are direct shunts between branches of the external carotid artery or meningeal branches of the cerebral vessels and dural sinuses. They are thought to be acquired and may be due to prior venous thrombosis. The clinical presentation depends on their location and venous drainage pattern.[176,177] Lesions shunting into the cavernous sinus commonly present with proptosis. Shunting into the transverse or sigmoid sinus may cause pulsatile tinnitus. Intracranial haemorrhage, which may be intracerebral, subarachnoid or subdural, usually occurs in lesions that reflux into cortical veins. They may go undetected on MRI or CT unless there are enlarged dural sinuses or cortical veins. MRA or CTA may show abnormal vessels more clearly but intra-arterial angiography is still required to make a definitive diagnosis (Fig. 62-36).

Angiography for an AVM or dural fistula should include injections of all possible feeding vessels using a high frame rate to improve delineation of the nidus, which otherwise can be obscured by overlying veins in rapidly shunting lesions. There may be associated aneurysms, either on the feeding arteries or within the nidus and venous drainage may be via deep and/or superficial systems. There may be venous varices or stenoses. There is an increased risk of haemorrhage in AVMs with the presence of intranidal aneurysms, a single draining vein, deep venous drainage and venous stenoses.[177–179] CTA and MRA show the components of an AVM[177] and increasingly dynamic contrast-enhanced MR and CT angiography can provide the temporal information only previously available from DSA.[173,174,180,181]

The treatment options for cerebral AVMs include surgery, radiosurgery and endovascular embolisation. More than one technique may be used in combination.

Cavernous angiomas are mulberry-like lesions consisting of vascular spaces with little intervening tissue and haemorrhage of different ages. The incidence of clinically symptomatic haemorrhage remains uncertain, but is less frequent than with cerebral AVMs or dural fistulae. A previous bleed and infratentorial location are the main prognostic factors for recurrent haemorrhage. Lesions in

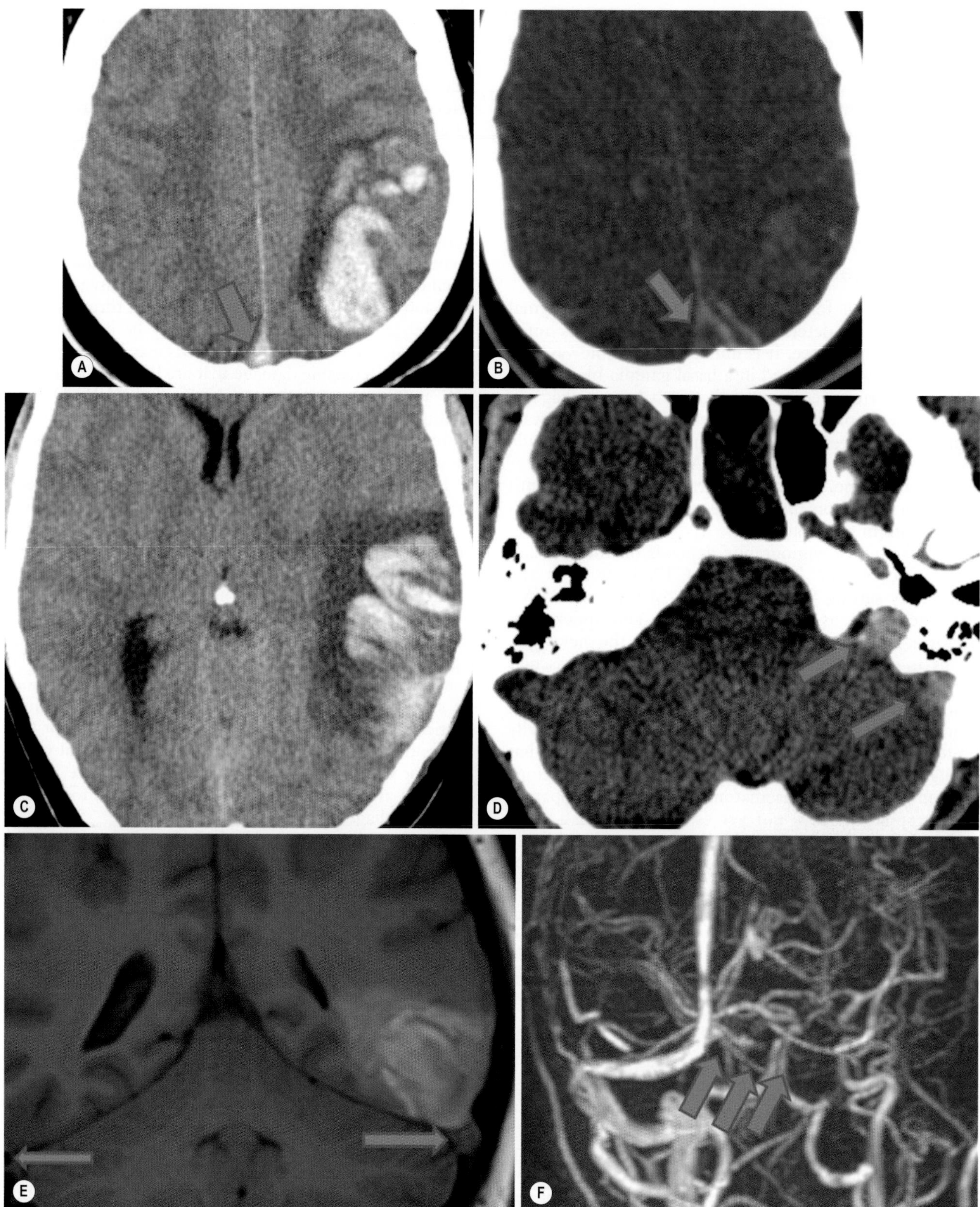

FIGURE 62-34 ■ (A) Fragmented parenchymal haemorrhage in dural venous sinus thrombosis (DVST). Note the hyperdense superior sagittal sinus on the NCET. (B) The venographic study shows absence of contrast enhancement within the sinus 'empty delta sign'. (C) The parieto-temporal location suggests lateral venous sinous/vein of Labbé thrombosis. (D) The hyperdense left lateral transverse sinus and sigmoid sinus is seen on the NCET. (E) Same patient as (C, D): coronal T1 FSE with parenchymal T1 shortening in keeping with haemorrhage. Note the attenuated left-sided venous sinus flow void (arrows). (F) The 3D MRV does not demonstrate any flow with the left transverse or sigmoid sinus. This can be a normal variant which should be confirmed with structural MRI imaging. In DVST there will be attenuation of the normal dural sinus flow void and it is usually hyperintense on the T2-dependent sequences although this is dependent on the age of the blood products. CT will also demonstrate the presence of a sinus grooving the occipital bone rather than showing true hypoplasia.

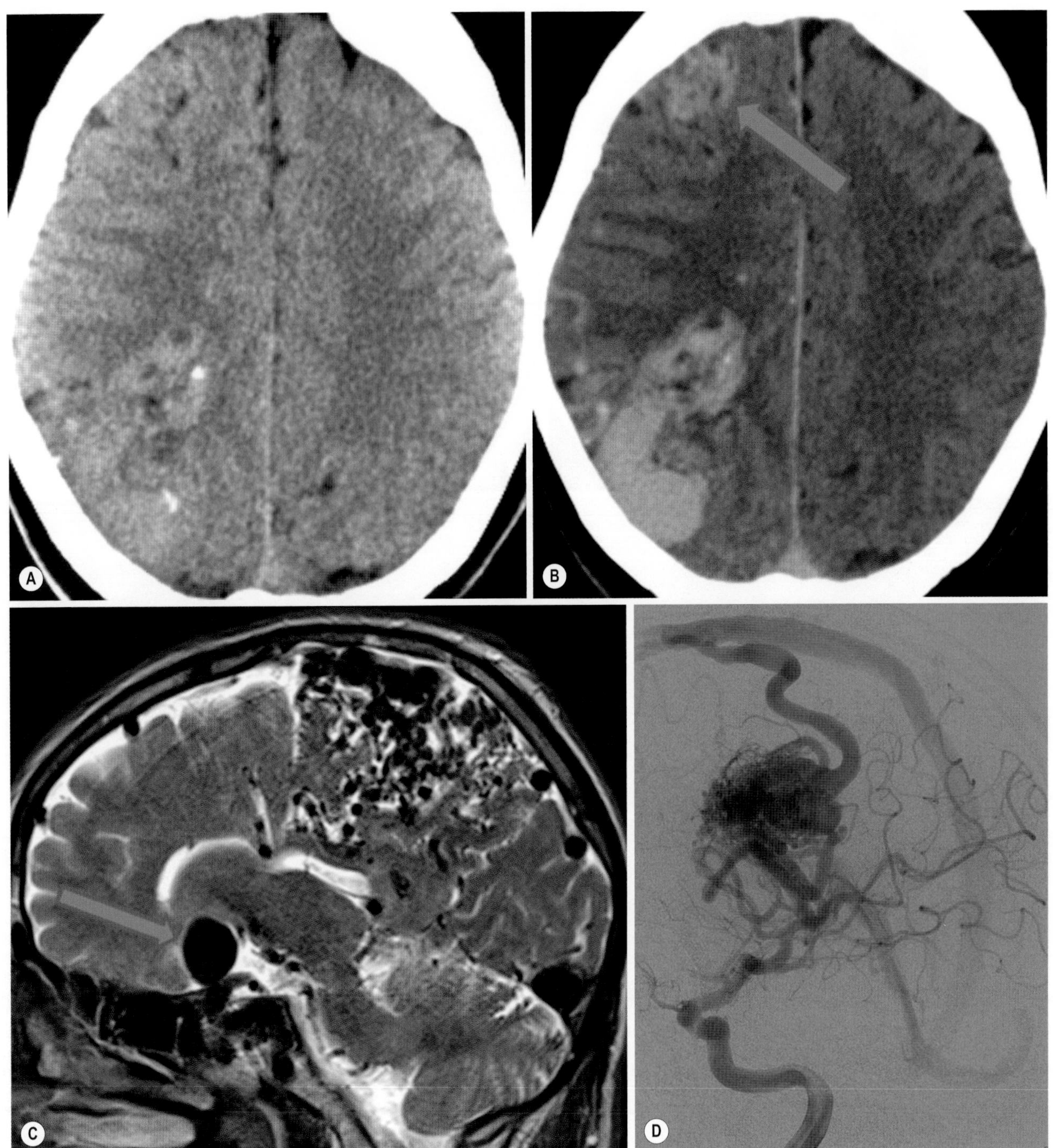

FIGURE 62-35 ■ CT in a young female patient who presented with a seizure. (A) Unenhanced study shows lobulated hyperdensity with focal areas of calcification. (B) Following contrast administration there is avid enhancement in two distinct areas of the right frontal and parietal lobes. The appearances are typical of an AVM. Multiple AVMs suggest hereditary haemorrhagic telangiectasia (HHT). In this case there was no parenchymal haemorrhage. (C) MRI in a different patient shows a diffuse parietal AVM with large superficial draining veins. Note the large flow aneurysm related to the terminal ICA (arrow). (D) DSA shows an AVM with a compact nidus. It is supplied by branches of the middle cerebral artery and drains via both the superficial and deep venous systems.

or close to the cerebral cortex may cause epilepsy. They are occasionally intraventricular or arise on a cranial nerve. They appear as relatively well-defined, dense or calcified lesions on CT, which may show patchy contrast enhancement. On MRI they appear multilobular with mixed but predomiantly elevated T2 signal intensity centrally surrounded by a dark haemosiderin rim.[182] Not surprisingly, susceptibility-based sequences are the most sensitive.[171,172] They may be multiple, particularly in familial cases.[183] In many clinical situations the discovery of a cavernoma represents an incidental finding (Fig. 62-37).

Developmental venous anomalies are not malformations but represent a benign variation in venous

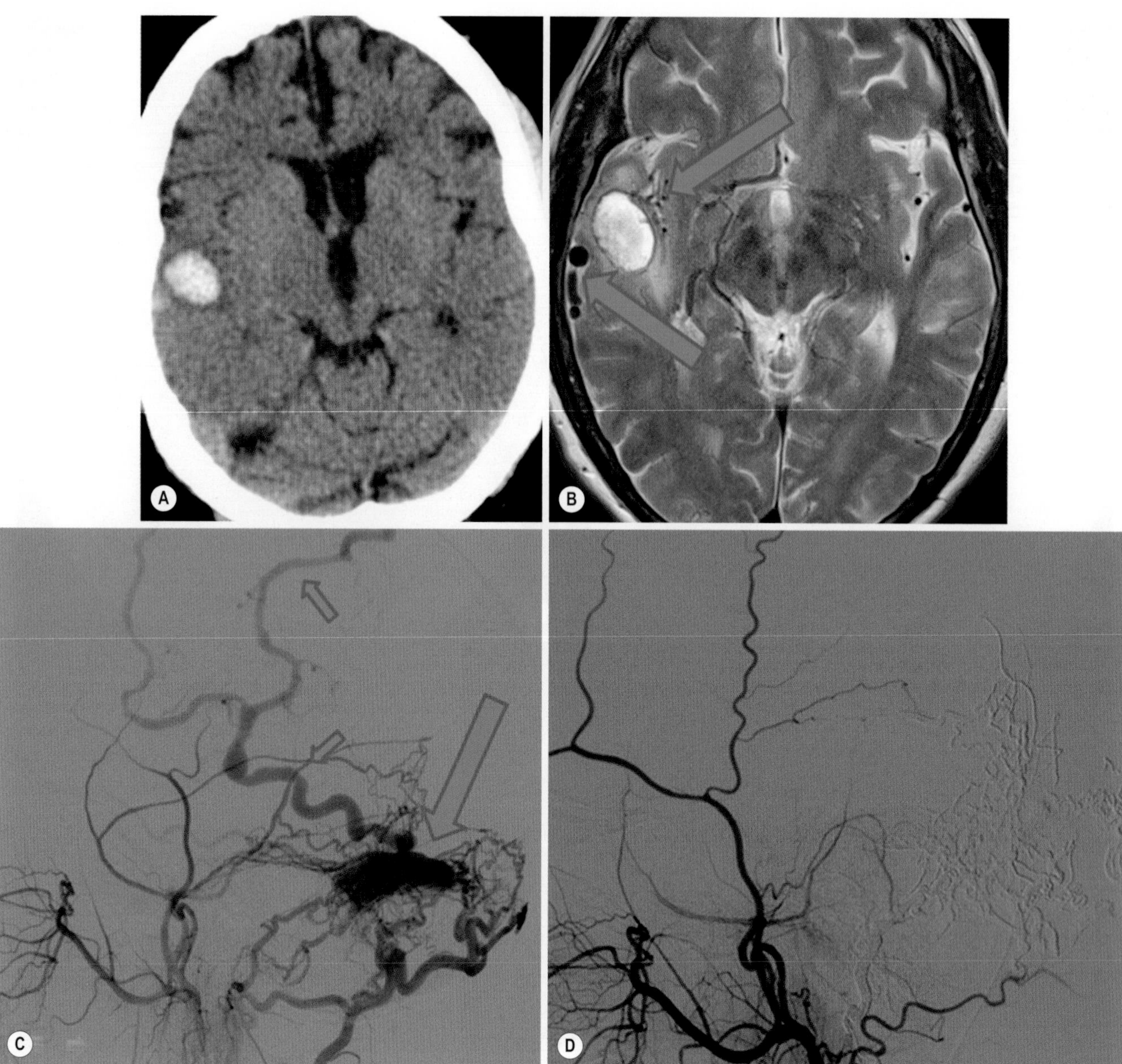

FIGURE 62-36 ■ (A) CT demonstrates small right temporal haemorrhage. (B) T2W MRI shows the haemorrhage but also demonstrates the presence of prominent local vessels (arrows). (C) DSA injection of the external carotid circulation shows a fistulous connection between ECA branches (occipital and meningeal) with an isolated transverse sinus (long arrow). There is retrograde venous drainage via a hyprotrophied vein of Labbé and the vein of Trolard (short arrows) into the superior sagittal sinus. (D) The fistula has been embolised using a liquid embolic agent.

drainage. They may be found with cavernomas. They consist of radially arranged, dilated transmedullary veins that have a typical 'caput medusa' appearance on the venous phase of conventional angiograms. They may drain into the superficial or deep venous system. They are readily diagnosed by contrast-enhanced CT or MRI.[182]

Capillary telangiectasias are benign nests of dilated capillaries with normal brain tissue in between. They are usually found on postmortem examinations and are occasionally visible on MRI as areas of very subtle T2 hyperintensity or ill-defined enhancement. They do not cause haemorrhage.

SUBDURAL AND EXTRADURAL HAEMORRHAGE

Acute subdural and extradural haematomas are almost always post-traumatic.

Occasionally, rupture of a cerebral aneurysm may cause an acute subdural haematoma, most frequently a posterior communicating artery aneurysm lying next to the free edge of the tentorium cerebelli. A dural arteriovenous fistula may also bleed into the subdural space. Angiography is therefore indicated following a spontaneous acute subdural haematoma, particularly in a young patient.

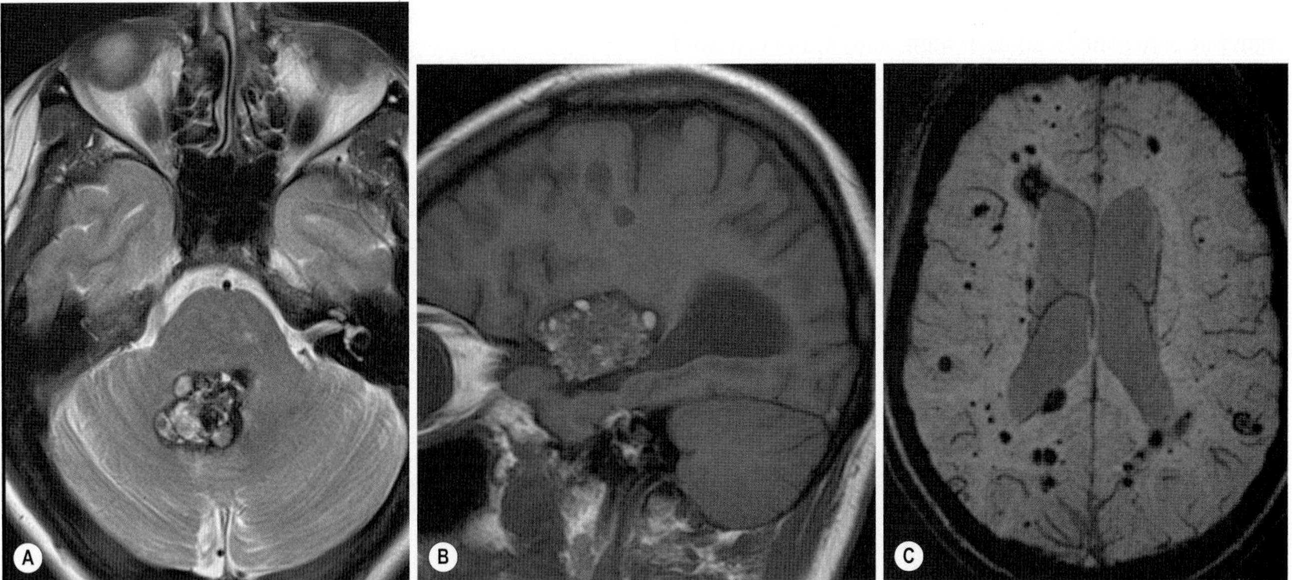

FIGURE 62-37 ■ (A) Posterior fossa cavernoma has a 'popcorn' appearance with a peripheral haemosiderin ring. (B) Sagittal T1W image again shows peripheral haemosiderin ring. There are locules of T1 shortening in keeping with blood degradation products. (C) SWI image demonstrates numerous areas of susceptibility 'blooming' related to blood products from multifocal cavernomas.

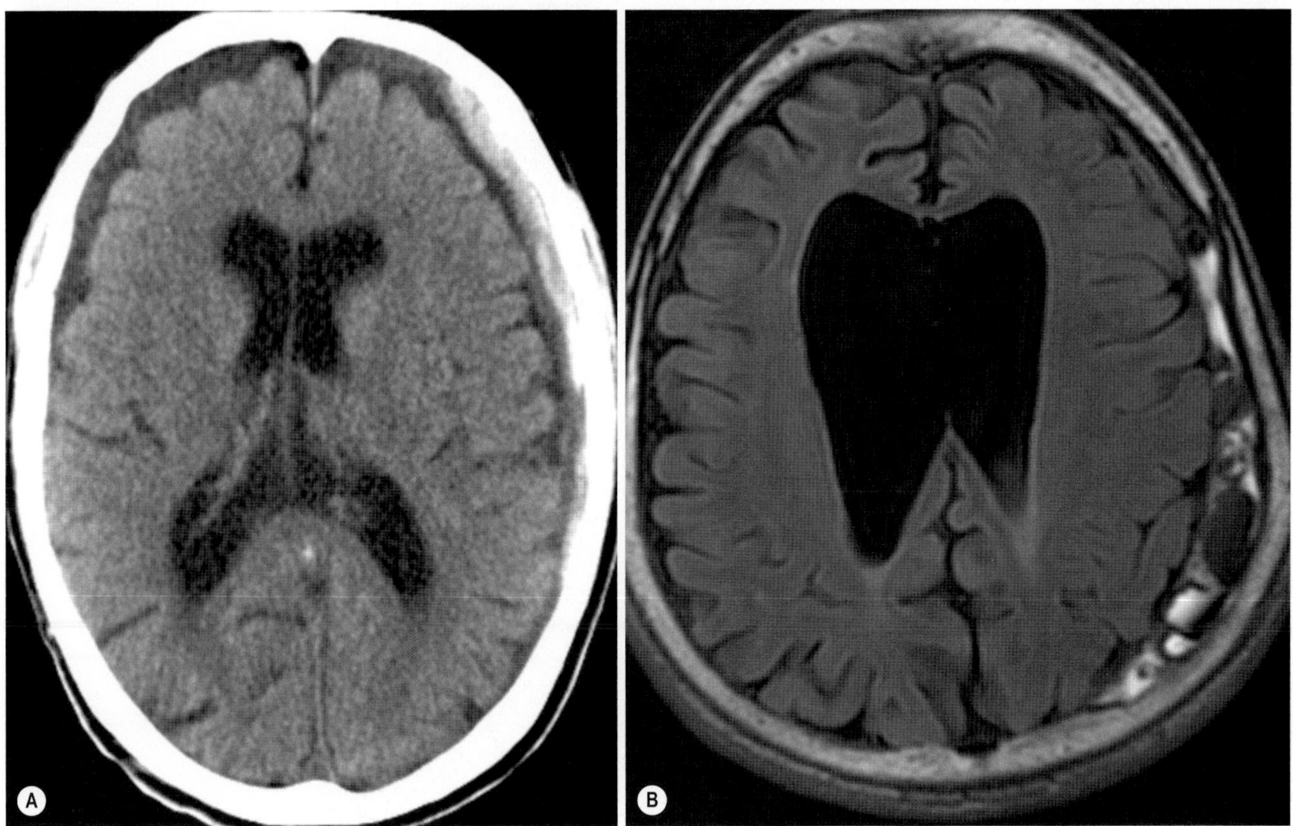

FIGURE 62-38 ■ (A) Shallow bilateral convexity chronic subdural haematomas. The increased density over the left convexity suggests a more acute component. (B) A larger left convexity chronic subdural haematoma on FLAIR. Note the local left hemispheric sulcal effacement.

Chronic subdural haematomas represent a different entity. These are frequently bilateral and occur in elderly patients or alcoholics with underlying brain atrophy, patients on anticoagulants or following shunting for hydrocephalus. The underlying mechanism is thought to be leakage from bridging cortical veins following minor trauma. They may present with increasing confusion and a reduction in conscious level. Burr holes for drainage of a chronic subdural collection, sometimes under a local anaesthetic, are one of the few neurosurgical operations performed on the very elderly (Fig. 62-38).

On CT they appear to be of lower density than the brain but may contain areas of high density, or even fluid levels, due to more recent haemorrhage. The MRI appearance evolves in a similar pattern to intraparenchymal haemorrhage. Chronic subdural haematomas continue to give high signal on T2-weighted images, while returning low signal on T1-weighted images, without becoming isointense to CSF, because of their higher protein content. Repeated episodes of bleeding can produce variable changes of signal intensity analogous to the variable density changes on CT. A pseudomembrane, which forms around chronic subdural haematomas, may show marked contrast enhancement or haemosiderin staining.

Shallow subdural fluid collections and occasionally overt haemorrhage may also develop around the cerebral hemispheres and cerebellum secondary to mild brain descent in the low CSF volume syndrome.[184] In this condition patients usually present with postural headache that is worse on standing and relieved by lying down. There is sometimes a history of vigorous Valsalva, lumbar puncture or other spinal intervention. The MRI features, other than subdural collections, are diffuse dural thickening shown best on FLAIR or contrast-enhanced T1-weighted images and mild cerebellar ectopia. These changes resolve after successful treatment.

For a full list of references, please see ExpertConsult.

FURTHER READING

8. Markus HS. Cerebral perfusion and stroke. J Neurol Neurosurg Psychiatry 2004;75:353–61.
10. Powers WJ. Cerebral hemodynamics in ischemic cerebrovascular disease. Ann Neurol 1991;29:231–40.
13. Marchal G, Young AR, Baron JC. Early postischemic hyperperfusion: Pathophysiologic insights from positron emission tomography. J Cereb Blood Flow Metab 1999;19:467–82.
27. Barber PA, Hill MD, Eliasziw M, et al. Imaging of the brain in acute ischaemic stroke: comparison of computed tomography and magnetic resonance diffusion-weighted imaging. J Neurol Neurosurg Psychiatry 2005;76:1528–33.
39. Liang L, Korogi Y, Sugahara T, et al. Detection of intracranial hemorrhage with susceptibility-weighted MR sequences. AJNR Am J Neuroradiol 1999;20:1527–34.
49. Davis SM, Donnan GA, Parsons MW, et al. Effects of alteplase beyond 3 h after stroke in the Echoplanar Imaging Thrombolytic Evaluation Trial (EPITHET): a placebo-controlled randomised trial. Lancet Neurol 2008;7:209–309.
107. Chappell FM, Wardlaw JM, Young GR, et al. Accuracy of noninvasive tests for carotid stenosis—an individual patient data meta-analysis. Radiology 2009;251:493–502.
144. White PM, Wardlaw JM, Easton V. Can noninvasive imaging accurately depict intracranial aneurysms? A systemic review. Radiology 2000;217(2):361–70.
169. Bradley WG Jr. Hemorrhage and hemorrhagic infections in the brain. Neuroimaging Clin North Am 1994;4:707–32.

CHAPTER 63

Intracranial Infections

Daniel J. Scoffings • Julia Frühwald-Pallamar • Majda M. Thurnher • H. Rolf Jäger

CHAPTER OUTLINE

BACTERIAL INFECTIONS

Bacterial Meningitis

The causes of bacterial meningitis are age-dependent; in adults the most common causes are *Streptococcus pneumoniae* and *Neisseria meningitidis*. Bacteria can reach the meninges by haematogenous dissemination, spread from an adjacent focus of infection (such as sinusitis or otomastoiditis) or through congenital or acquired structural defects in the skull. Clinical manifestations include fever, headache, photophobia, lethargy and confusion. Imaging is frequently normal in patients with uncomplicated bacterial meningitis and is not necessary for its diagnosis, which requires analysis of a sample of cerebrospinal fluid (CSF) obtained by lumbar puncture (LP). The issue of whether neuroimaging is necessary before LP can be a matter of dispute between referring clinicians and radiologists. Although computed tomography (CT) can show findings that contraindicate LP, such as effacement of the basal cisterns and cerebellar tonsillar herniation, a normal CT does not imply that LP can be performed without the risk of causing tonsillar herniation.[1] The guidelines of the National Institute for Health and Clinical Excellence (NICE) in the United Kingdom are that CT is indicated when there are focal neurological signs or with a reduced or fluctuating level of consciousness, but that treatment should not be delayed in order to obtain imaging.[2]

Imaging is often normal in patients with uncomplicated bacterial meningitis but some abnormalities may be observed. Subtle distension of the subarachnoid spaces by inflammatory exudate has been reported, but can be difficult to appreciate in the very young and in older subjects, both of whom have relatively prominent basal cisterns. Leptomeningeal contrast enhancement, which follows the surface of the brain and extends into the sulci and basal cisterns, may be seen and is better detected by contrast-enhanced magnetic resonance imaging (MRI) than by contrast-enhanced CT. Leptomeningeal enhancement can be difficult to distinguish from contrast enhancement in normal blood vessels and the detection of abnormal enhancement of the leptomeninges may be improved by the use of a post-contrast fluid-attenuated inversion recovery (FLAIR) sequence, which is less sensitive to vascular enhancement.[3] An unenhanced FLAIR sequence may also show increased signal intensity in the subarachnoid spaces, most often over the frontal convexities and in the sylvian fissures, as a result of increased protein concentration in the CSF, causing failure of signal suppression by the inversion pulse (Fig. 63-1).[4] This FLAIR hyperintensity is non-specific, however, and can also be seen with subarachnoid haemorrhage, with malignant meningitis and in patients receiving large doses of supplemental oxygen. In a minority of cases (probably less than 10%) diffusion-weighted imaging (DWI) can show multiple foci of high signal intensity in the subarachnoid spaces; these are typically nodular and are associated with increased signal intensity on the FLAIR sequences in most cases. The finding of subarachnoid high signal on DWI has been reported to be associated with a poor prognosis.[5]

Complications of bacterial meningitis include hydrocephalus, most often of the communicating type, brain abscess, subdural empyema and ventriculitis (see below). Focal parenchymal lesions may also be observed on DWI, principally secondary to vasculopathy of arteries surrounded by inflammatory exudate, and have been classified into four patterns: large vessel territory infarcts, perforator territory infarcts, multiple bilateral lesions in the cortex and subcortical white matter and multiple bilateral lesions restricted to the cerebral cortex.[6]

Cerebritis and Brain Abscess

In immunocompetent patients most brain abscesses are bacterial, streptococci accounting for the majority. In 20–40% no causative organism is identified. Brain abscesses arise by haematogenous dissemination, penetrating trauma or direct spread from contiguous infection. The site of an abscess depends on its cause: frontal sinusitis will result in an abscess in or beneath the adjacent frontal lobe, whereas mastoiditis will give rise to a temporal lobe or cerebellar lesion. Blood-borne infection can occur

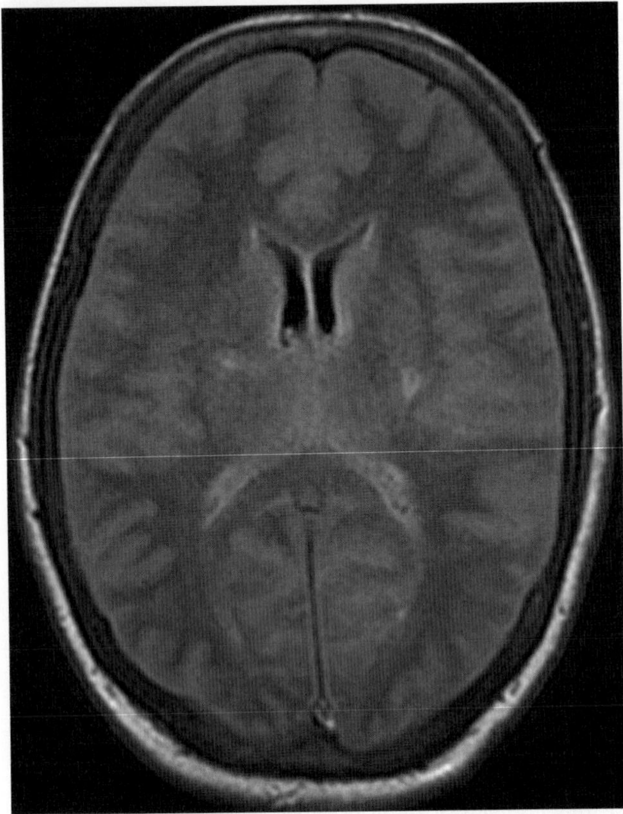

FIGURE 63-1 ■ *Listeria* meningitis in a renal transplant recipient. Axial fluid-attenuated inversion recovery (FLAIR) image shows failure of CSF suppression in the sulci as a result of pus in the subarachnoid space, manifesting as abnormal high signal intensity.

anywhere in the brain, but has a predilection for the territory of the middle cerebral arteries, particularly the frontoparietal region. A thorough search for a predisposing factor should be made; a cardiac cause is frequently overlooked (occult endocarditis and septal defects). Abscesses are frequently subcortical or periventricular. Four stages of development are described: early and late cerebritis and early and late capsule formation. Patients present with fever (in 50%), headache and focal neurological deficits. Brain abscesses are multiple in 10–50%.[7]

On CT, cerebritis appears as ill-defined low attenuation; enhancement is usually absent at the early stage but can appear irregular and peripheral in late cerebritis and may progress centrally on delayed images. With capsule formation the abscess shows central low attenuation, because of pus or necrotic debris and a rim of slightly higher attenuation surrounded by low-attenuation vasogenic oedema. After contrast medium, a ring of enhancement corresponds to the capsule. The enhancing rim typically has a smooth inner margin and shows thinning of its medial aspect.[8] In contrast to cerebritis, the centre of the abscess never enhances on delayed images. The degree of enhancement is diminished in patients who are immunocompromised or are on corticosteroid therapy.[9] Abscesses rarely contain gas; when present this is most often caused by surgical intervention or communication with a cranial air space such as the paranasal sinuses or mastoid air cells. It is only rarely because of a gas-forming organism.

On MRI, the signal of the abscess centre is intermediate between that of CSF and white matter on T1-weighted images and iso- or slightly hyperintense to CSF on T2-weighted images. On T2 sequences the abscess rim is relatively hypointense (Fig. 63-2); it may be slightly hyperintense to white matter on T1 images.[10] The abscess rim often appears markedly hypointense on susceptibility-weighted imaging (SWI); this is thought to be the result of free radicals produced by phagocytosis.[11] A 'dual rim' sign of concentric outer hypointensity and inner hyperintensity relative to the abscess core can also be seen on SWI.[12] The pattern of rim enhancement is similar to that shown by CT, the outer margin rim more often being smooth than lobulated.[13] Surrounding vasogenic oedema is of low signal on T1 and high signal on T2 images. The abscess centre is of high signal on DWI and low signal on maps of apparent diffusion coefficient (ADC), because of restricted diffusion in the viscous pus (Fig. 63-2). The degree of restriction of diffusion is inversely correlated with the viable cell count within the abscess centre.[14]

Though typical, the appearance of a brain abscess as a rim-enhancing mass is non-specific and may be mimicked by metastasis, glioblastoma and resolving haematoma. A thick, irregular rind of enhancement is more suggestive of tumour. Abscesses are more likely to show small satellite lesions. Despite initial hopes that restricted diffusion would reliably distinguish abscess from tumour, reduced ADC has been subsequently reported in metastases and glioblastomas. Dynamic contrast-enhanced perfusion MRI may help distinguish between brain abscess and tumour; abscesses have a lower relative cerebral blood volume in their enhancing rim than gliomas.[15]

The management of brain abscesses can require both medical and neurosurgical therapy. CT diagnosis has been responsible for a marked reduction in the mortality of brain abscesses. Follow-up imaging is recommended at biweekly intervals or when new symptoms arise. Sufficient treatment is indicated by resolution of rim enhancement or disappearance of the low signal rim on T2 images. Treatment response may be better assessed with DWI than conventional MRI; low signal on DWI correlates with a good clinical response, whereas increasing signal implies reaccumulation of pus.[16]

Epidural Abscess and Subdural Empyema

An intracranial epidural abscess is a collection of pus between the inner table of the skull and the endosteum of the skull, which forms the outer layer of the dura mater. Abscesses mainly arise by direct spread from a contiguous focus of infection, most often sinusitis or otomastoiditis, less often as a complication of dental sepsis or after craniotomy. *Streptococcus milleri* is the most frequent causative organism. As intracranial epidural abscesses are typically slow-growing, the clinical presentation is often insidious, usually with fever and headache. CT and MRI show a lentiform collection of fluid constrained by the dura at the sites of cranial sutures. Accordingly, when anteriorly located as a complication of frontal

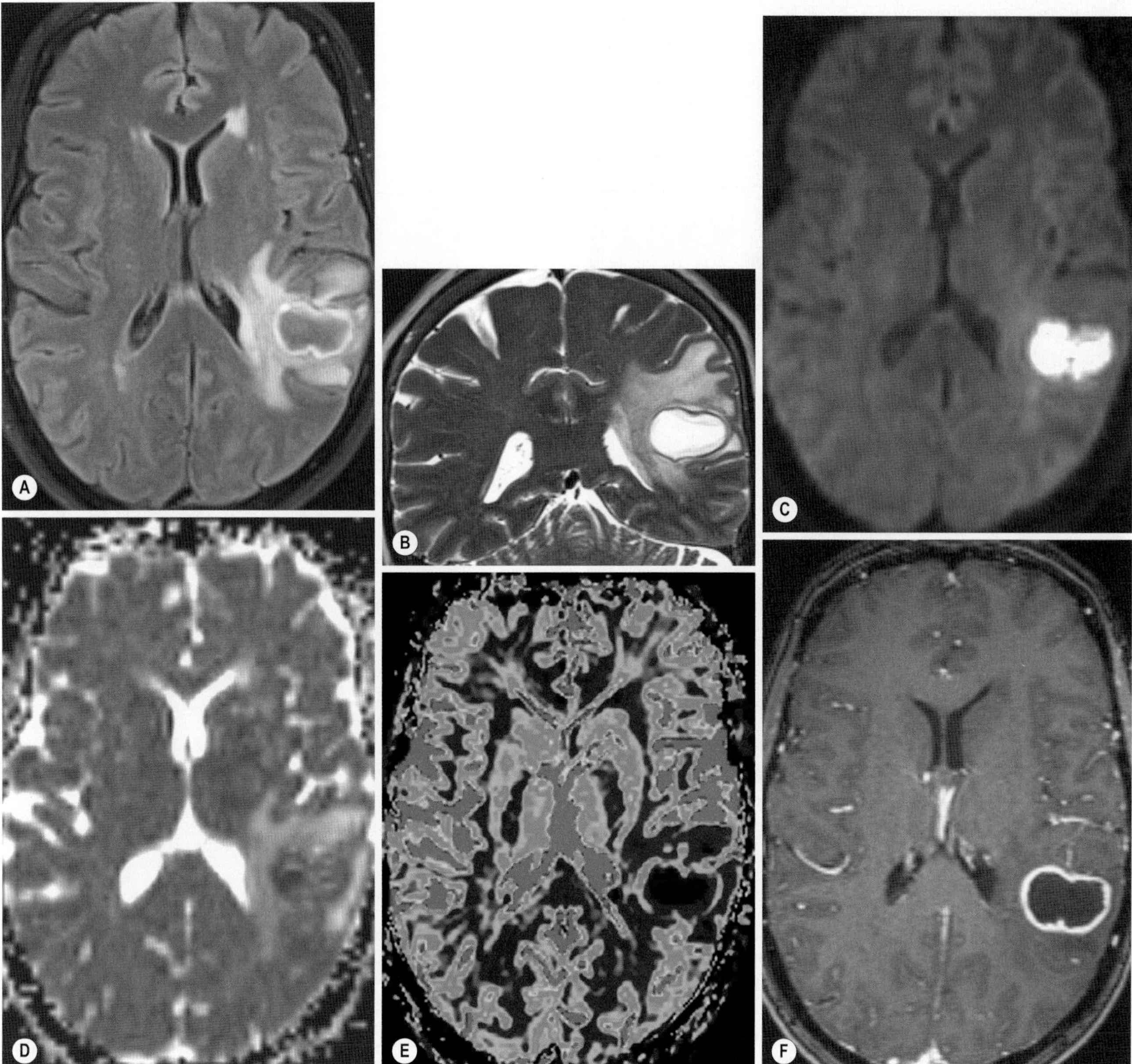

FIGURE 63-2 ■ Pyogenic brain abscess in a 40-year-old female patient. (A) Axial FLAIR image shows a ring-like low-signal-intensity lesion with marked perifocal oedema in the left hemisphere. (B) Coronal T2 image shows the lesion has a high-signal-intensity centre with a low-signal-intensity capsule. (C, D) On trace DWI (C), high signal was detected in the abscess cavity, with relatively low ADC values (D). (E) On the perfusion MRI, low relative cerebral blood volume (rCBV) was seen in the cavity, with a thin rim of increased perfusion in the capsule. (F) On post-contrast T1, a peripheral ring-like enhancement was observed.

sinusitis they can cross the midline, in contrast to subdural empyemas which do not cross the midline. The fluid within the epidural abscess is of slightly higher attenuation than CSF on CT and is hyperintense on T2 and FLAIR images and is slightly hyperintense compared to CSF on T1.[17] The dura at the deep margin of an epidural abscess typically shows thick and slightly irregular contrast enhancement (Fig. 63-3). Similar to cerebral abscesses, the pus within an epidural abscess can show restricted diffusion, appearing hyperintense on DWI and hypointense on ADC maps.[18] In patients with fever after a neurosurgical operation, normal and expected sterile fluid collections in the epidural space can be hard to distinguish from an epidural abscess, but a serial increase in the attenuation of the fluid suggests infection. DWI has been found to be less sensitive and specific in the postoperative setting.[19]

A subdural empyema is a collection of pus in the potential space between the inner layer of the dura mater and the arachnoid mater. Empyemas occur more commonly than epidural abscesses. As with epidural abscesses, the most frequent predisposing causes are sinusitis and otogenic infection; head trauma, surgery and haematogenous spread are less common. Headache, fever, focal neurological deficit and meningism are the most frequent clinical features at presentation. The CT and MRI

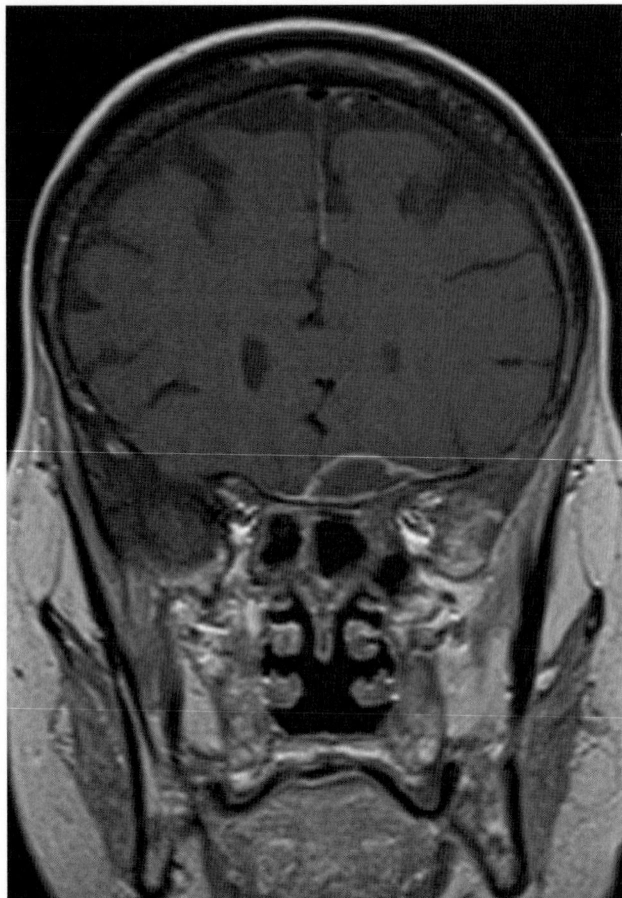

FIGURE 63-3 ■ **Epidural abscess.** Coronal T1 spin-echo image shows a left subfrontal epidural fluid collection surrounded by an enhancing rim of dura.

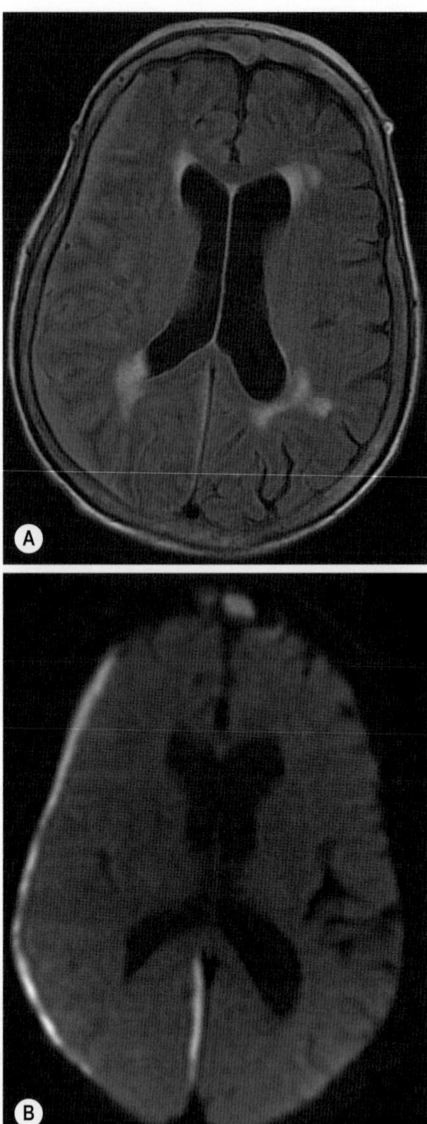

FIGURE 63-4 ■ **Subdural empyema.** (A) Axial FLAIR image shows a right cerebral convexity and posterior parafalcine fluid collection of higher signal intensity than ventricular CSF. (B) DWI shows restricted diffusion within the subdural collection.

appearances of subdural empyema are of a crescentic fluid collection overlying the cerebral convexity or in the interhemispheric fissure alongside the falx cerebri. The margins of the collection may be irregular and scalloped, as a result of loculation. Although contrast enhancement at the deep margin of a subdural empyema is a characteristic finding, it can be subtle or absent in the early stages of infection. The adjacent brain may show oedema or cortical contrast enhancement. The CT attenuation and MRI signal characteristics of a subdural empyema are the same as for an epidural abscess (Fig. 63-4).

Ventriculitis

Ventriculitis is uncommon. Causes include trauma, intraventricular rupture of an abscess, shunt infection and haematogenous spread of infection to the ependyma or choroid plexus. The most frequent imaging finding is intraventricular debris, which is slightly hyperattenuating compared to CSF on CT and is of increased signal on FLAIR and DWI sequences with low signal intensity on ADC maps (Fig. 63-5). Periventricular and subependymal high signal and enhancement of the ventricular margins are less common although are still present in most cases.[20,21] The affected ventricles are usually dilated.

Tuberculosis

Involvement of the central nervous system (CNS) occurs in 5% of cases of tuberculosis; most patients are younger than 20 years. Of patients with CNS tuberculosis, the chest radiograph is abnormal in 45–60%.[7] Tuberculous meningitis is the most frequent manifestation of tuberculous CNS infection. In the early stages of the disease a diffuse pattern of leptomeningeal enhancement is common, with a later predilection for the basal leptomeninges, most frequently in the interpeduncular cistern of the midbrain.[22] CT shows obliteration of the basal cisterns by isoattenuating or slightly hyperattenuating exudate, which enhances diffusely after IV contrast medium. The most sensitive and specific CT criteria for tuberculous meningitis are linear enhancement of the middle cerebral artery cisterns, obliteration by contrast of the CSF spaces around normal vascular enhancement,

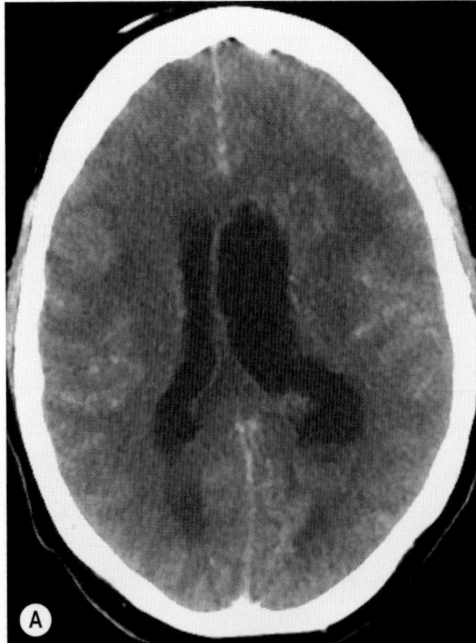

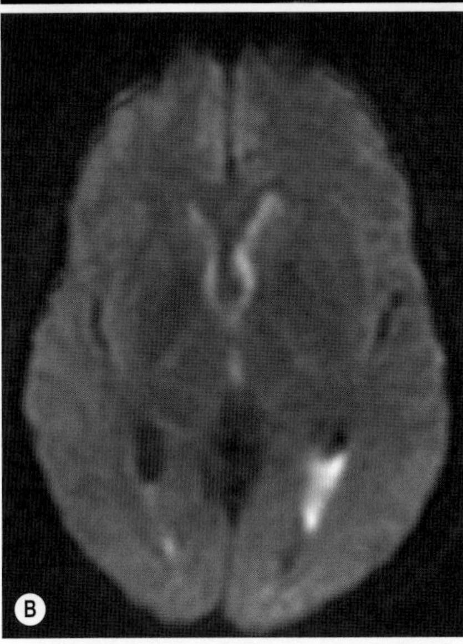

FIGURE 63-5 ■ Pyogenic ventriculitis. (A) Axial CT shows dilated lateral ventricles that contain intermediate attenuation debris. There is a rim of low-attenuation interstitial oedema surrounding the ventricles. (B) DWI at a more caudal level shows restricted diffusion in the debris.

Y-shaped enhancement at the junction of the suprasellar and middle cerebral artery cisterns and asymmetry of enhancement.[23] The meningeal exudate obstructs the resorption of CSF and so causes communicating hydrocephalus, resulting in dilatation of the lateral, third and fourth ventricles. This is seen in 50% of adults and 85% of children.[7] Less often, non-communicating hydrocephalus can occur because of obstruction of the outlet foramina of the fourth ventricle. Arteritis of the penetrating arteries within the subarachnoid space affected by areas of tuberculous meningitis can result in infarctions of the basal ganglia, internal capsules and brainstem. With healing, calcification of the affected meninges may be seen rarely.

MRI depicts the basal meningeal enhancement, hydrocephalus and perforator territory infarcts with greater sensitivity than CT (Fig. 63-6). The differential diagnosis for tuberculous meningitis includes fungal meningitis, neurosarcoid and carcinomatous meningitis.

Tuberculomas (parenchymal granulomas) occur most often at the junction of white and grey matter (Fig. 63-7). On CT they appear as small rounded lesions isoattenuating or hypoattenuating to normal brain, with variable amounts of surrounding vasogenic oedema. Contrast enhancement is homogeneous when lesions are solid and shows rim enhancement when central caseation or liquefaction occurs. The 'target sign' of central high attenuation with rim enhancement is not pathognomonic for tuberculoma. On MRI small, non-caseated, tuberculomas show low signal intensity on T1 sequences and high signal on T2 sequences. Caseation of tuberculomas results in low signal intensity on T2 (Fig. 63-7). On DWI tuberculomas may show elevated or restricted diffusion. Tuberculomas may calcify when healed, but, as with meningeal disease, this is uncommon.[24]

Tuberculous abscesses are uncommon; they may resemble tuberculomas but are usually larger and have a thinner enhancing rim. The enhancing rim of a tuberculous abscess is more often lobulated than smooth, whereas, similar to pyogenic abscesses, the non-enhancing core of a tuberculous abscess typically shows restricted diffusion.[13]

Neurosyphilis

CNS involvement can occur at any stage of syphilis; in human immunodeficiency virus (HIV) infection its course may be more aggressive. Meningovascular syphilis causes a small-vessel endarteritis that appears as arterial segmental 'beading' on angiography, with associated infarcts in the basal ganglia. Cerebral gummas are rare, typically arise from the meninges and appear as mass lesions with variable MR signal characteristics and enhancement.[25]

FUNGAL INFECTIONS

Fungal infections of the CNS are uncommon in immunocompetent patients, occurring most frequently in patients with acquired immunodeficiency syndrome (AIDS) or in transplant recipients. As with bacterial infections, fungi can cause meningitis (Fig. 63-8), epidural abscess or subdural empyema, cerebritis (Fig. 63-8), brain abscesses (Fig. 63-9) and granulomas. The imaging appearances of these manifestations are for the most part non-specific and do not suggest fungal infection as the cause. Fungal abscesses are a possible exception; one study found fungal abscesses to show intracavitary projections from their walls which were not present in bacterial or tuberculous abscesses. Unlike the bacterial and tuberculous abscesses, none of the fungal abscesses showed restricted diffusion in their non-ehancing core.[13] The type of CNS involvement has been reported to vary with the fungal species; meningitis is more common with small unicellular organisms such as *Candida* and *Cryptococcus* (Fig. 63-8), whereas cerebritis, granulomas and abscesses are more frequently caused by hyphal organisms such as *Aspergillus*.[26]

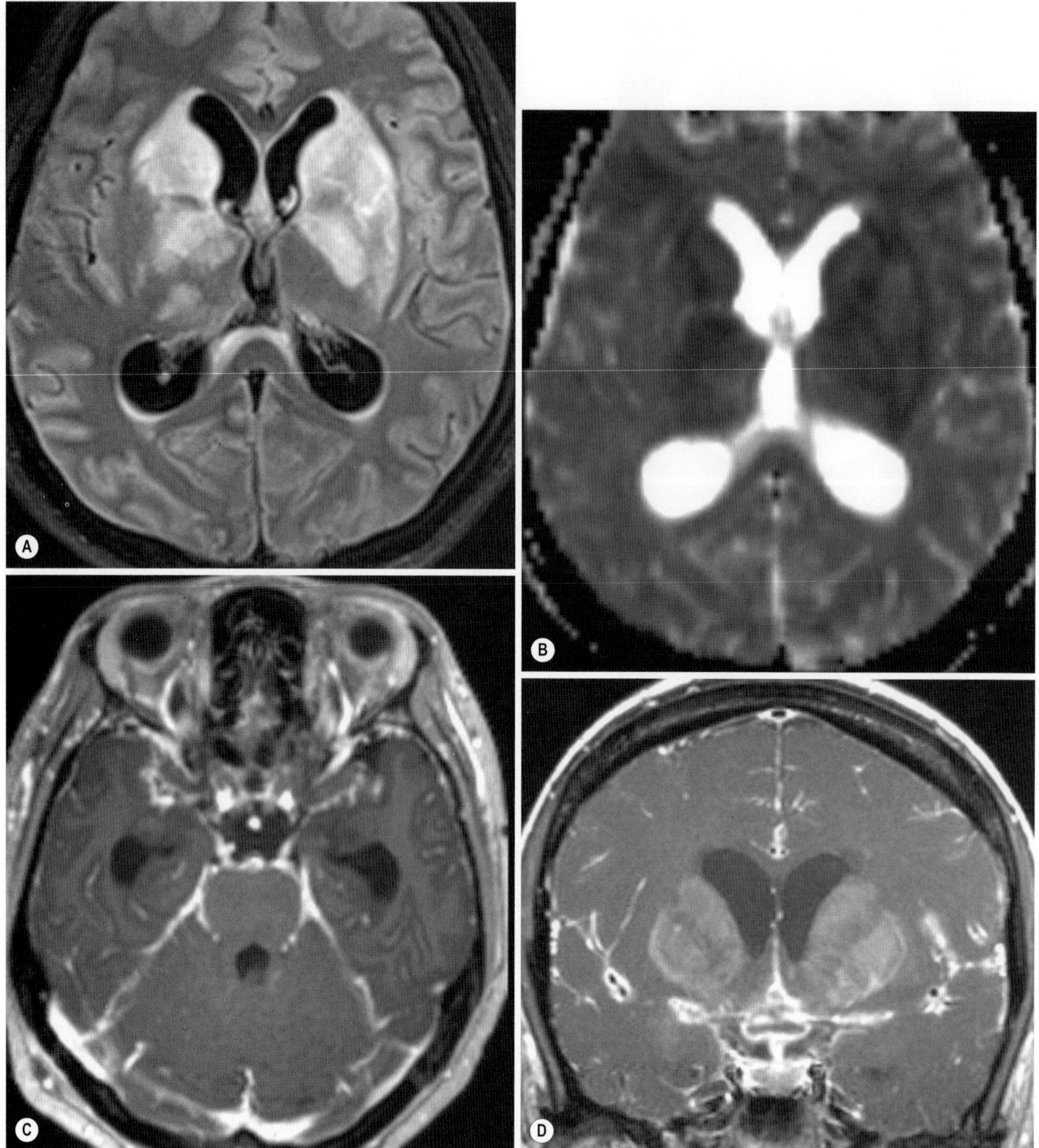

FIGURE 63-6 ■ Cerebral tuberculosis in a 27-year-old female patient. (A) Axial FLAIR image shows bilateral high-signal-intensity abnormalities in the basal ganglia regions. The ventricular system is mildly enlarged. (B) On the ADC map, low ADC values were measured, indicating restricted diffusion in the subacute infarctions. (C, D) On axial (C) and coronal (D) post-contrast T1 images, marked meningeal enhancement was detected, consistent with tuberculous meningitis.

VIRAL INFECTIONS

Herpes Simplex Encephalitis

Herpes simplex type 1 is the most frequent cause of viral encephalitis in adults and is often fatal without treatment. It results from reactivation of latent infection in the trigeminal ganglion or from reinfection by the olfactory route. Although early reports observed that CT appears normal in the first 3 to 5 days after onset, a more recent study with modern CT equipment showed that abnormalities were visible in the majority of patients within 3 days.[27] CT shows low attenuation and swelling in the anteromedial temporal lobe and inferior frontal lobe, with less frequent involvement of the insula and cingulate gyrus. The abnormalities are initially unilateral but often progress to become bilateral. Haemorrhage is seen as a late feature and not usually a prominent finding. Contrast

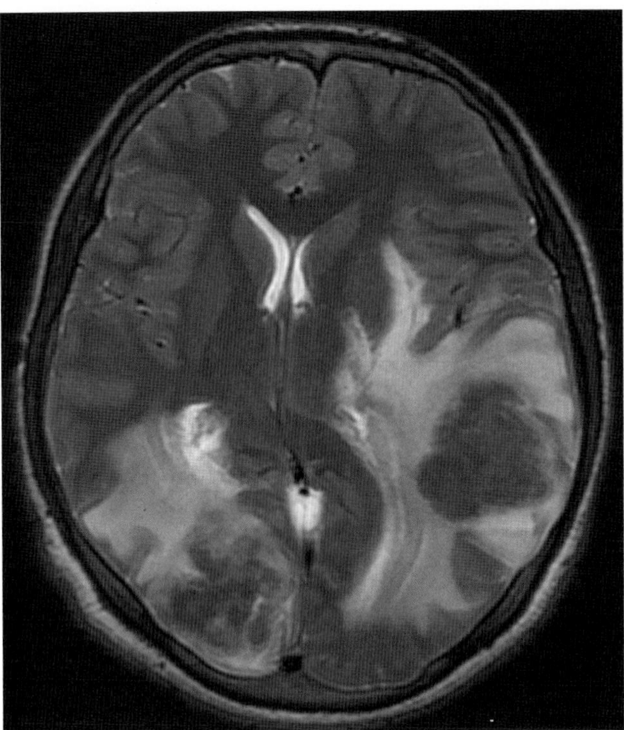

FIGURE 63-7 ■ **Tuberculomas.** Axial T2 fast spin-echo image shows large, hypointense, bilateral caseating granulomas. The extensive surrounding high signal in the cerebral white matter is caused by vasogenic oedema.

enhancement within the affected areas may be patchy or gyriform. MRI is more sensitive; T2 and FLAIR sequences show high signal and swelling within 2 days of onset (Fig. 63-10). The abnormal signal is mainly cortical, with secondary involvement of the subjacent white matter. MRI is also more sensitive than CT to foci of haemorrhage, particularly with the use of T2* gradient echo or SWI. Diffusion-weighted imaging shows cortical hyperintensity with greater sensitivity than conventional MRI.

Other Viral Encephalitides

Imaging appearances in most other viral encephalitides are less characteristic than in the case of herpes simplex encephalitis. Japanese encephalitis, caused by a flavivirus, is an exception and most often manifests as areas of hyperintensity on T2 and FLAIR sequences in the thalami, basal ganglia and brainstem—particularly in the substantia nigra. Other viral infections of the CNS, such as West Nile virus and tick-borne encephalitis, have a predilection for the basal ganglia, thalami and brainstem but, like the clinical presentation, the imaging is often non-specific and does not suggest a particular virus.[28]

Human Immunodeficiency Virus (HIV) and Acquired Immunodeficiency Syndrome (AIDS)

Infection by HIV merits a more detailed coverage in view of its high prevalence and global importance. Here we discuss the direct impact of the HIV on the brain and the associated complications of progressive multifocal leukoencephalopathy (PML) and immune reconstitution inflammatory syndrome (IRIS). Opportunistic infections, which can occur in AIDS, such as cryptococcal infection and toxoplasmosis, are discussed under the headings of 'Fungal Infections' and 'Parasitic Infections', respectively.

The HIV/AIDS pandemic is now in its fourth decade and UNAIDS estimates that, in 2011, a total of 34.2 million people were living with HIV infection. Prognosis has dramatically improved since the introduction of combination antiretroviral therapy (cART) and HIV/AIDS has been transformed from a death sentence into a manageable illness. However, in 2011, still less than 25% of all HIV-infected people had access to antiretroviral therapy or had virologic suppression from receipt of such therapy.[29]

Opportunistic infections (OIs) are still of concern in undiagnosed and untreated patients with HIV/AIDS. For those with access to cART, there has been a dramatic decline in the incidence of OIs and neurocognitive and vascular CNS complications of HIV have become the major causes of morbidity.

HIV Encephalopathy

The HIV virus invades peripheral macrophages, endogenous microglial cells and astrocytes. Direct neuronal invasion is very rare and neuronal injury, which may be partially reversible, occurs as a consequence of the release of toxic viral gene products as well as pro-inflammatory cytokines, including tumour necrosis factor, quinolinic acid and platelet activating factor.[30]

The neuroradiological correlates of HIV encephalopathy (HIVE) are areas of hyperintense signal on T2 and FLAIR images which can be either ill-defined, diffuse and symmetrical (Fig. 63-11), or patchy and scattered; involvement of the deep grey matter is also seen (Fig. 63-11).[30] The MRI appearances are thought to reflect an increase of water content and serum proteins in the brain parenchyma as a result of increased vascular permeability in the presence of circulating cytokines and/or a loss of myelin.

Advanced MRI techniques such as diffusion tensor imaging, MR perfusion imaging and MR spectroscopy can be used to investigate more subtle effects of HIV on the brain parenchyma and provide quantitative measures.[31]

Brain volume loss is a feature of more advanced HIVE and was one of the most prominent imaging features in the pre-cART era. Cerebral atrophy caused by HIV is not diffuse but has a predilection for specific regions such as the basal ganglia, thalamus, corpus callosum and frontal lobes.[32]

HIVE is typically associated with various degrees of cognitive impairment and a new classification of HIV-associated neurocognitive disorders (HAND) was proposed in 2007,[33] distinguishing the following:

1. Asymptomatic neurocognitive impairment (ANI) where patients have abnormal neuropsychological tests but are not impaired in their everyday life.
2. Mild cognitive impairment (MND) with mildly impaired functioning.

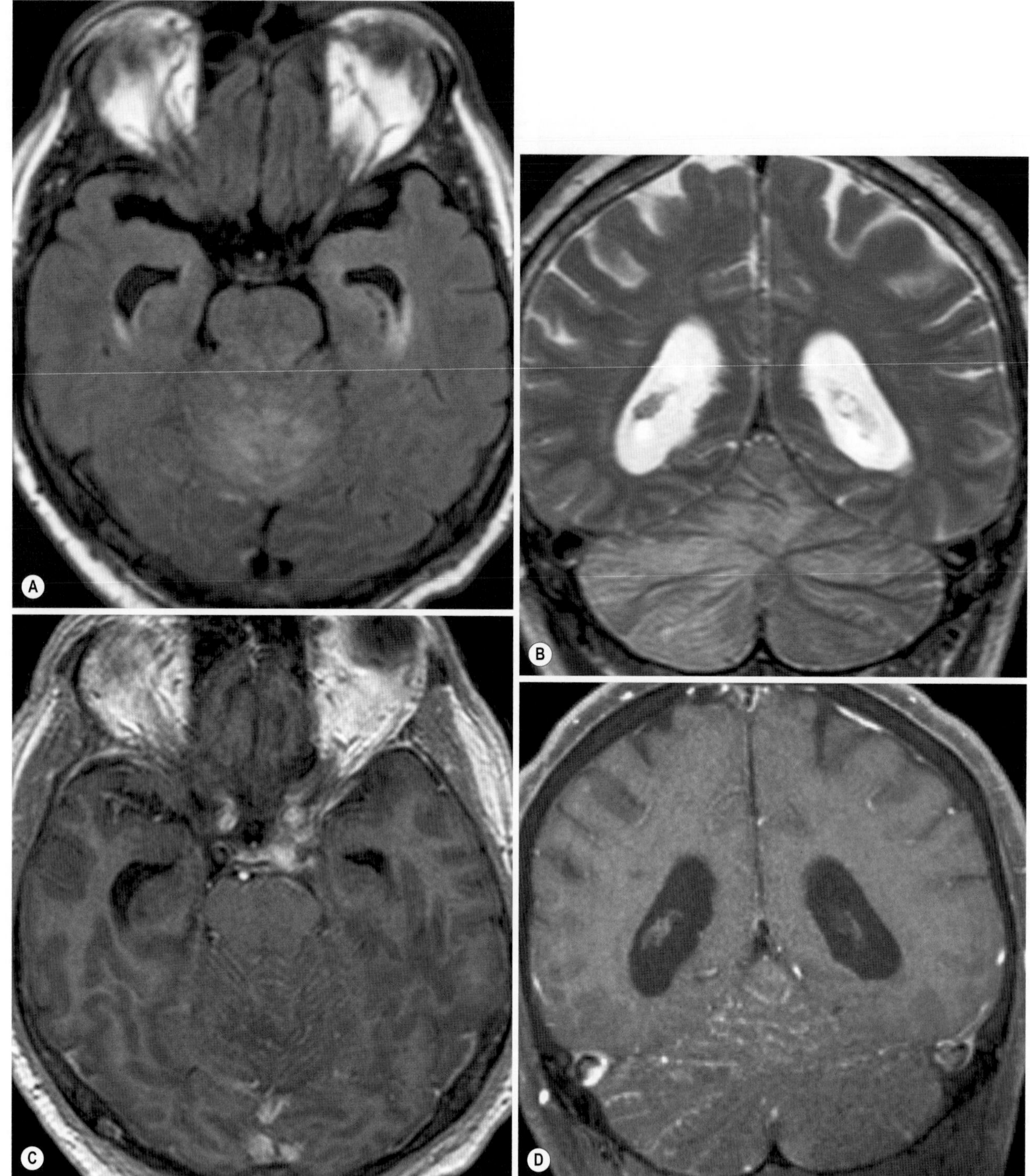

FIGURE 63-8 ■ ***Crypotcoccus neoformans* meningitis and cerebellitis in a renal transplant recipient.** (A) Axial FLAIR images show high signal intensity of the subarachnoid spaces in the region of the cerebellar vermis. (B) High signal in the cerebellum on both sides was demonstrated on the coronal T2 MR image. (C, D) Strong leptomeningeal enhancement is nicely shown on axial and coronal post-contrast T1 images.

3. HIV-associated dementia (HAD), which corresponds to the former AIDS dementia complex.

Before the introduction of cART, the prevalence of HAD was around 16%, with an annual incidence of 7% among patients with advanced HIV infection. In the era of cART, this is now rare but milder forms of cognitive impairment present a major cause of morbidity.

HIV and Vascular Disease

HIV patients have an increased risk of stroke and ischaemic stroke is far more frequent than haemorrhagic stroke.[34] There is a cumulative increase in risk according to the duration of cART.[35] Several mechanisms contribute to the increase of non-haemorrhagic stroke in HIV

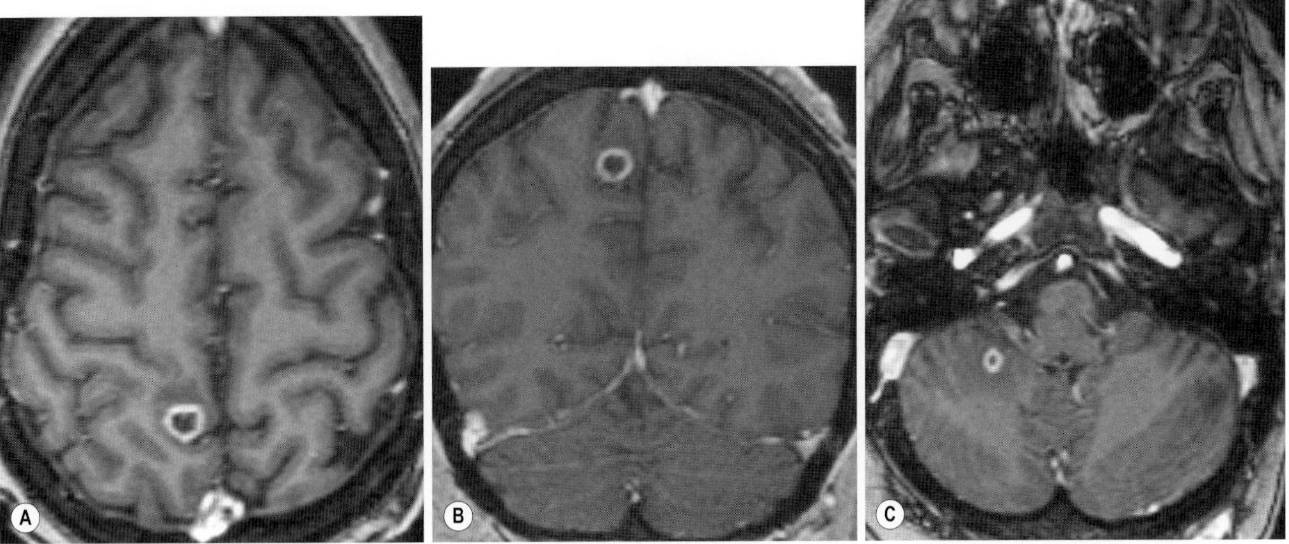

FIGURE 63-9 ■ Multiple fungal abscesses in an 8-year-old bone marrow transplant recipient. On axial (A, C) and coronal (B) post-contrast T1 MR images, FLAIR ring-like enhancing focal lesions were detected in the right cerebellum and right parietal region.

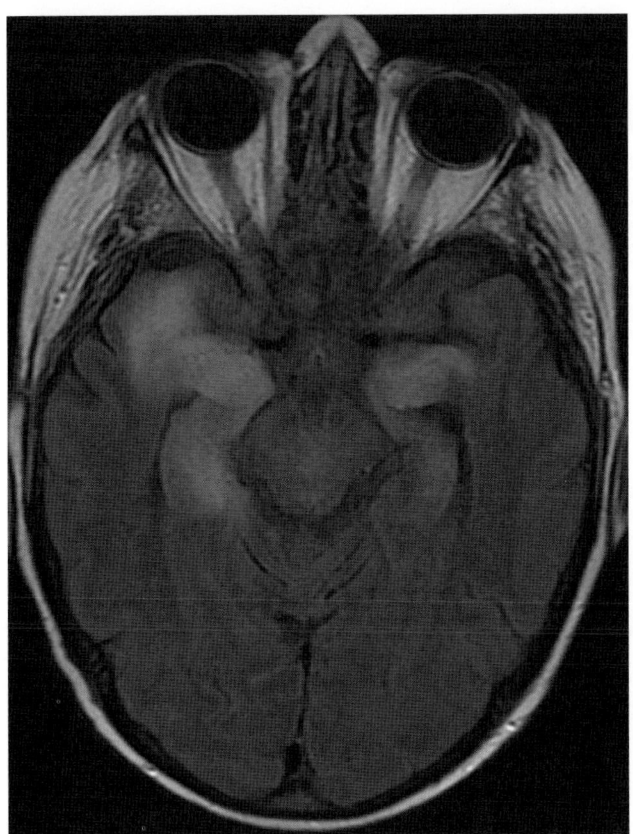

FIGURE 63-10 ■ Herpes simplex encephalitis. Axial FLAIR image shows asymmetrical swelling and increased signal intensity in the anteromedial temporal lobes, more severe on the right.

including endothelial dysfunction in the presence of chronic inflammation, coagulopathies, such as HIV-associated thrombocytopaenia and the atherogenic effect of certain antiretroviral drugs. HIV infection can cause accelerated atherosclerosis and/or vasculitis of the extracranial and intracranial vessels. Immune-mediated vascular damage can also lead to the formation of aneurysms, which are more common in young male patients (Fig. 63-12).

Progressive Multifocal Leukoencephalopathy

PML is a form of progressive demyelination caused by reactivation of a latent *John Cunningham virus* (*JC papovavirus*) infection in immunocompromised patients, typically seen in HIV patients with a CD4 count less than 100/mm^3. PML can also occur in other forms of immunocompromise and in patients receiving immunosuppressive drugs.[36] Clinical presentation can be with gradual cognitive impairment and personality disturbances, or acutely with focal neuropathy and seizures.

The lesions are typically hyperintense on T2 and FLAIR images and hypointense on T1-weighted images, have ill-defined borders and involve predominantly the subcortical or cerebellar white matter. DWI shows a characteristic peripheral hyperintense rim corresponding to the front line of active demyelination around a central area of necrosis (Fig. 63-13). Grey matter involvement and lesion enhancement have been demonstrated, particularly in patients in immune recovery.

Immune Reconstitution Inflammatory Syndrome (IRIS)

Immune reconstitution inflammatory syndrome (IRIS) is defined as a paradoxical deterioration in clinical status attributable to the recovery of the immune system during cART.[37] HIV/AIDS treatment with cART leads to an increase in CD4 cell count/function, and a recovery of the immune system, which can instigate an intense inflammatory response to dead or latent organisms, days to months after commencement of treatment. CD8 cell infiltration in the leptomeninges, perivascular spaces,

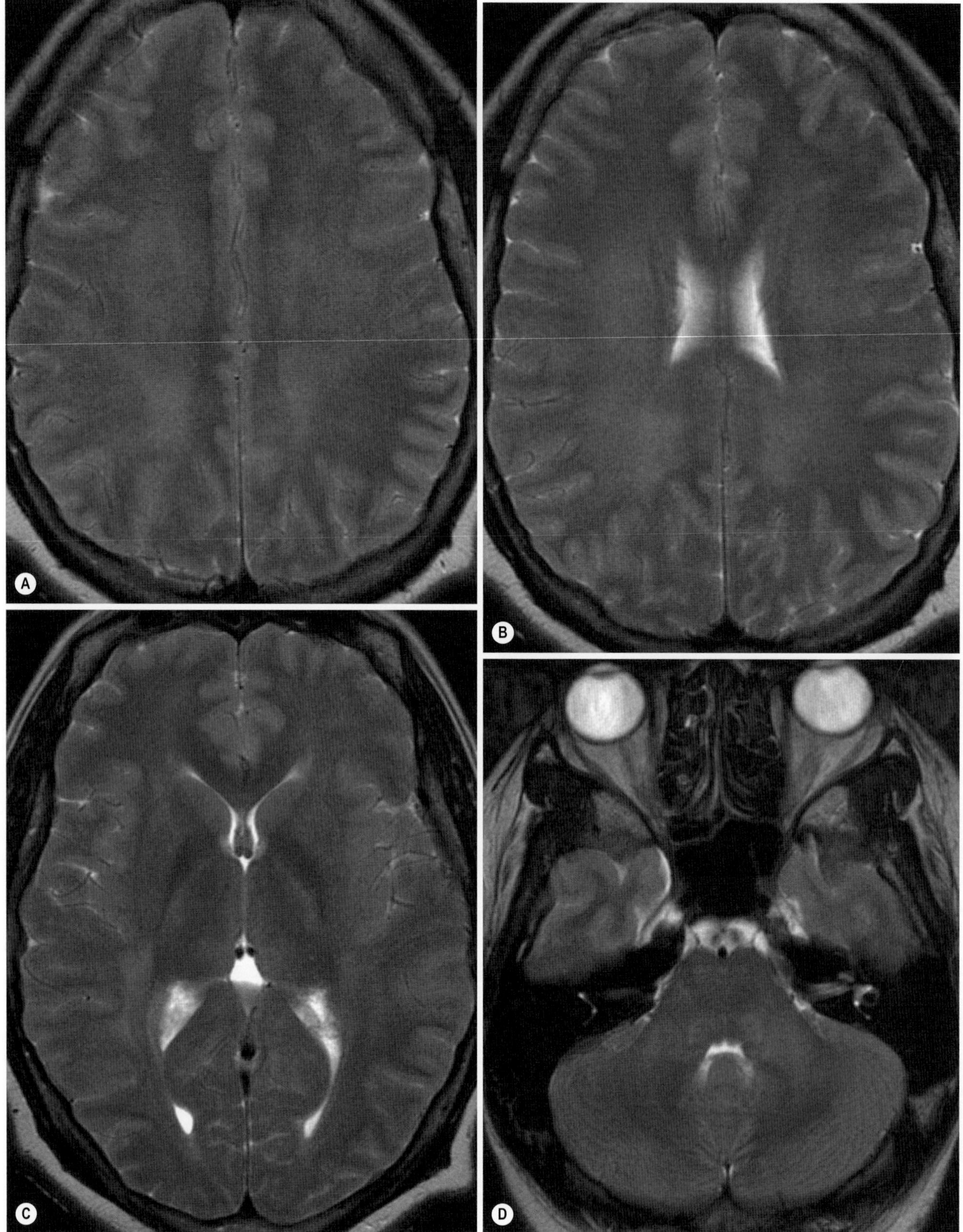

FIGURE 63-11 ■ HIV encephalopathy. T2 images showing a diffuse, ill-defined, symmetrical signal intensity increase of the white matter in the centrum semiovale (A), in periventricular white matter (B), in the thalami, caudate nuclei, right optic radiation and internal capsules (C) and in the middle cerebellar peduncles (D). These appearances are typical for HIVE and are potentially reversible with cART.

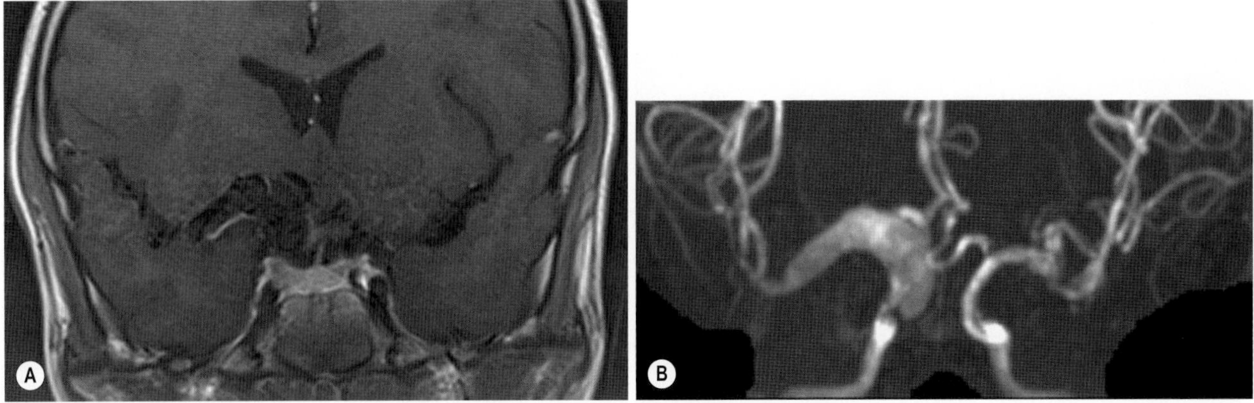

FIGURE 63-12 ■ **HIV vasculitis in a 15-year-old man with vertically transmitted HIV infection.** The coronal contrast-enhanced T1 (A) shows fusiform dilatation of the right distal internal carotid artery and of both middle cerebral arteries with some enhancement of the wall of the right middle cerebral artery. The extent of fusiform aneurysmal dilatation of the intracranial vessels is well demonstrated on the time-of-flight MRA (B).

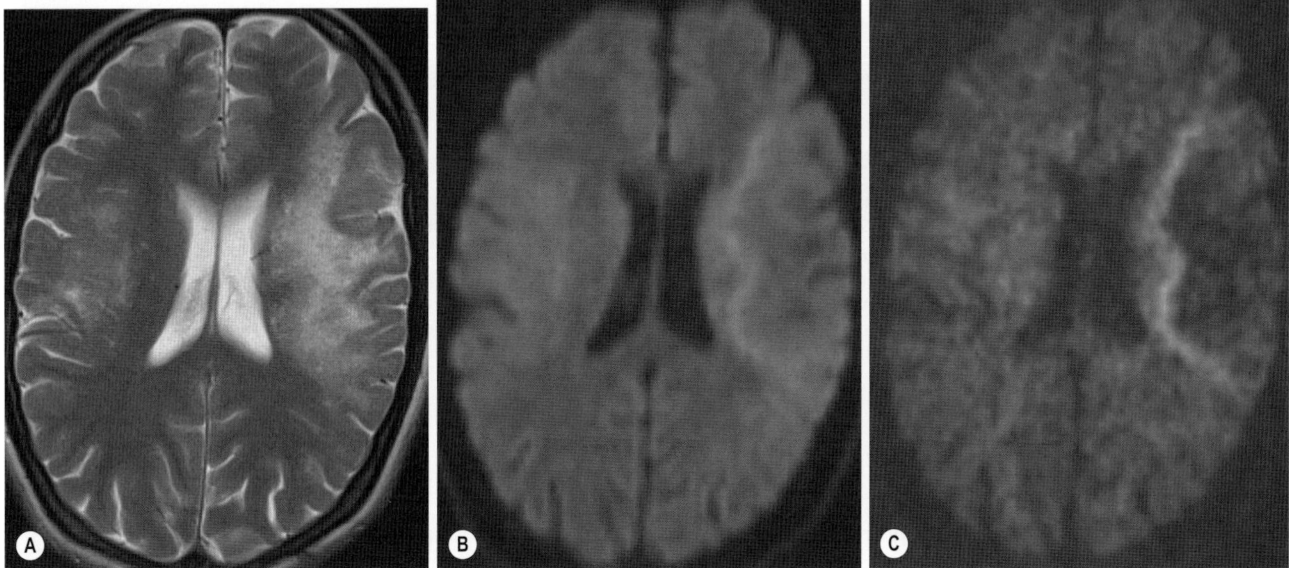

FIGURE 63-13 ■ **Progressive multifocal leukoencephalopathy (PML).** The T2 image (A) demonstrates widespread hyperintense signal change in the left, and to a lesser extent, right corona radiata. The involvement of the subcortical U fibres is typical for PML. DWI with $b = 1000$ (B) demonstrates a hyperintense edge of the lesion medially, particularly on the left, which is more clearly seen on the DWI with $b = 3000$ (C) and corresponds to the zones of active demyelination.

blood vessels and parenchyma is the pathological hallmark of CNS-IRIS. Risk factors include a rapid drop in viral load or increase in CD4 count and young age. The most commonly associated organisms are the JC virus (PML-IRIS) and *Cryptococcus* but an inflammatory response to other viruses (varicella-zoster virus, cytomegalovirus, HIV), *Candida*, *Mycobacterium tuberculosis* or *Toxoplasma gondii* can also occur.

Clinical presentation is diverse and depends upon the associated OI and extent of disease. Any patient who has commenced cART within the preceding 8 weeks presenting with new CNS symptoms or progressive cognitive dysfunction despite good viral control should be investigated for HIV-related IRIS. Recognition of IRIS in cART-treated patients allows adaptation of medical management, which can improve outcome and prevent death from IRIS-related illness, overall improving prognosis.[37]

Imaging features of CNS-IRIS are a transient increase in parenchymal high signal on FLAIR and T2 sequences, or hypoattenuation on CT, and contrast enhancement (Fig. 63-14). Mass effect and restricted diffusion can also occur. CNS-IRIS is associated with an improved long-term outcome if the acute inflammatory response can be contained.

PARASITIC INFECTIONS

There are many parasitic infections which can involve the brain. Some of these are very rare and only the most important parasitic infections will be discussed here.

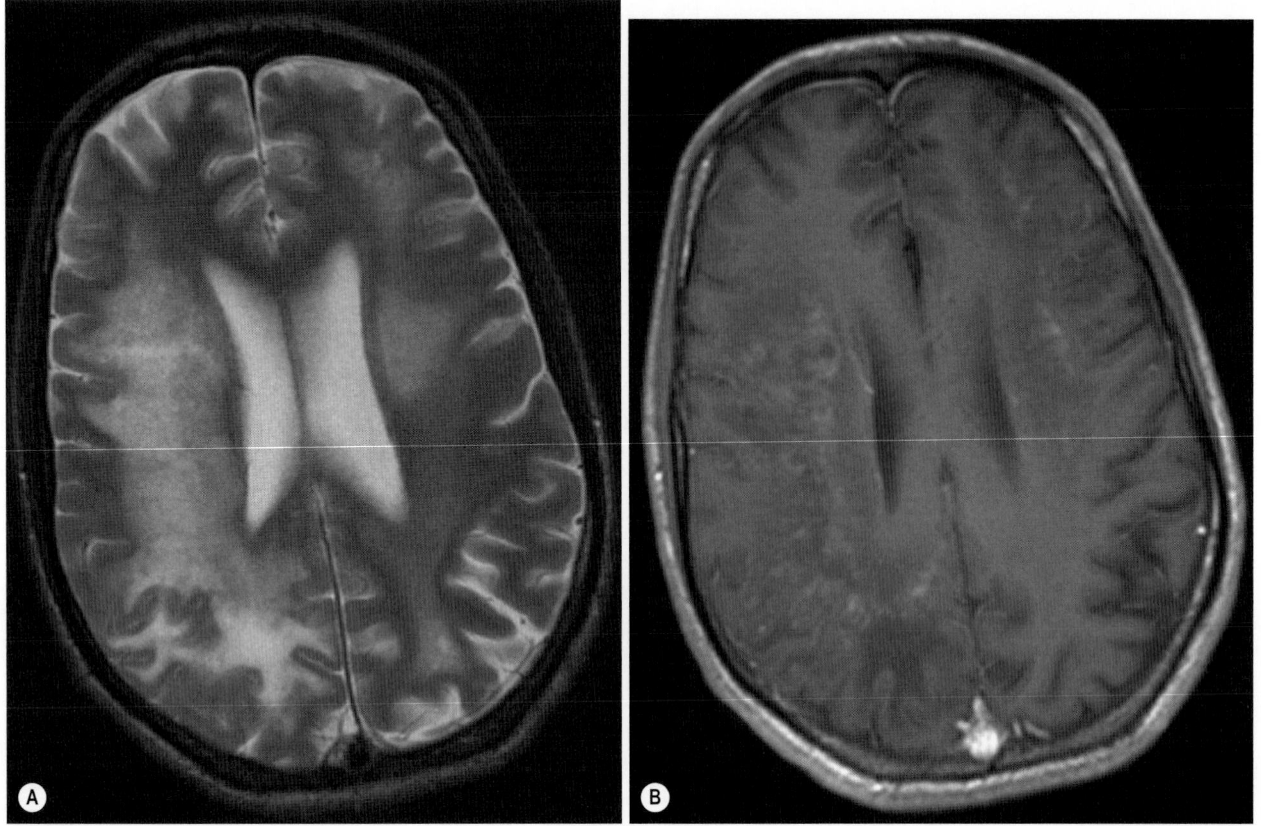

FIGURE 63-14 ■ Immune reconstitution inflammatory syndrome (PML-IRIS) in a 40-year-old HIV-infected patient with PML and low CD4 count at presentation. MRI was performed 8 weeks after treatment with cART. The T2 image (A) demonstrates widespread, confluent hyperintense signal change in the white matter of both cerebral hemispheres, extending into the subcortical U fibres, which is typical for PML. The contrast-enhanced T1 (B) demonstrates hypointense lesions with ill-defined enhancement that is more marked around the periphery and consistent with inflammatory response of a partially recovered immune system.

Toxoplasmosis

Toxoplasma gondii is an intracellular protozoan that infects humans via direct contact with feline excrement or ingestion of raw or undercooked vegetables, pork or lamb. In healthy patients, the acute infection is asymptomatic and becomes latent within the neuroparenchyma. The latent infection is reactivated in patients with a compromised immune system, most commonly in HIV patients with a low CD4 count (below 100 cells/mm^3).

Typical CT and MRI findings are ring-enhancing abscesses centred in the basal ganglia, thalamus and at the corticomedullary junction, with variable degrees of perilesional oedema and mass effect (Fig. 63-15). Enhancement can also be nodular or can be absent if the patient is severely immunocompromised. On non-enhanced MRI, the abscesses appear hyperintense on T2/FLAIR sequences and hypointense on T1 images, unless there has been haemorrhage which causes peripheral T1 shortening. The characteristic 'target sign' of toxoplasmosis on T2 images is caused by central hyperintensity (fluid), peripheral hypointensity (mural blood) and an outer ring of hyperintense perilesional oedema.

The main radiological differential diagnosis is primary CNS lymphoma of the immunocompromised. Lymphoma shows typically restricted diffusion on DWI, whereas toxoplasmosis has a wide range of diffusion characteristics, which can overlap with lymphoma. The latter shows also a much higher tracer uptake on thallium-201 SPECT and ^{18}F-FDG. In clinical practice, the diagnosis of toxoplasmosis is often made by the response to empirical treatment with pyrimethamine–sulfadiazine and folic acid, which should lead to a decrease of lesion size within 10 days.

Cysticercosis

Neurocysticercosis is the most important parasitic disease of the CNS worldwide and is common in Central and South America, India, Africa and Eastern Europe. It is caused by the encysted larvae of the tapeworm *Taenia solium*, which develop after ingestion of eggs in undercooked pork or faeco-oral transmission between humans. Larvae are disseminated by haematogenous spread to neural, muscular and ocular tissues. Symptoms occur approximately 5 years after initial infection and are non-specific, 50–70% presenting with epilepsy.

Neurocysticercosis larvae can spread to the brain parenchyma, subarachnoid space and ventricles. The parenchymal form is the most common, followed by the intraventricular form; mixed types can occur.[38]

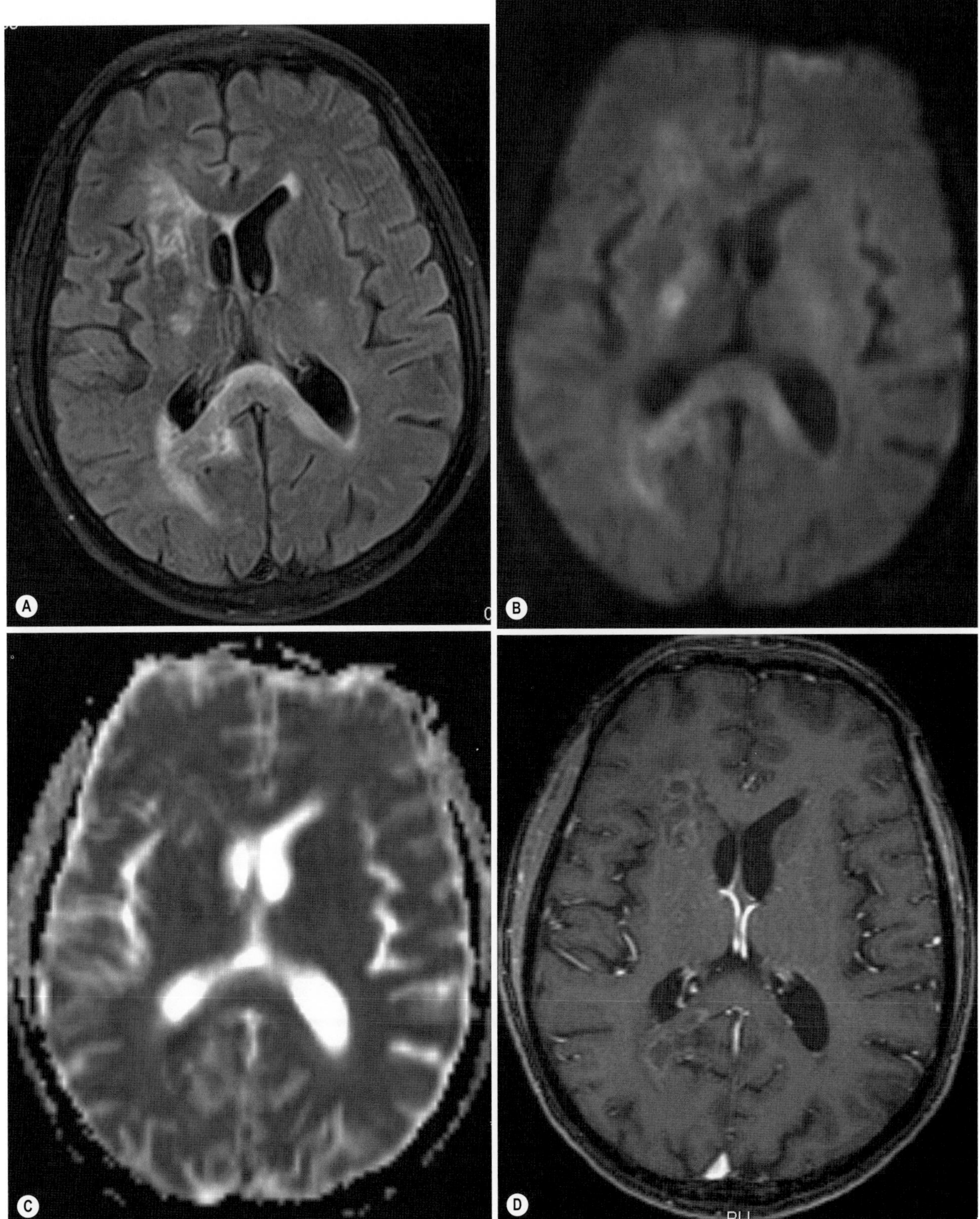

FIGURE 63-15 ■ Cerebral toxoplasmosis in a 50-year-old, HIV-infected male patient. (A) Axial FLAIR image shows signal intensity abnormalities in the right frontal periventricular region, as well as in the right part of the splenium of the corpus callosum. (B, C) High signal was noted on the trace DWI (B), with relatively low ADC values (C). (D, E) Peripheral, irregular enhancement of the lesions was demonstrated on axial (D) and coronal (E) post-contrast MR images.

Continued on following page

On imaging, one can distinguish four stages of *parenchymal neurocysticercosis*:[39]

1. *Vesicular stage*. This stage consists of a viable larva with a scolex (worm head). The cysts are thin-walled and show no or little enhancement and there is no perilesional oedema. The cyst fluid has similar signal characteristics to CSF and water diffusion is unrestricted. The scolex can appear hyperintense on T1, FLAIR and DWI images (Fig. 63-16).
2. *Colloidal vesicular stage*. This is the stage where larva breaks down and an immune response from the host is instigated. Ring-enhancing lesions with perilesional oedema and mass effect are typical imaging findings (Figs. 63-17A, B). Compared to the vesicular stage, the cyst content is more proteinaceous and appears consequently more hyperintense on T1 and FLAIR images.
3. *Granular nodular stage*. As the larva dies, the cyst collapses and the host response is marked with thick enhancing cyst walls and progression of surrounding oedema (Figs. 63-17C, D).
4. *Calcified nodular stage*. This is the non-active form of neurocysticercosis. The oedema resolves and small calcified lesions of 2–10 mm diameter are seen. Contrast enhancement and oedema are unusual for this stage but may occur in the context of seizure activity.

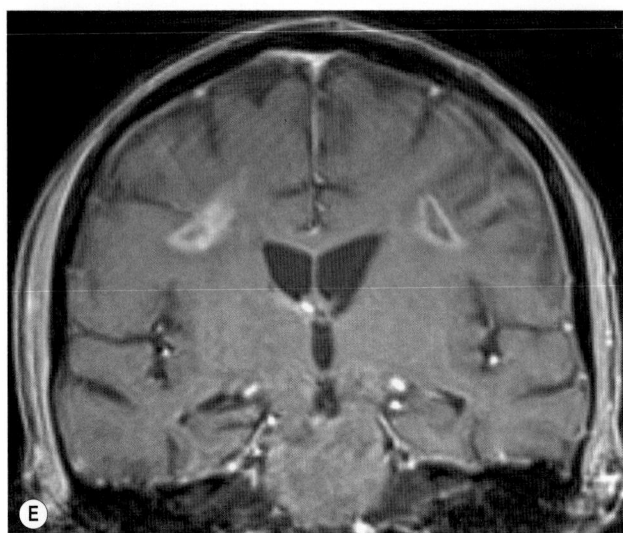

FIGURE 63-15, Continued

Intraventricular cysticercosis is the second most common form of neurocysticercosis and larvae are more frequently found in the fourth and third ventricles than in the lateral ventricles. Intraventricular cysts can cause obstruction to the CSF flow and hydrocephalus, which may present acutely. *Subarachnoid cysticercosis* can involve the basal cisterns, sylvian fissures and cerebellopontine angle regions. *Racemose cysticercosis* is a rare form of subarachnoid cysticercosis where multiple clustered cysts are separated by septae, causing a 'bunch of grapes' appearance. The racemose form can lead to large cystic lesions, which may be associated with local meningeal nodular enhancement.[39]

Echinococcus (Hydatid Disease)

There are two main types of hydatid disease: cystic echinococcosis and aveolar echinococcosis, the latter being much less common. Carnivores such as dogs are

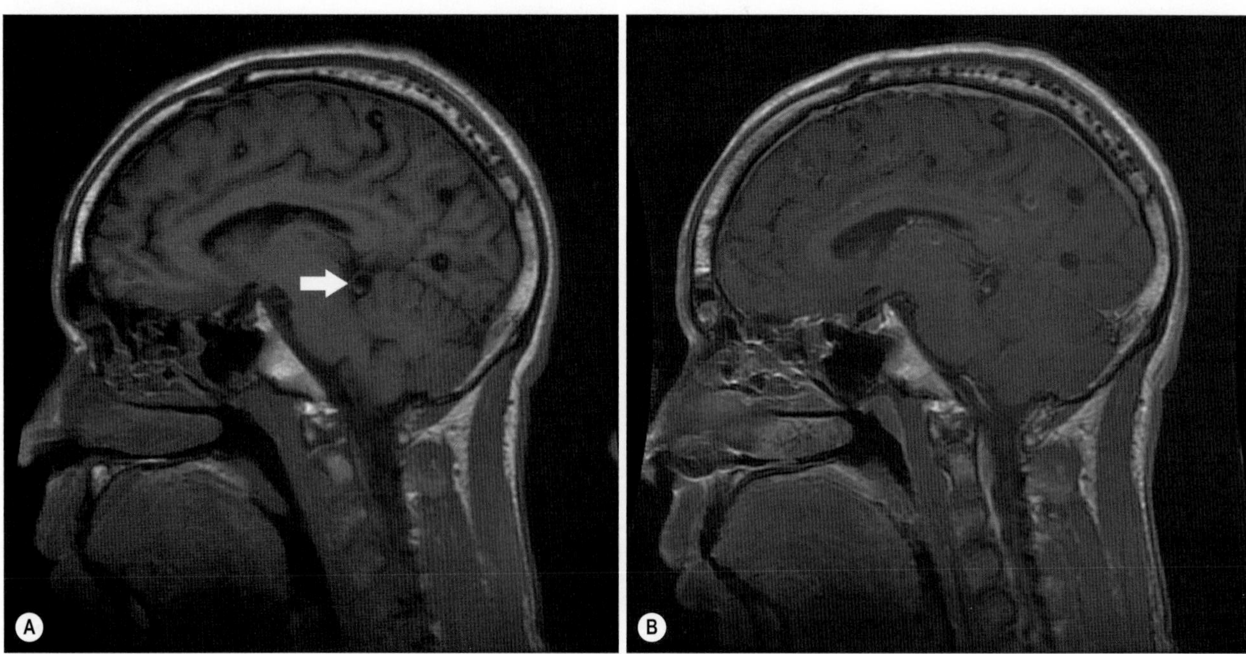

FIGURE 63-16 ■ **Neurocysticercosis.** Sagittal T1 (A), contrast-enhanced T1 (B), axial T2 (C) and coronal FLAIR image (D) in a patient with extensive parenchymal and subarachnoid (arrows) cysticercosis. Most of the lesions are in the vesicular stage showing thin-walled cysts with little or no enhancement and a scolex (worm head) in the centre of the cyst. There is no oedema.

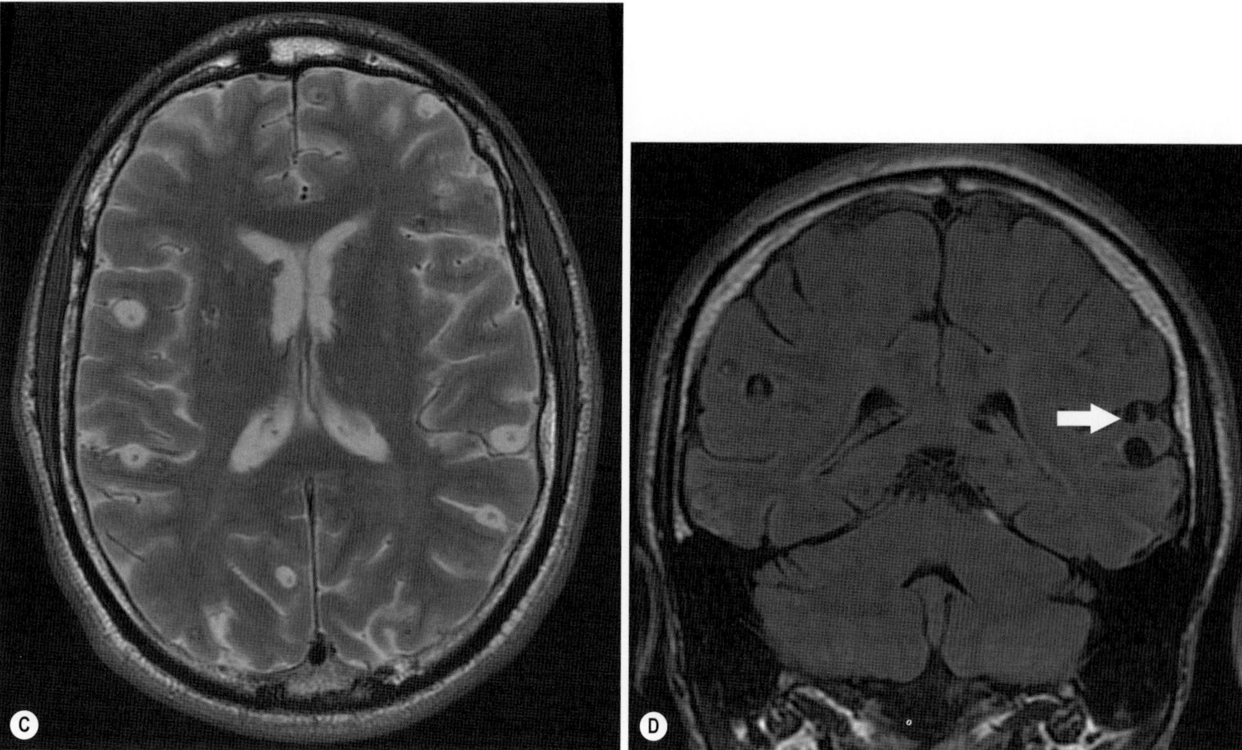

FIGURE 63-16, Continued

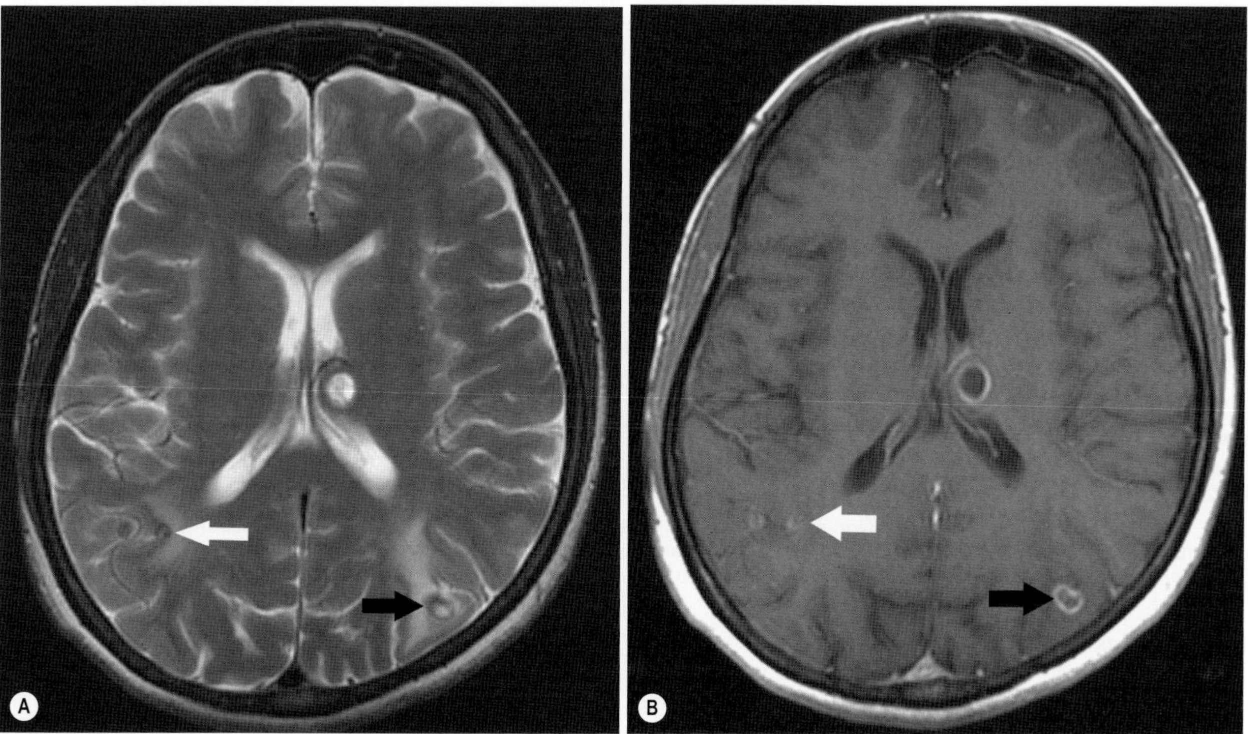

FIGURE 63-17 ■ **Neurocysticercosis.** T2 image (A) and contrast-enhanced T1 image (B) showing the vesicular stage (lesion in the left lateral ventricle), colloidal vesicular stage (black arrows) and calcified nodular stage (white arrows) of cysticercosis.

Continued on following page

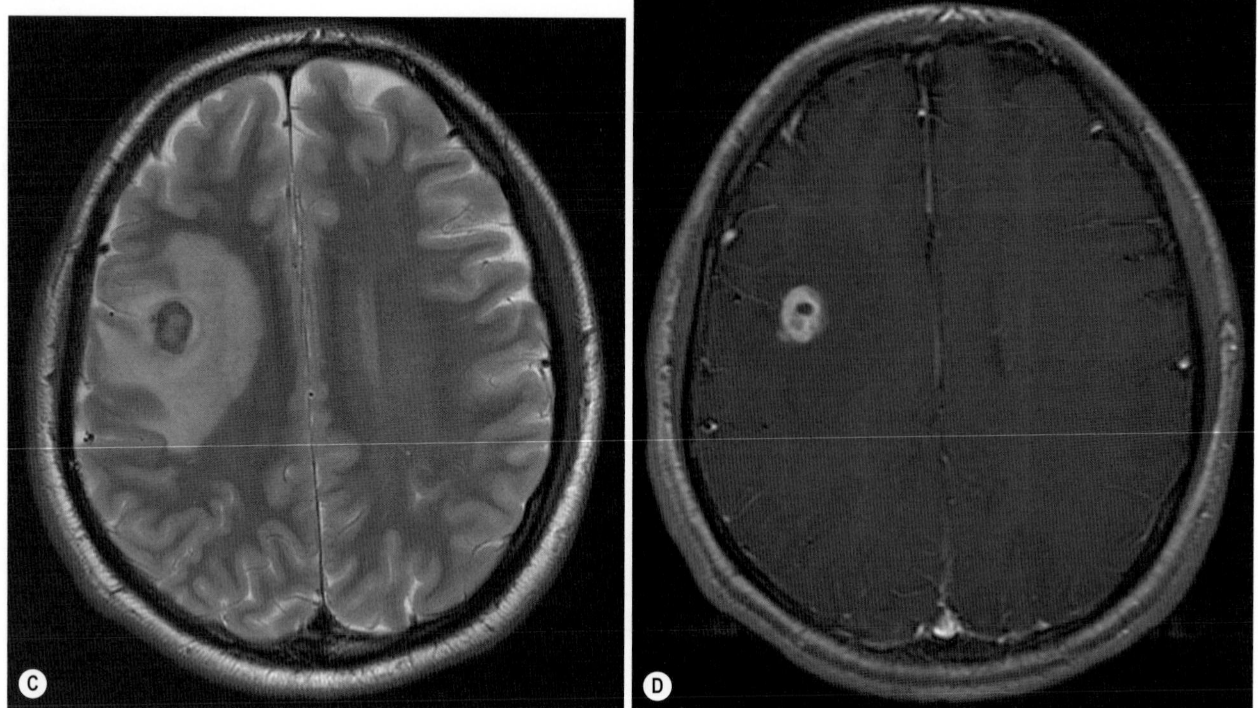

FIGURE 63-17, Continued ■ T2 image (C) and enhanced T1 image (D) demonstrating the granular nodular stage with a partially collapsed cyst associated with marked immune reaction from the host evidenced by a thick enhancing wall and marked surrounding oedema.

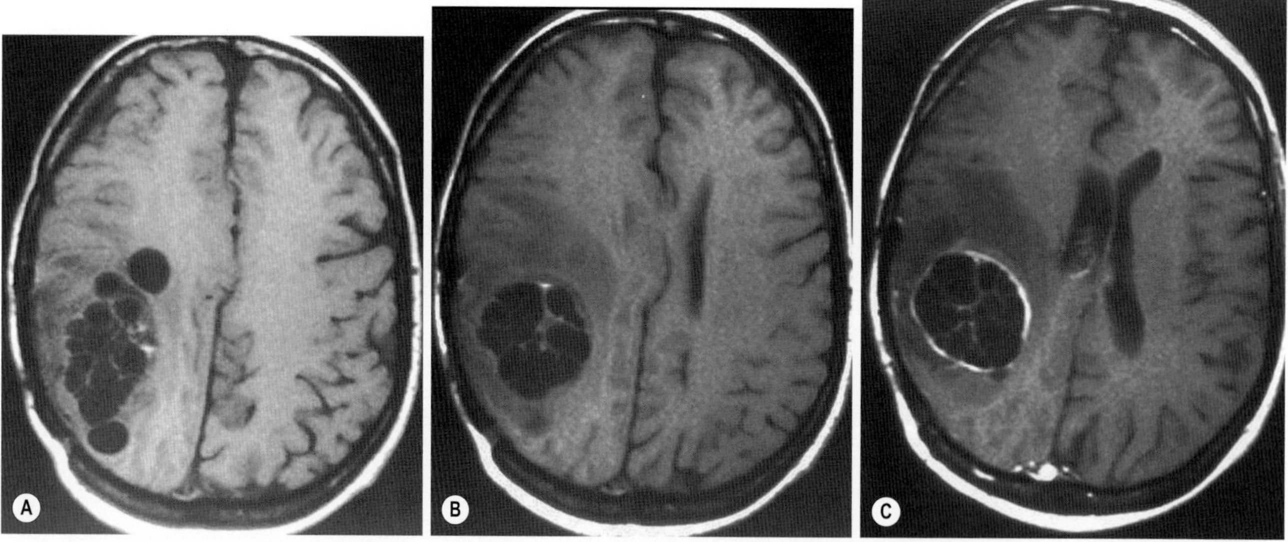

FIGURE 63-18 ■ ***Echinococcus* (hydatid).** Non-enhanced T1 (A, B) show multiple well-defined cysts corresponding to a hydatid cyst with multiple daughter cysts. There is also some associated oedema which appears hypointense. The contrast-enhanced T1 (C) demonstrates a thin outer rim of enhancement, which together with the oedema indicates that this is an active hydatid cyst.

definitive hosts to the *Echinococcus* (or hydatid) tapeworm. Herbivores such as sheep and cattle are intermediate hosts and humans are accidental hosts, infected by faeco-oral transmission. CNS involvement is seen in approximately 4% of patients with primary hepatic or pulmonary infestation.

Cystic echinococcosis in the brain is usually the result of haematogenous spread of embryos from the gastrointestinal tract and usually manifests itself as large, isolated, unilocular, well-defined and relatively thin-walled cysts. Small daughter cysts may be arranged peripherally within a large maternal cyst and this is considered to represent a pathognomonic sign of a hydatid cyst.[38] The cyst fluid appears similar to CSF on CT and MRI. In active cysts, a thin rim of enhancement and surrounding oedema may be detectable on MRI (Fig. 63-18). At a late stage CT may show calcification, which is an indicator that the cyst is dead.

Alveolar echinococcosis has a high mortality rate and the imaging features are of numerous irregular

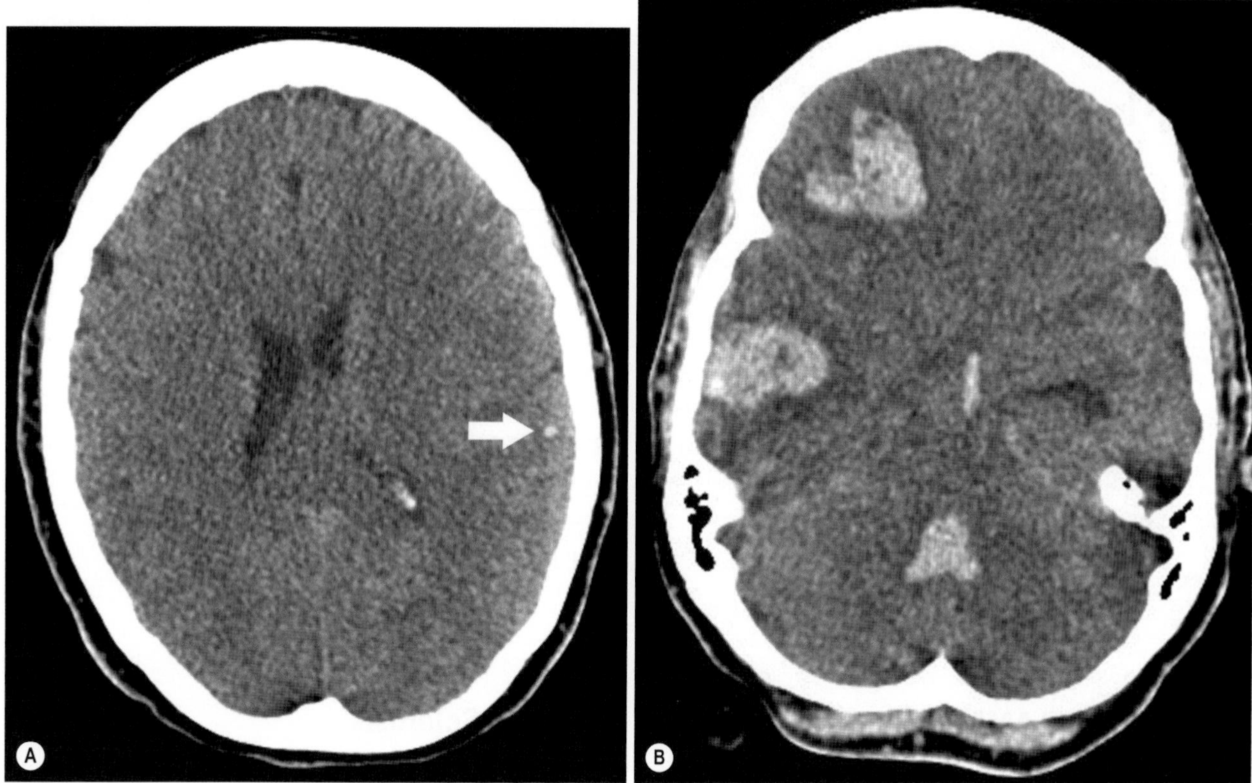

FIGURE 63-19 ■ Cerebral *Plasmodium falciparum* malaria in a 40-year-old woman with a state of confusion with reduced conscious level. The initial CT (A) performed on admission shows a small bleed peripherally in the left frontal lobe (arrow). An emergency CT performed 24 h later (B) shows multiple intraparenchymal and intraventricular haemorrhages and brain swelling with obliteration of the basal cisterns.

small cysts. Heterogeneous, nodular and cauliflower-like enhancement has been reported.

Malaria

With increasing travel to endemic regions, one must be aware of cerebral involvement in malaria, which occurs in about 2% of patients with *Plasmodium falciparum* infection. Cerebral malaria is a serious and life-threatening condition with a mortality rate of 20–50%. Early diagnosis and treatment are essential. Symptoms are often non-specific and include raised intracranial pressure, seizures, altered consciousness and stroke.

The infected erythrocytes cause occlusion of the cerebral capillaries and imaging findings include cortical and subcortical ischaemic lesions, cerebral oedema, microhaemorrhages, which are best seen on susceptibility-weighted imaging,[40] and macrohaemorrhages (Fig. 63-19).

For a full list of references, please see ExpertConsult.

FURTHER READING

1. Hughes DC, Raghavan A, Mordekar SR, et al. Role of imaging in the diagnosis of acute bacterial meningitis and its complications. Postgrad Med J 2010;86:478–85.
5. Kawaguchi T, Sakurai K, Hara M, et al. Clinico-radiological features of subarachnoid hyperintensity on diffusion-weighted images in patients with meningitis. Clin Radiol 2012;67:306–12.
6. Katchanov J, Siebert E, Endres M, Klingebiel R. Focal parenchymal lesions in community-acquired bacterial meningitis: a clinico-radiological study. Neuroradiology 2009;51:723–9.
11. Lai PH, Chang HC, Chuang TC, et al. Susceptibility-weighted imaging in patients with pyogenic brain abscesses at 1.5T: characteristics of the abscess capsule. Am J Neuroradiol 2012;33:910–14.
13. Luthra G, Parihar A, Nath K, et al. Comparative evaluation of fungal, tubercular and pyogenic brain abscesses with conventional and diffusion MR imaging and proton MR spectroscopy. Am J Neuroradiol 2007;28:1332–8.
19. Farrell CJ, Hoh BL, Pisculli ML, et al. Limitations of diffusion-weighted imaging in the diagnosis of postoperative infections. Neurosurgery 2008;62:577–83.
20. Fujikawa A, Tsuchiya K, Honya K, et al. Comparison of MRI sequences to detect ventriculitis. Am J Roentgenol 2006;187:1048–53.
26. Mathur M, Johnson CE, Sze G. Fungal infections of the central nervous system. Neuroimaging Clin N Am 2012;22:609–32.
28. Rath TJ, Hughes M, Arabi M, Shah GV. Imaging of cerebritis, encephalitis and brain abscess. Neuroimaging Clin N Am 2012;22:585–607.
31. Thurnher MM, Donovan Post MJ. Neuroimaging in the brain in HIV-1-infected patients. Neuroimaging Clin N Am 2008;18:93–117.
37. Post MJD, Thurnher MM, Clifford DB, et al. CNS-immune reconstitution inflammatory syndrome in the setting of HIV infection, part 1: overview and discussion of progressive multifocal leukoencephalopathy-immune reconstitution inflammatory syndrome and cryptococcal-immune reconstitution inflammatory syndrome. Am J Neuroradiol 2013;34:1297–307.
38. Abdel Razek AA, Watcharakorn A, Castillo M. Parasitic diseases of the central nervous system. Neuroimaging Clin N Am 2011;21:815–41.

CHAPTER 64

Inflammatory and Metabolic Disease

Alex Rovira • Pia C. Sundgren • Massimo Gallucci

CHAPTER OUTLINE

IDIOPATHIC INFLAMMATORY-DEMYELINATING DISORDERS OF THE CENTRAL NERVOUS SYSTEM

Idiopathic inflammatory-demyelinating diseases (IIDDs) represent a broad spectrum of central nervous system disorders that can be differentiated on the basis of severity, clinical course and lesion distribution, as well as imaging, laboratory and pathological findings. The spectrum includes monophasic, multiphasic and progressive disorders, ranging from highly localised forms to multifocal or diffuse variants.

Relapsing-remitting and secondary progressive multiple sclerosis (MS) are the two most common forms of IIDDs.[1] MS can also have a progressive course from onset (primary progressive and progressive relapsing MS). Fulminant forms of IIDDs include a variety of disorders that have in common the severity of the clinical symptoms, an acute clinical course and atypical findings on MR imaging. The classic fulminant IIDD is Marburg's disease. Baló's concentric sclerosis, Schilder's disease and acute disseminated encephalomyelitis can also present with acute and severe attacks.

Some IIDDs have a restricted topographical distribution, such as Devic's neuromyelitis optica, which can have a monophasic or, more frequently, a relapsing course. Other types of IIDDs occasionally present as a focal lesion that may be clinically and radiographically indistinguishable from a brain tumour. It is difficult to classify these tumefactive or pseudotumoural lesions within the spectrum of IIDDs. Some cases have a monophasic, self-limited course, while in others the tumefactive plaque is the first manifestation or appears during a typical relapsing form of MS. MR imaging of the brain and spine is the imaging technique of choice for diagnosing these disorders, and, together with the clinical and laboratory findings, can accurately classify them.[2]

Multiple Sclerosis

MS is a chronic, persistent inflammatory-demyelinating disease of the central nervous system (CNS), characterised pathologically by areas of inflammation, demyelination, axonal loss and gliosis scattered throughout the CNS. MS has a predilection for the optic nerves, brainstem, spinal cord and cerebellar and periventricular white matter.

MS is one of the most common neurological disorders and the second cause of disability in Western countries in young adults of Caucasian origin. It is relatively common in Europe, the United States, Canada, New Zealand and parts of Australia, but rare in Asia, and in the tropics and subtropics of all continents. Multiple sclerosis is twice as common in women as in men; men have a tendency for later disease onset, with a poorer prognosis. The incidence of MS is low in childhood, increases rapidly after the age of 18, reaches a peak between 25 and 35, and then slowly declines, becoming rare at 50 and older.[3]

The aetiology of MS is still unknown, but it most likely results from an interplay between as-yet unidentified environmental factors and susceptibility genes.

The clinical course of MS can follow different patterns over time, but is usually characterised by acute episodes of worsening (relapses, bouts), gradual progressive deterioration of neurological function, or a combination of both these features (relapsing MS). In a relatively small percentage of patients, the disease has a progressive course from onset, without acute relapses (primary progressive MS).

Relapsing MS accounts for 85% of all MS. This clinical form typically presents as an acute clinically isolated syndrome attributable to a monofocal or multifocal CNS demyelinating lesion. The presenting lesion usually affects the optic nerve (optic neuritis), spinal cord (acute transverse myelitis), brainstem (typically an internuclear ophthalmoparesis) and cerebellum (clumsiness and gait ataxia). Over the following years, patients usually experience episodes of acute worsening of neurological function, followed by variably complete recovery (relapsing-remitting (RR) course). Clinical and subclinical activity is frequent in this form. After several years of the RR course, more than 50% of untreated patients will develop progressive disability with or without occasional relapses, minor remissions and plateaus (secondary progressive (SP) course).[1]

As long as the aetiology of MS remains unknown, causal therapy and effective prevention are not possible. Immunomodulatory drugs such as beta-interferon, glatiramer acetate, natalizumab and fingolimod can alter the course of the disease, particularly in the RR form, by reducing the number of relapses and the accumulation of lesions as seen on MR imaging, and by influencing the impact of the disease on disability. Patients with the SP form of MS, continuing relapses of activity and pronounced progression of disability may also benefit from immunomodulatory or immunosuppressive therapy.

Primary progressive forms (PPMS) comprise approximately 10% of MS cases. This form of MS begins as a progressive disease with occasional plateaus and relapses, and temporary minor improvements. Progressive-relapsing MS follows a progressive course like PPMS, but shows clear acute relapses that may or may not be followed by full recovery.[1] Compared to patients with the more frequent relapsing forms of MS, patients with PPMS have smaller T_2 lesion loads, smaller T_2 lesions, slower rates of new lesion formation and minimal gadolinium enhancement on brain MRI, despite their accumulating disability. The presence of extensive cortical damage, diffuse white matter tissue damage and prevalent involvement of the spinal cord may partially explain this discrepancy between the MR abnormalities and the severity of the clinical disease. Because patients with PPMS may have less inflammation than those with relapsing MS, they may be less likely to respond to immunomodulatory therapies.

MR Imaging

Brain. MR imaging is the most sensitive imaging technique for detecting MS plaques throughout the brain and spinal cord. Proton density (PD) or T_2-weighted MR images show areas of high signal intensity in the periventricular white matter in 98% of MS patients. MS plaques are generally round to ovoid in shape and range from a few millimetres to more than 1 cm in diameter. They are typically discrete and focal at the early stages of the disease, but become confluent as the disease progresses, particularly in the posterior hemispheric periventricular white matter (Fig. 64-1). MS plaques tend to affect the deep white matter rather than the subcortical

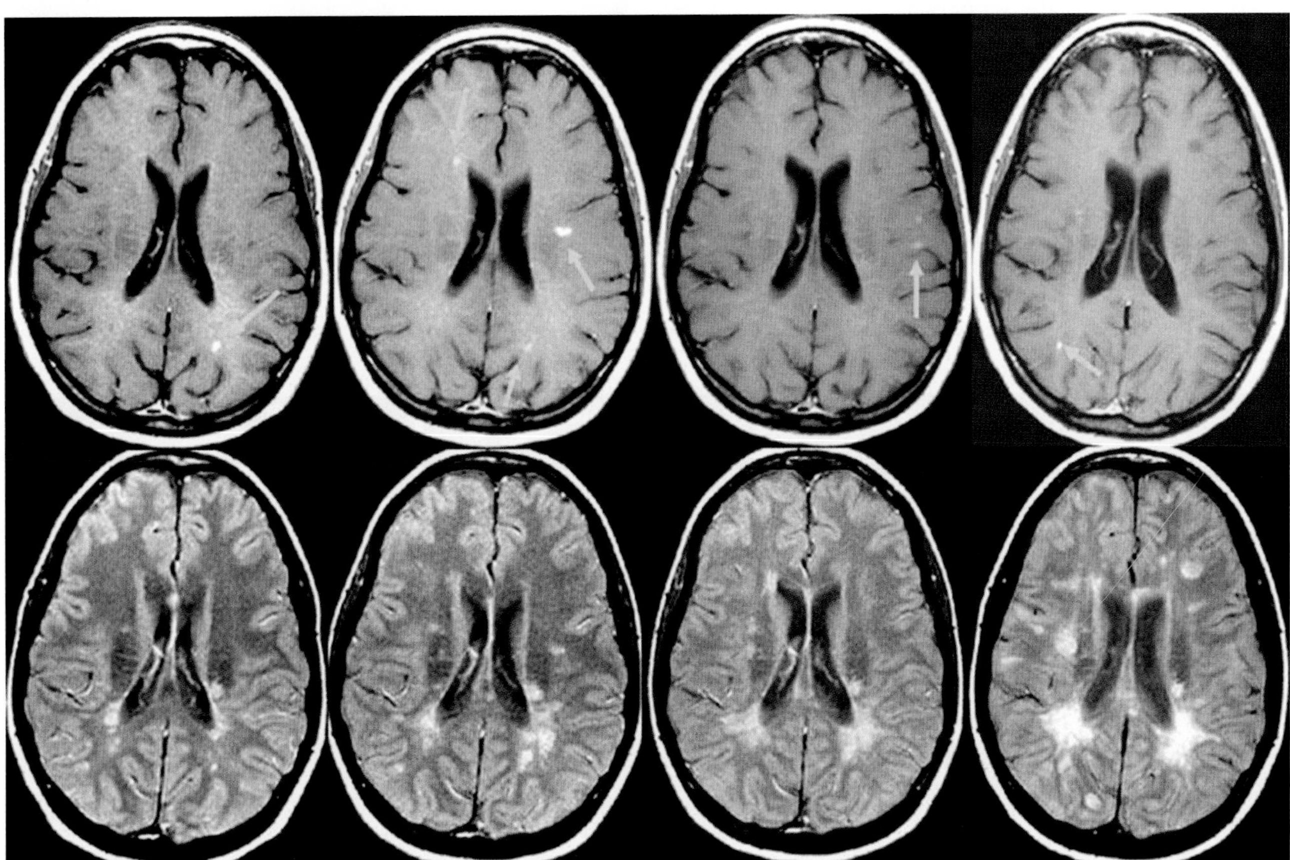

FIGURE 64-1 ■ **Relapsing form of multiple sclerosis.** Serial, contrast-enhanced T_1-weighted (top row) and FLAIR (bottom row) MR images of the brain obtained yearly in a patient with a typical relapsing form of MS and progressive disability. Note the new lesions that appeared during this three-year follow-up, some of them showing gadolinium enhancement (arrows).

white matter, whereas small vessel ischaemic lesions tend to involve the subcortical white matter more than the periventricular white matter.[4,5] The total T_2 lesion volume of the brain increases by approximately 5 to 10% each year in the relapsing forms of MS.[6]

Both acute and chronic MS plaques appear bright on PD- and T_2-weighted sequences, reflecting their increased tissue water content. The signal increase indicates oedema, inflammation, demyelination, reactive gliosis and/or axonal loss in proportions that differ from lesion to lesion. The vast majority of MS patients have at least one ovoid periventricular lesion, whose major axis is oriented perpendicular to the outer surface of the lateral ventricles (Fig. 64-2). The ovoid shape and perpendicular orientation derive from the perivenular location of the demyelinating plaques (Dawsons' fingers).

Multiple sclerosis lesions tend to affect specific regions of the brain, including the periventricular white matter situated superolateral to the lateral angles of the ventricles, the callososeptal interface along the inferior surface of the corpus callosum, the cortico-juxtacortical regions, and the infratentorial regions. Focal involvement of the periventricular white matter in the anterior temporal lobes is typical for MS and rarely seen in other white matter disorders (Fig. 64-3). The lesions commonly found at the callososeptal interface are best depicted by sagittal fast-FLAIR images; so this sequence is highly recommended for diagnostic MR imaging studies (Fig. 64-4).

Histopathological studies have shown that a substantial portion of the total brain lesion load in MS is located within the cerebral cortex. Presently available MR imaging techniques are not optimal for detecting cortical lesions because of poor contrast resolution between normal-appearing grey matter (NAGM) and the plaques in question, and because of the partial volume effects of the subarachnoid spaces and CSF surrounding the cortex. Cortical lesions are better visualised by 2D or 3D fast-FLAIR sequences and newer MR techniques such as 3D double inversion recovery (DIR) MR sequences which selectively suppress the signal from white matter and cerebrospinal fluid (Fig. 64-5).[7]

Juxtacortical lesions that involve the 'U' fibres are seen in two-thirds of patients with MS. They are a rather characteristic finding in early stages of the disease, and are best detected by fast-FLAIR (Fig. 64-6) sequences.

Multiple sclerosis frequently affects the brainstem and cerebellum, leading to acute clinical syndromes, such as trigeminal neuralgia, internuclear ophthalmoplegia, vertigo and ataxia. Later on, chronic damage to the

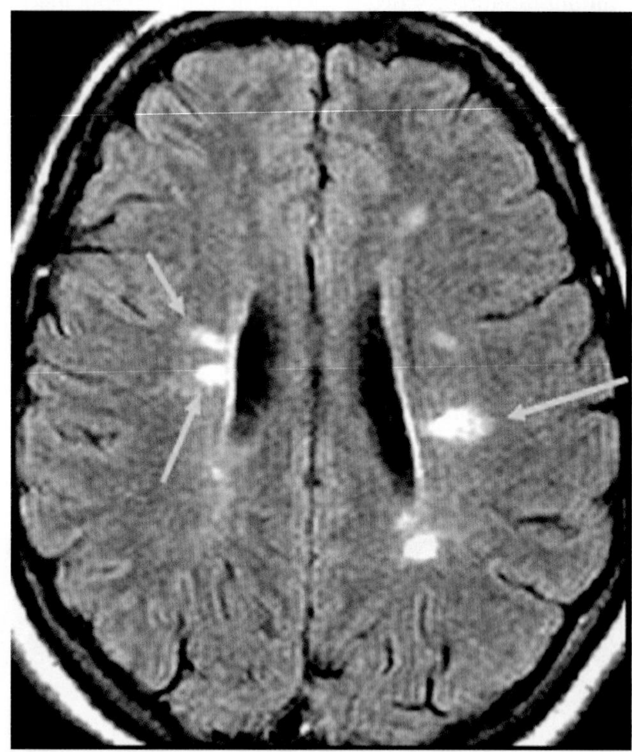

FIGURE 64-2 ■ Relapsing-remitting MS. Transverse fast-FLAIR MR image shows typical ovoid demyelinating plaques (arrows), whose major axis is perpendicular to the ventricular wall.

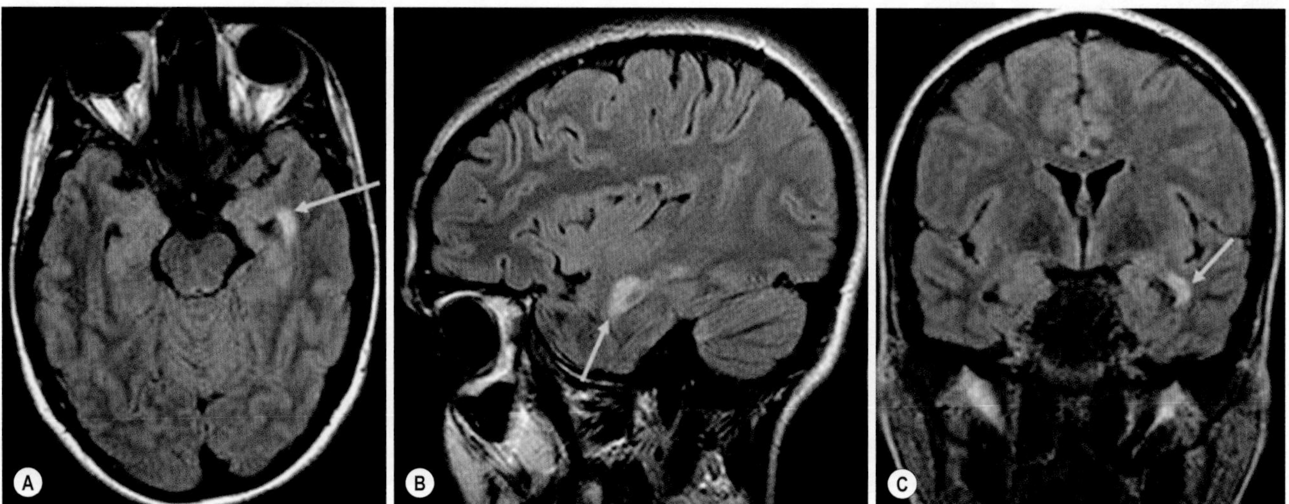

FIGURE 64-3 ■ (A–C) Relapsing-remitting MS. Transverse, sagittal and coronal fast-FLAIR MR images depict typical demyelinating plaques affecting the anterior temporal periventricular white matter on the left side (arrows).

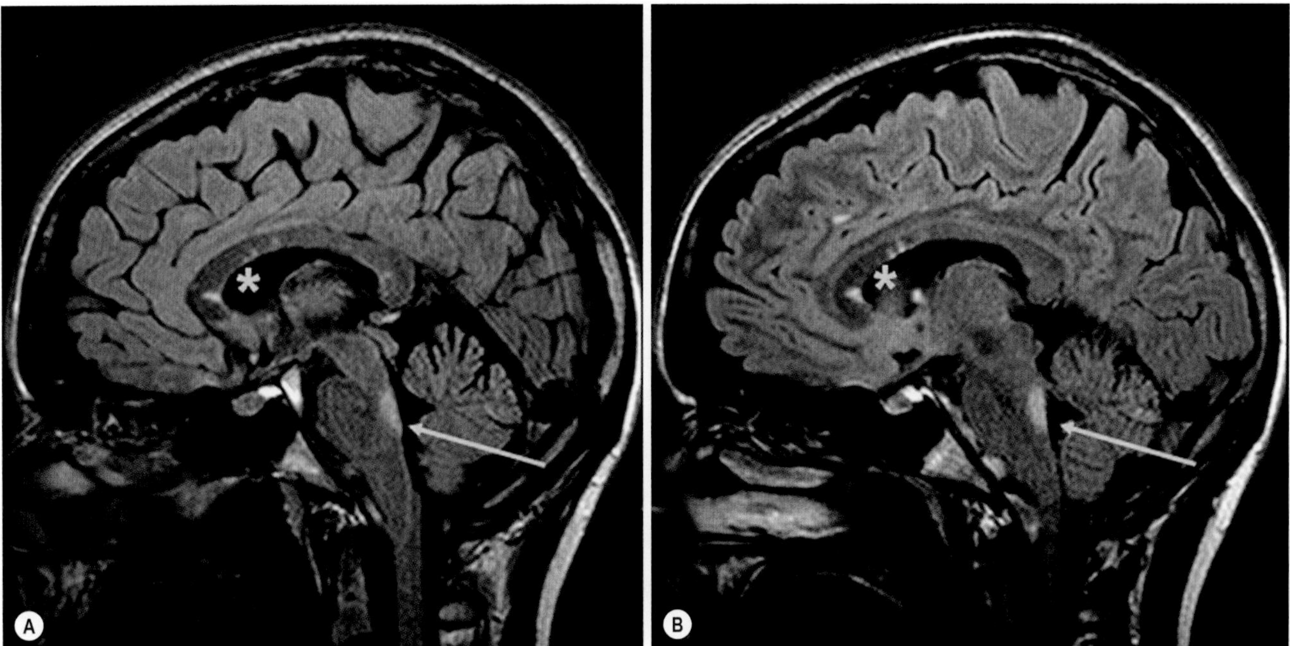

FIGURE 64-4 ■ **(A, B) Clinically isolated syndrome of the brainstem (internuclear ophthalmoplegia).** Sagittal fast-FLAIR MR images show the symptomatic lesion located in the floor of the IV ventricle (arrows), and subclinical lesions on the callososeptal interface (asterisks).

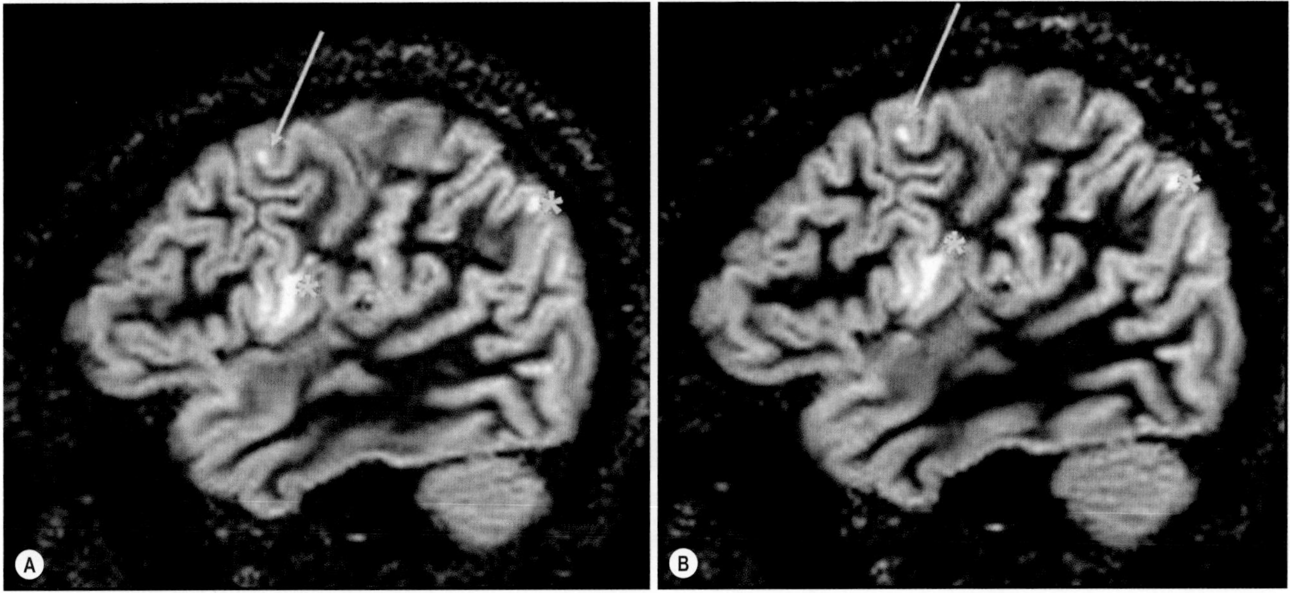

FIGURE 64-5 ■ **(A, B) Relapsing-remitting MS.** Sagittal double inversion recovery MR images show small hyperintense lesions involving the posterior frontal cortex (arrow) and multiple juxtacortical lesions affecting the inferior frontal and parietal lobes (asterisks).

posterior fossa causes chronic disabling symptoms such as ataxia and oculomotor disturbances. Acute symptomatic lesions appear as well-defined, hyperintense focal lesions that enhance with contrast administration on T_1-weighted images (Fig. 64-7).

Posterior fossa lesions preferentially involve the floor of the fourth ventricle, the middle cerebellar peduncles and the brainstem. Most brainstem lesions are contiguous with the cisternal or ventricular cerebrospinal fluid spaces, and range from large confluent patches to solitary, well-delineated paramedian lesions or discrete 'linings' of the cerebrospinal fluid border zones. Predilection for these areas is a key feature that helps to identify MS plaques and to differentiate them from focal areas of ischaemic demyelination and infarction that preferentially involve the central pontine white matter. Because of their short acquisition time and greater sensitivity, PD- and T_2-weighted fast spin-echo sequences are preferred over conventional spin-echo or fast-FLAIR sequences for detecting posterior fossa lesions.

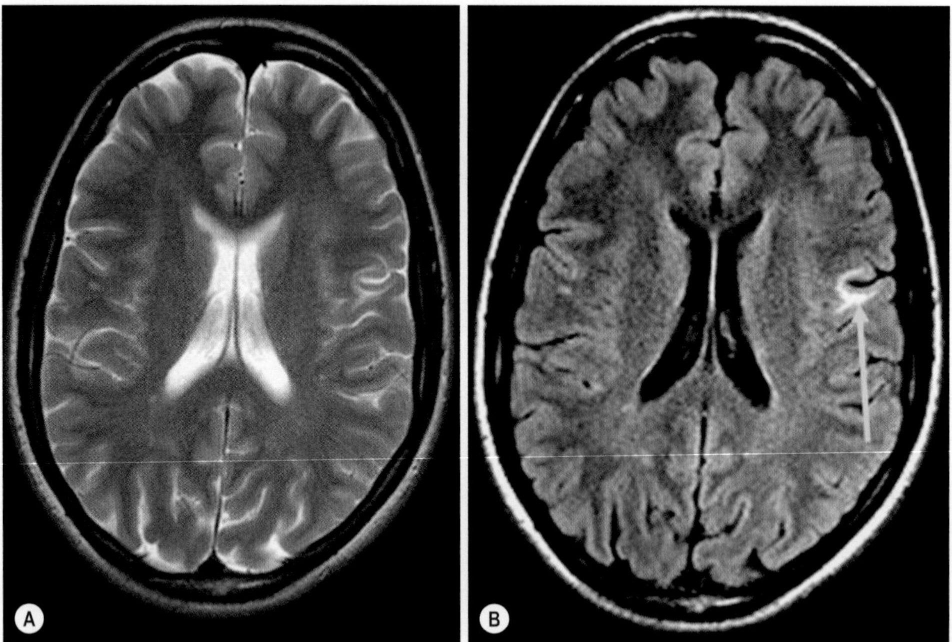

FIGURE 64-6 ■ **Relapsing-remitting MS.** Transverse fast spin-echo T_2-weighted (A) and fast-FLAIR (B) MR images. A juxtacortical lesion involving the inferior frontal lobe is better depicted on the fast-FLAIR image as compared to the fast spin-echo image (arrow).

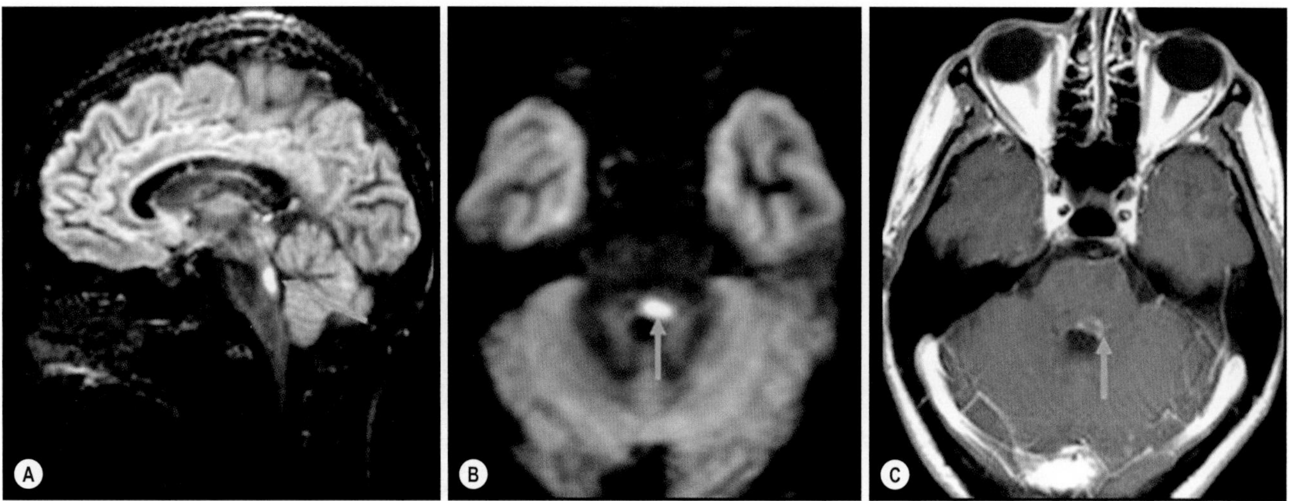

FIGURE 64-7 ■ **Clinically isolated syndrome of the brainstem (internuclear ophthalmoplegia).** Sagittal (A) and transverse (B) double inversion recovery (DIR) and contrast-enhanced T_1-weighted (C) MR images. The symptomatic lesion is clearly seen on the DIR sequence as a well-defined focal hyperintense area affecting the left medial longitudinal fasciculus and showing contrast uptake (arrows).

Approximately 10–20% of T_2 hyperintensities are also visible on T_1-weighted images as areas of low signal intensity compared with normal-appearing white matter. These so-called 'T_1 black holes' have a different pathological substrate that depends, in part, on the lesion age. The hypointensity is present in up to 80% of recently formed lesions and probably represents marked oedema, with or without myelin destruction or axonal loss. In most cases the acute (or wet) 'black holes' become isointense within a few months as inflammatory activity abates, oedema resolves and reparative mechanisms like remyelination become active. Less than 40% evolve into persisting or chronic black holes,[8] which correlate pathologically with the most severe demyelination and axonal loss, indicating areas of irreversible tissue damage. Chronic black holes are more frequent in patients with progressive disease than in those with RR disease (Fig. 64-8), and are more frequent in the supratentorial white matter as compared with the infratentorial white matter. They are rarely found in the spinal cord and optic nerves.

MS lesions of the spinal cord resemble those in the brain. The lesions can be focal (single or multiple) or diffuse, and mainly affect the cervical cord segment. On sagittal images, the lesions characteristically have a cigar shape and rarely exceed two vertebral segments in length. On cross-section they typically occupy the lateral and

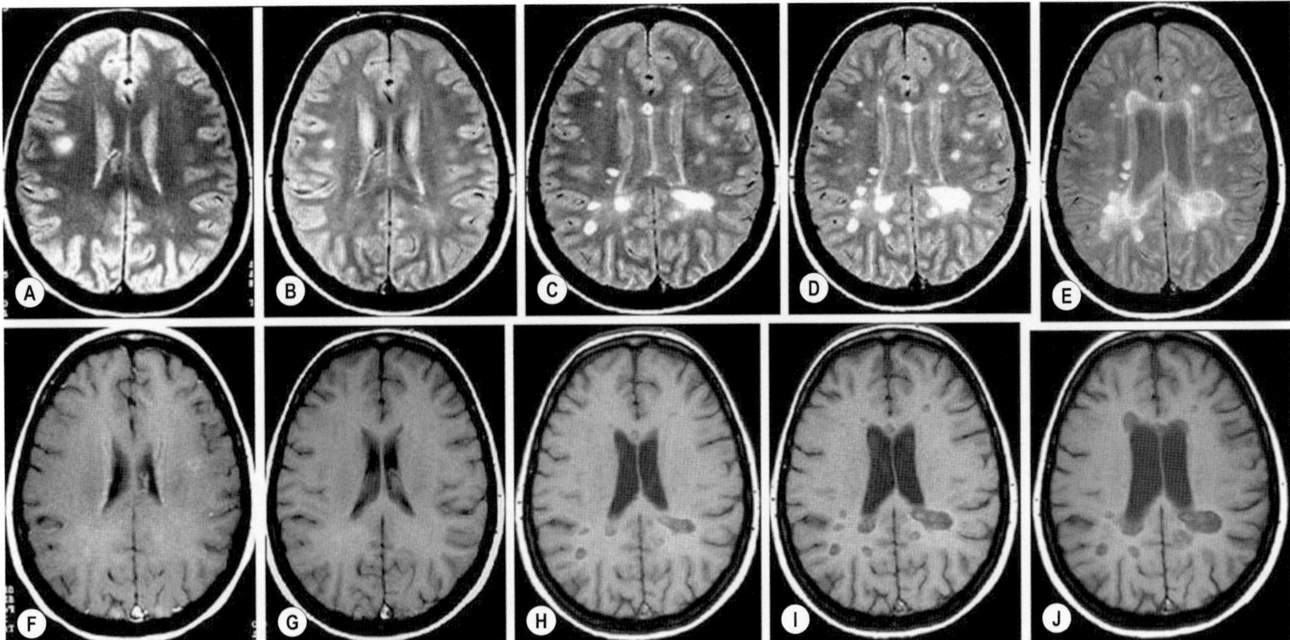

FIGURE 64-8 ■ Serial MR images obtained on a biyearly basis in a patient with a relapsing form of MS. Transverse proton-density-weighted (A–E) and T_1-weighted (F–J) MR images. In addition to the increasing number of plaques within the hemispheric white matter, observe the increase in number and size of irreversible black holes and progressive brain volume loss.

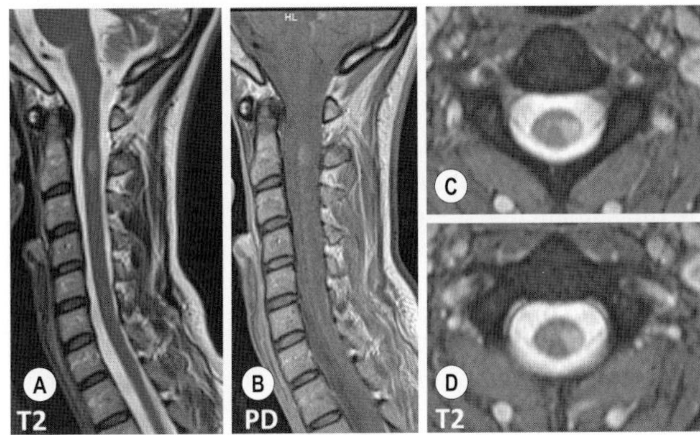

FIGURE 64-9 ■ (A–D) Relapsing-remitting MS with plaques in the cervical spinal cord. Sagittal T_2 and proton-density and transverse T_2 MR images. Observe the small focal lesion that does not exceed two vertebral segments in length and does not affect more than half the cross-sectional area of the cord.

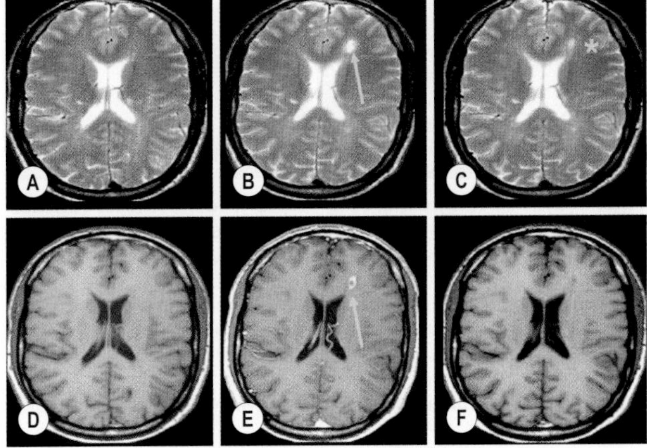

FIGURE 64-10 ■ Relapsing-remitting MS with new brain plaque formation. Transverse T_2-weighted (A–C) and contrast-enhanced T_1-weighted (D–F) brain MR images obtained serially at monthly intervals. Observe formation of a new plaque in the left frontal white matter showing transient contrast uptake (arrows). With cessation of inflammatory activity, the T_2 lesion decreased in size, but left a persistent hyperintense footprint on the T_2-weighted image (asterisk).

posterior white matter columns, extend to involve the central grey matter, and rarely occupy more than one-half the cross-sectional area of the cord[9] (Fig. 64-9).

Acute spinal cord lesions can produce a mild-to-moderate mass effect with cord swelling and may show contrast enhancement. Active lesions are rarer in the spinal cord than the brain, and are almost always associated with new clinical symptoms. The prevalence of cord abnormalities is as high as 74–92% in established MS, and depends on the clinical phenotype of MS. In clinically isolated syndromes, the prevalence of spinal cord lesions is lower, particularly if there are no spinal cord symptoms. Nevertheless, asymptomatic cord lesions are found in 30–40% of patients with a clinically isolated syndrome. In relapsing-remitting MS, the spinal cord lesions are typically multifocal. In secondary progressive MS, the abnormalities are more extensive and diffuse and are commonly associated with spinal cord atrophy. In primary progressive MS, cord abnormalities are quite extensive as compared with brain abnormalities. This discrepancy may help to diagnose primary progressive MS in patients with few or no brain abnormalities.

Longitudinal and cross-sectional MR studies have shown that the formation of new MS plaques is often associated with contrast enhancement, mainly in the acute and relapsing stages of the disease[10] (Fig. 64-10).

The gadolinium enhancement varies in size and shape, but usually lasts from a few days to weeks, although steroid treatment shortens this period. Incomplete ring enhancement on T_1-weighted gadolinium-enhanced images, with the open border facing the grey matter of the cortex or basal ganglia, is a common finding in active MS plaques and is a helpful feature for distinguishing between inflammatory-demyelinating lesions and other focal lesions such as tumours or abscesses[11] (Fig. 64-11).

Focal enhancement can be detected before abnormalities appear on unenhanced T_2-weighted images, and can reappear in chronic lesions with or without a concomitant increase in size. Although enhancing lesions also occur in clinically stable MS patients, their number is much greater when there is concomitant clinical activity. Contrast enhancement is a relatively good predictor of further enhancement and of subsequent accumulation of T_2 lesions, but shows no (or weak) correlation with progression of disability and development of brain atrophy.

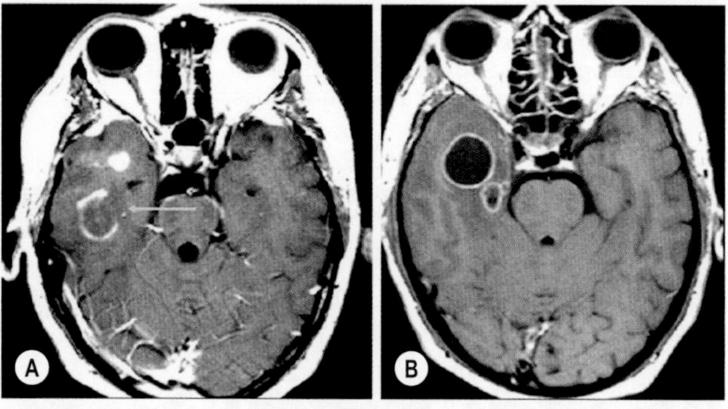

FIGURE 64-11 ■ Ring-enhancing pattern of contrast uptake. Contrast-enhanced T_1-weighted MR images obtained in a patient with relapsing-remitting MS (A) and a patient with glioblastoma multiforme (B). Both patients have focal lesions in the right temporal lobe. However, an incomplete ring-enhancing pattern of contrast uptake with the open margin facing the cortical grey matter of the hippocampus (arrow) is only seen in the patient with MS. In glioblastoma, the multiforme lesions show a complete ring of enhancement, despite contact with the cortical grey matter.

In relapsing-remitting and secondary progressive MS, enhancement is more frequent during relapses and correlates well with clinical activity. For patients with primary progressive MS, serial T_2-weighted studies show few new lesions and little or no enhancement with conventional doses of gadolinium, despite steady clinical deterioration.[12] Contrast-enhanced T_1-weighted images are routinely used in the study of MS to provide a measure of inflammatory activity in vivo. The technique detects disease activity 5–10 times more frequently than clinical evaluation of relapses, suggesting that most of the enhancing lesions are clinically silent. Subclinical disease activity with contrast-enhancing lesions is four to ten times less frequent in the spinal cord than the brain, a fact that may be partially explained by the large volume of brain as compared with spinal cord. High doses of gadolinium and a long post-injection delay can increase the detection of active spinal cord lesions.

Optic neuritis (ON) can usually be diagnosed clinically. MR imaging is not necessary to confirm the diagnosis, unless there are atypical clinical features (e.g. no response to steroids, long-standing symptoms). In these situations, brain and optic nerve MR imaging should be performed to rule out an alternative diagnosis, such as a compressive lesion.[13] Coronal fat-saturated T_2-weighted images are the most sensitive MR technique for depicting signal abnormalities. Focal thickening of the affected optic nerve reflects demyelination and inflammation (Fig. 64-12), which may persist for long periods despite improvements in vision and visual-evoked potential findings. Intense optic nerve enhancement seen on fat-suppressed contrast-enhanced T_1-weighted images is a consistent feature of acute ON (Fig. 64-12). The length of the enhancing optic nerve segment on axial images correlates with the severity of visual impairment, but does not predict the degree of visual recovery. In MS, signal abnormalities may also be seen in the absence of acute attacks of ON.

Atrophy of the brain and spinal cord is an important part of MS pathology, and a clinically relevant component of disease progression.[14] Although this process is more severe in the progressive forms of the disease, it

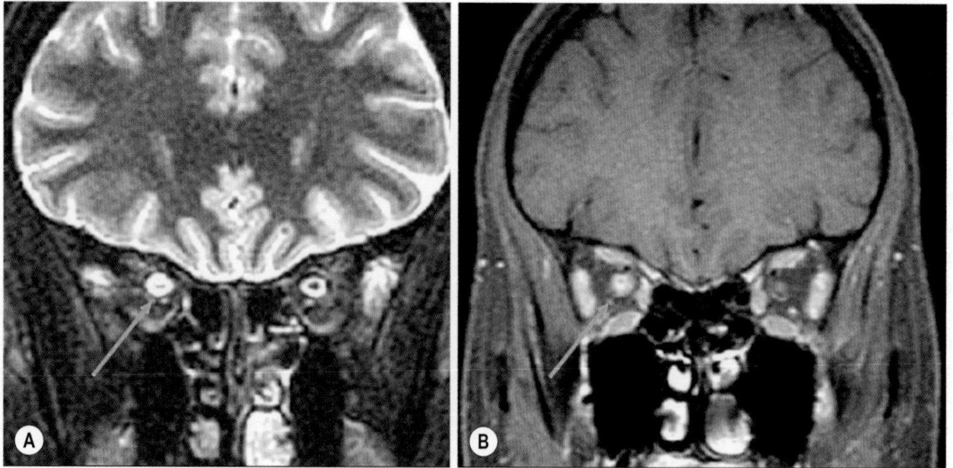

FIGURE 64-12 ■ Right optic neuritis. Coronal fat-suppressed T_2-weighted fast spin-echo (A) and fat-suppressed contrast-enhanced T_1-weighted MR images. There is hyperintensity of the right optic nerve, with diffuse enhancement (arrows) (B).

may also occur early in the disease process (Fig. 64-8). In fact, early atrophy seems to predict subsequent development of physical disability better than do measures of lesion load. The aetiology of CNS atrophy is multifactorial and likely reflects demyelination, Wallerian degeneration, axonal loss and glial contraction. CNS atrophy, which involves both grey and white matter, is a progressive phenomenon that worsens with increasing disease duration, and progresses at a rate of 0.6–1.2% of brain loss per year. Quantitative measures of whole-brain atrophy, acquired by automated or semi-automated methods, display this progressive loss of brain tissue bulk in vivo in a sensitive and reproducible manner. Subcortical brain atrophy is particularly well correlated to neuropsychological impairment, which can be explained by a disruption of frontal-subcortical circuits. Spinal cord atrophy is better correlated with motor disability.

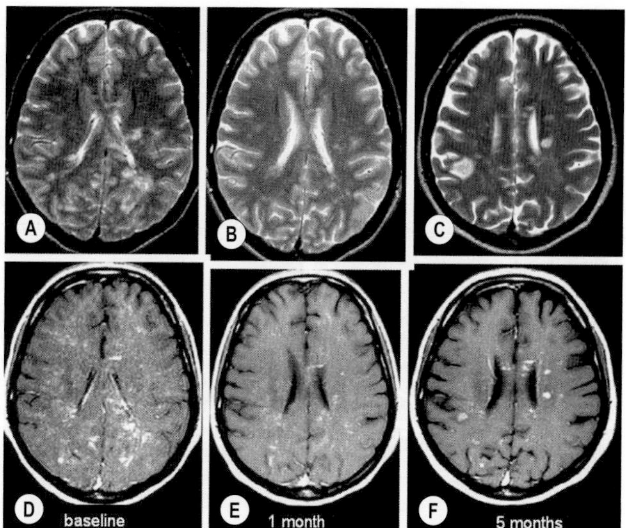

FIGURE 64-13 ■ **Marburg's disease.** Serial T_2-weighted (A–C) and contrast-enhanced T_1-weighted (D–F) MR images of the brain obtained in a patient with a final diagnosis of fulminant IIDD. Note multiple contrast-enhanced focal lesions diffusely involving the cerebral white matter. Some of the lesions are persistent, whereas others are new. The patient died 5 months after symptoms onset.

Multiple Sclerosis Variants

Marburg's Disease

Marburg's disease (MD) (also termed malignant MS) is a rare, acute MS variant that occurs predominantly in young adults. It is characterised by a confusional state, headache, vomiting, gait unsteadiness and hemiparesis. This entity has a rapidly progressive course with frequent, severe relapses leading to death or severe disability within weeks to months, mainly from brainstem involvement, or mass effect with herniation. Most of the patients who survive subsequently develop a relapsing form of MS. Because MD is often preceded by a febrile illness, this disease may also be considered a fulminant form of acute disseminated encephalomyelitis, if has a monophasic course. Pathologically, Marburg's lesions are more destructive than those of typical MS or acute disseminated encephalomyelitis and are characterised by massive macrophage infiltration, acute axonal injury and tissue necrosis. Despite the destructive nature of these lesions, areas of remyelination are often observed. In MD, MRI typically shows multiple focal T_2 lesions of varying size, which may coalesce to form large white matter plaques disseminated throughout the hemispheric white matter and brainstem (Fig. 64-13). Mild-to-moderate perilesional oedema is often present and the lesions may show peripheral enhancement.[2] A similar imaging pattern is also seen in acute disseminated encephalomyelitis.

Schilder's Disease

Schilder's disease (SD) is a rare acute or subacute disorder that can be defined as a specific clinical-radiological presentation of IIDD. It commonly affects children and young adults. The clinical spectrum of SD includes psychiatric predominance, acute intracranial hypertension, intermittent exacerbations and progressive deterioration. Imaging studies show large ring-enhancing lesions involving both hemispheres, sometimes symmetrically, and located preferentially in the parieto-occipital regions. These large, focal demyelinating lesions can resemble a brain tumour, an abscess or even adrenoleucodystrophy. MR features that suggest possible SD include large and relatively symmetrical involvement of brain hemispheres, incomplete ring enhancement, minimal mass effect, restricted diffusivity and sparing of the brainstem (Fig. 64-14).[2] Histopathologically, SD consistently shows well-demarcated demyelination and reactive gliosis with relative sparing of the axons. Microcystic changes and even frank cavitation can occur. The clinical and imaging findings usually show a dramatic response to steroids.

Baló's Concentric Sclerosis

Baló's concentric sclerosis (BCS) is thought to be a rare, aggressive variant of MS that can lead to death in weeks to months. The pathological hallmarks of the disease are large demyelinated lesions showing a peculiar pattern of alternating layers of preserved and destroyed myelin. One possible explanation for the concentric alternating bands in this variant of MS may be that sublethal tissue injury is induced at the edge of the expanding lesion, which would then stimulate the expression of neuroprotective proteins to protect the rim of periplaque tissue from damage, thereby resulting in alternative layers of preserved and non-preserved myelinated tissue.[15]

These alternating bands can be identified with T_2 MR imaging, which typically shows concentric hyperintense bands corresponding to areas of demyelination and gliosis, alternating with isointense bands corresponding to normal myelinated white matter (Figs. 64-15 and 64-16). This pattern can appear as multiple concentric layers (onion skin lesion), as a mosaic, or as a 'floral' configuration. The centre of the lesion usually shows no layering because of massive demyelination. Contrast enhancement and decreased diffusivity are frequent in the outer rings (inflammatory edge) of the lesion (Fig. 64-16). On MR imaging, this Baló pattern can be isolated, multiple or

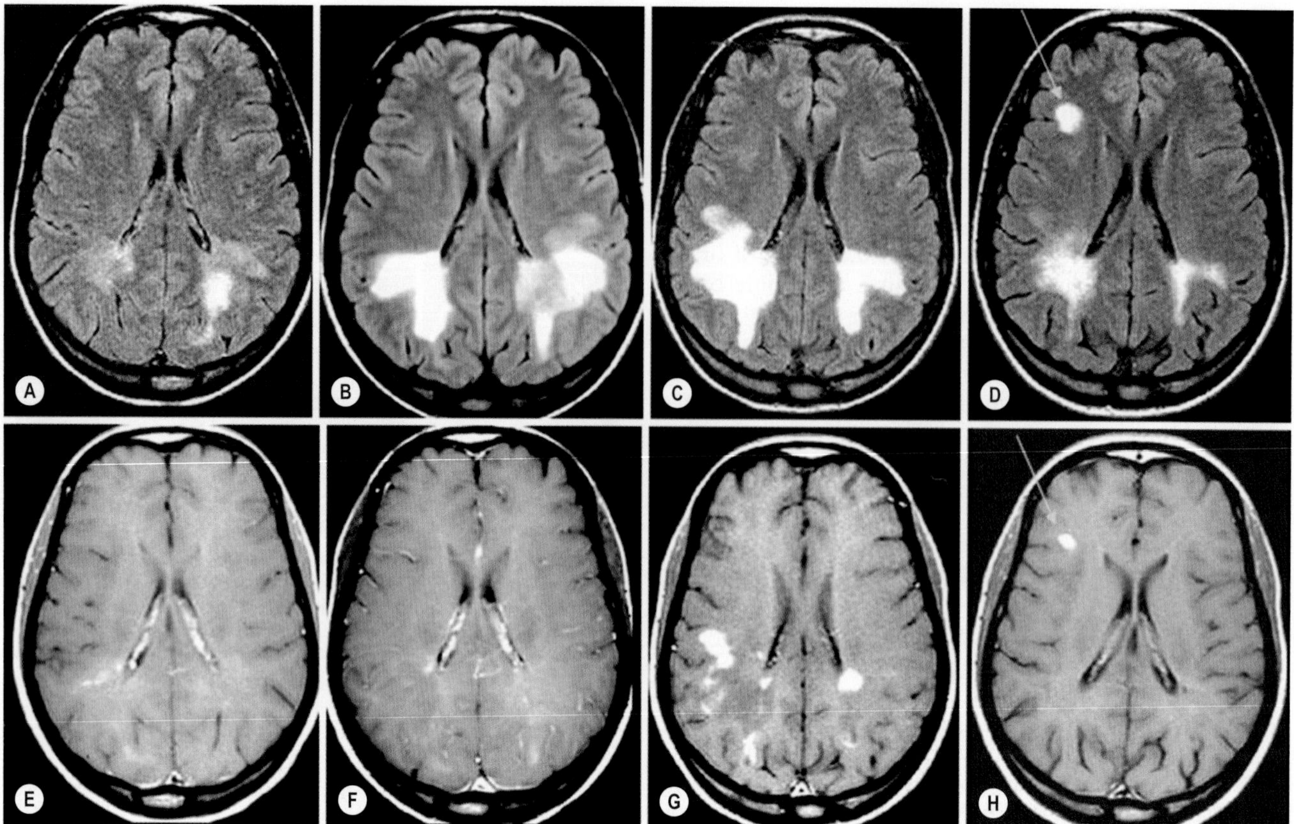

FIGURE 64-14 ■ **Schilder's disease.** Serial brain MR images in a patient with Schilder's disease who later developed clinically definite MS. Transverse fast-FLAIR images (A–D) and contrast-enhanced T_1-weighted (E–H) images obtained serially over 6 months. Note the progressive appearance of large, bilateral, almost symmetrical lesions in the posterior periventricular white matter. Despite considerable extension of the lesions, there is no mass effect. The 6-month image obtained during an episode of optic neuritis shows a new contrast-enhancing lesion in the right frontal white matter (arrows). A final diagnosis of relapsing-remitting MS was established.

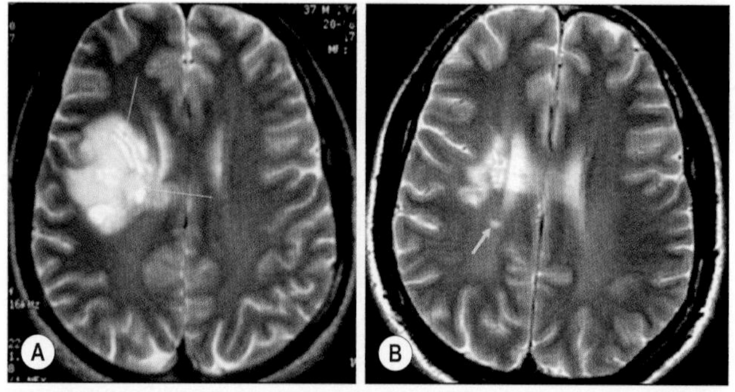

FIGURE 64-15 ■ **Baló-like lesion in a patient who converted to MS.** Transverse T_2-weighted MR image of the brain shows a large focal lesion within the right frontal white matter. The striking lamellated pattern of alternating bands of demyelination and relatively normal white matter, reflecting either spared or remyelinated regions, is clear in this image (arrows) (A). Note partial resolution of the large hemispheric lesion in a follow-up MR image obtained 4 years after symptoms onset, and the presence of a new T_2 lesion (arrow) (B).

mixed with typical MS-like lesions. Although Baló's concentric sclerosis was initially described as an acute, monophasic and rapidly fatal disease that resembled Marburg's disease, large Baló-like lesions are frequently identified on MR imaging in patients with a classical acute or chronic MS disease course, or in acute disseminated encephalomyelitis, with a non-fatal course.

Tumefactive or Pseudotumoural IIDDs

Infrequently, IIDDs present as single or multiple focal lesions that can be clinically and radiographically indistinguishable from a brain tumour. This situation represents a diagnostic challenge, and may require biopsy for definitive diagnosis, despite the clinical suspicion of demyelination. Given the hypercellular nature of these lesions, however, even the biopsy specimen may resemble a brain tumour. Large reactive astrocytes with fragmented chromatin (Creutzfeldt–Peters cells) are often present.

In some cases, pseudotumoural IIDDs are the first clinical and radiological manifestation of MS. More commonly, tumefactive demyelinating plaques affect patients with a known diagnosis of MS (Fig. 64-17). In rare cases, pseudotumoural IIDDs have a relapsing course, with single or multiple pseudotumoural lesions appearing over time in different locations. On CT or MR imaging the pseudotumoural plaques usually present as large, single or multiple focal lesions within the cerebral hemispheres. Clues that can help to differentiate these lesions from a brain tumour are the relatively minor mass effect and the presence of *incomplete* ring enhancement on

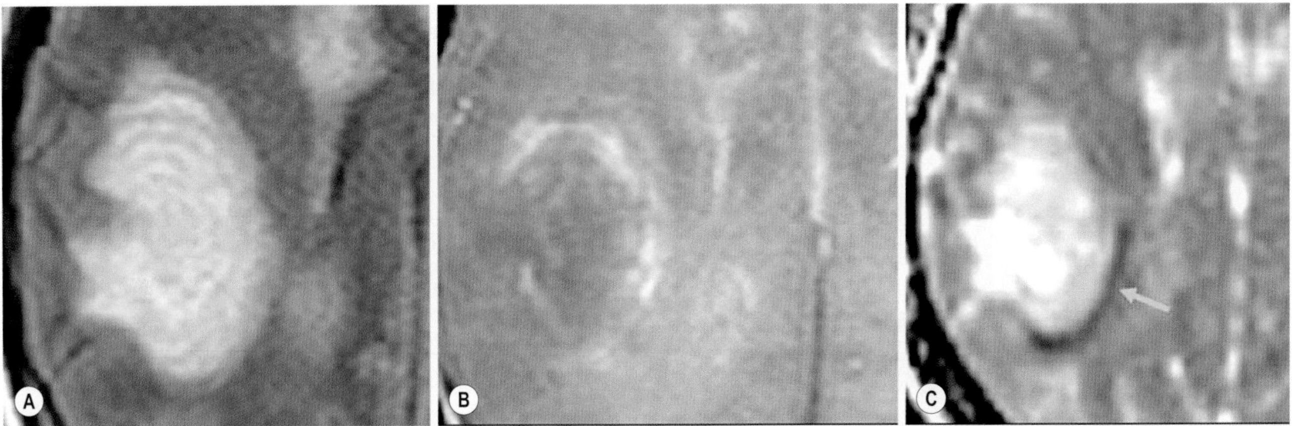

FIGURE 64-16 ■ **Baló-like lesion in patients with acute disseminated encephalomyelitis.** Transverse T_2-weighted (A) and contrast-enhanced T_1-weighted (B) MR images, and apparent diffusion coefficient (ADC) map. Observe the alternating concentric bands, peripheral contrast uptake and decreased peripheral diffusivity (C).

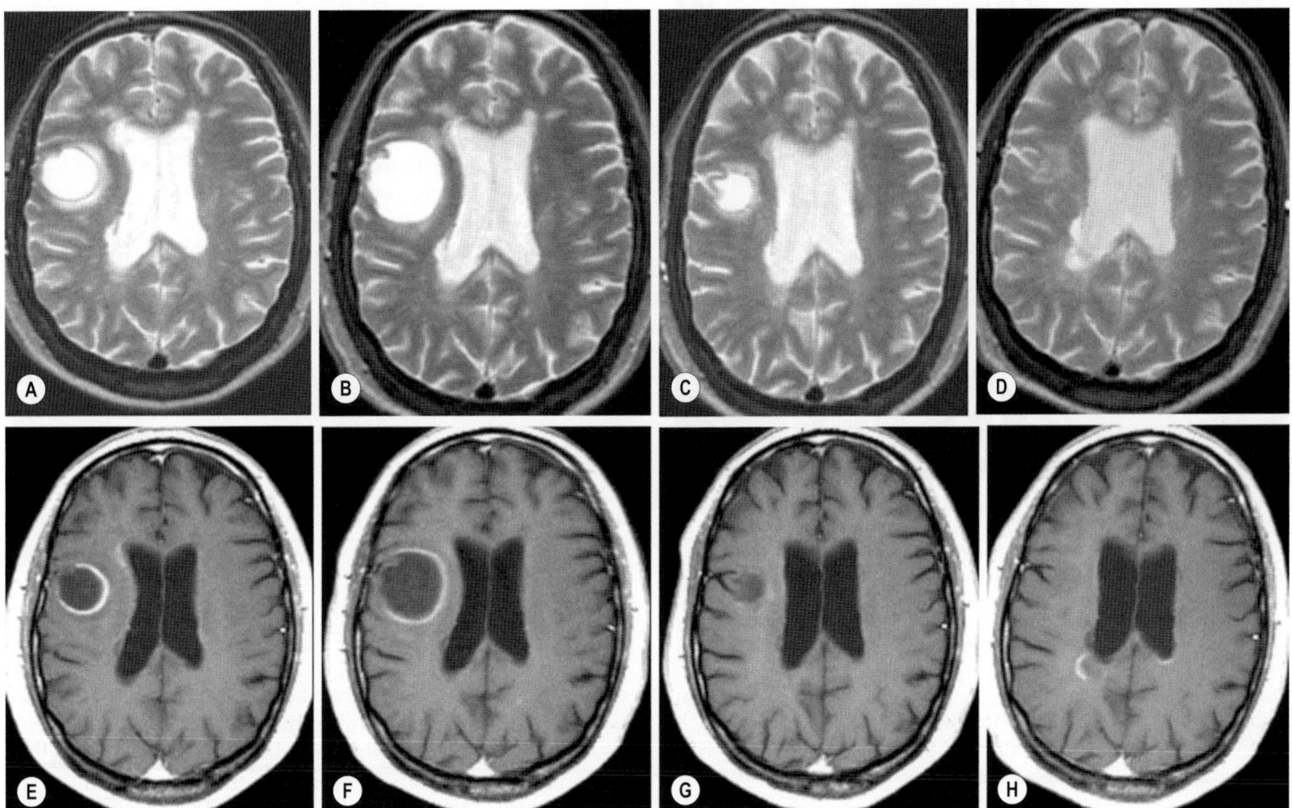

FIGURE 64-17 ■ **Tumefactive form of relapsing-remitting MS.** T_2-weighted (A–D) and contrast-enhanced T_1-weighted (E–H) serial MR images of the brain acquired over 12 months in a patient with the relapsing-remitting form of MS. Note the initial increase, and later decrease in size of the right frontal lobe pseudotumoural lesion, which is almost imperceptible on the 12-month imaging. The lesion shows an open ring-enhancing pattern of contrast uptake, with the open margin facing the grey matter. This pseudotumoural lesion was asymptomatic.

gadolinium-enhanced T_1-weighted images, with the open border facing the grey matter of the cortex or basal ganglia (Fig. 64-18),[16] sometimes associated with a rim of peripheral hypointensity on T_2-weighted sequences.

Devic's Neuromyelitis Optica

Devic's neuromyelitis optica (NMO) is an uncommon and topographically restricted form of IIDD that is best considered to be a distinct disease rather than a variant of MS. NMO is characterised by severe unilateral or bilateral optic neuritis and complete transverse myelitis, which occur simultaneously or sequentially within a varying period of time (weeks or years), without clinical involvement of other CNS regions. The incidence and prevalence of NMO are unknown, but the condition likely accounts for less than 1% of IIDDs in Caucasians. NMO affects females almost exclusively.

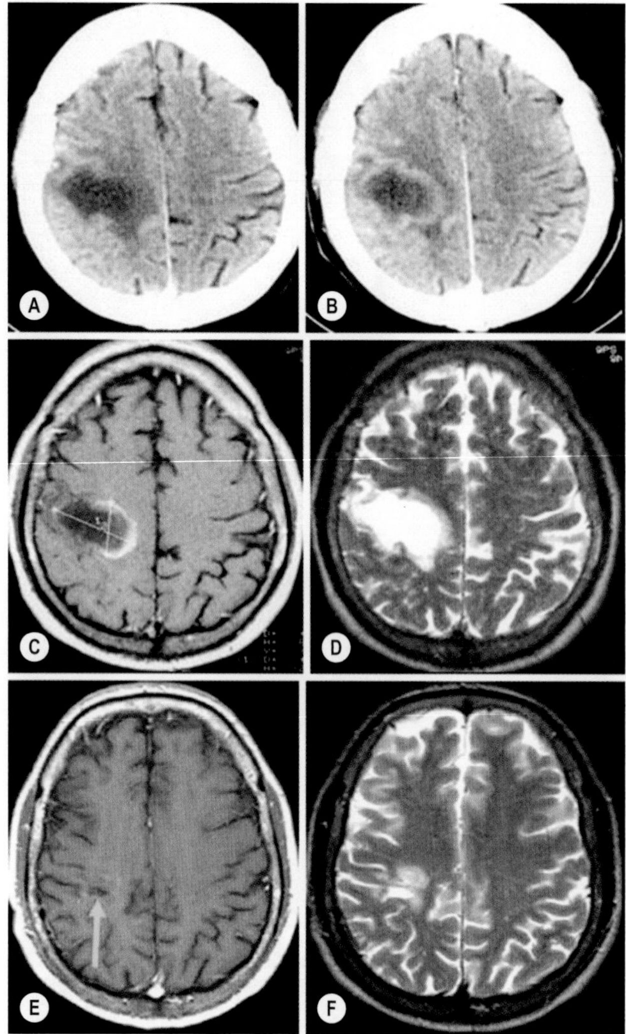

FIGURE 64-18 ■ Tumefactive inflammatory demyelinating lesion. Unenhanced and contrast-enhanced brain CT (A, B) and T_2-weighted and contrast-enhanced T_1-weighted MR images (C, D) show a posterior frontal lesion with minimal surrounding vasogenic oedema and no mass effect. Observe the ring-enhancing pattern of contrast uptake, with the open margin facing the cortical grey matter. A follow-up brain MR imaging performed one year later (E, F) shows almost complete resolution of the lesion. The necrotic focus (arrow) in the subcortical white matter corresponds to the site of a brain biopsy, which confirmed the diagnosis of inflammatory demyelinating lesion.

Approximately 85% of patients have a relapsing course with severe acute exacerbations and poor recovery, accumulating increasing neurological impairment and a high risk of respiratory failure and death due to cervical myelitis.[17]

Clinical features alone are insufficient to diagnose NMO; CSF analysis and MR imaging are usually required to confidently exclude other disorders. Cerebrospinal fluid pleocytosis (>50 leucocytes/mm^3) is often present, while CSF oligoclonal bands are seen less frequently (20–40%) than in MS patients (80–90%).

A serum autoantibody marker for NMO (NMO-IgG) has been recently developed. The target antigen of NMO-IgG is aquaporin-4, a water channel located on the foot process of the astrocyte. It is associated with tight endothelial junctions and cerebral microvessels and plays a critical role in maintaining fluid homeostasis in the CNS. This autoantibody is reported to have a sensitivity of 73% and a specificity of 91% for NMO. It may be helpful for distinguishing this form of IIDD from MS and may predict relapse and conversion to NMO in patients presenting with a single attack of longitudinally extensive myelitis. Wingerchuk et al. have proposed a revised set of criteria for diagnosing NMO (Table 64-1).[18] These new criteria remove the absolute restriction on CNS involvement beyond the optic nerves and spinal cord, allow any interval between the first events of optic neuritis and myelitis, and emphasise the specificity of longitudinally extensive spinal cord lesions on MR imaging and NMO-IgG seropositive status.

TABLE 64-1 **Revised Diagnostic Criteria for Devic's Neuromyelitis Optica (NMO)[18]**

Definite NMO:
- Optic neuritis
- Acute myelitis
- At least two of three supportive criteria:
  - Contiguous MRI spinal cord lesion extending over ≥3 vertebral segments
  - Brain MRI findings do not meet diagnostic criteria for multiple sclerosis
  - NMO-IgG seropositive status

Devic's neuromyelitis optica is a B-cell-mediated disorder that can coexist with diverse systemic autoimmune diseases, such as systemic lupus erythematosus, Sjögren's syndrome and autoimmune thyroiditis. The presence of prodromal factors such as fever, infections and autoimmune abnormalities suggest that previous infectious-inflammatory events may be involved in the pathogenesis of the disease.[19]

MR imaging of the spinal cord shows extensive cervical or thoracic tumefactive myelitis, involving more than three vertebral segments on sagittal and much of the cross-section on axial T_2-weighted images, which sometimes enhance with gadolinium for several months (Fig. 64-19). In some cases, the spinal cord lesions are small at the onset of symptoms, mimicking those in MS, and then progress in extent over time. These lesions are usually located centrally, can progress to atrophy and necrosis, and may lead to syrinx-like cavities on T_1-weighted images (Fig. 64-20). MR imaging of the brain can demonstrate unilateral or bilateral optic nerve enhancement during acute optic neuritis. In contrast to MS, white matter lesions are absent or few in the early stages, and are non-specific. Over the next years serial studies may reveal an increasing number of cerebral white matter lesions but < 10% ever meet MR imaging criteria for MS. Paediatric cases sometimes show diencephalic (hypothalamic), brainstem, or cerebral hemispheric lesions, which should be considered atypical for MS[20] (Fig. 64-21). Hypothalamic lesions seem to be relatively specific for NMO, and may be associated with clinical and laboratory evidence of hypothalamic endocrinopathy.

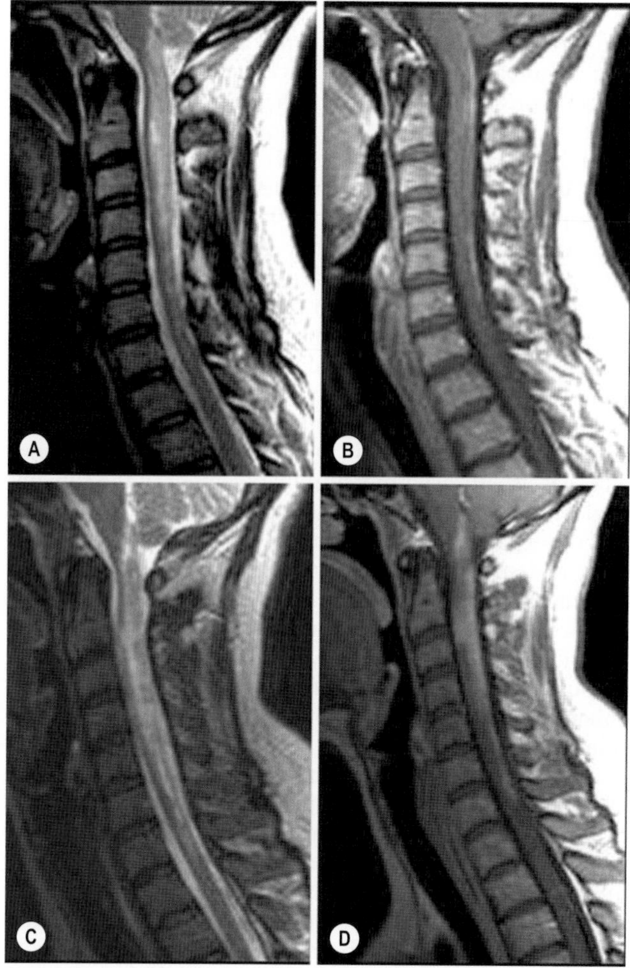

FIGURE 64-19 ■ **Devic's neuromyelitis optica (NMO).** Sagittal fast spin-echo T_2-weighted and contrast-enhanced T_1-weighted MR images of the cervical spinal cord obtained serially over a period of 4 months. Baseline examination (A, B) shows a large spinal cord lesion extending to the brainstem. Follow-up MR image acquired 4 months later (C, D) shows lesion extension to the thoracic cord and persistent and more extensive contrast uptake.

Acute Disseminated Encephalomyelitis

Acute disseminated encephalomyelitis (ADEM) is a severe, immune-mediated inflammatory disorder of the CNS that is usually triggered by an inflammatory response to viral or bacterial infections and vaccinations.[21] It predominantly affects the white matter of the brain and spinal cord. In the absence of specific biological markers, the diagnosis of ADEM is based on the clinical and radiological features (Table 64-2). Although ADEM usually has a monophasic course, recurrent or multiphasic forms

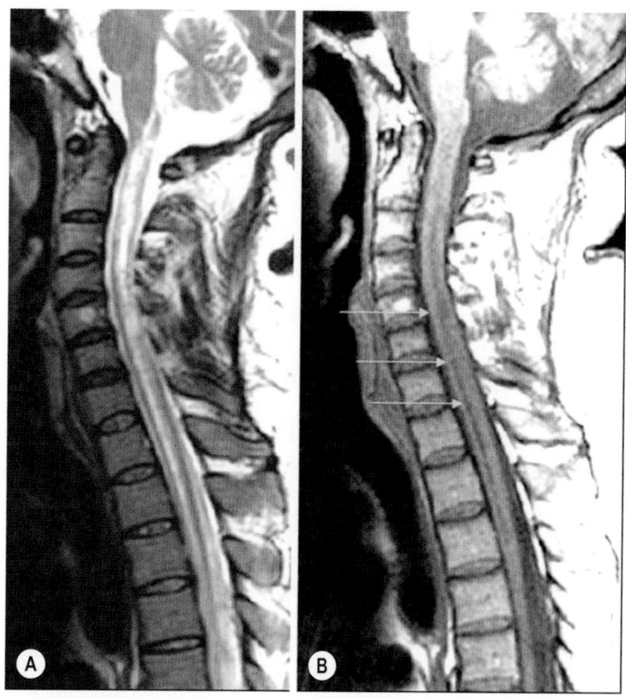

FIGURE 64-20 ■ **(A, B) Devic's neuromyelitis optica (NMO).** Sagittal T_2-weighted and T_1-weighted MR images of the cervicodorsal spinal cord showing a long syrinx-like spinal cord lesion extending to the lower medulla (arrows).

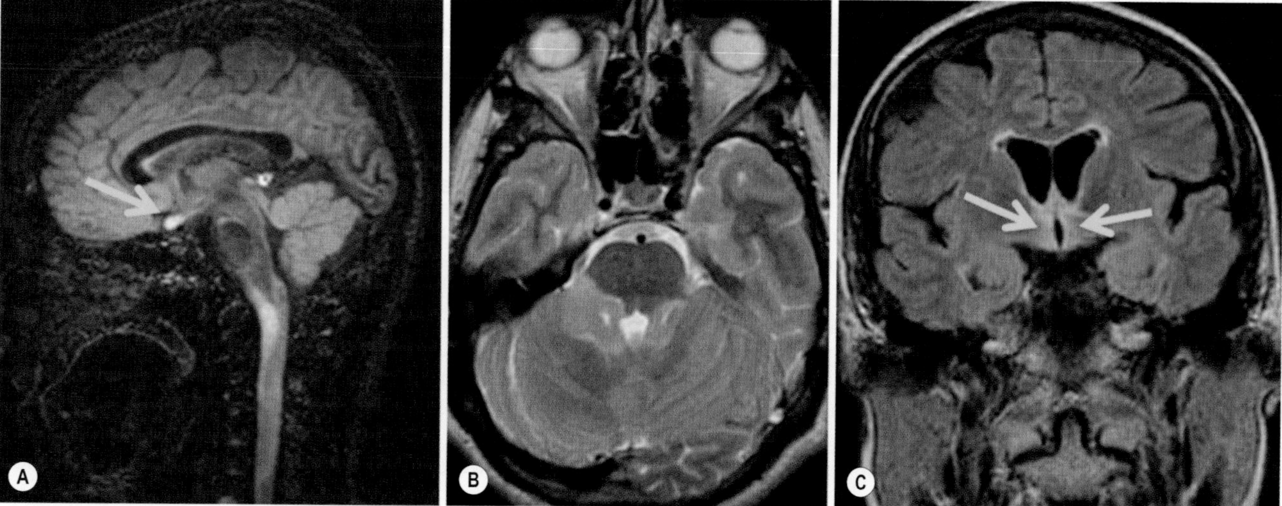

FIGURE 64-21 ■ **Devic's neuromyelitis optica (NMO).** Brain MRI showing hyperintense T_2 lesions (arrows) involving the optic chiasm and proximal segment of the cervical cord (A), the brainstem (B) and hypothalamic region (C).

TABLE 64-2 **Clinical, Biological and Radiological Differences between Acute Disseminated Encephalomyelitis (ADEM) and Multiple Sclerosis (MS)**

	ADEM	MS
Age	≤10 years	>10 years
Gender	Male = female	Male < female
Prior flu	Very frequent	Variable
Encephalopathy	Required	Rare
Attacks	Fluctuate over 3 months	Separated by >1 month
Large MRI lesions	Frequent	Rare
Lesion margins	Poorly defined	Well defined
Deep grey matter	Frequently involved	Rarely involved
Spinal cord lesions	Extensive	Small
Longitudinal MRI	Resolution	New lesions
CSF white blood cell count >50	Frequent	Very rare
CSF oligoclonal bands	Variable	Frequent

have been reported, raising diagnostic difficulties in distinguishing these cases from MS.

Acute disseminated encephalomyelitis affects children more commonly than adults, and in contrast to MS, shows no sex preponderance. The estimated incidence is 0.8 per 100,000 population per year. In 50–75% of cases, the clinical onset of disease is preceded by viral or bacterial infections, usually non-specific upper respiratory tract infections. ADEM may also develop following a vaccination (postimmunisation encephalomyelitis). Although ADEM is relatively rare, it is becoming increasingly important, since vaccination schedules have expanded over the past years, particularly for children. Typically, there is a latency of 7 to 14 days between a febrile illness and the onset of neurological symptoms. In the case of vaccination-associated ADEM, this latency period may be longer.

Patients commonly present with non-specific polyfocal symptoms, which developed subacutely over a period of days, frequently associated with encephalopathy that is relatively uncommon in MS and defined as an alteration in consciousness (e.g. stupor, lethargy) or behavioral change unexplained by fever, systemic illness or postictal symptoms. In general, the disease is self-limiting and the prognostic outcome favourable. Neurological symptoms usually developed subacutely over a period of days and lead to hospitalisation within a week. Although ataxia, altered level of consciousness and brainstem symptoms are frequently present in both paediatric and adult cases, certain signs and symptoms appear to be age-related. In childhood ADEM, long-lasting fever and headaches occur more frequently, while in adult cases, motor and sensory deficits predominate. According to the International Most of ADEM have a monophasic course, although a small proportion (<4%) of patients have a multiphasic course defined as a new encephalopathic event consistent with ADEM, separated by three months after the initial illness but not followed by any further events. The second ADEM event can involve either new or a re-emergence of prior neurologic symptoms, signs and MRI findings. Relapsing disease following ADEM that occurs beyond a second encephalopathic event is no longer consistent with multiphasic ADEM but rather indicates a chronic disorder, most often leading to the diagnosis of MS or NMO (22). Not infrequently, an ADEM attack is the first manifestation of the classical relapsing form of MS. In fact, 30% of patients who meet the ADEM criteria at initial presentation ultimately receive a diagnosis of MS. Hence, ADEM is likely to be overdiagnosed on the basis of the initial clinical presentation and MR findings. For this reason, presumptive diagnoses of ADEM mandates close clinical and MR imaging follow-up.

Unlike lesions in MS, the lesions of ADEM are often large, patchy and poorly marginated on MR imaging. There is usually asymmetrical involvement of the subcortical and central white matter and cortical grey–white junction of cerebral hemispheres, the cerebellum, brainstem and spinal cord (Fig. 64-22). The grey matter of the thalami and basal ganglia is frequently affected, particularly in children, typically in a symmetrical pattern.[23] Lesions confined to the periventricular white matter and corpus callosum are less common than in MS. Contrast enhancement is not a common feature in ADEM. The spinal cord is involved in less than 30% of ADEM patients,[23] predominantly in the thoracic region (Fig. 64-22). The cord lesion is typically large, causes swelling of the cord and shows variable enhancement. Most ADEM patients show partial or complete of the MR imaging abnormalities within a few months after treatment. This evolution is positively associated with a final diagnosis of ADEM. Because ADEM is usually a monophasic disease, the focal lesions would be expected to appear and mature simultaneously and to resolve or remain unchanged, with no new lesions on follow-up MR images. Not infrequently, however, new lesions are seen on follow-up MRI within the first month after the initial attack. Most MR lesions appear early in the course of the disease, supporting the clinical diagnosis, In some cases there may be a delay of more than 1 month between the onset of symptoms and the appearance of lesions on MR imaging. Therefore, a normal brain MR imaging obtained within the first days after the onset of neurological symptoms suggestive of ADEM does not exclude this diagnosis.

Acute Disseminated Encephalomyelitis Variants

Bickerstaff's Encephalitis. Bickerstaff's encephalitis is a rare acute syndrome considered to be a subgroup of ADEM, in which inflammation appears to be confined to the brainstem.[24] The syndrome consists of localised encephalitis of the brainstem, commonly preceded by a febrile illness, and has a benign prognosis. T_2-weighted MR imaging usually shows an extensive high-signal-intensity lesion involving the midbrain, the pons and sometimes the thalamus. The clinical outcome is good and parallels resolution of the MR imaging lesions (Fig. 64-23). The pathogenesis of Bickerstaff's encephalitis is uncertain; however, the absence of CSF oligoclonal bands

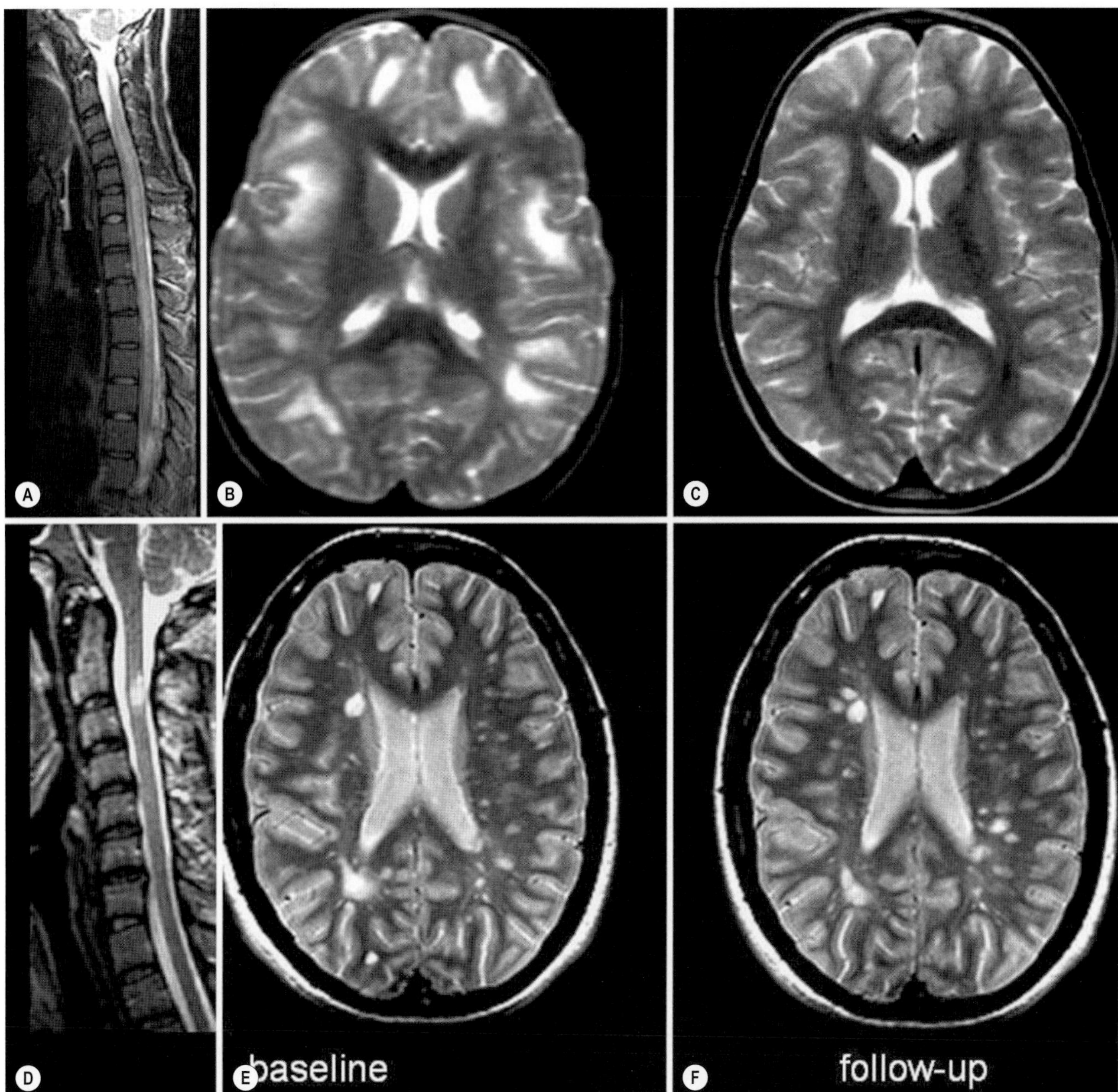

FIGURE 64-22 ■ **MR imaging differences between acute disseminated encephalomyelitis (ADEM) (A–C) and multiple sclerosis (MS) (D–F).** Spinal cord lesions are extensive in ADEM and are usually associated with large, poorly defined subcortical white matter lesions on brain MR imaging. In MS, symptomatic cord lesions are usually small and commonly associated with subclinical white matter brain lesions of the type seen in MS. In ADEM, longitudinal studies usually show resolution of lesions, while in MS, new lesions appear (arrows).

and resolution of the clinical symptoms and MR imaging lesions suggest an inflammatory origin and make demyelination unlikely.

Acute Disseminated Necrohaemorrhagic Leucoencephalitis. Acute disseminated necrohaemorrhagic leucoencephalitis (acute haemorrhagic encephalomyelitis or Hurst's disease) is an uncommon condition that has been observed in patients of all ages. It is thought to be a hyperacute form or the maximal variant of ADEM. This usually fatal disease manifests clinically with abrupt onset of fever, neck stiffness, hemiplegia or other focal signs, seizures and decreasing level of consciousness.[21] At autopsy, the brain is congested and swollen, sometimes asymmetrically, and herniation is frequent. Multiple petechial haemorrhages are distributed diffusely throughout the brain. The perivascular lesions chiefly consist of ball-like or ring haemorrhages surrounding necrotic venules, sometimes with fibrinous exudates within the vessel wall or extending into adjacent tissue. Perivenous demyelinating lesions, identical to those occurring in ADEM, may also be present. Perivascular cuffs of mononuclear cells, often with neutrophils, are seen. T_2*-weighted MR sequences show large regions

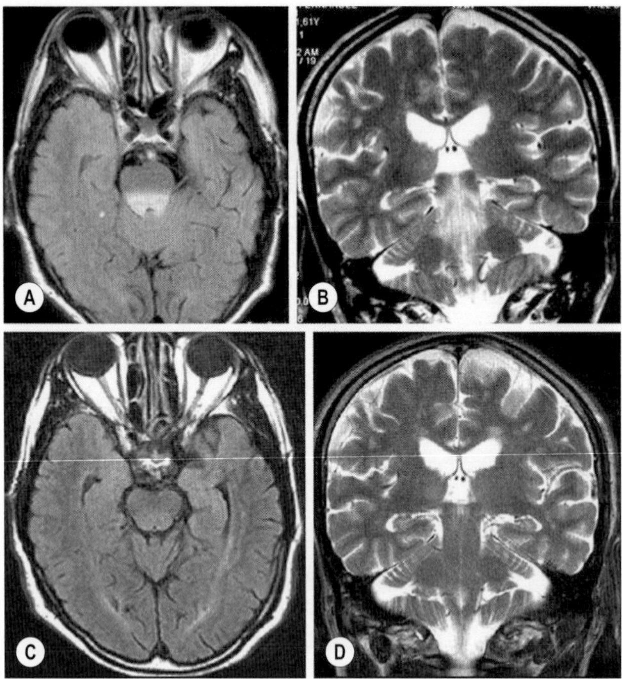

FIGURE 64-23 ■ Bickerstaff's encephalitis. Initial brain MR imaging (transverse fast-FLAIR and coronal fast spin-echo T_2-weighted sequences) shows an extensive brainstem lesion (A, B) that fully resolved in a follow-up study obtained 2 months later (C, D).

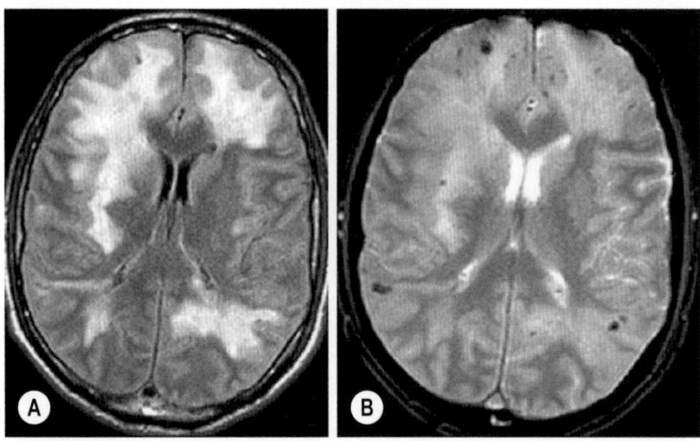

FIGURE 64-24 ■ Acute haemorrhagic leucoencephalitis (Hurst's encephalitis). Axial FLAIR MR image shows an extensive abnormal signal affecting the periventricular and subcortical white matter (A), with acute haemorrhagic foci visualised as markedly hypointense areas within the white matter lesions on the T_2*-weighted gradient-echo MR image (B).

of demyelination and petechial haemorrhages in the peripheral white matter of both cerebral hemispheres (Fig. 64-24).

PRIMARY AND SECONDARY VASCULITIS

Central Nervous System Vasculitis

There are many different causes of central nervous system (CNS) vasculitis and the diagnosis should always be suspected in patients who present with severe headache, focal or multifocal neurological dysfunction, altered cognition or consciousness, and non-specific MR or CT imaging findings. More often the angiographic picture is more convincing but the definitive diagnosis can only be made after confirmation by CNS biopsy. Since the distribution of the CNS vasculitis can be segmented and focal, a positive biopsy is enough to confirm the diagnosis, while one single negative biopsy does not exclude it.[25] Vasculitis has been reported to be responsible for 3–5% of strokes occurring in patients younger than 50 years of age. The CNS vasculitis can be divided into primary and secondary. There are no exact numbers of the incidence rate of either the primary or secondary vasculitides of the CNS. However, primary CNS vasculitis is relatively uncommon but has a generally poor prognosis.

Primary Central Nervous System Vasculitis

Primary angiitis of the CNS (PACNS) is a rare and severe idiopathic disorder limited to the central nervous system that results in multifocal inflammation of predominantly small arteries, but can also involve medium-sized leptomeningeal, cortical and subcortical arteries, and veins of the cortex and leptomeninges.

Its hallmark is a striking inflammatory alteration of the affected vessel wall. The mean age of onset is 50 years, and men are affected twice as commonly as women. The most frequent initial symptoms of PACNS are headaches and encephalopathy. Strokes or persistent neurological deficits occur in 40% of patients with PACNS, and transient ischaemic attacks have been reported in 30–50% of patients but occur in less than 20% of patients at the onset of disease.[26] Less commonly, seizures may also occur as the presenting symptom. MRI of the brain is abnormal in more than 90% of patients, but the patterns are not specific and are seen predominantly in the subcortical white matter, followed by the deep grey and white matter, and the cerebral cortex (Fig. 64-25). Other less common findings are infarcts, mass lesions, and confluent white matter lesions, which can be mistaken for multiple sclerosis, or cortical laminar necrosis. However, intracranial haemorrhages are infrequent.[27] Parenchymal and leptomeningeal enhancement can be seen in up to 35% of patients. The cerebrospinal fluid (CSF) analysis is abnormal in 80–90% of the patients with modest, non-specific elevations in total protein level or white blood cell count. Angiography has a low sensitivity and low specificity. Common findings are those seeing in other forms of vasculitis, including single or multiple areas of segmental narrowing and dilatations along the course of a vessel, and vascular occlusions (Fig. 64-26).

The most frequent mimic of PACNS is a group of disorders known collectively as the reversible cerebral vasoconstriction syndromes (RCVS). Features that are more suggestive of RVCS are acute thunderclap headache, with normal CSF analysis. The final diagnosis of PACNS is established by brain biopsy. The typical biopsy specimen reveals segmental inflammation of small arteries and arterioles, intimal proliferation and fibrosis, with sparing of the media, and in some cases multinucleate

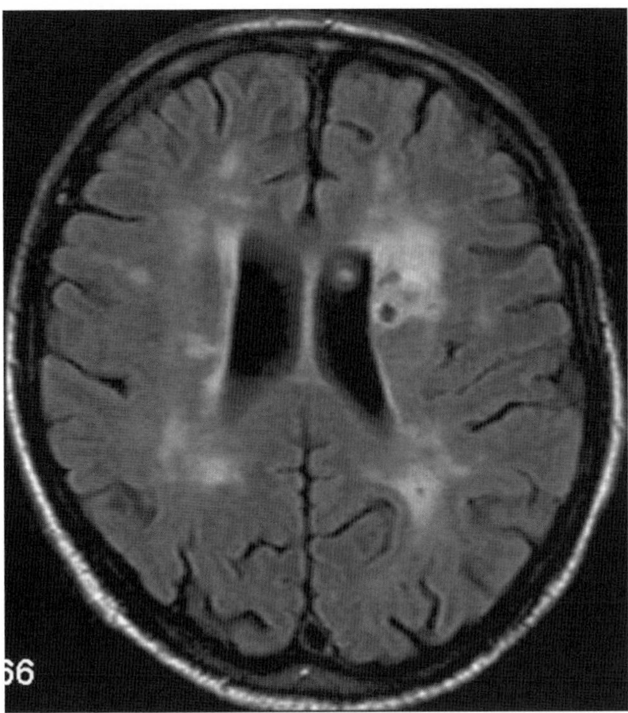

FIGURE 64-25 ■ Axial fluid-attenuated inversion recovery (FLAIR) image demonstrating diffuse increased signal in the periventricular, deep and subcortical white matter in a patient diagnosed with primary angiitis of the CNS (PACNS).

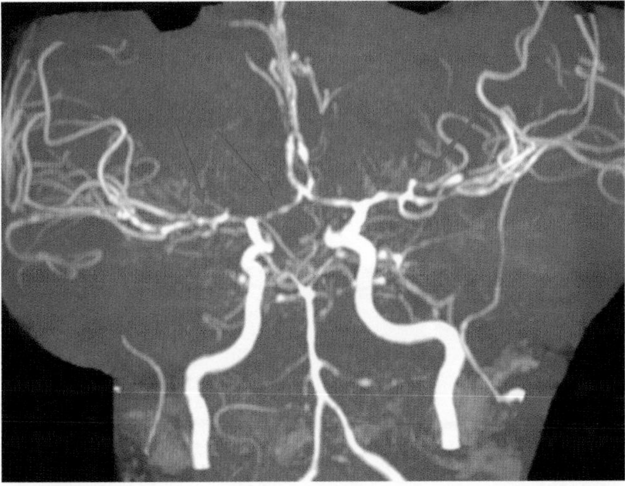

FIGURE 64-26 ■ MR angiography (MRA) of the intracranial vessels demonstrates narrowing and irregularities of the right middle cerebral artery and of other medium-sized intracranial vessels.

giant Langerhans cells.[28] Since PACNS is fatal if untreated, patients with biopsy-proven PACNS are treated with cyclophosphamide and prednisone.

Secondary Central Nervous System Vasculitis

Secondary CNS vasculitis of the nervous system caused by an underlying disease is more commonly seen than the primary vasculitides and may involve either the CNS or the peripheral nervous system (PNS) or both. They can be further classified into a systemic disorder or infection with or without evidence of systemic vasculitis. One of those related to infection is the one caused by the varicella-zoster virus that might present fever, headache, seizures or stroke-like symptoms due to with encephalitis secondary to vasculitis in large or small vessels. MRI might demonstrate multiple areas of ischaemic and haemorrhagic infarcts of varying size, involving both the grey and white matter. Human immunodeficiency virus and herpes virus infections are other less common viral causes of secondary CNS vasculitis. Uncommonly, CNS vasculitis has been reported in association with some malignant conditions and drug abuse, including amphetamines and related sympathomimetic agents, cocaine and opioids.

Primary Systemic Vasculitis with Central Nervous System Involvement

CNS vasculitis can occur as a systemic manifestation of other primary small, medium or large vessel vasculitits such as giant cell arteritis, Takayasu's arteritis, Kawasaki's disease, Wegener's granulomatosis, polyarteritis nodosa, and Churg–Strauss syndrome.

Giant Cell Arteritis. The most common form of primary systemic vasculitis is giant cell arteritis (temporal arteritis) defined as a granulomatous arteritis of the aorta and its major branches often involving the extracranial branches of the carotid artery such as the temporal artery. It usually occurs in patients older than 50 years. Most common neurological complications are retinal ischaemia, ischaemic optic neuropathy and diplopia secondary to ischaemia of the extraocular muscles. Stroke might occur, even if uncommon, secondary to the involvement of the posterior intracranial circulation. There is a known association with polymyalgia rheumatica and the combination of increased CRP value with an elevated ESR has a high diagnostic specificity.[29] A daily dose of corticosteroids is the classic treatment.

Takayasu's Arteritis. Takayasu's arteritis is a granulomatous arteritis of the aorta and its major branches and is considered a form of giant cell arteritis, affecting younger individuals under 50 years of age. CNS involvement is fairly common and is seen in up to one-third of the patients secondary to carotid artery stenosis, and cerebral hypoperfusion.

Kawasaki's Disease. Kawasaki's disease, generally affecting infants and children, is an acute febrile vasculitis that predominantly involves medium-sized arteries. However, large, and small arteries might also be affected. Its aetiology is still unknown even if an infectious cause has been suggested. Neurological symptoms include seizures, facial palsy and, rarely, cerebral infarction.

Wegener's Granulomatosis. Wegener's granulomatosis is an inflammatory multisystem disorder characterised by necrotising granulomas in the upper and lower respiratory tract, with or without focal segmental glomerulonephritis and a systemic necrotising vasculitis, affecting small-to-medium-sized vessels. Neurological involvement has been reported, with the most common symptoms being mononeuritis multiplex, followed by distal symmetric sensorimotor neuropathy. Less common is involvement of the brain and meninges that can present as intracerebral or subarachnoid haemorrhage, and cerebral arterial or venous thrombosis. Typical CNS findings such as diffuse linear or focal dural thickening and enhancement, infarcts, non-specific white matter changes, an enlarged pituitary gland with infundibular thickening and enhancement, granulomatous lesions and atrophy are well presented on MRI.[30]

Polyathritis Nodosa. A classic systemic necrotising vasculitis that affects medium-sized and small vessels is polyarteritis nodosa (PAN). Neurologically, both CNS and PNS occur in PAN. CNS involvement is seen in up to 40% of patients and may occur as diffuse encephalopathy with cognitive decline and seizures secondary to the involvement of small arteries. Stroke-like symptoms with focal or multifocal findings are seen secondary to involvement of medium-sized arteries. Other uncommon findings are cranial nerve palsies, intracerebral or subarachnoid haemorrhages or spinal cord involvement secondary to vasculitis of the spinal arteries.

NEUROSARCOIDOSIS

Sarcoidosis is a multisystem disease process of unknown aetiology whose pathogenesis involves formation of an inflammatory lesion known as a granuloma. The lungs are affected most frequently, but other organs like the eyes, the CNS, heart, kidneys, bones and joints may also be affected. CNS involvement—neurosarcoidosis—is seen in approximately 25% of patients with systemic sarcoidosis, although it is subclinical in most of these cases. In over 80% of established cases of neurosarcoidosis the chest radiograph is abnormal. Neurosarcoidosis is slightly more common in women than men. Cranial neuropathy, particularly facial nerve palsy, often multifocal with other neuropathies, is the most common clinical presentation. Other clinical presentations of neurosarcoidosis include encephalopathy, peripheral neuropathy with muscle weakness and sensory loss, meningitis, seizure, cerebellar ataxia, psychiatric disorders, spinal cord dysfunction and myopathy. MRI is the method of choice in the diagnostic evaluation and follow-up of patients with neurosarcoidosis and both FLAIR images and images after administration of gadolinium are recommended to increase sensitivity. The most frequent finding is meningeal disease with dural thickening and masses that can mimic meningioma and enhancement of the basal and suprasellar meninges. Other common MRI findings include non-enhancing lesions with high signal on T_2-weighted images in the periventricular white matter and brainstem that might mimic MS lesions, multiple small contrast-enhancing granulomas often located superficially in brain parenchyma bordering the basal cisterns (Fig. 64-27), enhancement of the optic nerve and other cranial nerves, and intramedullary spinal cord lesions[31] (Fig. 64-28). Less often, subependymal granulomatous infiltration causes hydrocephalus (Fig. 64-29). There is no known cure for sarcoidiosis. Treatment is indicated if symptoms are severe or progressive and might include prednisone to reduce inflammation, hormone replacement and immunosuppressive treatment if needed. The goal of treatment is to reduce symptoms.

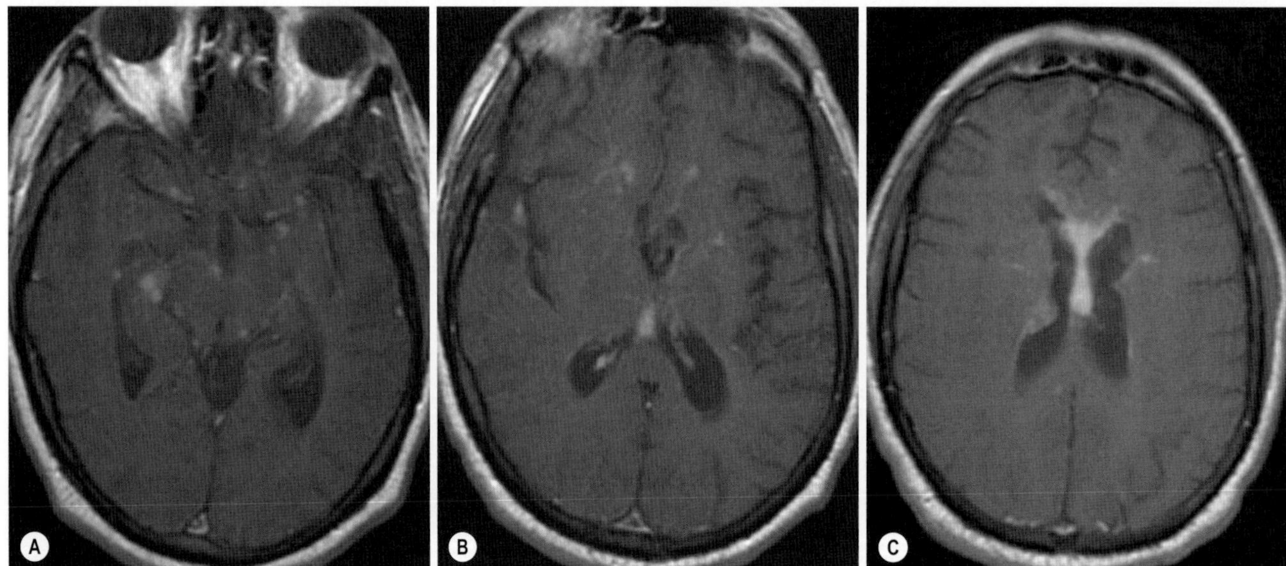

FIGURE 64-27 ■ Axial post-contrast-enhanced T_1-weighted images of the brain in a 40-year-old woman with neurosarcoidosis demonstrate multiple contrast-enhancing lesions on the leptomenginal surfaces (A), and subependymal lesions (B, C) with slight enlargement of the lateral ventricles (C).

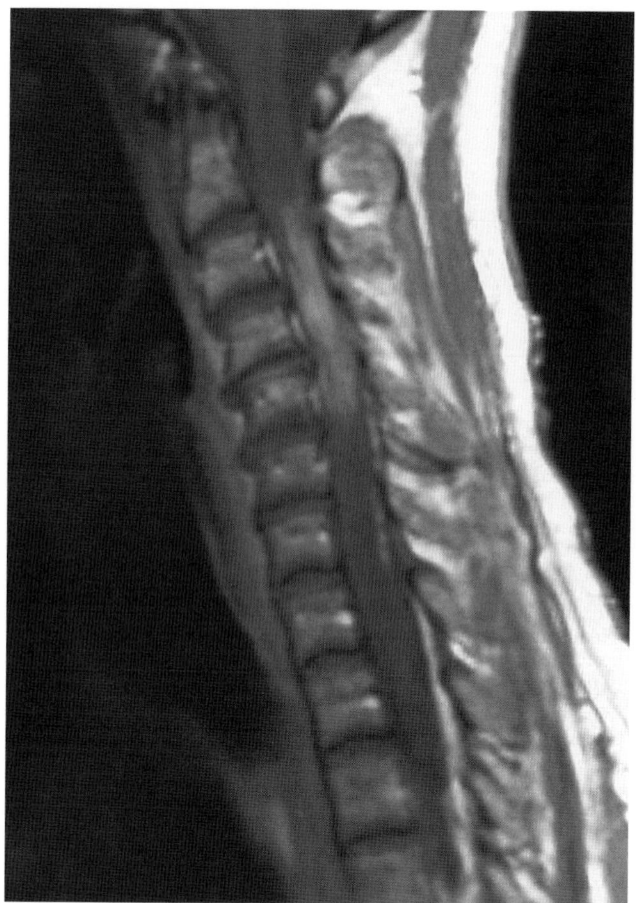

FIGURE 64-28 ■ Sagittal post-contrast-enhanced T_1-weighted image in a patient with known neurosarcoidosis demonstrates en focal pathological enhancing intramedullary lesion in the cervical cord.

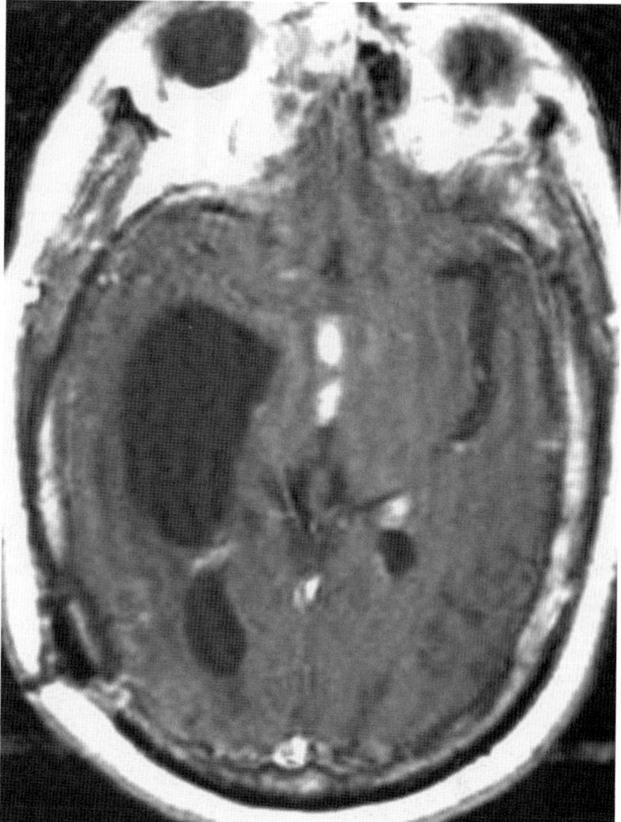

FIGURE 64-29 ■ Transverse contrast-enhanced T_1-weighted image demonstrates multiple enhancing subependymal granulomatous infiltrative lesions causing obstructing hydrocephalus with enlargement of the temporal horn of the right lateral ventricle.

BEHÇET'S DISEASE

Behçet's disease (BD) is a multisystemic, vascular inflammatory disease of unknown origin involving the larger vessels that may present with a classic triad of oral and genital ulcerations with uveitis. Patients present with different focal or multifocal neurological problems. The most common neurological symptom is severe headache; other common symptoms are weakness, and different cognitive and behavioural changes. Isolated optic neuritis, aseptic meningitis and intracranial haemorrhage secondary to ruptured aneurysms are rare manifestations of the disease. Neurological involvement in BD is a cause of major morbidity, and approximately 50% of the patients are moderate-to-severely disable after 10 years of disease.[32] CNS involvement most often occurs as a chronic meningoencephalitis.[9] MRI is very sensitive to demonstrate the typical reversible inflammatory parenchymal lesions generally located within the brainstem, occasionally with extension to the diencephalon, or within the basal ganglia, the periventricular and subcortical white matter[33,34] (Fig. 64-30). Rarely, the lesions may resemble those seen in MS. Brainstem atrophy is seen in chronic cases. Neuro-BD is treated with either oral or intravenous prednisolone until improvement.

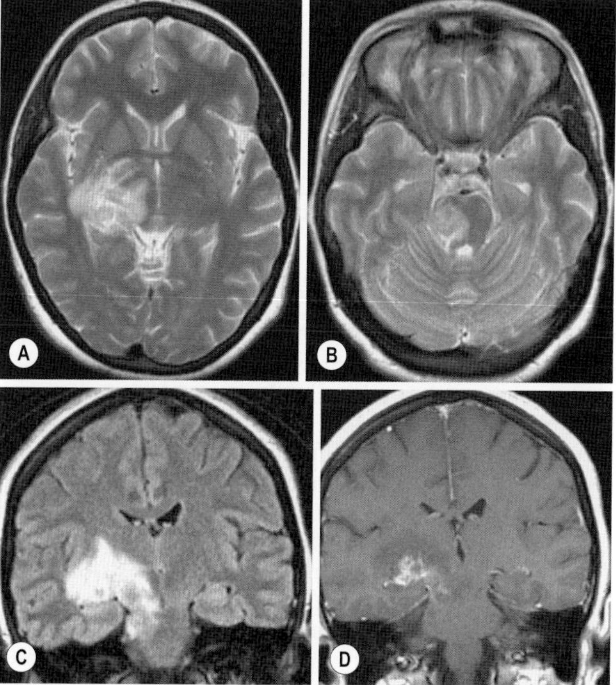

FIGURE 64-30 ■ **Neuro-Behçet's disease.** Transverse T_2-weighted images (A, B) and coronal T_2 FLAIR and contrast-enhanced T_1-weighted images (C, D). Observe the contrast-enhancing right pontomesencephalic lesion that extends to the basal ganglia. (Courtesy of Dr. A. Rovira-Gols, UDIAT-Parc Tauli, Sabadell. Spain.)

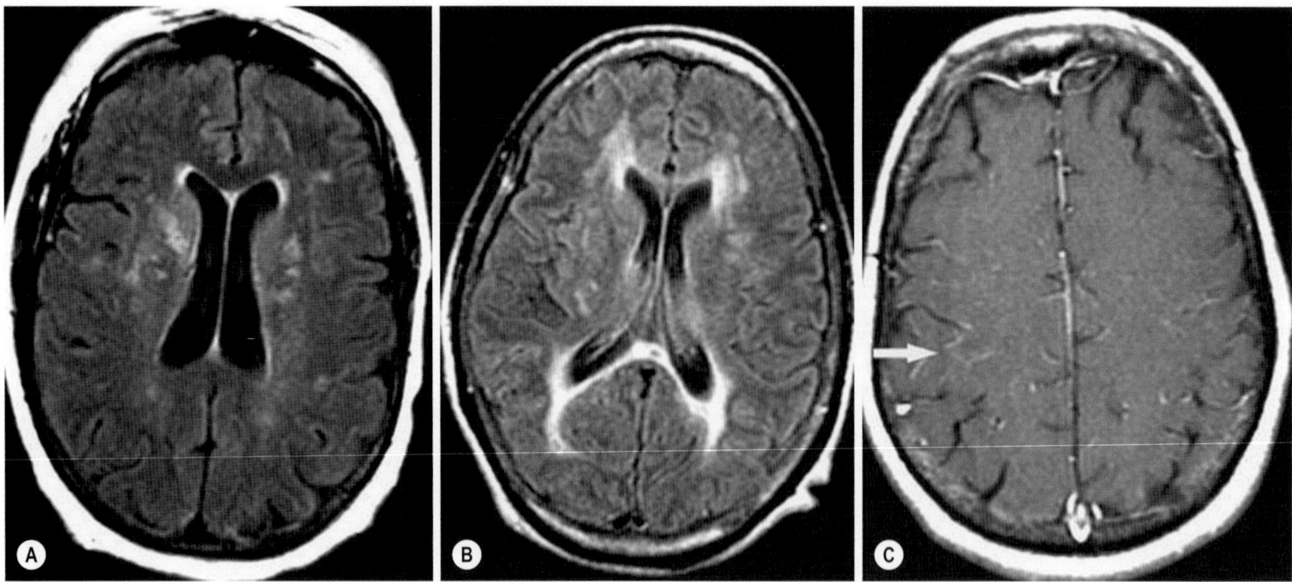

FIGURE 64-31 ■ Brain MRI in a 45-year-old woman with SLE. Axial fluid-attenuated inversion recovery (FLAIR) demonstrates small foci of increased signal in the periventricular and deep white matter (A) and more confluent areas of increased signal in the periventricular white matter (B). Axial post-contrast-enhanced image demonstrates diffuse faint pathological contrast enhancement (arrow) in a systemic lupus erythematosus female patient with vasculitis (C).

SYSTEMIC LUPUS ERYTHEMATOSUS

Systemic lupus erythematosus (SLE) is an autoimmune disorder with an annual incidence of 2.0–7.6 per 100,000 and with myriad manifestations. One of those manifestations is neuropsychiatric systemic lupus erythematosus (NPSLE), which occurs in 25–70% of patients with SLE and is associated with increased morbidity and mortality. Unfortunately, NPSLE patients have a worse prognosis and more cumulative damage than patients with SLE alone. Currently, the underlying causes as to why patients develop NPSLE are still unknown and unclear. Investigators speculate that CNS damage is secondary to autoantibody production, microangiopathy, atherosclerosis, or intrathecal production of proinflammatory cytokines.[35] Histopathologically, patients with NPSLE might show multifocal microinfarcts, cortical atrophy, gross infarcts, haemorrhage, ischaemic demyelination and patchy multiple sclerosis-like areas of demyelination. The clinical manifestations of NPSLE include psychosis, stroke and epilepsy, in addition to more subtle symptoms such as headache and neurocognitive dysfunction.[36] Patients with concomitant antiphospholipid antibodies (APL-ab) are at additional risk for neuropsychiatric events. Lupus patients are also at increased risk for a wide range of CNS events related to immunosuppressive therapy, including infection and drug toxicity, hypercoagulability and accelerated atherosclerosis. CNS vasculitis and/or cerebritis represent a potentially severe form of NPSLE and may present with seizures, movements disorders, altered consciousness, stroke and coma.[37] While CNS inflammation is uncommon in SLE, this diagnosis must be entertained any time a lupus patient presents with CNS signs or symptoms. Although clinical assessment is the keystone in the diagnosis of NPSLE, the diagnosis is often difficult and remains presumptive in some patients. MR findings are variable and in some cases the MRI is unremarkable. However, abnormal conventional MRI findings are common in both SLE and NPSLE patients and range from non-specific small punctate focal lesions in white matter (present in the majority of NPSLE patients, but not specific) (Fig. 64-31) to more severe findings such as cortical atrophy, ventricular dilation, cerebral oedema, cerebral infarctions, intracranial haemorrhage and signs of vasculitis[38–40] (Fig. 64-32). These findings are attributed to different mechanisms, including thrombosis, vasculitis and antibody-mediated neuronal injury imaging. Several MR spectroscopy studies have demonstrated a decrease in *N*-acetylaspartate (NAA), known as a neuronal marker, and an increase in the choline peak, a marker for cell membrane turnover and activity.[40] These changes in metabolic activity are suggestive of neuronal loss and axonal damage that, based on recent studies, might be in part reversible after treatment. Another metabolite, *myo*-inositol (mI), has been found to be elevated early in the course of an active flare of NPSLE prior to changes on MRI. Studies using diffusion-weighted imaging and magnetic transfer have demonstrated that NPSLE patients have increased whole-brain diffusivity as well as differences in grey and white matter compared to healthy individuals.[41,42] Altogether, these findings are suggestive of the presence of subtle and widespread damage in the brain parenchyma. Reduced structural integrity in the brain, such as axonal loss and/or demyelination, is a possible aetiology for this widespread damage.

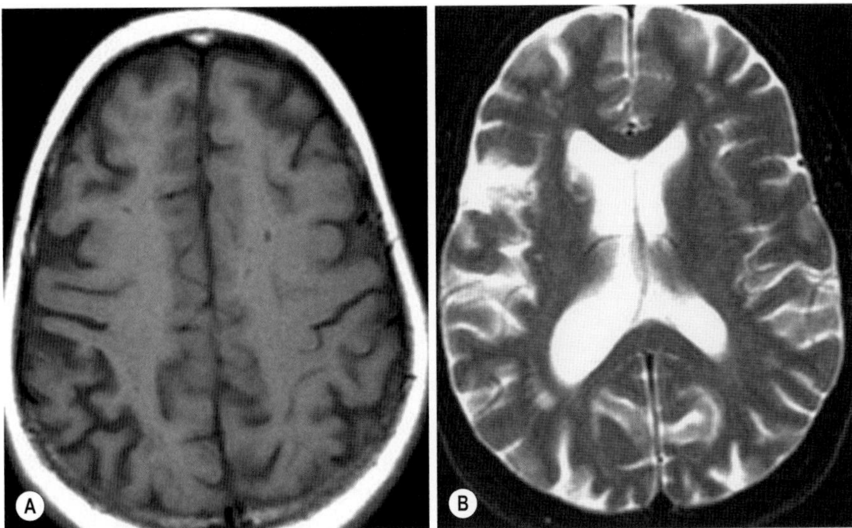

FIGURE 64-32 ■ Axial T_1-weighted (A) and T_2-weighted (B) MR images demonstrate mild-to-moderate cortical atrophy in a 35-year-old woman with long-standing systemic lupus erythematosus.

METABOLIC AND TOXIC DISORDERS IN THE ADULT

While in childhood metabolic diseases are in most cases congenital on inherited bases, toxic and metabolic diseases are usually acquired disorders in adults. CNS exposure to toxic factors can be endogenous or exogenous, and happens when metabolic toxins or exogenous toxic substances circulate in high concentrations in the blood and accumulate in the CNS, causing intoxication. Structures with high metabolic activity are mainly involved. This may be the reason of the predominant involvement of basal ganglia and brainstem, without or with cortical involvement. White matter involvement may be present, but is usually less noticeable than in hereditary metabolic diseases.

Ethanol Intoxication

Brain abnormalities in alcoholics include atrophy, Marchiafava–Bignami disease, Wernicke's encephalopathy, osmotic myelinolysis, and consequences of liver cirrhosis such as hepatic encephalopathy and coagulopathy.[43,44] All the reported entities are not specific to alcohol and can be found in many other toxic or metabolic conditions. Ethanol direct brain toxicity is caused by under-regulation of receptors of *N*-methyl-D-aspartate, abnormal catabolism of homocysteine, resulting in an increased susceptibility to glutamate excitatory and toxic effects. Moreover, immune response occurs mediated by lipid peroxidation products that bind to neurons, resulting in neurotoxicity.[45] Neuroimaging studies show a characteristic distribution of loss of volume: initially there is infratentorial predominance with atrophy of the vermis and the cerebellum. Frontal and temporal atrophy is subsequently evident, followed by diffuse atrophy of the brain. The possibility of partial reversibility of these alterations is also observed. In pregnancy, ethanol determines inhibition of maturation of Bergmann's fibres of cerebellum, with consequential marked cerebellar atrophy (Fig. 64-33).

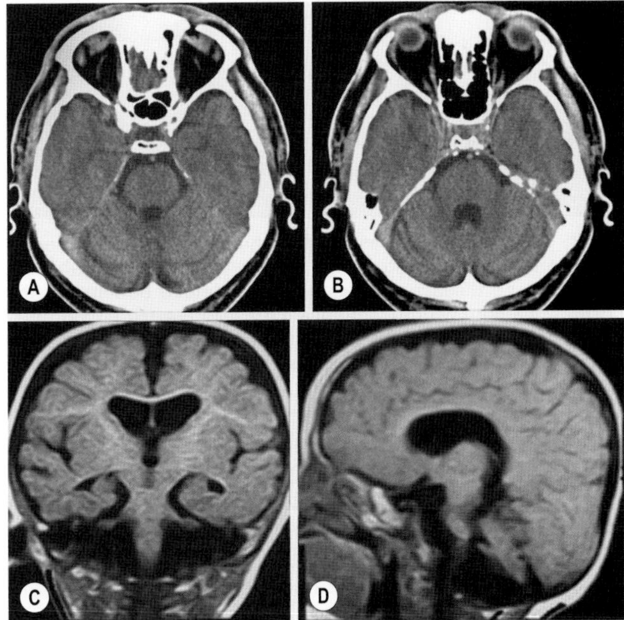

FIGURE 64-33 ■ (A, B) CT demonstrates atrophic changes selectively involving the cerebellum in a chronic alcoholic subject. In the initial stages, volume reduction is caused by water loss and brain tissue shrinkage, and is therefore reversible. (C, D) T_1-weighted MRI images show global cerebellar hypotrophy in a baby born from an alcoholic. Alcohol inhibits development of Bergmann's fibres and consequently impairs processes of neuroblastic migration and normal cerebellar development.

Marchiafava–Bignami Disease

Marchiafava–Bignami disease is a rare complication of chronic alcoholism, characterised by demyelination and

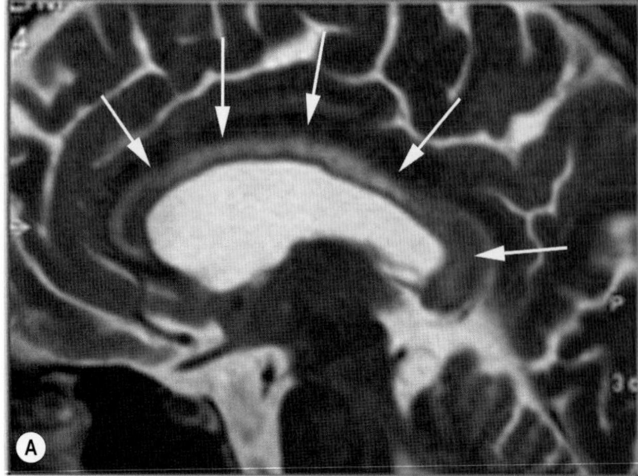

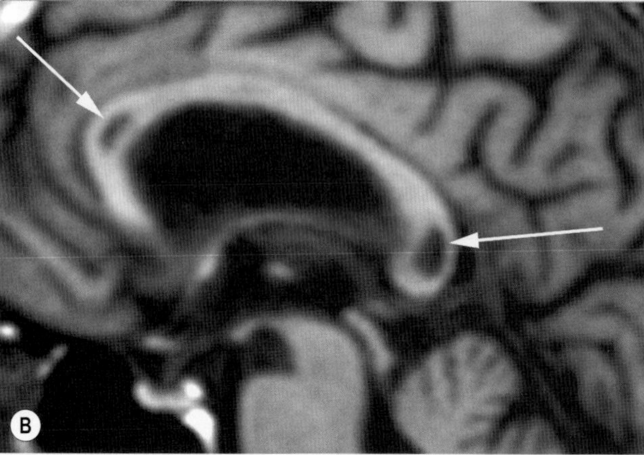

FIGURE 64-34 ■ **Two cases of Marchiafava–Bignami disease.** (A) Sagittal T_2-weighted image shows typical acute–subacute aspect of the disease, characterised by diffuse oedema of the corpus callosum without significant mass effect. (B) T_1-weighted image obtained in chronic phase, showing typical necrotic cavities selectively involving the genu and splenium.

necrosis of the corpus callosum, with rare involvement of extracallosal regions. Aetiology remains unknown but is believed to be caused by toxic agents in low-quality red wine and deficiency of Group B vitamins. Rarely, it has also been reported in non-alcoholic patients. Symptoms are mainly represented by cognitive deficits, psychosis, hypertonia and interhemispheric disconnection, until coma and death. Typical features at MRI in the acute phase are corpus callosum hyperintensity on T_2-weighted sequences and FLAIR, without significant mass effect, with peripheral enhancement. Diffusion is restricted due to cytotoxic oedema. In chronic forms, necrosis of the genu and splenium can be detected[46] (Fig. 64-34).

Wernicke's Encephalopathy

Wernicke's encephalopathy (WE) is an acute condition first described by the French ophthalmologist Gayet in 1875, and later by the German neurologist Wernike in 1881, caused by a deficiency of vitamin B_1 (thiamine). WE develops frequently but not exclusively in alcoholics. Other potential causes include extended fasting, malabsorption, digitalis poisoning and massive infusion of glucose without vitamin B_1 in weak patients. The autoptic incidence is reported to be 0.8–2% in random autopsies, and 20% in chronic alcoholics.[47] The classic clinical triad of ocular dysfunctions (nystagmus, conjugate gaze palsy, ophthalmoplegia), ataxia and confusion is observed only in 30% of cases. Treatment consists of thiamine infusion, and avoids irreversible consequences like Korsakoff's dementia or death. Memory impairment and dementia are related to damage of the mamillary bodies, anterior thalamic nuclei and interruption of the diencephalic-hippocampal circuits. Depletion of thiamine leads to failure of conversion of pyruvate to acetyl-CoA and α-ketoglutarate to succinate, altered pentose monophosphate shunt and the lack of Krebs cycle, with cerebral lactic acidosis, intra- and extracellular oedema, swelling of astrocytes, oligodendrocytes, myelin fibres and neuronal dendrites. Neuropathological aspects include neuronal degeneration, demyelination, haemorrhagic petechiae, proliferation of capillaries and astrocytes in periacqueduct grey substance, mamillary bodies, thalami, pulvinar, III cranial nerves nuclei and cerebellum.[47,48] At MRI, bilateral and symmetrical hyperintensities on T_2-weighted sequences and FLAIR are evident at the level of the already-mentioned structures, mainly mamillary bodies and thalami[49,50] (Fig. 64-35). Rarely, cortex of the forebrain can be involved.[50] DWI shows areas of high signal with ADC signal reduced due to cytotoxic oedema (Fig. 64-35), although the ADC can sometimes be high due to the presence of vasogenic component.[50] Rarely T_1-weighted images show bleeding ecchymotic haemorrhages in the thalami and mamillary bodies, a sign considered clinically unfavourable (Fig. 64-35). In 50% of cases, contrast enhancement is present in periacqueductal regions. Marked contrast enhancement of mamillary bodies is evident in 80% of cases, even prior to the development of visible changes in T_2-weighted sequences, and is considered highly specific for WE[51] (Fig. 64-35). In chronic forms, change of signal in T_2-weighted sequences becomes less prominent due to the diffuse brain atrophy, more pronounced at the level of mesencephalon and mamillary bodies.

Subacute Combined Degeneration

This disorder of the spinal cord, also known as funicular myelitis or Putnam–Dana syndrome, occurs in patients with vitamin B_{12} deficiency, and is characterised by a slight-to-moderate degree of gliosis in association with spongiform degeneration of the posterior and lateral columns. Clinical presentation consists in spastic paraparesis and spinal ataxia. At MRI, T_2-weighted hyperintensities are detected in the spinal cord posterior and lateral columns.[52] These lesions can be reversible after adequate vitamin B_{12} administration, or evolve towards atrophy. In some cases hyperintensity can be also detected along the spinothalamic tracts and lemnisci mediali (Fig. 64-36).

Osmotic Myelinolysis

Osmotic myelinolysis (OM) usually occurs in patients with hyponatremia that is too quickly corrected. This causes destruction of the blood–brain barrier with

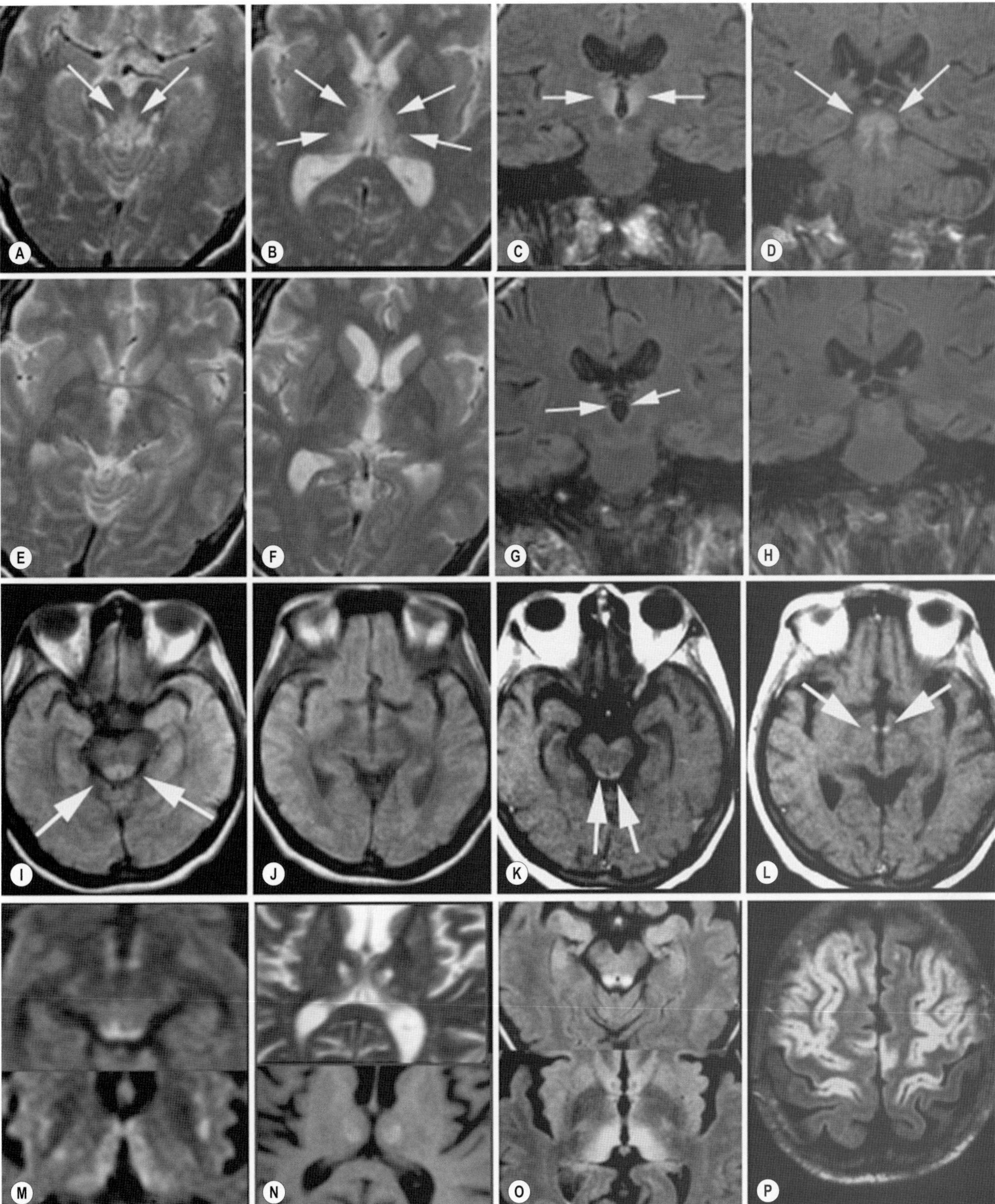

FIGURE 64-35 ■ **Different cases of Wernicke's encephalopathy.** (A–D) Typical case studied in the acute phase: prolongation of T_2 involves periacqueductal grey matter, colliculi, mid-thalamic and pulvinar regions. (E–H) Same case after therapy: normalisation of signal with mild atrophic changes (III ventricle dilatation). (I–L) Colliculi and mamillary bodies are involved and there is a clear contrast enhancement in both structures. (M) DWI of a different case with restricted diffusion in mamillary bodies, mesencephalic roof and thalami. (N) Lethal case with petechial haemorrhages in thalami. (O, P) Typical lesions associated with diffuse cortical involvement.

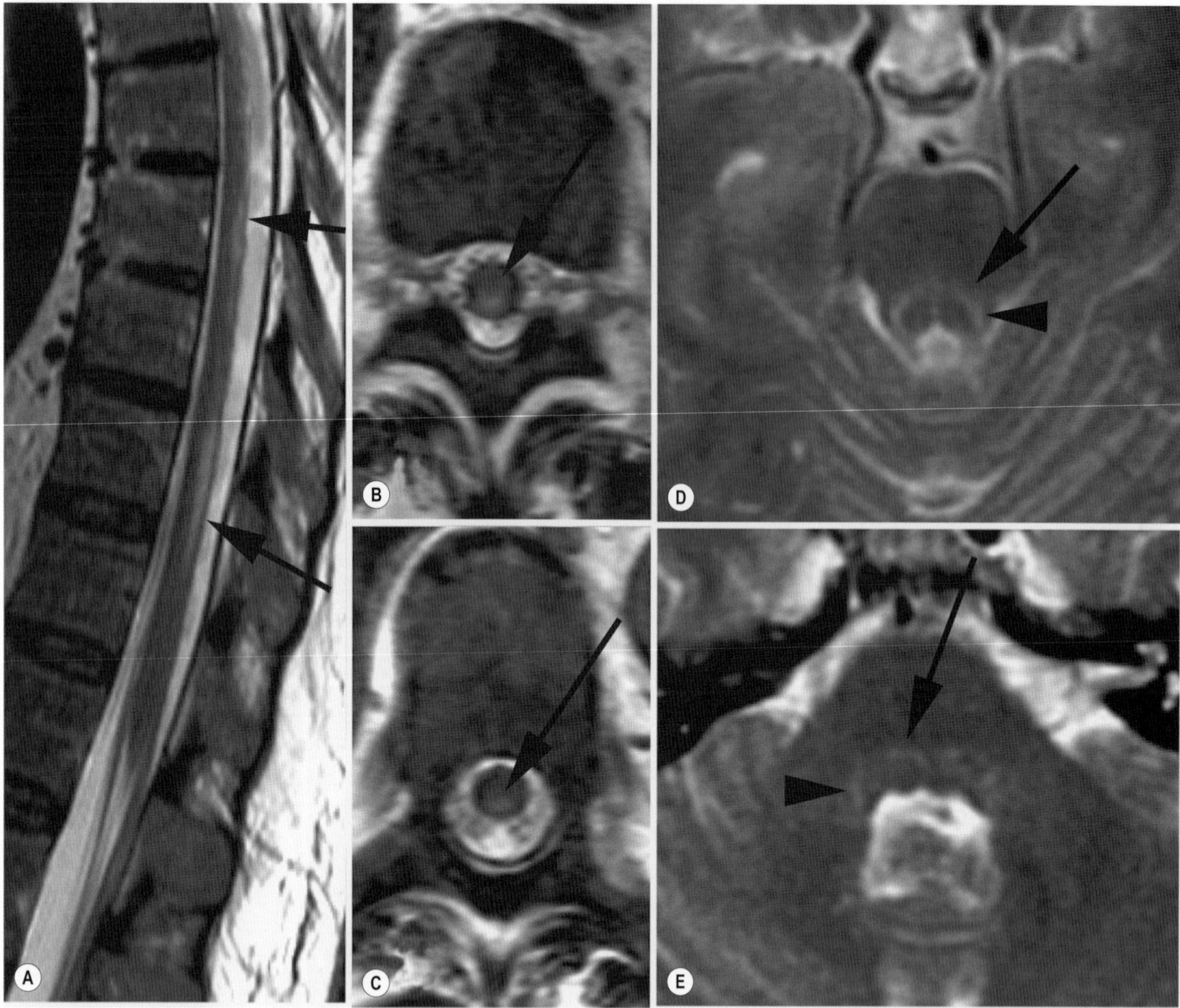

FIGURE 64-36 ■ **Two cases of combined sclerosis.** (A–C) Sagittal and axial T_2-weighted sequences show hyperintensities selectively involving the posterior columns in a young vegan female patient suffering from progressive spinal ataxia. (D, E) A different case in which hyperintensities extended to ascending sensitive pathways: lemniscus medialis (arrows) and spinothalamic tracts (arrowheads).

hypertonic fluid accumulation in extracellular space, resulting in a non-inflammatory demyelination. The most common damage is in the pontine fibres.[53,54] OM is observed in alcoholics with nutritional deficiency. The most common symptoms include paralysis, dysphagia, dysarthria and pseudobulbar palsy. Death is frequent. Rarely, OM affects other regions, especially basal ganglia, thalami and deep white matter. MRI usually shows an area of high signal on T_2-weighted sequences and FLAIR in the central part of the pons, sparing ventrolateral portions and corticospinal tracts.[53] The lesion is moderately hypointense in T_1 and may show positive contrast enhancement (Fig. 64-37). If the patient survives, the acute phase can evolve in a cavitated pontine lesion.

Methanol Poisoning

Acute methanol poisoning usually occurs after drinking counterfeit alcoholic beverages or following accidental ingestion of solvents and coolants. Toxic effects are due to formic acid, the main metabolite of methanol, which causes metabolic acidosis; the more susceptible structures are putamen, and symptoms occur within hours after ingestion and are characterised by headache, visual disturbances, nausea and vomiting. Coma, respiratory arrest and death can occur typically 6–36 hours after the poisoning.

Putaminal necrosis appears hypodense on CT and hyperintense on T_2-weighted sequences[55] (Fig. 64-38). More than 10% of cases are associated with putaminal ecchymotic haemorrhages, appearing hyperintense on T_1-weighted sequences. Alterations may also involve pallidum and centrum ovale.

Diethylene Glycol

Diethylene glycol is commonly used as a solvent for paints, antifreeze and other chemicals. About 12 hours

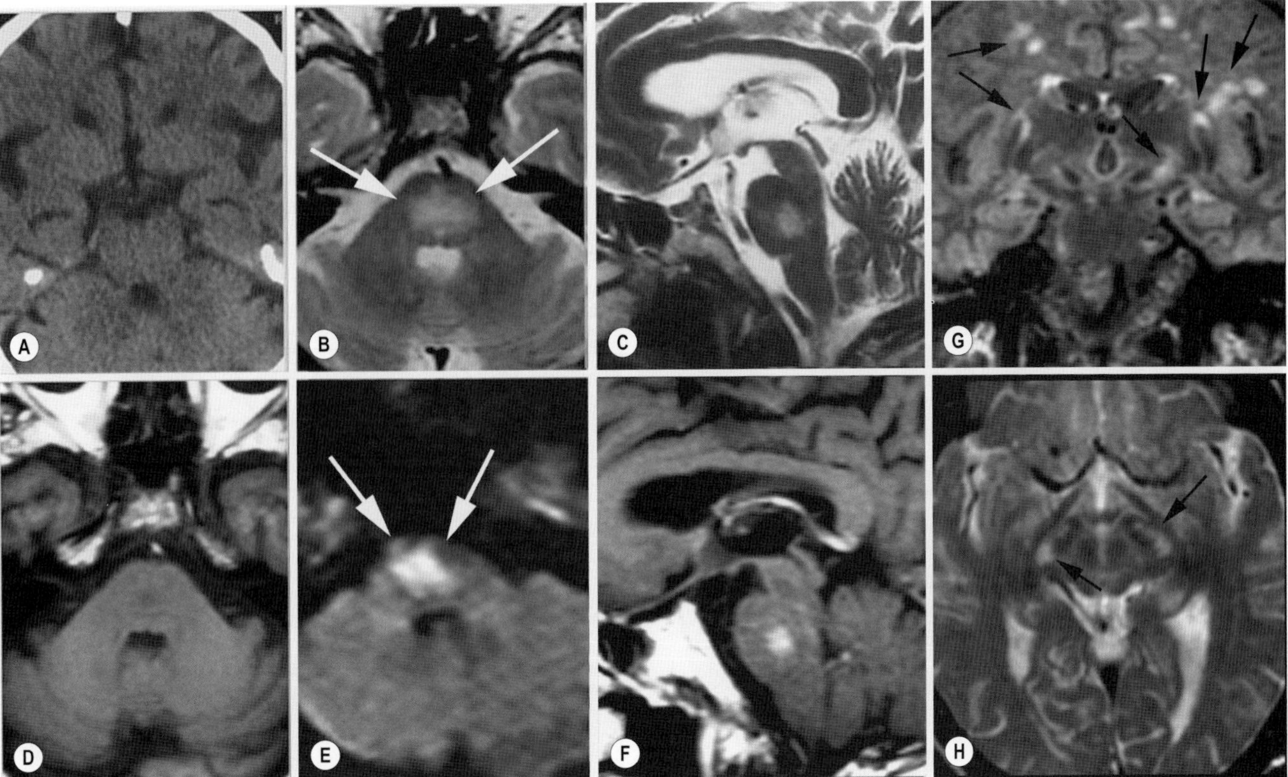

FIGURE 64-37 ■ **Osmotic myelinolysis.** (A–F) Typical pontine localisation in an alcoholic patient (central pontine myelinolysis, CPM). CT does not show any abnormality. MR shows a tegmental pontine lesion, hyperintense on T_2-weighted images, central, with restricted diffusivity (E), and positive contrast enhancement (F). (G, H) Different case affected by post-dyalitic extrapontine osmotic myelinolysis. Lesions are located in the basal ganglia (putamina and substantia nigra) and supratentorial white matter.

after ingestion patients develop fulminant hepatorenal insufficiency, coma and seizures. MRI shows brain oedema initially widespread; then after 24–48 hours frontal white matter necrosis, basal ganglia, thalami and brainstem involvement appear[56] (Fig. 64-38).

Hepatic Encephalopathy

The term *hepatic encephalopathy* (HE) includes a spectrum of neuropsychiatric abnormalities occurring in patients with liver dysfunction. Most cases are associated with cirrhosis and portal hypertension or portal-systemic shunts, but the condition can also be seen in patients with acute liver failure and, rarely, in those with portal-systemic bypass and no associated intrinsic hepatocellular disease. Although HE is a clinical condition, several neuroimaging techniques, particularly MR imaging, may eventually be useful for the diagnosis because they can identify and measure the consequences of CNS increase in substances, which, under normal circumstances, are efficiently metabolised by the liver. Classical MR abnormalities in chronic HE include high signal intensity in the globus pallidum on T_1-weighted images, likely a reflection of increased tissue concentrations of manganese (Fig. 64-39), and an elevated glutamine/glutamate peak coupled with decreased *myo*-inositol and choline signals on proton MR spectroscopy, representing disturbances in cell-volume homeostasis secondary to brain hyperammoniemia.[57] Recent data have shown that white matter abnormalities, also related to increased CNS ammonia concentration, can also be detected with several MR imaging techniques: magnetisation transfer ratio measurements show significantly low values in otherwise normal-appearing brain white matter, fast-FLAIR sequences reveal diffuse and focal high signal intensity lesions in the hemispheric white matter and diffusion-weighted images disclose increased white matter diffusivity. All these MR abnormalities, which return to normal with restoration of liver function, probably reflect the presence of mild diffuse interstitial brain oedema, which seems to play an essential role in the pathogenesis of HE.

In acute HE, bilateral symmetric signal-intensity abnormalities on T_2-weighted images, often with associated restricted diffusion involving the cortical grey matter, are commonly identified (Fig. 64-40). Involvement of the subcortical white matter and the basal ganglia, thalami and midbrain may also be seen. These abnormalities, which can lead to intracranial hypertension and severe brain injury, reflect the development of cytotoxic oedema secondary to the acute increase of brain hyperammoniemia.[58]

Carbon Monoxide

Carbon monoxide (CO) is a source of accidental acute intoxication with relatively frequent high mortality. CO

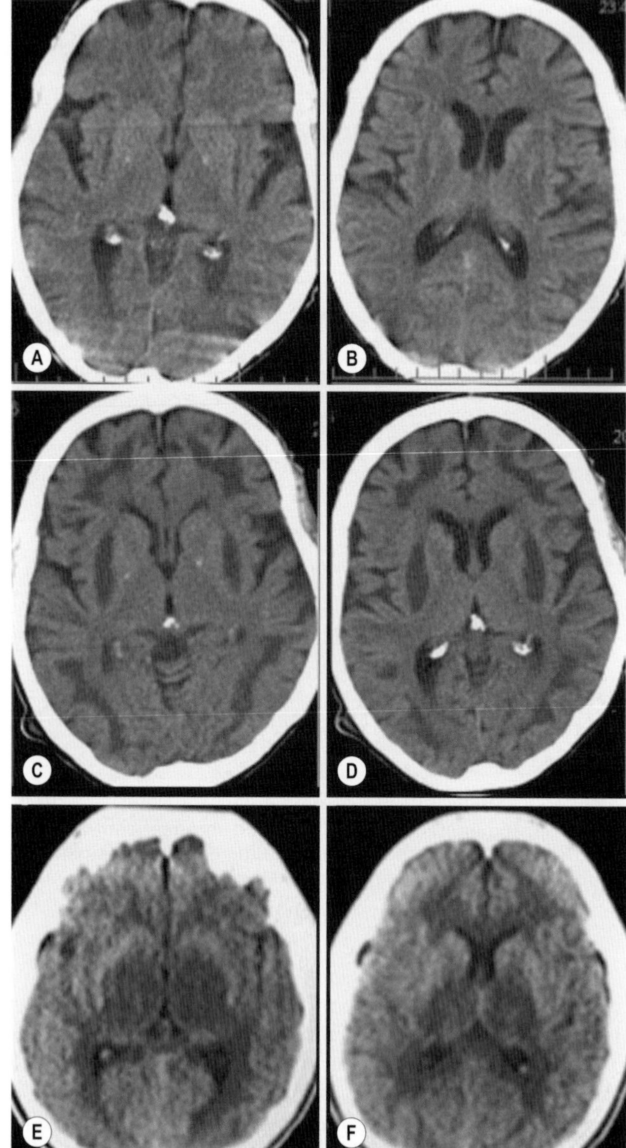

FIGURE 64-38 ■ (A, B) Methanol intoxication: CT examination performed in the acute phase. Oedema of the putamen and external capsule is becoming evident. (C, D) Same case after 24 hours: clear hypodense lesions in both putamen extended in the subcortical white matter with prevalence in frontal and occipital regions. (E, F) Diethylene glycol intoxication in subacute phase. Oedema is mostly localised in thalami, internal capsules and pallidi.

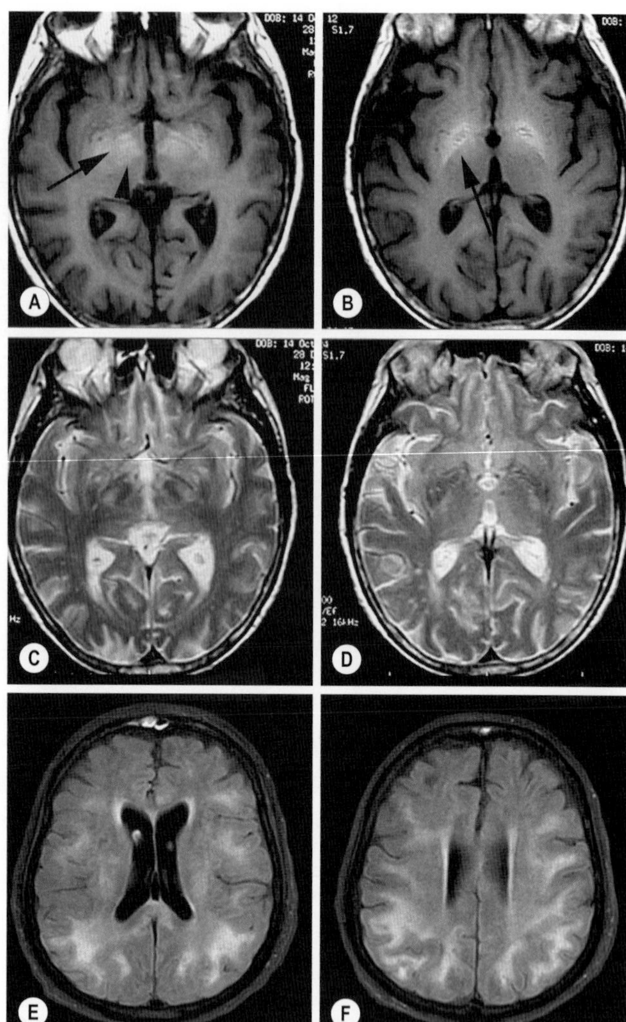

FIGURE 64-39 ■ **Hepatic encephalopathy.** Typical hyperintense signal on T_1-weighted sequences involves substantia nigra (arrow in A), red nucleus (arrowhead in A), and pallidum (arrow in B). These alterations are visible even though less prominent on T_2-weighted sequences (C, D). (E, F) A different case with diffuse white matter oedema. ((E, F) Courtesy of Dr. T. Krings, Toronto Western Hospital, Canada.)

determines a neurological hypoxic damage. In fact, CO has an affinity for haemoglobin 250 times greater than oxygen, with whom it competes. CO attaches to haemoglobin, resulting in the formation of carboxyhaemoglobin, and thereby reducing the ability of haemoglobin to transport oxygen. Clinically, CO poisoning causes headache, tinnitus, dizziness and nausea, then progressive disorders of consciousness arise until death; the survivors often have severe extrapyramidal disorder or dementia.

CO poisoning causes bilateral globus pallidus necrosis, sometimes extended to lenticular nuclei and caudate; more rarely involved are thalami and hippocampus. Sometimes distal frontal white matter involvement is also evident. Selective damage of pallidi is probably not only from hypoxia but also from specific toxic phenomena. At MRI, bilateral signal alteration of the pallidi is evident. The basal ganglia affected usually have low signal on T_1 and high on T_2. Sometimes, the presence of microbleeding determines inhomogeneous signal. Hyperintensity in the subcortical white matter can be present in most severe cases.[59] Temporal involvement is rare. In the acute phase, diffusion-weighted imaging shows diffusion restriction in the basal ganglia, and may also show reduced diffusivity in areas with normal signal at the conventional sequences (Fig. 64-41). The lesions tend gradually to evolve towards cavitation and atrophy.

Heavy Metal Poisoning

Some heavy metals are rare due to acute or chronic intoxication, usually professionally exposed workers are

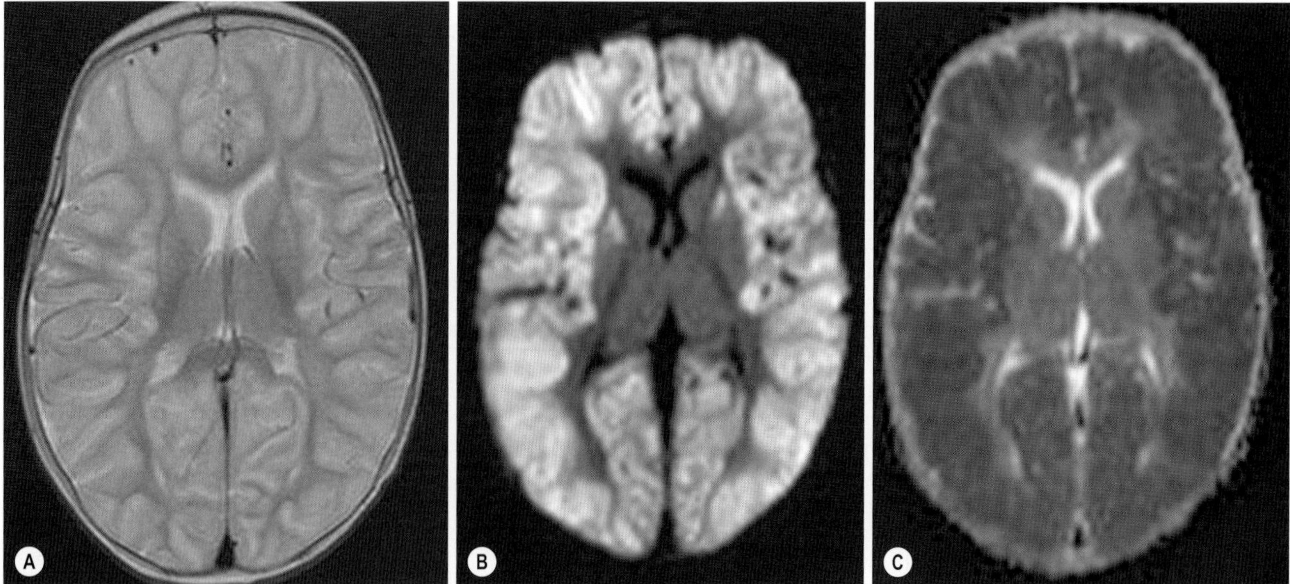

FIGURE 64-40 ■ **Acute hepatic encephalopathy.** A 7-month-old boy with acute hepatic failure. Brain MRI imaging shows symmetric and diffuse abnormal high signal intensity on T_2-weighted images involving the cortical grey matter (A). This abnormality showed increased signal intensity on the isotropic diffusion-weighted image (B) and low signal on the apparent diffusion coefficient map (C) which corresponds to cytotoxic oedema.

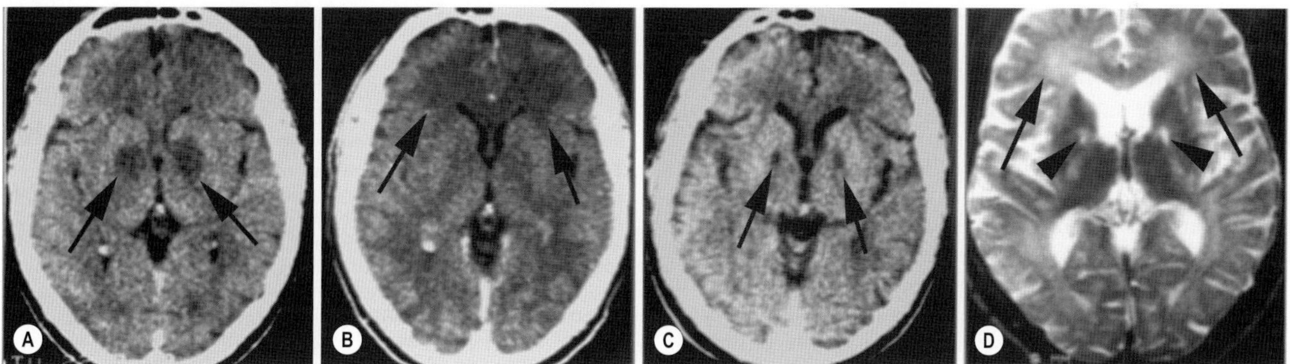

FIGURE 64-41 ■ **Carbon monoxide intoxication.** (A, B) CT imaging performed in acute phase; oedema of both pallidi and frontal deep and subcortical white matter. In chronic phase, CT (C) shows necrotic degeneration of pallidi and hypodensity of the frontal white matter. T_2-weighted sequences (D) confirm diffuse hyperintensity of the frontal white matter and both pallidi.

victims. Manganese poisoning can affect workers in the mining industry, patients in chronic parenteral nutrition and, rarely, patients who abuse ephedrine. Chronic poisoning causes accumulation of manganese and neuronal loss in the basal ganglia; the main symptoms include dementia, hallucinations and extrapyrimidal disorders. The accumulation of manganese appears at MRI as bilateral hyperintensity on T_1-weighted sequence of pallidi nuclei, sometimes extended to other nuclei and cerebral peduncles.[59] T_2 signal is usually normal. Mercury poisoning mainly affects miners or consumers of fish caught in contaminated water. The metal accumulates mainly in the cerebellar vermis and visual cortex, and manifests as a signal hypointense on T_1, iso- and hypointense on T_2 and hypointense on T_2*-weighted sequences.

Lead intoxication can cause alteration of the signal in subcortical and thalamic regions. Aluminium can intoxicate patients undergoing dialysis and is characterised by elective involvement of the limbic system.

Organic Solvent Poisoning

This particular poisoning occurs among people who inhale glue. Toluene and other organic solvents are readily transported by air to the blood, cross the blood–brain barrier and enter the central nervous system. This poisoning manifests as neurological impairment and cognitive decline. Pathological studies reveal axonal loss with diffuse cerebral white matter demyelination and cerebellar degeneration and gliosis. At MRI, diffuse T_2 increase in cerebellar and cerebral white matter is registered, often with a slight shortening of T_2 in the putamen. In some cases it may be a shortening of T_2, also in the thalamus and in the cerebral cortex.[60]

Cocaine

Cocaine acts by blocking reuptake of catecholamines. This causes a short-lived intense feeling of euphoria, increased energy and alertness. Acute neurotoxic effects include agitation and convulsions. Most commonly, cocaine is inhaled in the form of cocaine hydrochloride; its alkaline base (crack) can be smoked.

Most of the central nervous system complications induced by cocaine are ischaemic and haemorrhagic strokes. Bleeding related to cocaine can be localised in the subarachnoid space or intracerebral, and is twice more frequent than infarctions. Approximately 50% of patients are bearers of a concomitant pathology as cerebral arteriovenous malformations or aneurysms, which break consequently to increased blood pressure and heart rate caused by cocaine-induced sympathetic effects. In cases where it is not possible to document the presence of concomitant vascular pathology, intraparenchymal bleedings are most commonly located in the basal ganglia and thalami; the risk of bleeding increases with alcohol abuse.

While the pathogenetic mechanisms of haemorrhagic stroke are clear, the causes of ischaemic stroke are diverse and include vasoconstriction induced by cocaine and vasculitis (by additives/contaminants added to cocaine) (Fig. 64-42). Cocaine increases the platelet response to arachidonic acid with a increased level of thromboxane that increases platelet aggregation, resulting in thrombosis and heart and/or brain infarcts. Brain lesions are mostly located in the subcortical white matter or in the middle cerebral artery territory (Fig. 64-42). Mesencephalic infarcts seem to be more frequent when cocaine is used in conjunction with amphetamine. Angiography may show focal constrictions of the main arteries, while contrast enhancement of the vessel wall indicates the presence of vasculitis. Cerebral atrophy is observed in patients who are chronic abusers of cocaine. The frontal lobe is typically more severely involved, followed by the temporal. Chronic ischaemia may be the causative mechanism of the atrophy.[61]

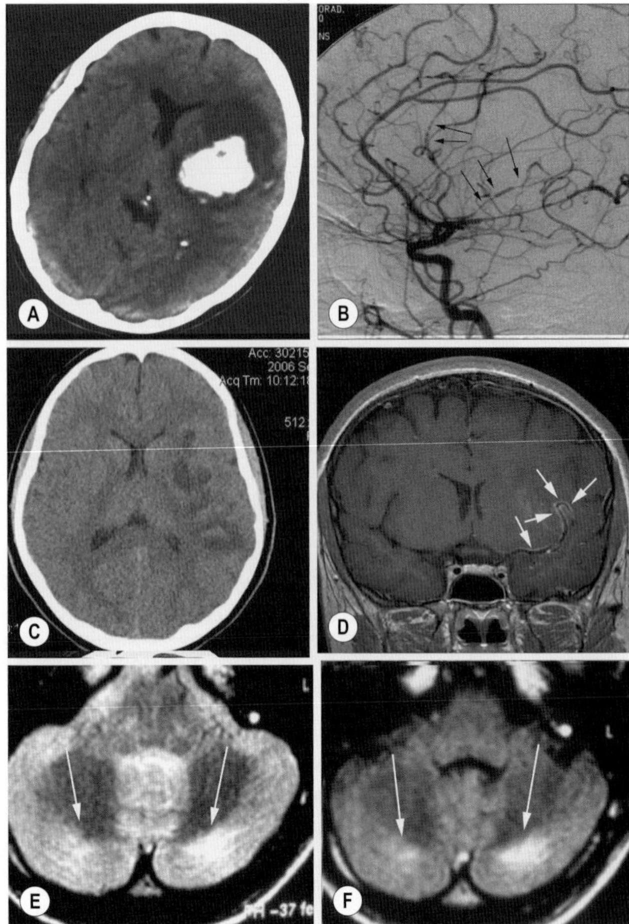

FIGURE 64-42 ■ Different cases of vascular disease: consequences of illegal drugs administration. (A, B) Capsulolenticular haemorrhage in a cocaine abuser with clear angiographic 'pearl and string signs' along different branches of middle cerebral artery, suggesting vasculitis. (C, D) A different case of vasculitis in a cocaine user, with ischaemic stroke in the territory of the left middle cerebral artery. (D) Contrast-enhanced T_1-weighted image shows positive enhancement of the perivascular leptomeninges, and the vessel walls, indicating active inflammation. (E, F) Acute bilateral cerebellar infarction in a cocaine consumer. ((A–D) Courtesy of Dr. T. Krings, Toronto Western Hospital, Canada.)

Ecstasy

Ecstasy or 3,4-methylenedioxymethamphetamine (MDMA), a drug derived from methamphetamine, is known as a party drug that has stimulatory and moderately hallucinatory effects. In the acute phase the subject experiences euphoria, increased self-esteem and sensory perceptions and hyperthermia, tachycardia, and sometimes acute psychosis and lockjaw. These effects disappear in 24–48 hours and are accompanied by muscle aches, depression, fatigue and decreased concentration. MDMA causes a sharp and quick release of 5-hydroxytryptamine (5-HT), a serotonin receptor, with a powerful vasoconstriction, and determines an increase of synaptic dopamine in different brain areas. Although the permanent neurotoxicity is still a matter of debate, there is evidence that the stimulation of the 5-HT 2A receptors in the small vessels results in prolonged vasospasm and necrosis of brain regions is involved. The occipital cortex and the globus pallidus are the most vulnerable areas to high levels of 5-HT.[61]

Opioids and Derivatives

Heroin is the most common drug among those in this group, and is also the one responsible for more neurological side effects. Other derivatives include morphine, hydrocodone, oxycodone, hydromorphine, codeine and other opiates (i.e. fentanyl, pethidine and methadone). Both acute and chronic effects of heroin on the brain have been reported. These include neurovascular disorders, leucoencephalopathy and atrophy. Moreover, beyond the direct effects of heroin, complications secondary to the addition of additives should be considered, as lipophilic substances (cutting of heroin) or crystalline impurities. Ischaemic strokes are the most frequent

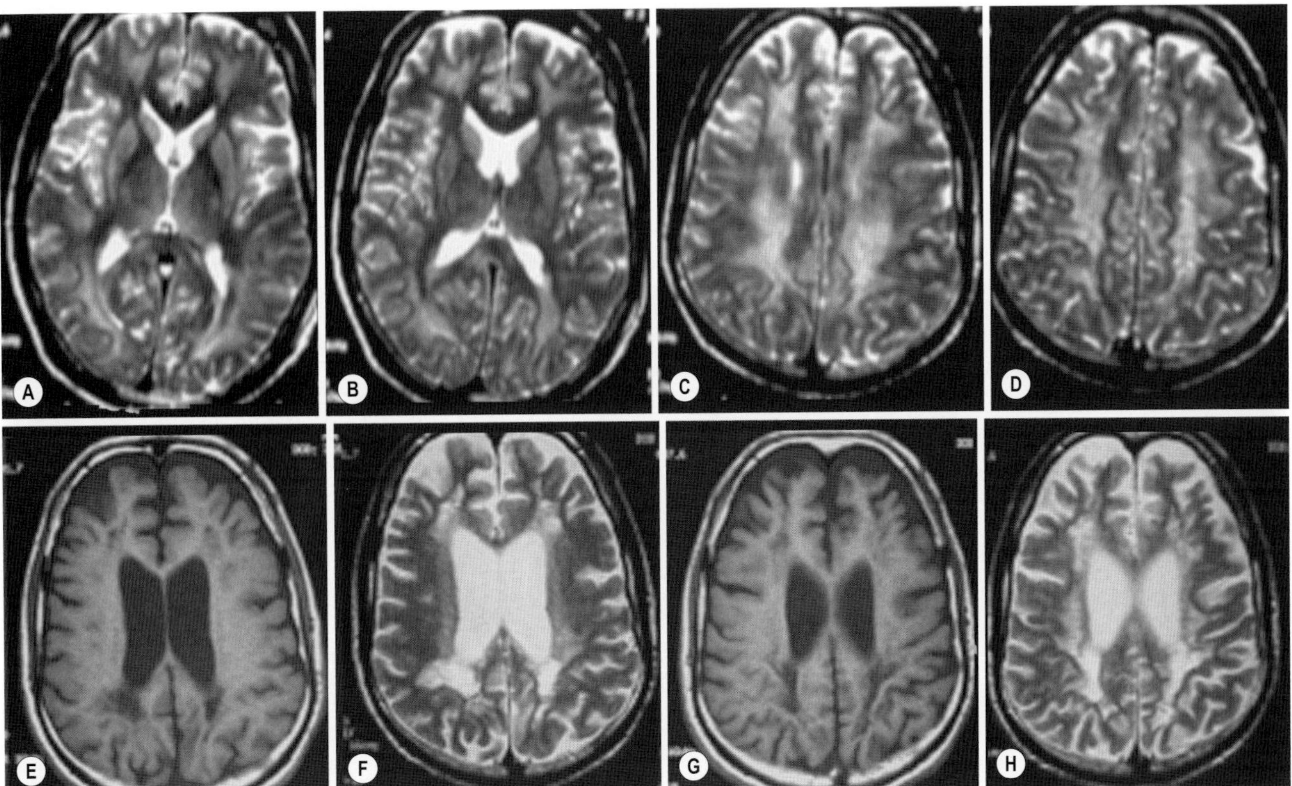

FIGURE 64-43 ■ (A–H) Delayed post-hypoxic leucoencephalopathy (DPHL) in a 29-year-old heroin user. In the upper row, T_2-weighted images show diffuse oedema of the supratentorial white matter 4 hours after prolonged cardiac arrest following intravenous drug injection. In the lower row, a follow-up brain MR obtained 1 year later. Extensive necrotic degeneration of the white matter is evident, while the cortex is spared.

heroin complication. The pathogenetic mechanisms proposed are similar to those for cocaine, and can be reversible: vasospasm, immune-mediated vasculitis, embolic events for crystalline additives. Ischaemia is more frequently observed in patients who take heroin intravenously than by oral ingestion or inhalation. Globus pallidus is most frequently involved (5–10% of subjects chronically abusing heroin). In chronic abuse, white matter changes from microvascular pathology can be seen. These aspects are, however, generally less severe than in cocaine chronic abuse. Haemodynamic cerebral infarcts are also possible in consequence of cardiac arrest (Fig. 64-43). A major heroin-induced complication is the leucoencephalopathy. It occurs in the process of inhalation, when the drug is heated on a piece of tin, and the fumes inhaled. Presumably, leucoencephalopathy associated with generalised oedema is the consequence of activation of a substance not yet known.[61]

The chronic form of subacute encephalopathy is characterised by spongiform degeneration of the corticospinal tracts associated with vacuolar degeneration of oligodendrocytes. Symptoms progress from cerebellar and extrapyramidal, to diffuse spasms and palsy, which ultimately can lead to death. Radiological aspects on MRI are quite specific and consist of hyperintense lesions on T_2, mainly localised in the supratentorial white matter, the cerebellar hemispheres and the posterior limb of the internal capsule, sparing the anterior one and the subcortical white matter. In the acute phases, diffusion is restricted by cytotoxic oedema, while subacute phases are associated with an increased prevalence of myelin damage (Fig. 64-44).

The most common secondary complications from heroin abuse are infections. Up to 45–58% of patients with localised endocarditis develop neurological sequelae from septic embolism (mycotic aneurysms, brain abscesses).

Excytotoxic Oedema

Among the category of toxic encephalopathies, the so-called 'excytotoxic' forms are also considered. These are due to altered metabolism of glutamate related to various aetiology, resulting in an altered 'uptake' of this metabolite that accumulates in the synaptic region, thus determining an increase of post-synaptic excitatory activity followed by cytotoxic oedema, in most cases reversible. These conditions are detectable in hepatic insufficiency and in some forms of status epilepticus, particularly in cases associated with the use of opiates.[62] In those cases, the epileptogenic effect of an additive, acetylcodeine, is considered responsible (Fig. 64-45). Similar conditions can be also detected as a consequence of pharmacological intoxication (valproate) or sudden

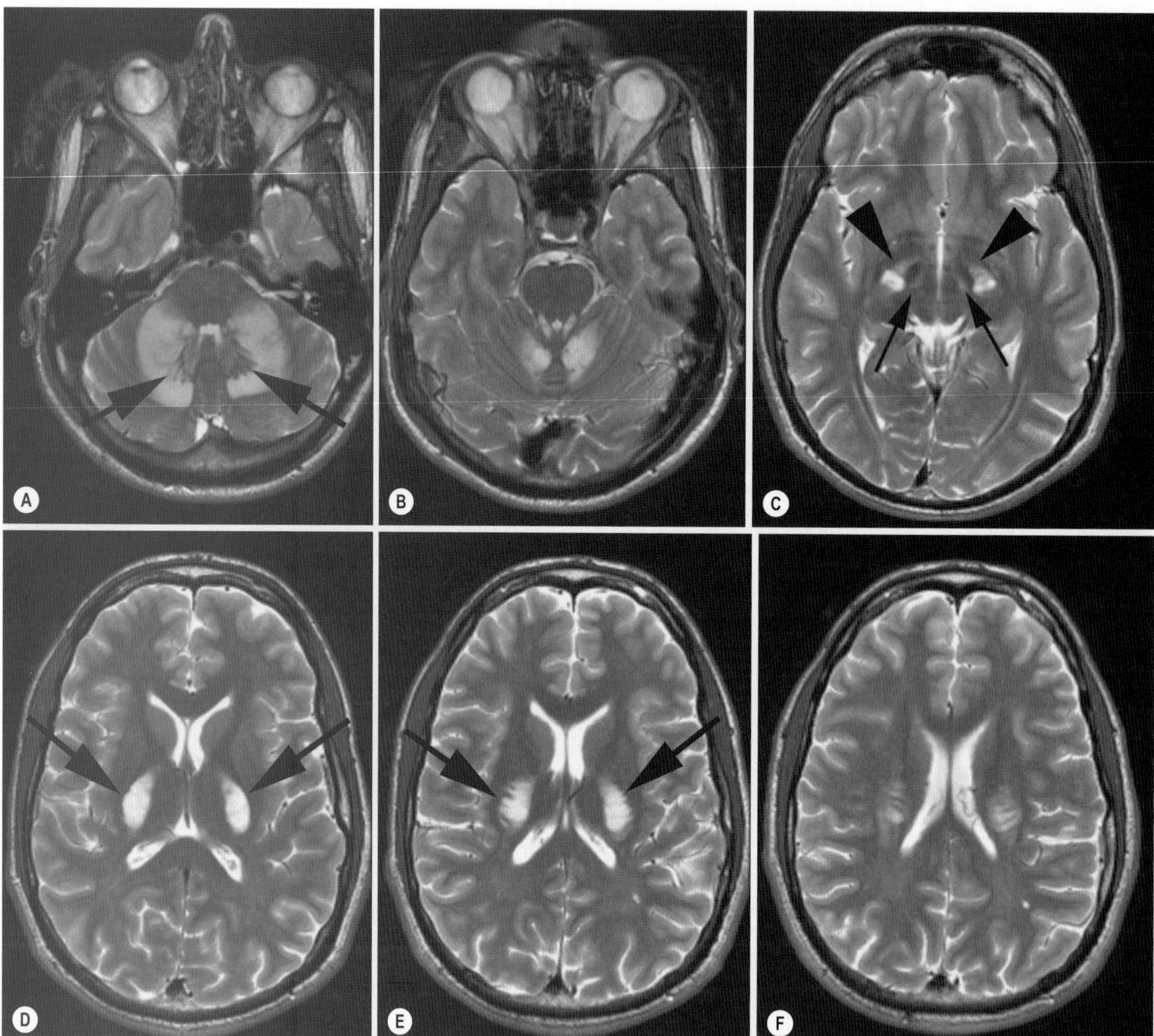

FIGURE 64-44 ■ Extensive myelin degeneration after inhalation of heroin (so-called 'chasing the dragon'). Diffuse white matter changes are present, involving the posterior limb of the internal capsule (arrows in D, E), with sparing of the dentate nuclei (arrows in A) and the cerebellar cortex, and involvement of the corticospinal tracts (arrowheads in C) and medial lemnisci (arrows in C). (Courtesy of Dr. T. Krings, Toronto Western Hospital, Canada.)

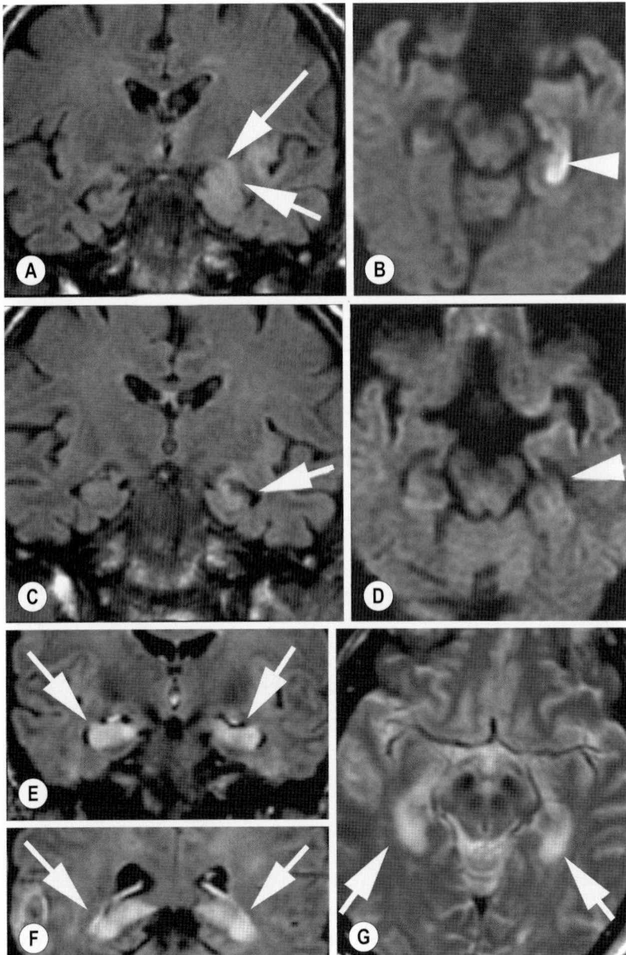

FIGURE 64-45 ■ Two different examples of hippocampal excytotoxic oedema as a consequence of exogenous intoxication. (A, B) A case of delirium tremens in alcohol withdrawal. (C, D) Same case in the chronic phase. Hippocampal signal is normalised and atrophic changes are evident with dilatation of the temporal horns. (E, F) Status epilepticus after heroin injection. This condition is probably related to epileptogenic addictives (such as acetylcodeine). Bilateral hippocampal oedema is clearly evident on both FLAIR (E, F) and T_2-weighted sequences (G).

withdrawal of alcohol or antiepileptic drugs. In this last case, the splenium of the corpus callosum can be selectively involved.[63]

For a full list of references, please see ExpertConsult.

FURTHER READING

2. Rovira Cañellas A, Rovira Gols A, Río J, et al. Idiopathic inflammatory-demyelinating diseases of the central nervous system. Neuroradiology 2007;49:393–409.
4. Rovira A, León A. MR in the diagnosis and monitoring of multiple sclerosis: an overview. Eur J Radiol 2008;67:409–14.
5. Filippi M, Rocca MA. MR Imaging of Multiple Sclerosis. Radiology 2011;259:659–81.
9. Lycklama G, Thompson A, Filippi M, et al. Spinal-cord MRI in multiple sclerosis. Lancet Neurol 2003;2:555–62.
14. Bermel RA, Bakshi R. The measurement and clinical relevance of brain atrophy in multiple sclerosis. Lancet Neurol 2006;5: 158–70.
18. Wingerchuk DM, Lennon VA, Pittock SJ, et al. Revised diagnostic criteria for neuromyelitis optica. Neurology 2006;66:1485–9.
22. Krupp LB, Tardieu M, Amato MP, et al. International Pediatric Multiple Sclerosis Study Group criteria for pediatric multiple sclerosis and immune-mediated central nervous system demyelinating disorders: revisions to the 2007 definitions. Mult Scler 2013;19: 1261–7.
27. Salvarani C, Brown RD Jr, Calamia, KT, et al. Primary Central Nervous System Vasculitis: Analysis of 101 Patients. Ann Neurol 2007;62:442–51.
40. Sundgren PC, Jennings J, Attwood TJ, et al. MRI and 2D-MR CSI spectroscopy of the brain in the evaluation of patients with acute onset of Neuropsychiatric Systemic Lupus Erythematosus. Neuroradiology 2005;47:576–85.
43. Geibprasert S, Gallucci M, Krings T. Alcohol-induced changes in the brain as assessed by MRI and CT. Eur Radiol 2010;20: 1492–501.
57. Rovira A, Alonso J, Cordoba J. MR imaging findings in hepatic encephalopathy. AJNR Am J Neuroradiol 2008;29:1612–21.
61. Geibprasert S, Gallucci M, Krings T. Addictive Illegal Drugs: Structural Neuroimaging. AJNR Am J Neuroradiol 2010;31: 803–8.

CHAPTER 65

Neurodegenerative Diseases and Epilepsy

Beatriz Gomez Anson • Frederik Barkhof

CHAPTER OUTLINE

AGEING AND DEMENTIA—INTRODUCTION AND CLINICAL

With the rising age of the population, both normal ageing phenomena in the brain and neurodegenerative disorders become more prevalent. While exceptionally the brain may not be affected by age (successful ageing), the more typical or unusual ageing involves general involutionary alterations, which may mimic or herald neurodegenerative disease. Clinically, mild memory loss and reduced processing speed are considered normal for age, and can only be objectively established with extensive neuropsychological testing.

Dementia is a clinical syndrome that is defined as an acquired condition involving multiple cognitive impairments that are sufficient to interfere with activities of daily living, and often is progressive. Alzheimer's disease (AD) is the most common cause of dementia and often presents with memory impairment, but in other diseases like frontotemporal dementia (FTD), behavioural or language problems may prevail. Diagnosis is critically dependent on careful history taking from patient and informant, followed by clinical and cognitive examination supported by ancillary investigations, of which neuroimaging is one of the most important.

The a priori chance of a particular disease being present is dependent on age. In younger patients, more rare disease may occur and FTD is relatively common, although AD is still the most prevalent disorder. In the older patients, AD, dementia with Lewy bodies (DLB) and vascular disease are the most common. Mixed AD and vascular disease is the most frequent pathology in the elderly (>85 years). Genetic causes of dementia are important in FTD, but only explain 1–2% of (presenile) AD cases. Neoplasms rarely present with cognitive decline.

Ancillary investigations in the work-up of suspected dementia are quite important, since clinical diagnosis has a relatively low accuracy compared to histopathology. Cerebrospinal fluid (CSF) analysis plays an important role by examining levels of β-amyloid and (phosphorylated) tau. Neuroimaging is the most important ancillary investigation in the work-up of suspected dementia, and should be combined with clinical, neuropsychological and laboratory data in a multidisciplinary conference to enhance diagnostic accuracy. Despite the absence of definitive treatment for most disorders, establishing a correct nosological disorder is important in terms of counselling and planning, and identifying relevant (vascular) comorbidity.

NORMAL AGEING PHENOMENA IN THE BRAIN

Normal ageing may be subdivided into successful ageing (without any discernible changes) and the more commonly observed typical (usual) ageing. Typical ageing includes a variety of changes, including overall brain shrinkage, but also local alterations, such as white matter changes. Many of these 'normal' ageing phenomena have been linked to risk factors (e.g. vascular) and although cognitive function may seem intact, subtle abnormalities may be detected on detailed neuropsychological testing.

TABLE 65-1 **Brain Alterations Observable during Typical/Usual Ageing**

Mild-to-moderate brain volume loss:
- Ventricular enlargement, including third ventricle
- Sulcal enlargement mostly affecting frontal and parietal lobes
- Mild medial temporal lobe atrophy and hippocampal sulcus cavities

Enlarged perivascular (Virchow–Robin) spaces on/in the:
- Basal ganglia region, near the anterior commissure (large ones seen on CT)
- White matter of centrum semiovale, near the vertex (MRI only)
- Mesencephalon (MRI only)

Changes of the vascular wall:
- Elongation and tortuosity (e.g. basilar artery)
- Wall-thickening and calcification (e.g. carotid siphon or vertebral artery)

Vascular changes (better visible on MRI than CT):
- Punctiform or early confluent ischaemic white matter changes
- Lacunar infarcts and microbleeds

Iron accumulation on MRI in the:
- Globus pallidus, putamen, dentate nucleus

Calcifications on CT in the:
- Globus pallidus, pineal gland, choroid plexus (esp. foramen of Luschka)
- Cerebral falx, sometimes with bony transformation

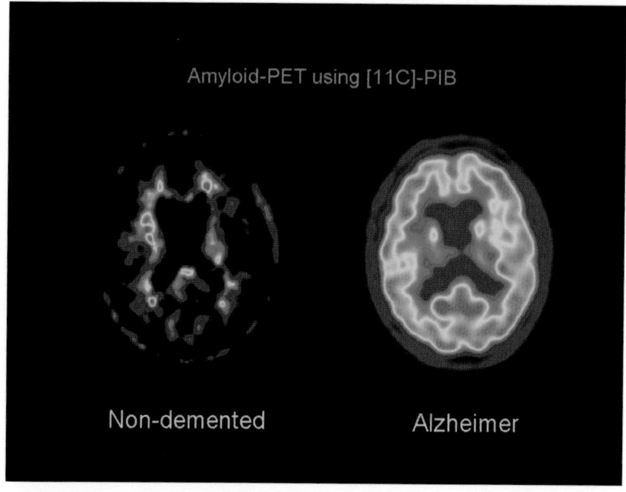

FIGURE 65-1 ■ Amyloid-PET using [^{11}C]-PIB in a healthy control (left) and patient with Alzheimer's disease (right). Note low physiological binding to the white matter only in the control and widespread cortical tracer uptake in AD. (Image courtesy of Bart van Berckel.)

Such relationships are often only discernible on a group level, and predictions in individual subjects are difficult to provide.

Table 65-1 lists the alterations observable in typical/usual ageing.

DEMENTIA—IMAGING APPROACH

Indications for Imaging

The focus of imaging in suspected dementia has shifted from an exclusionary to an inclusionary approach.[1] Exclusion of a (surgically) treatable cause of dementia (e.g. tumour or subdural haematoma) can be ascertained by using computed tomography (CT), but demonstration of positive disease markers (e.g. hippocampal atrophy for AD) becomes increasingly more relevant and magnetic resonance imaging (MRI) adds positive predictive value to the diagnosis in dementia. Catheter angiography (DSA) is hardly ever indicated, except perhaps for suspicion of vasculitis. While MRI is the modality of choice for investigating dementia, multislice CT offers a reasonable alternative, with coronally reformatted images enabling examination of the medial temporal lobe. However, CT is still clearly inferior to MRI, for example, in subjects suspected of having some rare disorders causing dementia, such as encephalitis or Creutzfeldt–Jakob disease (CJD).

When structural imaging is equivocal or does not lead to the diagnosis, functional imaging may add diagnostic value.[2] Second-line investigations include metabolic information obtained by using single-photon emission computed tomography (SPECT) or positron emission tomography (PET), or physiological information obtained by using diffusion or perfusion MRI. For example, in the early stages of frontotemporal lobar degeneration (FTLD) without discernible atrophy, fluorodeoxyglucose PET (FDG-PET) or hexamethylpropyleneamine oxime SPECT (HMPAO-SPECT) may already demonstrate decreased metabolism or hypoperfusion. Molecular imaging provides even more early and specific information, e.g. amyloid-PET in Alzheimer's disease (Fig. 65-1) and dopaminergic tracers in Lewy-body dementia.

Protocol for CT and MRI

Sructured reporting is essential in dementia[3] and should consider:

- Exclusion of mass lesion, haematoma or hydrocephalus.
- Vascular pathology: territorial infarcts, lacunes, thalamic lesions, white matter lesions.
- Focal atrophy:
  - Medial temporal lobe and hippocampus or precuneus (AD)
  - Frontal lobe and temporal pole (FTLD)
  - Mesencephalon (progressive supranuclear palsy)
  - Pons (multisystem atrophy).

ALZHEIMER'S DISEASE AND OTHER PRIMARY NEURODEGENERATIVE DEMENTIAS

Alheimer's Disease

The disease is named after Aloïs Alzheimer, who first described senile plaques and neurofibrillary tangles in a 51-year-old woman in 1906. Although the aetiology of AD is uncertain, the amyloid cascade predicts that

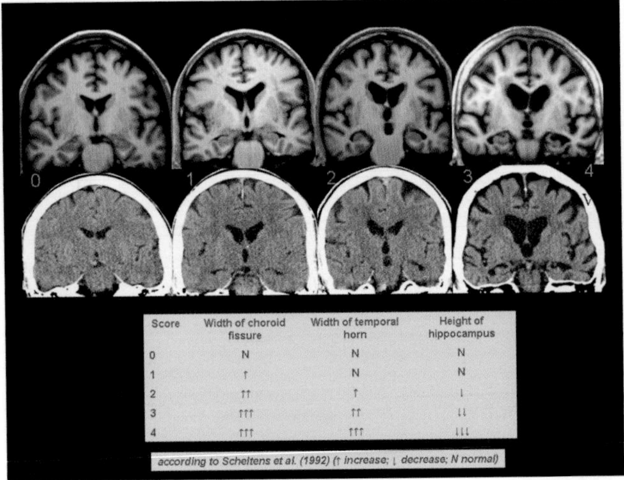

Score	Width of choroid fissure	Width of temporal horn	Height of hippocampus
0	N	N	N
1	↑	N	N
2	↑↑	↑	↓
3	↑↑↑	↑↑	↓↓
4	↑↑↑	↑↑↑	↓↓↓

according to Scheltens et al. (1992) (↑ increase; ↓ decrease; N normal)

FIGURE 65-2 ■ Visual rating of medial temporal lobe atrophy (MTA). In these same-day studies a perfect similarity between MRI and CT is noted for assessment of the medial temporal lobe for visual rating of MTA. (Modified with permission from Radiology 2009;253:174–183.)

FIGURE 65-3 ■ In this patient with onset of Alzheimer's disease at the age of 62, there is little hippocampal atrophy (green circle) but more severe atrophy of the precuneus, including the posterior cingulate (red circle).

abnormal aggregation of amyloid leads to impaired nerve function, formation of extracellular amyloid (neuritic) plaques and subsequent formation of intracellular neurofibrillary tangles, leading to neuronal loss and atrophy. The process usually starts in the medial temporal lobe (entorhinal cortex and hippocampus) or the posterior cingulate, and then spreads to the tempoparietal cortex. In <1% of cases, a mutation in genes encoding for amyloid-processing enzymes is found; however, most cases are sporadic, with APOE4 genotype increasing the risk of AD moderately. Age and cardiovascular risk factors are important predictors as well.

The clinical manifestations of AD are episodic memory impairment, but in younger patients visuospatial disturbances may prevail, and even language problems can be seen. While a clinically probable AD diagnosis requires interference in at least two separate domains, biomarkers such as CSF amyloid, PET and MRI can be useful in the prodromal stage of mild cognitive impairment (MCI) by providing evidence of amyloid pathology and subsequent neurodegeneration. The conversion rate from MCI to AD is 10–15% per year and this risk increases markedly when MRI shows atrophy suggestive of AD, e.g. hippocampal atrophy.

MRI and CT are both useful for excluding surgically treatable disorders and demonstrate focal atrophy suggestive of AD.[4] Coronal images perpendicular to the long axis of the temporal horn should be used to determine the amount of hippocampal and medial temporal lobe atrophy (MTA). Since volumetric analysis of the hippocampus is quite time-consuming, MTA can best be analysed using a visual rating scale depicted in Fig. 65-2.

A score of 2 is considered abnormal under the age of 75, and a score of 3 above that age. Strong asymmetry between left and right side should trigger a suspicion of FTD, which can be recognised by concomitant atrophy of the temporal poles and frontal lobes. In younger subjects with AD, the hippocampus may be spared, with pathology dominating in the precuneus (including posterior cingulate) and parietal cortex (Fig. 65-3).

Vascular changes and AD are common and therefore coexisting pathologies in the elderly. The combination of infarcts and Alzheimer pathology is the strongest predictor of dementia in population-based autopsy studies. Atherosclerosis may lead to ischaemic brain damage and probably also accelerates the formation of Alzheimer pathology. In individual patients, it may be difficult to pinpoint their respective relevance, but vascular alterations, especially white matter lesions on MRI, provide an independent target for treatment. Treatment of vascular risk factors may not only prevent further vascular pathology but also benefit progress of AD.

FRONTOTEMPORAL LOBAR DEGENERATION

The term FTLD describes a group of disorders with tau pathology presenting with language and behavioural symptoms. FTLD is the third most common degenerative cause of dementia after AD and dementia with Lewy bodies, accounting for about 5–10% of all cases of dementia and, in younger patients, it is second in frequency after AD. Arnold Pick first described patients with focal atrophy of the frontal and temporal lobes in 1892, including patients with both personality change and language impairment.

The Lund-Manchester criteria recognise three main subtypes of FTLD:

- behavioural variant frontotemporal dementia (bvFTD);
- progressive non-fluent aphasia (PNFA); and
- semantic dementia (SD).

Less commonly, patients with right-sided FTLD present with difficulty recognising faces. It should be noted that language and behavioural disturbances can also be seen

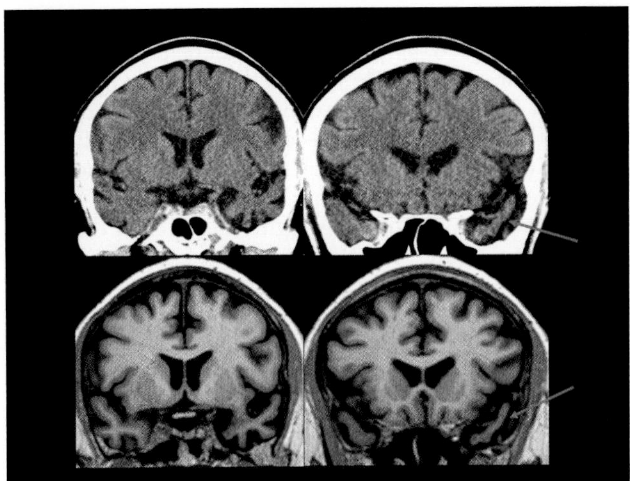

FIGURE 65-4 ■ Coronal CT and MR in a patient with semantic dementia, part of the FTLD spectrum. Note that the coronal reformats of the multidetector CT (top) are quite comparable to the coronal MR (bottom) images in showing left more than right anterior temporal atrophy in the same patient. (Images courtesy of Mike Wattjes.)

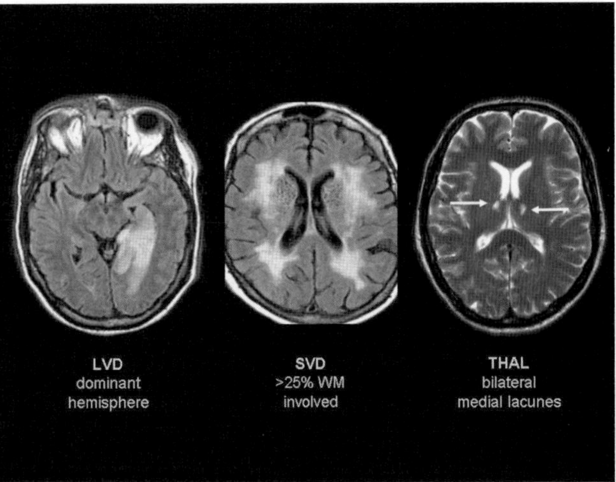

FIGURE 65-5 ■ Vascular dementia is a heterogeneous group of disorders that can be caused by large-vessel infarcts in strategic locations (mostly in the dominant hemisphere), by extensive small-vessel disease and/or by bilateral thalamic lesions. Large-vessel vascular disease (LVD), small-vessel vascular disease (SVD), thalamic disease (THAL).

in (atypical) AD cases and corticobasal degenration (CBD) and progressive supranuclear palsy (PSP).

In contrast to AD, a significant proportion of patients with FTLD have an autosomal dominant family history, sometimes linked to chromosome 17, which can be due to mutations in the microtubule-associated protein tau (MAPT) or progranulin. Other mutations can be found as well, especially in patients with increasingly recognised overlap syndromes with motor neuron disease and amyotrophic lateral sclerosis (ALS).

The hallmark imaging finding in FTLD is atrophy of the temporal and frontal lobes, often (initially) asymmetrical (Fig. 65-4). The patients presentating with the language variant SD often have marked left temporal lobe atrophy (temporal pole more than hippocampus), but in patients with bvFTD, atrophy of the frontal lobes can be mild at the time of presentation. In particular, in these patients, FDG-PET and perfusion MRI can be useful detect functional changes, although care should be taken to exclude depression, which may be similar clinically and on imaging.

VASCULAR DEMENTIA

Vascular dementia (VaD) is the second most common type of dementia after AD, especially in the elderly (where they often coexist and even reinforce one another). The term VaD implies the existence of dementia; however, it is often hard to prove dementia is indeed secondary to cerebrovascular disease (only). Furthermore, VaD is a heterogeneous entity and comprises various conditions due to small- or large-vessel involvement:

- Diffuse confluent age-related white matter changes (ARWMC):
  - also referred to as subcortical arteriosclerotic encephalopathy (SAE).
- Multilacunar state ('état lacunaire').
- Multiple (territorial) infarcts.
- Strategic cortical–subcortical or borderzone infarcts.
- Cortical laminar necrosis (granular cortical atrophy).
- Delayed post-ischaemic demyelination.
- Hippocampal sclerosis.

Clearly, not every vascular pathological finding seen on brain MRI or CT is sufficient to associate with occurrence of dementia in a given patient.[5] The NINDS-AIREN (National Institute of Neurological Disorders and Stroke and Association Internationale pour la Recherché et l'Enseignement en Neurosciences) criteria are the most strict ones for VaD and detail various causes of small- and large-vessel pathology that are likely to cause dementia (Fig. 65-5), which we will discuss in the following sections.

Large-Vessel VaD

Dementia may result from multiple or single cortical–subcortical or subcortical (e.g. borderzone) cerebrovascular lesions (infarcts) involving strategic regions of the brain, such as the hippocampus, paramedian thalamus and the thalamocortical networks, especially if they occur in the dominant hemisphere.

Small-Vessel VaD

Also referred to as leukoaraïosis or subcortical arteriosclerotic encephalopathy, extensive small-vessel disease due to microangiopathy is the most common form of VaD. Most of these cases are idiopathic or sporadic; i.e. there is no proven or specific/genetic cause that can be identified, although many patients will have a history of cardiovascular risk factors. Within the group of small-vessel VaD, the following subtypes exist:

- extensive white matter lesions—confluent hyperintensities involving >25% of WM;

- multiple lacunes—at least two lacunes in basal ganglia and centrum semiovale each; and
- bilateral thalamic lesions—small infarcts in both medial thalami.

Fluid-attenuated inversion recovery (FLAIR) is most suited for detecting small-vessel disease and is able to differentiate (hyperintense) white matter lesions from (hypointense) lacunes. Thalamic lesions, however, are better seen on T2 than FLAIR images. Recent white matter lesions can be bright on diffusion-weighted imaging (DWI), suggesting recent 'lacunar' infarction (i.e. involving a single perforating arteriolar territory). White matter lesions with more severe tissue destruction become T1 hypointense and are better appreciated on CT and tend to correlate better with clinical severity. The white matter lesions in small-vessel VaD involve most of the deep white matter of frontal and parietal lobes, but tend to spare the U-fibres (in contrast to multiple sclerosis) and the temporal lobes (in contrast to multiple sclerosis and CADASIL; see below). The basal ganglia and the central pons are also frequently affected.

CADASIL, Fabry's Disease and CAA

While no specific cause can be identified in most cases of small-vessel VaD, there are few examples of inherited/genetic diseases that can be identified readily using MRI:

- cerebral autosomal dominant arteriopathy with subcortical infarcts and leukoencephalopathy (CADASIL);
- Fabry's disease; and
- cerebral amyloid angiopathy (CAA).

CADASIL is caused by a mutation in the gene *notch-3* and may present with headache and presenile dementia. In presymptomatic mutation carriers, the white matter of the temporal poles is often affected in mid-life, and by the time patients become symptomatic, very extensive white matter changes extending into the U-fibres at the convexity are present (Fig. 65-6). Lacunes and microbleeds are common.

Fabry's disease is an X-linked recessive vasculopathy resulting from α-galactosidase A deficiency. Since it accounts for ~1% of male strokes, there should be screening for it in young male patients. The imaging findings are mostly non-specific small- and large-vessel pathology on CT or MRI. A relatively specific MRI finding is hyperintensity of the pulvinar on T1-weighted images, with hypointensity on T2*-weighted images in the more severe cases, related to calcification on CT.

Several rare genetic causes of CAA exist in small genetic clusters. Most CAA cases, however, are sporadic and present with lobar haemorrhaging and extensive white matter lesions and (silent) infarcts. Less advanced cases may present with multiple cerebral microbleeds (MBs) only, which can be visualised with T2* gradient-echo images or susceptibility-weighted images (Fig. 65-7). Such MBs are a risk factor for subsequent bleeding and stroke in CAA, but also in more typical cases of stroke. CAA is due to β-amyloid deposition in the media and adventitia of small- to medium-sized cerebral arteries and is linked to Alzheimer pathology in a substantial number of cases.

Systemic Causes of VaD

In addition to ischaemia caused by vascular wall changes, as discussed in the preceding sections, systemic disorders can also cause ischaemia and lead to cognitive dysfunction and ultimately dementia. Systemic causes of ischaemia include cellular dysfunction (mitochondrial disease), but also clotting disorders (e.g. sickle-cell disease) and anaemia/hypotension.

Differential Diagnosis of WM Disorders in Dementia

While most white matter lesions in ageing and dementia are of vascular origin, there is a long differential diagnosis that might be considered, especially in young-onset cases.

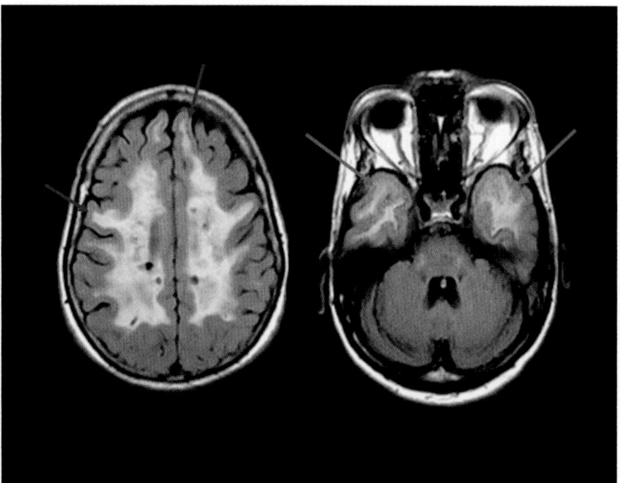

FIGURE 65-6 ■ White matter lesions in CADASIL differ from those in common small-vessel disease by involving the temporal poles (red arrows) and U-fibres at the convexity (blue arrows).

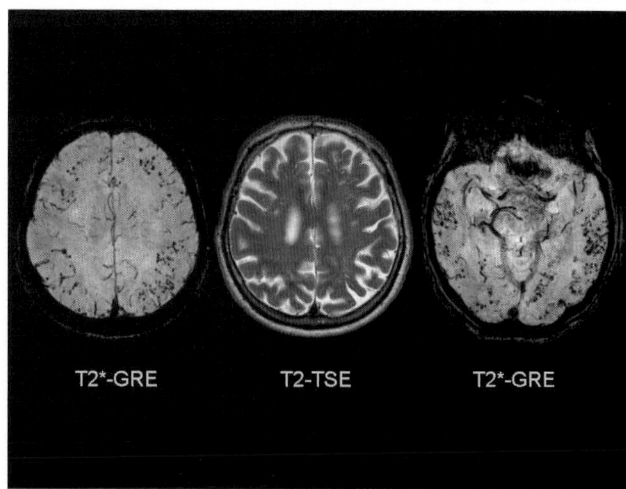

FIGURE 65-7 ■ Gradient-echo (GRE) T2*-weighted images reveal hundreds of small lobar microbleeds not seen on routine T2 spin-echo (TSE) images due to the blooming effect caused by haemosiderin in vessel walls, which became fragile due to amyloid deposition in this patient with Alzheimer's disease.

For example, multiple sclerosis may first present with cognitive impairment, especially when juxtacortical lesions are abundant. Other autoimmune disorders that tend to impair cognition include SLE. Several metabolic disorders may first present in adulthood, e.g. vanishing white matter disease and adult polyglucosan body disease. These typically present with symmetric confluent white matter abnormalties and should be differentiated from toxic disorders. Finally, several infections can manifest with dementia, e.g. HIV encephalitis and progressive multifocal leukoencephalopathy (PML), which will be discussed in the next section.

RAPIDLY PROGRESSIVE AND OTHER ATYPICAL DEMENTIAS

Infectious and Inflammatory Disease

HIV and PML

HIV may affect the brain in several ways. First, direct infection may lead to HIV encephalitis. Secondly, opportunistic infections, such as toxoplasmosis, CMV and PML, may occur. HIV encephalitis is best demonstrated on FLAIR images that may show an ill-defined and often symmetrical hyperintensity in the cerebral white matter, with no typical predilection—the subcortical U-fibres are characteristically spared. PML is an opportunistic infection that occurs in up to 5% of AIDS patients, and has a very poor prognosis, even with treatment. PML is caused by the JC papovavirus, a ubiquitous DNA virus that infects oligodendrocytes in immunocompromised patients and leads to massive demyelination with rapidly progressive clinical presentation. CT may reveal multifocal lesions with swelling and marked hypodensity with little contrast enhancement. MRI is more sensitive and shows multiple focal T2 hyperintense and markedly T1 hypointense lesions, located in the subcortical white matter, with gyral swelling mostly sparing the cortical ribbon—so-called 'scalloping out' of the grey–white border. Gadolinium enhancement is rare and, if it occurs, is patchy.

Prion Disease

Prions are protein-like structues that may cause disease in an infectious manner, especially in those that are genetically susceptible. Prion diseases include:

- Creutzfeldt–Jakob disease (CJD)—sporadic, familial and iatrogenic forms;
- variant CJD (vCJD)—sporadic (and possibly iatrogenic);
- Gerstmann–Sträussler–Scheinker (GSS) syndrome—only familial;
- fatal familial insomnia (FFI)—familial and sporadic; and
- kuru—only sporadic.

CJD usually presents in the fifth to seventh decade, and is sporadic in the vast majority of cases. Presentation typically is with a triad of subacute dementia, myoclonus and motor disturbances (extrapyramidal or cerebellar) with a characteristic EEG pattern consisting of triphasic waves and CSF abnormalities (increased tau and/or 14-3-3 protein).

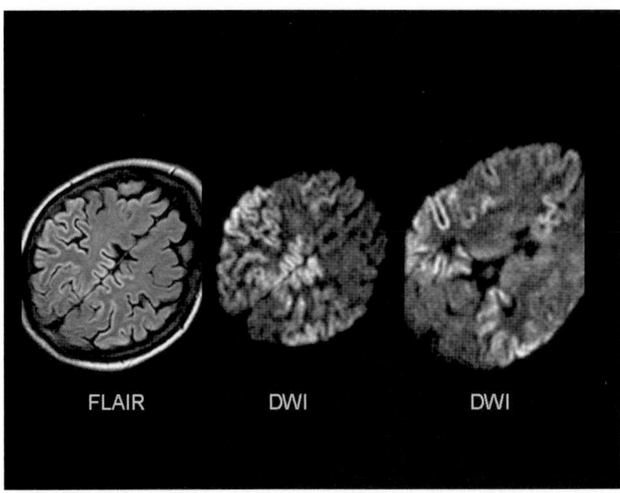

FIGURE 65-8 ■ In this patient with rapid cognitive decline due to CJD, FLAIR images show mildly increased signal intensity in multiple areas of the neocortex, which are much more prominent on DWI.

MRI should include DWI; images after contrast material administration are useful for ruling out alternative disorders. FLAIR sequences may show increased signal in the striatum, especially the putamen, or discontinous involvement of the neocortex (Fig. 65-8). Abnormal DWI may be especially prominent in early phases of the disease when vacuoles are small, leading to restricted diffusion (which may disappear in late stages). Sometimes there is a combination of neocortical and subcortical involvement. Usually the pattern of involvement is bilateral, but it may be unilateral as well (initially).

Autoimmune Limbic Encephalitis

Non-infectious limbic encephalitis occurs in patients presenting with a subacute onset of memory impairment and confusion, focal, usually medial temporal lobe seizures. Classically, this occurs in the context of a distant malignancy (mostly lung cancer) through a variety of antibodies. However, non-neoplastic variants exist as well, with a similar autoimmune basis. These include antibodies against voltage-gated potassium channels or the NMDA-receptor, but may also involve antibodies that are gluten-sensitivity or thyroid-related (Hashimoto's encephalitis). Typically, the hippocampus is involved with hyperintensity and swelling on coronal FLAIR images, but more extensive abnormalities may involve the basal ganglia as well (e.g. in Hashimoto's encephalitis). The differential diagnosis includes herpes simplex encephalitis, which is often unilateral and involves the insula as well.

Toxic/Metabolic Disorders

Toxic encephalopathies include vitamin B deficiencies, dialysis dementia, CO intoxication, delayed post-hypoxic demyelination, organic solvents (including toluene) and heroin intoxication. Wernicke's encephalopathy mostly occurs in alcoholics due to vitamin B_1 deficiency and typical MRI findings comprise T2/FLAIR hyperintensity in the medial thalamus, mamillary bodies, periaqueductal grey matter and colliculi. Increased signal on T1 may occur due to microhaemorrhages and diffusion can be restricted in the acute phase. In vitamin B_{12} deficiency, brain MRI may show diffuse supratentorial areas of T2 hyperintensity in the periventriclular and deep white matter, while brainstem and the cerebellar white matter are relatively spared. Spinal cord MRI may show a mild swelling and signal abnormalities in the dorsal and lateral columns. Contrast enhancement is not observed.

Most leukodystrophies are genetically determined and present early in life and lead to dementia in a later phase. However, some leukodystrophies present later in life and do have cognitive decline as a characteristic feature, e.g vanishing white matter, mitochondrial disease and cerebro-tendinous xanthomatosis. The cardinal imaging feature of the leukodystophies is involvement of the white matter, with hyperintensity on T2-weighted and FLAIR images. Involvement usually occurs in a strictly symmetric fashion, except in mitochondrial disorders such as mitochondrial encephalomyopathy, lactic acidosis and stroke-like episodes (MELAS). The corticospinal tracts and cerebellum are frequently involved structures. Important diagnostic clues can be obtained from the family history, and from involvement of the peripheral nervous system, the eyes, adrenal glands, tendons or other organs. The most common genetic disorder is fragile X-associated tremor/ataxia syndrome (FXTAS), which presents mostly in men after the age of 50 with intention tremor or gait ataxia; bilateral hyperintensity of the middle cerebellar peduncles is one of the diagnostic criteria.

PARKINSON'S DISEASE AND RELATED DISORDERS

Idiopathic Parkinson's Disease and Differential Diagnosis

Idiopathic Parkinson's disease is caused by abnormal accumulation of α-synuclein protein in grey matter of the brainstem and basal ganglia. The symptoms include bradykinesia, rigidity, tremor and loss of postural reflexes. The disease process starts in the substantia nigra in the mesencephalon and by the time patients become symptomatic, 90% of neurons have disappeared. The dopaminergic deficit itself can be demonstrated using PET or SPECT.

Since parkinsonism can be caused by other pathological features leading to the same dopaminergic deficit, structural imaging should aim to rule out:

- Secondary parkinsonism caused by focal pathological features in the basal ganglia:
  - especially vasculoischaemic lesions (Fig. 65-9).
- Parkinson-plus syndromes: progressive supranuclear palsy (PSP) and multiple system atrophy (MSA):
  - selective atrophy in the mesencephalon (PSP) and pons (MSA).
  - Typical hyperintensities on MRI in the middle cerebellar peduncles and midpons in the cerebellar form of MSA (MSA-C), and along the lateral aspects of the putamina in the parkinsonian form of MSA (MSA-P).

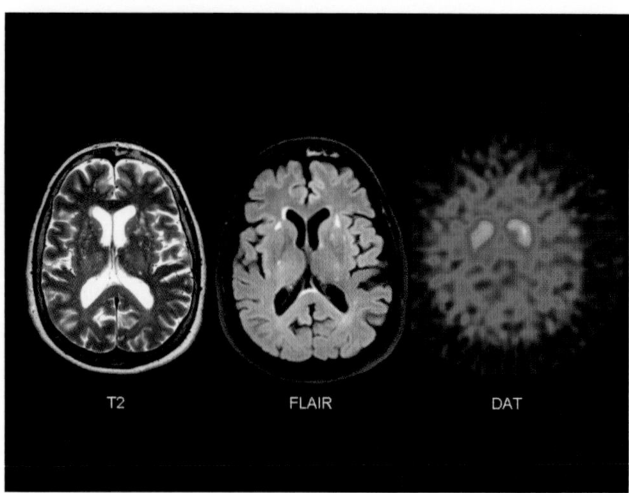

FIGURE 65-9 ■ This case of parkinsonism was secondary to vascular lesions in the basal ganglia seen on MRI, while a DAT-SPECT revealed normal striatal tracer uptake, which rules out primary Parkinson's disease.

Dementia with Parkinsonism

A number of neurodegenerative diseases present with a combination of cognitive impairment and parkinsonism. In many of these conditions additional phenotypic features such as dysautonomia, gaze palsies, cerebellar and pyramidal signs may suggest one pathological process over another, but none are pathognomonic for PSP, MSA or corticobasal degeneration (CBD).

Lewy body disease is the most common cause of progressive cognitive decline with parkinsonism. DLB and Parkinson's disease dementia (PDD) are regarded as ends of a continuous spectrum—the former with an initial presentation with dementia, the latter presenting with parkinsonism followed by dementia after more than a year, but ultimately both have widely distributed Lewy bodies in the cerebral cortex.

Imaging findings in dementia with parkinsonism (Fig. 65-10) include:

- DLB—normal hippocampi on MRI, abnormal dopamine SPECT;
- PSP—mesencephalic atrophy on MRI ('hummingbird' sign); and
- MSA—pontine atrophy and 'hot-cross bun' sign.

Neurodegeneration and Other Movement Disorders

Non-parkinsonian movement disorders can be found in a rare number of other neurodegenerative disorders. For example, amyotrophic lateral sclerosis (ALS)-like phenotypes can be seen in FTD.

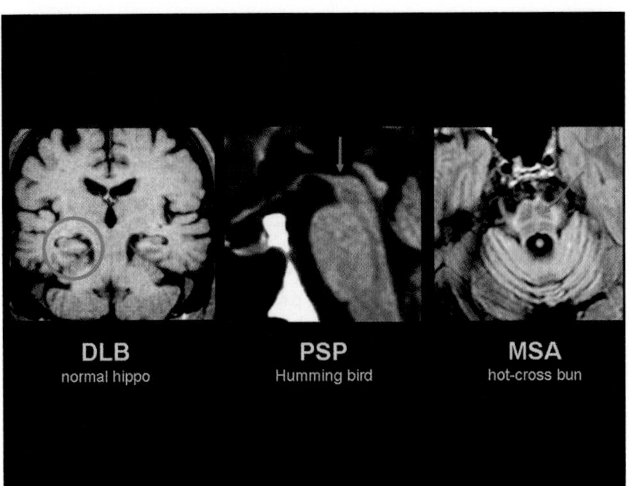

FIGURE 65-10 ■ MRI findings in patients with dementia and parkinsonian features. In DLB, a normal hippocampus helps to rule out Alzheimer's disease. In progressive supranuclear palsy (PSP), severe mesencephalic atrophy occurs, giving the appearance of a hummingbird on mid-sagittal images. In multisystem atrophy (MSA), there is severe atrophy of the pons, sometimes with a hot cross bun-like pattern on FLAIR and T2-weighted images.

Neuroimaging can help in the following diseases:

- Neurodegeneration with brain iron accumulation (NBIA, formerly Hallervorden–Spatz disease):
  - low signal on T2* images in the basal ganglia.
- Huntington's disease: atrophy of the caudate nucleus; and
- Wilson's disease: T2 hyperintensity in the mesencephalon.

EPILEPSY—INTRODUCTION AND CLINICAL

Epilepsy is defined as a chronic neurological condition of patients having spontaneous, recurrent seizures as a result of increased neuronal discharges. It has a prevalence of 0.4 to 1% in the population.[6] Epilepsy syndromes can be divided into two groups: generalised and focal (partial). In generalised syndromes seizures originate simultaneously from both cerebral hemispheres, which can either occur primarily or as a consequence of focal seizures extending to the rest of the brain (secondary generalisation).

Focal seizures/epilepsy syndromes start in a localised area of the brain and are classified as simple partial seizures, if the patient does not suffer any loss of consciousness during the seizure, or complex partial seizures, which are always associated with loss of consciousness.

Classification of Seizures

- Generalised
  - Primary generalised
  - Secondarily generalised
- Focal (partial)
  - Simple partial
  - Complex partial

Initial treatment of epilepsy is medical, with a large variety of antiepileptic drugs currently available in clinical practice. Most patients with generalised seizures respond to antiepileptic drug treatment. Although about 30% of patients with partial seizures are resistant to medical treatment,[7] further treatment options are available, the most effective being surgical resection of the brain region/lesion causing the seizures.

Appropriate classification of patients with seizures, and especially those having medically refractory epilepsy, is crucial for improving management and care of patients. Imaging tools, especially MRI, play a substantial role in detecting pathological features underlying the seizure origin. However, the ability of MRI to detect underlying brain lesions/abnormalities in patients with epilepsy varies and depends on the patient groups studied. In general, MRI has a greater sensitivity for lesion detection in patients with intractable epilepsy, amounting to about 85%.[8] The value of MRI in patients with idiopathic, generalised epilepsy is very little. However, with advances in technology, improved knowledge of neuroradiologists and more dedicated epilepsy clinics, the value of imaging will certainly increase, especially when MRI is combined with functional imaging techniques, including nuclear medicine (PET and SPECT).

EPILEPSY—IMAGING APPROACH

Indications for Imaging

Current published guidelines for management of patients with epilepsy include that MRI should always be performed in a non-urgent setting, excluding those patients with idiopathic, generalised seizures. In the urgent setting, especially if there are focal neurological signs, or associated fever or trauma, CT remains the examination of choice.

The main role of MRI in a patient with epilepsy is to identify an underlying brain abnormality that relates to the patient's symptoms and that helps to define the clinical syndrome. MRI helps in characterising underlying pathological substrates, and in defining their relationship to functional brain areas, such as those related to motor or language tasks. Concordance of the lesion seen on imaging with either clinical or electrophysiological data, indicating a possible origin of the seizures (lateralisation to one cerebral hemisphere), is crucial for appropriate patient assessment. Finally, MRI also helps in defining surgical treatment options in patients with intractable epilepsy, and in the postsurgical setting. In this regard, MRI, either alone or combined with other functional imaging techniques, such as PET, may provide further insight in patients having poor response to surgery, identifying remaining epileptogenic areas.[9]

Imaging Protocol

Appropriate MRI of the brain in patients with epilepsy should include high-resolution volumetric T1, high-resolution T2 (Fig. 65-11) and FLAIR images covering the entire brain. Coronal images are very helpful in

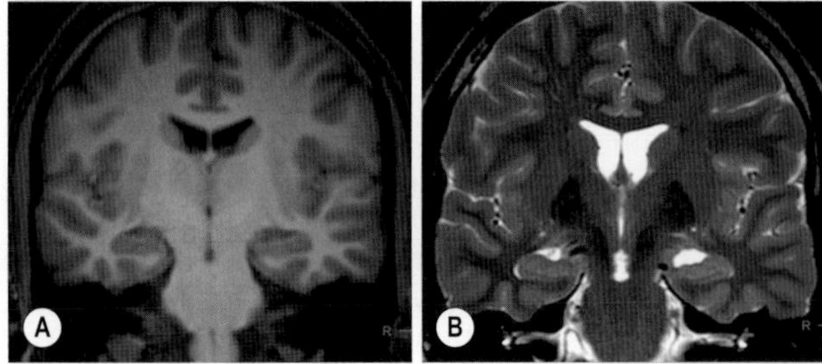

FIGURE 65-11 ■ Dedicated MRI to study patients with epilepsy. High-resolution T1 coronal (A) and T2 (B) images, covering the entire brain, and allowing detailed assessment ot the medial temporal lobes, should be obtained.

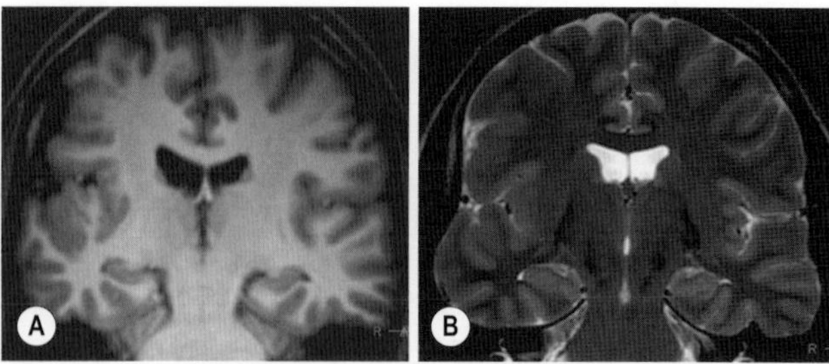

FIGURE 65-12 ■ MRI findings in a patient with an abnormality of cortical development. There is abnormal cortex, with abnormal gyri, around the right sylvian fissure (A), faint cortical T2 hyperintensity and blurring of the normal grey–white matter differentiation in the right insula (B).

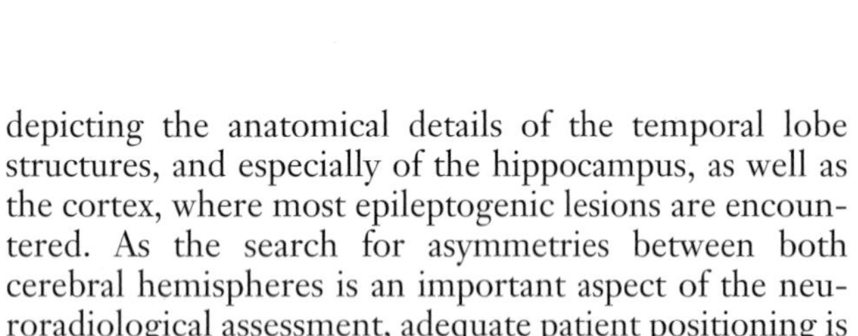

depicting the anatomical details of the temporal lobe structures, and especially of the hippocampus, as well as the cortex, where most epileptogenic lesions are encountered. As the search for asymmetries between both cerebral hemispheres is an important aspect of the neuroradiological assessment, adequate patient positioning is crucial. As a general rule, both internal auditory meati should be identified on the same MR image.

Most common causes for epilepsy identified on MRI include post-traumatic brain lesions, tumours, vascular malformations and infections. Additionally, MRI is particularly helpful in identifying further entities, more commonly seen in patients with intractable epilepsy, such as hippocampal sclerosis, abnormalities of cortical development, syndromes associating with several intracranial abnormalities, such as the phacomatoses, and other less common abnormalities, including non-specific areas of gliosis.

EPILEPSY—CONGENITAL DISORDERS

Migration and Gyration Disorders

Developmental disorders have been increasingly recognised on MRI in children and young adults with epilepsy, accounting for up to 50% of paediatric cases of intractable epilepsy, and about 25% of those in young adults.[10] Disorders altering neuronal and glial proliferation, migration or organisation of the cortical layers are now grouped together as abnormalities of cortical development and further subclassified, depending on the most relevant underlying pathogenesis.

These abnormalities include the following entities, which may also coexist in the same patient, and involve different brain regions simultaneously:

- cortical dysplasia
- focal cortical dysplasia (FCD)
- agyria/pachygyria
- polymicrogyria
- heterotopias
- schizencephaly
- hamartomas, or cavernous malformations (according to some authors).

Typical MRI findings are the presence of abnormal cortex, which may be thickened, or have few or too many, abnormal gyri. There may also be abnormal sulci, cortical signal abnormalities and abnormalities in the underlying white matter, with blurring and loss of the normal cortical–subcortical differentiation on MRI (Fig. 65-12).

Abnormalities of cortical development, especially in focal cortical dysplasia, are characterised by areas of abnormal lamination of the cortex, and abnormal 'balloon neurons' on histology. MRI features include thickened cortex, which may be slightly hyperintense on T2 images, and blurring of the cortical–subcortical boundaries. The patients may have further abnormalities in the ipsilateral, or even contralateral medial temporal lobe structures on MRI, including changes in the hippocampi with loss of hippocampal volume and T2 signal change, reflecting neuronal loss and gliosis, as shown on epilepsy surgery specimens.[11] Abnormalities of cortical metabolism on FDG-PET may be larger than the abnormal area on structural MRI, indicating that abnormalities in the brain of patients with FCD are more extensive than previously thought. The significance of these findings with respect to patients' symptoms is unclear, but they may potentially indicate additional areas of epileptogenesis.[12,13]

Heterotopias are characterised by the presence of normal neurons in abnormal locations, and they are usually divided into three types based on clinical and imaging features: subependymal/periventricular, subcortical and band/laminar. Heterotopias typically show the same signal as cortical grey matter on all sequences, and they may be associated with other abnormalities of cortical development, such as schizencephaly. Band heterotopias (Fig. 65-13) are considered as a mild form of lissencephaly (smooth brain) by some authors, and have recently been associated with several different genes.[14]

In general, many abnormalities of cortical development are indeed epileptogenic, but the extent of the epileptogenic area may be greater than the lesion seen on MRI, or the epileptogenic area may not precisely correlate with the malformation itself. As mentioned already, FDG-PET can show more widespread areas of abnormal metabolism in the brain than those seen on structural MRI.[15] For these reasons imaging information always needs to be considered within the context of all patient investigations, taking into account clinical and electrophysiological data, especially if patients are being considered as surgical candidates.

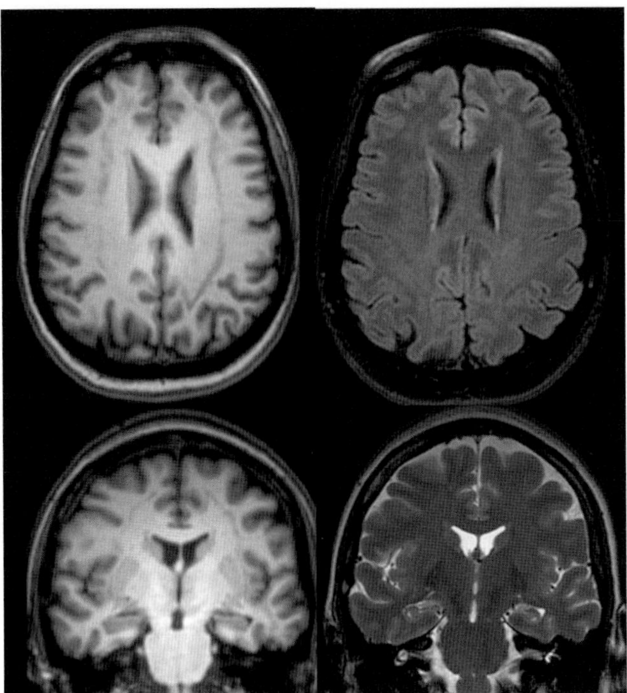

FIGURE 65-13 ■ MRI findings in a patient with band heterotopias in both cerebral hemispheres. Axial and coronal T1 (left top and bottom, respectively), axial FLAIR (right top) and coronal T2 (right bottom) images. There are band-like appearances of grey matter signal on all sequences within the white matter of both cerebral hemispheres which are most conspicuous on the T1 images.

Genetic Syndromes

Several genetic and congenital syndromes are associated with epilepsy, including some of the better known neurocutaneous syndromes, such as tuberous sclerosis and Sturge–Weber syndrome.

Tuberous sclerosis complex is a multisystem congenital syndrome with widespread CNS anomalies. Neurological manifestations include epilepsy and cognitive impairment, and approximately 90% of patients have seizures, with intractable epilepsy developing in 25–30% of patients. Typical imaging findings include cortical or subcortical tubers, subependymal nodules, subependymal giant cell astrocytomas and white matter radial migration lines (Fig. 65-14). On T2-weighted and FLAIR MR images, tubers typically appear as areas of increased signal intensity in the cortical and subcortical regions. Subependymal nodules are found on the walls of the lateral ventricles. Subependymal giant cell astrocytomas can grow, eventually resulting in ventricular obstruction and hydrocephalus. Radial migration lines are believed to represent heterotopic glia and neurons along the expected path of cortical migration. Radial migration lines are primarily located in the subcortical white matter and are occasionally seen in relation to tubers.

Patients with the Sturge–Weber neurocutaneous syndrome present typically with a facial angioma in the trigeminal nerve distribution and ipsilateral meningeal angiomatosis. Clinically, patients have intractable seizures, hemiparesis, hemianopsia and mental retardation.

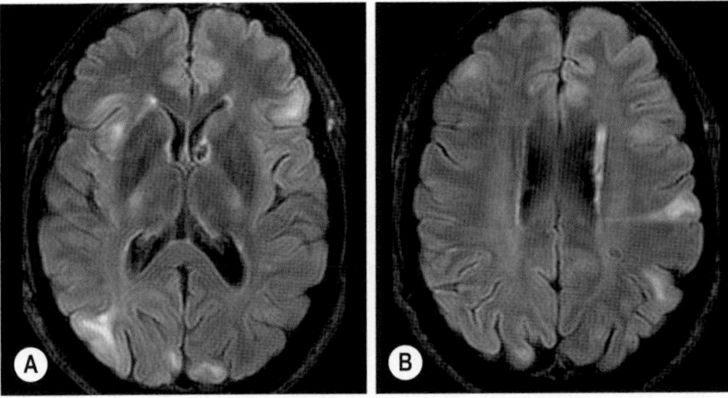

FIGURE 65-14 ■ MRI findings in a patient with tuberous sclerosis. Axial FLAIR image (A) shows several hyperintense cortical–subcortical tubers in both cerebral hemispheres, a subependymal tumour at the level of the foramen of Monroe on the left and signal change areas in the white matter representing radial migration lines, reaching the left lateral ventricle (B).

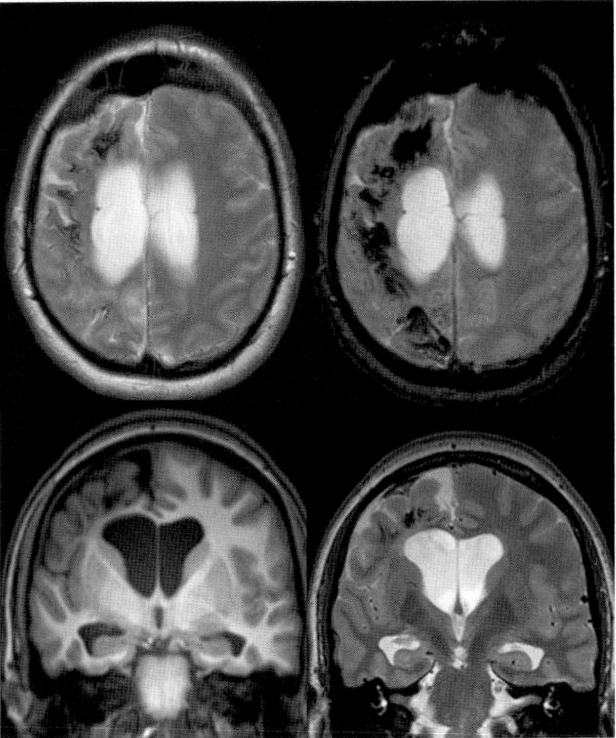

FIGURE 65-15 ■ Typical MRI findings in a patient with Sturge–Weber syndrome. The predominantly hypointense pial angioma is seen in the right cerebral hemisphere, which has a smaller volume. T2* gradient-echo images show the signal change associated with the pial angiomata more clearly (above right side).

MRI findings in these patients may include (Fig. 65-15):

- pial angiomata in the parieto-occipital regions;
- cortical calcifications subjacent to the cortex and white matter, typically in the parieto-occipital region;
- enlarged choroid plexus;
- atrophy of the ipsilateral cerebral hemisphere (angioma side);
- enlarged and elongated globe of the eye; and

- prominent enlarged subependymal and medullary veins, and secondary signs of cerebral atrophy involving the paranasal sinuses, mastoid cells and calvarium.

EPILEPSY—ACQUIRED DISEASES

Hippocampal Sclerosis

This is the most common abnormality found in temporal lobe resections of patients with intractable epilepsy undergoing surgery. On pathology, this entity is defined by the presence of neuronal loss and gliosis. Typical MRI findings[16] are hippocampal volume loss and increased T2 signal within the abnormally small hippocampus (Fig. 65-16).

Further imaging findings on MRI in patients with hippocampal sclerosis include:

- loss of the internal architecture of the hippocampus;
- atrophy of the ipsilateral mamillary body and fornix; and
- dilatation of the adjacent temporal horn.

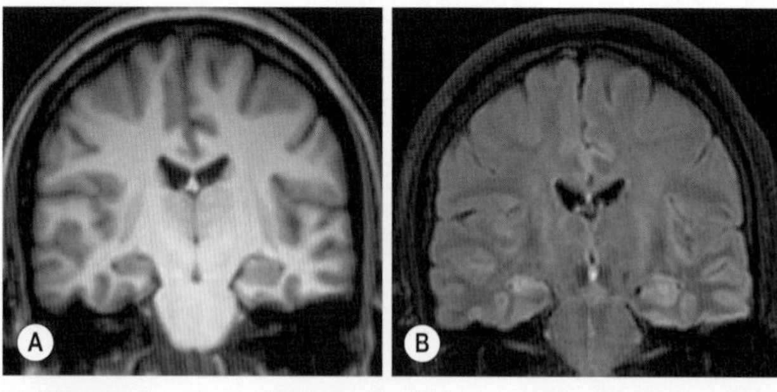

FIGURE 65-16 ■ MRI findings in hippocampal sclerosis. There is loss of volume of the right hippocampus seen on high-resolution T1-weighted images (A), as well as increased T2 signal within it on coronal FLAIR images (B), reflecting neuronal loss and gliosis, respectively.

MRI identifies up to 90% of the cases of hippocampal sclerosis. Hippocampal sclerosis may also occur bilaterally in up to 20% of the cases. Some patients may have an additional epileptogenic area, either temporal extra-hippocampal or even extratemporal, which is referred as 'dual pathology'. The most common association occurs between cortical dysplasia and hippocampal sclerosis. Surgery is curative in up to 70% of patients with hippocampal sclerosis, especially in those not having dual pathology, and where there is a concordance in lateralisation among clinical, electrophysiological and MRI information.[17]

Neoplasms

A tumour is found in about 4% of patients having epilepsy. About 70% of those tumours causing epilepsy are found in the temporal lobes and in most cases near the cortex. MRI is particularly helpful in defining the relationship of tumours to functionally eloquent areas of the brain, as complete resection of the tumour and overlying cortex results in complete control of seizures in many cases, and improves the patient's outcome.

In patients with seizures, the tumours most frequently found include low-grade astrocytomas, gangliogliomas, dysembryoplastic neuroepithelial tumour (DNET), oligodendroglioma, pleomorphic xanthoastrocytoma and metastasis.[16] The precise characterisation of these tumour types is not always straightforward. Gangliogliomas are usually found in the temporal lobes in young adults, are partly solid and partly cystic and are located in the cortex. They may show calcification and contrast enhancement. DNETs are low-grade, multicystic tumours, also located in the cortex, or middle temporal lobe structures, usually occurring in children and young adults. Their radiological appearance is variable, and there may be calcification, bleeding and contrast enhancement in up to a third of cases (Fig. 65-17).

In patients with tumours, functional MRI techniques have proven to be useful for surgical planning. Using different paradigms, such as a motor or verbal task, eloquent areas of the brain and their relationship to the

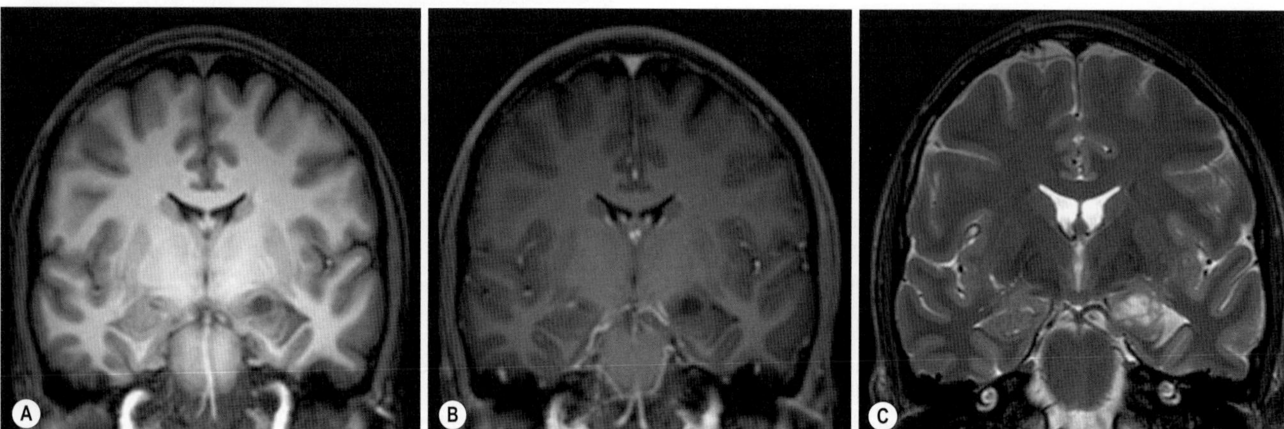

FIGURE 65-17 ■ MRI findings in a patient with a DNET in the left medial temporal lobe, involving the hippocampus. The mass appears heterogenously T1 hypointense with a cystic component (A), and no contrast enhancement (B), as well as heterogeneous T2 hyperintense (C).

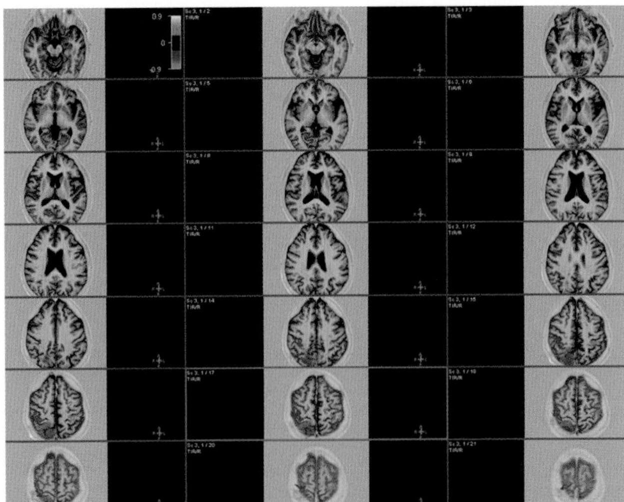

FIGURE 65-18 ■ fMRI using a motor task (opposition of all digits, alternating both hands). The primary motor cortex of both cerebral hemispheres is shown. The right hemisphere tumour lies posterior to the right-sided primary motor area, being adjacent to it, but not in close contact. The risk for motor-deficit postsurgically exists, but is less than with a tumour attached to or involving the functional area.

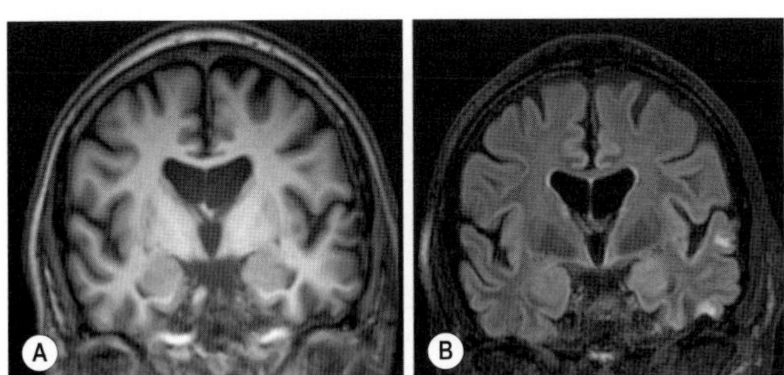

FIGURE 65-19 ■ MRI findings in a patient with post-traumatic epilepsy. There is an abnormal left superior temporal gyrus, showing cortical thinning and signal change, which is hypointense on T1 images (A), and hyperintense on FLAIR images (B), in keeping with mature damage (encephalomalacia).

tumour can be identified, allowing a better assessment of potential for focal deficits after surgery (Fig. 65-18).

Post-Traumatic Epilepsy

This is not an uncommon condition. Head injuries can cause damage to the cortex, most frequently in the frontal lobes or in the temporal regions, due to the underlying, adjacent bony structures. Cerebral contusions at these sites may leave haemosiderin deposits and gliosis, which are known to be involved in seizure generation and propagation. Several risk factors have been identified for late post-traumatic epilepsy, such as early seizures, severe brain injury, depressed skull fractures, penetrating injuries or brain contusions. MRI is very helpful in showing acute and chronic haemorrhage, diffuse axonal injury and gliosis (Fig. 65-19).

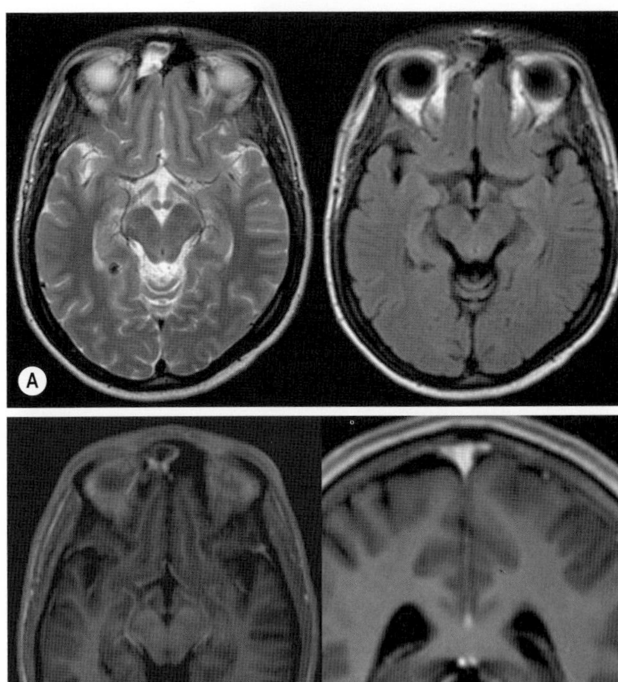

FIGURE 65-20 ■ MRI findings in a patient with cysticercosis. There is a small, rounded lesion in the right posterior part of the medial temporal lobe, of low signal on T2 and FLAIR images (A) region, which enhances only very minimally (B). The appearances are consistent with a partially calcified nodular stage of cysticercosis.

Infections

Bacterial, viral, fungal, mycobacterial or parasitic infections may cause seizures, both in the acute phase (being the early clinical presentation), as well as in the chronic stage, as a result of gliosis. Among these, cysticercosis frequently presents with seizures, and can be identified on imaging studies. In the active phase, cysticercosis appears as thin-walled, non-enhancing cysts that may have an eccentrically located nodule (scolex) within them. Death of the parasite causes inflammatory changes in the adjacent brain, with vasogenic oedema and enhancement. In the final stages, calcification occurs (Fig. 65-20).

Rasmussen encephalitis is a chronic encephalitis characterised by partial motor seizures and progressive neurological and cognitive deterioration, mostly seen in children. MRI demontrates involvement of one cerebral hemisphere, with increased T2 signal in the cortex and subcortical white matter, progressing to atrophy in the late stages.

For a full list of references, please see ExpertConsult.

CHAPTER 66

Orbit

Stefanie C. Thust • Katherine Miszkiel • Indran Davagnanam

CHAPTER OUTLINE

THE ORBIT

INTRODUCTION

The orbit represents a key element of the visual pathway. Diseases of the orbit, particularly those affecting vision, may be severely debilitating and impact on many aspects of the affected individual's life. Owing to its complex structure and specialised function, there are several pathologies, which are specific to the orbit. Alternatively, the orbit may be involved in a variety of systemic processes including diseases of the retro-orbital visual pathway.

ORBITAL ANATOMY

The shape of the orbit can be likened to that of an elongated pyramid, whereby the base lies anteriorly and the apex posteriorly. The orbit has four walls: a roof, floor, medial and lateral wall, all of which converge posteriorly at the orbital apex. The medial orbital walls run virtually parallel, but due to the shape of the orbits, their long axes diverge at approximately 45°.[1] The roof of the orbit is composed of the frontal bone anteriorly and the lesser wing of sphenoid posteriorly. The orbital roof forms the floor of the frontal sinus and part of the anterior cranial fossa. At the anterior margin of the orbital roof, a small notch or sometimes a complete foramen can be found, which transmits the supraorbital nerve, a branch of the ophthalmic division (V1) of the trigeminal nerve. The floor of the orbit is made up of the zygomatic bone laterally and the maxilla medially, with a small contribution from the orbital process of the palatine bone; it contains a small canal for the infraorbital nerve, a branch of the maxillary division of the trigeminal nerve. The orbital floor forms the roof of the maxillary sinus and is relatively thin, thus susceptible to blow-out fracture or spread of severe sinus infection. The medial orbital wall is composed of several bones (maxilla, frontal, ethmoid, lacrimal and sphenoid) and separates the orbit from the ethmoid air cells. It is a very thin wall, also referred to as the lamina papyracea, and can easily be injured. The lateral wall of the orbit is formed by the frontal and zygomatic bones. It runs obliquely from lateral to medial posteriorly, separating the orbit from the temporal fossa anteriorly and from the middle cranial fossa posteriorly.

The following apertures can be found in the orbit posteriorly: the superior orbital fissure lies between the lateral orbital wall and roof and contains the cranial nerves (CN) III, IV, V1 and VI and the ophthalmic veins, which drain into the cavernous sinus; the optic nerve canal lies at the junction of the roof and medial wall and contains the optic nerve and ophthalmic artery; the inferior orbital fissure lies between the lateral wall and floor of the orbital and contains the infraorbital nerve.

There are six extraocular muscles: namely, four rectus muscles and two oblique muscles. The four rectus muscles arise from the annulus of Zinn, a fibrous tendon ring which surrounds the optic nerve at the orbital apex, and inserts into the globe. The superior oblique muscle runs from the orbital apex to the superior orbital border, where it loops around the trochlea and then passes posteriorly to insert in the globe. The inferior oblique muscle originates anteriorly from the orbital floor and inserts on the back of the globe. The lateral rectus muscle is innervated by the abducens nerve (CN VI) and the superior oblique muscle by the trochlear nerve (CN IV). All other extraocular muscles and also the levator palpebrae are supplied by the oculomotor nerve (CN III). The rectus muscles with their fascial layers form the *orbital cone*, a landmark which can be used to divide the orbit into three compartments: the *extraconal* compartment, which comprises all structures *peripheral* to the cone, the *conal* compartment and the *intraconal* compartment, which comprises all structures central to muscle. A compartmental approach is very useful when defining the anatomical location of orbital pathology, as this may significantly narrow the list of potential differentials. Even in cases of a multi-compartmental lesion, defining the epicentre of an abnormality may still be useful.

The orbital septum is an important anatomical boundary, which can be found anterior to the globe. It is an incomplete fibrous membrane continuous with the levator palpebrae superioris superiorly and the tarsus inferiorly and forms a barrier between the orbit and subcutaneous tissues. This can be relevant for the spread of infection.

The globe is divided into three major tissue layers. These are:

- the sclera and cornea, which constitute the outer layer;
- the middle layer representing the uvea, which consists of the choroid, the iris and ciliary body; and
- the inner layer, the retina.

The globe is divided by the lens and iris into an anterior chamber filled with aqueous humour and a posterior chamber filled with vitreous humour.

The optic nerve (CN II) consists of four segments: a very short intraocular portion, an intraorbital, intracanalicular and intracranial segment. Embryologically, it is not a true cranial nerve, but rather an extension of brain parenchyma; it is myelinated by oligodendrocytes and not Schwann cells. This explains why pathologies such as gliomas and meningiomas affect the optic nerve, whereas schwannomas and neurofibromas occur in other cranial nerves. Arterial supply to the optic nerve is via the retinal artery (a branch of the ophthalmic artery), which runs inside the nerve to the globe. Further branches of the ophthalmic artery which supply the orbit are the frontal, lacrimal and nasociliary branches. The superior and inferior ophthalmic veins represent the main venous drainage pathways of the orbit.

IMAGING OF THE ORBIT

Plain film radiography was historically performed as an initial assessment in suspected bony trauma, but had limited sensitivity and does not reliably assess the intraorbital soft tissues. Ultrasound, including colour Doppler sonography, can be very useful in evaluation of the globe, particularly of the retina and anterior chamber but is also useful in assessing vascularity in ocular tumours and directional flow through the superior ophthalmic veins. However, it has only limited benefit in assessing structures beyond the globe itself.

Computed tomography (CT) is readily available at most institutions and offers quick multiplanar orbital imaging. The different densities of orbital structures (bone, fat, muscles and vitreous humour) provide good natural contrast resolution. CT is useful in trauma to identify orbital and periorbital injuries, especially fractures, which are best identified on thin-section multiplanar bone reconstructions. The main role of contrast-enhanced CT of the orbits lies in evaluation of suspected infiltrative, inflammatory and neoplastic disease. Reconstruction is usually performed in the axial, coronal and sagittal planes, both with a soft-tissue and a bone reconstruction algorithm and a slice thickness of 1–3 mm (depending on equipment and local protocol) or less depending on equipment and the clinical question. Axial imaging should be acquired parallel to the orbital axis to allow visualisation of the optic nerve, medial and lateral rectus muscle on a single image. Coronal imaging must be perpendicular to the optic axis.[1]

Magnetic resonance imaging (MRI) has superior soft-tissue contrast to CT and is the most accurate technique in characterising orbital mass lesions. Like CT, MRI is capable of multiplanar imaging; however, these require usually separate acquisitions rather than reconstructions in at least two planes (usually axial and coronal). A typical orbital MRI protocol includes pre-contrast T1 and T2 fat-suppressed imaging and post-contrast imaging with at least one fat-suppressed sequence, all at a slice thickness of 3 mm or less. At minimum, a T2 sequence of the whole brain should also be performed to not miss coexisting intracranial pathology.

ORBITAL PATHOLOGY

Congenital Disease

Coats' Disease

Coats' disease is a congenital vascular malformation of the retina, which results in telangiectasis and aneurysm formation. Due to endothelial damage, leakage of exudative lipoproteniaceous fluid and blood product into the subretinal space occurs and results in progressive thickening of the retina and subsequent retinal detachment. The disease is usually unilateral and presents in childhood age. The most common presenting feature is leukocoria, but visual impairment, pain, secondary glaucoma and strabismus may occur.[2] The nature of the disease is progressive, with loss of vision over a variable length of time. CT findings include increased attenuation along the subretinal space or even filling the entire vitreous. MR imaging may demonstrate increased T1 and T2 signal due to presence of lipoproteinaceous material (Fig. 66-1). There is typically no contrast enhancement.

Persistent Hypertrophic Primary Vitreous (PHPV)

In embryogenesis, the primary vitreous connects the posterior aspect of the lens with the retina. As it is gradually being replaced by the definitive vitreous, the primary vitreous regresses into a band-like fibrovascular structure between the posterior lens surface and retina. A central hyaloid artery can remain present within this. There may

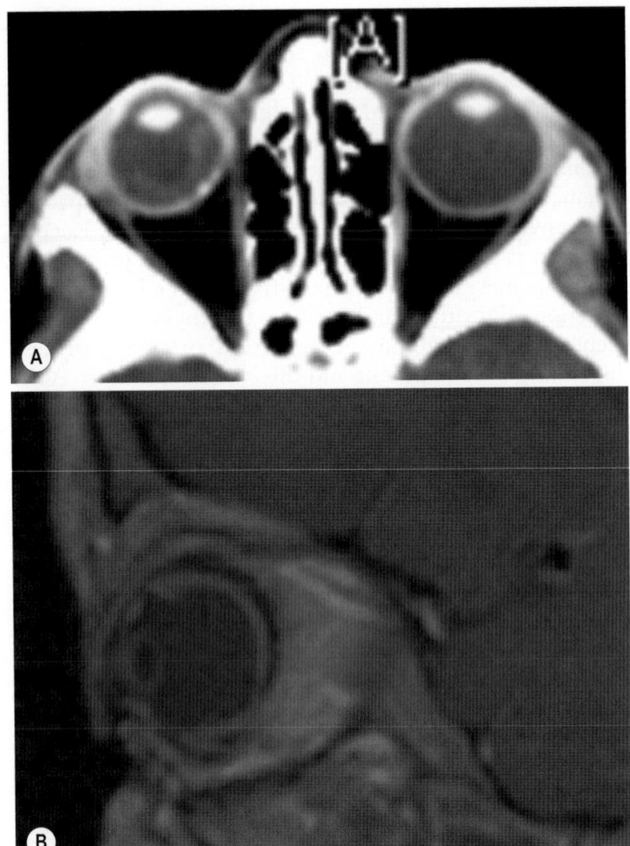

FIGURE 66-1 ■ **Coats' disease.** Axial CT of the orbits (A) demonstrates a right posterior hyloid detachment and filling of the posterior hyloid space which appears T1W hyperintense on the sagittal MRI of the orbits (B) representing accumulation of lipoproteniaceous fluid. Note that the right globe is small.

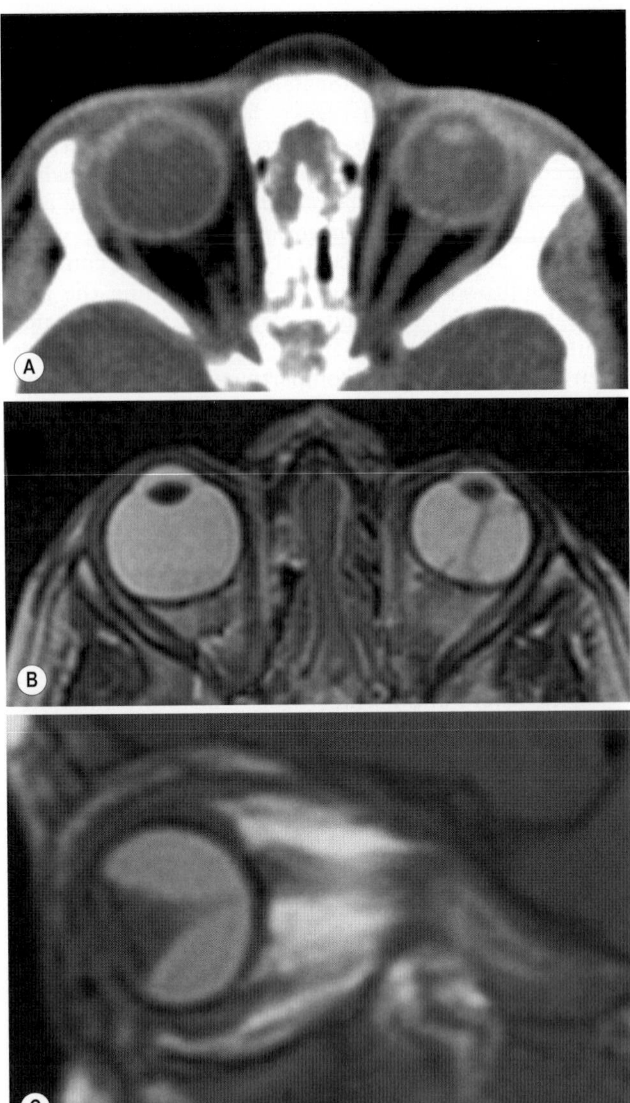

FIGURE 66-2 ■ **Persistent hypertrophic primary vitreous.** Axial CT of the orbits demonstrates a small left globe with a V-shaped retrolental density (A). On the MRI of the orbits on the axial T2W this confirms the presence of a retrolental hypointense fibrovascular band (B). The sagittal T1W (C) shows retinal detachment with T1W hyperintense subretinal haemorrhage.

be an associated defect in the posterior lens capsule resulting in complications such as lens swelling and destruction or cataract formation. Secondary retinal detachment is common and may appear as a V-shaped structure within the globe on axial imaging (owing to the retina being relatively fixed bilaterally at the ora serrata and posteriorly at the optic disc). Recurrent haemorrhage or glaucoma are indications for enucleation surgery.[2] On imaging, PHPV demonstrates a cone or band-shaped structure at the posterior aspect of the lens and is usually associated with microphthalmia. Blood product including fluid–fluid levels within the globe can be present if there has been recent haemorrhage. The presence of a linear septum extending from the lens to the retina is diagnostic (Fig. 66-2). The primary vitreous may demonstrate contrast enhancement. Surgical intervention with preservation of the eye is an option in patients with disease confined to the anterior portion of the globe, but not infrequently PHPV progresses to phthisis bulbi or requires enucleation.

Retinopathy of Prematurity

This has also been termed *retrolental fibroplasia* and represents a condition which occurs secondary to excessive oxygen therapy to treat premature lungs. This results in the arrested development of the retinal vasculature, which then recommences in a disorganised fashion with the growth of new vessels and fibrous tissue that may contract to cause retinal detachment. With the introduction of surfactant therapy to aid lung maturation, retinopathy of prematurity is becoming less common. Simultaneous periventricular leukomalacia may be encountered on brain imaging.

Coloboma

Congenital coloboma represents an anomaly of the optic nerve head, occurring during development of the eye. This may take the form of small optic pits to colobomas

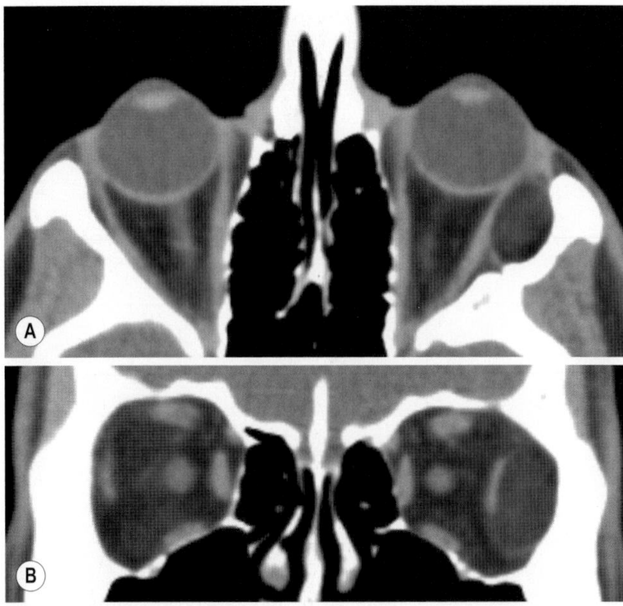

FIGURE 66-3 ■ **Dermoid tumour.** Axial (A) and coronal (B) CT reconstructions of the orbits demonstrating a well-circumscribed fatty density mass occupying the temporal aspect of the extraconal space of the left orbit. Note the scalloping of the overlying bone.

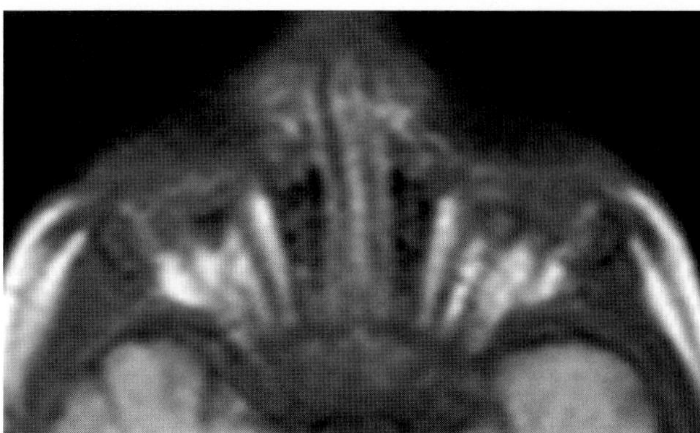

FIGURE 66-4 ■ **Anophthalmia.** The T1W MRI examination demonstrates an infant with no recognisable ocular structures in either orbit.

which involve the entire optic disc, the latter known as 'morning-glory papilla', and may involve the retina, the choroid/iris and the lids. Diagnostic imaging plays no direct role in the assessment of optic nerve coloboma; however, it may represent an associated finding in CHARGE, Patau's, Joubert's or Warburg's syndrome.

Dermoid

Dermoid cysts are the most common congenital mass lesion of the orbit[3] and are usually situated within the extraconal space. They result from inclusion of ectodermal components within the developing orbit and demonstrate slow growth over time with associated bony remodelling or focal erosion. Dermoids are most commonly found at the superolateral orbital margin in the region of the frontozygomatic suture and medially near the frontoethmoidal suture.[3,4] They may be an incidental imaging finding; however, symptomatic presentation occurs particularly following rupture. Fatty elements are a useful diagnostic feature on CT and MR imaging; fat-fluid levels or calcification may also be observed (Fig. 66-3).

Disorders of Globe Size or Shape

When assessing ocular size, it is necessary to determine which is the abnormal side taking into account the possibility of bilateral pathology. Macrophthalmia is defined as generalised enlargement of the globe, which can be congenital or acquired. This is most commonly due to myopia, i.e. axial elongation of the globe resulting in convergence of light anterior to the retina with the patient being shortsighted. Macrophthalmia also occurs in collagen vascular disorders such as Marfan's, Ehlers-Danlos syndrome and homocystinuria.

Microphthalmia is defined as a small globe; if this is congenital or acquired in early childhood an associated small bony orbit will be evident on imaging. Causes include PHPV, Coats' disease, coloboma, previous infection, trauma or radiotherapy and syndromes associated with hemifacial hypoplasia. Anophthalmia refers to complete absence of the embryological formation of an optic vesicle globe in the presence of ocular adnexae, although 'clinical anophthalmia' refers to the absence of a clinically identifiable globe on examination or imaging (Fig. 66-4). In some cases, there may be remnants of globe tissue in the orbit only detectable on histological examination.

Buphthalmos (*bous* = Greek for ox, cow) refers to generalised globe enlargement due to increased intraocular pressure, which is typically seen in children rather than adults as the infantile sclera is relatively elastic, allowing the globe to expand under pressure.[5] Buphthalmos occurs in paediatric glaucoma and is also seen in association with neurofibromatosis 1 (NF1). Apparent globe enlargement may also be due to exophthalmos secondary to an intraorbital mass; therefore imaging should be mandatory, especially if symptoms are rapidly progressive. Staphyloma is a term used to describe a focal protrusion in the sclera, which can occur anywhere along the globe surface, but is most commonly seen posteriorly on the temporal side of the optic disc.[5] The latter is frequently associated with myopia, but staphyloma can also be idiopathic, caused by previous infection, trauma or surgery (Fig. 66-5).

Degenerative Disease

Drusen

Drusen are deposits of lipoproteinaceous material between the basal lamina of the retinal pigment epithelium and the inner collagenous layer of Bruch's membrane. They are commonly asymptomatic and found as a normal feature in aging eyes but also in association with age-related macular degeneration.[6] On funduscopy, drusen can be a cause of blurring of the optic disc margin

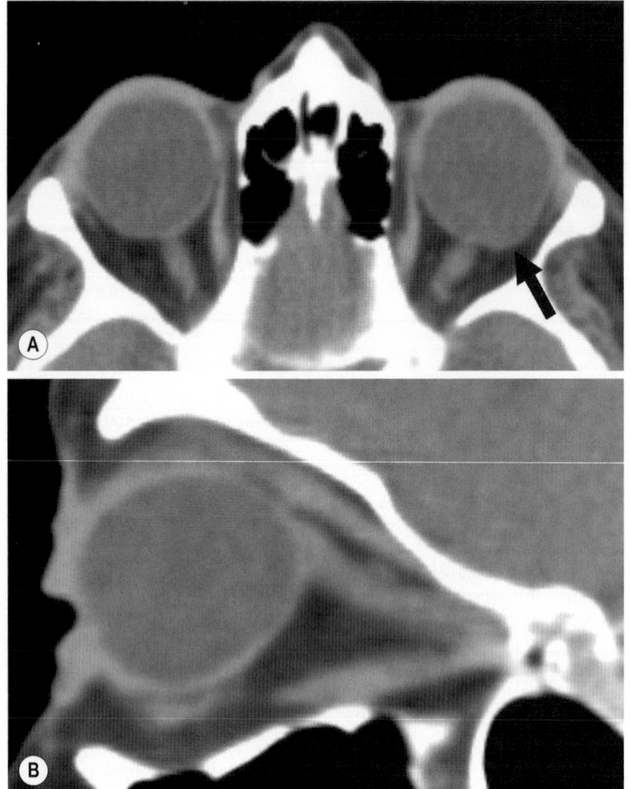

FIGURE 66-5 ■ Staphyloma in myopia. Axial (A) and sagittal (B) CT reconstructions of the orbit demonstrating axial elongation of the left globe with a focal outpouching of the posterior sclera just lateral to the optic nerve head (black arrow).

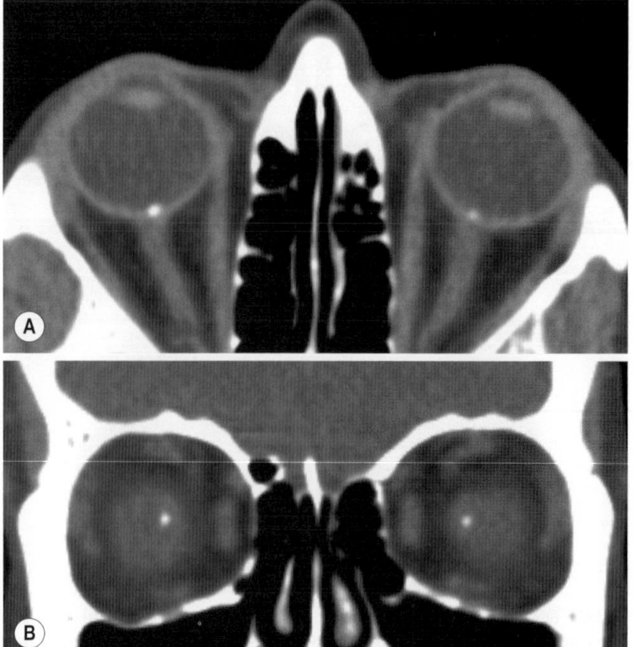

FIGURE 66-6 ■ Drusen. Axial (A) and coronal (B) CT reconstructions of the orbits demonstrating bilateral calcific foci at the optic nerve heads.

and hence may be mistaken for papilloedema. The classic CT appearances are those of small punctate and often bilateral calcific foci at the optic nerve heads (Fig. 66-6).

Orbital Inflammatory Disease

Idiopathic Orbital Inflammation

Idiopathic orbital inflammation (also known as *idiopathic orbital pseudotumour*) is a non-infective disease of unknown cause. Pseudotumour can affect individuals of any age with no clear sex predilection, but most commonly occurs around the fifth decade. It is the most common cause of a painful orbital mass in adults and represents approximately 10% of all orbital mass lesions.[7,8] An immune-modulated aetiology has been postulated, and although orbital pseudotumour mostly occurs in isolation, it can be associated with systemic autoimmune inflammatory conditions such as vasculitis and collagen-vascular disorders. Pseudotumour is usually a diagnosis of exclusion, which relies on a combination of clinical and radiological findings. Patients may present with proptosis, chemosis, painful restricted eye movements, diplopia and occasionally associated cranial nerve palsy. The disease often presents acutely, but can be more insidious. Approximately 80% of patients show good response to first-line treatment with steroids.[9] Recurrent or chronic pseudotumour may result in fibrosis, which has a worse prognosis. Radiotherapy may be useful in patients who poorly respond to steroids or in those with rapidly progressive disease. Methotrexate is an option in patients who are refractory to conventional treatment.

The anatomical pattern of orbital pseudotumour may vary significantly between individuals. Any orbital structure can be affected; however, the lacrimal gland is most frequently involved.[3] A classic feature is tubular enlargement of the extraocular muscles, including the tendon, an important distinction from thyroid orbitopathy, in which the tendon is spared. Unilateral involvement of a single muscle is most common (Fig. 66-7) and in order of frequency this typically affects the medial rectus, superior rectus, lateral rectus and inferior rectus. Manifestation of pseudotumour at the orbital apex and in the cavernous sinus may be indistinguishable on imaging from *Tolosa–Hunt syndrome*.

CT is mostly sufficient in demonstrating features of orbital pseudotumour such as muscle enlargement, lacrimal gland involvement and infiltration of the orbital fat. However, MRI may be useful in complex cases, particularly if there is concern regarding intracranial extension and to delineate fibrosis, which is characterised by reduced T1 and T2 signal.[7]

Thyroid Orbitopathy

Thyroid eye disease is an immune-mediated disorder, which most commonly presents in association with hyperthyroidism in Graves' disease. However, it may be seen in euthyroid or even hypothyroid individuals. Importantly, orbitopathy may precede the actual thyroid disease. Thyroid orbitopathy occurs with a female-to-male ratio of 4 : 1 and a peak in the fourth to fifth decade.[4]

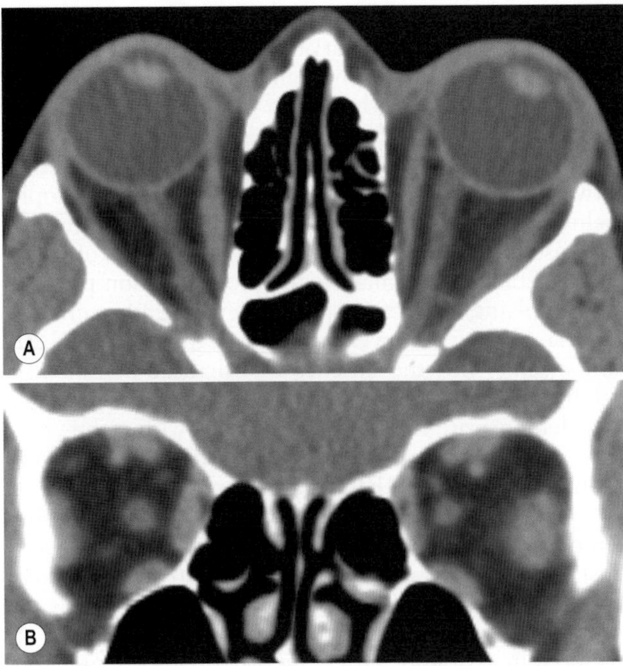

FIGURE 66-7 ■ Idiopathic orbital inflammation (orbital pseudotumour). Axial (A) and coronal (B) CT reconstructions of the orbits demonstrating asymmetrical swelling of the left lateral rectus muscle and tendon. Note the stranding of the adjacent orbital fat indicative of an active inflammatory process.

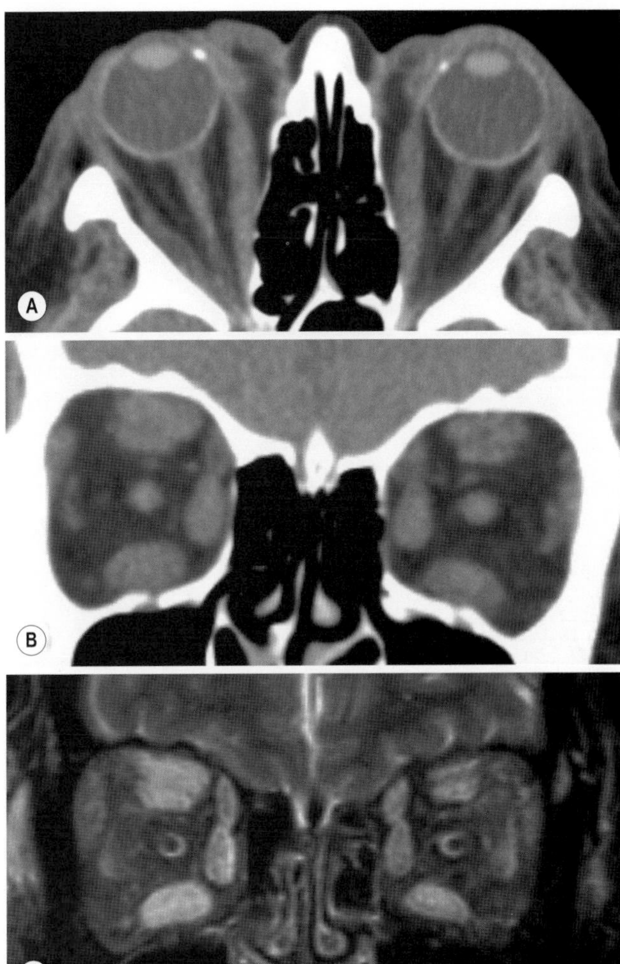

FIGURE 66-8 ■ Thyroid orbitopathy. Axial (A) and coronal (B) CT reconstructions of the orbits as well as a corresponding coronal STIR MRI (C). There is bilateral proptosis, extraocular muscle enlargement, intraorbital fat stranding and expansion as well as thickening of the eyelids.

It is the most common cause of bilateral or unilateral proptosis. Bilateral involvement is the most frequent presentation; in fact in some individuals, 'unilateral' proptosis may represent bilateral asymmetrical disease. Histologically, there is deposition of mucopolysaccharides, namely hyaluronic acid, within the extraocular muscles. This results in a classic imaging appearance of fusiform muscle enlargement with sparing of the muscular tendon. In descending order of frequency, the inferior, medial, superior and lateral recti are most commonly affected. Isolated lateral rectus involvement is rare and should prompt consideration of an alternative diagnosis.[3] There may be an increase of intraorbital fat, and fat stranding with a 'dirty' appearance on imaging (Fig. 66-8).

Systemic Inflammatory Diseases with Orbital Involvement

A variety of systemic autoimmune conditions such as vasculitides, sarcoidosis, connective tissue disorders and inflammatory bowel disease may show associated ocular inflammation. Episcleritis is a benign idiopathic condition which represents inflammation of the superficial sclera layer only. This is usually self-limiting and does not require imaging.[10] Scleritis, however, is more serious and can occur either in isolation or associated with a host of autoimmune conditions as listed above. Posterior scleritis may be evident on imaging as scleral thickening (Fig. 66-9) and can result in complications such as necrosis, retinal or choroidal detachment. Uveitis represents inflammation of the vascular layer of the globe and can be seen in both autoimmune disease, for example rheumatoid, seronegative arthropathies and sarcoid but also in infection.[10] Retinal vasculitis may result in ischaemia, microaneurysm formation and haemorrhages.[11] The majority of pathologies confined to the globe may be more readily appreciated on ophthalmological examination rather than cross-sectional imaging. However, there may be imaging evidence of inflammation in the form of fat infiltration, necrotising features or inflammatory masses.

Sjögren's syndrome, either in isolation or on a background of rheumatoid arthritis, involves the lacrimal gland and clinically results in dry eyes. Sarcoidosis is a disorder of multisystemic inflammation which commonly affects the respiratory tract, skin and eyes. Ocular involvement occurs in as many as 50–80% of patients and may present as non-caseating granulomas of the conjunctiva, uveitis or lacrimal gland infiltration.[12,13] Orbital sarcoid is typically bilateral and tends to respond to steroid treatment. Imaging features may be non-specific, ranging from diffuse infiltration to mass-like appearances

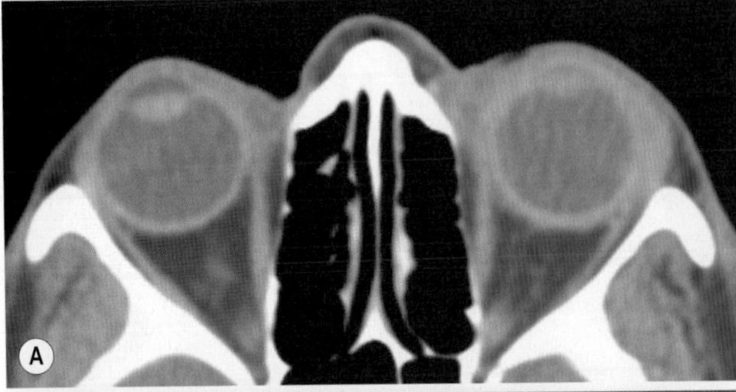

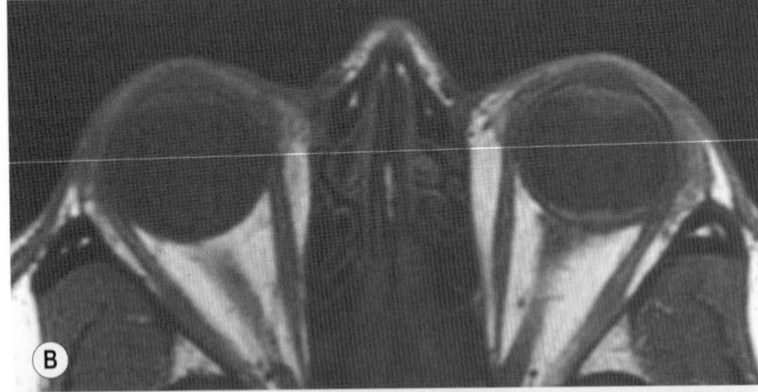

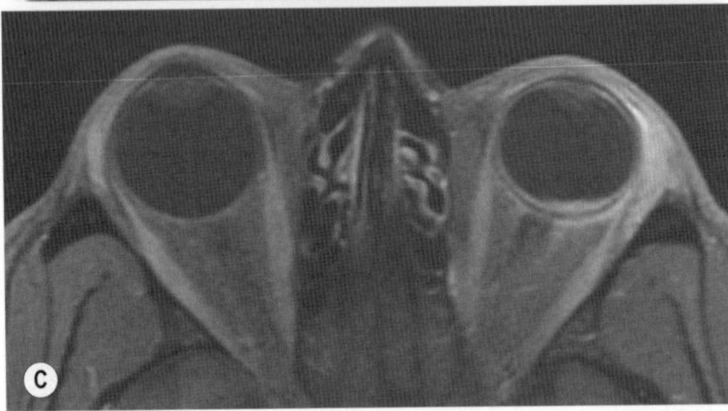

FIGURE 66-9 ■ Posterior scleritis. Axial (A) CT of the orbits demonstrating thickening of the left posterior sclera and associated subtle stranding of the retrobulbar fat suggestive of inflammation. Axial pre- (B) and post-gadolinium (C) fat-saturated contrast MRI of the orbits demonstrating thickening and enhancement of the left posterior sclera and retrobulbar fat.

(Fig. 66-10). Lacrimal gland enlargement with enhancement is a typical feature.[13] Chest imaging may provide a hint to the underlying sarcoidosis, but not infrequently histological sampling is required to conclusively establish the diagnosis.

Wegener's granulomatosis (now known as *granulomatosis with polyangiitis)* is a multisystem small-vessel necrotising granulomatous vasculitis. This most commonly involves the respiratory tract and the renal system of patients. Involvement of ocular and orbital structures may be present 40–50% of patients.[14] Orbital disease is commonly associated with sinus disease with bony erosions (Fig. 66-11). As with other granulomatous disease, orbital disease may appear hypointense on T2 MRI.

Orbital Infection

Toxocara endophthalmitis (also known as *ocular larva migrans*) results from infection with the nematode *Toxocara cani* or *T. cati* via ingestion of eggs in faecally contaminated soil or sandboxes. The source is from domestic dogs or cats. Larvae hatch from the ingested eggs and transgress the human intestinal wall into the bloodstream, whereby they reach various end organs such as the liver, lungs, brain and eyes.[15] Infection typically occurs in childhood and ocular disease tends to present between the ages of 5 and 10 years. *Toxocara* endophthalmitis is the result of a granulomatous immune response to retinal infiltration with larvae. Loss of vision due to retinal detachment is the most common presenting complaint; other non-specific signs include pain, leukocoria and a red eye. Imaging features are mostly non-specific, but the absence of calcification can be a helpful distinguishing feature from retinoblastoma. CT may demonstrate increased attenuation within the vitreous, representing protein leakage from retinal and choroidal vessels.[10] MRI signal is variable, especially on T2 sequences, where both hyper- and hypointensity can occur depending on the degree of fibrosis with contrast enhancement usually present.[16] Untreated, *Toxocara* invariably leads to blindness.

Endophthalmitis can also be fungal (*Candida* sp.) or bacterial in aetiology with *Staphylococcus aureus*, *Staphylococcus epidermidis*, *Streptococcus* sp. representing the most common pathogens.[10] Infectious uveitis may be bacterial, viral, fungal or parasitic (e.g. toxoplasmosis, Lyme disease, leptospirosis) in nature. Orbital tuberculosis is rare, even in endemic areas, and most commonly occurs in children. Clinically, the disease may be indolent with non-specific symptoms, only mild pain and proptosis. The lacrimal gland and orbital walls are most commonly affected, extending from adjacent paranasal sinus inflammatory/infective disease, and can be associated with simultaneous intracranial disease.[17] Imaging features include inflammatory soft-tissue masses and retrobulbar or subperiosteal abscess formation (Fig. 66-12).

A serious complication of intraorbital infection spread usually via paranasal sinus infection is superior ophthalmic vein thrombosis, which can be further complicated by cavernous sinus thrombosis (Fig. 66-13).

Benign Neoplasms and Mass-Like Lesions

Pleomorphic Adenoma

Pleomorphic adenoma is the most common tumour of the lacrimal gland, comprising over half of all epithelial gland tumours.[18] Imaging findings may vary from a homogeneous mass to a more heterogeneous appearance with cystic or necrotic elements. On MRI, small lesions tend to be of relatively uniform low T1 and high T2 signal, whereas larger lesions typically show heterogeneous signal, sometimes also containing haemorrhagic elements (Fig. 66-14). Similar to its behaviour in the parotid gland, lacrimal pleomorphic adenoma has a propensity for malignant transformation, making excision desirable.

Nerve Sheath Tumour

Schwannoma is the most common nerve sheath tumour in the orbit. It is a slow-growing benign peripheral nerve

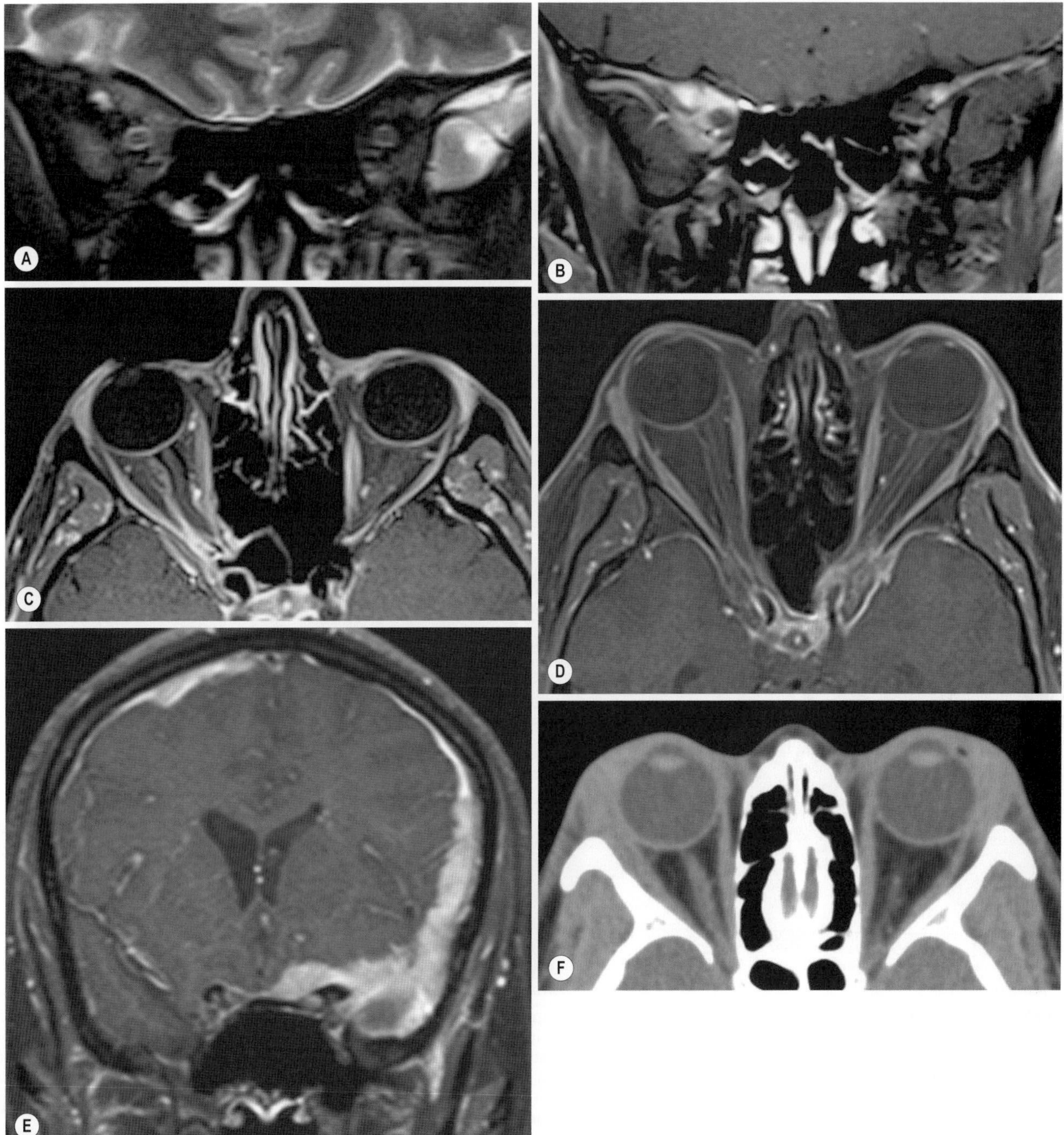

FIGURE 66-10 ■ Orbital sarcoid. Coronal STIR (A), coronal (B) and axial (C) T1-weighted post-gadolinium fat-suppressed MRI of the orbits demonstrating T2-weighted hyperintensity and enhancement at the right orbital apex. Axial T1-weighted post-gadolinium fat-suppressed MRI of the orbits (D) in another patient demonstrating thickening and enhancement of both optic nerve sheaths in a sarcoid perineuritis resembling the 'tram-track sign'. The corresponding T1-weighted post-gadolinium fat-suppressed MRI of the brain (E) demonstrates extensive convexity dural thickening and enhancement, predominantly on the left. Note the extension through the left optic canal and superior orbital fissure. CT of the orbits (F) in a patient with proptosis and bilateral lacrimal gland enlargement.

sheath tumour and is mostly seen in adults. Painless progressive proptosis is a classic, although not specific, presentation. Schwannomas frequently arise from sensory branches of the ophthalmic nerve (V1), namely the supraorbital, supratrochlear or lacrimal nerve, which explains their sometimes extraconal position within the superior portion of the orbit.[19] On MRI, these tumours tend to be hypointense on T1- and hyperintense on T2-weighted sequences (Fig. 66-15). Imaging features also depend on the histological tumour composition, whereby so-called Antoni A lesions with densely packed cells demonstrate more homogeneous enhancement than

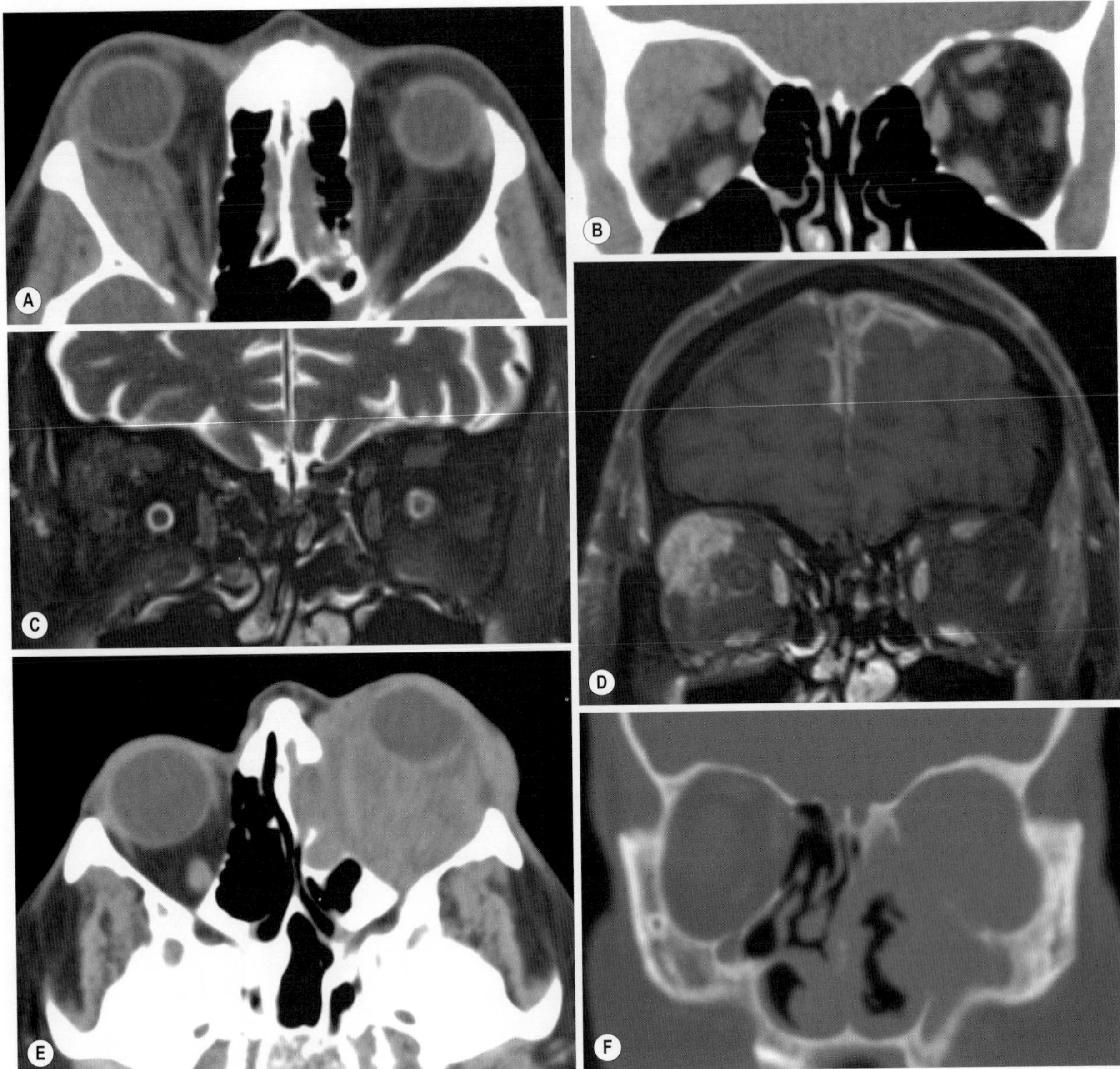

FIGURE 66-11 ■ **Wegener's granulomatosis (granulomatosis with polyangiitis).** Axial (A) and coronal (B) CT of an inflammatory mass occupying the upper temporal quadrant of the right orbit causing right proptosis. The corresponding coronal STIR (C) and T1-weighted post-gadolinium fat-suppressed MRI (D) of the orbits demonstrates T2-weighted intermediate signal inflammatory mass with enhancement in that location. Note the dural involvement along the falx cerebri. CT of another patient with a large inflammatory mass occupying the left orbit causing left proptosis on the soft-tissue windows (E) as well as bony erosion with extension of the inflammatory mass through the lamina papyracea and nasal septum on the coronal reformats on bone windows (F).

Antoni B lesions.[3] Neurofibroma may also occur in the orbit and can have similar imaging features to schwannoma. It can arise either in isolation or in the context of neurofibromatosis 1 (NF1). Plexiform neurofibroma is associated with hypoplasia of the greater wing of sphenoid in NF1 patients. Calcification may be present in some neurofibromata and can help distinguish this from schwannoma, which rarely calcifies.

Optic Nerve Glioma

This intrinsic tumour predominantly presents in young patients, with a peak in the first decade. Bilateral optic nerve glioma is virtually diagnostic of NF1. Histologically, pilocytic astrocytoma (WHO grade 1) is the most common and may show little or no progression over time. Visual loss is more common in non-NF patients than in neurofibromatosis.[20] The rarer adult form of optic nerve glioma can be more aggressive when of a corresponding histology of anaplastic glioma (WHO grade 3) or glioblastoma multiforme (WHO grade 4) and has a rapidly progressive clinical course. On imaging, there may be fusiform enlargement of the optic nerve, with associated expansion of the optic canal. MRI is the most accurate at demonstrating optic nerve glioma, which appears isointense to hypointense on T1 and

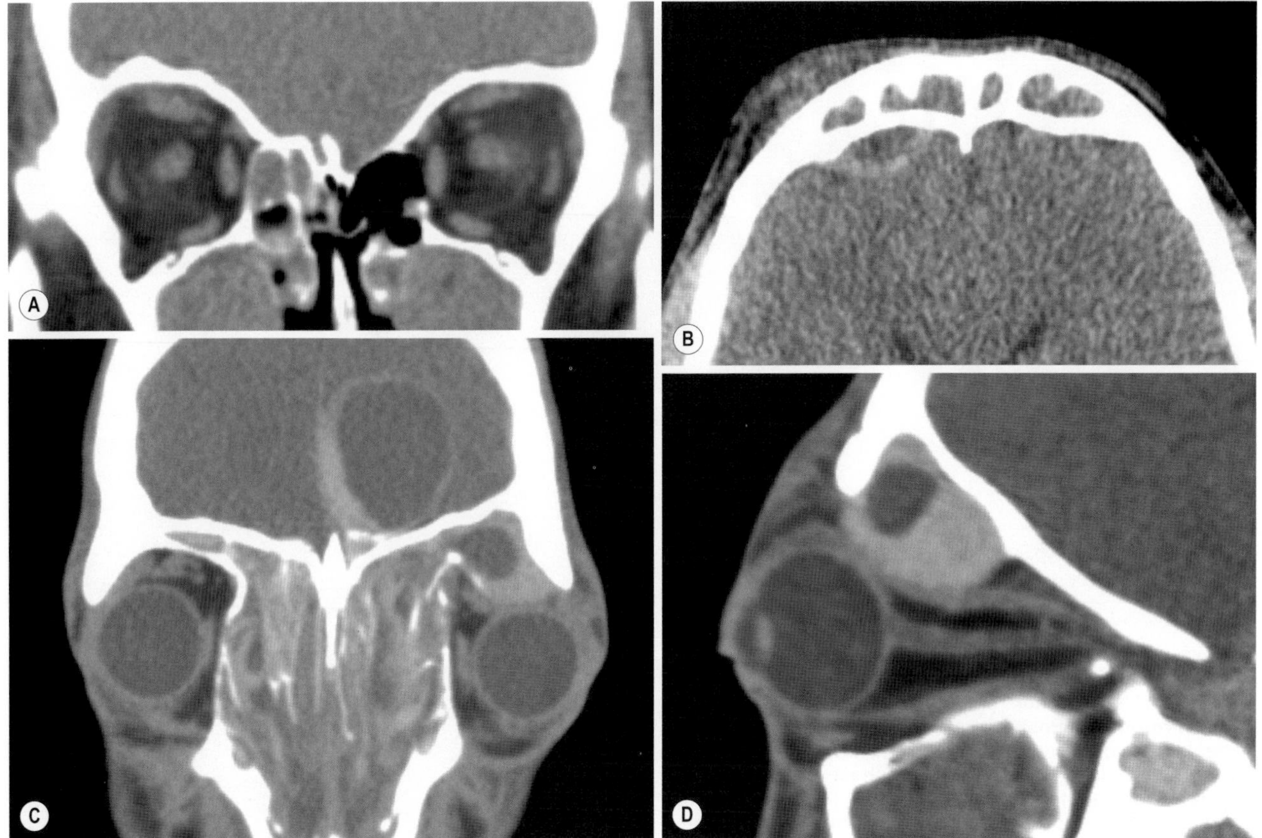

FIGURE 66-12 ■ **Orbital infection.** Coronal CT of the orbits (A) in a patient with right orbital cellulitis, demonstrating subtle stranding of the intraorbital fat on the right with asymmetric swelling of the superior-rectus levator complex and a soft-tissue inflammatory mass superior to it. Note the extensive opacification of the maxillary antra and right ethmoidal air cells. Axial CT of the brain in this patient (B) revealed an empyema subjacent to opacified frontal sinuses and right forehead cellulitis. Coronal (C) and sagittal (D) reformatted post-contrast CT of a patient with severe chronic fungal sinusitis. Proptosis and hypoglobus on the left is seen secondary to displacement of the left frontal sinus pyocele. Note the left frontal cerebral abscess and the gross expansion and opacification of the paranasal sinuses.

hyperintense on T2 sequences with variable contrast enhancement (Fig. 66-16).

Optic Nerve Sheath Meningioma

Primary optic nerve sheath meningioma arises from the arachnoid sheath of the optic nerve and should be distinguished from secondary meningioma, which has spread from an intracranial tumour either centred on the anterior clinoid process or sphenoid wing to involve the orbit via the optic canal or the orbital fissure (Fig. 66-17). Both occur most frequently in middle-aged women. Bilateral optic nerve sheath meningiomas are a feature of neurofibromatosis 2 (NF2). On imaging, generalised circumferential or fusiform enlargement of the optic nerve-sheath complex are the most common, but focal eccentric masses can also occur. CT may be useful for demonstrating calcification within the meningioma, a relatively specific finding, which occurs in 20–50% of cases and is not observed in optic nerve glioma. Another feature of optic nerve meningioma is the so-called tram-track sign, which is defined as relative hypoattenuation of the optic nerve on CT or reduced signal on fat-suppressed post-gadolinium MRI due to peripheral enhancement of the tumour around the nerve. This is not a specific appearance, however, and can be seen in other pathologies, including pseudotumour, optic neuritis, sarcoid (e.g. Fig. 66-10D), lymphoma and metastatic disease.[21]

Vascular Lesions of the Orbit

Cavernous Haemangioma

Cavernous haemangioma is the most common primary orbital tumour in adults, representing approximately 6% of all orbital masses.[22] The classification as a tumour is actually a misnomer; in fact, this lesion type represents an angiographically silent venous malformation consisting of endothelial-lined vascular spaces with a fibrous pseudocapsule. It is usually centred on the intraconal compartment and may contain phleboliths on imaging (Fig. 66-18). Frank haemorrhage is atypical, but haemosiderin staining may occur. Rarely, cavernous haemangiomas can be intraosseous and therefore extraconal. The

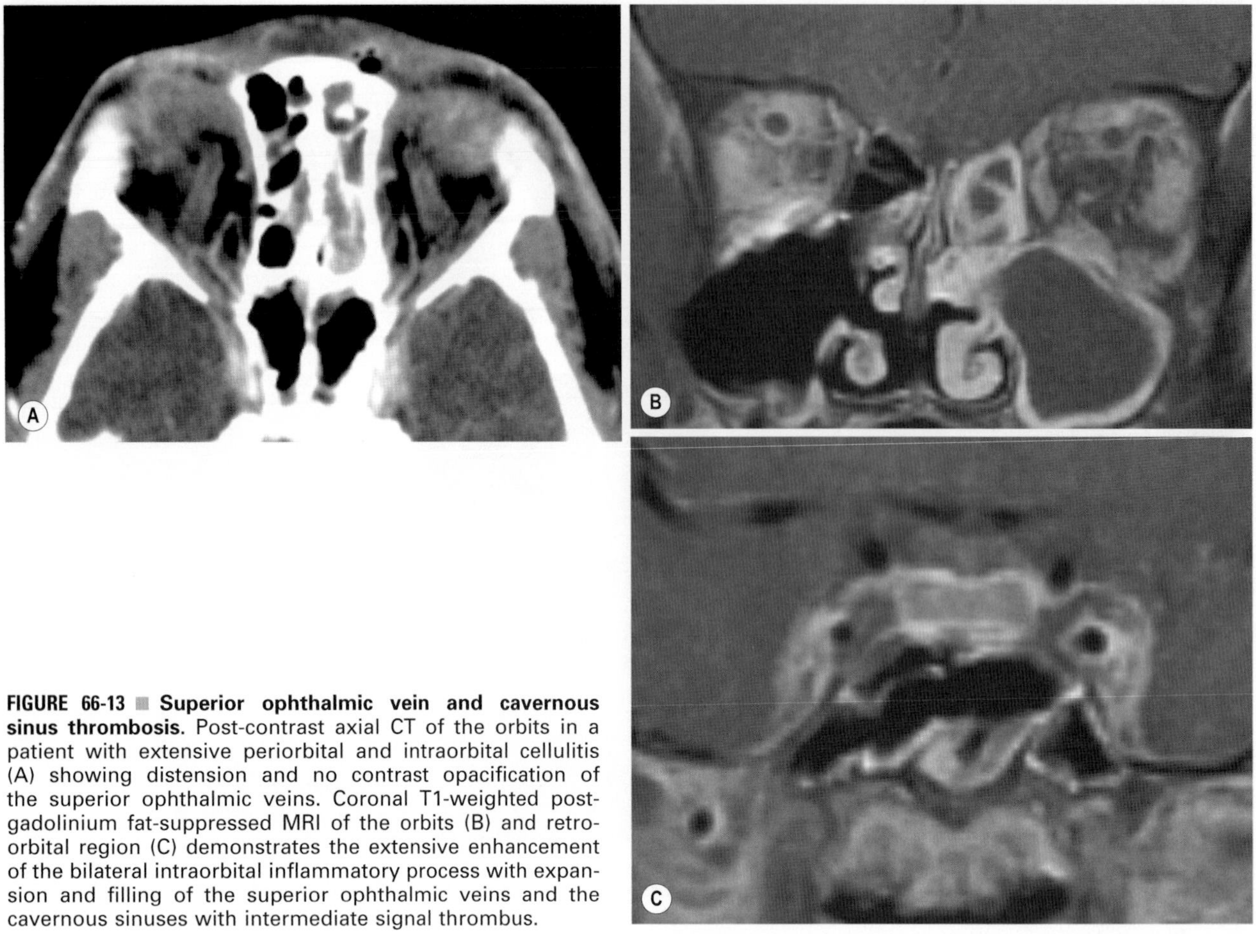

FIGURE 66-13 ■ Superior ophthalmic vein and cavernous sinus thrombosis. Post-contrast axial CT of the orbits in a patient with extensive periorbital and intraorbital cellulitis (A) showing distension and no contrast opacification of the superior ophthalmic veins. Coronal T1-weighted post-gadolinium fat-suppressed MRI of the orbits (B) and retro-orbital region (C) demonstrates the extensive enhancement of the bilateral intraorbital inflammatory process with expansion and filling of the superior ophthalmic veins and the cavernous sinuses with intermediate signal thrombus.

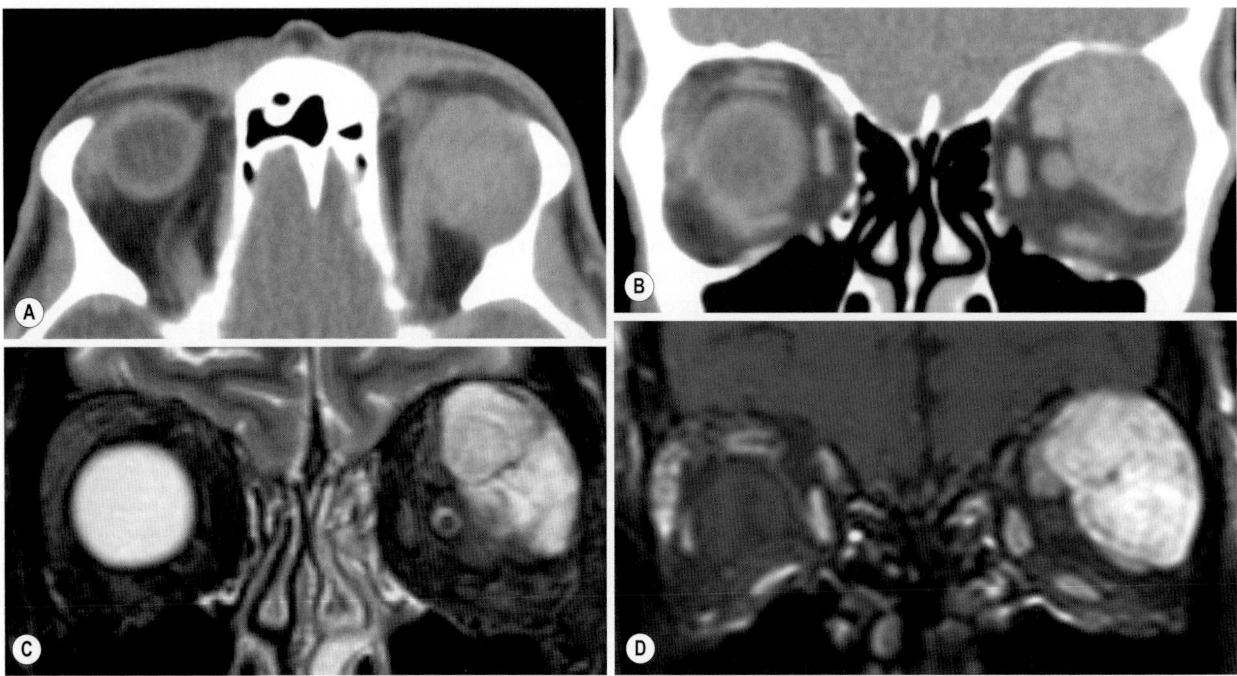

FIGURE 66-14 ■ Pleomorphic adenoma. Axial (A) and coronal (B) CT of the orbits demonstrating a well-circumscribed soft-tissue mass in the superior-temporal quadrant of the left orbit, causing remodelling of the overlying sphenoid bone. The coronal STIR (C) and T1-weighted post-gadolinium fat-suppressed (D) MRI of the mass reveals avid and homogeneous enhancement.

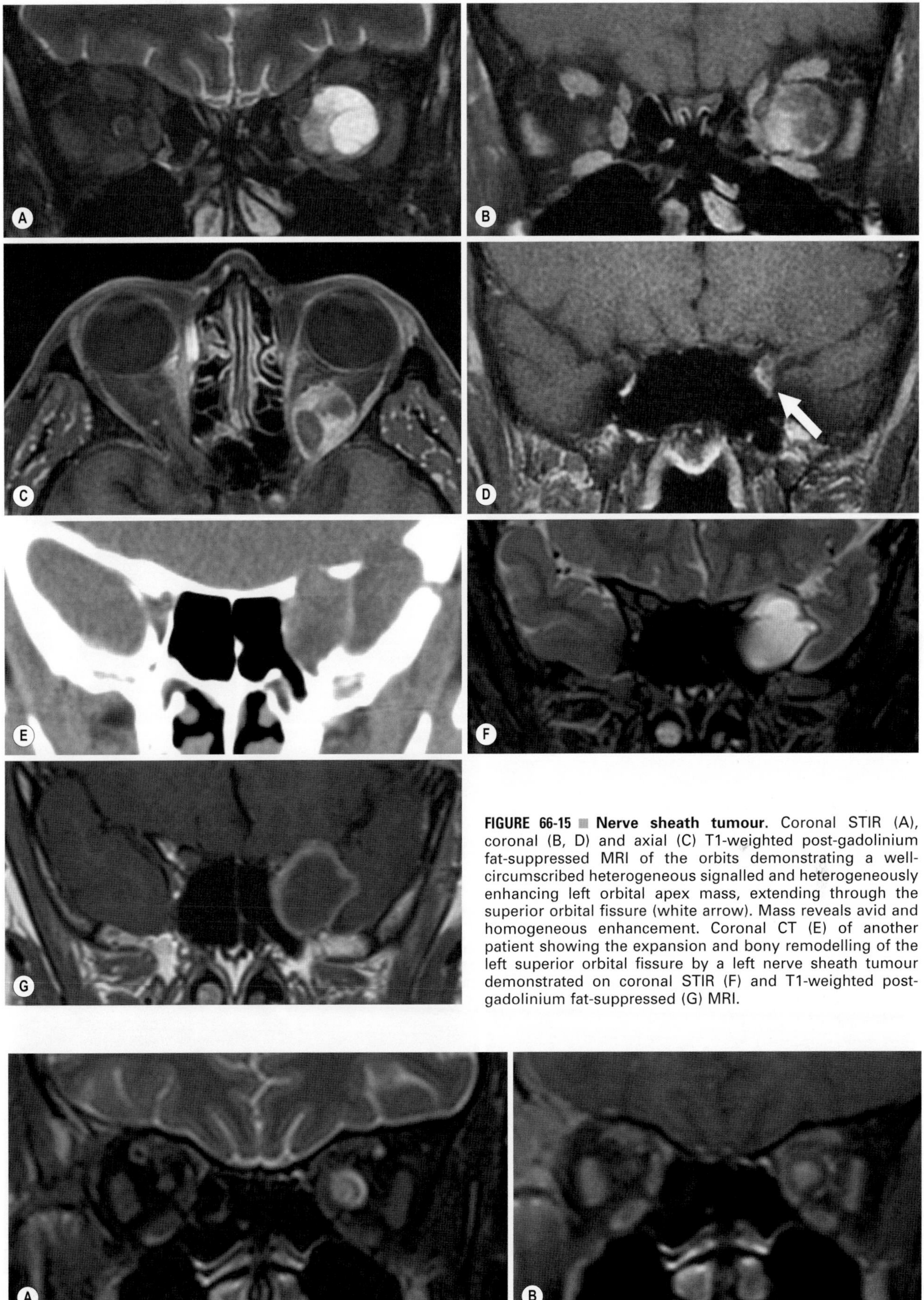

FIGURE 66-15 ■ **Nerve sheath tumour.** Coronal STIR (A), coronal (B, D) and axial (C) T1-weighted post-gadolinium fat-suppressed MRI of the orbits demonstrating a well-circumscribed heterogeneous signalled and heterogeneously enhancing left orbital apex mass, extending through the superior orbital fissure (white arrow). Mass reveals avid and homogeneous enhancement. Coronal CT (E) of another patient showing the expansion and bony remodelling of the left superior orbital fissure by a left nerve sheath tumour demonstrated on coronal STIR (F) and T1-weighted post-gadolinium fat-suppressed (G) MRI.

FIGURE 66-16 ■ **Optic nerve glioma.** Coronal STIR (A), coronal (B) and axial (D) T1-weighted post-gadolinium fat-suppressed and axial T2-weighted (C) MRI of the orbits demonstrating expansion and enhancement of the intraorbtial and canalicular segments of the left optic nerve through an expanded left optic canal (white arrow). The retro-orbital intracranial segment and optic chiasm are also involved.

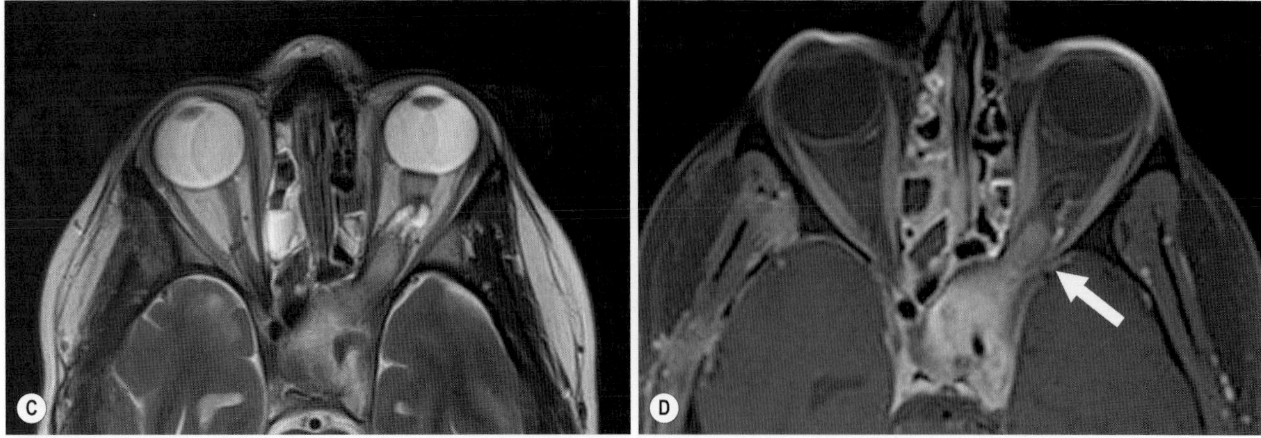

FIGURE 66-16, Continued

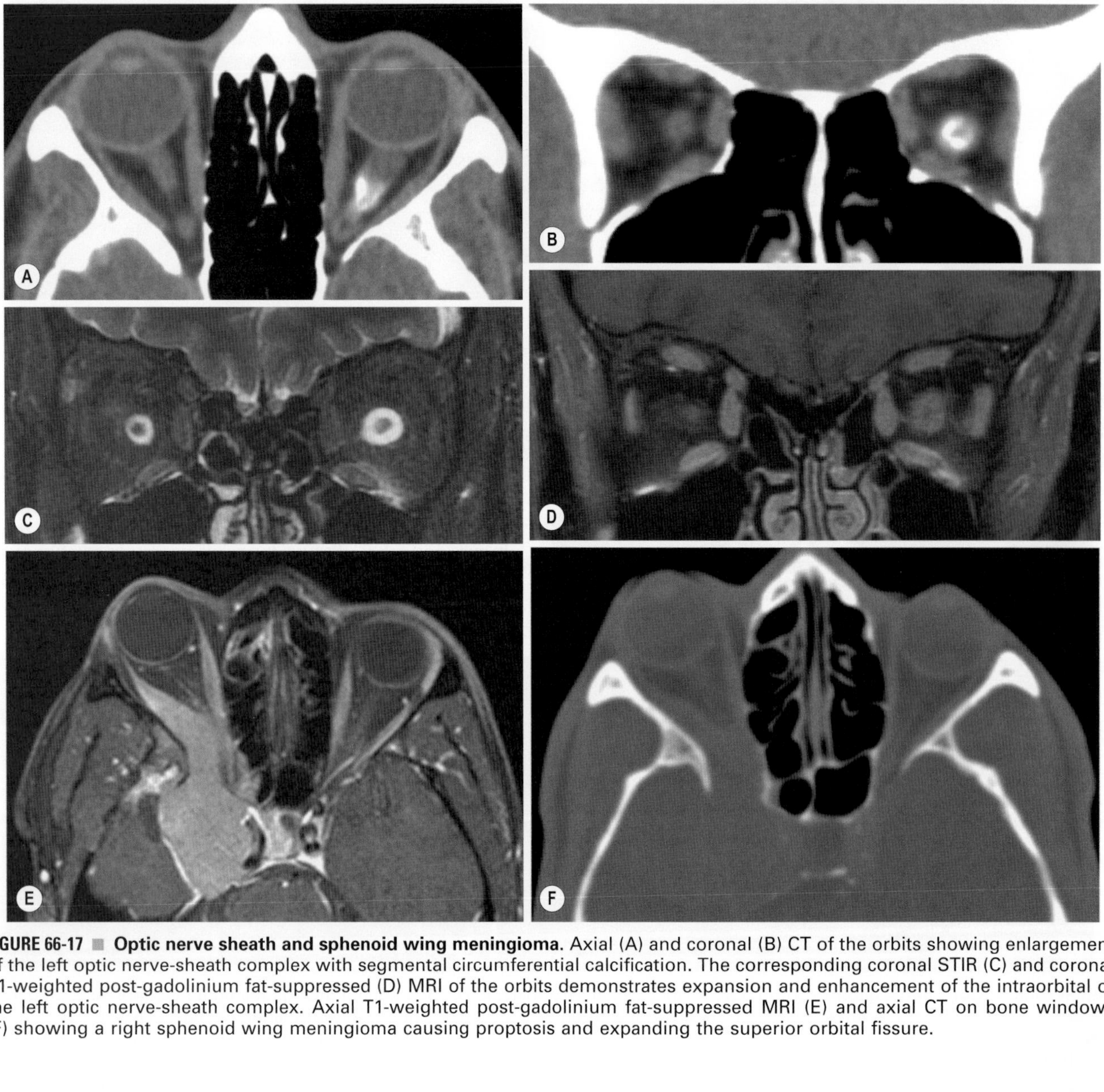

FIGURE 66-17 ■ **Optic nerve sheath and sphenoid wing meningioma.** Axial (A) and coronal (B) CT of the orbits showing enlargement of the left optic nerve-sheath complex with segmental circumferential calcification. The corresponding coronal STIR (C) and coronal T1-weighted post-gadolinium fat-suppressed (D) MRI of the orbits demonstrates expansion and enhancement of the intraorbital of the left optic nerve-sheath complex. Axial T1-weighted post-gadolinium fat-suppressed MRI (E) and axial CT on bone windows (F) showing a right sphenoid wing meningioma causing proptosis and expanding the superior orbital fissure.

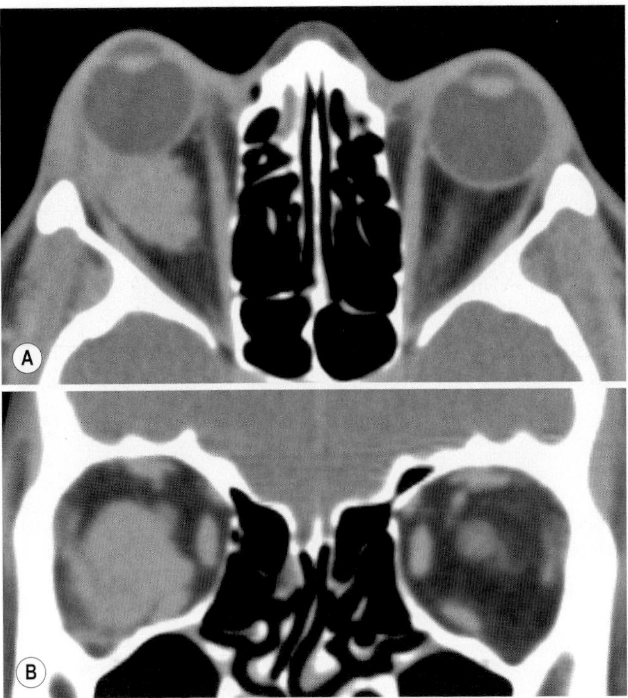

FIGURE 66-18 ■ **Cavernous haemangioma.** Post-contrast axial (A) and coronal (B) CT examination of a well-circumscribed retrobulbar enhancing mass causing right proptosis.

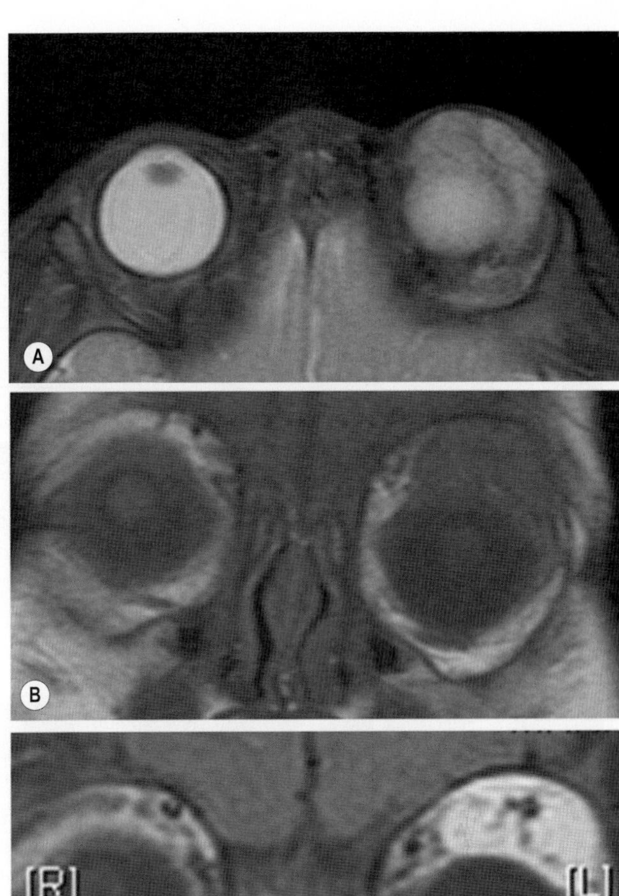

FIGURE 66-19 ■ **Capillary haemangioma.** Axial STIR (A), coronal pre- (B) and fat-suppressed post-gadolinium (C) T1-weighted orbital MRI of a child demonstrating a left anterior and superior lobulated enhancing orbital mass causing proptosis and hypoglobus.

clinical presentation is that of painless slowly progressive proptosis and diplopia. Increased growth may occur in pregnancy or following trauma.[3] On MR, cavernous haemangioma mostly demonstrates low T1 signal and high T2 signal with variable enhancement and progressive spread of enhancement from a single point or small component of the mass on dynamic post-gadolinium MRI; the latter is a characteristic feature of cavernous haemangioma, similar to progressive 'filling-in' of cavernous haemangioma in the liver.[22–24] This is relevant as, in some of these lesions, a conservative approach and monitoring may be favoured over surgical resection.

Capillary Haemangioma

This is a different entity of vascular malformation, which should not be confused with cavernous haemangioma. Capillary haemangioma presents in the paediatric population soon after birth and demonstrates rapid growth during the first year of life with often subsequent involution approximately by the age of 10.[4] There is an association with cutaneous facial malformations, the presence of which may aid the diagnosis. Capillary haemangioma is most commonly found in the extraconal compartment anteriorly and within the superomedial orbital quadrant[3] (Fig. 66-19). Irregularity of the mass and spread to the intraconal compartment can mimic malignancy. On T2 MR imaging, low signal flow voids can be a helpful differentiating feature. These result from arterial flow supply via the external or internal carotid branches. Retinal haemangioblastoma (also termed retinal capillary haemangioma) is a further lesion category and occurs in association with von Hippel–Lindau disease (VHL) and familial cancer syndromes.

Venous Varix

A varix is defined as an abnormally dilated vein or cluster of veins. Although sometimes cited as part of the orbital lymphovascular malformation spectrum, orbital varices are now thought to represent a discrete entity.[3] Varices can occur at any age, but are most common in the second and third decade with no gender predilection.[25] The hallmark of an orbital varix is enlargement under pressure, resulting in a sometimes dramatic proptosis, for example during a Valsalva manoeuvre or when the patient bends forward. Importantly, varices may not always be evident on standard supine cross-sectional imaging and therefore may require a provocation manoeuvre during imaging (Fig. 66-20). On CT, varices may demonstrate increased

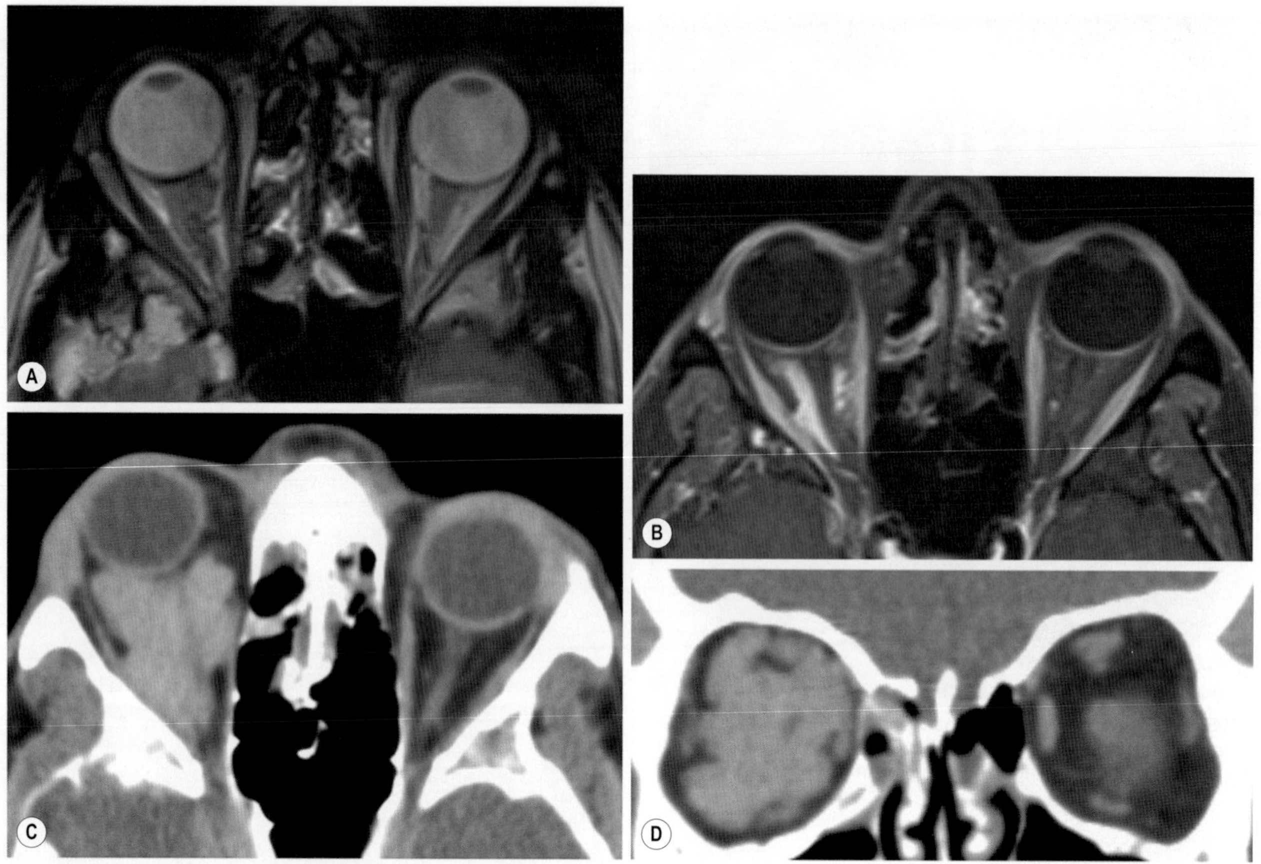

FIGURE 66-20 ■ **Orbital varices.** Axial T2-weighted (A) and fat-suppressed post-gadolinium T1-weighted (B) orbital MRI demonstrating a right proptosis from a left retrobulbar enhancing lesion surrounding the optic nerve-sheath complex. A subsequent post-contrast axial (C) and coronal (D) CT examination with the patient performing a Valsalva manoeuvre illustrates the characteristic enlargement of the mass and worsening proptosis due to venous engorgement.

attenuation due to blood product and, if present, calcified phleboliths are pathognomonic. T2-weighted MRI may reveal flow voids, but these can be absent, especially if there is variceal thrombosis. Haemorrhage is also a potential complication and may result in acute painful proptosis.

Venous Lymphatic Malformation

This type of lesion is sometimes referred to as *lymphangioma*, but it does not represent a neoplasm. Venous lymphatic malformations may manifest at birth or in early childhood and typically demonstrate slow growth or no growth at all. Clinically, they can result in proptosis, restriction of ocular movements and occasional haemorrhage. Unlike a varix, a venous lymphatic malformation does not enlarge under Valsalva-type stress. MRI (Fig. 66-21) is the most sensitive method of characterising these lesions, which may show proteinaceous and haemorrhagic components with fluid–fluid levels and typically enhance poorly.[25]

Arteriovenous Malformations (AVMs)

Congenital arteriovenous malformations purely involving the orbit are extremely rare, resulting in visible cutaneous stigmata due to congestive changes within the periorbital soft tissues and orbit. They may also involve the bony orbit. The arterial supply of these AVMs is typically from the anterior ethmoidal rami off the ophthalmic artery or the internal and external maxillary arteries (Fig. 66-22). When these AVMs involve the retina and midbrain (Fig. 66-23), the terms *congenital unilateral retinocephalic vascular malformation syndrome* or *Bonnet–Dechaume–Blanc syndrome* or *Wyburn-Mason syndrome* describe a neurocutaneous syndrome characterised by these AVMs.[1,26]

Carotid-Cavernous Fistula

A carotid-cavernous fistula represents an abnormal direct or indirect connection between one or more branches of the internal or external carotid artery and the cavernous sinus. This can occur spontaneously, most frequently in the context of a collagen vascular disorder, but more commonly is the result of trauma, surgery, previous thrombosis or aneurysm rupture.[4,25] Middle-aged to elderly women are most frequently affected. The clinical findings are those of pulsatile exophthalmos, conjunctival injection and there may be an auscultatory bruit. Imaging features (Fig. 66-24) include dilatation of the superior ophthalmic vein, proptosis, fullness of the cavernous sinus and extraocular muscle congestion.[25]

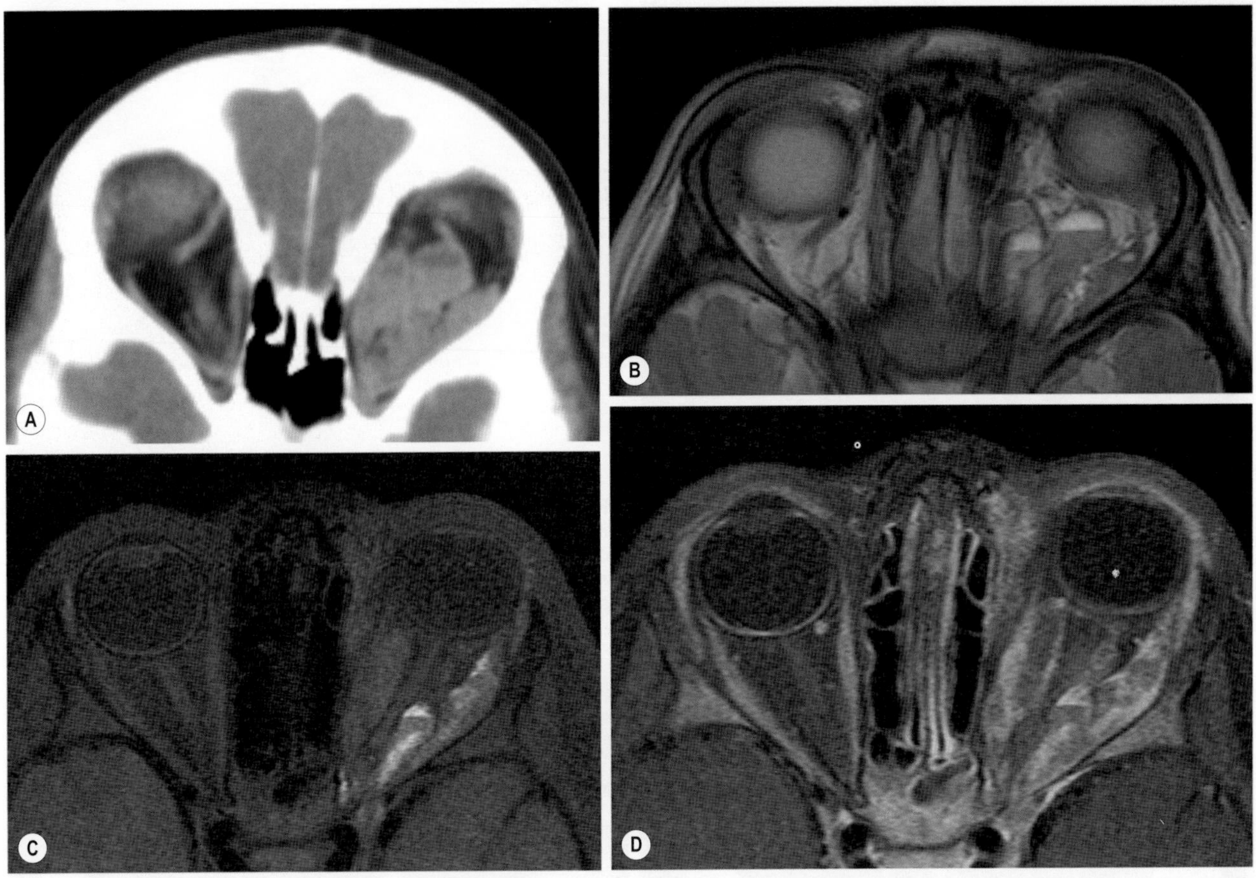

FIGURE 66-21 ■ Orbital venous lymphatic malformation. Post-contrast axial CT (A), axial T2-weighted (B) and pre- (C) and post- (D) fat-suppressed T1-weighted orbital MRI demonstrating a left superior orbital complex heterogeneously enhancing mass causing left proptosis and containing multiple fluid–fluid levels representing proteinaceous and haemorrhagic components.

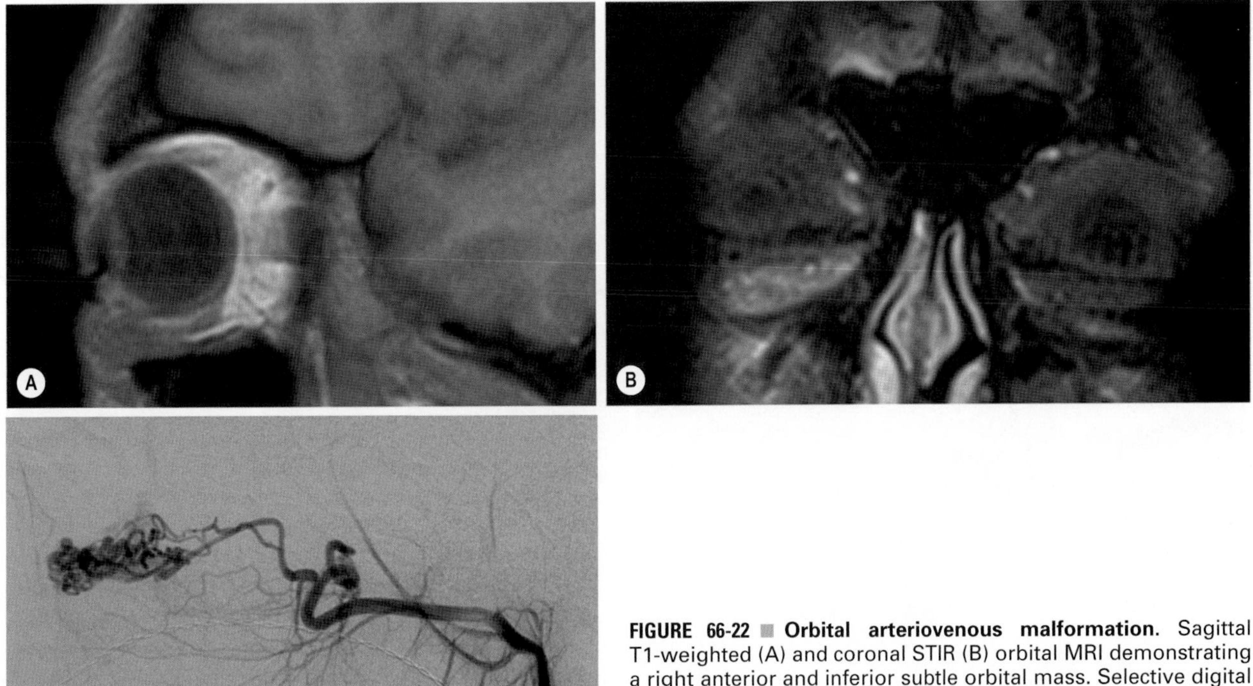

FIGURE 66-22 ■ Orbital arteriovenous malformation. Sagittal T1-weighted (A) and coronal STIR (B) orbital MRI demonstrating a right anterior and inferior subtle orbital mass. Selective digital subtraction angiography (DSA) of the right internal maxillary artery (C) demonstrates arteriovenous shunting through the mass through a tangle of abnormal vessels representing the nidus of an AVM.

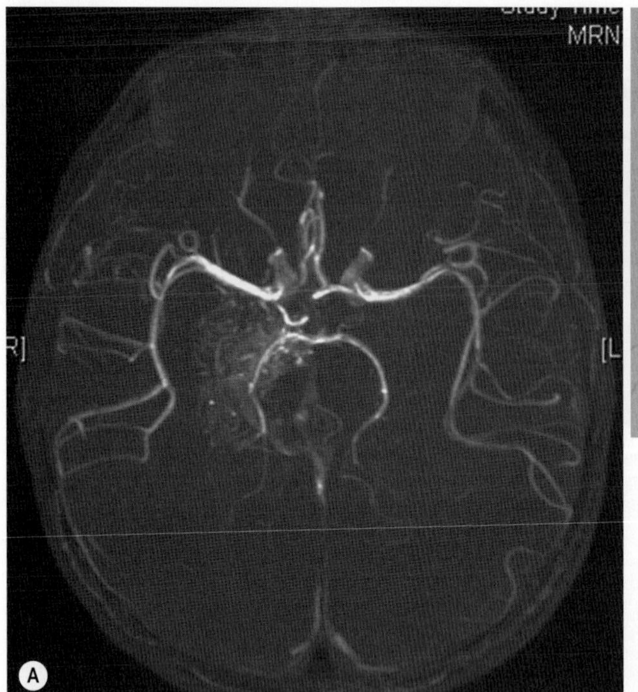

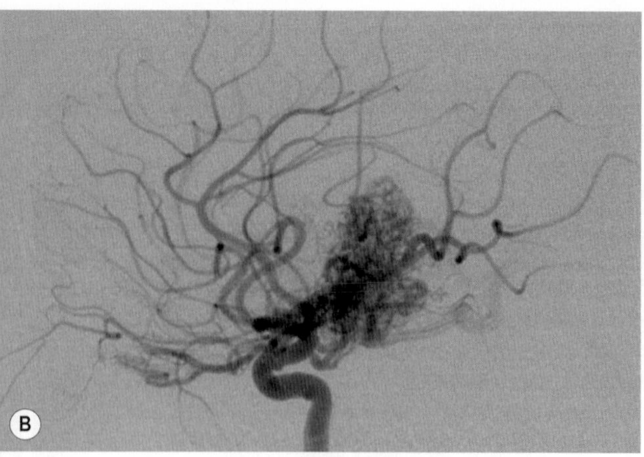

FIGURE 66-23 ■ **Congenital unilateral retinocephalic vascular malformation syndrome (Wyburn-Mason syndrome).** Time-of-flight MR angiography (A) and selective digital subtraction angiography of the right internal carotid artery (B) demonstrating a right mesencephalic AVM in a patient with a known right retinal AVM.

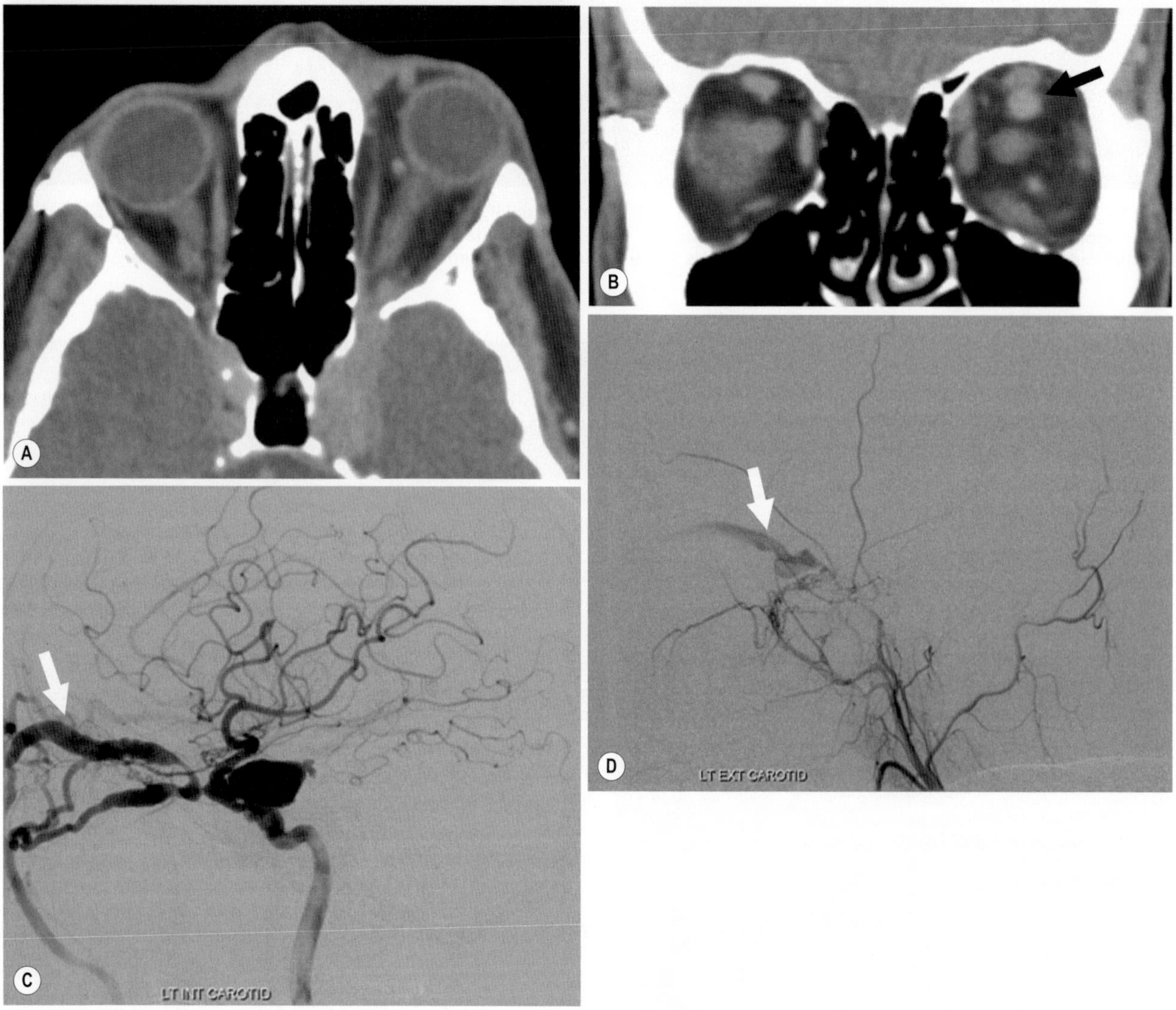

FIGURE 66-24 ■ **Carotid-cavernous fistula.** Post-contrast axial (A) and coronal (B) CT examination demonstrating left proptosis, stranding of the intraorbital, swelling of the extraocular muscles as well as asymmetric bulkiness of the left cavernous sinus and dilatation of the left superior ophthalmic vein (black arrow). Selective digital subtraction angiography of the left (C) internal and (D) external carotid arteries in two different patients demonstrating a direct and indirect arteriovenous fistula with early filling and retrograde flow through the superior ophthalmic vein (white arrows).

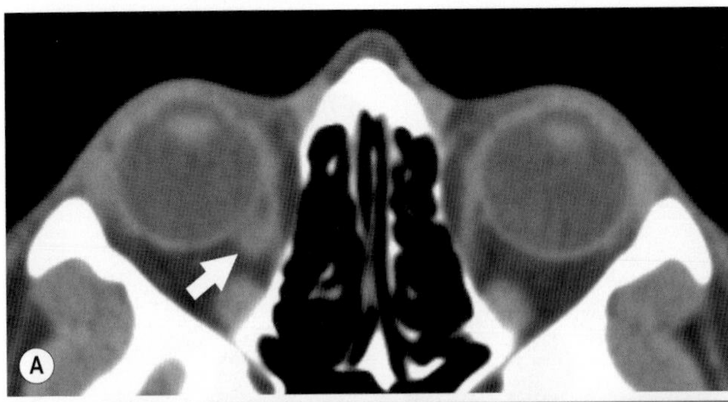

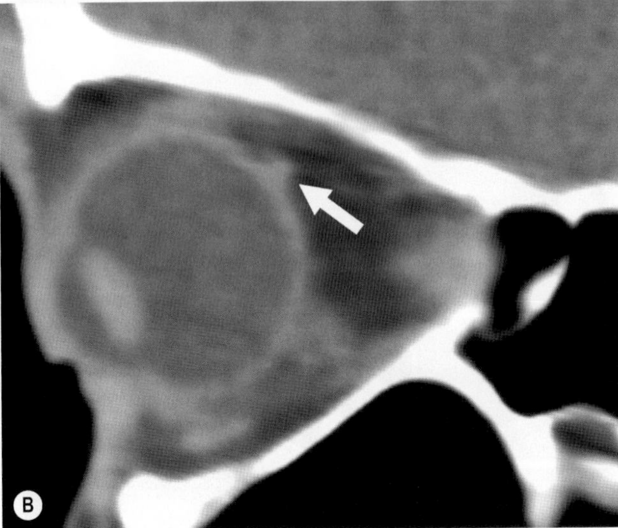

FIGURE 66-25 ■ **Uveal exophytic melanoma.** Post-contrast axial (A) and right sagittal (B) reformats of a CT examination of the orbits demonstrating a small enhancing nodule on the posterior nasal aspect of the right globe (white arrows).

Malignant Neoplasms

Uveal Melanoma

Uveal melanoma is the commonest intraocular primary malignancy in adults[10,20] and commonly presents with progressive visual loss. Extensive spread beyond the globe is common, even in the presence of only a small ocular lesion,[10] resulting in the typical *'collar button'* lesion. Tumour morphology can vary from nodular (Fig. 66-25) to plaque-like lesions and diffuse infiltration. Ophthalmological examination and ultrasound typically form part of the initial work-up. Cross-sectional imaging, particularly MRI, is useful to evaluate for optic nerve involvement and extraocular spread. Increased attenuation on CT as well as T1 shortening (paramagnetic effect) on MRI may be observed due to the presence of melanin. There may also be avid lesional contrast enhancement.

Metastatic Disease

Metastases from extraorbital cancers are most frequently located within the uveal layer, but can involve any intraorbital or adexal structure (Fig. 66-26). Breast, lung cancers and cutaneous melanoma are the most common primaries.[10,27] Prostate cancer is also relatively common, with a propensity for the bony orbit. Rapidly worsening proptosis and globe displacement, diplopia and pain are typical clinical presentations. In children, neuroblastoma commonly metastasises to the orbit. Of note, metastases from sclerosing carcinoma types such as scirrhous breast cancer or gastric carcinoma can result in enophthalmos. Simultaneous brain metastases may provide an important clue on imaging and can be present in up to two-thirds of patients with orbital metastatic disease.[3]

Lymphoproliferative Malignancy

Orbital lymphoma and leukaemia constitute a large share of orbital malignant neoplasms.[28] Orbital involvement can occur in the context of spread from systemic non-Hodgkin's lymphoma (NHL), although only a minority (<2%) of patients with systemic lymphoma demonstrate secondary orbital involvement.[29] Primary orbital lymphoma most frequently represents low-grade mucosa-associated lymphoid tissue (MALT) lymphoma. This commonly affects the lacrimal gland or orbital adnexa and occurs in the absence of systemic disease. Alternatively, orbital involvement may be the initial presentation of systemic lymphoma; therefore, supplementary body imaging as well as appropriate follow-up should be considered in patients with apparently isolated orbital disease. Orbital lymphoma predominantly affects the older population, with a peak of 50–70 years, but can occur at a younger age, especially in immunosuppressed individuals.[30] Clinical symptoms are often insidious, including painless proptosis, diplopia or visual disturbances. Malignant lymphoma may demonstrate hyperdensity on CT both pre- and post-contrast[31] (Fig. 66-27). Decreased signal on T1 and variable signal on T2 MR imaging may be observed. Bone destruction is rare, but can occur in high-grade lesions. Imaging can be non-specific or even negative in early disease, if there is isolated ocular or adnexal involvement.[29,31] Intermediate T1 and T2 signal, post-contrast gadolinium enhancement on MRI and, importantly, PET positivity can be features of adnexal lymphoma.[32]

Orbital involvement in leukaemia is rare but has been described in both in myeloid and lymphoblastic leukaemias. Any orbital structure can be involved, whereby leukaemic infiltration of the optic nerve constitutes an oncological emergency because of the threat to vision. Leukaemia may present as a diffuse infiltrate or mass. In particular, acute myeloid leukaemia (AML) can be associated with mass formation, which is referred to as *chloroma* or *granulocytic sarcoma*. The most common eye complication of leukaemia is retinal haemorrhage secondary to thrombocytopenia.[28]

Adenoid Cystic Carcinoma

This represents the most common malignant epithelial neoplasm of the lacrimal gland and most commonly is the result of malignant transformation of a benign mass, i.e. carcinoma ex pleomorphic adenoma rather than a de novo malignancy.[18] Unless there are convincing aggressive features (Fig. 66-28), this type of lesion may be difficult to distinguish from other lacrimal gland pathologies

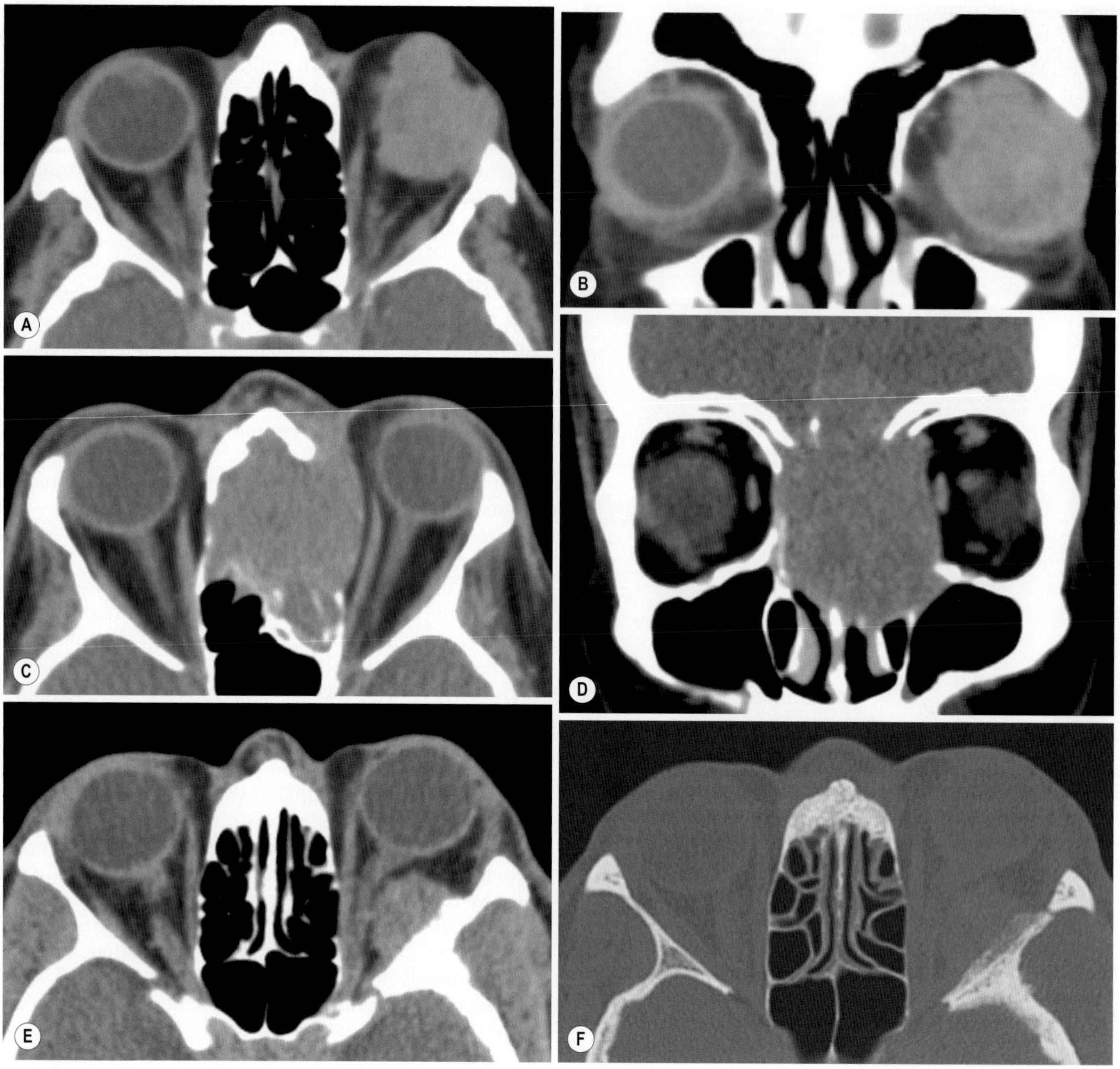

FIGURE 66-26 ■ Ocular and orbital metastases. Post-contrast axial (A) and coronal (B) CT examination demonstrating an enhancing left orbital metastatic lesion involving the entire left globe. Post-contrast axial (C) and coronal (D) CT examination showing an extensive paranasal sinus carcinoma with local invasion into the nasal aspect of the left orbit and intracranially through the cribriform plate and frontal sinuses. Post-contrast axial CT examination on soft-tissue (E) and bone (F) algorithms demonstrating a prostatic carcinoma metastatic deposit of the left sphenoid trigone causing expansion and sclerosis of the bone as well as an associated soft-tissue component occupying the temporal aspect of the left orbit resulting in left proptosis.

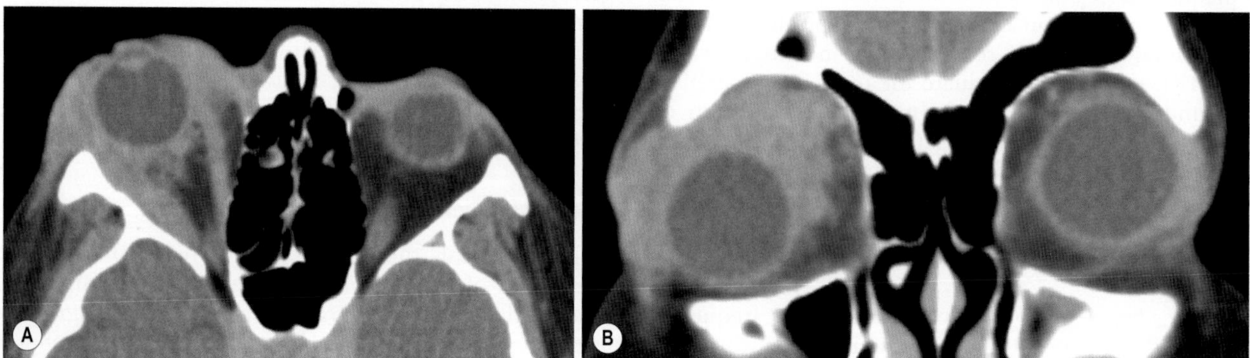

FIGURE 66-27 ■ Orbital lymphoma. Post-contrast axial (A) and coronal (B) CT examination demonstrating enhancing soft tissue encasing the subtotal circumference of the right globe and extending into the retrobulbar and temporal aspects of the right orbit, causing proptosis and hypoglobus.

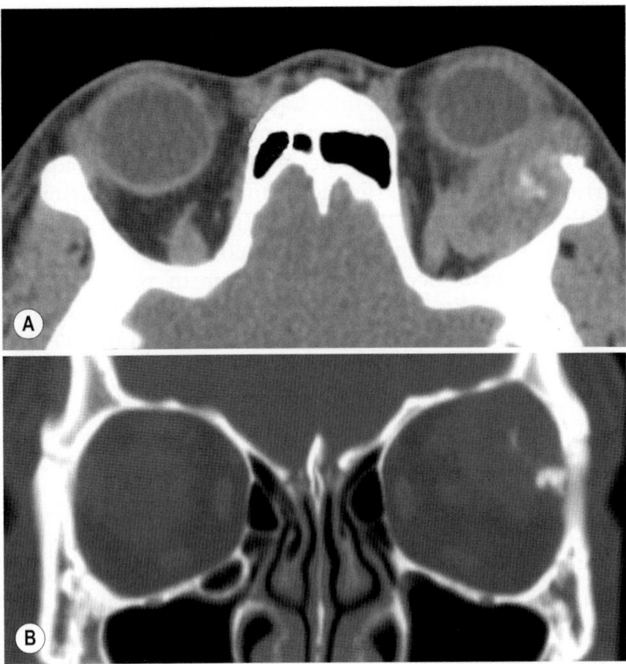

FIGURE 66-28 ■ **Adenoid cystic carcinoma.** Post-contrast axial CT on a soft tissue (A) and coronal CT on a bone (B) algorithms demonstrating a heterogeneous, peripherally enhancing left orbital mass with central coarse calcification indistinguishable from the lacrimal gland. Note the proptosis, deformation of the posterotemporal aspect of the left globe and left lateral orbital wall erosion and bony remodelling by the mass.

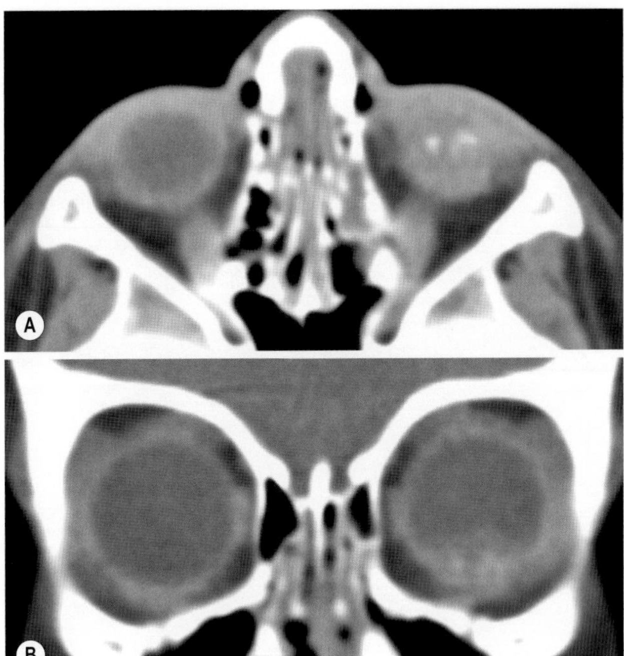

FIGURE 66-29 ■ **Retinoblastoma.** Axial (A) and coronal (B) CT examination in a child demonstrating a lesion involving the inferior aspect of the globe, extending into the vitreous and containing areas of fine punctate calcification.

such as dacryoadenitis, adenoma or lymphoma on imaging alone.

Paediatric Neoplasms

Retinoblastoma

Retinoblastoma is an aggressive malignant neoplasm, which arises from the immature retina. It is the most common intraocular tumour of childhood and usually manifests by the age of 5. Sporadic cases, heritable de novo mutations and familial cases have been reported. The underlying pathomechanism is damage to the RB1 tumour suppressor gene on the long arm of chromosome 13 with subsequent uncontrolled cell proliferation. Patients with inherited retinoblastoma tend to present at a younger age than those with sporadic tumours. Multifocal or bilateral tumours are generally associated with inherited disease. These patients are also at increased risk of associated neuroblastic tumours of the sellar or pineal region, a constellation which is referred to as *trilateral retinoblastoma*. Additionally, patients with inherited retinoblastoma demonstrate an increased incidence of somatic tumours such as osteosarcoma, melanoma and carcinomas. The most common clinical presentation is with leukocoria, i.e. loss of the normal red reflex of the affected eye. Secondary signs include pain, visual disturbance, heterochromia of the iris, glaucoma and retinal detachment. Some retinoblastomas elicit a periocular inflammatory response, which may simulate orbital cellulitis and delay diagnosis.[15] Histologically, endophytic, exophytic and mixed forms are recognised and may demonstrate varying imaging appearances.

The most common finding is that of a nodular lesion arising from the retina. CT is the initial imaging technique of choice and typically demonstrates a hyperattenuating mass in the posterior globe with calcification in 95% of cases[33] (Fig. 66-29). MR imaging is the most sensitive method to delineate intracranial spread and should always include dedicated orbital and whole-brain sequences. Retinoblastoma follows the signal intensity of grey matter on MRI and generally demonstrates contrast enhancement. Prognosis has much improved over the years, resulting in a shift from preservation of life to preservation of sight. However, decreased survival is associated with delayed diagnosis, extraocular extension and distant metastatic disease, usually to lung and bone.

Rhabdomyosarcoma

Rhabdomyosarcoma is the most prevalent extraocular malignancy in children, accounting for approximately 5% of all childhood cancers.[2,34] Approximately a third of paediatric rhabdomyosarcomas arise in the orbit, most often in the first decade, with a peak age around 7 years. It presents as a rapidly progressive unilateral proptosis with or without globe displacement and there may be periorbital swelling, particularly lid swelling, which can lead to misdiagnosis as cellulitis. An aggressive course is typical, with invasion of bone and surrounding soft tissues including the paranasal sinuses. Intracranial spread does occur but is less common.

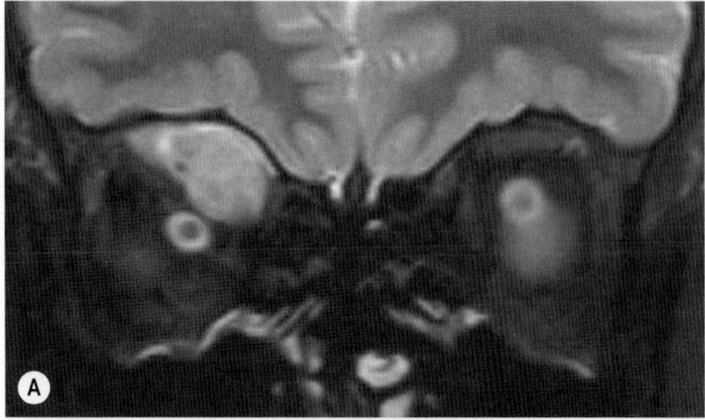

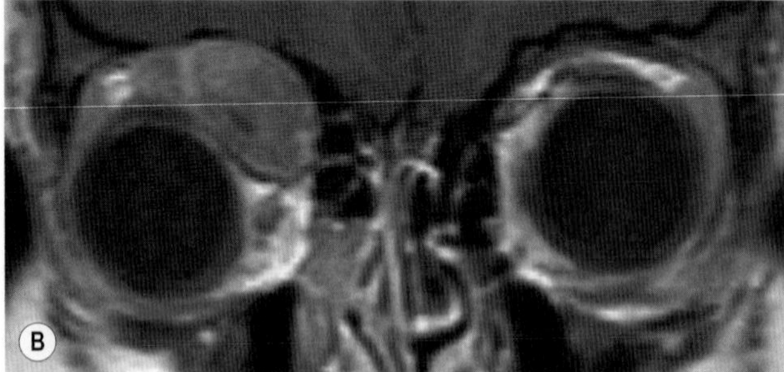

FIGURE 66-30 ■ **Rhabdomyosarcoma.** Coronal STIR (A) and post-contrast T1-weighted (B) orbital MRI in a child demonstrating a superonasal enhancing mass and inferotemporal displacement and some distortion of the right globe.

Metastases are typically haematogenous, with lung and bone involvement being the most common. Cross-sectional imaging is used both for staging and follow-up, whereby CT is most useful to identify bony invasion and MRI is very sensitive at delineating intracranial spread. On CT, the neoplasm may show attenuation similar to muscle or brain, with relatively homogeneous contrast enhancement. The tumour itself does not calcify, but occasionally may contain hyperdense foci if it had infiltrated through bone. On MRI, rhabdomyosarcoma tends to be isoattenuating to muscle on T1 and mildy hyperattenuating on T2 sequences[2,4,34] (Fig. 66-30).

Medulloepithelioma

This is a rare embryonal tumour, which arises from the medullary epithelium of the ciliary body and usually occurs around the age of 5 years, although it can occasionally manifest later, even in adulthood. Benign and malignant variants have been described. On CT imaging, the tumour may demonstrate increased attenuation, sometimes with dystrophic calcifications or cartilaginous components. Localisation of the neoplasm within the ciliary body may be an important clue; however, medulloepithelioma may also arise from or spread to the retina, thus becoming indistinguishable from retinoblastoma on imaging alone.

Ischaemia

Ischaemia of the retina or optic nerve may result in transient (*amaurosis fugax*) or permanent loss of vision. This is commonly caused by a stenosis or occlusion of the ipsilateral internal carotid artery with secondary retinal emboli.[20] Anterior ischaemic optic neuropathy (AION) as the term implies results in ischaemia damage of the optic nerve and constitutes one of the major causes of seriously impaired vision among the middle-aged and elderly, particularly the non-arteritic form (NAION).[35] Arteritic AION is secondary to temporal (giant cell) arteritis, a medium-vessel inflammatory vasculopathy.

Retinal vein occlusion may occur in patients with hypercoaguability; for example, systemic lupus erythematosus and antiphospholipid syndrome.[36] Migraine is also a differential for transient loss of vision, particularly in young patients with a relevant history.

ORBITAL TRAUMA

Injury to the orbital region represents a significant proportion of emergency department attendances and is common in patients with multisystem trauma: for example, following motor vehicle accidents. To date, trauma remains a leading cause of monocular blindness. Certain eye injuries, such as superficial lacerations and a proportion of globe ruptures, may be evident on clinical examination. However, imaging plays a major role in assessing for occult injuries, evaluation of the bony orbit, deep orbital structures and in identifying foreign bodies.

Plain radiography has limited sensitivity in identifying orbital fractures and cannot reliably assess the intraorbital soft tissues. Ultrasound (US) may be of value when there is concern regarding intraocular injury such as traumatic retinal detachment, but it is contraindicated in suspected globe rupture. The technique of choice for the evaluation of suspected orbital injury is thin-section (0.625–1.25 mm slice thickness) CT with multiplanar bone and soft-tissue reconstructions. MR imaging is less commonly employed in acute trauma and is inferior to CT in identifying fractures. Owing to its soft-tissue contrast, it can be useful in complex cases. It must be borne in mind that MR is contraindicated whenever a metallic foreign body is present.

Within the bony orbit, an orbital floor fracture may be a cause of ophthalmoplegia as a result of herniation of fat or muscle into a defect and para/anaesthesia of the maxillary division of the trigeminal nerve when involving the infraorbital canal/nerve. The lamina papyracea is another common site for fractures, as it consists of very thin bone. In addition to a functional deficit, orbital wall fractures may have cosmetic impact: for example, when there is hypoglobus. Care should be taken to review the orbital apex, where a small fracture can be associated with optic nerve injury and require urgent surgical intervention.[37] Evaluation of the orbital soft tissues may reveal fat stranding, haematoma or gas as signs of significant injury (Fig. 66-31).

Metallic and glass orbital foreign bodies are of increased attenuation and best delineated on CT. The appearance of wood on CT can be of similar attenuation to air, thus mimicking intraorbital gas (Fig. 66-32). A wood or organic foreign body should be suspected when there is a low attenuation collection with a geometric

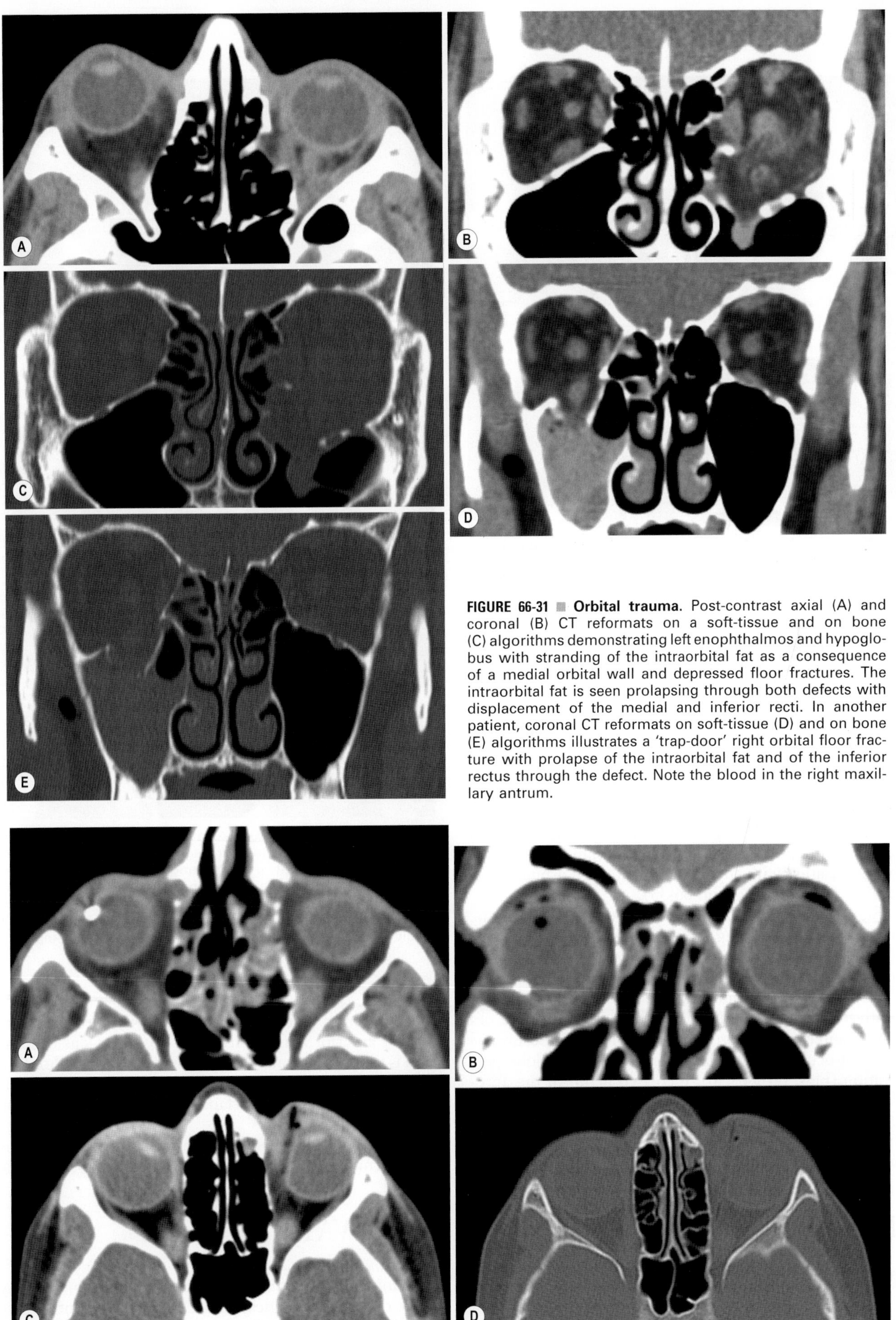

FIGURE 66-31 ■ **Orbital trauma.** Post-contrast axial (A) and coronal (B) CT reformats on a soft-tissue and on bone (C) algorithms demonstrating left enophthalmos and hypoglobus with stranding of the intraorbital fat as a consequence of a medial orbital wall and depressed floor fractures. The intraorbital fat is seen prolapsing through both defects with displacement of the medial and inferior recti. In another patient, coronal CT reformats on soft-tissue (D) and on bone (E) algorithms illustrates a 'trap-door' right orbital floor fracture with prolapse of the intraorbital fat and of the inferior rectus through the defect. Note the blood in the right maxillary antrum.

FIGURE 66-32 ■ **Ocular foreign bodies.** Axial (A) and coronal (B) CT showing a metallic radiodense intraocular penetrating foreign body and vitreal air. Axial CT on soft-tissue (C) and bone (D) algorithms demonstrating a linear hypodensity, resembling air, traversing the nasal aspect of the left globe in a patient with penetrating injury from a wooden splinter. A small locule of air is also seen in the anterior chamber of the eye.

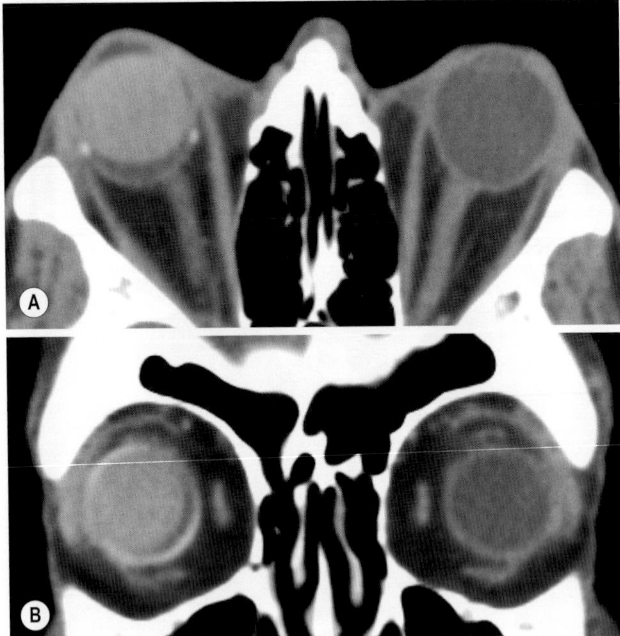

FIGURE 66-33 ■ Axial (A) and coronal (B) CT of a right scleral banding and silicone tamponade as treatment of retinal detachment.

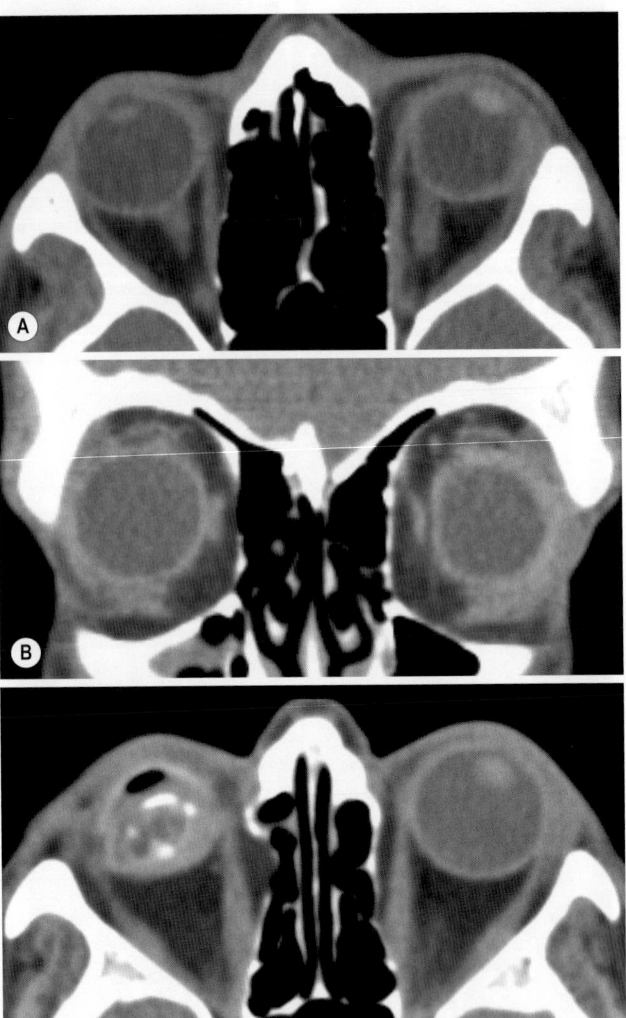

FIGURE 66-34 ■ **Globe rupture.** Axial (A) and coronal (B) CT demonstrating some vitreal haemorrhage in a relatively smaller left globe in a patient with a penetrating injury of the left globe. Note the flattening of the nasal aspect of the globe resembling a 'flat tyre' reflecting globe hypotonia. Axial CT (C) in a patient with previous traumatic injury to the right eye illustrating a small non-functioning calcific right globe or phthisis bulbi.

margin.[38] Within days of the injury, the attenuation of a wooden foreign body may increase, approaching that of water.[39] In challenging cases, T2-weighted and post-contrast fat-suppressed MR imaging can be a potential aid in delineating an inflammatory reaction around the foreign body.[37] Potential mimics of penetrating injury with presence of gas include previous gas injections and placement of low-attenuation silicone sponges for the treatment of retinal detachment. A high-attenuation scleral band around the globe, also a treatment for retinal detachment, can be mistaken for a foreign body; therefore correlation with any previous history of orbital intervention is mandatory (Fig. 66-33).

Signs of globe rupture include loss of globe volume and contour (excluding non-traumatic causes such as coloboma or staphyloma), the *flat tyre* sign and intraocular gas. Retinal detachment shows as a characteristic V-shape structure within the globe, because the retina is relatively fixed at the optic disc posteriorly and at the ora serrata anteriorly. Choroidal detachment can occur as a result of ocular pressure loss: for example, in globe perforation (Figs. 66-34A, B). Increased depth of the anterior chamber is a more subtle sign of open globe injury. *Hyphaema* is defined as blood within the anterior chamber; this may be seen as a blood–fluid level on clinical inspection or as increased attenuation on CT. Decreased depth of the anterior chamber may occur due to corneal laceration or anterior lens subluxation. Posterior lens dislocation is more common, however. Bilateral lens subluxation or dislocation is rare and should raise suspicion of a collagen disorder such as Marfan's, Ehlers-Danlos syndrome or homocystinuria.

Phthisis bulbi refers to a shrunken calcified globe as long-term sequelae of (penetrating) injury (Fig. 66-34C).

THE RETRO-ORBITAL VISUAL PATHWAY

INTRODUCTION

Various diseases have potential to affect the retro-orbital visual pathway, whereby the clinical deficit is usually determined by the anatomical location of the abnormality more than its histological nature. Because the optic nerve is a fibre tract of the brain rather than a true cranial nerve, it may be affected by the same disease processes as the brain and meninges.[40] We provide a brief overview of retro-orbital visual pathway anatomy and pathology according to the respective lesion location.

ANATOMY

Where the intracanalicular optic nerve exits intracranially from its canal, it becomes the intracranial optic nerve. This prechiasmatic segment is approximately 10 mm long, lies below the A1 segment of the anterior cerebral artery and above the internal carotid artery.[40] The optic chiasm is located in the midline at the floor of the third ventricle in close relation to the pituitary stalk and diaphragm sellae. At the optic chiasm, nerve fibres from the nasal aspect of both retinas (carrying information from the temporal visual fields) decussate, whereas fibres from the lateral retina (carrying information from the nasal visual fields) do not decussate. The partially decussated fibre tracts, which emerge dorsally from the chiasm, are termed optic tracts, each containing axons from the ipsilateral temporal and contralateral nasal retina, respectively.

From the chiasm, the optic tracts run dorsolaterally and slightly upwards on each side, passing anterolateral to the tuber cinereum of the hypothalamus towards the lateral geniculate nucleus (LGN) of the thalalmus. Most of the axons from the optic tracts terminate in the LGN, with a few fibres terminating in the superior colliculus of the midbrain. Additional neural connections exist between the LGN and the superior colliculus.[1,41] From the LGN, the optic radiation arises with approximately half of its fibres running posterolaterally, forming part of the superolateral wall of the lateral ventricles. The other half of the optic radiation passes first forward and then backwards along the lateral aspect of the temporal and occipital horns, forming a loop, also known as *Meyer's loop*.

The optic radiation fans out into the primary visual cortex of the occipital lobes. This is sometimes referred to as the striate cortex (named after the *stria of Gennari*, a relatively thick myelinated band within layer 4 of the visual cortex) or V1. The striate cortex is located in the occipital lobe along the banks of the calcarine fissure and at the occipital pole. As a result of the partial decussation and anatomical distribution of nerve fibres, the primary visual cortex of each cerebral hemisphere receives information from the contralateral visual field and visual information is projected upside down; i.e. visual signals from the caudal retina are projected into the cranial aspect of the visual cortex and vice versa (Fig. 66-35). The primary

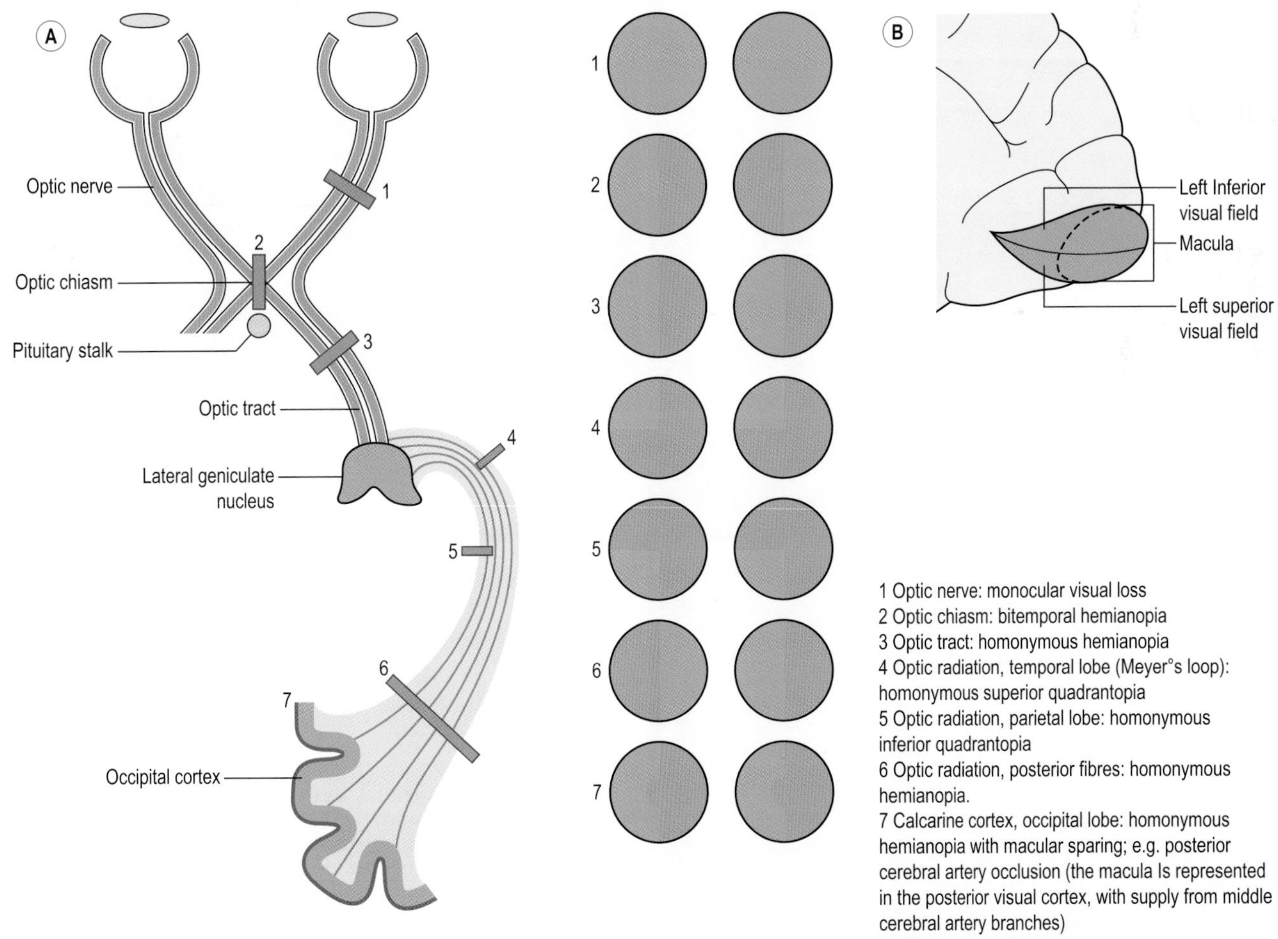

FIGURE 66-35 ■ Schematic diagram of the visual pathway and the associated field defects with its disruption at different points on the pathway. (Reproduced from Butler P, Mitchell A, Healy J 2012 Applied Radiological Anatomy 2nd edn. Cambridge University Press, Cambridge, UK.)

visual cortex (V1) is surrounded by several areas of visual association cortex (V2, V3, etc.). Fundamentally, some functions of the associate visual cortical regions overlap with those of the striate cortex, whereas others are involved in higher visual processing such as complex pattern recognition and visual memory formation. To deal with higher visual function in detail would be beyond the scope of this chapter, but for further reading see references 1 and 42.

Vascular supply to the primary visual cortex is predominantly via the posterior cerebral artery, which gives rise to the calcarine artery. Small medial and lateral choroidal branches arise from the P2 segment. Rarely, when these are occluded in isolation, this can result in specific deficits of the central post-chiasmatic visual pathway such as sector anopsia.[43]

PATHOLOGIES OF THE ANTERIOR VISUAL PATHWAY (OPTIC NERVES, CHIASM AND OPTIC TRACTS)

Congenital

Hypoplasia, or in severe cases aplasia, of the optic nerve can occur for several reasons. Examples are chromosomal abnormalities, sporadic mutations, intrauterine insult such as maternal drug intake, but also advanced maternal age.[44] The imaging findings are those of a reduced-calibre nerve without pathological enhancement, usually best appreciated on coronal T2W and STIR MR images (Figs. 66-36A–D).

Septo-optic dysplasia represents a symptom complex featuring a variable combination of midline defects.

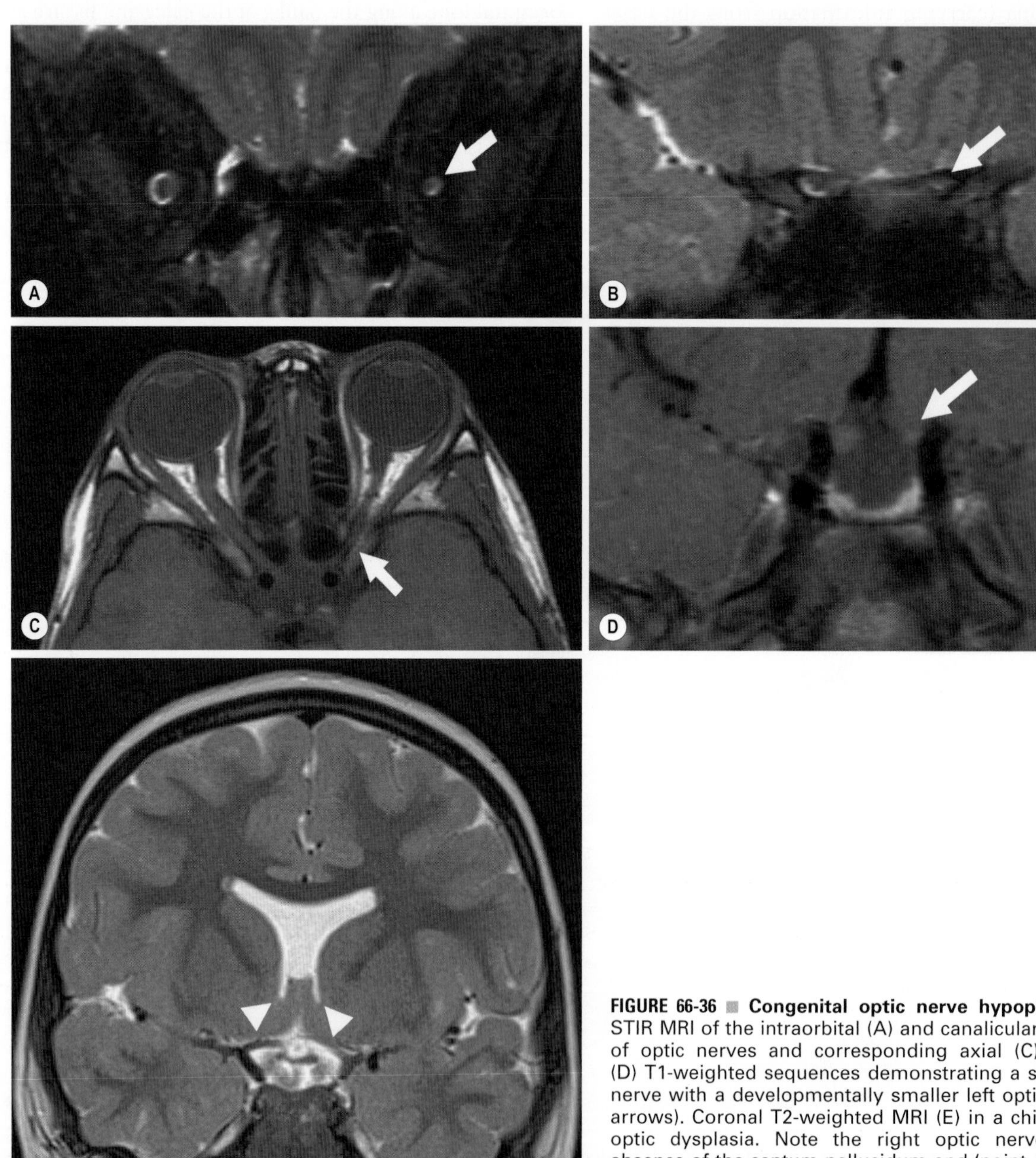

FIGURE 66-36 ■ **Congenital optic nerve hypoplasia.** Coronal STIR MRI of the intraorbital (A) and canalicular (B) segments of optic nerves and corresponding axial (C) and coronal (D) T1-weighted sequences demonstrating a small left optic nerve with a developmentally smaller left optic canal (white arrows). Coronal T2-weighted MRI (E) in a child with septo-optic dysplasia. Note the right optic nerve hypoplasia, absence of the septum pellucidum and 'point-down' appearance of the frontal horns of the lateral ventricles (white arrowheads).

These typically include hypoplasia of the optic nerves, hypoplasia or absence of the septum pellucidum and dysplasia/dysfunction of the hypothalamus–pituitary axis (Fig. 66-36E). Clinical signs consist of visual dysfunction, hormonal abnormalities and varying degrees of learning impairment. Septo-optic dysplasia can be associated with other brain abnormalities such as corpus callosum dysplasia, schizencephaly or cortical dysplasia. In a recent study, 75% of children with septo-optic dysplasia showed associated brain malformations on imaging.[45] Cross-sectional coronal MRI is particularly useful for depicting abnormal optic nerves and sagittal images may demonstrate low-lying fornices if the septum pellucidum is absent.[33]

Intrinsic Tumours

As described in 'The Orbit' section, most intrinsic gliomas are of low grade (pilocytic astrocytoma) and involve the optic nerve in young patients, with a peak in the first decade. Some of these tumours extend to involve the optic chiasm (Fig. 66-18) and approximately 7% of gliomas are confined to the chiasm exclusively.[46] Mortality increases if there is additional hypothalamic involvement. High-grade optic pathway glioma occurs in adult patients and is universally fatal.

Cavernoma is an angiographically occult venous malformation and can occur in any brain parenchymal structure, including the anterior visual pathway. This may be discovered incidentally or present due to slow expansion or haemorrhage, although the latter is rarely clinically apparent.[46] MRI appearances are often diagnostic with the classic 'popcorn' appearance and blooming artefact due to haemosiderin staining and/or calcification visible on gradient-echo and susceptibility-weighted imaging (Fig. 66-37).

Inflammatory/Demyelinating Lesions

Retrobulbar optic neuritis is the initial manifestation of multiple sclerosis in 15–20% of patients and up to half of patients with an episode of optic neuritis will eventually develop MS.[40] Although optic neuritis can be asymptomatic, painful loss of vision with a relatively acute onset over days is more common. MRI is the most sensitive imaging technique for assessing suspected optic neuritis. There may be swelling of the optic nerve with associated signal increase of the nerve on T2 and STIR imaging and post-gadolinium enhancement (Fig. 66-38). Neuromyelitis optica (NMO, also known as *Devic's disease*) should be considered as a differential for bilateral optic neuritis, both on imaging and clinically. NMO may be associated with spinal cord abnormality, which typically affects a longer cord segment (three or more vertebral segments) than MS-type demyelination. Of note, positivity for aquaporin-4 antibodies is a specific finding associated with NMO.

Less commonly, granulomatous inflammation in TB or sarcoidosis (Fig. 66-39) may involve the anterior visual pathway. Imaging abnormalities include nodular or smooth enhancement along the optic nerve or chiasm, and occasionally nerve swelling may be observed.[40] However, these features are not specific and may be difficult to distinguish from a neoplasm on imaging alone. Metastatic disease is also a differential to be considered in this imaging scenario.

Extrinsic Compression

Extrinsic compression of the optic chiasm is more common than intrinsic lesions of this region. Compressive symptoms can occur secondary to a host of different intracranial pathologies such as pituitary macroadenoma, craniopharyngioma, Rathke's cleft cyst, meningioma, germinoma, chordoma, metastases and aneurysms (Fig. 66-40). The classic deficit arising from midline chiasmatic compression is a bitemporal hemianopia. In contrast, a lesion compressing the chiasm laterally is more likely to cause a nasal visual field defect due to compression of nerve fibres supplying the temporal retina.

PATHOLOGIES OF THE POSTERIOR VISUAL PATHWAY (LATERAL GENICULATE NUCLEUS, OPTIC RADIATION AND VISUAL CORTEX)

Although there are no diseases which specifically target the LGN, this may be involved by intracranial pathology in its proximity. Isolated LGN pathology is rare, but this is known to produce a specific visual deficit of homonymous sector defects on the horizontal meridian.[47]

Equally, the optic radiation and visual cortex can be compromised by intracranial pathology of any nature nearby. The clinical picture and visual deficit will be dictated predominantly by the lesion location. Posterior cerebral artery (PCA) infarction is a common central cause for acute-onset visual impairment, with the field defect being determined by location and extent of ischaemia. If involving the entire primary visual cortex, bilateral PCA infarction may lead to 'cortical blindness' or *Anton–Babinski syndrome*. A large infarct may be evident on CT within hours of onset, but generally MRI, including diffusion-weighted imaging, is the most sensitive method, particularly for the detection of small infarcts, and MR is able to demonstrate imaging abnormality earlier than CT (Fig. 66-41).

Space-occupying masses may produce symptoms either due to direct infiltration or secondary to compression of neural structures. Intrinsic primary brain tumours, but also intracranial metastases (commonly breast, lung or melanoma) or lymphoma, are typical examples. Infection, including abscess formation, can involve any intracranial structure and should be considered particularly in immunosuppressed patients. Other aetiologies, which may be encountered along the posterior visual pathway, include encephalitis, abscesses, posterior reversible encephalopathy syndrome (PRES), progressive multifocal leukencephalopathy (PML) and arteriovenous malformations (Fig. 66-42). For a more detailed description of intracranial pathologies, please see Chapter 60.

Text continued on p. 1589

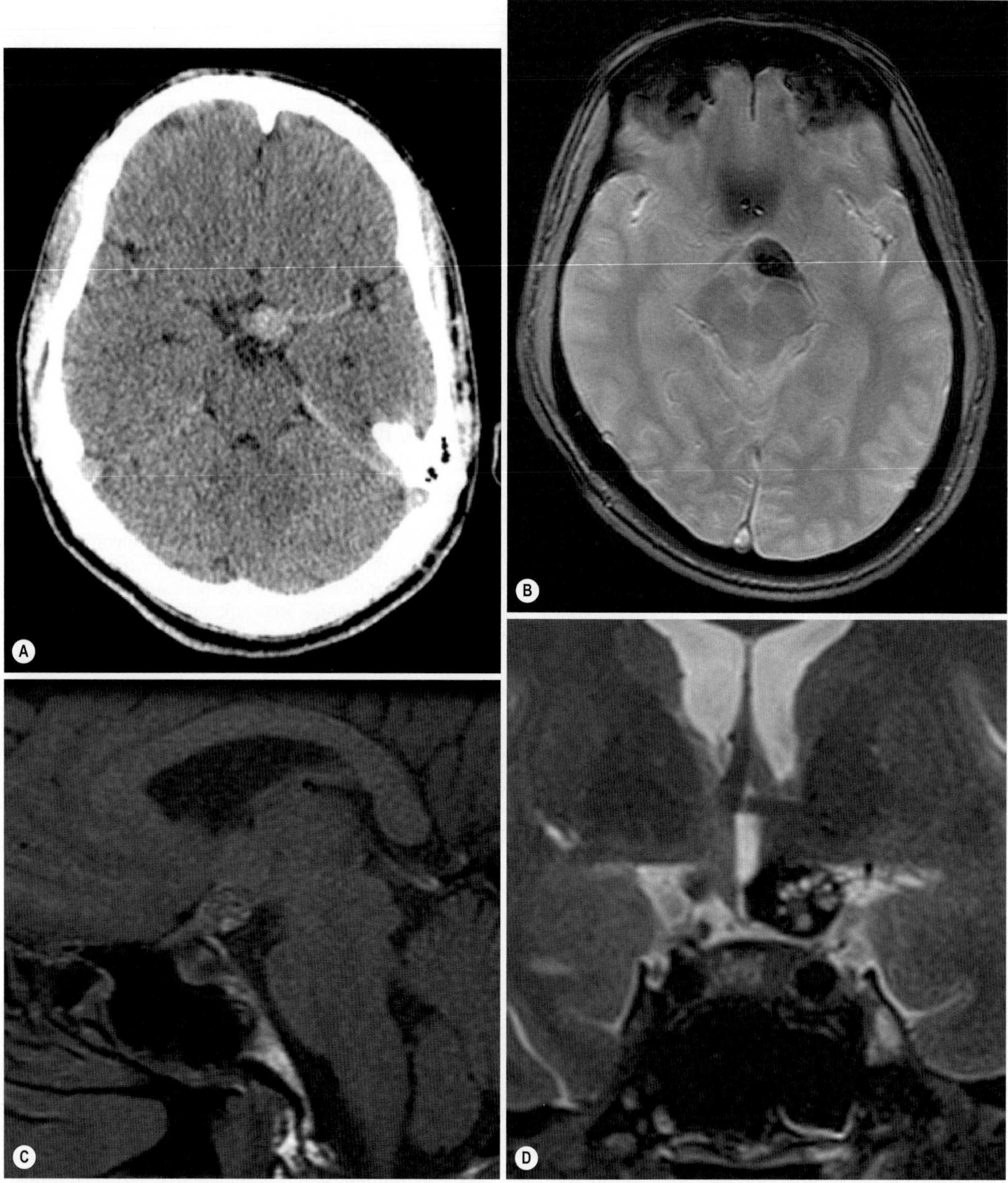

FIGURE 66-37 ■ **Optic pathway cavernoma.** Post-contrast axial CT (A) showing a hyperattenuating mass in the left suprasellar cistern, thought initially to be an aneurysm. Corresponding axial T2*- (B), sagittal T1- (C) and coronal T2-weighted (D) MRI demonstrating the classic 'popcorn' appearance of a cavernoma intrinsic to the left optic chiasm and tract.

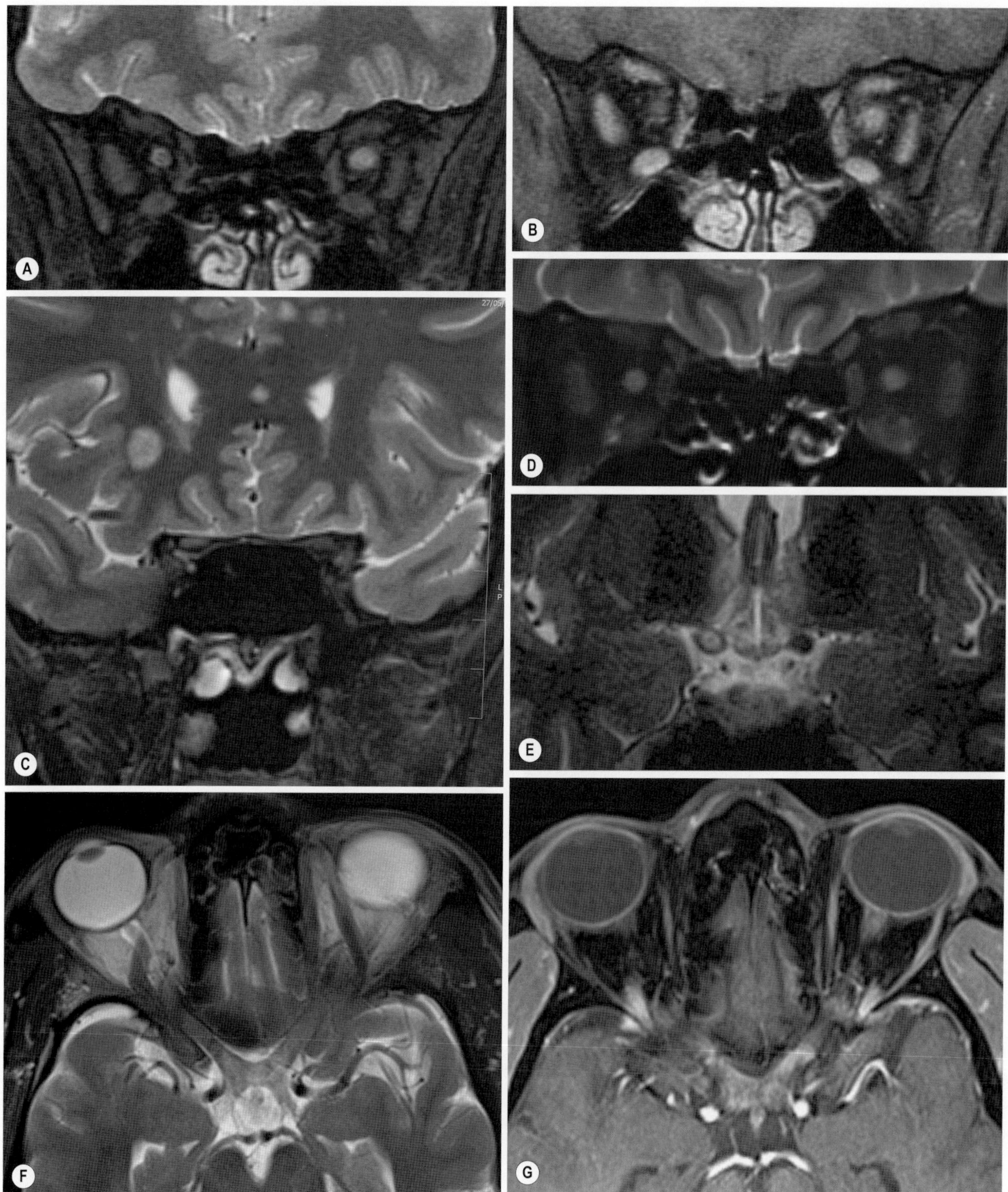

FIGURE 66-38 ■ Optic neuritis in multiple sclerosis. Coronal STIR (A) and post-contrast fat-suppressed T1-weighted (B) MRI of the orbits demonstrating hyperintensity, swelling and enhancement of the intraorbital segment of the left optic nerve in a patient presenting with left optic neuritis. Coronal STIR images through the canalicular (C) and intraorbital (D) segment of the optic nerves and of the optic tracts (E) in two other patients. In (C), there is hyperintensity and swelling of the canalicular right optic nerve and demyelinating lesions in the white matter of the frontal lobes. Neuromyelitis optica: In (D, E), bilateral inflammation involving the intraorbital segment of the optic nerves and the right optic tract. Note the associated hypothalamic inflammation. The axial T2- (F) and post-contrast fat-suppressed T1-weighted (G) MRI of the orbits as well as a sagittal T2-weighted image of the upper spinal cord (H) demonstrate inflammation and enhancement of the optic chiasm as well as a contiguous segmental myelitis of the upper thoracic spinal cord.

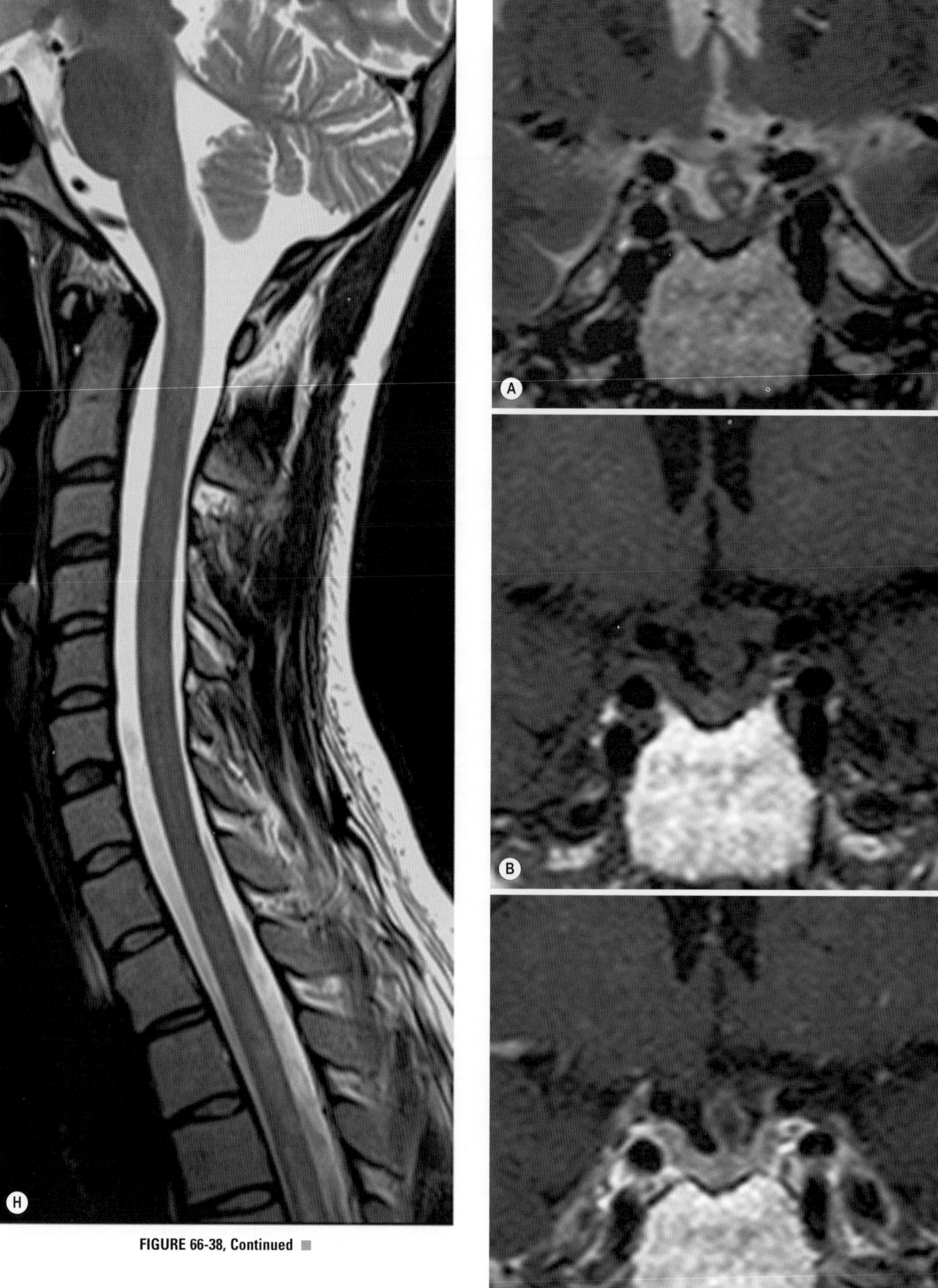

FIGURE 66-38, Continued ■

FIGURE 66-39 ■ **Optic pathway granulomatous inflammation.** Coronal T2- (A), T1- (B) and post-contrast coronal (C) and sagittal (D) T1- weighted MRI of an enhancing inflammatory process of the pituitary infundibulum and the optic chiasm in a patient with sarcoidosis. *Continued on following page*

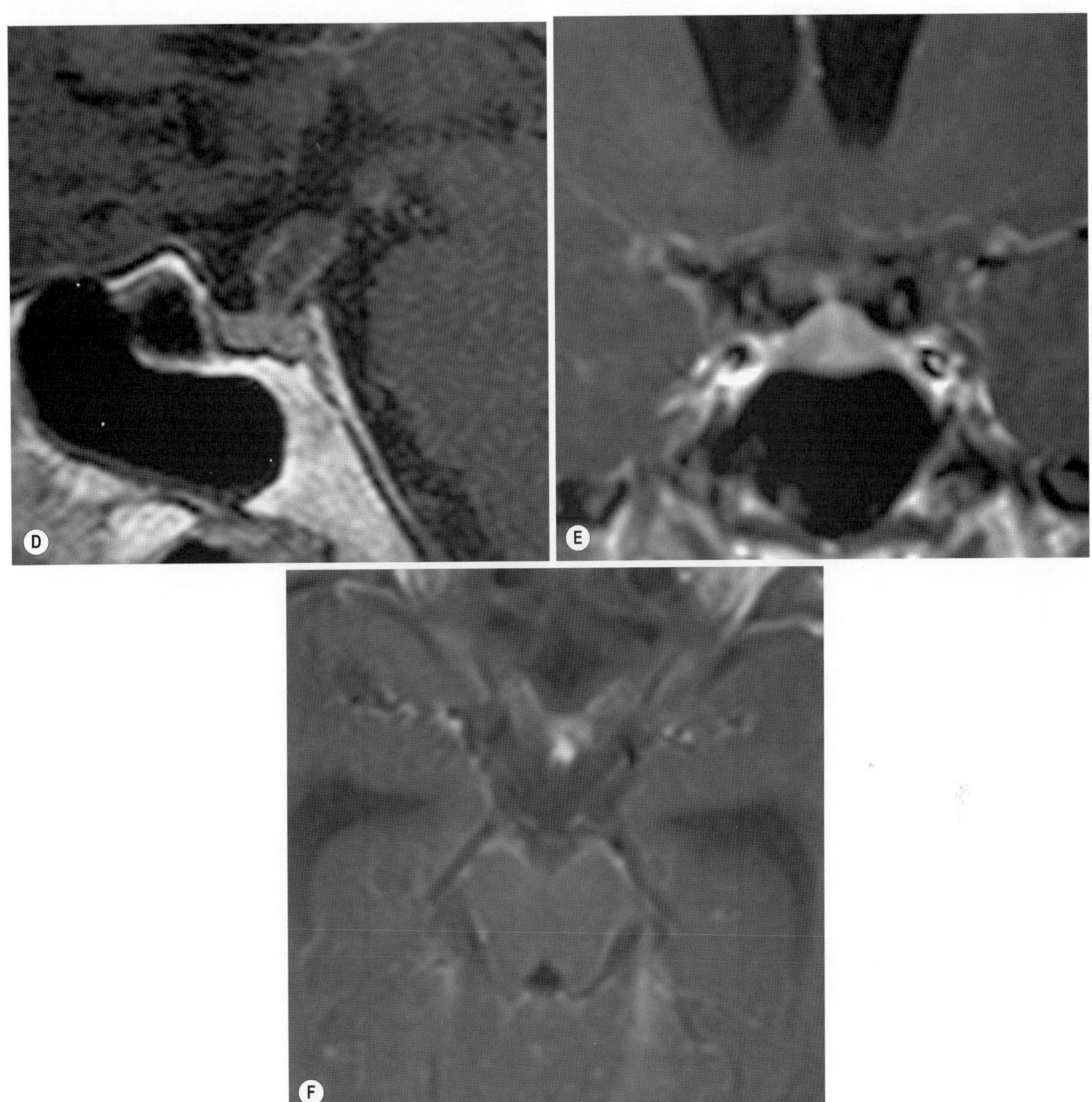

FIGURE 66-39, Continued ■ Post-contrast coronal (E) and axial (F) T1-weighted MRI demonstrating a diffuse enhancing leptomeningeal process affecting the intracranial optic nerves and optic chiasm in a patient with tuberculous basal meningitis.

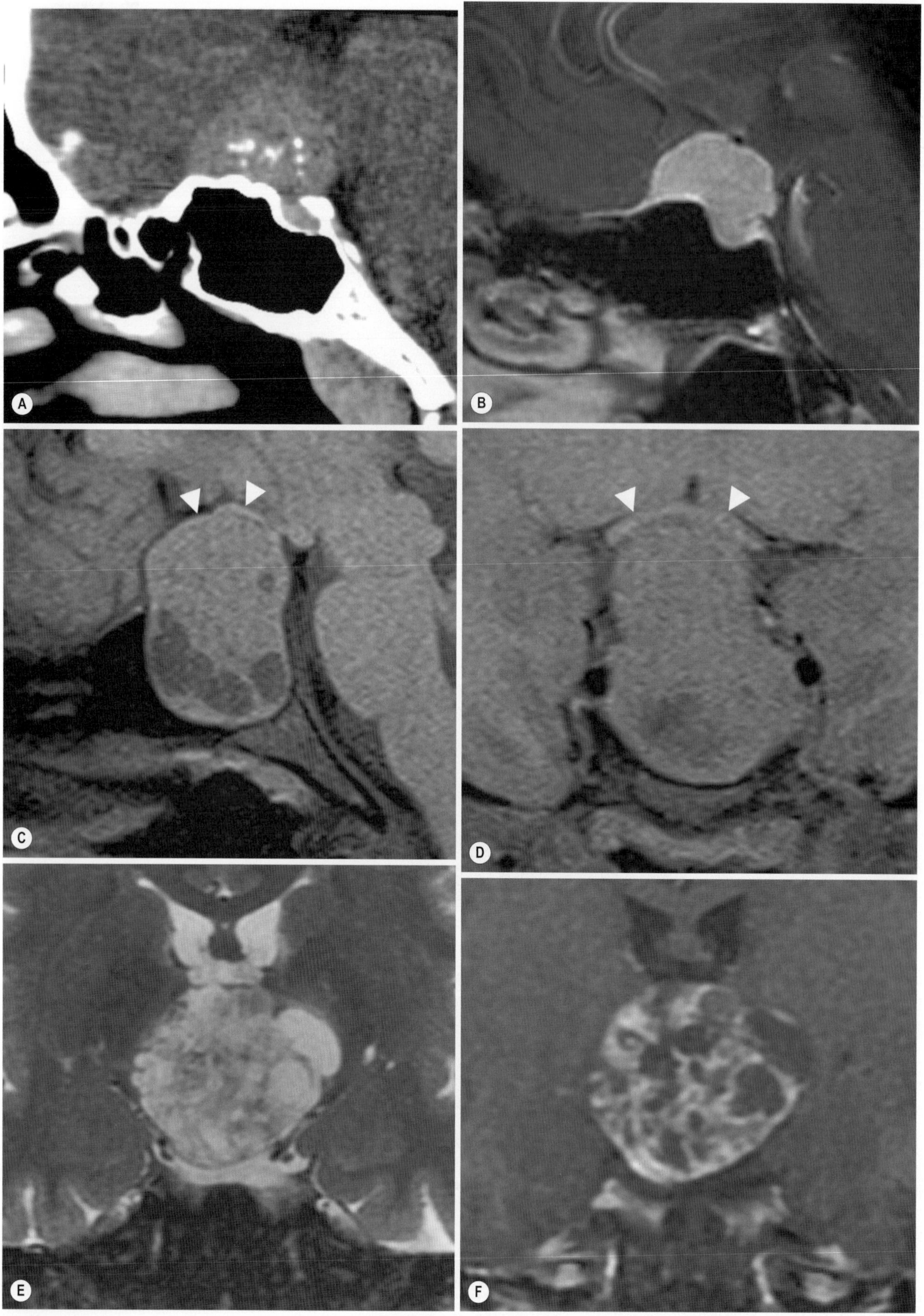

FIGURE 66-40 ■ **Optic pathway compressive tumours.** Sagittal reformatted post-contrast CT (A) and post-contrast sagittal T1-weighted MRI (B) of an enhancing calcific meningioma of the planum sphenoidale, compressing the optic chiasm. Sagittal (C) and coronal (D) T1-weighted MRI of a pituitary macroadenoma compressing the optic chiasm. Note the optic chiasm draped over the suprasellar component of the tumour (white arrowheads). Coronal T2- (E) and post-contrast T1-weighted (F) MRI of a craniopharyngioma causing similar compression.

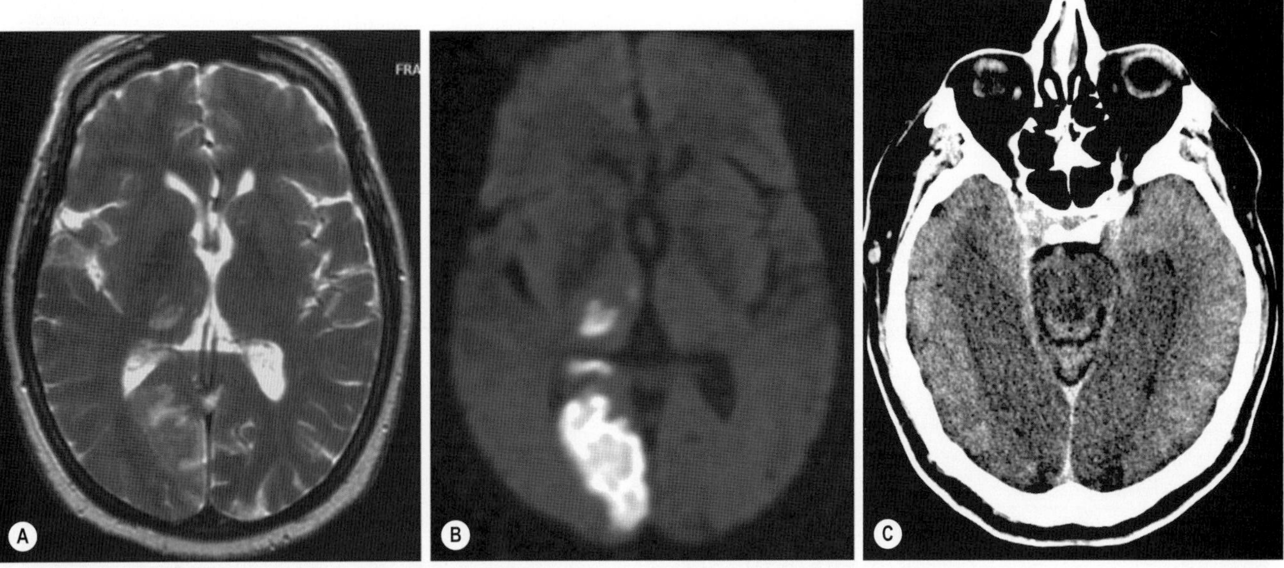

FIGURE 66-41 ■ Posterior cerebral artery (PCA) infarction. Axial T2- (A) and diffusion-weighted (B) MRI illustrating an acute right occipital and thalamic infarct with restriction on DWI. Axial CT (C) of a basilar artery thrombosis with pontine and bilateral PCA territory hypodense infarcts.

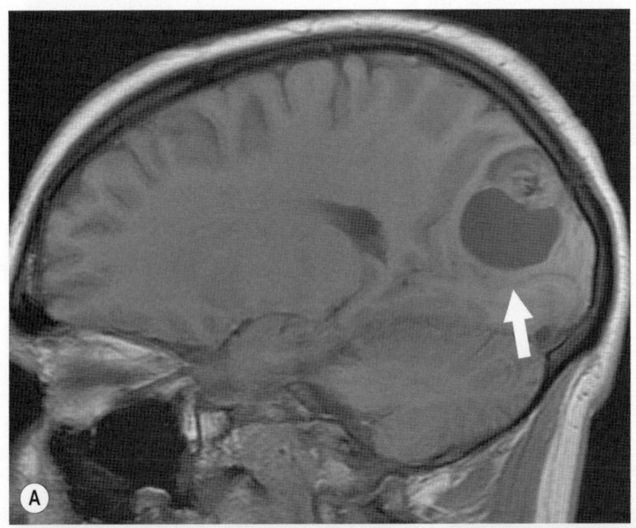

FIGURE 66-42 ■ Lesions of the posterior visual pathway. Sagittal T1-weighted MRI (A) of an intrinsic glioma of the cuneus of the occipital lobe. Note the displaced calcarine sulcus (white arrow). Axial T2- (B) and post-contrast T1-weighted (C) MRI of enhancing primary CNS lymphoma in a periventricular distribution. Axial T2- (D) and post-contrast T1-weighted (E) MRI of enhancing metastases from a lung primary.

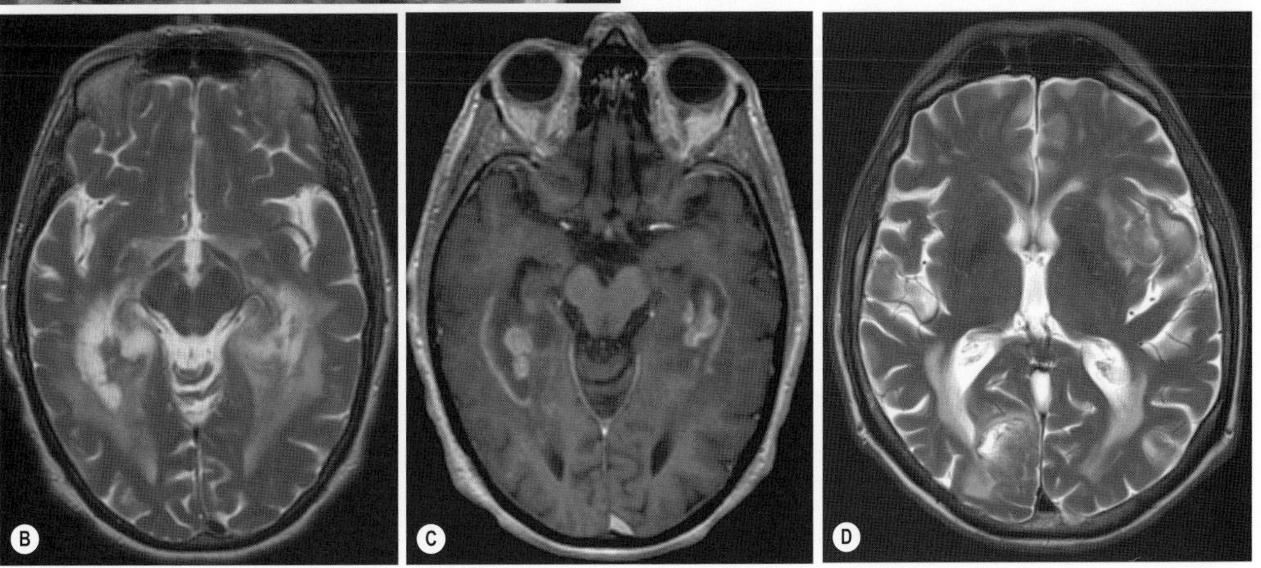

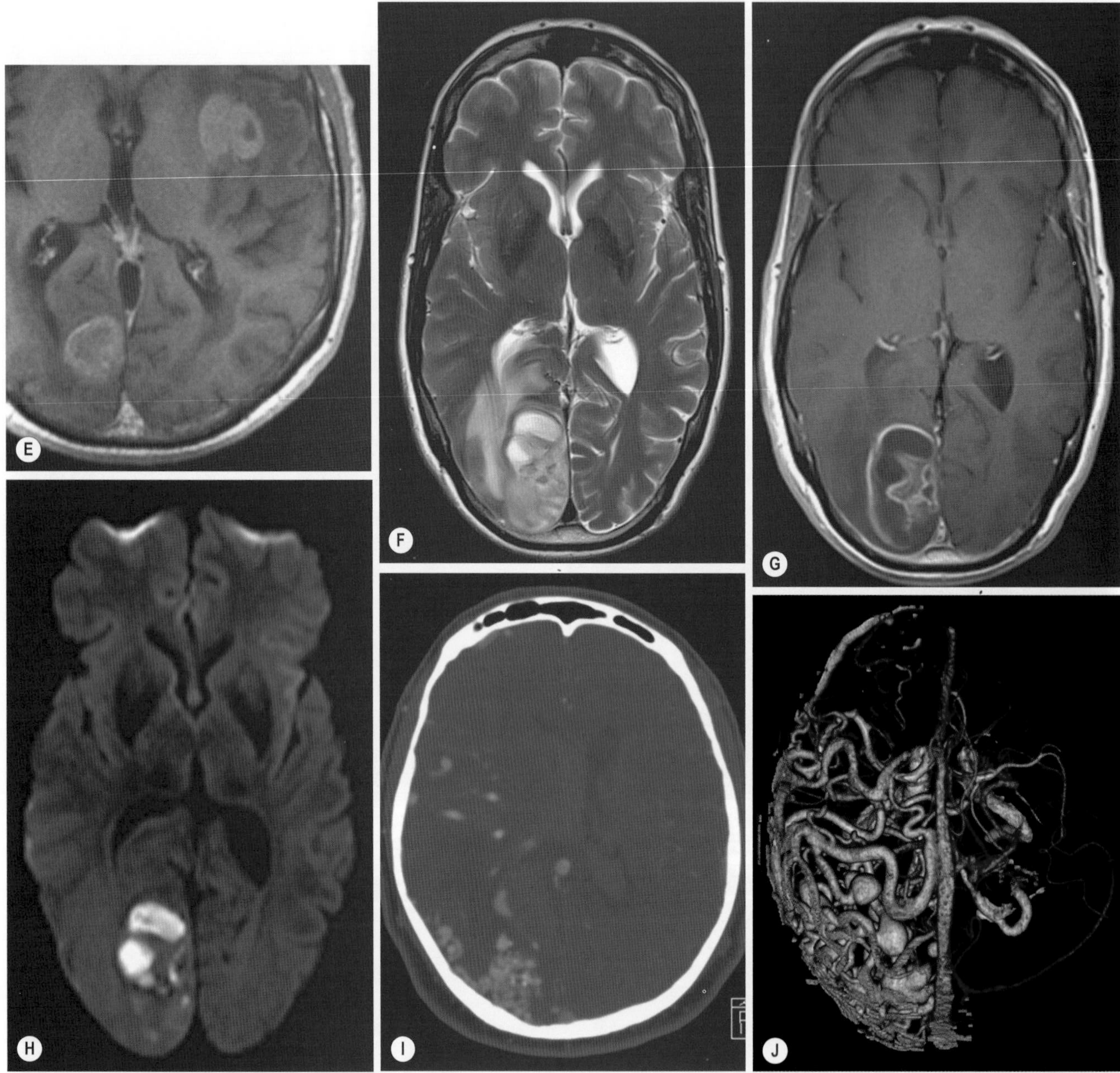

FIGURE 66-42, Continued ■ Axial T2- (F), post-contrast T1- (G) and diffusion-weighted (H) MRI of a right occipital lobe abscess. Axial CT angiogram (I) and 3D surface-rendered reconstruction (J) of a large right occipital lobe arterio-venous malformation.

OTHER NEURO-OPHTHALMOLOGICAL CONDITIONS

Idiopathic Intracranial Hypertension

Idiopathic intracranial hypertension (previously known as *pseudotumour cerebri*) is a disease of unknown aetiology, typically affecting young obese women and producing a syndrome of raised intracranial pressure that is not related to an intracranial disorder, a meningeal process or cerebral venous thrombosis.[48] Associated imaging findings include tortuosity and ectasia of the optic nerve sheaths, flattening of the posterior globes (Fig. 66-43), which correlate with the clinical observation of papilloedema, an expanded empty sella turcica and narrowing of the distal transverse venous sinuses.

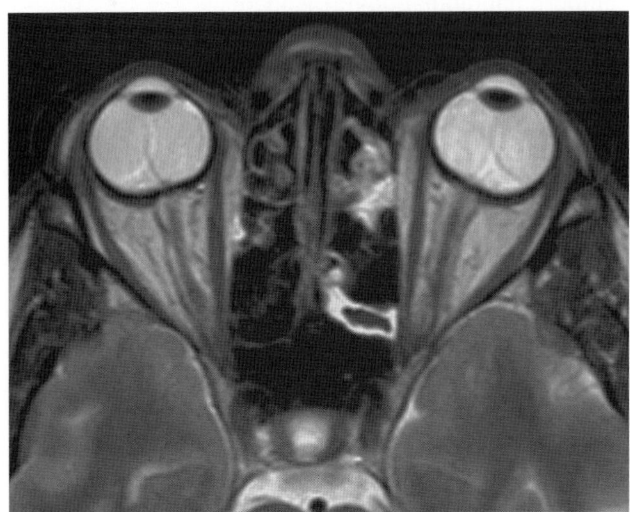

FIGURE 66-43 ■ **Papilloedema in idiopathic intracranial hypertension.** Axial T2-weighted MRI of the orbits demonstrating ectasia of the optic nerve sheaths, posterior globe flattening and protrusion of the optic nerve heads into the globes.

Recurrent Ophthalmoplegic Cranial Neuropathy

Recurrent ophthalmoplegic cranial neuropathy (*ophthalmoplegic migraine*) is a rare and poorly understood neurological syndrome which usually presents in children, but can persist in adulthood. It is characterised by recurrent bouts of head pain and ophthalmoplegia which recovers in most patients within days to weeks, but a small proportion of patients affected are left with persistent neurological deficits. The oculomotor nerve is most commonly affected, at times associated with mydriasis and ptosis. This can be associated with thickening and enhancement of the third (in approximately 75%) or rarely the fourth and/or sixth cranial nerve on contrast-enhanced MRI.[49]

For a full list of references, please see ExpertConsult.

FURTHER READING

1. Baert AL, Sartor K, Mueller-Forell WS, editors. Imaging of the Orbital and Visual Pathway. Springer; 2002.
3. Aviv RI, Miszkiel K. Orbital imaging: Part 2. Intraorbital pathology. Clin Radiol 2005;60:288–307.
20. Jaeger HR. Loss of vision: Imaging the visual pathways. Eur Radiol 2005;15(3):501–10.
33. Barkovich AJ. Pediatric Neuroimaging. 4th ed. Philadelphia: Lippincott & Williams; 2005.
42. Aminoff M, Boller F, Swaab D, editors. Handbook of Clinical Neurology, vol. 102. Neuro-ophthalmology. Elsevier; 2011.
46. Mueller-Forell W. Intracranial pathology of the visual pathway. Eur J Radiol 2004;49:143–78.

CHAPTER 67

ENT, Neck and Dental Radiology

Timothy Beale • Jackie Brown • John Rout

CHAPTER OUTLINE

INTRODUCTION

The anatomy of the head, neck and dental regions is complex. The continued advances in imaging (in particular computed tomography (CT), cone beam computed tomography (CBCT) and magnetic resonance imaging (MRI)) with ever faster imaging times and higher resolution studies have resulted in more anatomical detail revealing itself, none more so than in the head, neck and dental region where identifying subtle changes in the normal anatomy such as middle ear ossicular erosion in cholesteatoma, widening of the cranial nerve foramina in perineural/intracranial extension of disease and subtle erosion of the laryngeal cartilages in squamous cell carcinoma (SCC) of the larynx is crucial in the accurate diagnosis and staging of head and neck pathology and the planning of appropriate treatment. Knowledge of the normal anatomy and anatomical variants is the essential foundation required to support the recognition and accurate assessment of pathology in this complex region, even more so with the advent of more targeted treatment such as intensity-modulated radiotherapy (IMRT), brachytherapy or proton beam therapy.

THE EAR, PARANASAL SINUSES AND NASAL CAVITY

THE AURICLE AND EXTERNAL AUDITORY CANAL

Anatomy

The auricle and external auditory canal (EAC) funnel the sound to the tympanic membrane. The EAC is approximately 25 mm in length, lined by squamous epithelium, has an S-shaped course and consists of a fibrocartilaginous lateral third and an osseous medial two-thirds (Fig. 67-1). In cross-section the canal has an oval configuration. The fibrocartilaginous portion is deficient inferiorly (fissures of Santorini) that act as conduits for infection and malignancy (see below).

Pathology

High-resolution axial CT (HRCT) or cone beam CT CBCT with multiplanar reformats (MPR) in the coronal and sagittal planes is essential for assessing the bony EAC.

Chronic Stenosing Otitis Externa

Recurrent otitis externa (Fig. 67-2) may result in a fibrotic band of soft tissue occluding the medial EAC. It is important for the radiologist to answer the following questions: Is there any erosion of the adjacent bony walls to suggest a more aggressive process? What is the depth of the occluding soft tissue? Does the fibrotic tissue extend to involve the tympanic membrane (TM)? Is there a normally pneumatised middle ear cleft deep to the occluding soft tissue? Always review the contralateral side as this pathology is commonly bilateral.

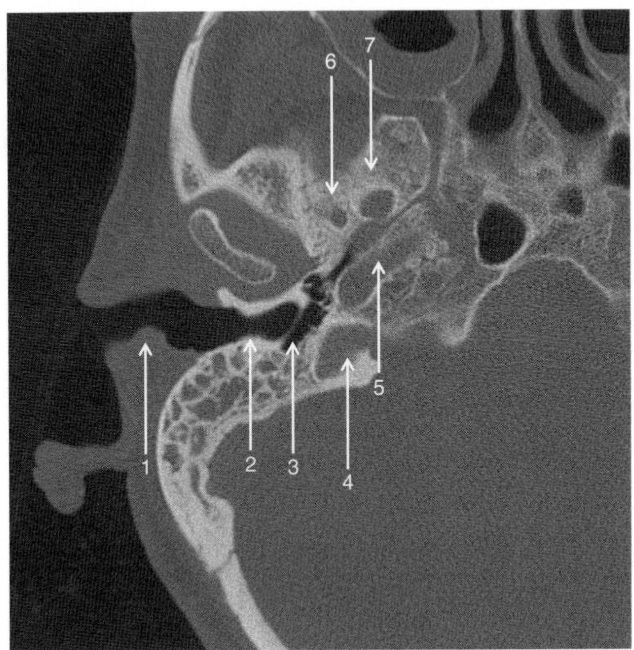

FIGURE 67-1 ■ Axial CT of right petrous temporal bone. 1 = fibrocartilaginous EAC; 2 = isthmus bony EAC; 3 = tympanic membrane (TM); 4 = jugular bulb; 5 = intrapetrous ICA (horizontal segment); 6 = foramen spinosum; 7 = foramen ovale.

Exostoses and Osteoma of the External Auditory Canal

The EAC osteoma usually arises spontaneously, but exostoses are associated with repeated exposure to cold water and are also known as 'surfer's ear'. The two pathologies (Fig. 67-3) cannot be distinguished histopathologically; however, exostoses are usually broad-based and bilateral, whereas osteoma are pedunculated, unilateral and lateral to the bony isthmus of the canal. They may cause sufficient narrowing of the EAC to require surgery. It is important when assessing EAC exostoses and osteoma to answer the following questions: What is the maximum depth and transverse diameter of the exostosis? What is the exact site of origin of the osteoma? What is the distance between the medial aspect of the exostosis and the TM and the deep aspect of the exostosis and the descending facial nerve canal? Are there any associated obstructed secretions in the medial EAC and is the middle ear cleft normally pneumatised?

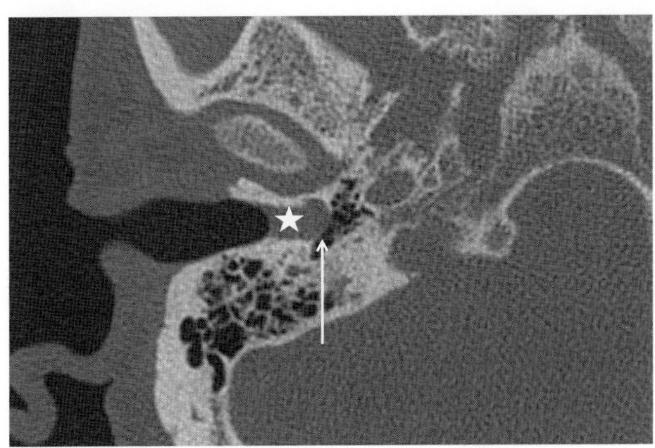

FIGURE 67-2 ■ Axial CT of right petrous temporal bone. Star = fibrotic band occluding EAC; arrow = tympanic membrane.

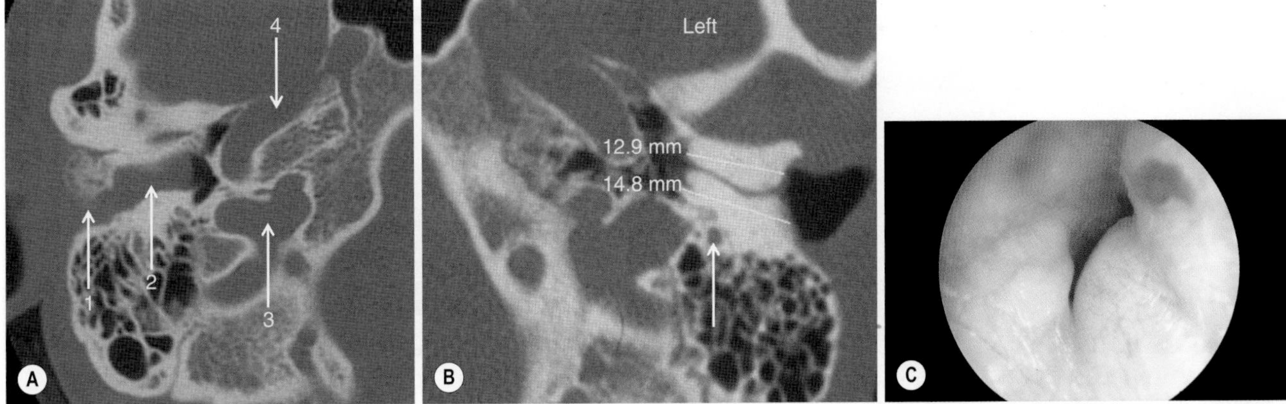

FIGURE 67-3 ■ (A) Axial CT of right petrous temporal bone: 1 = pedunculated osteoma; 2 = soft tissue filling bony EAC medial to obstructing osteoma; 3 = jugular foramen; 4 = intrapetrous ICA (horizontal segment). (B) Axial CT of left petrous temporal bone: arrow = descending (mastoid) segment facial nerve canal. The measurements are of the transverse distance of the broad-based exostoses. (C) Otoscopic view of exostoses narrowing the EAC.

Keratosis Obturans

Keratosis obturans (Fig. 67-4) is usually a bilateral accumulation of keratin within the EAC. The CT appearances are of soft tissue filling the EAC that may be associated with expansion of the canal and remodelling but not erosion of the bony canal walls. Keratosis obturans is associated with otalgia and conductive hearing loss and most frequently occurs in young men.

External Auditory Canal Cholesteatoma

An EAC cholesteatoma (Fig. 67-5) can be differentiated from keratosis obturans as it is associated with erosion of the floor/posterior wall of the bony EAC and is usually seen in an older population (>40 years).

It may be indistinguishable on CT from SCC and otoscopy ± biopsy is suggested.

Necrotising Otitis Externa (NOE)

Also known as malignant otitis externa, a misleading term used because of what used to be the high mortality associated with this condition. The pathology is a necrosis usually of the walls and in particular floor of the EAC at the bony cartilaginous junction typically in the elderly diabetic patient who presents with severe otalgia. *Pseudomonas* is the usual organism. The infection commonly extends inferiorly via the fissures of Santorini (see the section 'Anatomy', above), causing a skull base osteomyelitis, and involves the soft tissues inferior to the skull base where the lower cranial nerves (VII to XII) may be affected (Fig. 67-6). Anterior extension into the temporomandibular joint may cause destruction of the mandibular condyle.

HRCT of temporal bone is the usual initial imaging technique. MR will more clearly assess any soft-tissue involvement, meningeal enhancement or oedema of the bone marrow. Nuclear medicine (gallium 67) is helpful in confirming the location of the infection and monitoring its response to treatment.

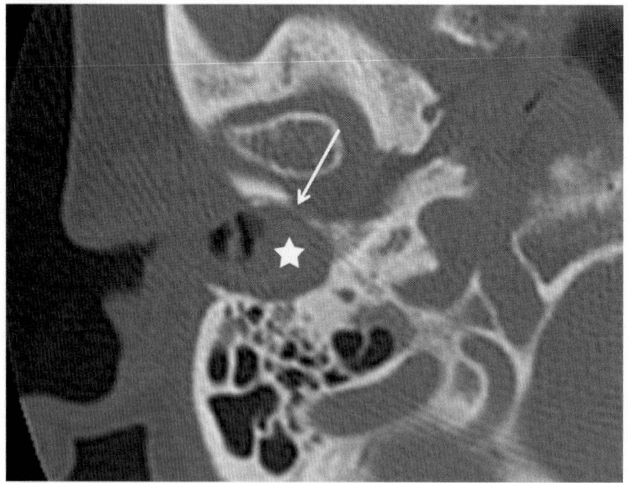

FIGURE 67-4 ■ Axial CT of right petrous temporal bone. Star = soft tissue expanding and remodelling walls of bony EAC; arrow = focal dehiscence of anterior wall of bony EAC.

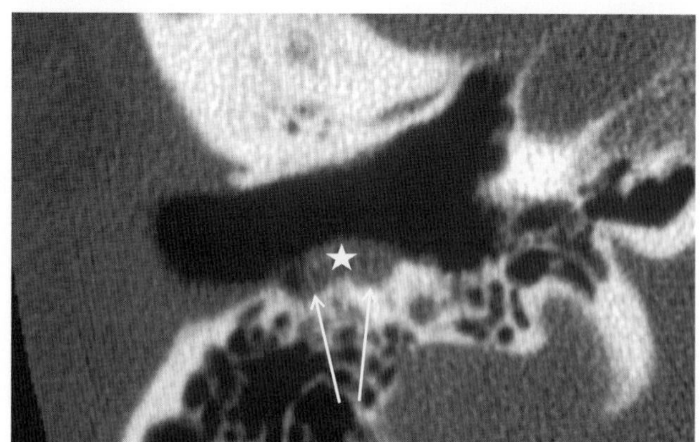

FIGURE 67-5 ■ Axial CT of right petrous temporal bone. Star = lobulated cholesteatoma eroding underlying posterior wall; arrows = highlight areas of focal erosion.

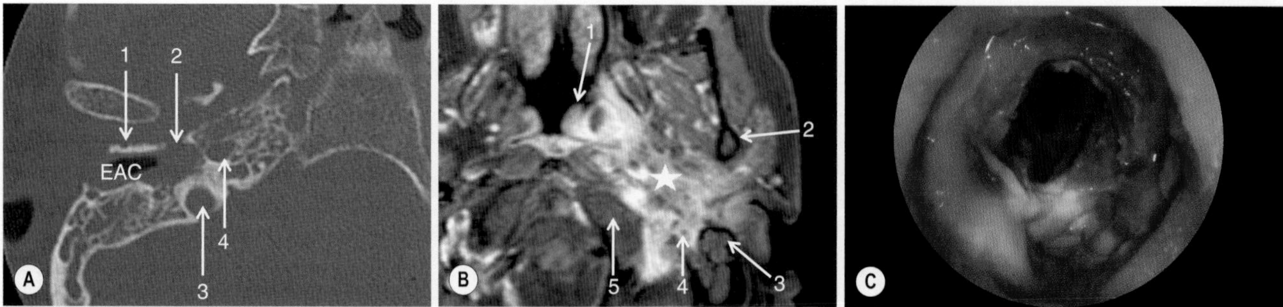

FIGURE 67-6 ■ (A) Axial CT of right petrous temporal bone: Note soft-tissue lining the EAC and the opacified middle ear cleft. 1 & 2 = Eroded anterior wall of bony EAC; 3 = jugular bulb; 4 = posterior genu intrapetrous ICA. (B) Axial T1W fat-saturated post gadolium MR of the soft tissues just inferior to the left EAC. Star = centre of ill-defined enhancing soft tissue extending from the stylomastoid foramen and facial nerve posteriorly to the nasopharynx medially. 1 = torus of nasopharynx; 2 = neck of condyle; 3 = opacified mastoid process; 4 = facial nerve in stylomastoid foramen; 5 = occipital condyle. (C) Otoscopic view of necrotising otitis externa. Note necrotic slough replacing the normal mucosa.

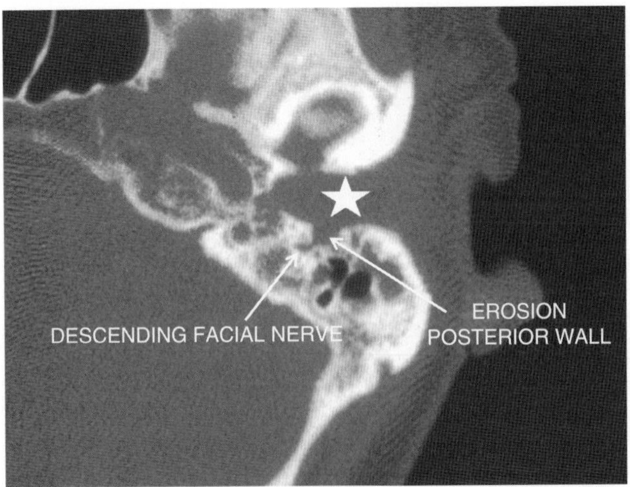

FIGURE 67-7 ■ Axial CT of left petrous temporal bone. Star = soft tissue filling the EAC. Note the bony erosion of the posterior wall extending up to the mastoid (descending) segment of the facial nerve canal.

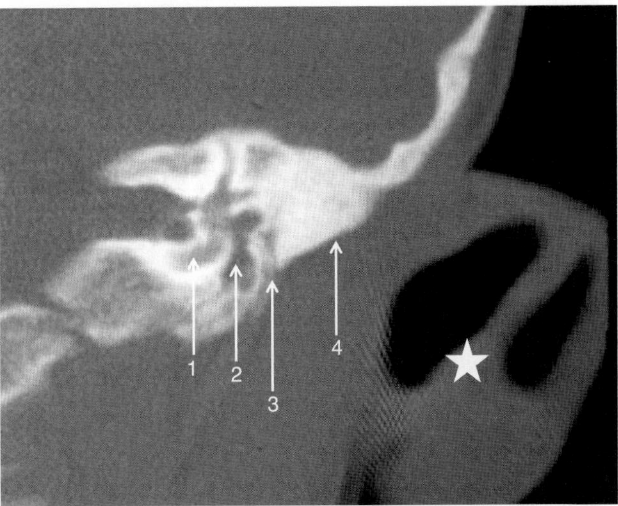

FIGURE 67-8 ■ Coronal CT of left petrous temporal bone. Patient with Treacher Collins syndrome: star = deformed auricle; 1 = basal turn of cochlea; 2 = small opacified middle ear cleft; 3 = displaced (anterior and laterally positioned) mastoid segment of the facial nerve canal; 4 = atretic bony plate.

It is important to answer the following questions when assessing patients with NOE: Is there any erosion of the bony walls of the EAC? Is there any inflammatory change in the soft tissues inferior to the skull base, in particular around the stylomastoid opening of the facial nerve, and is there involvement/effacement of the normal parapharyngeal fat? Is there erosion of the skull base (look for loss of the normal dense line of the bony cortex of the clivus, petroclival region and petrous apex)? Is there anterior extension to involve the mandibular condyle or involvement of the contralateral side via the prevertebral and retropharyngeal soft tissues anterior to the clivus? Has the differential of an SCC of the EAC or a nasopharyngeal tumour with extension to the skull base been excluded?

Squamous Cell Carcinoma of the Auricle and External Auditory Canal

These are rare tumours presenting in the elderly (F > M) with a painful, discharging ulcerative lesion of the EAC that most frequently extends inferiorly. CT is the usual imaging technique (Fig. 67-7), but MRI is recommended if there is suspected superior extension into the middle cranial fossa or medial extension into the middle ear cleft (both are rare).

It is important to answer the following questions: As with all soft tissue noted within the bony EAC, is there any associated bony erosion? Is there extension outside of the EAC? Is there any nodal involvement (in particular, review the intraparotid and upper deep cervical nodes)?

Congenital Atresia/Stenosis of the External Auditory Canal

The EAC may be stenosed or completely atretic (absent). The atresia may be membranous, bony or a mixture of the two. The atresia is usually unilateral in non-syndromic and bilateral in syndromic patients (Fig. 67-8). The rule of thumb is the more severe the EAC abnormality, the greater the auricular deformity (microtia/anotia). The inner ear structures are usually not affected unless there is severe EAC atresia with an absent auricle, small middle ear cleft and absent ossicles. If surgery is being considered it is important to assess the following on CT:

- The severity and type of the atresia.
- The size and degree of pneumatisation of the middle ear cleft.
- The appearance of the ossicles, in particular:
  - Is a stapes superstructure present?
  - Is the oval window atretic?
- The course of the tympanic segment of the intrapetrous facial nerve as the posterior genu (junction of tympanic and descending segments) is often more anteriorly and laterally positioned than normal and therefore at risk during surgery.

THE MIDDLE EAR

Anatomy and Physiology

The tympanic membrane (TM) is inclined at an angle of 140° in relation to the superior border of the EAC, measures 9–10 mm in diameter and separates the middle ear from the external ear (Fig. 67-9). The lateral (short) process of the malleus is attached to the TM at the malleal prominence and the handle at the umbo. Extending both anterior and posterior from the malleal prominence are folds separating the TM into a superior, thinner and more flexible pars flaccida and the more inferior pars tensa. The middle ear cleft is divided from superior to inferior into epitympanum (attic), mesotympanum and hypotympanum and contains three ossicles (the malleus, incus and stapes), two muscles (tensor tympani attached to the neck of the malleus and stapedius to the head of

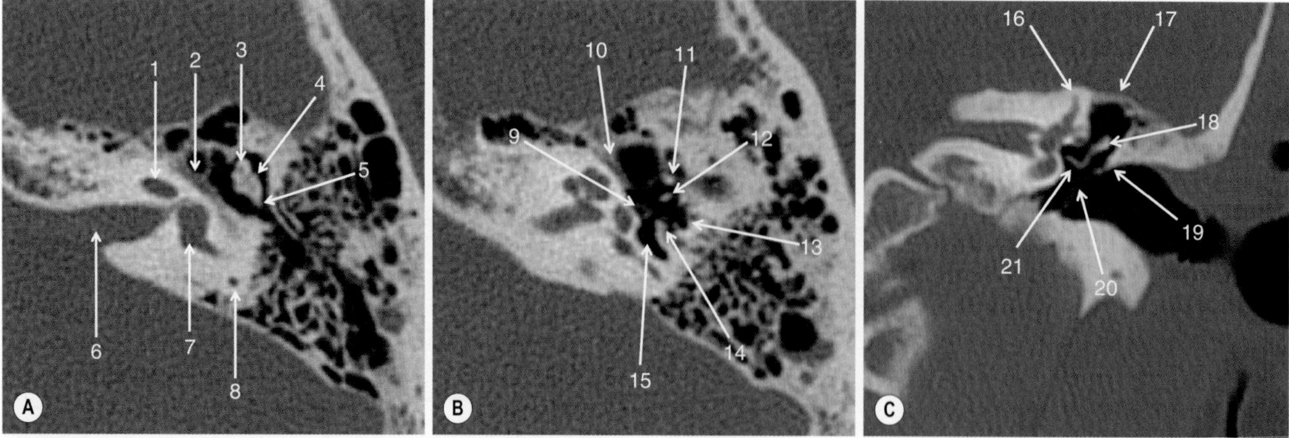

FIGURE 67-9 ■ (A, B) Axial and (C) coronal CT of left petrous temporal bone. 1 = cochlea (middle turn); 2 = facial nerve (tympanic segment); 3 = malleus (head); 4 = incus (body); 5 = incus (short process); 6 = IAC; 7 = vestibule; 8 = posterior SCC; 9 = stapes superstructure; 10 = tensor tympani muscle; 11 = malleus (neck); 12 = incus (long process); 13 = facial recess; 14 = pyramidal eminence; 15 = sinus tympani; 16 = superior SCC; 17 = tegmen tympani; 18 = incus (body); 19 = scutum; 20 = tympanic membrane; 21 = incus (lenticular process).

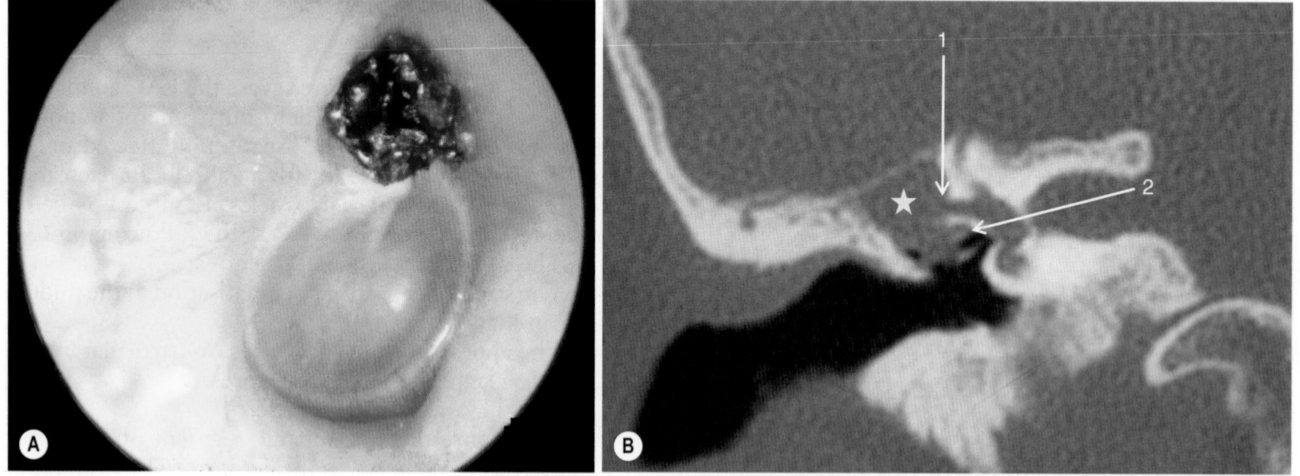

FIGURE 67-10 ■ (A) Otoscopic view showing a retraction pocket in pars flaccida of TM. (B) Coronal CT of right petrous temporal bone. Star = cholesteatoma in attic; 1 = eroded otic capsule over lateral SCC; 2 = facial nerve (tympanic segment).

the stapes). Part of the intrapetrous course of the facial nerve and one of its branches (the chorda tympani) also pass through the middle ear cleft.

HRCT including CBCT is the most common technique used for assessing the middle ear cleft usually in the clinical setting of conductive or mixed hearing loss. MRI is a complementary investigation used to assess possible intracranial complications arising from middle ear pathology, the rare middle ear tumours such as glomus tympanicum or where a recurrence of cholesteatoma is suspected (see below).

Pathology

Cholesteatoma

Cholesteatoma is a poor term for this pathology as it neither is a tumour nor does it contain cholesterol. It is actually skin in the wrong place. There are two types: the common acquired (98%) and the rarer congenital (2%) cholesteatoma. In acquired cholesteatoma, as a consequence of negative middle ear pressure, a retraction pocket develops usually in the more flexible pars flaccida (superior aspect) of the TM (Fig. 67-10A), but occasionally in the pars tensa (inferior aspect). Desquamated skin accumulates in the retraction pocket and can enlarge, causing bony destruction most frequently of the scutum and long process of the incus, but may extend to involve the otic capsule overlying the lateral semicircular canal (Fig. 67-10B), that may be associated with symptoms of dizziness, the tegmen tympani and the tympanic facial nerve canal (causing facial palsy).

Usually the diagnosis of cholesteatoma is apparent from the otoscopic appearances of a retraction pocket in acquired and a retrotympanic 'pearl' of cholesteatoma behind an intact TM in congenital cholesteatoma

(Fig. 67-11). The clinician needs to know how extensive the cholesteatoma is, which can be assessed by the degree of ossicular or bony erosion.

In particular, answer the following questions:

- Is the bony roof (tegmen tympani or mastoideum) eroded?
- Is the otic capsule overlying the lateral semicircular canal eroded?
- Is there ossicular erosion (in particular, is the stapes eroded)?
- Does the cholesteatoma abut the tympanic facial nerve canal?
- Are there anatomical variants such as a low-lying tegmen or a lateralised sigmoid sinus that may affect the surgical approach?

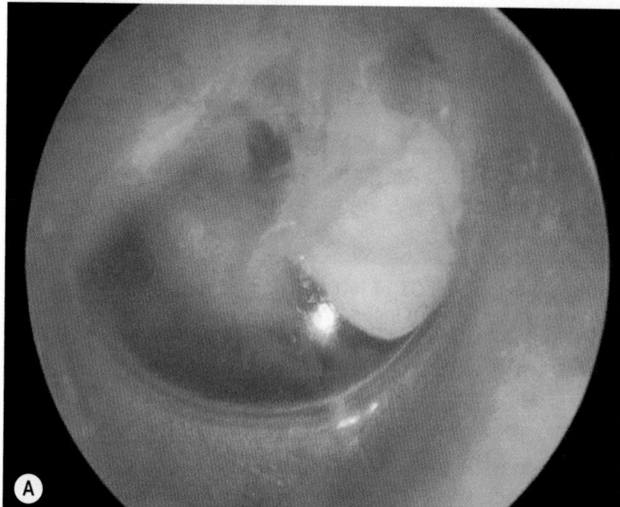

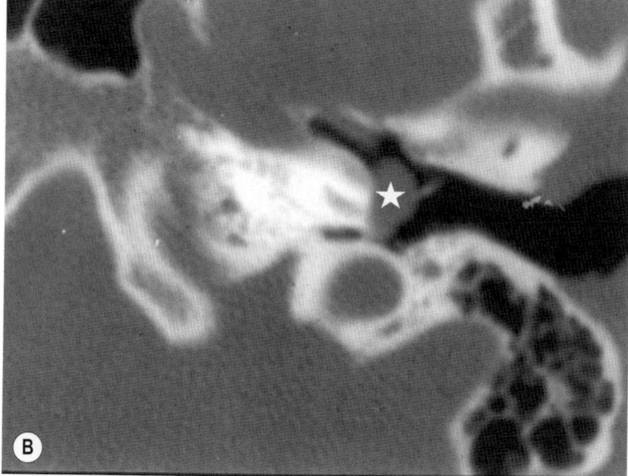

FIGURE 67-11 ■ (A) Otoscopic view of cholesteatoma (pearl) behind intact TM. (B) Star = congenital cholesteatoma overlying cochlear promontory.

A pars flaccida cholesteatoma is identified by a mass in the attic (epitympanium) lateral to the head of malleus and body of incus associated with ossicular erosion in 70%. A pars tensa cholesteatoma is identified as soft tissue in the posterior mesotympanum often extending medial to the ossicles. HRCT is used for assessing any bony involvement. Non-echo planar diffusion-weighted MR (non-EPI DWI) is increasingly used for assessing whether there is any recurrent or residual cholesteatoma in patients who have undergone canal wall preservation surgery where otoscopy provides limited visualisation. Cholesteatoma consisting of desquamated skin shows markedly restricted diffusion (Fig. 67-12) and can be differentiated from other soft tissue (granulation tissue, etc.).

Tympanosclerosis

The CT appearance is of foci of calcification, punctate or web-like in the middle ear cleft (Fig. 67-13) and tympanic membrane. Usually this is associated with a long history of otitis media (OM). The suspensory ligaments and muscles may also calcify. There is varying conductive hearing loss depending on the degree of ossicular fixation. If the tympanic membrane only is involved (calcified), the condition is known as myringosclerosis.

Otosclerosis

The diagnosis is usually suggested clinically. The hearing loss may be conductive, mixed or sensorineural. Otospongiosis is a term also used and describes the spongiform changes within the involved bone. In patients with otosclerosis the normal dense bone is replaced by foci of spongy less dense bone. Patients usually present in the third decade. The CT appearances are commonly bilateral (85%) and there may be a family history. There are two main types: fenestral and retrofenestral.

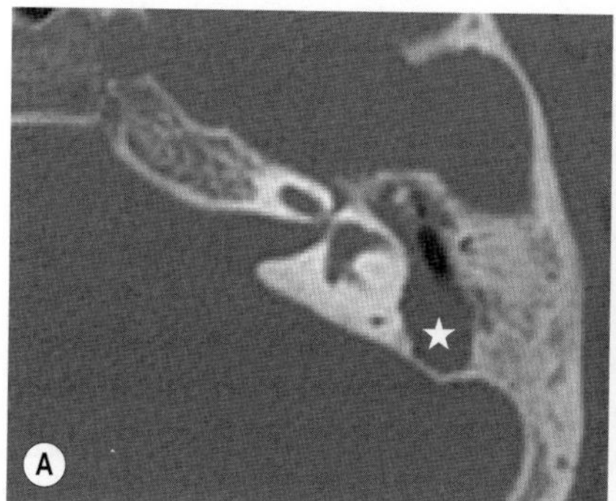

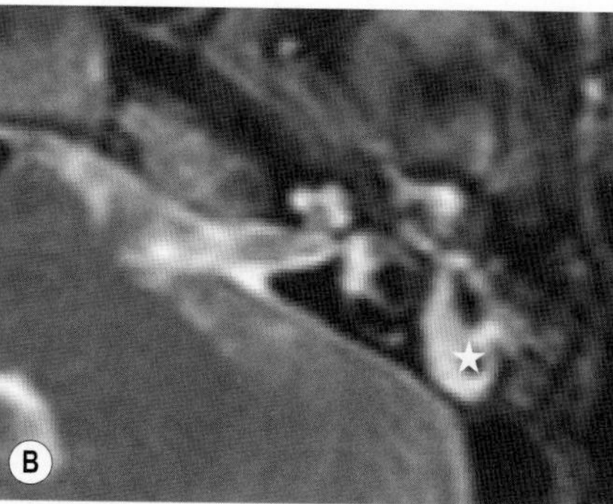

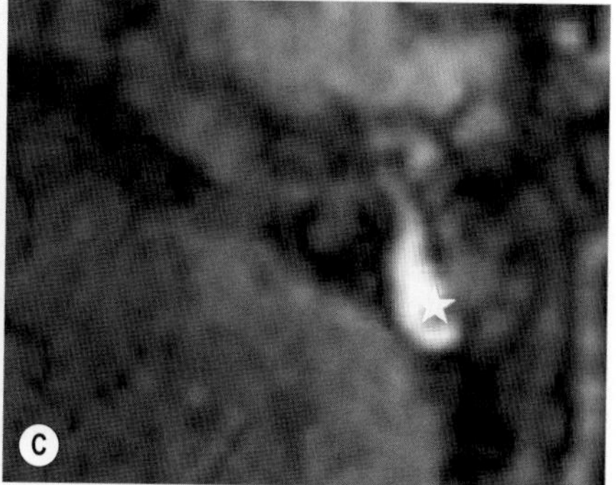

FIGURE 67-12 ■ (A) Axial CT of left petrous temporal bone and (B, C) equivalent T2W and non-EPI diffusion weighted b1000 MR images showing cholesteatoma (star) in mastoid antrum.

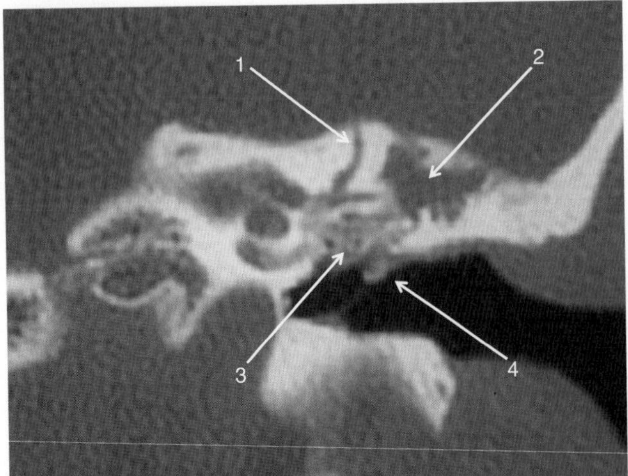

FIGURE 67-13 ■ **Coronal CT of left petrous temporal bone.** 1 = superior SCC; 2 = opacified attic; 3 = densely calcified soft tissue (tympanosclerosis) surrounding ossicles; 4 = calcified TM.

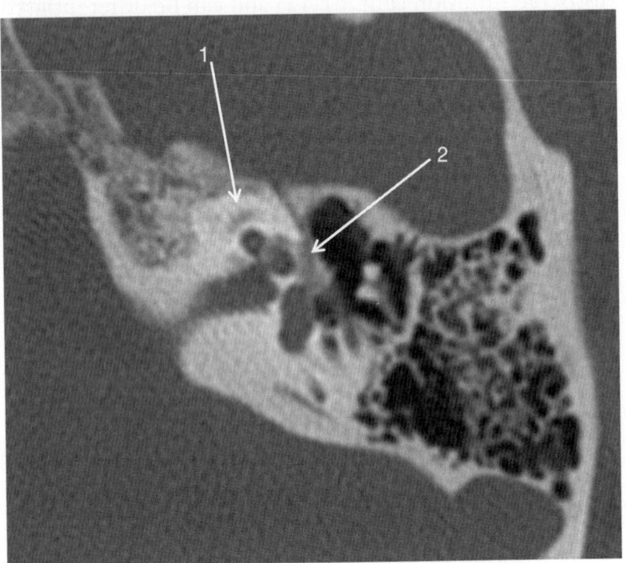

FIGURE 67-14 ■ **Axial CT of left petrous temporal bone.** 1 = pericochlear; 2 = fenestral otospongiosis.

Fenestral. The spongiotic foci occur in the lateral wall of the otic capsule in the fissula antefenestram (anterior to the oval window; Fig. 67-14) where it extends posteriorly to involve the footplate, fixing the anterior crus of the stapes causing CHL. The round window and cochlear promontory may also be involved.

Retrofenestral or Cochlear. Spongiotic foci replace the normal dense bone of the otic capsule surrounding the cochlea (Fig. 67-14) and may encroach on the cochlea and, less commonly, the vestibule and semicircular canals, causing mixed or sensorineural hearing loss. The most frequent location for a spongiotic focus is between the middle turn of the cochlea and the anterior aspect of the lateral internal auditory canal. In severe cases the cochlea is encircled, giving the appearance is of a cochlea within a cochlea. CT is used for assessing otosclerosis although

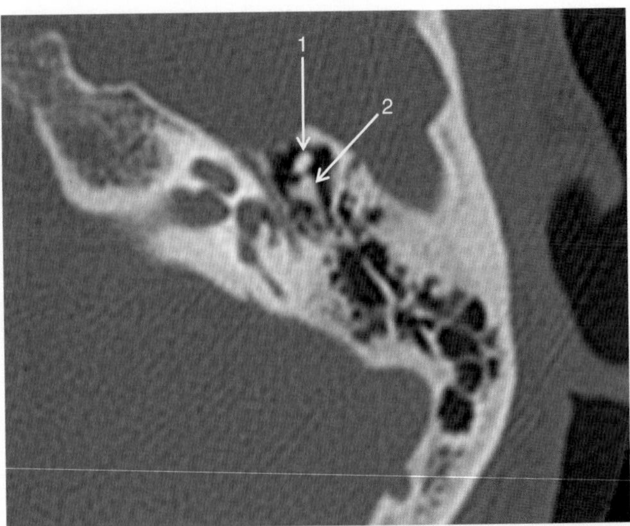

FIGURE 67-15 ■ **Axial CT of left petrous temporal bone.** 1 = head of malleus; 2 = body of incus. Note the malleoincudal separation and compare with normal anatomy in Fig. 67-9A.

the foci may be visible on MR as high signal areas on T2 that enhance post-gadolinium.

Cochlear otosclerosis is rare in the absence of fenestral disease.

Questions to answer when reviewing the CT are the following:

- Is there fenestral or pericochlear otosclerosis or both?
- Is there bilateral involvement (in 85% on CT) that may only be clinically evident on one side?
- Is the round window also involved? Round window involvement may reduce the effectiveness of surgery.
- Is the whole oval window involved and what is the depth of involvement? A markedly thickened footplate will alter the surgical technique and reduce the likelihood of a successful outcome.
- Is the facial nerve dehiscent as this may complicate surgery?

Ossicular Disruption

Nearly all ossicular disruption is associated with a temporal bone fracture. Incudostapedial joint (ISJ) disruption is the commonest derangement. Malleoincudal disruption results in loss of the normal 'ice cream cone' appearance on axial images of the head of malleus articulating with the body of the incus (Fig. 67-15). Complete dislocation of the incus is the next most common finding. Much more rarely found are fractures of the individual ossicles. The incus is the ossicle most frequently disrupted as the malleus is supported by three ligaments and the tensor tympani muscle and the stapes by the annular ligament and the stapedius muscle.

When assessing ossicular trauma, look first for the normal 'ice cream cone' appearance of the malleoincudal joint and then closely assess the alignment of the distal long process of the incus with the head of stapes at the ISJ and compare with the normal contralateral side.

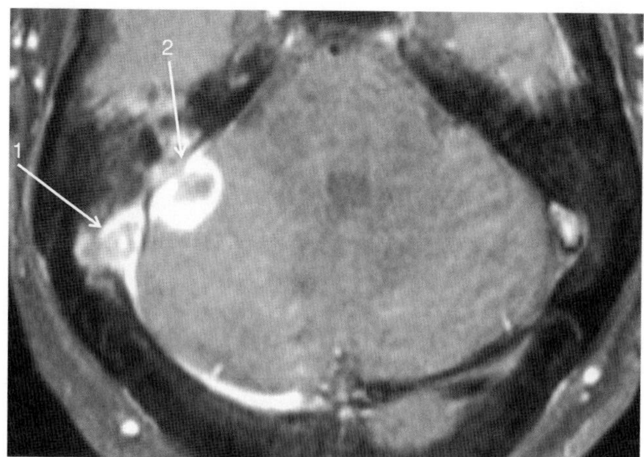

FIGURE 67-16 ■ Axial T1W MR post-gadolinium image posterior fossa. 1 = Thrombus in sigmoid sinus; 2 = epidural abscess.

Venous Sinus Thrombosis

The sigmoid sinus is an immediate posterior relation to the mastoid air cells and mastoiditis may result in sinus thrombosis with occasionally severe intracranial complications (Fig. 67-16). The transverse sinus and jugular bulb may also be involved, although the latter is usually thrombosed due to retrograde extension from the neck.

Always assess the bony dural sinus plate overlying the sigmoid sinus if adjacent air cells are opacified. If there is bony erosion, MRV or CT venography may be helpful to exclude thrombosis.

Intracranial Complications

Fortunately, intracranial complications from petromastoid infection are now rare. The commonest is extradural empyema in the posterior fossa often associated with sigmoid sinus thrombosis. Very rarely subdural empyema and intracranial abscesses may occur.

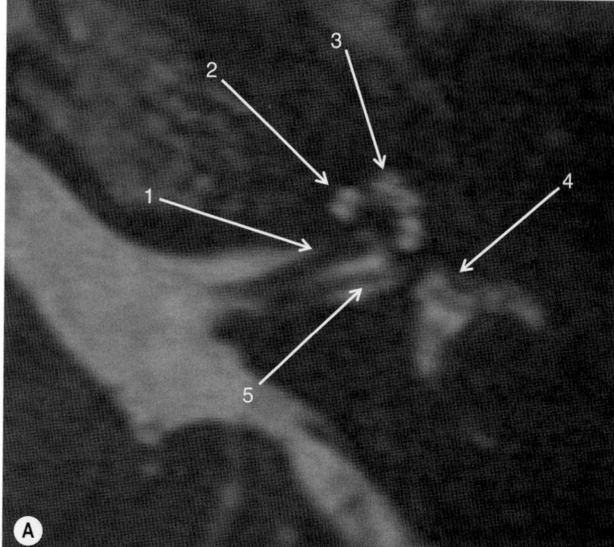

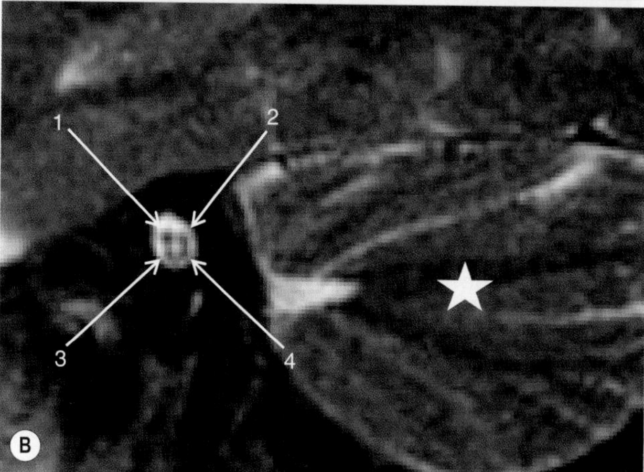

FIGURE 67-17 ■ (A) Axial T2W MR image of IAMs. Normal anatomy: 1 = cochlear nerve; 2 = cochlea (middle turn); 3 = cochlea (distal turn); 4 = vestibule; 5 = vestibular nerve (inferior). (B) Sagittal oblique T2W MR image through IAC. Star = cerebellar hemisphere; 1 = facial nerve; 2 = vestibular nerve (superior); 3 = cochlear nerve; 4 = vestibular nerve (inferior). Note 'seven-up and coke down' to remember position of nerves in IAC.

THE INNER EAR

Anatomy and Physiology

The inner ear consists of endolymph containing the functional sensory epithelium surrounded by perilymph and covered by a bony labyrinth (otic capsule). Sound is transmitted from the TM via the ossicles to the oval window. The mechanical vibrations via the vestibule then pass to the perilymph containing scala vestibuli up to the apical turn of the cochlea, returning via the perilymph containing scala tympani to the round window (Fig. 67-17A). Both perilymph scala surround the endolymphatic scala media or cochlear duct that contains the hair cell receptors of the organ of Corti. It is movement of these hair cells that generates electronic impulses in the cochlear nerve fibres. Higher frequencies up to 20 kHz are perceived in the basal turn and 20 Hz at the apex. The range of intensity of sound is huge and is expressed in alogorithmic decibel scale of 0–120 dB. A quiet whisper is 30 dB, a lawnmower is 90 dB and a jet plane take-off is 120 dB.

The electrical output of the hair cells passes to the spiral ganglion in the cochlea and then the cochlea division (Fig. 67-17B) and main trunk of the vestibulocochlear nerve to enter the brainstem in the upper lateral medulla synapsing with two cochlear nuclei, the latter forming a bulge in the lateral recess of the fourth ventricle and the foramen of Luschka. Within the brainstem, nerves pass in ipsi- and contralateral pathways to the inferior colliculus of the mid-brain, medial geniculate body of the thalamus and from there to the posterior aspect of the superior temporal gyrus. Ipsilateral hearing loss results when there is damage to the auditory pathway between the hair cells in the cochlea and the brainstem nuclei and bilateral hearing loss between the brainstem nuclei and inferior colliculi.

The semicircular canals consist of three rings, each orthogonal to the others, again containing perilymph bathing the endolymph. The superior and lateral canals are innervated by the superior vestibular nerve and the posterior by the inferior vestibular nerve. The semicircular canals form the kinetic labyrinth as they respond to rotational movement and acceleration. The dilated component of the semicircular canals called ampullae contains the hair cells forming the electronic impulses.

The vestibule consists of the utricle and macule (static labyrinth) and detects the position of the head relative to gravity.

Pathology

Vestibular Schwannoma

Vestibular schwannomas are the most common cerebellopontine angle (CPA) tumour and the most common pathology causing asymmetrical sensorineural hearing loss (SNHL). The majority are centred within the internal auditory canal, or at the porus acusticus and occur sporadically. When bilateral they indicate the diagnosis of neurofibromatosis type 2. Only a minority (approximately 2.5%) of patients who present with tinnitus or asymmetrical hearing loss have a vestibular schwanomma. There is no relationship between the size of the tumour and degree of hearing loss. The management approach is 'wait and scan' for the majority of vestibular schwannomas as approximately 60–70% do not increase in size on follow-up (MR) imaging. Those that require intervention have two options: surgery via retrosigmoid, translabyrinthine or subtemporal middle cranial fossa approach, or gamma-knife (radiation) treatment.

MRI is the imaging technique of choice when assessing patients for a possible vestibular schwannoma, but the protocols vary. A high-resolution T2-weighted imaging is the most commonly used sequence with pre- and post-gadolinium-enhanced T1-weighted sequences reserved for the small percentage of patients where a neuroma is identified and requires confirmation (Fig. 67-18) or other pathology requires clarification.

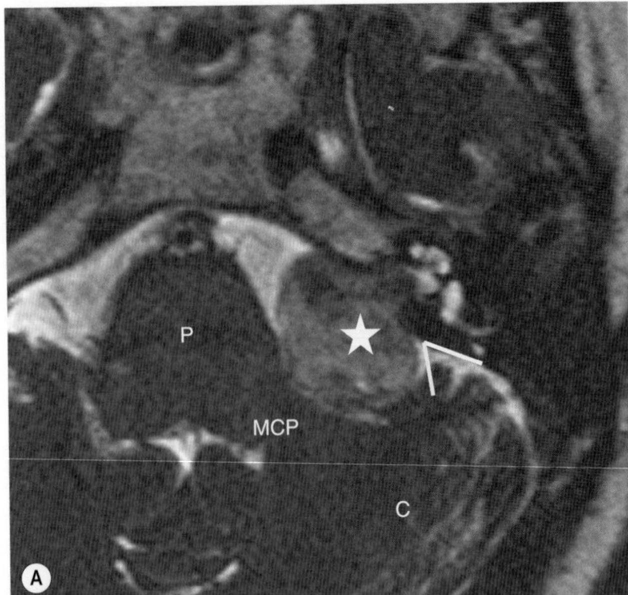

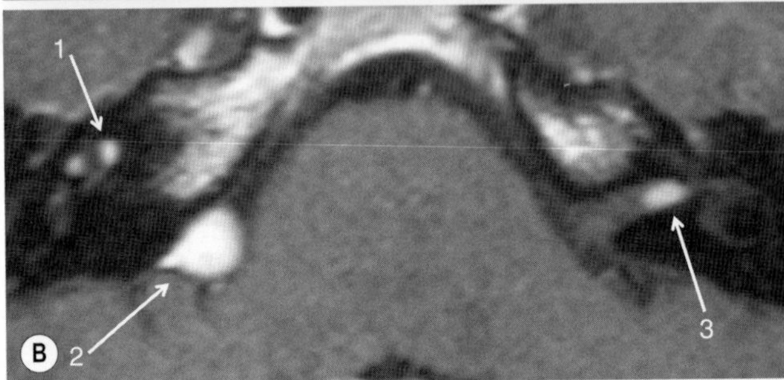

FIGURE 67-18 ■ (A) Axial T2W MR image of posterior fossa. Star = vestibular schwannoma (VS); white line shows acute angle between VS and posterior surface of petrous bone which helps differentiate between VS and posterior fossa meningioma with the latter having an obtuse angle; P = pons; MCP = middle cerebellar peduncle; C = cerebellar hemisphere. (B) Axial T1W MR post-gadolinium image of through posterior fossa. 1 = intracochlear schwannoma (in middle turn); 2 = right CPA schwannoma; 3 = left intracanalicular schwannoma.

Trauma

Skull base fractures involving the petrous bone are uncommon, but are important to identify as they may be associated with cerebrospinal fluid (CSF) otorrhoea or rhinorrhoea, facial nerve palsy or ossicular disruption.

In patients undergoing CT for head trauma HRCT reconstructions of the skull and skull base are frequently part of the routine imaging protocol. Assessing any intracranial trauma is the initial priority, but identifying skull base and, indeed, upper cervical fractures is also essential.

Classically, petrous temporal fractures have been divided broadly into transverse fractures (20%) usually secondary to occipital or frontal trauma or longitudinal fractures (80%) secondary to temporoparietal trauma. However, the fracture line frequently takes an oblique course and prognostically it is more important to accurately describe its course and the structures involved.

When reviewing the image for a possible petrous fracture, remember that transverse fractures usually start at sites of weakness such as the jugular foramen (Fig. 67-19) or vestibular aqueduct and longitudinal fractures

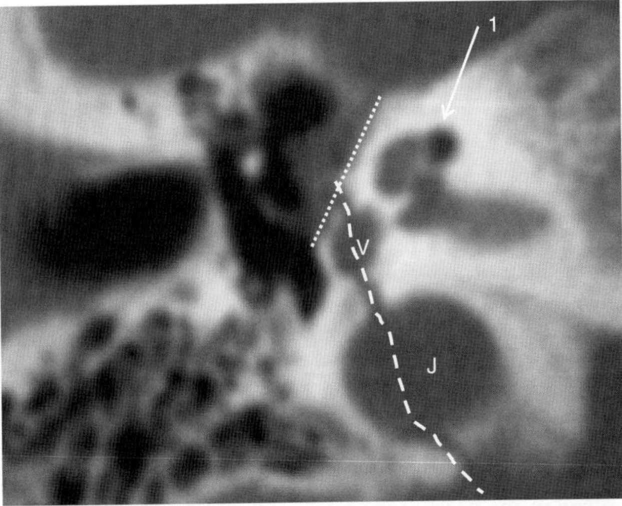

FIGURE 67-19 ■ **Axial CT of right petrous temporal bone.** Interrupted line = transverse fracture; dotted line is facial nerve (tympanic segment); 1 = air in cochlea (pneumolabyrinth); J = jugular bulb; v = vestibule.

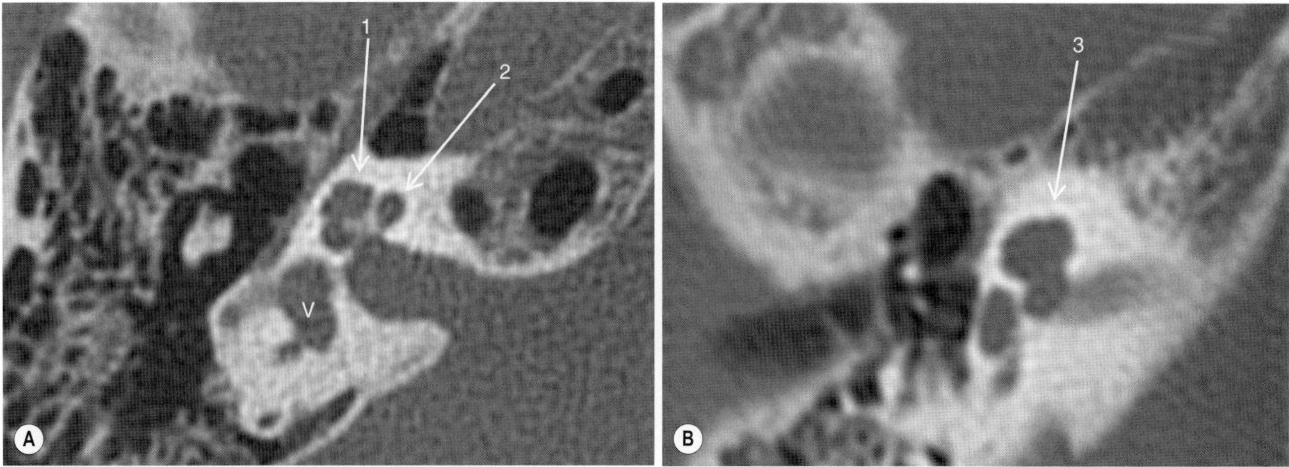

FIGURE 67-20 ■ **Axial CT of right petrous temporal bone.** (A, B) 1 and 2 = normal partitioning of distal and middle turns of cochlea, 3 = incomplete partitioning in image B; V = vestibule.

frequently involve the EAC, extending to the middle ear cleft or more inferiorly the posterior genu of the intrapetrous internal carotid artery, but usually sparing the facial nerve and inner ear structures.

Please note: CSF rhinorrhoea may be secondary to a petrous temporal fracture, with CSF passing along the eustachian tube into the postnasal space and this area should be reviewed as a recognised but rarer cause of CSF rhinorrhoea along with the anterior and central skull base and sinonasal regions. There is a 10% annual risk of meningitis in patients with CSF rhinorrhoea.

In patients with post-traumatic facial nerve palsy it is important to identify the exact site of trauma as it will alter both the surgical approach and repair technique.

As noted in the earlier section 'The Middle Ear', the commonest ossicular disruption is of the incudostapedial joint followed by the malleoincudal joint and then incus dislocation. The malleus and stapes are rarely involved as they are more firmly held in place both by a muscle (tensor tympani and stapedius) and several ligaments.

Congenital Malformations

Congenital malformation of the cochlea and/or labyrinth may be genetic (alone or as part of a syndrome) or non-genetic.

The inner ear and middle/external ear have independent embryological developments, but still approximately 10% of patients with EAC atresia have inner ear deformities. The inner ear structures develop between the third and twenty-second week of intrauterine life and inner ear malformations are usually classified according to severity from the rare Michel deformity (arrest at third week and complete absence of the inner ear) to mild dysplasia of the lateral semicircular canal (twenty-second week).

CT and MR are complementary investigations and, although this subject is outside the scope of this chapter, the following checklist needs to be gone through:

- Cochlea: Is there a normal basal turn? Is the modiolus present (Fig. 67- 20)? Are there a normal number of turns?
- Vestibule: is it enlarged? Is it separate from the cochlea?

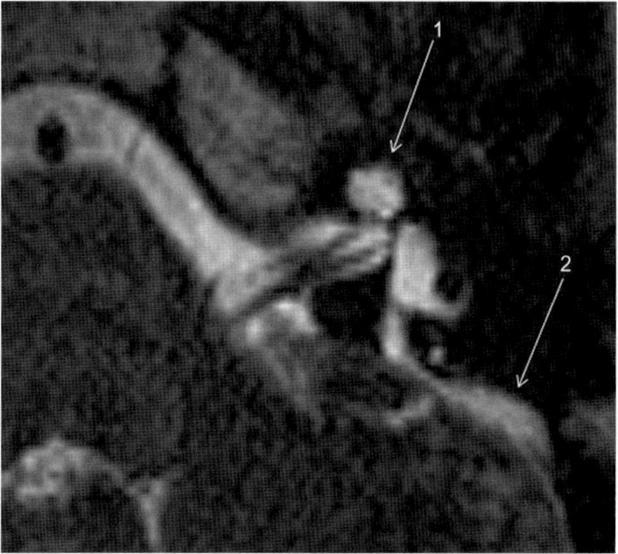

FIGURE 67-21 ■ **Axial T2W MR image of posterior fossa.** 1 = incomplete partitioning of cochlea (compare with Fig. 67-17A); 2 = enlarged vestibular aqueduct and endolymphatic sac.

- Semicircular canals: Are they present or dysplastic?
- Oval and round windows: Are they normal, narrowed, atretic?
- Vestibular aqueduct: Is the vestibular aqueduct and endolymphatic sac enlarged? This is the most common imaging finding in patients with sensorineural hearing loss dating to infancy and is frequently missed with serious clinical consequences (Fig. 67-21).
- Cochlear nerve: Is the nerve present and of normal size?
- Facial nerve: Does the nerve take a normal course? Is it dehiscent?

Facial Palsy

Acute facial palsy is usually secondary to Bell's palsy or trauma. Bell's palsy is frequently seen clinically but is

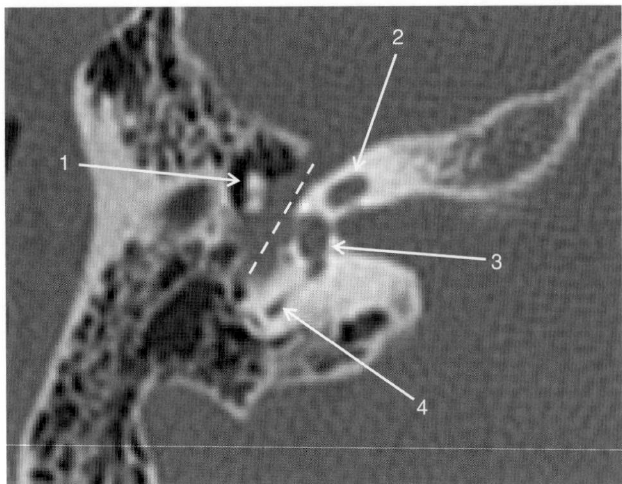

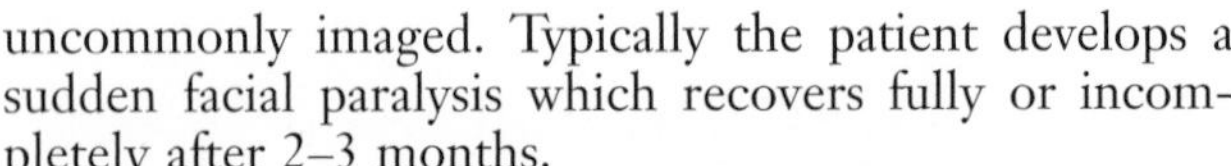

FIGURE 67-22 ■ **Axial CT of right petrous temporal bone.** There is a diffuse enlargement of the facial nerve (tympanic segment) = interrupted white line; 1 = malleus (neck); 2 = cochlea (middle turn); 3 = vestibule; 4 = posterior SCC.

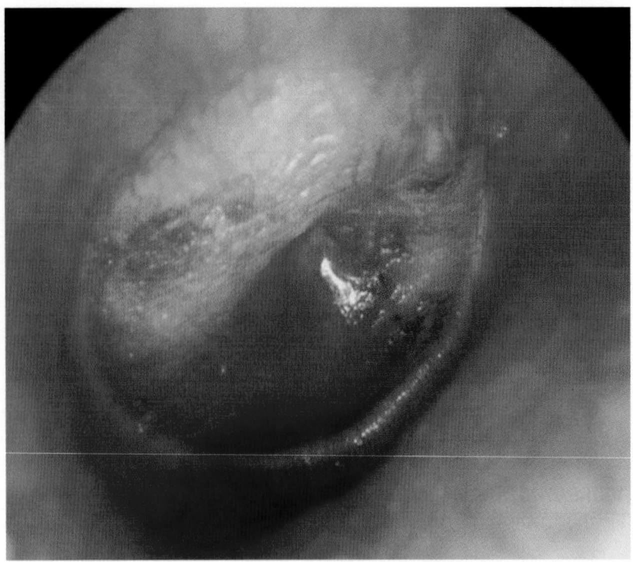

FIGURE 67-23 ■ **Otoscopic view of a retrotympanic vascular mass in a patient with a glomus tympanicum.**

uncommonly imaged. Typically the patient develops a sudden facial paralysis which recovers fully or incompletely after 2–3 months.

Imaging is mandatory for atypical cases: i.e. progressive or recurrent facial palsy (Fig. 67-22). CT and MRI are complementary. MRI is preferred but CT is usually performed if pathology such as cholesteatoma or otomastoiditis is suspected on otoscopy. Both the intra- and extracranial course of the facial nerve must be covered or pathology such as an impalpable malignant parotid tumour will be missed. On MRI, enhancement of the facial nerve within the geniculate ganglion, tympanic and mastoid segments is normal. Abnormal enhancement includes intense enhancement of the labyrinthine and mastoid segments. Enhancement of the facial nerve in the fundus of the internal auditory canal is always pathological.

Glomus Tumours (Paragangliomas)

Paragangliomas are the most common tumours causing pulsatile tinnitus and glomus tympanicum and glomus jugulotympanicum are the most common tumours of the middle ear and the second most common tumours of the temporal bone after vestibular schwannoma. It is vital to distinguish the two types. Glomus tympanicum arise on the medial wall of the middle ear cavity on the cochlear promontory and can be removed via a mastoid approach (Fig. 67-23). Glomus jugulotympanicum are tumours arising in the jugular foramen that extend into the middle ear cleft usually requiring preoperative embolisation followed by skull base surgery.

HRCT and MRI are complementary. When the tumour extends into the adjacent bone such as in a glomus jugulotympanicum or extensive glomus tympanicum, there is a characteristic permeative bony destruction seen on HRCT. MRI demonstrates an intensely enhancing tumour that on the unenhanced T1-weighted sequence may demonstrate a 'salt and pepper' appearance with the salt representing subacute haemorrhage and the pepper representing flow voids in large tumour vessels (Fig. 67-24).

Cochlear Electrode Implantation

Implantable cochlear electrodes offer a chance of hearing for some individuals, typically those whose hearing has been damaged by childhood meningitis. An array of electrodes (usually 12, 16 or 22 depending on the device) are inserted into the scala tympani of the proximal basal turn. MRI and HRCT are usually both requested preoperatively to assess for the patency of the cochlea, the size of the cochlea nerve and any malformation or anatomical variant that might alter the surgical approach or technique. Assessment of implant position can be made intraoperatively or in the early postoperative period with plain X-ray (reverse Stenver's view), HRCT or CBCT. Early studies suggest CBCT can assess whether the electrodes are within the scala tympani or vestibuli (Fig. 67-25). Cochlear implantation is now commonly bilateral and may be performed in patients with unilateral hearing loss and debilitating tinnitus.

THE PARANASAL SINUSES AND NASAL CAVITY

Anatomy and Physiology

The external nose consists of bone superiorly (frontal process of maxilla and nasal bones) and alar cartilage inferiorly. The arterial supply is via facial and ethmoidal arteries and venous drainage into the angular vein up to the medial canthus of the eye, which explains one route of how nasal sepsis can spread to involve the cavernous sinus.

The nasal cavity extends from the vestibule anteriorly to the choanae posteriorly divided by the midline nasal

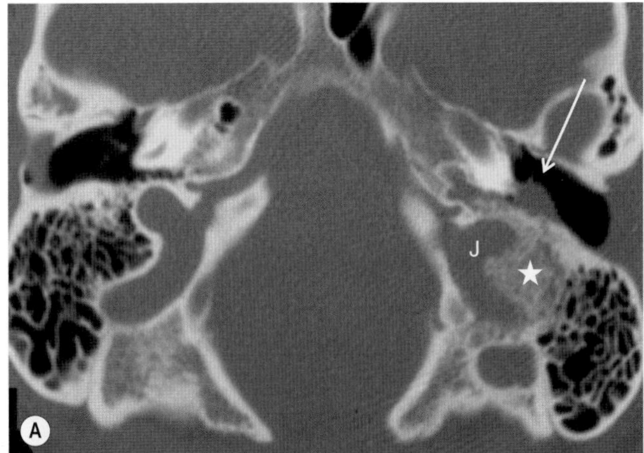

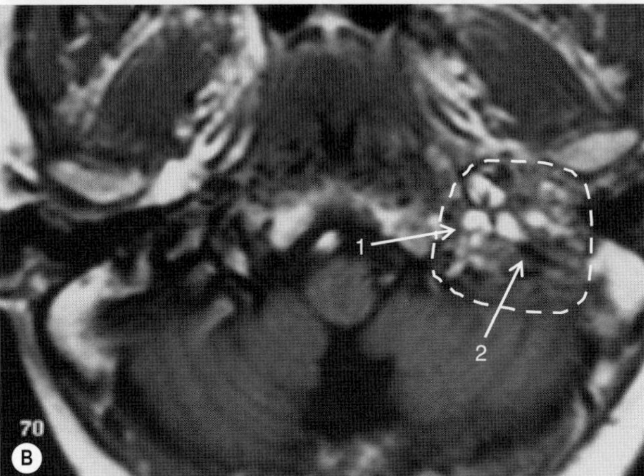

FIGURE 67-24 ■ (A) Axial CT of petrous temporal bone. Star = classic permeative appearance of a glomus tumour. Note also the loss of the dense cortical line of the jugular foramen (J). The tumour extends into the middle ear (white arrow), which is the tip of the iceberg of a large glomus jugulotympanicum (GJT). (B) Axial T1W MR image of the same patient. Interrupted white line outlines the GJT. The 'salt and pepper' appearance of the tumour is shown. 1 = T1W high signal of foci of haemorrhage; 2 = signal void of large feeding vessel.

septum. The anterior cartilaginous septum fuses posteriorly with the bony septum consisting of the vomer inferiorly and perpendicular plate of ethmoid superiorly. The roof of the nasal cavity is formed by the cribriform plate part of the anterior skull base and the floor is the hard palate. The lateral wall is more complex and supports the three turbinates (superior, middle and inferior) and their associated airway or meatus.

The middle meatus is functionally the most important and receives drainage from the maxillary sinus via the infundibulum, the anterior ethmoidal air cells via individual ostia and the frontal sinus via the frontal recess. The ostiomeatal unit is the complex anatomical region where these three mucociliary drainage pathways (frontal, anterior ethmoidal and maxillary) meet (Fig. 67-26).

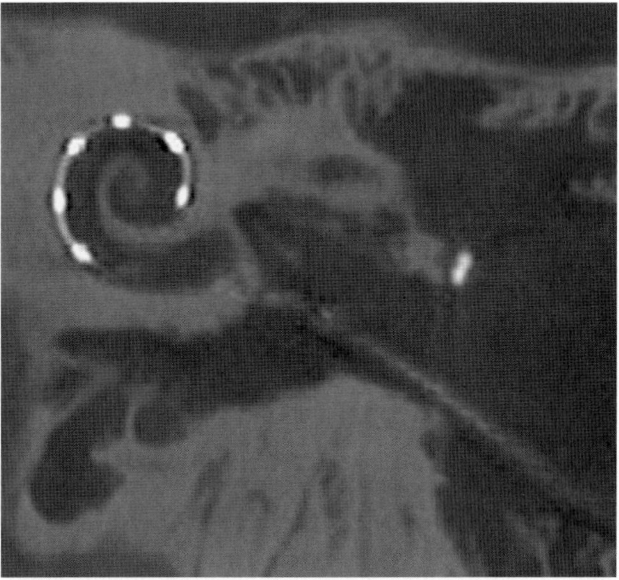

FIGURE 67-25 ■ **CBCT showing six-electrodes of the cochlear implant (CI) in the scala tympani of the cochlea.**

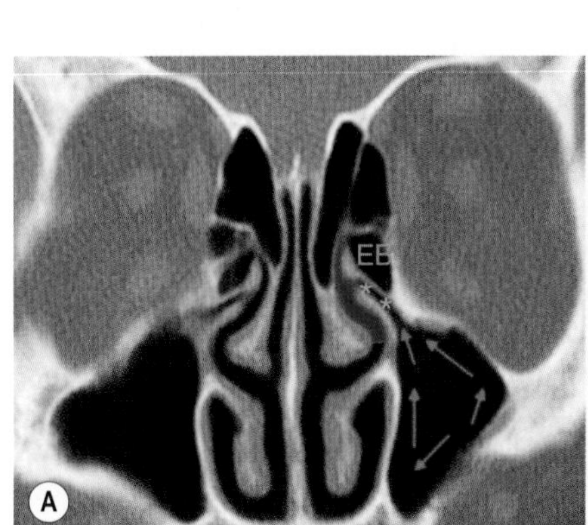

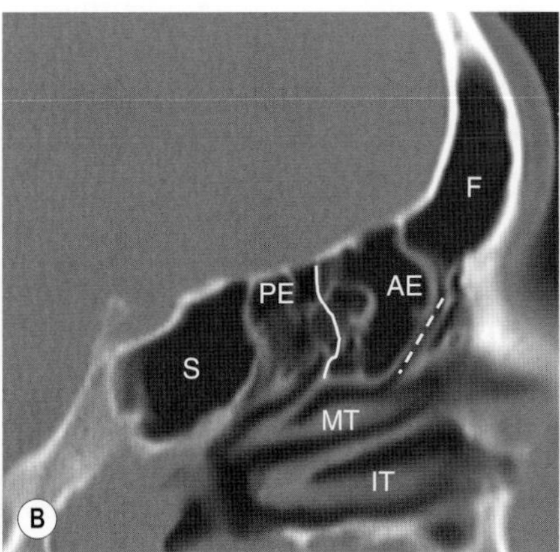

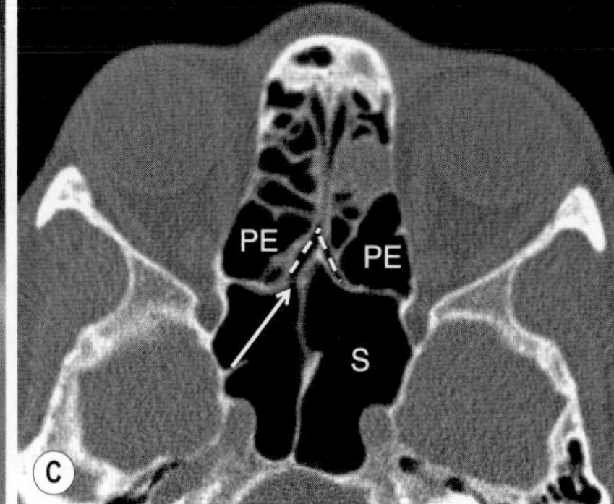

FIGURE 67-26 ■ (A) Coronal CT of paranasal sinuses and nasal cavity. Red arrows = mucociliary flow in left antrum pointing towards the infundibulum (green stars). Blue = middle meatus. EB = ethmoidal bulla (the ethmoidal air cell superior to the infundibulum or outflow). (B) Sagittal CT of paranasal sinuses and nasal cavity. F = frontal sinus; interrupted white line = frontal sinus drainage pathway; AE = anterior ethmoidal air cell; PE = posterior ethmoidal air cell; white line = basal lamella that divides AE from PE air cells; S = sphenoid sinus; MT = middle turbinate; IT = inferior turbinate. (C) Axial CT of paranasal sinuses and nasal cavity. S = sphenoid sinus; PE = posterior ethmoidal air cells; white arrow = sphenoid sinus ostium; interrupted white line = sphenoethmoidal recess (common drainage pathway for S and PE air cells).

The inferior meatus receives drainage from the nasolacrimal duct and the superior meatus the posterior ethmoidal air cells, the latter then draining into the sphenoethmoidal recess along with the sphenoid sinus.

It is important to understand the mucociliary drainage pathways and their common anatomical variants as the aim of functional endoscopic sinus surgery (FESS) is to restore these pathways.

The lining of the nose is pseudostratified ciliated columnar epithelium common to the respiratory tract. A specialised sensory epithelium lies on either side of the septum immediately beneath the cribriform plate (the olfactory niche).The specialised non-myelinated neurons connect in the olfactory niche with olfactory bulbs in the anterior cranial fossa via a perforated bone (lamina cribrosa). The commonest cause of anosmia is mucosal thickening. Other causes include frontal trauma and rarely neoplasia (olfactory neuroblastoma, subfrontal meningioma).

The sinonasal cavity serves a number of functions:

- smell;
- respiration (mouth breathing usually only required in exercise);
- air conditioning (heat exchange, humidification and cleaning);
- immune response to antigen (antibodies in nasal mucosa first line of defence); and
- sound quality (listen to anyone with a cold, the sinonasal cavity acts as a resonant chamber).

Radiology and Pathology

Low-dose CT and, increasingly, CBCT are indicated when the patient has failed medical treatment, FESS is being considered or there is an acute presentation such as orbital cellulitis or mucocoele. MRI is a problem solver and is used to differentiate tumour from inflammation, assess tumour extent and exclude non-sinonasal causes of anosmia.

Rhinosinusitis

This is an extremely common condition usually treated medically. There are a number of common causes:

- Allergic: very common and may develop into polyposis.
- Vasomotor: a disorder of autonomic regulation of mucus production.
- Infective: as in the common cold.
- Ciliary disorders: Kartagener's syndrome.
- Iatrogenic: overuse of nasal congestants.

When medical treatment has failed, surgery (FESS) is aimed at widening the mucociliary pathways with procedures such as an uncinectomy (± bullectomy) to widen the ostium of the maxillary antrum.

CT or CBCT should be performed in the axial plane with coronal and sagittal reformatted images and soft-tissue reconstruction. Radiological assessment should include the following:

- Identification of relevant anatomical variants such as deviated nasal septum and septal spur, concha bullosa or paradoxical turn to the turbinates, hypoplasia or enlargement of normal structures (maxillary antrum, frontal sinus, ethmoidal bulla, etc.) and the presence of anomalous air cells (frontoethmoidal, sphenoethmoidal and infraorbital).
- Identification of the extent of disease in relation to the mucociliary pathways. For example, does the antral inflammation extend to the ostium, infundibulum or middle meatus or is the whole ostiomeatal unit involved? Does the frontal or sphenoid sinus disease extend to the ostium or further into the frontal and sphenoethmoidal recess, respectively? Are there fluid levels to suggest an acute component (Fig. 67-27)? The extent of disease will guide the extent of surgery.
- Identification of bony thickening suggesting chronicity, or bony erosion/destruction suggesting a more aggressive process.
- Identification of dental disease that may cause a reactive inflammatory change in the overlying antra and be the underlying cause of the patient's symptoms (Fig. 67-28).
- Identification of orbital or, rarely, intracranial extension.
- Assessment of the postnasal space.
- Identification of previous surgery including extent.
- Review of soft-tissue reconstructed images in order to identify fungal disease (Fig. 67-29), desiccated secretions or tumour and pathology extending outside the sinonasal region (pre- and postantral, pterygopalatine fossa, orbit), suggesting a more aggressive process, of particular importance in immunocompromised patients.

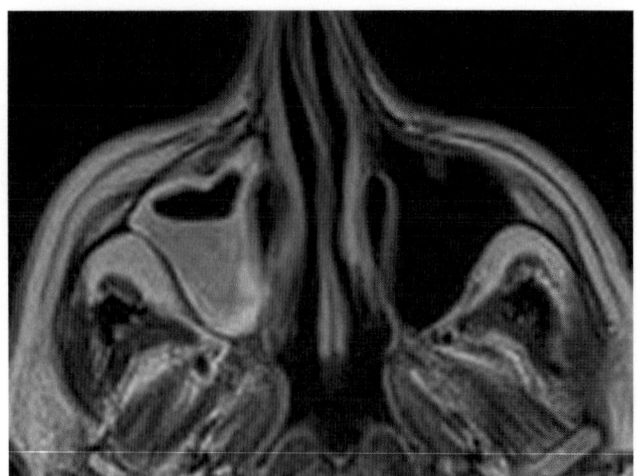

FIGURE 67-27 ■ Axial T2W MR image of the maxillary antra showing a fluid level in the right antrum and surrounding high signal mucosal thickening.

Because of the high inherent contrast in the paranasal sinuses and nasal cavity, a low-dose technique can be used. The anterior ostiomeatal unit is best assessed in the coronal plane, the frontal sinus drainage pathway in the sagittal plane and the sphenoethmoidal recess in the axial plane (Fig. 67-26).

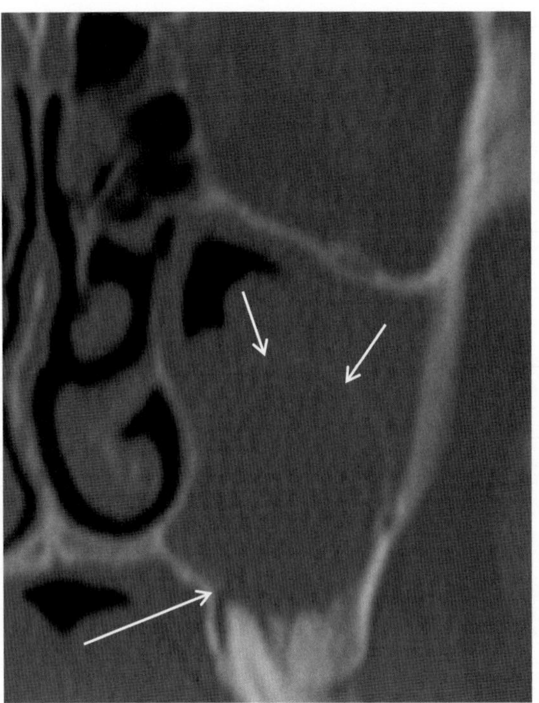

FIGURE 67-28 ■ Magnified coronal CT of left antrum. Note almost completely opacified antrum. Short white arrows = roof of radicular cyst arising from palatal root of left upper molar (long white arrow).

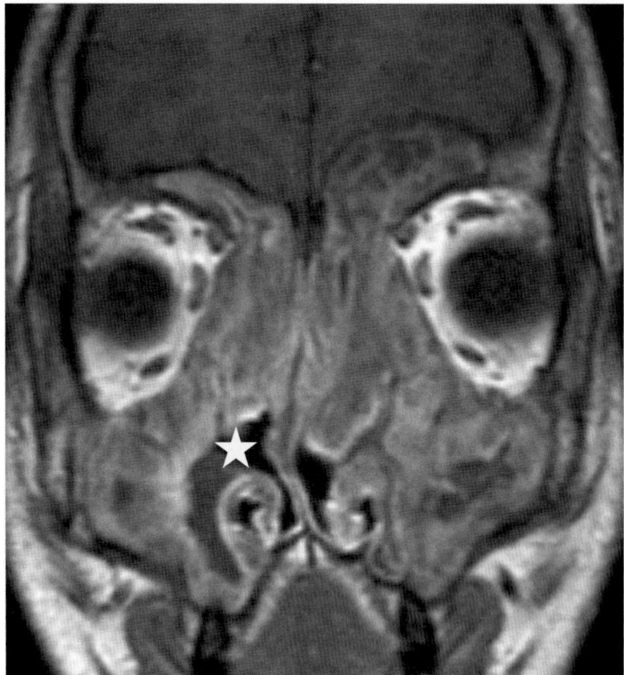

FIGURE 67-30 ■ Coronal T1W MR post-gadolinium image of the anterior osteometal unit region. Note completely opacified antra, frontal sinuses and AE air cells secondary to polypoidal mucosal thickening obstructing the outflow. Star = previous right middle meatal antrostomy.

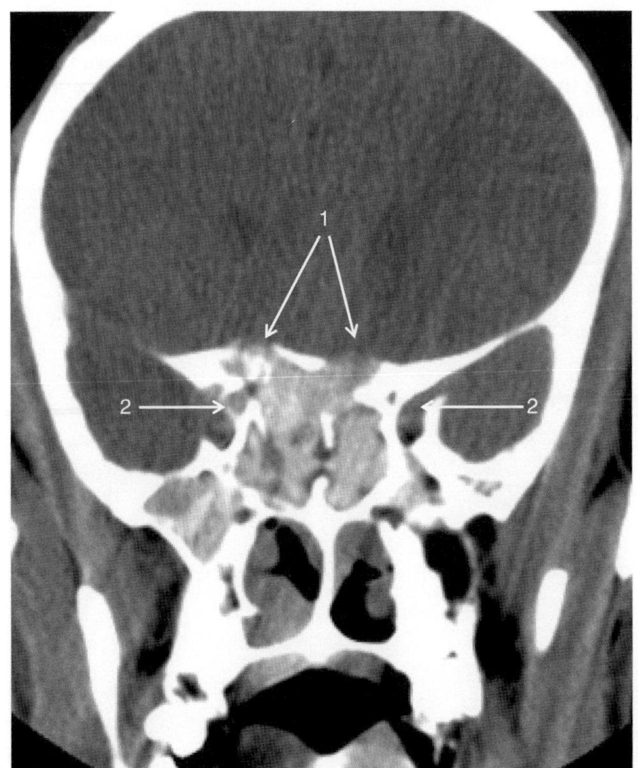

FIGURE 67-29 ■ Coronal CT of the sphenoid sinus (soft-tissue recons). Note high attenuation material filling the sphenoid sinus in keeping with fungal infection eroding the roof (1). Note close relation with the optic nerve (2).

Common problems requiring imaging include nasal polyps, antrochoanal polyp, mucocoeles, fractures, epistaxis, nasal and paranasal sinus tumours.

Nasal Polyposis

Nasal polyposis is a common condition in adults, but if seen in children cystic fibrosis should be considered as a possible cause. Nasal polyps are usually located in the middle meati, roof of nasal cavity and ethmoidal regions; they are multiple and bilateral and involve both the nasal cavity and sinuses. They are secondary to inflammatory swelling of the sinonasal mucosa which forms polyps (Fig. 67-30).

Please note that if a superior nasal cavity polyp is observed, careful review of the anterior skull base is mandatory to exclude a meningocoele or encephalocoele (Figs. 67-31 and 67-32).

Please also note that unilateral polyps require direct inspection ± biopsy to exclude neoplasia. Polyps are usually treated medically, but surgery (FESS) is frequently required.

Antrochoanal Polyp

An antrochoanal polyp is a solitary dumbbell-shaped polypoid mass that largely fills the antrum and extends through a widened accessory sinus ostium or infundibulum into the nasal cavity and from there posteriorly through the choana into the postnasal space and even the oropharynx (Fig. 67-33). These polyps are most commonly seen in young adults.

Although the imaging features and patient age are usually characteristic, nasal endoscopy is important in any patient with unilateral sinus disease to exclude underlying sinister pathology such as an inverted papilloma or other neoplasia.

Mucocoeles

The important features are a completely opacified, expanded sinus with smoothly thinned walls (Fig. 67-34). Approximately 90% occur in the frontal and ethmoidal sinuses. Mucocoeles are usually painless but present when the mass effect becomes critical. Frontal mucocoeles may present with frontal swelling or more rarely headache secondary to posterior extension into the anterior cranial fossa. Frontal and anterior ethmoidal mucocoeles may extend into the orbit, giving rise to proptosis. Mucocoeles are usually sterile but can become infected with a dramatic clinical presentation of rapid onset of pain and fever requiring urgent surgical drainage.

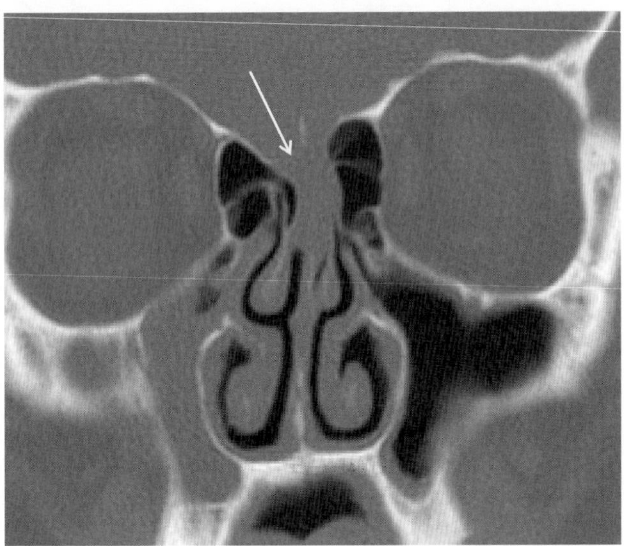

FIGURE 67-31 ■ Coronal CT of paranasal sinus and nasal cavity. Patient referred with nasal 'polyp'. Note defect in anterior skull base (white arrow). MR therefore organised (Fig. 67-32).

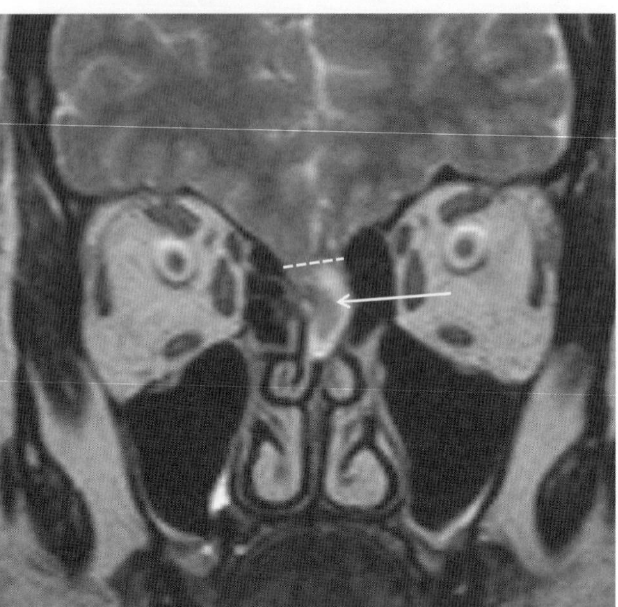

FIGURE 67-32 ■ Coronal T2W MR images of paranasal sinuses and nasal cavity. Interrupted white line = anterior skull base. Note that the 'polyp' seen in Fig. 67-31 is a meningoencephalocoele of the right gyrus rectus (white arrow).

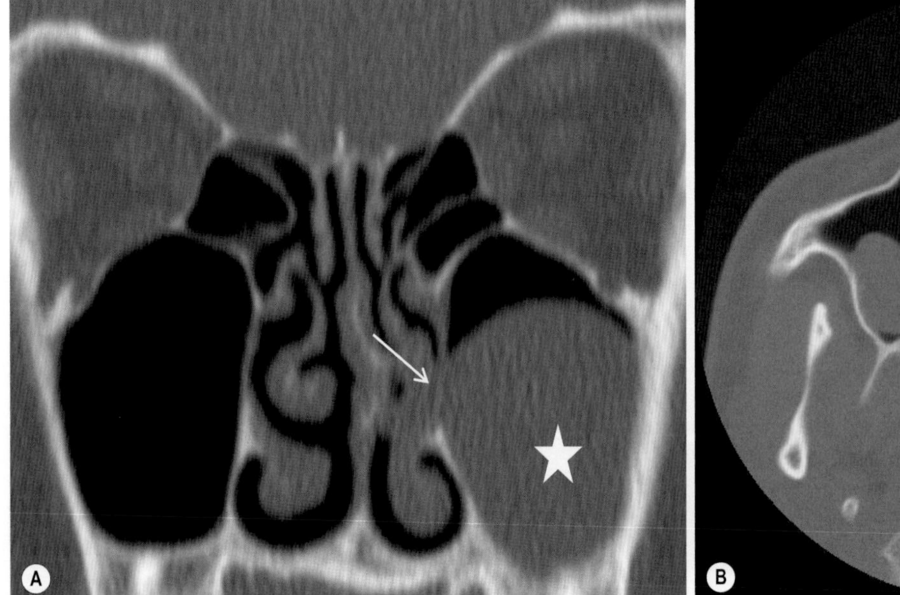

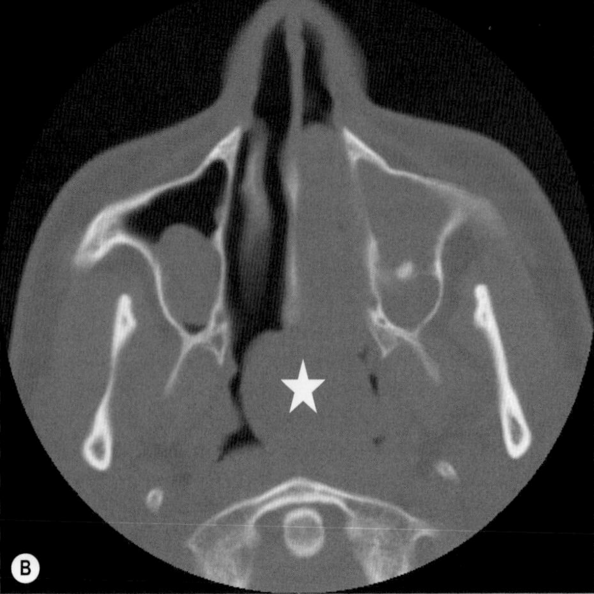

FIGURE 67-33 ■ (A) Axial CT of paranasal sinuses and nasal cavity. Star = polyp within left antrum extending through accessory sinus ostium into middle meatus (white arrow). (B) Axial CT of paranasal sinus and nasal cavity. Note polyp filling the left side of the nasal cavity and extending through the choana to fill the postnasal space (star) in keeping with an antrochoanal polyp.

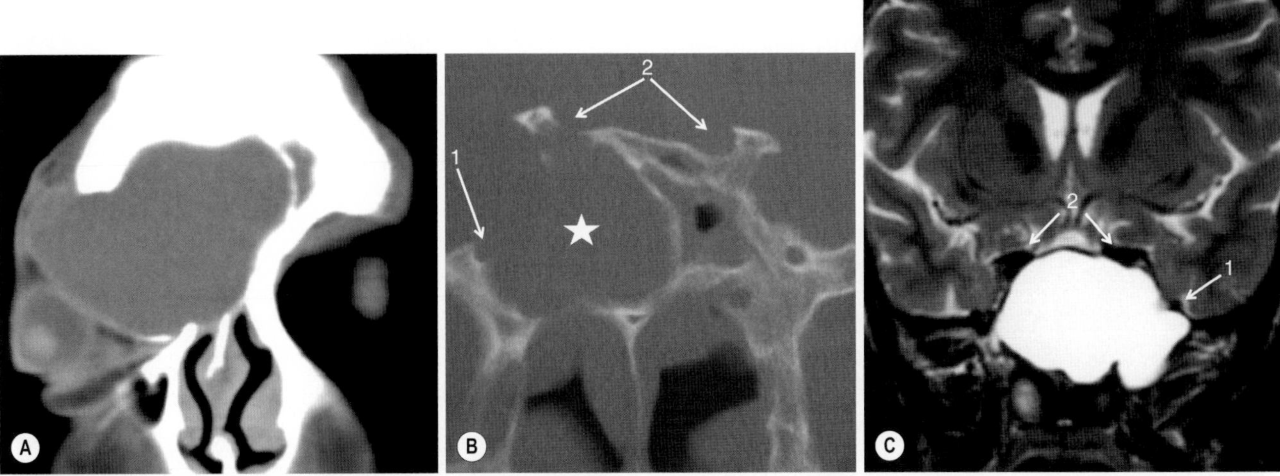

FIGURE 67-34 ■ (A) Coronal CT of frontal sinus. Note a markedly expanded and opacified right frontal sinus with extensive dehiscent inferolateral wall and secondary displacement and proptosis of the right globe in keeping with a frontal mucocoele. (B) Magnified coronal CT of sphenoid sinus. Note opacified expanded right side of the sphenoid sinus (star) with dehiscent lateral wall and close relation with the maxillary division of the trigeminal nerve (1) and the optic nerves (2). (C) Coronal T2W MR image of sphenoid sinus. Note expanded opacified sphenoid sinus filled with T2 high signal material and again the close relation to the maxillary division of the trigeminal nerve (1) and the optic nerves (2).

Epistaxis

Epistaxis does not usually require imaging, but if the bleeding is profuse or recurrent then a source for the bleeding may require investigation usually with CT post IV contrast medium performed in the arterial phase. Severe uncontrolled epistaxis may be life-threatening. Contrast angiography and selective embolisation of bleeding vessels may be life-saving.

Nasal and Paranasal Sinus Tumours

Sinonasal tumours are often advanced at presentation as the early symptoms are similar to chronic sinusitis and because tumours enlarge within hollow cavities, thus not exerting pressure effects. Early diagnosis requires a high index of suspicion in patients who have unilateral or recurrent symptoms and do not respond to medical treatment.

Early symptoms of malignancy include unilateral facial pain, nasal obstruction, unilateral nasal discharge and epistaxis. Late symptoms include altered sensation in the V2 distribution, proptosis, epiphora and trismus.

There are three main prognostic factors in sinonasal malignancy: tumour type, intracranial and orbital involvement. The radiologist's role is defining extent rather than histological diagnosis. Tumours vary from indolent to very malignant.

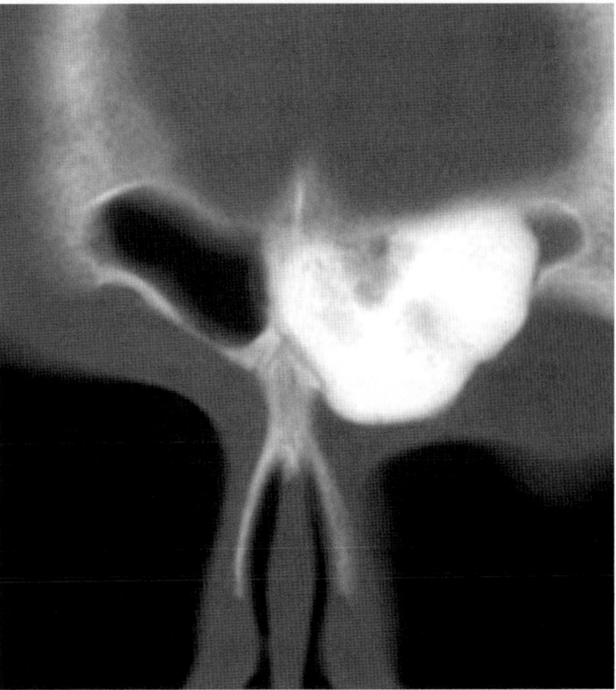

FIGURE 67-35 ■ **Coronal CT of left frontal sinus osteoma.** Note well-defined dense bony lesion filling most of left frontal sinus and bulging into the superomedial left orbit.

Osteoma

These are the most common tumour of the paranasal sinuses usually noted as an incidental finding. They are well-defined, sessile or pedunculated lesions arising from a wall of the frontal sinus (80%), ethmoidal sinus (20%) or rarely maxillary and sphenoid sinuses (Fig. 67-35). They are slow growing and often not requiring treatment although surgery is considered if the osteoma is compromising the drainage pathway or >50% of the sinus volume.

Inverted Papilloma

They are frequently present as a middle meatal mass causing unilateral nasal obstruction usually in an ostiomeatal pattern. The sex ratio is M.F 4:1. Ten per cent demonstrate calcification at the site of tumoural attachment. They have a characteristic lobulated outline on CT and a cerebriform pattern on MRI (Fig. 67-36). Surgery must include subperiosteal resection at the site of attachment to avoid recurrence. Assessment with CT is usually satisfactory, with MRI used mainly to assess recurrence.

Juvenile Angiofibroma

Adolescent boys with heavy epistaxis characterise the disease. This benign, locally invasive mass originates at the sphenopalatine foramen, widens the pterygopalatine fossa (PPF), extends into the nasal cavity and erodes the adjacent medial pterygoid plate and skull base in the region of the vidian canal aperture (Fig. 67-37). The

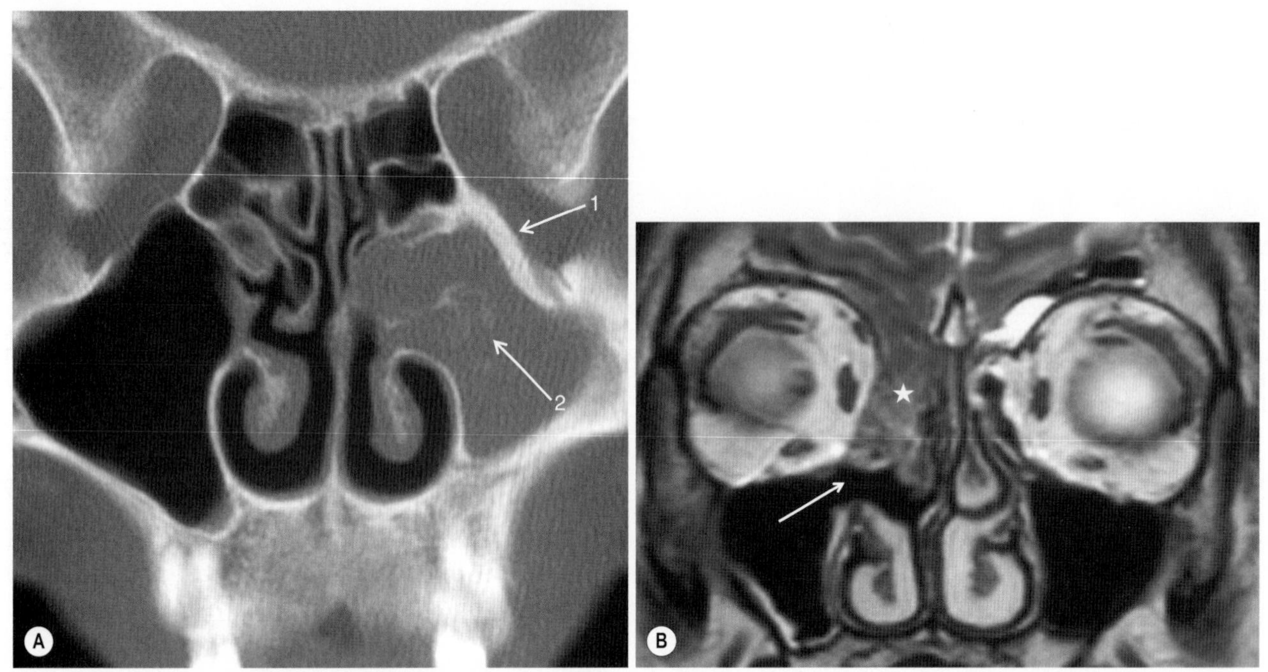

FIGURE 67-36 ■ (A) Coronal CT image of anterior osteometal unit (OMU). Note the unilateral opacified left antrum expanding into the middle meatus associated with bony thickening of the roof (1) and calcification (2). (B) Coronal T2W MR image of anterior OMU. Note (white arrow) the previous middle meatal antrostomy (MMA) and (white star) the intermediate signal of the recurrent inverted papilloma.

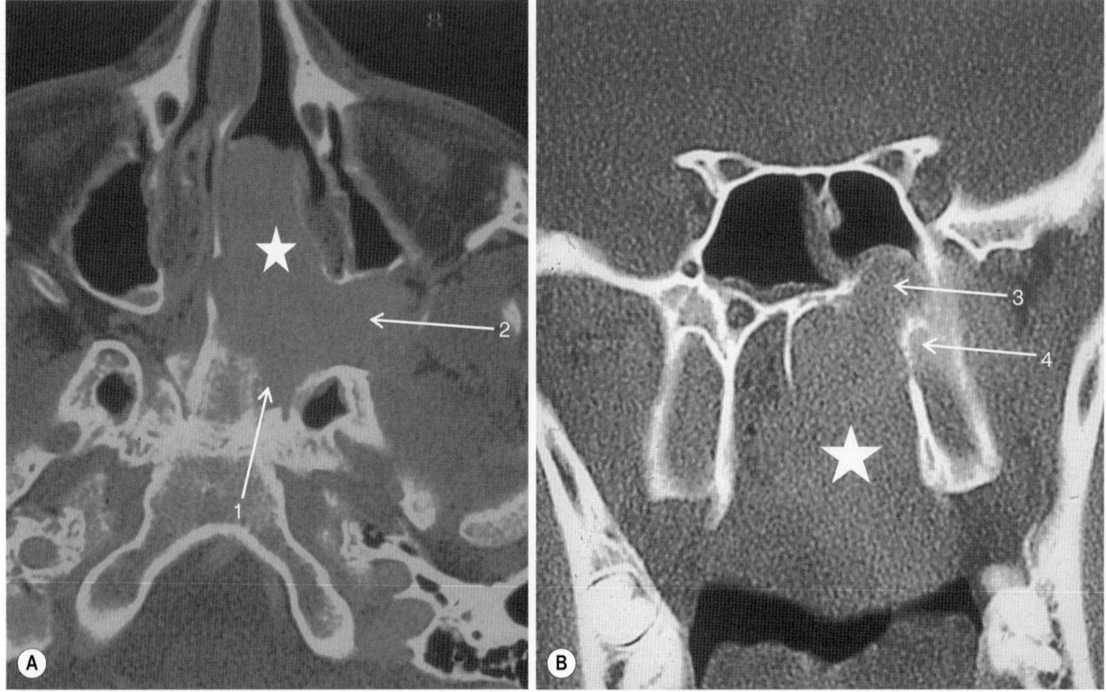

FIGURE 67-37 ■ (A) Axial and (B) coronal CT images. Note the angiofibroma (white star) filling and expanding the nasal cavity, eroding the sphenoid in the region of the vidian canal aperture (1 & 3), widening the PPF (2) and eroding the medial pterygoid plate (4).

presence of a nasal mass and a widened PPF in an adolescent male is pathognomonic. Contrast-enhanced MR is usually required and is complementary to CT for accurate preoperative assessment. Preoperative embolisation may be used to reduce blood loss.

Sinonasal Malignancy

Sinonasal malignancy is rare and there is a wide differential; however, approximately 80% are SCC (Fig. 67-38), with adenocarcinoma, adenoid cystic carcinoma and lymphoma comprising most of the remainder. Rarer sinonasal malignancies include olfactory neuroblastoma, melanoma and sarcomas. About 30% arise in the nasal cavity and most of the remainder arise in the antroethmoidal region, with < 5% arising in the frontal or sphenoid sinuses. The role of radiology is to define the tumour extent to form the basis of any treatment planning with, in particular, careful assessment of any intracranial, orbital, PPF, palatal or nodal involvement. Multiplanar MR is the technique of choice with fat-saturated sequences post-gadolinium helpful for assessing any orbital, dural involvement or perineural extension.

When assessing the anterior skull base, it is necessary to assess whether there is any skull base erosion, dural involvement or extension through the dura (Fig. 67-39).

When assessing the orbit it is important to identify whether there is erosion of the lamina papyracea, involvement of the orbital periosteum or extension through the periosteum. The lamina papyracea may be eroded on CT, but the low signal line of the orbital periosteum still preserved on MRI (Fig. 67-40). In equivocal cases frozen sections may be performed at the time of surgery, but the tendency is towards preserving the globe.

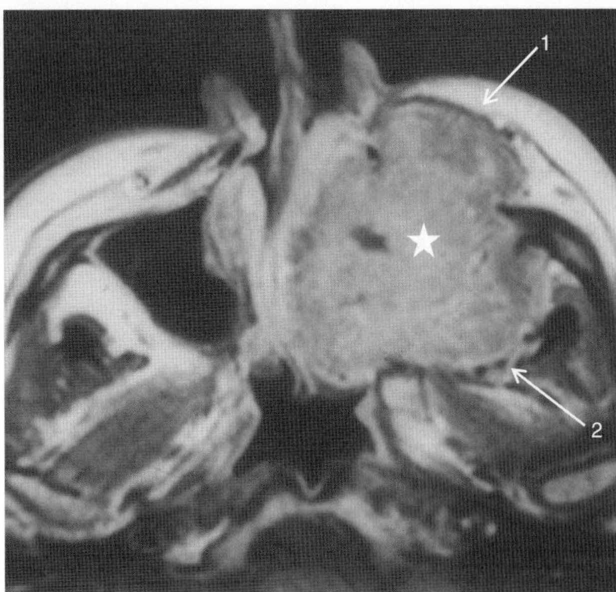

FIGURE 67-38 ■ **Axial T1W MR post-gadolinium image.** Note the expansile destructive mass (white star) centred on the left antrum extending into the pre- (1) and retroantral (2) soft tissues.

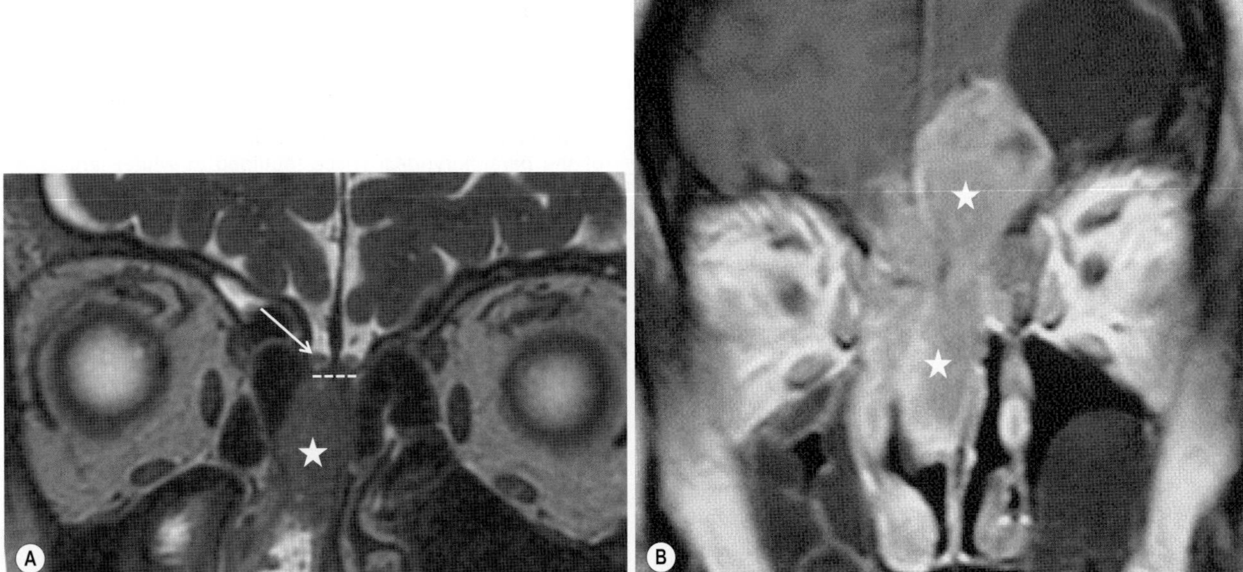

FIGURE 67-39 ■ (A) Magnified T2W coronal MR image. Note the mass (white star) filling and expanding the right olfactory niche but not eroding the cribriform plate (interrupted white line) or invading the more superior olfactory bulbs (white arrow). (B) Coronal T1 MR post-gadolinium image. There is a large dumbbell-shaped olfactory neuroblastoma (ON) (white stars), with both a large intracranial and superior nasal cavity component and a waist at the anterior skull base. Note also the peritumoural cyst occasionally seen in ON.

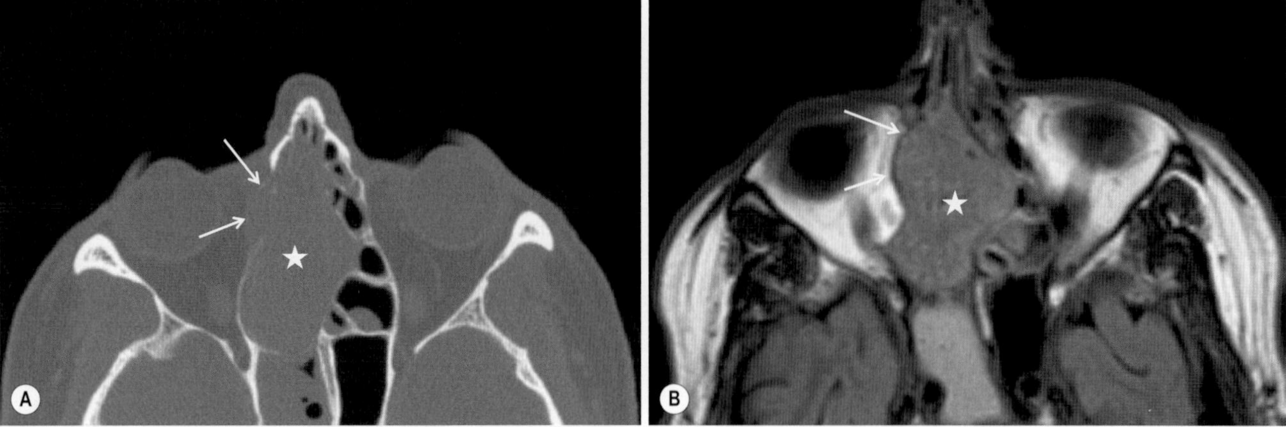

FIGURE 67-40 ■ **(A) Axial CT and (B) axial T1W MR post-gadolinium images.** Note the eroded lamina papyracea on CT, but the preserved orbital periosteum on MRI (white arrows). Tumour = white star.

THE NECK

THE SUPRAHYOID NECK

Anatomy

The suprahyoid neck is divided into spaces delineated by the three layers of deep cervical fascia. This is a logical method for reviewing this region as the fascial layers act as a barrier to the spread of disease and by localising the pathology to a particular space the differential diagnosis is simplified.

The following spaces in the suprahyoid neck are recognised (Fig. 67-41): the parapharyngeal space (PPS), the parotid space (PS), the retropharyngeal and danger spaces (RPS and DS), the masticator space (MS), the carotid space (CS), the pharyngeal mucosal space (PMS) and the perivertebral space (PVS).

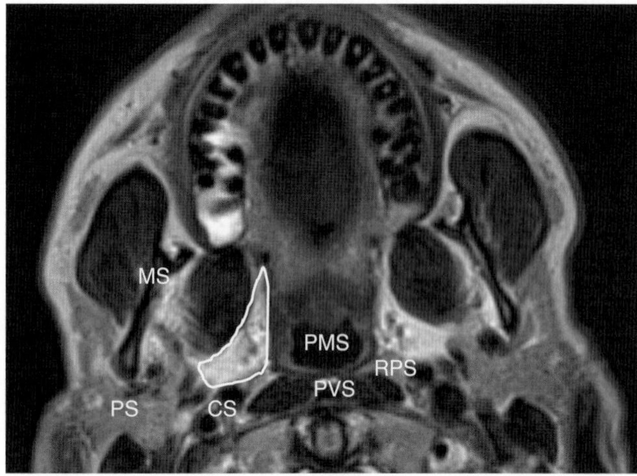

FIGURE 67-41 ■ **Axial T2W MR image.** Note the central location of the parapharyngeal space (outlined in white) largely filled with fat and therefore readily visible on both CT and MR relative to the other spaces of the suprahyoid neck: MS = masticator space, PS = parotid space, CS = carotid space, PVS = perivertebral space, RPS = retropharyngeal space. (The danger space (DS) has not been included as it cannot be separated on imaging from the RPS.)

The Parapharyngeal Space

The PPS is the key to the suprahyoid neck as it is centrally located and consists almost entirely of fat and therefore is easily identified on CT and MR (Fig. 67-41). This space was previously known as the prestyloid parapharyngeal space. It is rare for pathology to arise within the PPS (occasionally a salivary tumour from a salivary rest); however, the direction of displacement of the PPS fat helps the radiologist identify the adjacent suprahyoid space of origin of the pathology.

The Parotid Space

Anatomy and Radiology. The parotid space contains the parotid salivary gland, lymph nodes, facial nerve, retromandibular vein and external carotid artery enclosed by the superficial layer of deep cervical fascia (Fig. 67-42).

Ultrasound is the first-line imaging technique for salivary masses and may be combined with fine-needle aspiration cytology (FNAC). The important questions to ask on imaging are the following:

- Is the swelling arising in or adjacent to the parotid? Differentiation of an upper cervical lymph node from a tail of parotid lesion can be difficult.
- Is the swelling centred in the superficial and/or deep aspects of the gland? This is very important with regard to surgical planning and potential risk of iatrogenic facial nerve damage.
- Is the swelling ill-defined or well-defined, cystic or solid? That is, does it have features suggestive of malignancy or an inflammatory/infective process?

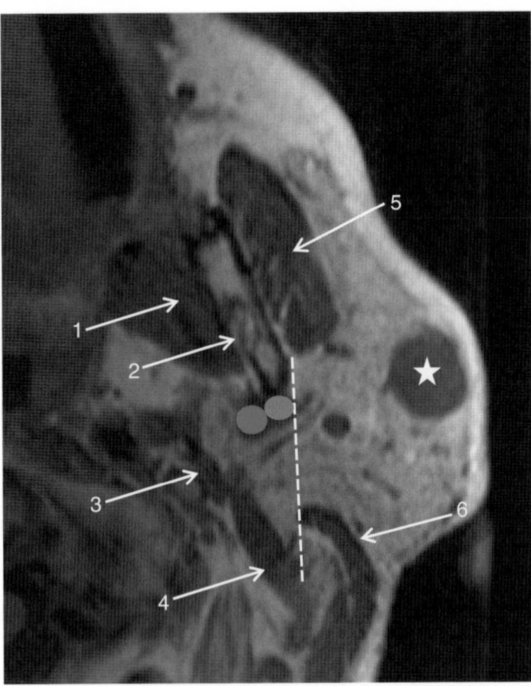

FIGURE 67-42 ■ **Axial/TW1 MR image of left parotid.** 1 = medial pterygoid muscle, 2 = inferior alveolar nerve (branch of V3), 3 = styloid process, 4 = posterior belly digastric muscle, 5 = masseter muscle, 6 = sternocleidomastoid muscle. Interrupted white line = junction of superficial and deep parotid (from lateral border of posterior belly digastric muscle to angle of mandible). Blue circle = retromandibular vein, red circle = external carotid artery (ECA), star = tumour in the superficial parotid (a pleomorphic salivary adenoma (PSA) in this patient).

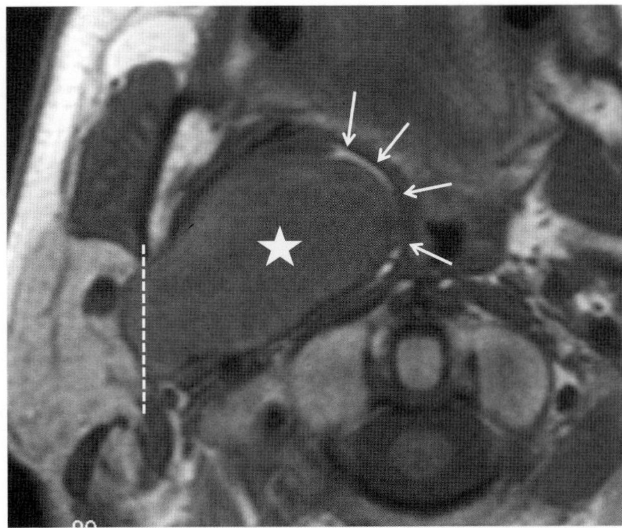

FIGURE 67-43 ■ **Axial T1W MRI of right parotid.** Interrupted white line = approximate junction superficial and deep parotid, white star = deep lobe of parotid tumour (PSA in this patient), white arrows = displaced PPS.

- Is the swelling single or multiple, unilateral or bilateral? If multiple, consider intraparotid nodes, benign lymphoepithelial lesions and chronic inflammatory pathology. If bilateral, consider the above and also a Warthin's tumour, in particular, in an elderly male smoker.
- Is there adjacent lymphadenopathy?

MRI is complementary to US and is used to assess local extent, in particular when there is proven malignancy on fine-needle aspiration (FNA) or in the parotid suspected deep lobe involvement (Fig. 67-43) or to assess perineural infiltration. Contrast-enhanced CT (CECT) does not differentiate the tumour from adjacent normal salivary tissue as clearly as MRI, but is helpful in assessing infection associated with sialolithiasis. MR sialography can be helpful in chronic inflammatory conditions such as Sjögren's syndrome (Fig. 67-44).

The Retropharyngeal and Danger Spaces (RPS and DS)

Anatomy. These are potential spaces centred posterior to the pharynx and anterior to the prevertebral muscles extending from the skull base to T4 in the superior mediastinum. The more posterior DS and RPS cannot be differentiated from each other on imaging. The importance of the RPS and DS is that disease, in particular infection in both spaces, can extend into the mediastinum.

The RPS contains a medial and lateral group of nodes from the skull base to hyoid bone, i.e. suprahyoid. Therefore, pathology in the suprahyoid RPS tends to be unilateral/asymmetrical.

Pathology. The radiological importance of the RPS is in two main areas: infection and malignancy.

The radiologist must try and differentiate between an RPS abscess that tends to distend the RPS and demonstrates wall enhancement from fluid that does not cause significant mass effect. It is important in all cases of an RPS abscess to include the superior mediastinum in the imaging field and to differentiate from pathology in the prevertebral part of the perivertebral space (PVS) by confirming that the pathology is anterior to the prevertebral muscles.

The RPS may be involved in malignancy, most frequently secondary to involved lymph nodes (in particular this region should always be reviewed when staging nasopharyngeal, oropharyngeal and the rarer posterior hypopharyngeal wall malignancy) and less commonly from direct posterior extension from the posterior pharyngeal wall (Fig. 67-45). The radiologist must try and identify whether the thin fatty density line of the RPS is preserved.

The Masticator Space

The masticator space, including the muscles of mastication, mandible and the inferior alveolar nerve (a branch of V3), is covered in the Jaw and Dental section of this chapter, as is the oral cavity.

The Carotid Space

Anatomy. The carotid space consists of the carotid arteries, internal jugular vein, sympathetic plexus and

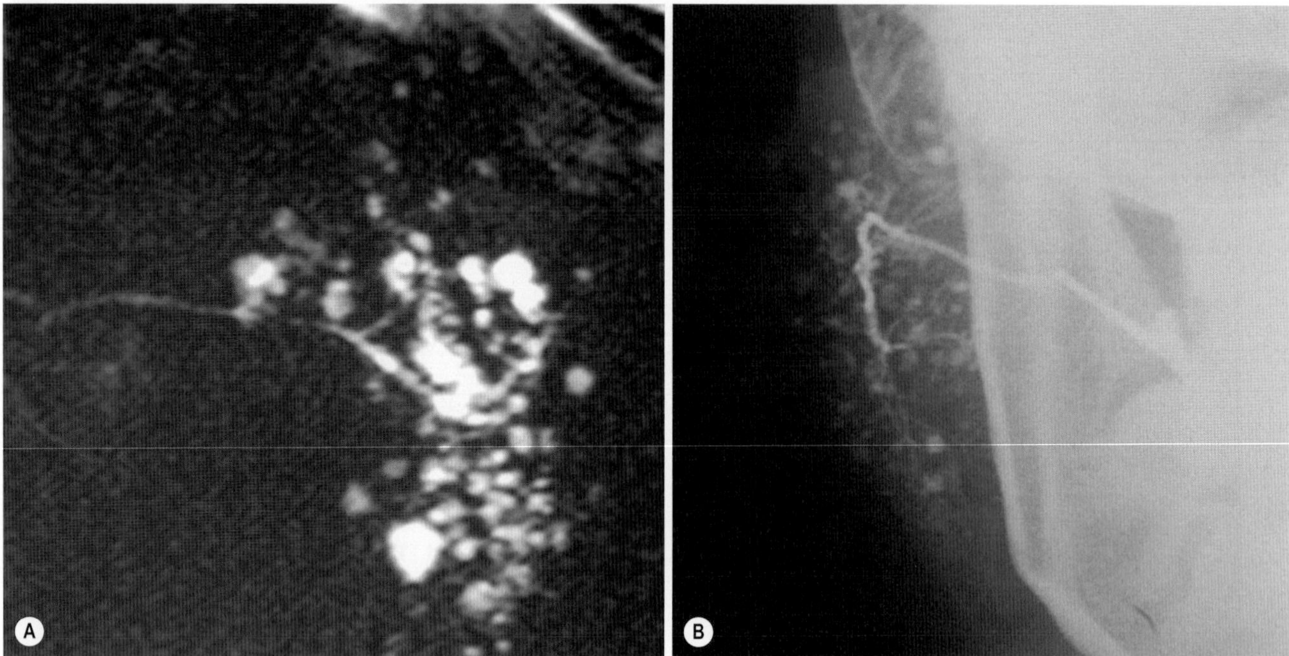

FIGURE 67-44 ■ (A) MR and (B) conventional sialogram in a patient with Sjögren's syndrome. Note the multiple punctate cystic spaces more marked in the MR sialogram.

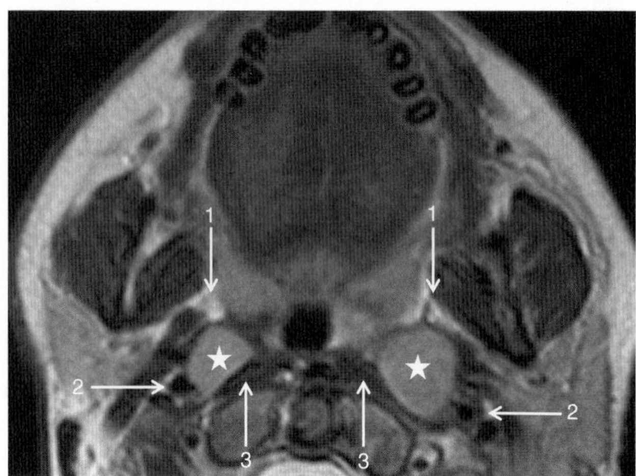

FIGURE 67-45 ■ T1W MR post-gadolinium image at the level of the oropharynx. Note the bilateral enlarged retrophayngeal lymph nodes (white stars) and their relation to the PPS (1), ICA (2) and prevertebral muscles (3).

cranial nerves IX–XII in the suprahyoid neck and cranial nerve X in the infrahyoid neck. It also used to be known as the retrostyloid parapharyngeal space.

The most common 'lesion' is the pseudolesion of the ectatic carotid artery or normal asymmetry of the internal jugular veins.

In infection of the deep neck it is important to exclude thrombosis of the internal jugular vein and when assessing malignant lymhadenopathy to assess whether there is invasion of the carotid or internal jugular vein. Loss of the fat plane or >180° of circumferential involvement of the carotid is suggestive of tumour involvement.

Pathology

Carotid Artery Dissection. The extracranial internal carotid artery is the most commonly involved site and is best demonstrated on axial T1 MRI with fat saturation where the intramural haematoma is of high signal.

Carotid and Vagal Paragangliomas. Paragangliomas (also known as glomus tumours) are vascular lesions that classically have a 'salt and pepper' appearance on T1 where the high signal foci represent subacute blood and the low signal flow voids from large tumour vessels. Carotid paragangliomas (or carotid body tumours) arise in the carotid bifurcation and characteristically splay the ICA and ECA (Fig. 67-46). Vagal paragangliomas are centred more superiorly posterior to and between the carotid and internal jugular vein. It is important to always review whether there is extension into the jugular foramen and whether there is a second synchronous lesion (5%–10%).

Schwannoma. These are well-defined, usually homogeneously enhancing, fusiform-shaped masses (Fig. 67-47) that occasionally, when large, demonstrate cystic change. They may, if vascular, be indistinguishable from a paraganglioma although if they extend into the jugular foramen they can be distinguished from paragangliomas as they remodel/expand the foramen rather than cause the classic permeative erosion of a paraganglioma.

The Pharyngeal Mucosal Space (PMS)

Anatomy. The PMS is deep to the middle layer of deep cervical fascia which surrounds the pharyngobasilar fascia

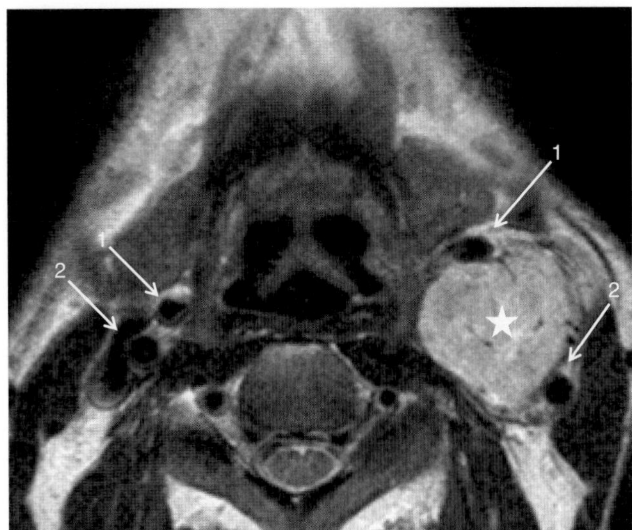

FIGURE 67-46 ■ **Axial T2W MR image.** Note the high signal carotid body tumour (white star) with flow voids splaying the ECA (1) and ICA (2) and compared to the right side. Remember up to 10% are bilateral.

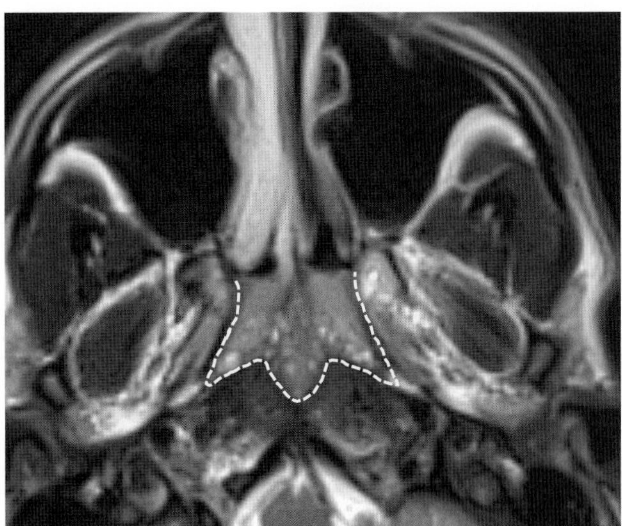

FIGURE 67-48 ■ **Axial T2W MR image.** The interrupted line outlines the pharyngobasilar fascia which has the appearance of an upturned crown. It separates the lymphoidal tissue within the PMS from the PPS laterally and the PVS posteriorly.

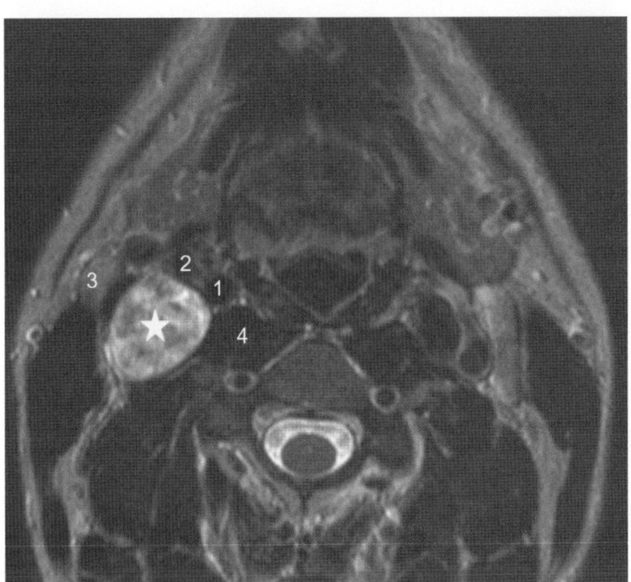

FIGURE 67-47 ■ **Axial T2W MR image.** The high signal vagal schwannoma separates the ICA (1) and ECA (2) from the compressed internal jugular vein (3) and is within the carotid space lateral to the prevertebral muscle (4).

(Fig. 67-48) and the superior and middle constrictors. The contents of the PMS include the mucosa of the nasopharynx and oropharynx (the more inferior hypopharynx is in the visceral space of the infrahyoid neck, which is an inferior continuation of the PMS), lymphatic tissue of Waldeyer's ring (in the nasopharynx adenoids and in the oropharynx faucial tonsils laterally and lingual tonsils, part of the tongue base, anteriorly) and minor salivary glands. The volume of this lymphatic tissue decreases with age.

The most important pathology in this region is SCC arising in the oropharynx and undifferentiated carcinoma in the nasopharynx.

A multidisciplinary team (MDT) approach including ENT, maxillofacial and plastic surgeons, oncologists, pathologists, cytopathologists, radiologists, radiotherapists, speech and language therapists, dietitians and specialist nurses is essential for treating malignant disease in this region. Benign disorders will also be discussed as a benign differential diagnosis is often considered even when malignant disease is suspected.

The PMS can be divided into the nasopharynx and oropharynx.

Nasopharynx

Anatomy. The nasopharynx is the superior division of the pharynx whose boundaries are the skull base superiorly, anterior arch of C1 posteriorly, the superior surface of the soft palate inferiorly, the nasal choanae anteriorly and the lateral pharyngeal wall including the prominence of the torus tubarius with anteriorly the eustachian tube opening and posteriorly the fossa of Rosenmüller.

Radiology and Pathology

Nasopharyngeal Malignancy. MR is superior to CT for assessing the nasopharynx.

Almost all nasopharyngeal malignancies are carcinomas (NPC) that are divided into keratinising, non-keratinising and undifferentiated. The differential includes non-Hodgkin's lymphoma (NHL) arising from lymphoidal tissue and minor salivary gland malignancy. The role of radiology is to define the extent for radiotherapy planning. Accurate assessment is of increasing importance with the advent of more targeted (intensity-modulated) radiotherapy or IMRT.

NPC usually arises in the lateral pharyngeal recess (of Rosenmüller). NPC is the most common tumour that

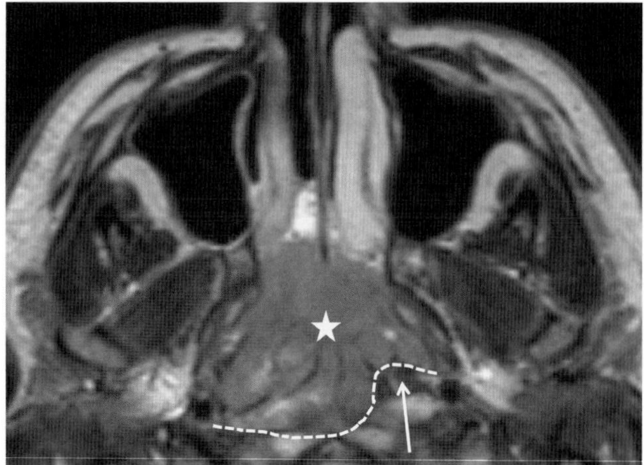

FIGURE 67-49 ■ **Axial T2W MR image.** The nasopharyngeal tumour (white star) has extended posteriorly (interrupted white line) and on the right laterally to invade the PVS and PPS. Note the remaining partially invaded left prevertebral muscle medial to the ICA (white arrow).

invades the skull base. Intracranial extension is most commonly via perineural spread through foramen ovale along the mandibular division of the trigeminal nerve (V3). Nodal metastases are present in 90% at presentation. There is a strong association with the Epstein–Barr virus (EBV) and EBV titres can be used as a marker of tumour response. NPC is the commonest cancer in Asian males. Treatment is radiotherapy or chemoradiotherapy, with surgery for recurrence following treatment.

The commonest differential of nasopharyngeal malignancy (Fig. 67-49) is adenoidal hypertrophy, which can usually be differentiated as the latter is symmetrical and contains visible folds of mucosa. Other benign pathology seen in the nasopharynx includes the Tornwaldt cyst (a benign midline developmental cyst) and a retention cyst, both of which are well defined and covered with normal mucosa. If there is still concern on nasal endoscopy, biopsy is suggested.

Oropharynx

Anatomy. The oropharynx is divided into the following subsites: the tongue base (largely comprising the lingual tonsils) and the valleculae anteriorly (the valleculae form the inferior boundary between oropharynx and hypopharynx), laterally the glosso-tonsillar sulcus and faucial tonsils, superiorly the soft palate (that separates oropharynx from nasopharynx) and posteriorly the posterior pharyngeal wall. Please note that the tongue base is included in the oropharynx and *not* the oral cavity.

Radiology and Pathology. The most common reason for imaging the oropharynx is to query tonsillar or peritonsillar abscess (quinsy). On contrast-enhanced CT (CECT) a tonsillar abscess is shown as a swollen tonsil with central low attenuation and rim enhancement. A peritonsillar abscess occurs when there is spread to adjacent spaces, commonly parapharyngeal masticator and submandibular spaces. If trismus is present, then suspect involvement of the masticator space muscles.

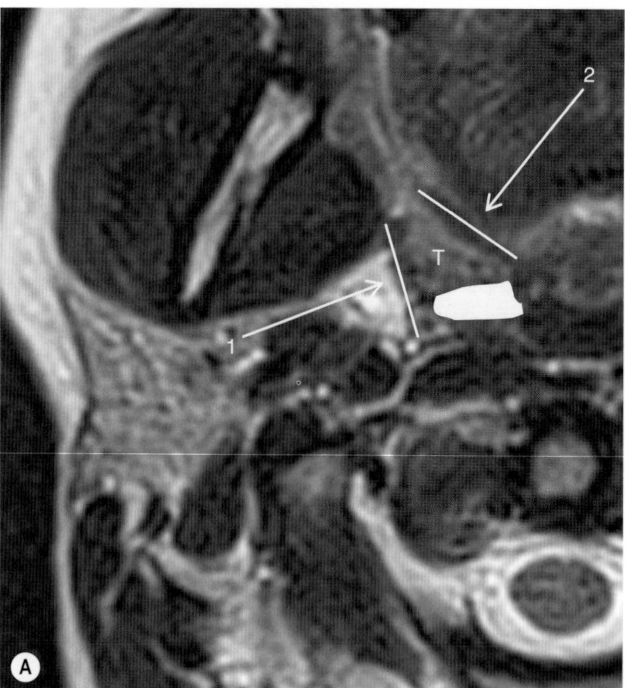

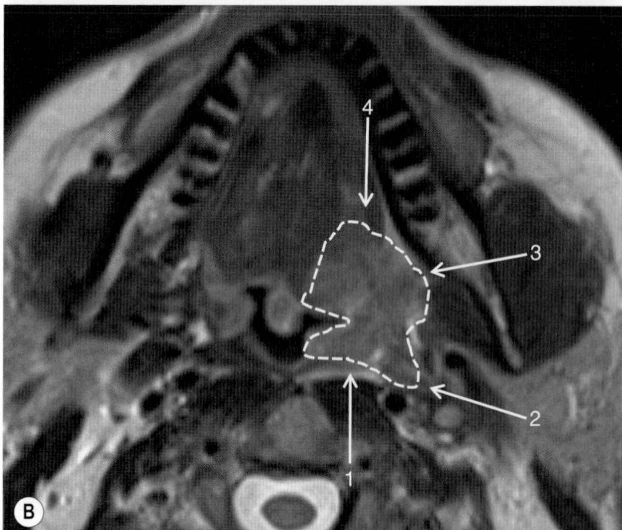

FIGURE 67-50 ■ (A) Axial T2W MR image of right faucial tonsil normal anatomy. T = faucial tonsil with the following relations: lateral border (1) = constrictors, anterior border (2) = palatoglossus muscle of the anterior tonsillar pillar and posterior border (filled in white area) = larger palatopharyngeus muscle of the posterior tonsillar pillar. (B) Axial T2W MR image of left tonsillar SCC. Note the left tonsillar SCC (interrupted white line) invading the following areas: 1 = posterior pharyngeal wall, 2 = RPS, 3 = PPS abutting the medial pterygoid muscle, 4 = tongue.

Nearly all oropharyngeal malignancy is SCC; the commonest site is the faucial tonsil and anterior tonsillar pillar (Fig. 67-50), followed by the lingual tonsil. The anterior tonsillar pillar (the palatoglossus muscle covered by mucosa) acts as a conduit for spread superiorly to the palate and inferiorly to the tongue base. MR imaging delineates oropharyngeal tumours better than CECT, but both lingual and faucial tonsillar tumours may be difficult to identify clinically and are two of the sites for an occult 'hidden' head and neck primary, the other sites being the fossa of Rosenmüller in the nasopharynx and the piriform fossa in the hypopharynx. As in the nasopharynx, rarer oropharyngeal tumours include non-Hodgkin's lymphoma (NHL) and minor salivary tumours (the latter usually arising at the junction of the hard and soft palate).

The following questions should be answered in patients with faucial tonsillar SCC:

- Is there extension laterally through the constrictors (Fig. 67-50B)?
- Is there superior extension to the palate or inferior extension to the tongue base (Fig. 67-50B)?
- Is there retropharyngeal and cervical lymphadenopathy?

The following areas should be reviewed in patients with lingual tonsillar SCC:

- Is there extension across the midline?
- What is the depth of invasion?
- Are the extrinsic tongue muscles involved?
- Is there inferior extension into the supraglottic larynx?

Fifteen per cent of patients with oropharyngeal SSC will have a second primary in the head and neck, and 60% have malignant lymphadenopathy at presentation.

Perivertebral Space (PVS)

This region is described in the neuroimaging chapters. The important point is to identify that when pathology arises in the prevertebral part of the perivertebral space it displaces the prevertebral muscles anteriorly, whereas an RPS mass is centred anterior to the prevertebral muscles, which are therefore displaced posteriorly. The commonest pathology in this region is a prevertebral abscess and metastatic disease.

THE INFRAHYOID NECK

Anatomy

As in the suprahyoid neck, the infrahyoid neck is divided into spaces defined by the layers of deep cervical fascia. There are five spaces but only one, the visceral space, is found solely in the infrahyoid neck. The other spaces are the carotid space (CS), retropharyngeal (RPS) and perivertebral spaces, which are discussed in the suprahyoid section above, and the posterior cervical space, which, as it only includes the accessory nerve, fat and lymph nodes, will not be discussed further except to note that the accessory nerve is sometimes sacrificed in neck dissection, resulting in a weak shoulder.

The visceral space includes the hypopharynx (a continuation of the pharyngeal mucosal space), the larynx and trachea, the thyroid and parathyroid glands, the recurrent laryngeal nerve and lymph nodes.

Hypopharynx

Anatomy. The hypopharynx, along with the larynx, is located within the visceral space of the infrahyoid neck and is divided into the pyriform fossae, the post-cricoid region and the posterior pharyngeal wall. The inferior aspect of the pyriform fossa is the apex. The hypopharynx and larynx are intimately associated. Surgery to the hypopharynx usually therefore involves surgery to the larynx.

Radiology and Pathology. Nearly all hypopharyngeal tumours are SCC (or very rarely minor salivary gland).

The majority arise in the pyriform fossa (Fig. 67-51A), followed by the post-cricoid area (Fig. 67-51B), and rarely the posterior hypopharyngeal wall. Patients tend to present late and approximately 50% have nodal involvement at presentation. There is a strong association with smoking and drinking. Critical observations to make are the following:

- Is there posterolateral extension into adjacent soft tissues and/or involvement of the posterior thyroid lamina?

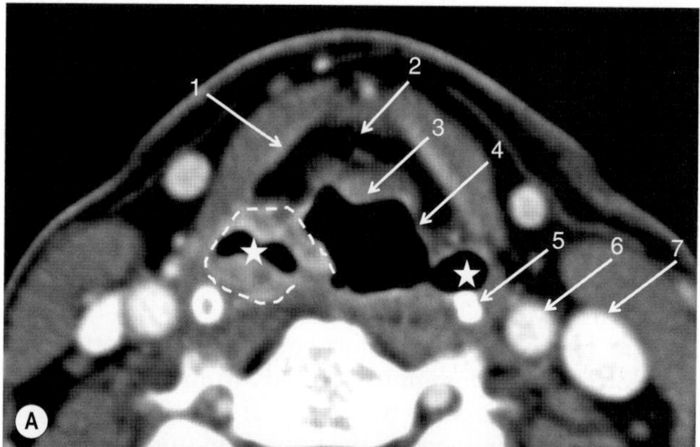

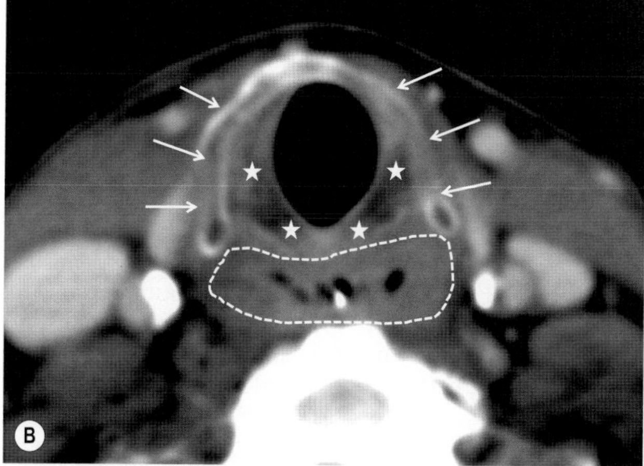

FIGURE 67-51 ■ (A) Axial CT post IV contrast through hypopharynx. Note the tumour (interrupted white line) arising in the piriform fossa (white stars). 1 = lamina of thyroid cartilage, 2 = pre-epiglottic fat, 3 = epiglottis, 4 = aryepiglottic fold, 5 = superior horn thyroid cartilage, 6 = CCA, 7 = IJV. (B) Note the circumferential post-cricoid and posterior hyppoharyngeal wall tumour (interrupted white line) containing a nasogastric tube posterior to the cricoid cartilage (white stars) and lamina of thyroid cartilage (white arrows).

- Is there inferior extension into the cervical oesophagus? Correlate with swallowing studies and endoscopic assessment.
- Is there retropharyngeal nodal involvement?

Larynx

Anatomy and Physiology. The larynx has two main functions:

1. Airway protection.
2. Sound generation.

The larynx sits on the cricoid cartilage, which resembles a signet ring with its face situated posteriorly. The larger V-shaped thyroid cartilage protects the vocal cords and consists of two lamina fused anteriorly and open posteriorly. Posteriorly there are superior and inferior extensions of the thyroid laminae called superior and inferior horns. The inferior horns articulate with the cricoid cartilage.

The arytenoid cartilages sit on the cricoid lamina protected by the thyroid laminae. The vocal cords arise from the anterior vocal processes of the arytenoid cartilage, meet anteriorly at the anterior commissure and are controlled by the intrinsic muscles of the larynx—cricoarytenoid abductors and thyroarytenoid adductors.

The epiglottis is attached inferiorly to the larynx at the petiole and to the hyoid by the hyoepiglottic ligament. It folds posteriorly over the laryngeal vestibule during swallowing, preventing aspiration.

The superior laryngeal nerve—a branch of the vagus—conveys sensation and cricothyroid motor function. All other functions are conveyed by the recurrent laryngeal nerve, also a branch of the vagus.

The larynx is divided into supraglottis, glottis and subglottis. The supraglottis extends from the epiglottic tip inferiorly to include the laryngeal ventricle and has a rich lymphatic drainage to the upper and mid deep cervical nodes. The glottis includes the true vocal cords. The subglottis extends from the undersurface of the true cords to the inferior cricoid cartilage. The glottis and subglottis have a poorer lymphatic drainage and drain to prelaryngeal, lower deep cervical and paratracheal nodes.

Radiology and Pathology

Laryngeal Malignancy. Nearly all laryngeal malignancy (98%) is SCC; other rarer tumours such as chondrosarcoma (Fig. 67-52) and adenoid cystic carcinoma will be discussed briefly. CT and MR are both useful for assessing the larynx. CT should be performed in quiet breathing with reconstructed images parallel to the true cords.

Laryngeal SCC. The role of the radiologist is to accurately stage both the primary tumour and nodal disease. Sixty per cent are glottic and usually present early due to the effect on the voice. Nodal involvement of SCC localised to the glottis is rare. Thirty per cent arise in the supraglottis and are often diagnosed late. In addition, because of the rich lymphatic network, approximately 50% of supraglottic tumours have nodal involvement at presentation. True subglottic tumours are rare. The subglottis is usually involved by inferior extension from the glottis. Transglottic tumours are so-called when tumour involves all three divisions of the larynx.

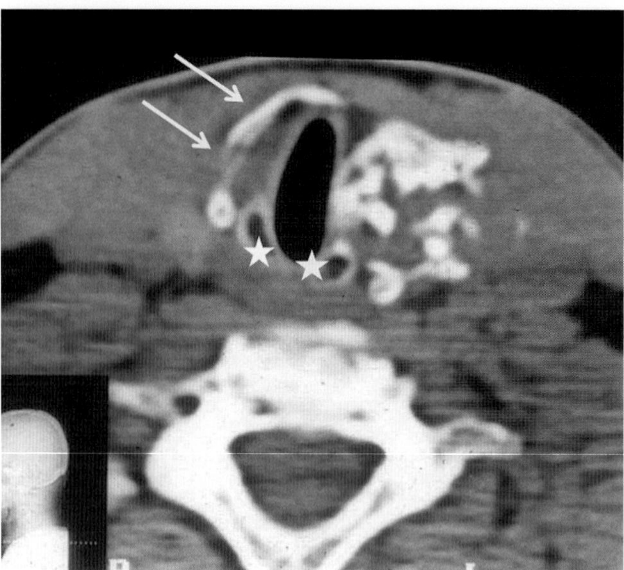

FIGURE 67-52 ■ **Axial unenhanced CT of larynx.** Note the classical coarse (popcorn) calcification of the chondrosarcoma arising from the left thyroid lamina. White arrows = right thyroid lamina, stars = cricoid cartilage.

Critical observations to make are the following:

- Does the tumour involve the anterior commissure?
- At the anterior commissure soft tissue only < 1 mm should be visible.
- Does tumour cross the midline?
- Is there subglottic extension?
- There should be no soft tissue visible within the cricoid ring.
- Is there supraglottic extension?
- In particular, is there involvement of the tongue base?
- Is there cartilage invasion?
- MRI is more sensitive than CT in difficult cases.

Chondrosarcoma. These are rare slow-growing tumours arising from laryngeal cartilage (usually cricoid); they show characteristic coarse calcification and are treated with local resection (Fig. 67-52).

Adenoid Cystic Carcinoma. These classically arise in the minor salivary glands of the subglottis and should be considered in the differential of a subglottic mass.

Laryngocoele. A laryngocoele is a dilatation of the laryngeal saccule that arises from the laryngeal ventricle and may be acquired or congenital. The laryngeal ventricle is a lateral out-pouching between the false and true cords. An internal laryngocoele is confined within the larynx and is visible as a smooth submucosal supraglottic swelling; an external laryngocoele extends through the thyrohyoid membrane at the site of the superior laryngeal vessels and may be visible as a neck swelling. The laryngocoele is usually air-filled but an air–fluid level or a completely fluid-filled structure may be present if the neck is obstructed (Fig. 67-53). It is important to exclude an obstructing SCC within the laryngeal ventricle.

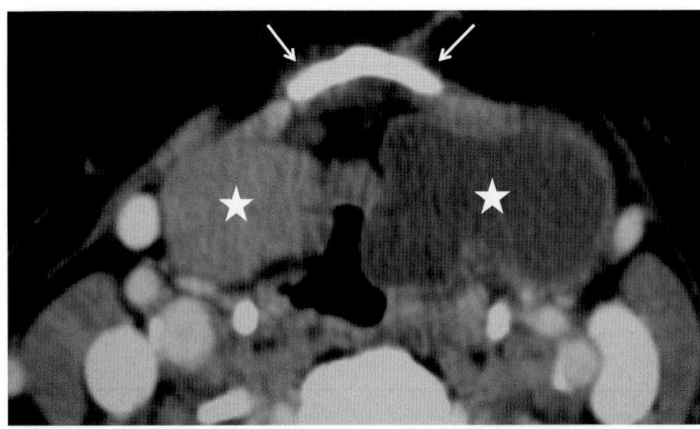

FIGURE 67-53 ■ Axial CT post IV contrast at level of hyoid bone (white arrows). Note the bilateral fluid-filled external laryngocoeles (white stars). The higher density of the right laryngocoele is due to its denser contents.

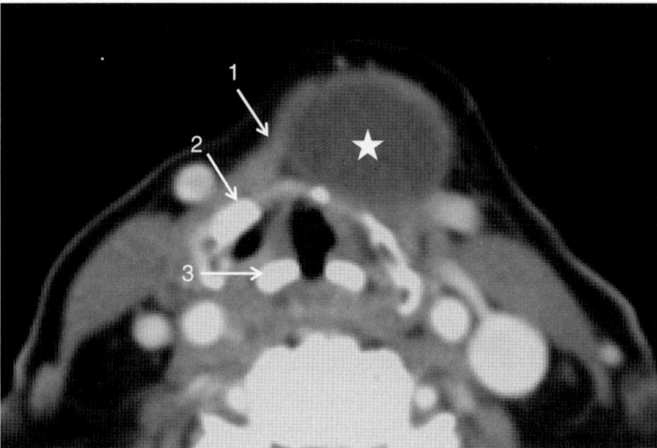

FIGURE 67-55 ■ Axial CT post IV contrast. Star = paramedian thyroglossal cyst centred anterior to the laminae of the thyroid cartilage (2) and elevating the sternohyoid muscle (1). 3 = arytenoid cartilage.

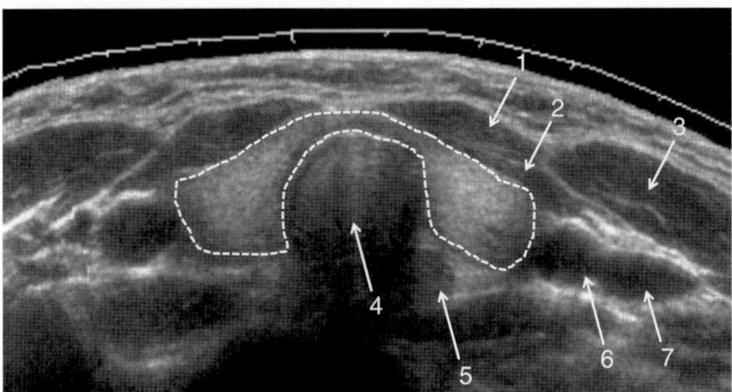

FIGURE 67-54 ■ Panoramic transverse ultrasound image through the thyroid gland (interrupted white line). 1 = sternohyoid muscle, 2 = sternothyroid muscle, 3 = sternocleidomastoid muscle, 4 = trachea, 5 = cervical oesophagus, 6 = CCA, 7 = IJV.

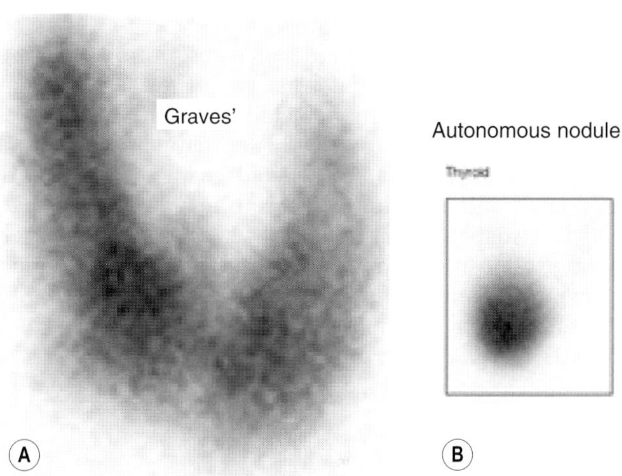

FIGURE 67-56 ■ ^{99m}Tc-pertechnetate image. Note the diffuse increased uptake in a patient with Graves' disease (A) and the second image (B) showing an autonomous (hot) nodule.

Thyroid and Parathyroid

Anatomy. The thyroid gland is also located within the visceral space (VS) of the infrahyoid neck and consists of two lobes on either side of the proximal cervical trachea connected by an isthmus (Fig. 67-54). The thyroid gland descends during development from the foramen caecum in the midline of the tongue base. Rarely there is arrested descent, resulting in a lingual thyroid, but more commonly a pyramidal lobe persists, best demonstrated on ultrasound as a tongue of thyroid tissue extending superiorly from the isthmus sometimes as far as the hyoid bone. Occasionally a remnant remains that presents as a midline or paramedian anterior neck swelling in the thyrohyoid region usually following a cold: a thyroglossal cyst (Fig. 67-55).

There are usually four, but occasionally up to six parathyroid glands located along the thymopharyngeal tract that extends from the level of the carotid bifurcation to the lower anterior mediastinum. They are most frequently located posterior to or just inferior to the mid-to-inferior aspect of the lobes of the thyroid.

Radiology

Ultrasound. Ultrasound is the primary imaging technique for both the thyroid and parathyroid because of the superficial location of these glands and provides the highest resolution of any technique. Ultrasound also can be combined with FNAC if required.

Nuclear Medicine. Diagnostic isotope studies (usually ^{99m}Tc-pertechnetate and iodine-123) are used less frequently in thyroid imaging as anti-thyroid autoantibodies such as anti-thyroperoxidase (TPO) antibody (a non-specific test for thyroiditis) and a more specific TSH receptor antibody for Graves' disease have largely replaced their use. They are still used sometimes in two clinical scenarios: to assess for an autonomous nodule in patients with a nodular thyroid and suppressed TSH (Fig. 67-56), and in suspected thyroiditis where the blood tests have proven unhelpful. Therapeutic I-131 treatment of Graves' disease is still widely used. ^{99m}Tc-sestamibi, usually in combination with ultrasound, is used for assessing patients with primary hyperparathyroidism.

MRI and CT. Cross-sectional imaging with CT and MRI is used to assess the degree of retrosternal extension and tracheal compression in multinodular goitre or invasion of adjacent structures in thyroid malignancy. CT with intravenous contrast must not be used if a papillary carcinoma is suspected as the use of iodinated contrast will preclude radioiodine treatment for approximately 2 months.

Thyroid Pathology

Thyroiditis. Hashimoto's thyroiditis (chronic lymphocytic) is the commonest. In the early stage on ultrasound the thyroid has a heterogeneous, hypoechoic echotexture in a slightly enlarged lobulated gland. At a later stage the gland commonly decreases in size and develops echogenic linear fibrotic septae, but remains heterogeneous (Fig. 67-57). In Graves' disease patients present with a diffusely enlarged hypoechoic thyroid demonstrating markedly increased colour flow called a thyroid inferno (Fig. 67-58).

Thyroid Malignancy. A detailed description is beyond the scope of this chapter. The vast majority (90%) are differentiated carcinomas, including papillary 70–80% (Fig. 67-59) and follicular 10–20%. Medullary carcinoma compromising 5–10% of thyroid malignancy may be associated with multiple endocrine neoplasia (MEN 2A and B). Anaplastic carcinoma (1–2%) has an extremely poor prognosis and presents in the elderly as a rapidly growing mass invading adjacent structures (Fig. 67-60). Primary thyroid lymphoma (NHL) is rare but has a 70–80× increased risk in patients with thyroiditis.

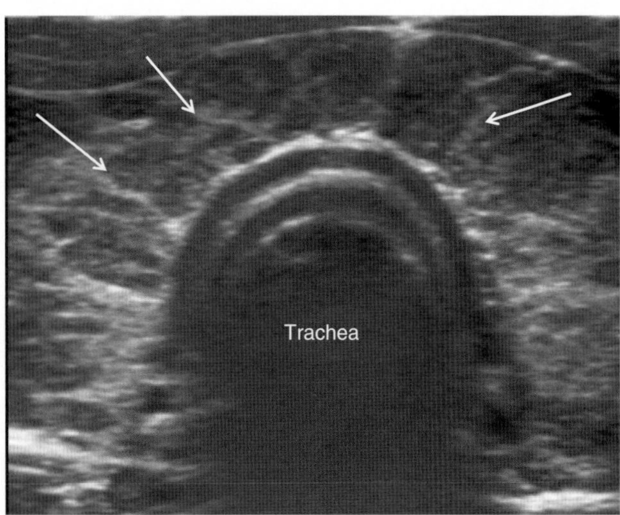

FIGURE 67-57 ■ **Transverse US of thyroid.** Note the diffusely heterogeneous hypoechoic (dark) thyroid containing hyperechoic lines (white arrows) in chronic thyroiditis and compare with Fig. 67-54.

Parathyroid Pathology. The most commonly clinical scenario is primary hyperparathyroidism usually investigated with a combination of ultrasound and ^{99m}Tc-sestamibi. The most frequent cause is a solitary parathyroid adenoma (80%), but parathyroid hyperplasia

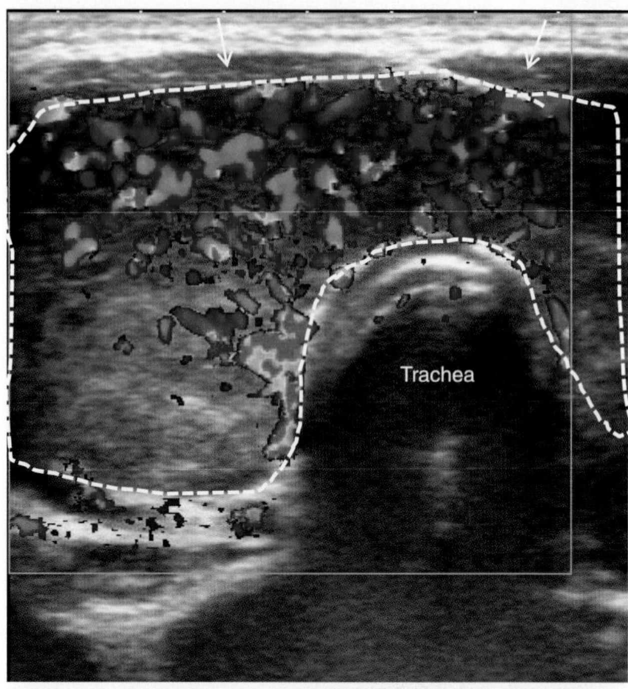

FIGURE 67-58 ■ **Transverse US of thyroid.** Note the swollen hypoechoic (dark) and hypervascular thyroid in Graves' disease. The appearance is called a thyroid inferno.

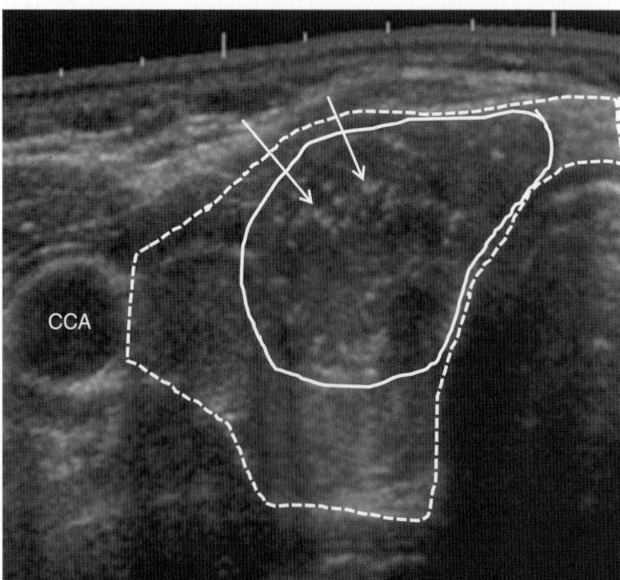

FIGURE 67-59 ■ **Transverse US of right thyroid.** The papillary tumour (continous white line) located within the medial right lobe of the thyroid is hypoechoic (dark) and contains characteristic echogenic foci (white arrows). Interupted white line = outline of right lobe and isthmus of the thyroid. CCA = Common carotid artery.

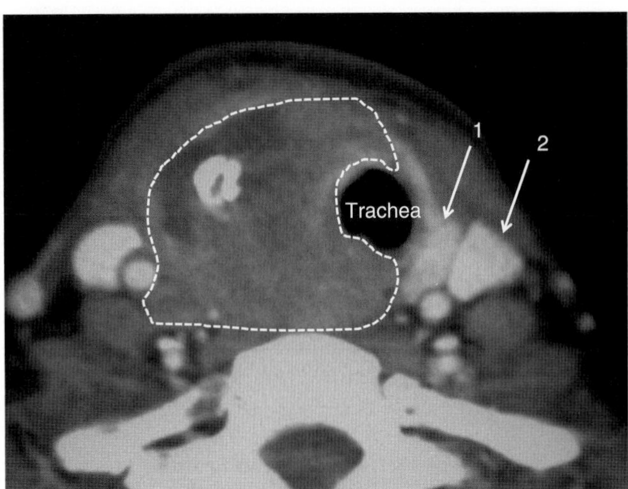

FIGURE 67-60 ■ **Axial CT of thyroid post IV contrast.** The ill-defined anaplastic tumour (interrupted white line) has replaced the whole right lobe and isthmus of the thyroid invading the overlying strap muscles and oesophagus. 1 = left lobe thyroid, 2 = IJV.

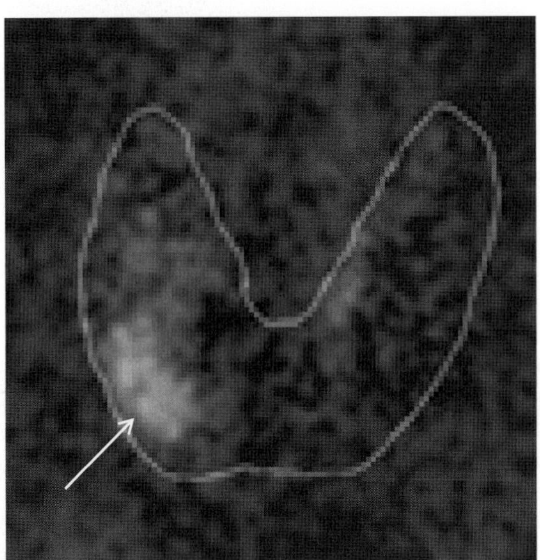

FIGURE 67-61 ■ ^{99m}Tc-sestamibi image showing focal uptake on delayed images in keeping with overactive parathyroid gland posterior to right lower pole of the thyroid.

is seen in 10–15%, multiple adenomas in 2–3% (Fig. 67-61) and parathyroid malignancy in approximately 1%.

The typical finding on ultrasound is a well-defined hypoechoic mass posterior or inferior to the thyroid (Fig. 67-62). Sestamibi will usually identify those adenomas not visible on ultrasound, i.e. located in the superior mediastinum or posterior to the trachea. CT, MRI and venous sampling is used in complex cases.

Recurrent Laryngeal Nerve. The course of the recurrent laryngeal nerve requires imaging when patients present with vocal cord palsy. Imaging must extend superiorly to include the medulla. On the left side the recurrent laryngeal nerve extends into the mediastinum, passing under the aortic arch, whereas on the right the recurrent laryngeal nerve remains within the neck passing under the right subclavian artery and only the neck, requires imaging.

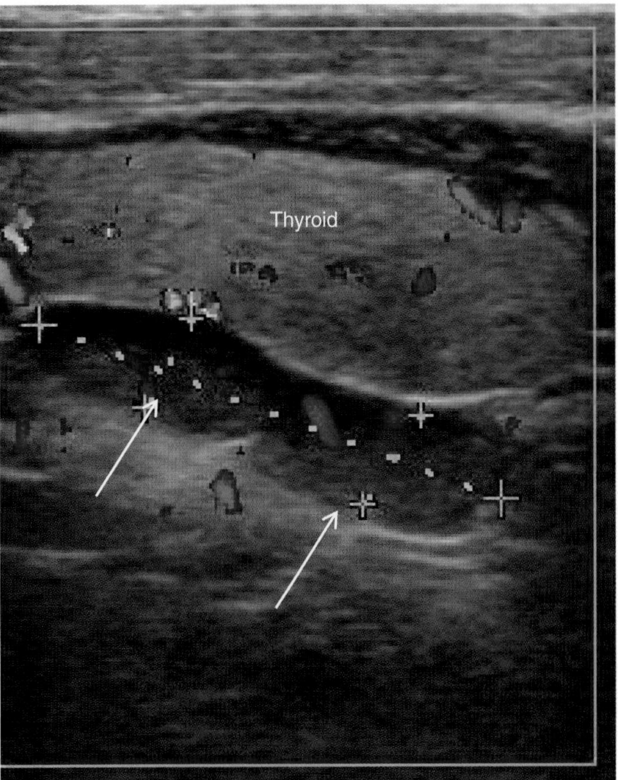

FIGURE 67-62 ■ **Longitudinal US of thyroid/parathyroid.** Note the two adjacent enlarged hypoechoic (dark) parathyroid glands (white arrows) posterior to the thyroid.

Cervical Lymph Nodes

Generalised lymphadenopathy is a common clinical presentation. If widespread and painful, glandular fever or other viral infections can be considered. If focal and painful, a bacterial lymphadenitis may be the aetiology. If painless spread from a head and neck malignancy, lymphoma or atypical bacterial infection may be the cause.

Radiology and Pathology. In the context of a head and neck malignancy pathological nodes are described as belonging to one of seven levels: Level 1 (a and b) submental and submandibular, 2 (a and b) upper, 3 middle and 4 lower deep cervical, 5 posterior triangle, 6 anterior cervical and 7 superior mediastinal (Fig. 67-63). These levels, however, do not include the retropharyngeal, intraparotid and facial lymph nodal groups.

Accurate nodal staging in head and neck SCC is vital for appropriate treatment and prognosis. The diagnosis

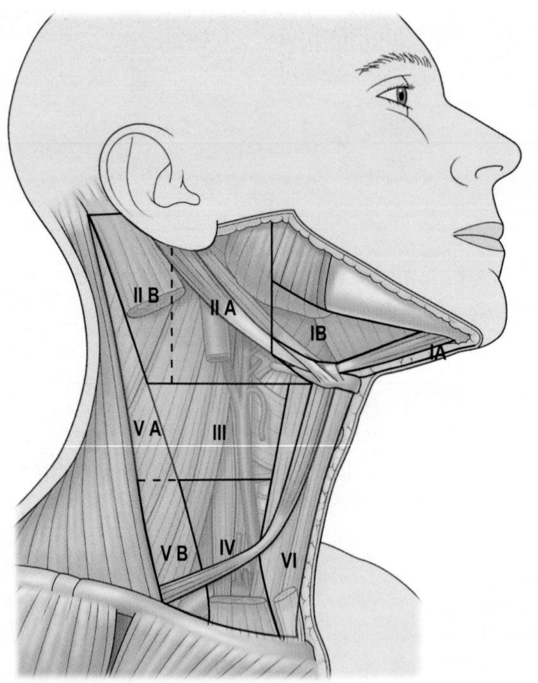

FIGURE 67-63 ■ Drawing of the right side of the neck with the sternocleidomastoid muscle and right submandibular salivary gland removed and the IJV tied off, demonstrating the nodal levels (1–6). Level 7 (superior mediastinum) has not been covered.

of an involved ipsilateral node, a contralateral node and extracapsular spread each decrease the long-term survival by 50%.

Ultrasound is the technique of choice for assessing a patient with a neck lump suspected to be secondary to lymphadenopathy and can be combined with FNAC or Tru-Cut biopsy. Often the ultrasound is performed on the same initial visit to the ENT clinic as a 'one-stop' procedure.

There are a number of imaging criteria for assessing whether a lymph node is pathological. These cannot be covered in detail in this chapter but the most important are size, shape, echotexture (on ultrasound), evidence of cystic change and abnormal or absent colour flow (ultrasound). A non-pathological lymph node should have a short axis of <1 cm and a long:short axis ratio of >2, i.e. a rugby ball rather than a round (football) shape. A darker or hypoechoic appearance on ultrasound is concerning.

DENTAL AND MAXILLOFACIAL

DISORDERS OF BONE

Developmental Disorders

Fibro-Osseous Lesions

This is a spectrum where normal bone is replaced in a benign process, extending from the purely fibrotic lesion at one end to a dysplastic bony lesion at the other. They include the ossifying fibroma, a well-defined expansile mass with a fibrous central area surrounded by a calcified rim, fibrous dysplasia and the osseous dysplasias.

Fibrous dysplasia is a localised expansile lesion in which cancellous bone is replaced initially by radiolucent fibrous tissue which matures with varying amounts of calcified tissue to a mixed-density lesion or as a radiopacity, typically with orange peel or ground-glass texture (Figs. 67-64 and 67-65). The maxilla is involved twice as frequently as the mandible. The margins blend with adjacent bone. It may displace teeth or prevent their eruption, and large lesions may cause considerable facial deformity. Seventy per cent of lesions are monostotic. Radiographically, it can resemble an ossifying fibroma, which is better defined and encapsulated, chronic sclerosing osteomyelitis and an osteosarcoma, which has ill-defined and destructive margins.

Periapical osseous dysplasia and florid osseous dysplasia are similar conditions, with the latter being the more extravagant and larger version. They mainly occur in women, particularly of Afro-Caribbean and Asian origin, after 25 years of age. Both conditions are characterised by the formation of multiple deposits around vital tooth roots, usually in the mandible. In periapical osseous dysplasia, radiolucent lesions forming at the apices of clinically sound teeth resemble periapical granulomas. Gradually, cemental-like tissue is deposited within it, becoming increasingly radiopaque and when mature is almost totally radiopaque except for a thin, peripheral radiolucent zone, which helps distinguish it from sclerosing osteitis.

Cherubism is a rare dysplasia of bone that develops during the first decade of life. It occurs bilaterally in both jaws, but more commonly affects just the mandible. It develops in the posterior aspects of the jaws as a multilocular, honeycombed, expansile radiolucency. Tooth displacement is common. It regresses spontaneously after skeletal growth ceases.

Inflammatory Disorders

Osteomyelitis of the jaws is uncommon, which is surprising considering the frequency of dental sepsis. It may

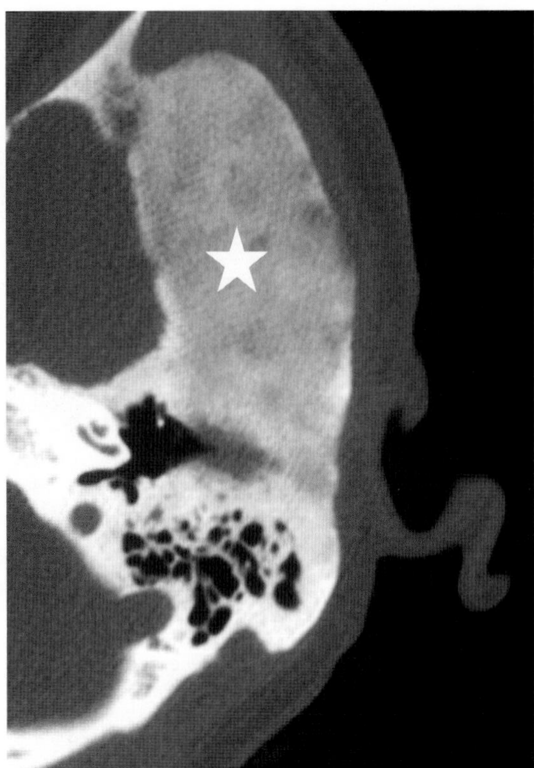

FIGURE 67-64 ■ Axial CT of left petrous temporal bone. Note markedly expanded squamous component of the temporal bone that has a ground-glass appearance in keeping with fibrous dysplasia (star).

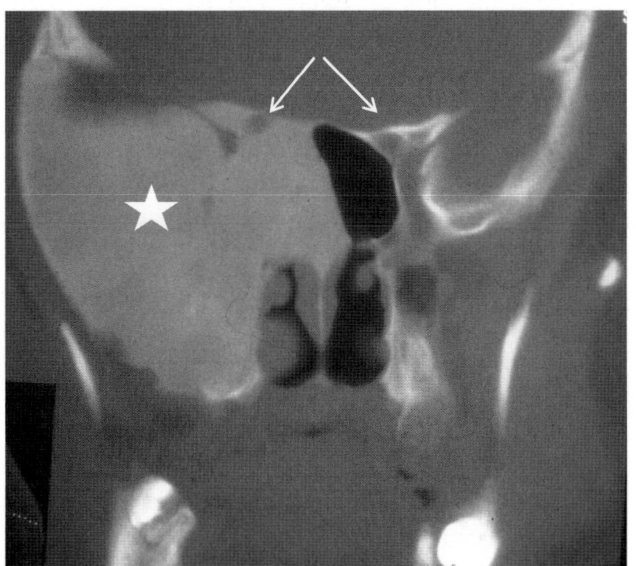

FIGURE 67-65 ■ Coronal CT through the sphenoid bone. The right side of the sphenoid is markedly expanded, with involvement of the body, greater and lesser wings, pterygoid plates, anterior clinoid process and the squamous component of the right petrous temporal bone (star). Note the close relation of the optic nerves (white arrows).

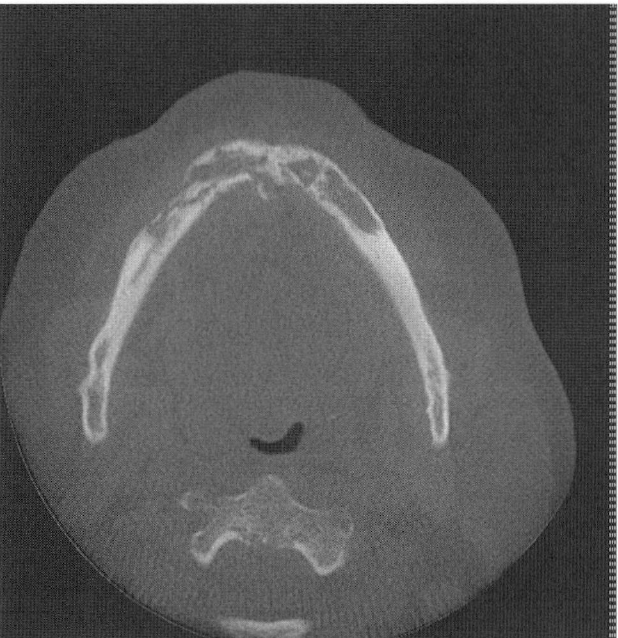

FIGURE 67-66 ■ Axial CBCT of mandible showing acute osteomyelitis of the anterior part of the mandible. The bone shows several dense bony sequestrae and lytic areas with destruction and perforation of the buccal and lingual cortical plates.

develop from a dental abscess, tooth extraction or jaw fracture. In acute osteomyelitis, there is thinning and discontinuity of the bony trabeculae to produce ill-defined, patchy areas of radiolucency. With time, bony sequestrae form and are recognised as irregularly shaped islands of bone set against a region of radiolucency (Fig. 67-66). The features of osteomyelitis are best visualised on CT or CBCT, which may also show periosteal bone formation. On MRI, the marrow usually shows a low signal intensity on T1 and high signal on T2-weighted images. If the disease becomes chronic, the bone becomes diffusely affected and extensively involved with sclerosis of the marrow spaces. CT or CBCT will demonstrate the internal structure and the presence of sequestration.

Diffuse sclerosing osteomyelitis is more common than acute osteomyelitis, from which it may develop. The bone becomes increasingly dense and radiopaque as a result of a proliferative response to low-grade infection. Bone deposition results in reduction in the size of the marrow spaces with gradual spread through the mandible; however, lytic areas are also seen. MRI shows a thickened cortex.

Bisphosphonate-Related Osteonecrosis of the Jaws (BRONJ)

This relative new condition can follow dental extraction or jaw infection of patients taking bisphophonates for osteoporosis or in the management of malignant tumours affecting the bone. Orally prescribed bisphosphonates result in a low incidence (1 in 10,000–50,000) of BRONJ, but when administered intravenously the incidence is much higher, being approximately 1 to 10%. Areas of

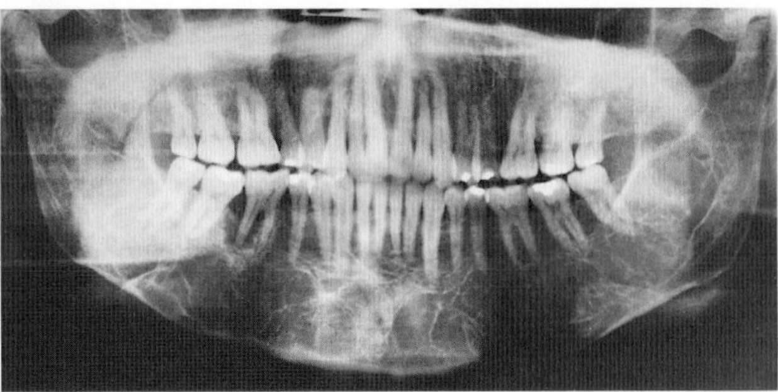

FIGURE 67-67 ■ **Panoramic radiograph of a case of thalassaemia.** There is marked increase in the height of the mandible, which is composed of coarse trabeculae enclosing large marrow spaces and the small maxillary sinuses. Note the generalised loss of the lamina dura and the periodontal abscess on the distal root of the lower right first molar.

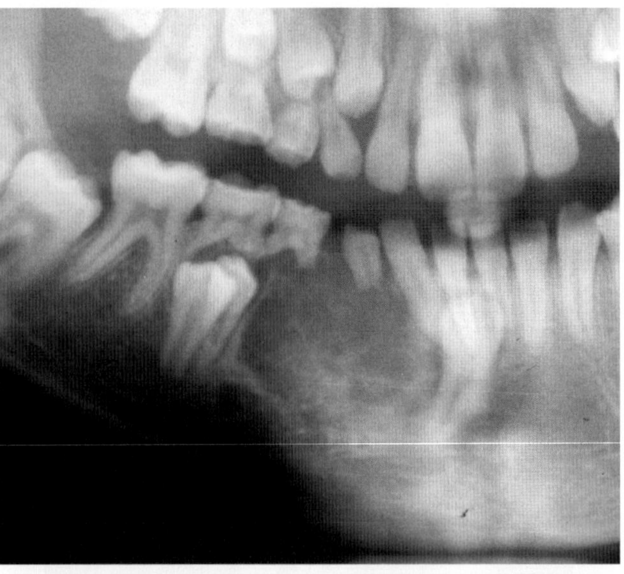

FIGURE 67-68 ■ Part of a panoramic radiograph of a **central giant-cell granuloma** of the right side of the mandible, which appears as a well-defined radiolucency containing numerous coarse bony trabeculae. There has been displacement of the premolar teeth posteriorly and the canine anteriorly.

necrotic bone develop and become exposed to the oral environment, leading to persistent chronic inflammation of the jaws. The radiographic features are of both acute and chronic osteomyelitis.

Osteoradionecrosis is an inflammatory condition that can affect the mandible if included in the radiation field after a dose of 45–50 Gy. It is a clinical diagnosis and presents as areas of exposed necrotic bone. The radiographic features resemble those of chronic osteomyelitis.

Metabolic, Endocrine and Haematological Disorders of Bone

Osteoporosis affects the jaws as elsewhere in the skeleton. The mandible becomes osteopenic, as the marrow spaces enlarge and the trabeculae thin. The cortical outline of the inferior alveolar canal becomes inconspicuous and the lower border of the mandible becomes thinner than normal, with endosseous radiolucencies.

The classical appearance of **hyperparathyroidism** is now seen less frequently because of improved diagnosis and management. However, when it affects the jaws it results in a general demineralisation of the bone, creating a ground-glass appearance, loss of the lamina dura and subperiosteal erosions at the angle. Brown tumours develop in the facial bones in approximately 15% of cases, particularly in long-standing cases and appear radiolucent and loculated, with margins that may be ill-defined or cystic.

Haematological replacement disorders may affect the jaws, the radiological manifestations depending on the severity of the condition. In moderate-to-severe thalassaemia, the jaws become radiolucent with coarse trabeculations due to marrow hyperplasia and the maxillary antrum is reduced in size (Fig. 67-67). The skull takes on a granular appearance, with thickening of the diploic spaces and occasionally a 'hair-on-end' appearance.

In sickle cell disease similar manifestations to thalassaemia are apparent; however, several sclerotic areas are seen as a consequence of dystrophic mineralisation of small thrombi.

Paget's disease of bone, a once frequently encountered disorder, is now rarely seen in the jaws, but when present affects a whole bone of the face or skull. The radiographic appearance depends on its stage of development, progressing from an initial radiolucent stage to a more granular or ground-glass appearance with loss of lamina dura. Bony trabeculae become coarse and arranged in a horizontal linear pattern and finally the bone becomes distorted and patchily radiopaque with focal collections of dense bone creating a 'cotton wool' appearance. Hypercementosis is a notable dental feature and skull changes are described as 'osteoporosis circumscripta', typically starting in the frontal bone.

Central giant cell granuloma is probably a reactive lesion and not neoplastic. It is most often detected during the first three decades of life, with twice as many being discovered in the mandible as the maxilla. The lesion is usually multilocular, is often well defined and lacks cortication, but some have ill-defined borders suggestive of a destructive lesion. Although largely radiolucent, the internal appearance varies from being almost devoid of any internal structures to those containing wispy septae (Fig. 67-68).

TUMOURS OF BONE

Ossifying fibroma is a tumour of bone but it can also be considered as a fibro-cemento-osseous lesion. Its behaviour varies from those showing slow growth to others being quite aggressive. It occurs mainly in young adults, mostly in the body of the mandible. The radiographic appearance depends on its degree of mineralisation, and typically contains a wispy or tufted bony trabecular pattern (Fig. 67-69). The lesion is encapsulated and so

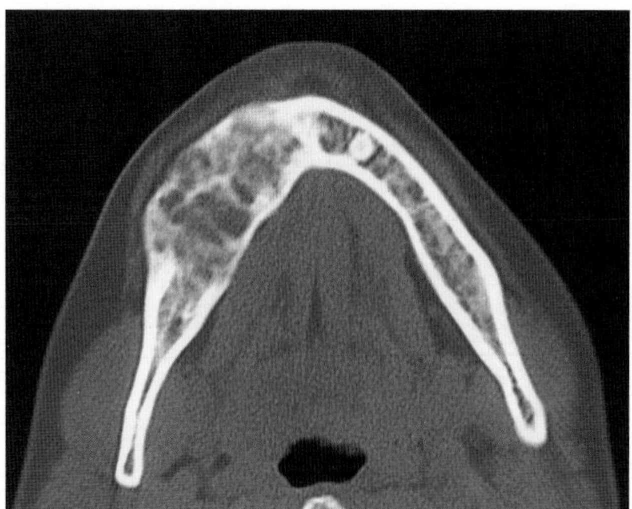

FIGURE 67-69 ■ Bone window setting of an axial CT of a **ossifying fibroma** of the mandible showing mainly buccal expansion and thinning of both cortical plates, which remain intact. The lesion is of mixed attenuation as it contains areas of fibrosis, mineralisation and coarse bony trabeculations.

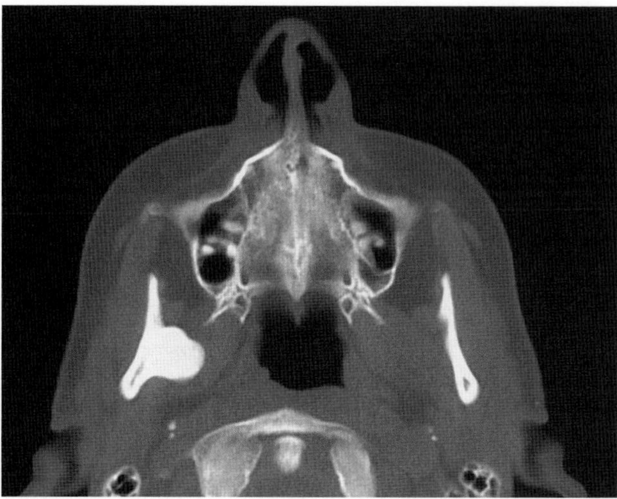

FIGURE 67-70 ■ Bone window setting of an axial CT showing a dense (compact) osteoma arising from the medial aspect of the ramus of the right mandible.

appears well defined, helping to distinguish it from fibrous dysplasia.

Osteomas of the maxillofacial bones and jaws are usually slow-growing, painless and thus discovered by chance. However, a large osteoma in the frontal sinuses may obstruct the drainage pathway and cause secondary infection. In the jaws, osteomas more commonly affect the mandible than the maxilla and, although any site can be involved, they tend to be found posteriorly on its medial aspect (Fig. 67-70). CT shows the site of origin and provides three-dimensional (3D) topographic detail. Multiple osteomas are a feature of Gardner's syndrome (familial adenomatous polyposis) and precede the formation of intestinal colonic polyposis.

Osteosarcoma is uncommon in the jaws, accounting for only 7% of all osteosarcomas. Although it can occur in early life, it most commonly presents in the jaws around 30 years of age, over 10 years later than osteosarcoma of the long bones. The mandible is more frequently affected than the maxilla. Maxillary lesions tend to arise from the alveolar ridge, and mandibular ones in the body. It has a destructive appearance and its density varies from being radiolucent, to patchily radiopaque or predominantly sclerotic. An important early dental radiographic sign is widening of the periodontal ligament space due to tumour spread along the periodontal ligament; however, this feature is also seen in other sarcomas (e.g. fibrosarcoma Ewing's sarcoma) and in a similar manner may also widen the inferior alveolar canal. Occasionally when the periosteum is elevated, a hair-on-end, sunray or onion skin appearance may be visible. CT is required to demonstrate accurately tumour calcification, bone destruction and bone reaction (Fig. 67-71), whereas MRI (T1- and T2-weighted images) will provide better information on the intramedullary and extraosseous components of the tumour.[1]

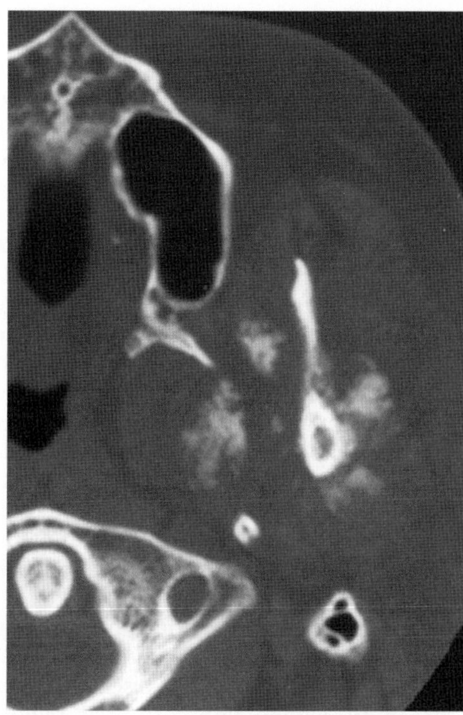

FIGURE 67-71 ■ **Bone window setting of an axial CT of osteogenic sarcoma of the left mandibular ramus.** There is bone destruction in the region of the sigmoid notch. The lesion contains areas of neoplastic bone formation and extends medially towards the lateral pterygoid plate, posteriorly to the styloid process and laterally resulting in facial swelling. (Courtesy of Mr S. Dover, Birmingham.)

Primary carcinoma of the overlying oral mucosa can invade the jaws to produce an ill-defined (but sometimes well-defined), non-corticated saucerised area of bone destruction (Fig. 67-72). Bone loss around the tooth roots may give an appearance of teeth floating in space,

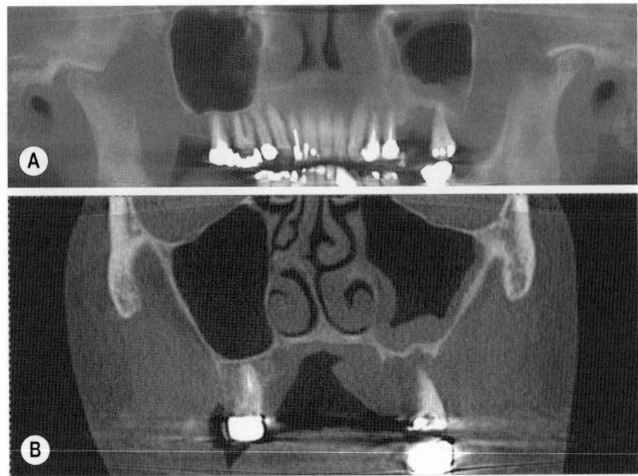

FIGURE 67-72 ■ (A) Panoramic style MPR from a CBCT and (B) coronal slice through posterior maxilla showing a primary SCC of the left maxillary palatal gingivae in the molar region in a patient presenting with a palatal swelling. It has caused alveolar bone destruction, although the antral floor remained intact. There is soft-tissue swelling in the base of the left antrum which was found to be inflammatory.

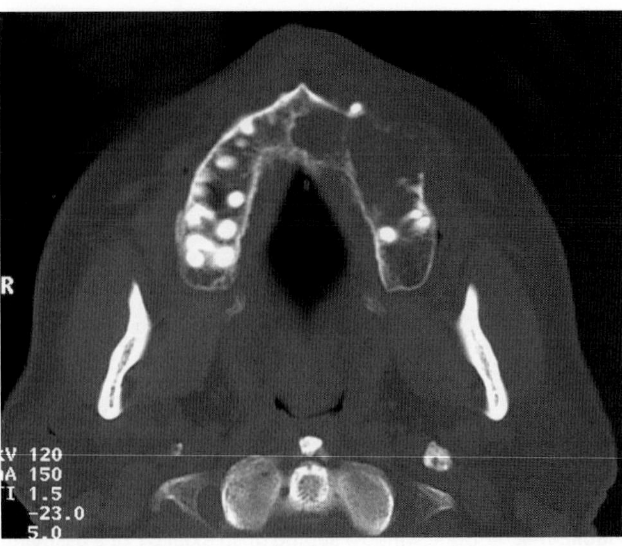

FIGURE 67-73 ■ **Extranodal lymphoma** of the maxilla shown on a bone window setting axial CT at the level of the alveolus. Although a few areas of the lesion are well defined, the overall appearance is destructive, with loss of much of the buccal alveolar plate.

also seen in Langerhans' histiocytosis. Very rarely, carcinoma may arise from malignant transformation of a cyst lining or epithelial residues within the jaw bone to produce an ill-defined osteolytic lesion. It affects older patients usually in the sixth or seventh decade of life.

Metastatic tumour involvement of the jaws is uncommon, mainly arising from breast, kidney, lung, colon and prostate. They form predominantly in the posterior aspects of the mandible, resulting in loss of the outline of the inferior alveolar canal and destruction of the cortical plates. Typically their outline is moderately to poorly defined, with irregular margins that appear destructive without new bone formation. Some metastatic deposits are characterised by the development of several areas, often small, of bone destruction. Although most lesions that metastasise to the jaws are lytic, others, notably from the prostate, can produce bone and appear diffusely radiopaque.

Extranodal lymphoma may affect the head and neck, with the sinonasal area being a common site. When it affects the jaws it can mimic other diseases. It generally appears as an ill-defined non-corticated radiolucency with destruction of cortical bony outlines (Fig. 67-73). **Langerhans' cell histiocytosis**, including eosinophilic granuloma, are occasionally found in the jaws, where they may mimic dental periapical or periodontal disease. The margins are usually well-defined but lack cortication. **Multiple myeloma** is a disseminated disease particularly affecting males over the age of 60 years. About 30% of patients with multiple myeloma may have jaw lesions, with the posterior body and angle region of the mandible being the most frequent site. The typical radiographic feature is of a well-defined radiolucency that lacks a cortical margin and so appears punched out, but some have ragged margins. It usually appears destructive on CT or CBCT.

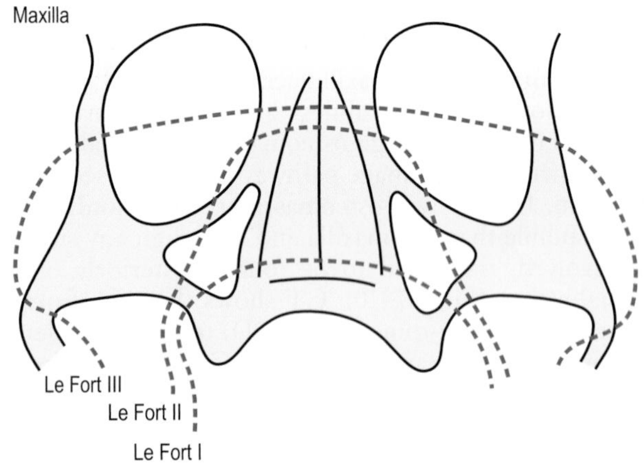

FIGURE 67-74 ■ **Fracture lines in Le Fort I, II, and III fractures.**

FRACTURES OF THE FACIAL SKELETON

The facial skeleton is a complex arrangement of bones, air cavities and soft tissues attached to the skull base. Fractures involving the facial bones are still classified according to the system described by Le Fort in 1900, who defined three principal types of fractures after applying blunt trauma to the faces of cadavers. The classification is contentious because fractures do not always follow the exact pattern he described (Fig. 67-74). Plain films form the initial assessment, but many of these injuries are complicated and require evaluation with axial and coronal CT or cone beam CT.

In **Le Fort I fracture** (Fig. 67-75), the tooth-bearing part of the maxilla is separated from the rest of the maxilla by trauma to the lower part of the face. The fracture line runs from the piriform fossa posteriorly to the pterygoid

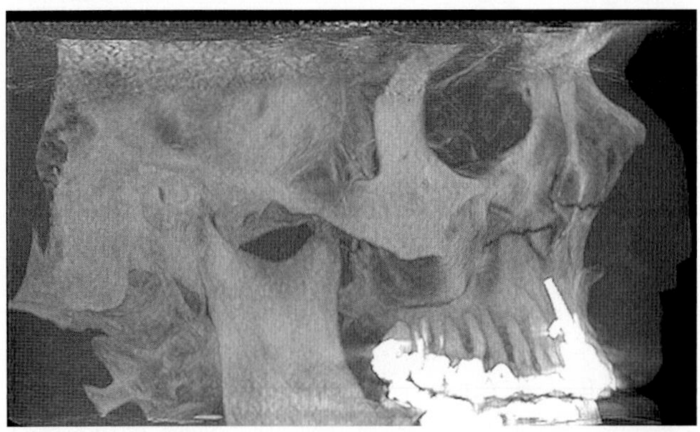

FIGURE 67-75 ■ **Le Fort I fracture.** CBCT ray-sum image of the right side showing an undisplaced fracture running from just above the piriform fossa, below the root of the zygoma to the pterygoid plate. A similar fracture was present on the left side.

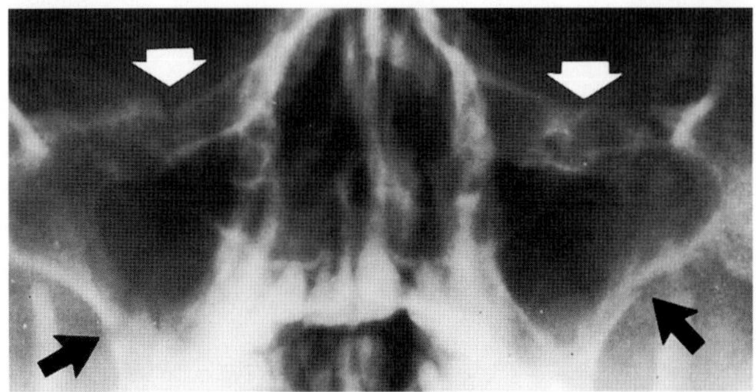

FIGURE 67-76 ■ **Le Fort II fracture.** The fractures of the inferior margins of the orbits and of the lateral walls of the maxillary sinuses have been arrowed. The fracture of the nasal bone is not visible on this projection.

plates, resulting in detachment of the dentoalveolar fragment from the remaining maxilla. The posterior portion may drop, resulting in an open bite, and this is a useful diagnostic feature, as the Le Fort I fracture can often be difficult to detect on radiographs.

Le Fort II fracture (Fig. 67-76) runs along the nasal bridge, through the lacrimal bones, across the medial orbital walls and orbital rims, to involve the anterior and posterolateral wall of the maxillary sinuses and pterygoid plates, where there may be a step deformity. The nasal septum is fractured at a variable level.

In **Le Fort III or suprazygomatic fracture** (Fig. 67-77), there is complete separation of the midface from the cranial base, resulting in clinical lengthening of the face. The fracture line runs through the nasal bones, the frontal processes of the maxilla, posterolaterally through the medial and lateral orbital walls, and through the zygomatic arches. The nasal septum is fractured superiorly.

In practice, many fractures do not exactly fit these descriptions. Fractures caused by sharp-edged objects can produce comminuted fractures of the maxilla (Fig. 67-78) without affecting the tooth-bearing alveolar bone, and some fractures are not symmetrical. For instance, Le Fort I, II and III fractures may be unilateral (Fig. 67-79), or a

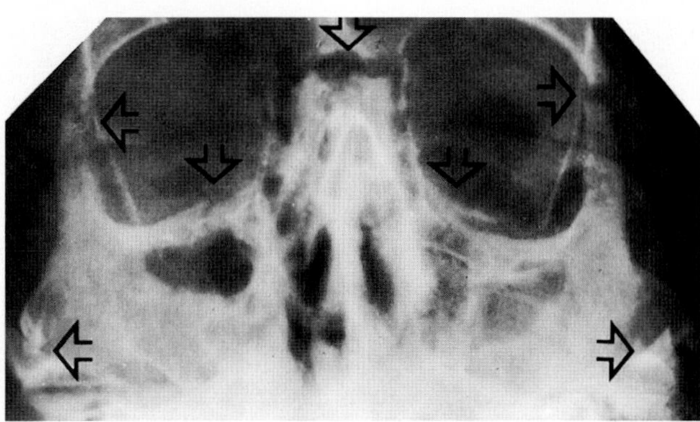

FIGURE 67-77 ■ **Combined Le Fort II and III fractures.** There are fractures of the nasal bones, lateral orbital margins, inferior orbital margins and zygomatic arches. All have been marked with arrows. There is a fluid level in the right maxillary sinus and opacification of the left maxillary sinus.

Le Fort I or II may coexist with a Le Fort III (Fig. 67-77). Nevertheless, the Le Fort classification is still widely used as it allows these complicated fractures to be described simply.

Fractures of the Zygomatic Complex

The zygomatic bone contributes to the lateral and inferior margins of the orbit, the lateral wall of the maxillary sinus and the anterior end of the zygomatic arch (Fig. 67-80) usually with fractures in the region of the zygomatico-frontal suture, zygomatico-temporal suture, infraorbital rim and the lateral wall of the antrum. As not all of the fractures are always visible on a single film, the presence of even one fracture should raise the suspicion that other fractures are present and, dependent upon clinical findings, further imaging may be required. CT is helpful in assessing comminuted fractures of the zygomatic complex as a result of severe trauma (Fig. 67-81). The zygomatic arch may be fractured in association with a fracture of the zygoma as described earlier, or it may be fractured alone as a result of direct trauma to the side of the head and is seen as three points of fracture (Fig. 67-81).

Orbital Blow-Out Fractures

Blunt trauma to the front of the orbit causing a blow-out leads to enophthalmos and possibly diplopia due to muscle entrapment, e.g. inferior rectus. The inward displacement of the eyeball temporarily increases orbital pressure, resulting in outward fracture of the thin bone of the orbital floor or medial wall (lamina papyracea of the ethmoid), but leaving the orbital rim intact. The orbital soft tissues herniate through the defect into the maxillary sinus. This shows as soft-tissue opacity in the upper aspect of the sinus on an occipitomental radiograph and sometimes a fluid level when blood is present. CT is helpful in defining the extent of the defect of the orbital floor and involvement of the external ocular muscles in the fracture (Fig. 67-82 and Fig. 67-83). Coronal and sagittal reformats are helpful. Orbital

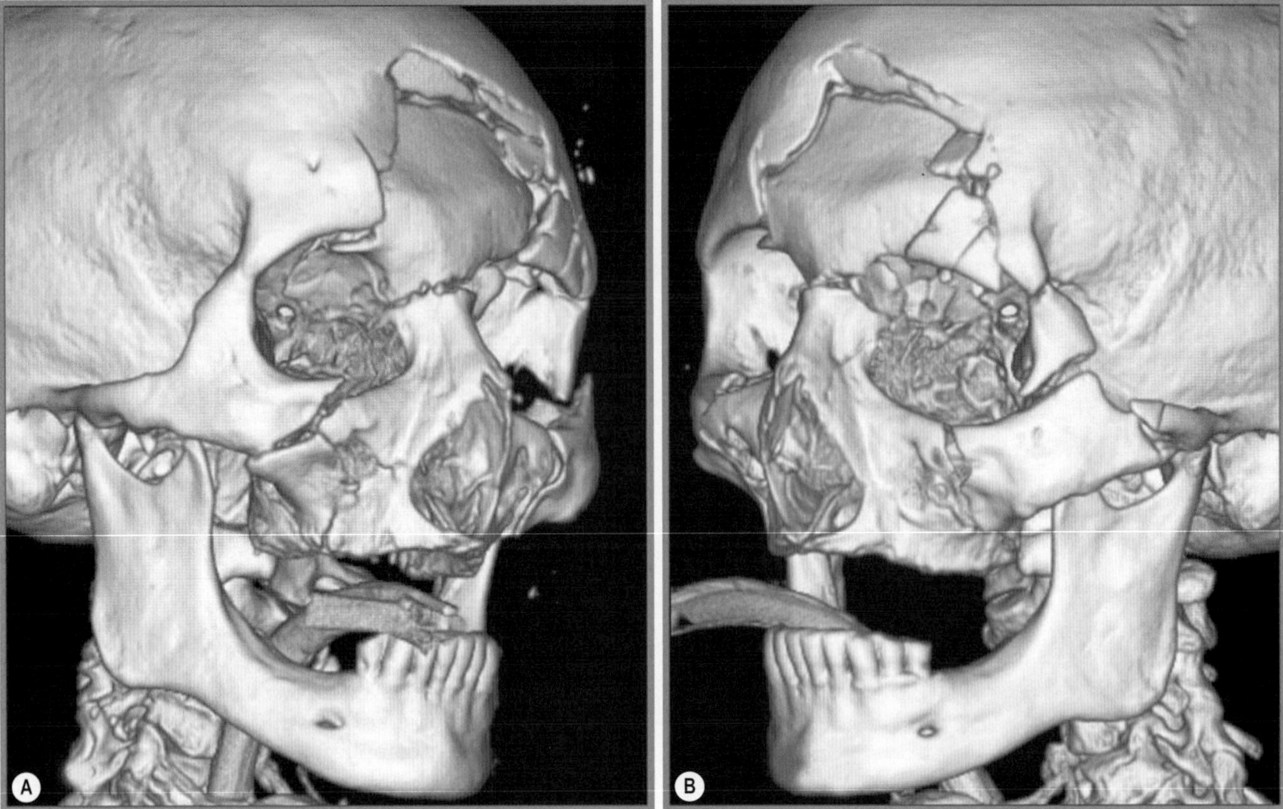

FIGURE 67-78 ■ Three-dimensional CT images showing multiple fractures of the facial bones (Le Fort II and unilateral Le Fort III) and depressed fracture of frontal ethmoidal complex. Note the asymmetrical pattern of the fractures, with the more severe injury involving the left side.

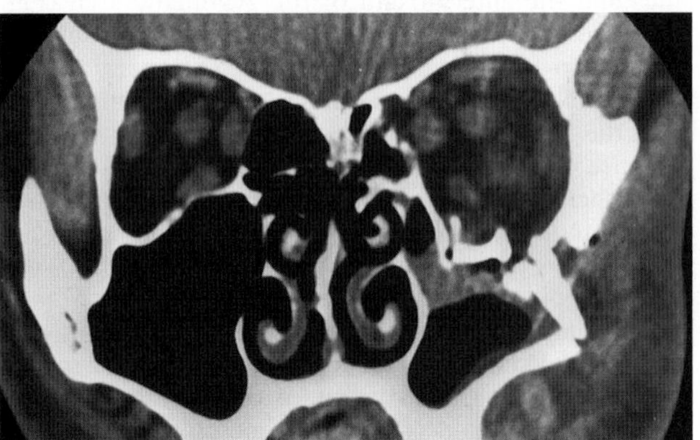

FIGURE 67-79 ■ Coronal CT of a unilateral left-sided Le Fort II fracture. There are fractures of the medial wall of the orbit, the floor and inferior rim of the orbit, and the anterior wall of the maxillary sinus.

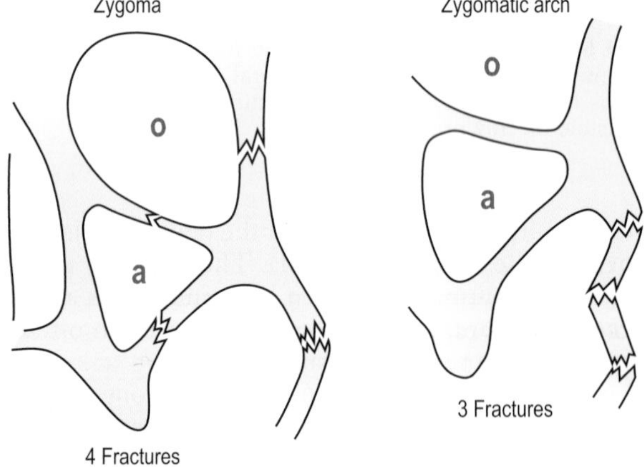

FIGURE 67-80 ■ Diagram of the usual sites of fracture of the zygoma and of the zygomatic arch. o = orbit, a = antrum.

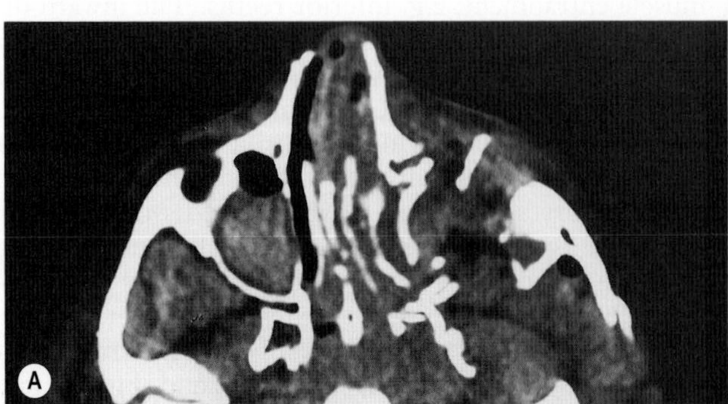

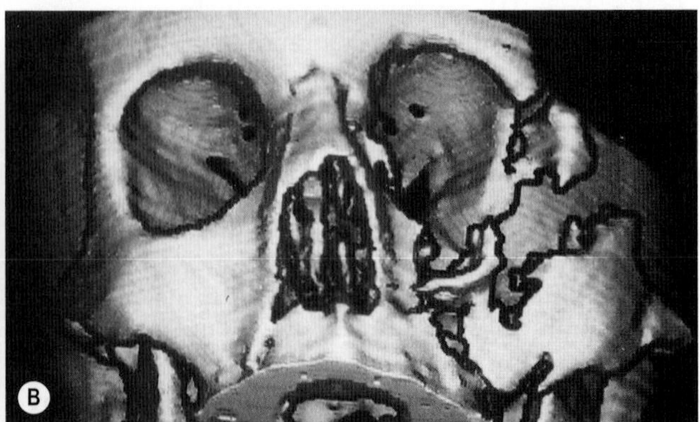

FIGURE 67-81 ■ Comminuted fracture of the left zygoma on axial CT. (A) There are multiple fractures of the anterior, posterolateral and medial walls of the maxillary sinus. There is air in the soft tissues of the cheek and infratemporal fossa. (B) Three-dimensional CT reconstruction of a comminuted fracture of the left zygoma (same case as A).

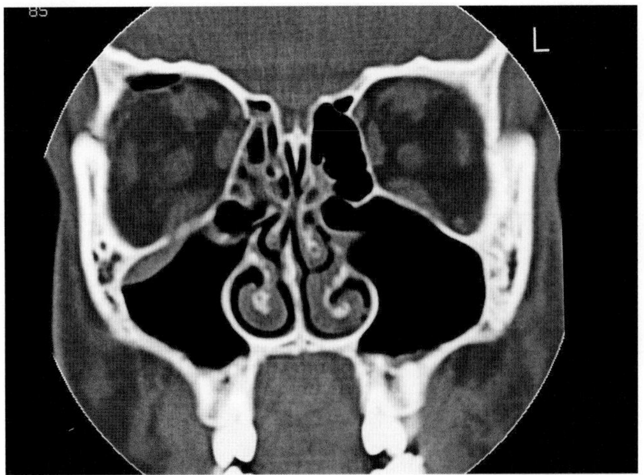

FIGURE 67-82 ■ Coronal CT showing a blow-out fracture of the floor of the right orbit. Fractures of the lamina papyracea (with blood within the ethmoid complex) and orbital floor (with herniation of orbital contents and air within orbital cavity).

ultrasound (US) may also detect orbital wall and orbital rim fractures.[2] Treatment is governed by the extent of the fracture and diplopia if it does not resolve spontaneously. Failure of recognition of a blow-out fracture or fusion of malpositioned bony fragments may lead to entrapped tissues, fibrosis and diplopia.

RADIOLOGICAL INVESTIGATION OF MAXILLARY FRACTURES

A standard occipitomental view is initially indicated, and delayed until the patient is cooperative. Oedema may obscure fracture detail. Fractures of the zygomatic arches are usually apparent on occipitomental (OM) projections, but may be better visualised on an underpenetrated submentovertical view. These views may be supplemented by other radiographs, CBCT, or CT particularly in the more severely injured patient. In CT, thin slices are desirable for good bone detail and need not be contiguous unless 3D reconstruction is planned. CT or CBCT with 3D reconstruction can graphically demonstrate fractures of the facial skeleton (Fig. 67-78 & Fig. 67-83) and 3D data are used in modelling for repair of residual traumatic deformities that require reconstructive surgery.

Questions to answer when reviewing CT: amount of displacement or rotation of the fractured fragments, injury to the globes, optic nerve compression from bone fragments, fracture of the cribriform plate and the possible presence of foreign bodies.

Fractures of the Mandible

Fractures of the mandible tend to occur at specific sites, as shown in Fig. 67-84. They are best demonstrated on a dental panoramic radiograph (Fig. 67-85; or right and left oblique lateral mandibular views), together with a PA mandible radiograph. Parasymphyseal fractures may require intraoral views, which are also useful where the

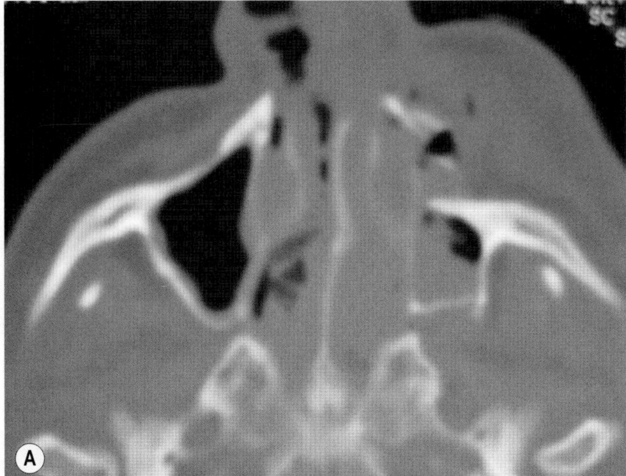

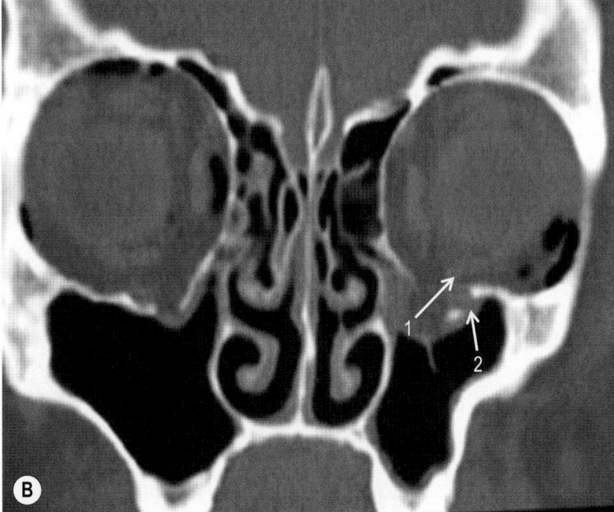

FIGURE 67-83 ■ (A) Axial CT of facial bones. Note depressed rotated left zygomatico-maxillary fracture. (B) Coronal CT of orbits. Note bilateral orbital floor fractures and orbital emphysema. 1 = inferior rectus muscle; 2 = infraorbital nerve.

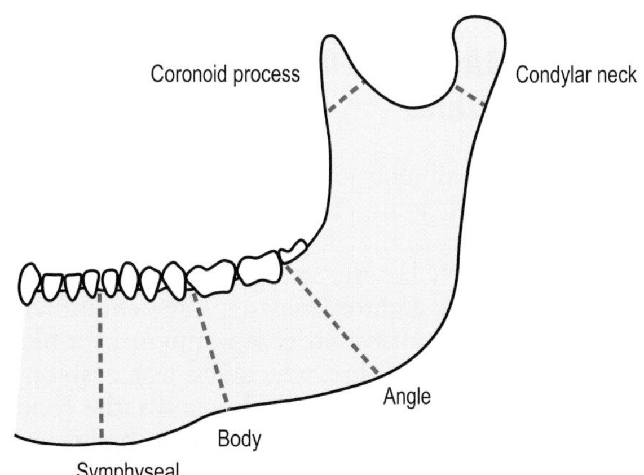

FIGURE 67-84 ■ Line diagram showing common sites of fracture of the mandible.

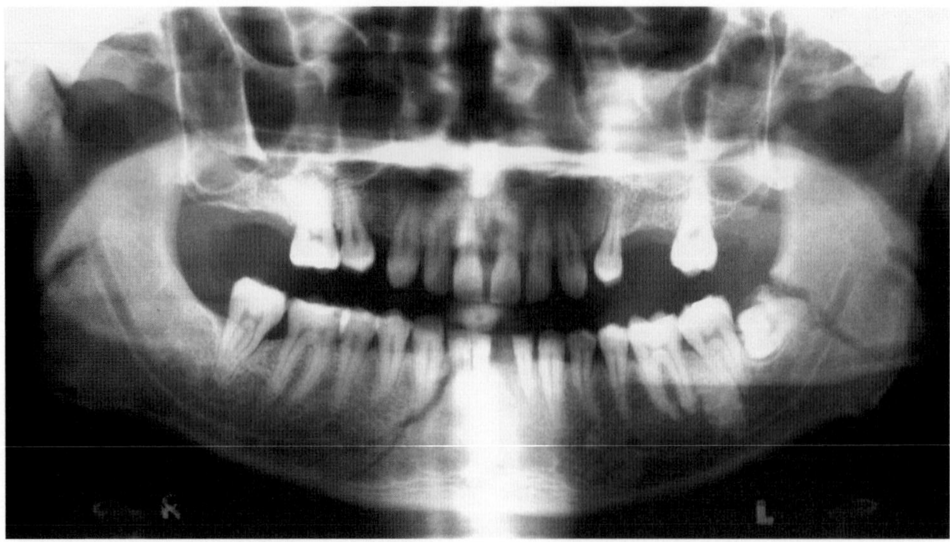

FIGURE 67-85 ■ Panoramic radiograph showing bilateral fractures of the mandible in the right canine region and left wisdom tooth region.

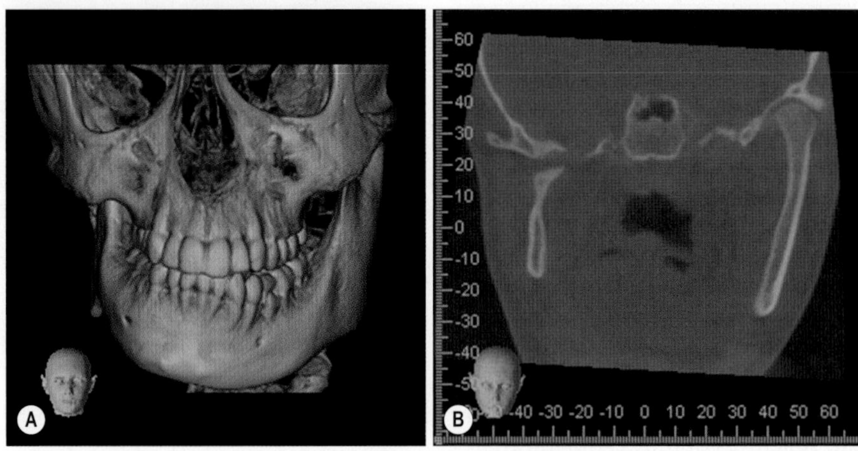

FIGURE 67-86 ■ (A, B) CBCT images of hemifacial microsomia. On the right side the ramus of the mandible and condyle is underdeveloped, resulting in flattening on the right side with facial asymmetry. The right glenoid fossa is shallow when compared with the left side.

anterior teeth are also thought to be fractured. A fracture of the body of the mandible is accompanied by a contralateral fracture in approximately 50% of cases, particularly of the condylar neck.

TEMPOROMANDIBULAR JOINT DISODERS

The temporomandibular joint (TMJ) is a complex diarthrodial, synovial joint. It contains the mandibular condyle, which sits in the glenoid fossa when the mouth is closed. Anteriorly lies the articular eminence and posteriorly the external auditory meatus. The joint is divided into an upper and lower joint compartment by a biconcave, fibrocartilagenous disc, which acts as a cushion for the mandibular condyle. The disc lies above the condyle and is attached posteriorly by fibroelastic tissue to the base of the skull, neck of the mandibular condyle and elsewhere to the fibrous joint capsule. The capsule is lined by a synovial membrane and encloses the joint. Fibres of the lateral ptergyoid muscle insert into the anterior aspect of the capsule and articular disc as well as to the anterior aspect of the condylar neck.

The TMJ is susceptible to conditions that affect other joints including developmental abnormalities, arthritic, traumatic and neoplastic disease.

Developmental Abnormalities

These usually affect the temporal and condylar components, mainly consisting of changes in size and form, and usually result in alteration in the growth of the affected side of the mandible.

Hypoplasia of the mandibular condyle is failure of the condyle to attain full size during its development. It may be confined to the joint or can be part of a local disorder such as hemifacial microsomia, which results in underdevelopment and deformity of the lower half of the face including the ears, mouth and mandible, with a reduced vertical height to the ramus on the affected side (Fig. 67-86).

Condylar hyperplasia causes enlargement of the mandibular condyle due to continued but temporary growth of the cartilaginous growth centre beyond puberty. It produces either a posterior open bite on the affected side or a centre line shift of the mandible relative to the maxilla. Radionuclide imaging may be required to demonstrate whether growth of the condylar cartilage is active prior to corrective treatment. In Hurler's syndrome (gargoylism) the articular surface of the condyle is usually concave instead of convex, an appearance thought specific for this syndrome.

Bifid condyle is believed to result from obstructed blood supply during its development or trauma at an early age. There are no clinical features but radiographically it appears as a notch or indentation of the condylar head.

Temporomandibular Joint Dysfunction

Temporomandibular joint dysfunction is a common condition and consists of myofascial pain, resulting in muscle tenderness, facial discomfort and/or internal derangement of the articular disc. Myofascial pain occurs in all age groups but is particularly common in young female patients. It presents as muscle tenderness, jaw stiffness and headaches, and is associated with stress and anxiety, tooth clenching or other parafunctional habits and occlusal disharmony. The condition is a type of fibromyalgia and as the bony tissues are not affected it has no specific radiological changes.

Internal derangement is an abnormality of the position of the articular disc, which may also show an altered morphology. The normal disc position in relation to the mandibular condyle is illustrated in Fig. 67-87. When the disc becomes displaced, it does so usually in an anteromedial, medial or sometimes lateral position relative to the condylar head. The condition may be painful and cause clicking or jaw locking; however, several studies have shown displaced discs in individuals without symptoms. Discomfort, tenderness and trismus are more prevalent in patients with disc displacement without reduction, particularly in combination with osteoarthrosis and bone marrow oedema.

The diagnosis is made from the clinical findings and in most cases the condition improves or resolves with or without non-surgical intervention. When this fails and more aggressive treatment is planned, or when the diagnosis is uncertain, the disc position can be demonstrated with MRI and the mouth in fully open and closed positions.[3]

Typically the joint is imaged using proton density (or T1) and T2 sequences using 3-mm parasagittal slices, the angulation being determined by the medial angulation of the condylar head. On MRI, the disc appears as a biconcave (bow tie-shaped) structure of low attenuation sandwiched between the anterior aspect of the articulating surface of the condyle and the glenoid fossa. Anterior disc displacement with reduction of the disc is shown in Fig. 67-88. When the mouth is opened, the anteriorly displaced disc reduces or moves back to a normal position relative to the condylar head; this manoeuvre often results

(A) Normal disc relationship

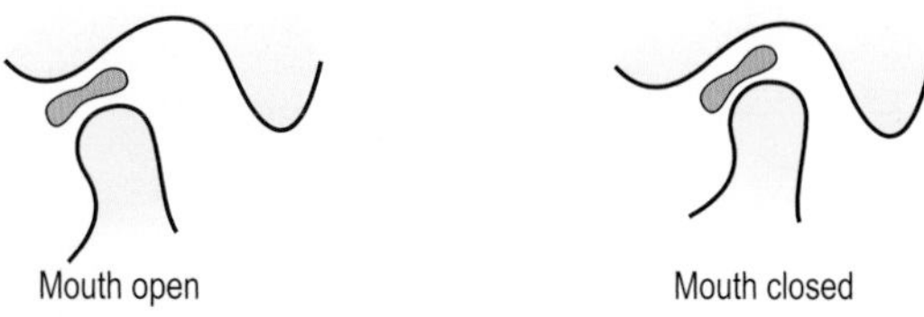

(B) Anterior disc displacement with reduction

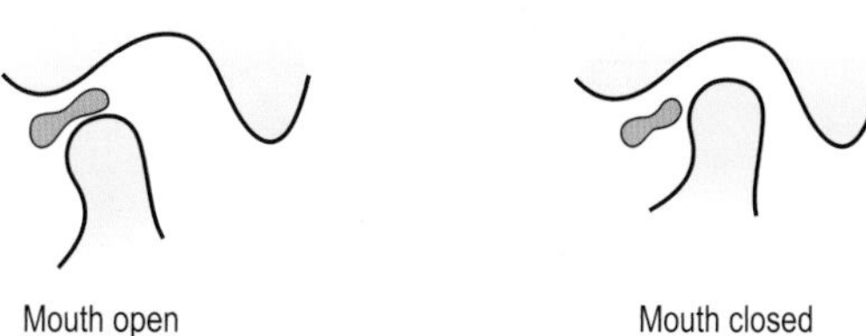

(C) Anterior disc displacement without reduction

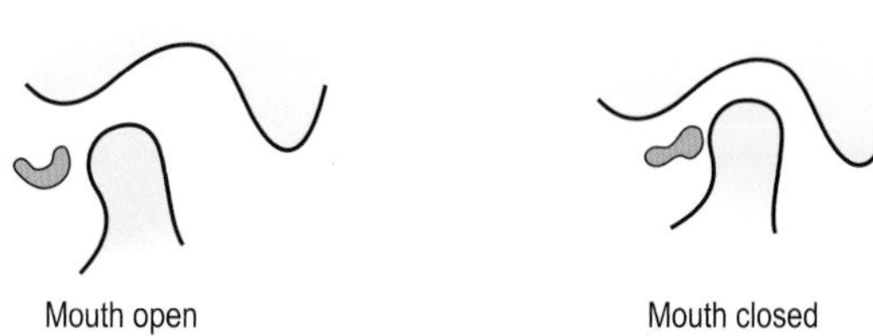

FIGURE 67-87 ■ Diagrammatic representation of the articular disc (shaded). (A) In a normal position in relationship to condylar head, (B) in an anteriorly displaced position with reduction on opening and (C) with a non-reducing disc.

in a click, which can be apparent to the patient and palpated by the clinician. However, if the disc remains anteriorly displaced (Fig. 67-89) it may interfere with forward translation of the condyle, resulting in locking and restricted mouth opening, and pressure on the disc may cause it to become distorted.

T2-weighted images can be used to show joint effusions and inflammatory change. The significance of joint effusion is controversial as it can occur in the non-painful joint. However, it is observed more often in joints with more advanced stages of disc displacement, i.e. non-reducing discs, and it is thought to represent the presence of synovitis.[4] Images taken in a coronal plane demonstrate disc displacement medially or laterally; this view is useful for showing degenerative changes to the articular surface. Using plain radiographs to assess joint space as a predictor of disc displacement has been shown to have a low predictive value.[5]

Arthritides

Degenerative joint disease (osteoarthritis) can develop at any age but its incidence increases with age. It is thought to occur when the joint is unable to adapt to remodelling forces. There may be no symptoms or there may be discomfort and joint tenderness similar to TMJ but crepitus is often present. The radiographic features are diagrammatically illustrated in Fig. 67-90, and include

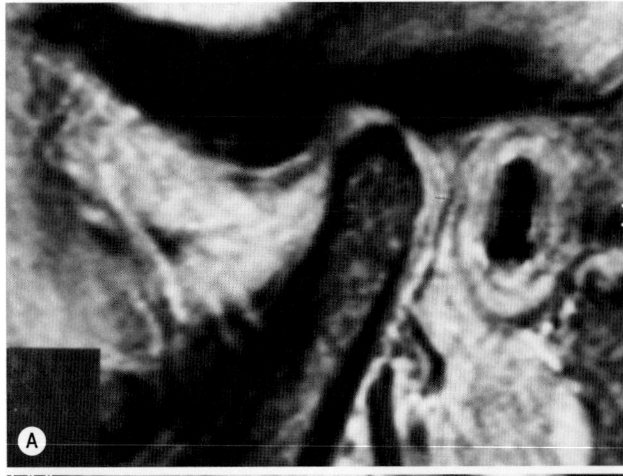

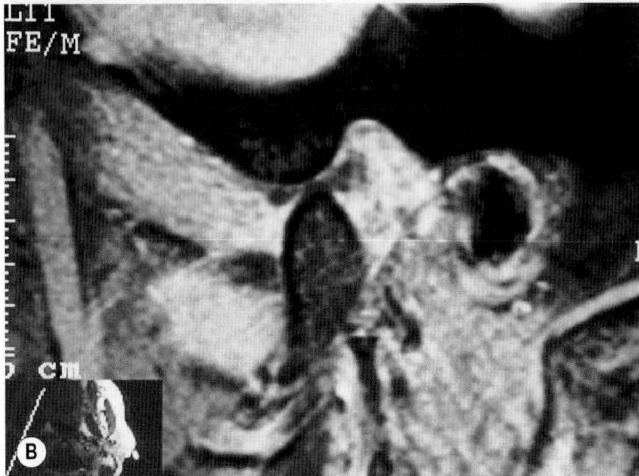

FIGURE 67-88 ■ Anterior reducible subluxation of disc. Fast-field echo (FFE) MRI parasagittal images showing an anteriorly positioned disc (A), which reduces on opening (B) to lie over the condyle.

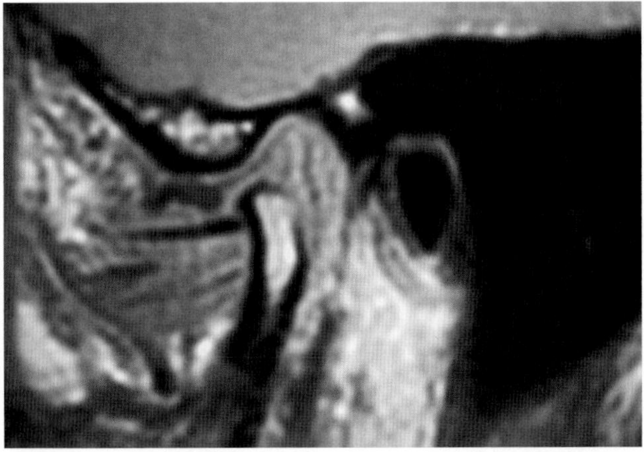

FIGURE 67-89 ■ Parasagittal T1-weighted MRI image with the mouth open showing a non-reducing, anteriorly displaced disc.

flattening and irregularity of the condylar surface, sclerosis and osteophyte formation, which is seen mainly on the anterosuperior condylar surface (Fig. 67-91). Dental panoramic radiography (OPG) demonstrates the mandibular condyles but sometime it is obscured by superimposition of the skull base. Small-volume CBCT provides excellent bony detail of the joint and may be indicated in those suspected of arthritic change not responsive to conventional management.

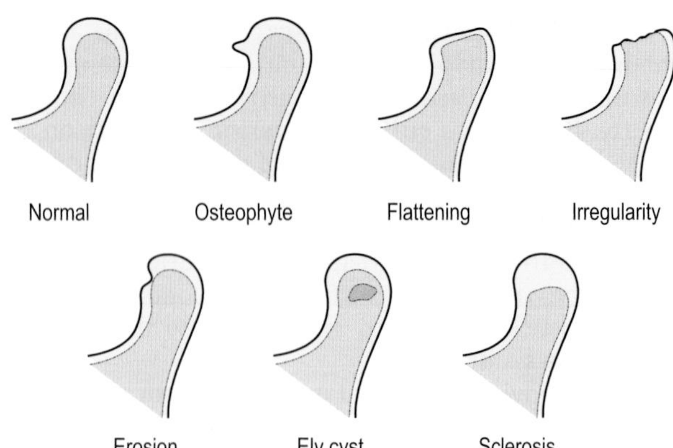

FIGURE 67-90 ■ Diagrammatic representation showing various degenerative changes that affect the mandibular condyle.

Rheumatoid arthritis (inflammatory arthritis) is a common condition in which the TMJ becomes involved in about half of cases. Symptoms include pain, swelling and jaw stiffness. Radiographic changes consist of loss of bone density and formation of erosions leading to a somewhat pointed condylar head. MRI T2-weighted coronal images are valuable for demonstrating the presence of joint inflammation. Other inflammatory arthritides may affect the joint, including systemic lupus, systemic sclerosis, psoriasis, Reiter's syndrome, juvenile chronic arthritis and synovial osteochondromatosis, which results in joint swelling and the presence of numerous loose calcific bodies (Fig. 67-92).

Juvenile chronic arthritis occurs during the first two decades of life and is characterised by intermittent synovial inflammation. It causes pain and tenderness of one or both joints and if severe will affect mandibular growth. The condyle becomes radiolucent and its surface develops erosions and irregularity.

Injury

Isolated fractures of the condylar neck can occur but often accompany fractures of the mandible, especially following a blow to the chin, and are usually visible on a dental panoramic radiograph and a PA condylar view. The slender condylar neck acts as a stress breaker, reducing the likelihood of the condyle being driven up into the middle cranial fossa. Fractures of the condylar neck may be simple and undisplaced or displaced with the condyle being pulled forwards and medially by the lateral pterygoid muscle (fracture dislocation). Intracapsular fractures are difficult to demonstrate on plain films and if suspected may require evaluation with CT if symptoms persist. Haemarthrosis and ankylosis may complicate recovery.

Acute dislocation of the TMJ occurs following a blow to the mandible when the mouth is open. It is diagnosed from the clinical presentation. The role of

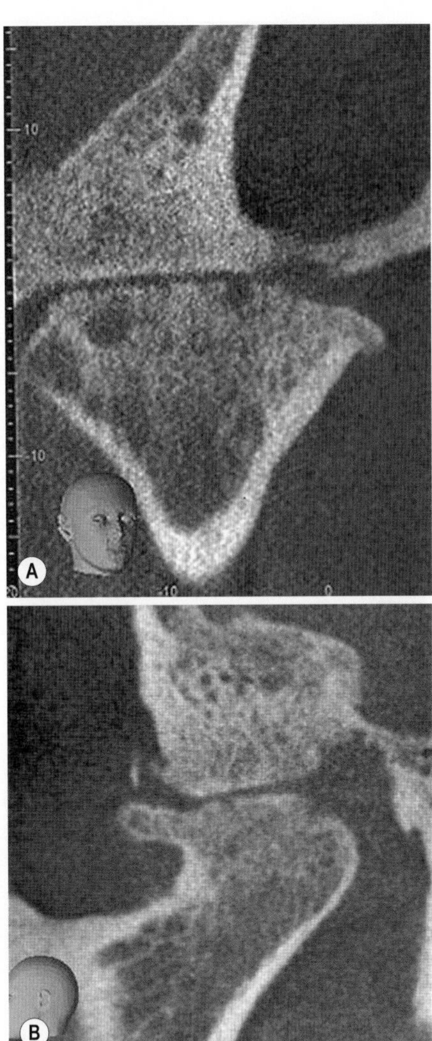

FIGURE 67-91 ■ TMJ degenerative arthritis shown on CBCT imaging. (A) Coronal slice and (B) parasagittal slice, both showing sclerosis of the condylar head with osteophyte formation and focal subchondral radiolucencies (Ely's cysts), slight irregularity of both articular surfaces and a narrowed joint space.

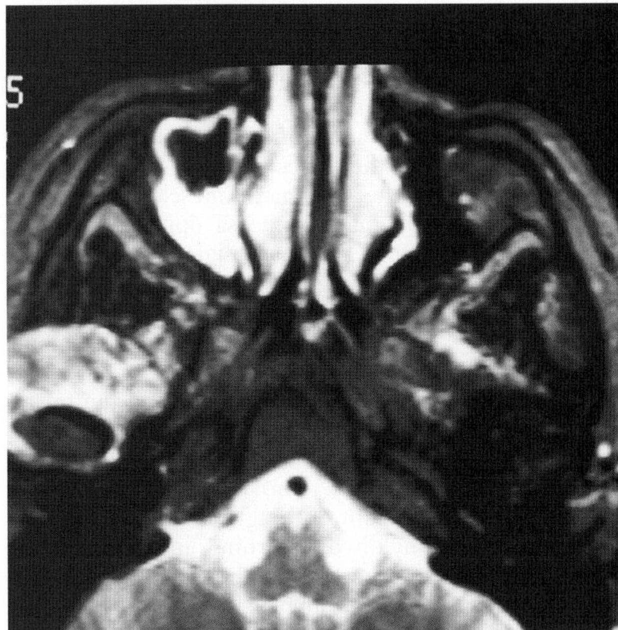

FIGURE 67-92 ■ Osteochondromatosis of the TMJ. Axial T2W MR view showing mass draped around the right condyle.

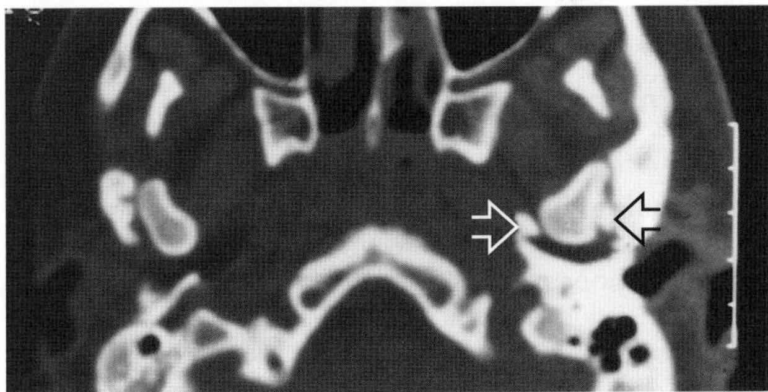

FIGURE 67-93 ■ Bony ankylosis of the left TMJ on axial CT. There are two bone fragments (arrows) between the mandibular condyle and the glenoid fossa, and there is partial bone union between the lateral bone fragment, the condyle and the glenoid fossa. Both mandibular condyles are rotated due to the fractures of the condylar necks. The patient had developed permanent trismus following an accident in childhood. (Courtesy of Dr Otto Chan.)

radiology is to exclude a fracture or other contributing disease. Recurrent dislocation can develop spontaneously and may be a feature of Marfan's syndrome and Ehlers–Danlos syndrome.

Ankylosis of the TMJ may follow a traumatic haemarthrosis or infective arthritis. When this happens in childhood, it may result in hypoplasia of the condyle secondary to concurrent damage to the epiphyseal growth centre. CT or CBCT is required to show the extent of the ankylosis (Fig. 67-93).

Neoplasms of the temporomandibular joint are uncommon and include osteoma, osteochondroma, chondrosarcomas and, rarely, metastatic deposits.

SALIVARY GLAND DISORDERS

There are three paired major salivary glands—the parotid, submandibular and sublingual glands—and numerous minor salivary glands supplying saliva to lubricate, cleanse and aid early digestion within the mouth.

Anatomy

The **parotid gland** lies between the posterior border of the mandibular ramus and the sternomastoid muscle attaching to the mastoid process. It is enclosed in deep cervical fascia and traversed by the retromandibular vein, external carotid artery and facial nerve. The retromandibular vein is easily visible on all forms of cross-sectional imaging and indicates the plane of the dividing plexus of the facial nerve lying just laterally, which divides the gland into a larger superficial and smaller deep portion.

While tumours are more common in the superficial lobe, surgical approach to the deep lobe involves dissection of the nerve branches, with attendant risk of nerve damage. The parotid gland drains through Stensen's duct, running horizontally forward approximately 1 cm below the zygomatic arch on the surface of masseter to turn medially, perforate the buccinator muscle and emerge on a papilla on the buccal mucosa opposite the first maxillary molar tooth. The sharp sigmoid bend in the anterior portion of the parotid duct is a common site for impaction of small salivary stones and is the location of the proposed 'buccinator window anomaly', a possible obstructive phenomenon.

The **submandibular gland** wraps around the posterior free border of the mylohyoid muscle, medial to the posterior body of mandible and descends for 2–3 cm into the suprahyoid neck. The main Wharton's duct passes up from the hilum of the gland, around the posterior margin of mylohyoid, turning anteriorly in the floor of the mouth to open through a small papilla situated on either side of the lingual frenulum, behind the lower incisor teeth.

The almond-sized **sublingual glands** lie anteriorly in the floor of mouth above the mylohyoid muscle. Each gland opens by a single Bartholin's duct or by multiple ducts into the floor of mouth or terminal part of Wharton's duct.

Radiological Techniques and Their Application

Plain radiographs are of limited value in salivary gland disease. An intraoral true mandibular occlusal view detects radiopaque salivary calculi in the anterior submandibular duct, of which 60–80% are radiopaque, while an inflated or puffed out PA view of the cheek may detect the 20–40% of parotid stones that are radiopaque. A negative result does not preclude obstruction.

Sialography has limitations in demonstrating parenchymal disease but remains a highly sensitive test of ductal abnormalities. Cannulation of the parotid duct is normally straightforward but the submandibular duct orifice may be very fine and difficult to identify and usually requires a sialogogue or gland massage to release a bolus of saliva to open the duct orifice. Occasionally the sublingual duct and gland may be incidentally demonstrated on sialography. Direct visualisation of ductal filling under fluoroscopy, particularly using digital subtraction techniques (Fig. 67-94), has benefits over the traditional plain film method and water-soluble contrast media should be used to avoid the permanent foreign body reaction sometimes seen when oily media are extravasated from the ductal system. Sialography has no place in the investigation of mass lesions and is indicated primarily for symptoms directly related to the ductal system such as obstruction and sialectasis. It has the advantage of dislodging mucus plugs and so frequently brings about symptomatic relief.

Interventional sialography offers a minimally invasive alternative to formal surgical sialadenectomy or sialolithectomy. Small mobile stones may be extracted from the duct system by Dormia basket or balloon catheter, and duct strictures dilated by angioplasty balloon (Figs. 67-95 and 67-96).[6,7]

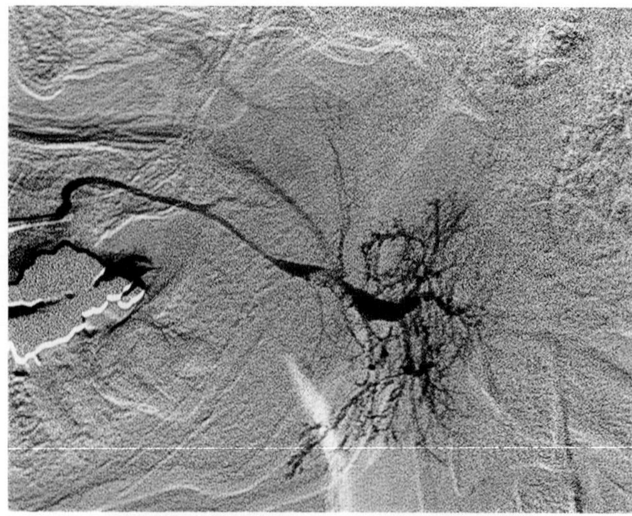

FIGURE 67-94 ■ **Collection of calculi at hilum of parotid gland.** There is minor sialectasis (irregularity of calibre of some intraglandular ducts).

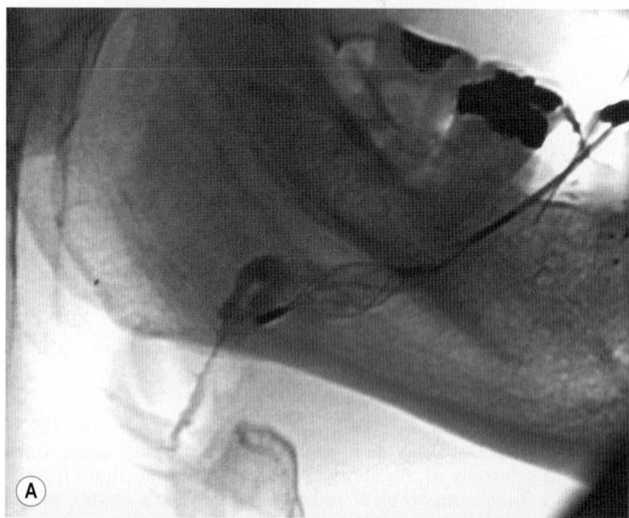

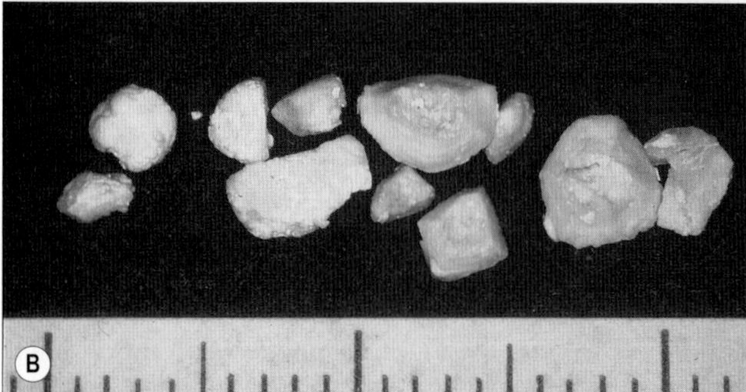

FIGURE 67-95 ■ (A) An intraoperative sialogram showing an **open Dormia basket within the submandibular duct** during removal of a salivary stone. (B) Resultant fragmented salivary stone removed from submandibular gland shown in (A).

Ultrasound (US) has become the first-line investigation for a mass within the salivary glands and for inflammatory salivary gland disease and can readily assess duct dilatation, facilitated by administering a sialogogue prior to investigation (Fig. 67-97). It is highly sensitive

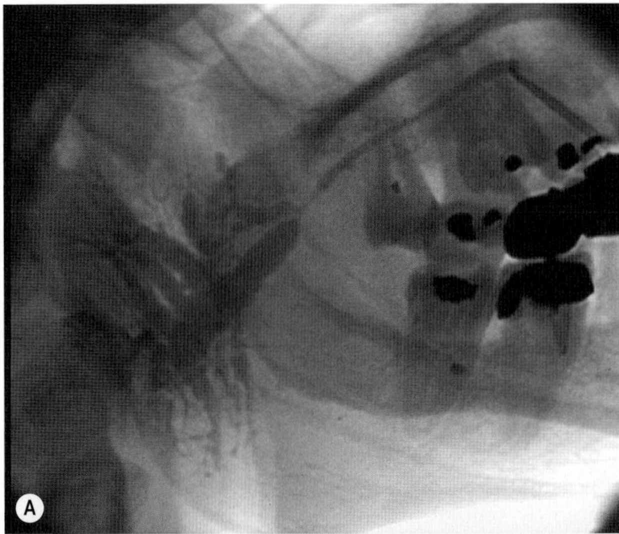

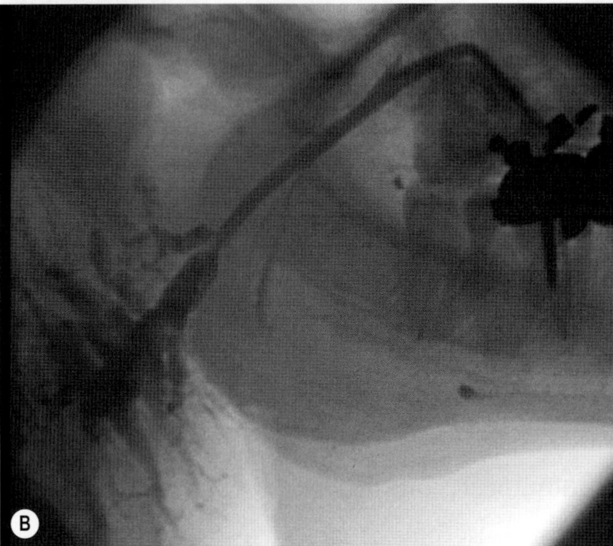

FIGURE 67-96 ■ (A) Sialogram showing a **diffuse stricture at the entrance to the hilum** of the parotid gland. (B) Postoperative sialogram showing dilatation of duct stricture following balloon ductoplasty.

for the 70–80% of tumours located within the superficial parotid gland when compared with CT, though it has limitations when imaging the deep pole where a curvilinear probe may be helpful.

CT is sensitive for the detection of salivary calculi though not resolving enough to show details of duct morphology in obstruction. **MRI** has largely superseded it for tumour assessment though it can be useful in imaging early involvement of cortical bone. The technique of CT sialography has been displaced by MR sialography.

MRI has major advantages for salivary gland imaging, particularly related to its high soft-tissue contrast and multiplanar data acquisition. Gadolinium enhancement is not required in uncomplicated cases, but can be of major importance in the assessment of recurrent tumours (Fig. 67-98).

Magnetic resonance sialography using heavily T2-weighted sequences (Figs. 67-99 and 67-100) allows noninvasive assessment of obstructive disease by imaging stimulated ductal saliva and correlates well with or even

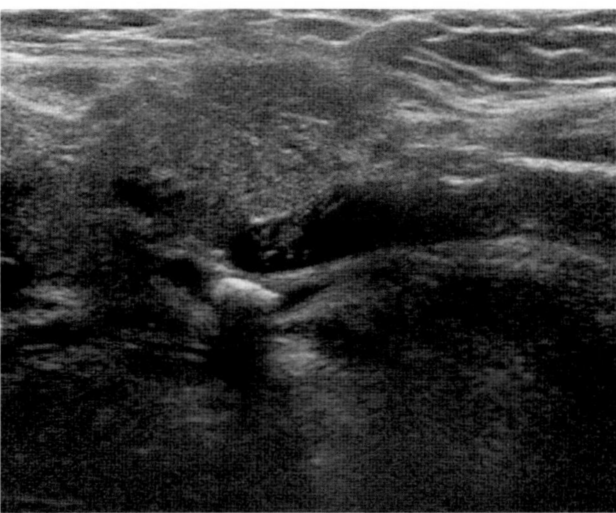

FIGURE 67-97 ■ **Ultrasound image of a salivary stone in the proximal portion of the submandibular duct.**

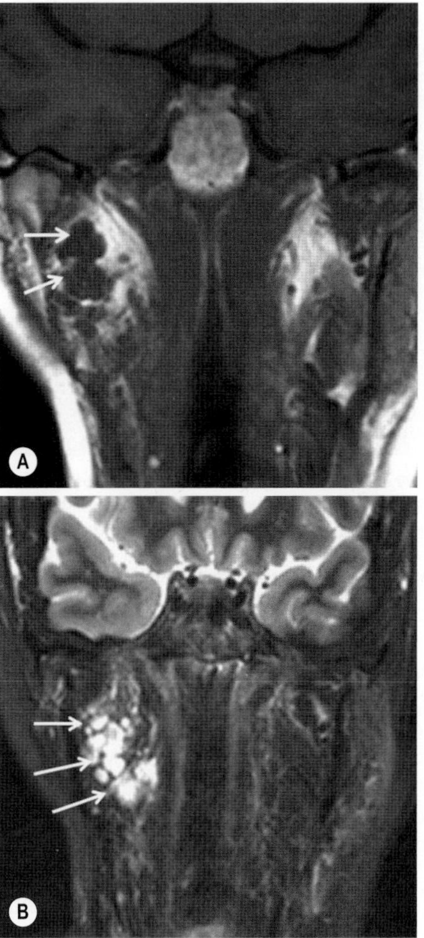

FIGURE 67-98 ■ T1W and STIR coronal MR (A and B) demonstrating multiple recurrent pleomorphic adenoma in parotid bed and parapharyngeal space (white arrows).

improves on conventional sialography in conditions such as **Sjögren's syndrome**.[8,9]

Radionuclide radiology has a limited role in salivary gland disease but may occasionally be used to assess glandular function in obstruction and inflammatory conditions. Low resolution and lack of uptake of ^{99m}Tc-sodium

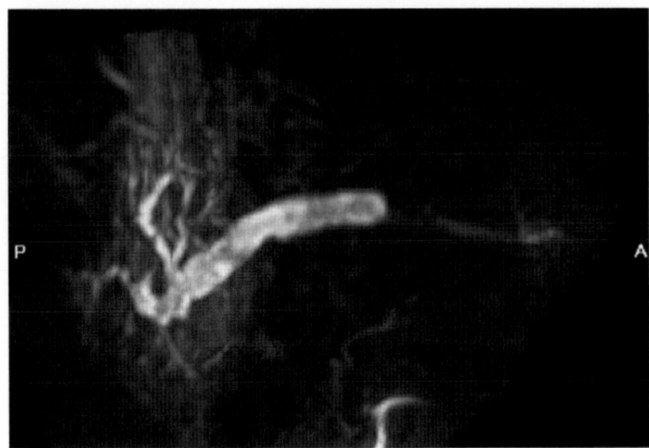

FIGURE 67-99 ■ MR sialography image showing gross dilatation of the main duct and some of the secondary ducts. Areas of low signal in the main duct are due to the presence of several large stones. The distal part of the duct is normal. (Courtesy of Dr M. Becker, Geneva.)

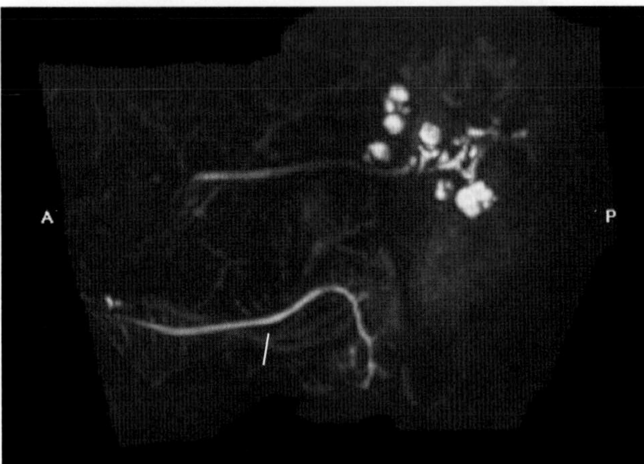

FIGURE 67-100 ■ MR sialography image showing chronic sialadenitis of the parotid gland with focal globular high signal areas of sialectasis within the parenchyma of the gland. The main duct appears normal. The submandibular duct and gland (arrow) (seen later) appear normal. (Courtesy of Dr M. Becker, Geneva.)

pertechnetate in adenolymphomas (**Warthin's tumours**) limits its value in tumour imaging.

Positron emission tomography has been used to image salivary gland tumours but, while being actively taken up by growing neoplasms, it is also concentrated in lymphoid tissue and salivary glands. It has higher uptake in both malignant tumours and in the benign Warthin's tumour.[10] The most commonly used glucose analogue is secreted in saliva, so small tumours may be missed. PET has strengths in assessing the post-treatment neck but may not distinguish tumour from acute infection or early wound healing.[11]

Calculi and Duct Strictures

Calculi cause partial obstruction of the salivary glands, typically resulting in mealtime-related swelling of the affected gland and a predisposition to infection, sialectasis and eventual gland atrophy. They are more common in the submandibular duct system (around 85%) where 60–80% are radiopaque. They may be found close to the duct opening, in the mid duct, at the genu of the submandibular duct or within the gland where they can reach a significant size. Only 20–40% of parotid calculi are radiopaque and are normally detected in the parotid hilum or main duct overlying the masseter muscle. CT is highly sensitive for small stones but US is a convenient and effective way of detecting the majority of salivary calculi (89–94% sensitivity, 100% specificity), except those lying in the most anterior parts of each duct. Single and multiple calculi may be found in dilated duct segments and may be associated with distally placed strictures. Mucus plugs also cause temporary duct obstruction but are radiolucent.

Strictures of the salivary ducts result from inflammation caused by infection or calculi and are best demonstrated by sialography or MR sialography.[12] These may appear point or diffuse with proximal dilatation of the duct system. Approximately 24% of salivary obstructions are due to strictures.[13] 'Sialadochitis' describes the combination of duct dilatation and stenosis that follows obstruction complicated by infection.

Sialectasis

Sialectasis develops in sialadenitis and radiologically demonstrates degenerative changes seen within the terminal salivary ducts and acini as a result of obstruction, infection and other conditions such as Sjögren's syndrome (see later). Progression from widened and tortuous ductules to frank cavitation is seen (cavitatory sialectasis).

Inflammatory Conditions

Infective sialadenitis of viral or bacterial origin causes generalised glandular enlargement on cross-sectional imaging with heterogeneous reduced echogenicity on US, increased uptake on contrast CT and high signal on T2-weighted MRI. Abscess formation is shown as an ill-defined hypoechoic area on US, with equivalent changes on CT and MR; acute inflammation is also evidenced by inflammatory stranding through the gland to the overlying tissues.

Focal chronic sclerosing sialadenitis (**Küttner's tumour**) presents as a localised area of hypoechoic tissue in the submandibular gland on US and may be mistaken for tumour.[14] Sialography is indicated in cases of recurrent infection in order to demonstrate any underlying calculus or duct stricture.

Sjögren's syndrome causes damage to intercalated salivary duct walls, allowing leakage of contrast media during sialography and creating a characteristically fine punctate sialectasis in approximately 70% of cases. This is evenly distributed throughout salivary gland tissue—normally a parotid gland is chosen to demonstrate involvement. Similar abnormalities have been described in association with other connective tissue disorders such as rheumatoid arthritis, systemic lupus erythematosus, ankylosing spondylitis, Reiter's disease, polyarteritis nodosa and scleroderma where, in the absence of clinical

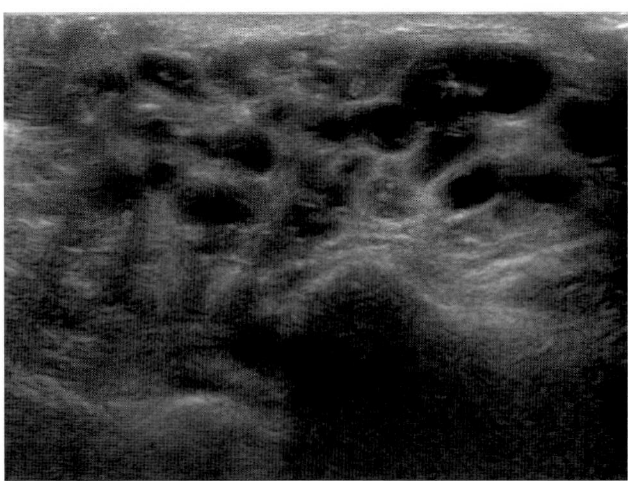

FIGURE 67-101 ■ Ultrasound image of the parotid gland showing the honeycomb pattern of hypoechogenic change in Sjögren's syndrome.

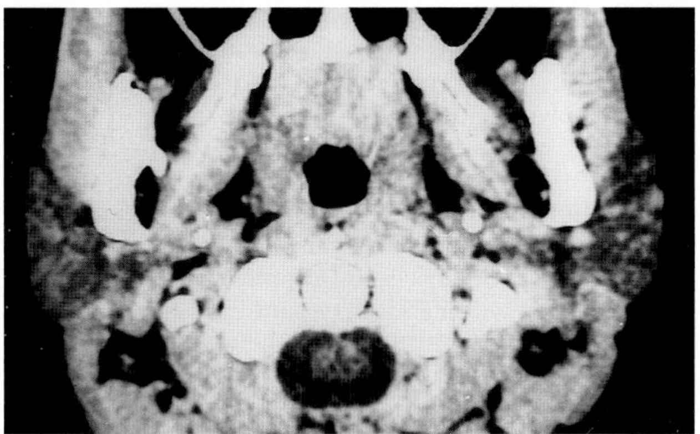

FIGURE 67-102 ■ Sarcoid of the parotid glands. There is generalised glandular enlargement and multiple small areas of decreased attenuation.

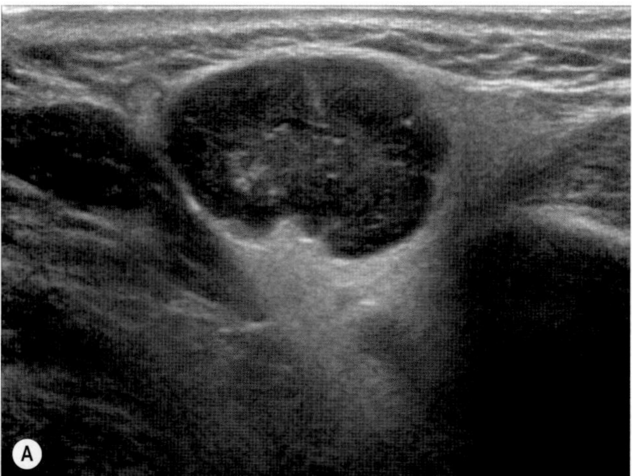

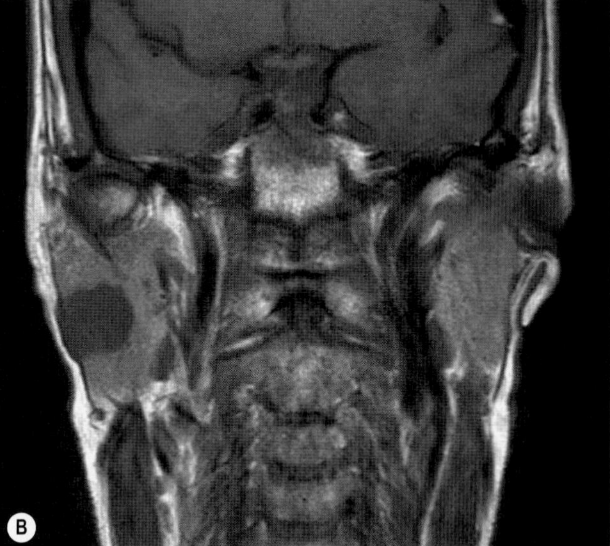

FIGURE 67-103 ■ Pleomorphic adenoma of the right parotid gland (A) on ultrasound and (B) on coronal T1W MRI.

features of Sjögren's syndrome, sialographic signs are estimated to exist in 5–15% of cases. MRI shows a speckled honeycomb appearance in moderately affected cases on both T1- and T2-weighted images, which is said to be specific and similar appearances may be found in the lacrimal glands. MR sialography has shown improved sensitivity and 100% specificity over conventional sialography in diagnosis of Sjögren's syndrome.[9] US shows a heterogeneous reticular pattern of small low-reflective foci (Fig. 67-101) and has a role in monitoring for lymphoma development, which may complicate late Sjögren's syndrome. Sjögren's syndrome sufferers have up to a 44× greater risk of developing mucosal-associated lymphoid tissue (**MALT**) lymphoma.[15]

Sarcoid results in generalised glandular enlargement with multiple small granulomatous areas of low attenuation on CT (Fig. 67-102), giving a reticular hypoechoic pattern or intraglandular nodal enlargement on US and diffuse high signal on MRI. There is, in common with all inflammatory conditions, high activity on ^{67}Ga scintigraphy.

Human immunodeficiency virus (HIV)-associated salivary gland disease is a spectrum of disorders that affects approximately 20% of children and 0.5% of adults with HIV, and includes lymphoepithelial infiltration that may progress to lymphoma. The combination of multiple intraparotid cysts and cervical lymphadenopathy should alert the radiologist to this syndrome, which can occur at any stage from early post infection to full-blown acquired immune deficiency syndrome (AIDS).

Salivary Gland Tumours

Most salivary gland tumours are benign and can develop at any age. Of these tumours, 80% are found in the parotid glands, 5% in the submandibular, 1% in the sublingual and the remaining 15% in the minor salivary glands. The overall incidence of malignancy is 10–20%, and the smaller the major gland, the higher the rate of malignancy.

Benign pleomorphic adenomas (benign mixed tumours) account for around 80% of salivary tumours and typically arise in the superficial portion of the parotid gland, being most common in middle-aged women. These appear uni- or mildly loculated hypoechoic lesions on US and characteristically give a low signal on T1- but high signal on T2-weighted MRI (Fig. 67-103). Although this tumour is benign, if left untreated for many years it has a tendency to become malignant.

The commonest malignant epithelial salivary tumours are mucoepidermoid and adenoid cystic carcinomas. Mucoepidermoid carcinomas have a variable behaviour depending on their degree of differentiation (well, intermediate or poor). Adenoid cystic carcinomas, in particular, have a propensity for insidious perineural spread. MRI can usually identify the presence, but underestimates the extent, of perineural spread. Mucoepidermoid tumours are the commonest malignancy in children.

Other salivary tumours include the benign **adenolymphoma (Warthin's tumour)**, and **lipoma**, and the malignant **acinic cell carcinoma** and **NHL**. Warthin's tumours are notably found in the parotid tail of older men and may be multiple (20%) and occasionally bilateral (approximately 15%). **Lipomas** give a characteristic hypoechoic appearance with numerous layered highly reflective internal strands on US and markedly low attenuation on CT.

Distinction between benign and malignant tumours is based upon criteria, some of which are common to all cross-sectional imaging, others being specific to a particular technique. Benignity is best identified by the presence of a capsule or well-defined outline; however, notably, many salivary malignancies are relatively low grade and are well defined in the early stages. Beyond this, CT may not be particularly discriminating, since many lesions show similarly increased attenuation, though more recently MRI diffusion studies have allowed better differentiation.

MRI has a sensitivity of about 75% for identifying benign features; this can be improved by using gadolinium enhancement. Ultrasound normally depicts benign lesions as well-defined and hypoechoic without regional lymphadenopathy. Additionally, colour flow Doppler indicates vascularity and may present evidence of neoangiogenesis common in malignant tumours. Ultrasound is further used to guide FNA to accurately target non-palpable lesions, but requires experienced cytopathology support to complete an effective diagnostic process and thus alter management.

Concurrent inflammatory change or haemorrhage can be confused with malignancy here. Contrast-enhanced MRI remains preferable for demonstrating recurrent tumour in areas that may be inaccessible to US and that give only non-specific soft-tissue change on CT. Whereas sialography is not recommended for the assessment of mass lesions, the incidental finding of distortion or amputation of intraglandular ducts should arouse concern as to the presence of a benign or malignant tumour, respectively.

Trauma

Laceration of the main parotid duct or of a larger intraglandular branch occasionally results from a penetrating facial injury, or is a rare complication of surgery. In recent injury, US may detect a fluid collection and sialography will show extravasation of contrast from the duct system into the soft tissues. Later, healing frequently results in duct stenosis.

Disorders of Function

Salivary gland function may be quantified by time–activity curves with ^{99m}Tc-pertechnetate scintigraphy and may distinguish between the functioning, the obstructed and the non-functional gland; however, the effective dose is relatively high. This may supplement sialography or be undertaken when sialography is not possible, and has been used to demonstrate recovery of salivary function following removal of an obstructing calculus.[16]

SOFT TISSUES

Effective near-field imaging, and colour flow and power Doppler ultrasound, combined with its established values of high soft-tissue contrast and use in guided biopsy, have led to US being seen as the first-line investigation for masses in the superficial soft tissues of the maxillofacial region. Some operator variability with US and difficulty in interpreting archived static images are reasons why CT remains widely used, as it demonstrates most lesions and assesses their relationship to adjacent structures, although IV contrast is often required for the accurate assessment of cervical lymphadenopathy. MRI, by virtue of its high soft-tissue contrast and multiplanar capabilities, will show most masses with similar or greater ease and has the additional advantage that different sequences may contribute information about the nature of a lesion.

US improves on the clinical examination of the parotid, submandibular and cervical regions, and is a rapid and accurate means of distinguishing between cervical lymphadenopathy, salivary and other soft-tissue neck lesions. Patterns suggestive of malignant involvement of cervical lymph nodes include a round shape (a short-axis measurement over 1 cm becoming significant), absence of hilus, irregular outline, heterogeneous internal pattern including coagulation or cystic necrosis, disorganised peripheral colour flow pattern on Doppler US, nodal clusters and fusion of nodes.[17] US has been found to be better than CT at detecting malignant cervical nodes but has the disadvantage of being unable to access deep nodes such as those within the retropharyngeal region. Identification of these features in combination with US-guided FNAC gave 100% accuracy compared with CT (77–89%), MR (88%) and US alone (83–98%).[18]

Infection in the head and neck region is characterised by spread along fascial-bound compartments (mucosal, parapharyngeal, carotid, masticator, retropharyngeal and prevertebral). CT or MRI both demonstrate such spread (Fig. 67-104).

Malignant tumours within the oral cavity and environs are predominantly squamous cell carcinomas. MRI has become the first-choice examination for imaging both the extent of the local tumour and any regional lymphadenopathy, but may be oversensitive in the assessment of recurrent disease. MRI is also useful for assessing marrow involvement and is steadily encroaching on CT's superiority in demonstrating cortical bone involvement from tumours such as those in the floor of the mouth (Fig. 67-105). The imaging of primary lesions is relatively straightforward, but controversy remains surrounding the place of imaging in the assessment of lymph node

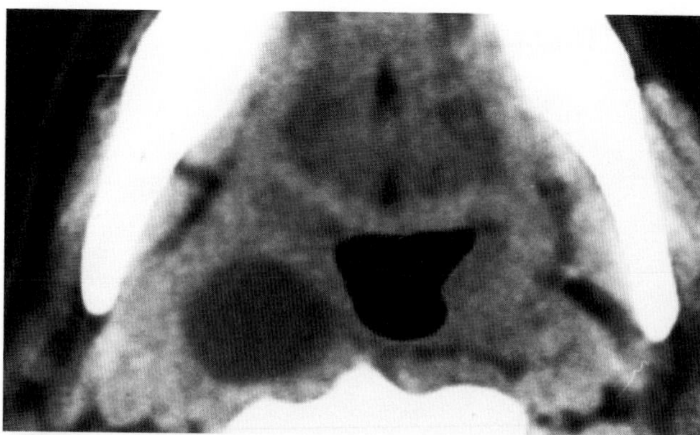

FIGURE 67-104 ■ Abscess in the right oropharyngeal region on axial CT. The patient had received antibiotic treatment for recurrent throat infections and sterile pus was subsequently aspirated from the lesion.

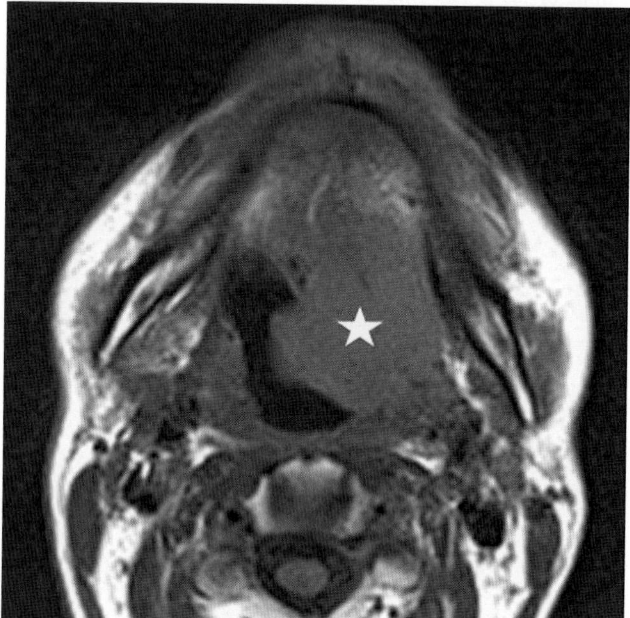

FIGURE 67-105 ■ Carcinoma of the left side of the tongue and oropharynx, T1-weighted axial MRI. The tumour (white star) extends to the midline.

involvement. Some studies state categorically that MRI lacks sufficient sensitivity and specificity to replace elective neck dissection for both staging and prognostic purposes,[19] but more recently imaging has shown increased sensitivity in detecting nodal metastases using US and combinations of PET and sentinel node biopsy. MRI has successfully predicted those patients in need of neck dissection,[20] and has successfully revealed micrometastases (described as intranodal tumour deposits of less than 2 mm diameter at any level of sectioning).[19,21] Positron emission tomography (PET), utilising either ^{18}F-fluorodeoxyglucose (FDG-PET) or ^{11}C-tyrosine (TYR-PET), has a similar sensitivity (72%) to CT (89%) for the detection of lymph node metastases, but this may be improved by co-registration with CT (96% sensitivity, 98.5% specificity), or by supplementary sentinel node biopsy.[20,22] PET and PET-CT are currently viewed as particularly promising techniques for the detection of

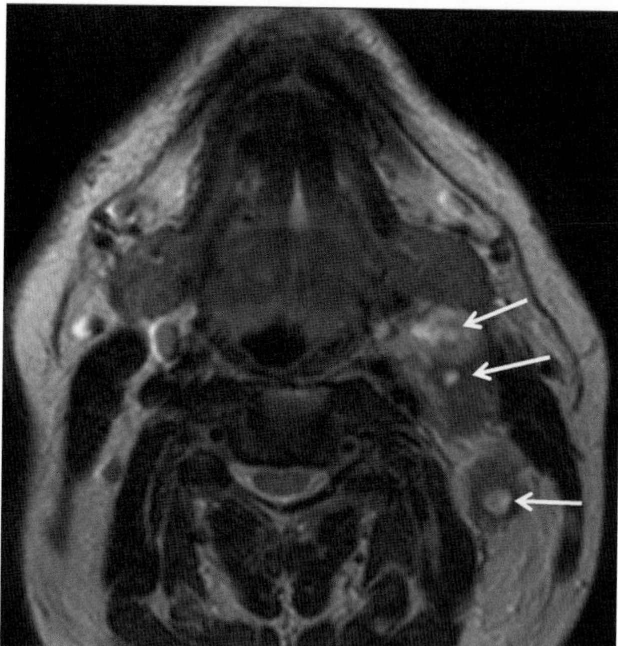

FIGURE 67-106 ■ Axial T2 MR demonstrating multifocal nodal recurrence in the left upper deep cervical region. Note the central T2 high signal in keeping with necrosis (white arrows).

occult primary lesions and along with diffusion weighted MR tumour recurrence especially in the post-radiotherapy situation. Recurrent neck disease, even when subclinical, may, however, be predicted with US and US-guided FNAC. The propensity for regional metastases from SCC to present late after treatment of the primary lesion is an indication for prolonged follow-up (Fig. 67-106). Lymphomas may arise in Waldeyer's ring and the salivary glands, including the minor glands.

Benign tumours of the soft tissues that require imaging in adults are relatively rare other than some dermoids, which present at lines of embryonic fusion; vascular abnormalities, which may grow extremely large, leading to secondary growth disturbances; and salivary gland tumours, as already discussed. Colour flow Doppler US and magnetic resonance angiography may be helpful in assessment, but conventional angiography may be necessary, particularly prior to embolisation. Phleboliths within such lesions may be apparent on plain films.

A wide spectrum of lesions present in newborns, infants and children often as benign vascular abnormalities (Figs. 67-107 and 67-108) but other hamartomas (Fig. 67-109) and malignant tumours may be seen.

Thyroglossal and branchial cysts have characteristic anatomical locations. Thyroglossal cysts arise from epithelial tissue trapped during the embryonic descent of the thyroid gland, and present as defined midline cystic structures lying on a line between the base of the tongue and the thyroid gland (Fig. 67-110). Branchial cysts arise from epithelium trapped during incorporation of the second branchial arch, and present as ovoid fluid-containing lesions lying deep to the sternomastoid muscle, protruding anterior to its anterior border.

Masseteric hypertrophy may be unilateral or bilateral, and often concurrently involves the pterygoid muscles. US is valuable for diagnosis.[23]

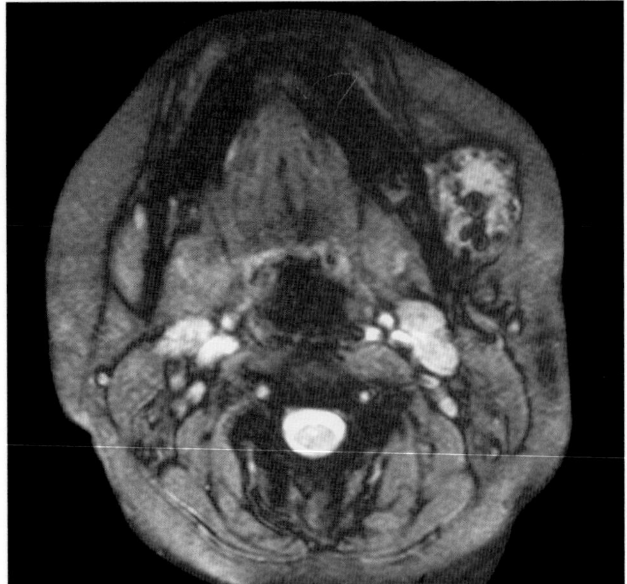

FIGURE 67-107 ■ **Axial MRI of a venous vascular malformation within the masseter muscle of a 10 year old.** Low signal areas represent calcific deposits (phleboliths).

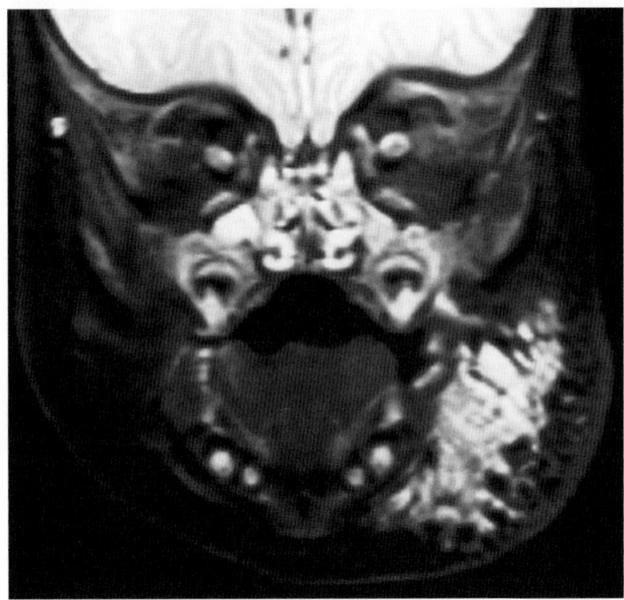

FIGURE 67-108 ■ **Lymphangioma in an infant.** Coronal STIR MRI.

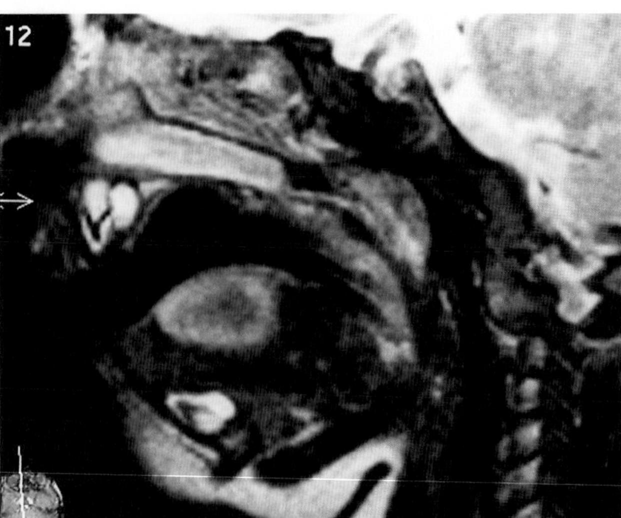

FIGURE 67-109 ■ **Fibroma of the tongue in an infant.** Sagittal T1-weighted MRI.

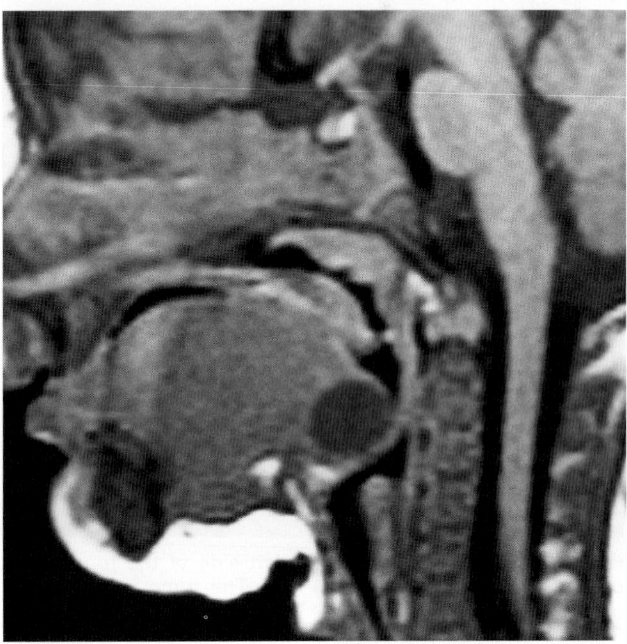

FIGURE 67-110 ■ **Thyroglossal cyst at base of tongue.** Sagittal T1-weighted MRI.

Calcification is occasionally seen in the walls of the facial and lingual arteries in patients with hypercalcaemia or renal failure. Small areas of subcutaneous calcification have been reported in Gorlin's syndrome and Ehlers–Danlos syndrome, and in acne and calcinosis cutis.

ANATOMY OF TEETH AND SUPPORTING STRUCTURES

Introduction

In the primary dentition, there are normally 20 teeth and 32 adult teeth. Both dentitons are identified using one of two systems illustrated in Table 67-1. The Zsigmondy system uses single digits for the permanent dentition and letters for the primary (deciduous) teeth, and the Fédération Dentaire Internationale (FDI) notation assigns double digits for each individual tooth (Figs. 67-111 and 67-112).[24]

Anatomy

All teeth consist of a crown and a root, which may be single or multiple (Fig. 67-113). The crown is covered with a layer of enamel, which is 97% mineral, and thus the most radiopaque tissue in the body. The bulk of the tooth consists of dentine, which is 70% mineralised. The

TABLE 67-1 **The Zsigmondy (Single Digit) and FDI (Double Digit) Systems of Tooth Identification**

Permanent Dentition

Upper Right								*Upper Left*							
(18)	(17)	(16)	(15)	(14)	(13)	(12)	(11)	(21)	(22)	(23)	(24)	(25)	(26)	(27)	(28)
8	7	6	5	4	3	2	1	1	2	3	4	5	6	7	8
8	7	6	5	4	3	2	1	1	2	3	4	5	6	7	8
(48)	(47)	(46)	(45)	(44)	(43)	(42)	(41)	(31)	(32)	(33)	(34)	(35)	(36)	(37)	(38)
Lower Right								*Lower Left*							

Primary Dentition

Upper Right					*Upper Left*				
(55)	(54)	(53)	(52)	(51)	(61)	(62)	(63)	(64)	(65)
E	D	C	B	A	A	B	C	D	E
E	D	C	B	A	A	B	C	D	E
(85)	(84)	(83)	(82)	(81)	(71)	(72)	(73)	(74)	(75)
Lower Right					*Lower Left*				

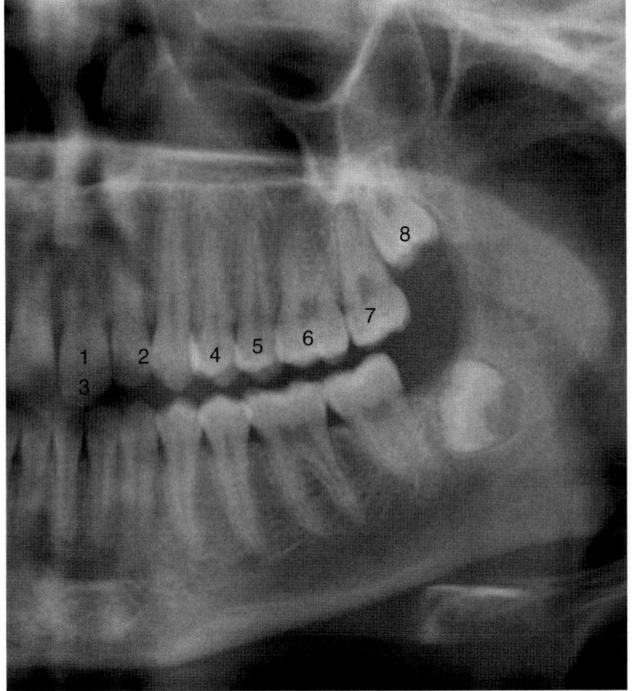

FIGURE 67-111 ■ Part of a panoramic radiograph showing the permanent dentition of a normal 18 year old. The teeth in the upper left quadrant have been numbered 1–8. The third molars are unerupted, incompletely formed and impacted.

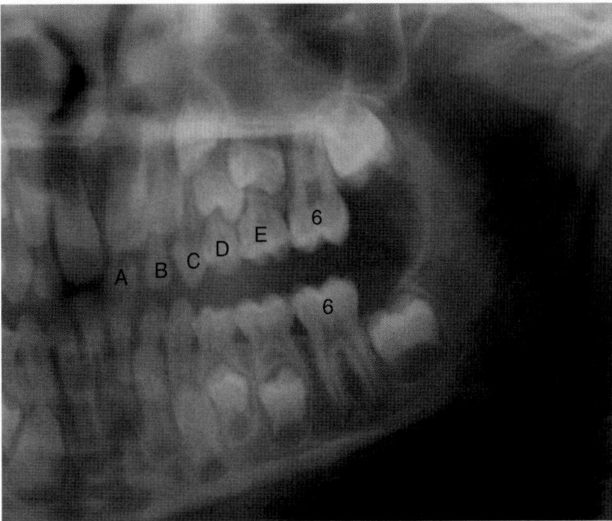

FIGURE 67-112 ■ Part of a panoramic radiograph showing the dentition in an 8 year-old child. The deciduous teeth in the upper left quadrant have been labelled A–E and the erupted first permanent molars (labelled 6).

root is covered by a thin layer of cementum, which has a radiodensity similar to that of dentine and so is indistinguishable from it. Lying within the centre of the tooth is the radiolucent soft tissue of the pulp, which runs from the pulp chamber within the crown along each root canal to the root apex, through which enter the neurovascular bundles. The tooth is supported in the jaws by the periodontal ligament, which consists largely of collagen fibres and appears as a narrow radiolucent line following the contours of the root. These fibres are inserted into a thin layer of dense cortical bone lining the tooth socket (lamina dura), which appears as a linear radiopaque structure, and is continuous with the cortical bone of the alveolar crest.

TOOTH ERUPTION

Normal Eruption

The normal eruption times are shown in Table 67-2. The primary teeth erupt between 6 and 24 months and the permanent teeth between 6 and 21 years. Root formation is not complete until 1.5–2 years and 2–3 years after eruption for the primary and permanent teeth, respectively.

Disorders of Tooth Eruption

The commonest cause for failure of full eruption is insufficient room in the dental arch to accommodate the erupting tooth. This particularly affects mandibular third molars and to a lesser extent maxillary canines. Alternatively a tooth may be prevented from erupting by, for example, a tumour, cyst or supernumerary tooth. Delayed

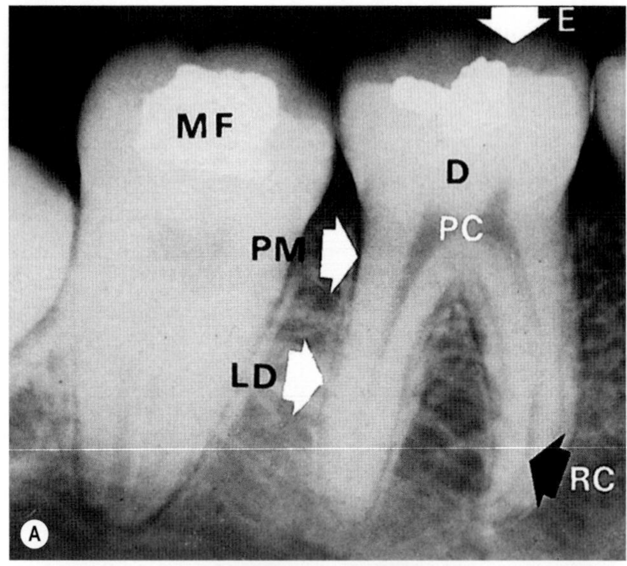

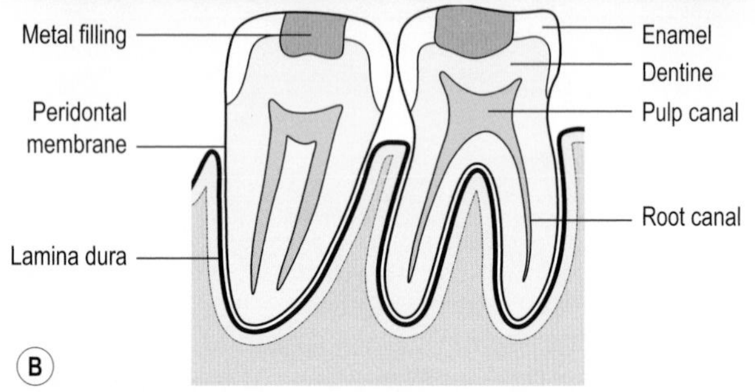

FIGURE 67-113 ■ (A) Periapical radiograph labelled to show a tooth and its supporting structures. E = enamel, D = dentine, PC = pulp chamber, RC = root canal, PM = periodontal membrane (periodontal ligament space), LD = lamina dura, MF = amalgam filling. (B) Corresponding line diagram.

TABLE 67-2 **Approximate Dates of Eruption of the Primary and Permanent Teeth**

Tooth	Designation	Age (months)
Primary Dentition		
Central incisors	A	6–8
Lateral incisors	B	7–10
Canines	C	16–20
First molars	D	10–14
Second molars	E	20–30
		Age (years)
Permanent Dentition		
Central incisors	1	6–7
Lateral incisors	2	7–9
Canines	3	9–12
First premolars	4	10–12
Second premolars	5	10–12
First molars	6	6–7
Second molars	7	11–13
Third molars	8	17–21

eruption occurs in certain endocrine disorders, e.g. hypothyroidism and some genetic abnormalities, e.g. Down's syndrome. Multiple failure of eruption of the permanent dentition is found in cleidocranial dysplasia (Fig. 67-114).

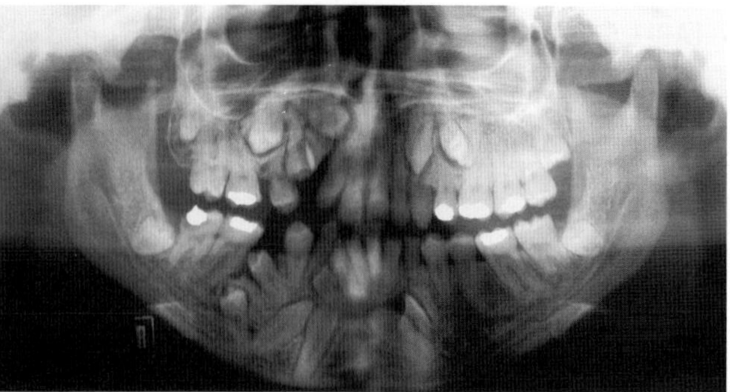

FIGURE 67-114 ■ **Panoramic radiograph of cleidocranial dysplasia in an adult.** There are numerous unerupted teeth including several supernumeraries.

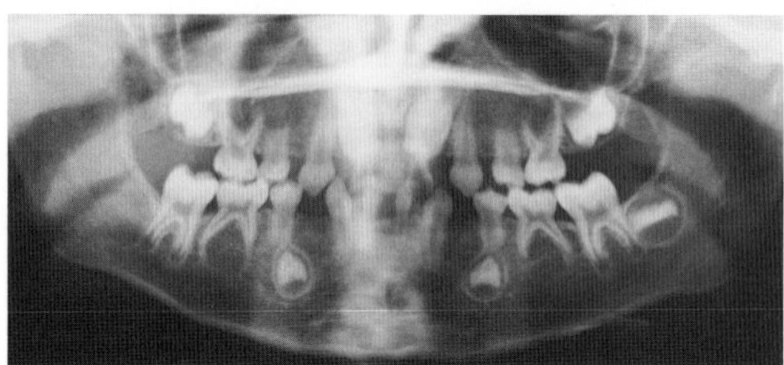

FIGURE 67-115 ■ **Panoramic radiograph showing a marked example of hypodontia involving both the primary deciduous and permanent dentitions in an 8 year-old child.** All four lateral incisors are missing from the primary deciduous dentition and 19 permanent teeth are also absent. Note that wisdom tooth formation normally starts between 9 and 13 years of age.

Disorders of Tooth Development

Variation in Tooth Number

Hypodontia is the absence of one or more teeth and anodontia (rare) where there is complete absence of teeth. Hypodontia most often affects third molars, mandibular second premolars and maxillary lateral incisors (Fig. 67-115). It is seen in association with cleft lip and palate, Ellis–van Creveld (chondroectodermal dysplasia) and facial-digital syndromes. Marked absence of teeth is seen in hypohydrotic ectodermal dysplasia.

Hyperdontia are teeth additional to the normal series and presents as either supplemental or supernumerary teeth. A supplemental tooth is an extra tooth identical in shape and form to an adjacent permanent one and is most frequently found in the lower premolar region. The commonest supernumerary teeth are mesiodens and tuberculates, which form in the maxillary midline. Mesiodens, which are small conical teeth, form chronologically after the primary upper central incisors and occasionally erupt. Tuberculate supernumeraries develop shortly after the formation of the permanent upper central incisors and usually impede their eruption. Marked hyperdontia in the permanent dentition is seen in cleidocranial dysplasia (Fig. 67-114).

Variation in Tooth Size

A tooth that is larger than normal is termed a macrodont and when smaller, a microdont, the latter being more common and typically affecting maxillary lateral incisors and upper wisdom teeth. Radiotherapy and/or chemotherapy can affect tooth development, resulting in arrested development such that they appear smaller than normal with short, spiculated roots (Fig. 67-116).

Variation of Tooth Form

Disturbance of tooth form can affect either the crown or root, or both, and may be developmental or acquired. A dens in dente is due to an infolding or invagination of the enamel into the underlying dentine towards the root, creating the appearance of a tooth within a tooth. A markedly hooked root is called dilaceration. It typically affects a maxillary central incisor either following traumatic intrusion of the primary incisor, which displaces the unerupted developing permanent incisor, or as a developmental anomaly. In taurodontism the pulp chamber is markedly elongated. A tooth that appears particularly enlarged may have split during its development (gemination) or may have become fused with an adjacent tooth.

DISTURBANCES IN STRUCTURE OF TEETH

Enamel

Enamel hypoplasia may affect a single tooth, following a localised periapical infection of its primary precursor (Turner's tooth). But a more generalised form occurs as a complication of severe childhood infections or a nutritional deficiency with the manifestation depending on the time of the insult (chronological hypoplasia).

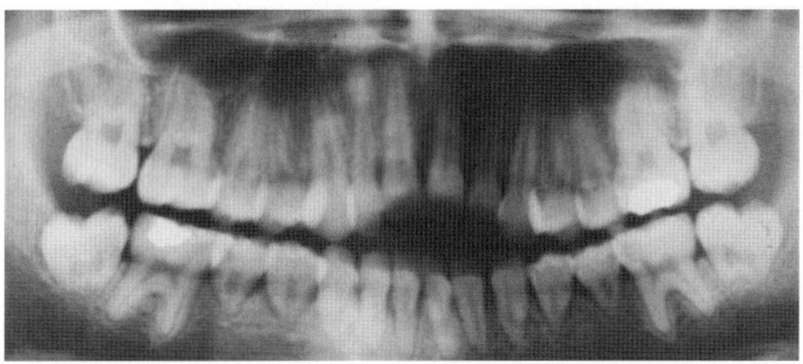

FIGURE 67-116 ■ Panoramic radiograph of a child aged 12 who received radiation to the neck for lymphoma when aged 5 years. The extent to which the roots have failed to form depends on their stage of development at the time of irradiation; thus the lower incisors, which had nearly completed root formation, are relatively unharmed. The lower first molars are slightly stunted and the premolars and second molars extensively shortened. Such teeth do not suffer from excessive mobility.

Amelogenesis imperfecta is a developmental disorder of enamel formation affecting all or most of the teeth in both dentitions. The enamel may show varying degrees of hypoplasia from being pitted (Fig. 67-117), to almost complete absence of enamel when the crown appears angular. Alternatively, the enamel may be of normal thickness but be hypomineralised such that its radiographic density is similar to that of dentine.

Dentine

Dentinogenesis imperfecta is a developmental anomaly of collagen formation that affects the dentine of both dentitions. The teeth are discoloured, having a brown or purple hue. The enamel readily chips away from the dentine so that the teeth rapidly wear down by attrition. The initial radiographic appearance shows bulbous crowns and large pulp chambers, which soon calcify with abnormal dentine formation so that little or none of the root canal is visible (Fig. 67-118). Although the teeth may appear sound, they are prone to infection, resulting in pulpal necrosis and periapical radiolucencies. The appearance of the bone of the mandible and maxilla remains normal, although type IV is associated with osteogenesis imperfecta.

Dentinal dysplasia resembles dentinogenesis imperfecta but is less common. In type I the crowns look normal in colour and shape but the roots of the primary and permanent teeth are short and abnormally shaped, and the pulp chambers become obliterated with dentine prior to eruption. In type II, loss of the pulp chamber and narrowing of the root canals occurs after tooth eruption. In some cases the pulp chambers may be thistle shaped.

Cementum

Hypercementosis describes the deposition of excessive amounts of cementum, typically around the apical half of the root so that it appears bulbous. Usually it is localised to one or two teeth as it is caused by chronic dental infection or occlusal overloading; however, it occurs in Paget's disease of the jaws (Table 67-3) and acromegaly where it is generalised.

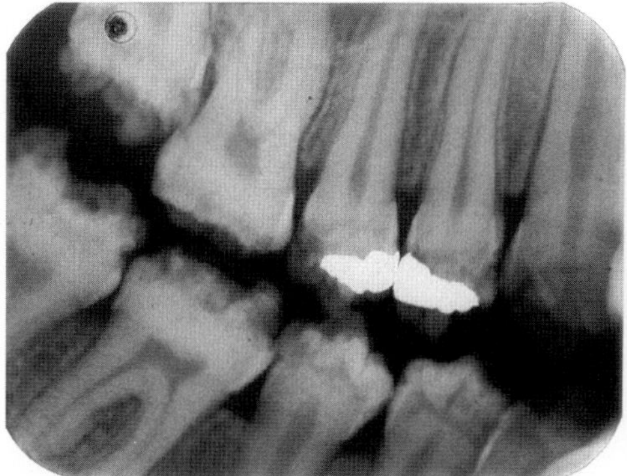

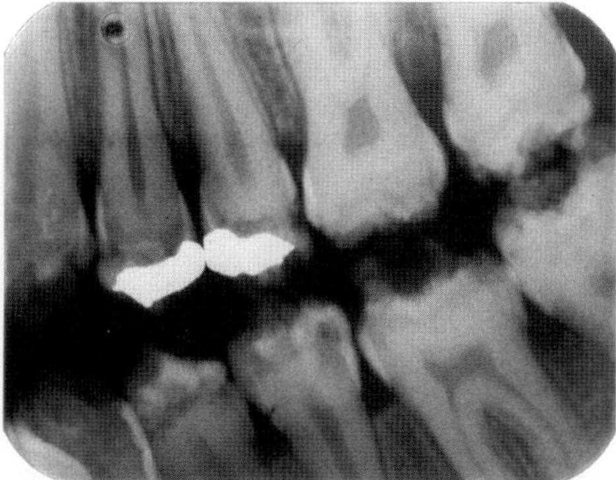

FIGURE 67-117 ■ Intraoral (bitewing) radiographs showing marked hypoplasia and pitting of the enamel, while the dentine appears normal. Several of the teeth are carious.

Miscellaneous Conditions

In **hypophosphataemia (vitamin D-resistant rickets)**, the pulps of the primary and permanent teeth are enlarged with pulp horns that extend towards the enamel/dentine junction, making the pulps susceptible to infection so that the teeth frequently become abscessed. Similar dental features are noted in hypophosphatasia but there is often premature loss of the primary teeth. In both conditions the jaws usually appear osteoporotic (osteopenic).

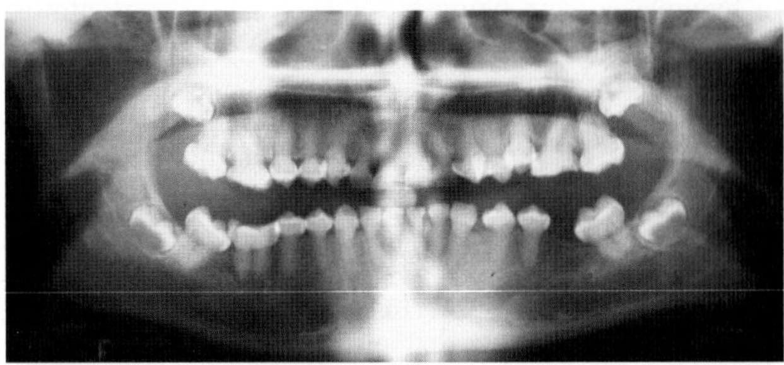

FIGURE 67-118 ■ A panoramic radiograph of a young adult with dentinogenesis imperfecta. The teeth have bulbous crowns, short stumpy roots and sclerosis of the root canals.

DENTAL CARIES

Dental caries is caused by microbial action on sugar with the formation of acid, which causes progressive demineralisation of the teeth, initially of the enamel, and then the dentine, with destruction of their organic components. If left untreated, it leads to the breakdown of the crown and subsequent bacterial infection of the pulp. It develops on the occlusal surfaces of the posterior teeth, on the approximal and cervical regions of the crown or root (if exposed), and as recurrent caries beneath restorations. The rate of mineral loss depends on a number of factors including the amount of sugar in the diet, the lack of effective oral hygiene, the presence of areas of food stagnation and

TABLE 67-3 **Differential Diagnosis of Localised Radiolucent and Radiopaque Lesions of the Jaws**

Unilocular Radiolucent	Multilocular Radiolucent	Radiopaque	Mixed Density
Common			
Alveolar abscess Apical granuloma Radicular cyst (apical) Residual cyst Dentigerous cyst Nasopalatine duct cyst Odontogenic keratocyst	Odontogenic keratocyst Central giant cell granuloma Ameloblastoma	Root fragment Dense bone island Mandibular torus Periapical sclerosing osteitis Hypercementosis Supernumerary tooth Sclerosing osteitis	Fibrous dysplasia (early) Cemento-ossifying fibroma Periapical cemento-osseous Compound odontome Complex odontome Florid cemento-osseous dysplasia Benign cementoblastoma (cementoma)
Uncommon			
Stafne's bone cavity Fibrous scar Fibrous dysplasia (early) Periapical cemento-osseous dysplasia (early) Osteomyelitis Giant cell tumour of hyperparathyroidism Central giant cell granuloma Ameloblastoma Lateral periodontal cyst Paget's disease (early) Brown's tumour of hyperparathyroidism	Giant cell tumour of hyperparathyroidism Ameloblastic fibroma Odontogenic myxoma	Fibrous dysplasia (late) Periapical cemento-osseous dysplasia Florid cemento-osseous dysplasia Ossifying fibroma (late) Complex odontome Compound odontome Paget's disease (late) Osteoma/exostosis	Chronic osteomyelitis Osteosarcoma Paget's disease
Rare			
Carcinoma Metastatic carcinoma Haemangioma Osteosarcoma Odontogenic myxoma Burkitt's lymphoma Lymphoma Eosinophilic granuloma Chondroma and chondrosarcoma Neurofibroma Neurilemmoma Odontogenic fibroma Ewing's tumour Myeloma	Aneurysmal bone cyst Haemangioma Cherubism Glandular odontogenic cyst	Metastatic carcinoma of prostate Cementoblastoma Osteosarcoma Chronic sclerosing osteomyelitis Chronic osteomyelitis Osteochondroma	Calcifying epithelial-odontogenic tumour (CEOT) Calcifying odontogenic cyst Osteoradionecrosis Adenomatoid odontogenic tumour Ameloblastic fibro-odontoma

the health of the individual. It is particularly rapid in those with reduced saliva production following radiation damage to the salivary glands.

The detection of dental decay requires images with good contrast and resolution. Bitewing radiographs are valuable in the detection and monitoring of dental decay, particularly on surfaces not easily visualised and for occult occlusal caries, which can be extensive beneath an apparently intact enamel surface. Panoramic radiographs can be used for gross and widespread dental decay.

A carious lesion appears as a radiolucent zone, corresponding to an area of demineralisation. An initial approximal lesion develops in the enamel just below the contact point with an adjacent tooth appearing as a small triangular shape with the apex pointing towards the dentine. As the lesion progresses, its advancing surface broadens as it extends along the enamel–dentine junction but also penetrates into the dentine, this margin being ill defined (Fig. 67-119). Adjacent carious lesions commonly develop on contiguous tooth surfaces. If left untreated, the caries reaches the pulp chamber and the weakened crown eventually crumbles away. A similar progression is seen on other tooth surfaces. The radiographic detection of dental caries can be difficult, particularly when the crown remains intact and the carious lesion is only marginally more radiolucent relative to the surrounding dentine.

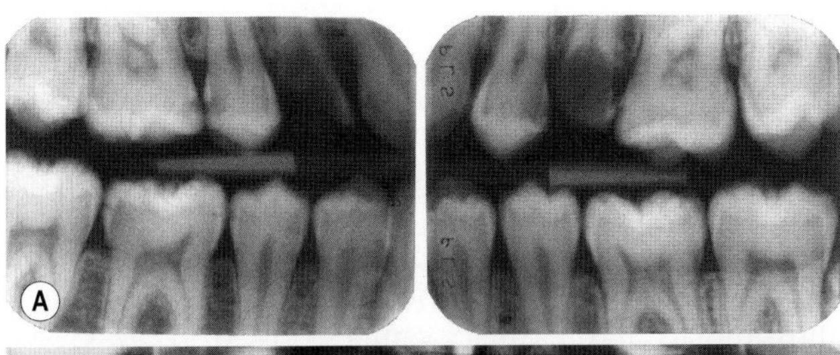

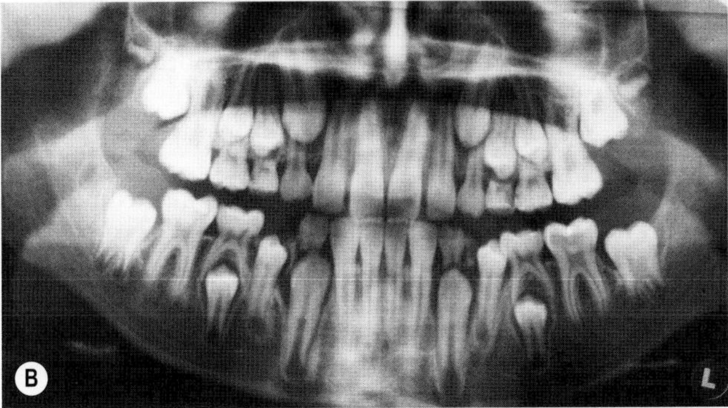

FIGURE 67-119 ■ (A) Bitewing radiographs showing gross caries with crown destruction affecting the upper right first and upper left second premolars. There is approximal caries, shown as radiolucencies of the crowns, at the contact points of the other remaining upper premolars, upper and lower right first molars and occlusal caries in the upper left first molar. (B) Panoramic radiograph of a child aged 10 in the mixed dentition. There is early approximal caries in the upper right deciduous first and second molars. There is gross caries distally in the upper left deciduous first molar, which has complete root resorption by the erupting successional premolar. The lower left permanent first molar has gross recurrent occlusal caries beneath a very small restoration. There is less extensive recurrent caries in the lower right permanent first molar. Both these teeth show periapical bone changes, most obviously the widening of the periodontal ligament space on the mesial root of the lower left permanent first molar, consistent with periapical periodontitis.

DISORDERS OF THE PULP

When dental decay extends to the pulp it usually results in acute inflammation (acute pulpitis), causing severe toothache, but has no radiological manifestations. Chronic pulpitis is much less painful or asymptomatic and results in regressive changes of the pulp due to chronic irritation such as calcific deposits (pulp stones) and sclerosis (narrowing) of the root canals. Generalised pulp sclerosis is a feature of renal osteodystrophy and prolonged corticosteroid therapy. Internal resorption of the root canal or external resorption of the outer root surface may occur following pulp death.

Periapical Periodontitis

Pulpal necrosis results from acute pulpitis (see earlier) or from dental trauma causing interruption of the pulp's blood supply. Bacterial action on the necrotic pulp within the root canal leads to the production of endotoxins, which exit the root apex and incite a periapical inflammatory response within the periodontal membrane (periodontitis) and dental abscess formation. When this is acute, the patient suffers severe discomfort and the offending tooth is tender to touch. Apical periodontitis presents as a widened periodontal ligament space, which appears more prominent than normal. However, the condition may also be chronic and continued progression of the chronic inflammatory process eventually leads to loss of the apical lamina dura and the formation of a discrete periapical radiolucency (Fig. 67-120) due to development of a focal inflammatory lesion, either a granuloma, radicular cyst or chronic abscess. When small, all three conditions have a similar radiographic appearance: i.e. a periapical radiolucency that is circular or oval, usually well defined, the outline being continuous with the remaining lamina dura around the root. Conversely, lower-grade stimulation from a non-vital tooth may result in reactive bone formation (sclerosing osteitis), which appears as an irregularly shaped, largely uniform area of dense bone at the root apex (Fig. 67-121).

CYSTS OF THE JAWS

Cysts occur in the jaws more frequently than in any other bone because of the numerous epithelial cell residues left after tooth formation. Generally they are slow growing and painless unless infected; however, some may reach a considerable size before detection.

Cysts of the jaws are divided into odontogenic, when they arise from epithelial residues of the tooth-forming tissues, or non-odontogenic, these being uncommon and mainly developmental, arising from epithelium not involved with tooth formation. The four most common

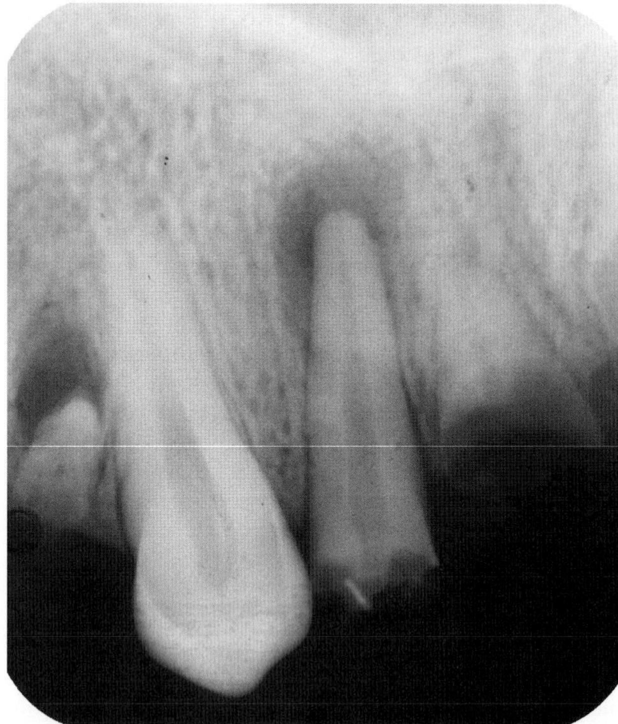

FIGURE 67-120 ■ Periapical granuloma at the apex of the grossly decayed upper right lateral incisor. Although well defined, its margins are not corticated. Note the loss of the lamina dura at the tooth apex. There is a similar but smaller lesion at the apex of the exfoliating upper right first premolar root and the upper right central incisor is markedly carious.

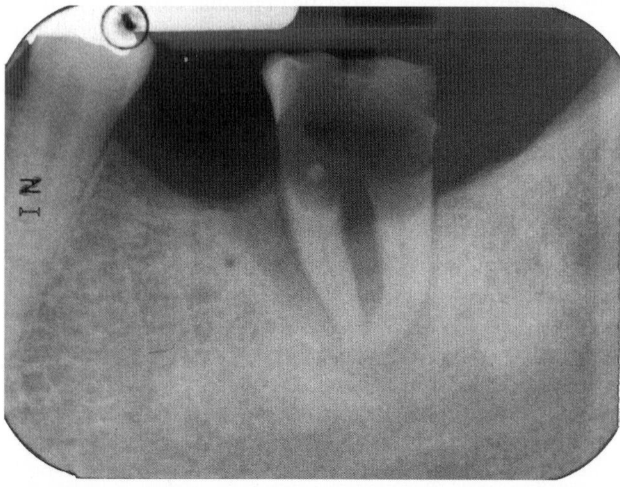

FIGURE 67-121 ■ Periapical radiograph showing sclerosing osteitis. The lower left molar is grossly decayed and its root is surrounded by a zone of radiolucency beyond which the bone is dense as shown by the lack of trabecular spaces.

odontogenic cysts are the inflammatory radicular (dental) and residual cysts, and the developmental dentigerous cyst and odontogenic keratocyst now called the keratocystic odontogenic tumour.

Odontogenic and non-odontogenic cysts have a number of radiological features in common that are characteristic of slow-growing lesions; i.e. they are radiolucent, well defined and often have a cortical margin. With the exception of the odontogenic keratocyst, they have raised intracystic pressure and expand by tissue fluid transudation, and so appear as circular or oval in shape. When large, the bony cortex of the jaws becomes thinned, expanded and then perforated. Jaw cysts tend to displace structures such as tooth roots, unerupted teeth, the inferior alveolar canal and the antral floor.

Odontogenic Cysts

Radicular cyst is the most common (over 50%) of the odontogenic cysts and develops at the apex of a non-vital tooth (see above periapical periodontitis). It arises from the cell rests of Malassez, which are epithelial remnants of root formation found in the periodontal ligament. Any tooth can be affected, but the majority are found on the permanent anterior teeth or first molars. When small (less than 15 mm in diameter) they resemble periapical granulomas but, unlike granulomas, can enlarge well beyond this size (Fig. 67-122). In the upper jaw they expand in to the maxillary sinus, displacing the antral floor.

In many cases extraction of the causative tooth brings about resolution, but when this does not happen, the cyst is then termed a '**residual cyst**'. Thus a residual cyst found in an edentulous part of the jaw has a well-defined, circular radiolucency usually with a cortical margin. A number may regress without treatment and some show dystrophic mineralisation.

Dentigerous cysts (follicular cysts) arise from the reduced enamel epithelium, the tissue which surrounds the crown of an unerupted tooth. They are thus found only on teeth that are buried, particularly mandibular third molars and maxillary canines (Fig. 67-123). Cystic enlargement of the tooth follicle produces a pericoronal radiolucency, which is attached to the tooth at its neck, with the crown appearing to lie within the cyst lumen; however, with large cysts this relationship may not be apparent.

Previously known as the **odontogenic keratocyst**, the WHO now recommend this lesion is called **keratocystic odontogenic tumour** because of its aggressive behaviour, high mitotic activity and association with chromosomal mutation of the PTCH gene. It arises from remnants of the dental lamina, the precursor of the tooth germ. The cyst is thought to enlarge by mural growth, thus behaving more like a benign neoplasm. It appears as a unilocular or multiloculated, elongated, irregularly shaped radiolucency with a scalloped, well-defined margin (Fig. 67-124). It lacks the more rounded characteristics of other odontogenic cysts appearing elongated, an important diagnostic feature. Keratocysts occur most often in the lower third molar/ramus region, where they may displace an unerupted wisdom tooth and resemble a dentigerous cyst. Recurrence is common, being 5–20%, so radiographic follow-up is necessary for at least 5 years. On non-enhanced CT, attenuation values of cyst fluid vary and although most are low the value can range from 30 to 200 Hounsfield units (HU), depending on the proteinaceous content with long-standing, multilocular cysts

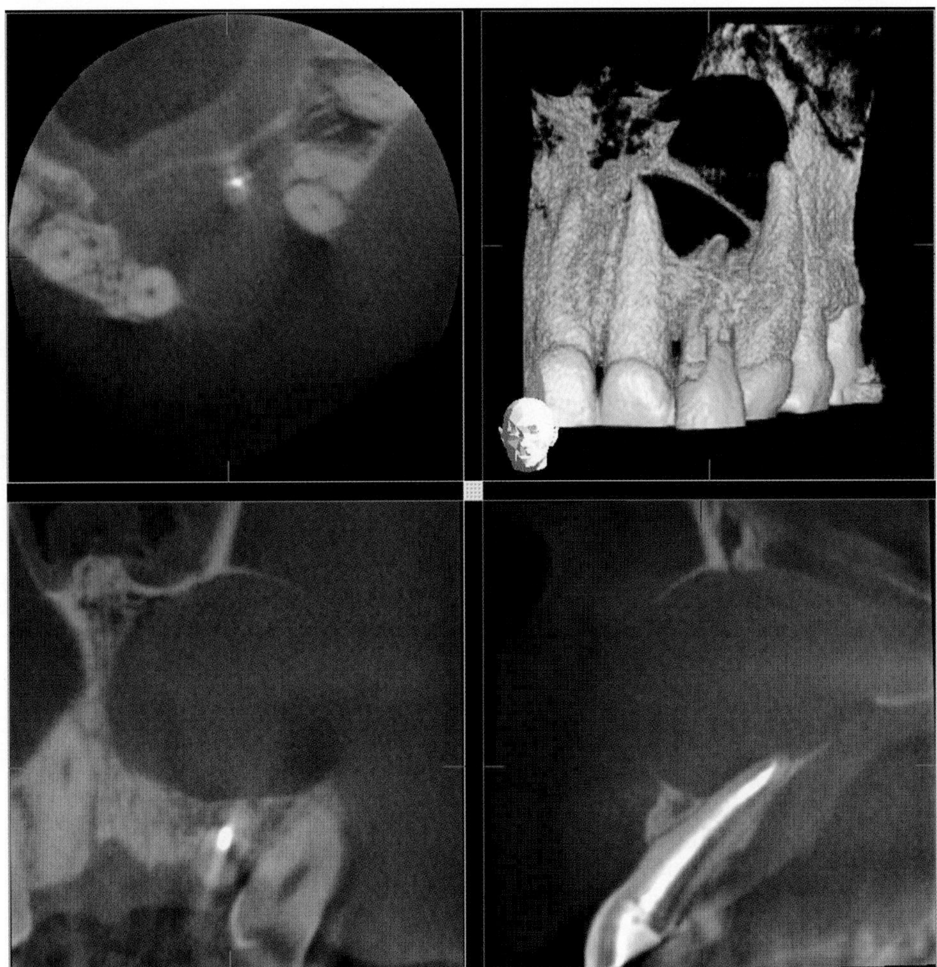

FIGURE 67-122 ■ CBCT sections in three planes showing a corticated radiolucent lesion associated with the **apex** of a root-filled upper left lateral incisor, causing expansion and thinning of the bone buccally and palatally, and of the nasal floor.

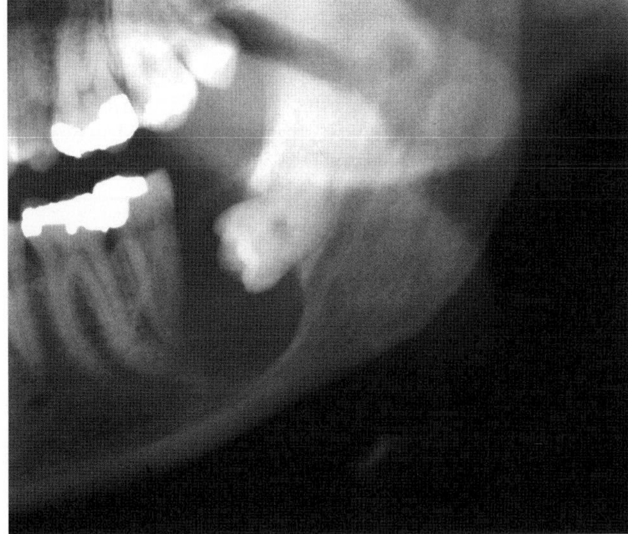

FIGURE 67-123 ■ Part of a panoramic radiograph of a dentigerous cyst arising on a lower left wisdom tooth, which is unerupted and lying horizontally. It appears as a well-defined, circular radiolucency attached to the tooth at its neck. The inferior alveolar canal has been displaced inferiorly.

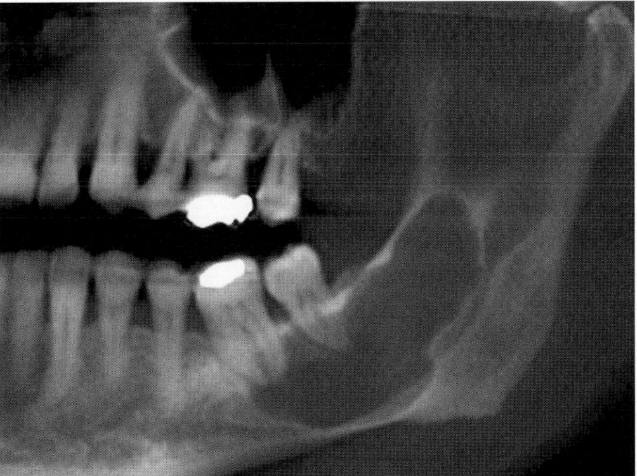

FIGURE 67-124 ■ Part of a panoramic-style MPR on CBCT of an odontogenic keratocyst which appears as an elongated, loculated radiolucency extending from the mandibular foramen to the lower first molar region. There is thinning of the bony cortices but no jaw expansion, a feature associated with odontogenic keratocysts.

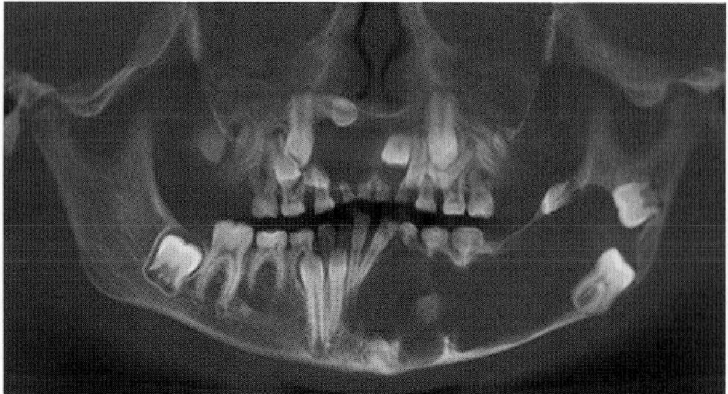

FIGURE 67-125 ■ Panoramic-style MPR on CBCT showing odontogenic keratocysts in the left mandible and anterior maxilla consistent with **Gorlin–Goltz syndrome**. There is marked displacement of teeth by the cysts, which show minimal expansion.

having the higher value.[25] On MRI the lesion has a low or intermediate signal in T1 but a high T2 signal.

Multiple odontogenic keratocysts are a feature of Gorlin–Goltz syndrome (naevoid basal cell carcinoma syndrome; Fig. 67-125), which also includes multiple basal cell naevi, calcification of the falx, bifid ribs, synostosis of the ribs, kyphoscoliosis, temporal and parietal bossing, hyperptelorism and shortening of the metacarpals.

There are several other less common odontogenic cysts. The lateral periodontal cyst is found on the lateral surface of a vital tooth root between two adjacent teeth, usually the lower incisor or canine teeth. The glandular odontogenic cyst (sialo-odontogenic cyst) mainly occurs in the anterior body of the mandible, as a multilocular or lobular, often large radiolucency that may cross the midline and has a tendency to recur.

Non-Odontogenic Cysts

The **nasopalatine cyst** is probably the commonest non-odontogenic cyst that is believed to arise from epithelial residues in the nasopalatine canal. It appears as a round, well-defined, midline radiolucency between, but not associated with, the upper central incisor teeth.

Cyst-Like Lesions

Three other lesions are now described that also resemble jaw cysts but have no epithelial lining. The solitary bone cyst occurs during the first two decades of life, mainly in the premolar/molar regions of the mandible. Its margin is less well defined than those of odontogenic cysts and its superior border typically arches up between the roots of the adjacent teeth (Fig. 67-126). Tooth displacement and root resorption is uncommon. At surgery an empty cavity is found, which subsequently heals after bleeding has been induced.

The **aneurysmal bone cyst** is considered to be a reactive lesion of bone and is characterised by a fibrous connective tissue stroma containing many cavernous blood-filled spaces. It is rare and occurs mainly in the young, with over 90% occurring before 30 years of age.

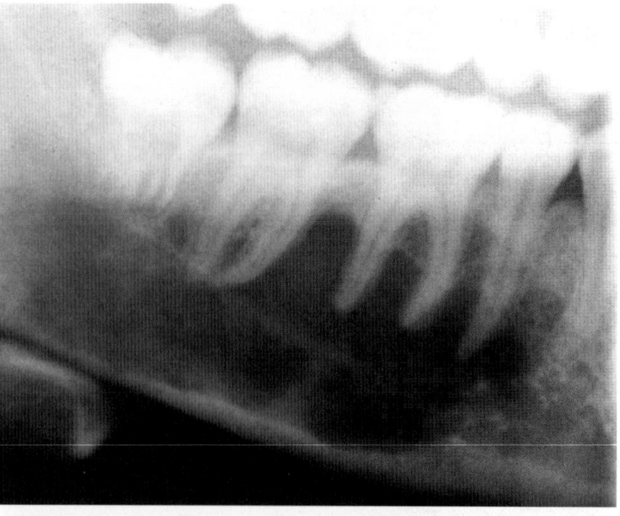

FIGURE 67-126 ■ Part of a panoramic radiograph showing a partially corticated radiolucency in the right mandible involving the apices of the second premolar and first and second molars diagnosed as a solitary bone cyst. Note the characteristic scalloping between the roots of the first and second molars.

It is typically found in the posterior region of the mandible as a well-defined, multilocular, often septated, circular radiolucency. It has a tendency to produce marked cortical expansion. On MRI it has a low-to-intermediate signal on T1- and T2-weighted images. A useful but nonexclusive feature is fluid levels due to blood-filled cavities which are more easily seen on MRI than with CT.

Stafne's bone cavity is asymptomatic and typically found in men over the age of 35 years. It forms a depression in the lingual cortex of the mandible just in front of the angle and below the inferior dental canal. Its origin is controversial and it has been postulated that it arises from pressure from the submandibular salivary gland; however, whereas some may contain salivary gland tissue, a number develop anterior to the gland. On plain radiographs, it appears as a well-defined, punched-out, dense radiolucency which rarely exceeds 2 cm in diameter (Fig. 67-127). Its appearance is characteristic and so does not require further imaging or biopsy. However, if CT or MRI is performed, the cavity is often found to contain fat.

DISEASE OF THE PERIODONTIUM

Introduction

There are several disorders that affect the support for the teeth, the **periodontium**, and these are referred to as periodontal disease. Intraoral views (bitewings and periapical films) are helpful in assessing the amount of remaining bone support for the teeth, the pattern of bone loss, the detection of subgingival calculus and local aggravating factors such as poorly contoured dental restorations. Dental panoramic radiography can be used for widespread advanced disease, although it does not demonstrate the anterior teeth particularly well.

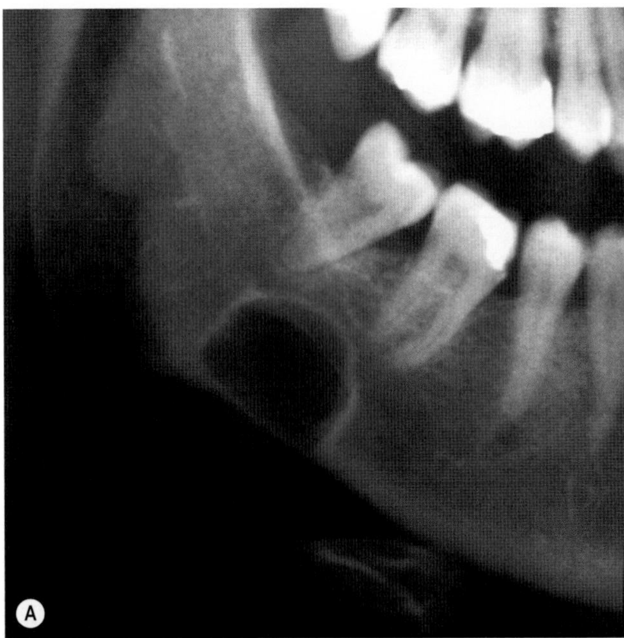

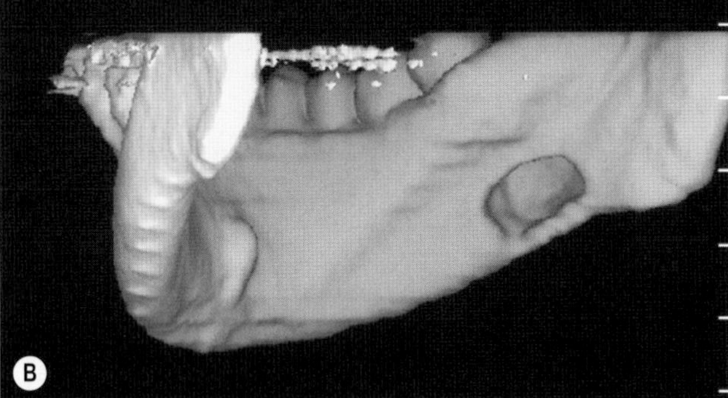

FIGURE 67-127 ■ (A) Part of a panoramic radiograph showing a corticated radiolucency between the inferior alveolar canal and the lower border of the mandible due to the presence of a Stafne's bone cavity. The 3D CT (B) shows the depression on the lingual aspect of the mandible.

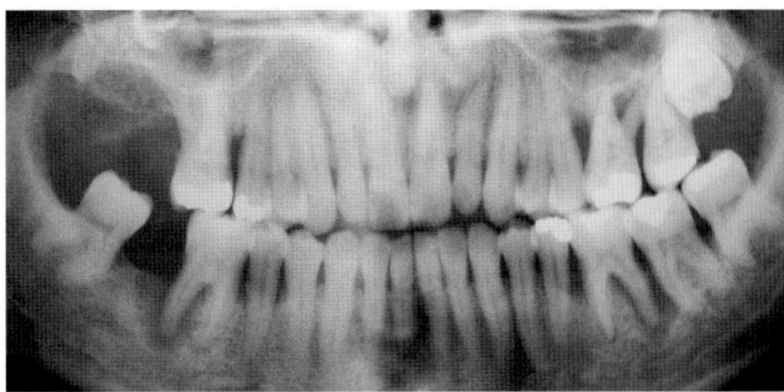

FIGURE 67-128 ■ **Part of a panoramic radiograph of a man aged 40 with smoking-related aggressive chronic periodontal disease.** There is furcation involvement of the upper left first molar and loss of up to 70% of the bony attachment between the upper right first molar and second premolar and similarly on the upper left side. Combined periodontal–endodontic lesions affect both lower first molars.

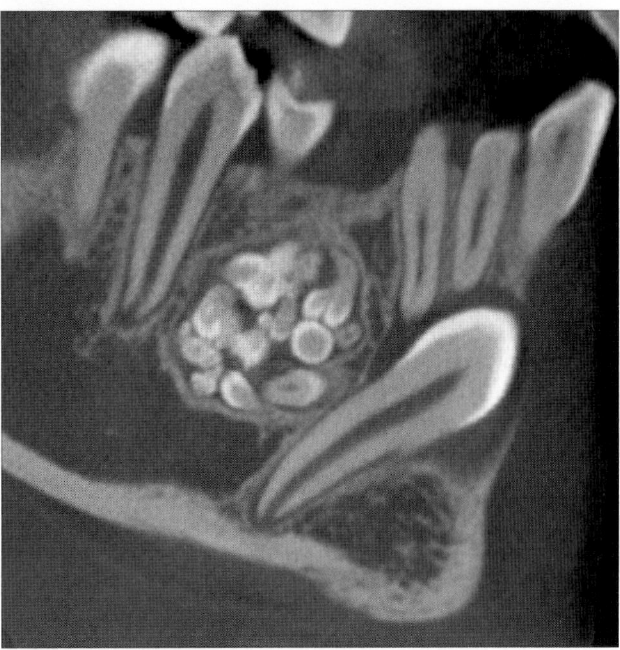

FIGURE 67-129 ■ **CBCT parasagittal slice showing a compound odontome consisting of numerous small teeth (denticles).** The odontome has displaced and prevented the lower right canine from erupting.

Chronic periodontitis results from the accumulation of dental plaque on the teeth, initially causing low-grade inflammation of the gingivae (gingivitis) with subsequent progression to involve the periodontal tissues. Gingivitis, which causes bleeding of the gums during tooth brushing, has no radiological features. Chronic periodontitis is a painless condition that affects almost all adults to a greater or lesser extent and results in slow but gradual horizontal bone loss from the alveolar crest so that the teeth lose their support. Advanced periodontitis affects 10–15% of the population, with smoking and poor oral hygiene being specific risk factors. A particularly aggressive form called rapidly progressive periodontitis occurs in young adults, where several teeth are affected by vertical bone loss resulting in angular bony defects that extend down towards the tooth apex (Fig. 67-128). Symmetrical widening of the periodontal ligament space affecting several teeth is sometimes seen in progressive systemic sclerosis or as irregular localised widening as an early feature of osteosarcoma of the jaws.

ODONTOMES AND ODONTOGENIC TUMOURS

As a generalisation, odontogenic disorders occur or are centred upon the tooth-bearing parts of the jaws, whereas lesions not involving the jaw alveolus, e.g. those lying predominantly below the inferior dental canal, are usually non-odontogenic.

Odontomes are developmental malformations or hamartomas consisting of dental hard tissues or tooth-like structures. Most are diagnosed in the second decade of life and frequently impede tooth eruption. There are two main types. The compound odontome consists of a collection of small discrete teeth called denticles (Fig. 67-129) and is found typically in the anterior region of

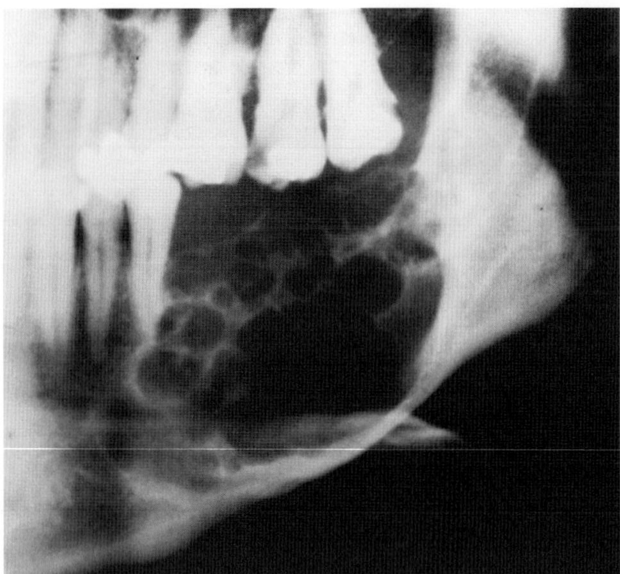

FIGURE 67-130 ■ Part of a panoramic radiograph showing an ameloblastoma, which appears as an expansile, multilocular radiolucency involving the left body of the mandible.

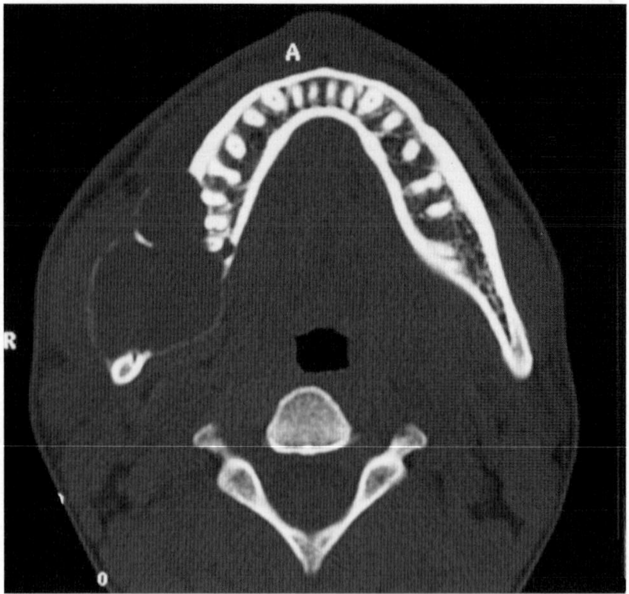

FIGURE 67-131 ■ An axial CT on bone window settings of a large cystic ameloblastoma of the right side of the mandible showing marked thinning and expansion of the bone. Note the presence of root resorption.

the maxilla, whereas the complex odontome consists of a randomly arranged mass of enamel, dentine and cementum and is found mostly in the lower premolar/molar region. Both types are densely radiopaque due to the presence of tooth enamel and are surrounded by a thin radiolucent capsular space and radiopaque cortical margin. There are several minor developmental anomalies also classified as odontomes that can resemble teeth.

Odontogenic tumours are uncommon, mostly benign and arise either from the odontogenic epithelium, odontogenic epithelium and ectomesenchyme, or primarily from ectomesenchyme. The **ameloblastoma** accounts for 11% of all odontogenic tumours. It occurs mainly in patients between 30 and 50 years of age, with most (80%) forming in the molar/ramus region of the mandible. When the maxilla is involved, it has the potential to spread insidiously to involve the infratemporal fossa, orbit and skull base; thus a thorough assessment is essential. The ameloblastoma has a variable radiographic appearance, being a unilocular or multilocular radiolucency, but typically contains septa or locules of variable size to produce a soap bubble appearance (Fig. 67-130). The margin is well defined, often corticated but, when large, produces jaw expansion with perforation of the bony cortex. A useful diagnostic feature is knife-edge resorption of the tooth roots by the tumour, which can be quite marked.

The lesion is locally aggressive and requires a wide excisional margin, so accurate presurgical assessment of the bone integrity is necessary. Contrast-enhanced CT will show the tumour–bone interface but has poor soft-tissue delineation. Multislice CT can be used to differentiate ameloblastoma from keratocystic odontogenic tumours which they resemble, because of higher-density increase during the arterial phase.[26] On T1-weighted images with gadolinium enhancement and T2-weighted images, there is good conspicuity of the tumour margin with the soft tissues, the lesion having a moderate-to-high signal. There is a rare malignant variety in which the ameloblastoma probably undergoes malignant transformation, with metastases most often occurring in the lungs.[27] The unicystic ameloblastoma occurs around the age of 20 years and often causes marked bony expansion (Fig. 67-131).

The **odontogenic myxoma** is a benign but locally aggressive tumour of odontogenic mesenchyme occurring mainly in those younger than 45 years of age. Most occur in the mandible in the premolar/molar region. The lesion is usually well defined, is unilocular and contains a variable number of straight internal coarse trabeculations to produce a reticular pattern.

There are many types of odontogenic tumour; however, two lesions that are well defined and contain variable amounts of focal mineral deposits are the calcifying epithelial odontogenic tumour and the adenomatoid odontogenic tumour. The former is more common in men, occurs in middle life and is found mainly in the premolar/molar region of the mandible. The latter mainly affects females in the second decade of life and typically occurs anteriorly, especially in the maxilla, and is associated with an unerupted tooth. The cementoblastoma is the only neoplasm of cementum; it is rare and mainly affects young males. It appears as an encapsulated radiopaque mass attached to the root, usually of a lower posterior tooth.

IMAGING IN IMPLANTOLOGY

Dental implants are placed into the jaws to replace missing teeth or give anchorage for dental prostheses. These have gained considerable popularity since the discovery, by Branemark, that endosseous titanium implants

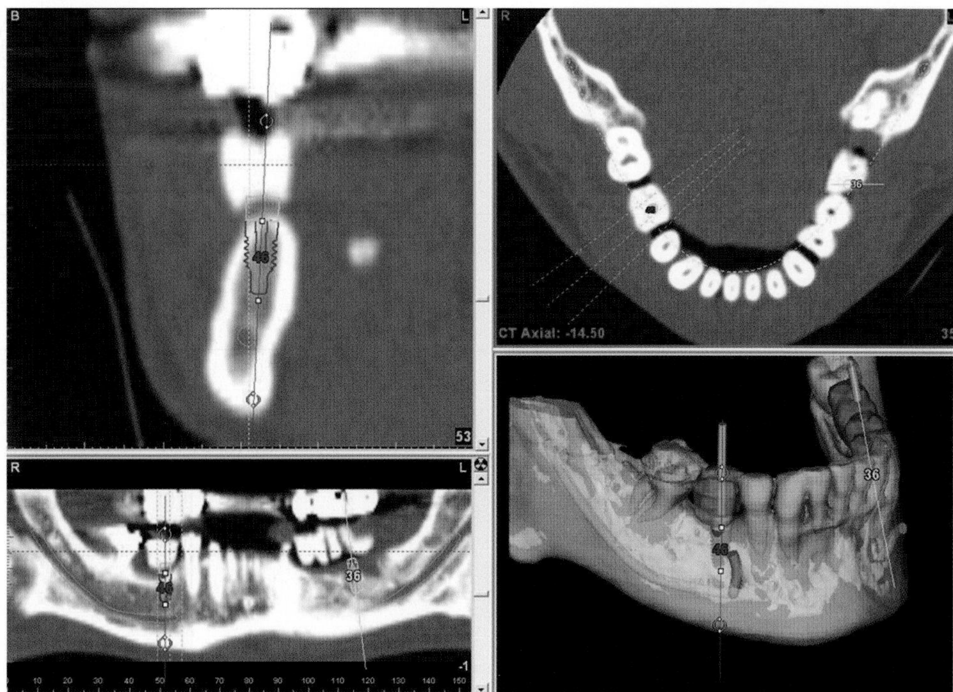

FIGURE 67-132 ■ Images reconstructed from fine axial CT slices of an implant site within the mandible (SimPlant). An original axial slice is cross-referenced with a cross-sectional slice, a panoramic-like reconstruction and 3D surface-rendered views. The software allows precise planning of implant placement to avoid injury to adjacent structures and helps predict the aesthetic outcome. (Courtesy of Mr Sean Goldner.)

could successfully integrate with bone. Imaging plays an essential role in pre-implant assessment, defining the volume and quality of recipient bone, identifying the location of relevant anatomical structures such as the inferior dental canal, the floor of the nose and maxillary antrum, and in assessing the status of adjacent teeth. Postoperatively, imaging is necessary to examine the degree of healing and monitor osseointegration.[28]

Intraoral periapical and dental panoramic radiography are valuable for initial preoperative assessment but cannot identify volume of a recipient bone site or accurately localise key structures and are prone to distortion. Cross-sectional imaging provides accurate information in all three planes and is particularly indicated in complex cases. CT data from multiple contiguous 1- to 2-mm slices taken parallel to the maxillary hard palate or lower border of mandible are reformatted by dedicated multiplanar reconstruction programmes to give cross-sectional slices cross-referenced with axial plan views of the dental arch. CBCT offers a similar imaging capability but with better resolution and substantially lower radiation exposure, due to use of exclusively hard tissue imaging parameters. Dedicated software packages depict the course of the inferior alveolar canal and allow 'trial placement of virtual implants' to assist with optimum implant location (Fig. 67-132). National and European selection or referral guidelines are available for the use of CBCT and implant assessment.[29,30] MRI has also been shown to be a feasible alternative to CT.[31] A radiographic localisation plate (stent) is generally needed for any form of cross-sectional imaging to indicate chosen implant sites—this may be metallic (tomography), gutta percha or brass (CT) or gadolinium (MRI).

In the postoperative phase intraoral periapical radiographs taken perpendicular to the implant, are most useful, monitoring osseointegration and identifying peri-implant bone loss, especially at the neck, which may indicate early failure of integration.

TRAUMA

Teeth

The teeth, particularly the upper incisors, are frequently involved in traumatic injuries to the face. They may be partially or completely avulsed or the crowns or roots may be fractured. Crown fractures may just involve the enamel, or the enamel and dentine, or if at a lower level expose the pulp. Root fractures occur less frequently and if undisplaced can be difficult to detect on radiographs when two different angled views may be required. Dental trauma can be associated with a localised dento-alveolar fracture in which a block of bone becomes detached containing several teeth. Intraoral radiographs best demonstrate traumatic injuries of the teeth.

For a full list of references, please see ExpertConsult.

FURTHER READING

Ahuja A, Evans R. Practical Head and Neck Ultrasound. Greenwich Medical Media; 2000.

Harnsberger HR. Handbook of Head and Neck Imaging. 2nd ed. Mosby; 1994.

Harnsberger HR. Diagnostic Imaging Head & Neck. Lippincott; 2010.

Hermans R. Head and Neck Cancer Imaging. Springer; 2012.

Swartz JD, Loevner LA. Imaging of the Temporal Bone. 4th ed. Thieme; 2009.

TRAUMA

Teeth

FURTHER READING

SECTION G

ONCOLOGICAL IMAGING

Section Editors: Vicky Goh • Andreas Adam

CHAPTER 68

Principles of Oncological Imaging

David MacVicar • Vicky Goh

CHAPTER OUTLINE

INTRODUCTION

Cancer is one of the major causes of death in the Western world, costing an estimated US$125 billion in 2010. There were 1.6 million projected new cancer cases and 577,190 cancer deaths in the USA alone in 2012.[1] The incidence of cancer is also increasing in developing countries, related to factors such as smoking, and shifts towards a more Western lifestyle. The commonest cancers include lung, bowel, breast and prostate cancers. In recent years there have been major advances in the approach to the assessment and treatment of cancer: for example, the introduction of screening, genomic testing and multimodality treatment, including:

- Conventional chemotherapy and novel targeted drugs, e.g. antiangiogenic drugs, such as bevacizumab, an anti-vascular endothelial growth factor agent;
- Radiotherapy, including 3D conformal radiotherapy, intensity-modulated radiotherapy, stereotactic radiosurgery (cyberknife, gamma knife) and proton therapy; and
- Surgery, with the emphasis on maintaining a good quality of life and reducing morbidity.

The subspeciality of oncological imaging has evolved in tandem with this. Oncological imaging now forms a significant proportion of the workload of a radiology department.[2] Imaging plays a major role at different stages along the patient pathway. Cross-sectional imaging is used widely for diagnosis, staging, assessment of treatment response and surveillance. A variety of anatomical and functional imaging techniques are available in clinical practice currently. High-resolution cross-sectional imaging techniques such as computed tomography (CT) and magnetic resonance imaging (MRI), which allow the whole body to be imaged with high accuracy, remain the mainstay of imaging practice. However, physiologically based functional imaging techniques that assess different aspects of tumour biology such as diffusion-weighted MRI (water diffusion; a surrogate of tissue cellularity) and dynamic contrast-enhanced CT or MRI (tumour perfusion and vascular leakage; a surrogate of angiogenesis) have been applied increasingly in clinical practice to improve tumour detection, staging and response assessment.

Molecular imaging techniques such as positron emission tomography (PET) provide more targeted imaging of tumour physiology and biology, with excellent anatomical localisation as hybrid imaging modalities (PET/CT and PET/MRI). While ^{18}F-fluorodeoxyglucose (FDG), an analogue of glucose, remains the commonest radio-labelled tracer in clinical use, allowing assessment of glucose metabolism, other tracers including ^{18}F-fluorothymidine (FLT), ^{11}C-choline, ^{18}F-misonidazole (FMISO), ^{18}F-FAZA, ^{61}C- or ^{64}Cu-ATSM and ^{11}C-acetate provide relevant information on tumour proliferation, hypoxia and lipogenesis, respectively. Each imaging modality has advantages and disadvantages (Table 68-1) and the 'best' imaging strategy will depend on the tumour type, tumour site, clinical indication (diagnosis, staging, treatment response assessment or surveillance), and availability and cost of the imaging technique.

A consequence of these advances in assessment and treatment has been improvements in patient outcome: this is especially so for early-stage disease, although survival for patients with advanced disease remains relatively poor. Another has been the recognition of the need for local, regional and national changes in the organisational aspects of cancer care. Typically in the United Kingdom, all new presentations of cancer are now assessed at a multidisciplinary meeting, and managed by a multidisciplinary team of specialists (including doctors (surgeons, medical and clinical oncologists, physicians, radiologists, pathologists), nurses, dieticians and physiotherapists) that are experienced in their cancer type in order to optimise clinical management. For a radiologist, this provides the opportunity to ensure the most suitable investigations are performed in a timely fashion at diagnosis, during treatment and in subsequent follow-up. This chapter will introduce key concepts in the imaging of patients with

TABLE 68-1 **The Different Imaging Techniques Available for Clinical Cancer Imaging**

Technique	Mechanism	Advantages	Disadvantages
Anatomical			
Plain film	Attenuation of X-rays by tissue structures	Availability Low cost	Limited resolution
Ultrasound	Attenuation of sound waves by tissue structures	Availability Low cost No radiation burden	Dependent on observer expertise
Computed tomography	Attenuation of X-rays by tissue structures	Availability Cross-sectional ability High spatial resolution	Radiation burden Relatively low contrast resolution
Magnetic resonance imaging	Absorption of radiowaves by atomic nuclei (most commonly hydrogen)	Cross-sectional ability High spatial and contrast resolution No radiation burden	Magnetic field effects and heating (particularly with high field systems)
Functional			
Diffusion-weighted MRI	Diffusion of water molecules	High spatial and contrast resolution No radiation burden Surrogate marker of tumour cellularity	Magnetic field effects and heating
Dynamic contrast-enhanced MRI	Kinetic modelling of gadolinium-based contrast agent to quantify vascular leakage	High spatial and contrast resolution No contrast burden Surrogate marker of angiogenesis	Magnetic field effects and heating
Blood oxygen level-dependent MRI	Paramagnetic effect of deoxyhaemoglobin	Surrogate marker of hypoxia (hypoxic blood volume)	Magnetic field effects and heating
Dynamic contrast-enhanced CT	Kinetic modelling of iodine-based contrast agent to quantify perfusion and vascular leakage	High spatial resolution Surrogate marker of angiogenesis and hypoxia	Radiation burden
Fluorodeoxyglucose (FDG) positron emission tomography	Uptake of ^{18}F-FDG, analogue of endogenous glucose	Cross-sectional ability May be combined with CT or MRI Quantification of tumour metabolic activity possible	Radiation burden Spatial resolution poorer than that of CT or MRI Relatively high cost

cancer. The role of imaging in diagnosis, staging, response assessment and surveillance will be described.

DIAGNOSIS

Primary Diagnosis

In the majority of cases, a patient will present with symptoms and signs related to the cancer, and appropriate investigations will be arranged, including imaging. Usually there are only a few diagnoses that can be made with confidence from imaging characteristics: for example, an ovarian dermoid, or other fat-containing tumours, and lesions that are obviously cystic. In most cases there is a differential diagnosis, requiring pathological confirmation of the diagnosis.

Confirmation of Diagnosis

Confirmation of a diagnosis may be undertaken using a variety of techniques, including cytological examination of fine needle aspiration samples, tumour specimens from automatic cutting needles and surgical biopsies (Figs. 68-1 and 68-2). Core biopsies yield a higher tumour volume than fine needle aspiration, and may be more suited for tumour biomarker analysis, often required by clinical trials.

Certain principles should be followed when needle aspiration or percutaneous core biopsy is being planned:

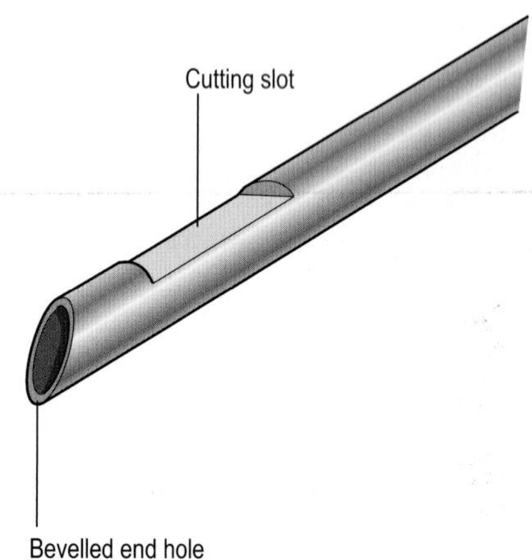

FIGURE 68-1 ■ **Diagram of Westcott-type needle.** This is used for aspiration of cytology samples. There is an end hole and a cutting side hole. Vacuum is applied when a central trocar is withdrawn following satisfactory placement of needle.

- The chosen technique should acquire sufficient tissue for a pathological diagnosis.
- The technique should be safe: for example, patient coagulation parameters should be checked and appropriate measures taken to minimise the risk of haemorrhage.
- For cytological specimens, a cytologist should be present to ensure enough material is present and to stain and interpret the cytology samples immediately.

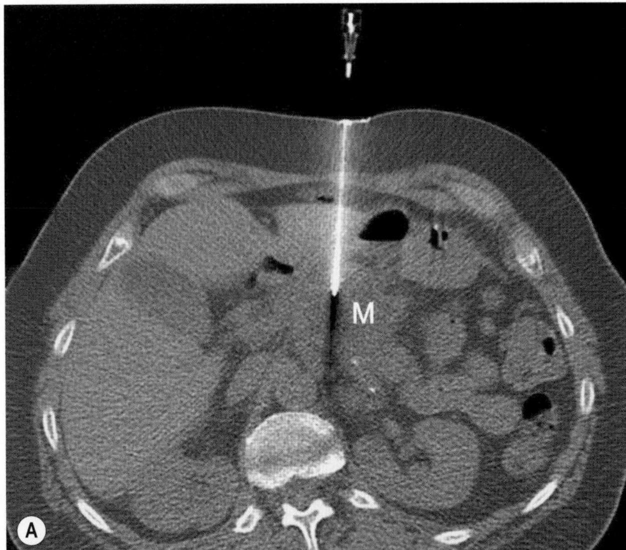

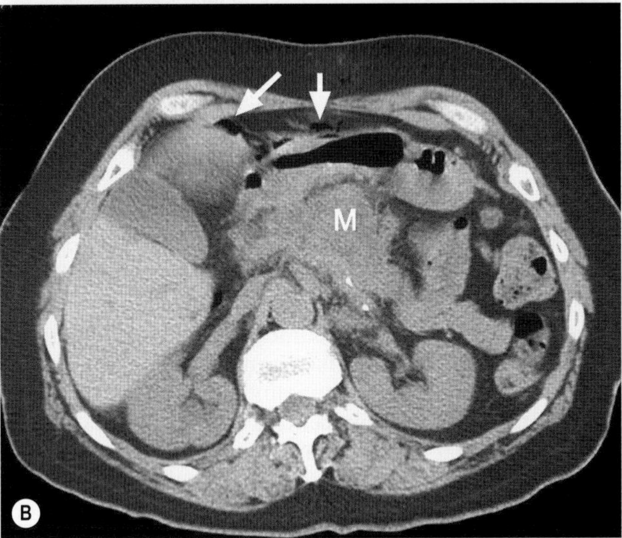

FIGURE 68-2 ■ Coaxial system for biopsy. (A) A coaxial needle has been introduced into a pancreatic mass (M) through the gastric antrum. Dense artefact is present at the tip of the trocar. Once the trocar is withdrawn, an automatic cutting needle of appropriate length is introduced through the cannula left in situ, and multiple biopsies can be obtained by angling in a variety of directions. (B) Once the system is withdrawn, limited free gas is present outside the stomach (arrows). No clinical symptoms developed and the patient was discharged 6 hours after the procedure.

- For core biopsies, specimen preparation should be discussed with the examining pathologist. Most specimens can be placed in formalin but others may require preparation for special staining techniques.
- If image-assisted tissue diagnosis is inconclusive, consideration of further percutaneous attempts or of open surgical biopsy should take into account the reason for diagnostic failure. For example, some tumours such as pancreatic carcinoma may have few malignant cells. The degree of risk involved in repeat biopsy, the technical ease with which the specimen was obtained and the likelihood of achieving positive tissue diagnosis on the second attempt should all be considered.

Several types of cutting needles may be used for core biopsy. The Tru-Cut needle has a central trocar that makes the initial movement forward, exposing a slot. The sheath is then advanced over the slot, cutting a piece of tissue into the slot, and the entire apparatus is withdrawn, with a core specimen contained in the slot. Coaxial systems enable multiple tumour cores to be obtained via a single puncture site. The principle involves placement of a needle from which the sharpened trocar is removed to leave a hollow unsharpened cannula in the mass for biopsy. An automatic cutting needle can then be placed down the cannula. Several cores can then be obtained, and different parts of the lesion may be sampled by angling the cannula slightly in a variety of directions. Since only one puncture is made of the skin and intervening tissue planes, more tissue is obtained without increasing the risk of track seeding. In some circumstances percutaneous needle techniques should not be used to avoid malignant seeding of the percutaneous biopsy track.

STAGING

Once the diagnosis of cancer has been confirmed, it is important for the subsequent management of a patient to stage the tumour, i.e. to assess the locoregional extent of the tumour as well as the presence/absence of distant metastatic disease.

The aims of a staging system are:

- To allow rational selection of primary therapy and assessment of the necessity for (neo)adjuvant treatment;
- To give some indication of the likely prognosis;
- To assist in the evaluation of results of treatment;
- To enable exchange of information between cancer treatment centres; and
- To contribute to the continuing investigation of human cancer.

Staging systems describe the anatomical extent of a tumour, and provide highly relevant information to guide appropriate therapy at diagnosis, although decision-making will be influenced also by other factors, including the histological grade of the tumour, its expected biological behaviour and the age and general fitness of a patient.[3] While clinical examination continues to have a significant role in the initial assessment of patients, imaging has a major role to play in the staging of cancer.

Staging Systems

An ideal staging system should be simple, precise, consistent and applicable to all clinical circumstances in oncology, and convey some prognostic information to facilitate best practice. Over the years, many staging systems have borne the name of eminent doctors (e.g. the Robson staging classification of renal tumours or Dukes' staging classification of colorectal cancer), institutions (e.g. the Royal Marsden Hospital staging classification for testicular germ cell tumours) or organisations (e.g. the Fédération Internationale de Gynécologie et d'Obstétrique (FIGO) classification systems for cervical, uterine and other gynaecological neoplasms). More recently, the tumour–node–metastasis (TNM system), espoused by the American Joint Committee on Cancer (AJCC) and the Union Internationale Contre le Cancer (UICC), has been adopted widely.

The TNM classification of malignant tumours and the AJCC cancer staging handbook are now in their seventh editions.[4] The system was originally devised by Pierre Denoix in the 1940s and has been modified over the subsequent decades. The 'T' category entails evaluation of local tumour extent. The 'N' category entails evaluation of nodal involvement. The 'M' category entails evaluation of disease at distant sites. The 'T' category, which may have the prefix 'c' to indicate 'clinical' staging, although this is frequently omitted, has several standard forms of notation: Tx indicates that primary tumour cannot be assessed; Tis indicates in situ disease with no evidence of invasion; T0 indicates no visible evidence of primary tumour; T1–T4 indicates increasing degrees of local tumour extent. These divisions may be adapted with the addition of subdivisions indicated by letters (e.g. 'a' or 'b') for greater flexibility in different tumour types. Although staging of the primary from T1 to T4 follows broad principles and there are some similarities between tumour types, refinements and adaptations for individual tumours are needed usually.

The 'N' category has similar notation. Direct spread of the primary tumour into an adjacent lymph node is classified as nodal spread. Nx is where regional lymph nodes cannot be assessed, N0 is where no regional lymph node metastases are present and N1, N2 and N3 indicate increasing involvement of regional lymph nodes. Likewise, these divisions may include subdivisions indicated by letters (e.g. 'a' or 'b'). The'M' category assesses distant metastasis where Mx indicates that distant metastasis cannot be assessed, M0 indicates there are no distant metastases and M1 indicates the presence of distant metastasis. The category M1 may be further specified indicating which organs are involved. For example, PUL indicates pulmonary metastases, OSS indicates osseous metastases and HEP indicates hepatic metastases. Again, subdivisions may be indicated by letters (e.g. 'a' or 'b').

All tumours must be confirmed pathologically. A number of general rules apply when using the clinical TNM staging system. Clinical stage is assigned by physical examination, imaging and other relevant investigations, but may be amended as pathological information becomes available, and given the prefix pTNM stage where microscopic extent of disease is known. If there is doubt what stage should be assigned, the lower category should be used. Therefore, an imaging investigation that is suspicious but not diagnostic of spread to the pelvic sidewall will be disregarded unless supplemented by further imaging or confirmation by histopathology.

Once assigned, the pre-treatment TNM stage is recorded in the patient's records and remains unchanged through subsequent treatment. For multiple synchronous primary tumours, the tumour with the highest 'T' category is used for staging purposes. For synchronous primary tumours arising in paired organs, each tumour should be assigned a separate TNM stage. In modern usage the TNM system has the advantages of clarity of communication, but is complex. This has led to a further system of stage grouping, which is published within the AJCC system. Stage groups of 0–4 are assigned as tumour becomes more extensive and widespread.

National bodies, such as the Royal College of Radiologists in the United Kingdom, have published recommendations or guidelines on the choice of staging investigation (CT, MRI or PET/CT), recognising that local availability of advanced imaging techniques and the preference and experience of individual radiologists are important considerations.[5] A potential effect of advances in imaging technology over time is stage migration, e.g. via improvements in tumour detection, resulting in upstaging, and artefactual improvement in subgroup prognosis, although overall survival will remain stable unless more effective treatment is given.

PRINCIPLES OF STAGING INVESTIGATIONS

Primary Tumour Staging

The principles of staging are illustrated in this section, with the following examples of some of the most common cancers.

Rectal Cancer

Rectal cancer is a good example of a tumour in which a staging system has evolved and changed over a period of more than 70 years, and technical refinement of surgery over the past 20 years has gone hand-in-hand with increasingly sophisticated imaging of the primary tumour such that imaging is now central to decision-making. It remains true that the vast majority of patients with rectal cancer should be offered surgery, as local symptoms due to growth within the pelvis are associated with severe pain that can be difficult to palliate. However, the timing of surgery and the role of neoadjuvant chemotherapy and radiotherapy depend on the local tumour stage at the time of diagnosis.

In 1932, Dukes highlighted the importance of extramural spread in the prediction of local recurrence and survival. He also observed that lymph node invasion was present in 14% of patients with tumours confined to the bowel wall and 43% of patients with tumours extending beyond the serosa.[6] A number of other prognostic indicators have subsequently been identified, including the pattern of local spread (a well-circumscribed margin implies a better prognosis than a widely infiltrated tumour with ill-defined borders). Spread beyond the peritoneal membrane results in a high incidence of both local recurrence and transcoelomic dissemination; invasion of extramural veins by tumour and extent and number of tumour-involved lymph nodes are all independent predictors of a poor prognosis.

For many years the preferred operation for rectal cancer was synchronous combined abdominoperineal excision of rectum (AP resection). However, total mesorectal excision has become the gold standard since its introduction in the 1970s.[7] In this technique, the surgeon dissects from above and finds the mesorectal plane. As

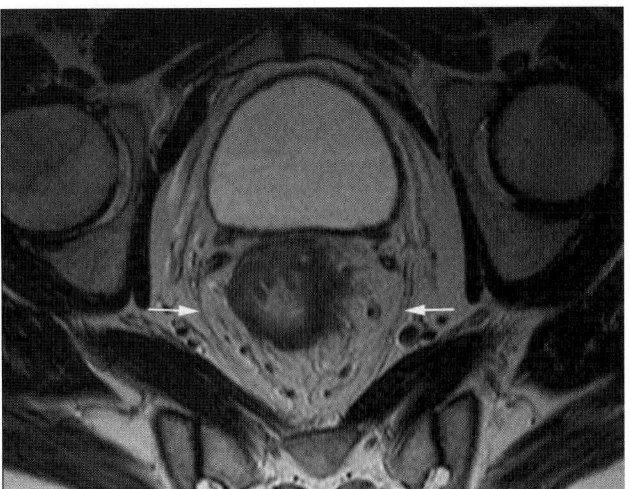

FIGURE 68-3 ■ T2-weighted MRI of the rectum. This axial image demonstrates a low signal adenocarcinoma predominantly involving the rectal wall to the left of the midline. There is evidence of spread into the mesorectum and extramural vascular invasion. The mesorectal fascia is clearly demonstrated (arrows). Neoadjuvant treatment with chemotherapy and radiotherapy may help to downstage the tumour prior to consideration of surgery.

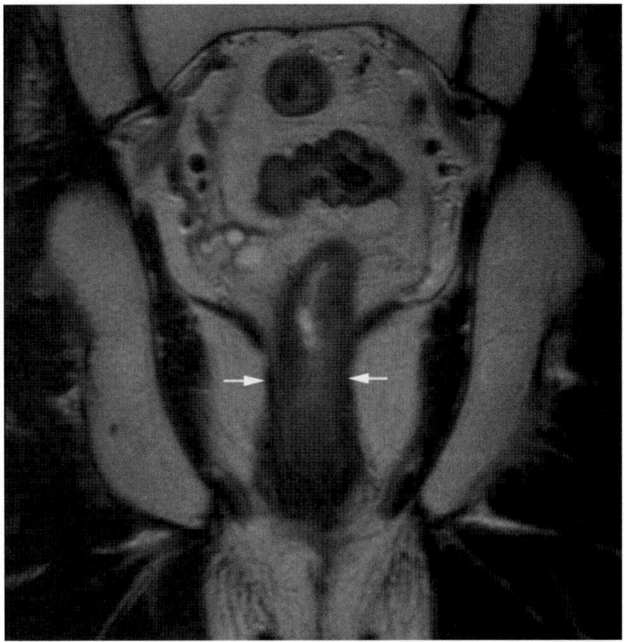

FIGURE 68-4 ■ T2-weighted MRI of a low rectal tumour. This coronal image demonstrates a tumour extending inferiorly to involve the anal sphincter complex (arrows). Sphincter-preserving surgery and re-anastomosis will not be technically possible.

the lymphatic vessels and nodes draining the tumour are located throughout the mesorectum, if this is divided or disrupted during surgical excision, spillage of malignant cells may occur and involved nodes may be left in situ. This increases the likelihood of local recurrence, and excision of the rectum is best achieved by dissection down the mesorectal fascia, allowing the mesorectum and rectum to be removed en bloc without disruption of the presacral fascia and the underlying venous plexus. The surgically excised specimen may then be sectioned transversely and the circumferential resection margin (CRM) examined for tumour involvement. The presence of tumour at the extremity of the resection margin is a major prognostic factor.[8]

In recent years, MRI has been shown to be the investigation of choice in demonstrating spread of tumour within the mesorectum and the mesorectal plane itself (Fig. 68-3). It is possible to demonstrate the relationship of the tumour to the anal canal, indicating the potential for sphincter-preserving surgery (Fig. 68-4). Criteria have been developed in pathologically correlated series for staging of the primary tumour and nodes within the mesorectum. Effectively, MRI can provide a 'road map' for the surgeon and studies have shown that the pathological status of the CRM can be predicted.[9,10] Other prognostic factors such as extramural venous invasion and peritoneal penetration can be demonstrated. If locally advanced disease with mural penetration is demonstrated, chemotherapy and radiation therapy may be employed to downstage the primary before an attempt at surgery, allowing a more tailored preoperative strategy.

Studies from the Royal Marsden Hospital have demonstrated that the incidence of tumour at the circumferential resection margin is only 2% in patients diagnosed by MRI as likely to have a safe resection margin for immediate surgery. Overall incidence of positive resection margins in those patients seen by the MDT, including those who had undergone preoperative chemotherapy and radiotherapy for disease diagnosed by MRI to be locally advanced at initial presentation, was 8.5%. In a group of patients not assessed by the MDT, positive resection margins were present in 24%.[11] The implication is clear: all patients newly diagnosed with rectal cancer should be assessed by a multidisciplinary team, within the framework of a cancer network, to ensure that up-to-date investigation and treatment is available.

Non-Small Cell Lung Cancer

Lung cancer, the most common cause of cancer mortality worldwide, is a good example of a multimodality staging approach to optimise patient management. Plain radiographs, CT, MRI, endobronchial or endoluminal ultrasound (EBUS or EUS) and PET/CT are part of the diagnostic algorithm in patients with suspected lung cancer[12] (Fig. 68-5). For patients with an early-stage lung cancer, surgery offers the best chance of cure, provided co-morbidity and the patient's lung function do not preclude this. Accurate staging of locoregional and distant metastatic disease optimises the selection of patients for curative treatment and reduces futile thoracotomy rates compared to standard staging.[13,14]

Breast Cancer

Breast cancer is a good example of a disease where surgical techniques have undergone frequent revision, from the days of very radical surgery in the 1950s, to lumpectomy favoured in the 1970s and more recent regimens involving wide local excision or quadrantectomy followed by radiotherapy. Although many primary breast tumours can be staged by clinical examination, local management may benefit from imaging planning. When multifocal disease is suspected or tumour is diffuse, contrast-enhanced MRI has very high sensitivity for lesion detection (Fig. 68-6). However, specificity is lower as areas of gadolinium enhancement within the breast do not necessarily represent cancer. Ultrasound has the advantage of being able to stage the primary tumour, detecting abnormal lymph nodes in the axilla and facilitating fine-needle aspiration for cytology if abnormal nodes are detected.

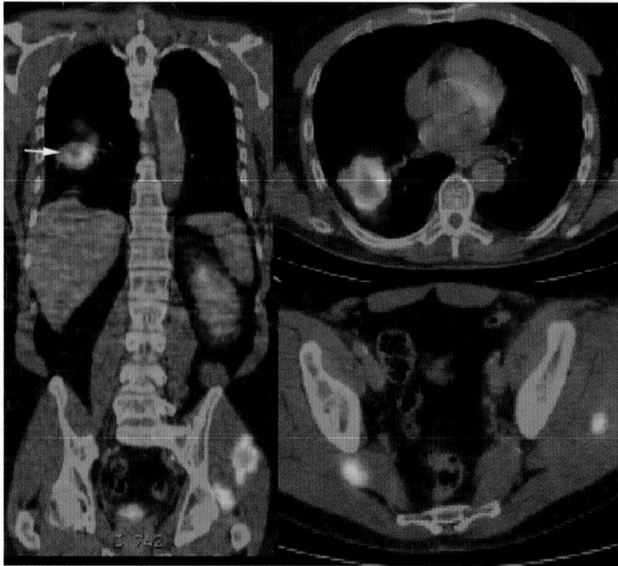

FIGURE 68-5 ■ ^{18}F-FDG PET/CT of a non-small cell lung cancer. This montage shows a right lung tumour with distant metastases within the gluteal muscles, precluding the patient from primary surgery.

The concept of sentinel-node detection prior to surgery also involves imaging. The principle is that the first lymph node in a nodal bed draining from a tumour will show metastatic disease if lymphatic spread has occurred. Absence of metastatic disease in a sentinel node in patients with breast cancer has been reported to have a negative predictive value for axillary nodal disease of 98%.[15] A combined technique using injected blue dye and an isotope, which is then localised by gamma camera imaging before surgery and with an intraoperative gamma probe during surgery, is usually recommended.

Prostate Cancer

Since the Radiologic Diagnostic Oncology Group (RDOG) demonstrated that both MRI and endorectal ultrasound show higher accuracy than clinical staging, and that MRI demonstrates higher sensitivity and specificity than endorectal ultrasound[16,17] for detection of extracapsular spread of prostate cancer, MRI assessment of prostate cancer has evolved. A multiparametric imaging approach, combining T1- and T2-weighted sequences with diffusion-weighted MRI, dynamic contrast-enhanced MRI and MRI spectroscopy, is utilised (Fig. 68-7). This has resulted in improvements in tumour detection and delineation of the extent of disease.[18,19] Nevertheless, it has been difficult to demonstrate a clear impact of using

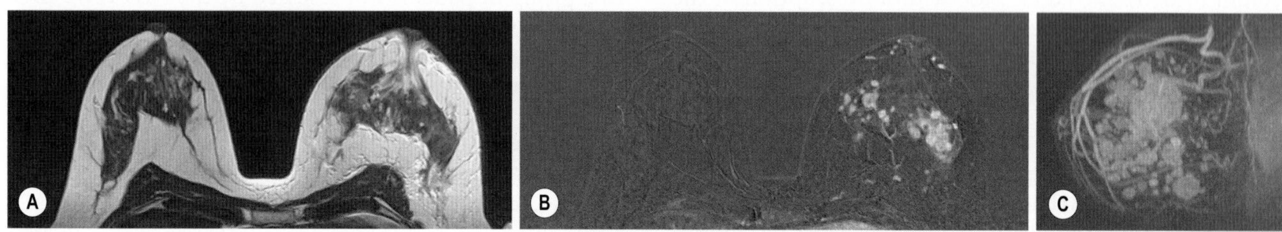

FIGURE 68-6 ■ MRI of a primary breast cancer. Axial T2-weighted (A), axial early subtracted dynamic contrast-enhanced T1-weighted MRI (B) and sagittal MIP image (C) of a left breast cancer showing an enhancing multifocal tumour.

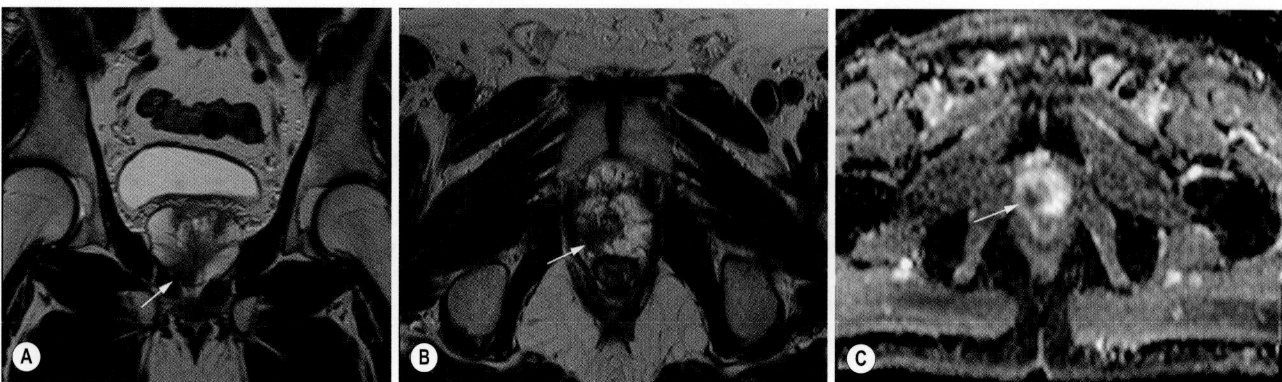

FIGURE 68-7 ■ MRI of a primary prostate cancer. T2-weighted coronal (A) and axial (B) images show there is low signal right apical peripheral zone tumour. The tumour extends to the capsular margin (arrow) but there is no confirmatory evidence of extracapsular spread indicating T2 disease. Diffusion-weighted imaging demonstrates restriction within this tumour, depicted as a low signal intensity area on the apparent diffusion coefficient map (C).

high-technology imaging on patient health. One of the reasons for this is that the natural history of the disease is heterogeneous and the optimal treatment of prostate cancer remains controversial.[20,21]

Staging Distant Metastatic Disease

Staging for distant metastatic disease remains an important facet in the management of cancer where a curative approach is being considered, e.g. surgery or radical radiotherapy. While CT remains the mainstay for staging distant metastatic disease, there is a role for other more sensitive modalities, i.e. ^{18}F-FDG PET/CT in certain cancer types, e.g. primary lung and oesophageal cancer.[13,22,23] The presence of metastatic disease does not necessarily contraindicate resection of the primary tumour, as local control will be necessary for symptomatic relief. Small-volume metastatic disease in liver and lungs may also be amenable to surgery ('metastectomy').

ASSESSMENT OF TREATMENT RESPONSE

The Role of Imaging

Imaging is used widely to demonstrate changes in tumour size with treatment but findings should be interpreted within the context of other response markers such as biochemical tumour markers, and the patient's clinical well-being on toxic therapy. In specialist cancer centres, the majority of patients are on clinical trials, which may stipulate the timing and technique of follow-up investigations. Nevertheless, even if the patient is not on a clinical trial, it is important to have some reproducible and objective technique that will allow directly comparable measurements to be made.

CT remains the most frequently used follow-up technique, although US, MRI and PET/CT can be used. It is important to ensure consistency at each attendance, i.e. that the same imaging protocol and sequences are used. The frequency of follow-up investigations depends on the perceived likelihood of response, and toxicity of treatment. The frequency may also be stipulated by clinical trials or physician preference: it is noticeable that some clinicians adopt shorter follow-up intervals for similar treatment regimens. There is also some pressure from the pharmaceutical industry to document reduction in tumour size: while overall survival rate remains the best objective parameter of efficacy of treatment, demonstration of some form of objective response earlier in the course of disease encourages development of certain drugs.

Objective Response Assessment

Effective systemic chemotherapy and cross-sectional imaging developed side by side during the 1970s, and it became clear that a common language and definition of guidelines for the assessment of objective tumour response was necessary. The World Health Organisation (WHO) proposed a system that remains in limited use today.[24,25] Miller et al[25] recommended that a partial response should be designated when bi-dimensional measurement of a single lesion shows greater than 50% reduction in cross-sectional area (perpendicular diameters should be measured). Separate categories are available where one-dimensional measurements only are obtainable, but no consideration is given to calculation of tumour volumes. It also states that objective response can be determined clinically, radiologically, biochemically or by surgical/pathological restaging.

The WHO criteria have been superseded since by other criteria. The response evaluation criteria in solid tumours (RECIST) were proposed by the European Organisation for Research and Treatment of Cancer (EORTC) in collaboration with the National Cancer Institute in the USA and the National Cancer Institute of Canada Clinical Trials Group,[26] and were updated in 2010.[27] The RECIST criteria allow one-dimensional measurement of target lesions and the sum of these, rather than the product of two perpendicular linear measurements, is used. A partial response is defined of at least a 30% decrease in the sum of the longest diameter of target lesions, taking as a reference the baseline sum of longest diameters (Table 68-2 and Fig. 68-8).

The aim of the RECIST criteria was to simplify the way in which information was gathered and recorded, and not necessarily to increase precision. The fundamental problem of observer variability and subjectivity remains. It is still the responsibility of an investigator to select lesions for measurement, but one of the important recommendations of the RECIST Group was that results of trials claiming response by measurement should be validated by an independent review committee.

It remains important to assess size alterations within the context of the clinical state of the patient and the natural history of the disease. It is also important to be aware that anatomical measurement criteria will fail to take account of functional changes within tumours. Likewise, cyst formation and necrosis within tumours will not be assessed using size criteria alone. To this end, more

TABLE 68-2 **RECIST Criteria for the Assessment of Therapeutic Response**

Target Lesion*	Complete Response	Partial Response	Stable Disease	Progressive Disease
Up to 5 target lesions with a maximum of 2 lesions/organ	Resolution of all target lesions	At least 30% reduction in mean sum longest diameter target lesions	Response not fulfilling PR or PD category	At least 20% increase in mean sum longest diameter target lesions or new lesions

*Target lesion: Any measurable lesion within an organ that is >1 cm in longest dimension. For lymph nodes the measurement is the shortest dimension (short axis) and this should be >1.5 cm for the node to be considered as a target lesion.

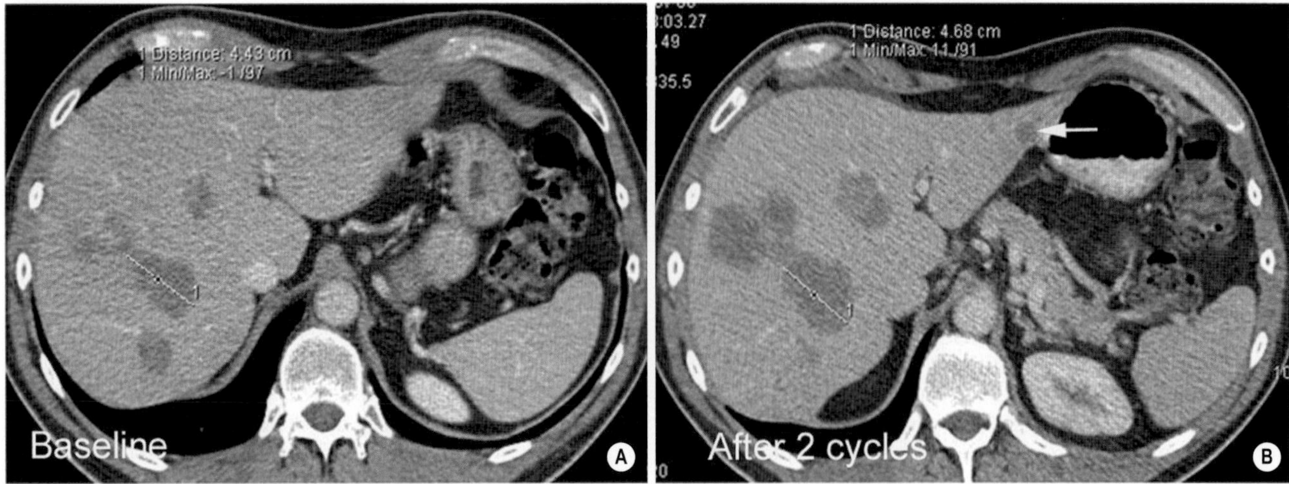

FIGURE 68-8 ■ **RECIST 1.1 assessment.** The target lesion chosen was a liver metastasis. Despite treatment there was disease progression with enlargement of existing metastases and development of a new metastasis (arrow).

recently criteria which take into account contrast enhancement change as well as size, as applied to gastrointestinal stromal tumours (Choi criteria)[28] and also to renal cell carcinoma[29,30] (modified Choi criteria), or which take areas of necrosis into account, as applied to non-small cell lung cancer, have been proposed.[31]

Imaging Residual Masses

A post-treatment residuum is frequently seen in several solid tumours, such as lung cancer, lymphoma and metastatic non-seminomatous germ cell tumours (NSGCT). Imaging techniques have been applied in an attempt to predict the likelihood of recurrence in these residual masses. Investigation has been most intensive in lymphoma. Enlargement of a residual lymphoma mass on CT is strong evidence of disease recurrence, but it is hoped that it will be possible to identify residual or recurrent disease earlier using functional techniques. There is good evidence of a high sensitivity for ^{18}F-FDG PET/CT in detection of residual disease. There are theoretical reasons for using ^{18}F-FDG PET/CT as a routine surveillance procedure following treatment. However, at the time of writing, there is no clear evidence to support this strategy.

MRI has also been evaluated in the investigation of residual lymphoma masses.[32] Reduction in signal intensity on T2-weighted images during treatment is taken as a sign of successful treatment, leaving a fibrotic residuum. However, MRI has not become a routine investigation because of high false-negative and false-positive rates. Imaging features suggestive of residual disease may help to select patients for repeat biopsy or further treatment, for example, with adjuvant radiotherapy. However, as treated cancer can leave abnormal tissue detectable by imaging, imaging alone is unreliable in predicting the pathological nature of the residuum.

Imaging of Treatment Toxicity

Radiotherapy and/or chemotherapy can affect all tissues of the body. Imaging features and the timing of their appearance vary from organ to organ. Radiotherapy causes acute change by a direct physical inflammatory process and later effects as a result of an ischaemic insult. Anticancer drugs have direct cytotoxic effects, but may also cause hypersensitivity reactions. Some organs are more susceptible to tissue damage than others, although observed imaging changes are not always of clinical importance. Interpretation is facilitated by knowledge of the type and timing of treatment.

Lung

A radiological diagnosis of radiation pneumonitis is made when there is evidence of acute radiotherapy change in the lungs, but this is always accompanied by clinical symptoms. Radiation pneumonitis usually appears 6–8 weeks after completion of treatment with 35–40 Gy, but is not generally seen at radiation doses below 30 Gy. It is almost always seen at doses over 40 Gy and will appear earlier than 6 weeks. It becomes most extensive 3–4 months after completion of radiotherapy. The histological appearance is of diffuse alveolar damage. At a later stage, an organising fibrosis develops, which becomes complete 9–12 months after termination of therapy. The histological appearances are non-specific, but the distinguishing feature on plain film radiography and CT is a straight edge corresponding to a radiation field. When there is significant volume loss, traction effects occur and there may be bronchiectatic changes.

Neoadjuvant cytotoxic chemotherapy enhances the effect of radiation, causing earlier radiation pneumonitis and more severe fibrosis. Drugs most commonly implicated include dactinomycin, doxorubicin, bleomycin, cyclophosphamide, mitomycin and vincristine. There is a growing list of cytotoxic drugs that are recognised to cause pulmonary parenchymal damage independent of radiation therapy. Bleomycin is used in the treatment of NSGCT, lymphoma and squamous cell carcinoma. The toxic effect is dose-dependent and exacerbated by the use of other agents in combination chemotherapy, adjuvant radiation therapy and oxygen therapy. Early radiographic abnormality is typically a reticular nodular pattern of interstitial disease, which is most severe in the basal segments. Lung damage may be progressive, leading to pulmonary fibrosis, which may be severe and cause traction pneumothorax and pneumomediastinum (Fig. 68-9).

Busulfan, which is used in haematological malignancy, causes interstitial lung damage. Methotrexate is responsible for a hypersensitivity reaction, which results in alveolar shadowing and sometimes in mediastinal adenopathy. If methotrexate therapy is prolonged, the lung damage may progress to fibrosis. Treatment-related lung toxicity can usually be seen on plain radiography, but CT is more sensitive.[33,34]

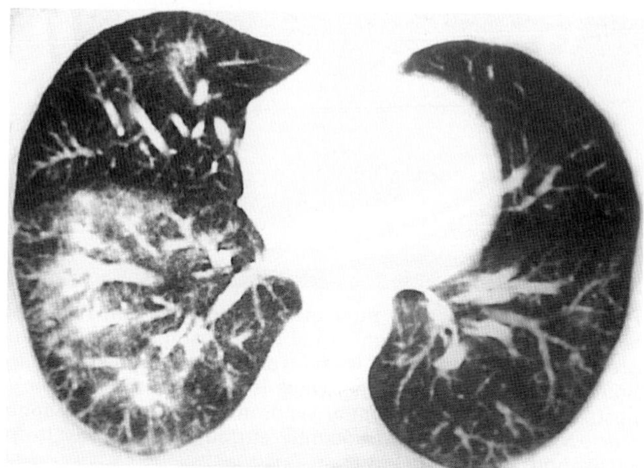

FIGURE 68-9 ■ CT of acute bleomycin toxicity. This shows widespread predominantly basal interstitial change.

Bone and Bone Marrow

Osseous changes in response to radiation were first described by Ewing as long ago as the 1920s. Local demineralisation and osteopenia are the earliest and often the only post-radiation changes noted on plain radiography. Later changes include mixed lytic and sclerotic areas and trabecular coarsening, which may develop 2 or more years after radiotherapy. Spontaneous fractures and aseptic necrosis can occur, but, in general, radiation damage to bone is becoming less common as a result of high-energy mega-voltage radiotherapy and more accurate dose distribution. However, the effect on bone marrow is frequently seen on MRI at relatively low doses, from 15 to 20 Gy. Haemopoietic bone marrow converts to fatty marrow, resulting in a high signal on T1-weighted sequences. Following treatment of metastatic bone disease or primary bone tumour with radiotherapy or chemotherapy, the marrow can take on a bizarre appearance on MRI that is virtually uninterpretable. For example, following treatment of lymphoma or neuroblastoma diffusely involving the bone marrow, the latter will usually alter its appearance, sometimes reverting to normal, but often leaving an array of mixed residual signal changes (Fig. 68-10).

Neurotoxicity

Therapeutic radiation to the brain induces an ischaemic insult, which is manifested as abnormality within the deep cerebral white matter. This is best demonstrated by MRI, where diffuse high signal is present on T2-weighted images or using the fluid attenuation inversion recovery

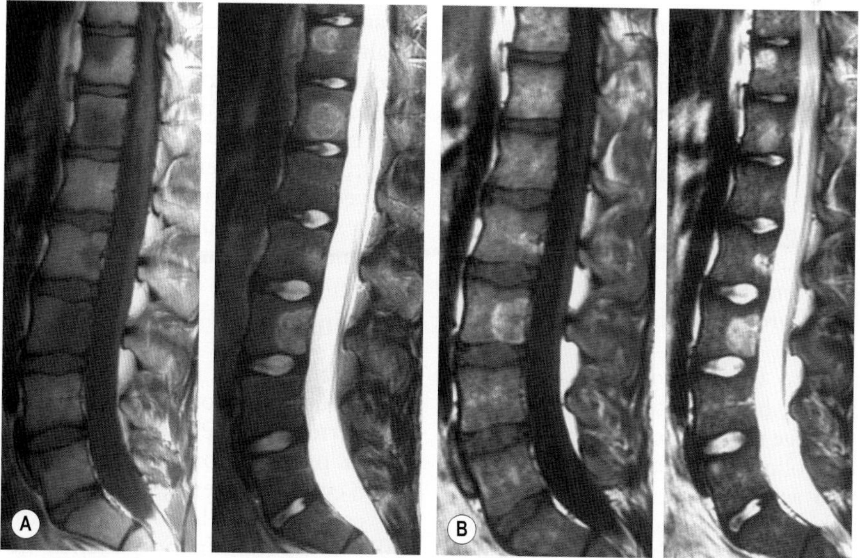

FIGURE 68-10 ■ Lymphoma of lumbar spine pre- and post-treatment. (A) Sagittal MRI of lumbar spine showing lymphoma in bone marrow. On T1-weighted sequence (left) low signal is returned from the marrow cavity of T11, 12, L2, 3 and 5. Corresponding focal areas of high signal are identified on the T2-weighted sequence (right). Uptake of ^{18}F-fluorodeoxyglucose (^{18}F-FDG) on PET was increased in these vertebrae. (B) Following chemotherapy, the T1-weighted sequence (left) shows a generalised increase of signal in the marrow cavities and focal high signal corresponding to previous tumour-involved areas. The signal is also increased on T2-weighted imaging (right) at these sites, although uptake of ^{18}F-FDG was normal. Although clearly abnormal, this MRI appearance was interpreted as successful treatment of lymphoma, and the patient remained disease-free 12 months after completion of therapy.

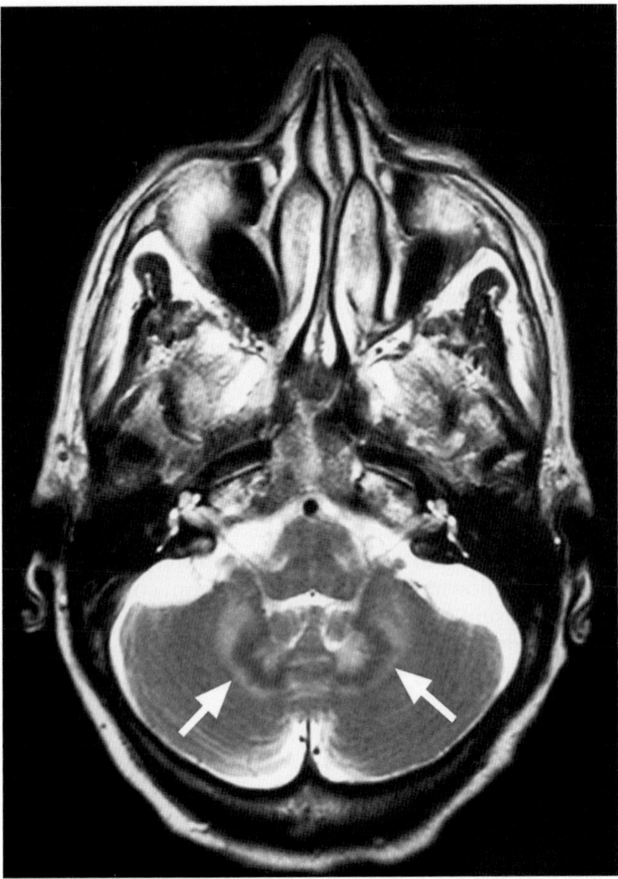

FIGURE 68-11 ■ T2-weighted MRI of posterior fossa. This shows diffuse high signal in cerebellum (arrows) following treatment with fluorouracil.

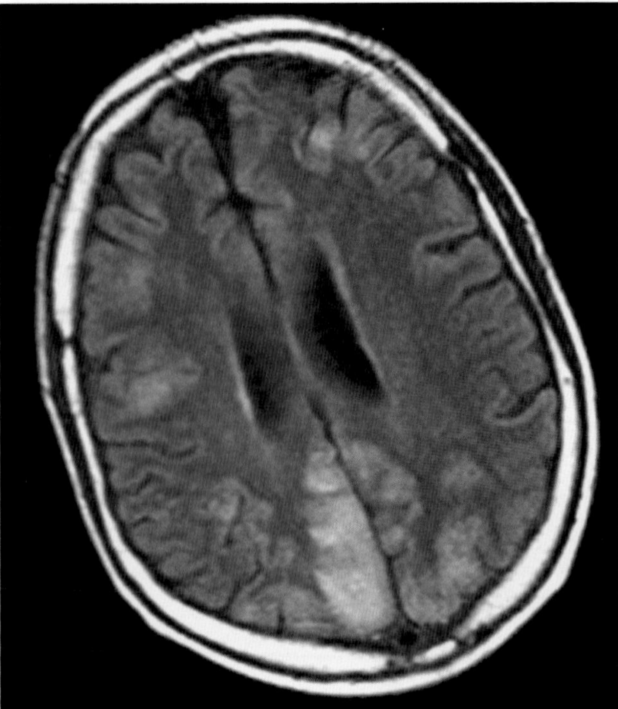

FIGURE 68-12 ■ MRI axial fluid attenuation inversion recovery sequence. This shows high signal in the parafalcine posterior grey and white matter with isolated areas of abnormal signal in both frontal lobes. This appearance is typical of the reversible posterior leukoencephalopathy syndrome seen following bone marrow transplantation, frequently attributed to toxicity from ciclosporin.

(FLAIR) sequence. Similar changes may be seen within the spinal cord as a result of radiation myelitis. White matter changes may also be identified with cytotoxic medications (Fig. 68-11), including fluorouracil, levamisole and intrathecal methotrexate. As with lung toxicity, a growing number of cytotoxic agents have been implicated in central neurotoxic events. Following bone marrow transplantation, immunosuppressive drugs, including ciclosporin, cause a reversible posterior leukoencephalopathy syndrome (RPLS), which has a characteristic distribution of grey and white matter change (Fig. 68-12).

Peripheral neuropathy is common with cytotoxic agents such as vincristine, but has no imaging features. However, radiation damage to the brachial plexus is occasionally encountered following treatment for breast cancer. This is due to an ischaemic insult to the vasa nervorum of the brachial plexus. Thickening of the elements of the brachial plexus within the radiation field is best demonstrated by MRI. This may be difficult to distinguish from the infiltrative forms of recurrent breast cancer. However, if there is no mass lesion, and if appropriate symptoms and clinical signs are present, MRI is an accurate way of diagnosing radiation-induced brachial plexopathy.[35]

Hepatic Toxicity

Many cytotoxic chemotherapy regimens induce abnormality of liver function. The change most frequently observed on imaging is hepatic steatosis. This may be reversible even if treatment is continued, which can be a source of confusion as contrast parameters within the liver in the presence of metastases can alter radically between examinations. It is, therefore, important to continue using the same imaging protocols throughout the treatment regimen.

Cardiotoxicity

Radiation to the thorax may cause acute and chronic pericarditis, cardiomyopathy and, in the long term, coronary artery disease and valvular dysfunction. A more frequent problem for the cancer patient is cardiotoxicity from cytotoxic agents; for example, doxorubicin is known to cause some degree of myocardial dysfunction in 50% of asymptomatic patients. In extreme cases, life-threatening congestive cardiac failure can develop. Circulatory problems may also develop due to fluid overload during hyper-hydration, which is necessary in a number of treatment regimens. Agents such as asparaginase can precipitate abnormalities of coagulation, resulting in venous thrombosis.

SURVEILLANCE AND RESTAGING

Surveillance of Asymptomatic Patients

Following the diagnosis and treatment of a primary tumour, decisions need to be made on how extensive the search for metastases should be, and how long imaging surveillance should continue. The approach differs between tumour types, and depends on the initial local (T) staging and tumour biology. Another factor to consider is whether there is a biochemical marker for the tumour, a rise in which would indicate the likelihood of a relapse that could subsequently be anatomically demonstrated by imaging. A good example of a tumour in which surveillance programmes are appropriate is NSGCT of the testis. Following orchidectomy, CT staging of chest, abdomen and pelvis is usually undertaken. Seventy per cent of patients will have no lymph node, pulmonary or other metastatic spread and will not relapse subsequently. However, 30% of patients with a normal CT study at the time of orchidectomy will relapse: 80% of this group will relapse within 1 year and 95% will relapse within 2 years. Two-thirds of these have a rise in tumour markers, but the remainder will be marker-negative. Cytotoxic chemotherapy for relapse is effective, with cure rates in excess of 90%. It is, therefore, justifiable to continue CT surveillance for 2 years; while some institutions practice a high-frequency surveillance programme, there is no definite evidence that a lower CT surveillance frequency at 6-monthly or even yearly intervals worsens prognosis. However, if large-volume disease is allowed to develop, this has an adverse prognostic significance, so shortening the inter-examination interval empirically makes sense.[36]

A further example where imaging is used to detect asymptomatic disease is colorectal carcinoma. Surgery in patients with resectable hepatic metastatic disease gives a 40% 5-year survival, compared with survival rates close to 0 in untreated patients.[37] Current strategies now aim to reduce the volume of hepatic metastatic disease so that previously non-resectable disease may undergo surgery with curative intent.[38] There is growing evidence that intensive follow-up that incorporates monitoring of carcinoembryonic antigen (CEA) and CT of chest, abdomen and pelvis contributes to detection of metastatic disease in patients who subsequently proceed to potentially curative resection.[39,40] CT has adequate sensitivity for detection of hepatic and pulmonary metastases, but ultrasound and MRI have a role in characterising liver lesions (Fig. 68-13).

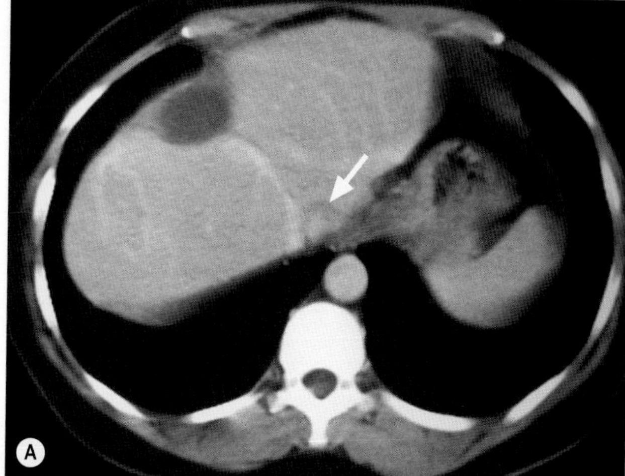

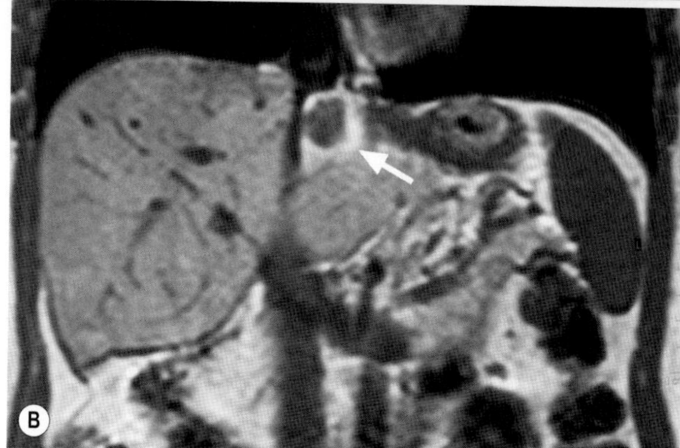

FIGURE 68-13 ■ **CT and MRI of a patient following hepatic metastectomy.** (A) Follow-up CT in a patient after hepatic metastectomy (low-attenuation post-surgical defect shown anteriorly). There is an intermediate attenuation abnormality in the upper liver close to the diaphragmatic surface (arrow). (B) Further investigation with mangafodipir trisodium (Mn-DPDP)-enhanced liver imaging shows perilesional enhancement on T1-weighted MRI 24 hours after administration of the contrast agent. This appearance is typical of a metastasis (arrow).

^{18}F-FDG PET and ^{18}F-FDG PET/CT may prove to be valuable in early detection of metastatic disease, particularly in areas where CT alone lacks sensitivity such as the peritoneal cavity (Fig. 68-14). ^{18}F-FDG PET/CT is a valuable problem-solving technique when CEA is rising, and other imaging techniques fail to demonstrate the site of recurrence. The frequency and duration of imaging follow-up is controversial, but is influenced by factors such as the T stage of the colorectal primary, histology and factors that help to predict relapse, such as positive CRM and vascular invasion. These principles may be applied to any tumour type, and should be influenced by the likelihood of detection of metastatic disease.

Following treatment of primary breast cancer, there is considerable variation in practice. Some surgeons request chest radiography, liver ultrasound examination and radionuclide bone examination, whereas others request whole-body CT. In T1 and T2 primary tumours (less than 5 cm) the incidence of metastatic disease at the time of diagnosis is extremely low. In a series of almost 500 consecutive patients who were imaged at diagnosis with chest radiograph, liver ultrasound examination and radionuclide bone examination, no metastases were found in patients with T1 tumours. In patients with T4 tumours, the rate of detection of metastases was 18%. Overall, distant metastases were found at the time of primary diagnosis in 3.9% of patients.[41] However, there is limited evidence that detection of metastatic breast cancer in asymptomatic patients improves 5-year survival.[42,43] In testicular NSGCT, relapse is eminently treatable with cytotoxic chemotherapy. In colorectal cancer, surgery for

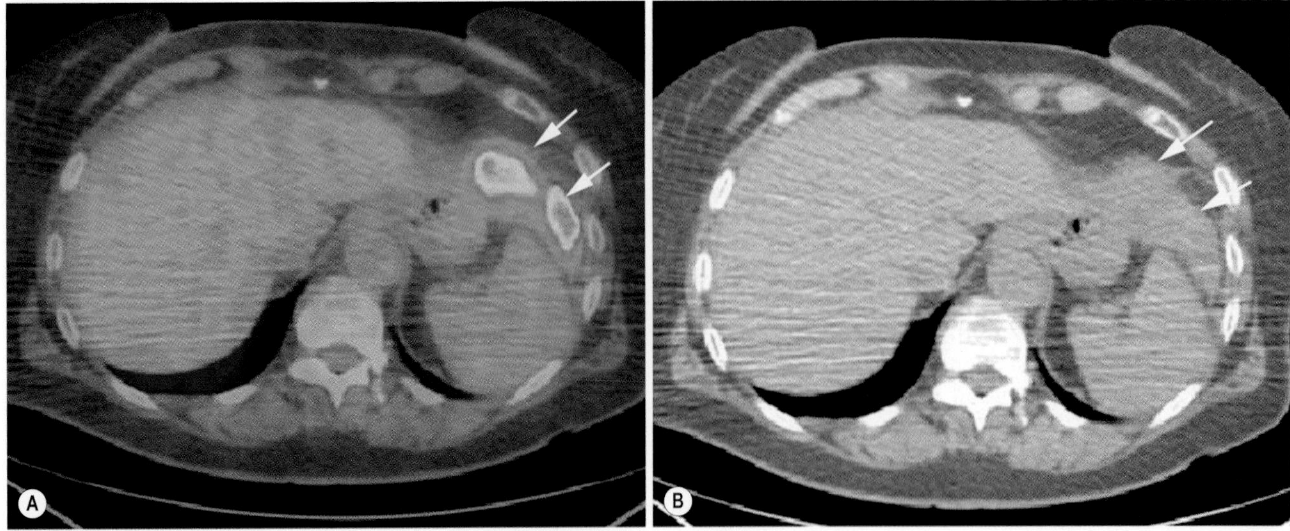

FIGURE 68-14 ■ **^{18}F-FDG PET/CT in a patient with rising CEA a year after resection of a colonic carcinoma.** PET/CT demonstrates evidence of peritoneal disease within the left upper quadrant (arrow) lying anterior to the stomach.

metastatic disease is beneficial, but in breast cancer surveillance protocols are less useful, owing to the natural history of the disease. Such factors need to be considered for each individual tumour type before embarking on prolonged and costly investigation.

Restaging of Symptomatic Patients

Once a patient has been diagnosed with a malignancy it often becomes the most important element of their medical history. Any prolonged or persistent complaint will usually precipitate a search for recurrence. Lethargy, fatigue and weight loss are frequent symptoms, but imaging investigation is easier to direct when there are localising symptoms such as abdominal pain or distension, dyspnoea, bone pain or a neurological event. The choice of investigation should be directed appropriately; for example, patients with abdominal pain should first be investigated with an ultrasound examination of the abdomen. A knowledge of the pattern of disease spread will assist choice and interpretation of investigations. With a history of colorectal cancer, hepatic pain from metastatic disease is likely, whereas ovarian tumours are more likely to disseminate through the peritoneal cavity, causing poorly localised abdominal pain and ascites.

Acute bone pain can be investigated with plain radiography, but more frequently radionuclide bone examinations are used. Most tumours can metastasise to bone, but breast, prostate, lung, kidney and thyroid do so particularly frequently. However, some metastases are not detectable by radionuclide bone examination, because of their failure to excite sufficient osteoblastic response. For example, in breast cancer 7% of patients with a normal skeletal scintigram have metastatic bone disease on MRI (Fig. 68-15).[44]

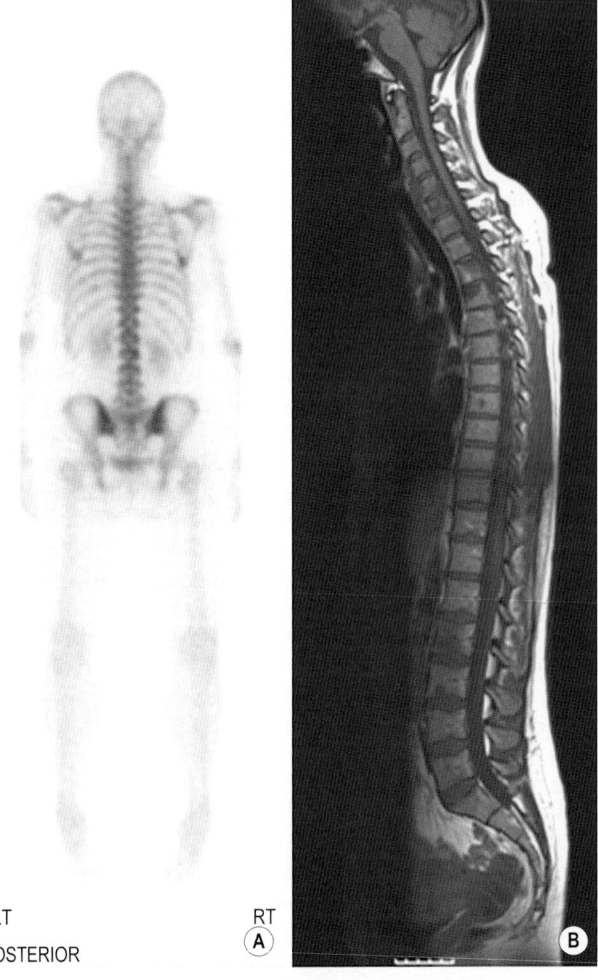

FIGURE 68-15 ■ **Patient previously diagnosed with breast cancer presenting with back pain.** (A) Skeletal scintigram. There are no focal areas of abnormal uptake in the skeleton. (B) T1-weighted sagittal MRI study of spine demonstrating multiple areas of low signal in the vertebral bodies consistent with bony metastases. Mechanical cord compression is threatened in the upper thoracic area. MRI was performed a week after scintigraphy.

A neurological presentation, such as a convulsion in a patient with a previous diagnosis of cancer, is best investigated with CT or MRI of the brain. The cause of dyspnoea may be diagnosed using chest radiography. There is a trend towards whole-body imaging to search for metastases, and CT of the thorax, abdomen and pelvis is often requested without any real attempt to investigate the presenting symptom. Whole-body CT is a widely available test, but some authors have suggested whole-body PET or whole-body MRI using the short tau inversion recovery (STIR) sequence.[45,46] Potentially, the greatest disadvantage of whole-body imaging techniques is that they will generate false-positive findings, or diagnose recurrence for which treatment is not possible or not necessary. It should always be borne in mind when investigating symptoms in a patient with a history of cancer that the diagnosis of metastatic disease is a major blow for the patient, and the diagnosis should only be made when there is a high degree of certainty. The imaging findings should be consistent with the known patterns of metastatic spread for the relevant tumour. If the imaging features are unconvincing or atypical, it is preferable to delay a positive finding of metastatic disease rather than to overdiagnose.

CONCLUSION

Oncological imaging is a rapidly evolving subspeciality of radiology, and forms a large proportion of imaging performed within a radiology department. It demands a sound knowledge of anatomy and understanding of patterns of spread and biological behaviour of individual tumour types. In these respects it is similar to other imaging specialities, but there are also many toxic effects of treatment and associated conditions, which must be discriminated from manifestations of the underlying malignancy. An accurate clinical history and a high level of multidisciplinary cooperation greatly enhance the practice of oncological imaging.

For a full list of references, please see ExpertConsult.

FURTHER READING

6. Dukes CE. The classification of cancer of the rectum. J Path Bact 1932;35:323.
7. Heald RJ. Total mesorectal excision is optimal surgery for rectal cancer: a Scandinavian consensus. Br J Surg 1995;82:1297–9.
8. Quirke P, Durdey P, Dixon MF, et al. Local recurrence of rectal adenocarcinoma due to inadequate surgical resection. Histopathological study of lateral tumour spread and surgical excision. Lancet 1986;2:996–9.
9. Beets-Tan RG, Beets GL, Vliegen RF, et al. Accuracy of magnetic resonance imaging in prediction of tumour-free resection margin in rectal cancer surgery. Lancet 2001;357:497–504.
10. The MERCURY study group. Diagnostic accuracy of preoperative magnetic resonance imaging in predicting curative resection of rectal cancer: prospective observational study. BMJ 2006;333:779.
11. Burton S, Brown G, Daniels IR. MRI directed multidisciplinary team preoperative treatment strategy: the way to eliminate positive circumferential margins? Br J Cancer 2006;94:351–7.
12. NCCN website. http://www.nccn.org/professionals/physician_gls/f_guidelines.asp.

CHAPTER 69

The Breast

Jonathan J. James • A. Robin M. Wilson • Andrew J. Evans

CHAPTER OUTLINE

Breast cancer is the most common malignant tumour in the UK with over 48,000 diagnoses annually—80% of cases are in women over the age of 50. It accounts for over 12,000 deaths per annum. Imaging is essential for the early detection and accurate diagnosis of breast cancer. Population screening with mammography aims to reduce mortality by detecting the disease at an earlier stage, before it has spread beyond the breast. Mammography and ultrasound are the first-line imaging investigations in women with breast symptoms. Magnetic resonance imaging (MRI) is established as an adjunctive diagnostic tool because of its high sensitivity for invasive breast cancer. Percutaneous image-guided breast biopsy is used for the pathological assessment of breast lesions. The combination of imaging, clinical examination and needle biopsy—known as 'triple assessment'—is the expected standard for breast diagnosis.

METHODS OF EXAMINATION

Mammography

Mammography remains one of the principal imaging modalities for diagnosis, although its use is rarely indicated in women under the age of 35. The main indications for mammography are:

- evaluation of breast symptoms and signs, including masses, skin thickening, deformity, nipple retraction, nipple discharge and nipple eczema;
- breast cancer screening;
- follow-up of patients with previously treated breast cancer; and
- guidance for biopsy, or localisation of lesions not visible on ultrasound.

Mammography places stringent demands on equipment and image quality. The breast is composed predominantly of fatty tissue and has a relatively narrow range of inherent densities. Consequently, special X-ray tubes are required to produce the low-energy radiation necessary to achieve high tissue contrast, enabling the demonstration of small changes in breast density. High spatial resolution is required to identify tiny structures within the breast, such as microcalcifications measuring in the order of 100 μm; and short exposure times are necessary to limit movement unsharpness. Where the breasts are thicker or are composed of denser glandular tissue, higher energy radiation is required, although radiation dose must be kept to a minimum.

X-ray tubes produce a spectrum of radiation energies, which are determined by the target and filter combination and the peak kilovoltage (kVp). A molybdenum target is used because it produces a low-energy spectrum with peaks of 17.5 and 19.6 keV, providing high contrast. A tungsten target is less desirable because it produces higher energies (Fig. 69-1). The spectrum is refined further by adding a filter to reduce the proportion of radiation above and below the desired range. Commercially available target/filter combinations include molybdenum/molybdenum, molybdenum/rhodium, rhodium/rhodium, tungsten/molybdenum and tungsten/rhodium. Molybdenum/molybdenum is the most frequently used combination.

To achieve the required spatial resolution, mammography tubes must have an extremely small focal spot, 0.3 mm for routine mammography. For magnification mammography a smaller focal spot of 0.1 mm is required. Tube current should be as high as possible in order to keep exposure times short. Movement unsharpness may occur when exposure times exceed 1 second. Grids are used routinely for all mammographic studies. These reduce scattered radiation and so increase contrast, especially in the dense or thick breast. Modern mammography machines have a facility for automatic selection of target/filter combination, kVp and tube current according to the breast density and the thickness of the compressed breast. In addition, automatic exposure control devices detect the amount of radiation striking the detector and terminate the exposure at a preset level.

Standard Projections

There are two standard mammographic projections: a mediolateral oblique (MLO) view and a craniocaudal

(CC) view (Fig. 69-2). Correct positioning is crucial to avoid missing lesions situated at the margins of the breast. The MLO view is taken with the X-ray beam directed from superomedial to inferolateral, usually at an angle of 30–60°, with compression applied obliquely across the chest wall, perpendicular to the long axis of the pectoralis major muscle (Fig. 69-3A). The MLO projection is the only projection in which all the breast tissue can be demonstrated on a single image. A well-positioned MLO view should demonstrate the inframammary angle, the nipple in profile, and the nipple positioned at the level of the lower border of the pectoralis major, with the muscle across the posterior border of the film at an angle of 25°–30° to the vertical (Fig. 69-2A).

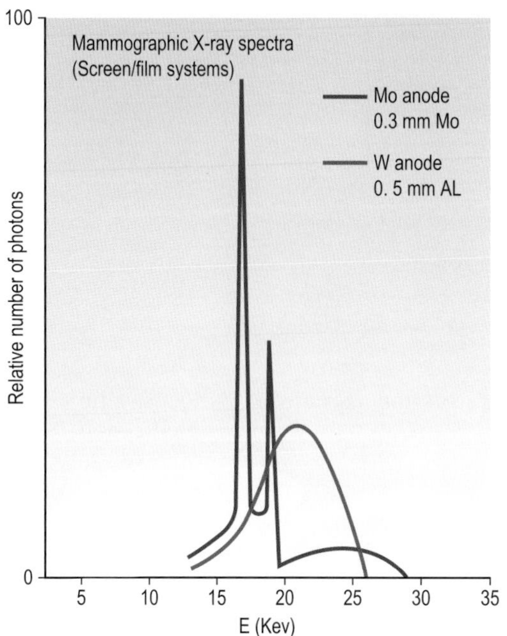

FIGURE 69-1 ■ X-ray spectra obtained from a molybdenum (Mo) target tube set at 29 kVp and a tungsten (W) target tube set at 26 kVp. (With permission from Haus A G, Metz C E, Chiles J T, Rossman K 1976 The effect of X-ray spectra from molybdenum and tungsten target tubes on image quality in mammography. Radiology 118: 705–709.)

For the CC view, the X-ray beam travels from superior to inferior. Positioning is achieved by pulling the breast up and forward away from the chest wall, with compression applied from above (Fig. 69-3B). A well-positioned CC view should demonstrate the nipple in profile. It should demonstrate virtually all of the medial tissue and most of the lateral tissue except the axillary tail of the breast. The pectoralis major is demonstrated at the centre of a CC film in approximately 30% of individuals and the depth of breast tissue demonstrated should be within 1 cm of the distance from the nipple to the pectoralis major on the MLO projection (Fig. 69-2B).

Additional Projections

Supplementary views may be taken to solve specific diagnostic problems.[1,2] For example, the CC view can be rotated to visualise either more of the lateral or medial aspect of the breast, compared to the standard CC projection. Localised compression or 'paddle views' can be performed. This involves the application of more vigorous compression to a localised area using a compression paddle (Fig. 69-4). These views are used to distinguish real lesions from superimposition of normal tissues and to define the margins of a mass. A true lateral view may

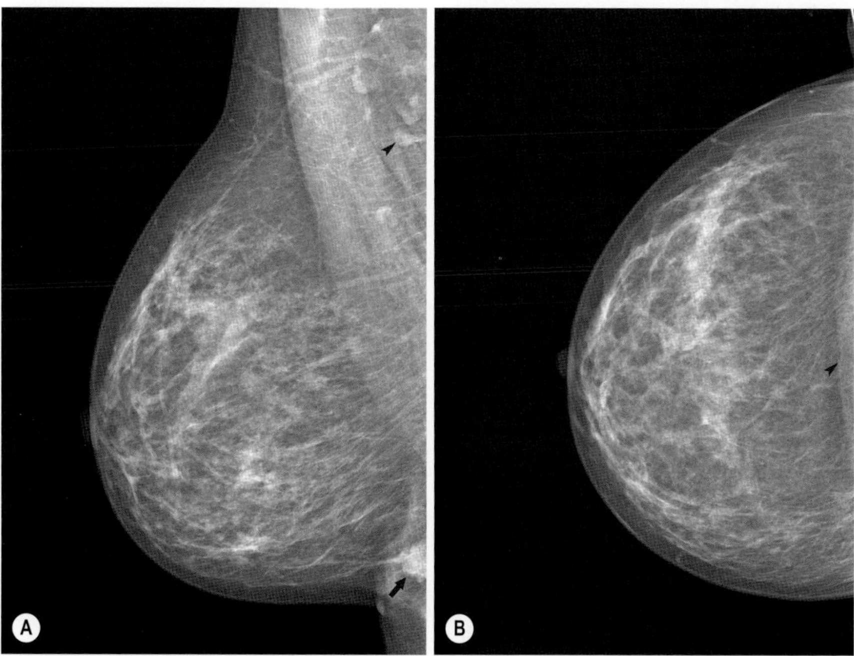

FIGURE 69-2 ■ A standard set of mammograms consists of the mediolateral oblique (MLO) view (A) and the craniocaudal (CC) view (B). (A) A cancer is seen in the inframammary area on the MLO view (arrow), illustrating the importance of correct positioning to avoid missing lesions. Normal lymph nodes (arrowhead) are frequently seen on the MLO projection. (B) The cancer is not demonstrated on this correctly positioned CC view, with pectoral muscle visualised at the back of the mammogram (arrowhead).

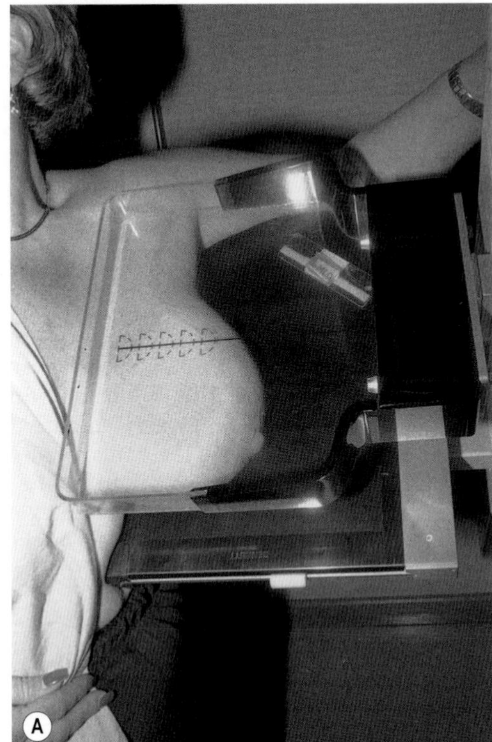

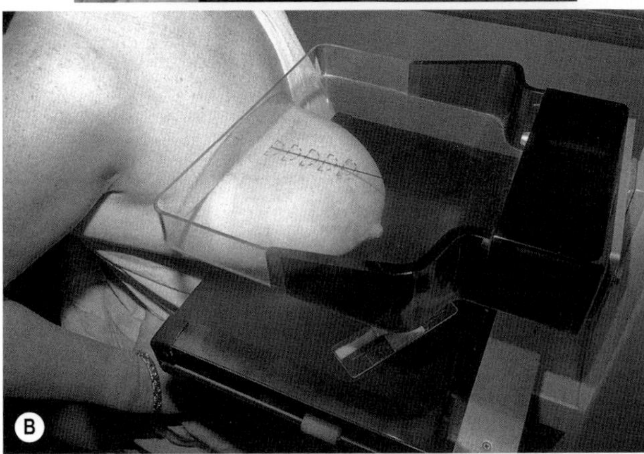

FIGURE 69-3 ■ **Breast positioning.** Positioning for the (A) mediolateral oblique and (B) craniocaudal views.

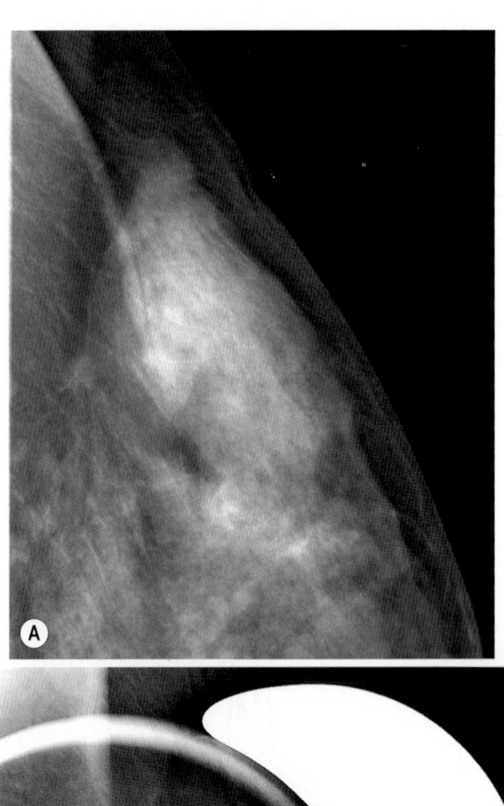

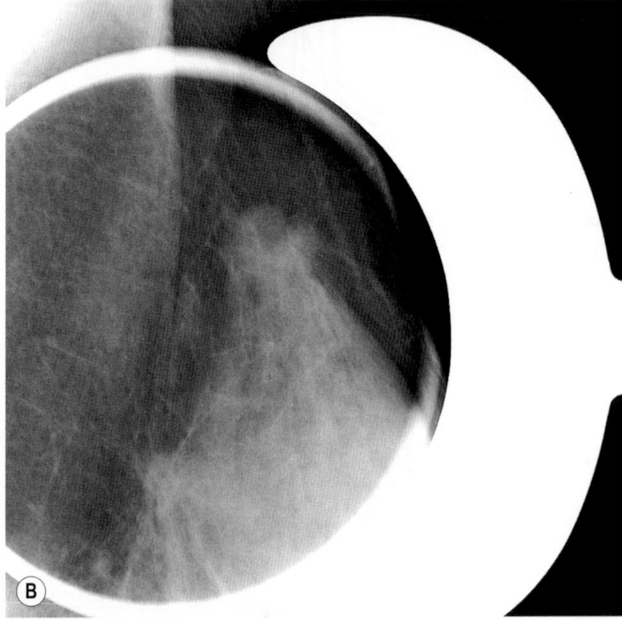

FIGURE 69-4 ■ **Additional mammographic views.** (A) An area of concern was identified in the lateral aspect of the left breast on initial mammography. (B) A 'paddle view' was performed and two suspicious spiculate mass lesions were demonstrated much more clearly. Both proved to be invasive carcinomas on subsequent biopsy.

be used to provide a third imaging plane in order to distinguish superimposition of normal structures from real lesions or to increase the accuracy of wire localisations of non-palpable lesions. The true lateral view is performed with the mammography unit turned through 90° and a mediolateral or lateromedial X-ray beam.

Magnification views are most frequently performed to examine areas of microcalcifications within the breast, to characterise them and to establish their extent. Magnification views are typically performed in the craniocaudal and lateral projections. The magnified lateral view will demonstrate 'teacups' typical of benign microcalcifications, described later in the chapter. Mammographic technique may need to be modified in women with breast implants. Silicon and saline implants are radio-opaque and may obscure much of the breast tissue. Consequently, mammography is of limited diagnostic value in some women. The Eklund technique can be employed to displace the implant posteriorly, behind the compression plate, maximising the volume of breast tissue that is compressed and imaged.[3] Mammography-induced implant rupture has not been reported to date.

Breast Compression

Compression of the breast is essential for good mammography, for the following reasons:

- It reduces geometric unsharpness by bringing the object closer to the film.

- It improves contrast by reducing scatter.
- It diminishes movement unsharpness by permitting shorter exposure times and immobilising the breast.
- It reduces radiation dose, as a lesser thickness of breast tissue needs to be penetrated and scatter is reduced.
- It achieves more uniform image density: a homogeneous breast thickness prevents overexposure of the thinner anterior breast tissues and underexposure of the thicker posterior breast tissues.
- It provides more accurate assessment of the density of masses. As cysts and normal glandular tissue are more easily compressed, the more rigid carcinomas are highlighted.
- It separates superimposed breast tissues so that lesions are better seen.

Radiation Dose

Mammography uses ionising radiation to image the breast. The risks of ionising radiation are well known and any exposure needs to be justified, with doses kept as low as possible. The radiation dose for a standard two-view examination of both breasts is approximately 4.5 mGy.[4] The average effective dose of radiation from mammography is equivalent to 61 days of average natural background radiation.[5]

Dose is more of an issue in a population screening programme, where women who may never develop breast cancer are being exposed to radiation. It has been estimated that the risk of inducing a breast cancer in women screened in the United Kingdom National Health Service Breast Screening Programme (NHSBSP) is 1 in 100,000 per mGy. A risk–benefit calculation has established that the benefits of screening far outweigh the risk of inducing a cancer, with the ratio of lives saved to lives lost calculated as approximately 100 : 1.[4]

Digital mammography systems have the potential to reduce patient dose without loss of image quality.

The Detector

Traditionally, the mammographic image has been recorded on film, but this has been superseded by digital technology. Manufacturers have developed a number of different approaches to producing a digital mammogram. The first type of digital system developed for mammography used photostimulable phosphor computed radiography (CR). This uses an imaging plate coated with a phosphor to replace the traditional screen/film mammography cassette. The imaging plate, stored in a conventional-looking cassette, is exposed in the usual fashion in a conventional (analog) mammography machine. A latent image is stored in the phosphor after exposure. The imaging plate is scanned by a laser beam in a plate reader and light is emitted in proportion to the absorbed X-rays. The emitted light is then detected by a photomultiplier system and the resulting electrical signal is digitised to produce the image.

More recently, full-field flat-panel detectors have been developed. One type of detector consists of a phosphor layer coated onto a light-sensitive thin-film transistor (TFT) array composed of amorphous silicon. Charge from the TFT array produced in response to the light emission from the phosphor is measured and digitised. The above digital systems require multiple conversion steps in the acquisition of the image: X-ray energy is converted into light energy, which is then converted into electrical energy. Multiple conversion steps are inefficient and have the potential to degrade image quality. Systems that avoid these conversion losses are described as being more 'direct'. Some manufacturers use amorphous selenium or silicon dioxide in the detector, allowing the energy of the X-ray photon to be directly converted into electrical energy.

Digital Mammography in Clinical Practice

There are clear logistical advantages to digital mammography, including the potential to improve patient throughput, as traditional screen/film mammography is labour intensive, with time taken in handling cassettes, loading/unloading film and processing. Digital mammography equipment interfaces directly with picture archiving and communication systems (PACS), leading to further increased efficiencies associated with image storage and display, with soft-copy reporting from high-resolution (5 megapixel) monitors.

It is important to establish whether an improvement in image quality can translate into an improvement in cancer detection. A powerful test of the potential of digital mammography to improve cancer detection rates is in a screening setting. Several early studies found that digital mammography was at least equivalent to screen/film mammography in terms of cancer detection rates.[6,7] The larger Oslo II study, which randomised over 25,000 women to either conventional or digital mammography, showed an increase in cancer detection in the women undergoing a digital mammogram, but this did not quite reach statistical significance ($p = 0.053$).[8]

To detect significant differences between the two techniques, the population size needs to be large, as the cancer detection rate in a screening population is around 6 per 1000 women screened. The North American Digital Mammographic Imaging Screening Trial (DMIST) enrolled 49,500 women.[9] This study found that overall the diagnostic accuracy of digital and conventional mammography was similar. However, there were some groups of women where digital mammography outperformed screen/film mammography, showing significantly improved diagnostic accuracy. These were women under the age of 50, those with dense breast parenchyma and women who were pre- or perimenopausal. Encouragingly, it is in these groups of women that conventional screen/film mammography had shown reduced sensitivity for detecting breast cancer.

Computer-Aided Detection

Computer-aided detection (CAD) is a software system that is designed to assist the film reader by placing prompts over areas of concern, to reduce observational oversights. CAD systems are highly sensitive for detecting cancers on screening mammograms. CAD will correctly prompt around 90% of all cancers, with 86–88% of all masses and 98% of microcalcifications correctly marked. Specificity is much more of a problem with a high rate of false-positive prompts. The number of false prompts will vary according to the level of sensitivity at which the system is set; typically, there are between two and four false prompts per standard set of mammogram images.[10–12]

The routine use of CAD remains controversial and there is no consensus in the literature as to whether CAD improves film reader performance; despite this, CAD is used in the interpretation of screening mammograms in around 75% of cases in the United States.[13] Some prospective studies of the use of CAD in the screening setting have shown a significant improvement in a single film reader's performance when CAD software is applied, whereas others have shown no effect on cancer detection rates.[12,14] A large multicentred retrospective review of the use of CAD in the interpretation of screening mammography in the United States found its use associated with a decrease in the specificity of screening, with an increase in recall rates for only a very minimal improvement in sensitivity, largely the result of a non-significant increase in the detection of ductal carcinoma in situ.[13]

It is difficult to extrapolate the findings of these studies to the UK breast screening programme (NHSBSP), where virtually all films are double read by two readers. Double reading is known to increase cancer detection rates by 4–14% compared to single reading, and so the question is whether one reader using CAD could produce results equivalent to double reading and whether CAD is a more cost-effective solution to recruitment problems than training non-medically qualified film readers. The Computer-Aided Detection Evaluation Trial (CADET II) was a large prospective trial of over 30,000 women that reported a comparable cancer detection rate for single reading with CAD to double reading but with a small but significant increase in recall rate.[15] A further sub-analysis has suggested that at the present time CAD is not a cost-effective alternative to double reading in the NHSBSP in view of the increase in recall rates.[16]

Digital Breast Tomosynthesis

One of the limitations of mammography is that it produces a two-dimensional (2D) radiographic view of a three-dimensional structure and, as a consequence, a cancer may not be detected due to overlapping normal glandular tissue obscuring the presence of a tumour. Lesions may be simulated by the superimposition of normal tissue, leading to unnecessary recalls following screening mammography. These factors result in a reduction in the sensitivity and specificity of mammography. Breast tomosynthesis is an emerging digital mammographic technique where thin slices through the breast are reconstructed from multiple low-dose projections acquired at different angles of the X-ray tube. The resulting thin sections can be scrolled through by the reporting radiologist, with the potential to alleviate the effects of tissue superimposition.

The role of tomosynthesis is still being defined, and there is debate surrounding its use as an adjunct or replacement for conventional 2D digital mammography. Its role in diagnosis and screening requires clarification. It has the potential to be an additional tool, for the work-up of screen-detected abnormalities replacing traditional 'paddle' views.[17] When used as a screening tool, studies show an improvement in specificity, with a reduction in recall rates of up to 11%; improvements in sensitivity over conventional 2D mammography are not so clear.[18]

Ultrasound

The main indications for ultrasound are:

- characterisation of palpable mass lesions;
- assessment of abnormalities detected on a mammogram;
- primary technique for the assessment of breast problems in younger patients; and
- guidance for biopsy and wire localisations.

Breast ultrasound requires high-quality, high-resolution grey-scale imaging, using linear probes with high frequencies typically between 7.5 and 15 MHz. Higher frequencies result in greater resolution, but as the frequency increases, the ability of the ultrasound beam to penetrate to deeper breast tissue decreases. Consequently, the frequency selected has to be appropriate for the size of the breast to be examined. Parameters such as harmonics and compounding are available on modern ultrasound machines and can be applied to enhance the displayed image. Their use is subject to operator preference. Techniques such as colour flow imaging (Doppler) and elastography may also have a role in lesion characterisation.

Elastography is an ultrasound technique that can provide additional information based on tissue stiffness or hardness. The concept that malignant lesions feel firmer or stiffer than the surrounding breast tissue is well recognised from clinical palpation. There are two methods of producing an elastography image or elastogram: strain elastography, where the operator gently manually compresses the breast tissue, and shear wave elastography, where pulses are generated by the transducer producing transverse shear wave propagation through the breast tissue. The main advantage of shear wave elastography is that the technique is quantitative and highly reproducible. Information regarding stiffness can be displayed as a black and white or colour overlay onto the grey-scale image (Fig. 69-5). Features on the elastogram that can be measured include quantitative elasticity (stiffness) in kPa and size ratios relative to conventional grey-scale imaging. In general, breast cancers tend to be stiff, with benign lesions or normal tissue appearing softer (elasticity <80 kPa). Invasive breast cancers often produce areas of stiffness that are larger than the grey-scale abnormality, likely due to changes in the tumour-associated stroma. Elastography has the potential to improve the specificity of breast ultrasound for differentiating benign from malignant masses, reducing the number of benign biopsies. In a recent study, the use of shear wave elastography resulted in a significant improvement in the specificity of breast mass assessment from 61.1 to 78.5%.[19]

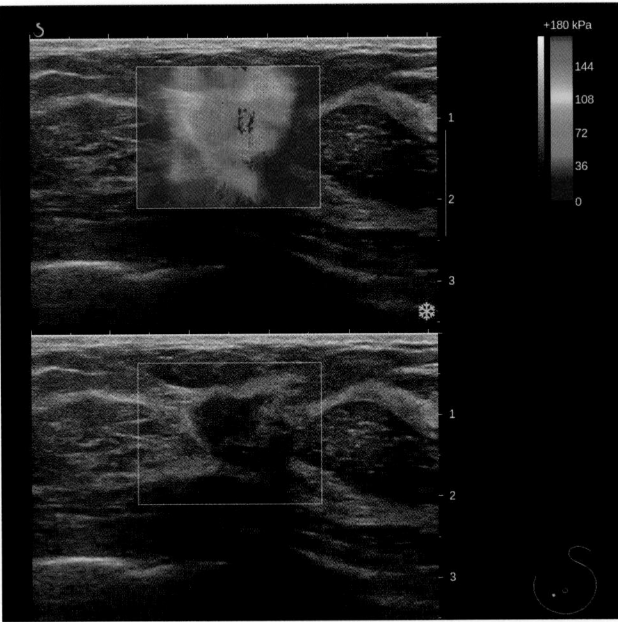

FIGURE 69-5 ■ Elastography. A hypoechoic mass is demonstrated in the left breast. Shear wave elastography is displayed simultaneously as a colour overlay. The colour scale is seen to the right and set to a maximum of 180 kPa. The zone of stiffness is larger, irregular and heterogeneously stiff, with elasticity values in the yellow to red end of the spectrum (108–180 kPa). All these features are suspicious of malignancy, with biopsy confirming an invasive ductal carcinoma.

Ultrasound Technique

The patient is examined in the supine position with the ipsilateral arm placed behind the patient's head. When imaging the outer portion of the breast it helps to turn the patient into a more oblique position. The aim is to flatten the breast tissue against the chest wall, reducing the thickness of breast tissue to be imaged. It is best to image the breast tissue in two planes perpendicular to each other. A transverse and a sagittal plane is a common combination, but some authors advocate examining the breast in a radial and anti-radial direction. The theory behind this method is that the ducts of the breast are positioned in a radial direction, running towards the nipple rather like the spokes of a bicycle wheel. Most breast cancers begin in the ducts and so tumours extending along the ductal system may be better visualised in this plane.[20]

NORMAL ANATOMY

The breast lies on the chest wall on the deep pectoral fascia with the superficial pectoral fascia enveloping the breast. Suspensory ligaments—called Cooper's ligaments—connect the two layers, providing a degree of support to the breast and giving the breast its shape (Fig. 69-6). Centrally, there is the nipple–areolar complex. Collecting ducts open onto the tip of the nipple. There are sebaceous glands within the nipple–areolar complex called Montgomery's glands. Small raised nodular structures called Morgagni's tubercles are distributed over the areola, representing the openings of the ducts of Montgomery's glands onto the skin surface.[21] Deep to the nipple–areolar complex, the breast is divided into 15–25 lobes, each consisting of a branching duct system leading from the collecting ducts to the terminal duct lobular units (TDLUs), the site of milk production in the lactating breast.

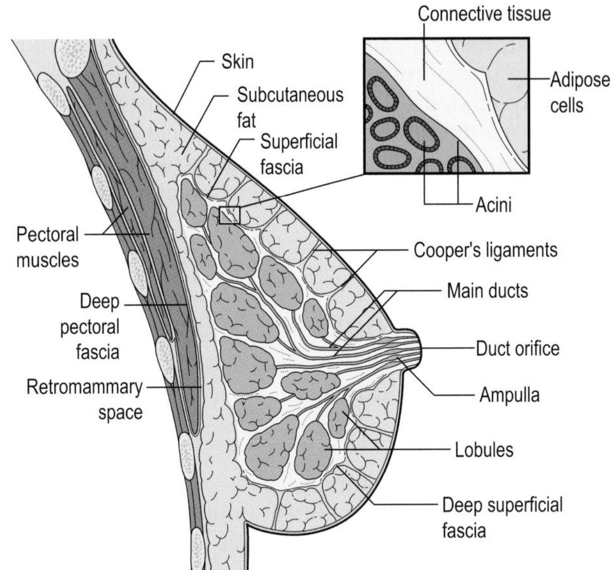

FIGURE 69-6 ■ Gross anatomy of the breast.

The number of TDLUs per lobe varies according to age, lactation, parity and hormonal status. At the end of reproductive life there is an increase in the amount of adipose tissue and, although the main duct system is preserved, there is considerable loss of lobular units. These changes in breast composition are manifested by changes in the breast density on mammography.

Younger women tend to have denser glandular breast tissue. In older women, the mammographic density tends to decrease, with replacement of the glandular tissue by fatty tissue. Classification systems have been developed to describe the density of breast tissue on mammography. One of the best known is the Wolfe classification:[22]

- Wolfe N1 refers to a breast containing a high proportion of fat;
- Wolfe P1 refers to a predominantly fatty breast with <25% visible glandular tissue;
- Wolfe P2 refers to a breast with >25% visible glandular tissue; and
- Wolfe DY refers to extremely dense breast tissue.

Similarly, the American College of Radiology (ACR) breast imaging reporting and data system (BIRADS) lexicon defines four patterns of increasing density, where 1 is almost entirely fatty and 4 is extremely dense.[23]

Mammographic density is a risk factor for the development of breast cancer, with a dense background pattern associated with a higher than average risk of developing breast cancer and more aggressive tumour characteristics.[24] The mechanism through which increased density contributes to breast cancer risk remains unclear. In addition, dense breast tissue may hide abnormalities in the breast, making cancer detection more difficult. The sensitivity of mammography for detecting breast cancer is directly related to the density of the breast tissue. In general, mammography is more sensitive at detecting breast cancer in older, postmenopausal women because the breast tends to be composed of greater amounts of fatty tissue.

BREAST PATHOLOGY

Benign Mass Lesions

Cysts

Cysts are the most common cause of a discrete breast mass, although they are often multiple and bilateral. They are common between the ages of 20 and 50 years, with a peak incidence between 40 and 50 years. Simple cysts are not associated with an increased risk of malignancy and have no malignant potential.

On mammography they are seen as well-defined, round or oval masses (Fig. 69-7A). Sometimes a characteristic halo is visible on mammography. Ultrasound also demonstrates well-defined margins, with an oval or round shape. There is an absence of internal echoes indicating the presence of fluid. The area of breast tissue behind a cyst appears bright on ultrasound (posterior enhancement) due to improved transmission of the ultrasound beam through the cyst fluid (Fig. 69-7B). When these features are present, a cyst can be diagnosed with certainty. Aspiration is easily performed under ultrasound guidance to alleviate symptoms or when there is diagnostic uncertainty. Cytology on cyst fluid is not routinely performed unless there are atypical imaging features or the aspirate is bloodstained.

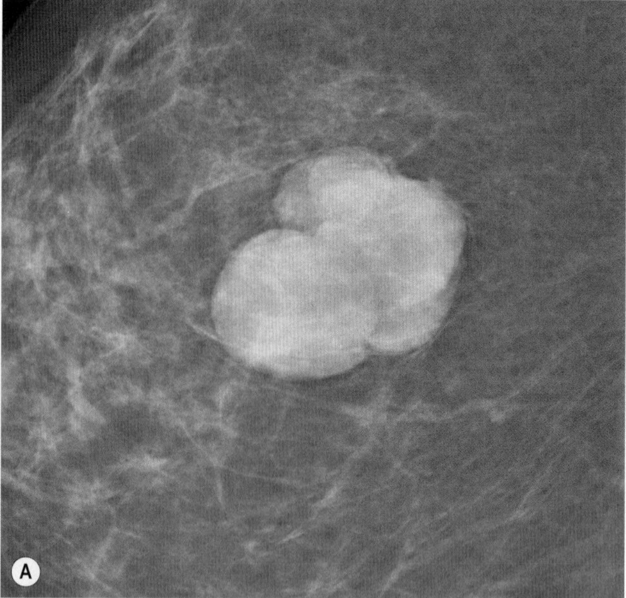

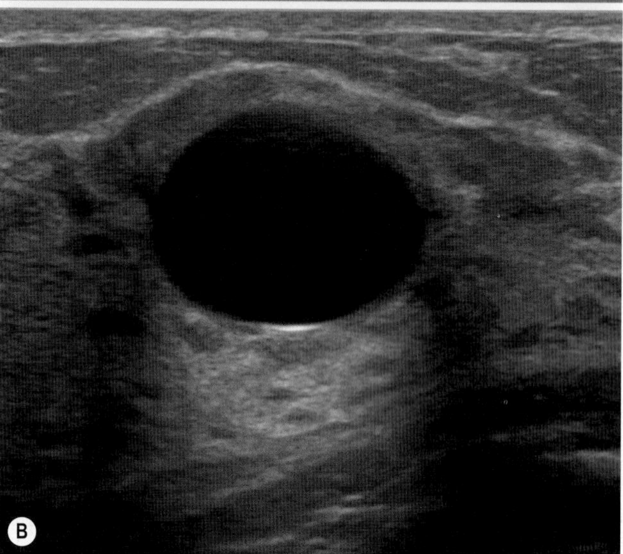

FIGURE 69-7 ■ **Cyst.** (A) A well-defined rounded mass, with an associated lucent halo typical of a cyst. (B) The absence of internal echoes and the posterior enhancement of the ultrasound beam are diagnostic of a cyst.

Fibroadenomas and Related Conditions

Fibroadenomas are the most common cause of a benign solid mass in the breast. They present clinically as smooth, well-demarcated, mobile lumps. They are most frequently encountered in younger women with a peak incidence in the third decade. With the advent of screening, many previously asymptomatic lesions are detected.

On mammography, fibroadenomas are seen as well-defined, rounded or oval masses (Fig. 69-8A). Coarse calcifications may develop within fibroadenomas, particularly in older women (Fig. 69-9).

Ultrasound features have been described that are characteristic of benign masses.[20] These include hyperechogenicity compared with fat, an oval or well-circumscribed lobulated or gently curving shape and the presence of a thin echogenic pseudocapsule. If these features are present with no features suggestive of malignancy, then a mass can be confidently classified as benign.

These features are demonstrated by fibroadenomas (Fig. 69-8B). Most fibroadenomas are isoechoic or mildly hypoechoic relative to fat, with an oval shape and lobulated contour. A thin echogenic pseudocapsule may be seen. Percutaneous biopsy may be avoided in women under the age of 25, where the risks of any mass being malignant are very small;[20] however, in most cases, even though the mass appears benign, percutaneous biopsy is undertaken to confirm the diagnosis.

Fibroadenomas must be distinguished from well-circumscribed carcinomas; this is done by percutaneous biopsy. Phyllodes tumour can also have a similar appearance to fibroadenoma, leading to diagnostic difficulties (Fig. 69-10). The pathological characteristics can also be similar to those of large fibroadenomas. Most phyllodes tumours are benign, but some (less than 25%) are locally aggressive and may even metastasise.[21] When a diagnosis of phyllodes tumour is made, surgical excision must be

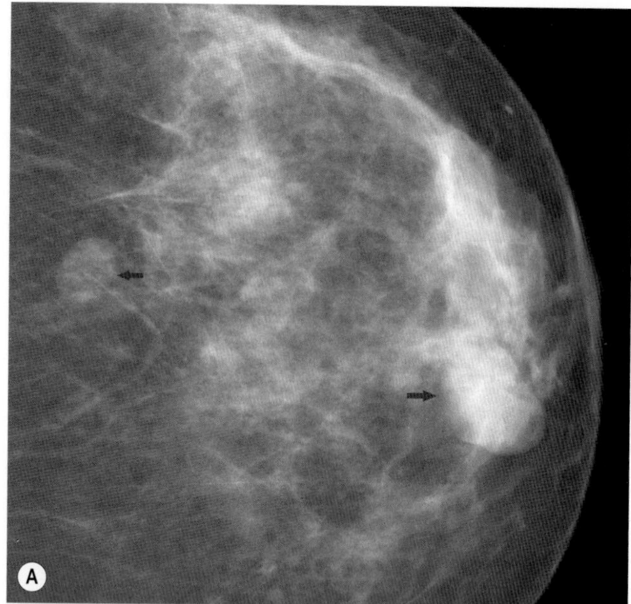

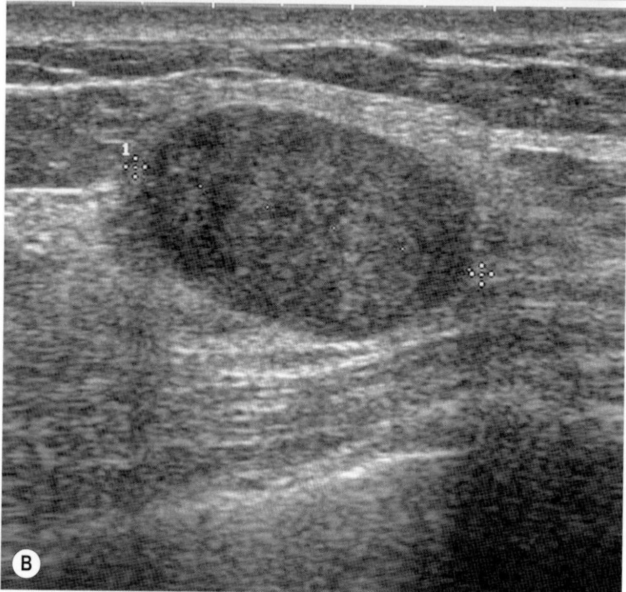

FIGURE 69-8 ■ **Fibroadenoma.** (A) Two well-defined masses on mammography (arrows). (B) Ultrasound of the lesion nearer the nipple showed a well-defined oval mass. Both lesions were confirmed as fibroadenomas on ultrasound-guided core biopsy.

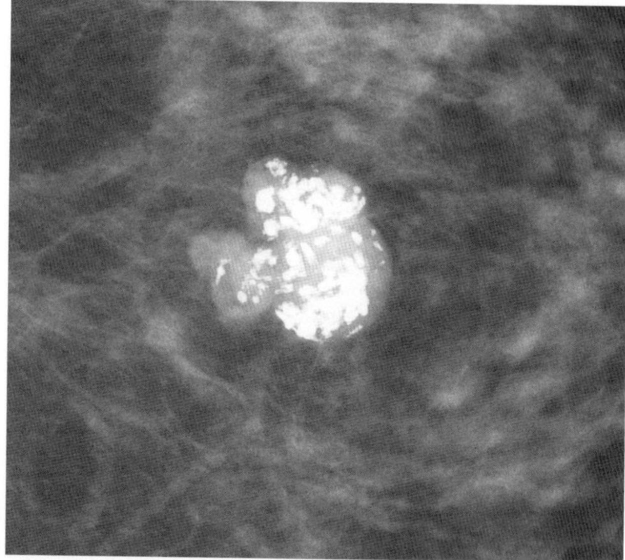

FIGURE 69-9 ■ **Fibroadenomas.** Fibroadenomas may develop coarse 'popcorn'-type calcifications.

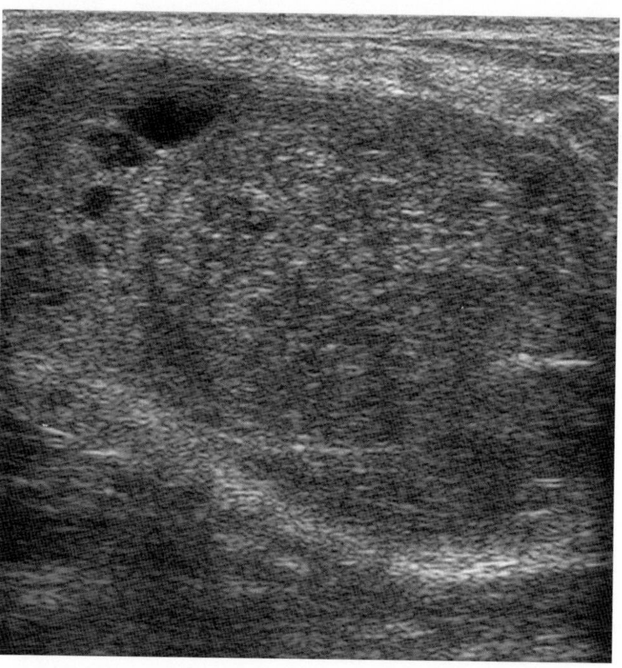

FIGURE 69-10 ■ **Phyllodes tumour.** The presence of several cystic spaces within this large, well-defined mass suggested the possibility of a phyllodes tumour. This was confirmed on core biopsy and surgical excision.

complete with clear margins to prevent the possibility of recurrence. Many larger fibroadenomas (over 3 cm) and those that show a rapid increase in size are excised in order to avoid missing a phyllodes tumour.

Papilloma

Papillomas are benign neoplasms, arising in a duct, either centrally or peripherally within the breast. Many papillomas secrete watery material, leading to a nipple discharge. As they are often friable and bleed easily, the discharge may be bloodstained.

On mammography, they may be seen as a well-defined mass, commonly in a retroareolar location (Fig. 69-11A). Sometimes the mass is associated with microcalcifications. On ultrasound, they typically appear as a filling defect within a dilated duct or cyst (Fig. 69-11B). On aspiration, any cyst fluid may be bloodstained. As it is impossible to differentiate papillomas from papillary carcinomas on imaging criteria, percutaneous biopsy is required.

Papillomas are associated with an increased risk of malignancy, particularly if they are multiple or occur in a more peripheral location within the breast.

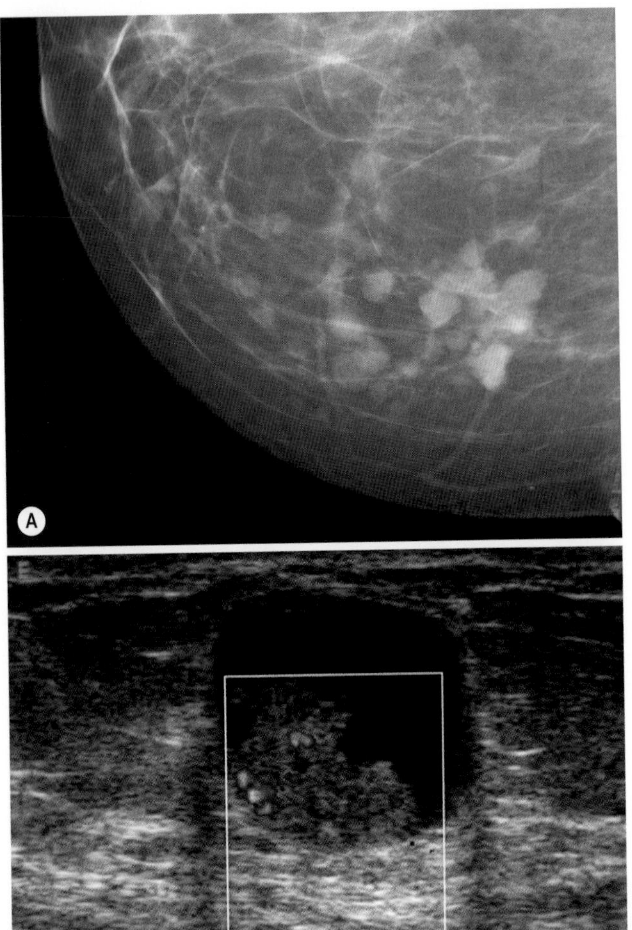

FIGURE 69-11 ■ Multiple small papillomas. (A) Papillomas are frequently well defined on mammography, although part of the mass may have an irregular or ill-defined contour. (B) On ultrasound, the presence of a filling defect within a cystic structure suggests the diagnosis. Colour Doppler can be useful for distinguishing debris within a cyst from a soft-tissue mass.

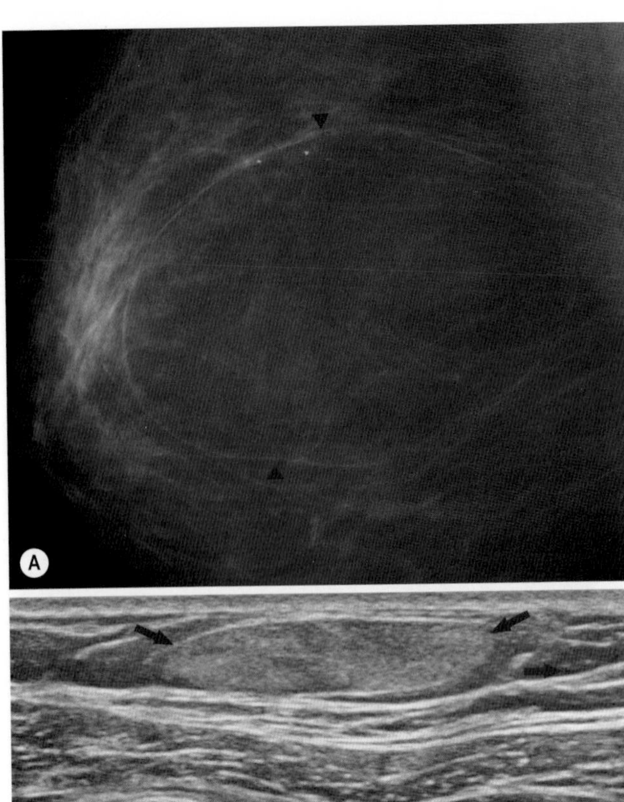

FIGURE 69-12 ■ Lipoma. (A) On mammography, a lipoma may be seen as a well-defined mass of fat density, contained within a thin capsule (arrowheads). (B) On ultrasound, a well-defined hyperechoic lesion characteristic of a lipoma is seen (arrows).

Consequently, excision of papillary lesions is desirable and may be therapeutic in cases of nipple discharge. In situations where percutaneous biopsy shows no evidence of cellular atypia, an alternative to surgical excision is piecemeal percutaneous excision using a vacuum-assisted biopsy device.

Lipoma

Lipomas are benign tumours composed of fat. They present clinically as soft, lobulated masses. Large lipomas may be visible on mammography as a radiolucent mass (Fig. 69-12A). On ultrasound their characteristic appearance is that of a well-defined lesion, hyperechoic compared with the adjacent fat (Fig. 69-12B).

Hamartoma

Hamartomas are benign breast masses composed of lobular structures, stroma and adipose tissue—the components that make up normal breast tissue. They occur at any age. On imaging they may be indistinguishable from other benign masses, such as fibroadenomas. Sometimes large hamartomas are detected on screening mammograms and are impalpable (Fig. 69-13). On mammography they classically appear as large, well-circumscribed masses containing a mixture of dense and lucent areas, reflecting the different tissue components present. Diagnostic difficulty may be encountered because percutaneous biopsy specimens may be reported as normal breast tissue.

Invasive Carcinoma

Breast carcinomas originate in the epithelial cells that line the terminal duct lobular unit (TDLU). When malignant cells have extended across the basement

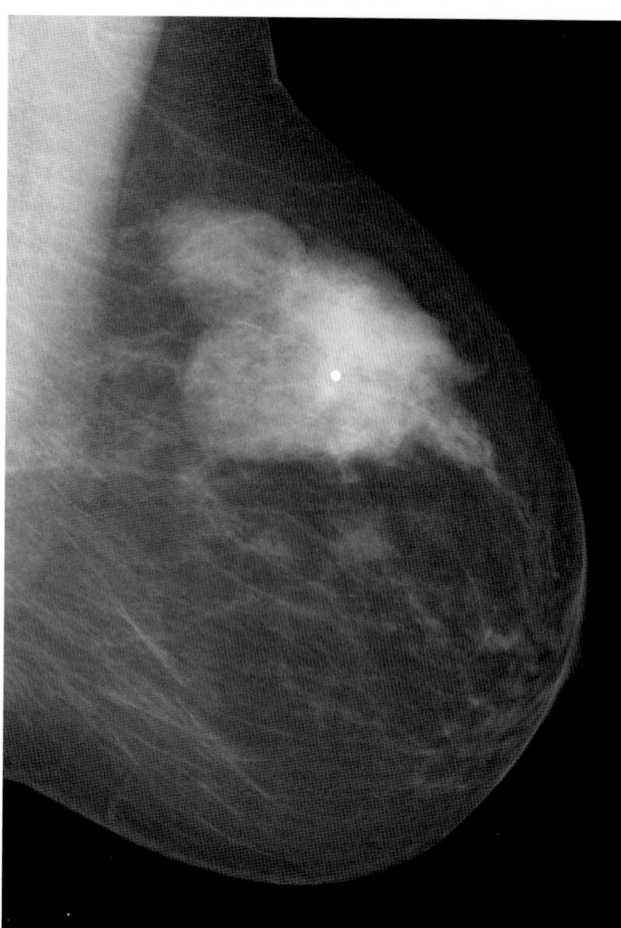

FIGURE 69-13 ■ **Hamartoma.** Hamartomas are frequently encountered on screening mammograms as large, lobulated masses with areas of varying density reflecting the presence of elements which are of fat and soft-tissue density.

membrane of the TDLU into the surrounding normal breast tissue, the carcinoma is invasive. Malignant cells contained by the basement membrane are termed non-invasive or in situ.

Classification of Invasive Breast Cancer

There is much confusion regarding the classification of breast cancer. Some tumours show distinct patterns of growth, allowing certain subtypes of breast cancer to be identified. Those with specific features are called invasive carcinoma of special type, while the remainder are considered to be of no special type (NST or ductal NST). Special-type tumours include lobular, medullary, tubular, tubular mixed, mucinous, cribriform and papillary. Different types of tumour have different clinical patterns of behaviour and prognosis. It should be understood that when a tumour is classified as of a special type this does not imply a specific cell of origin, but rather a recognisable morphological pattern.[21,25]

Histological grade has implications for tumour behaviour, imaging appearances and prognosis. The morphological features on which histological grade is based are tubule formation, nuclear pleomorphism and frequency of mitoses.[25] Low-grade tumours that are well differentiated are less likely to metastasise.

Imaging Appearance of Invasive Breast Cancer

Mammography. Carcinomas typically appear as ill-defined or spiculate masses on mammography (Figs. 69-14A, B). Lower-grade cancers tend to be seen as spiculate masses, due to the presence of an associated

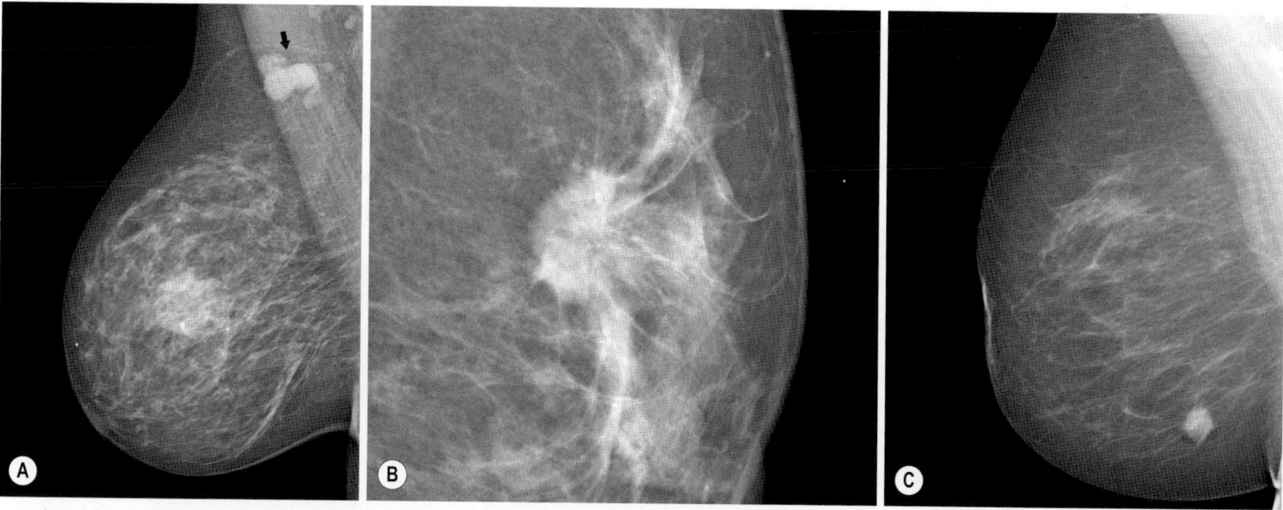

FIGURE 69-14 ■ **Mammographic appearances of invasive carcinoma.** Ill-defined and spiculate masses are typical of malignancy. (A) There is an ill-defined mass lying centrally in the right breast, containing some microcalcifications. Calcifications, representing DCIS, may be found in association with invasive carcinoma. There are also several enlarged lymph nodes in the axilla (arrow) which were proven to contain tumour on ultrasound-guided biopsy. (B) A spiculate mass that proved to be a ductal NST tumour of intermediate histological grade on ultrasound-guided biopsy. (C) Sometimes high grade tumours that exhibit rapid growth may appear well defined.

desmoplastic reaction in the adjacent stroma. Higher-grade tumours are usually seen as an ill-defined mass, but sometimes a rapidly growing tumour may appear relatively well defined, with similar appearances to a benign lesion such as a fibroadenoma (Fig. 69-14C).

Many breast cancers arise from areas of ductal carcinoma in situ (DCIS) and are associated with microcalcifications on mammography (Fig. 69-14A). This is particularly true for high-grade invasive ductal carcinomas that are often associated with high-grade DCIS.[26]

Special-type tumours can have particular mammographic characteristics:

- Lobular carcinomas can be difficult to perceive on a mammogram due to their tendency to diffusely infiltrate fatty tissue. Compared with ductal NST tumours, lobular cancers are more likely to be seen on only one mammographic view, are less likely to be associated with microcalcifications and are more often seen as an ill-defined mass or an area of asymmetrically dense breast tissue.[27]
- Tubular and cribriform cancers often present as architectural distortions or small spiculate masses.[28]
- Papillary, mucinous and medullary neoplasms may appear as new or enlarging multilobulated masses and may be well defined, simulating an apparently benign lesion.[29,30]

Sometimes the only clue to the presence of an invasive tumour may be abnormal trabecular markings, known as an architectural distortion, or the presence of microcalcifications, which tend to be visible even when the breast parenchyma is dense. The ability to perceive small or subtle cancers on a mammogram is improved by having the two standard mammographic views available and seeking out previous studies for comparison. An increase in the size of a mass or the presence of a new mass is suspicious of malignancy, whereas a lesion that remains unchanged over many years is invariably benign. Multiple masses in both breasts would favour a benign disease such as cysts or fibroadenomas.

Ultrasound. There are characteristic malignant features on ultrasound:[20]

- Carcinomas are seen as ill-defined masses and are markedly hypoechoic compared with the surrounding fat (Fig. 69-15).
- Carcinomas tend to be taller than they are wide (the anterior to posterior dimension is greater than the transverse diameter).
- There may be an ill-defined echogenic halo around the lesion, particularly around the lateral margins, and distortion of the adjacent breast tissue may be apparent, analogous to spiculation on the mammogram.
- Posterior acoustic shadowing is frequently observed, due to a reduction in the through transmission of the ultrasound beam in dense tumour tissue.

Poorly differentiated, high-grade tumours are more likely to be well defined, without acoustic shadowing (Fig. 69-15B); hence, the importance of carrying out a biopsy of solid masses even when the ultrasound appearances are benign. Microcalcifications are sometimes observed, associated with high-grade tumours arising in areas of DCIS, although this is less frequently encountered than with mammography (Fig. 69-15C). Lobular carcinomas can be difficult to demonstrate on ultrasound. They may produce vague abnormalities, such as subtle alterations in echotexture, or the ultrasound findings may even be normal.

Doppler imaging and elastography can help differentiate benign from malignant masses. Doppler may show abnormal vessels that are irregular and centrally penetrating in a malignant mass. Conversely, benign lesions such as fibroadenomas tend to show displacement of normal vessels around the edge of a lesion. Shear wave elastography of malignant lesions tends to demonstrate areas of increased elasticity, with the area of increased tissue stiffness larger than the grey-scale abnormality (Fig. 69-5).

Ultrasound is a useful tool in the local staging of breast cancer preoperatively. It tends to be a better predictor of tumour size than mammography and may detect intraductal tumour extension. Ultrasound may also detect small satellite tumour foci not visible on mammography (Fig. 69-16).

It has long been recognised that involvement of axillary lymph nodes is one of the most important prognostic factors for women with breast cancer. Traditionally, the axilla has been staged at the time of surgery by lymph node sampling procedures, sentinel node biopsy or clearance of the axillary lymph nodes. Surgical clearance of

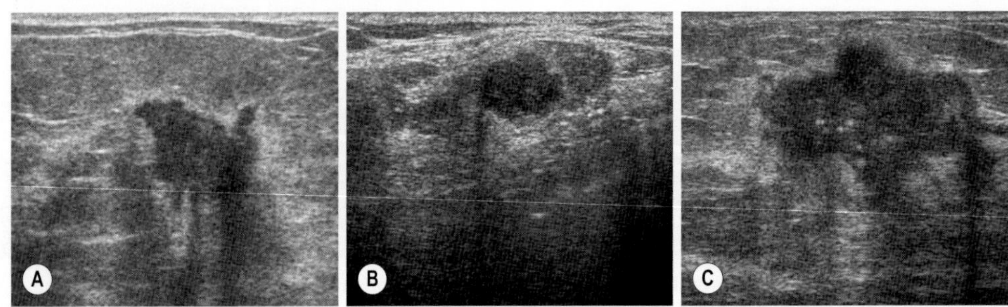

FIGURE 69-15 ■ **Ultrasound appearances of invasive carcinoma.** (A) This irregular hypoechoic mass with acoustic shadowing and an echogenic halo is typical of a carcinoma. (B) Occasionally, high-grade tumours may appear well defined, mimicking benign lesions. This shows the importance of performing a core biopsy even on apparently benign-appearing mass lesions. (C) Small echogenic foci of microcalcification associated with malignant lesions may be identified.

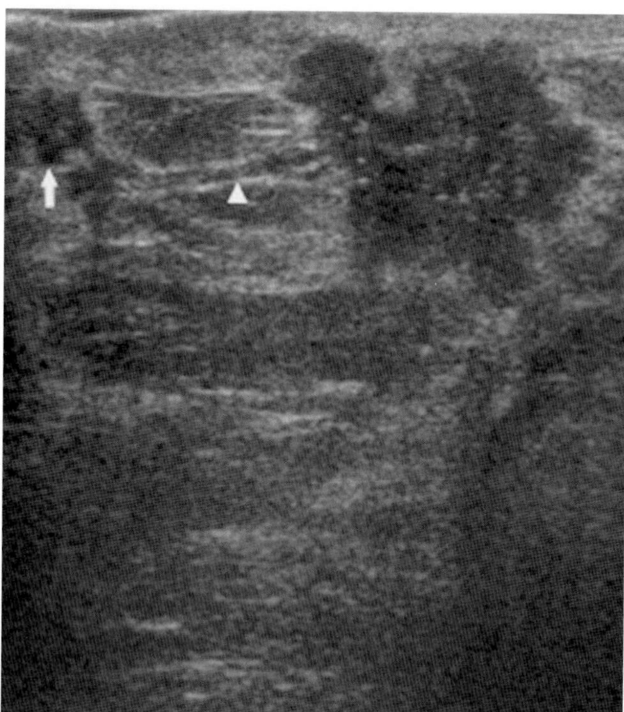

FIGURE 69-16 ■ A small satellite tumour focus. A small satellite tumour focus (arrow) is visible adjacent to the main tumour mass. A duct can be appreciated extending between the two lesions (arrowhead).

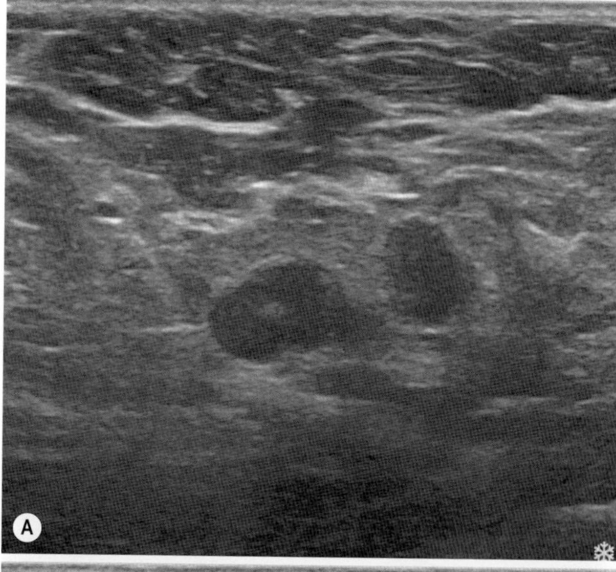

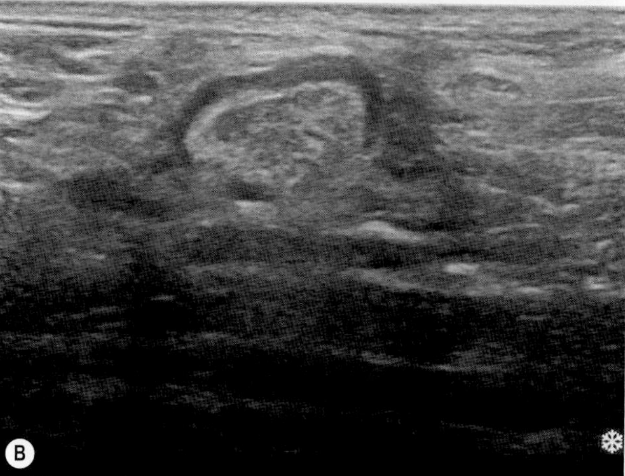

FIGURE 69-17 ■ Axillary lymph nodes. Axillary lymph nodes can be assessed on the basis of shape and the morphology of the cortex. (A) Nodes are likely to contain tumour if their longitudinal-to-transverse diameter ratio is less than 2 (the node appears round rather than oval). Nodes are more likely to contain tumour if the cortex is thickened to more than 2 mm. (B) This node has a normal shape, but the cortex has a thickness of 3 mm. Ultrasound-guided biopsy showed tumour containing lymph nodes in both cases.

axillary lymph nodes carries the risk of significant postoperative morbidity, with some women developing disabling lymphoedema in the arm. Ultrasound can identify abnormal nodes preoperatively that can then be biopsied percutaneously under ultrasound guidance (Fig. 69-17), allowing a preoperative diagnosis of lymph node involvement to be made in just over 40% of patients who are lymph node positive.[31] This enables the more radical axillary clearance to be targeted to those patients with a preoperative diagnosis of axillary disease, with the sampling or sentinel node procedures reserved for those patients with a much lower risk of axillary involvement.

The Differential Diagnosis of Malignancy

Many apparently suspicious findings seen on mammography or ultrasound can be caused by benign disease or even normal breast tissue. A surgical scar may result in a spiculate mass or an architectural distortion (Fig. 69-18). Radiographers should be encouraged to record the presence and position of any scars when performing a mammogram to aid image interpretation by the film reader.

Infection and inflammatory processes in the breast can be mistaken for malignancy on mammography and ultrasound. Breast abscesses are typically encountered in young lactating women. Treatment is with antibiotics and aspiration of the pus, frequently under ultrasound guidance. Inflammation in a non-lactating breast is a more worrying feature, although infections and more unusual inflammatory conditions such as granulomatous mastitis can occur. Skin erythema and oedema may be caused by an underlying carcinoma, termed 'inflammatory carcinoma'. In this situation, skin thickening and oedema may be the only signs of malignancy recognised on the mammogram. In any case of unexplained inflammation, or when infection fails to resolve, percutaneous biopsy is required to make the diagnosis or exclude malignancy.

Radial scars, also called complex sclerosing lesions, can produce a spiculated lesion, indistinguishable from malignancy on both mammography and ultrasound (Fig. 69-19). Many of these lesions are asymptomatic and are encountered on screening mammography. Epithelial atypia, DCIS and invasive carcinoma are found in association with radial scars.

Superimposition of normal breast tissue may produce apparent masses, distortions or worrying asymmetric densities on mammography. These summation shadows

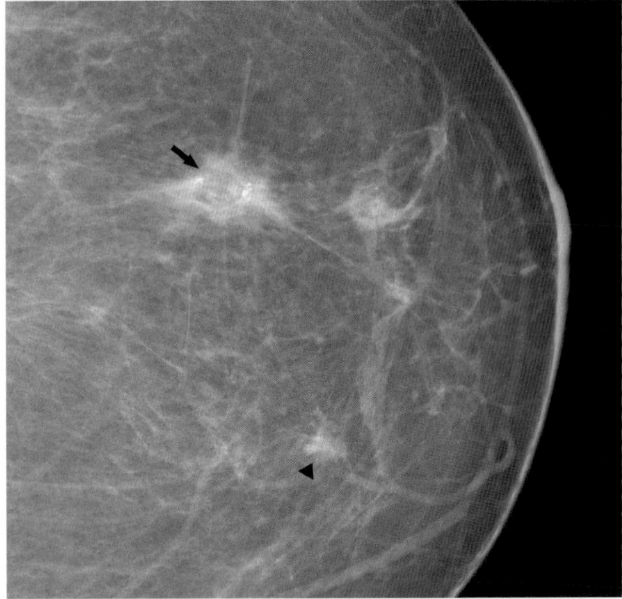

FIGURE 69-18 ■ **Postoperative scar.** A surveillance mammogram on a patient who has undergone a previous wide excision for a screen-detected cancer. The surgical scar (arrow) contains an area of lucency and coarse calcifications indicating associated fat necrosis. A small spiculate mass is demonstrated adjacent to the surgical scar (arrowhead); this was found to be recurrent tumour on ultrasound-guided biopsy.

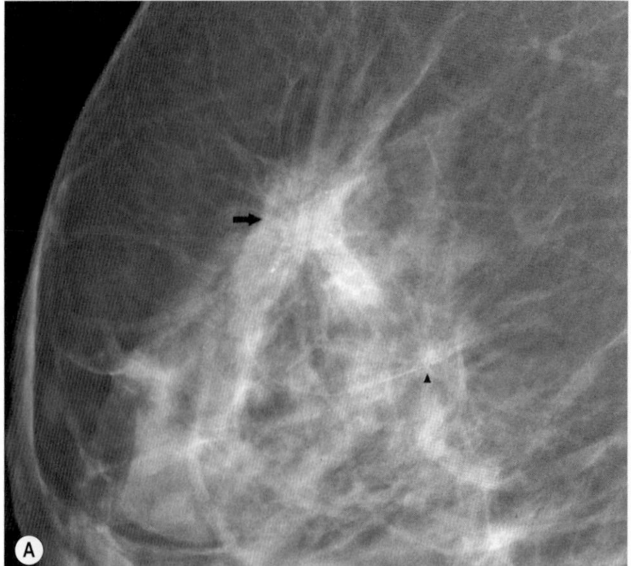

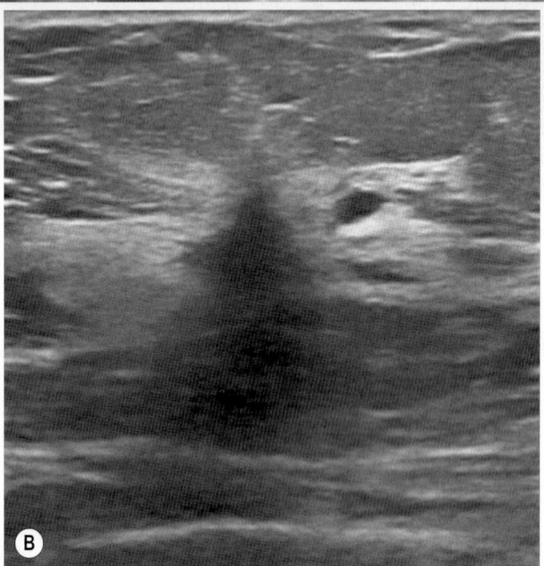

FIGURE 69-19 ■ **Radial scars.** Radial scars can mimic the appearance of malignancy on mammography and ultrasound. (A) A large spiculate mass (arrow) with an adjacent smaller lesion (arrowhead) is demonstrated on mammography. (B) Both were visible on ultrasound and were found to be radial scars on biopsy.

are usually evaluated with additional mammographic views. Localised compression or paddle views are particularly helpful in deciding whether a lesion is real or just a summation shadow. Ultrasound of the area of mammographic concern can help to determine whether a lesion is truly present.

Microcalcifications

Microcalcifications are frequently encountered on routine screening mammograms. In many cases these microcalcifications turn out to be benign, but occasionally are an important feature of DCIS. Some calcifications have a characteristic benign appearance and require no further action. There is a considerable overlap between the appearance of benign and malignant microcalcifications, necessitating percutaneous biopsy in many cases.

Benign Microcalcifications

Many benign processes in the breast can cause microcalcifications, including fibrocystic change, duct ectasia, fat necrosis and fibroadenomatoid hyperplasia. Fibroadenomas and papillomas can also become calcified. Sometimes normal structures, such as the skin or small blood vessels, calcify. Calcifications can also develop in atrophic breast lobules or normal stroma.

Vascular calcifications have a characteristic 'tramline' appearance caused by calcification in both walls of the vessel (Fig. 69-20). Similarly, duct ectasia has a classical appearance that rarely causes diagnostic difficulty. In this condition, coarse rod and branching calcifications are recognised due to calcification of debris within dilated ducts. These calcifications have been described as having a 'broken needle' appearance and are usually bilateral (Fig. 69-21A). Sometimes the debris may extrude from the ducts into the adjacent parenchyma, leading to an inflammatory-type reaction. Fat necrosis may then occur and the calcifications take on a characteristic 'lead-pipe' appearance (Fig. 69-21B). In many cases the diagnosis is obvious, but sometimes biopsy may be required, particularly if the calcifications are unilateral or focal.

Fibrocystic change is a common cause of microcalcifications (Fig. 69-22). On a lateral magnification view, layering of calcific fluid contained within microcysts can be appreciated, producing a characteristic 'teacup' appearance. However, in many cases, percutaneous biopsy is required to exclude DCIS.

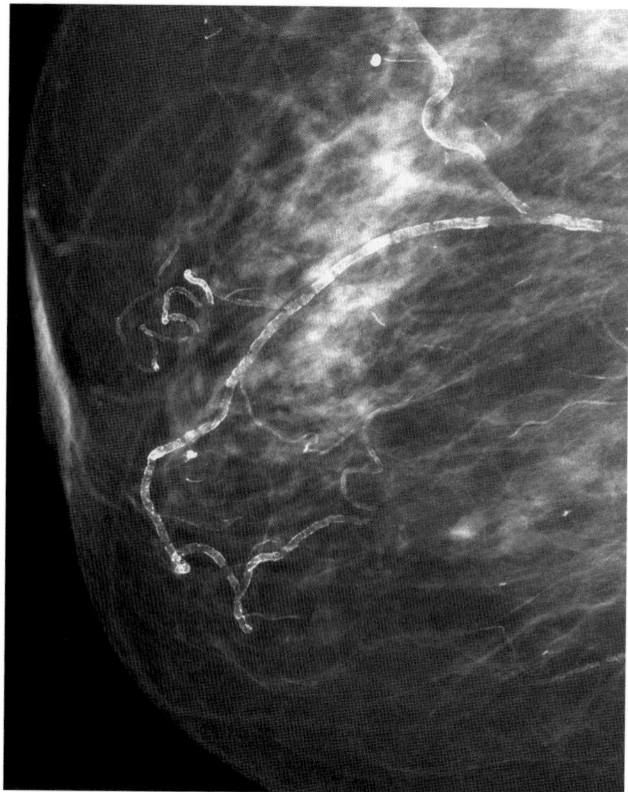

FIGURE 69-20 ■ **Vascular calcifications.**

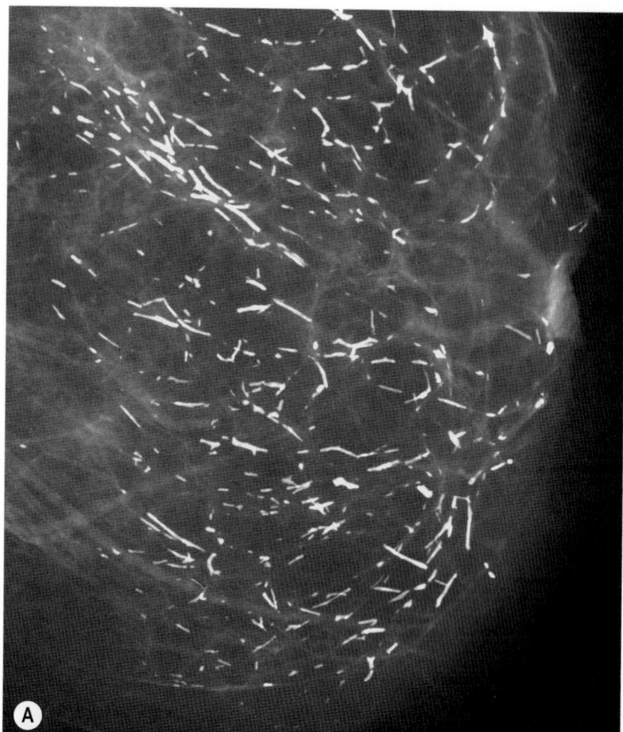

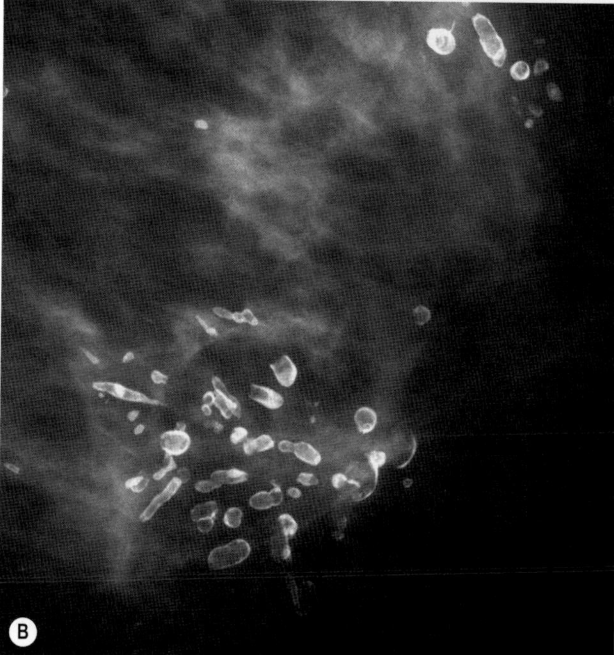

FIGURE 69-21 ■ **Duct ectasia.** (A) Broken needle appearance, typical of duct ectasia. (B) Sometimes thicker, more localised calcifications can be seen, giving a 'lead-pipe' appearance.

Fat necrosis is a frequently encountered cause of benign calcifications, particularly when there is a history of trauma or previous surgery (Fig. 69-23). It may present as 'egg shell' calcifications within the wall of an oil cyst or as coarse dystrophic calcifications associated with areas of scarring (Fig. 69-18).

Fibroadenomas may become calcified, particularly after the menopause. Classically, the calcifications have a coarse, 'popcorn' appearance (Fig. 69-9). However, they can be small and punctate, necessitating a biopsy to establish the diagnosis. Fibroadenomatoid hyperplasia is an increasingly common cause of microcalcifications detected during screening. Histologically, there are features of a fibroadenoma and fibrocystic change. There is usually no associated mass lesion and in many cases biopsy is required to exclude DCIS (Fig. 69-24).

Skin calcifications are characteristically round, well defined, have a lucent centre and are very often bilateral and symmetrical. Talcum powder or deodorants on the skin, as well as tattoo pigments, can mimic microcalcifications.

Malignant Microcalcifications

Microcalcifications are found associated with invasive breast cancer and DCIS. Calcifications are more likely to be malignant if they are clustered rather than scattered throughout the breast, if they vary in size and shape (pleomorphic), and if they are found in a ductal or linear distribution. Malignant microcalcifications associated with high histological grade DCIS are classically rod shaped and branched. These calcifications are known as casting or comedo microcalcifications and represent necrotic debris within the ducts; hence, their linear, branching structure (Fig. 69-25). Approximately one-third of malignant microcalcification clusters have an invasive focus within them at surgical excision.[32] The greater the number of flecks of microcalcification associated with an area of DCIS, the greater the risk of invasive disease.[32]

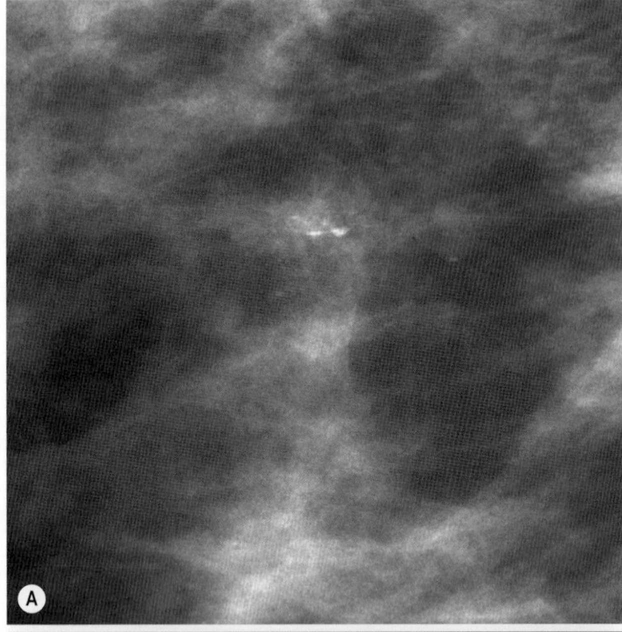

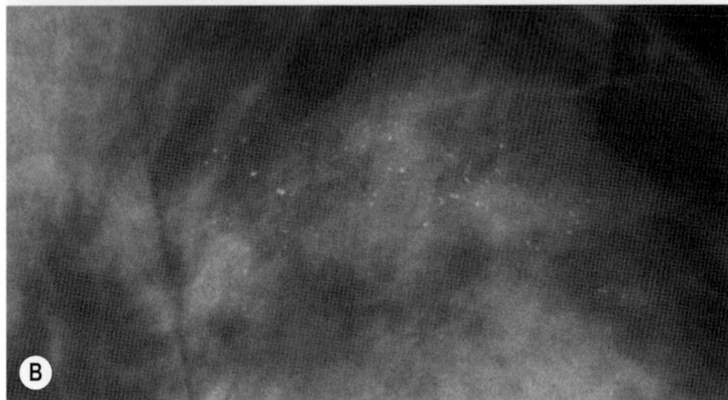

FIGURE 69-22 ■ **Fibrocystic change.** (A) 'Teacups' representing the layering out of calcific material in the dependent portion of microcysts on a lateral magnification view. (B) As calcifications associated with areas of fibrocystic change may not exhibit this characteristic appearance, stereotactic core biopsy is required.

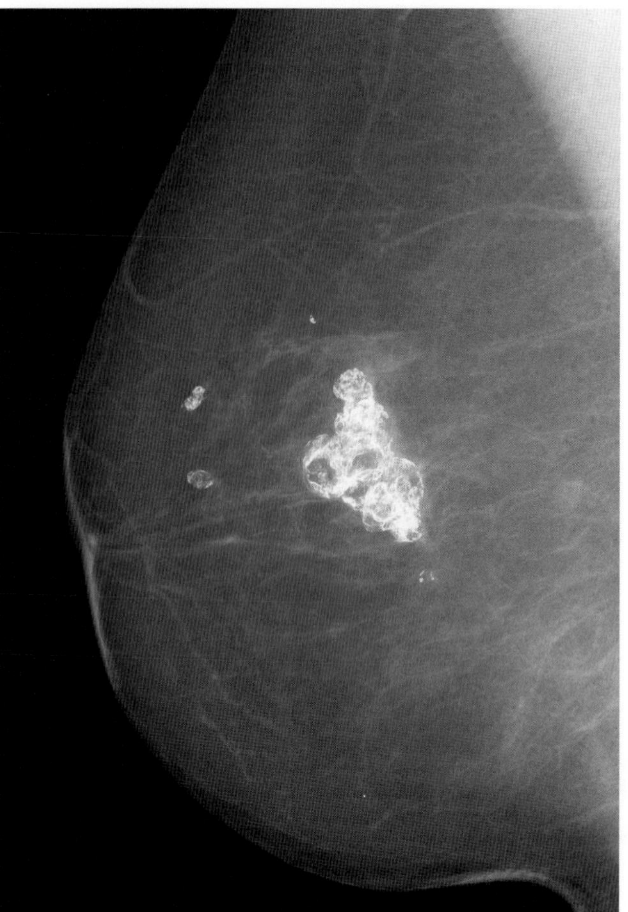

FIGURE 69-23 ■ **'Egg shell' calcifications of fat necrosis.**

In the screening setting, it is often the presence of mammographically visible calcifications associated with high-grade DCIS that leads to the diagnosis of small, high-grade cancers.[33] Calcifications are much less frequently found in low-grade DCIS, as there is usually no intraductal necrosis. When they do occur, they are clustered, but otherwise have a non-specific appearance.

The sensitivity of ultrasound for detecting DCIS is significantly lower than that of mammography, which is one of the reasons why ultrasound is not a useful screening test for breast cancer. However, ultrasound may be able to identify areas of microcalcifications seen on a mammogram, aiding percutaneous biopsy.

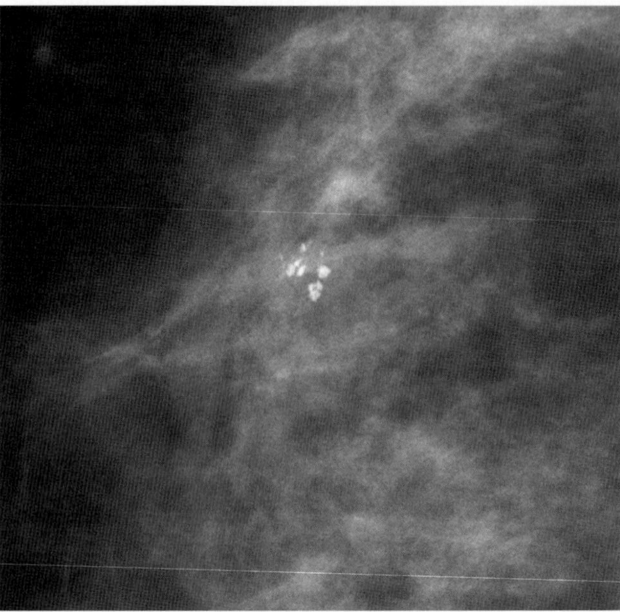

FIGURE 69-24 ■ **Small cluster of indeterminate microcalcifications.** Stereotactic biopsy revealed fibroadenomatoid change.

ADDITIONAL IMAGING TECHNOLOGIES

Magnetic Resonance Imaging

Although mammography and ultrasound remain the most frequently used techniques for imaging the breast,

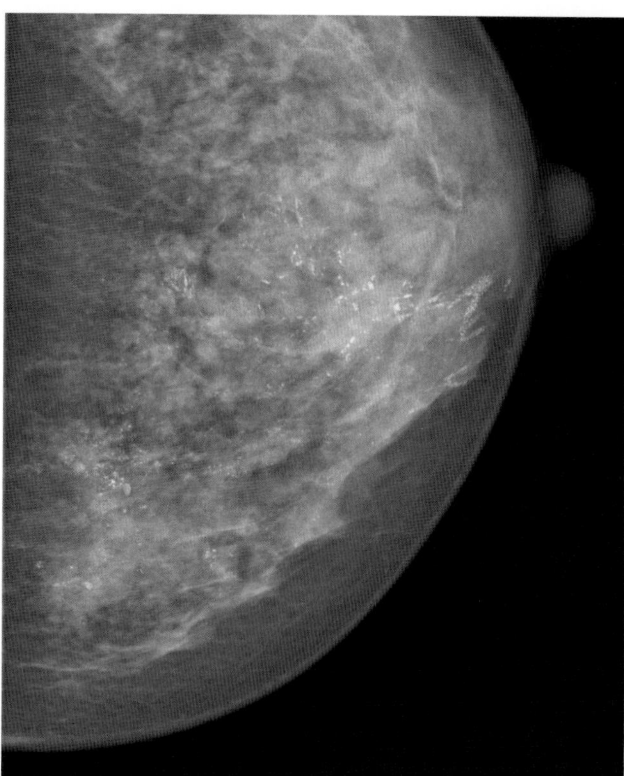

FIGURE 69-25 ■ Ductal carcinoma in situ (DCIS). Mammography shows the segmental distribution of pleomorphic microcalcifications. Granular, rod-shaped and branching calcifications can be identified. The appearances are typical of high-grade DCIS.

contrast-enhanced MRI is becoming increasingly important, largely because of its high sensitivity for detecting invasive breast cancer, which approaches 100% in many studies. MRI is the technique of choice for assessing the integrity of breast implants. It is more accurate than mammography, ultrasound or clinical examination in identifying implant failure.

Technique

Successful breast MR studies require at least a 1.5-tesla system and the use of a dedicated breast coil. Some breast coils have inbuilt compression devices to stabilise the breast and reduce the number of slices required to cover the whole of the breast. Patients are examined in the prone position, with the breast hanging down into the coil. The intravenous injection of gadolinium-based contrast agent is required; it is the presence of abnormal vasculature within the lesion that enables detection.

Some method of eliminating the signal from fat is needed as an enhancing lesion and fat display similar high signal on a T1-weighted image. Fat suppression may be active or passive: active fat suppression is typically achieved by the use of spectrally selective pulse sequences to suppress the signal from fat; passive fat suppression involves subtraction of the unenhanced images from the enhanced images. Subtraction allows faster imaging, with good spatial and temporal resolution, but it requires no patient movement between the two sets of images. Methods of active fat suppression, such as parallel imaging, allow fat suppression to be achieved with shorter examination times while maintaining good spatial and temporal resolution.

Fast 3D gradient-echo pulse sequences provide the optimum method for imaging small lesions. Temporal resolution is important because the optimum contrast between malignancy and normal breast tissue is achieved in the first 2 min following the injection of gadolinium. Later, normal breast tissue may start to show non-specific enhancement, masking the presence of disease. Other signs of malignancy, such as a rapid uptake of contrast agent followed by a 'washout' phase, may only be apparent if images are acquired dynamically every minute over a period of 6–7 min after the gadolinium injection.

A higher temporal resolution allows rapid dynamic imaging but at the expense of spatial resolution or the volume of the breast imaged. Good spatial resolution can only be achieved at the expense of an increased examination time. With modern equipment it should be possible to achieve a slice thickness of <3 mm while maintaining a temporal resolution of 60–90 s, covering the whole of both breasts.

At 3 tesla there is an increase in the signal-to-noise ratio, leading to potential improvements in image quality. There are issues with field inhomogeneity at 3 tesla that can lead to problems, particularly with fat suppression.

Newer MRI techniques, such as diffusion-weighted imaging (DWI) and spectroscopy, are being investigated to try and improve the specificity of breast MRI. DWI is an unenhanced echoplanar sequence which measures the mobility of water molecules within the breast tissue. Cancers generally have a higher cellular density and extracellular water is less able to diffuse; thus values of apparent diffusion coefficient (ADC) are lower (typically $<1.5 \times 10^{-3}$ mm^2/s) compared to benign lesions or normal breast tissues (typically $>1.6 \times 10^{-3}$ mm^2/s). There is overlap between the ADC values of benign and malignant lesions, but the use of DWI has the potential to increase the specificity of breast MRI.[34,35]

Spectroscopy provides metabolic information about a tumour. Choline is an important substrate of phospholipid synthesis and so is a marker of membrane biosynthesis. Consequently, choline levels are elevated in rapidly proliferating breast cancer cells. The presence or absence of a choline peak on the MR spectra has been used as a way of differentiating malignant from benign lesions, although sometimes choline can be detected in benign or normal tissue. MRI spectroscopy can be performed as a single-voxel or multi-voxel technique enabling information to be gathered from a large volume of tissue. Multi-voxel techniques, also referred to as spectroscopic or chemical shift imaging, have the ability to provide quantitative information of choline concentration.[36] MR spectroscopy is dependent on the signal-to-noise ratio of the examination and so the accuracy of spectroscopy is improved when imaging at field strengths of 3 tesla and above.

Lesion Characterisation

There are two main approaches to image interpretation: the first relates to lesion morphology and the second to assessment of enhancement kinetics. The architectural features that indicate benign and malignant disease are similar to those already described for mammography and ultrasound. Benign lesions tend to be well defined with smooth margins, whereas malignant lesions are poorly defined and may show spiculation or parenchymal deformity.

Malignant lesions tend to enhance rapidly following the injection of contrast agent and may show characteristic ring enhancement. Dynamic contrast-enhanced MRI enables more detailed enhancement curves to be calculated to aid characterisation. Malignant lesions usually show a rapid uptake of contrast agent in the initial phase of the examination, followed by a washout or plateau in the intermediate and late periods after injection, whereas benign lesions exhibit a steady increase in signal intensity throughout the time course of the examination.[37] There is some overlap in the enhancement characteristics of benign and malignant lesions. One of the strengths of breast MR imaging is that invasive cancer can be effectively excluded with a high degree of certainty if no enhancement is seen.

Investigators use a combination of architectural features and enhancement kinetics to differentiate benign from malignant lesions. The use of the breast imaging reporting and data system (BIRADS) lexicon aids reporting.[23] Using this system, lesions can be characterised into one of three morphological groups: (1) a focus (a lesion <5 mm, rarely worthy of further investigation); (2) a mass (>5 mm); and (3) non-mass enhancement (an area of enhancement without a morphological correlate). Further descriptors can then be used to describe the shape, margin and enhancement characteristics of mass lesions and the distribution and internal enhancement characteristics of non-mass lesions. Enhancement kinetics are helpful in the assessment of mass lesions, but are not useful in the assessment of non-mass enhancement where DCIS and lobular carcinoma are part of the differential diagnosis.

Normal breast tissue may enhance and this enhancement is in part dependent on the phase of the menstrual cycle. The optimum time for performing a breast MRI is during the second week of the menstrual cycle (between days 7 and 13) when background glandular enhancement should be least intense.[38] Timing the MRI examination with the second week of the menstrual cycle may not be possible for patients undergoing cancer staging, but should be undertaken for screening and follow-up studies.

Recent surgery or radiotherapy can interfere with image interpretation. Enhancement patterns return to normal between 3 and 6 months after radiotherapy.[39] Percutaneous breast biopsy (FNAC, core, or vacuum-assisted biopsy) rarely interferes with MRI interpretation.

Indications for Breast MRI

Contrast-enhanced breast MRI is used for local staging of primary breast cancer. MRI is the most accurate technique for sizing invasive breast carcinomas and will sometimes show unsuspected multifocal disease in the same breast or even additional tumour foci in the contralateral breast. MRI can be expected to show additional tumour foci in the affected breast away from the primary tumour site in around 16% of cases[40] and additional disease in the contralateral breast in around 4% of cases.[41] This may lead to a change in the therapeutic approach, potentially avoiding inappropriate breast-conserving surgery or unnecessary mastectomies. The routine use of MRI for the preoperative staging of primary breast cancer remains controversial and so careful patient selection is important. MRI is usually reserved for patients where estimating tumour size is proving difficult by conventional methods, including mammographically occult lesions, patients with mammographically dense breasts, and where there is significant discrepancy between size estimations at mammography, ultrasound and clinical examination.

Another group of patients who benefit from preoperative staging with MRI are those whose carcinomas have lobular features. Lobular carcinomas are more likely to be multifocal compared with ductal NST tumours. They are more difficult to detect and their size is more difficult to measure by conventional methods because of their infiltrating growth pattern. In approximately 50% of such patients MRI will show more extensive tumour (Fig. 69-26).[42]

Another important role of MRI is identifying an occult primary tumour in women presenting with malignant axillary lymphadenopathy with a normal mammogram and breast ultrasound. In this situation, MRI is highly sensitive for identifying an occult primary. MRI is also useful in the postsurgical breast, differentiating surgical scarring from tumour recurrence.

MRI can help to assess the response to treatment in women receiving neoadjuvant chemotherapy for locally advanced primary breast cancers. It can recognise responders to treatment earlier than other imaging methods by demonstrating a reduction in lesion size, or a change in the enhancement pattern, with the level of enhancement reducing or taking on a more benign appearance. Neoadjuvant chemotherapy can also be used to downstage large breast cancers to enable breast-conserving surgery to become a treatment option. MRI can be used to plan the extent of surgical resection in positive responders, with successful breast conservation possible in around 59% of women where mastectomy would have been necessary.[43]

MRI has become an important tool for screening younger women with a high familial risk of breast cancer. Some of these women (e.g. known gene mutation carriers) have a lifetime risk of developing breast cancer of around 85%. In these younger women the sensitivity of mammography for detecting malignancy is low, largely due to the presence of mammographically dense breast parenchyma. Screening with MRI is superior to mammography in detecting invasive breast cancer in such women, although mammography remains more sensitive for detecting DCIS.[44,45]

Managing MRI-Detected Lesions

Lesions detected at MRI require proper work-up, including histological diagnosis where appropriate. Findings should be correlated with mammography, but probably most useful is a targeted, second-look ultrasound of the

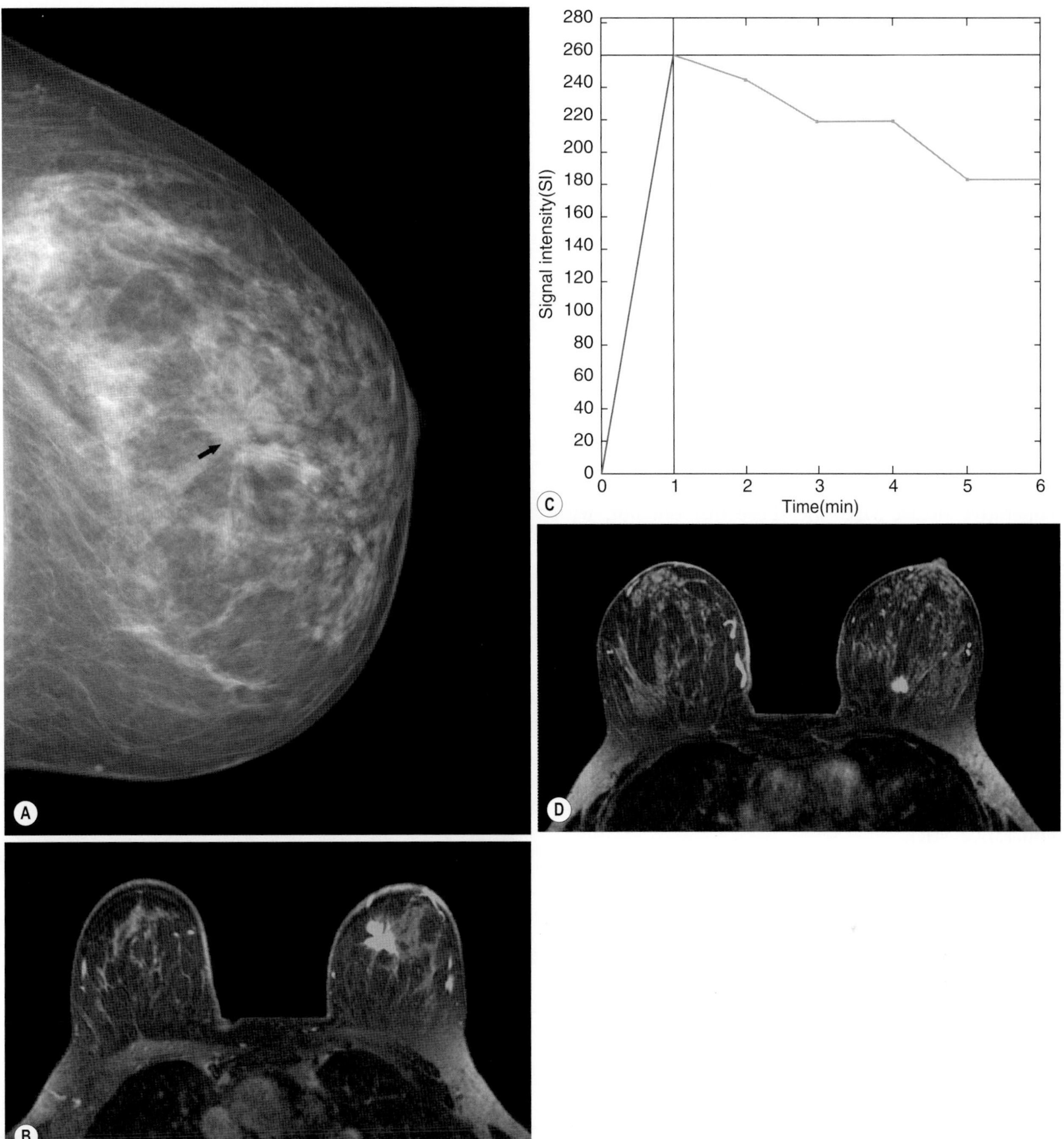

FIGURE 69-26 ■ MRI for local tumour staging. This patient presented with a mass in the left breast. Mammography showed a spiculate lesion (arrow) lying centrally within the breast, best appreciated on the CC view (A). Biopsy indicated a carcinoma with lobular features. MRI confirmed the presence of a malignant spiculate lesion (B) with a typically malignant enhancement curve (rapid uptake of contrast agent followed by a washout phase) (C). An additional tumour focus was identified away from the primary tumour site (D). This was confirmed at biopsy.

area. In many cases, ultrasound will identify any additional lesions and facilitate image-guided biopsy. Lack of an ultrasound correlate makes the chances of malignancy much less likely. In one study, carcinoma was found in 43% of MRI lesions that had an ultrasound correlate compared with 14% of MRI lesions that lacked an ultrasound correlate.[46] An ultrasound correlate is more likely for invasive carcinoma compared with DCIS.[46] However, where MRI lesions are suspicious or indeterminate, the absence of a corresponding ultrasound abnormality does not negate the need to pursue a histological diagnosis and MRI-guided biopsy should be considered. For lesions that are considered low risk, follow-up MRI after a suitable period of time, typically one year, is acceptable.

When MRI is used for staging breast cancer, problems arise when additional enhancing lesions are detected away from the primary tumour site. The same principles of mammographic review and second-look ultrasound apply. Surgical management should not be changed unless additional enhancing lesions are histologically proven to represent malignancy.

Controversies Surrounding the Use of Breast MRI

It would seem reasonable to assume that the identification of additional tumour foci in the breast at the time of diagnosis should improve surgical planning and long-time patient outcomes with a decrease in both tumour recurrence rates and the incidence of contralateral disease in the years following treatment. No robust evidence is yet available to support these assumptions. If the use of MRI for surgical planning is effective, a reduction in surgical re-excision rates would be expected in women who underwent preoperative MRI. A randomised controlled trial (COMICE, Comparative Effectiveness of MRI in Breast Cancer) found no significant difference in the re-excision rates between the group who underwent preoperative breast MRI and those that did not, with re-excision rates of 18.8 and 19.3%, respectively.[47] There is also very little evidence that MRI improves long-term outcomes for patients. In one study, local recurrence rates and the incidence of contralateral disease were assessed over an 8-year period in women who had undergone breast-conserving surgery: no significant difference was observed in women who underwent preoperative MRI compared with those who did not.[48] There is evidence that MRI does lead to changes in surgical treatment, typically from breast-conserving surgery to mastectomy. A recent meta-analysis has shown more extensive surgery than initially planned in 11.3% of women who underwent preoperative MRI.[40]

There are two factors to consider when explaining why routine preoperative staging MRI has not been shown to affect outcomes in breast cancer patients. The first relates to the specificity of MRI and the second to a form of overdiagnosis. Although MRI is very sensitive for detecting malignancy, reported specificities are lower, varying between 81 and 97%. Consequently, it is very important that any additional lesions identified at MRI are proven to be malignant before management changes are made, avoiding potential unnecessary mastectomies. Obtaining a tissue diagnosis can increase the number of percutaneous biopsies performed and the diagnostic uncertainty may precipitate some women choosing more radical surgery. The second, more important, factor is the clinical significance of any additional disease identified. There is no doubt that breast MRI does find additional disease, but some of this disease may not be clinically relevant in patients undergoing breast-conserving surgery followed by radiotherapy, chemotherapy and hormone treatments. It is well established that these adjuvant treatments are effective at reducing local recurrence rates by controlling foci of residual disease not excised at the time of breast-conserving surgery.

MRI for Imaging Breast Implants

MRI is the technique of choice for assessing the integrity of breast implants, with a sensitivity and specificity of over 90%. When imaging breast implants, no contrast agent is required unless malignancy is suspected. Imaging should be performed in the prone position using a dedicated breast coil. The main goal is to determine whether the implant has ruptured and, if so, to establish the location of the leaked filler (usually silicon).

When implants fail, the rupture may be either intracapsular or extracapsular: intracapsular rupture occurs when silicon has escaped from the plastic shell of the implant, but is contained within the fibrous implant capsule (Fig. 69-27); signs of intracapsular rupture include the 'wavy line', 'linguini', 'key-hole' and 'salad oil' signs.[49] False-positive interpretations can be made when normal implant folds are mistaken for signs of rupture.

Extracapsular rupture is diagnosed when silicon is demonstrated outside the fibrous capsule. In this situation, ultrasound can be diagnostic, demonstrating free silicon, silicon granulomas or silicon-containing axillary lymph nodes (Fig. 69-28).

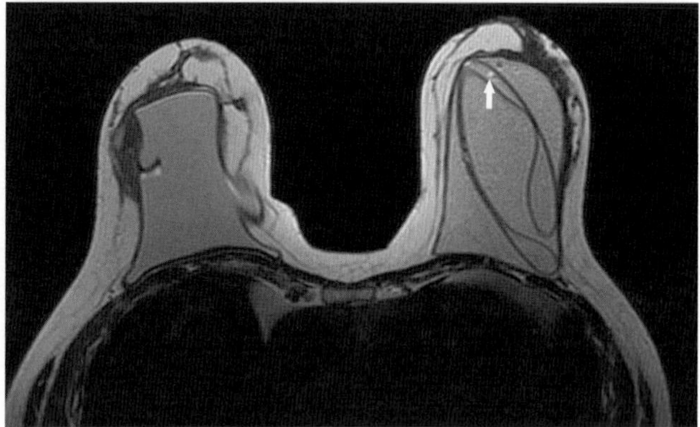

FIGURE 69-27 ■ Intracapsular implant rupture. On these T2-weighted fast spin-echo images, the plastic shell of the left breast implant can be seen floating within the silicon, producing a 'wavy line' or 'linguini' sign. Note the presence of a bright dot of water-like material (arrow), the 'salad oil' sign.

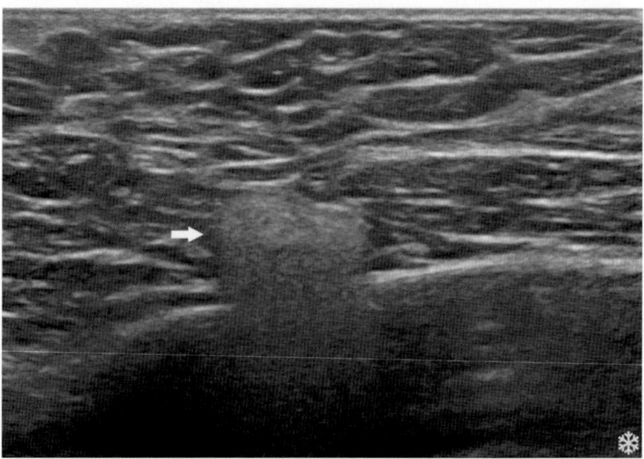

FIGURE 69-28 ■ Extracapsular implant rupture. A small silicon granuloma is visible, lying adjacent to a breast implant (arrow). The silicon granuloma has a characteristic 'snow storm' appearance.

Nuclear Medicine Techniques

Sestamibi imaging using ^{99m}Tc-MIBI and PET imaging techniques using ^{18}F-FDG have been developed following the observation that many breast cancers show uptake of these isotopes. Breast-specific gamma imaging (sometimes referred to as scintimammography) and FDG positron emission mammography (PEM) have significantly improved in recent years with the development of high-resolution mini-camera detectors designed specifically for imaging the breast. Indications for use overlap with those for MRI, including local staging, searching for a mammographically occult primary, particularly where there is dense mammographic background pattern, and detecting recurrence in the postsurgical breast. Research is continuing, but so far these techniques have failed to establish a place in routine practice.

BREAST CANCER SCREENING

Introduction

Breast cancer mortality in the UK is amongst the highest in the world. The causes of breast cancer are not well understood and, in the absence of any effective preventative measures, much effort and health care resources have been focused on the quest to reduce breast cancer mortality by early detection through screening. A number of randomised controlled trials (RCTs) and case control studies carried out since the mid-1960s have shown that screening by mammography can reduce breast cancer mortality.

The UK National Health Service Breast Screening Programme was set up following the publication of the Forrest Report in 1986.[50] This document, commissioned by the UK Department of Health under the chairmanship of Professor Sir Patrick Forrest, reviewed the scientific evidence for population breast cancer screening. It recommended the immediate introduction of screening by mammography in the UK.

Within a year of publication, population breast cancer screening, free at the point of delivery, was introduced into the UK National Health Service. This was the first population-based breast screening programme in the world. Currently in the UK, breast cancer screening by mammography is provided for all women over the age of 50. Women between the ages of 50 and 70 are invited every 3 years. Two-view mammography is used for all screens and the mammograms are double read. Women over 70 are not invited but are encouraged to attend by self-referral. There is an ongoing trial to assess the possible mortality benefits of extending the screening invitation from 47 to 73.

The Evidence for Screening

Data from RCTs provide the strongest evidence of the efficacy of screening in reducing breast cancer mortality. The design of RCTs enables the elimination of lead-time bias. Most of the RCTs of screening were carried out in Sweden. An overview of these trials was published in 2002 and included data from Malmo, Gothenburg, Stockholm and the Ostergotland arm of the Two Counties study.[51] Almost a quarter of a million women were included in these studies, with approximately half being invited for screening and the other half making up the control group. The median trial time was 6.5 years and the median follow-up 15.8 years. The overall results indicated a 21% reduction in breast cancer mortality. The mortality reduction was largest in women aged 60–69 (33%).

Due to continuing criticisms of RCTs of breast screening, which suggested that the overall mortality may be higher in those screened because of adverse effects of treatment, this study also looked at total cause mortality. This showed a relative risk of dying of any cause in the study arm of 0.98, which was of borderline statistical significance.[51] The precise mortality reduction attributable to screening is controversial, as RCTs may underestimate the benefit of screening due to non-attendance and contamination (mammography occurring within the control group). It has been suggested that regular attendance for mammographic screening may result in a 63% reduction in breast cancer deaths.[52]

Which Age Groups Should be Screened?

There is definite evidence from RCTs of a reduction in mortality in women aged 55–69; previous meta-analyses have supported the introduction of screening at age 50 but these data are based on 10-year age bands. Data analysis based on 5-year age bands of screening women aged 50–55 has never shown a mortality benefit in this age group. The reasons for this are unclear but it has been postulated that this may be due to the unusual behaviour of breast cancer in perimenopausal women.

There is no evidence from RCTs to support the screening of women over the age of 70. However, the number of women over the age of 70 in these studies is low. Although the mammograms of older women are easy to read and the incidence of cancer is high, there would be a significant risk of overdiagnosis and consequently overtreatment in this age group. Overdiagnosis is the detection and treatment of cancers that would not become clinically apparent or threaten life. Overdiagnosis probably occurs in about 10% of cancers detected when screening women aged 50–70, with significantly higher rates in women aged over 70 years. Pathological lesions that might be considered overdiagnosed and treated are low-grade DCIS and invasive tubular cancers. A number of studies are now addressing this issue by suggesting either less invasive treatment or a watch and wait policy for such lesions.

A recent meta-analysis of RCTs screening women aged 39–49 at random has shown a statistically significant mortality reduction of 17%.[53] The Malmo and Gothenburg studies have both shown statistically significant mortality reductions in this age group.[54,55] As breast cancer is only half as common in women in their 40s compared with women in their fifties, some authors have suggested that presenting data in terms of percentage reduction in population mortality may be misleading. On the other hand, preventing breast cancer deaths in younger women will result in a larger number of life years gained and it has been shown that breast cancers arising in women in their 40s account for 34% of life years lost to breast cancer.

The RCTs of screening were not designed to look at particular age groups and such subanalysis has been criticised. In particular, a proportion of the screening episodes occurring in women aged 40–49 at randomisation actually occurred when women were over the age of 50. In addition, women in the control groups of these studies were not always screened at 50. Therefore, it is possible that part of the mortality benefit demonstrated in these women may be due to screening episodes over the age of 50.

There are other issues to consider when screening women in their 40s. The lower cancer incidence results in the specificity of both recall and biopsy being lower than that in older women. The sensitivity of mammography for detecting malignancy is also lower for women in their 40s, although the introduction of digital mammography should substantially improve screening performance in this age group.[9]

The interval at which a screening mammogram needs to be repeated is determined by lead-time, which is age related. The lead-time of screening is that time between mammographic detection of breast cancer and clinical presentation. The lead-time of screening in women under the age of 50 in the Gothenburg screening trial was 2.2 years.[55] This suggests the ideal screening interval for women under the age of 50 is either every 18 or 12 months. The high frequency of screening required in younger women and the lower incidence of breast cancer have led to questions being raised regarding the cost-effectiveness of screening in this age group. These disadvantages may be partly negated by the large number of life years gained per life saved. On the other hand, the lead-time of screening for older women aged over 50 is 3–4 years, so the 3-year screening interval in the UK would seem appropriate. However, reducing the screening interval to 2 years for the over-fifites may be beneficial as a high rate of interval cancers are seen in the UK in the third year after screening.[56]

The Screening Process and Assessment

Screening mammograms are carried out by female radiographers, either at static sites or using mobile vans. In the UK, interpretation of screening mammograms is limited to practitioners who read a high volume of images (greater than 5000 examinations per year). Evidence suggests that high-volume readers have a significantly increased sensitivity for detection of breast cancer compared to medium- and low-volume readers.[57] In the UK, there has been a national shortage of breast screening radiologists. This has led to the introduction of radiographer film readers. Radiographers have been shown to have identical sensitivity and specificity when compared with screening radiologists once they have been trained.

Double reading is standard practice in the UK screening programme, with consensus or arbitration adopted to deal with discordant double-reading opinions. For consensus double reading, disparate opinions are discussed by the two film readers and a consensus achieved. Arbitration involves a third reader independently reviewing the mammograms and deciding whether recall is necessary. Data from the UK screening programme have shown that double reading with arbitration results in the best small invasive cancer detection rate with acceptable recall rates.[58]

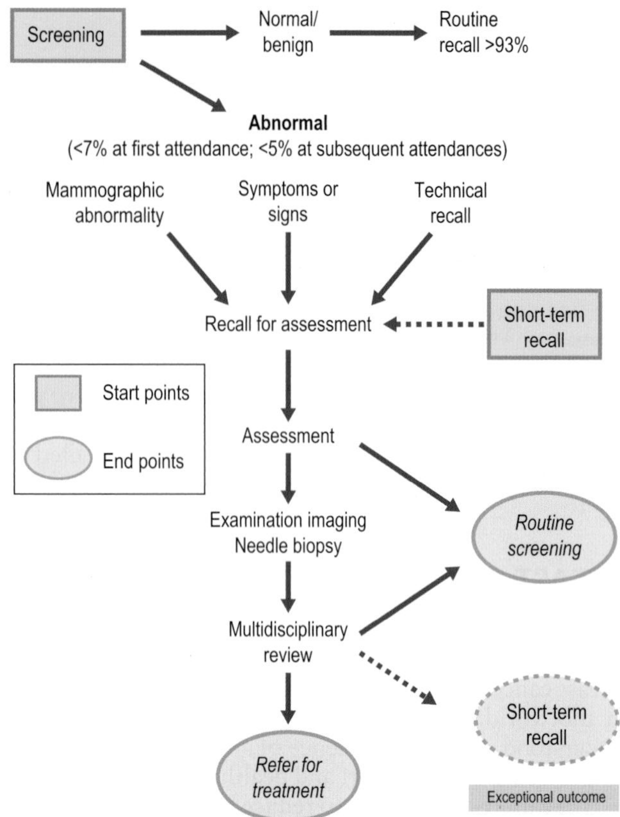

FIGURE 69-29 ■ The screening assessment process.

Approximately 5% of women are called back for assessment. Figure 69-29 outlines the assessment process; typically it involves a combination of extra mammographic views, ultrasound and physical examination. Approximately one in seven of those recalled have breast cancer.

Interval Cancers

These are cancers that arise symptomatically in women who have had a normal screening mammogram before their next invitation to screening. Interval cancer analysis helps assess the effectiveness of a screening programme and enables radiologists to learn by reviewing the screening mammograms of women who later present with symptomatic cancers. Interval cancers have a prognosis similar to symptomatic cancers in the non-screening population, which is worse than that of cancers detected at screening.

Interval cancers in the NHSBSP are now divided into three subtypes:

- Type 1 interval cancers are cancers where the previous screening mammograms show no evidence of malignancy, even in retrospect.
- Type 2 interval cancers are cancers where the previous screening mammograms show uncertain features when viewed retrospectively.
- Type 3 interval cancers are cancers where there are malignant features on the previous screening mammograms.

The mammographic features most frequently missed or misinterpreted on screening mammograms are calcification and architectural distortion.[59]

How Does Mammographic Screening Reduce Breast Cancer Mortality?

Most of the benefit of mammographic screening is due to detection of small lymph node-negative invasive cancers. Finding high-grade invasive breast cancer less than 10 mm in size is particularly useful as the prognosis of such tumours is excellent, whereas grade 3 invasive breast cancers presenting symptomatically have a very poor prognosis.[60] However, some of the low-grade tubular cancers detected at screening are so indolent that a number of these lesions may never threaten life and mammographic screening in these instances may lead to overdiagnosis and overtreatment.[61]

Approximately 25% of cancers detected by mammographic screening are DCIS. High-grade DCIS is accepted by most authorities to be a precursor of high-grade invasive disease. Most DCIS diagnosed through screening is high-grade and so detection is beneficial. The merit of detecting low-grade DCIS is more controversial, with only approximately 40% of cases eventually developing low-grade invasive breast cancer.

Quality Assurance (QA)

In the UK, local performance is monitored by regional QA teams with the data collected centrally by the Department of Health. This is a statutory requirement and the teams are responsible for screening-unit performance monitoring and for individual performance appraisal. Some of the recent national performance figures are shown in Table 69-1. The standardised detection ratio is the actual number of cancers detected expressed as a ratio of the predicted number of cancers that need be detected to achieve a mortality reduction of 25%.

Interventional Breast Radiology

Breast radiology requires skills in interventional techniques, particularly ultrasound and X-ray stereotactic-guided needle sampling, percutaneous excision of benign lesions and localisation of abnormalities for surgical excision. Eighty per cent of abnormalities detected by screening mammography are impalpable and need to be biopsied and localised using image-guided techniques.

Needle biopsy is highly accurate in determining the nature of most breast lesions and is now used in place of open surgical biopsy. For patients with breast cancer, needle biopsy provides accurate information on the nature of malignant disease, such as histological type and grade, and allows assessment of tumour biology, cell markers and genetics.

TABLE 69-1 **UK National Health Service Breast Screening Programme Performance 2008–2010**

	2008/2009	2009/2010
Number of women invited	2,702,876	2,754,885
Acceptance rate (% of invited)	73.7%	73.3%
Number of women screened (invited)	1,990,534	2,018,403
Number of women screened (self-referred)	87,661	84,467
Total number of women screened	2,078,195	2,102,870
Number of women recalled for assessment	91,395	89,164
Women recalled for assessment (%)	4.4%	4.2%
Number of benign open surgical biopsies	1746	1646
Number of cancers detected	16,535	16,476
Cancer detected per 1000 women screened	7.96	7.84
Number of in situ cancers detected	3438	3257
Number of invasive cancers less than 15 mm	6791	6939
Standardised detection ratio	**1.45**	**1.44**

Source: NHSBSP Annual Review 2011, NHSBSP Publications, Sheffield, UK.

The methods available for breast tissue diagnosis are:

- fine-needle aspiration for cytology (FNAC);
- needle core biopsy for histology;
- vacuum-assisted biopsy (VAB); and
- open surgical biopsy.

Fine-Needle Aspiration for Cytology and Needle Core Biopsy

FNAC involves the manual passage of a small-bore needle (usually 23 gauge) repeatedly through an abnormality to shear off clumps of cells into the needle lumen. This is usually performed while applying suction to the aspiration needle. The aspirate is then either smeared onto a microscope slide or washed into a buffer solution ready for cytological assessment. FNAC can be performed freehand on a palpable abnormality or carried out under image guidance. The procedure is quick to perform and associated with minimal morbidity. However, it is associated with significant false-positive and false-negative results, is operator dependent and relies greatly on the experience and skill of the cytopathologist.[62] It also does not provide reliable information about whether a cancer is in situ or invasive or the pathological type and grade.

Core biopsy of breast tissue is carried out using a 14G diameter needle with a 20-mm sample notch attached to an automated spring-loaded device. Smaller-gauge needles give less reliable results. The needle retrieves a core of tissue, approximately 15–20 mg in weight, which is suitable for histological assessment. This technique is less operator dependent than FNAC and breast tissue histological expertise is much more widely available. Core needle biopsy is associated with fewer false-positive and false-negative results than FNAC and is the technique of choice for routine use in breast diagnosis. FNAC is still favoured by some operators for sampling axillary lymph nodes, although most abnormal nodes lie low in the axilla, away from vascular structures, and are amenable to 14G core biopsy.[31]

The better overall performance of core biopsy compared with FNAC is illustrated in the performance of the NHS Breast Screening Programme in the UK. At the start of the programme, needle sampling by FNAC was almost universal but fewer than 10% of the 90 screening units were able to achieve the target of 90% preoperative diagnosis of breast cancer. After transferring to core biopsy, all of these units now routinely achieve greater than 90% preoperative diagnosis of breast cancer.

Vacuum-Assisted Biopsy

The predominant reasons for failure to achieve accurate diagnosis by needle biopsy are sampling error and failure to retrieve sufficient representative material. Vacuum-assisted biopsy (VAB) addresses these issues. Systems typically use 7 to 11G needles to obtain multiple cores, each weighing up to 300 mg.

VAB significantly improves the diagnostic accuracy for borderline breast lesions and lesions at sites in the breast difficult to biopsy using other techniques. The use of VAB to biopsy microcalcifications halves the risk of missing a coexisting invasive cancer in an area of DCIS compared with 14G core biopsy.[63] VAB is indicated for:

- very small mass lesions;
- architectural distortions;
- failed 'conventional' core biopsy;
- microcalcifications;
- papillary and mucocele-like lesions;
- diffuse non-specific abnormality;
- excision of benign lesions; and
- sentinel node sampling.

VAB can be used under ultrasound, stereotactic or MRI guidance. After needle placement in the breast, suction is applied pulling tissue into a sampling chamber. A rotating or cutting inner cannula automatically advances. In most systems, suction is then used to retrieve the specimen so that multiple cores can be obtained without the need to remove the needle from the breast. Contiguous core biopsies can be obtained by rotating the probe through 360°. Unlike core biopsy, the VAB probe does not have to pass directly through the area being sampled as the suction can be used to draw the abnormality into the sampling chamber, allowing a satisfactory sample to be obtained by placing the probe close to rather than through the abnormality. Ultrasound-guided hand-held vacuum-assisted devices can be used as an alternative to surgery to completely excise benign lesions, such as fibroadenomas, and to widely sample lesions that may be associated with an increased risk of malignancy, such as radial scars and papillary lesions.

Guidance Methods for Breast Needle Biopsy

Ultrasound guidance is the method of choice for biopsy of both palpable and impalpable breast lesions, as it provides real-time visualisation of the biopsy procedure and visual confirmation of adequate sampling. Between 80 and 90% of breast abnormalities that need to be biopsied are visible on ultrasound. For impalpable abnormalities not visible on ultrasound, stereotactic X-ray-guided biopsy is required. A few lesions are visible only on MRI and require MR-guided biopsy.

X-ray-guided stereotactic biopsy is used for impalpable lesions that are not visible on ultrasound. Most microcalcifications and mammographic architectural distortions need to be biopsied under X-ray guidance. There are two types of stereotactic equipment: add-on devices that attach to a conventional upright mammography machine and dedicated prone table devices (Fig. 69-30). Prone table devices are expensive and can only be used for breast biopsy; they require a room in the breast imaging department dedicated for this purpose. The main advantage of this type of device is that the patient cannot see the biopsy procedure while it is being done and vasovagal episodes are said to be less frequent.

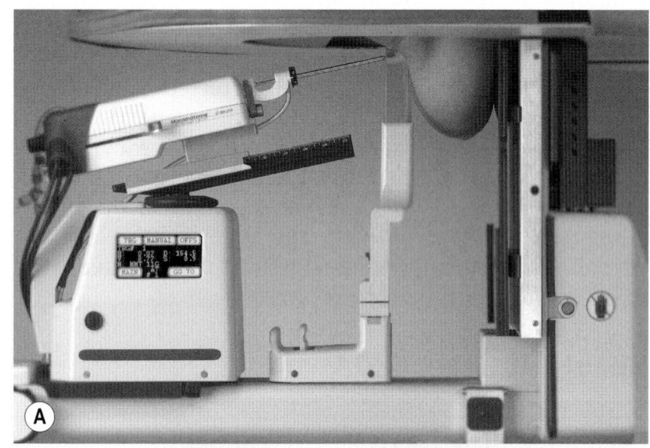

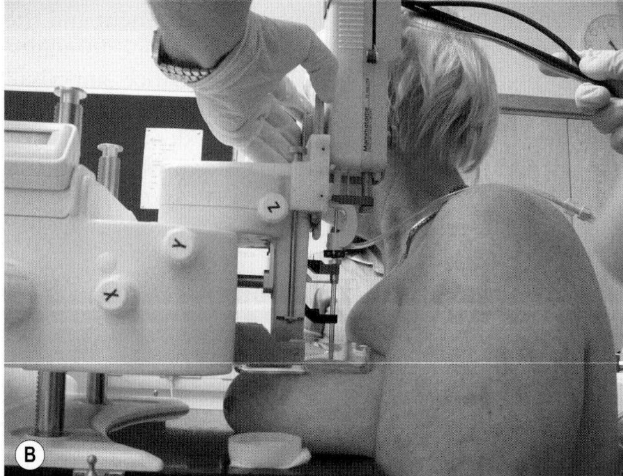

FIGURE 69-30 ■ **Stereotactic breast biopsy.** (A) A prone stereotactic X-ray breast biopsy table. (B) An upright add-on breast biopsy device showing vacuum-assisted biopsy being performed with vertical positioning of the biopsy needle.

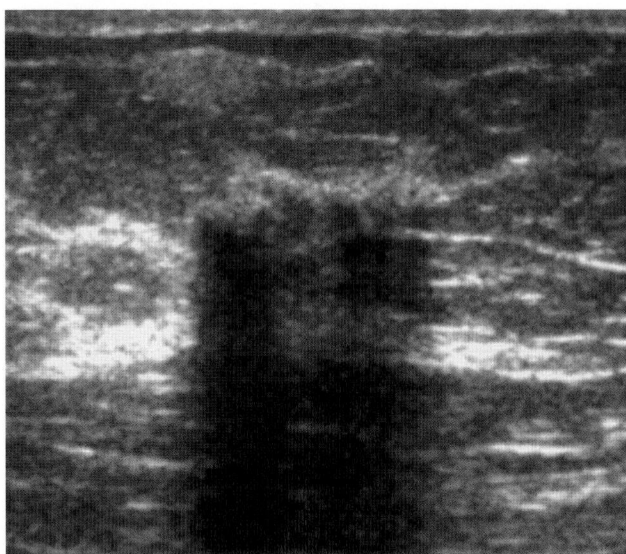

FIGURE 69-31 ■ Ultrasound visible biopsy marker. An ultrasound image of breast tissue containing gel pellets placed at the site of a stereotactic biopsy showing how the mass effect with distal shadowing allows the biopsy site to be easily identified on ultrasound.

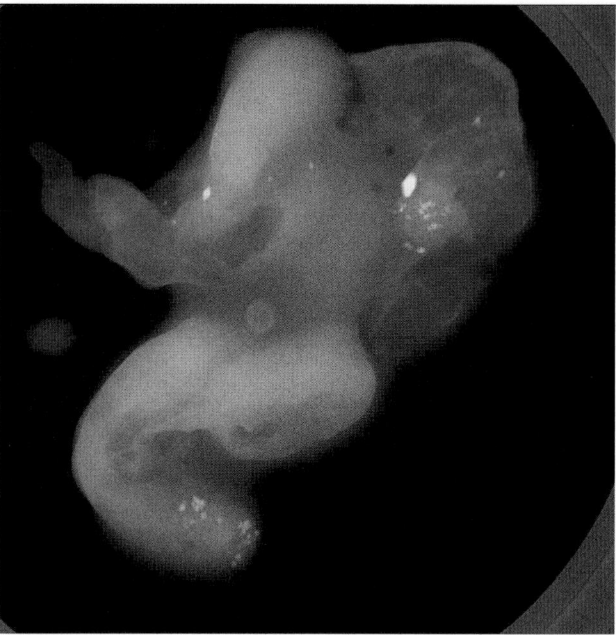

FIGURE 69-32 ■ Core specimen radiography. A specimen radiograph showing a good yield of microcalcifications in several vacuum-assisted biopsy samples.

Add-on devices can be attached to a mammography machine that is otherwise available for routine mammography. These are less expensive and do not require dedicated space. The two methods have equally high levels of accuracy (95% retrieval of representative material) and both are associated with low levels of morbidity and few complications. Vasovagal episodes can be minimised by giving the patient an anxiolytic agent such as sublingual Lorazepam 30 min before the procedure. Upright add-on systems can also be used with the patient lying in the lateral decubitus position.

Both the add-on and prone table stereotactic devices allow precise localisation of the lesion by acquiring two images, 15° on either side of the central axis of the X-ray gantry. The x, y and z coordinates of the lesion are calculated from the relative positions of the target lesion on the two stereotactic images compared with a fixed reference point. After injection of local anaesthetic, the biopsy needle is advanced into the breast via a small skin incision through a needle holder that guides it to the correct depth.

It is possible, particularly after VAB, that the whole of the mammographic abnormality may have been removed, so a marker should be placed at the biopsy site. A variety of metal clip and gel pellet markers are available for this purpose; combined gel and metal markers are ideal as these render the biopsy site ultrasound-visible, allowing subsequent localisation procedures to be carried out under ultrasound rather than stereotactic guidance (Fig. 69-31).

Number of Samples

Sufficient material must be obtained but it is unnecessary to take multiple cores as a matter of routine. For ultrasound-guided biopsy, a minimum of two core specimens is recommended. Stereotactic biopsy is typically used for abnormalities that are more difficult to define or sample, and so a minimum of five core specimens should be obtained. Core specimen radiography is performed when sampling microcalcifications to prove that representative material has been obtained (Fig. 69-32). The identification of microcalcifications in at least three separate cores and/or a total of five separate flecks of calcification in the biopsy specimen should allow an accurate diagnosis to be made.[64] When diagnostic uncertainty remains, larger-gauge VAB can be used to obtain greater tissue volumes (approximately 300 mg per core). The aim is to obtain at least 2 g of tissue.

MRI-Guided Biopsy

A few breast lesions are only visible with MRI and therefore have to be biopsied under MRI guidance. A number of different approaches have been developed for this procedure, but the most widely used system involves the patient lying prone within the breast coil with the breast immobilised between compression plates, one of which is in the form of a grid (Fig. 69-33A). Vacuum-assisted biopsy is the preferred method of tissue sampling under MRI guidance.

Compression is important to stabilise the breast and keep a lesion's location fixed once initially localised. It is important to avoid over-compression, as this can interfere with lesion conspicuity. A vitamin E capsule is placed over the expected lesion position and sagittal imaging performed following intravenous gadolinium injection. The position of the lesion within the breast relative to the skin can then be determined by reference to the skin marker and the gridlines; depth is calculated on the basis

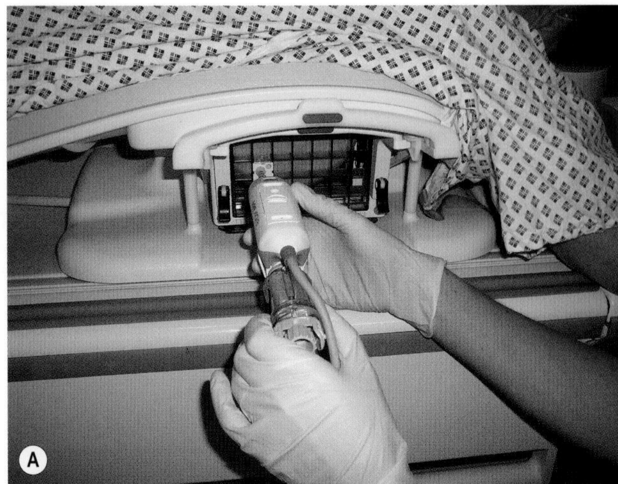

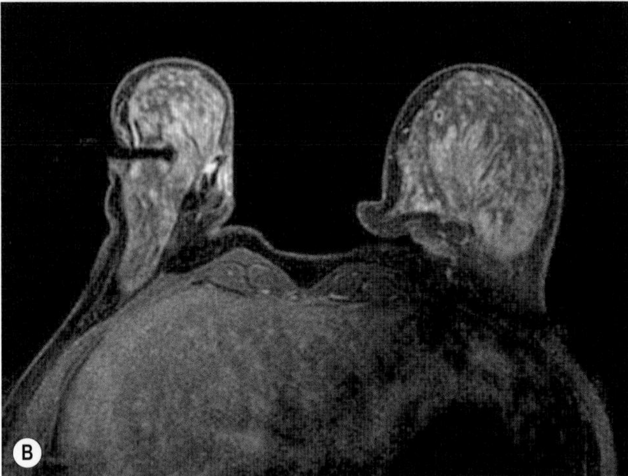

FIGURE 69-33 ■ MRI-guided breast biopsy. (A) The breast being biopsied is immobilised by the grid compression plate and the vacuum biopsy device inserted via the introducing cannula. (B) The introducing cannula is visible on this axial MRI image, enabling the position to be checked before the biopsy.

of the slice thickness and the number of slices between the skin and the lesion. Following the injection of local anaesthetic, an introducing cannula is inserted through a needle guide into the breast with the correct position confirmed by further imaging (Fig. 69-33B). The biopsy device is inserted through the introducing cannula and the biopsy samples obtained (Fig. 69-33A). The patient is re-imaged to ensure that the correct area has been sampled and a biopsy marker deployed.

MRI-guided biopsies are more challenging than other breast biopsies, due to lesion access and visibility. Most modern breast coils enable the breast to be accessed from both the medial and lateral directions, but problems can be encountered with posterior lesions that cannot be captured within the compression grid. Lesion visibility tends to decrease with time following the injection of gadolinium due to a combination of contrast washout from the lesion and increased background enhancement. Despite these limitations, vacuum-assisted MRI-guided biopsy offers a safe and accurate way of obtaining a tissue diagnosis from MRI-only-visible breast lesions.

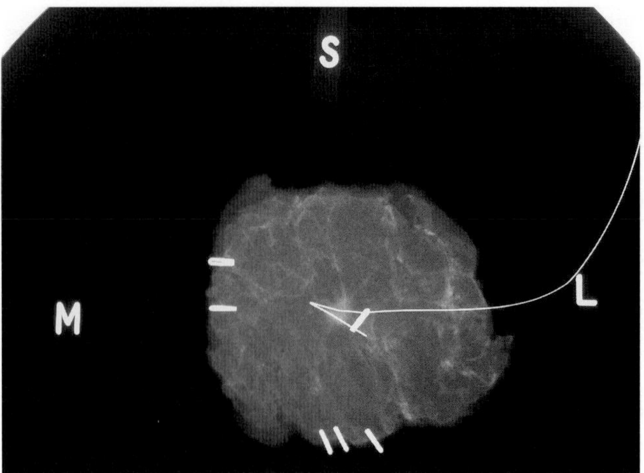

FIGURE 69-34 ■ Surgical specimen radiograph. A specimen radiograph of a marker localisation surgical biopsy showing the hook wire through the small mass lesion. The specimen is orientated by surgical clips showing the superior (S), lateral (L) and medial (M) margins. The radiograph shows clear margins of excision.

Managing the Result of Needle Biopsy

It is important that the result of needle breast biopsy is correlated with the imaging and clinical findings. This is best achieved by reviewing each case at a multidisciplinary meeting at which the imaging, clinical and pathological findings are reviewed and management decisions and choices to be offered are discussed and agreed before the patient is seen with the results.

Preoperative Localisation of Impalpable Lesions

The purpose of preoperative localisation is to ensure that an impalpable lesion is accurately marked, facilitating complete surgical excision. For malignant lesions, the aim is to remove a minimum of 5 mm (and preferably 10 mm) of surrounding normal tissue at all margins. Without localisation, much larger volumes of tissue may be removed, with the potential to cause unnecessary deformity of the breast. Specimen radiography is used to confirm that the lesion has been removed and that adequate margins have been achieved (Fig. 69-34). The specimen is orientated using radio-opaque markers to identify the margins. If excision appears inadequate, further margin excision can be carried out at the same operation.

There are a number of methods available for preoperative localisation. These include simple skin marking over the lesion, insertion of a wire, or injection of carbon dye or radioisotope-labelled colloid. Ultrasound is the preferred method of image guidance.

The ideal wire is easy to deploy, maintains a stable position in the breast and is flexible enough to allow check mammography to take place following insertion. Several types of hook wire systems are available. All use an introducing needle through which the wire is advanced into the breast. For mass lesions and small clusters of microcalcification, the wire should be placed directly through the lesion or area, with the tip of the wire just beyond it. For a larger area of microcalcifications, several wires may be used to 'bracket' the area to be removed. Check mammograms should be performed to confirm that the correct area has been localised; these should be available to the surgeon.

Impalpable lesions can be localised using radio-labelled high-molecular-weight colloid. This technique is known as radio-opaque lesion localisation (ROLL). ^{99m}Tc-labelled colloid is injected under image guidance into the immediate vicinity of the tumour and the surgeon then localises the lesion using a fine-tipped gamma probe. The colloid must be large enough not to diffuse away from the injection site; the type of colloid used for lung scintigraphy is ideal.

CONCLUSION

Mammography and ultrasound continue to be the primary imaging tools for the assessment and diagnosis of breast disease. The development of digital mammography and high-resolution ultrasound has led to improvements in image quality and breast cancer detection. MRI is an important additional tool for local staging of breast cancer in carefully selected cases, aiding surgical planning.

The modern breast radiologist requires interventional radiology skills, with biopsies performed under ultrasound, X-ray and MRI guidance. Accurate preoperative diagnosis with image-guided percutaneous core biopsy is crucial in the management of breast disease, with surgery reserved for treatment rather than diagnosis. Increasingly sophisticated vacuum-assisted biopsy devices are available to improve the yield of representative tissue during biopsy, further improving preoperative diagnosis rates.

The past 20 years have seen a reduction in breast cancer mortality despite increasing incidence of the disease. Population-based breast cancer screening with mammography aims to reduce mortality by early detection. This remains a controversial area, but the benefits of screening in reducing mortality continue to outweigh the risks of overdiagnosis and overtreatment.

For a full list of references, please see ExpertConsult.

FURTHER READING

9. Pisano ED, Gatsonis C, Hendrick E, et al. Diagnostic performance of digital versus film mammography for breast-cancer screening. N Engl J Med 2005;353:1846–7.
15. Gilbert FJ, Astley SM, Gillan MGC, et al. Single reading with computer-aided detection for screening mammography. N Engl J Med 2010;359:1675–84.
19. Berg WA, Cosgrove DO, Doré CJ, et al. Shear-wave elastography improves the specificity of breast US: The BE1 multinational study of 939 masses. Radiology 2012;262:435–49.
20. Stavros AT, Thickman D, Rapp CL, et al. Solid breast nodules: use of sonography to distinguish between benign and malignant lesions. Radiology 1995;196:123–34.
23. American College of Radiology. Breast Imaging Reporting and Data Systems Atlas (BI-RADS Atlas). Reston, VA: American College of Radiology; 2003.
31. Damera A, Evans AJ, Cornford EJ, et al. Diagnosis of axillary nodal metastases by ultrasound-guided core biopsy in primary operable breast cancer. Br J Cancer 2003;89:1310–13.
47. Turnbull LW, Brown SR, Harvey I, et al. Comparative effectiveness of MRI in breast cancer (COMICE) trail: a randomized control trial. Lancet 2010;375:563–71.
48. Solin LJ, Orel SG, Wei-Ting H, et al. Relationship of breast magnetic resonance imaging after breast-conservation treatment with radiation for women with early-stage invasive breast carcinoma of ductal carcinoma in situ. J Clin Oncol 2008;26:386–91.
51. Nystrom L, Andersson I, Bjurstam N, et al. Long-term effects of mammographic screening: update overview of the Swedish randomised trials. Lancet 2002;359:909–19.
63. Brennan ME, Turner RM, Ciatto S, et al. Ductal carcinoma in situ at core-needle biopsy: meta-analysis of underestimation and predictors of invasive cancer. Radiology 2011;260:119–28.

CHAPTER 70

RETICULOENDOTHELIAL DISORDERS: LYMPHOMA

Sarah J. Vinnicombe • Norbert Avril • Rodney H. Reznek

CHAPTER OUTLINE

The lymphomas are complex, but may be divided into two broad groups: Hodgkin's lymphoma (HL) and non-Hodgkin's lymphoma (NHL). The overall incidence of NHL has increased steadily since 1960, with age-adjusted incidence rates being highest in more developed countries. It is estimated that there will be 70,000 new cases in 2012, an age-adjusted incidence of 19 per 100,000 persons per year, representing a 73% increase since the early 1970s.[1] This is due in part to secondary lymphoma arising in the setting of acquired immune deficiency syndrome (AIDS), though the incidence had started to increase before the AIDS epidemic. In the corresponding period, the incidence of HL has remained relatively steady at around 3 per 100,000.

EPIDEMIOLOGY

Age

HL has a peak incidence in the 20–30-year age group, with a second peak in the elderly population. The incidence of NHL increases exponentially with age after 20 years. The subtypes of lymphoma encountered differ in frequency between adult and paediatric groups, with a strong bias towards precursor B- and T-lymphoblastic lymphoma and Burkitt's lymphoma (BL) in childhood. Lymphomas with less typical age distribution include mediastinal large B-cell lymphoma, which has a peak incidence between 25 and 35 years, and mantle cell lymphoma, which is more common in those over 60 years.

Infectious Agents

Oncogenic lymphotrophic viruses have been implicated in many types of NHL. The single most important agent in this regard is Epstein–Barr virus (EBV). The EBV genome was first detected in cultured African Burkitt's lymphoma cells and is present in over 90% of such cases. EBV is important as a trigger for lymphoproliferations/lymphomas occurring in congenital immunodeficiencies, immunosuppressed organ transplant recipients, patients receiving maintenance chemotherapy and patients receiving combined immunosuppressive therapy for collagen disorders. EBV is also found in HL (mostly the mixed cellularity type); patients who have had infectious mononucleosis are at increased risk of HL. The retrovirus human lymphotropic virus type 1 (HTLV–1) is implicated in the causation of adult T-cell lymphoma, which is endemic in certain areas of East Africa, the Caribbean, southwest Japan and New Guinea. Human herpesvirus 8 (HHV–8) has been implicated as a cause of primary effusion lymphoma, a rare type of large cell lymphoma confined to serous-lined body cavities, which occurs with highest frequency in the HIV-positive population. Bacterial overgrowth can also promote lymphomagenesis. In gastric lymphoma of mucosa-associated lymphoid tissue (MALT) type, *Helicobacter pylori* infection has been shown to be necessary for the development and early proliferation of the lymphoma.

Immunosuppression

A variety of NHL is associated with pre-existing immunosuppression. The degree of immunosuppression is important in determining the lymphoma type that may emerge. In organ-specific autoimmune diseases, such as Hashimoto's thyroiditis and Sjögren's syndrome, extranodal marginal zone lymphomas of MALT type can arise within the affected organ. In severe immunodeficiency states, such as the congenital immunodeficiencies, AIDS and after organ transplantation, the lymphomas are very often EBV-driven large B-cell lymphomas. Infection with human immunodeficiency virus (HIV) explains much of the massive increase in the incidence of NHL in the past two decades. In the setting of systemic collagen diseases, there is an increase in haematological malignancy and patients receiving immunosuppressive therapy for these conditions are at still greater risk. The types of haematological malignancy that arise are quite varied, but there is a slight excess of myeloma and small B-lymphocytic lymphoma.

Genetic Factors

It is known that the risk of developing haematological malignancy is increased in patients with a family history of disease. This increased risk does not extend to the histological type or lineage of the tumours in question, such that one family member may have HL whereas a relative may have NHL or myeloid leukaemia.

Gender and Race

There is a slight predominance of NHL and HL in men (1.1–1.4 to 1). The incidence of NHL and HL varies by race, with higher frequencies in whites than blacks or Asians. Certain NHL types cluster according to race: for example, the natural killer (NK) T-cell lymphomas are most frequently encountered in oriental populations.

HISTOPATHOLOGICAL CLASSIFICATION

Hodgkin's Lymphoma

Biological studies have shown that HL is a true lymphoma. The defining malignant cell of HL is the Reed–Sternberg cell, a large, binucleated blast cell. Mononuclear counterparts are called Hodgkin's cells. The Reed–Sternberg cells and their variants form a minority population within any involved lymph node. The balance is made up of reactive non-neoplastic T cells, histiocytes, plasma cells, eosinophils and fibroblasts, varying in proportion according to the histological subtype. Since the 1960s, so-called classical HL has been subclassified into four histological types, indicated below along with their relative frequencies in Western populations:

- Lymphocyte-rich—5%
- Mixed cellularity (MC)—20–25%
- Nodular sclerosing (NS)—70%
- Lymphocyte-depleted (LD)—<5%.

In the nodular sclerosing type, substantial fibroblastic activity results in segmentation of involved nodes into cellular nodules separated by thick bands of collagen. It typically presents as a bulky mediastinal mass. In mixed cellularity HL, classical Reed–Sternberg cells are mixed with sheets of inflammatory elements. It is commoner in developing countries and in patients with HIV infection, as is the rare lymphocyte-depleted HL. Both have an aggressive clinical course. All four classical subtypes share the same immunophenotype and together constitute 95% of all cases of HL. A second distinct entity is nodular lymphocyte predominant HL, which was probably misdiagnosed as lymphocyte-rich classical HL in the past. It has a different morphology, immunophenotype and clinical course from classical HL; latent EBV infection is not a feature.

Non-Hodgkin's Lymphoma

Many of the difficulties that beset early taxonomists in the classification of NHL have been overcome with improved immunological and molecular methods of diagnosis. The Revised European–American Lymphoma (REAL) classification in 1994 depended on a triad of morphology, immunophenotype and molecular methods as well as clinical features for defining disease entities,[2] differentiating it from earlier morphologically based classifications. The scheme forms the backbone of the World Health Organisation (WHO) classification of tumours of haematopoietic and lymphoid tissues.[3] A summary of the WHO classification (4th edition) is given in Table 70-1. The WHO classification stratifies neoplasms by lineage into clinically distinct disease entities and is a real advance in the ability to identify disease accurately and consistently. Further, it can be refined so as to improve patient management.[4] For example, it has recently been shown that gene expression profiling in diffuse large B-cell lymphoma (DLBCL) enables recognition of discrete subsets (germinal centre B-cell type and activated B-cell type) which have independent prognostic significance, and this has been included in the 4th edition of the classification.[3] Other additions include paediatric follicular lymphoma, primary DLBCL of the central nervous system (PCNSL), and two so-called 'grey zone' lymphomas: B-cell lymphoma with features intermediate between DLBCL and classical HL, and B-cell lymphoma with features intermediate between DLBCL and BL.

STAGING, INVESTIGATION AND MANAGEMENT

Hodgkin's Lymphoma

Clinical Features and Staging

Most patients present with lymph node enlargement, most often in the cervical chains. Up to 40% have B symptoms (fever, drenching night sweats and weight loss of more than 10% of the person's bodyweight). Other constitutional symptoms can occur, such as pruritus, fatigue, anorexia and rarely alcohol-induced pain at the site of enlarged lymph nodes. Clinical examination usually reveals lymphadenopathy, most commonly in the neck. Axillary nodal enlargement occurs in up to 20% and inguinal disease in up to 15%, although exclusive infradiaphragmatic nodal disease is seen in up to 10% of patients at presentation. Splenomegaly may be evident on clinical examination in up to 30%.

Tissue biopsy is essential to make the diagnosis. Though a diagnosis of lymphoma may be made from a cutting needle biopsy, surgical excision biopsy of an entire node is preferable, so that the architecture of the node can be evaluated. Investigations will comprise a

TABLE 70-1 WHO Classification of Lymphoid Neoplasms

Neoplasm	Percentage of NHL*
B-CELL NEOPLASMS	85.0
Precursor B-cell neoplasms	
Precursor B-lymphoblastic leukaemia/ lymphoma	
Mature B-cell neoplasms	
CLL/small lymphocytic lymphoma	6.7
B-cell prolymphocytic leukaemia	
Lymphoplasmacytic (lymphoplasmacytoid) lymphoma	1.2
Splenic marginal zone lymphoma	<1.0
Hairy cell leukaemia	
Plasma cell myeloma	
Solitary plasmacytoma of bone	
Extraosseous plasmacytoma	
Extranodal marginal zone B-cell lymphoma of mucosa-associated lymphoid tissue (MALT)	7.6
Nodal marginal zone lymphoma	1.8
Follicular lymphoma	22.0
Mantle cell lymphoma	6.0
Diffuse large B-cell lymphoma (BCL)	32.0
Mediastinal (thymic)	2.4
Intravascular	
Primary effusion lymphoma	
Burkitt's lymphoma/leukaemia	1.0
B-CELL PROLIFERATIONS OF UNCERTAIN MALIGNANT POTENTIAL	
Lymphomatoid granulomatosis	
Post-transplant lymphoproliferative disorder, polymorphic	
T-CELL AND NK-CELL NEOPLASMS	14.0
Precursor T-cell neoplasms	
Precursor T-lymphoblastic lymphoma/ leukaemia	1.7
Blastic NK-cell lymphoma	
Mature T-cell and NK-cell neoplasms	
T-cell prolymphocytic leukaemia	
T-cell large granular lymphocytic leukaemia	
Aggressive NK-cell leukaemia	
Adult T-cell leukaemia/lymphoma	2.4
Extranodal NK-/T-cell lymphoma, nasal type	<1.0
Enteropathy-type T-cell lymphoma	
Hepatosplenic T-cell lymphoma	<0.001
Subcutaneous panniculitis-like	1.0
T-cell lymphoma	
Mycosis fungoides	
Sézary syndrome	1.2
Primary cutaneous anaplastic large cell lymphoma	
Peripheral T-cell lymphoma, unspecified	
Angioimmunoblastic T-cell lymphoma	7.0
Anaplastic large cell lymphoma	
T-CELL PROLIFERATIONS OF UNCERTAIN MALIGNANT POTENTIAL	
Lymphoid papulosis	
HODGKIN'S LYMPHOMA	
Nodular lymphocyte-predominant HL	
Classical HL	
Nodular sclerosis classical HL	
Lymphocyte-rich classical HL	
Mixed cellularity classical HL	
Lymphocyte-depleted classical HL	

*Approximate frequency—refers to lymph node biopsies in adults, with 1% accounting for the very rare entities.

TABLE 70-2 Cotswold's Modification of the Ann Arbor Staging Classification of Hodgkin's Disease

Stage	Classification
I	Involvement of a single lymph node region (I) or a single extralymphatic organ or site (IE)
II	Involvement of two or more lymph node regions on the same side of the diaphragm (II) or one or more lymph node regions plus an extralymphatic site (IIE)
III	Involvement of lymph node regions on both sides of the diaphragm (III) (the spleen is included in stage III) subdivided into: III(1): involvement of spleen and/or splenic hilar, coeliac and portal nodes III(2): with para-aortic, iliac, or mesenteric nodes
IV	Involvement of one or more extralymphatic organs, e.g. lung, liver, bone, bone marrow, with or without lymph node involvement
Additional qualifiers denote the following:	A: asymptomatic B: fever, night sweats and weight loss of >10% body weight X: bulky disease (defined as a lymph node mass >10 cm in diameter or, if involving the mediastinum, a mass greater than one-third of the intrathoracic diameter at the level of T5 E: involvement of a single extranodal site, contiguous with a known nodal site

blood count and erythrocyte sedimentation rate (ESR), together with liver biochemistry, renal function and serum urate. A staging computed tomography (CT) or a diagnostic positron emission tomography (PET)/CT imaging with 2-[F-18]fluoro-2-deoxy-D-glucose (FDG) is mandatory and may show involvement of intrathoracic, abdominal or pelvic lymph nodes. The so-called Cotswold's modification[5] of the original Ann Arbor staging classification (Table 70-2) was designed to take into account prognostic factors such as the volume of lymph node masses as identified with CT. A bone marrow aspirate and trephine biopsy should be performed in all patients except those with stage I disease, in whom the likelihood of bone marrow infiltration is negligible.

Prognosis and Treatment

For HL a poorer prognosis is noted with:

- Older patients
- Tumour subtype
- Raised ESR
- Mutiple sites of disease
- Bulky mediastinal disease
- B symptoms.

Treatment is almost invariably given with curative intent. The choice of treatment will depend predominantly on stage, and the presence/absence of adverse prognostic factors. HL is highly radiosensitive, and until recently many patients were treated with 'mantle' radiotherapy, which encompassed the cervical nodal chains, the axillae and the mediastinum down to the level of T10. However, there has been a steady trend towards the avoidance of radiotherapy in young patients because of the significant increase in secondary cancers, notably of the thyroid and breast (areas included in the radiotherapy field), and death through coronary artery disease.

Localised Disease (Stages IA and IIA). The majority of patients with early-stage favourable disease (non-bulky) are treated with combination chemotherapy. The use of interim FDG/PET imaging may allow escalation or de-escalation of therapy, with the goal of avoiding radiotherapy in patients who have a good response to combination chemotherapy and who are therefore in a very good prognostic group.

Advanced Disease (Stages IIB, IIIA/B and IVA/B). Patients presenting with a large mediastinal mass (i.e. a mass greater than 10 cm in diameter at CT) are generally treated with more intense chemotherapy initially, so as to shrink the mass. Consolidative radiotherapy may then be given. For advanced-stage disease, treatment comprises extensive combination chemotherapy, with or without subsequent consolidatory radiotherapy to sites of 'bulky' disease.

Failure to achieve an initial complete or almost complete response to first-line treatment and recurrence in the first year are both associated with a poor prognosis. Patients who develop recurrent HL more than once will generally ultimately die of the disease. By comparison, patients who develop recurrent HL some years after receiving treatment for localised disease can be given further combination chemotherapy and still be cured.

Non-Hodgkin's Lymphoma

Accurate diagnosis requires adequate tissue biopsy and an experienced histopathologist. Some lesions, for example, retroperitoneal, mediastinal and mesenteric masses, may be amenable to ultrasound or CT-guided core-needle biopsy, which may safely yield adequate tissue for histological diagnosis and immunophenotyping[6] but, as with HL, an entire lymph node is preferable for diagnosis.

Clinical Features and Staging

Most patients present with painless lymph node enlargement, but B symptoms are less frequent compared to HL, occurring in approximately 20%. In contradistinction to HL, the histological subtype of NHL is the major determinant of treatment rather than the stage. Nonetheless the stage of the disease has strong prognostic significance, a more advanced stage being associated with a significantly worse prognosis.[7] As with HL, the modified Ann Arbor staging system is generally used. Around 80% of patients will have advanced disease (stage III or IV) at presentation, so all newly diagnosed patients should undergo detailed physical examination, including examination of the fauces and testes. As with HL, CT or FDG-PET/CT of the neck, chest, abdomen and pelvis is mandatory, together with a bone marrow aspirate and trephine biopsy, owing to the propensity of most NHL to infiltrate the bone marrow at presentation. Depending on the pattern of symptoms, other radiological investigations such as MRI may be indicated, especially for central nervous system lymphoma.

Prognosis and Treatment

The prognosis of NHL varies tremendously, depending upon the histological subtype. In order to evaluate therapies better and to choose the most appropriate treatment for a given patient, the International Prognostic Index (IPI) was developed.[7] The IPI is strictly speaking only applicable to aggressive lymphomas such as diffuse large B-cell lymphoma (DLBCL). Five factors were statistically associated with significantly inferior overall survival:

- Age >60 years
- Elevated serum lactate dehydrogenase (LDH)
- Performance status >1 (i.e. non-ambulatory)
- Advanced stage (III or IV)
- Presence of >1 extranodal site of disease.

A similar prognostic index (FLIPI) has been developed for more indolent follicular lymphoma (FL), where the important factors are considered to be:

- Age >60 years
- Elevated serum LDH
- Haemoglobin <12 g/dL
- Advanced stage (III or IV)
- More than four nodal sites of disease.

A recent modification (FLIPI 2) includes elevated serum β_2-microglobulin and longest diameter of the largest involved lymph node over 6 cm.[8]

The histological subtype determines not only the type of treatment but also when treatment should start. For asymptomatic patients with FL, surveillance alone may be appropriate until symptoms develop or transformation to a more aggressive DLBCL occurs. On the other hand, patients with relatively localised DLBCL require treatment with multi-agent anthracycline-containing chemotherapy immediately. Standard treatment for DLBCL and higher-grade FL comprises cyclophosphamide, doxorubicin, vincristine and prednisone (CHOP) combined with rituximab, a chimeric monoclonal antibody against the CD20 receptor, expressed by over 95% of B-cell NHL (CHOP-R). Radiotherapy alone is considered for the small proportion of patients with stage I disease and no adverse factors, in whom surgical excision alone is considered inappropriate.

LYMPH NODE DISEASE IN LYMPHOMA

In HL, lymph node involvement is usually the only manifestation of disease, whereas in NHL nodal disease is frequently associated with extranodal involvement. There are differences in the patterns of lymph node involvement in HL and NHL at presentation. Lymph nodes tend to be larger in NHL than HL; indeed, in nodular sclerosing and lymphocyte-depleted HL, nodal enlargement may be minimal. Typically, involved nodes tend to displace adjacent structures rather than invade them, except in the case of primary mediastinal large B-cell lymphoma (PMBL), which is characterised by local invasion of adjacent structures.

Imaging Nodal Disease

At present, size is the only criterion by which lymph nodes demonstrated on CT or MRI are considered to be involved, though clustering of multiple small lymph nodes, for example within the anterior mediastinum or the mesentery, is suggestive. A maximum short-axis diameter of 10 mm is taken to be the upper limit of normal, depending upon the exact site within the neck, thorax, abdomen, or pelvis. There are exceptions: normal neck jugulodigastric node can measure up to 13 mm short-axis diameter; nodes in the gastrohepatic ligament and porta hepatis are considered abnormal if they measure more than 8 mm in diameter; retrocrural nodes greater than 6 mm are taken as enlarged;[9] and in the pelvis the upper limit of normal is 8 mm.[10] Lymph nodes at some sites, such as the splenic hilum, presacral and perirectal areas, are not usually visualised on cross-sectional imaging and, whenever demonstrated, are likely to be abnormal.

Enlarged lymph nodes in both HL and NHL are usually homogeneous, of soft-tissue density on CT. Mild or moderate uniform enhancement occurs after intravenous injection of contrast medium. Calcification is uncommon but may be seen on post-treatment images. Necrosis is rarely seen in large nodal masses in both HL (particularly nodular sclerosing HL) and aggressive NHL, more frequently after treatment. On MRI, involved lymph nodes have low-to-intermediate signal intensity on T1-weighted images, and they may have very high signal intensity on fat-suppressed T2-weighted and short tau inversion recovery (STIR) sequences. Though the signal intensity of involved nodes and the presence of necrosis do not appear to have much prognostic significance, there is some evidence that within large lymphomatous masses, heterogeneous T2 signal at magnetic resonance imaging (MRI), or heterogeneous enhancement at CT, is associated with a worse outcome.

Choice of Imaging Technique

CT has been the technique of choice for the staging and follow-up of lymphoma for some time, and enables localisation of the most appropriate lesion for consideration of percutaneous image-guided biopsy. Ultrasound has no value in whole-body staging. Ultrasonographic appearances of lymphomatous nodal disease are non-specific, though the pattern of vascular perfusion as demonstrated by power Doppler interrogation may suggest the diagnosis, lymphomatous nodes having rich central and peripheral perfusion. The main value of ultrasound in lymphoma lies in confirming the nature of a palpable mass and assessing the major viscera. The accuracy of MRI in detecting lymph node involvement is equal to that of CT (and is better in some areas such as the supraclavicular fossa and within the pelvis), but it has no particular advantage over CT in this respect and its role is essentially adjunctive, to solve problems or monitor response to treatment. Recent advances in MRI technology (high field strength magnets and parallel imaging) have enabled MRI to be used for whole-body staging: the role of whole-body diffusion-weighted imaging in staging and response assessment is a field of active research.[11] Major advantages in patients with HL in particular (who are often young) include the lack of ionising radiation.

Detection of disease in normal-sized nodes is not possible with cross-sectional imaging, nor is it possible to differentiate between nodal enlargement secondary to lymphoma or reactive hyperplasia. Functional imaging is often able to make this distinction. The superior diagnostic accuracy and more favourable imaging characteristics of PET with FDG and, latterly, PET/CT, has resulted in a dramatic decline in the use of gallium-67 scintigraphy, which no longer has a role as an isolated tool in the staging of lymphoma.

Numerous studies have shown that FDG-PET is at least as accurate as CT in the depiction of nodal and extranodal disease[12,13] and more sensitive than Ga-67 scintigraphy. It results in clinically significant upstaging in up to 10–20% of patients compared to CT, which may result in changes in therapy, particularly in HL.[14] Most NHLs are FDG-avid, though false-negative studies can occur with low-grade lymphomas such as small lymphocytic lymphoma, cutaneous lymphoma, some peripheral T-cell lymphomas and MALT types. For these subtypes, contrast-enhanced CT remains the standard of care. The development of PET/CT with accurate co-registration means that both morphological and functional abnormalities can be assessed simultaneously with improved diagnostic performance of FDG-PET as a result.[15] It is important to recognise that lymphomatous involvement of certain organs can be very difficult to recognise with FDG-PET/CT, because of physiological uptake—for example, in the stomach and central nervous system.[16] Debate continues as to whether it is necessary to carry out a full diagnostic CT imaging as part of the PET/CT study and often a low-dose CT, for the purposes of attenuation correction and anatomical correlation, is sufficient.[17,18]

Neck

Between 60 and 80% of patients with HL present with cervical lymphadenopathy. The spread of the disease is most frequently to contiguous nodal groups, with involvement of the internal jugular chain and spread to other deep lymphatic chains in the neck. Patients with supraclavicular or bilateral neck adenopathy are at increased risk of infradiaphragmatic disease.

Cervical adenopathy is less common in NHL, but commonly occurs in association with extranodal disease in Waldeyer's ring. Approximately 40–60% of patients who present with head and neck involvement will have disseminated NHL. Involved nodal groups tend to be non-contiguous. Central necrosis within a lymph node is rarely seen. Imaging with contrast-enhanced CT or MRI has a useful role in evaluating the neck in patients with lymphoma, as it may identify enlarged nodes which are impalpable. It is helpful in response assessment, particularly in patients treated with radiotherapy, where post-treatment fibrosis renders clinical assessment difficult.

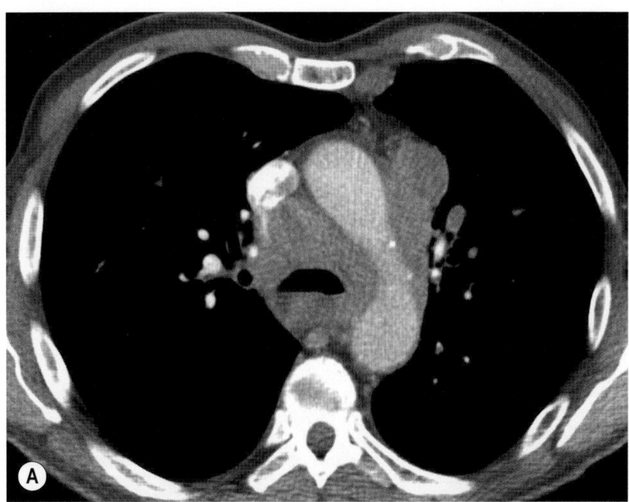

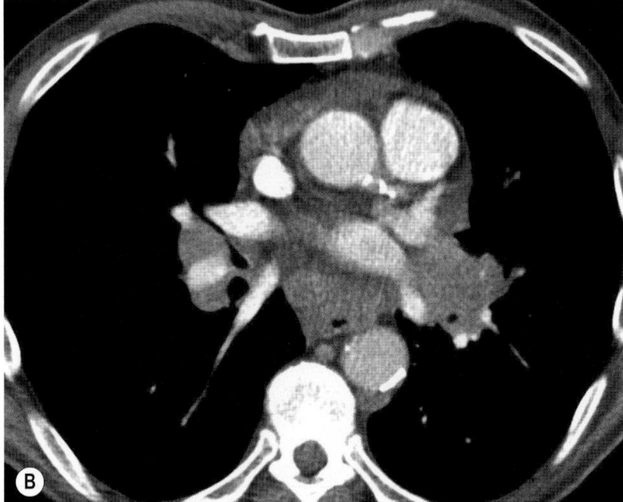

FIGURE 70-1 ■ Anterior and middle mediastinal nodal disease. (A) Contrast-enhanced CT showing marked confluent enlargement of the middle mediastinal nodes, extending laterally into the aortopulmonary window and extending into the prevascular left para-aortic region. (B) Subcarinal, bilateral hilar and para-aortic nodal involvement in the same patient.

Thorax

Intrathoracic nodes are involved at presentation in 60–85% of patients with HL and 25–40% of patients with NHL.[19] Nodes larger than 1 cm short-axis diameter are considered enlarged. Any intrathoracic group of nodes may be affected, but all the mediastinal sites other than paracardiac and posterior mediastinal nodes are more frequently involved in HL than NHL. Nearly all patients with nodular sclerosing HL have disease in the anterior mediastinum. The frequency of nodal involvement in HL is as follows:[19] prevascular and paratracheal—84% (Fig. 70-1); hilar—28% (Fig. 70-1); subcarinal—22% (Fig. 70-1); others—5% (aortopulmonary, anterior diaphragmatic, internal mammary (Fig. 70-2)). In NHL involvement of the hilar and subcarinal groups is rarer, occurring in 9 and 13%, respectively, whereas superior mediastinal nodes are involved in 35%.[20]

The great majority of cases of HL show enlargement of two or more nodal groups, whereas only one nodal group is involved in up to half of the cases of NHL. Hilar nodal enlargement is rare without associated mediastinal involvement, particularly in HL. Although paracardiac and internal mammary nodes are rarely involved at presentation in HL, they may be involved in recurrent disease, as they are not included in the classical 'mantle' radiation field. In HL and NHL, large anterior mediastinal masses usually represent thymic infiltration as well as a nodal mass (Fig. 70-3). A large anterior mediastinal mass in HL is recognised as an adverse prognostic feature and, as such, defines the need for more aggressive initial therapy. CT will demonstrate unsuspected mediastinal nodal enlargement despite a normal chest radiograph in 10% of patients with HL, and these patients have a poorer prognosis. CT of the chest has been shown to alter management in up to 25% of patients with HL. The therapeutic impact is less in patients with NHL, who are likely to receive chemotherapy regardless of stage. Impalpable axillary nodal enlargement is also frequently detected on CT in HL and NHL.

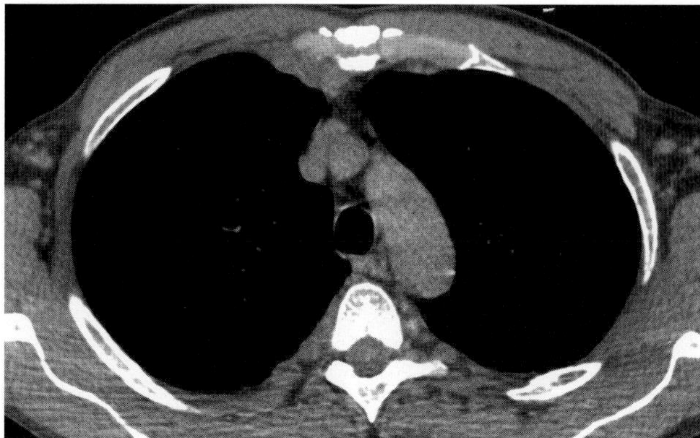

FIGURE 70-2 ■ Internal mammary lymphadenopathy. Axial CT showing marked enlargement of the right internal mammary lymph nodes. Note the minimal bilateral axillary lymph node enlargement and paravertebral extrapleural disease bilaterally.

Abdomen and Pelvis

At presentation the retroperitoneal nodes are involved in 25–35% of patients with HL but up to 55% of patients with NHL.[21] Mesenteric lymph nodes are involved in more than half the patients with NHL and less than 5% of patients with HL.[21] Other sites such as the porta hepatis and splenic hilum are also less frequently involved in HL than NHL (Fig. 70-4). In HL, nodal spread is predictably from one lymph node group to another through directly connected lymphatic pathways. Nodes are frequently of normal size or only minimally enlarged. Spread from the mediastinum occurs through the lymphatic vessels to the retrocrural nodes, coeliac axis and so on. Around the coeliac axis, multiple normal-sized nodes may be seen, which can be difficult to evaluate because involved, normal-sized nodes are frequent in HL[22] (Fig. 70-4). The coeliac axis, splenic hilar and porta hepatis nodes are involved in about 30% of patients and splenic hilar nodal involvement is almost always associated with diffuse splenic infiltration (Fig. 70-4). The node of the foramen of Winslow (porta caval node), lying between

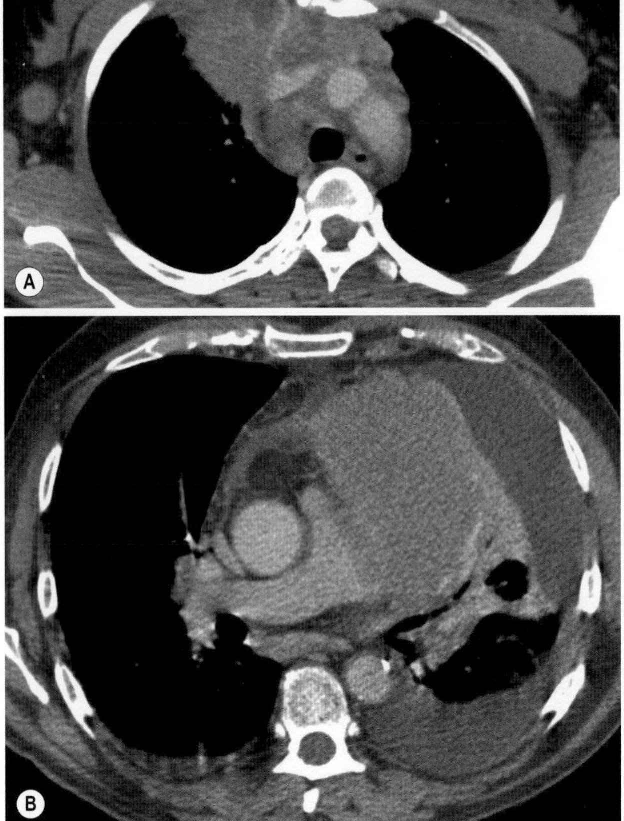

FIGURE 70-3 ■ **Mediastinal masses in lymphoma.** (A) Contrast-enhanced CT showing a large anterior mass involving the chest wall in a young patient with Hodgkin's lymphoma. Note the right axillary nodal disease. (B) Contrast-enhanced CT in a patient with primary mediastinal large B-cell lymphoma (PMBL) in the anterior and middle mediastinum. Note the pericardial involvement, compressive atelectasis of the left upper lobe and large left pleural effusion.

the portal vein and the inferior vena cava, is important, as it is often overlooked and may be the only site of disease relapse. It has a triangular shape; its normal long-axis diameter is up to 3 cm and in the anteroposterior plane is approximately 1 cm.

In NHL, nodal involvement is frequently non-contiguous and bulky and is more frequently associated with extranodal disease. Discrete mesenteric nodal enlargement or masses may be seen with or without retroperitoneal nodal enlargement. Large-volume nodal disease in both mesentery and retroperitoneum may give rise to the so-called 'hamburger' sign, in which a loop of bowel is compressed between two large nodal masses (Fig. 70-5). Multiple normal-sized mesenteric nodes should be regarded with suspicion for the diagnosis of lymphoma and lymphoma is a recognised cause of the 'misty mesentery'. In NHL, regional nodal involvement is frequently seen in patients with primary extranodal lymphoma involving an abdominal viscus. Involved nodes tend to enhance uniformly and the presence of multilocular enhancement should suggest an alternative diagnosis such as tuberculosis or atypical infection.

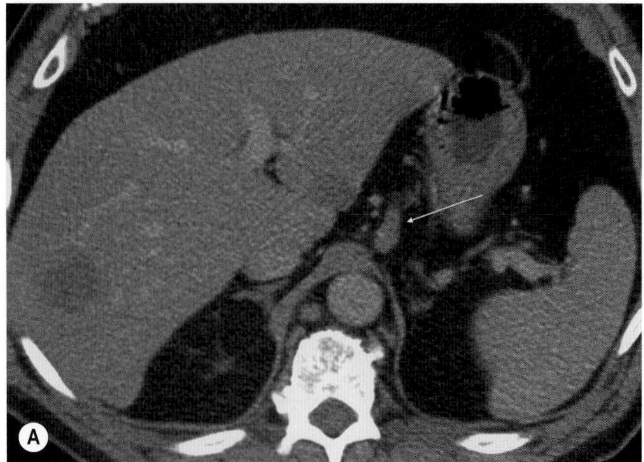

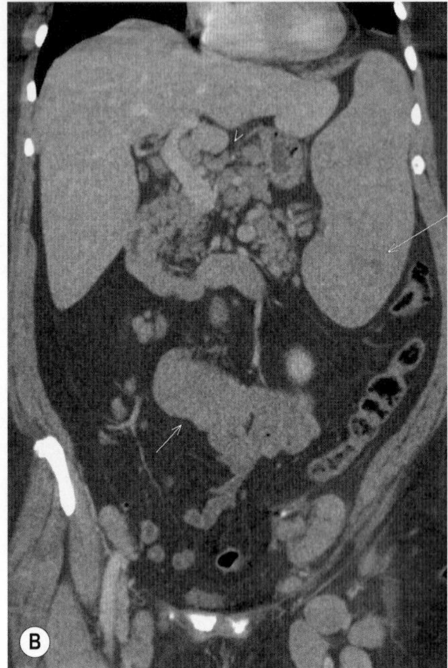

FIGURE 70-4 ■ **Upper abdominal lymph node enlargement.** (A) Contrast-enhanced CT showing an enlarged lymph node in the gastrohepatic ligament (arrow). Minimal lymph node enlargement (exceeding 6 mm) is also seen in the right retrocrural region Two liver deposits are present in this patient with HL. (B) Coronal reformatted contrast-enhanced CT showing lymph node enlargement around the coeliac axis and porta hepatis (arrowhead), the splenic hilum, the mesentery (short arrow), the left external iliac chain and both inguinal regions. There is splenomegaly and a focal splenic lesion (long arrow).

In the pelvis, any nodal group may be involved in both HL and NHL. Presentation with enlarged inguinal or femoral lymphadenopathy is seen in less than 20% of HL, and its presence should prompt close scrutiny of the pelvic nodal groups. In patients with massive pelvic disease, MRI is helpful for delineating the full extent of tumour and the effect on the adjacent organs.

EXTRANODAL DISEASE IN LYMPHOMA

Involvement of extranodal sites by lymphoma usually occurs in the presence of widespread advanced disease elsewhere. Such secondary involvement is a recognised

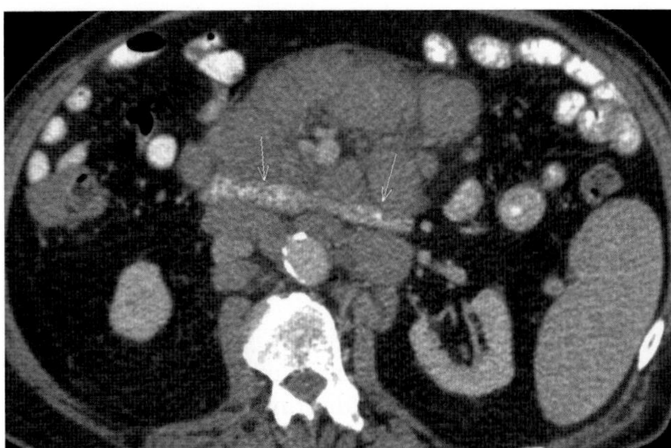

FIGURE 70-5 ■ **Extensive mesenteric nodal disease.** Nodal enlargement in the mesentery and the retroperitoneum in a patient with NHL, compressing the third part of the duodenum (arrows) resulting in the hamburger sign.

adverse prognostic feature in HL and NHL but is much commoner in the latter. However, in approximately 35% of cases of NHL, primary involvement of an extranodal site occurs, with lymph node involvement limited to the regional lymph nodes: stages I–IIE. Primary extranodal HL is extremely rare and rigorous exclusion of disease elsewhere is essential before this diagnosis can be made. The incidence of extranodal involvement in NHL depends on factors such as the age of the patient, the presence of pre-existing immunodeficiency and the pathological subtype of lymphoma. Extranodal disease is commoner in children, (particularly in the gastrointestinal tract, the major abdominal viscera and extranodal locations in the head and neck)[23] and in the immunocompromised host. The high incidence of extranodal involvement in these patient groups is a reflection of the fact that such lymphomas are usually aggressive histological subtypes.

The incidence of extranodal NHL is rising faster than that of nodal NHL. For example, primary lymphomas of the CNS were increasing in frequency at a rate of 10% per annum until the introduction of highly active antiretroviral therapies.[24] Of the various pathological subtypes of NHL, mantle cell (a diffuse B-cell lymphoma), lymphoblastic lymphomas (80% of which are T-cell), BL (small cell non-cleaved) and MALT lymphomas demonstrate a propensity to arise in extranodal sites.

CT generally performs well in the depiction of extranodal disease, though there are certain instances where other techniques are preferable. FDG-PET is more sensitive than CT chiefly because of its ability to identify splenic and bone marrow infiltration[13] (Fig. 70-6). PET or PET/CT can upstage as many as 40% of cases, though the CT component remains essential: for example, in low-grade lymphoma and in the lungs, where small nodules may be below the resolution of PET technology.

Thorax

Pulmonary Parenchymal Involvement

Several categories of lung involvement can be identified including:

- lymphomatous involvement associated with existing or previously treated intrathoracic nodal disease;
- lymphomatous involvement associated with widespread extrathoracic disease;
- primary pulmonary HL; and
- primary pulmonary NHL.

Some authors also separate out AIDS-related lymphoma (ARL) and the post-transplant lymphoproliferative disorder (PTLD),[25] both of which commonly affect the lungs.

Lung involvement at presentation occurs in just under 4% of patients with NHL, but in approximately 12% of patients with HL. It is usually secondary to direct extension of nodal disease into the adjacent parenchyma, hence its paramediastinal or perihilar location. In this circumstance there is no effect on stage; the 'E' lesion. Patients with HL presenting with an intrapulmonary lesion in the absence of demonstrable mediastinal disease are unlikely to have lymphomatous disease of the lung unless there has been previous mediastinal or hilar irradiation, when recurrence may be confined to the lungs. Conversely, in NHL, nodal disease is absent in 50% of those patients with pulmonary or pleural involvement. As nodal disease progresses or relapses, lung involvement becomes commoner in HL and NHL, such that 30–40% of patients with HL have pulmonary involvement at some stage during the course of the disease.

The radiographic appearances are extremely variable, but the commonest pattern is of one or more discrete nodules, with or without cavitation, which tend to be less well defined than those of primary or metastatic carcinoma, which they otherwise resemble (Figs. 70-7 and 70-8).[26] The disease often spreads along lymphatic channels and involves lymphoid follicles around bronchovascular divisions, resulting in peribronchial nodulation spreading out from the hila, which can result in streaky shadowing visible on chest radiographs and at CT (Fig. 70-7).

Less commonly, lymphomatous cells fill the pulmonary acini, producing rounded or segmental areas of consolidation with air bronchograms (Fig. 70-8). Nodulation along the bronchial wall may enable differentiation from infective consolidation. A rare pattern of disease is widespread interstitial reticulonodular shadowing, producing a lymphangitic picture. Another rare manifestation is atelectasis, which usually results from endobronchial lymphoma rather than extrinsic compression by nodal disease.

The differential diagnosis of pulmonary involvement in lymphoma is extensive, and includes drug-induced changes, the effect of radiotherapy, and opportunistic infection during or following chemotherapy, particularly in patients with antecedent immunosuppression. Precise clinical correlation is essential in determining the most likely diagnosis.

Primary Pulmonary Lymphoma

Primary pulmonary lymphoma accounts for less than 1% of all lymphomas and is usually low-grade B-cell NHL, arising from MALT or bronchus-associated lymphoid tissue (BALT). BALT lymphomas tend to occur in the fifth to sixth decades, have an indolent course with 5-year survivals of over 60% and tend to remain extranodal, although lymph node involvement can occur with advanced disease.[27] Many patients will have a prior history of inflammatory or autoimmune disease, such as Sjögren's syndrome, collagen vascular disease and dysgammaglobulinaemia.[28] The imaging findings are non-specific with the single commonest manifestation being a solitary nodule. Multiple nodules, or one or more rounded or segmental areas of consolidation,[29] are also seen. These can persist unchanged for long periods. Pleural effusions are seen in up to 20% of cases.[28]

In the remaining 15–20% of patients, primary lung lymphoma is due to high-grade NHL. The most common finding on a chest radiograph is of a solitary or multiple pulmonary nodules, which characteristically grow rapidly. Chest wall and nodal involvement occurs more frequently than with pulmonary MALT-type lymphomas.[27] Primary pulmonary HL is extremely rare. The most frequently described finding is single or multiple nodules with upper zone predominance and a relatively high incidence of cavitation.

Pleural Disease

Pleural effusions are usually accompanied by mediastinal lymphadenopathy (Fig. 70-9) and may be detected on CT in 50% of patients with mediastinal nodal disease. They are usually exudates secondary to central lymphatic or

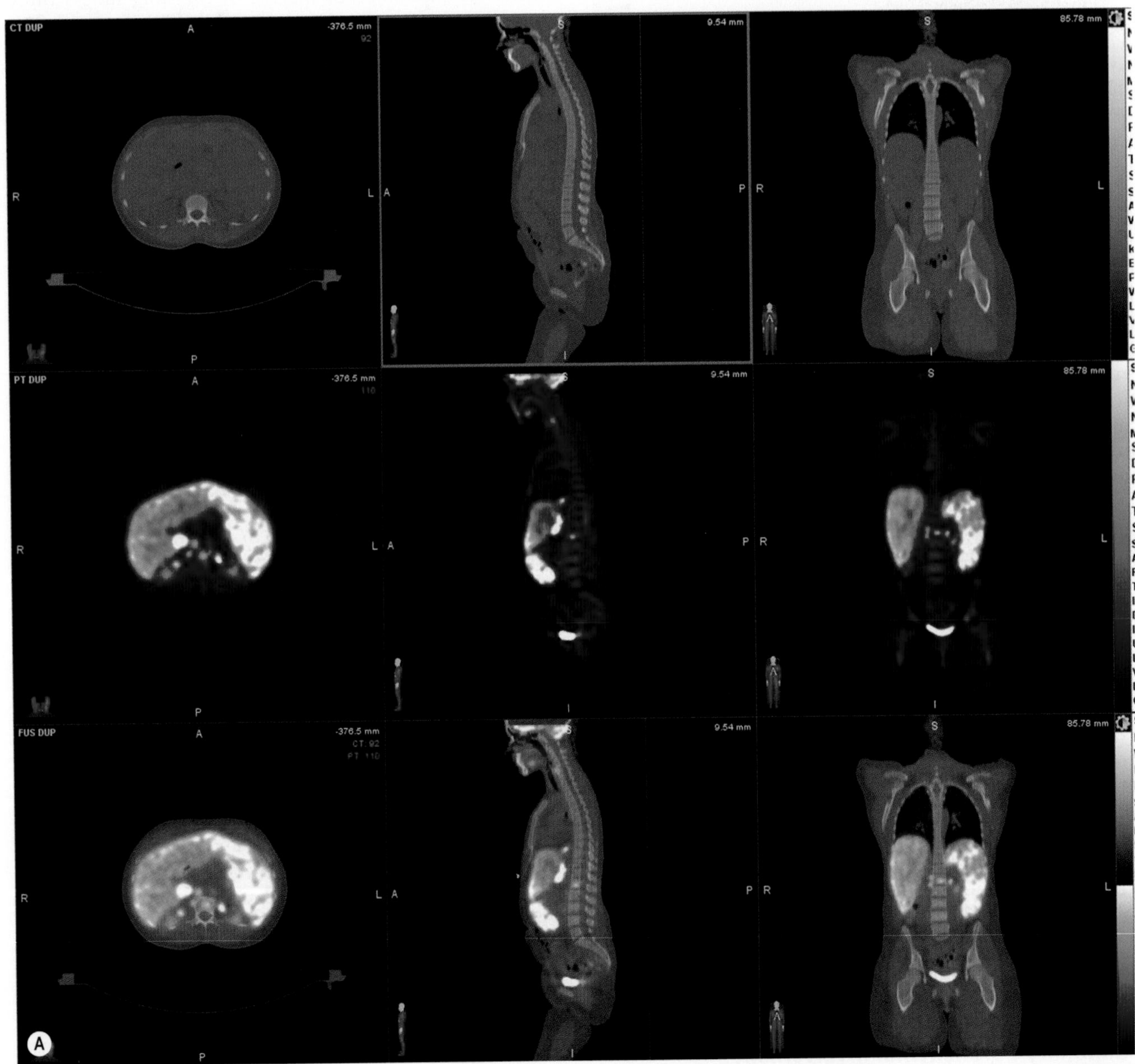

FIGURE 70-6 ■ PET/CT image resulting in upstaging. There is metabolically active disease in lymph nodes above and below the diaphragm with splenomegaly, but the PET/CT also demonstrates disease in the liver and the body of L1, making this stage IV disease.

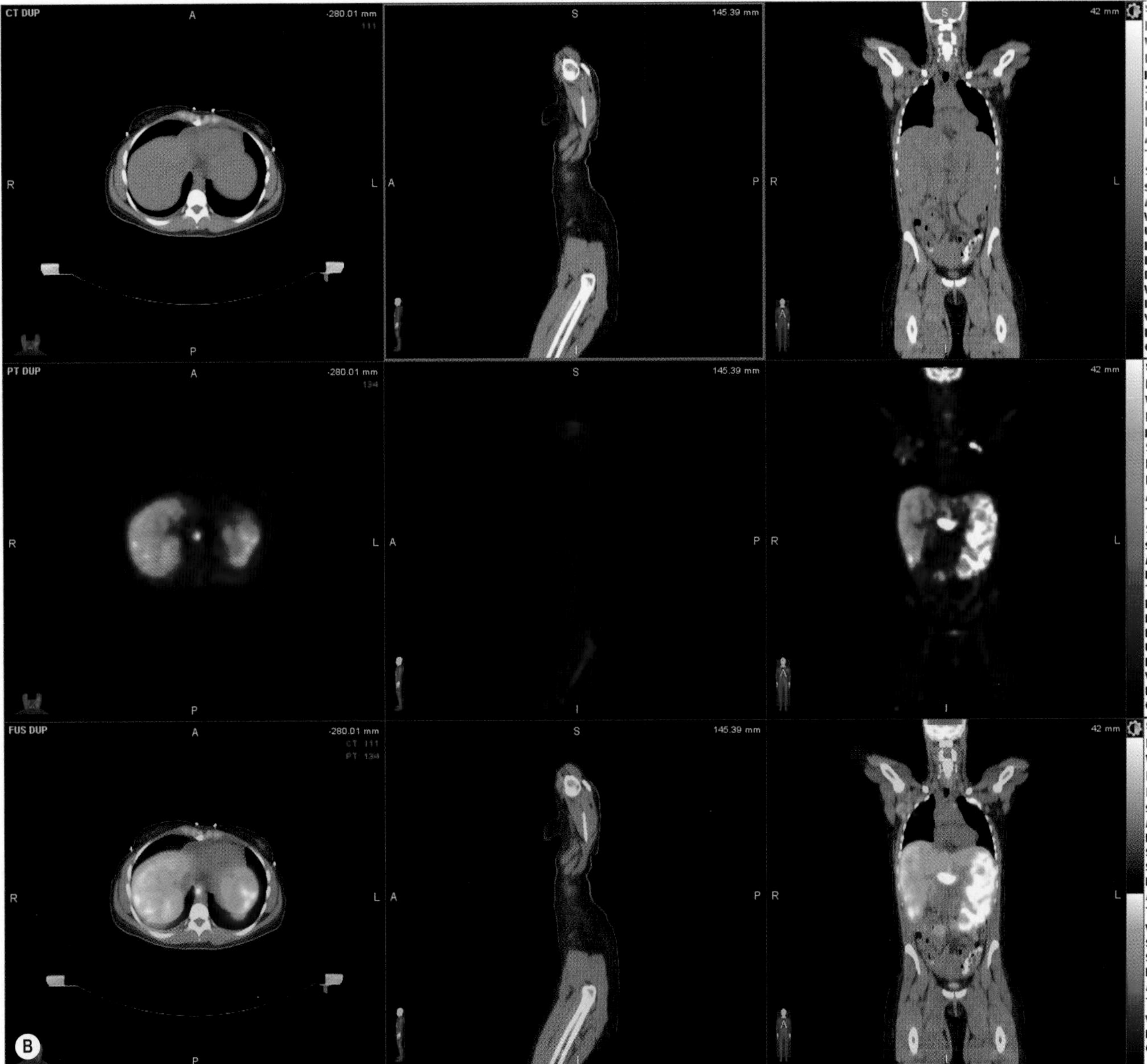

FIGURE 70-6, Continued

venous obstruction and therefore clear promptly with treatment of the mediastinal disease. Pulmonary involvement need not be present. Focal pleural masses do occur at presentation but are more commonly seen in recurrent disease, when they are generally accompanied by an effusion.

Pericardium and Heart

Direct pericardial and cardiac involvement can occur with high-grade peripheral T-cell and large B-cell lymphomas. It is rare at presentation, except in patients with AIDS-related lymphoma (ARL) and PTLD who may present with acute onset of heart block, tamponade, or congestive cardiac failure. Pericardial effusions occur in 6% of patients with HL at the time of presentation and are associated with large masses adjacent to the heart. They are also common in primary mediastinal large B-cell lymphoma (PMBL) (Fig. 70-3B). Effusions are regarded as evidence of pericardial involvement, although this does not alter disease stage. Small pericardial effusions of uncertain aetiology are often seen at CT during treatment. They usually resolve with time, although some pericardial thickening may persist.

Thymus

Thymic involvement by HL in association with mediastinal nodal disease occurs in around 30% of patients at presentation. PMBL characteristically involves the thymus, occurring typically in young women between the ages of 25 and 40 years (Fig. 70-3B). Rapidly growing bulky disease is usual and up to 40% have superior vena caval obstruction, which is rare with other lymphomas.

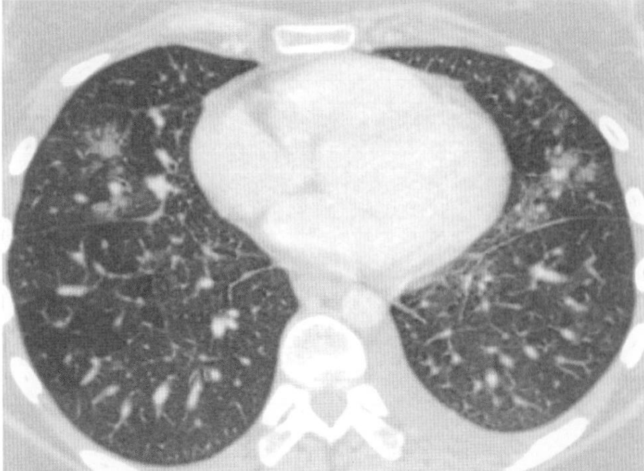

FIGURE 70-7 ■ Pulmonary involvement in a patient with Hodgkin's lymphoma. CT performed at the time of presentation, showing widespread ill-defined intrapulmonary nodular shadowing scattered throughout both lungs with a bronchocentric distribution. Note also the abnormal thickened interlobular septae and patchy ground-glass opacity.

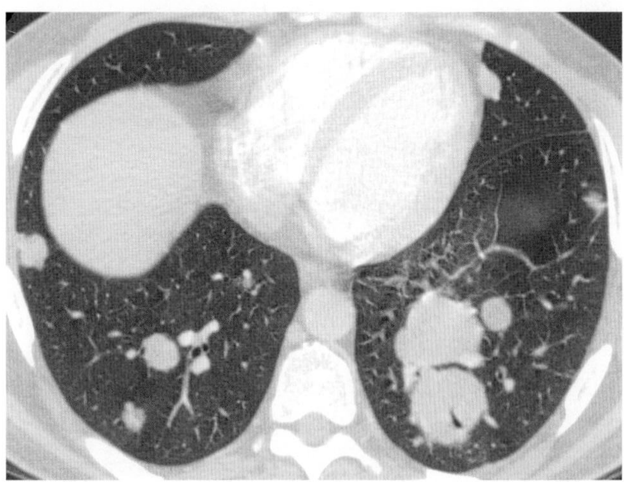

FIGURE 70-8 ■ Lung involvement in recurrent Hodgkin's lymphoma. CT showing multiple rounded nodules: the left lower lobe nodule is beginning to cavitate.

On CT, differentiation of enlarged mediastinal lymph nodes from thymic involvement is often difficult as the thymus involved by lymphoma usually has a homogeneous soft-tissue density or a heterogeneous nodular appearance. On MRI as well, the gland is often of mixed signal intensity similar to that of involved nodes. Nodal masses tend to be more lobulated, whereas thymic involvement is generally diffuse. Cystic change can be recognised at CT and MRI with PMBL and HL. These cysts can persist or even increase in size following regression of the rest of the involved gland with successful treatment. Calcification may be present at the outset or may develop during treatment.[30] Benign thymic rebound hyperplasia can develop after completion of chemotherapy, and can be difficult to differentiate from recurrent disease. Unfortunately, functional imaging with FDG-PET may not always differentiate between the two and clinical correlation combined with follow-up studies may be necessary.

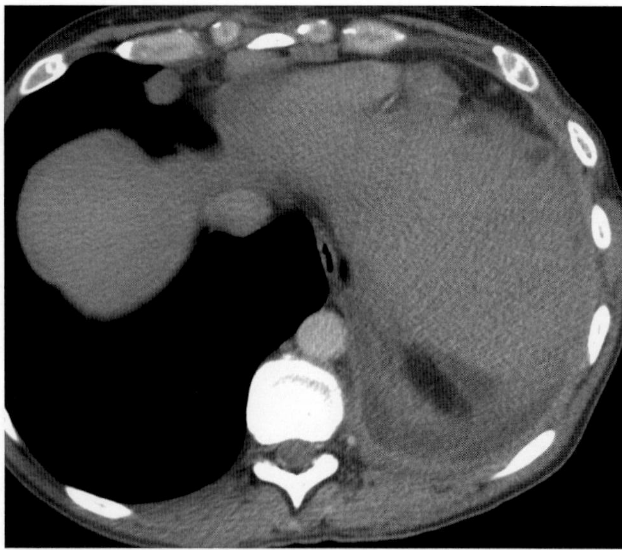

FIGURE 70-9 ■ Pleural disease in lymphoma. CT showing a typical appearance of pleural involvement in a patient with NHL. There is uniform pleural thickening with an accompanying pleural effusion. Note also the right and left paracardiac lymph node enlargement.

Chest Wall

In HL, spread into the chest wall usually occurs by direct infiltration from an anterior mediastinal mass, especially from the internal mammary chain. However, chest wall masses can arise de novo, especially in NHL. Bony destruction is rare and should suggest an alternative diagnosis. Thoracic wall disease is better shown by MRI than CT, particularly on T2-weighted or STIR sequences, where there is excellent contrast between the mass and normal low signal intensity muscle. PET/CT can also demonstrate chest wall involvement and these techniques may facilitates more accurate planning of radiotherapy portals.[31]

Breast

Lymphoma of the breast is usually associated with widespread disease elsewhere. There may be multiple nodules, with associated large-volume adenopathy. Primary NHL of the breast is rare, accounting for approximately 2% of all lymphomas and under 1% of all breast malignancies. The age distribution is bimodal, with the first peak occurring during pregnancy and lactation, often high-grade or Burkitt's lymphoma (BL) and affecting both breasts diffusely with an inflammatory picture at ultrasound and mammography.[32] There is a second peak at around 50 years when patients present with discrete masses which are usually solitary, but multiple masses occur and disease is bilateral in over 10%. The masses are usually fairly well defined, with little accompanying architectural distortion. Calcification has not been described.

Hepatobiliary System and Spleen

Liver

Liver involvement is present in up to 15% of adult patients with NHL at presentation. This figure is higher in the paediatric population and in recurrent disease. In HL, liver involvement occurs in about 5% of patients at presentation, almost invariably in association with splenic HL. Pathologically, diffuse microscopic infiltration around the portal tracts is the most common form of involvement. CT and MRI are therefore insensitive in the detection of liver involvement. However, hepatomegaly strongly suggests the presence of diffuse infiltration (in contradistinction to the significance of splenomegaly). Larger focal areas of infiltration are present in only 5–10% of patients with hepatic lymphoma. Cross-sectional imaging may demonstrate miliary nodules or larger solitary or multiple masses, resembling metastases (Fig. 70-10) and with entirely non-specific features on all forms of cross-sectional imaging. At MRI, as with metastases, deposits have moderate T2 hyperintensity. Superparamagnetic iron oxide particles and hepatocyte-specific contrast agents can increase the conspicuity of focal deposits. Occasionally, especially in children, periportal infiltration is manifest as periportal low-attenuation tissue at CT (Fig. 70-11).

True primary hepatic lymphoma, indistinguishable radiologically from hepatocellular carcinoma, is rare but the incidence is rising, up to 25% of affected patients being hepatitis B or C positive. Non-Hodgkin's lymphoma of the bile ducts and gallbladder is rare but occurs with relatively high frequency in patients with ARL.

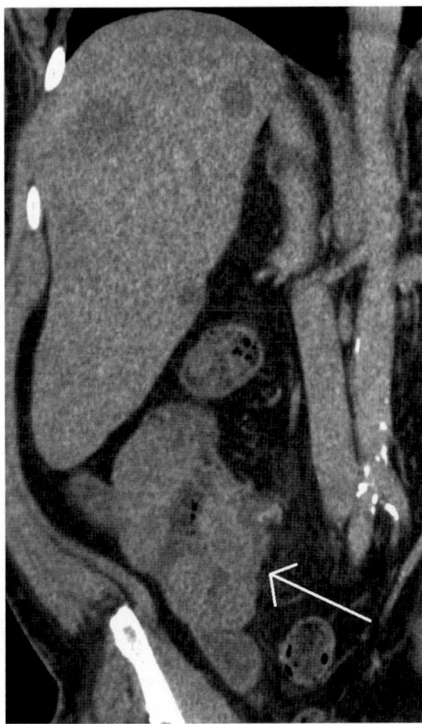

FIGURE 70-10 ■ Lymphomatous infiltration of the liver. There are multiple poorly defined low-density lesions in the liver in this patient with T-cell NHL of the small bowel (arrowed).

Spleen

The spleen is involved in 30–40% of patients with HL at the time of presentation, usually in the presence of nodal disease above and below the diaphragm (stage III), but in a small proportion it is the sole focus of intra-abdominal disease (designated stage IIIS). In the majority of patients, the involvement is microscopic and diffuse and thus particularly difficult to identify on cross-sectional imaging. Splenomegaly is an unreliable sign of involvement; 33% of patients have splenomegaly without infiltration and, conversely, 33% of normal-sized spleens are found to contain tumour following splenectomy. Measurements of splenic volume and splenic indices are not generally utilised.

Focal splenic deposits occur in only 10–25% of cases and may be demonstrated by any form of cross-sectional imaging when they are more than 1 cm in diameter (Fig. 70-4B). Up to 40% of patients with NHL have splenic involvement at some stage. Imaging findings include a

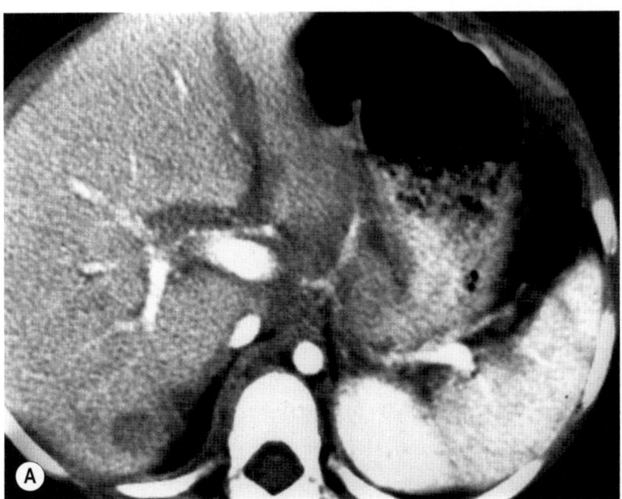

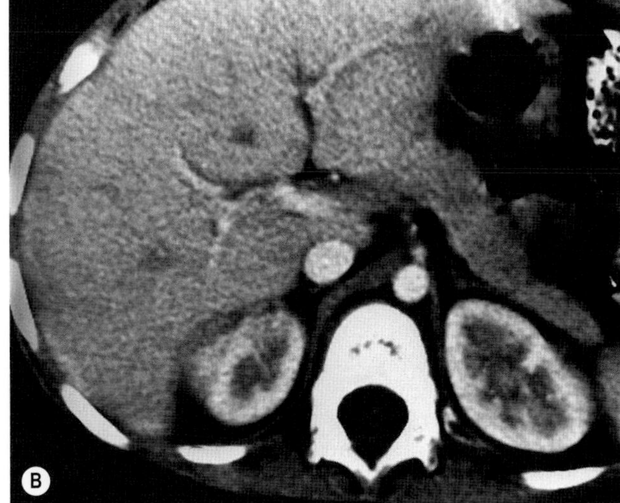

FIGURE 70-11 ■ Periportal lymphoma. (A) Contrast-enhanced CT in a child with NHL, showing infiltration of low-density lymphomatous tissue from the porta hepatis, encasing the main portal vein, extending alongside the right portal vein. A solitary focal abnormality is seen posteriorly within the liver. (B) Follow-up after chemotherapy shows complete resolution of the disease.

solitary mass, miliary nodules or multiple masses, all of which have a non-specific appearance. The differential diagnosis of multiple masses includes opportunistic infection and granulomatous disease.

In early studies, the sensitivity of ultrasound and CT for the detection of splenic involvement was extremely low (about 35%). Detection of small nodules has improved with the advent of contrast-enhanced multidetector CT (MDCT) with optimisation of splenic parenchymal opacification. MRI with superparamagnetic iron oxide may improve diagnostic accuracy but is seldom undertaken outside the research arena. However, FDG-PET can detect splenic disease more accurately than either CT or gallium scintigraphy.[33] In the past, the poor sensitivity of imaging for the detection of splenic involvement in HL necessitated staging laparotomy with splenectomy, but the development of effective combination chemotherapy with good salvage regimens has led to this practice being abandoned.

Primary splenic NHL is rare, accounting for 1% of all patients with NHL. Patients present with splenomegaly, often marked and focal masses are usual. Splenic involvement is also a particular feature of certain other pathological subtypes of NHL, such as mantle cell lymphoma and splenic marginal zone lymphoma. Infarction is a well-recognised complication.

Gastrointestinal Tract

The gastrointestinal (GI) tract is the commonest site of primary extranodal NHL, accounting for 30–45% of all extranodal presentations and constituting about 1% of all GI tumours. It is the initial site of lymphomatous involvement in up to 10% of all adult patients and up to 30% of children.[23] As elsewhere, primary HL of the gastrointestinal tract is most unusual. Secondary involvement of the gastrointestinal tract via direct extension from involved mesenteric or retroperitoneal lymph nodes is extremely common, and consequently multiple sites of involvement occur.

Primary lymphomas arise from lymphoid tissue of the lamina propria and the submucosa of the bowel wall and occur most frequently below the age of 10 years (usually BL) and in the sixth decade (MALT type and enteropathy-associated T-cell type). Primary gastrointestinal lymphoma is usually unifocal.

Accepted criteria for the diagnosis of primary disease include:

- No superficial or intrathoracic lymph node enlargement
- No involvement of the liver or spleen
- A normal white cell count
- No more than local regional lymph node enlargement.

In both primary and secondary cases, the stomach is most frequently involved (50%), followed by the small bowel (35%) and large bowel (15%).

Stomach

Primary lymphoma accounts for about 2–5% of all gastric tumours.[34] It originates in the submucosa, affecting the antrum more commonly than the body or cardia. Radiologically the appearances reflect the gross pathological findings; common appearances are multiple nodules, some with central ulceration, or a large fungating lesion with or without ulceration. About a third of patients have diffuse infiltration, with marked thickening of the wall and narrowing of the lumen, sometimes with extension into the duodenum, indistinguishable from linitis plastica. Only about 10% are characterised by diffuse enlargement of the gastric folds, similar to the pattern seen in hypertrophic gastritis (Fig. 70-12).

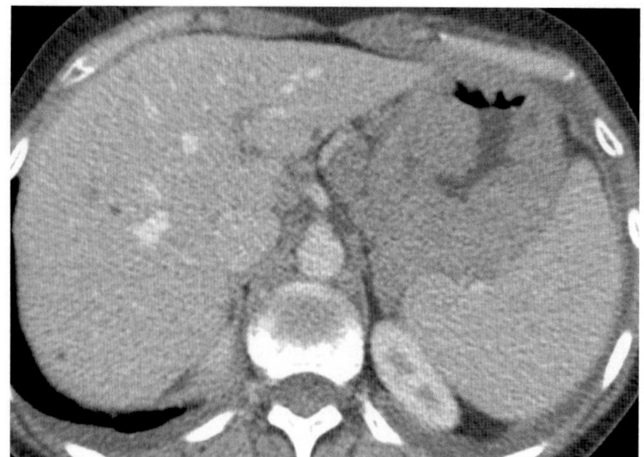

FIGURE 70-12 ■ **Gastric lymphoma.** Axial contrast-enhanced CT showing gross gastric mural and rugal thickening with adjacent enlarged gastrohepatic lymph node.

As the disease originates in the submucosa, the signs described above are best demonstrated on barium studies or endoscopically, but CT better reflects the true extent of gastric wall thickening and accompanying nodal involvement. Typically, infiltration of adjacent organs is unusual but it may occur in DLBCL. In gastric MALT lymphomas, mural thickening may be minimal; CT is of limited value even with dedicated studies, and endoscopic ultrasound with biopsy is more useful in staging, prognostication and assessment of response (Fig. 70-13). Low-grade MALT lymphoma is more likely to cause shallow ulceration and nodulation, whereas high-grade lymphoma can produce more massive gastric infiltration and polypoid masses (Fig. 70-11).

Small Bowel

Lymphoma accounts for up to 50% of all primary tumours of the small bowel, occurring most frequently in the terminal ileum, and becoming progressively less frequent proximally; duodenal lymphomas are rare (Fig. 70-14). In children, the disease is almost exclusively ileocaecal. Most bowel lymphomas are of B-cell lineage. The disease is multifocal in up to 50% of cases; mural thickening with constriction of bowel segments is typical. Patients commonly present with obstructive symptoms. Bowel wall thickening is well demonstrated on CT (Figs. 70-10 and 70-15). With progressive tumour spread through the submucosa and muscularis mucosa, aneurysmal dilatation of long segments of bowel can develop, presumably due

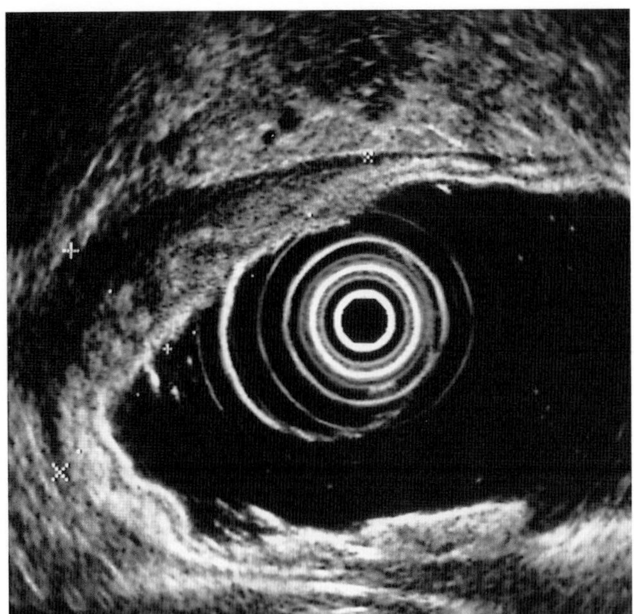

FIGURE 70-13 ■ MALT lymphoma. Endoscopic ultrasound showing a narrow sheet of low echogenic tissue in the submucosa (arrowed). (Image courtesy of Dr A. McLean, Department of Diagnostic Imaging, St Bartholomew's Hospital, London.)

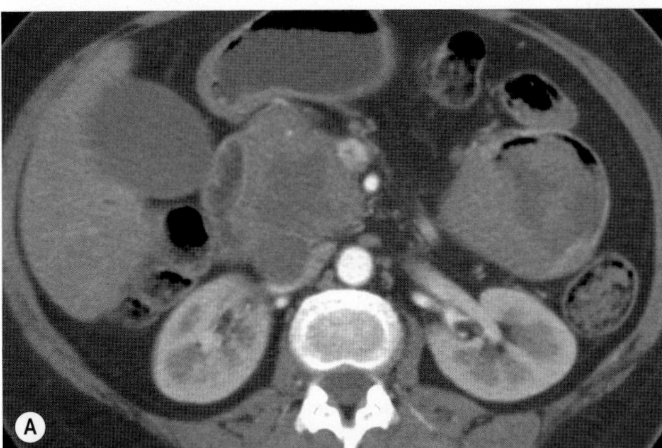

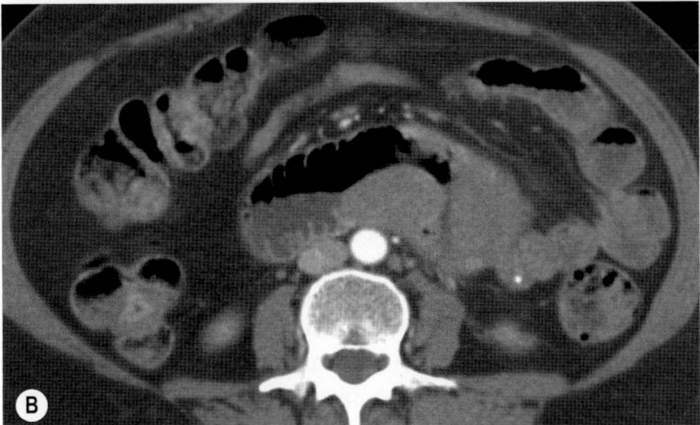

FIGURE 70-14 ■ Burkitt's lymphoma involving the duodenum. (A, B) There is a large mass in the head of the pancreas and the wall of the second part of the duodenum, causing obstruction of the common bile duct posteriorly, with involvement of the fourth part of the duodenum. (B) Disease involving the third part of the duodenum.

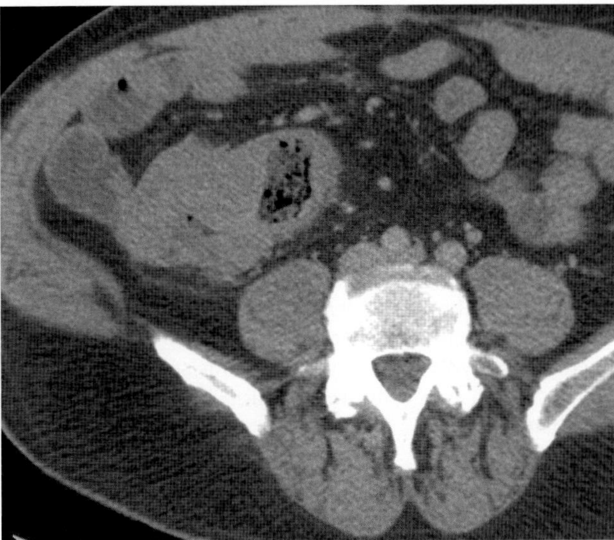

FIGURE 70-15 ■ Involvement of large bowel in non-Hodgkin's lymphoma. CT showing marked and extensive diffuse thickening of the wall of the caecum and ascending colon.

to infiltration of the autonomic plexus. Alternating areas of dilatation and constriction are a common manifestation of infiltration and are well demonstrated by CT.

If lymphomatous infiltration is predominantly submucosal, multiple nodules or polyps of varying size result, mostly in the terminal ileum. It is this form of lymphoma that typically causes intussusception, usually in the ileocaecal region. Lymphoma is the commonest cause of intussusception in children older than 6 years.

Enteropathy-associated T-cell lymphoma and immunoproliferative small intestinal disease (alpha-chain disease) commonly present with clinical and imaging features of malabsorption, but acute presentations with perforation are common. Often the whole small intestine is affected, especially the duodenum and jejunum. In the small bowel (and colon), MALT lymphoma is manifest as mucosal nodularity, which can be appreciated in barium studies. Secondary invasion of the small bowel is commonly seen when large mesenteric lymph node masses cause displacement, encasement or compression of the bowel. Peritoneal disease identical to that seen with ovarian carcinoma generally occurs late in advanced disease, although it may be seen at presentation in BL.

Colon and Rectum

Primary colonic lymphomas are usually of Burkitt's or MALT subtypes, but account for under 0.1% of all colonic neoplasms, most arising in the caecum and rectum (Fig. 70-15). The most common pattern of disease is a diffuse or segmental distribution of small nodules 0.2–2.0 cm in diameter, typically with intact mucosa. A less common form of the disease is a solitary polypoid mass, often in the caecum, indistinguishable from carcinoma on imaging unless there is concomitant involvement of the terminal ileum.

In advanced disease, there may be marked thickening of the colonic or rectal folds, resulting in focal strictures, fissures or ulcerative masses with fistulation. Lymphomatous strictures are generally longer than carcinomatous strictures and irregular excavation of the mass strongly suggests lymphoma. Involvement of the anorectum is a feature of ARL. Patients usually present with obstruction and rectal bleeding.

Oesophagus

Involvement of the oesophagus is extremely unusual and begins as a submucosal lesion, usually in the distal third of the oesophagus. Ulceration is a later phenomonem. Secondary involvement by contiguous spread from adjacent nodal disease is more common but rarely results in dysphagia.

Pancreas

Primary pancreatic lymphoma accounts for only 1.3% of all pancreatic malignancies and 2% of patients with NHL. It usually presents with a solitary mass, often in the head of the pancreas, indistinguishable from primary adenocarcinoma on US, CT, or MRI.[35] Biliary or pancreatic ductal obstruction can occur (Fig. 70-14). Calcification and necrosis are rare. Less commonly, diffuse uniform enlargement of the pancreas is seen. Involvement is far more common in NHL than in HL. Secondary pancreatic involvement usually results from direct infiltration from adjacent nodal masses, either focal or massive.

Genitourinary Tract

The genitourinary tract is not commonly involved at the time of presentation (<5%); however, >50% of patients will have involvement of some part of the genitourinary tract at autopsy. The testicle is the most commonly involved organ, followed by the kidney and the perirenal space; only rarely are the bladder, prostate, uterus, vagina or ovaries involved. True primary genitourinary lymphoma is rare, as there is normally very little lymphoid tissue within the genitourinary tract.

Kidneys

CT is sensitive in the diagnosis of lymphomatous renal masses, but since renal involvement is generally a late phenomenon, renal involvement is identified in only around 3% of patients undergoing staging CT. Close to 90% of cases are associated with high-grade NHL and detection of renal involvement rarely alters the disease stage. In over 40% of patients the disease occurs at the time of recurrence only and renal function is usually normal.[36]

The commonest pattern of disease, seen in 60%, is multiple masses (Fig. 70-16). On CT, the masses may show a typical 'density reversal pattern' before and after administration of contrast medium, lesions being more dense than the surrounding parenchyma before contrast medium administration and less dense after. A solitary renal mass is seen in only 5–15% of cases and may be indistinguishable from renal cell carcinoma (Fig. 70-17).[36]

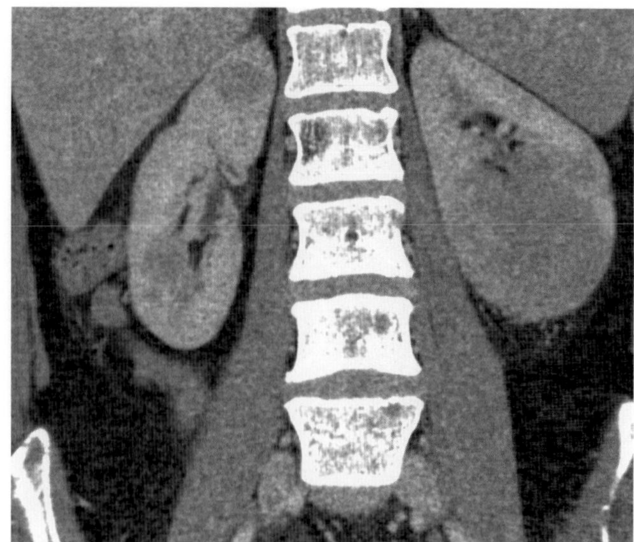

FIGURE 70-16 ■ Multiple lymphomatous renal masses. Coronal reformatted CT showing multiple masses, hypodense compared with the normally enhancing adjacent renal parenchyma. There are also multiple lytic bone lesions in this patient with NHL.

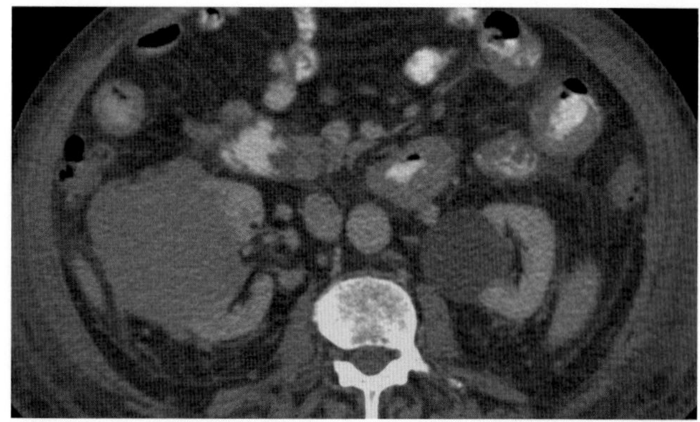

FIGURE 70-17 ■ Renal lymphomatous mass. A large right renal mass extends into the perinephric space on contrast-enhanced CT in a patient with NHL. There is also a lymphomatous mass in the left perinephric space; multiple peritoneal and retroperitoneal nodules; mesenteric nodal disease and extensive small bowel involvement.

Importantly, in over 50% of lymphomatous renal masses, there is no accompanying retroperitoneal lymph node enlargement on CT.

Direct infiltration of the kidney by contiguous retroperitoneal nodal masses is the second most common type of renal involvement, occurring in 25% of cases. Associated encasement of the renal vessels and extension into the renal hilum and sinus is common and radiologically this pattern can closely resemble transitional cell carcinoma of the renal pelvis. In a further 10%, soft-tissue mass(es) are seen in the perirenal space, occasionally encasing the kidney without any evidence of invasion of the parenchyma (Fig. 70-17).

Diffuse intrinsic infiltration of the kidney resulting in global enlargement is the least common manifestation of renal lymphomatous involvement. This pattern can occur with high-grade and paediatric lymphomas such as BL.

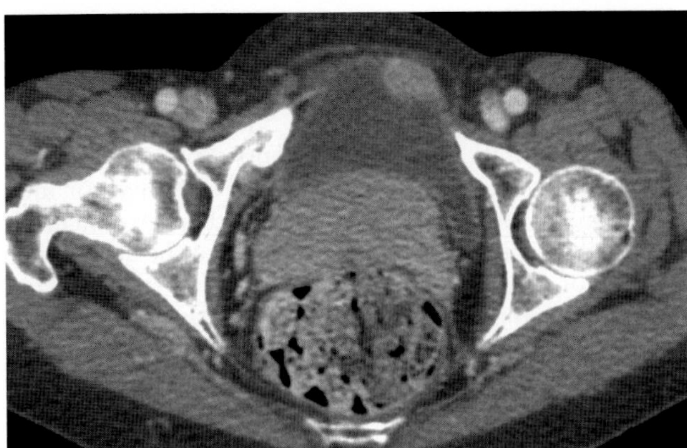

FIGURE 70-18 ■ **Bladder lymphoma.** Contrast-enhanced CT of the pelvis in a female patient showing a polypoid soft-tissue mass arising from the wall of the bladder. There is involvement of the vagina.

On ultrasound, the kidneys are diffusely enlarged and uniformly hypoechoic. On CT, the appearance following intravenous injection of contrast medium is variable, but usually the normal parenchymal enhancement is replaced by homogeneous non-enhancing tissue.

Bladder

The urinary bladder is a rare site of primary extranodal involvement, accounting for less than 1% of all bladder tumours.[37] Small cell and MALT types are seen, the latter often in middle-aged women with a history of recurrent cystitis. Large multilobular submucosal masses with minimal or no mucosal ulceration are typical (Fig. 70-18). Transmural spread into adjacent pelvic organs can occur and is well demonstrated on cross-sectional imaging. The prognosis is generally good. Secondary lymphoma of the bladder is found in 10–15% of patients with lymphoma at autopsy, resulting from contiguous spread from adjacent involved pelvic lymph nodes. Microscopic involvement is far more common than gross infiltration, but both can be associated with haematuria. On CT the appearances are usually non-specific and indistinguishable from transitional cell carcinoma, producing either diffuse widespread thickening of the bladder wall or a large nodular mass.

Prostate

Primary prostatic lymphoma is also extremely rare, but in contradistinction to primary bladder NHL it carries a very poor prognosis. It is generally intermediate-to-high grade and histological examination usually shows diffuse infiltration with spread into the periprostatic tissues. More frequently, prostatic involvement is secondary to spread from the adjacent nodes in the setting of advanced disease.

Testis

Testicular lymphoma accounts for about 5% of primary testicular tumours overall and is the commonest primary tumour in patients over the age of 60 years. It is vanishingly rare in HL but is seen at presentation in approximately 1% of all patients of NHL, usually with DLBCL or BL. There is an association with lymphoma of Waldeyer's ring, the skin and central nervous system. Patients usually present with a painless testicular swelling and in up to 25% of cases the involvement is bilateral. Relapse can occur in the contralateral testis. Ultrasonically, the lesions usually have a non-specific appearance, with focal areas of decreased echogenicity, or a more diffuse decrease in reflectivity of the testicle without any focal abnormality. Because of the association with disease elsewhere, staging must always include ultrasonic evaluation of the contralateral testis and whole-body cross-sectional imaging. Cranial CT or MRI, and CSF examination should also be considered.

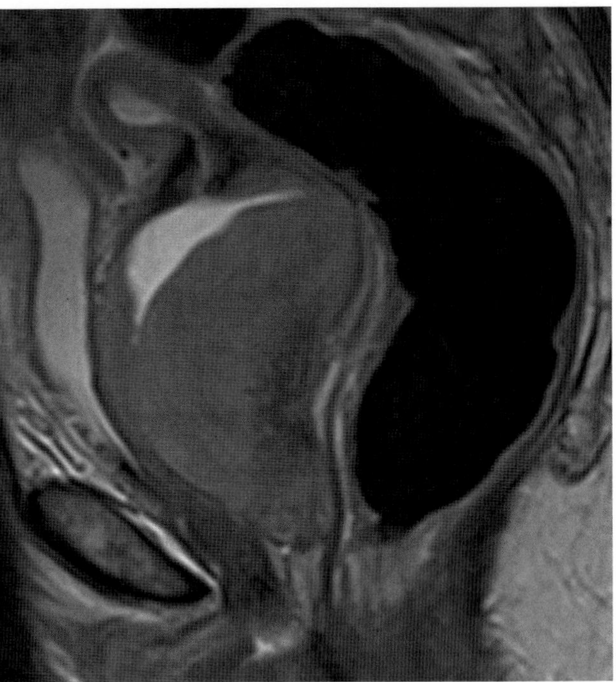

FIGURE 70-19 ■ **Lymphoma involving the vagina.** Sagittal T2-weighted MRI of the patient described in the legend to Fig. 70-18 demonstrates a large intermediate-to-high signal intensity mass, substantially larger than seen usually in a squamous carcinoma of the cervix. Biopsy showed an aggressive B-cell lymphoma.

Female Genital Tract

Isolated lymphomatous involvement of the female genital organs is rare, accounting for approximately 1% of extranodal NHL. Nearly 75% of women affected are postmenopausal and present with vaginal bleeding. The cervix is affected more frequently than the uterus and vagina. Involvement of the gynaecological tract is best demonstrated by MRI, where primary lymphoma of the cervix and/or vagina is characterised by a large soft-tissue mass with homogeneous intermediate-to-high T2 signal intensity (Fig. 70-19).[38] Involvement of the uterine body usually produces diffuse enlargement, often with a lobular contour similar to a fibroid. Characteristically,

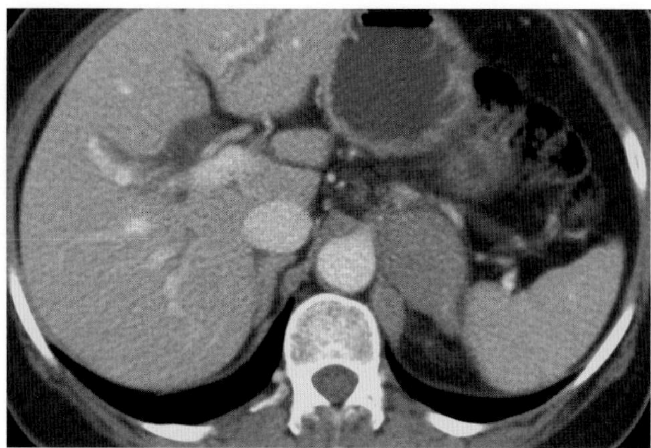

FIGURE 70-20 ■ **Adrenal lymphoma.** Contrast-enhanced CT showing a large homogeneous left adrenal mass. Note biliary obstruction which was secondary to a mass in the duodenum and head of the pancreas (same patient as that described in the legend to Fig. 70-14).

the mucosa and underlying junctional zone are intact. Primary uterine lymphoma has a good prognosis and MRI can demonstrate complete resolution after treatment. Primary ovarian lymphoma, by contrast, has a very poor prognosis as it often presents late and disease is frequently bilateral. It is less common than uterine lymphoma. The usual pathological subtypes are DLBCL or BL. Imaging appearances are identical to those of ovarian carcinoma, although haemorrhage, necrosis and calcification are relatively rare.

Adrenal Glands

Primary adrenal lymphoma is extremely rare, usually occurring in men over the age of 60. Secondary involvement of the adrenals is detected in about 6% of patients undergoing routine abdominal staging CT, usually in the presence of widespread retroperitoneal disease. Adrenal insufficiency is unusual, even with bilateral disease. The appearance on cross-sectional imaging is indistinguishable from that of metastases (Fig. 70-20). Bilateral adrenal hyperplasia in the absence of metastatic involvement is also recognised.[39]

Musculoskeletal System

Involvement of the bone, bone marrow and skeletal muscles can occur in both HL and NHL. Bone and bone marrow are particularly important sites of disease relapse and any skeletal symptoms following previous treatment for lymphoma should always raise the suspicion of bone disease. Involvement of osseous bone does not necessarily imply bone marrow involvement and the two have different prognostic implications. Neither skeletal radiography nor isotope bone imaging have any predictive value in determining marrow involvement.

Bone Marrow

Since the bone marrow is an integral part of the reticuloendothelial system, lymphoma may arise within the marrow as true primary disease, which is then categorised as stage IE disease. More often, however, the marrow is involved as part of a disseminated process, when it is categorised as stage IV disease. In NHL, marrow involvement is present in 20–40% of patients at presentation and is associated with a poorer prognosis than liver or lung involvement. Bone marrow biopsy is therefore included in the staging of NHL and will increase the stage in up to 30% of cases, usually from stage III to stage IV.[40] In FL infiltration is often paratrabecular rather than diffuse, whereas in high-grade NHL the marrow is more likely to be affected focally; hence the increased incidence of marrow positivity with bilateral iliac crest biopsies. In HL, marrow involvement at presentation is rare but will develop during the course of the disease in 5–15% of patients. Bone marrow biopsy, therefore, is not considered necessary as part of the initial staging of patients with clinical early-stage HL.

Magnetic resonance imaging is extremely sensitive in detecting bone marrow involvement, involved areas having low signal intensity on T1-weighted images and high signal on STIR sequences; T1-weighted sequences are the most sensitive.[41] It can upstage as many as 30% of patients with negative iliac crest biopsies and a positive MRI study appears to confer a poorer prognosis regardless of bone marrow biopsy status. Whole-body diffusion-weighted imaging with background suppression (DWIBS) can be used to stage and monitor treatment,[11] though limited availability has precluded widespread adoption of this technique in the UK.

FDG-PET is moderately sensitive for bone marrow involvement at presentation,[42] upstaging a similar proportion of patients as MRI when compared to bone marrow biopsy. However, as with MRI, false-negative studies occur especially with microscopic infiltration (under 5%) and low-grade lymphoma which is FDG-PET negative elsewhere.[43] On the other hand, diffuse or heterogeneously increased uptake in a pretreatment image may indicate reactive marrow hyperplasia rather than infiltration. FDG-PET/CT can also be used to assess treatment response, though reactive marrow hyperplasia can limit specificity, especially where granulocyte colony stimulating factors have been administered. Neither MRI nor FDG-PET can replace histological examination of the bone marrow, firstly because of their relatively low negative predictive value (NPV) and secondly because composite lymphomas are not infrequent.

Bone

True primary lymphoma of bone is nearly all NHL and accounts for almost 1% of all NHL and 5% of extranodal lymphoma. The criteria for the diagnosis of primary lymphoma of bone require that:

- only a single bone is involved;
- there is unequivocal histological evidence of lymphoma;
- other disease is limited to regional areas at the time of presentation; and
- the primary tumour precedes metastases by at least 6 months.

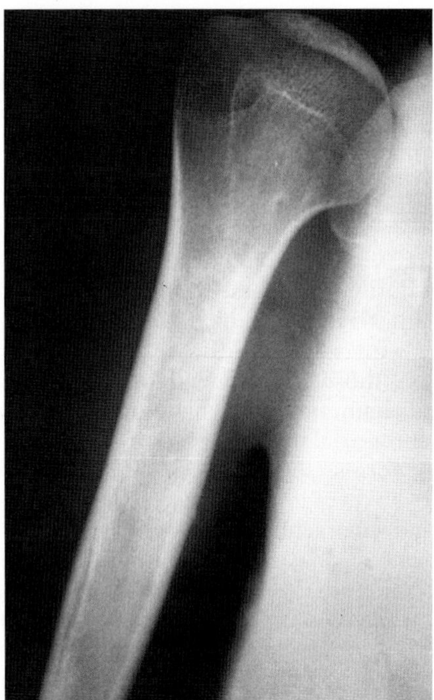

FIGURE 70-21 ■ Primary non-Hodgkin's lymphoma of bone. Plain radiograph of the humerus of a 14-year-old child showing a poorly defined sclerotic lesion in the proximal humerus. Further investigation revealed no other sites of lymphomatous disease.

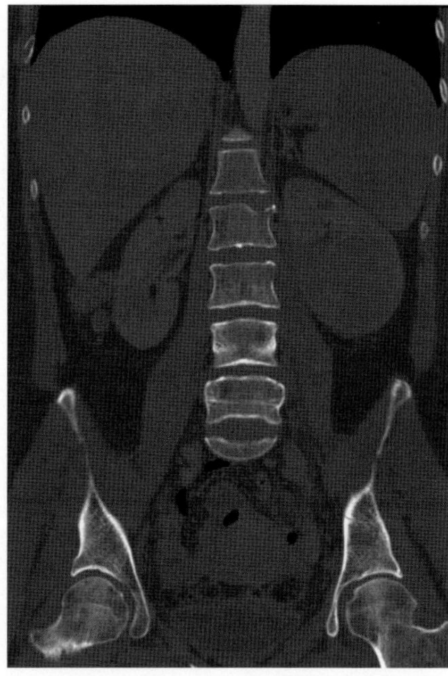

FIGURE 70-22 ■ Non-Hodgkin's lymphoma of bone. Coronal CT on bone settings (same patient as that described in the legend to Fig. 70-16) showing multiple lytic lesions throughout the visualised skeleton with pathological fractures in a right rib, L2 and the right iliac blade.

The diagnosis of true primary bone lymphoma is made less often than in the past, probably because better imaging has allowed detection of synchronous disease elsewhere, indicating that the apparent 'primary' osseous involvement is in fact secondary. This is particularly the case in children. The median age at presentation is 40–50 years with a slight male predominance and usually occurs in the pelvis or appendicular skeleton, involving the femur, tibia and humerus in descending order of frequency.[44]

Infiltration of bone can also occur secondarily by direct invasion from adjacent soft-tissue masses. Radiographic evidence of secondary bone involvement is present during the course of the disease in 20% of patients with HL, appearing in 4% at initial presentation. Secondary involvement of bone is present in 5–6% of patients with NHL, although it is more frequent in children with NHL.[23] The axial skeleton is much more commonly affected than the appendicular skeleton.

Whether primary or secondary, bone lesions in NHL are permeative and osteolytic in just under 80% of cases, sclerotic in only 4% and mixed in 16% (Fig. 70-21).[45] By comparison, HL typically gives sclerotic or mixed sclerotic and lytic lesions (86%) and is far less frequently lytic (14% of cases). In HL, most lesions are found in the skull, the spine and the femora. The classic finding is the sclerotic 'ivory' vertebra. Nevertheless, radiographically, primary and secondary NHL, HL and other bone tumours (such as Ewing's sarcoma and other small round cell tumours) may be indistinguishable. Soft-tissue disease typically may involve adjacent bones; anterior mediastinal and paravertebral masses not infrequently involve the sternum and vertebrae, respectively, resulting in scalloping or destruction.

CT will often demonstrate bony disease if there is a prominent lytic or sclerotic process (Fig. 70-22). Screening for bone involvement is reserved for patients with specific complaints. Radionuclide radiology has a sensitivity of close to 95% in the detection of bone involvement, but is of limited value compared with FDG-PET or PET/CT. MRI depicts primary bone lymphoma in exquisite anatomical detail (Fig. 70-23), and is the method of choice in local staging of primary bone lymphoma,[46] often demonstrating a greater extent of associated extra-osseous involvement and degree of marrow infiltration. It is also of value in the assessment of response to treatment, but there is some evidence that FDG-PET can demonstrate response to treatment earlier and more accurately than conventional techniques including MRI.[47]

Central Nervous System

Primary

Primary CNS lymphoma (PCNSL) is restricted to the cranio-spinal axis, with no evidence of systemic disease and is nearly always intracranial. It increased dramatically in incidence in the 1990s, and accounts for over 3% of all primary brain tumours and up to nearly 30% of cases of NHL in some series. The increase in younger adults can be explained by the association with AIDS and iatrogenic immunosuppression and until the advent of highly active antiretroviral therapy up to 6% of patients with AIDS could be expected to develop PCNSL during the course of the disease. However, the incidence is also rising steadily in the over 60 year olds, for reasons

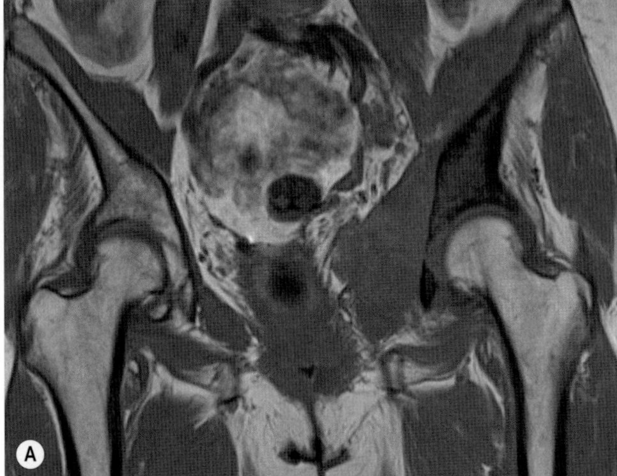

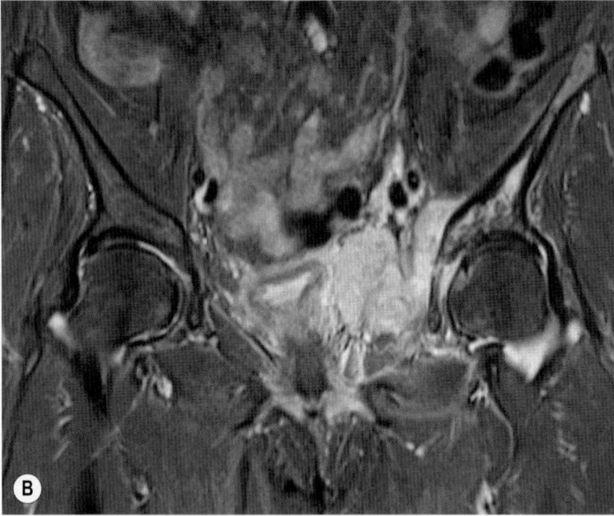

FIGURE 70-23 ■ Non-Hodgkin's lymphoma of bone. Coronal T1-weighted (A) and STIR (B) images of a patient with NHL of the left hemipelvis involving the adjacent obturator internus muscle and bladder. There is extensive involvement of the left hemipelvis manifest as low T1 and high T2 signal. Note exquisite depiction of the extent of bony and soft-tissue involvement with this combination of sequences.

unknown. Peak incidence is in the fifth and sixth decades. Presentation is that of an intracranial space-occupying lesion or personality changes, as the lesions are often frontal.[48] Fits are rare, but are reported.

More than 50% of tumours occur within the cerebral white matter, close to or within the corpus callosum[49] and often abutting the ependyma. A butterfly distribution with spread across the corpus callosum is a typical finding. The deep grey matter of the thalamus and basal ganglia is affected in about 15% (Fig. 70-24). Only approximately 10% arise in the posterior fossa, usually near the midline. In about 15% of cases the disease is multifocal, though the incidence of multifocality is much higher in AIDS-related PCNSL.

Up to 70% of tumour masses are typically isodense or hyperdense on unenhanced CT and in 90% of cases, enhance homogeneously[49] (Fig. 70-24). Calcification virtually never occurs and there is relatively little surrounding vasogenic oedema or mass effect.[50] On MRI, the masses are typically isointense on T1- and T2-weighted sequences. As at CT, there is homogeneous enhancement after the administration of gadolinium-DTPA (Fig. 70-23), though atypical forms with rim enhancement can occur with AIDS-related PCNSL.[51]

Secondary

Secondary CNS involvement is exceptionally rare in HL but occurs during the course of the disease in 10–15% of patients with NHL. Certain groups are known to be at risk: those with stage IV disease, testicular or ovarian presentation; those with high-grade histology (lymphoblastic and immunoblastic histologies) and also BL. Although intra-axial masses do occur, appearing identical to primary forms, secondary involvement much more commonly involves the extracerebral spaces (epidural, subdural and subarachnoid) as well as the spinal epidural and subarachnoid spaces. Presentation with cranial nerve palsies is common. MRI with intravenous injection of gadolinium-based contrast medium is superior to CT in the detection of such subdural and leptomeningeal disease, which is seen as enhancing plaques over the cerebral convexities and around the basal meninges.[52]

Contrast-enhanced MRI can also demonstrate spinal leptomeningeal disease, but there is a significant false-negative rate, higher than that for leptomeningeal carcinomatosis.[53] Disease in the spinal epidural space can cause spinal cord compression and cauda equina syndromes. This is a late manifestation of HL, but can be the presenting feature of NHL (Fig. 70-25). Epidural extension of tumour into the spinal canal from a paravertebral mass is the commonest cause, resulting in a so-called 'dumb-bell' tumour. The dura itself usually acts as an effective barrier to the intrathecal spread of tumour, and disease may be limited to the neural foramen. Less commonly, vertebral involvement results in epidural spread and extrinsic compression of the theca. Though all these patterns of epidural spread can occasionally be depicted at CT, subtle disease is readily missed unless actively sought and is much better demonstrated by MRI.

Orbit

Primary orbital lymphomas are nearly all NHL, which constitutes the most common primary orbital malignancy in adults, accounting for 10–15% of orbital masses and 4% of all primary extranodal NHL. They occur most commonly in patients between 40 and 70 years of age and typically present as a slow-growing, diffusely infiltrative tumour for which the main differential diagnosis is from the non-malignant condition, orbital pseudotumour. Secondary orbital involvement occurs in approximately 3.5–5.0% of both HL and NHL. Any component of the orbit can be involved and in both the primary and secondary forms, the clinical manifestations will depend on the site of involvement. Retrobulbar lymphoma infiltrates around and through the extraocular muscles, causing proptosis and ophthalmoplegia, but rarely disturbing visual acuity. Lacrimal gland involvement displaces the globe downwards and is bilateral in 20% of cases. Bilaterality does not appear to alter prognosis, which is generally good in

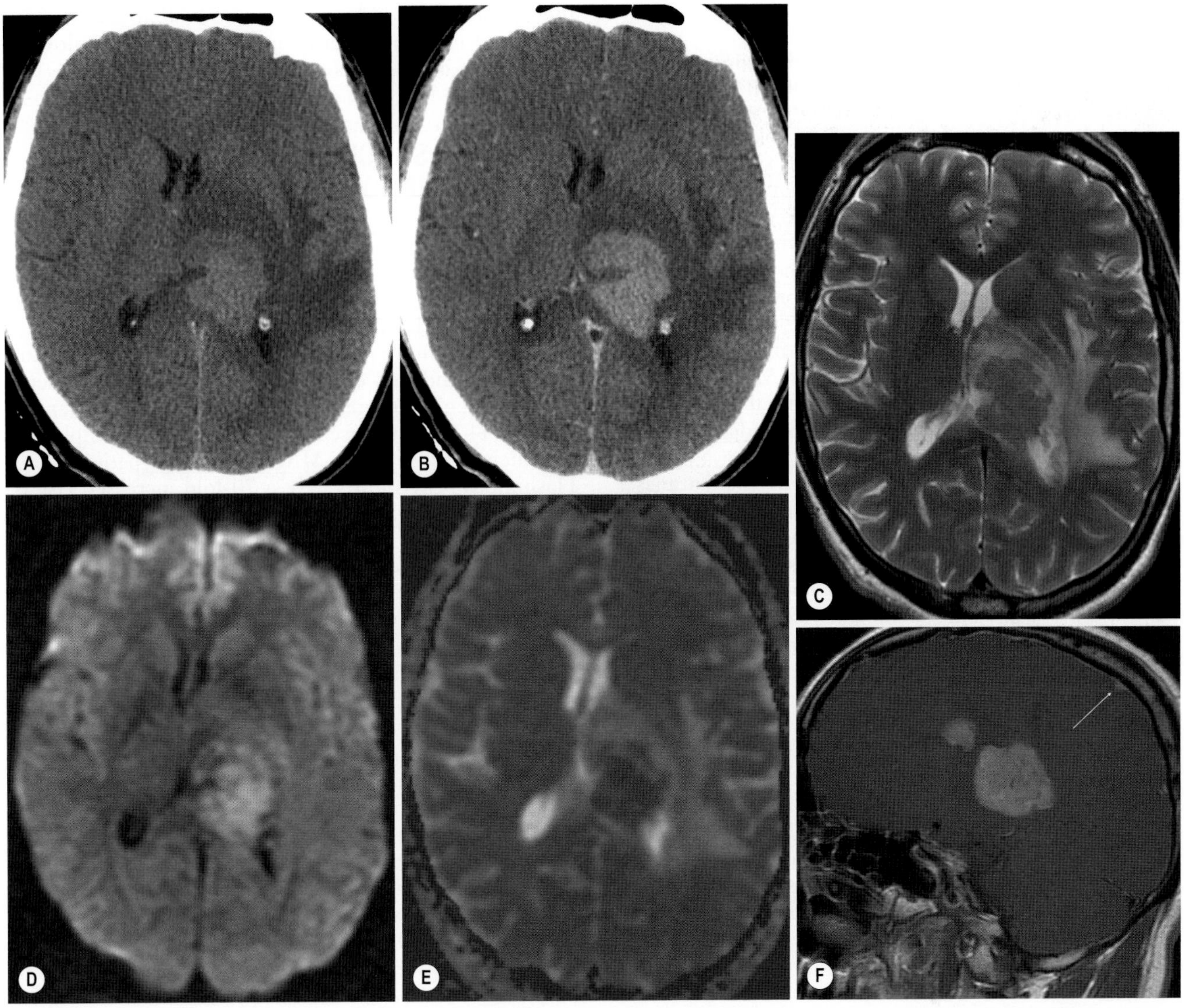

FIGURE 70-24 ■ **Cerebral non-Hodgkin's lymphoma.** (A) Unenhanced axial CT showing a hyperdense mass in the left thalamus extending into the splenium of the corpus callosum. (B) Post-contrast image demonstrating uniform enhancement of the mass. (C) Axial T2-weighted MRI image demonstrating the typical location of the lymphomatous mass and moderate surrounding vasogenic oedema. (D, E) Diffusion-weighted image (b800) and ADC map showing restriction of diffusion within the mass. (F) Sagittal T1-weighted MRI image post-intravenous gadolinium demonstrates a second intraventricular mass and dural involvement (arrow).

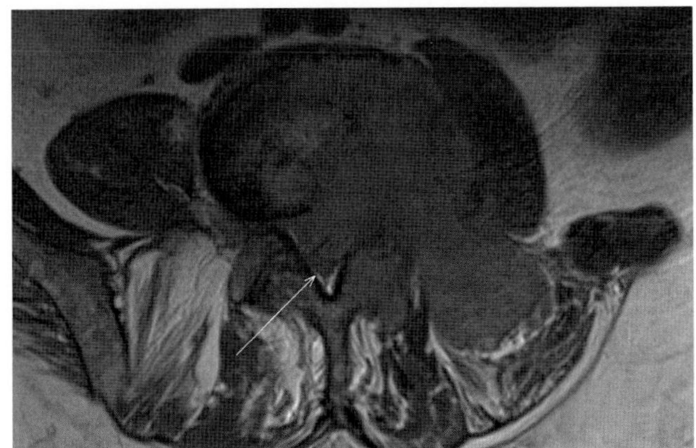

FIGURE 70-25 ■ **Epidural lymphoma.** T2-weighted axial MRI showing a mass of intermediate-to-high signal intensity in the paravertebral soft tissues, extending into the vertebral body and into the spinal canal as well as the paraspinal musculature. The mass is displacing and compressing the theca (arrowed).

all the primary forms. MALT lymphomas of the lacrimal glands can present as a mass or periorbital swelling. CT and MRI depict uni- or bilateral enhancing masses with a non-specific appearance. In patients with an orbital lymphomatous mass, about half will be found to have an extracentral nervous system primary site of origin. MRI best depicts the extent of disease and the presence, if any, of intracranial extension.

Head and Neck Lymphoma

Although HL typically involves the cervical lymph nodes as the presenting feature, true extranodal involvement of sites in the head and neck region with HL is rare. In contrast, 10% of patients with NHL present with extranodal head and neck involvement. About half of these will prove to have disseminated lymphoma. Extranodal NHL accounts for approximately 5% of head and neck cancers.

Waldeyer's Ring

Waldeyer's ring comprises lymphoid tissue in the nasopharynx, oropharynx, the faucial and palatine tonsil and the lingual tonsil. It is the commonest site of head and neck lymphoma and there is a close link with involvement of the gastrointestinal tract, either synchronous or metachronous, possibly reflecting the fact that up to 20% of these NHL are the MALT type. Accordingly some centres include endoscopy as well as whole-body cross-sectional imaging as part of staging, since up to 30% of patients will have advanced disease at presentation. The tonsils are most commonly affected, the commonest pattern being asymmetrical thickening of the pharyngeal mucosa, which is well shown by CT and MRI. A diagnosis of NHL is suggested by circumferential involvement or multifocality. Secondary invasion from adjacent nodal masses is also common.

NHL comprises 8% of tumours of the paranasal sinuses. In the West, the disease affects middle-aged men and the maxillary sinus is most commonly involved, commonly by DLBCL, whereas the aggressive diffuse T-cell type (that forms part of the 'lethal midline granuloma' syndrome) typically affects younger Asians and is linked to EBV. Paranasal sinus involvement often presents with acute facial swelling and pain, and disease often spreads from one sinus to the other in a contiguous fashion, though bony destruction is considerably less marked than in squamous cell carcinomas. These tumours are locally aggressive; spread through the skull base into the cranium is seen in up to 40%. Thus prophylactic intrathecal chemotherapy is often administered. MRI is the preferred imaging technique for evaluating head and neck lymphoma. Multiplanar fat-suppressed T1-weighted images pre-and post-intravenous gadolinium-based contrast medium are the most helpful in defining the full extent of disease and depicting tumour spread into the cranial cavity from the infratemporal fossa and skull base foramina.

Salivary Glands

All the salivary glands may be involved in lymphoma but the parotid gland is most frequently affected, usually by MALT lymphoma. Single or multiple well-defined masses are seen, which are of higher density than the surrounding gland on CT, hypoechoic on ultrasound and of intermediate signal intensity on T1- and T2-weighted MRI sequences. Many of the patients are middle-aged women and a history of Sjögren's disease is common.

Thyroid

NHL accounts for 2–5% of malignant tumours of the thyroid. MALT-type lymphomas arise in women in association with Hashimoto's disease. Presentation is with diffuse enlargement or large discrete nodules. However, DLBCL and anaplastic forms also occur, such patients presenting with a rapidly growing mass and obstructive symptoms. Direct spread of tumour beyond the gland and involvement of adjacent lymph nodes is common. At ultrasound these masses are relatively hypoechoic. At CT they usually have a lower attenuation than the normal gland and may show peripheral enhancement following injection of intravenous contrast medium.

MUCOSA-ASSOCIATED LYMPHOID TISSUE LYMPHOMAS

The MALT lymphomas arise from mucosal sites that normally have no organised lymphoid tissue, but within which acquired lymphoid tissue has arisen as a result of chronic inflammation or autoimmunity. Examples include Hashimoto's thyroiditis, Sjögren's syndrome and *Helicobacter*-induced chronic follicular gastritis. Patients with Sjögren's syndrome (lymphoepithelial sialadenitis) are at a 44-fold increased risk of developing lymphoma, of which over 80% are MALT type, and patients with Hashimoto's thyroiditis have a 70-fold increased risk of thyroid lymphoma. The histological hallmark of MALT lymphoma is the presence of lymphomatous cells in a marginal zone around reactive follicles, which can spread into the epithelium of glandular tissues to produce the characteristic lymphoepithelial lesion. In up to 30%, transformation to large cell lymphoma occurs.

Adults with a median age of 60 are most often affected, with a female preponderance. Most patients present with stage IE or IIE disease, which tends to be indolent. Bone marrow involvement is unusual (occurring in around 10%) but the frequency varies depending on the primary site. Multiple extranodal sites are involved in up to 25%, but this does not appear to have the same poor prognostic import as in other forms of NHL. Nonetheless, extensive staging investigations may be necessary.[54]

The commonest site of involvement is the gastrointestinal (GI) tract (50%) and within the GI tract, the stomach is most often affected (around 85% of cases) (Fig. 70-13). The small bowel and colon are involved in immunoproliferative small intestinal disease (IPSID), previously known as alpha-chain disease. Other sites commonly affected include the lung, head, neck, ocular adnexae, skin, thyroid and breast.

BURKITT'S LYMPHOMA

Burkitt's lymphoma (BL) is a highly aggressive B-cell variant of NHL, associated with EBV in a variable proportion of cases. Three clinical variants are recognised:

- Endemic (African) type
- Sporadic (non-endemic)
- Immunodeficiency associated.

Though these tumours are extremely aggressive and rapidly growing, they are potentially curable with intensive combination chemotherapy. They account for only 2–3% of NHL in immunocompetent adults, but 30–50% of all childhood lymphoma is BL. Immunodeficiency-associated BL is seen chiefly in association with HIV infection and may be the initial manifestation of AIDS. EBV is identified in up to 40% of cases. Extranodal disease is common and all three variants are at risk for CNS disease.

In the endemic form, the jaws and orbit are involved in 50% of cases, producing the 'floating tooth sign' on plain radiography. The ovaries, kidneys and breast may be involved. The sporadic forms have a predilection for the ileocaecal region and patients can present with acute abdominal emergencies such as intussusception (Fig. 70-14). Again, ovaries, kidneys and breasts are commonly involved. Retroperitoneal and paraspinal disease can cause paraplegia, the presenting feature in up to 15%. Disease is confined to the abdomen in approximately 50% of patients[55] and thoracic disease is relatively rare. Leptomeningeal disease can be seen at presentation, and as a site of relapse.

LYMPHOMA IN THE IMMUNOCOMPROMISED

The WHO classification recognises four broad groupings associated with an increased incidence of lymphoma and lymphoproliferative disorders:[3]

- lymphoproliferative diseases associated with primary immune disorders;
- lymphomas associated with HIV infection;
- post-transplant lymphoproliferative disorders; and
- other iatrogenic immunodeficiency-associated lymphoproliferative disorders.

The development of lymphoma in these settings is multifactorial, but mostly related to defective immune surveillance, with or without chronic antigenic stimulation.

Lymphomas Associated with HIV

The incidence of all subtypes of NHL is increased 60- to 200-fold in patients with HIV. However, the risk has declined markedly since the introduction of highly active antiretroviral therapy (HAART). Despite the lower risk with HAART, lymphoma is more often the first AIDS-defining illness. Prior to the advent of HAART, the incidence of PCNSL and BL was increased 1000-fold compared with the general population. Most are aggressive B-cell lymphomas and various types are seen, including those seen in immunocompetent patients, such as BL and DLBCL. Others occur much more frequently in the HIV population (e.g. primary effusion lymphoma and plasmablastic lymphoma of the oral cavity). The incidence of HL is also increased up to eightfold and has increased further since HAART was introduced. DLBCL tends to occur later, when CD4 counts are under $100 \times 10^{6-}$ L^{1}, whereas BL occurs in less immunodeficient patients. EBV positivity occurs in a variable proportion; PCNSL is associated with EBV in over 90% of cases and EBV positivity is seen in nearly all cases of HL associated with HIV.

Most tumours are aggressive, with advanced stage, bulky disease and a high serum LDH at presentation. Most have a marked propensity to involve extranodal sites, especially the GI tract, CNS (less frequent with the advent of highly active antiretroviral therapy), liver and bone marrow. Multiple sites of extranodal involvement are seen in over 75% of cases.[56] Peripheral lymph node enlargement is relatively uncommon.

In the chest, NHL is usually extranodal; pleural effusions and lung disease are common, with nodules, acinar and interstitial opacity being described. Hilar and mediastinal nodal enlargement is generally mild. There is a wide differential diagnosis and in one study the presence of cavitation, small nodules under 1 cm in diameter and nodal necrosis predicted for mycobacterial infection rather than lymphoma. Within the abdomen, the GI tract, liver, kidneys, adrenal glands and lower genitourinary tract are commonly involved. Mesenteric and retroperitoneal nodal enlargement is less common than in immunocompetent patients, but there are no real differences in the CT features of patients with or without AIDS.

Regarding PCNSL, certain features such as rim enhancement and multifocality are seen more often than in the immunocompetent population. This can cause confusion with cerebral toxoplasmosis, though the location of PCNSL in the deep white matter is suggestive. Quantitative FDG-PET uptake can help in the differentiation of PCNSL, toxoplasmosis and progressive multifocal leucoencephalopathy.

Post-transplant Lymphoproliferative Disorders

These occur in 2–4% of solid organ transplant recipients depending on the type of transplant, the lowest frequency being seen in renal transplant recipients (1%) and the highest in heart–lung or liver–bowel allografts (5%). Marrow allograft recipients are at low risk (1%). Most appear to represent EBV-induced monoclonal or, more rarely, polyclonal B- or T-cell proliferation as a consequence of immune suppression and reduced T-cell immune surveillance.[3] The clinical features are variable, correlating with the type of allograft and type of immunosuppression. PTLD develops earlier in patients receiving ciclosporin rather than azathioprine (mean interval 48 months). EBV-positive cases occur earlier than EBV-negative cases, the latter occurring 4–5 years after transplantation. In all cases, extranodal disease is disproportionately commoner, though CNS disease is rare. Involvement of the allograft itself is commoner in early-onset EBV-driven PTLD. In patients who have received ciclosporin, the GI tract is frequently affected. The bone marrow, liver and lung are often involved, with multiple intrapulmonary masses, pleural effusions, involvement of multiple segments of bowel and the transplanted organ all being reported.[57]

MONITORING RESPONSE TO THERAPY

Achievement of complete response after treatment is the most important factor for predicting prolonged survival in both HL and NHL. A complete response is designated when there is no clinical or radiological evidence of disease after treatment. Imaging plays a critical role in monitoring response and the advent of FDG-PET and FDG-PET/CT has resulted in a paradigm shift in response assessment in lymphoma. For large-volume intrathoracic disease, the chest radiograph remains useful

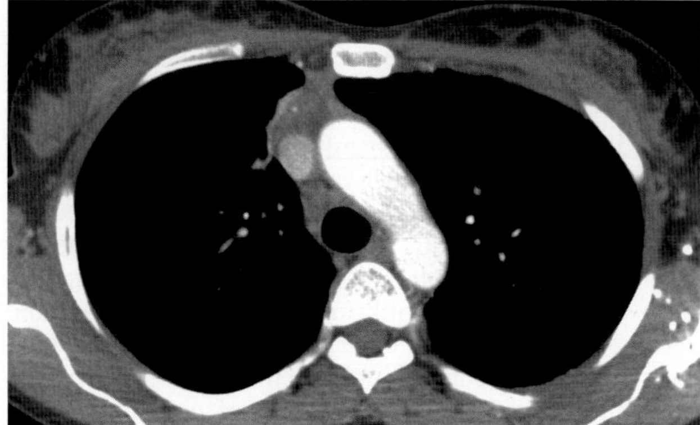

FIGURE 70-26 ■ Thoracic residual mass in Hodgkin's lymphoma. This is the same patient as that described in the legend to Fig. 70-3A. After treatment, follow-up CT at 6 months shows a residual anterior mediastinal mass; the right axillary lymph node has completely resolved. The mass has been stable for 2 years.

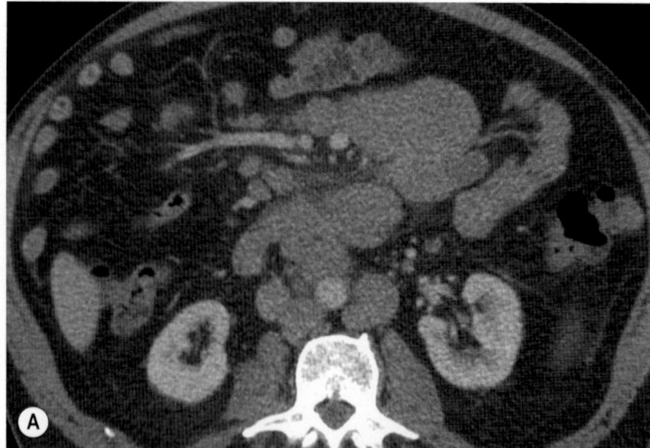

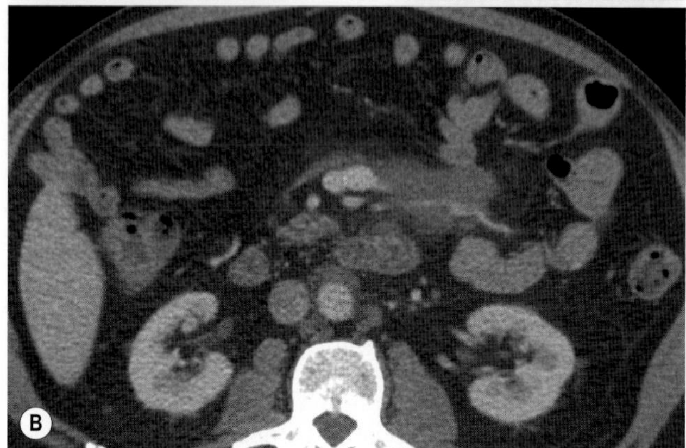

FIGURE 70-27 ■ Mesenteric residual mass. (A) Contrast-enhanced CT in a patient with NHL presenting with a large mesenteric nodal mass and bilateral para-aortic nodal disease. (B) Follow-up CT performed 1 year after treatment shows a persistent low-density soft-tissue mass within the mesentery encasing the mesenteric vessels, whilst the retroperitoneal nodal enlargement has resolved.

in assessing early response. However, changes due to radiotherapy, rebound thymic hyperplasia or thymic cyst formation make the mediastinum difficult to assess on a chest radiograph, particularly in children. Therefore, cross-sectional imaging is essential in final assessment of response in the chest, as well as the abdomen and pelvis (Figs. 70-26 and 70-27). Assessment of response requires the measurement of a number of marker lesions before, during and after therapy, for which the reproducibility and reliability of contrast medium-enhanced CT is a great advantage. Since there is significant interobserver variation in the measurement of masses, wherever possible well-defined regular masses above and below the diaphragm should be assessed.[58] Many centres favour an interim CT or FDG-PET/CT study after two cycles of chemotherapy for certain lymphomas, especially HL, and this is mandatory in many clinical trials. The optimal timing of final response assessment depends on the technique chosen and the availability of resources. Most centres assess patients with CT one month after completion of therapy, but if FDG-PET/CT is used, a longer interval is required (6–8 weeks for chemotherapy alone and 12 weeks if radiotherapy has been given).

Prognostication

Numerous studies have shown that an interim FDG-PET imaging yields much more prognostic information than CT alone, since FDG-PET can detect and quantify changes in functional/metabolic activity long before structural changes have taken place (Fig. 70-28). Interim FDG-PET also has a role to direct further treatment (escalation or de-escalation of treatment) and to avoid potential toxicity from an ineffective therapy. FDG-PET performed after one to three cycles of chemotherapy appears to predict progression-free and overall survival in 'aggressive' NHL more accurately than PET at the end of treatment and more accurately than conventional imaging.[59,60] The same is true of HL,[61,62] even after only one cycle of chemotherapy.[63] A large body of evidence shows that the NPV of the test exceeds 80% in patients with aggressive NHL and 90% in patients with HL. In one multicentre study of patients with HL, the 2-year progression-free survival for interim PET-negative and -positive patients was 95% and 12%, respectively.[62] This suggests that early FDG-PET imaging could allow response-adapted modification of treatment, but it is as yet unknown whether this will translate into overall survival benefits. There are currently five ongoing trials evaluating de-escalation of therapy in early responders with limited-stage HL (for example, the RAPID trial, a quality-assured multicentre trial designed to establish whether interim PET can identify early responders, who may not require radiotherapy).[64] For NHL, the data are more heterogeneous, and therefore interim imaging is only recommended in the context of clinical trials.

It is recommended that the time from chemotherapy to imaging should be as close as possible to the next cycle to reduce the risk of false-negative results due to the 'tumour stunning'. Various response criteria have been proposed for interim PET images, including a category of 'minimal residual uptake' (MRU) lower or equal to that in the liver, but a semi-quantitative standardised uptake value approach may be more useful.[65]

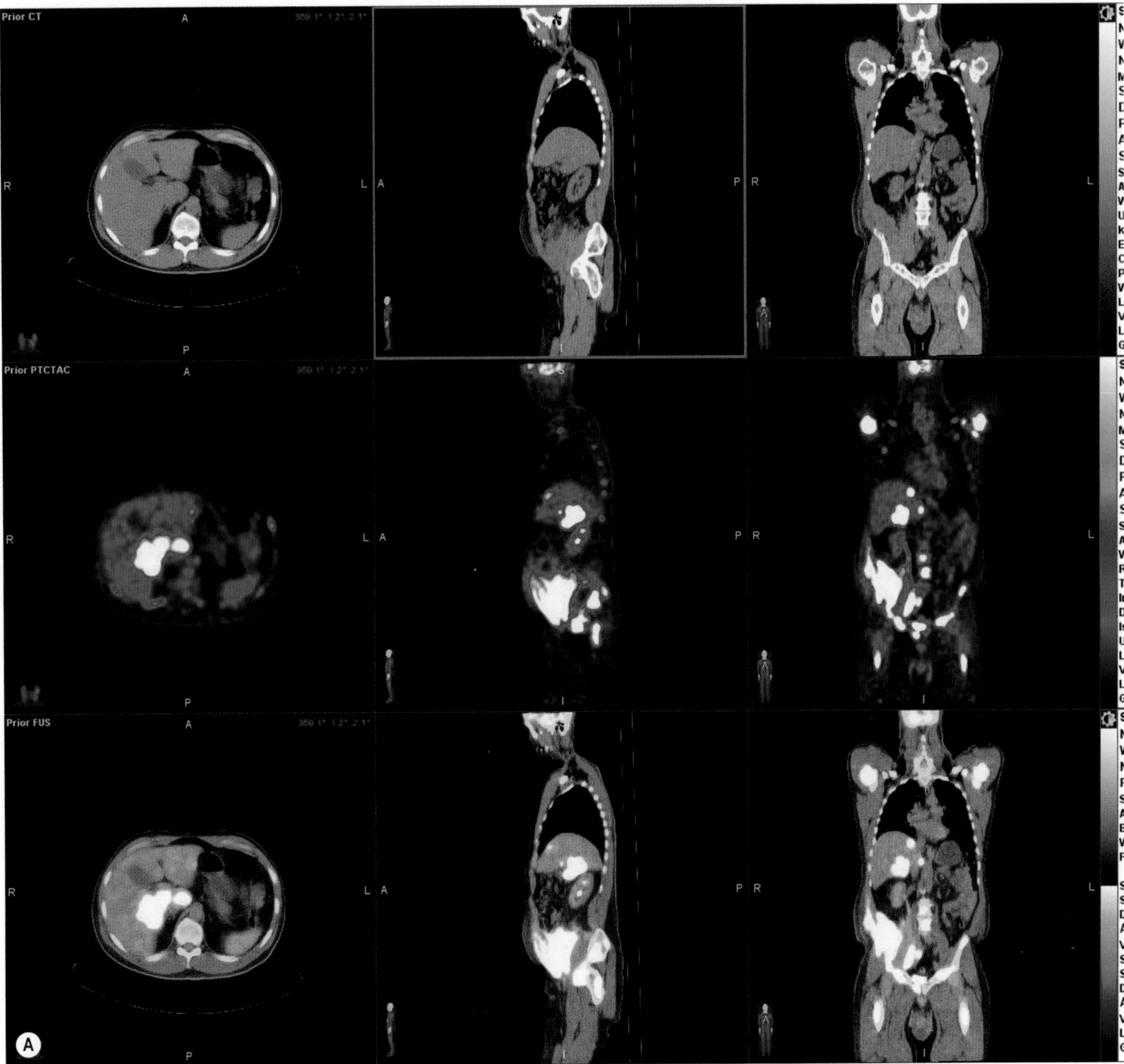

FIGURE 70-28 ■ PET/CT in interim response assessment. (A) Initial staging PET/CT in a patient with stage IVB DLBCL. Unenhanced CT, PET and fused images demonstrate extensive bony disease, a large confluent nodal mass in the right hemipelvis and hepatic involvement.

Response Criteria

Standardised response criteria are essential for clinical research and comparison of different therapies. In 1999, a report set out standardised international criteria for assessment of response in NHL, similar to those already in use for HL.[66] The International Working Group (IWG) radiological criteria are essentially morphological and are as follows.

Complete Remission (CR)

- Complete disappearance of all radiological evidence of disease.
- All nodal masses to have decreased to normal: (A) < 1.5 cm in greatest transverse diameter for nodes that were > 1.5 cm pretherapy; (B) nodes initially between 1 and 1.5 cm must have decreased to 1 cm or less.
- The spleen, if previously enlarged on CT, must be normal in size and any focal deposits should have resolved.

Complete Remission, Unconfirmed (CR_u)

- A residual mass > 1.5 cm short-axis diameter (SAD) which has regressed by more than 75% of the sum of the products of the greatest diameters (SPD) of the original mass.

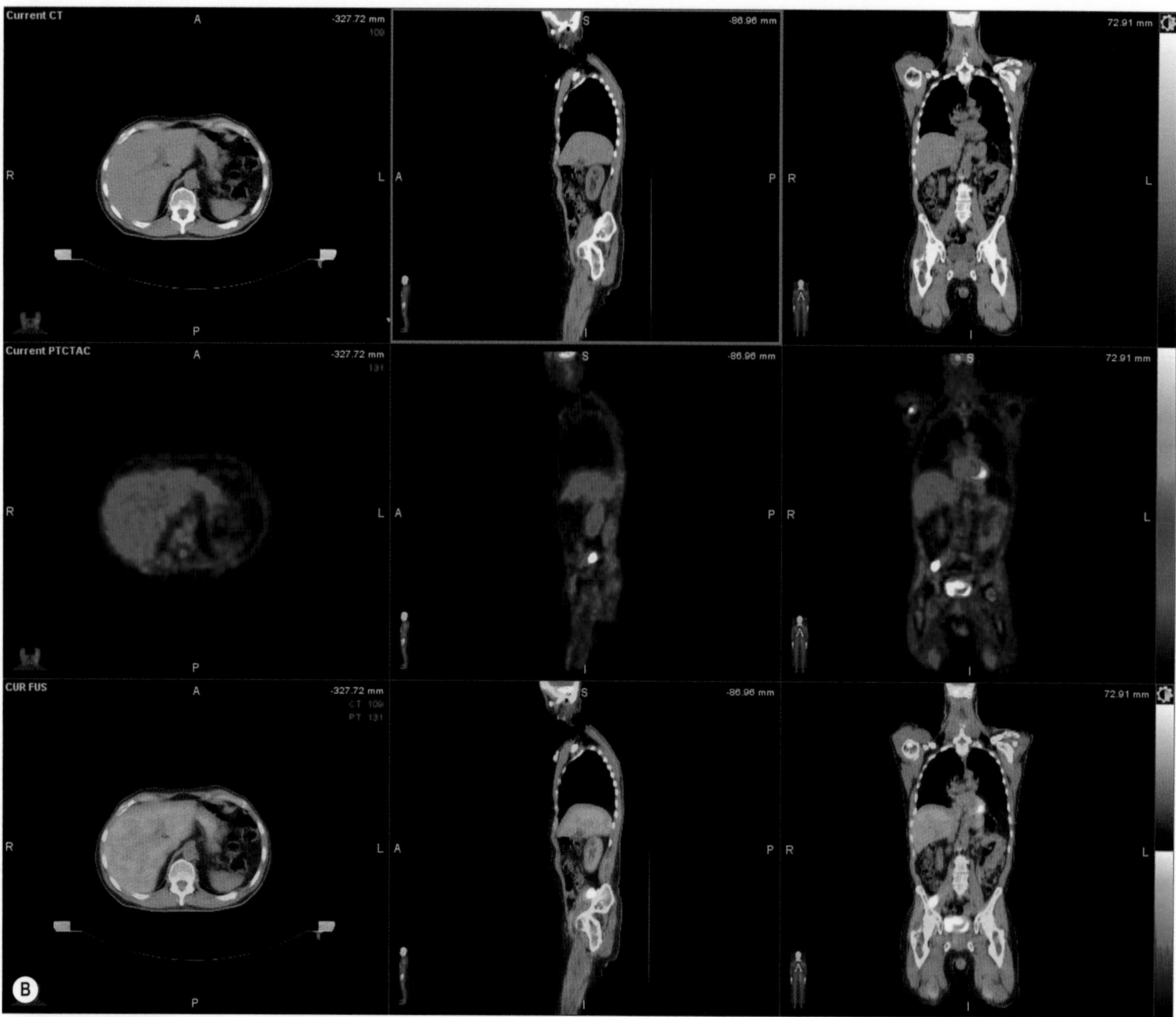

FIGURE 70-28, Continued ■ (B) After two cycles of CHOP-R, there has been a marked response to treatment with resolution of the disease in the liver and the right hemipelvis. Some osseous disease persists, especially in the right humerus (SUV reduced from 16.8 pre-treatment to 10.5).

Partial Response (PR)

- > 50% decrease in the SPD of largest nodes/masses.
- No increase in size of spleen, liver or lymph nodes.
- Splenic or hepatic nodules decreased by 50%.

Stable Disease (SD)

- No evidence of progressive disease.
- Decrease in SPD less than 50%.

Progressive Disease (PD)

- ≥50% increase from nadir in the SPD of an established node/mass.
- Appearance of a new lesion during or at the end of therapy.

Residual Masses

Successfully treated, enlarged nodes often return to normal size in both HL and NHL. However, a residual mass of fibrous tissue can persist in up to 80% of patients treated for HL (usually within the mediastinum) and 20–60% of patients with NHL[30,67] who are in clinical CR (Figs. 70-26, 70-27 and 70-29). Residual masses occur more frequently in patients with bulky disease but how often such masses lead to relapse is uncertain. Until the advent of FDG-PET, determination of the nature of a residual mass was a major challenge in oncological radiology.

Computed Tomography

CT cannot distinguish between fibrotic tissue and residual active disease on the basis of density or size; hence the consistently low specificity and positive predictive

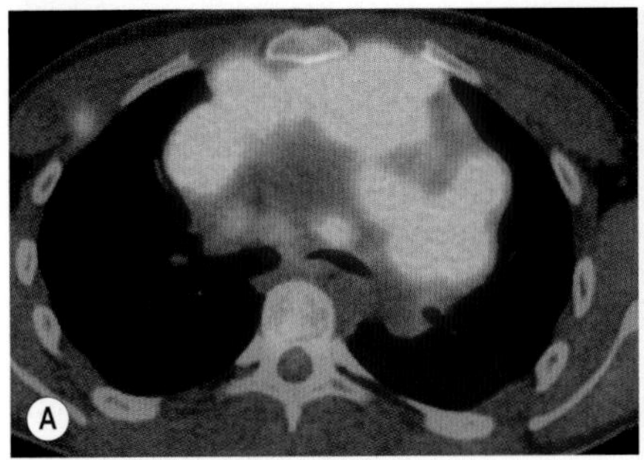

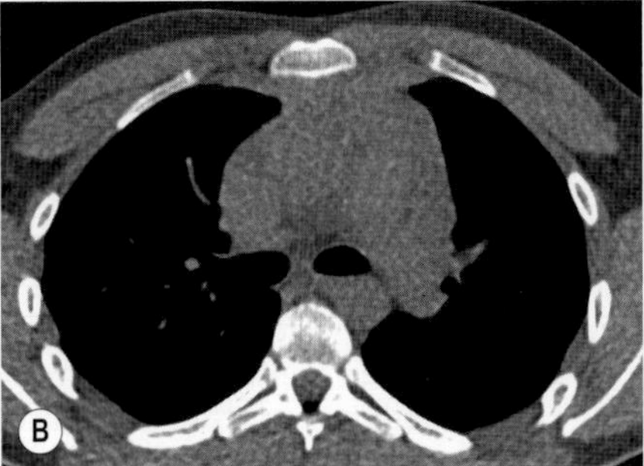

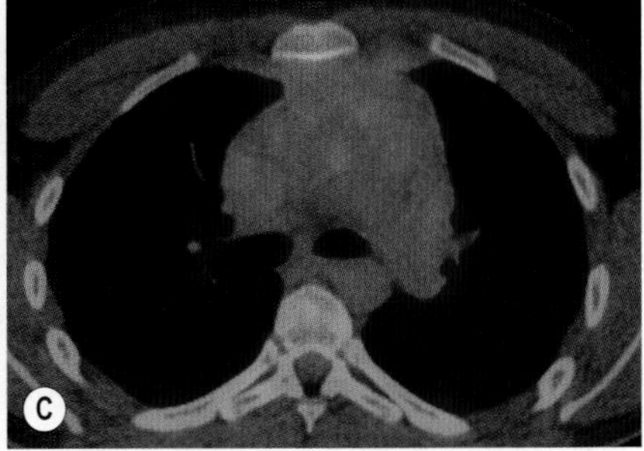

FIGURE 70-29 ■ **PET in assessment of the residual mass.** (A) Fused PET/CT image demonstrating a large metabolically active anterior/middle mediastinal mass and metabolically active but normal-sized right subpectoral lymph node. (B) Post-treatment CT shows a residual anterior mediastinal mass. (C) The mass has normal levels of FDG uptake, identical to that of the remainder of the mediastinum (a metabolic CR by the IHP criteria).

value (PPV) of CT after treatment in determining the likelihood of relapse in the presence of a residual mass. Until recently, serial CT every 2–3 months was used and masses that remained stable for 1 year were considered inactive.

MRI

MRI may help to differentiate active tumour from a fibrotic mass. Most tumours have high T2-signal intensity, which diminishes in response to treatment. Persistent heterogeneous or recurrent high T2 signal suggests residual or recurrent disease, respectively. However, small foci of tumour can persist undetected within a residual mass; hence the fairly low sensitivity of MRI. In addition, false-positive studies are common, especially soon after treatment because of non-specific inflammation and necrosis. Evidence for the value of diffusion-weighted imaging and measurement of the apparent diffusion coefficient (ADC) is not compelling at present.

Functional Imaging

Although gallium–67 scintigraphy is a far better predictor of disease relapse in patients with a residual mass than CT alone, it has many drawbacks. Thus it has been superseded by FDG-PET. At the end of treatment, FDG-PET has a very high PPV for early relapse, with or without a residual mass at CT.[68–70] However, false-negative and false-positive images occur. Recent evidence suggests that the PPV of FDG-PET may be lower in patients treated with rituximab.[71] Therefore, clinical correlation is essential when interpreting FDG-PET results.[72]

FDG-PET in Response Assessment

FDG-PET is more accurate than CT in response assessment, with a PPV at least double that of CT. In one follow-up study, all PET-positive/CT-negative patients relapsed, whereas only 5% of PET-negative/CT-positive patients relapsed[73] (Fig. 70-29). The few studies directly comparing FDG-PET and gallium–67 suggest that FDG-PET is more sensitive and has a greater overall accuracy.[74] However, it should be recognised that FDG-PET predicts for early relapse and that false-negative studies do occur with late relapse.

The profound impact of PET on the IWG criteria was first evaluated by Juweid et al. in a retrospective analysis of 54 patients with aggressive NHL who underwent PET and CT after completion of treatment.[75] Patients with a PR by standard IWC who were PET-negative did as well as those who were in CR by IWC and IWC + PET, indicating superior discriminative ability with FDG-PET. As a result of such studies, an International Harmonisation Project was convened to revise the IWC criteria.[76] These guidelines support the use of FDG-PET for end-of-therapy response assessment in DLBCL and HL, but not for other NHL, unless the CR rate is a primary endpoint of a clinical trial. In the revised criteria, patients with any residual mass can be assigned to the CR category provided that it is FDG-PET negative at the end of treatment and was (or can reasonably expected to have been) PET positive before treatment. The CR_u category is eliminated. A PR exists when there is residual FDG-PET positivity in at least one previously involved site.

The group has also issued guidance on timing, performance and interpretation of FDG-PET images.[77] Specifically, simple visual assessment of tracer uptake is deemed sufficient and it is not necessary to measure the standardised uptake value (SUV) or utilise cut-off values. Mediastinal blood pool activity is recommended as the reference background activity to define PET positivity for a residual mass ≥ 2 cm in greatest transverse diameter, regardless of its location. A smaller residual mass or a normal-sized lymph node should be considered positive if its activity is above that of the surrounding background.[77] Imaging should be performed at least 3 weeks and preferably at 6 to 8 weeks after completion of chemotherapy or chemoimmunotherapy, and 8 to 12 weeks after radiation or chemoradiotherapy. FDG-PET is also extremely useful in prognostication for patients about to undergo high-dose treatment and autologous stem cell transplantation.[78] Patients commencing high-dose therapy with a positive pre-treatment PET image have a much poorer prognosis.

SURVEILLANCE AND DETECTION OF RELAPSE

Relapse after satisfactory response to initial treatment occurs in 10–40% of patients with HL and approximately

50% of patients with NHL. In HL, relapse usually occurs within the first 2 years after treatment and patients are followed up closely during this period, although CT is not required unless clinical features suggest the possibility of recurrence.

For patients who attain a CR, there is very little evidence for routine surveillance with imaging. A number of studies have shown that relapse is rarely identified by conventional imaging before patients become symptomatic.[79–82] Functional imaging is able to identify early relapse before CT and, indeed, before the development of clinical signs. However, there is as yet little evidence for the efficacy of FDG-PET in this role. In one series of a cohort of patients treated for HL, relapses were identified by FDG-PET before there was any other evidence of relapse[83] but the false-positive rate was high. In another study it was concluded that there was no benefit from surveillance studies for HL or aggressive NHL beyond 18 months.[84] In these and other studies, true positive images in the absence of clinical suspicion of relapse were rare. On the other hand, in suspected relapse, the development of a positive PET image is highly suggestive and in this situation PET-CT is likely to have a significant therapeutic impact, allowing image-guided biopsies which can target the most metabolically active lesion and thereby direct therapy by establishing relapse or transformation.[6]

CONCLUSION

Management of patients with lymphoma depends heavily on the imaging findings, which are vital in initial staging of the disease, prognostication and monitoring response to treatment. The radiologist needs to understand the fundamental aspects of tumour behaviour and must appreciate the factors that will influence therapy. The radiological report should document the number of sites of nodal disease; the presence and sites of bulky disease; the presence of any extranodal disease; and factors which may influence delivery of therapy, such as central venous thrombosis or hydronephrosis. FDG-PET/CT has revolutionised the imaging of lymphoma, providing unprecedented insight into the functional behaviour of this diverse group of tumours, but further research is needed to establish the precise roles of PET and PET/CT and their place in the investigative algorithm. For all of these reasons, the radiologist has become a pivotal member of the multidisciplinary team managing patients with lymphoma.

For a full list of references, please see ExpertConsult.

FURTHER READING

4. Jaffe ES. The 2008 WHO classification of lymphomas: implications for clinical practice and translational research. Hematology Am Soc Hematol Educ Program 2009;523–31.
11. Lin C, Luciani A, Itti E, et al. Whole-body diffusion magnetic resonance imaging in the assessment of lymphoma. Cancer Imaging 2012;12:403–8.
13. Moog F, Bangerter M, Diederichs CG, et al. Extranodal malignant lymphoma: detection with FDG-PET versus CT. Radiology 1998;206:475–81.
15. Kwee TC, Kwee RM, Nievelstein RA. Imaging in staging of malignant lymphoma: a systematic review. Blood 2008;111:504–16.
16. Chua SC, Rozalli FI, O'Connor SR. Imaging features of primary extranodal lymphomas. Clin Radiol 2009;64(6):574–88.
43. Elstrom R, Guan L, Baker G, et al. Utility of FDG-PET scanning in lymphoma by WHO classification. Blood 2003;101(10):3875–6.
54. Raderer M, Vorbeck F, Formanek M, et al. Importance of extensive staging in patients with mucosa-associated lymphoid tissue (MALT)-type lymphoma. Br J Cancer 2000;83:454–7.
63. Kostakoglu L, Goldsmith SJ, Leonard JP, et al. FDG-PET after 1 cycle of therapy predicts outcome in diffuse large cell lymphoma and classic Hodgkin disease. Cancer 2006;107(11):2678–87.
66. Cheson BD, Horning SJ, Coiffier B, et al. Report of an international workshop to standardize response criteria in non-Hodgkin's lymphoma. J Clin Oncol 1999;17:1244–53.
77. Juweid ME, Stroobants S, Hoekstra OS, et al. Use of positron emission tomography for response assessment of lymphoma: consensus of the Imaging Subcommittee of International Harmonization Project in Lymphoma. J Clin Oncol 2007;25:571–8.

CHAPTER 71

Bone Marrow Disorders: Haematological Neoplasms

Asif Saifuddin

CHAPTER OUTLINE

Chapters 71 and 72 deal with a variety of blood-related disorders that have a major influence on imaging of the skeletal system. The 2008 World Health Organisation (WHO) classification of myeloproliferative neoplasms is complex and includes a variety of conditions of differing malignant potential.[1] Only those that have significant radiological manifestations in the skeletal system will be discussed.

PRIMARY MYELOFIBROSIS[2]

Primary myelofibrosis (PMF) is a myeloproliferative neoplasm characterised by stem cell-derived clonal myeloproliferation resulting in bone marrow fibrosis, anaemia, splenomegaly and extramedullary erythropoiesis. The diagnosis is based on bone marrow morphology, showing evidence of fibrosis, and is supported by a variety of genetic abnormalities.

Clinical Features

It affects men and women equally, with an age range of 20–80 years (median age 60 years). The disorder presents insidiously with weakness, dyspnoea and weight loss due to progressive obliteration of the marrow by fibrosis or bony sclerosis, which leads to a moderate normochromic normocytic anaemia. Extramedullary erythropoiesis takes place in the liver and spleen, which become enlarged in 72 and 94% of cases, respectively, but is also reported in lymph nodes, lung, choroid plexus, kidney, etc. The natural history is one of slow deterioration, with death typically occurring 2–3 years after diagnosis. Progression to leukaemia is also a feature.

Radiological Features[3]

Bone sclerosis is the major radiological finding, being evident in approximately 30–70% of cases. Typically, this is diffuse (Fig. 71-1) but occasionally patchy, occurring most often in the axial skeleton and metaphyses of the femur, humerus and tibia. Sclerosis is due to trabecular and endosteal new bone formation, resulting in reduced marrow diameter. In established disease, lucent areas are due to fibrous tissue reaction. Periosteal reaction occurs in one-third of cases, most often in the medial aspects of the distal femur and proximal tibia. The skull may show a mixed sclerotic and lytic pattern.

MRI appearances vary depending upon the tissue contained in the marrow. Typically, the hyperintensity of marrow fat is replaced on both T1- and T2-weighted (T1W, T2W) sequences by hypointensity, which may be diffuse or heterogeneous (Fig. 71-2). Additional features include arthropathy due to haemarthrosis and secondary gout, occurring in 5–20% of cases. Also, infiltration of the synovium by bone marrow elements may result in polyarthralgia and polyarthritis. Leukaemic conversion may manifest radiologically by the development of an extraosseous soft-tissue mass (Fig. 71-3).

Radiological differentiation between other causes of increased bone density may be difficult, but the presence of anaemia and splenomegaly should suggest the diagnosis in this age group. Radiological differential diagnosis includes osteopetrosis, fluorosis, mastocytosis, carcinomatosis and adult sickle cell disease (SCD).

SYSTEMIC MASTOCYTOSIS[4]

Systemic mastocytosis represents a clonal disorder of mast cells, which is classified according to the WHO 2008 system into indolent mastocytosis, systemic mastocytosis with an associated haematological non-mast cell disorder, aggressive systemic mastocytosis and mast cell leukaemia. The majority of cases are associated with a pathological increase in the number of mast cells in both skin and extracutaneous tissues, although bone marrow involvement can occur without skin disease.

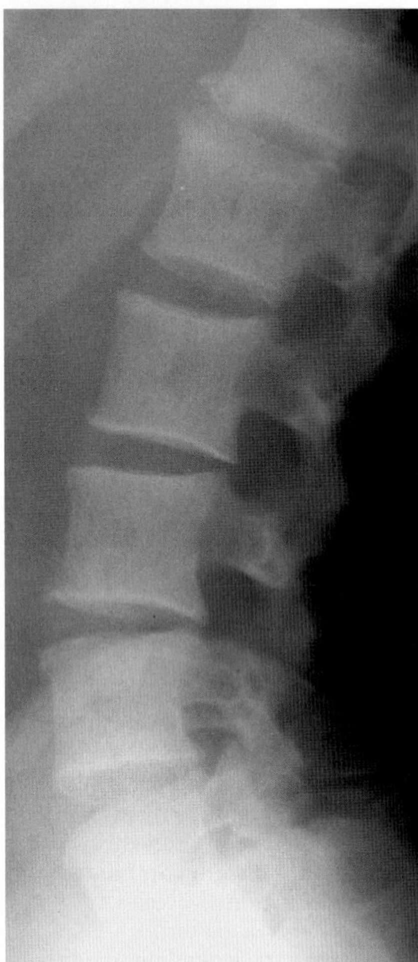

FIGURE 71-1 ■ **Myelofibrosis.** Lateral radiograph of the lumbar spine showing heterogeneous marrow sclerosis throughout the vertebral bodies.

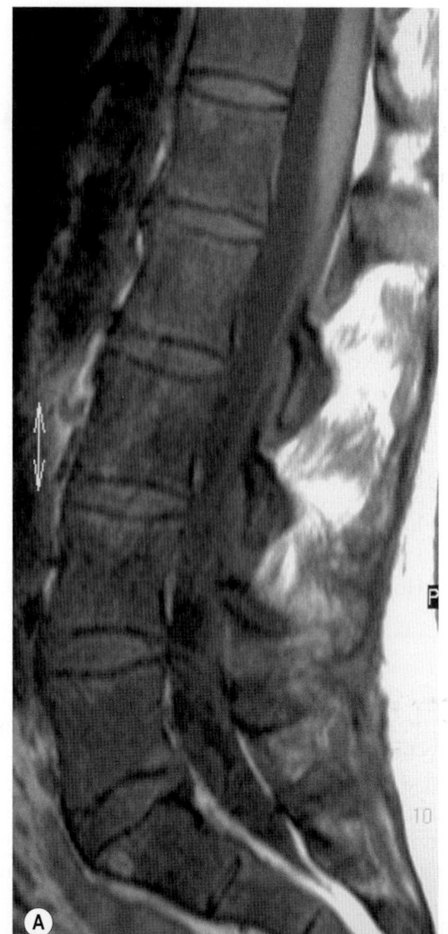

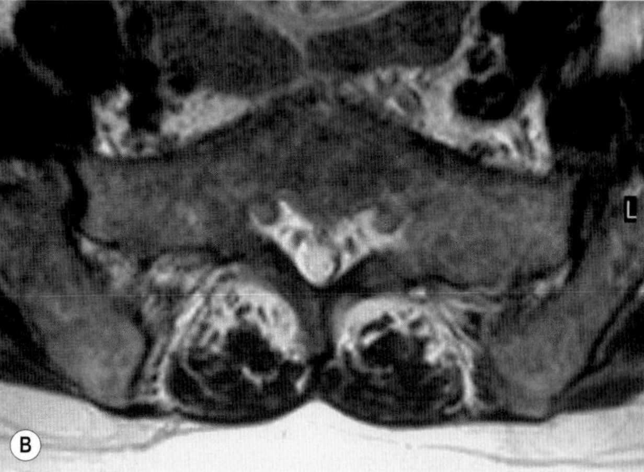

FIGURE 71-2 ■ **Myelofibrosis.** (A) Sagittal T1W SE and (B) axial T2W FSE MRI of the lumbar spine and sacrum showing heterogeneous reduction of marrow SI.

Clinical Features

The condition presents in the fifth to eighth decades with equal frequency in men and women. Bone marrow involvement is present in approximately 90% of cases and is often asymptomatic, but may produce thoracic and lumbar spinal pain and arthralgia. The condition may be associated with myelodysplastic syndromes, myeloproliferative neoplasia, leukaemia and lymphoma. The prognosis is variable.

Radiological Features

Imaging, including radiography, scintigraphy, bone densitometry, CT and MRI, plays a role in the diagnosis, staging and monitoring of the disease. Skeletal changes are due to both the direct effect of mast cells and the indirect effect of secreted mediators such as histamine, heparin and prostaglandins. They include both osteolytic and osteosclerotic lesions, which may be either diffuse or focal. Small (4–5 mm) lytic lesions may be surrounded by a rim of sclerosis and are most commonly seen in the spine, ribs, skull, pelvis and tubular bones. Diffuse osteopenia is a common pattern (Fig. 71-4), most commonly involving the axial skeleton, and may be complicated by pathological fracture in 16% of cases. Differential diagnosis includes cystic osteoporosis, Gaucher's disease, myeloma, hyperparathyroidism or thalassaemia.

Osteosclerosis produces trabecular and cortical thickening with reduction of the marrow spaces (Fig. 71-5), and multifocal sclerotic lesions simulating osteoblastic metastases (Fig. 71-6). Both Multidetector CT (Fig. 71-7) and MRI are more sensitive than radiography in

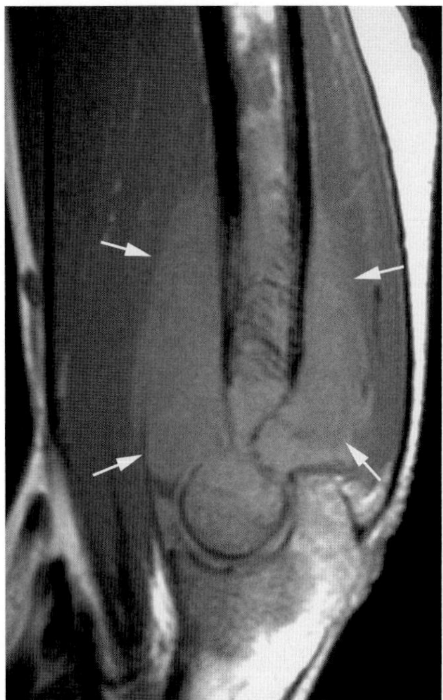

FIGURE 71-3 ■ **Myelofibrosis.** Sagittal T1W SE MRI of the distal humerus demonstrating heterogeneous reduction of marrow SI and a circumferential extraosseous mass (arrows) due to leukaemic transformation.

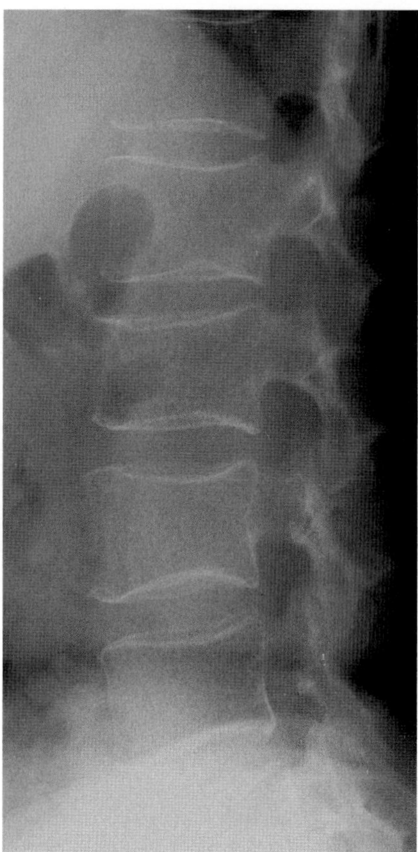

FIGURE 71-4 ■ **Mastocytosis.** Lateral radiograph of the lumbar spine showing diffuse osteopenia and multilevel mild compression fractures.

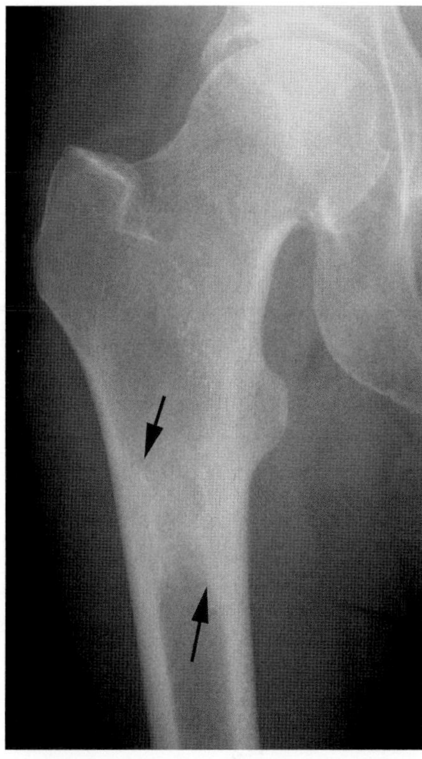

FIGURE 71-5 ■ **Mastocytosis.** AP radiograph of the right hip showing endosteal sclerosis in the proximal femur (arrows).

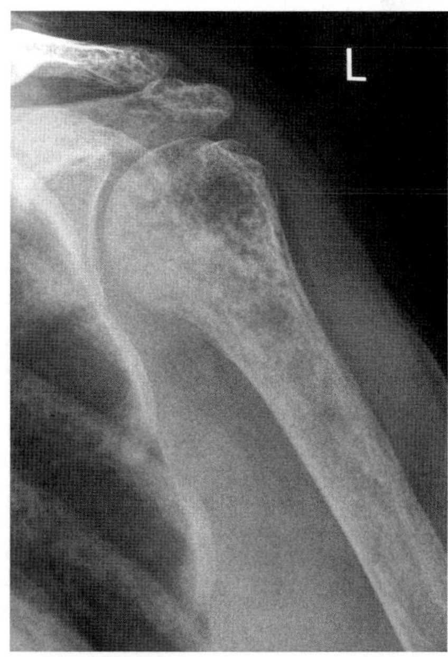

FIGURE 71-6 ■ **Mastocytosis.** AP radiograph of the left shoulder showing nodular sclerosis in the ribs and proximal humerus.

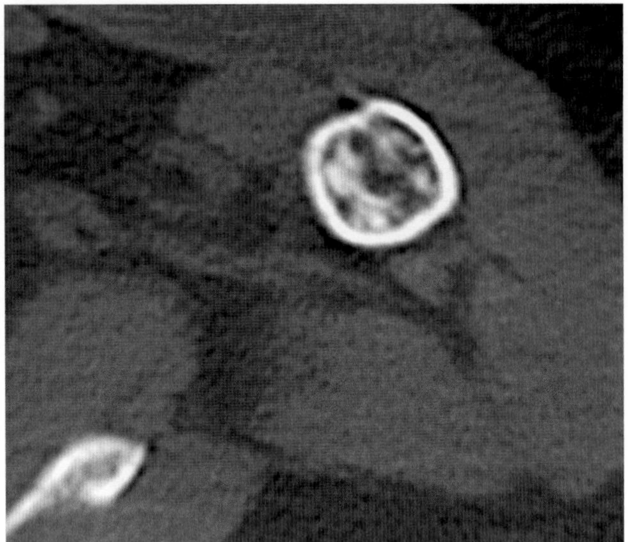

FIGURE 71-7 ■ **Mastocytosis.** CT of the left proximal humerus demonstrating multiple intramedullary sclerotic lesions.

the identification of marrow involvement. In mild cases, MRI may be normal. Otherwise, there is a generalised reduction of T1W signal intensity (SI), with variable T2W and short tau inversion recovery (STIR) SI, depending upon the degree of associated marrow fibrosis. Sclerotic lesions appear hypointense on all pulse sequences. The role of FDG-PET is unclear.

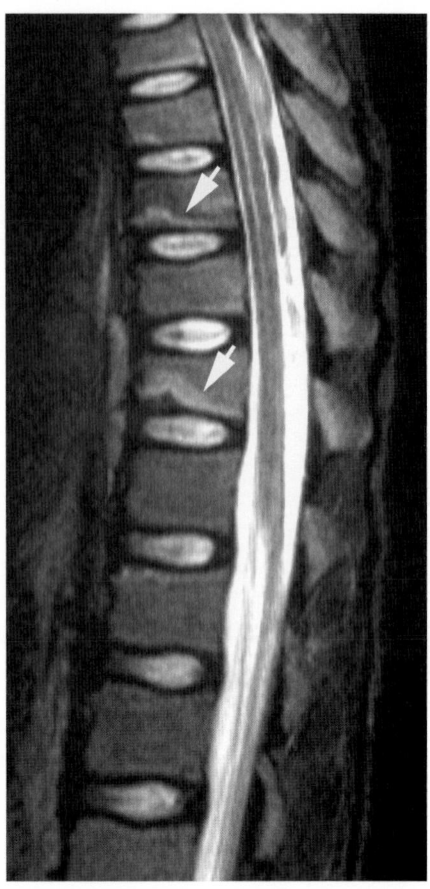

FIGURE 71-8 ■ **Acute leukaemia.** Sagittal T2W FSE MRI of the thoracolumbar junction showing multilevel end-plate fractures (arrows).

LEUKAEMIA[5]

Leukaemia accounts for approximately 25–33% of all childhood malignancy, the vast majority being the acute form. Acute lymphocytic leukaemia (ALL) accounts for 75%, acute myeloid leukaemia (AML) for 20% and other types for 5% of cases. Chronic leukaemias predominate in adults but sometimes terminate in an acute blastic form. While radiographic demonstration of bone lesions in children is relatively common, skeletal lesions in adults tend to be uncommon and focal, often simulating metastases.

Clinical Features

ALL usually presents in children at 2–3 years of age, while AML is most commonly seen in the first 2 years of life, and then also in adolescence. The acute disease is often insidious, with non-specific malaise, anorexia, fever, petechiae and weight loss. Limb pain and pathological fracture are common. Bone pain at presentation is five times more common in children than adults, being reported in over 33% of cases.

Adults are most commonly affected by ALL and chronic myeloid leukaemia (CML). Most skeletal lesions in adults affect sites of residual red marrow, the axial skeleton and proximal ends of the femora and humeri. Chronic lymphatic leukaemia (CLL) is a disease of the elderly, characterised by enlargement of the spleen and lymph nodes with skeletal involvement being rare, except as a terminal event.

Radiological Features

Radiological evidence of bone involvement in acute paediatric leukaemia is reported in approximately 40% at the time of presentation, the incidence of the various features being as follows: osteolysis (13.1%), metaphyseal bands (9.8%), osteopenia (9%), osteosclerosis (7.4%), permeative bone destruction (5.7%), pathological fracture (5.7%), periosteal reaction (4.1%) and mixed lytic–sclerotic lesions (2.5%).[6] However, such changes will be seen in up to 75% of children during the course of their disease.

Diffuse osteopenia is reported in 16–41% of cases and either may be metabolic in aetiology due to protein and mineral deficiencies or may be related to diffuse marrow infiltration with leukaemic cells. The effects of corticosteroids and chemotherapy also contribute to osteoporosis. Compression fractures occur in association with osteopenia of the spine (Fig. 71-8), while approximately 1% of children treated for leukaemia develop osteonecrosis.

Metaphyseal lucent bands primarily affect sites of maximum growth, such as the distal femur, proximal tibia and distal radius, but other metaphyses and the vertebral

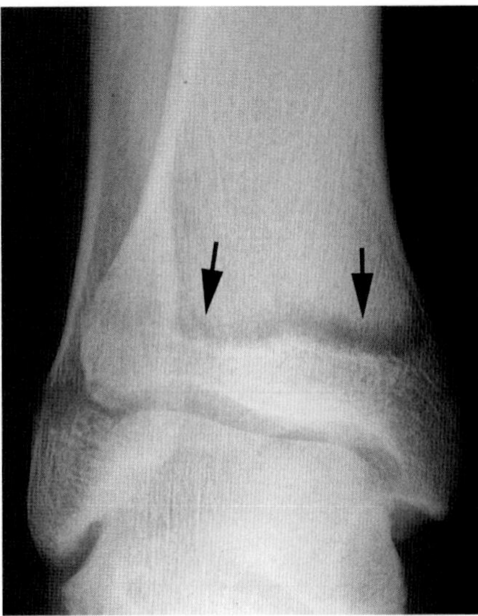

FIGURE 71-9 ■ **Acute leukaemia.** AP radiograph of the right ankle showing metaphyseal lucent bands (arrows).

bodies are affected later. They are typically 2–15 mm in width (Fig. 71-9). These changes are non-specific, with the differential diagnosis including generalised infection, although this is more common in infancy. In children over the age of 2 years, leukaemia is more likely.

More extensive involvement results in diffuse, permeative bone destruction (Fig. 71-10) similar to the spread of highly malignant tumours such as Ewing sarcoma. The cortex becomes eroded on its endosteal surface and may ultimately be destroyed. The permeative pattern is reported in 18% of leukaemic children and may indicate a poor prognosis.

Osteolytic lesions secondary to bone destruction typically have a moth-eaten appearance and most commonly affect the metaphyses of long bones. Such lesions are reported in 10–40% of patients and predispose to pathological fracture. A particular focal lesion in AML is granulocytic sarcoma (chloroma), which is usually located in the skull, spine, ribs or sternum of children. This is an expanding geographical tumour caused by a collection of leukaemic cells and is reported to occur in 4.7% of patients.

Osteosclerosis is rare, being reported in 6% of cases. Sclerotic changes in the metaphyses of long bones may occur spontaneously or as a result of therapy. Mixed

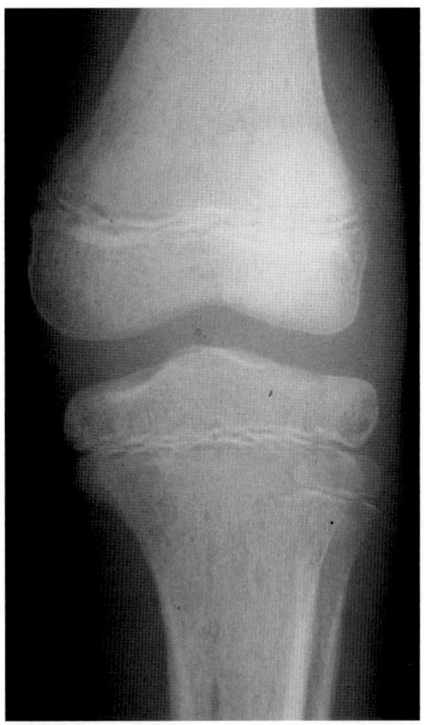

FIGURE 71-10 ■ **Acute leukaemia.** AP radiograph of the left knee showing permeative bone destruction in the distal femur and proximal tibia.

lytic–sclerotic lesions are identified in around 18% of children. Periosteal reaction is reported in 2–50% of cases and may occur in isolation or in association with destructive cortical lesions. It is due to haemorrhage or proliferation of leukaemic deposits deep to the periosteum. Non-specific cortical destruction may involve the medial aspect of the proximal humerus, tibia and sometimes femur.

In adults, skeletal lesions are less common and must be differentiated from metastases or a primary malignant bone neoplasm.

MRI typically demonstrates diffuse marrow infiltration with reduction of T1W SI in affected areas. A change from normal to nodular to diffuse low SI can be seen with disease progression, together with an increase in the extent of SI abnormality. Response to therapy is also demonstrable. MRI can identify complications of treatment such as osteonecrosis.

LYMPHOMA[7–9]

Lymphoma encompasses Hodgkin's and non-Hodgkin's disease, Burkitt's lymphoma and mycosis fungoides (cutaneous T-cell lymphoma), these lymphoreticular neoplasms primarily arising in extraskeletal locations with osseous involvement usually being secondary to hematogenous spread or by direct extension from surrounding involved lymph nodes or soft tissues. Secondary skeletal involvement implies stage IV disease and is usually identified during the course of the disease, or at staging or when it becomes symptomatic. Primary bone lymphoma is a relatively rare condition.

PRIMARY LYMPHOMA OF BONE[10,11]

Clinical Features

Primary lymphoma of bone (PLB) is a rare condition that has been described as lymphomatous involvement of the

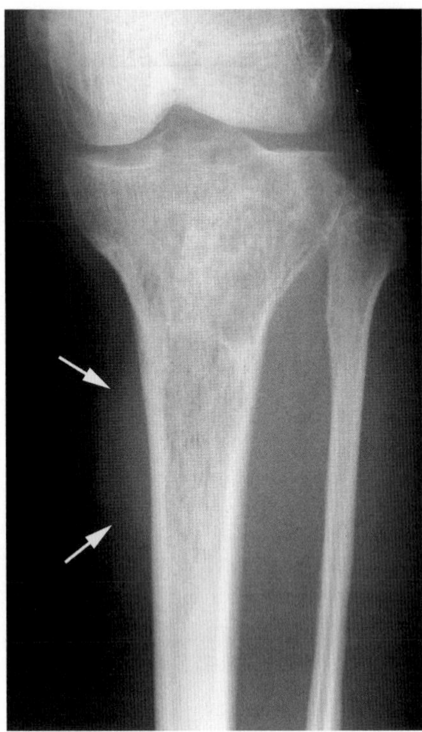

FIGURE 71-11 ■ Primary lymphoma of bone. AP radiograph of the proximal right tibia showing an extensive area of permeative bone destruction with an associated soft-tissue mass (arrows).

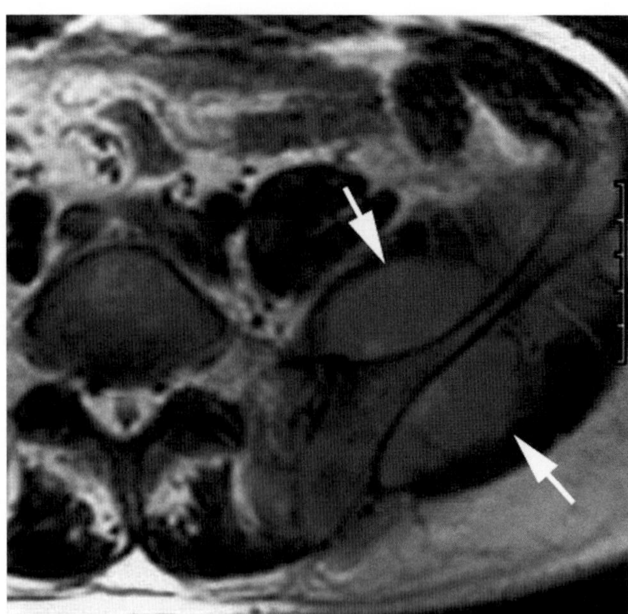

FIGURE 71-12 ■ Primary lymphoma of bone. Axial T2W FSE MRI of the left ilium shows relatively low SI of the extraosseous mass (arrows). Note also the relative preservation of the cortex.

bone marrow, which may be focal or multifocal (termed primary multifocal osseous lymphoma or multifocal PLB) and involve regional lymph nodes, but without distant disease at presentation or within 6 months of presentation. PLB accounts for 5% of all extranodal lymphomas. The majority are non-Hodgkin's lymphomas (NHLs) of the diffuse large B-cell subtype, with primary osseous involvement by Hodgkin's disease being very rare. Most patients present in the fifth to sixth decades of life (median age 42–54 years) with bone pain and/or a soft-tissue mass and the disease is more common in males (M:F ratio 1.5–2.3:1).

Radiological Features

Approximately 70% of PLB involves the major long bones (femur, tibia, humerus), usually arising in the metadiaphyseal region. However, epiphyseal lesions with joint involvement are also recognised. The flat bones and spine can also be involved. Disease limited to the marrow space may be radiologically occult, but the vast majority result in moth-eaten or permeative bone destruction (Fig. 71-11), with only 2% being osteoblastic. Pathological fracture occurs in 17–22% of cases. An aggressive periosteal reaction is seen in 50% and approximately 50–75% of patients will have an associated soft-tissue mass (Fig. 71-11), which is optimally demonstrated by MRI and is indicative of more aggressive disease with a worse prognosis. The combination of a large soft-tissue mass and relative preservation of the cortex is a well-recognised feature of bone lymphoma. MRI signal characteristics are non-specific,[12] but relatively low T2W SI is a recognised feature (Fig. 71-12).

Multifocal PLB accounts for 11–33% of cases and more commonly involves the spine (Fig. 71-13), the imaging characteristics being as described above. Multifocal disease can be detected by whole-body scintigraphy[13] or whole-body MRI.[14] Diffuse skeletal involvement results in a generalised reduction of T1W SI with increased marrow SI on STIR (Fig. 71-14). Enlarged regional lymph nodes may also be seen.

HODGKIN'S LYMPHOMA[7–9]

Clinical Features

Hodgkin's disease (HD) accounts for 25% of all lymphomas and is characterised by the Reed–Sternberg cell, which is usually a B cell. Between 1 and 4% of patients with HD present with a skeletal lesion, while 5–32% will develop bone involvement during the course of the disease.

Three-quarters of patients present between 20 and 30 years of age, with a second peak occurring after the age of 60 years. A slight male predominance (1.4:1) is found and the spine is the commonest site of involvement, from either direct lymph node extension or haematological spread. The pelvis, ribs, femora and sternum are the other commonly involved sites. HD presents as PLB in 6% of cases.

Radiological Features

Approximately one-third of skeletal lesions are solitary, and whole-body staging with scintigraphy or whole-body MRI is mandatory to identify further lesions. Osteolytic

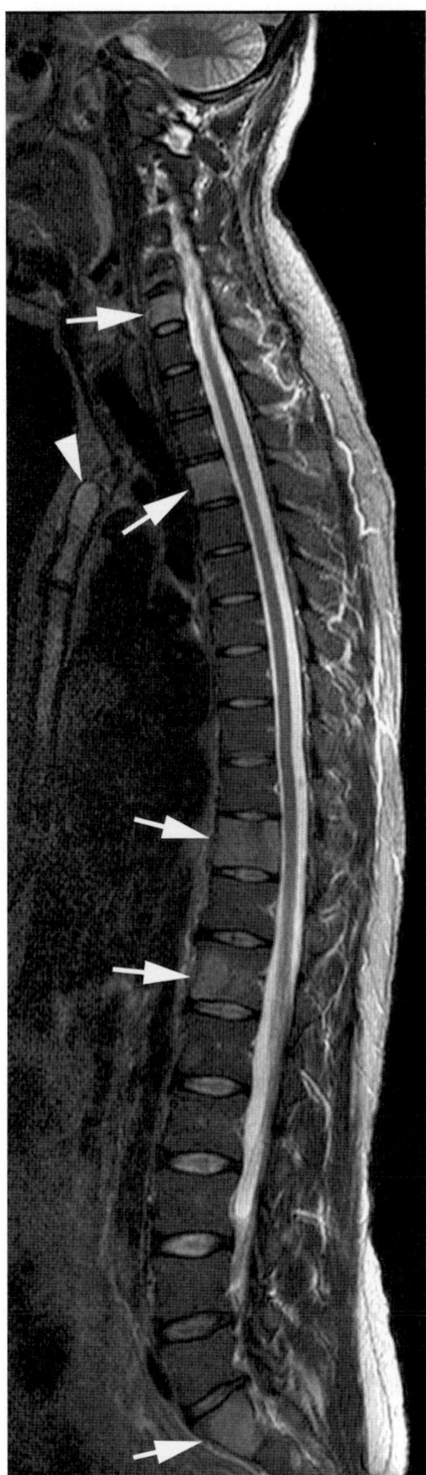

FIGURE 71-13 ■ Primary multifocal osseous lymphoma. Sagittal STIR MRI of the spine showing multilevel vertebral (arrows) and sternal (arrowhead) marrow infiltration.

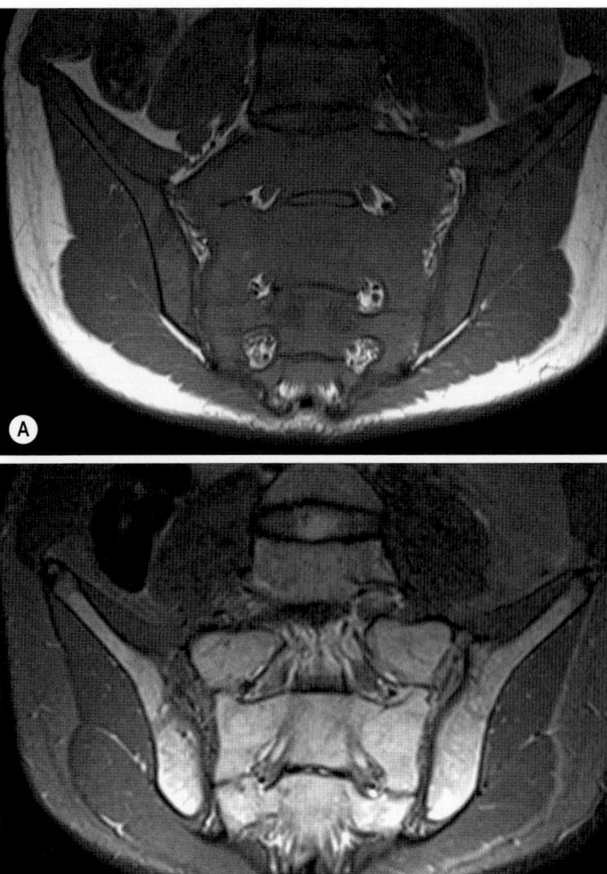

FIGURE 71-14 ■ Primary multifocal osseous lymphoma. (A) Coronal T1W SE and (B) STIR MRI showing diffuse reduction of T1W and increased STIR marrow SI.

lesions or mixed lytic–sclerotic lesions account for almost 90% of cases, the remainder being purely sclerotic.

In the spine, HD most commonly causes sclerosis, although it is an uncommon cause of 'ivory' vertebra. Vertebral collapse takes place early, with lytic lesions, occasionally producing vertebra plana. Erosion of the anterior border of one or more vertebral bodies is also found, possibly by direct spread from affected prevertebral lymph nodes. Such features are best shown with MRI. In the thoracic region, paravertebral masses may precede radiographic evidence of bony involvement, while mediastinal disease is a recognised cause of hypertrophic osteoarthropathy.

Rib involvement is common, with multiple lytic lesions associated with soft-tissue masses predominating. Occasionally the ribs appear expanded. In the pelvis, involved nodes may invade the bone directly, usually in the posterior half of the ilium. Mixed lesions are relatively common and the ischium and pubic rami may show expansion. Direct haematogenous involvement of the sternum is common. The typical lesion is lytic and expanding, associated with a soft-tissue mass.

CT clearly demonstrates all of the described radiological features, and in addition will show the associated extraosseous mass (Fig. 71-15). Sequestrum formation is also a recognised feature of bone lymphoma. Marrow involvement is most sensitively detected by MRI[13] and may be focal or diffuse. However, the SI characteristics are non-specific. In focal involvement, MR can be used to guide biopsy.

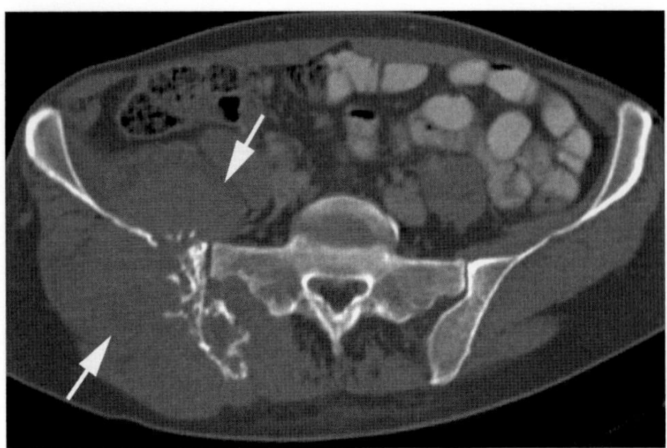

FIGURE 71-15 ■ **Hodgkin's disease.** CT of the pelvis showing an aggressive destructive lesion of the posterior right iliac blade with a large soft-tissue mass (arrows).

NON-HODGKIN'S LYMPHOMA[7–9]

Clinical Features

Non-Hodgkin's lymphoma (NHL) is the commonest haematopoietic neoplasm and comprises a variety of clinicopathological subtypes, the majority of which are of B-cell origin. Predisposing factors include AIDS and transplant-related immunosuppression. Skeletal involvement may be either primary (see above) or secondary. Secondary skeletal involvement occurs in 20–30% of children and 10–20% of adults with NHL, but detection of an osseous lesion at initial presentation is uncommon.

Radiological Features

The radiological features are similar to those described for HD. Children with generalised NHL tend to have widespread skeletal involvement manifesting as osteopenia. MRI may show multifocal marrow lesions before the diffuse infiltration of established disease. MRI may also be used to stage disease and will occasionally demonstrate marrow disease despite negative iliac crest biopsy. Although the MRI appearances are non-specific, the presence of a paravertebral soft-tissue mass with maintenance of the cortical outline of the vertebral body is highly suggestive of lymphoma.

BURKITT'S LYMPHOMA[15]

Burkitt's lymphoma is a high-grade NHL with distinctive clinical and histological features. A causative relationship to the Epstein–Barr virus and more recently HIV is probable. A 74% 4-year survival rate is reported.

Clinical Features

The disease shows a male: female ratio of 2 : 1, affecting mainly African children. Large tumours affect the jawbones and abdominal viscera. The mean age at presentation is 7 years, with a range of 2–16 years. Added to this endemic (African) group are the non-endemic (sporadic) cases, mainly in white children. The jaw is the initial focus in about 50% of patients, although less so in non-endemic cases. Other sites of involvement include the pelvis, long bones and bones of the hands and feet.

Radiological Features

The jaw lesion is generally destructive, starting in the medulla and later affecting the cortex. Bone destruction and dental displacement in the enlarging soft-tissue mass give the appearance of 'floating' teeth. Lesions in other bones show similar appearances and periosteal reaction may be present in all locations. Full assessment and staging is required for this multicentric neoplasm.

PLASMA CELL DISORDERS[16]

PLASMACYTOMA

Solitary plasmacytoma accounts for less than 5% of patients with plasma cell tumours. It may remain localised for many years but more than 30% progress quite rapidly to generalised myelomatosis.

Clinical Features

Presentation with pain is common and the age of presentation tends to be earlier than in multiple myeloma (MM). As plasma protein changes are related to the total tumour mass, protein electrophoresis is often normal and the erythrocyte sedimentation rate (ESR) is also normal or only slightly elevated.

Radiological Features

Plasmacytoma is typically lytic and destructive with sclerosis being rare. The lesion arises in the medulla and the radiological features suggest a relatively slow growth rate. The margin is often well defined and cortical thinning with expansion is usually present (Fig. 71-16). Apparent trabeculation or a 'soap bubble' appearance is common and an associated soft-tissue mass is frequently seen. Affected sites usually contain persistent red marrow and include the axial skeleton, pelvis, proximal femur, proximal humerus and ribs. Following the diagnosis of plasmacytoma, whole-body MRI is indicated to identify additional lesions,[17] which may be seen in up to 80% of cases. Occult lesions may also be demonstrated by FDG PET-CT.[18]

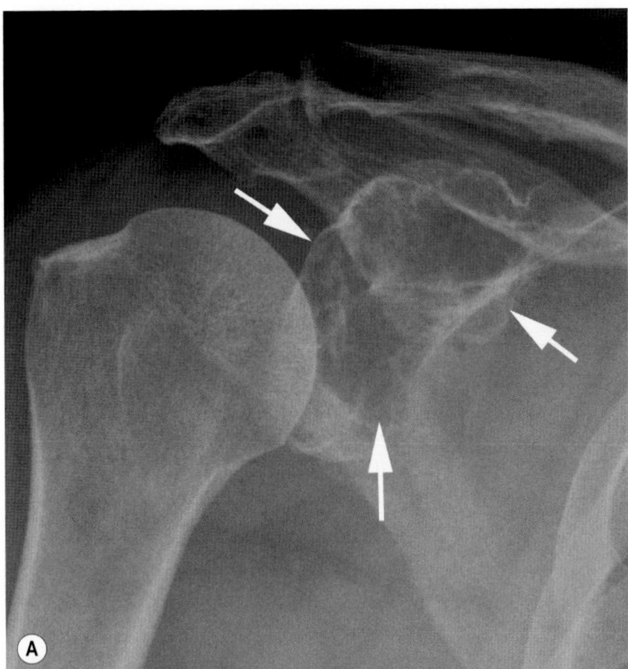

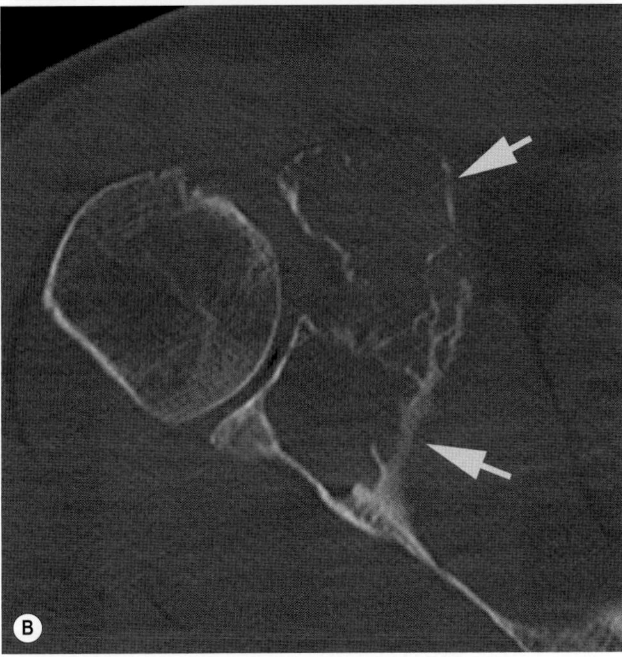

FIGURE 71-16 ■ **Plasmacytoma.** (A) AP radiograph of the shoulder showing a well-defined lytic lesion (arrows) in the bony glenoid. (B) Axial CT shows the expansile nature of the lesion with a thinned but largely intact cortex (arrows).

Involvement of a vertebral body is common, sometimes leading to early collapse. Extension across the disc space is a rare feature. The differential diagnosis includes metastatic carcinoma, which rarely destroys two or three bodies in continuity, and infection. A solitary plasmacytoma in the spine may show characteristic MRI features, particularly the presence of peripheral thickened trabeculae.[19] In long and flat bones, plasmacytoma may resemble an aneurysmal bone cyst or an expanding metastasis.

MULTIPLE MYELOMA[20–23]

Multiple myeloma (MM) is the most common primary malignant neoplasm of bone and is the predominant plasma cell neoplasm, accounting for approximately 1% of all malignant disease and 10% of haematological malignancies.

Symptomatic MM is diagnosed by the following: (1) >10% atypical plasma cells on bone marrow aspirate/biopsy or plasmacytoma; (2) monoclonal paraprotein present in blood or urine; and (3) myeloma-related organ or tissue impairment (including nephropathy, hypercalcaemia, anaemia and bone lesions). The presence of only the first two criteria represents asymptomatic (smouldering) myeloma, while isolated elevation of serum M-protein (<30 g/L) is termed monoclonal gammopathy of uncertain significance (MGUS).

Clinical Features

Three-quarters of affected patients are over 50 years of age (median age 65 years) and approximately 3% of patients present before the age of 40 years. There is a male predominance of up to 2 : 1. Widespread involvement of the skeleton is present in 80%, the axial skeleton and proximal ends of the long bones being particularly involved. Fever, pain, backache and weakness are common symptoms. Amyloidosis is reported in approximately 20% of patients with MM.

Radiological Features

The classical appearance of MM consists of well-defined 'punched-out' lesions throughout the skeleton (Fig. 71-17), most characteristic in the skull (Fig. 71-18). The only common differential diagnosis in this age group is metastatic disease. The presence of multiple small (up to 20 mm), well-defined round or oval lesions is more suggestive of MM.

Diffuse osteopenia usually involves the spine and may result in multiple compression fractures. Pathological fracture of the vertebrae affects approximately 50% of patients at some stage. Osteoblastic or mixed lesions are rare in untreated patients, but marginal sclerosis may be observed following radiotherapy. Purely sclerotic myeloma is recognised and may be associated with POEMS syndrome, a paraneoplastic condition due to an underlying plasma cell neoplasm. The major criteria for the syndrome are polyradiculoneuropathy, clonal plasma cell disorder (PCD), sclerotic bone lesions, elevated vascular endothelial growth factor and the presence of Castleman disease.[24]

Multidetector CT (MDCT) is more sensitive than radiography in detecting myeloma and a low-dose technique can be used to limit radiation to the patient. Sagittal reconstructions of the spine and coronal whole-body reconstructions are typically performed. Purely marrow lesions appear as focal areas of soft-tissue density, but the diffuse osteopenia of MM may be indistinguishable from other causes such as osteoporosis. Progressive disease results in endosteal scalloping (Fig. 71-19), cortical destruction and soft-tissue masses. Low-dose MDCT is

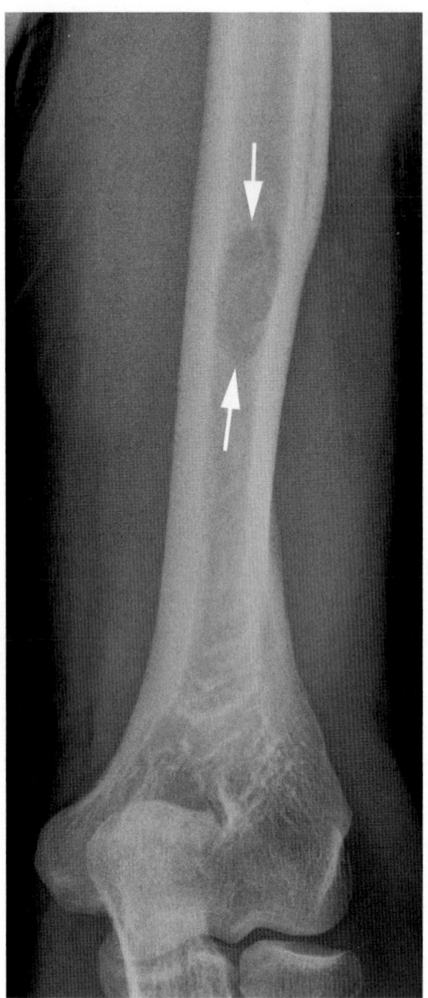

FIGURE 71-17 ■ **Multiple myeloma.** AP radiograph of the humerus demonstrating a well-defined lytic lesion (arrows) in the diaphysis.

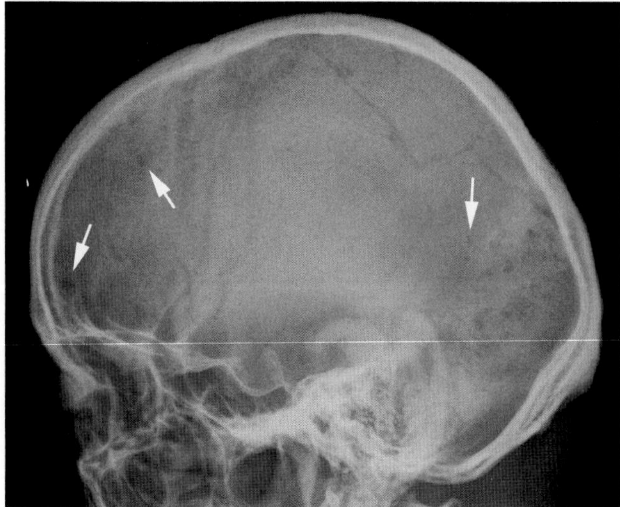

FIGURE 71-18 ■ **Multiple myeloma.** Lateral radiograph of the skull showing multiple small lytic lesions (arrows).

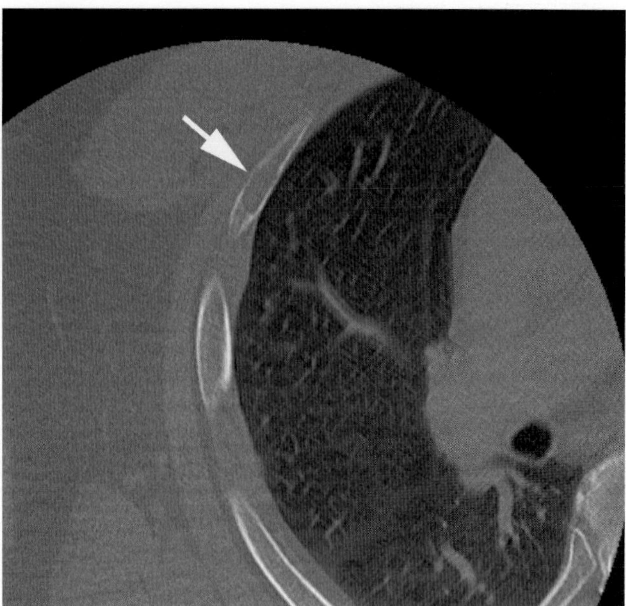

FIGURE 71-19 ■ **Multiple myeloma.** Axial CT showing a radiologically occult, well-defined oval lytic lesion, which is resulting in mild endosteal scalloping (arrow).

also valuable in excluding myeloma lesions in patients with MGUS.[25]

The MRI appearances in MM are variable, with five patterns described. A normal marrow pattern may be seen in patients with low-grade plasma cell infiltration of the marrow spaces, and occasionally in stage III disease. A focal pattern consists of localised areas of decreased SI on T1W images with corresponding increased SI on T2W and STIR images, seen in 30% of cases. Occasionally, focal lesions may be relatively hyperintense on T1W and identified only on fat-suppressed T2W images. The diffuse pattern manifests as generalised reduction of marrow SI on T1W, such that the intervertebral discs appear hyperintense compared with the vertebral bodies. The marrow appears hyperintense on fat-suppressed T2W and STIR images and shows diffuse enhancement following gadolinium. A combined focal and diffuse pattern may also be seen (Fig. 71-20). Finally, a 'variegated' pattern, which consists of multiple tiny foci of reduced SI on T1W and hyperintensity on T2W/STIR on a background of normal marrow (Fig. 71-21), is described. This pattern is seen almost always in early disease. These patterns have some prognostic value, in that patients with diffuse marrow abnormality on MRI will have a poorer outcome than those with a normal MRI pattern.

Whole-body MRI is far more sensitive than skeletal survey for the detection of lesions and can result in a significant change in the staging of the disease.[26] The Durie and Salmon PLUS staging system for MM now includes whole-body imaging information from MRI and FDG PET-CT, compared to the original Durie and Salmon staging system which relied on radiographic skeletal survey. MRI also allows assessment of response to therapy, with a normalisation of marrow SI being indicative of a good response.

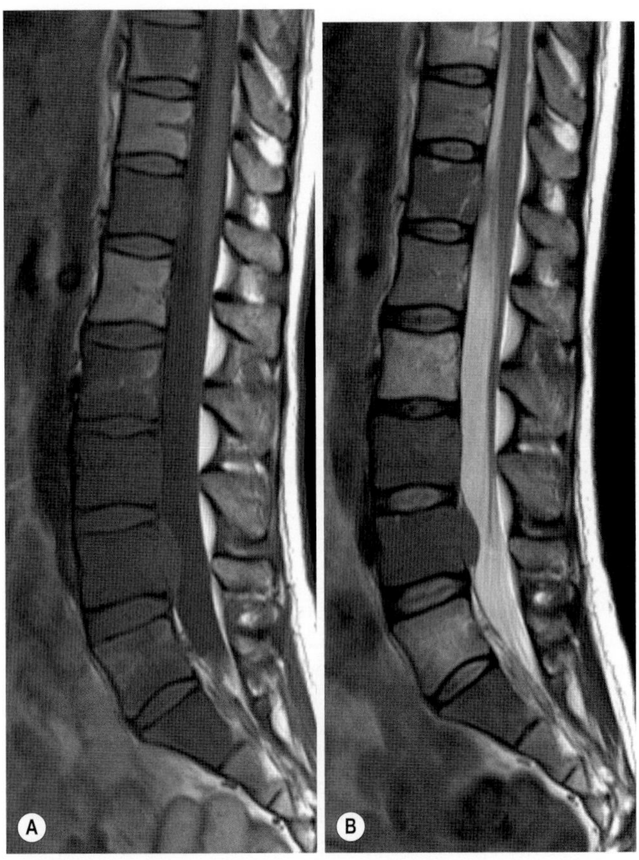

FIGURE 71-20 ■ Multiple myeloma. (A) Sagittal T1W SE and (B) T2W FSE MRI of the lumbar spine showing a combined pattern of diffuse and focal vertebral marrow infiltration.

Vertebral fractures in MM occur in 55–70% of cases and may be benign, due to diffuse osteopenia (~66%), or pathological due to tumour infiltration (~33%), the majority occurring in the thoracolumbar region. MRI is valuable in the differentiation of benign versus malignant collapse. MRI may also demonstrate other complications, such as steroid-induced marrow infarction.

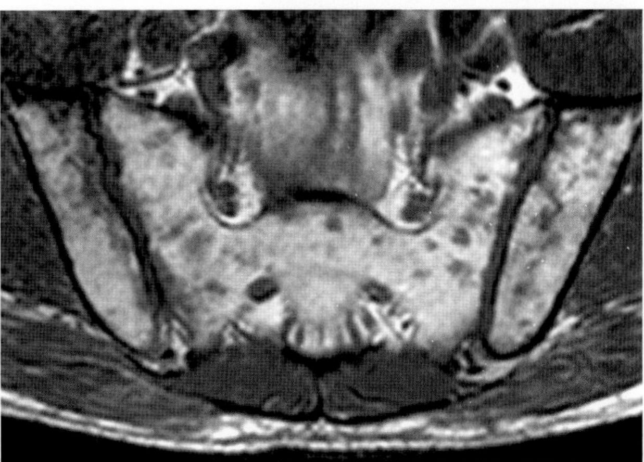

FIGURE 71-21 ■ Multiple myeloma. Axial T1W SE MRI of the sacrum showing the 'variegated' pattern of marrow infiltration.

For a full list of references, please see ExpertConsult.

FURTHER READING

3. Guermazi A, de Kerviler E, Cazals-Hatem D, et al. Imaging findings in patients with myelofibrosis. Eur Radiol 1999;9:1366–75.
4. Fritz J, Fishman EK, Carrino JA, Horger MS. Advanced imaging of skeletal manifestations of systemic mastocytosis. Skeletal Radiol 2012;41(8):887–97.
5. Guillerman RP, Voss SD, Parker BR. Leukemia and lymphoma. Radiol Clin North Am 2011;49:767–97.
14. Berger FH, van Dijke CF, Maas M. Diffuse marrow changes. Semin Musculoskelet Radiol 2009;13:104–10.
17. Terpos E, Moulopoulos LA, Dimopoulos MA. Advances in imaging and the management of myeloma bone disease. J Clin Oncol 2011;29:1907–15.
22. Shortt CP, Carty F, Murray JG. The role of whole-body imaging in the diagnosis, staging, and follow-up of multiple myeloma. Semin Musculoskelet Radiol 2010;14:37–46.
23. Hanrahan CJ, Christensen CR, Crim JR. Current concepts in the evaluation of multiple myeloma with MR imaging and FDG PET/CT. Radiographics 2010;30:127–42.

CHAPTER 72

Bone Marrow Disorders: Miscellaneous

Asif Saifuddin

Chapters 71 and 72 deal with a variety of blood-related disorders that have a major influence on imaging of the skeletal system.

DISORDERS OF RED CELLS

In late fetal life and infancy, the entire bone marrow is utilised for red blood cell (RBC) formation, supplemented by extramedullary erythropoiesis in the liver and spleen. As the child becomes older and RBC life span increases, erythropoiesis is withdrawn from the liver and spleen, then gradually from the diaphyses of the long bones, so that by the age of 25 years, active bone marrow is confined to the axial skeleton, the flat bones and the proximal ends of the femora and humeri.[1] This process of withdrawal will not occur with a need for extra erythropoiesis and reverses in the presence of increased RBC destruction.

The Anaemias

Only chronic anaemias affect the radiological appearances of bone. Anaemias that do not produce reactive erythropoiesis, such as aplastic anaemia, do not affect the skeletal radiograph, but may manifest on MRI as a generalised increase in fatty marrow signal intensity (SI).[1] Also, the myelodysplastic syndromes may manifest as diffuse reduction of T1-weighted (T1W) marrow SI due to marrow reconversion.[1] A variety of inherited syndromes, such as Fanconi's anaemia, may be associated with skeletal dysplasia, but these are not an effect of the anaemia per se and will not be discussed.

CHRONIC HAEMOLYTIC ANAEMIAS

The Haemoglobinopathies[1]

The haemoglobin molecule consists of a protein (globin) and four haem groups, each with four pyrrole rings surrounding an iron atom. The protein moiety consists of 574 amino acids arranged in four spiral polypeptide chains. The different chains are designated by letters of the Greek alphabet (α, β) and the three normal haemoglobins (Hbs) A, A2 and F each contain two α chains, differing only in their second pairs.

Three types of haemoglobinopathy are found:

1. Thalassaemia: an inherited defect of HbA synthesis with inadequate manufacture of α- or β-chains.
2. Haemoglobin variants: inherited defects of HbA synthesis producing abnormal α- or β-chains. All the variants differ from HbA by the substitution of only one amino acid in the chain: e.g. HbS (sickle-cell anaemia) where valine is substituted for glutamine at residue 6 in the β-chain.
3. Combination of thalassaemia and abnormal haemoglobin, e.g. HbS–thalassaemia.

Thalassaemia[1–3]

Thalassaemia is an inherited disorder and exists in two forms, the homozygous (thalassaemia major) and heterozygous (thalassaemia intermedia and thalassaemia minor), and may affect production of either α- or β-chains, resulting in α-thalassaemia or β-thalassaemia, respectively.

β-Thalassaemia is prevalent in the Mediterranean countries (Greece, southern Italy and the Mediterranean islands), while α-thalassaemia is encountered in those of West African descent.

Clinical Features. Thalassaemia major causes severe childhood anaemia with hepatosplenomegaly, extramedullary erythropoiesis and secondary skeletal deformity. Treatment is by regular blood transfusion in infancy to maintain a haemoglobin level of 9–10 g/dL, iron chelation with agents such as desferrioxamine (DFX) to prevent/reduce iron overload, and bisphosphonates to treat the associated osteoporosis. With the introduction of successful transfusion regimes, the skeletal changes due to the disorder itself are now less commonly encountered, but osseous complications related to repeated transfusion and the effects of DFX therapy must be recognised.

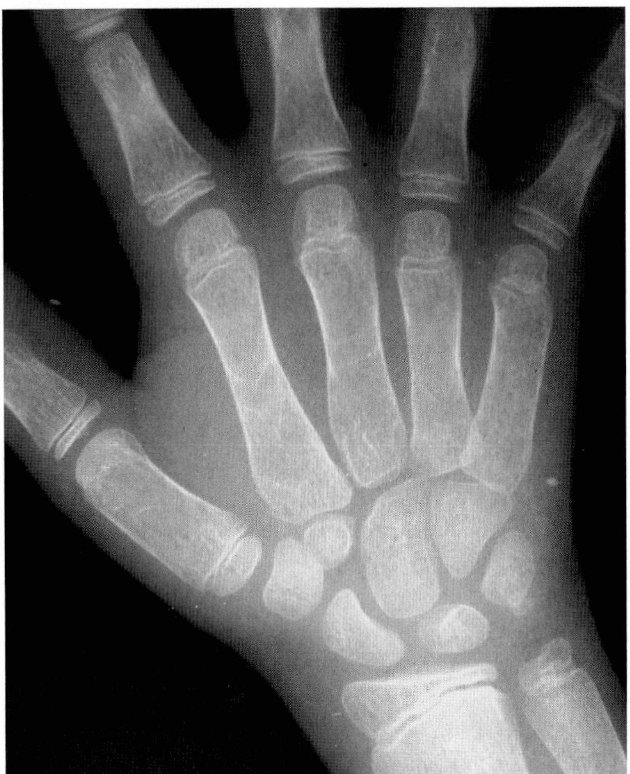

FIGURE 72-1 ■ **Thalassaemia.** AP radiograph of the hand demonstrates generalised osteopenia, medullary expansion with cortical thinning and coarse trabeculae.

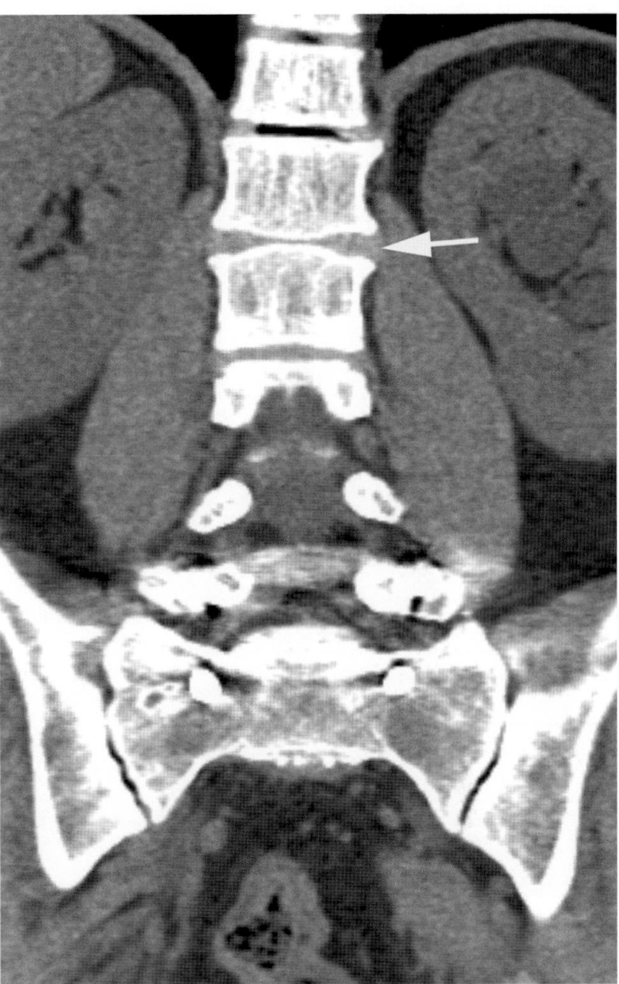

FIGURE 72-2 ■ **Thalassaemia.** Coronal CT MPR showing vertical trabecular thickening in the vertebral bodies, convexity of the end-plates adjacent to the L1–L2 disc (arrow) and advanced T11–T12 and T12–L1 disc degeneration with vacuum phenomenon.

Radiological Features[1,2]

Untreated Thalassaemia Major. Skeletal changes in untreated children are essentially the result of chronic anaemia and marrow hyperplasia (15–30 times normal) and are most commonly seen after the age of 1 year, affecting almost all regions of the skeleton. Medullary hyperplasia results in bony expansion and cortical thinning, which in long bones produces the characteristic Erlenmeyer flask appearance, also found in conditions such as Gaucher's disease. Within the medulla, trabecular thinning initially occurs, followed by trabecular coarsening due to new bone formation, the changes being most marked in the metacarpals and phalanges, which become cylindrical or even biconvex (Fig. 72-1). Trabecular coarsening may also be seen in the pelvis and vertebrae (Fig. 72-2). The ribs are similarly affected with club-like anterior ends, while a 'rib-within-a-rib' appearance also occurs due to subperiosteal extension of haematopoietic tissue through the rib cortex.

Extramedullary erythropoiesis occurs in severe cases surviving to adulthood, the most common sites being the thoracic paravertebral region by extension from the adjacent ribs, the mediastinum (Fig. 72-3) and presacral region (Fig. 72-4). Epidural extension from paraspinal extramedullary erythropoiesis may result in spinal cord compression. These features are optimally demonstrated by MRI, which also shows diffuse reduction in marrow signal intensity (SI) on T1W images caused by marrow reconversion (Fig. 72-4).

With severe childhood disease, the paranasal sinuses develop poorly and often contain red marrow, accounting for the facial abnormalities (seen in 17%) and dental malocclusion. The ethmoidal cells are spared since they contain no red marrow. The diploë of the skull vault are widened, except in the occiput. These changes occur earliest and most severely in the frontal bone, producing the classical 'hair-on-end' appearance (Fig. 72-5). Occasionally, well-defined lytic lesions may be seen in the skull.

Spinal changes consist of generalised osteopenia, resulting in compression fractures and biconcavity of the vertebral bodies. Despite optimised therapy, osteoporosis may still be seen in as many as 90% of cases based on DEXA studies. Scoliosis is reported in 20% of children with thalassaemia major, while early disc degeneration is also a feature (Fig. 72-2), optimally demonstrated by MRI.

Premature fusion of the growth plates may contribute to short stature. These radiological changes are reported in ~15% of patients, generally occurring after 10 years of age and most commonly affecting the proximal humerus and distal femur. Growth arrest lines may also be seen.

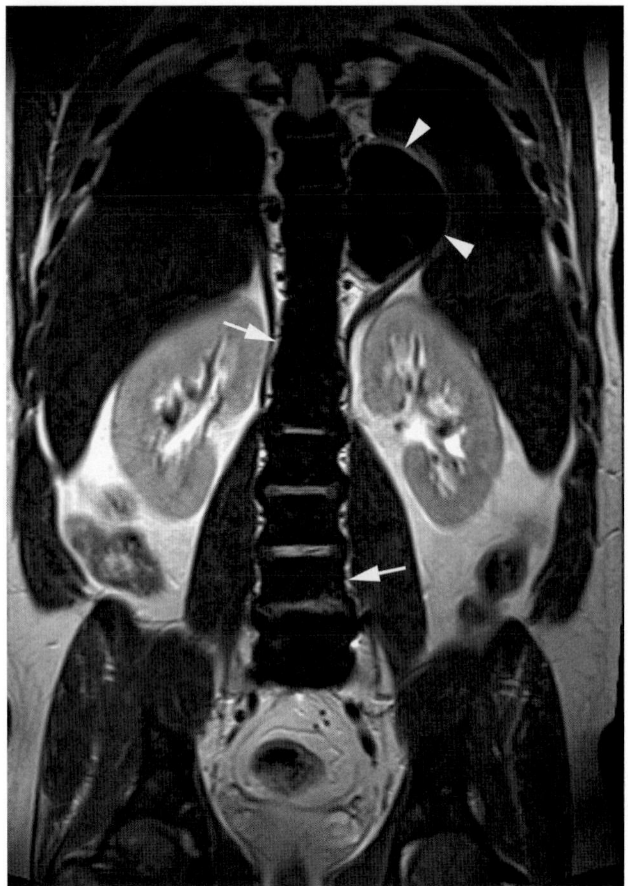

FIGURE 72-3 ■ **Thalassaemia.** Coronal T2W FSE MRI showing profound, diffuse reduction of marrow SI (arrows) and a large left paraspinal soft-tissue mass (arrowheads) due to extramedullary erythropoiesis.

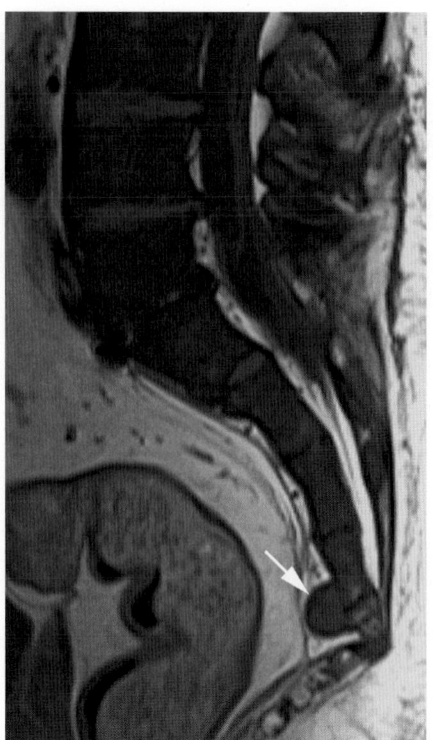

FIGURE 72-4 ■ **Thalassaemia.** Sagittal T1W SE MRI showing marked reduction of marrow SI (arrows) such that the discs appear hyperintense, and a small pre-sacral mass (arrowhead) due to extramedullary erythropoiesis.

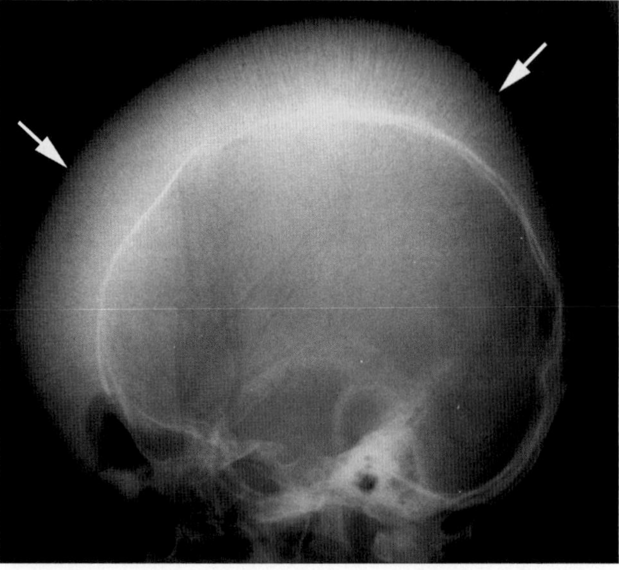

FIGURE 72-5 ■ **Thalassaemia.** Lateral radiograph of the skull showing marked thickening of the skull vault with a 'hair-on-end' appearance (arrows).

Hypertransfusion. Repeated transfusion therapy may produce iron overload and hyperuricaemia. Raised blood iron levels result in synovial and articular cartilage abnormalities, manifesting radiologically as symmetrical loss of joint space, cystic changes, subchondral collapse and osteophytosis. Chondrocalcinosis may also be seen and the larger joints tend to be more commonly affected than in primary haemochromatosis. Occasionally, the radiographic changes of gout may be evident and there is also a predisposition to osteonecrosis and osteomyelitis. Iron deposition within bone also contributes to osteoporosis and is a further cause of reduced marrow SI on MRI, particularly on T2-weighted (T2W; Fig. 72-3) and gradient-echo sequences. MRI may be used to estimate tissue siderosis.[4]

DFX Therapy. Iron chelation therapy is recognised as causing dysplastic changes in the spine and long bones, as well as growth retardation, especially when treatment is started before the age of 3 years and with higher doses. The incidence is unclear, since many cases are asymptomatic. Changes typically occur at the metaphysis/physis/epiphysis of the proximal humerus, distal femur, proximal tibia and distal radius and ulna.

Radiographs and MRI demonstrate irregularity of the metaphyseal–physeal junction with dense sclerotic metaphyseal bands, which may then extend in a 'flame-shaped' manner towards the diaphysis. Splaying of the metaphysis and widening of the growth plate are later features, which resemble rickets. Severe dysplasia at the proximal femur and around the knee may result in SUFE and genu varuma or valguma.

In the spine, platyspondyly and a biconvex contour to the vertebral bodies (Fig. 72-2) are seen and kyphosis may develop. DFX therapy also results in growth retardation, affecting both the axial and appendicular skeleton.

Deferiprone is an alternative treatment to DFX and has been associated with agranulocytosis and arthropathy, most commonly affecting the knees, resulting in effusion and synovitis, which can be demonstrated on MRI. Chronic changes include flattening of the femoral condyles, tibial plateau and patella.

Sickle-Cell Disease[1,5,6]

The clinical findings in sickle-cell disease (SCD) are explained by the physical properties of the abnormal haemoglobin. In situations of hypoxia, intracellular polymerisation of the HbS molecule occurs, rendering the RBC less flexible. Recurrent cycles of oxygenation and deoxygenation lead to irreversible membrane damage to the erythrocyte, causing the cells to become less deformable and sickle-shaped. Sickle cells obstruct small blood vessels, leading to stasis and tissue hypoxia/anoxia and eventually infarction. Sickle cells also have a much shorter circulating life (~1/10th normal), being removed from the circulation prematurely by the reticuloendothelial system, resulting in haemolytic anaemia.

The full clinical and radiological picture occurs in the homozygous sickle-cell subject (HbS-S). When only one parent carries the abnormal gene, the sickle-cell trait (HbS-A) occurs, without anaemia but with sickling to a lesser degree.

Clinical Features. SCD mainly affects people of African racial origin and approximately 8–10% of black Americans have sickle-cell trait, but only 0.2% have sickle-cell anaemia. People from the Middle East and Eastern Mediterranean are also affected. The anaemia of SCD is not as marked as in thalassaemia major. Homozygous SCD reduces average life expectancy by 25–30 years and most patients will die by the age of 50 years.

The most striking clinical features are due to vaso-occlusive sickle crises, which result in infarctions. Medullary infarction involving the small bones of the hands and feet, resulting in sickle-cell dactylitis or 'hand-foot' syndrome, is a common presentation of SCD in infants between 6 months and 2 years of age but is rare after 6 years. Presentation is with pain and swelling of the digits, together with fever, and affects approximately 50% of children with SCD. Marrow infarction may also involve the long bones, in which case it is difficult to differentiate from osteomyelitis, while infarction of the epiphyses results in avascular necrosis, most commonly of the femoral and humeral heads. SCD is the most common cause of osteonecrosis of the femoral head in children, while approximately 50% of all patients will develop osteonecrosis by the age of 35 years. Rib or sternal infarcts may simulate heart or lung disease, while soft-tissue involvement results in ulcers and muscle infarction, which are well demonstrated by MRI.

Osteomyelitis in SCD typically involves the long bone diaphyses and is most commonly due to various *Salmonella* species, with ~10% of cases being due to *Staphylococcus aureus*. The prevalence of osteomyelitis is reported as 18%, while septic arthritis is also relatively common in SCD, with a reported prevalence of 7%.

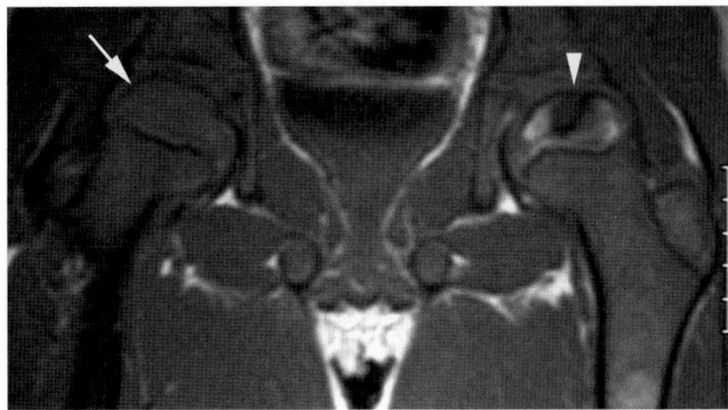

FIGURE 72-6 ■ **Sickle-cell disease.** Coronal T1W SE MRI of the hips in a child showing intermediate SI in the right femoral capital epiphysis (arrow) due to marrow hyperplasia and osteonecrosis on the left side (arrowhead).

Sickle variants show less anaemia with fewer crises. However, bone infarction, especially of the femoral head, affects patients with HbS-C disease five times more often than those with HbS-S, although the overall prevalence of HbS-C is only one-third that of the homozygous disease. This may reflect the longer survival in HbS-C disease. In sickle-cell trait (HbS-A), significant anaemia and bone infarction are rare.

Radiological Features. The changes in SCD and its variants are similar, varying only in degree. Changes can be divided into those due to marrow hyperplasia, bone infarction and secondary osteomyelitis.

Marrow Hyperplasia. This is more severe in the homozygous disease and the radiological features are as described for thalassaemia. Marrow reconversion is well demonstrated by MRI, with replacement of normal fatty marrow by intermediate SI on T1W images, which may extend to involve the epiphyses (Fig. 72-6). Persistence of red marrow predisposes to osteomyelitis and marrow infarction.

Bone Infarction. This is estimated to be at least 50 times more common than osteomyelitis in SCD. In children, sickle-cell dactylitis results in lytic medullary lesions with associated periostitis and soft-tissue swelling (Fig. 72-7). Asymmetrical shortening of tubular bones is a common sequelae to childhood sickling crises. In adolescents and adults, infarction occurs more in the metaphyses and epiphyses. The earliest radiological evidence of bone infarction is laminar periosteal reaction followed by patchy medullary destruction. Healing leads to reactive sclerosis. MRI shows medullary oedema on T2W and short tau inversion recovery (STIR) sequences with associated periostitis and adjacent soft-tissue inflammation, making differentiation from osteomyelitis difficult. With healing, these areas assume a low SI due to fibrosis and medullary sclerosis. Infarction of the metaphyses on either side of the knee is common and may lead to premature fusion of the growth plates.

Infarction of the vertebral body occurs in approximately 10% of patients and is usually due to venous

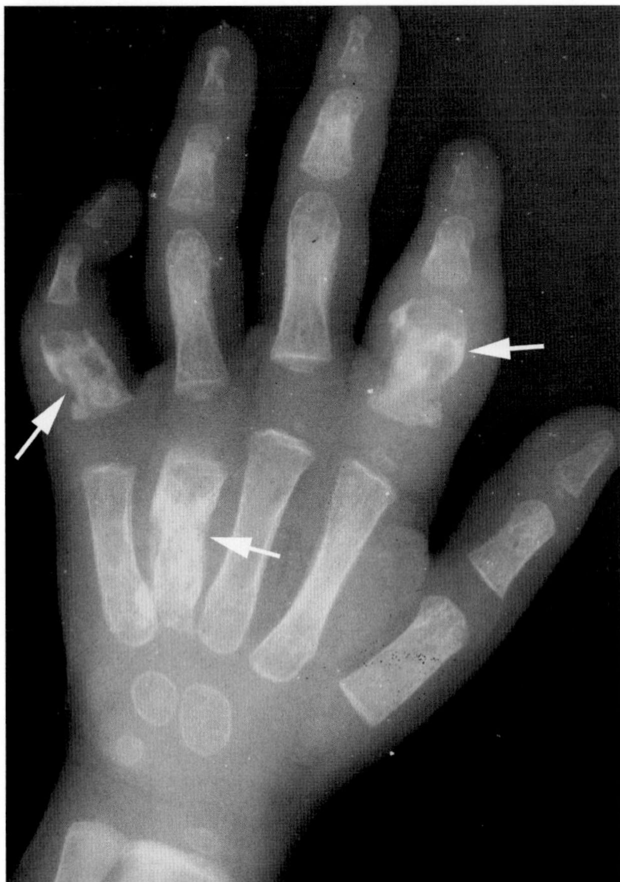

FIGURE 72-7 ■ **Sickle-cell disease: dactylitis.** Infarction in several of the metacarpals and proximal phalanges has resulted in bone destruction (arrows) and swelling of the soft tissues.

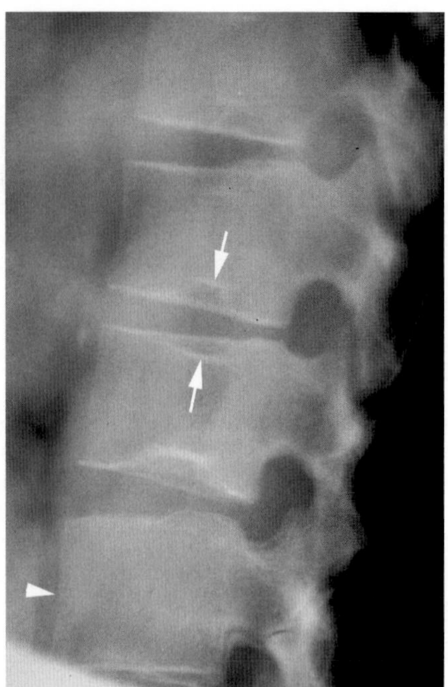

FIGURE 72-8 ■ **Sickle-cell disease.** The classical 'stepped depression' of the vertebral end-plates is seen (arrows), producing the 'H-shaped' vertebra. Note increased height of the adjacent 'tower' vertebra (arrowhead).

thromboembolism in the centre of the vertebral end-plate, with focal collapse producing the 'H-shaped' vertebra. The floor of the depression forms a flat sclerotic margin during healing (Fig. 72-8). This appearance is almost pathognomonic of SCD but has also been reported in Gaucher's disease. Overgrowth of an adjacent vertebral body, producing a 'tower' vertebra, is also reported (Fig. 72-8).

The earliest manifestation of osteonecrosis is epiphyseal oedema seen on MRI. Radiographic abnormalities include mixed lysis and sclerosis with a subchondral fracture being typical. Eventually, secondary osteoarthritis will supervene. Chronic ischaemia or multiple small infarctions in SCD may produce cortical thickening that is both endosteal and periosteal, with narrowing of the marrow cavity (Fig. 72-9). Splitting of the cortex may give rise to a 'bone-within-a-bone' appearance, while secondary myelofibrosis causes medullary sclerosis.

Osteomyelitis. Osteomyelitis usually complicates bone infarction and it may be difficult to distinguish clinically or radiologically between an infarct with infection and one without. *Salmonella* osteomyelitis is common in African children.

Osteomyelitis causes increased bone destruction with laminar or multilaminar periostitis (Fig. 72-10A) and eventual sequestration and involucrum formation. Early

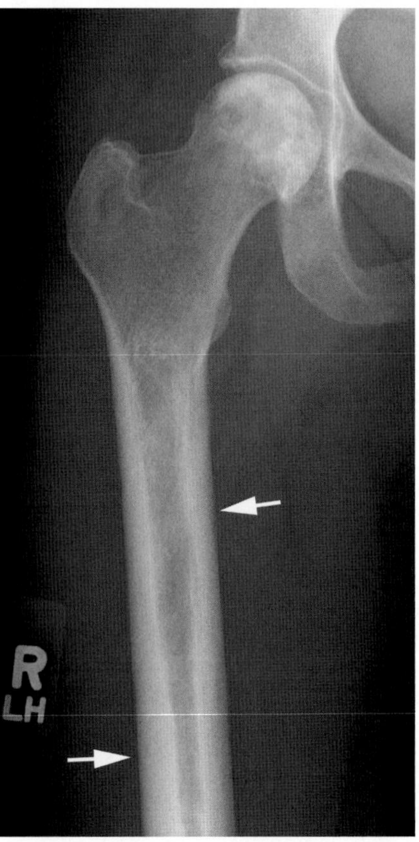

FIGURE 72-9 ■ **Sickle-cell disease.** AP radiograph of the right hip and femur showing heterogeneous femoral head sclerosis due to osteonecrosis and medullary endosteal sclerosis (arrows) due to healed medullary infarction.

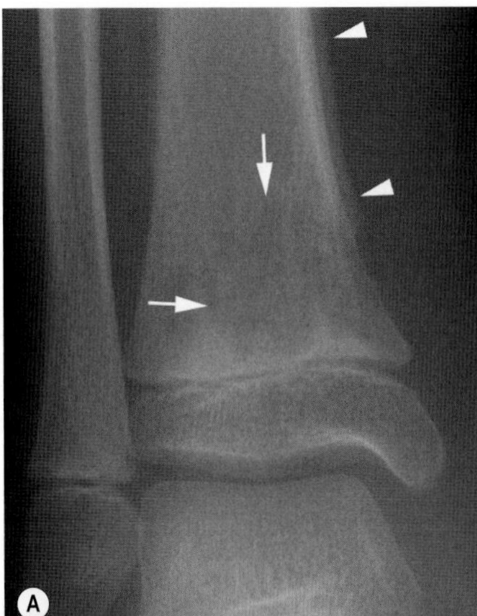

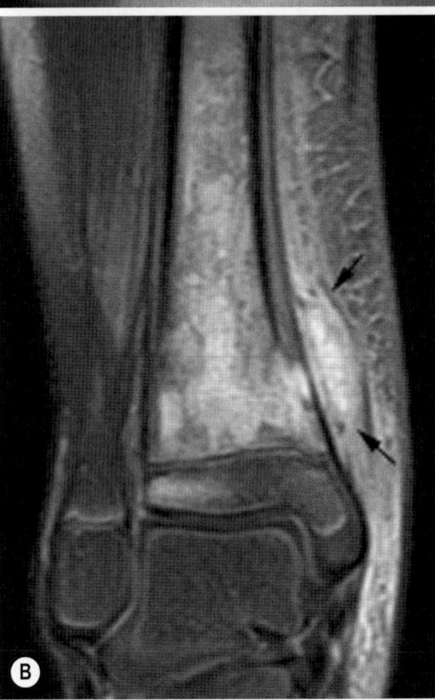

FIGURE 72-10 ■ Sickle-cell disease: osteomyelitis. (A) AP radiograph of the right ankle showing a poorly defined lytic lesion in the distal tibial metaphysis (arrows) and associated periostitis (arrowheads) consistent with acute osteomyelitis. (B) Coronal STIR MRI showing the irregular distal tibial bone abscess, which communicates with a soft-tissue abscess (arrows) through a cortical defect. Note also the marrow oedema and periosteal elevation.

diagnosis of bone infection is important. MRI typically demonstrates poorly defined marrow oedema, periostitis and soft-tissue oedema, which are also seen in acute infarction. However, the communication between a fluid collection in the medulla and surrounding soft tissues through a cortical defect is indicative of osteomyelitis (Fig. 72-10B). Also, the presence of geographic regions of marrow enhancement on fat-suppressed post-contrast T1W images is strongly associated with infection, while acute marrow infarcts tend to show serpentine peripheral enhancement. Ultrasound (US) may aid the diagnosis of infection by the guided aspiration of subperiosteal fluid collections.

MISCELLANEOUS DISORDERS

Gaucher's Disease[7,8]

Gaucher's disease is the commonest lipid storage disorder and is due to a genetic enzyme (glucocerebrosidase) deficiency, which results in the accumulation of the lipid glucocerebroside in the lysosomes of monocytes and macrophages. These engorged cells are called Gaucher cells and the accumulation of Gaucher cells within a variety of organ systems accounts for the symptoms of the disorder. Many of those affected are Ashkenazi Jews (~1/400–600), but all races are vulnerable. Three types are recognised: the common type 1, which is non-neuronopathic, and the rare neuronopathic types 2 (acute) and 3 (subacute).

The adult form mainly affects older children and young adults, but older adults are not exempt. Bone disease is the commonest cause of long-term morbidity, affecting up to 75% of patients. Both dull bone pain and acute painful crises occur. Bone crises are characterised by acute episodes of severe skeletal pain, fever, leucocytosis and raised erythrocyte sedimentation rate (ESR).

Radiological Features

Radiological features relate to lipid storage effects and bone necrosis. The large amounts of lipid in the marrow spaces cause osteopenia. Loss of normal modelling of the long bones in childhood results in the Erlenmeyer flask appearance of their ends (Fig. 72-11). However, this appearance is common to other marrow-expanding disorders. Lytic areas of varying size (Fig. 72-11A) and a 'soap bubble' appearance may be seen. The cortex is scalloped on its endosteal surface and becomes thinned. Osteopenia is associated with an increased risk of pathological fracture. Osteosclerosis may also occur as a healing response following bone infarction. Metaphyseal notching of the humerus is also a characteristic feature and is thought to be secondary to increased bone turnover.

Bone infarction is common and either due to interference of blood supply by lipid-laden cells or to fat embolism. Episodes of bone pain, fever and elevation of ESR may indicate osteonecrosis. Bone infarction involves particularly the subarticular bone of the femoral and humeral heads, the metaphyseal regions of long bones and the vertebral bodies, in which case vertebral collapse with or without cord compression may occur. Acute bone crises may show periosteal reaction on radiography, focal photopenic areas on scintigraphy and marrow oedema on MRI. The condition must be differentiated from osteomyelitis, which also complicates Gaucher's disease.

MRI is most useful in evaluating the extent of marrow infiltration, being manifest as either homogeneous or

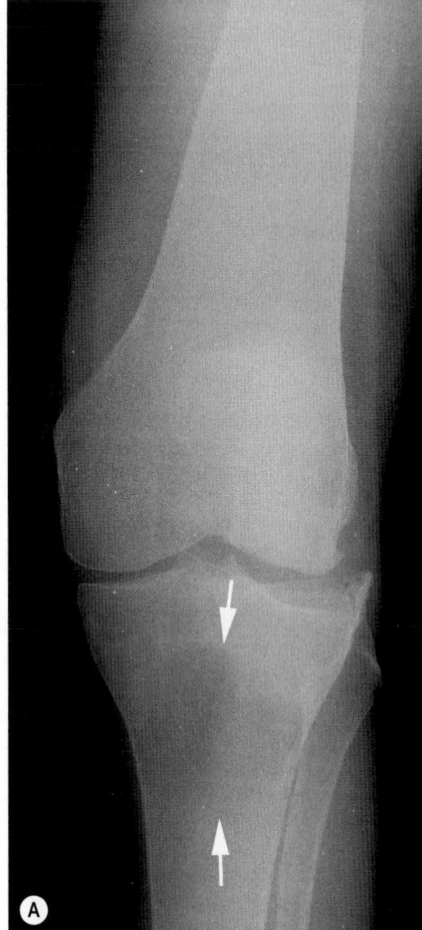

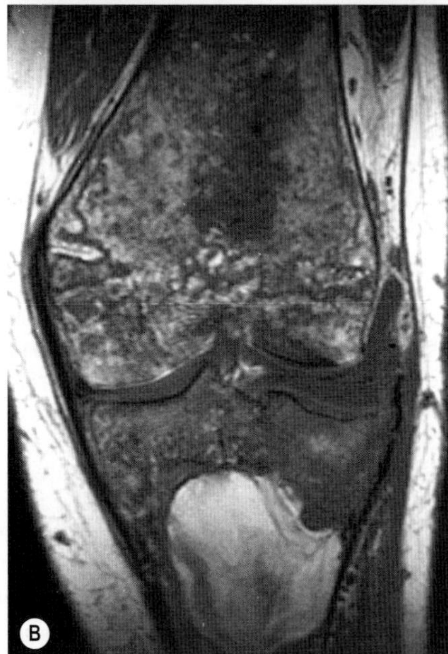

FIGURE 72-11 ■ **Gaucher's disease.** (A) AP radiograph of the left knee showing the Erlenmeyer flask deformity of the distal femoral and proximal tibial metaphyses, generalised osteopenia and a lytic lesion in the proximal tibia (arrows). (B) Coronal T1W SE MRI of the left knee showing heterogeneous reduction of marrow SI.

heterogeneous reduced SI on T1W (Fig. 72-11B) and T2W images. Such changes are always present in the spine. Complications such as bone infarction, osteomyelitis and fracture can also be assessed, while response to enzyme replacement therapy (ERT) is possible using specialised chemical shift imaging sequences.[9]

The prevalence of bone changes depends upon whether ERT has been administered. In the absence of ERT, 94% of patients will demonstrate some form of osseous radiological abnormality, including Erlenmeyer flask deformity (61%), osteopenia (50%), bone infarction and osteonecrosis (35%), fractures (26%) and lytic lesions (18%). All of these features are less common in patients receiving ERT.

DISORDERS OF BLOOD COAGULATION

Three major inherited disorders are considered:

1. classic haemophilia (haemophilia A)
2. Christmas disease (haemophilia B)
3. von Willebrand's disease.

All produce the same radiological appearances, the diseases differing only in the frequency and severity of the observed changes. Very occasionally, a patient of either sex may develop antibodies to antihaemophilic globulin and develop an acquired form of haemophilia. The prevalence of haemophilia A is estimated at 1 : 5000 and Christmas disease 1 : 30,000.

Haemophilia (Haemophilia A)[10–12]

Haemophilia A is an X-linked recessive disorder resulting from deficiency of factor VIII. Bleeding, which usually follows minor trauma, may occur in the first year of life and 70% of haemophiliacs have experienced haemarthrosis by the age of 2 years. Repeated haemarthroses result in chronic arthropathy and eventually premature osteoarthritis. Soft-tissue haemorrhage, often close to muscle attachments, produces another lesion characteristic of the disease, the haemophilic pseudotumour.

Christmas Disease (Haemophilia B)

Named after the first patient studied, this disorder is due to deficiency of factor IX and is also an X-linked recessive disease. It is less severe than haemophilia.

Von Willebrand's Disease

Inherited as a dominant character and affecting both sexes, von Willebrand's disease is due to both a capillary defect and a deficiency in factor VIII. The coagulation defect is mild and only occasionally causes significant skeletal abnormality. The severity of the disease relates to the level of factor VIII in the blood, which is variable.

Radiological Features

In patients with severe haemophilia, 85–90% of all bleeding events involve the joints. Radiologically, acute haemarthrosis appears as a tense joint effusion (Fig. 72-12) and associated periarticular osteoporosis may indicate previous episodes. MRI is more accurate than clinical examination at identifying haemarthrosis and US may also have a role in early detection. The most common joints involved are the knee, elbow, ankle, hip and shoulder. Repeated episodes of haemorrhage result in progressive joint damage referred to as haemophilic arthropathy.

Haemorrhage initially occurs into the synovium and eventually extends into the joint space. Recurrent haemarthrosis results in a chronic haemorrhagic synovitis and articular cartilage damage. Hyperaemia results in periarticular osteopenia, epiphyseal overgrowth and premature closure of the growth plates. Pannus similar to that occurring in rheumatoid arthritis causes marginal erosions. Loss of secondary trabeculae leads to a permanent coarsening of the trabecular pattern, while growth arrest lines indicate the episodic nature of the disorder. Fibrosis results in joint contracture and intraosseous haemorrhage produces subarticular cysts, which predispose to subchondral collapse. Synovial thickening together with osteopenia make the soft tissues appear radiographically denser. An absolute increase in the soft-tissue density may also occur due to concentration of haemosiderin by macrophages in the periarticular regions.

The knee is the most common joint involved. Radiological features include enlargement of the distal femoral and proximal tibial epiphyses, varus or valgus deformity, squaring of the inferior pole of the patella with patellar overgrowth and widening of the intercondylar notch. Eventually, advanced secondary osteoarthritis (OA) develops.

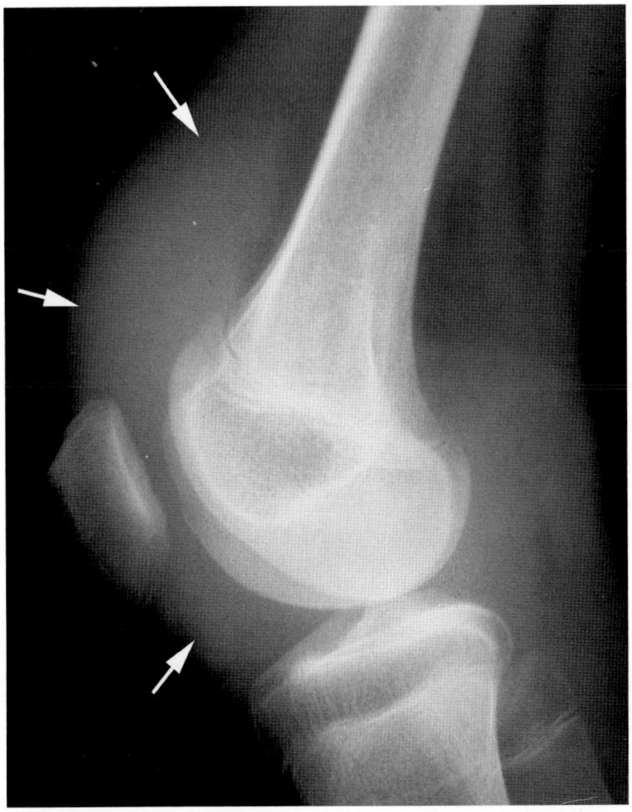

FIGURE 72-12 ■ **Haemophilia.** Lateral radiograph of the knee showing a prominent joint effusion (arrows) due to acute haemarthrosis.

In the elbow, chronic hyperaemia causes accelerated appearance of the ossification centres and overgrowth of the radial head. Pressure erosion of the radial notch of the ulna, large lytic lesions of the proximal ulna and erosion of the trochlear notch are also seen.

In the ankle, asymmetric growth of the distal tibial epiphysis results in medial tibiotalar slant. Marked flattening of the talar dome, a variety of ankle and foot deformities and, rarely, ankylosis of the ankle or subtalar joints may be seen.

Typical radiographic features of osteonecrosis may be evident in the hip and may simulate Perthes' disease, eventually resulting in coxa magna. Protrusio acetabuli and secondary OA are also seen, while haemorrhage into the growth plate may result in slipped epiphysis. Coxa valga may result from delayed weight-bearing.

Staging of haemophilic arthropathy has typically been with radiography, utilising the Pettersson score. However, radiography is insensitive to the earliest changes, which occur in soft tissue. US can demonstrate acute/chronic haemarthrosis and the resulting synovitis but is less able to assess the cartilage and subchondal bone. All of the pathological features of haemophilic arthropathy can be well demonstrated by MRI, which may demonstrate changes in the joint before any clinically evident episode of bleeding. MRI shows the earliest evidence of haemarthrosis as a low SI intra-articular blood clot within a hyperintense joint effusion. Fluid–fluid levels may also be seen. In chronic cases, the haemosiderin-laden synovium appears irregularly thickened and markedly hypointense

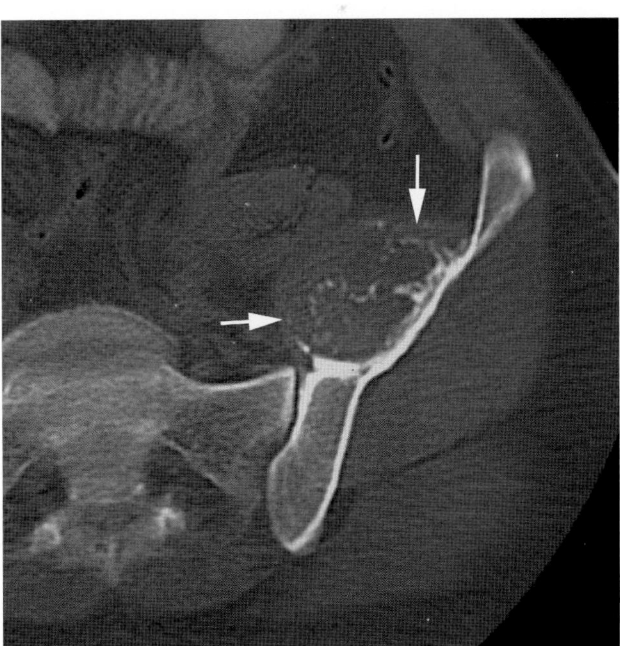

FIGURE 72-13 ■ **Haemophilic pseudotumour.** Axial CT study of the left ilium showing a calcified mass (arrows) in the left iliacus with chronic erosion of the adjacent iliac blade.

on T2W images, particularly gradient-echo sequences. Other features include focal cartilage defects and subchondral cysts.

Small soft-tissue haematomas are common and when repetitive may lead to contractures. Of more importance is the infrequent progressive haemorrhage close to muscle attachments, usually with no history of injury, resulting in the haemophilic pseudotumour. This is more common in adults, with a reported incidence of 1.56%. Most are reported in the pelvis, thigh, or calf. Subperiosteal or intraosseous haemorrhage causes pressure erosion of the bone, particularly the iliac blade in relation to the extensive origin of the iliacus muscle (Fig. 72-13) and the femur. Pathological fracture may be the first manifestation of a haemophilic pseudotumour of bone.

Radiographically, a haemophilic pseudotumour appears as a soft-tissue mass, which may be calcified. Bone lesions may show geographic lytic destruction with cortical thickening. CT identifies the thick, relatively hyperdense pseudocapsule with a hypodense centre. The MRI SI varies with the age of the contained blood, progressing from being isointense to muscle in the first week on T1W and subsequently becoming hyperintense on both T1W and T2W images. The wall tends to be hypointense because of its contained haemosiderin. Mural nodules provide a highly characteristic appearance. Treatment is by management of the haemophilia and exploratory operation is to be avoided.

For a full list of references, please see ExpertConsult.

FURTHER READING

1. Martinoli C, Bacigalupo L, Forni GL, et al. Musculoskeletal manifestations of chronic anemias. Semin Musculoskelet Radiol 2011;15:269–80.
2. Tyler PA, Madani G, Chaudhuri R, et al. The radiological appearances of thalassaemia. Clin Radiol 2006;61:40–52.
5. Ejindu VC, Hine AL, Mashayekhi M, et al. Musculoskeletal manifestations of sickle cell disease. Radiographics 2007;27:1005–21.
8. McHugh K, Olsen EOE, Vellodi A. Gaucher disease in children: radiology of non-central nervous system manifestations. Clin Radiol 2004;59:117–23.
10. Kerr R. Imaging of musculoskeletal complications of hemophilia. Semin Musculoskelet Radiol 2003;7:127–36.
11. Jelbert A, Vaidya S, Fotiadis N. Imaging and staging of haemophilic arthropathy. Clin Radiol 2009;64:1119–28.

CHAPTER 73

Imaging for Radiotherapy Planning

Peter Hoskin • Roberto Alonzi

CHAPTER OUTLINE

Radiation therapy has been used as a treatment for cancer for more than 100 years, with its earliest roots dating back to the discovery of X-rays in 1895. Its development in the early 1900s is largely due to the work of Marie Curie (1867–1934), who discovered the radioactive elements polonium and radium in 1898. Despite these distant origins, radiotherapy remains at the forefront of the treatment for cancer. Approximately 60% of cancer patients currently receive radiation therapy at some stage during their illness with 75% of these treated with curative intent.[1] Despite major advances in drug treatments for cancer, there has continued to be a steady annual increase in radiotherapy treatment that is unlikely to change within the next 10–20 years.[2]

As a result of advances in imaging and computer technology, radiotherapy has been transformed from 2-dimensional (2D) techniques to highly precise 3-dimensional (3D) conformal treatments that utilise axial tomographic images of the patient's anatomy to guide 3D intensity-modulated, image-guided therapy. Advances in imaging have allowed radiation oncologists to delineate and target tumours more accurately, thereby producing better treatment outcomes, improved organ preservation and fewer side effects. Furthermore, with the development of functional imaging techniques such as positron emission tomography (PET), dynamic contrast-enhanced computed tomography (CT) and multi-parametric magnetic resonance imaging (MRI) it is now possible to integrate biological information (for example, tumour oxygenation, cellular proliferation or tumour blood flow) into the radiotherapy planning process. Imaging is therefore critical at almost every stage in the practice of modern radiation delivery (Fig. 73-1).

TYPES OF RADIOTHERAPY

External Beam Radiotherapy

External beam radiotherapy constitutes the mainstay of radiation treatment in developed countries. External beam radiotherapy refers to any situation where the source of the radiation is located at a distance from the patient and the beam of radiation is then directed towards a defined treatment area. Approximately 85% of all therapeutic radiation exposures are delivered using external beam techniques. Various types and energies of radiation can be delivered in this way, including electromagnetic radiation such as X-rays and γ-rays, or particles such as electrons and protons. Higher energies of radiation penetrate deeper into body tissues. As a result low-energy X-rays (60–300 keV) are reserved for the treatment of skin cancers and superficial subcutaneous tumours. Most external beam radiotherapy treatments utilise megavoltage X-rays or electrons (6–18 MeV) generated by a linear particle accelerator (Fig. 73-2).

Conventional External Beam Radiotherapy

Conventional radiotherapy refers to techniques in which the treatment volume is defined by simple geometric parameters. In general, no attempt is made to delineate the tumour outline or to shape the radiation dose distribution to conform to the tumour volume. This is commonly practised for palliative treatments where long-term normal tissue toxicity is less relevant. The irradiated volume can be defined clinically but more often fluoroscopic or CT simulation is used. The radiation fields tend to run parallel to each other, creating a box-like treatment volume (Fig. 73-3).

Three-Dimensional Conformal Radiotherapy

The incorporation of axial imaging data allows 3D reconstruction of the tumour and surrounding organs. This provides more accurate localisation of the target volume and more information regarding the amount of normal tissue that will be irradiated. The radiotherapy planning computer software then utilises the attenuation coefficient information (Hounsfield units) derived from the CT image on a voxel-by-voxel basis to predict the attenuation of each therapeutic radiation beam as it passes through the body. As a result, the number and profile of the radiation beams can be orientated and shaped to fit the profile of the target from a beam's eye view using a

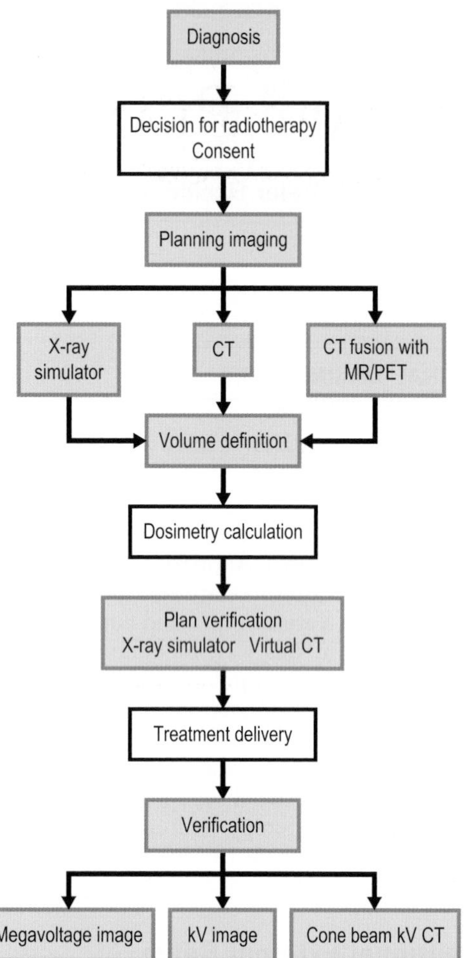

FIGURE 73-1 ■ The radiotherapy pathway. Processes outlined in green involve imaging.

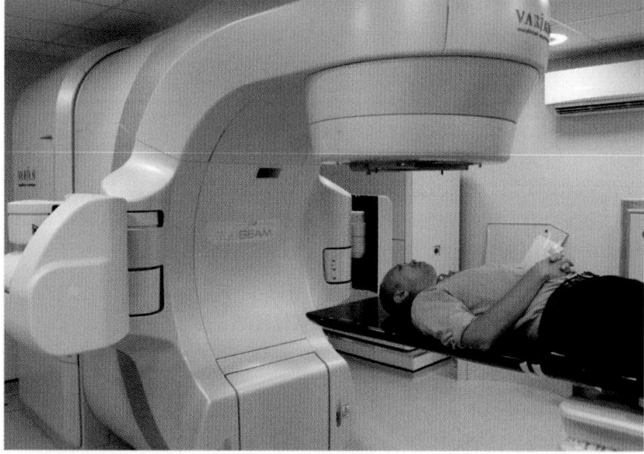

FIGURE 73-2 ■ External beam radiotherapy. A patient preparing to receive external beam radiotherapy on a linear particle accelerator.

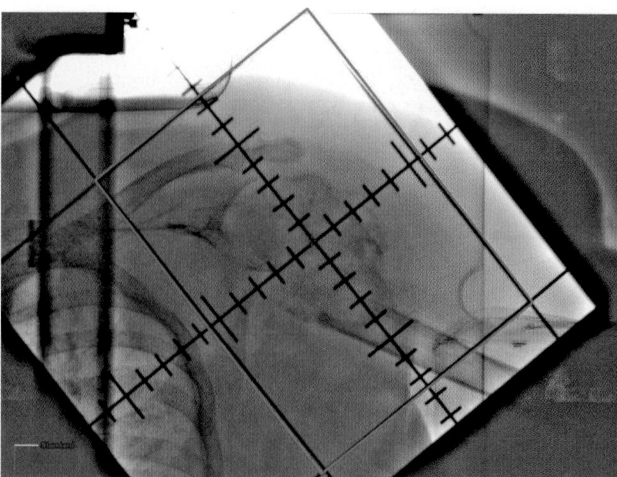

FIGURE 73-3 ■ Palliative conventional external beam radiotherapy for a destructive bone metastasis of the proximal humerus that has caused a pathological fracture. The edges of the treatment beam have been defined using fluoroscopy. For illustrative purposes the edges of the treatment field have been outlined in red. The treatment will be implemented using parallel opposed beams of radiation from the anterior and posterior directions, thereby creating a box-like treatment volume.

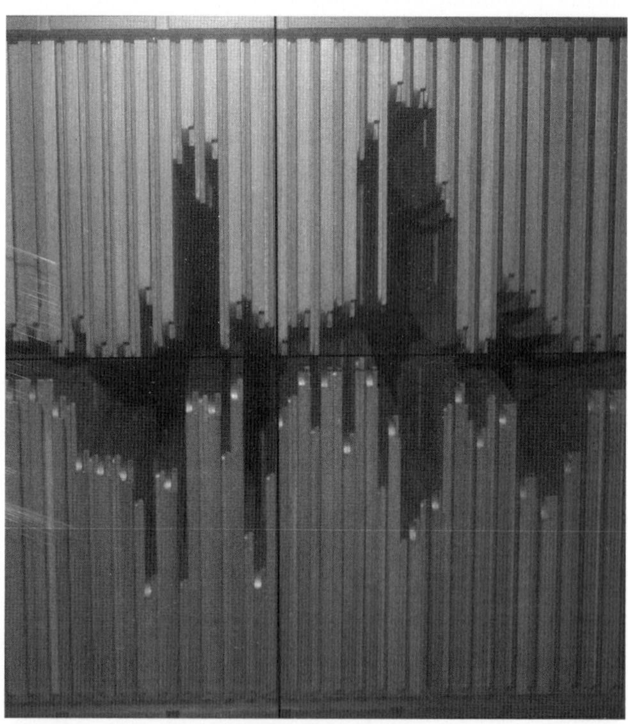

FIGURE 73-4 ■ A multileaf collimator (MLC). This is made up of individual 'leaves' of a high atomic numbered material, usually tungsten, which can move independently in and out of the path of a radiation beam in order to block it. This device is situated in the head of a linear accelerator to shape the treatment beam in order to match the borders of the target tumour. For intensity-modulated treatments the leaves of an MLC are moved across the field while the beam is on to create fluence modulation.

multileaf collimator (Fig. 73-4). The resulting radiotherapy plan can be displayed as a colour map of radiation dose overlaid onto the anatomical CT images so that the radiation oncologist can determine whether the tumour volume will receive sufficient irradiation with acceptable normal tissue dose sparing (Fig. 73-5). By reducing the irradiated volume and dose to the sensitive surrounding normal tissues, this technique facilitates the delivery of higher tumour radiation doses than would be achievable using conventional techniques.

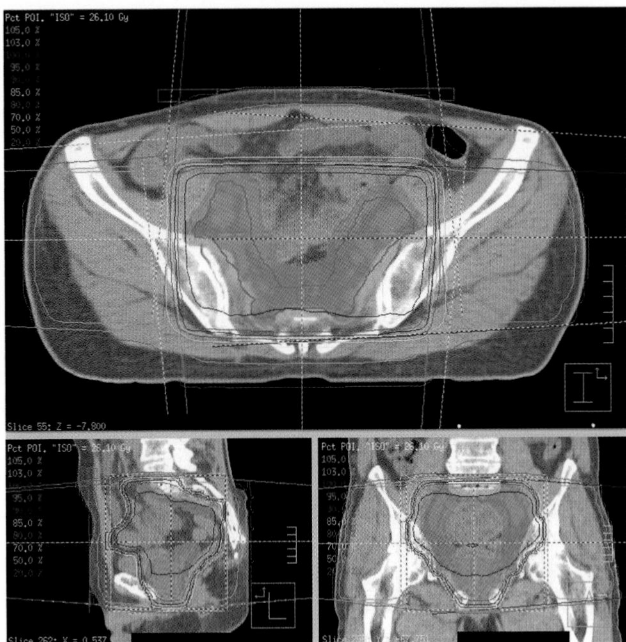

FIGURE 73-5 ■ A 3-dimensional conformal radiotherapy plan for treatment of the pelvic lymph nodes. The planning target volume is defined by the shaded green region. Four treatment beams (anterior, posterior, left and right lateral) overlap over the target volume to provide the desired dose in this region with reduced dose to surrounding normal structures. The coloured lines represent the dose gradient in a similar way to the contour lines on a map and correspond to the numbers in the top left corner. For example, the red line represents the 95% isodose (i.e. every point on this line will receive 95% of the prescribed radiation dose). The coronal and sagittal views show the shaping of the beam by the multileaf collimator (MLC). Despite the use of the static MLC, the transverse image clearly shows that the small bowel anterior to the horseshoe-shaped target volume will still receive the full radiation dose.

FIGURE 73-6 ■ An intensity-modulated radiotherapy (IMRT) plan for treatment of the left maxilla and bilateral lymph nodes. The primary tumour region has been outlined and is defined by the solid red line. This has been expanded to produce a planning target volume shown as the dark blue shaded region and will receive a radical dose to control the macroscopic tumour. The level II lymph nodes have also been defined and will be treated to a lower overall dose to control any microscopic disease spread. The use of intensity modulation has allowed shaping of the dose distribution to avoid the brainstem. The isodose lines can be seen to bend anteriorly around the brainstem, leaving this structure in a region of low radiation dose (between the green and blue isodose lines, which correspond to 50–70% of the prescribed dose, thereby taking the brainstem below its tolerance threshold).

Intensity-Modulated Radiotherapy (IMRT)

IMRT represents a further step in the development of high-precision radiotherapy delivery. The term refers to a variety of techniques in which the radiation beams are not only shaped and orientated to conform to the tumour volume but also the intensity of radiation is modulated across each treatment beam. This technique can produce dose distributions that conform highly to complex shapes, including treatment volumes that wrap around sensitive normal structures such as the spinal cord (Fig. 73-6), enabling high-dose delivery to the tumour volume whilst sparing dose to the normal structures.

IMRT can be achieved using a number of different technologies. Most commonly, several static radiation fields in the same plane of orientation are used, similar to the situation for 3D conformal radiotherapy, but with varying dose flux across the profile of the beam which is achieved by moving the leaves of the multileaf collimator across the beam at varying rates.[3] Alternatively, arc therapies utilise a number of non-coplanar beam arcs in which the radiation is delivered using multiple 'stop and shoot' beams or as a continuously moving field that varies in intensity throughout rotation.[4] Tomotherapy is another technique for achieving IMRT in which a megavoltage X-ray source is mounted in a similar fashion to a CT X-ray source (Fig. 73-7). The treatment volume is irradiated using the machine's continuously rotating beam that is modulated in intensity whilst the patient moves through the gantry bore.[5]

Stereotactic Body Radiotherapy (SBRT)

In SBRT the distribution of radiation beams is in three dimensions and not in two as in traditional radiotherapy.[6] It is based on a precise evaluation of the positioning of the tumour in real time and on the delivery of the dose by multiple beams (sometimes one hundred or more beams per treatment—Fig. 73-8). The treatment is based upon stereotactic radiosurgery methods for the treatment of intracranial tumours. However, it can only be used for selected, small extracranial lesions such as tumours of the lung and prostate or small solitary metastases. Even with small tumours, the complexity of the technique can sometimes result in treatment times of over an hour per fraction, thereby necessitating a small number of radiotherapy fractions to make a course of SBRT treatment

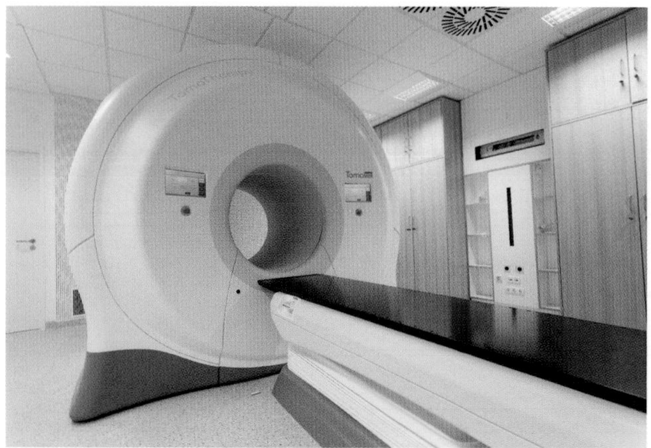

FIGURE 73-7 ■ **A tomotherapy unit.** Tomotherapy is essentially a combination of spiral CT and intensity-modulated radiation therapy technology. As with a CT unit, the patient moves through the unit, but instead of a kilovoltage diagnostic X-ray, hundreds of pencil beams of megavoltage therapeutic X-ray radiation spirally rotate around the patient. Each of these dynamically rotating beamlets vary in intensity to conform to the complex tumour shape.

clinically (and economically) feasible. Fortunately, the precision of SBRT allows high doses to be delivered in a very limited number of fractions. This is sometimes referred to as ultra-hypofractionation in which doses per fraction can be as high as 20 grays (conventional radiotherapy is delivered at 2 grays per fraction). There is current speculation that the mechanism of radiation-induced tumour cell killing may differ at such high doses per fraction. It has been hypothesised that radiation doses of more than 10 grays per fraction can cause rapid obliteration of the tumour vasculature, which cannot be achieved with the lower conventional doses, resulting in a biological advantage for ultra-hypofractionation.

Brachytherapy

Brachytherapy refers to a situation in which a radioisotope is placed onto or inside the patient. The radiation source is sealed in a protective capsule or wire which prevents the radioisotope from moving or dissolving in body fluids but allows the emission of ionising radiation

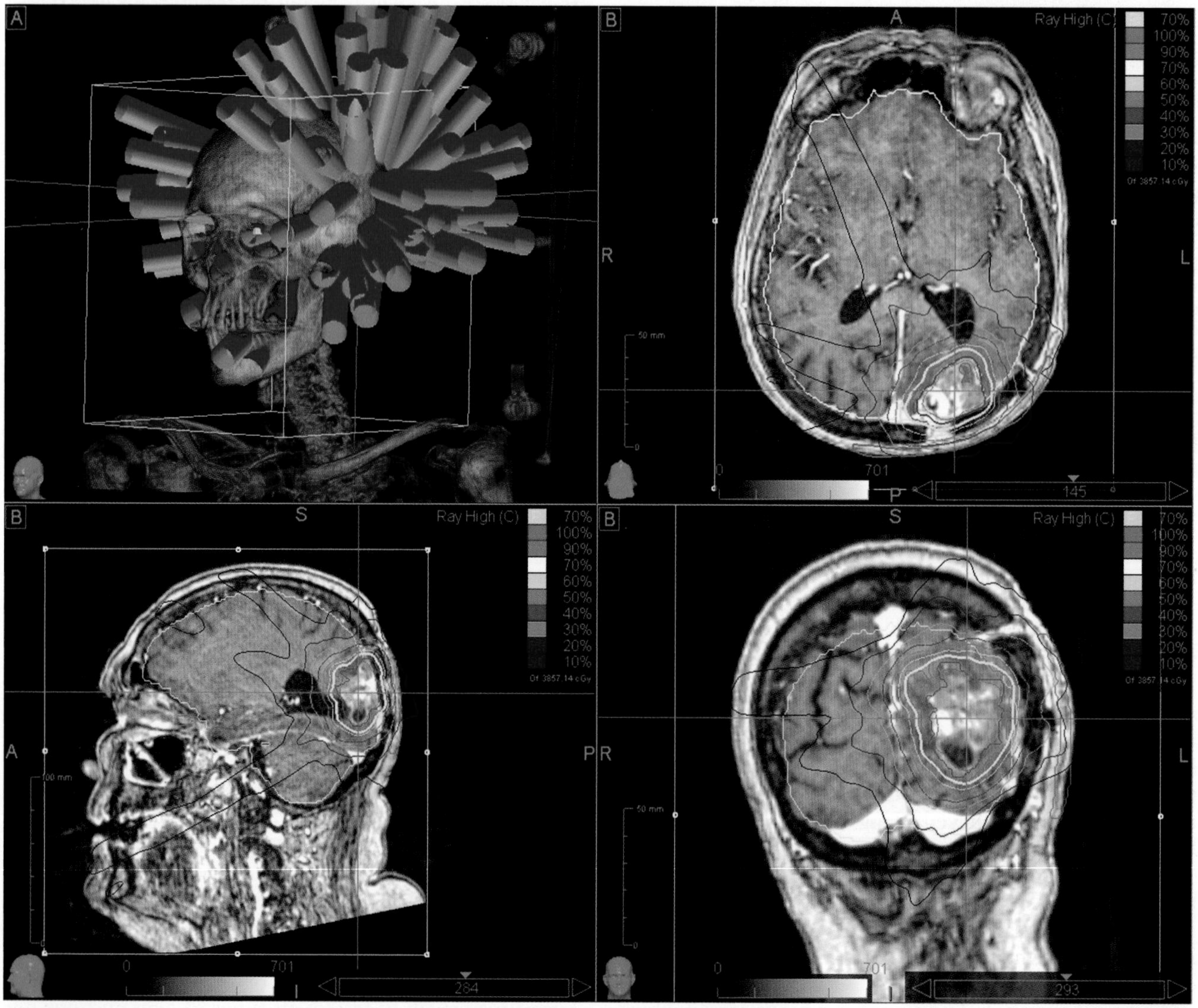

FIGURE 73-8 ■ **A stereotactic body radiotherapy plan using the CyberKnife robotic radiosurgery system to treat a recurrent glioblastoma of the occipital lobe.** Each of the blue cylinders represents a pencil beam of radiation that is controlled with extreme accuracy using image guidance. The machinery can correct for movements of the tumour caused by breathing or internal organ motion. The resulting dose distribution, which can be seen in the transverse, coronal and sagittal views, conforms extremely well with the tumour volume.

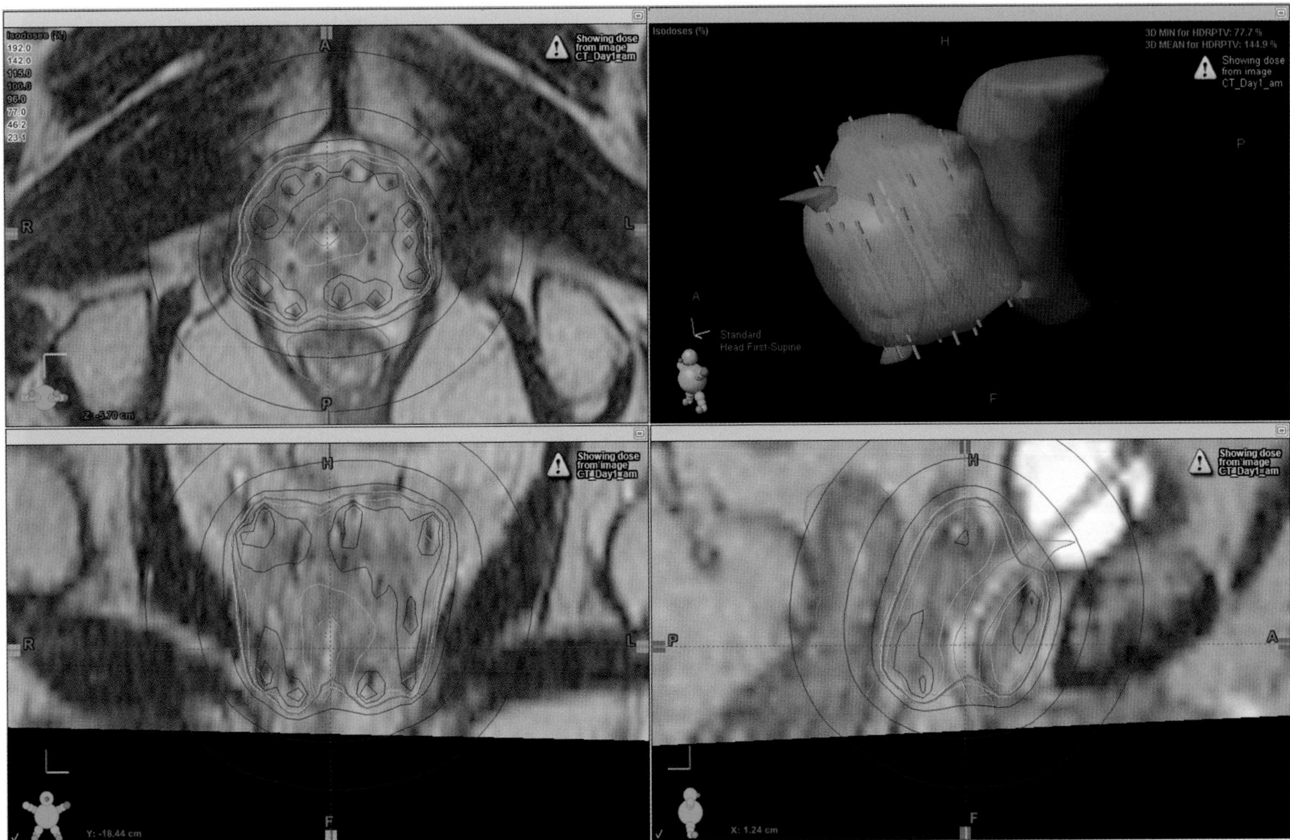

FIGURE 73-9 ■ **A high dose-rate brachytherapy plan for treatment of an intermediate-risk prostate cancer.** The 3-dimensional reconstruction in the top right panel shows the dwell positions of the ^{192}Ir source as it passes though each of the catheters that have been inserted through the prostate gland. The shaded light blue region on the transverse, sagittal and coronal images represents the target volume. The red isodose line is the prescribed dose (i.e. every voxel within this line will receive at least the prescribed radiation dose). Note how closely this line fits to the target volume. The outermost blue line represents 23.1% of the prescribed dose, showing that the dose falls off within very short distances from the target, thereby sparing the surrounding normal tissues.

(in the form of α, β, γ or X-radiation) to the surrounding tissues. The source can be placed into the target tissues or tumour itself such as the prostate or breast (interstitial brachytherapy), into a body cavity such as the uterine cavity, oesophagus or bronchus (intracavitary/intraluminal brachytherapy) or onto the skin surface to treat a cutaneous malignancy.

In certain situations brachytherapy offers some major advantages over external beam techniques. One of the key features of brachytherapy is that the irradiation only affects a very localised area around the radiation sources as dose falls off rapidly, obeying the inverse square law. As long as the sources are precisely placed within the tumour, there is minimal exposure to radiation of healthy tissues further away from the sources. This allows very high doses to be administered to the target volume (Fig. 73-9). Also, patient set-up and tumour motion are less relevant because the radiation sources move with the tumour and therefore retain their correct position; this increases the confidence that the radiation has been delivered in accordance with the required plan.

Due to the very short distances between the radiation source and the treatment volume, the absorbed tissue dose is almost entirely a function of the distance from the source, rather than due to the attenuation coefficient of the tissues that the radiation passes through (in contrast to the situation with external radiation). Radiation from a point source is inversely proportional to the square of the distance from the source. Tissues twice as far away receive only one-quarter of the dose in the same time period. As a result, brachytherapy techniques do not necessarily require Hounsfield number information from CT data to produce conformal treatment plans. As long as the position of the radiation sources can be reliably located, any imaging modality can be used for planning (Fig. 73-10).

Brachytherapy applicators have been adapted to enable better imaging. For example, CT- and MRI-compatible intrauterine tubes have been developed for gynaecological treatments. Seeds containing ^{125}I are commonly used to treat prostate cancer and have been designed with roughened and bevelled ends to maximise ultrasound visibility. Because precise reproduction of the source position is critical to brachytherapy dose calculations, any distortion or registration error may be critical and should be carefully quality-assured before incorporating in routine practice. Specific MR sequences may be developed to enable certain applications: for example, proton-rich sequences for identification of ^{125}I seeds in the prostate.[7] Imaging also has a crucial role in the

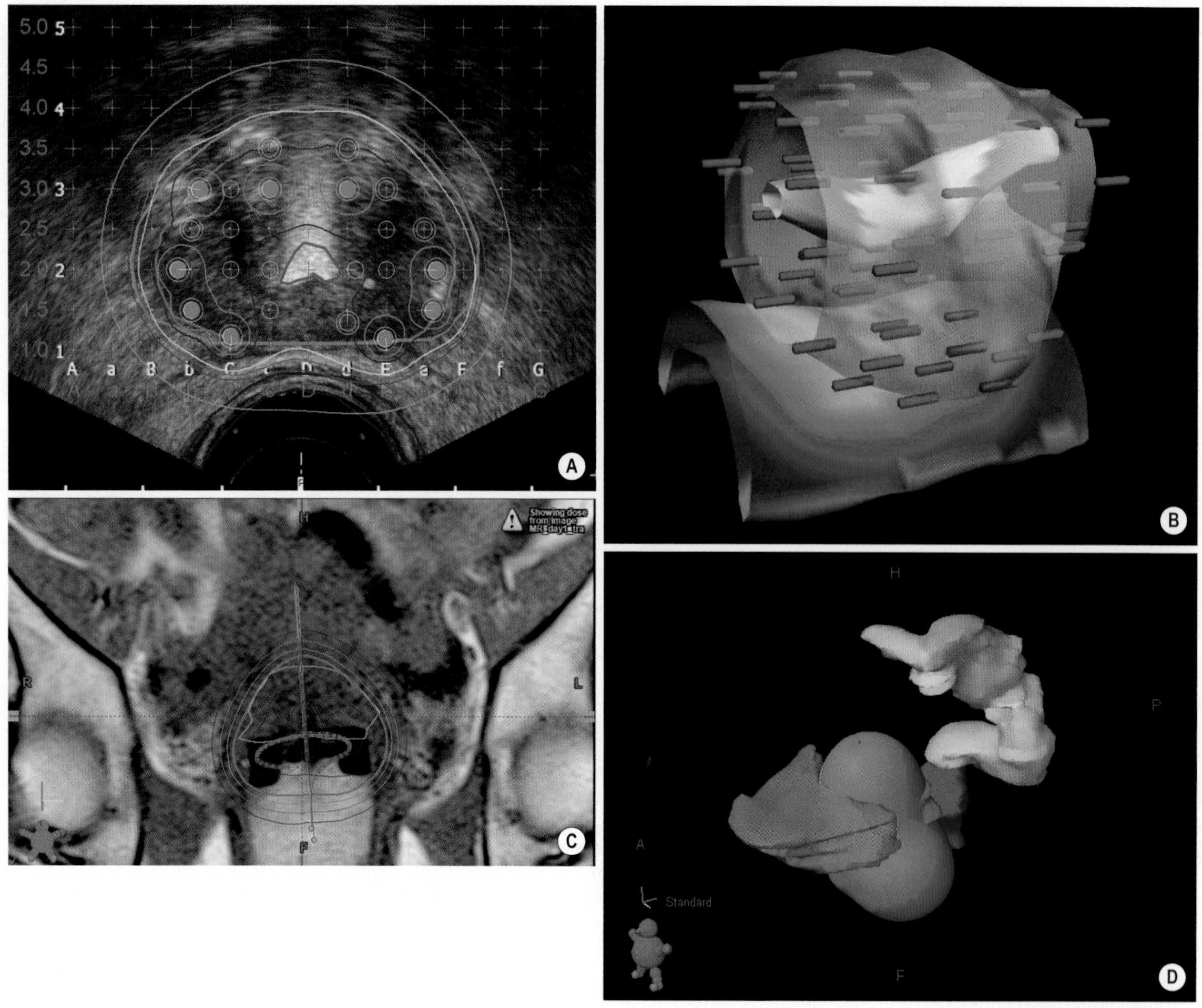

FIGURE 73-10 ■ **Brachytherapy planning without the use of CT.** (A) Pre-plan for an ^{125}I prostate seed implant: a transrectal ultrasound image has been acquired and the prostate margin (red), urethra (green) and rectum (dark blue) have been defined. The prostate margin has been expanded to produce the planning target volume (light blue). (B) The seeds can then be positioned to deliver the maximum dose to the prostate whilst minimising dose to the urethra and rectum. (C) High dose-rate brachytherapy planning for a cervical carcinoma using MRI. An intrauterine tube and cervical ring have been inserted under general anaesthetic and their position has been marked (green and pink segmented line). Each segment of the line represents a dwell position for the ^{192}Ir isotope. The time that the isotope remains at each dwell position determines the dose distribution, which is manipulated to maximise dose to the tumour and avoid normal structures. (D) The final dose distribution with the prescribed radiation isodose is represented by the light blue shaded region. The bladder (pink), rectum (green) and colon (yellow) are also shown.

accurate positioning of radiation sources or afterloading applicators for brachytherapy. Its flexibility and real-time imaging capability means that ultrasound is considered particularly valuable in this respect.

Brachytherapy is often defined by the rate at which the radiation dose is applied. Low-dose rate (LDR) brachytherapy sources emit radiation at a rate of up to 2 Gy·h^{-1}. These sources can be permanent, as is the case with LDR prostate brachytherapy (Fig. 73-11), or removed after several days, as for oral cavity tumours. High-dose rate (HDR) brachytherapy sources emit radiation at a rate of over 12 Gy·h^{-1}; however, the most commonly used HDR units with an ^{192}Ir source emit radiation at a much higher rate of between 60 and 100 Gy·h^{-1}. HDR sources are always afterloaded (instead of directly placing the source into the patient); hollow catheters are inserted and subsequently connected to the HDR unit which can be operated remotely to deliver the source into each catheter with the operator outside the shielded room (Fig. 73-12).

Particle Therapy

Also known as hadron therapy, particle therapy is an external beam technique in which highly energetic particles such as protons, neutrons or positive ions are directed at the tumour. Although electrons are particles, these are not usually considered in the category of particle therapy. The most common form of particle therapy uses protons that are accelerated by a cyclotron or synchrotron. Protons have several physical characteristics

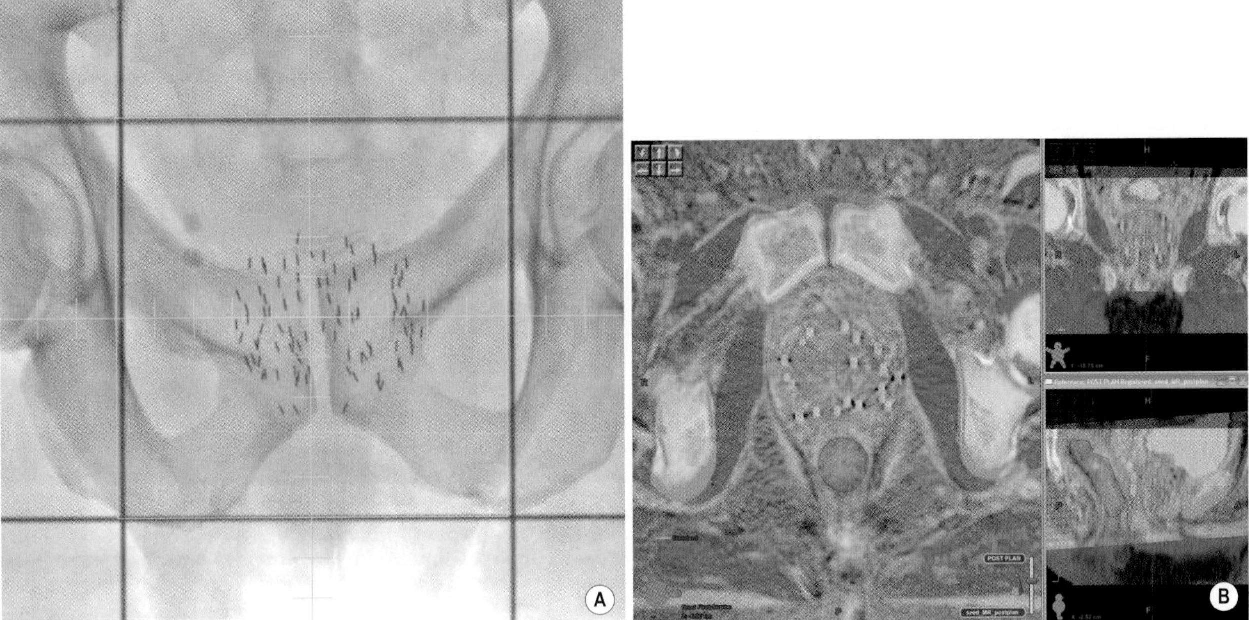

FIGURE 73-11 ■ Brachytherapy for a low-risk prostate cancer. (A) Plain radiograph of the pelvis taken a few minutes after ^{125}I seed implantation for a patient with low-risk prostate cancer. (B) Fused CT and MR imaging of the same patient on day 28 after the implant. The iodine seeds emit 35 kV X-radiation (maximum energy) and have a half-life of 59 days. As a result the prostate is irradiated over a period of months rather than weeks or days. Following the implant procedure there is often some migration of seed positions caused by bleeding and swelling from the trauma of implantation. It is therefore important to determine the final dose distribution from imaging a few weeks after seed insertion rather than from their initial position.

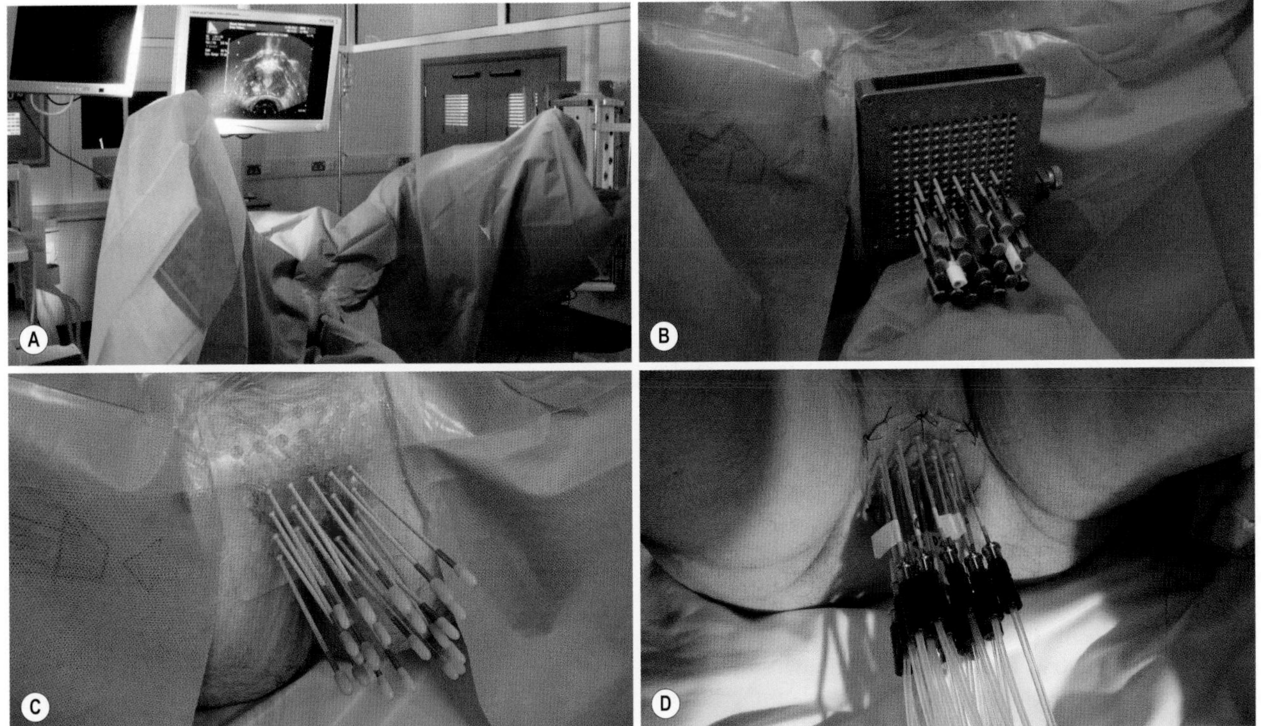

FIGURE 73-12 ■ Implantation technique for high dose-rate brachytherapy of the prostate. The procedure is carried out under general or spinal anaesthetic in the lithotomy position with a transrectal ultrasound probe mounted on a fixed stand with a template (A). Flexible plastic catheters are inserted through the perineum into the prostate in a parallel arrangement guided by the template (B). The catheters are left inside the patient whilst imaging (CT and/or MRI) and planning is performed (C). The catheters are then connected to the afterloading device, which robotically introduces the high activity radiation source through each catheter in turn in a pattern determined by the radiotherapy plan (D).

that provide an advantage over photon treatments. Protons penetrate deep into body tissues and deposit the majority of their energy in the last few millimetres of their range with virtually no radiation passing beyond this distance.[8] Therefore, varying the energy of the proton beam can control the depth of treatment.

For most treatments, protons of different energies are applied to treat the entire tumour. Also, due to their greater mass, protons scatter less and the beam remains focused with less broadening than photon beams. These properties translate into a clinical advantage when it is paramount to limit the radiation dose to critical normal structures that lie deep to the tumour. In particular, where there may be a critical normal tissue such as the spinal cord immediately behind the target, the minimal exit dose using proton therapy can prevent major long-term morbidity. This is particularly true for paediatric neoplasms such as medulloblastoma where there is convincing clinical data to show the advantage of sparing the developing brain and cord.[9–11]

There are only a few centres in the world that have the capability of treating patients with the other forms of particle therapy: namely, fast neutron therapy or carbon ion therapy. These techniques have physical advantages similar to that of protons, with sparing of tissues at depth, but in addition there are biological benefits. Both neutrons and carbon ions cause dense ionisation with much greater transfer of energy along the radiation track. This results in more radiation damage and cell death.[12] Furthermore, there is theoretical evidence that intensely ionising radiation of this sort can overcome the detrimental effects of tumour hypoxia, which is a major cause of treatment failure with standard radiotherapy.[13]

THE RADIOTHERAPY PROCESS

Radiotherapy Treatment Volume Definition

As radiotherapy dose delivery becomes more precise, the need for accurate diagnostic imaging that can be incorporated into the radiotherapy process increases. It is now possible to deliver radiation with near-millimetre accuracy. This puts considerable pressure on diagnostic technology to define tumour boundaries with similar accuracy. Because of the uncertainties inherent in the delineation of tumour volume, it is standard practice to incorporate a safety margin around the 'visible' gross tumour volume (GTV) to produce a clinical target volume (CTV) that accounts for extension of the tumour that is beyond the resolution of current diagnostic imaging capability. A further expansion is then made to account for set-up errors which occur due to the inherent variability in equipment geometry and beam alignment and intra-fraction tumour movement to produce a planning target volume (PTV) (Fig. 73-13). In order to further capitalise on the accuracy of modern radiotherapy equipment and make additional reductions in normal tissue toxicity whilst increasing dose to the tumour, this safety margin needs to be reduced. This can only occur if (1) there is a higher level of confidence in defining tumour volumes and (2) tumour movements during radiation delivery can be visualised and accounted for. Both of these require advanced imaging capabilities.

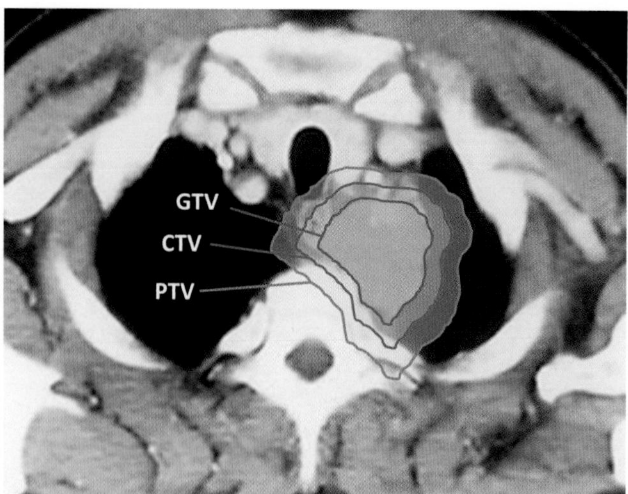

FIGURE 73-13 ■ Contrast-enhanced radiotherapy planning CT image. The gross tumour volume (GTV) of a lung tumour has been outlined (blue). The treatment planning computer software has been used to expand this volume into a clinical target volume (CTV) to account for the possible microscopic spread of tumour cells into surrounding tissues (orange). This volume has, in turn, been expanded into a planning target volume (PTV) to account for set-up error and tumour motion during treatment (green). The treatment plan will then be created to encompass the PTV with the required treatment isodose.

Clinical Volume Definition (Non-imaging-Based)

This is used for visible tumours or for palliative treatments where accurate tumour localisation is not required. For skin cancers, the visible tumour boundary is outlined and a margin for microscopic spread is marked on the skin surface (Fig. 73-14). For treatment to deeper structures the field borders can be defined using anatomical landmarks.

Conventional Simulation

The 'simulator' is a kilovoltage X-ray machine and detector that is designed to emulate the movements of a radiotherapy treatment machine (linear accelerator) to reproduce treatment conditions (Fig. 73-15). It has a couch that is capable of all the movements of a linear accelerator couch and a gantry that can be rotated through 360°. It produces 2D X-ray images, which can be viewed in real time on the screen. Palpable tumours can be marked with wire to aid localisation and contrast can be used to define some organs (for example, the bladder, rectum or oesophagus). Screening demonstrates organ and tumour movement to allow adjustment of the treatment fields. Field borders are defined on the screen and transferred to the patient using positioning lights that are aligned to the field edges. Skin tattoos act as

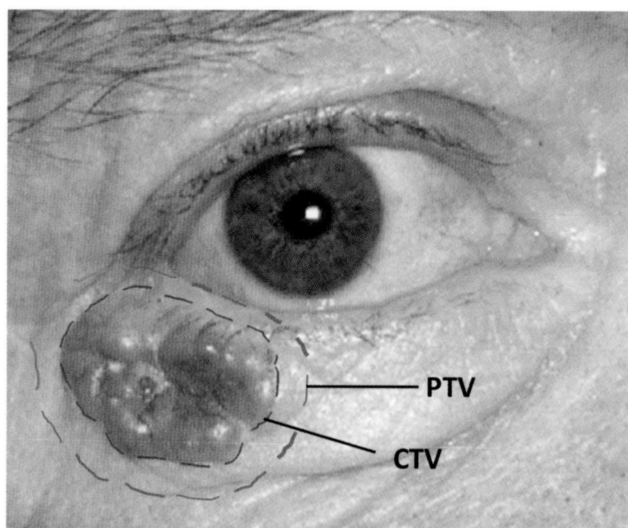

FIGURE 73-14 ■ **Clinical 'mark-up' for a nodular basal cell carcinoma.** The tumour boundary is defined visually and by palpation and marked onto the patient's skin (CTV). An expansion is made to account for microscopic extension and set-up error (PTV); this is also drawn on the skin. A lead cutout is then custom-made to shield the normal skin from the radiation beam.

reference points to aid identical set-up on the treatment machine.

Traditionally, the conventional simulator was used to plan all types of radiotherapy, including multiple beam treatments. In order to achieve this, anteroposterior and lateral images were taken together with a transverse outline of the body contour through the centre of the simulated volume, which the planning department could then convert into a 3D volume. However, the main limitation of this method was the inability to accurately define the tumour volume and adjacent normal structures due to poor soft-tissue contrast. As a result, treatment volumes were predominately defined by bony landmarks, producing generic treatment volumes without any reliable ability to estimate the dose and volume of normal tissue irradiated. Furthermore, the lack of tissue density information meant that the estimated doses delivered to the tumour and adjacent structures were purely based on the body contour, and the depth of tissue that the beam had to penetrate to deposit the radiation dose. Because of this, there is no longer a role for a conventional simulator in planning curative radiotherapy; the sale of such machines is now almost nonexistent in the UK and North America. The role of the conventional simulator is now restricted to checking radiotherapy plans and planning palliative treatments (Fig. 73-15).

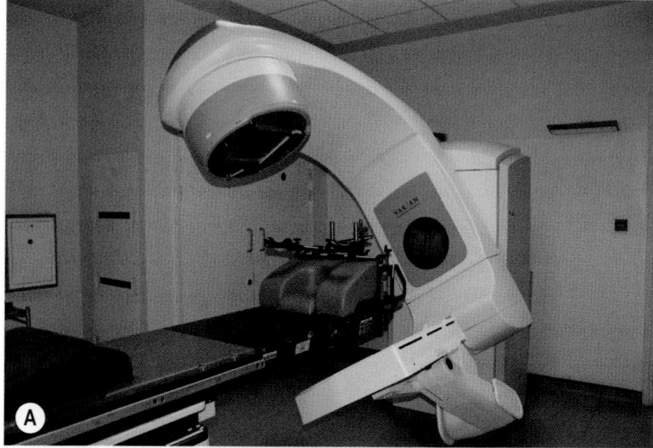

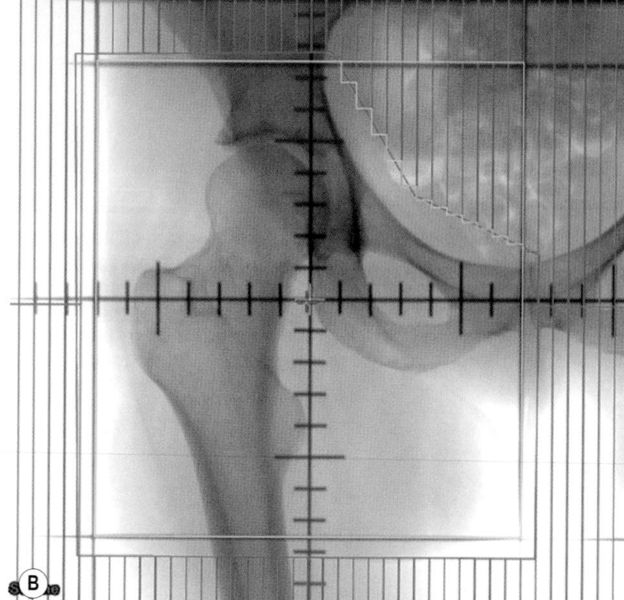

FIGURE 73-15 ■ **Conventional simulator.** (A) Photograph of a conventional simulator. The simulator is a kilovoltage X-ray machine and detector designed to emulate the movements of a linear accelerator which it resembles (compare with Fig. 73-2). Simple geometric treatment fields can be planned using this method. (B) Planning for palliative radiotherapy for metastases in the right proximal femur and pubic bones. A multileaf collimator has been used to partially shield some of the sensitive pelvic organs and bowel.

CT Simulation

CT simulation replaces the use of the conventional simulator with a CT imager to gather information. CT provides excellent bone and soft-tissue imaging as well as tissue density information, which is necessary for the accurate calculation of the dose distribution. CT simulation refers to the simulation process performed with data collected from the CT imaging. Data are downloaded onto a 3D treatment planning computer where the simulation can be performed. This technology provides the radiation oncologist with information on internal anatomy and the ability to view the patient's body in any plane with high soft-tissue and bone contrast. The software is capable of producing digitally reconstructed radiographs (DRRs), which are images that mimic a conventional radiograph in any field direction (Fig. 73-16). This information is then used in two ways to define the radiotherapy delivery:

- Virtual simulation in which the tumour volume may be outlined formally or simply viewed in three dimensions and the fields necessary to cover the

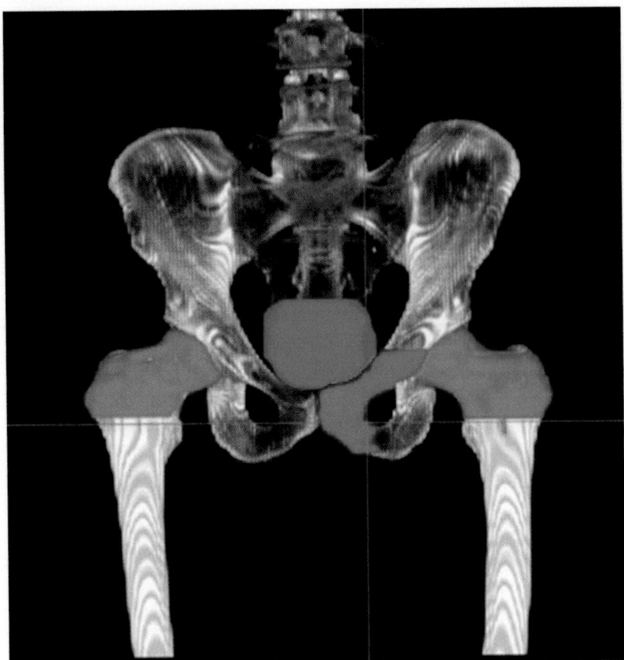

FIGURE 73-16 ■ Digitally reconstructed radiograph (DRR) of the bony anatomy. In this example the intended target is a bone metastasis in the left pubic bone (red). The organs at risk have also been defined. The bladder is shown in green. The head and neck of both femora have also been included as organs at risk (pink) due to the fact that excessive radiation can cause avascular necrosis of the femoral head and risk of subsequent fracture.

volume are simulated on the computer screen. This will typically be used for simple palliative treatments to internal organs or bones and use single or opposed fields for which the subsequent dose distribution can be calculated (Fig. 73-17).

- CT conformal planning in which the CT data are harnessed to a sophisticated planning system using computer software to calculate complex dose distributions. The target volume is defined by contouring directly onto the CT images and multi-field plans with varying tissue compensation may be employed to deliver a homogenous dose to the tumour volume and minimise dose to surrounding normal organs at risk (see Figs. 73-5 and 73-6).

The advantages of virtual simulation over conventional simulation include a faster simulation procedure, better soft-tissue imaging, the collection of tissue density information, more precise tumour localisation, more precise organ definition, the collection of 3D anatomy data and the facilitation of complex planning techniques.

Image Fusion

CT is the imaging platform for all modern radiation dosimetry planning systems. Tissue density information derived from the Hounsfield number of each voxel of the planning CT imaging is required for accurate estimation of the radiation dose distribution which can vary considerably where the treatment volume includes the lungs or other air cavities. However, whilst a CT image is always required for external beam planning it may not be the best imaging technique for tumour volume and organ at risk delineation. For example, pelvic and brain tumours are often more accurately defined using MRI and tumours of the head and neck and lung benefit from FDG-PET/CT for locating the tumour.[14–16] In order to capitalise on the performance of each imaging technique it is sometimes necessary to fuse imaging data sets to produce the best radiotherapy plan[17] (Fig. 73-18).

This process is not without its complications, as can be illustrated using the example of lung cancer. Bronchial tumours frequently cause collapse of some of the surrounding normal lung tissue. Using CT it is often difficult to define the true extent of the tumour because of a lack of contrast between the cancer and the adjacent collapsed lung. There is, therefore, a risk of missing tumour (if the radiotherapy field is made too small) or of irradiating an unnecessary volume of benign lung tissue (if the defined treatment volume incorporates collapsed lung as well as tumour). ^{18}F-FDG PET/CT is an important tool for the staging of lung cancer and can demonstrate the geographical distribution of the primary tumour and metastases. Many studies have attempted to fuse PET/CT images with the planning CT to aid tumour volume definition. However, the PET/CT image displayed is entirely dependent on the SUV thresholds chosen. Lower thresholds will increase the apparent tumour volume and higher thresholds will do the opposite. There is currently no consensus on how to define tumour borders using PET data. There are also other difficulties that occur when trying to fuse multi-technique imaging sets. These include variations in resolution, spatial distortions that can occur with certain methods (e.g. MRI), physiological and anatomical changes that occur during the time between the imaging acquisitions, increased workload and cost.

Treatment Planning and Verification

Once the planning target volume and normal organs have been defined in three dimensions, the optimum dose distribution for treating the tumour is sought. This is a multi-stage process. Initially, a beam energy must be chosen according to the depth of the target and the size of the patient. Low-energy beams give maximum dose close to the surface and penetrate less. Higher-energy beams give maximum dose deeper within tissues, thereby sparing the skin, and penetrate further into tissues but also give a higher exit dose beyond the target. Other factors to be considered include the quality of the beam, degree of lateral scatter, the availability of beam modification (such as multileaf collimators or the possibility of intensity modulation) and the facility for image guidance.

Next, the required dose to the tumour and the maximum allowable doses to normal organs must be specified. In principle, the aim is to achieve the highest possible dose to the tumour and the lowest possible dose to the normal structures, in particular the defined organs

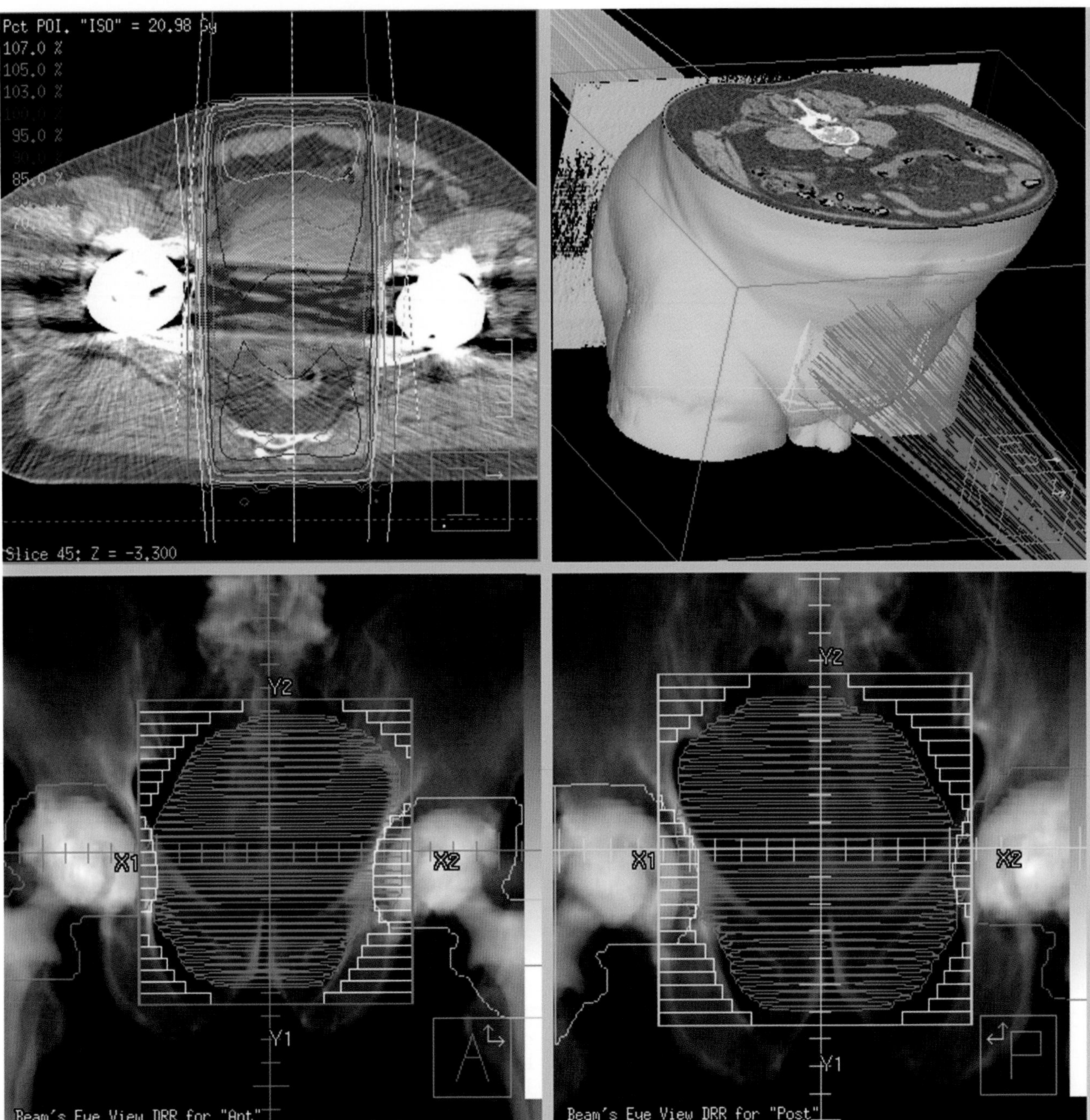

FIGURE 73-17 ■ Virtual simulation for treatment of an invasive bladder cancer in a patient with bilateral hip replacements. The hip prostheses prevent the use of lateral or oblique beam angles which would normally be used for pelvic treatments, allowing only anterior and posterior fields (top right). The bladder has been contoured on each CT slice (green). Anterior and posterior 'beam's eye view' digitally reconstructed radiographs are shown (bottom panels). On these views the beam has been shaped by the multileaf collimator. Despite the beam shaping, the fact that only two beams could be used results in a column of high dose through the pelvis in the anteroposterior direction without any possibility of sparing the rectum (top left panel).

at risk, which will be those with critical function nearest the target and those with low radiation tolerance. The results of clinical studies, as well as years of experience, have helped to define acceptable doses to the normal tissues and the minimum tumour dose required to destroy the tumour. It is then the job of the radiotherapist and dosimetrist to devise an acceptable compromise between the probability of tumour control and the chance of normal tissue toxicity. This is achieved by choosing the optimum beam arrangement (number, energy, size, weighting, angle of beam entry and beam modification using collimators or intensity modulation) and defining the normal tissue constraints, which are doses to specified volumes that will not be exceeded.

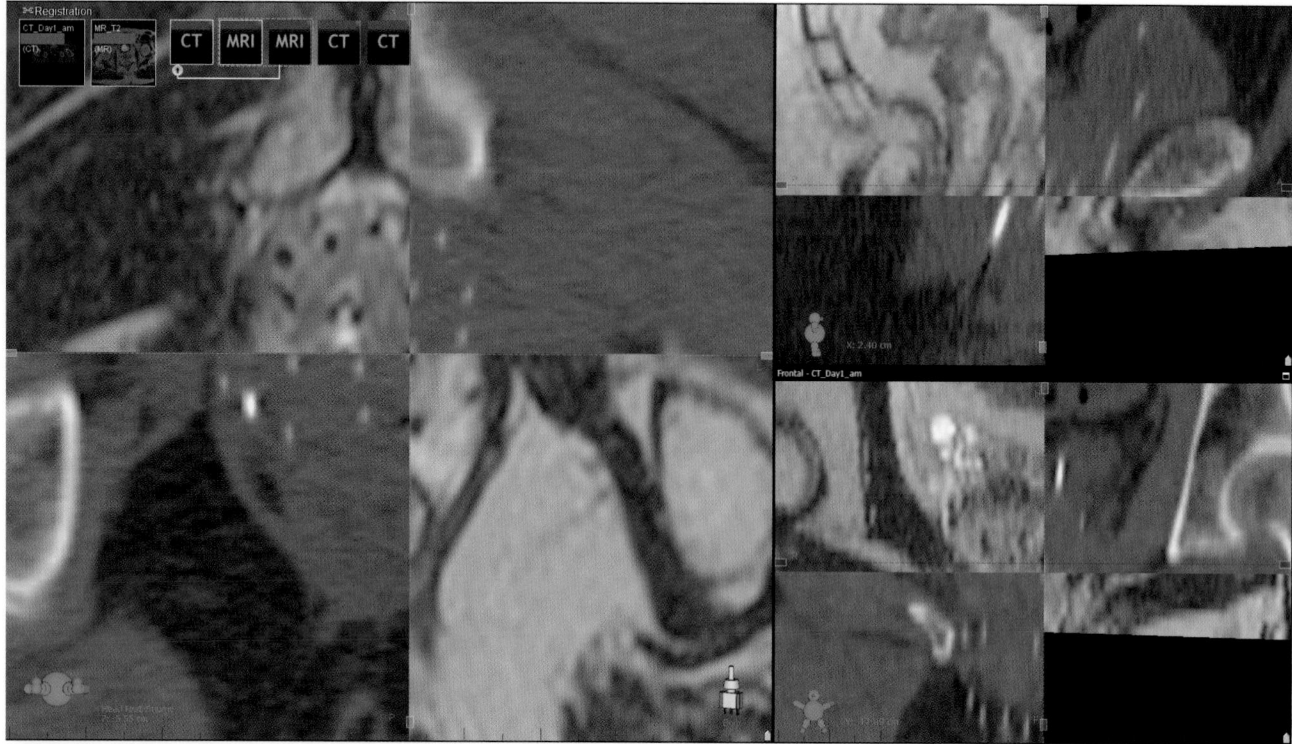

FIGURE 73-18 ■ CT-MR image fusion illustrated in a patient with brachytherapy catheters in the prostate. Automated registration software is now widely available but manual correction for more accurate registration is still sometimes required. Inaccuracies can occur if there has been patient or organ movement between the acquisition of the two imaging sets. Also, differences in resolution, spatial distortion and slice thickness can affect the reliability of fusion. Deformable registration programs, where one image is distorted to fit the other more precisely, are currently under evaluation.

Attenuation of an X-ray beam is affected by tissue density; for example, it is less in lung tissue, which is of low density, than in bone. This variation affects both the shape of the dose distribution and the amount of radiation absorbed. Density corrections are used to correct for dose inhomogeneity. If 2D planning is used, correction is only valid at the planned central slice of the target volume. For example, when treating the breast, CT-simulator slices may be used to measure the volume of lung in the tangential beam. For more accurate heterogeneity corrections, 3D planning is needed with localisation of lung tissue throughout the 3D volume using CT planning. Using CT, a pixel-by-pixel correction can be made to take account of all tissue densities within the body contour by conversion of CT numbers into relative electron densities using a predefined calibration.

Various computer algorithms are used to model the interactions between the radiation beam and the patient's anatomy to determine the spatial distribution of the radiation dose.[18–20] Different mathematical algorithms are necessary to account for the different types of radiation and computational complexity. With the increase in computational performance available today, improved algorithms are continually being developed. All external beam planning systems use X-ray-based image data as the density data are necessary for the dosimetry calculations.

Radiotherapy planning can be performed in two ways. In *forward* planning, the planning dosimetrist manually chooses beam parameters that are likely to maximise the tumour dose whilst sparing the normal tissues. The treatment planning system then calculates a predicted dose to the various predefined structures. If the dose to the tumour is insufficient or a normal tissue tolerance is exceeded, then the beam parameters are altered and the process repeated. After a number of iterations an acceptable plan is generated. This type of planning can only handle relatively simple cases in which the tumour has a simple shape and is not near any critical organs. For more sophisticated plans, *inverse* planning is used. With this technique the radiotherapist defines a patient's critical organs and tumour and gives target doses for each. A weighting can also be applied to each target dose to allow the computer to give precedence of one dose level over another. For example, 100% weighting may be given to the spinal cord dose where excessive radiation effects can be catastrophic, whilst a lower weighting may apply to the bladder which is much more radioresistant. Then, an optimisation programme is run to find the treatment plan which best matches all the input criteria.

Image Guidance during Radiotherapy Delivery

For external beam treatment, the radiotherapy plan is based on the planning CT images. This CT is a snapshot

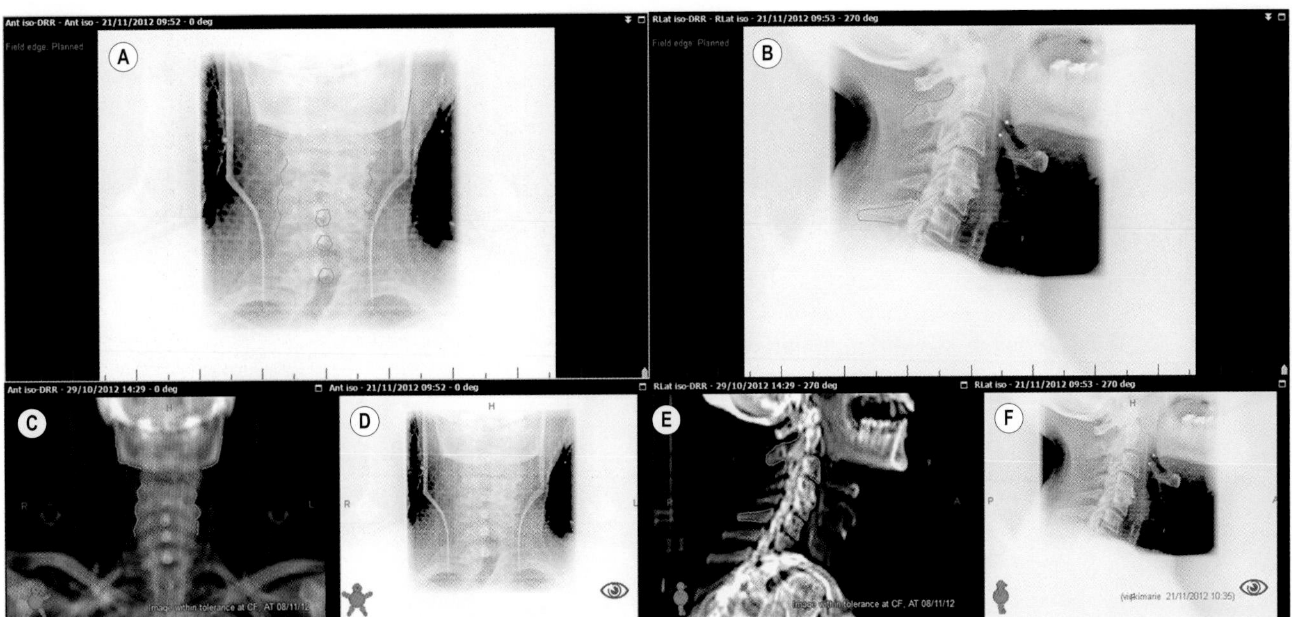

FIGURE 73-19 ■ **Planar (2-dimensional) image guidance.** Two static kilovoltage images have been acquired at 90° to each other using a linear accelerator-based on-board imaging device with the patient on the treatment couch and about to be irradiated (D, F). Bony landmarks have been outlined on the digitally reconstructed radiographs, which have been derived from the planning CT imaging (C, E). These outlines have been transposed onto the kilovoltage images in order to determine whether there has been any deviation from the planned treatment (A, B). In this case there is clearly a discrepancy of 3–4 mm in the craniocaudal direction. This is best seen on the anteroposterior image (A) where the mandible and spinous processes are notably higher than intended. To prevent an inaccurate exposure, either the patient will be repositioned or the fields will be delivered with the appropriate correction. This situation is not uncommon for head and neck cancer treatments where there is often weight loss during the therapy period and as a result the immobilisation head shell becomes loose fitting, allowing movement to occur.

of the patient's position and anatomy at a single point in time. All internal organs are subject to a degree of movement, which can occur daily (inter-fraction motion) or during the treatment delivery (intra-fraction motion). For some organs, such as the lung, the movement is predictable with a repetitive cyclical motion in 3 dimensions. For other organs, such as the bowel, random movements occur with the passage of gas and faeces. To account for this, larger margins are added to the planning target volume. However, the addition of margins to the tumour target volume increases the volume of normal tissue treated and can also increase the dose to organs at risk.

Image guidance refers to the process of locating the exact 3-dimensional position of the tumour and surrounding organs during treatment and then correcting for any deviation from the original plan. This will optimise the chance of accurately targeting the tumour and, thereby, over the entire course of fractionated treatment, maximise the tumour dose whilst minimising the dose to surrounding structures. As a result, the PTV margins can be substantially decreased, leading to a substantial reduction in the volume of radiation prescribed. Furthermore, with the ability of high-precision dose delivery and real-time knowledge of the target volume location, image-guided radiotherapy (IGRT) has opened the possibility for new indications for radiotherapy previously considered impossible. Research to improve image quality in radiotherapy is not new, but developments in computer software that quantify target localisation errors, on the basis of real-time imaging in the treatment room and hardware allowing automated set-up, have stimulated the mainstream clinical application of IGRT.

IGRT makes use of many different imaging strategies. IGRT techniques can be split into planar (2D) imaging, volumetric (3D) imaging or imaging over time (4D) during the radiotherapy treatment. In addition, for some anatomical sites implanted fiducial markers can be used to localise the treatment.[21]

Planar (2-Dimensional) Imaging

This is when two or more static images are acquired, usually at 90° to each other (i.e. anteroposterior and lateral) (Fig. 73-19). It allows comparison of the bony anatomy or of a target visible by plain X-ray (such as a lung tumour) in all three axes (superoinferiorly, laterally and anteroposteriorly). Planar imaging with megavoltage (MV) electronic portal imaging (EPI) is a standard feature on most conventional linear accelerators. However, images acquired at the energies used for radiotherapy (6–18 MeV) are not of diagnostic quality. In particular, the contrast between bone, soft tissue and air seen with conventional X-ray imaging (i.e. kV) is not seen at higher megavoltage energies. Planar 2D imaging with kilovoltage (kV) EPI is available on linear accelerators with a kV cone beam facility or may also be acquired using a system independent of the linear accelerator gantry: for example, a tube and detector system mounted on the floor and ceiling.

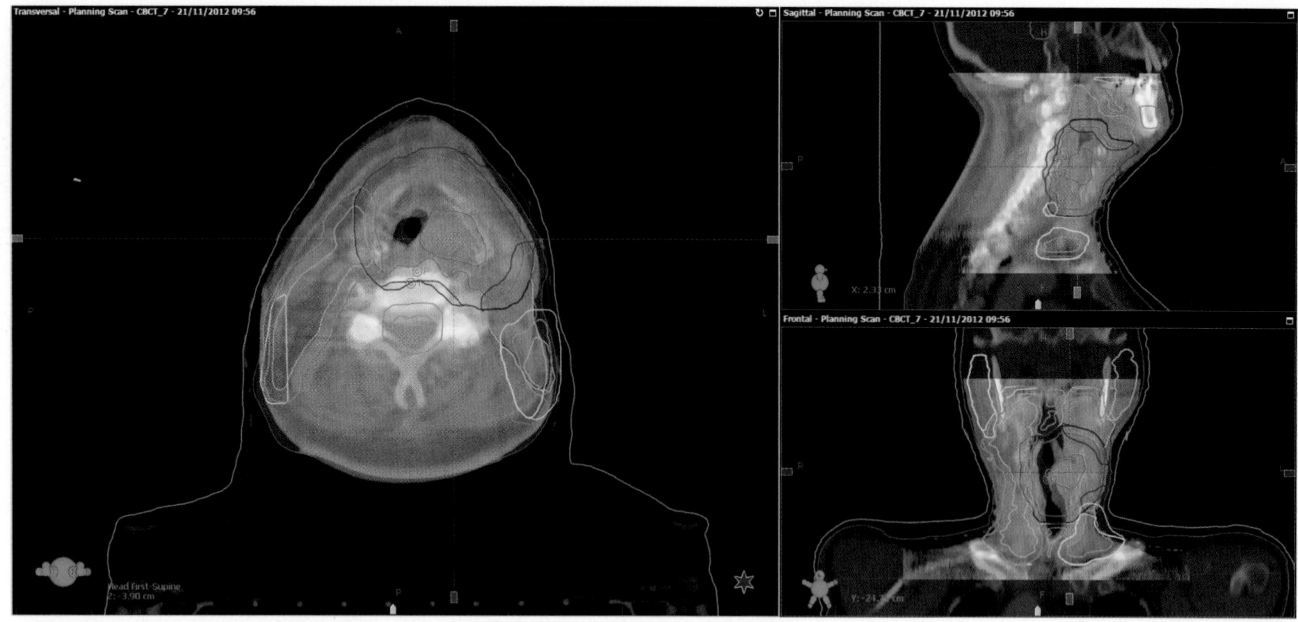

FIGURE 73-20 ■ Image guidance using cone beam CT. This patient is receiving treatment for a T4 laryngeal tumour. A cone beam CT image has been obtained with the patient on the treatment couch and about to be irradiated. The cone beam CT has been reconstructed in the transverse, sagittal and coronal planes and fused with the planning CT image. The fusion can be best seen on the sagittal and coronal images because the cone beam CT has been obtained for a shorter cranio-caudal length than the planning image. In contrast to the planar imaging (Fig. 73-19), the position of the soft tissues and the tumour itself can be clearly seen and contoured. Any discrepancy between the planning image and the cone beam CT can therefore be corrected in 3 dimensions to ensure tumour coverage and avoidance of normal tissues.

Volumetric (3-Dimensional) Imaging

Volumetric imaging allows for a 3D image to be acquired in the treatment position on the linear accelerator prior to or during radiotherapy. This enables the internal structures to be visualised including the target and surrounding normal tissues. There are four methods for obtaining a volumetric image on the linear accelerator:

- *Cone beam CT* (CBCT). For most standard linear accelerators volumetric imaging is available via cone beam CT technology, which is a kV tube mounted at 90° to the linear accelerator head and is rotated around the patient using the linear accelerator gantry. Both the treatment head (MV) and the CBCT system (kV) have an imaging capability (Fig. 73-20).
- *Megavoltage CT*. This technique uses a megavoltage energy fan beam to create a volumetric image for verification with helical imaging as used in conventional CT imaging.
- *CT on rails*. This consists of a CT unit in the same room as the linear accelerator. The patient couch can be rotated at 180° to transfer from the linear accelerator to the CT.
- *Ultrasound*. Ultrasound probes can provide volumetric images for IGRT in prostate cancer.

Four-Dimensional (4D) Imaging

This describes the process of imaging the tumour and relevant structures over a period of time. Before the advent of 4D image guidance, the gross tumour volume was expanded to create a clinical target volume to account for microscopic spread. An additional margin was then added for set-up variation (including any motion) to create the planning target volume (as described earlier). However, kilovoltage fluoroscopy or CBCT can be performed before the radiotherapy treatment to quantify tumour motion (Fig. 73-21). The gross tumour volume can then be defined at the extremes of motion and at the mid-point of the movement. These are then expanded for microscopic disease to create their respective clinical target volumes. The union of these clinical target volumes is then used to create an internal target volume with a smaller margin added for geometric set-up errors to create the planning target volume.

Alternatively, 4D kV or MV imaging can be used during radiotherapy to track the tumour, or more commonly, implanted fiducial markers, which are radio-opaque seeds or wires, can be placed in or near to the tumour, during treatment delivery. These can either provide additional points of reference in the images acquired, for example with CBCT, or be used as a surrogate for target position in planar imaging where soft-tissue information is not available. Once implanted, the fiducial markers will move with the tumour. Any displacement in 3 dimensions, as well as tilt and rotation, will be quantifiable by measuring the change in the relative positions of the markers and the radiotherapy plan can then be changed accordingly (Fig. 73-22).

Fiducial markers also enable real-time tracking during the delivery of the radiotherapy fraction. For example, the CyberKnife system (Accuray, Sunnyvale, CA, USA) uses a combination of X-ray imaging and optical tracking

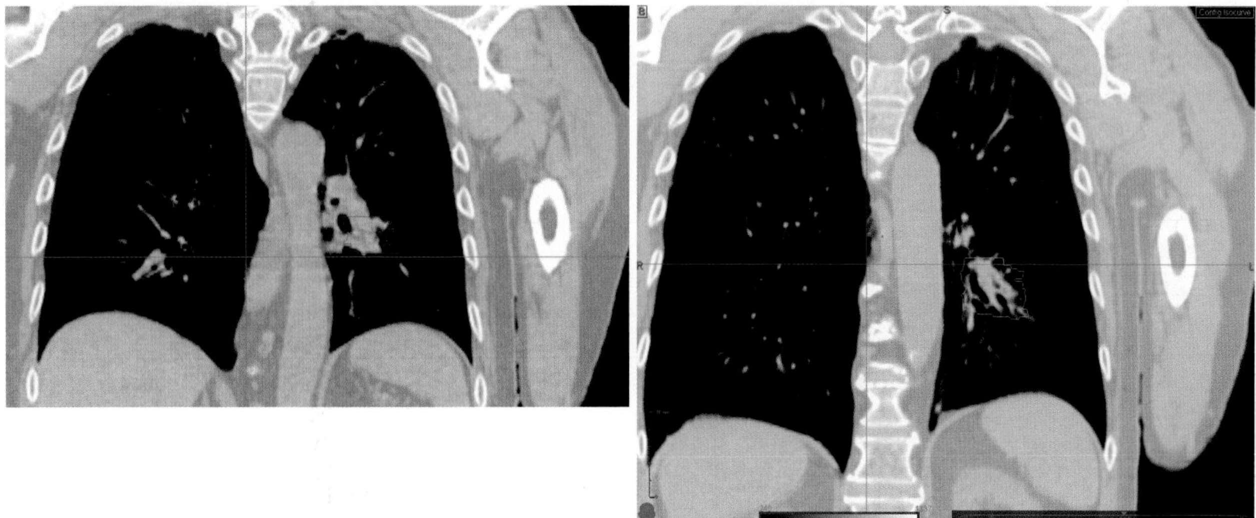

FIGURE 73-21 ■ **Cone beam CT being used to quantify the motion of a peripheral small lung tumour.** The degree of movement can be minimised by breath-holding techniques or by using mechanical methods to splint the diaphragm. Alternatively, respiratory gating can be used where the beam is automatically turned off when chest or tumour motion exceeds a predefined threshold.

in its motion tracking system.[22] Two kilovoltage X-ray tube and detector pairs are mounted in the treatment room at right angles. X-rays are taken periodically during treatment to determine the location of the fiducial markers within the target. For thoracic tumours there is also continuous optical tracking of the patient's skin to detect the breathing motion. These two data sources are then combined by the tracking software and a mapping function between the position of the external skin markers and the position of the internal target is computed. By knowing the motion of the internal target the Cyber-Knife robot arm can steer the radiation beam to follow that motion.

FUNCTIONAL IMAGING IN THE RADIOTHERAPY PROCESS

Inclusion of Biological Information to the Treatment Process

Several imaging techniques produce valid biomarkers for radio-biologically relevant tumour characteristics such as hypoxia, cellular proliferation, vascularity and clonogen density.[23–26] The ability to incorporate such biological information into radiotherapy planning allows the possibility of further manipulation of the radiation dose–distribution. Increasing the dose administered to relatively resistant tumour regions and moderation of the dose to sensitive areas should achieve better tumour control with less toxicity. Mathematical modelling studies have demonstrated theoretical advantages for biological conformality.[27–33] However, the translation of the theory into clinical practice has been limited.

Two factors must combine for biological radiotherapy planning to occur. Firstly, accurate and validated biological imaging must be available. Over recent years, this focus of imaging research has grown considerably. Many groups have used a variety of technologies to image numerous different tumour characteristics. However, it has been extremely difficult to prove whether the imaging data reliably reflect the biological process being studied or even whether the correct process is being measured at all. True validation requires simultaneous collection of imaging and physiological data, which is often impossible. As a result surrogate measures must be employed, each with its own set of assumptions and inaccuracies.

For example, one of the most important and relevant aspects of the tumour microenvironment that has a direct impact on the success of radiotherapy treatment is tumour oxygenation. Great efforts have been made to devise a method of imaging tumour oxygenation for the purpose of improving radiotherapy delivery, some of which have appeared to be promising. However, in order to prove that an imaging test is accurately measuring tumour oxygenation it must be compared with an established standard. This entails probing the tumour with oxygen-measuring electrodes or removal of the tumour for immunohistochemical assessment. Because oxygen levels vary over short periods of time, the imaging and direct oxygen measurement need to occur at the same time or at least only a few minutes apart. This poses a great challenge for experimental design. Furthermore, the 'gold-standards' with which the new imaging technology is being compared have inherent flaws. Polarographic electrodes have the unique ability to directly measure tissue pO_2. However, they can only sample a tiny proportion of a tumour and the position of the needle with regard to the tumour location is never known with certainty. Also, the trauma during needle insertion creates a non-physiological microenvironment from which the measurements are obtained. Tumour removal inevitably affects the oxygenation status, even if it is rapidly fixed. Therefore, immunohistochemical methods must be

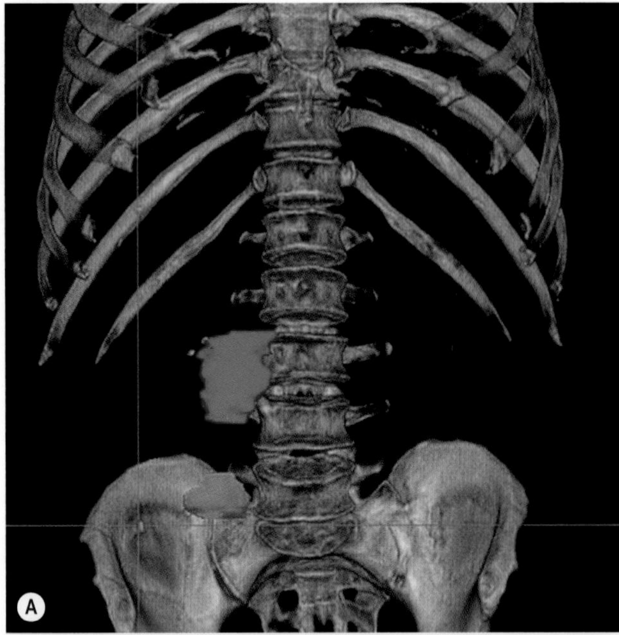

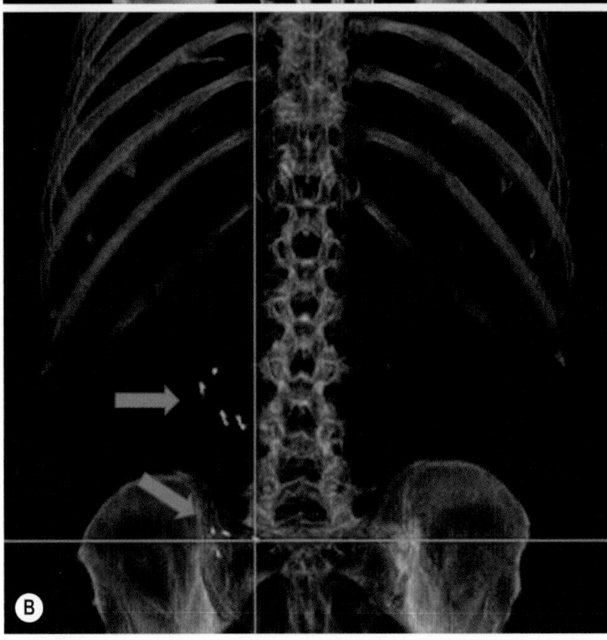

FIGURE 73-22 ■ Two areas of recurrent, chemotherapy refractory, metastatic testicular seminoma have been outlined in red (A). The intention is to treat these metastases with stereotactic body radiotherapy. In order to achieve accurate dose deposition, fiducial markers have been inserted into both tumours (arrows, B) so that any tumour motion can be tracked in real time during treatment delivery. (Image courtesy of Dr Peter Ostler, Mount Vernon Cancer Centre, UK.)

interpreted with caution. As a result it has been extremely difficult to prove that an imaging test accurately reflects the degree of tumour oxygenation. Individual validation experiments cannot give a definitive answer and these techniques must be intepreted in the context of the overall body of evidence.

There are a variety of techniques for imaging tumour hypoxia under evaluation; three warrant further discussion.[34]

^{18}F-Misonidazole Positron Emission Tomography

^{18}F-Fluoromisonidazole is a hypoxia imaging tracer with homogeneous uptake in most normal tissues and tumours. The initial distribution of ^{18}F-misonidazole is flow-dependent, as with any freely diffusible tracer, but local oxygen tension is the major determinant of its retention above normal background in tissues after 2 h. ^{18}F-Misonidazole accumulates in tissues by binding to intracellular macromolecules when the pO_2 is less than 10 mmHg. Retention within tissues is dependent on nitroreductase activity and accumulation in hypoxic tissues over a range of blood flows has been demonstrated.

Cu-ATSM Positron Emission Tomography

Several pre-clinical studies have evaluated and validated Cu-diacetyl-bis(N^4-methylthiosemicarbazone) for imaging hypoxia in tumours. The mechanism of retention of the reagent in hypoxic tissues is largely attributed to the low oxygen tensions and the subsequent altered redox environment of hypoxic tumours. Cu(II)ATSM is bioreduced (from Cu(II) to Cu(I)) once entering the cell. The reduced intermediate species is trapped within the cell because of its charge. This transient complex can then go through one of two competing pathways: reoxidation to the uncharged Cu(II) species (which can escape by diffusion), or proton-induced dissociation (which releases copper to be irreversibly sequestered by intracellular proteins). [Cu-ATSM] favours the reoxidation route because it is easily oxidised but chemically more resistant to protonation. Copper from Cu(II)ATSM is trapped reversibly as [Cu-ATSM]- (if oxygen is absent), with the possibility of irreversible trapping by dissociation over a longer period. Cu(II)ATSM is thus hypoxia-selective.

Blood Oxygenation Level-Dependent Magnetic Resonance Imaging (BOLD-MRI)

As in any magnetic resonance image, tissue contrast in BOLD images is affected by intrinsic tissue properties including spin–lattice and spin–spin relaxations. Additionally, BOLD MRI contrast is affected by blood flow and paramagnetic deoxyhaemoglobin within red blood cells (oxyhaemoglobin is not paramagnetic). Deoxyhaemoglobin increases the MR transverse relaxation rate (R_2*) of water in blood and surrounding tissues; thus, BOLD-MRI is sensitive to pO_2 within, and in tissues adjacent to perfused vessels. In order to decouple the effects of flow from deoxyhaemoglobin it is necessary to measure the T_2* relaxation rate (R_2*=1/T_2*), which can be done by using a multi-echo GRE sequence. Decoupling of flow from static effects on R_2* images occurs because the flow component can be thought of as affecting individual T_2* images of a multi-gradient echo sequence

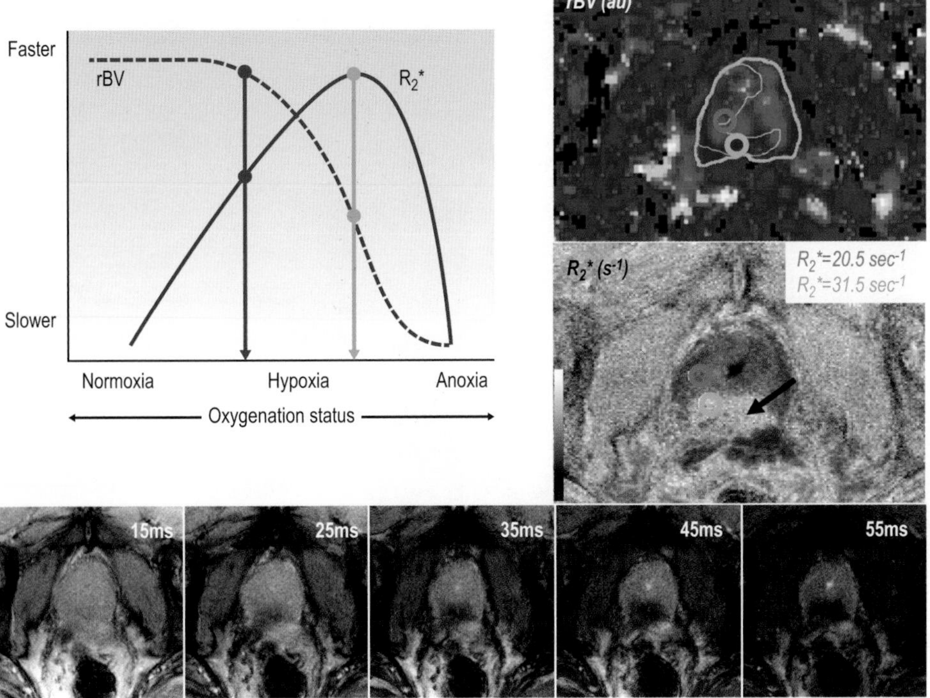

FIGURE 73-23 ■ **Blood oxygenation level-dependent (BOLD) MRI.** The graph shows the theoretical changes in R_2* and relative blood volume (rBV) with changes in oxygenation. Note that R_2* not only falls in well-oxygenated tissue but also in poorly oxygenated tissue where there is insufficient blood volume to produce the BOLD effect. The R_2* pixel map of the prostate was obtained using multiple spoiled gradient-echo images on a single central slice with increasing TE times (15–55 ms), using a 1.5-tesla MR system (bottom row of images). The dynamic susceptibility contrast (DSC) MRI rBV pixel map of the same patient was generated using T_2*-weighted data acquired every 2 s for 2 min with a 0.2 mmol/kg bolus of Gd-DTPA administered after 20 s. In this example the region of high R_2* (arrow) in the posterior peripheral zone corresponds to the region of low blood volume (orange circles and orange line on the graph) and the transition zone has high blood flow with low R_2* (green circles and green line on the graph).

equally. It is important to remember that, although synthetic R_2* images are free of the contribution of blood flow (that is, they mainly reflect deoxyhaemoglobin content and static tissue components), improving blood flow and vascular functioning will also increase tissue oxygenation, which can be seen by changes in R_2* images (Fig. 73-23).

The second factor that is required for successful biological radiotherapy planning is the ability to accurately vary the radiation dose over very short distances so that the radiation dose–distribution conforms to the distribution of the biological parameter in question. This has only been possible since the development of the modern radiotherapy techniques as described earlier. Many groups have concentrated on external beam intensity-modulated radiotherapy (IMRT), although there are still a number of technical limitations with this method. IMRT requires a motionless target if precise doses are to be administered to small regions within tumours. Immobilisation devices, respiratory gating and image guidance technology are becoming highly advanced and are approaching the levels of accuracy required for biological 'dose-painting'. However, biological targets within tumours are frequently only a few millimetres in diameter. The current degree of set-up error, as well as patient and internal organ movement during treatment with IMRT, makes the delivery of biological conformal radiotherapy using this method a considerable challenge.

High dose-rate (HDR) brachytherapy uses a radiation source placed within the tumour, which bypasses the need for immobilisation and image guidance during treatment delivery. It achieves high dose gradients, providing the most conformal dose distributions of all radiotherapy techniques. HDR brachytherapy is delivered over a period of 1–2 days rather than weeks. This reduces the effects of compensatory changes in tumour physiology that may alter the biological subvolume during treatment. It is for these reasons that with current levels of technology, HDR brachytherapy may be the optimal modality to explore the principle of biologically based treatment planning, although not suitable for all tumour types (Fig. 73-24).

In summary, radiotherapy requires close integration of both diagnostic and therapeutic radiation technology. Most of the advances in radiotherapy in recent years have been in response to better imaging, enabling accurate 3D image acquisition and the integration of physiological information with the morphological data. Modern radiotherapy represents sophisticated application of state-of-the-art imaging for diagnosis, target and organ at risk volume definition, tissue density measurements and verification of the therapeutic beam delivery.

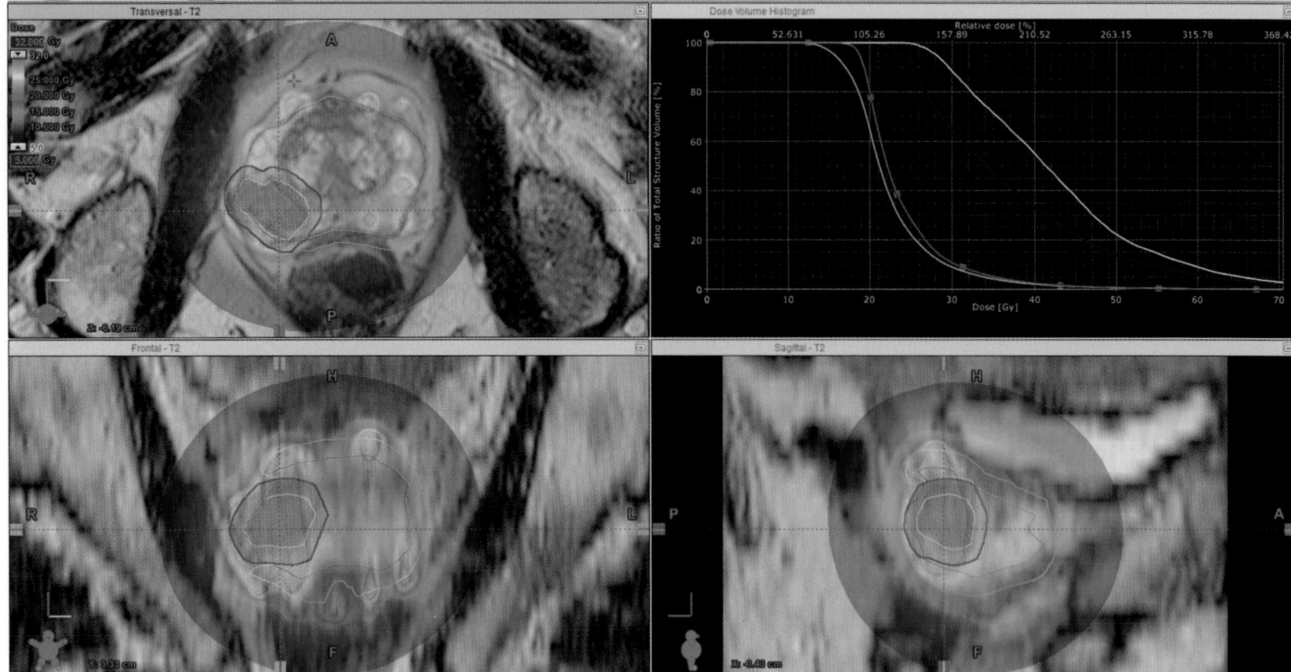

FIGURE 73-24 ■ **Biologically optimised radiotherapy.** A dominant intra-prostatic lesion (DIL) in the right posterolateral peripheral zone has been defined using multi-parametric MRI (black outline on the transverse, coronal and sagittal images). High dose-rate brachytherapy catheters have been inserted under general anaesthetic. The planning computer optimisation software has been programmed to maximise the radiation dose to the DIL and limit the dose to the rest of the prostate to a defined ceiling. The dose volume histograms (top left) demonstrate the dual dose levels. The DIL and DIL PTV (dark blue and yellow lines) receive a higher dose as a proportion of their volume than the non-dominant prostate and the non-dominant prostate PTV (light blue and red lines).

For a full list of references, please see ExpertConsult.

FURTHER READING

3. Staffurth J. A review of the clinical evidence for intensity-modulated radiotherapy. Clin Oncol (R Coll Radiol) 2010;22:643–57.
14. Padhani AR. Integrating multiparametric prostate MRI into clinical practice. Cancer Imaging 2011;11(Spec No A):S27–37.
16. Thorwarth D, Schaefer A. Functional target volume delineation for radiation therapy on the basis of positron emission tomography and the correlation with histopathology. Q J Nucl Med Mol Imaging 2010;54:490–9.
17. Webster GJ, Kilgallon JE, Ho KF, et al. A novel imaging technique for fusion of high-quality immobilised MR images of the head and neck with CT scans for radiotherapy target delineation. Br J Radiol 2009;82:497–503.
27. Bentzen SM. Theragnostic imaging for radiation oncology: dose-painting by numbers. Lancet Oncol 2005;6:112–17.
34. Padhani AR, Krohn KA, Lewis JS, et al. Imaging oxygenation of human tumours. Eur Radiol 2007;17:861–72.

CHAPTER 74

Functional and Molecular Imaging for Personalised Medicine in Oncology

Ferdia A. Gallagher • Avnesh S. Thakor • Eva M. Serrao • Vicky Goh

CHAPTER OUTLINE

PERSONALISED MEDICINE IN ONCOLOGY

The essence of oncological imaging is to detect and differentiate tumour from normal tissue. It is therefore necessary to understand the fundamental changes that occur within tissues or cells when a tumour forms, and how this can be used to generate tissue contrast. On the very simplest level, the differences in X-ray attenuation and water content between cancer and its surrounding tissues can be used to distinguish cancer from normal tissue using computed tomography (CT) and magnetic resonance imaging (MRI), respectively. Biological research in the field of oncology is increasingly revealing the fundamental tissue, cellular and molecular changes that form the hallmarks of cancer and this knowledge is now being applied to the development of new imaging biomarkers which will be more specific and sensitive for cancer detection than morphological information alone.[1] Examples include the use of CT and MRI contrast agents to probe angiogenesis, as well as positron emission tomography (PET) tracers to detect alterations in cellular energetics and proliferation within cancerous tissue.

In addition to identifying tumours, imaging biomarkers can be used to assess the efficacy of treatment such as chemotherapy and radiotherapy. Traditionally, this has been performed by identifying changes in tumour size using criteria such as the response evaluation criteria in solid tumours (RECIST); new imaging biomarkers which are more specific and sensitive for the detection of early response to treatment by detecting early cellular or molecular changes that predict long-term successful outcome are being developed. The introduction of therapies which have specific molecular targets (such as bevacizumab and sunitinib) has been problematic for traditional imaging approaches as improved clinical outcome with these drugs is often not accompanied by a significant change in tumour size; e.g. an anti-vascular drug may induce tumour necrosis with little change in the overall tumour diameter. Consequently, alternative imaging approaches are needed to identify a successful early response to therapy in this context; the concept of combining a specific targeted drug with an imaging biomarker that directly probes the cellular pathways affected by the drug is a very attractive approach for the future management of cancer patients.

These specific targeted imaging biomarkers also open up the possibility of detecting subtle differences in drug response between patients: a cellular pathway may be upregulated in one patient but downregulated in another in response to the same drug at the same dose. The old concept of a single treatment algorithm for all patients is increasingly being replaced by a personalised or patient-centred approach where drug therapy can be tailored to an individual patient. Modern medical practice is underpinned by an understanding of the molecular biology of disease processes; complementing this with new imaging techniques will be increasingly important. These molecular imaging methods can be defined as the visual representation, characterisation and quantification of biological processes at the cellular and subcellular levels within intact living organisms.[2] Functional imaging is more loosely defined and includes techniques which probe physiological processes such as blood flow, metabolism and features of the tumour microenvironment. There is some overlap between the two terms and often the combination of functional and molecular imaging is used to define a range of imaging techniques that are more specific than anatomical or morphological imaging and

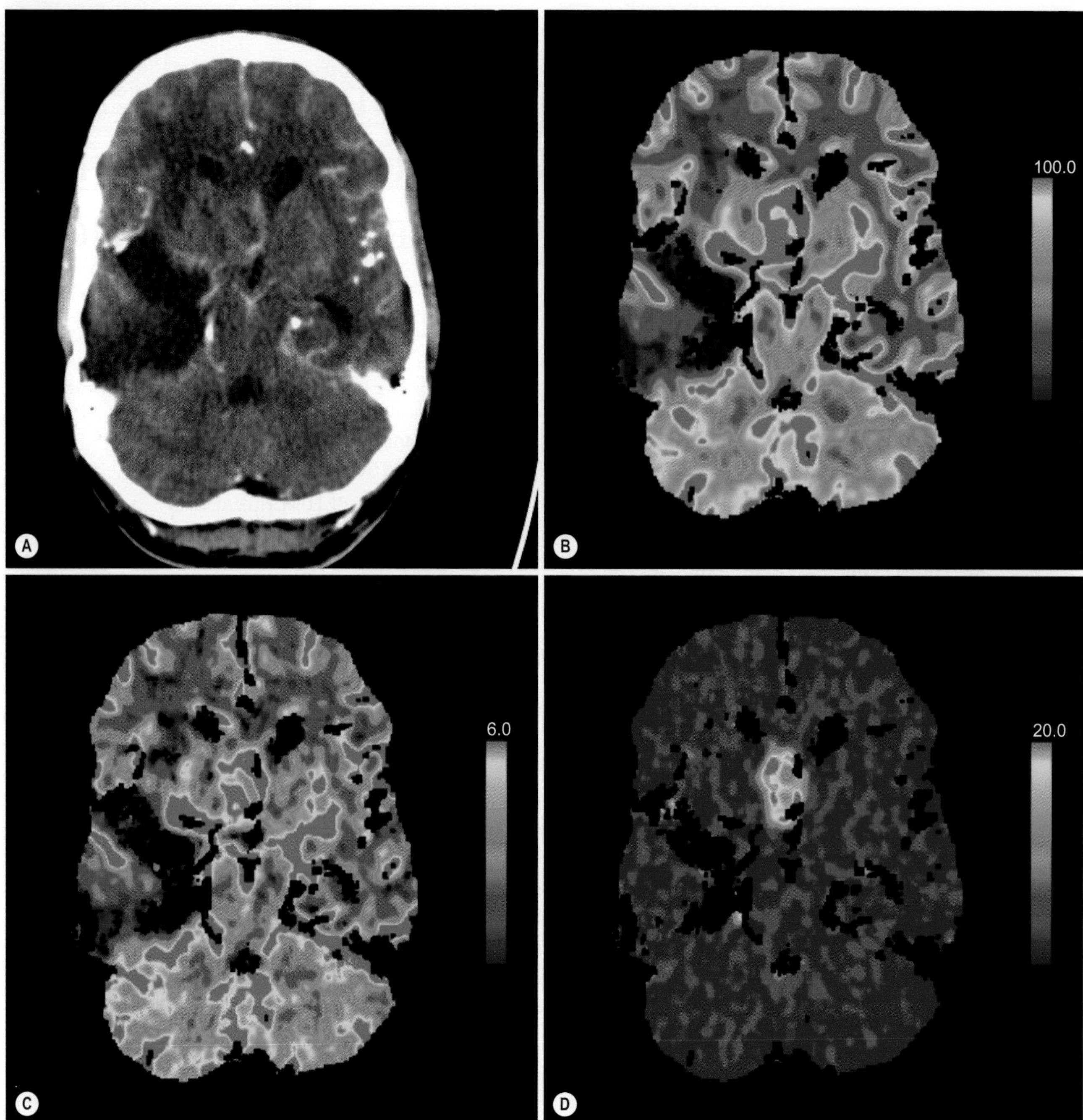

FIGURE 74-1 ■ Dynamic contrast-enhanced CT acquisition with parametric maps from a glioblastoma multiforme tumour. (A) Contrast-enhanced CT, (B) regional blood flow, (C) blood volume and (D) permeability–surface area product. The images demonstrate a vascular solid component with disruption of the blood–brain barrier best seen on the permeability–surface area product map.

probe processes from a tissue to a molecular level. This chapter will explore the use of these functional and molecular techniques in oncological imaging.

DYNAMIC CONTRAST-ENHANCED COMPUTED TOMOGRAPHY (DCE-CT)

There has been a recent resurgent interest in dynamic contrast-enhanced CT techniques for assessing the vasculature, which were first used in the early 1990s. This has been facilitated by technological advances allowing high temporal sampling acquisitions to be performed over a large volume (also known as *perfusion CT*) as well as therapeutic developments in stroke and cancer which have required an assessment of the functioning vasculature on an individual patient basis (Fig. 74-1).

Contrast Agent Kinetics

CT contrast agents used in clinical practice are low molecular weight contrast agents (< 1 kDa) with

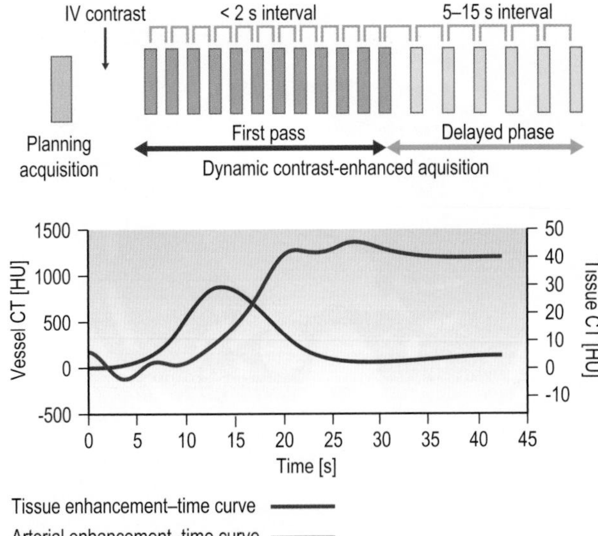

FIGURE 74-2 ■ Typical DCE-CT acquisition is shown, with the arterial (purple line) and tissue (green line) attenuation–time curves acquired for a lung cancer. Maximum enhancement reached within the aorta and tumour within the time period of the acquisition was 800 and 45 HU, respectively.

negligible serum protein binding and therefore a distribution similar to that of extracellular fluid. These agents are typically derivatives of iodobenzoic acid with an iodine concentration of at least 300 mg/mL. After intravenous injection (typically 4 mL/s or faster), the pharmacokinetic modelling can be approximated to a two-compartment model: the injected contrast agent initially remains within the intravascular compartment before diffusing into the extravascular and extracellular space (EES). The rate of this diffusion is determined by the perfusion of the organ, the vessel surface area and its permeability or leakiness; there is negligible transfer into the intracellular compartment (< 1%). The contrast agent then passes back from the EES into the intravascular compartment before being excreted predominantly by the kidneys; up to half of the administered dose is eliminated from the blood within the first two hours of injection.

By acquiring a rapid series of images following intravenous contrast agent administration, and assessing the changes in tissue and vessel attenuation during the acquisition, functional parameters can be derived (Fig. 74-2). These may be semi-quantitative (describing the 'curve shape' of the tissue attenuation–time graph), or quantitative parameters derived from kinetic modelling. As the change in measured CT attenuation is directly proportional to the concentration of iodine within the blood vessels or tissues, temporal changes in attenuation can be directly modelled to assess the tissue vascularity. The situation is somewhat different for MRI, where there is a complex relationship between MR signal intensity and the local tissue concentration of MR contrast medium. Acquisition is normally acquired over the 45 s of the perfusion phase and the larger the number of data acquisition points during this period, the better the data fitting. However, this has to be balanced against increasing radiation dose and the finite time required for each acquisition.[3] In general, at least five time points are acquired and the quantitative parameters are derived using a number of models, e.g. the Johnson–Wilson model, the Patlak method and the maximum slope model.[3–6] Further description of these techniques is given in Chapter 7.

The derived parameters include:

- regional tumour blood flow—blood flow per unit volume or unit mass of tissue;
- regional tumour blood volume—the proportion of tissue that comprises flowing blood;
- mean transit time—the average time for contrast material to traverse the tissue vasculature;
- extraction fraction—the rate of transfer of contrast material from the intravascular space to the EES;
- permeability–surface area product—which characterises the rate of diffusion of the contrast agent from the intravascular compartment to the EES.

The basis for the use of DCE-CT in oncology is that microvascular changes during angiogenesis are reflected in changes in the measured DCE-CT parameters; for example, permeability–surface area product is usually lower in normal tissue than in tumours (Fig. 74-3). DCE-CT measurements have been validated in a range of tumours in both animal models and human studies.[7,8] Measurements have been correlated positively with histological markers of angiogenesis and negatively with histological markers of hypoxia, indicating that these may be appropriate surrogates of fundamental biological processes during cancer formation.

In terms of characterisation, DCE-CT may distinguish benign from malignant lesions within the lung, pancreas and bowel though there is some overlap between malignant and inflammatory lesions, which reflects the generic nature of the vascular changes that can be probed.[9–12] In general, higher perfusion parameters have been reported in patients with tumours although there is variability between different types of tumours and even within the same tumour, which underlies the complexity of tumour heterogeneity. The major application of DCE-CT in routine clinical practice is in the assessment of the anti-vascular effects of conventional chemotherapies and interventional procedures, which target the vasculature. DCE-CT is also used to provide pharmacodynamic information in early-phase clinical trials in a variety of cancers (Table 74-1).[13–23] These have included anti-angiogenic and vascular disrupting agents, where DCE-CT is providing a direct imaging biomarker of the drug action and can be used to determine the appropriate drug dose. The wide availability of CT, the low cost of CT and the ease of standardisation of DCE-CT are advantages over MRI for its use in clinical practice despite the radiation burden. However, CT carries a significant radiation burden and there still remains a lack of data concerning the relationship between acute vascular reduction and long-term patient outcome.

In addition to identifying treatment response, DCE-CT may have an important role in risk stratification and as a predictive biomarker of treatment. The basis for the predictive value of DCE-CT in the setting of chemotherapy is likely to relate to reduced drug delivery, while in radiotherapy this is likely to represent a marker of the hypoxic environment, which in turn correlates with

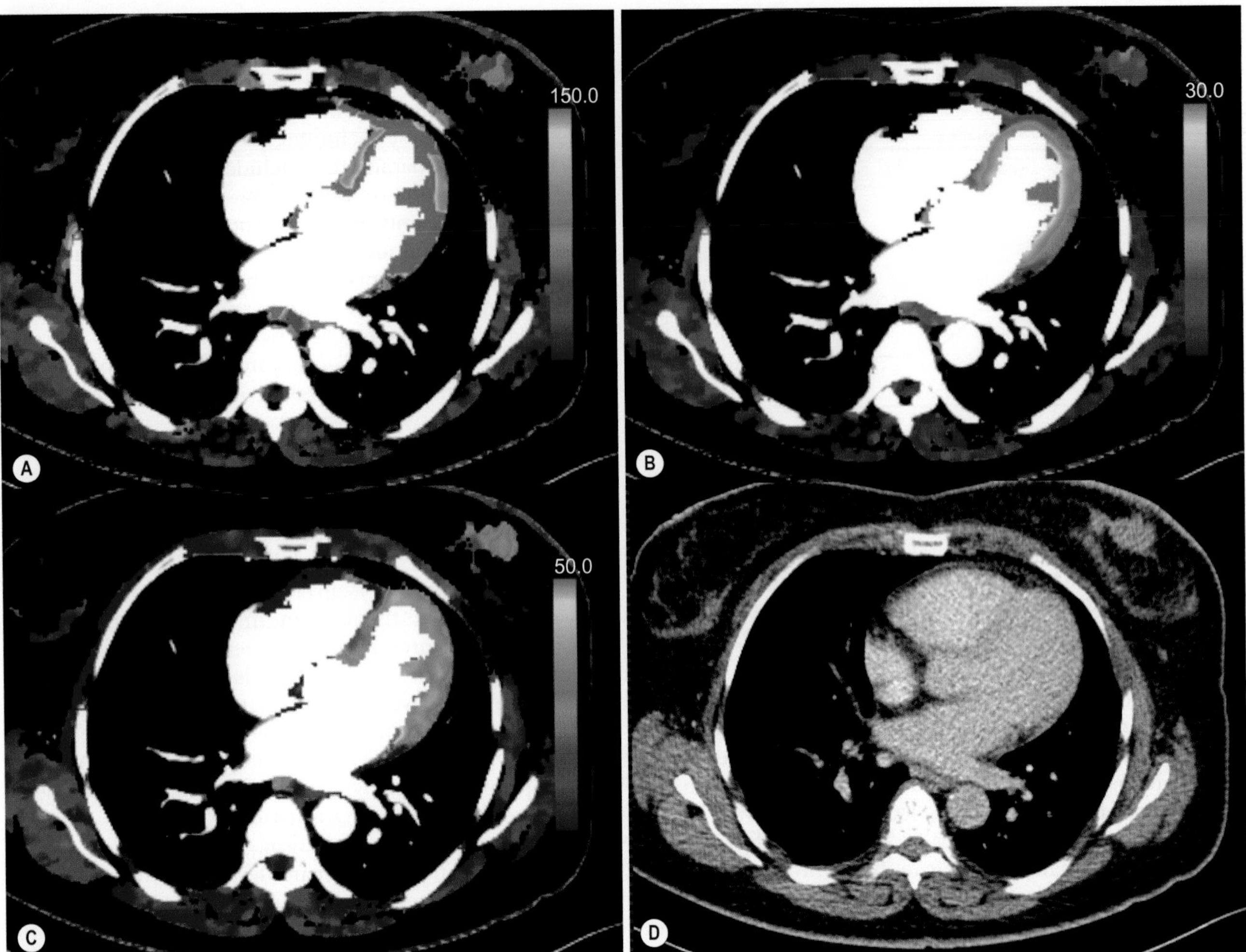

FIGURE 74-3 ■ DCE-CT parameter maps of a breast tumour. (A) Regional blood flow, (B) blood volume and (C) permeability–surface area product maps with corresponding (D) contrast-enhanced CT. The images demonstrate a higher vascularity within the tumour than within normal breast tissue.

TABLE 74-1 **Table of Clinical Trials Incorporating DCE-CT**[13–23]

Tumour	Therapy	Parameter	Author	Year
Solid tumours	Endostatin	BF, BV (decrease)	Thomas et al.[13]	2003
Rectal cancer	Bevacizumab	BF, BV (decrease)	Willett et al.[14]	2004
Solid tumours	SU6668	BF, BV (decrease)	Xiong et al.[15]	2004
Solid tumours	MEDI-522	MTT (increase)	McNeel et al.[16]	2005
Renal cancer	Thalidomide	BF, BV (decrease)	Faria et al.[17]	2007
Squamous cell carcinoma oropharynx	Cisplatin and 5FU	BF, BV (decrease in responders)	Gandhi et al.[18]	2006
Solid tumours	AZD2171 and gefitinib	BF (decrease)	Meijerink et al.[19]	2007
Non-small cell lung cancer	Combretastatin and radiotherapy	BV (decrease)	Ng et al.[20]	2007
Solid tumours	Nitric oxide synthase inhibitor	BV (decrease)	Ng et al.[21]	2007
Renal cell carcinoma	Tyrosine kinase inhibitors	BF, BV (decrease)	Fournier et al.[22]	2010
Non-small cell lung cancer	Erlotinib/sorafenib	BF (decrease)	Lind et al.[23]	2010

BF = regional blood flow; BV = regional blood volume; MTT = mean transit time.

resistance to radiotherapy. For example, in locally advanced squamous cell carcinoma of the head and neck treated with surgery and adjuvant chemoradiotherapy, pre-treatment primary tumour blood flow and permeability may be independent predictors of disease recurrence.[24] In pancreatic cancer, a low baseline volume transfer constant (K^{trans}) predicts for a poorer response to chemotherapy with gemcitabine and radiotherapy.[25] In colorectal cancer, tumours with a lower blood flow at staging are more likely to have nodal metastases and a poorer outcome; rectal tumours with a lower blood flow are also more likely to respond poorly to chemoradiation.[26,27]

The cancer risk associated with the radiation dose of DCE-CT has to be balanced against potential benefits of vascular quantification and must be judged in the context of the population under investigation. Typical effective radiation doses from a first-pass volumetric perfusion CT study of the thorax, abdomen or pelvis range from 13.7 to 28.7 mSv.[28] Using a risk estimate of 4.2% per Sv from the International Commission on Radiation Protection, the estimated lifetime risk of developing a cancer from a single such perfusion CT is approximately 1 in 1000.[29]

MAGNETIC RESONANCE IMAGING (MRI)

Dynamic Contrast-Enhanced MRI (DCE-MRI)

DCE-MRI consists of serial MRI acquisitions following injection of an intravenous contrast agent in a similar manner to that described above for DCE-CT. Clinical dynamic MRI is usually performed using low molecular weight gadolinium chelate-based contrast agents. These have paramagnetic ions that are known to interact with nearby hydrogen nuclei and lead to shortening of T1 (and T2) relaxation times, resulting in signal enhancement on T1-weighted images, thus producing positive contrast. The major advantages of MRI include the absence of ionising radiation, high contrast-to-noise ratio, high signal-to-noise ratio and the many mechanisms which can be utilised to produce tissue contrast.[30]

As with contrast-enhanced CT, contrast-enhanced MRI can either be used to provide a qualitative snapshot of tissue enhancement, as is used routinely in clinical practice, or more quantitatively in the form of DCE-MRI (Fig. 74-4). The latter permits a fuller depiction of contrast kinetics within lesions in much the same way as DCE-CT. DCE-MRI can be repeated over a course of treatment to monitor changes in tumour vascularity over time. Although the technique is reproducible when using a single clinical MRI system, the reproducibility of DCE-MRI studies between centres may be less robust, due to the differences in scanner hardware, contrast agent injection protocols, acquisition parameters, and kinetic models employed.[31]

DCE-MRI protocols most commonly involve T1-weighted image acquisition before, during and after the injection of the MR contrast agent (typically 0.1 mmol/kg with injection after 1 min and continuous data acquisition for up to 10 min); this provides an assessment of the different stages of tissue uptake and washout.[32,33] The contrast agents used are either low molecular weight agents (< 1 kDa) that rapidly diffuse into the extracellular space or larger macromolecular agents (> 30 kDa) that demonstrate prolonged intravascular retention.[30] Given the lack of ionising radiation in DCE-MRI, temporal data can be continuously acquired during the phases of tissue enhancement, unlike in DCE-CT. The concentration of the contrast agent in the vasculature allows an assessment of perfusion, and in the case of the low molecular weight agents, this is followed by rapid diffusion into the EES where it accumulates. As with DCE-CT, the rate at which this occurs is dependent on blood flow as well as vessel permeability and surface area.[30,34] However, MR signal intensity is not directly proportional to the contrast agent concentration and therefore more complex quantitative data analysis is required to convert the MR signal intensity into biologically meaningful quantitative parameters.[35–37]

A simple approach is to use the initial area under the curve (IAUC), which describes the shape of the graph of contrast agent concentration over time; although this is frequently used in trials, it is difficult to interpret physiologically.[38] Therefore, in clinical trials, assessment of the effect of an anti-angiogenic or vascular disrupting agent

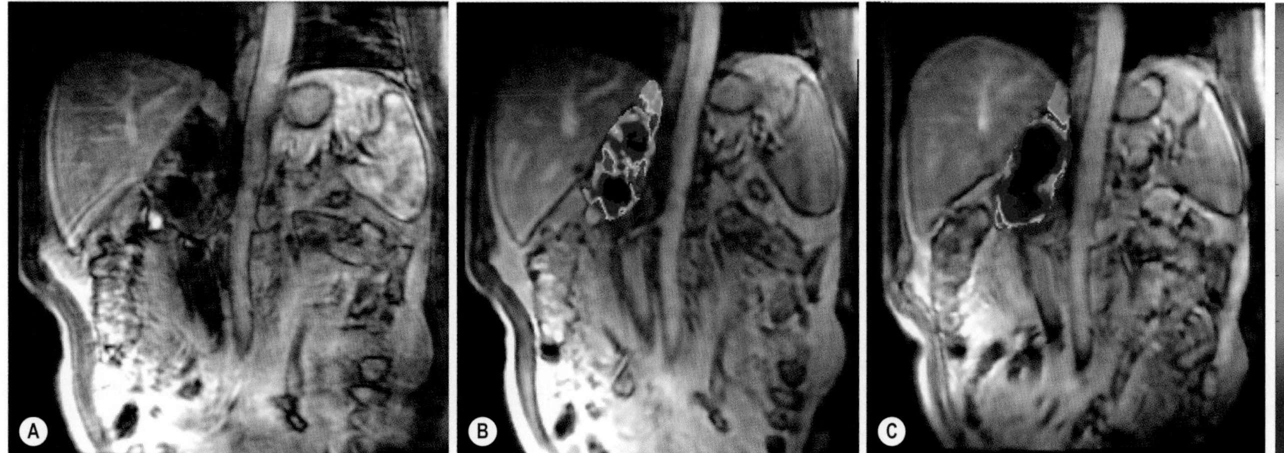

FIGURE 74-4 ■ Example parameter maps for a renal cell carcinoma metastasis. (A) Image from a dynamic contrast-enhanced acquisition, (B) initial area under the gadolinium curve (over 90 s; IAUGC90) map before treatment, (C) IAUGC90 map 48 h after treatment with an anti-angiogenic agent (bevacizumab), showing decrease in the tumour perfusion with colour scale. (Images courtesy of Andrew Gill, Dr Andrew Priest, Professor Duncan Jodrell and Professor Tim Eisen, Addenbrooke's Hospital, Cambridge.)

is often modelled using changes in K^{trans} (the volume transfer coefficient of contrast between the blood plasma and the EES, as described above for CT) and the volume of the EES (v_e).[39] The other commonly used pharmacokinetic variables are summarised in Tables 74-2 and 74-3.[32,40]

DCE-MRI and DCE-CT exploit the fact that the onset of many diseases is associated with an alteration in vascular density, vascular permeability and blood flow. In particular, tumours develop a network of new vessels as they grow, but unlike normal vasculature, tumour angiogenesis is chaotic and inefficient with permeable vessels.[41] Therefore, an increase in signal enhancement, vessel permeability, and flow is often demonstrated within tumours when compared with benign lesions or normal tissue.[42–45]

DCE-MRI has been used for tumour detection, characterisation, staging, and therapy monitoring. However, the meaning of an elevated K^{trans} is still controversial in terms of prognosis, as studies have shown conflicting results;[46,47] there is stronger evidence that K^{trans} can be used to demonstrate which tumours are responding to therapy as a pharmacodynamic biomarker of drug activity, particularly in the context of anti-angiogenic drugs or vascular disrupting agents.[38,48] Changes in K^{trans} have been shown to correlate both with the administration of vascular endothelial growth factor (VEGF, a signalling molecule that stimulates the growth of new blood vessels), as well as the administration of therapeutic monoclonal antibodies that block its effect.[49] Consequently, both DCE-MRI and DCE-CT can be used as a platform to understand drug and tumour interactions.[50]

Another emerging approach has been to use dynamic susceptibility contrast MRI (DSC-MRI), which also relies upon the serial acquisition of images after the injection of a contrast agent.[51,52] However, DSC-MRI measures induced alterations in the transverse relaxation times, T2 and T2*, resulting in signal loss and hence transient darkening of the tissues (thus acting as a negative contrast unlike that seen with T1-weighted imaging).[30] The degree of signal loss is dependent on the concentration of the agent as well as vessel size and density and therefore this can be used to estimate the relative blood volume (rBV) of the tissue under assessment.[53] Using this technique, changes in relative cerebral blood volume (rCBV) maps have been correlated with glioma grade and this approach can be used not only to understand the nature of tumour heterogeneity better but also to target biopsies to focal areas of vascular changes within a tumour, which may help to avoid sampling error.[54] The method has also been used to distinguish radiation necrosis from recurrent disease, evaluate response to therapy and as a prognostic marker.[55,56] Its application to extracerebral tumours (e.g. breast and prostate) is under investigation.[57,58]

The role of DCE-MRI in clinical practice has been limited by the relatively small number of patients in many published trials, the use of widely varying acquisition techniques and modelled parameters between centres, as well as the use of diverse disease endpoints. Current attempts to standardise DCE-MRI will help to address these issues in the future. Although DCE-MRI has shown much promise, it has yet to be incorporated into routine clinical practice (Table 74-4).[59–68]

TABLE 74-2 Most Common Pharmacokinetic Parameters Used in DCE-MRI Analysis[32,40]

Parameter (units)	Alternative Nomenclature	Definition
K^{trans} (min^{-1})	EF, K^{PS}	Volume transfer constant between blood plasma and EES
v_e (a.u.)	Interstitial space	EES volume per unit tissue volume
v_p (a.u.)		Blood plasma volume per unit tissue volume
k_{ep} (min^{-1})	k_{21}	Rate constant from EES to blood plasma $k_{ep} = K^{trans} / v_e$
k_{pe} (min^{-1})	k_{12}	Rate constant from blood plasma to EES
k_{el} (min^{-1})		Elimination rate constant
Amp (a.u.)	A	Amplitude of the normalised dynamic curve

Adapted from Yang et al.[40] and Tofts et al.[32]; a.u., arbitrary units.

TABLE 74-3 Model-Free Parameters Applied in DCE-MRI Analysis[32,40]

Parameter (Units)	Alternative Nomenclature	Definition
Area under the curve (min or mmol·min/L)	IAUC, AUC, AUGC, IAUGC	Area under the signal intensity or gadolinium dynamic curve
Relative signal intensity (a.u.)	RSI = $S_{(t)}/S_0$	Relative signal intensity at time (t)
Initial slope (min^{-1})	Enhancement slope, upslope, enhancement rate	Maximum or average slope in the initial enhancement
Washout slope (min^{-1})	Downslope, washout rate	Maximum or average slope in the washout phase
Peak enhancement ratio (a.u.)	Maximum signal enhancement ratio (SER_{max})	PER = $(S_{max} - S_0)/S_0$
T_{max} (s)	Time-to-peak (TTP)	Time to peak enhancement
Maximum intensity-time ratio (s^{-1})	MITR = PER/T_{max}	

Adapted from Yang et al.[40] and Tofts et al.[32]; $S_{(t)}$, MR signal intensity at time t; S_0, precontrast signal intensity; S_{max}, maximum signal intensity; a.u., arbitrary units.

TABLE 74-4 **Table of Some Clinical Studies Incorporating DCE-MRI**[59–68]

Tumour	Therapy	Parameter	Author	Year
Solid tumours	AG-013736	K^{trans}, IAUC	Lui et al.[59]	2005
Solid tumours	AZD2171	IAUC	Drevs et al.[60]	2007
Renal cell carcinoma	Sorafenib	K^{trans}	Flaherty et al.[61]	2008
Breast cancer	Neoadjuvant 5-fluorouracil, epirubicin and cyclophosphamide	K^{trans}, k_{ep}, v_e, rBV, rBF, MTT	Ah-See et al.[62]	2008
Primary liver tumours	Floxuridine and dexamethasone	K^{trans}, k_{ep}, AUC	Jarnagin et al.[63]	2009
Glioblastoma	Bevacizumab	K^{trans}, v_e	Ferl et al.[64]	2010
Breast cancer	Neoadjuvant therapy: 5-fluorouracil, epirubicin and cyclophosphamide	K^{trans}, v_e	Jensen et al.[65]	2011
Prostate cancer	Androgen deprivation therapy	K^{trans}, k_{ep}, v_p, IAUGC	Barrett et al.[66]	2012
Cervical cancer	Radiotherapy & cisplatin and 5-fluorouracil plus cisplatin	K^{trans}, k_{ep}, v_e	Kim et al.[67]	2012
Rectal cancer	FOLFOX and bevacizumab	K^{trans}, k_{ep}, v_e, AUC	Gollub et al.[68]	2012

Diffusion-Weighted Imaging (DWI)

Water molecules in the liquid phase undergo thermally driven random motions, a phenomenon known as Brownian motion or free diffusion, and it is these small motions—typically of the order of 30 μm—which can be probed and quantified using DWI.[69] These small molecular movements can be measured by spin-echo T2-weighted sequences, in which two equal diffusion sensitising gradients are applied before and after a 180° radiofrequency pulse.[69,70] The *b*-value (in s/mm^2) is a commonly applied term that allows the quantification of these gradients by pooling information from a number of variables. By measuring how far a molecule moves in a fixed time interval, the diffusion constant can be calculated.

In routine clinical practice, DWI can be used both qualitatively and quantitatively. Qualitative assessment identifies relative DWI changes compared to the surrounding normal tissue. Quantitative information can be obtained through the calculation of the apparent diffusion coefficient or ADC. This mathematical entity can be calculated from the slope of relative signal intensity (on a logarithmic scale) against a series of *b*-values.[71]

There is increasing evidence that the calculated ADC correlates with tissue cellularity. Within biological tissue, the small molecular movements of water are subject to restrictions, which are inherent to the medium due to the surrounding cells and constituency of the extracellular space. In the presence of few or no cells, there is high water diffusion and the molecules will diffuse further in a fixed time interval compared to water molecules within a high cellular environment. Tissues with low cellularity have lower DWI signal intensity and higher ADC values, while the opposite occurs in more solid tissues with a high cellularity, e.g. tumour, cytotoxic oedema, abscess and fibrosis.[70-72] Although the restricted diffusion seen within tumours is largely due to increased cellular density, other factors are likely to play a role such as the tortuosity of the extracellular space, extracellular fibrosis and the shape and size of the intercellular spaces.[73] Clinically, DWI is used to detect, characterise and stage tumours, distinguish tumour from surrounding tissues, predict and monitor response to therapy as well as evaluate tumour recurrence.[74-80] Successful treatment is generally reflected by an increase in the ADC value, although transient early decreases can occur following treatment.[7,11]

The development of stronger diffusion gradients, faster imaging sequences and improvements in hardware have allowed DWI to be extended to whole-body imaging applications, which has been particularly useful in oncology (Fig. 74-5).[72,81] Although many studies have shown its clinical potential as an imaging tool, protocol standardisation and larger clinical trials are necessary in the future.[81] In addition, further work is still required to understand the complicated interplay between ADC and the biophysical and cellular environment.

MR Spectroscopy (MRS)

Magnetic resonance spectroscopy is a technique that allows simultaneous non-invasive detection and measurement of several metabolites and chemicals found in tissue. The detection and identification of the metabolite peaks resides primarily on the subtle changes in the nuclear resonance frequency exerted by the atomic structure of its constituent molecule. For example, the two hydrogen nuclei (^{1}H or protons) in each molecule of water have a different resonant frequency from the hydrogen nuclei in fat and this can be exploited in fat-suppressed imaging. The measurement of the shift in frequency of a peak (in parts per million; ppm) relative to a standard such as water allows a molecule to be identified; the area under the curve of the peak gives an indication of the concentration of the molecule relative to the standard. Therefore, multiple endogenous metabolites can be simultaneously identified and an indication of their relative concentrations can be derived.

Proton MRS is often termed ^{1}H-MRS as the hydrogen nucleus contains a single proton. ^{1}H-MRS has been used to detect tumour metabolism since the 1980s and has a number of applications in the central nervous system.[82,83] Common metabolites that can be identified are choline-containing molecules (Cho), creatine (Cr), phosphocreatine (PCr) and *N*-acetylaspartate (NAA).[69] NAA is predominately present in neurons and the loss of NAA is associated with neuronal loss as occurs in stroke or in the

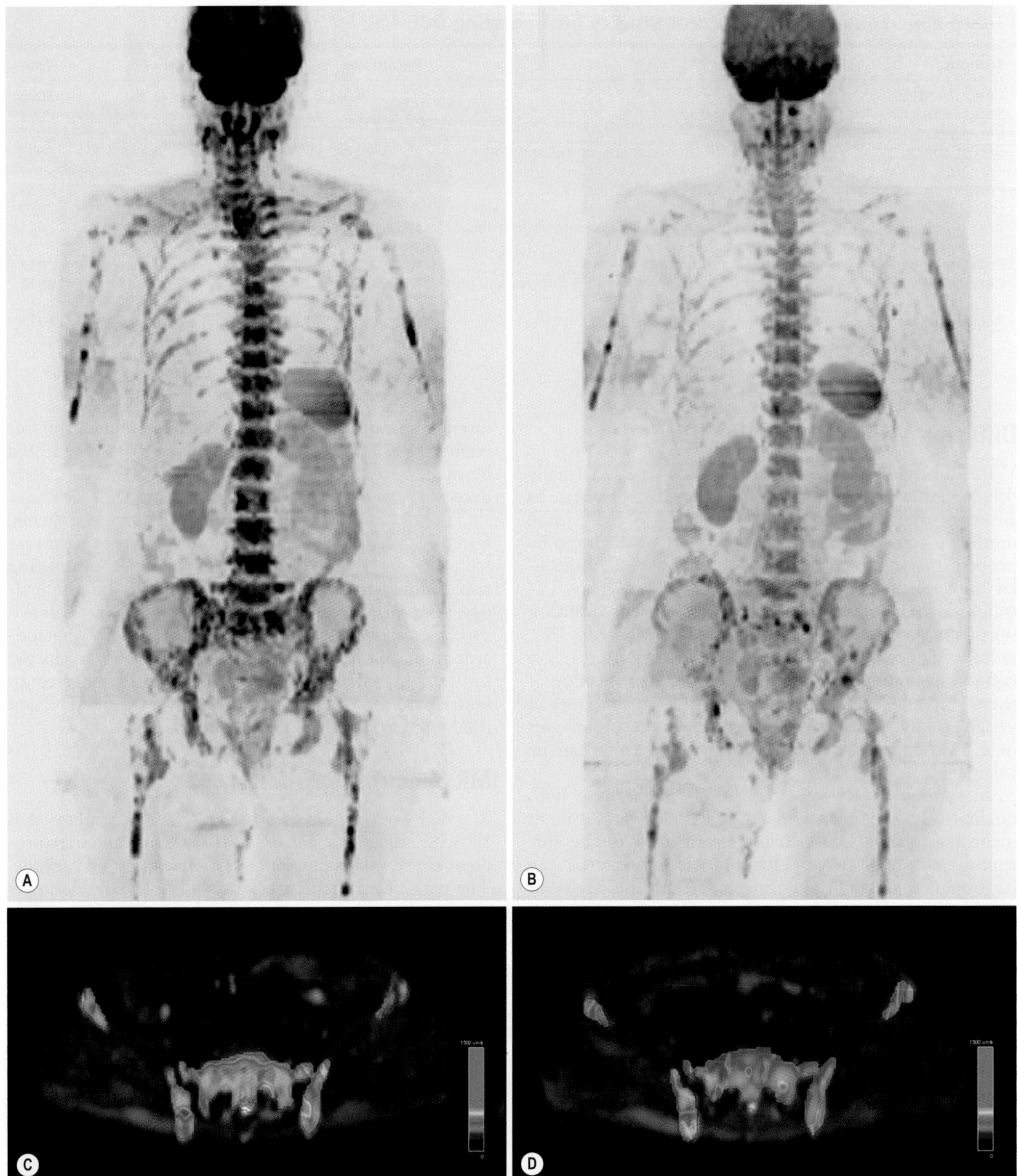

FIGURE 74-5 ■ Example of whole-body diffusion-weighted imaging. Serial changes in a 64-year-old woman with metastatic breast cancer treated with chemotherapy and bisphosphonates. (A) Inverted 3D maximum intensity projection (MIP) diffusion-weighted images showing widespread metastatic bone disease; (B) there is a subsequent decrease in the restricted diffusion and disease extent following treatment. (C) Colour ADC map of the pelvis in the same patient before treatment; (D) after treatment there is an increase in ADC, demonstrated by the colour change, indicating a response to treatment. (Images courtesy of Professor Anwar Padhani, Mount Vernon Cancer Centre, Northwood, Middlesex.)

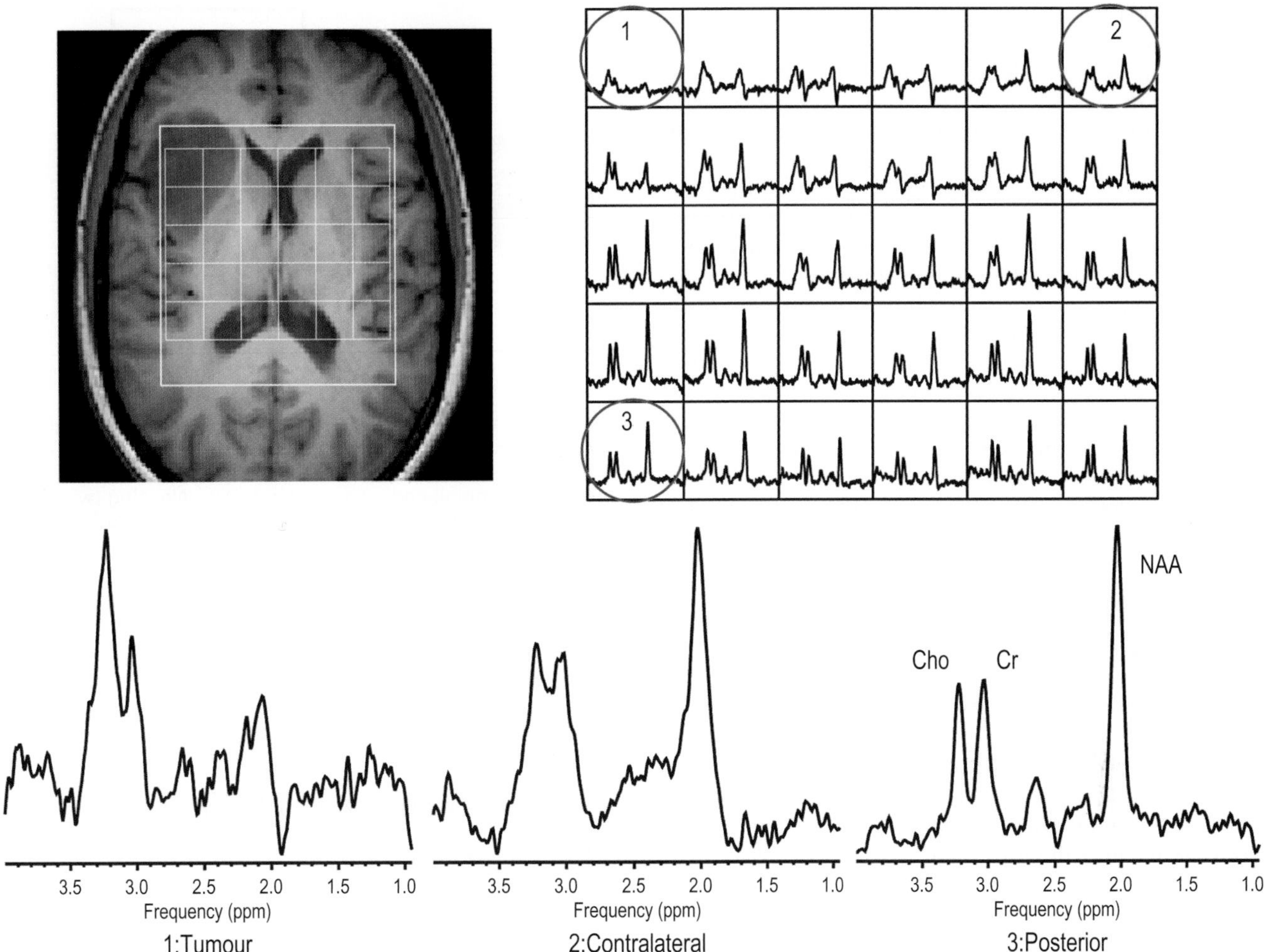

FIGURE 74-6 ■ Example of magnetic resonance spectroscopy (MRS) in a patient with a brain tumour. Localised spectroscopy has been acquired from a patient with a low-grade glioma. Three voxels have been enlarged to include: (1) tumour; (2) normal contralateral brain; and (3) normal ipsilateral brain. Common metabolites identified are: choline-containing molecules (Cho); creatine (Cr); and *N*-acetylaspartate (NAA). **NAA is present predominately in neurons and loss of NAA is associated with neuronal damage. The glioma demonstrates low levels of NAA and a Cho peak which is larger relative to the Cr peak.** (Images courtesy of Dr Mary McLean, Cancer Research UK, Cambridge Institute.)

presence of an intracranial tumour (Fig. 74-6).[84–86] Choline is part of the lipid biosynthesis pathway and because tumours contain a higher proportion of lipids than normal tissue, the choline-containing metabolite peak is a dominant feature of most tumour spectra.[69] Furthermore, a decrease may be seen following successful treatment with a chemotherapeutic agent.[87] As well as diagnosis and treatment response, applications of MRS in the clinical setting include tumour grading, identification of tumour margins for radiotherapy, and evaluation of local recurrence.[87–92]

MR spectroscopy can also be applied to other nuclei such as phosphorus-31 (^{31}P), fluorine-19 (^{19}F) and carbon-13 (^{13}C). ^{31}P-MRS is particularly suited to investigate cellular membrane metabolism and energy state, as it can detect the basic energy unit within the cell—adenosine triphosphate (ATP).[93] Tumours tend to have altered membrane metabolism, showing high levels of phosphomonoesters (PME) detectable by ^{31}P-MRS, which can be used as a marker of tumour aggressiveness as well as assessing the response to therapy.[93,94] Intracellular pH (pH$_i$) can also be determined by this technique using the pH-sensitive inorganic phosphate (P$_i$) peak; although alterations in intracellular pH occur in tumours, the major pH change demonstrated in cancer is an acidification of the extracellular space.[95–98] ^{19}F-MRS has been mainly used to ascertain the pharmacokinetics of fluorinated drugs, such as 5-fluorouracil.[93,99] Finally, ^{13}C-MRS is a technique used to study metabolism of carbon-containing molecules which are fundamental to most cellular processes such as the citric acid cycle; abnormalities in the processing of carbon-containing metabolites are an early hallmark of a number of disease processes.[100] The use of ^{13}C-MRS in clinical practice has been limited by its low sensitivity, due in part to the fact that carbon-13 represents approximately 1% of total carbon in the body.

MRS is an attractive method for non-invasive detection of the biochemical status of disease processes. It is a very powerful tool for distinguishing endogenous metabolites from each other; however, its routine use in the clinical arena has been hampered by inherent technical constraints: low sensitivity and low spatial resolution. Recently, new methods for helping overcome some of these limitations have been described; e.g. hyperpolarisation techniques which significantly increase the sensitivity of MRI are being developed. Hyperpolarised gases have been used to image the microstructure of the lungs and a method termed dynamic nuclear polarisation (DNP) has been applied to hyperpolarise carbon-13. The latter involves intravenous administration of a hyperpolarised ^{13}C-labelled molecule followed by imaging of the injected molecule and the metabolites formed from it.[101] This has been used to assess fundamental biochemical pathways and physiological processes within animals.[101] To date, the most promising molecule has been ^{13}C-labelled pyruvate, which has been used as an early treatment response biomarker in cancer and DNP has recently undergone its first clinical trial in prostate cancer.[102]

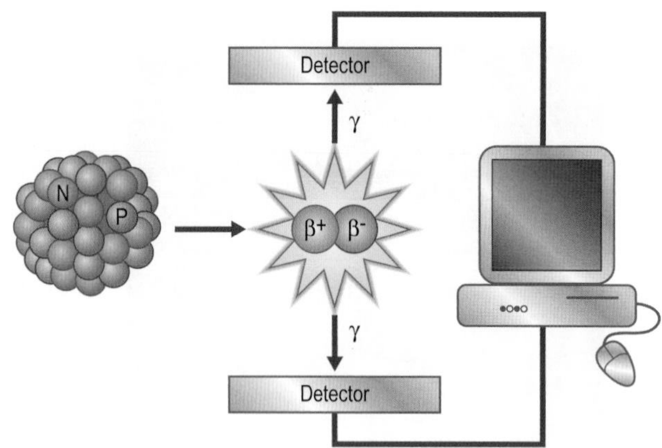

FIGURE 74-7 ■ **The principles of PET imaging.** The released positrons (β^+) from the nucleus of a radionuclide (e.g. the ^{18}F within FDG) travels a short distance (a), the *mean positron range*. The positron is annihilated by an electron (β^-), releasing two coincidence 511-keV photons (γ), which are then collected by detectors. N, neutron; P, proton.

POSITRON EMISSION TOMOGRAPHY (PET)

Positron emission tomography (PET) is based on the detection of an injected positron-emitting radioactive tracer. The positron (β^+) combines with an electron in the local tissue and, as a result of the annihilation, paired photons are simultaneously emitted 180° apart. These photons are subsequently detected outside of the patient by detectors that surround the patient and because they are 180° apart, the annihilation can be localised to a line connecting the two detectors. PET relies on the simultaneous or coincidence detection of the annihilation photons (γ) released when the radionuclides injected in the patient emit positrons that undergo annihilation with electrons. As collimators are not required to reconstruct the image, the sensitivity of PET imaging is generally very high. Furthermore, given that these radiolabelled tracers are often physiological or functional molecules, PET can obtain quantitative functional information of physiological or pathological processes. Although PET can identify the presence of a radiolabel with high sensitivity, it cannot differentiate individual species that are radiolabelled; i.e. an injected radiolabelled molecule may be metabolised into one or more molecules but the measured PET signal combines all of these together. Therefore image contrast with PET is generated from regional differences in radiolabel accumulation rather than the identification of individual metabolites as in MRS. The relatively low spatial resolution PET imaging is usually combined with high-resolution anatomical information acquired from CT or MRI, termed PET-CT or PET-MRI.

PET radiotracers or radiopharmaceuticals are compounds of biomedical interest, which are labelled with radionuclides such as fluorine-18 (^{18}F), carbon-11 (^{11}C) or oxygen-15 (^{15}O). The accumulation of a radioactively labelled tracer (and its metabolic products) can be used as a quantitative measure of the biological processes that are being probed (Fig. 74-7). Corrections can be applied for the weight of the patient and the injected dose to produce a standardised uptake value (SUV); the maximum tracer uptake of a single voxel within a region of interest is termed the SUV_{max} and this is commonly used in clinical practice as a simple metric of PET metabolism.

Fluorodeoxyglucose-PET (FDG-PET)

PET-CT has emerged as a promising technique in oncological imaging for diagnosis, staging, therapy response and evaluation of recurrence in a number of malignancies. Although there is an extensive array of clinical radiotracers available, the most widely used is ^{18}F-labelled 2-fluoro-2-deoxy-D-glucose (FDG), a fluorinated analogue of glucose. FDG is transported by the glucose transporters into the cell and phosphorylated by the enzyme hexokinase; no further metabolism occurs and the phosphorylated FDG becomes trapped and accumulates within the cell. The use of this tracer is based on the principle that the majority of malignant cells have upregulated glycolysis: i.e. increased glucose uptake and metabolism compared to normal cells. Upregulated glycolysis leads to an increased formation of lactate; lactate is produced in normal tissue in the presence of reduced oxygen levels but in tumours this occurs even in the presence of oxygen, a phenomenon termed aerobic glycolysis or the Warburg effect.[104,105] The phenomenon of aerobic glycolysis underlies the widespread use of ^{18}F-labelled FDG-PET in oncology. There is increasing evidence to support a role for FDG-PET in the management of oncology patients, as listed in Table 74-5.[106]

Non-FDG-PET Tracers

FDG is the leading clinical molecule for PET and many centres only use FDG as a clinical tracer in PET. The great versatility of PET is the large number of molecules that can be labelled to probe a wide range of biological processes. PET tracers can be broadly classified into markers of morphological structure, perfusion, altered metabolism, proliferation, cell death, hypoxia and cell surface protein expression, e.g. receptors (Fig. 74-8). Table 74-6 summarises the common non-FDG tracers used in clinical practice, the mechanisms that they probe and their clinical applications.[107–130] These tracers are at varying stages of development: there are a large number of preclinical tracers, a smaller number of experimental clinical probes and a relatively limited number of agents that are used routinely in clinical practice.

TABLE 74-5 Current Clinical Indications for Use of FDG-PET-CT in Oncology

- Evaluation of indeterminate lesions detected by another imaging method in order to help in the differential diagnosis between a benign and a malignant process
- Guidance of initial or subsequent treatment strategy in patients with a known malignancy
- Monitoring of treatment response
- Evaluation of residual post-treatment abnormalities detected by another imaging method in order to determine whether it represents persistent viable tumour or post-treatment changes
- Localisation of the primary site of a tumour when metastatic disease is the first manifestation of malignancy
- Establishment and localisation of disease sites as a cause for an elevated serum marker
- Guidance of clinical procedures, such as directed biopsies and radiation therapy planning

From the American College of Radiology and Society for Pediatric Radiology Guidelines 2012.[106]

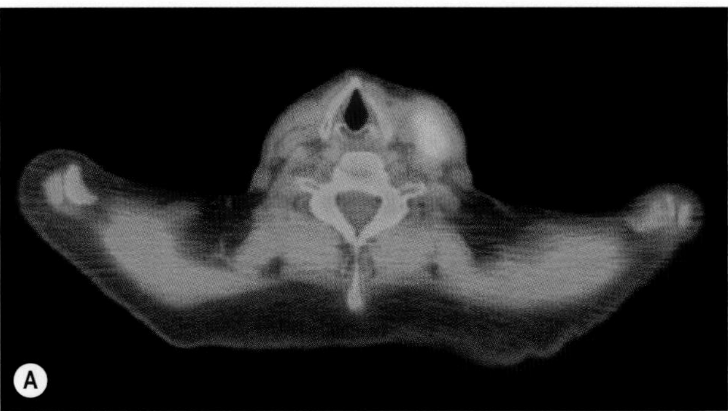

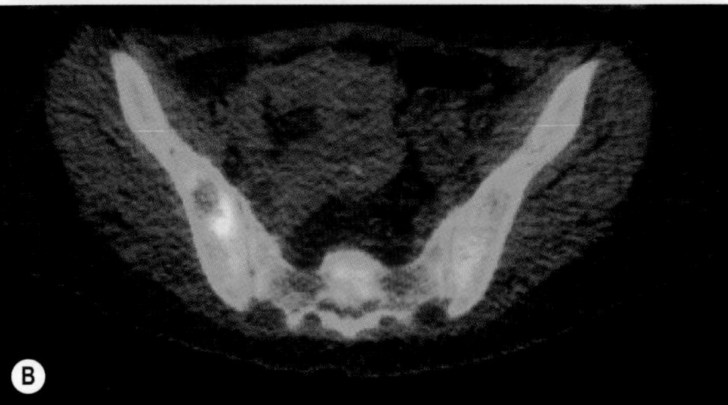

FIGURE 74-8 ■ Examples of non-FDG-PET imaging in metastatic renal cell carcinoma. (A) An ^{18}F-labelled FMISO PET-CT study showing focal retention of the tracer within a hypoxic left cervical metastasis. (B) ^{18}F-labelled sodium fluoride PET-CT in a different patient—there is focal uptake around a lytic bone metastasis within the right side of the pelvis. (Images courtesy of Dr John Buscombe, Addenbrooke's Hospital, Cambridge.)

TABLE 74-6 Summary of Non-FDG-PET Tracers Used in The Clinic[107–130]

Tracer	Radionuclide	Mechanism of Action Clinical Applications
Sodium fluoride	^{18}F	Uptake reflects blood flow and bone remodeling; Detects primary and secondary bone tumours[108]
FLT	^{18}F	Thymidine analogue; Detects cellular proliferation; Distinguishes malignant from benign lesions in lung, breast and colon[107]
Methionine	^{11}C	Radiolabelled amino acid; Tumour uptake reflects cellular proliferation and microvessel density; Used in grading of brain tumours, differential diagnosis and identifying recurrence[109–113]
FET	^{18}F	Radiolabelled amino acid; Detection of high-grade glioma[114]
FMAU	^{18}F	Proliferation probe; Detection of brain, prostate and bone tumours[115]
Acetate	^{11}C	Fatty acids precursor; Detection of prostate cancer and low-grade hepatic cancer[116–119]
FMISO	^{18}F	Hypoxia imaging probe; Predictor for local recurrence in head, neck and lung cancer[120,121]
FAZA	^{18}F	Hypoxia imaging probe; Predictor of successfully radiotherapy[122,123]
ATSM	^{62}Cu	Hypoxia imaging probe; Predictor of response to chemoradiotherapy[124]
^{15}O water	^{15}O	Perfusion probe; Evaluation of response to cytotoxics, anti-angiogenic and vascular disrupting agents in solid tumours[125–127]
Annexin V	^{68}Ga ^{18}F	Cell death probe; Treatment response marker[128]
DOTA-TATE	^{68}Ga	Binds to somatostatin receptors; Diagnosis of new lesions in patients with or suspected neuroendocrine tumours[129,130]

Abbreviations: FLT, 3-deoxy-3-[^{18}F]fluorothymidine; FET, O-(2-[^{18}F]fluoroethyl)-L-tyrosine; FMAU, [^{18}F]-1-(2′-deoxy-2′-fluoro-beta-D-arabinofuranosyl)thymine; FMISO, [^{18}F]-fluoromisonidazole; FAZA, [^{18}F]-fluoroazomycinarabinoside; ATSM, diacetyl-bis(N^{4}-methylthiosemicarbazone).

For example, a thymidine analogue, ^{18}F-labelled 3-deoxy-3-fluorothymidine (FLT), has been used to probe cellular proliferation and growth; it is phosphorylated by thymidine kinase and retained intracellularly with a small amount being incorporated into DNA.[131] FLT has been used to distinguish malignant from benign lesions in the lung, breast and in the colon and has shown promise as a tool for imaging cell growth.[107] Another example is the use of PET to image amino acid transport and metabolism: L-[methyl-^{11}C]methionine (MET) has shown high sensitivity (up to 95%) for the detection of glioma as well as providing prognostic information.[132] Other examples include ^{11}C-choline and ^{11}C-acetate, which have been used to probe tumour lipid metabolism, as well as to detect tumour recurrence after treatment.[133,134]

In summary, the great strength of PET is its very high sensitivity as a technique, which can be used in conjunction with a wide range of tracers to probe fundamental physiological and pathological processes. However, it remains an expensive method for the foreseeable future, involves a significant radiation burden, and certain short-lived radionuclides require an adjacent cyclotron facility which only a few sites have access to.

EMERGING MOLECULAR IMAGING TECHNIQUES AND THERANOSTICS

There are a very large number of emerging imaging methods that have been developed on animal imaging studies. The vast majority of new imaging approaches have been developed using animal models, before then being translated to patients, although there are some exceptions. There is an increasing trend towards *hybrid imaging* where two differing but complementary imagine techniques are combined to produce a test that is greater than the sum of its parts; for example, by combining the functional information acquired with PET with the anatomical CT data, PET-CT has proved to be a very powerful clinical tool. In addition, combining a diagnostic imaging test with a therapeutic approach which is closely related to the diagnostic test is another developing field which falls under the more general term of *theranostics*. Examples include the use of functional imaging combined with image-guided intervention as well as the use of radiolabelled molecules for both imaging and therapy.

Ultrasound

Ultrasound has been used in oncology for many decades not only to demonstrate tissue anatomy at very high resolution but also to reveal functional information about tissue perfusion and flow with the use of Doppler ultrasound. Although it is relatively limited as a molecular imaging tool, the generation of tissue contrast with microbubbles has opened up the possibility of its use on a molecular level. Microbubbles with a gaseous central core are injected intravenously and remain within the vasculature; local application of a resonant frequency ultrasound pulse at the area of interest causes the bubbles to burst and this significantly enhances the ultrasound signal measured, giving an enhanced image of the vascular space. By conjugating these bubbles to a targeted probe for a protein of interest (for example, VEGF), the image of the signal acquired when the bubbles are subsequently burst gives an indication of the spatial distribution of the protein of interest. The advantages of ultrasound are its very high spatial resolution and lack of ionising radiation, but, to date, it has been limited to the imaging of vascular structures and proteins. An emerging approach with ultrasound is the development of drug-containing microbubbles where the microbubbles are burst within the tissue of interest. This deposits the therapeutic agent at a high concentration where it is required while reducing the systemic dose and toxicity to normal tissues.

Optical Imaging

Optical imaging is a non-invasive and non-ionising technology that uses light to probe cellular and molecular function in living subjects. Visible light is a form of electromagnetic radiation, which has properties of both particles and waves. As light travels through tissue, photons can be absorbed, reflected or scattered, depending on the tissue composition. Different forms of optical imaging analyse these interactions to provide unique spectral signatures which can report on the molecular structure of the tissue in question. For example, fluorescence and phosphorescence depend on the emission of light following its absorption, and Raman spectroscopy analyses the inelastic scattering of light. Optical imaging has a very high spatial resolution in the nanometer (nm) range and can provide real-time and quantitative information. However, the main limitation of optical imaging is its limited penetration depth due to the strong scattering of light in biological tissues. This can be partly overcome by using fibreoptic endoscopic probes, which allow both tissue illumination and the collection of the emitted light from deep within the body. In addition, in the near-infrared (NIR) part of the electromagnetic spectrum, soft tissues show less scattering and absorption than in the visible band; hence, using NIR optical imaging enables the probing depth to be increased to a few centimetres.[135]

Fluorescence imaging describes the emission of light by a substance (i.e. a fluorophore) that has previously absorbed light. When a fluorophore absorbs light it enters an unstable excited state. Eventually fluorophores will return to the ground state, releasing any stored energy as light. In most cases the emitted light will have a lower energy (and hence a lower frequency) than the initial absorbed light due to some loss of energy during the transient excited lifetime (Fig. 74-9). Fluorophores can repeatedly undergo excitation and emission, allowing them to generate a signal multiple times, thereby making fluorescence a very sensitive technique. In contrast, bioluminescence imaging is the production and emission of light by a living organism whereby energy is released by a chemical reaction in the form of light. For example, luciferase is an enzyme that catalyses a reaction in which the chemical luciferin reacts with molecular oxygen to create light.

Clinically, optical spectroscopy has been shown to be useful in identifying and monitoring cancer since the characteristics of light emission change as cancer develops. During neoplastic transformation, there is (i) an increase in optical absorption due to an increase in nuclear size, DNA content and irregular chromatin clumping, (ii) an increase in optical scattering as a result of angiogenesis, which increases vessel density and haemoglobin concentration and (iii) changes in fluorescence—an increase in epithelial fluorescence (due to higher metabolic rates in pre-cancerous tissues), but a decrease in stromal fluorescence (due to changes in the extracellular matrix).[136] Intraoperative optical imaging using fluorescence has been used for tumour margin delineation and to identify malignant/sentinal nodes to ensure complete surgical resection of tumours. In addition, the use of fluorescence during routine endoscopic screening examinations in the gastrointestinal, bronchial and urinary tracts is also proving to be an invaluable tool to allow clinicians to detect occult dysplastic lesions (Fig. 74-10).[137]

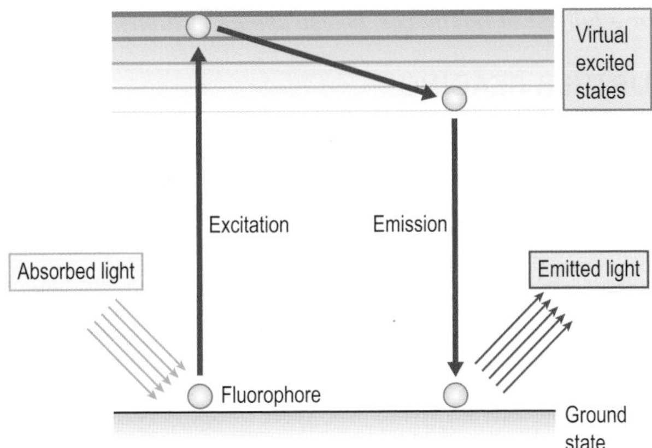

FIGURE 74-9 ■ Schematic showing the production of fluorescent light by an electron within a fluorophore. By absorbing light, the electron enters an excited state and, as it falls back to the lower-energy state again, it releases the stored energy as emitted light.

Optical imaging is frequently used as a gene reporter in preclinical tumour models—a gene encoding either a fluorescent protein (e.g. green fluorescent protein) or a bioluminescent protein (e.g. luciferase enzyme) is encoded with a regulatory sequence for another gene of interest; the expression of the gene of interest can be indirectly detected by the light emitted from the co-expressed reporter gene.[2] This approach is potentially very attractive for the detection of successful gene therapy, which is in its infancy in human studies.

Unlike fluorescence in which light is absorbed, Raman spectroscopy depends on the inelastic scattering of light. When monochromatic laser light is directed at a molecule, some of the photons will scatter; energy from the incident photon can be passed to the molecule, resulting in the photon being inelastically scattered and losing energy. This energy exchange between the incident light and the scattering molecule is known as the Raman effect. The molecular structure and composition of the material is encoded as a set of frequency shifts in the Raman scattered light, giving it a spectral signature, which acts as a reporter or fingerprint of the molecule in question.

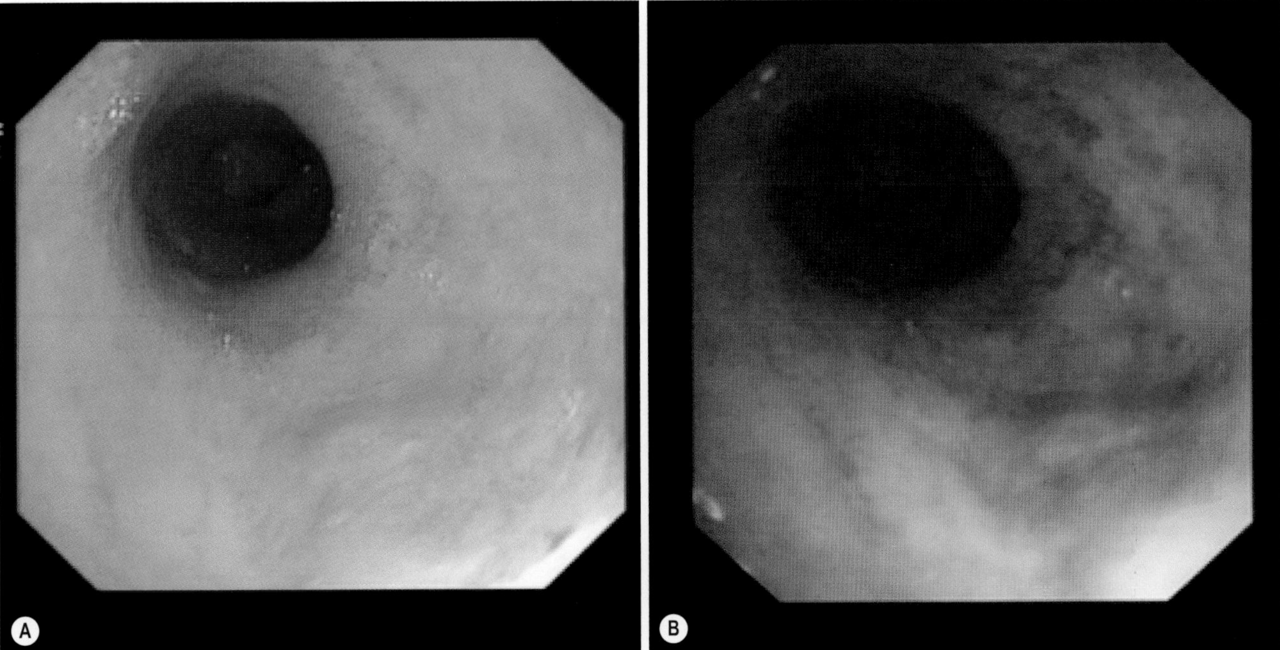

FIGURE 74-10 ■ Example of a clinical application of optical imaging: the detection of Barrett's oesophagus on endoscopy. (A) The Barrett's lesion is inconspicuous on standard white-light imaging; (B) autofluorescent imaging shows an abnormal purple area with normal surrounding green tissue; the abnormal area was confirmed histologically as low-grade dysplasia. Autofluorescence imaging is based on the detection of fluorescence emitted by endogenous molecules within tissue; changes in these molecules between normal and abnormal tissue can be exploited for the detection of dysplastic tissue that would otherwise be difficult to detect. (Images courtesy of Dr Rebecca Fitzgerald, Addenbrooke's Hospital, Cambridge.)

However, as the magnitude of the Raman effect is inherently very weak, this limits the sensitivity and hence its clinical application. In recent years, advances in nanobiotechnology have enabled the synthesis of nanoparticles which can overcome this problem by taking advantage of a phenomenon known as surface-enhanced Raman scattering (SERS) which can result in very high Raman signals at picomolar concentrations in deep tissue, thereby making it ideal as an in vivo imaging agent.[138] This very sensitive technique is being investigated as a technique to detect early tumour formation on endothelial surfaces such as the colon. The potential applications of SERS nanoparticles in tumour imaging are tremendous but concerns over toxicity need to be addressed before they will gain widespread clinical use.

In summary, molecular optical imaging offers many potential advantages, including high spatial resolution and sensitivity, although in general it demonstrates poor tissue penetration and is not used routinely in patients yet.

CONCLUSION: ROLE OF FUNCTIONAL AND MOLECULAR IMAGING IN ONCOLOGY

In general, functional and molecular techniques probe processes that require amplification for detection and therefore represent a compromise between spatial resolution and sensitivity. Instead of traditional high spatial resolution imaging, lower-resolution parameter maps or spectra are produced. Consequently, if these techniques are to find a place in routine clinical practice it is likely that functional and molecular images will be combined with traditional anatomical imaging in much the same way as in PET-CT. Many of these techniques described above are already used for clinical imaging and some of the more novel methods are undergoing clinical assessment. However, translating a preclinical tool into a routine clinical technique may take many years of development and longer to demonstrate clinical efficacy and cost-effectiveness; it requires collaboration between academics, clinicians, non-clinical scientists and industry. Functional and molecular imaging promises powerful tools to aid diagnosis, identify disease heterogeneity, predict outcome, target biopsies and determine treatment response non-invasively.

For a full list of references, please see ExpertConsult.

FURTHER READING

Barrett T, Kobayashi H, Brechbiel M, Choyke PL. Macromolecular MRI contrast agents for imaging tumor angiogenesis. Eur J Radiol 2006;60(3):353–66.

Choi KY, Liu G, Lee S, Chen X. Theranostic nanoplatforms for simultaneous cancer imaging and therapy: current approaches and future perspectives. Nanoscale 2012;4(2):330–42.

Gallagher FA. An introduction to functional and molecular imaging with MRI. Clin Radiol 2010;65(7):557–66.

Kapoor V, McCook BM, Torok FS. An introduction to PET-CT imaging. Radiographics 2004;24(2):523–43.

Kurhanewicz J, Bok R, Nelson SJ, Vigneron DB. Current and potential applications of clinical 13C MR spectroscopy. J Nucl Med 2008; 49(3):341–4.

Malayeri AA, et al. Principles and applications of diffusion weighted imaging in cancer detection, staging, and treatment follow-up. RadioGraphics 2011;31(6):1773–91.

McRobbie DW, et al. MRI from picture to proton. 2nd ed. Cambridge: Cambridge University Press; 2007. p. 406.

O'Connor JP, Jackson A, Parker GJ, Jayson GC. DCE-MRI. Biomarkers in the clinical evaluation of antiangiogenic and vascular disrupting agents. Br J Cancer 2007;96(2):189–95.

Qayyum A. MR Spectroscopy of the liver: principles and clinical applications. RadioGraphics 2009;29:1653–64.

SECTION **H**

PAEDIATRIC IMAGING

Section Editors: Catherine M. Owens • Jonathan H. Gillard

CHAPTER 75

Challenges and Overview of Special Features and Techniques

Catherine M. Owens • Carolyn Young • Øystein E. Olsen

CHAPTER OUTLINE

Ultrasound is the primary diagnostic technique for follow-up in paediatric imaging, and its application is described in the organ-specific chapters in this section. This chapter describes general principles for the application of radiography, computed tomography and magnetic resonance imaging in paediatric radiology.

Medical diagnostic imaging has evolved and rapidly improved over the past five decades as a result of novel development in diagnostic digital imaging and interventional techniques. With technical advances in computer processing power, along with high-resolution display monitors/workstations, together with increased computing power and electronic data archive systems, diagnostic imaging departments have transformed, from being labour-intensive analogue film-based imaging units into fully integrated digital environments.

However, with all this new technology readily available, there remains a lack of dedicated purpose-built equipment suitable for use in children and easily available on the market.

Although manufacturers are aware of the more important radiation implications pertaining to children, and have made inroads into lowering medical radiation doses, the ultimate responsibility remains with radiology technicians and radiologists, who control and operate diagnostic equipment, to adapt and adjust the (primarily adult-designed) techniques and protocols to suit the younger, more radiation-vulnerable population.

PROJECTION RADIOGRAPHY

The development of digital imaging in plain film radiography is advantageous within paediatric imaging. First introduced to computed radiography (CR) and later in direct readout radiography (DR) systems (utilising flat-panel detector (FD) technology), this technology helped provide greater efficiency in converting incident X-ray energy into image signal. This, together with its inherent wide dynamic range, greatly improved image quality, when compared with conventional screen-film-based systems, if equivalent exposure parameters were used. This has the potential for lowering radiation dosage for the patient and also reducing the risk of failed, i.e. non-diagnostic, exposure. Using post-processing capabilities, both bone and soft-tissue anatomy can now be optimally displayed on the same image, thus eliminating the need for repeated radiation exposure.[1–3]

However, care must be taken when setting exposure factors, as unlike with film-based techniques, overexposure can easily occur with digital imaging. This happens without adverse effect on image quality, and may not be recognised by the operator, as the image brightness can be freely adjusted, independent of exposure level.[4,5]

In general, FD technology is an efficient method for obtaining high-quality image data and enabling immediate image preview, storage and distribution over local area networks for viewing by clinicians, thus enhancing efficiency and productivity within high workflow departments.

Other applications of FD technology include digital tomosynthesis (or digital tomography), providing quasi 3-dimensional images, adapted for use in chest imaging. As a chest radiograph is a 2-dimensional image, sensitivity may be reduced when detecting underlying pathology because of overlapping anatomy. This can be overcome by CT applications but with an inherent increased radiation dose. Tomosynthesis evolved from conventional geometric tomography and was introduced as a low-dose alternative for chest radiographic examination in monitoring children with cystic fibrosis, and in the detection of pulmonary nodules.[6,7] This technique, involving the acquisition of a number of projection images at different angles during a single vertical motion of the X-ray tube (between a given angular range of −17.5° and +17.5°) directed at a stationary digital flat-panel detector, results in up to 60 coronal sectional images at an arbitrary depth.[6–8] Anatomical structures within each image section are sharply depicted, whilst structures located anteriorly and posteriorly are blurred. Spatial resolution is higher in tomosynthesis than in CT in the acquired imaging plane, but depth resolution is inferior, due to the limited angles used.

Further limitations to this imaging technique include the necessity of a 10-s acquisition time, increasing the likelihood of respiratory motion artefacts in non-compliant patients, which will exclude younger children who are unable to hold their breath. Although the radiation dose for tomosynthesis is much reduced compared with CT, it is three times higher than that for a frontal chest radiograph. This can be offset by a higher nodular detection rate than that seen with the plain radiograph, making this technique a possible alternative to CT examinations in some children.

FLUOROSCOPY

The introduction of digital fluoroscopy with its high-speed digitisation of the analogue video signal has revolutionised real-time fluoroscopy that relied on the use of image intensifier/TV systems to display the diagnostic image. Development of fluoroscopy FD technology with its fast digital readout and dynamic acquisition of image series at high frame rates (up to 60 frames per second) has become a well-established application in cardiac paediatric angiography. The other important application is within minimally invasive interventional procedures, due to their less invasive nature, when compared with conventional surgery. Advantages of FD compared with image intensifier systems that help minimise radiation dose include pulsed fluoroscopy, last-image hold and screen capture, which negate further diagnostic image exposures. Other features that improve image quality include homogeneous image uniformity with lack of geometric distortion across the entire image, reduced veiling glare, and a rectangular or square field-of-view, which utilises the full width of the image monitor. The small compact size of FD mounted on a dedicated C-arm system increases operational flexibility and ease of patient access, both features which are particularly pertinent within paediatric imaging.[2,3]

Modern C-arm angiography systems utilising FD technology are equipped with rotational angiography applications, providing 3-dimensional CT image capture (FD-CT) that is used mainly in interventional procedures. The ability to combine 2-dimensional fluoroscopic and 3-dimensional CT imaging within a single unit is advantageous for providing planning, guidance and monitoring of interventional procedures and intraoperative imaging.[9,10] The image quality is lower in FD-CT than in clinical CT, but in situations where a quick CT control diagnosis is required, an alternative lower spatial resolution image is acceptable. In addition, due to the slow rotation of FD-CT, patient movement and respiratory artefacts in body imaging further reduce spatial resolution. The radiation dose is noted to be higher in FD-CT due to lower detection efficiency, although the milliamperes per second (mAs) per single image acquisition is much lower. It is the cumulative dose of the procedure that is crucial in this instance, with variation seen in each individual investigation/treatment.

COMPUTED TOMOGRAPHY (CT)

CT is a proven essential diagnostic imaging technique and is considered the most sensitive method for evaluating airway diseases in children.

Two CT imaging configurations exist: namely, multi-detector CT (MDCT) with up to 320 detector rows and dual-source CT (DSCT) utilising MDCT technology. The increasing temporal and better spatial resolutions have extended the role of CT applications in young children to include cardiac imaging. Advantages of these systems include subsecond tube rotation times (down to 0.33 s). This increase in acquisition speed has the potential for reducing motion and respiratory artefacts and improving image quality. The overall reduction in examination acquisition time may also obviate the need for sedation in some children. The availability of small detector elements (0.5 mm) combined with thin-slice collimation provides isotropic resolution that allows image data to be manipulated/reformatted in any orthogonal plane and displayed as either 2- or 3-dimensional images that have the same spatial resolution as the base axial data set and with reduced partial volume artefact.

320-Row MDCT

The availability of 320-slice MDCT allows for larger volume coverage of up to 16 cm in the *z*-axis coverage. The advantage is that this coverage is well within the clinical range of thoracic length in neonates and young children. Therefore, imaging of the entire chest can be accomplished in a single-volume cone beam acquisition during one tube rotation of 0.35 s.[11] This is much faster than either helical MDCT or DSCT acquisition. Axial volumetric acquisitions have the potential of radiation dose saving. Due to the large nominal beam width used, the contribution of the penumbra effect is less prominent. Also, unlike in helical CT, over-ranging in the longitudinal axis is not applicable in this instance, as the exposed range corresponds exactly to the imaged range and therefore more effective usage of the radiation exposure for image formation. Axial volumetric acquisition can be applied to other clinical situations that include cardiac imaging in children, as when using prospective ECG-gating, the entire heart can be imaged within a single tube rotation.[11]

Dual-Source CT

The second-generation DSCT system (Siemens Flash, Forchheim, Germany) is currently the latest in CT technology. It incorporates two X-ray tubes each with corresponding 64-row detector systems (each contributing 128 slices by means of a *z* flying focal spot), mounted at an angular offset of 90° to each other. Designed for cardiac imaging, the two-tube detector system does not operate simultaneously, but in tandem, whereby data from the second detector system are collected a quarter of a rotation later following the first set of detectors. This allows gapless volume high-pitch CT (up to 3.2 pitch), avoiding overlapping slices with reduced radiation dose.[12,13] Together with a fast gantry rotation time of 0.28 s, a 75-ms temporal resolution is achieved, enabling helical prospective ECG-triggered cardiac imaging for the first time.[14] High heart rates are no longer a limiting factor when imaging children, and DSCT is invaluable for both the pre- and post-surgical assessment of a wide variety of congenital heart diseases, resulting in improved visualisation of the coronary arteries if data are captured in the systolic phase[15] even in younger children. Prospectively gated cardiac imaging is the preferred technique in young children, where often only morphological and proximal coronary artery detail is required. This negates the need for retrospectively gated imaging with its higher radiation burden. The sharp anatomical delineation between adjacent structures seen in prospective gating is superior to that seen in non-gated CTA studies, and with lower radiation dose levels.

Dual-Energy Dual-Source CT

The availability of two X-ray tubes allows simultaneous acquisition of two data sets at different tube potentials (80 and 140 kVp), during the same phase of contrast enhancement and excludes temporal changes and spatial misregistration. This technique takes advantage of differences between tissue and material composition and differences in their photon absorption characteristics. In particular, materials with a high atomic number (like iodine) exhibit a different degree of attenuation between the two tube potentials. By applying specific post-processing algorithms to the acquired data, virtual unenhanced and virtual angiographic data sets can be generated, based on the three-material composition principle;[16–18] e.g. within the abdomen, the materials analysed are soft tissue, fat and iodine, whilst in the chest, soft tissue, air and iodine are analysed. Application of the bone removal algorithm will display an angiographic data set without overlying bony structures, resulting in easier image interpretation. This eliminates the need for pre-intravenous contrast CT examinations imaging, as may be required if using a single tube device, for data subtraction purposes. Thus radiation doses are halved.

Overall radiation dose associated with dual-energy CT (DECT) is noted to be comparable to that of single-source MDCT systems. Other clinical dual-energy applications include characterisation of abdominal masses, chemical composition of renal calculi, myocardial and pulmonary perfusion imaging.

The depiction of iodine distribution for the detection of peripheral lung perfusion defects from suspected pulmonary emboli adds functional information to conventional pulmonary CT angiography. Its application in paediatrics is relevant in the evaluation of subsegmental pulmonary emboli.[17,19] By applying advanced post-processing software to the acquired data set, an iodine distribution map is generated and overlaid onto a grey-scale image. A normal perfusion image will show homogeneous colour distribution extending to the lung periphery and is displayed in a multiplanar format that can be manipulated manually. The presence of a filling or hypoperfusion is indicative of an obstructed vessel supplying the relevant lung segment. Review of the grey-scale image will help determine anatomical detail and location.

Other DECT applications include the use of xenon ventilation in chest imaging, as it is found to be more sensitive in the evaluation of regional and global airway and lung abnormalities in children.[20] Conventional CT investigation requires both inspiratory and expiratory acquisitions to demonstrate whether air-trapping exists. However, the use of xenon with the ability to demonstrate regional ventilation defects on inspiration obviates the need for an additional expiratory phase acquisition, with consequent radiation dose saving. In addition, the quantitative evaluation of lung density on CT is dependent on age and level of respiration. As this varies in young children, the use of xenon with its insensitivity to respiration level will provide more accurate measurements.

Radiation Dose Consideration

The increase in radiation burden associated with CT imaging and the potential risk to children cannot be ignored. CT requests must, therefore, be justified; a robust risk–benefit analysis should always be carried out before undertaking CT examination in children. Imaging techniques and dedicated paediatric protocols must be available to the operators, ensuring adherence to the ALARA principle. Adjustments to the CT parameters could be based on the patient's age, body weight or body diameter.

A list of guidelines for routine imaging are detailed in Tables 75-1 to 75-5. The use of 120 kVp is no longer

TABLE 75-1 Routine Chest Imaging

Indications	Airway disease Tumour masses and metastases Tracheomalacia Tracheobronchial stenosis Vascular anomalies
CT mode	Helical
CT parameter	Under 9 kg: 80 kVp, 60 ref mAs 10 kg and above: 100 kVp, 30-48 ref mAs
Tube rotation	0.5 s
Tube collimation	0.6 mm
Pitch	1
CT slice width	0.6 mm
Recon slice width	1 mm
Recon kernel	Medium-soft B30 and high-resolution B60
Contrast media	Omnipaque 300 2 mL per kg to a maximum of 100 mL
CT delay	Using pressure injector, 25 s from start of injection

TABLE 75-2 Routine Abdominal Imaging

Indications	Tumour masses Vascular anomalies
CT mode	Helical
CT parameter	100 kVp, 60–75 ref mAs
Tube rotation	0.5 s
Tube collimation	Under 15 kg: 0.6 mm 16 kg and above: 1.2 mm
Pitch	1
Tube current modulation	On
CT slice width	0.6 mm
Recon slice width	1 mm
Recon kernel	Medium-soft B30
Contrast media	Omnipaque 300 2 mL per kg to a maximum of 150 mL
CT delay	Using pressure injector, 45 s from start of injection

TABLE 75-3 **Routine Head Imaging**

Indications	Postoperative for tumour removal NAI Bleed/subdural Infection
CT mode	Sequential
CT parameter	120 kVp, 160–300 ref mAs
Tube rotation	1 s
Tube collimation	1.2 mm
Tube current modulation	On
CT slice width	1.2 mm
Recon slice width	5 mm, 2 mm if reformat required
Recon kernel	Medium-soft C30
Contrast media	Omnipaque 300 1 mL per kg to a maximum of 100 mL
CT delay	Hand injection, 3 min post-injection

TABLE 75-4 **Hydrocephalus Assessment**

Indications	Hydrocephalus Blocked shunt
CT mode	Sequential
CT parameter	Under 6 years: 100 kVp, 180–230 ref mAs 7 years and above: 120 kVp, 220 ref mAs
Tube rotation	1 s
Tube collimation	10 mm
Tube current modulation	On
CT slice width	10 mm
Recon slice width	10 mm
Recon kernel	Medium-soft C30
Contrast media	Not required

TABLE 75-5 **Low-dose 3-Dimensional Head Imaging**

Indications	Maxillofacial assessment
CT mode	Helical
CT parameter	Under 6 years: 100 kVp, 50 ref mAs 7 years and above: 120 kVp, 50 ref mAs
Tube rotation	1 s
Tube collimation	0.6 mm
Pitch	0.9
Tube current modulation	On
CT slice width	0.6 mm
Recon slice width	1 mm
Recon kernel	Soft C20
Contrast media	Not required

advocated in paediatric body imaging, and can be reduced to 80 or 100 kVp[21] without detriment to image quality, and, indeed, improves contrast resolution, thus allowing a smaller concentration of contrast medium to be administered. The tube current can also be reduced but at the detriment of increased image noise and reduced spatial resolution.[22] The degree of reduction is dependent on the level of 'tolerable' image noise deemed acceptable by the reporting radiologists. In general, image noise is less well tolerated in small children, due to the lack of inherent soft-tissue contrast (i.e. less fat), compared with adults, resulting in the necessity for proportional increase in milliamperes per second when imaging younger children. Utilisation of automatic tube current modulation (ATCM) with real-time ('on the fly') adaptation of tube current ensures that a constant image noise level is maintained across the area of interest, with the potential for reducing radiation dose. The disadvantage of this is that the tube current will increase, e.g. at the level of the shoulders, and at the lung base/diaphragm regions in thoracic imaging and across the pelvis in abdominal imaging. ATCM effectiveness is also debatable in younger children as they are more rounded in body shape, rendering angular tube current modulation futile.

More recent developments in radiation dose reduction strategies include exposure modulation over sensitive organs, where the radiation output is reduced when the X-ray tube is in the AP position over the breast and thyroid region. This eliminates the need for bismuth shielding that can increase tube current especially if ACTM is employed. The issue with over-ranging in the longitudinal axis, associated with helical imaging, has been overcome in modern devices by deployment of dynamic collimators at the start and end of the helical range, to block unnecessary radiation and reduce dose to the patient.

Iterative reconstruction is also widely available on modern CT systems. It allows use of lower exposure factors with significant reduction in image noise, without loss of diagnostic information, with a reported dose reduction of 35% noted in chest CT[23] and 23–66% in abdominal CT.[24]

Patient Care

Due to the speed of present-day CT machines, children over 3 years of age are usually compliant for their procedure, provided they are properly prepared through play therapy beforehand, using a mock-up toy of the machine to take the child and their parents through the imaging process. It is also a good opportunity to assess the child's ability to respond to breath-holding instructions; otherwise, gentle respiration is encouraged. A range of suitable sedatives may be prescribed to younger children, which include the light-acting sedative chloral hydrate at a dose of 50 mg/kg, or the short-acting midazolam hydrochloride at 0.1 mg/kg body weight.

Some centres prefer the more quick-acting sedative proprofol but this must be administered in the presence of an anaesthetist. The use of general anaesthesia is reserved only for non-compliant patients, or in cases where sedation had not been successful.

Dental Cone Beam CT

Diagnostic imaging is essential in clinical dental assessment and for those receiving orthodontic treatment.[25] This is accomplished by intra-oral projection radiography, and with rotational panoramic radiography (RPR) providing 2-dimensional images of what is really a 3-dimensional object, and often with inaccurate measurement due to inherent magnification and geometric distortion of the image. The development of low-dose cone beam computed tomography (CBCT) is a significant advancement in dental imaging, providing accurate high-resolution volumetric visualisation of the osseous structures in the maxillofacial region, and this has extended applications to treatment planning and image guidance for surgical procedures.[26]

There are various CBCT designs based on the available vertical height or field-of-view (FOV), ranging between 5 and 13 cm with coverage from a localised region to include the facial skeleton. It is important to select the correct equipment for the intended diagnostic task.

The systems operate in a similar fashion to RPR, utilising a divergent pyramidal-shaped source of radiation; the system rotates around the patient in a single 180° to 360° arc, acquiring multiple sequential planar projections directed onto the detector. The resultant number of base images is dependent on the frame rate, speed of rotation and completeness of the trajectory arc. These base images, similar in appearance to cephalometric radiographic images, are then integrated and displayed as a 3-dimensional volumetric data set.[26,27] Image quality is dependent to a certain extent on the acquired number of image projections, and can be improved by increasing the tube rotation from 180° to 360°, but with an increase in radiation dose. By way of limiting radiation dose and exposure to radiosensitive tissues (salivary gland and thyroid), the FOV should be adjusted in height and width to cover the area of interest only.

Using a large FOV, the base of skull and spinal anatomy is included in the resultant image. Thes images will require interpretation and reporting, and this in turn may not be within the remit of the dental practitioner, and will need to be coreported by a radiologist. This increases workload on reporting radiologists and needs to be reflected in optimal practice.

CBCT is comparable to conventional CT, and may be better at delineating bony details of the jaw and skull, but the system is unable to display soft-tissue structures. It is unsuitable for dental caries diagnosis in some cases, due to streak artefacts and dark bands across the image caused by beam hardening from data acquisition and from restored dentition. Radiation dose is much lower in CBCT than in CT, but higher than in conventional dental radiography.[28,29] A low-dose technique with 50% tube current reduction without loss of diagnostic quality can be applied for the purposes of orthodontic treatment and pre-surgical implant planning.[30] It is therefore important that exposure parameters used should be appropriate to the diagnostic task and to the size of the patient.

MAGNETIC RESONANCE IMAGING (MRI)

Apart from imaging of lung parenchyma and cortical bone, and in some cases of cardiovascular malformations and in trauma cases, MRI is the preferred cross-sectional imaging technique in children. This is due to the multitude of tissue contrasts inherent to this technique, and because there is no exposure to ionising radiation. Paediatric MRI is, in practice, somewhat different from the adult equivalent in that it requires particular attention to preparing the child, optimising the signal-to-noise ratio (SNR), handling motion artefacts and adjusting for differences in tissue contrast.

Patient Preparation

It may seem appealing to opt for the fastest pulse sequences in a potentially moving child; however, such a strategy may compromise the diagnostic performance of MRI. For example, whereas steady-state free-precession-type pulse sequences may be very useful for bowel imaging and for certain types of non-contrast-enhanced vascular imaging, they are in general not a good option for imaging tissues. Some of the best anatomical imaging sequences available, e.g. volumetric T2-weighted spin-echo, require a long acquisition time (in excess of 10 min). Since long acquisitions are usually required and because movement during the MR data acquisition is detrimental to the diagnostic quality of the resulting images, careful preparation is necessary.

A developmental age of less than 6–8 years in general means that sedation or general anaesthesia is required. General anaesthesia is considered safe, with reported fatal complications at 10 in 101,885 anaesthetic episodes (about 0.001%)—all related to pre-existing medical conditions.[31] Sufficient sedation is usually possible in children with bodyweight less than 15 kg; however, there are important contraindications such as airways being compromised.[32] Compared with general anaesthesia, sedation may be considered less safe (no airways protection), but this depends on the medical condition of the child and on local procedures for the safe selection of children for sedation. For the imager, sedation is less reliable (about 75% success rate in one study[33]) than general anaesthesia, and it does not allow breath-holding during the procedure. Sedation is hence often suboptimal for MRI of the chest and abdomen, but may suffice for neuro- and musculoskeletal MRI.

Postprandial sleep may sufficiently immobilise the young infant. The child is fed and gently swaddled (feed-and-wrap) to induce sleep. Acoustic shielding is then applied. Success is more likely if the feed follows 4 hours of fasting.[34]

In the older child, previous introduction to the imaging environment by means of a mock machine may improve compliance during the MRI examination.[35] Thorough briefing appropriate for the developmental stage of the child and availability of in-built entertainment systems are helpful.

Radiofrequency Coils

The coil is the single most important determinant of SNR. Multi-channel coils result in higher SNR.[36] A coil or coil combination that gives optimal coverage is essential.[37] The coverage should be about 1.5 times the size of the region of interest. A coil coverage that is too small would give insufficient signal reception, whereas a larger-than-required coverage would add noise. Therefore, a wide spectrum of coils needs to be available to allow selection of a coil combination that most appropriately fits the region of interest. This might, for example, mean using an adult knee coil for abdominal or chest MRI in a neonate.[38]

Motion Artefact Reduction

The amount of gross motion is managed by adequate patient preparation. Attenuation of peristalsis is important for T2-weighted spin-echo acquisitions, and is achieved with intravenous administration of glucagon or hyoscine-*N*-butylbromide. Physiological gating freezes periodic motion by only allowing readout during well-defined event-driven time windows. This window may be end-diastole for ECG-gated acquisitions and around end-expiration for ventilatory-gated acquisitions.

In chest imaging, a combination of ECG- and ventilation-gating is possible. Fast imaging techniques make dual gating practically more feasible. Physiological gating is less feasible for T1-weighted spin-echo sequences, but good fat suppression may partly compensate for this deficiency. Gating is not required for diffusion-weighted acquisitions.[39] When gating is impossible, one may consider: (1) targeted saturation and (2) advanced *k*-space trajectories.

Manipulation of *k* space may be as simple as changing the phase-encoding direction to direct any artefact away from an area of interest. For example, axial images of the thymus may be improved with a right-to-left phase-encoding direction. Some pulse sequences have *k*-space trajectories designed to reduce the impact of motion artefact. One example is a trajectory that uses several different readout directions (PROPELLER, BLADE, MultiVane, RADAR, JET). The result is that motion artefact is distributed over several radial directions and, hence, becomes less perceivable in the final image.

Tissue Contrast

Poor SNR is more tolerable if the image contrast is optimised. The principles for good image contrast are: (1) to always use a combination of different image weightings and (2) to use intravenous contrast media.

Most childhood tumours have restricted water diffusion,[40] so diffusion-weighted imaging is mandatory for imaging mass lesions in children. Fat suppression at T1-weighted imaging is useful for depicting the pancreas, and fat suppression also accentuates the enhancement following gadolinium administration. Non-fat-suppressed sequences need to be part of any MR protocol for two reasons: (1) for the detection of fat-containing lesions (e.g. teratoma, lipoblastoma) and (2) for the definition of anatomical planes.

Hyaline cartilage of epiphyses, epiphyseal equivalents and apophyses constitute a large and important portion of the skeleton in young patients. Cartilaginous defects may be constitutional (e.g. proximal focal femoral deficiency) or acquired (e.g. secondary to juvenile idiopathic arthritis). Cartilage has intermediate signal intensity on fat-suppressed T1-weighted images, on proton density spin-echo and on fat-suppressed (double-echo) balanced steady-state free-precession images.[37]

Intravenous gadolinium-based contrast media generally improve the diagnostic efficacy of MRI. In childhood tumours this is sometimes due to the negative contrast of a poorly enhancing tumour against normally enhancing surrounding tissues. Arterial or early portal venous phase volumetric spoiled gradient-echo acquisitions often show the perimeter of the lesion, and demonstrate important vascular (arterial, portal venous, renal venous) relations. As for adults, gadolinium should be used with caution in children with reduced renal function. Young infants (less than 6 months of age) have physiologically low renal function, and it may be recommended to routinely estimate GFR in these. There are also licensing restrictions to using gadolinium in children (as for many other pharmaceuticals), so institutional policies need to be in place.

Image Resolution

MRI measures signal intensity voxel by voxel. A voxel cannot be depicted if its signal intensity is lower than that of the background noise. Since a small voxel contains fewer hydrogen nuclei, it will have a lower MRI signal than a larger voxel. SNR is therefore proportional to the voxel volume. Hence, if decreasing the size of the field of view, one needs to revise the acquisition matrix or else risk suboptimal SNR. However, due to the finer anatomical landscape in children, it is often desirable to maintain a voxel size somewhat smaller than that in adult imaging. Either one must then accept a lower SNR (which may be tolerable if the contrast is good and if there is only minimal motion artefact) or one needs to compensate for the loss in SNR. Compensation may be achieved by averaging a higher number of acquisitions, decreasing the receiver bandwidth, reducing the parallel imaging factor and/or by oversampling *k* space.

Imaging Planes

Imaging planes are fundamentally arbitrary and may be ignored in volumetric imaging, where optimal planar reconstruction is left to the post-processing stage. Isotropic imaging has in the past been restricted to gradient-echo sequences, and to spin-echo sequences with very long echo times. The problem with intermediate echo times has been degradation from blurring of the contrast due to long echo trains. This problem is solved with the implementation of volumetric proton density and T2-weighted spin-echo sequences (SPACE, VISTA, CUBE) that use a scheme of variable flip-angle evolutions to assign different weights to readouts depending on their order.

However, 2-dimensional acquisitions may still be required, and for these the imaging planes need to be perpendicular to the most important anatomical planes, and at least two different planes need to be acquired. Generally, in the abdomen, axial imaging is most useful because the axial plane is perpendicular to the largest portions of the peritoneum and body wall, the aorta and inferior vena cava and the renal fossae, and perpendicular to the planes between most of the major organs. In the pelvis, the sagittal plane is most useful because it transects

TABLE 75-6 **Suggested Basic Protocol for Abdominal MRI in a Child with an Abdominal Mass Lesion**

Pulse Sequence or Event, Key Parameters	Image Volume	Voxel Size, mm (approx.)
Localisers		
Intravenous Administration of Hyoscine		
STIR coronal, ventilatory gated	Abdomen and pelvis	1.1 × 1.1 × 5.0
Volumetric T2-weighted spin-echo with variable flip-angles, ventilatory gated	Region of lesion	0.9 × 0.9 × 0.9
Diffusion-weighted imaging (*b* values, at least 0 and 1000) axial	Lesion	2.7 × 2.7 × 6.0
Fat-suppressed T1-weighted spin-echo axial	Region of lesion	1.0 × 1.0 × 6.0
Fat-suppressed volumetric spoiled gradient-echo, breath-hold	Abdomen	0.9 × 1.0 × 1.1
Administration of Gadolinium-Based Contrast Agent via Power Injector		
Fat-suppressed volumetric spoiled gradient-echo, breath-hold, early portal venous phase using bolus tracking	Abdomen	0.9 × 1.0 × 1.1
Fat-suppressed T1-weighted spin-echo axial	Region of lesion	1.0 × 1.0 × 5.0

the planes between the bladder, internal genital organs, the rectum and the anterior/posterior body walls. The sagittal image plane is also chosen for other midline structures, such as the thymus.

Practical Consequences

One protocol for abdominal MRI in a child with an abdominal mass lesion is suggested in Table 75-6. This protocol incorporates several image contrasts: water-sensitive sequences (STIR), diffusion-weighted imaging, non-fat-suppressed imaging (2-D or 3-D T2-weighted spin-echo) and contrast-enhanced acquisitions. Dynamic contrast-enhanced volumetric gradient-echo sequences are optional but improve the definition of vascular relations. A large FOV coronal STIR acquisition is included for lesion detection over a large anatomical region. Motion artefact is reduced by mostly using fat-suppressed sequences, by administration of hyoscine and by using respiratory gating whenever possible.

For a full list of references, please see ExpertConsult.

FURTHER READING

6. Vult von Steyern K, Bjorkman-Burtscher I, Geijer M. Tomosynthesis in pulmonary CF with comparison to radiography and CT: a pictorial review. Insights Imaging 2012;3:81–9.
7. Vikgren J, Zachrisson S, Svalkvist A, et al. Tomosynthesis and chest radiography for the detection of pulmonary nodules: human observer of clinical cases. Radiology 2008;249:1034–41.
8. Dobbins JT 3rd, Godfrey DJ. Digital x-ray tomosynthesis: current state of the art and clinical potential. Phys Med Biol 2003;48(19): R65–106.
9. Kalander WA, Kyriakou Y. Flat-detector computed tomography. Eur Radiol 2007;17:2767–79.
10. Hausegger KA, Furstner M, Hauser M, et al. Clinical application of flat-panel CT in the angio suite. Rofo 2011;183(12):1116–22.
11. Kroft LJM, Roelofs JJH, Geleijns J. Scan time and patient dose for thoracic imaging in neonates and small children using axial volumetric 320-detector row CT compared to helical 64, 32, and 16 detector row CT acquisition. Pediatr Radiol 2010;40:294–300.
12. Lell M, Marwan M, Schepis T, et al. Prospectively ECG-triggered high-pitch spiral acquisition for coronary CT angiography using dual source CT: technique and initial experience. Eur Radiol 2009;19:2576–83.

CHAPTER 76

THE NEONATAL AND PAEDIATRIC CHEST

Veronica Donoghue • Tom A. Watson • Pilar Garcia-Peña • Catherine M. Owens

CHAPTER OUTLINE

THE NEONATAL CHEST

NORMAL ANATOMY AND ARTEFACTS

The anteroposterior (AP) diameter of the neonatal chest is almost as great as its transverse diameter, giving the chest a cylindrical configuration. The degree of rotation is best assessed by comparing the length of the anterior ribs visible on both sides. As newborn chest radiographs are taken in the AP plane, the normal cardiothoracic ratio can be as large as 60%.

The thymic size is variable and may alter with the degree of lung inflation. It may blend with the cardiac silhouette, it may have an undulating boarder due to underlying rib indentation (Fig. 76-1) or it may exhibit the classic 'sail sign' more commonly seen on the right side. It may involute rapidly with prenatal or postnatal stress, for example in severe illnesses such as hyaline membrane disease or infections, or following corticosteroid treatment.

There are some well-recognised artefacts on a newborn chest radiograph. The hole in the incubator top may be confused with a pneumatocele or lung cyst. Skin folds may be visible over the chest wall and may mimic a pneumothorax. These can usually be seen to extend beyond the lung.

NORMAL LUNG DEVELOPMENT

The normal lung development is well described by Agrons et al.[1] During the embryonic phase of gestation (from 26 days to 6 weeks) the lung bud develops from the primitive foregut and divides to form the early tracheobronchial tree. During the pseudoglandular phase (6–16 weeks) there is airway development to the level of the terminal bronchioles, with a deficient number of alveolar saccules. Multiple alveolar ducts develop from the respiratory bronchioles during the cannicular or acinar phase (16–28 weeks). These ducts are lined by type II alveolar cells which can produce surfactant, and which differentiate into thin type I alveolar lining cells. At the end of this phase primitive alveoli form. Progressive thinning of the pulmonary interstitium allows gas exchange with approximation of the proliferating capillaries and the type I cells.

During the saccular phase (28–34 weeks) there is an increase in the number of terminal sacs, further thinning of the interstitium, continuing proliferation of the capillary bed and early development of the true alveoli.

The alveolar phase extends from approximately 36 weeks' gestation until 18 month of age, with most alveoli formed at 5–6 months of age.

IDIOPATHIC RESPIRATORY DISTRESS SYNDROME

Idiopathic respiratory distress syndrome (IRDS) or hyaline membrane disease (HMD) mainly affects the premature infant less than 36 weeks' gestational age. The primary problem in HMD is a deficiency of the lipoprotein pulmonary surfactant in association with structural immaturity of the lungs. The lipoproteins are produced in the type II pneumocytes, are concentrated in the cell lamellar bodies and then transported to the cell surface and expressed onto the alveolar luminal surface. These lipoproteins then combine with surface surfactant

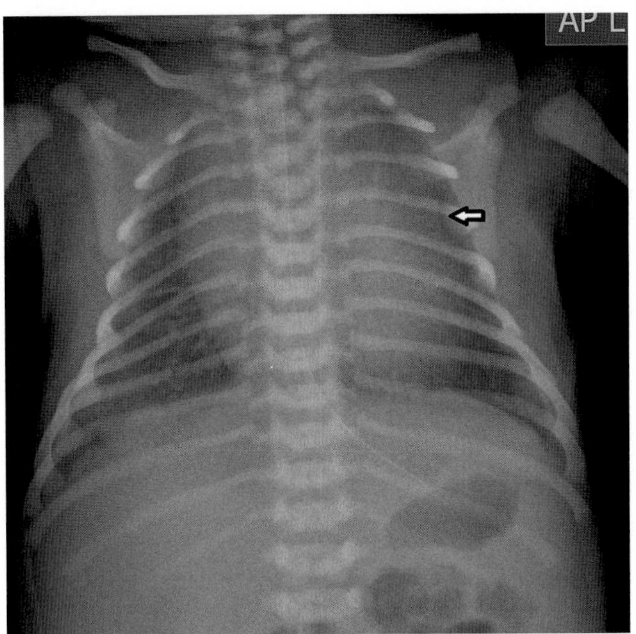

FIGURE 76-1 ■ There is mediastinal widening, due to normal thymic tissue. The undulated appearance of the left thymic border is due to rib indentation (arrow).

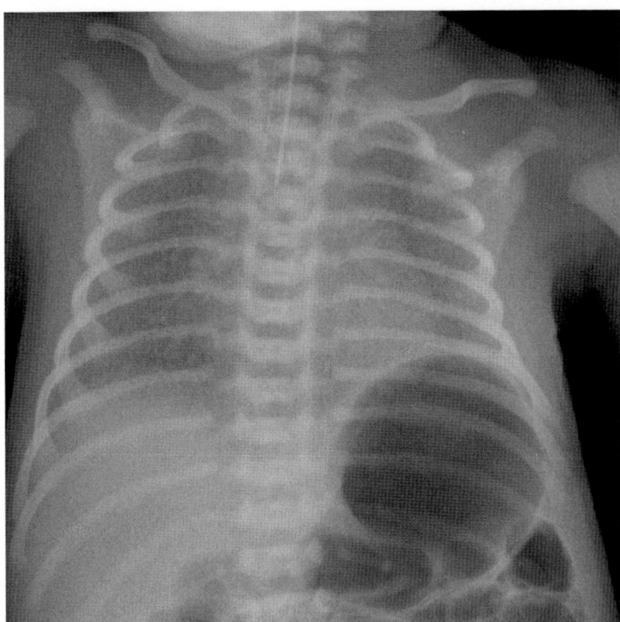

FIGURE 76-2 ■ Infant born at 26 weeks' gestation. There is poor lung inflation and aeration with mild diffuse granular opacification in keeping with IRDS.

proteins (A, B, C, D), which are also produced by the type II pneumocytes to form tubular myelin. This is the principal contributor at the alveolar air–fluid interface which lowers alveolar surface tension and prevents acinar collapse on expiration.[1] Without this, there is alveolar collapse and, as a result, poor gas exchange, hypoxia, hypercarbia and acidosis. The alveolar ducts and terminal bronchioles are distended and lined by hyaline membranes which contain fibrin, cellular debris and fluid, thought to arise from a combination of ischaemia, barotrauma and the increased oxygen concentrations used in assisted ventilation.[2] Hyaline membrane formation can also occur in other neonatal chest conditions requiring ventilation.

Clinically these premature infants are usually symptomatic within minutes of birth with grunting, retractions, cyanosis and tachypnoea. Chest radiographic findings may be present shortly after birth but occasionally the maximum features may not be present until 6–24 hours of life.

Before the commencement of treatment, the typical radiographic features include underaeration of the lungs, fine granular opacification, which is diffuse and symmetrical, and air bronchograms (Fig. 76-2), due to collapsed alveoli interspersed with distended bronchioles and alveolar ducts. When there is less distension, the granularity is replaced by more generalised opacification or complete white-out of the lungs (Fig. 76-3). Atelectasis is the main cause of this opacification, but in the very premature infant in particular, oedema, haemorrhage and occasionally superimposed pneumonia contribute.

Very premature infants, less than 26 weeks' gestation, may have clear lungs or mild pulmonary haziness initially. Their lungs are structurally and biochemically immature and require prolonged ventilatory support. Prenatal

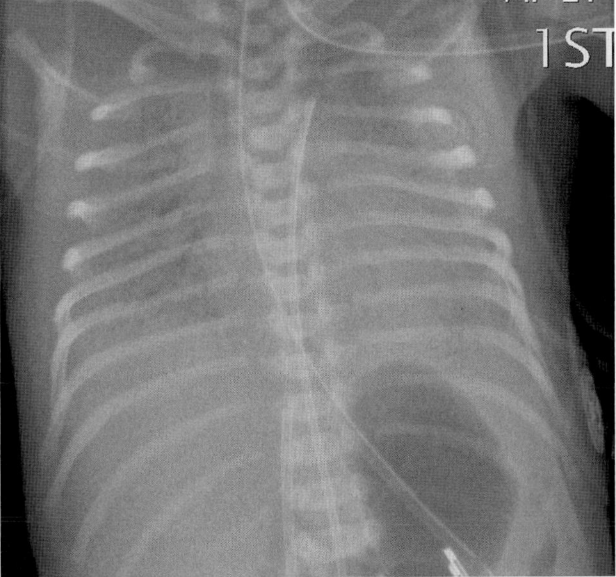

FIGURE 76-3 ■ Premature infant with severe IRDS. There is almost complete 'white-out' of the lungs with air bronchograms.

corticosteroid administration during the 2 days prior to delivery significantly reduces the incidence of IRDS in premature infants.

The clinical use of artificial surfactant, given as a liquid bolus through the endotracheal (ET) tube, has been a major therapeutic advance. It may not be evenly distributed throughout the lungs, leading to areas of atelectasis interspersed with areas of good aeration, and may produce radiographic findings similar to neonatal pneumonia or pulmonary interstitial emphysema (PIE) (Fig. 76-4).

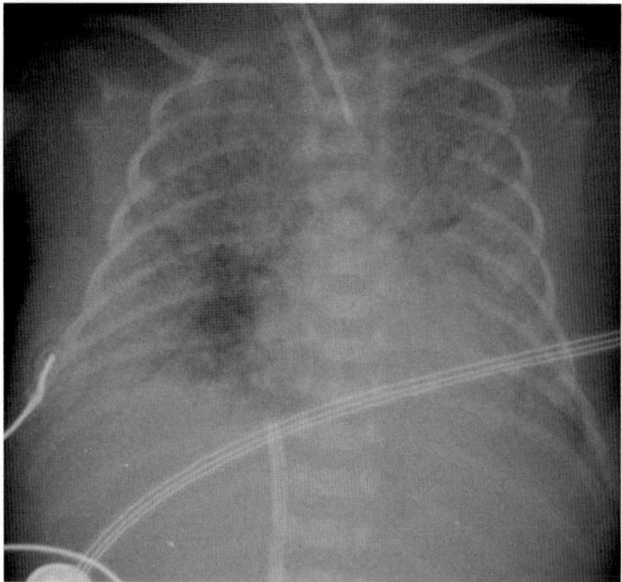

FIGURE 76-4 ■ **Uneven aeration following surfactant administration.** The appearances in some areas mimic those of PIE.

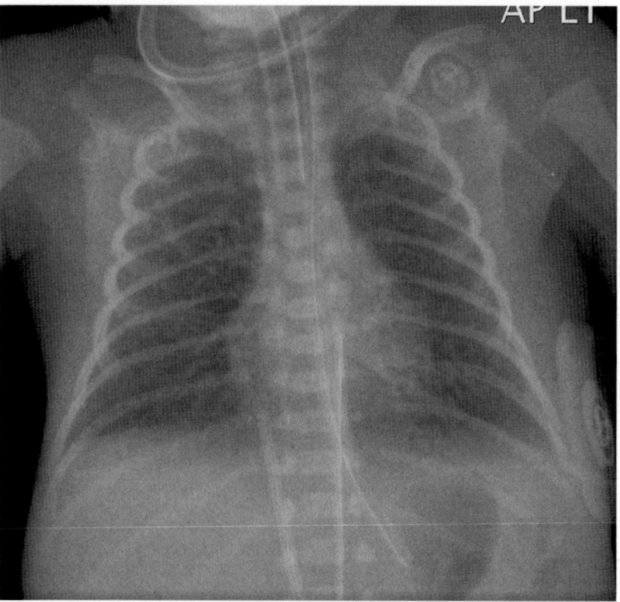

FIGURE 76-5 ■ **Very premature infant born at 24 weeks' gestation.** The chest radiograph at 24 hours demonstrates some hyperinflation, hazy and streaky opacification, similar to the changes seen in bronchopulmonary dysplasia.

Correlation with the clinical picture is, therefore, very important.

In general, infants greater than 27 weeks' gestation respond best to surfactant therapy. In the very premature infant, less than 27 weeks' gestation, the lungs become clear following surfactant administration, but they are still immature with fewer alveoli than normal. This results in inadequate gas exchange, leads to prolonged ventilation, hazy lung opacification and occasionally a picture similar to that seen in bronchopulmonary dysplasia (Fig. 76-5).

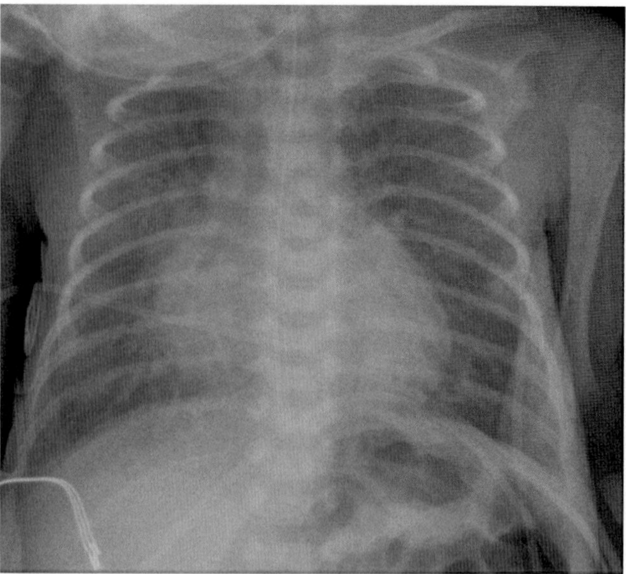

FIGURE 76-6 ■ There is cardiac enlargement, splaying of the carina indicating left atrial enlargement, prominent pulmonary vasculature and hazy opacification centrally, suggestive of a left-to-right shunt at PDA level.

A patent ductus arteriosus is frequent in the premature infant and contributes to the disease. The rigid lungs caused by IRDS and the associated hypoxia and hypercarbia may lead to right-to-left shunting through the ductus. With surfactant therapy and improved oxygenation there is reduced pulmonary resistance and as a result there may be left-to-right shunting. Initial treatment if required is with ibuprofen, which inhibits prostaglandin production, but surgery may occasionally be required.

The chest radiograph may demonstrate sudden cardiac enlargement, left atrial enlargement causing elevation of the left main bronchus and varying degrees of pulmonary oedema (Fig. 76-6). There is an increasing use of prophylactic continuous positive airway pressure (CPAP) ventilation in infants suspected of developing IRDS, which helps reduce the incidence of complications in these infants. High-frequency ventilation is also used to reduce the incidence of barotrauma, particularly in the very premature infant. In these infants the radiographs do not differ significantly from those infants receiving conventional ventilation. The chest radiograph is used to assess the degree of lung inflation. The dome of the diaphragm should project at the level of the 8th–10th posterior ribs if the mean airway pressure is appropriately adjusted.

The use of positive pressure ventilation in the newborn is the most common cause of pneumothorax, pneumomediastinum, pulmonary interstitial emphysema (Fig. 76-7) and pneumopericardium (Fig. 76-8). These complications have become much less common in infants who have been treated with surfactant and high-frequency ventilation. Areas of atelectasis can occur in surfactant deficiency and are frequently due to poor clearance of secretions (Fig. 76-9). Premature infants are at an increased risk of pneumonia, which may coexist with IRDS. Pulmonary haemorrhage resulting in airspace

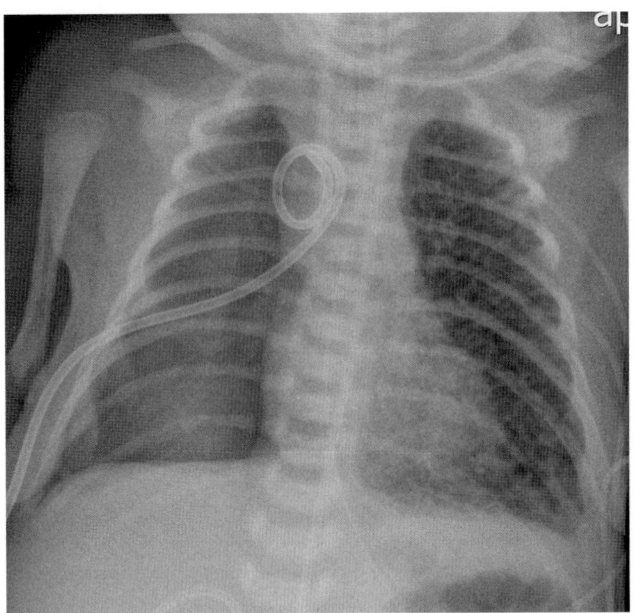

FIGURE 76-7 ■ **Left pulmonary interstitial emphysema.** On the right there is hyperlucency with a sharp mediastinal edge, a sharp right heart border and right hemidiaphragm indicating a right pneumothorax. There is a pigtail drainage catheter in situ.

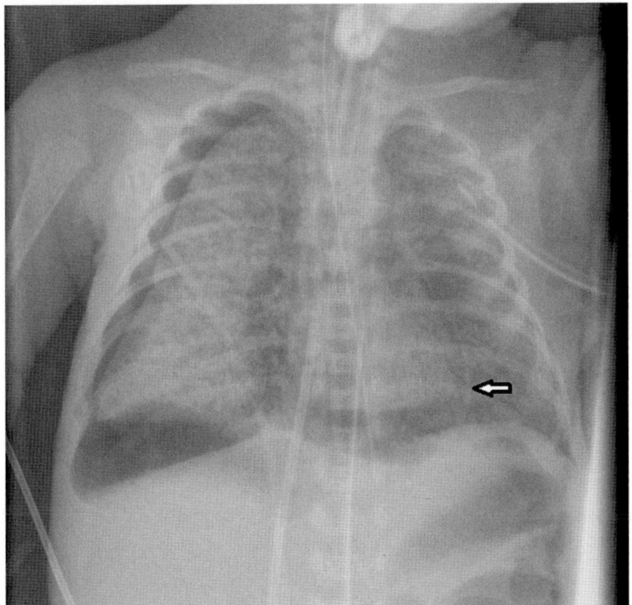

FIGURE 76-8 ■ There is a lucency surrounding the heart and the pericardial sac is visible as a white line (arrow), indicating a pneumopericardium. There is also a right pneumothorax.

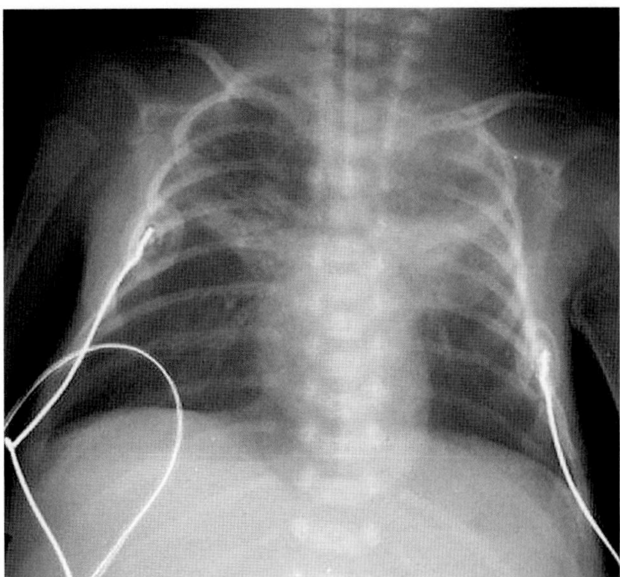

FIGURE 76-9 ■ **Bilateral upper lobe segmental atelectasis.**

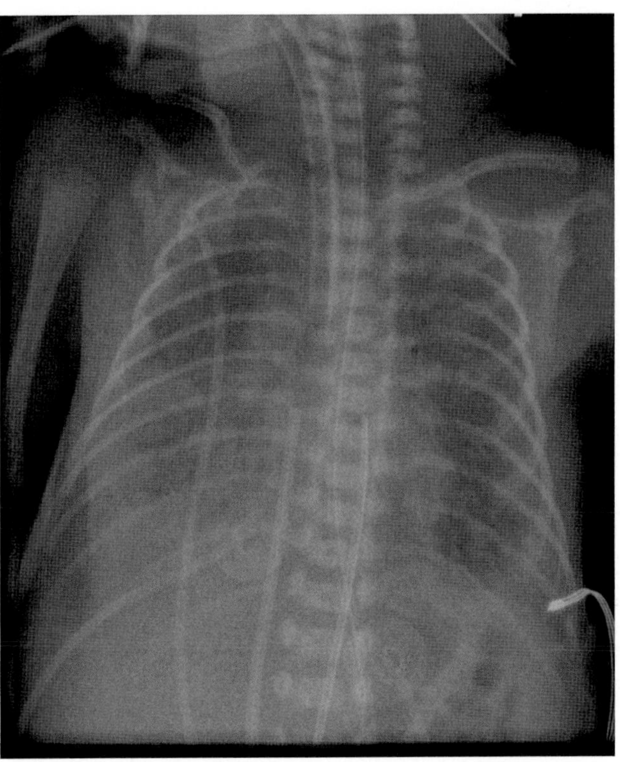

FIGURE 76-10 ■ **Infant born at 24 weeks' gestation.** The chest radiograph at 24 hours demonstrates airspace opacification in the right middle and both lower lobes due to intrapulmonary haemorrhage. Blood was seen to ooze from the ET tube prior to obtaining the radiograph.

opacification may also be a superimposed problem, and is usually due to severe hypoxia and capillary damage (Fig. 76-10). Bronchopulmonary dysplasia (BPD) or chronic lung disease is a significant long-term complication of IRDS. Because of the many advances in neonatal care, its incidence and severity have reduced significantly in infants born at 28 weeks' gestation or older. The unchanged overall incidence is due to the increased survival of the infants of extreme prematurity as they require more prolonged ventilation. Air leaks, patent ductus arteriosus and infection are contributing factors as they also prolong ventilation. A higher incidence of BPD has been demonstrated in infants with previous culture-proven *Ureaplasma urealyticum* pneumonitis.[3]

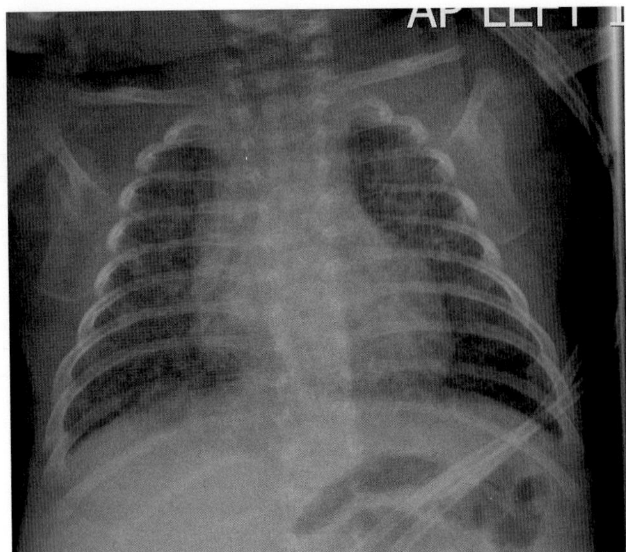

FIGURE 76-11 ■ **Premature infant ventilated for IRDS.** Chest radiograph at 4 weeks of age demonstrates hyperinflation, interstitial and alveolar opacification throughout both lungs in keeping with BPD.

The four classic stages of BPD described by Northway[4] are now very rarely seen. Nowadays the most common radiographic appearance is diffuse interstitial shadowing with mild-to-moderate hyperinflation of gradual onset (Fig. 76-11). A new type of BPD was described by Jobe in 1999[5] in immature infants with minimal lung disease at birth, and who become symptomatic during the first week of life. This entity seems inseparable from the condition described previously as Wilson–Mikity syndrome.

TRANSIENT TACHYPNOEA OF THE NEWBORN (TTN)

This condition is also referred to as retained fetal lung fluid or wet-lung syndrome. Normally fluid is cleared from the lungs at, or shortly after, birth by the pulmonary lymphatics and capillaries. In TTN the normal physiological clearance is delayed. The incidence is greater in infants delivered by Caesarean section, in hypoproteinaemia, hyponatraemia and maternal fluid overload. There is also an increased incidence in small, hypotonic and sedated infants who have had a precipitous delivery.

Typically the infants have mild-to-moderate respiratory distress without cyanosis in the first couple of hours. The process resolves rapidly with almost complete resolution in 48 hours. Treatment consists of supportive oxygen and maintenance of body temperature. Radiographically, the most common appearances are mild overinflation, prominent blood vessels, perihilar interstitial shadowing and fluid in the transverse fissure with occasional small pleural effusions (Fig. 76-12). There may be mild associated cardiomegaly. The appearances may be asymmetrical with right-sided predominance, which remains unexplained. The features may simulate

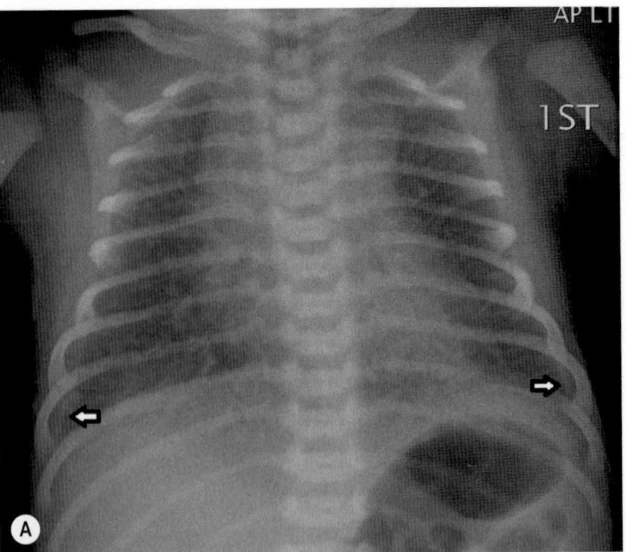

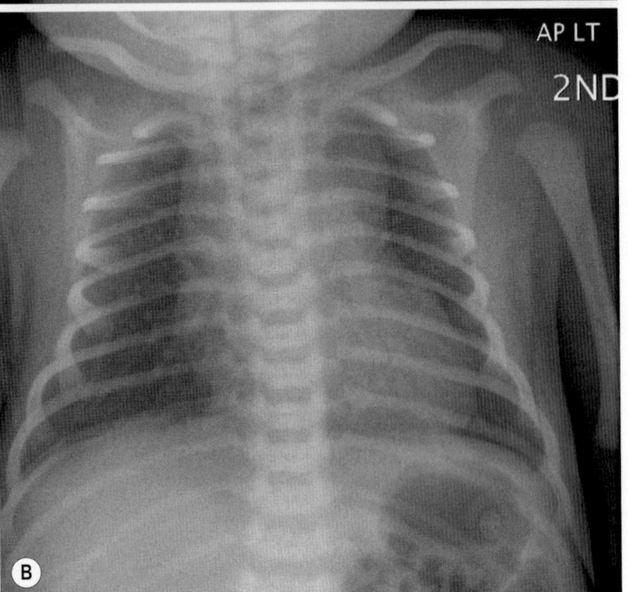

FIGURE 76-12 ■ (A) Term infant. Radiograph shows mild hyperinflation, prominent vasculature, interstitial opacification most marked in the lower lobes and small pleural effusions (arrows) suggestive of TTN. (B) There is almost complete resolution at 24 hours.

meconium aspiration syndrome and congenital neonatal pneumonia, particularly when severe.

MECONIUM ASPIRATION SYNDROME

The definition of meconium aspiration syndrome is an infant born through meconium-stained amniotic fluid where the symptoms cannot be otherwise explained.[6] It is thought that fetal hypoxia causes fetal intestinal hyperperistalsis and passage of meconium, which is aspirated by a gasping fetus. It is most common in infants who are post-mature. It is diagnosed by the presence of meconium below the level of the vocal cords.

The radiographic features may, in part, be due to the inhalation of meconium itself in utero or during birth.

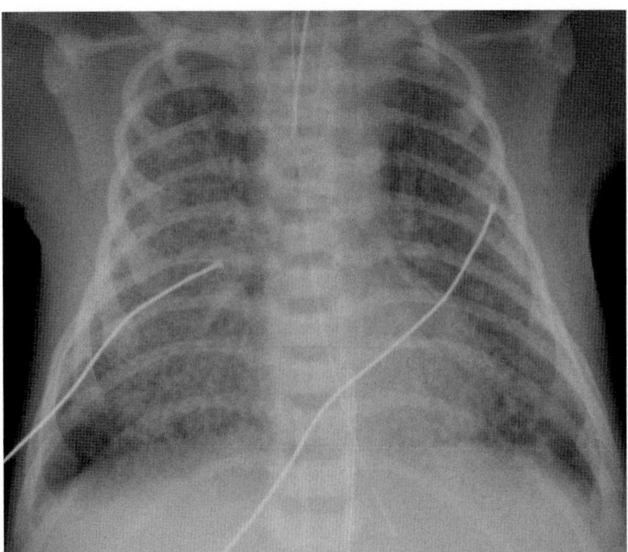

FIGURE 76-13 ■ Infant born at 42 weeks' gestation. There is bilateral asymmetrical coarse opacification in the lungs in keeping with meconium aspiration.

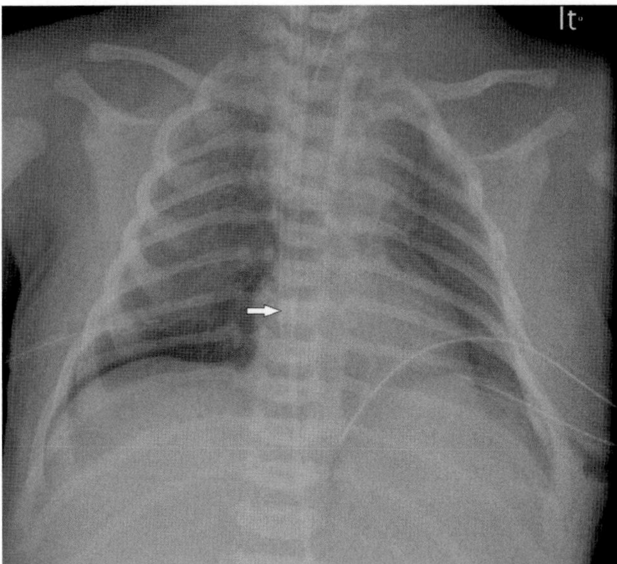

FIGURE 76-14 ■ Term infant with meconium aspiration undergoing ECMO. Radiograph obtained immediately following insertion of a veno-venous catheter in the right atrium (arrow). There are bilateral pneumothoraces with chest drains in situ bilaterally.

It is a thick viscous substance and may lead to areas of atelectasis and overinflation. It may migrate to the distal airways, causing complete or partial obstruction and lead to a 'ball-valve' effect. It may also cause a chemical pneumonitis (Fig. 76-13). There may be associated alterations in the pulmonary vasculature, leading to pulmonary arterial hypertension. Air leaks are common and small associated pleural effusions may be seen.

Approximately 30% of infants will require mechanical ventilation. The mortality rate has been improved by the use of inhaled nitric oxide, to treat severe pulmonary hypertension and also by extracorporeal membrane oxygenation (ECMO), which is used only in those infants where the conventional treatments have failed. The ECMO technique can be used either with the veno-arterial method, where one catheter is placed in the internal jugular vein and one in the carotid artery, or the veno-venous method, where a double lumen catheter is placed in the internal jugular vein, superior vena cava or right atrium (Fig. 76-14). The circulation bypasses the lungs, which are minimally inflated, and allows physiologic levels of oxygen saturation.

NEONATAL PNEUMONIA

Neonatal infections acquired transplacentally, such as TORCH (toxoplasmosis, rubella, cytomegalovirus, herpes), are rare and seldom develop pulmonary abnormalities. Infections acquired perinatally can occur via ascending infection from the vagina, transvaginally during birth or as a hospital-acquired infection in the neonatal period. Prolonged rupture of membranes prior to delivery is a major risk factor. It is thought that most cases of neonatal pneumonia occur during birth, when the infant may swallow and/or aspirate infected amniotic fluid or vaginal tract secretions. Group B streptococcus is the most common organism identified. The radiological features are non-specific.

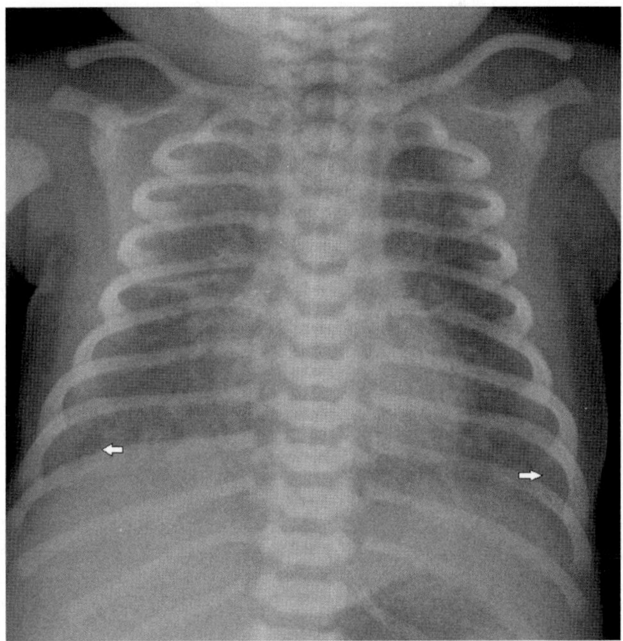

FIGURE 76-15 ■ Infant with group B streptococcus infection. There is bilateral asymmetrical coarse pulmonary opacification and small bilateral pleural effusions (arrows). The appearances are similar to those seen in meconium aspiration syndrome.

The most common features seen on the chest radiograph in term infants who present with severe acute symptoms in the first 24–48 h are coarse bilateral asymmetrical alveolar opacification with or without associated interstitial change (Fig. 76-15). In these infants the

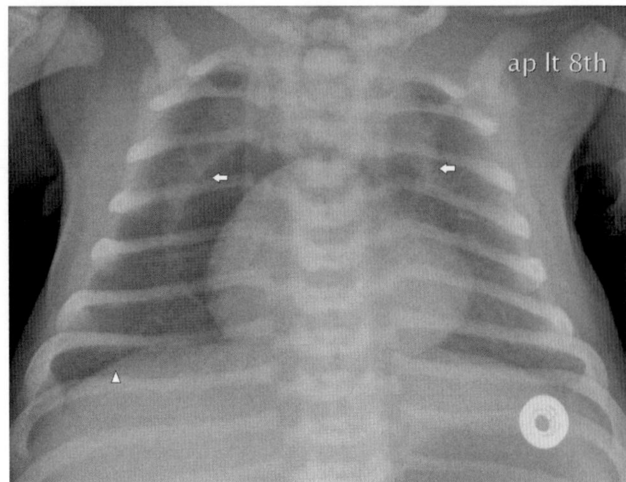

FIGURE 76-16 ■ Spontaneous pneumomediastinum outlining the thymus (arrows) and right pneumothorax (arrowhead).

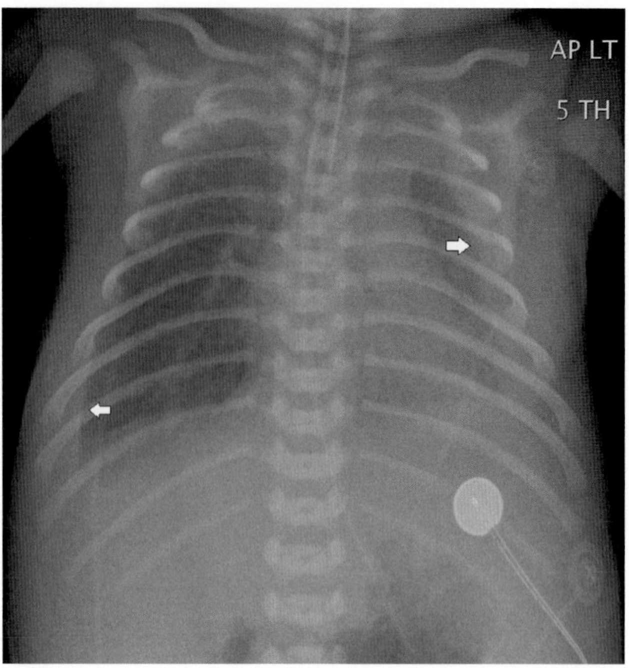

FIGURE 76-17 ■ **Newborn with bilateral chylothoraces.** Radiograph demonstrates bilateral pleural effusions (arrows).

radiographic changes may mimic meconium aspiration syndrome or severe transient tachypnoea. The presence of pleural effusions, pulmonary hyperinflation and mild cardiomegaly may not be helpful in differentiating pneumonia from these other conditions.

In the premature infant there maybe diffuse fine granular opacification, similar to the appearances seen in IRDS.[7] Some infants may have both IRDS and group B streptococcus pneumonia. Chlamydial infection classically presents first with conjunctivitis at 1–2 weeks after birth and the lung infection does not usually become evident until 4–12 weeks of age. Typically the radiograph demonstrates interstitial opacification with some hyperinflation.

The association of *Ureaplasma urealyticum* with neonatal pneumonia is increasingly recognised. These infants have a mild early course and develop features of BPD at an earlier age than would be expected in a premature infant.[8]

AIR LEAKS

Spontaneous pneumothorax and pneumomediastinum causes respiratory distress in the newborn infant. Many are transient and do not require intervention. A pneumothorax may be radiographically subtle in sick infants as supine radiographs are usually performed and free air accumulates over the lung surface, producing a hyperlucent lung and increased sharpness of the mediastinum (Figs. 76-7 and 76-14). A pneumomediastinum usually outlines the thymus (Fig. 76-16) and when there is a pneumopericardium the air surrounds the heart (Fig. 76-8).

PLEURAL EFFUSIONS

In infants who do not have hydrops, the most common cause of a congenital pleural effusion is chylothorax. The cause is unknown, and late maturation of the thoracic duct has been suggested as an aetiology. The abnormality is usually detected on antenatal ultrasound (US) and in utero drainage may be performed to prevent pulmonary hypoplasia. Postnatally, the chest radiograph demonstrates the pleural effusions (Fig. 76-17). Aspirated fluid will have a high lymphocyte count but will not have a milky appearance until such time as the infant is fed with fat. Resolution is usually complete but often after multiple aspirations.

SURFACTANT DYSFUNCTION DISORDERS

Disorders of surfactant deficiency due to a genetic abnormality in the surfactant protein B (SpB)[9] and C (SpC)[10] and the ATP-binding cassette transporter protein A3 (ABCA3) can lead to interstitial lung disease. Inherited mutations in the SpB and ABCA3 are autosomal recessive and may present immediately after birth with respiratory symptoms. Mutations in the SpC are autosomal dominant and may present later in infancy. The chest radiograph may show diffuse hazy opacification initially, with the later development of interstitial shadowing which may be progressive (Fig. 76-18A). Computed tomography (CT) demonstrates diffuse ground-glass opacification with septal thickening[11] and cystic change (Figs. 76-18B and C).

Pulmonary interstitial glycogenosis (PIG) may present in the preterm or term infant very soon after birth. It has been reported in isolation but is frequently associated

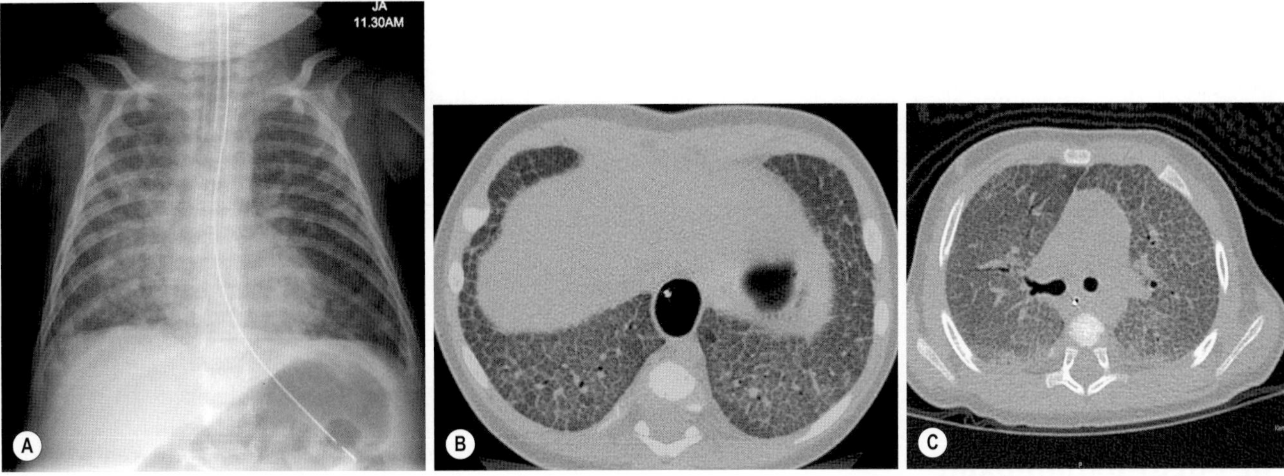

FIGURE 76-18 ■ **Infant with surfactant dysfunction disorder (ABCA3).** (A) CXR shows bilateral interstitial, granular and fluffy opacification. (B, C) Two axial CT slices demonstrate ground-glass opacification and septal thickening, giving a 'crazy paving' appearance similar to the pattern typically described in alveolar proteinosis.

with conditions that affect lung growth and the diagnosis is made by the pathological examination of lung tissue. The imaging features may be similar to those seen in the other disorders of surfactant deficiency.

LINES AND TUBES

The tip of an ET tube may vary considerably with head and neck movement and the correct position must therefore be assessed by taking the patient's head position and the tip of the tube into consideration.

The umbilical arterial line courses inferiorly in the umbilical artery, into the internal and common iliac arteries and then into the aorta. The tip should be positioned to avoid the origins of the major vessels, which are usually between T6 and T9 (Fig. 76-19) or in some institutions inferior to L3 vertebral bodies.

The umbilical venous line courses superiorly towards the liver. It enters the left portal vein, through the ductusvenosus and into the inferior vena cava (IVC). The ideal position is at the junction of the IVC and the right atrium (Fig. 76-19).

The correct position of central venous lines or peripherally inserted central catheters (PICC) is controversial. The position of PICC line tips inserted through the upper limbs is usually in the superior vena cava. The tips of those inserted through the lower limbs are usually positioned at the junction of the IVC and the right atrium. US may be particularly helpful in assessing a catheter's position and injection of very small amounts of intravenous water-soluble, low osmolar contrast medium may also be useful in checking the position of the tip.

Nasogastric tube tip positions should always be reported on, in order to avoid misplacement of nasogastric feeds.

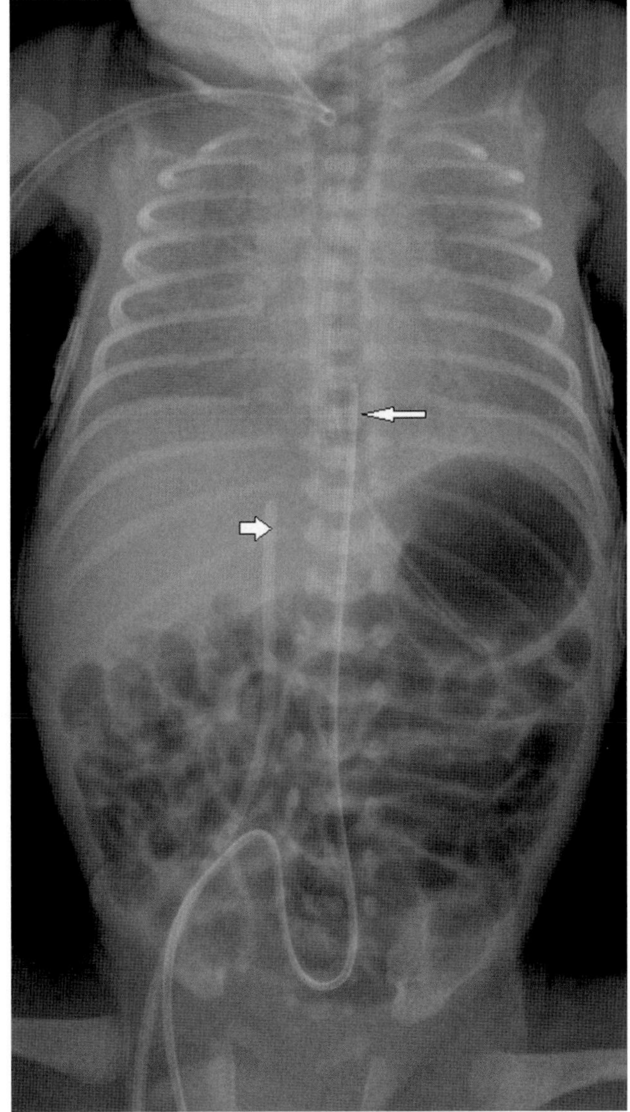

FIGURE 76-19 ■ **Umbilical arterial and venous catheters.** The tip of the umbilical arterial catheter is at T7 level (long arrow). The tip of the umbilical venous catheter is in the IVC (short arrow) and should ideally be placed more distally in the IVC close to the right atrium.

THE CHEST IN OLDER CHILDREN

Diseases of the respiratory tract occur frequently in children. These will range from the presentation of congenital abnormalities, infections through to complex immunodeficiency syndromes and malignancy.

The chest radiograph is the most frequently requested radiological investigation encountered within paediatric practice, and although pathological manifestations may mimic that seen in adults, a thorough knowledge of the variations within paediatric practice is vital to the general radiologist. In this section, we will cover some of the unique aspects of chest disease in the older child.

THE CHEST RADIOGRAPH

The plain chest radiograph remains the first radiological examination in use for the evaluation of the chest in children. Frontal chest radiographs are widely performed. Lateral views tend only to be performed after review of the frontal radiograph, when there are unanswered clinical questions.

A PA erect radiograph taken at full inspiration is optimal but difficult to obtain in uncooperative children; hence, an AP supine view is usually obtained in infants and small children. An inspiratory plain chest radiograph is considered adequate when the right hemidiaphragm is at the level of the eighth rib posteriorly. Poor inspiration may cause significant misinterpretation of the chest radiograph (Fig. 76-20). Radiographs obtained in expiration frequently show a rightward kink in the trachea, owing to the soft cartilage, relatively long trachea and the presence of a left aortic arch in the majority of children. Other features of an expiratory radiograph include some degree of ground-glass opacification of the lungs and relative enlargement of the heart. Rotation of the patient causes problems with interpretation, including apparent mediastinal shift/distortion of vasculature, the thymus and vessels mimicking a 'mass' (Fig. 76-21) and relative lucency of one lung compared to the other, simulating oligaemia/air trapping.

NORMAL VARIANTS

The normal thymus is a frequent cause of physiological widening of the anterior mediastinum occurring during the early years of life.

Normal thymic tissue is soft, malleable and compliant; hence, it often undulates beneath the overlying ribs, giving it a lobulated appearance known as the 'thymic wave'. The right thymic margin can often have a sharp 'sail-like' configuration (Fig. 76-1). The thymus may involute during periods of illness, severe stress or whilst on steroids or other chemotherapy. Rebound hyperplasia of the thymus may then occur following recovery or cessation of therapy, and this should not be confused with the development of a pathological mediastinal mass. If chest radiographic differentiation between normal thymus and pathology proves difficult on the radiograph, US can help distinguish intrathymic or adjacent masses within the anterior mediastinum from a normal isoechoic homogeneous thymus. Pathological tissue is heterogeneous, and may cause compression or indeed occlusion of adjacent airway or vasculature, something which never occurs with a normal thymus. In some cases where US is inconclusive, magnetic resonance imaging (MRI) is performed to differentiate a normal thymus from mediastinal pathology. On T2-weighted spin-echo sequences, the normal thymus has an intermediate signal similar to that of the spleen. On gadolinium-enhanced T1-weighted spin-echo sequences, the thymus should show only minimal enhancement.[12] Care should be taken to avoid confusing overlying plaits or braids of hair superimposed over the upper chest film as intraparenchymal lung pathology.

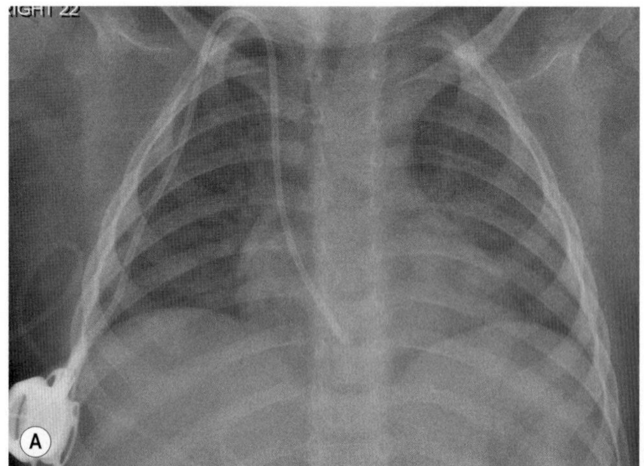

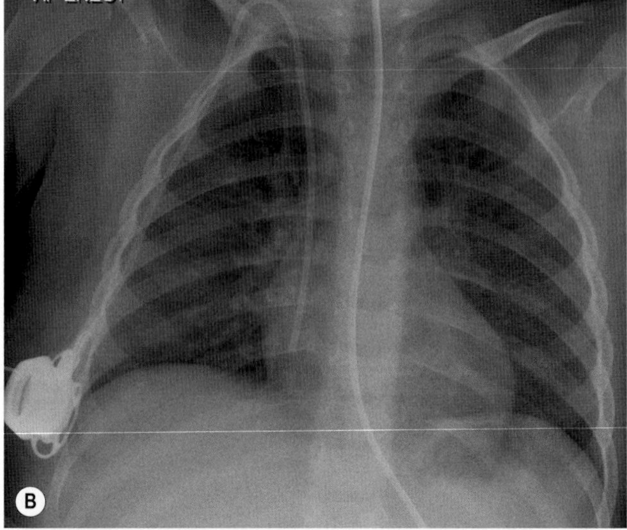

FIGURE 76-20 ■ The effect of inspiration. Two radiographs of the same patient highlight the problems in interpreting radiographs taken in poor inspiration. (A) The child's trachea is buckled and the heart appears enlarged; both phenomena are not shown on a subsequent radiograph (B) taken in good inspiration.

TABLE 76-1 **Asymmetric Lung Densities**

Respiratory Causes with Contralateral Mediastinal Shift	Respiratory Causes without Mediastinal Shift	Cardiac Causes
Foreign body aspiration—may be normal on inspiratory image, fluoroscopy can help	Unilateral hypoplastic lung	Pulmonary embolism—rare
Mucous plugging—asthmatics and ventilated patients	Congenital venolobar syndrome	Post-cardiac surgery—e.g. Blalock–Taussig shunt
Congenital lobar emphysema	Constrictive bronchiolitis—formerly known as Sywer–James syndrome	
External mass compression—mediastinal mass compressing a bronchus		
Bronchomalacia		
Endobronchial lesion—e.g. bronchial carcinoid		

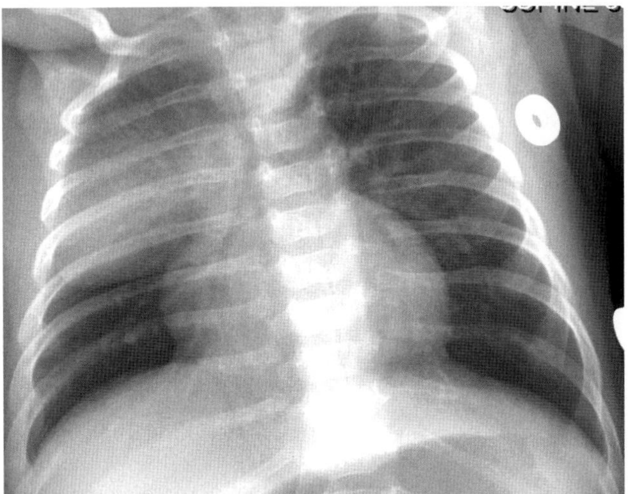

FIGURE 76-21 ■ **The effect of rotation.** A rotated patient showing a normal thymus (proven on subsequent radiograph) masquerading as a mediastinal mass.

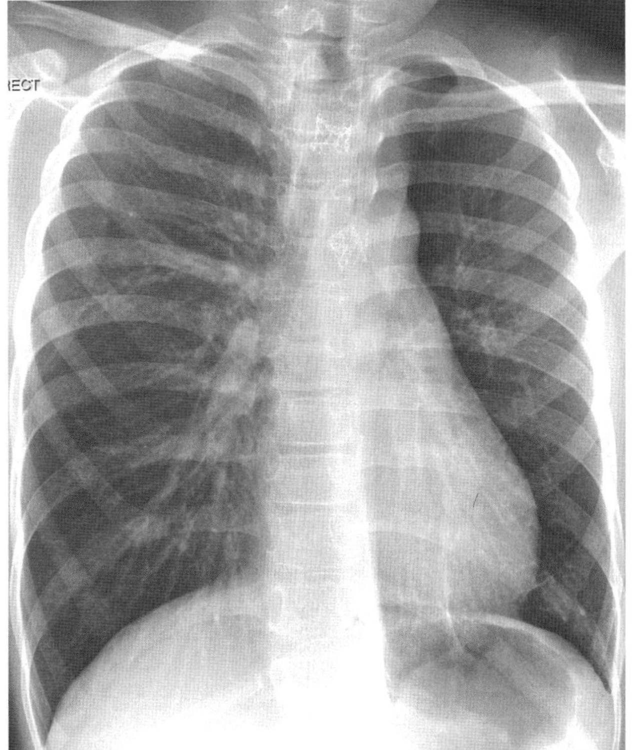

FIGURE 76-22 ■ **Assymmetric lung density.** The left lung is more hyperlucent than the right and there is a paucity of left-sided vascular markings. Tracheal and left main bronchus stents can be seen in this patient with known tracheobronchomalacia.

CARDIAC OR RESPIRATORY?

When the chest radiograph shows asymmetrical lung volumes, the lung with fewer vessels per unit area is usually the abnormal lung. The lack of, or reduction in, vascular markings is usually due to the presence of primary airways disease in children and the resultant homeostatic reflex vasoconstriction (Table 76-1) (Fig. 76-22). The presence of reduced vascularity in the hyperlucent areas resulting from a primary vascular pathological process, such as thromboembolism or pulmonary hypertension, is rare in children, although various congenital cardiac disorders can result in pulmonary oligaemia.

Prominent/enlarged generalised lung parenchymal vessels could indicate the presence of a left-to-right shunt at either intracardiac or great vessel level. Cardiac failure as a primary cause of pleural effusion in children is not common. In children, fluid overload tends to cause peribronchovascular oedema, which then results in overinflation of the lungs due to air trapping, along with perihilar infiltrate and upper lobe venous diversion.

THE LUNGS

Pulmonary Infection

Respiratory infections in children are the most frequent disorders encountered by paediatricians.[13] Chest radiography is the primary imaging technique used to evaluate acute lung disease.

Chest CT has, however, an important role in evaluating immunocompromised patients and both the acute and chronic complications of respiratory tract infection, such as empyema and bronchiectasis.[14] A frontal radiograph is usually adequate to confirm or exclude pulmonary infection/pneumonia.

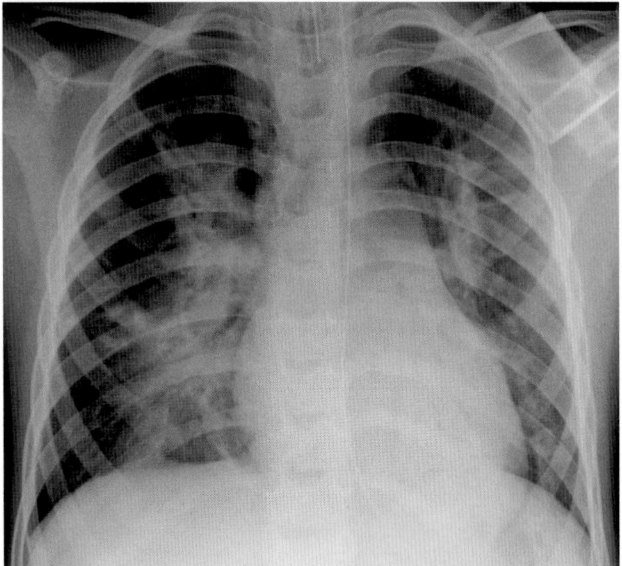

FIGURE 76-23 ■ Perihilar consolidation. This child was admitted to intensive care with severe respiratory distress due to influenza infection. The initial CXR shows extensive perihilar opacities with numerous air bronchograms, in keeping with severe influenza pneumonia.

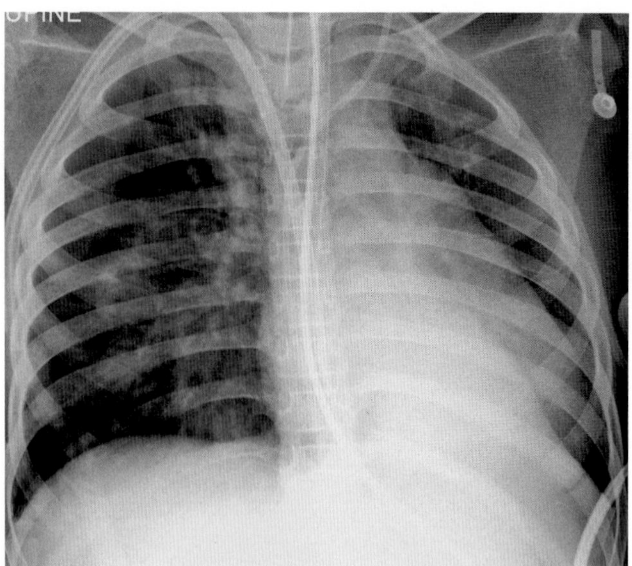

FIGURE 76-24 ■ Lobar consolidation. Left lower lobe consolidation/collapse in an intubated child.

Bacterial vs Viral

Within all age groups, viral infection is more common than bacterial. Viral infection usually affects the respiratory mucosa and airways, causing bronchial and bronchiolar oedema. This results in hyperinflation (due to air trapping as a result of partial bronchial obstruction as a result of peribronchial thickening), segmental and subsegmental atelectasis and small patches of consolidation frequently occurring in a perihilar location (Fig. 76-23).

Bacterial pneumonia, in general, causes inflammation within the acini, resulting in oedema and intra-alveolar exudate. This causes consolidation within the air spaces and results in the presence of 'air bronchograms' seen on radiographs. The typical location is lobar or segmental, and associated pleural (parapneumonic) effusions are not uncommon (Fig. 76-24). Although these patterns have traditionally been associated with viral and bacterial pathogens, studies indicate that prediction of causative pathogen using radiographic patterns is notoriously inaccurate.[15] In addition viral and bacterial infection may be present simultaneously, so these 'classic' radiographic patterns are not always accurate.

Features of Infection

Round Pneumonia

Round pneumonias occur frequently in young children, usually under 8 years of age, due to the presence of immature collateral ventilation pathways between the small airways (Fig. 76-25).[16] *Streptococcus pneumoniae* is the causative pathogen in >90% of normal hosts. Radiographs shows a rounded or spherical opacity with poorly defined margins, unlike a primary or metastatic chest tumour (which are usually very well circumscribed).[17]

Follow-up chest radiography to ensure resolution of pneumonia is not routinely necessary, in an otherwise previously healthy child. Follow-up should be reserved for those children who have persistent or recurrent symptoms, or have an underlying condition such as immunodeficiency. Causes of recurrent/persistent pneumonia include infection within a pre-existing lung abnormality, bronchial obstruction, aspiration associated with gastro-oesophageal reflux and rarely an H-type congenital trachea-oesophageal fistula (Fig. 76-26).

Necrotising/Cavitatory Pneumonia

Necrotising pneumonia with ensuing cavitatory necrosis has been described in association with staphylococcal pneumonias, and less frequently with *Klebsiella* infection. Areas of decreased or absent enhancement on contrast-enhanced CT indicate the presence of necrotising pneumonia with parenchymal ischaemia or infarction. Unlike the adult population, this is not such a poor prognostic indicator in children and good recovery of lung occurs with non-surgical therapy. Infected congenital bronchopulmonary foregut (cystic) malformations may sometimes have appearances very similar to that of cavity necrosis, and evaluation with CT may be helpful.[18] Thin-walled pneumatoceles are classic sequelae of staphylococcal infection (Fig. 76-27).[12] These commonly occurring lesions can be differentiated from lung abscesses by a lack of wall enhancement and their anatomical location within the interstitial spaces of the lungs.

Specific Infections

Tuberculosis

Tuberculosis remains an enormous worldwide public health issue. Within the traditionally 'low-risk' industrialised countries of western Europe, as a result of the

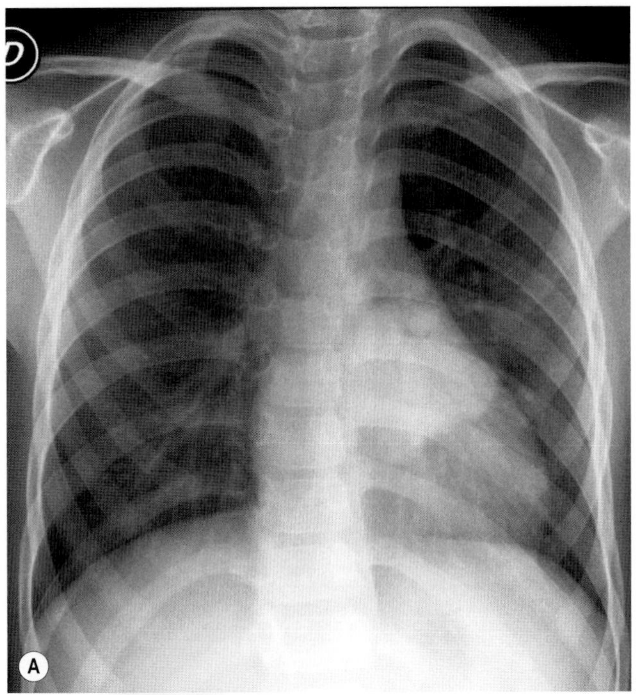

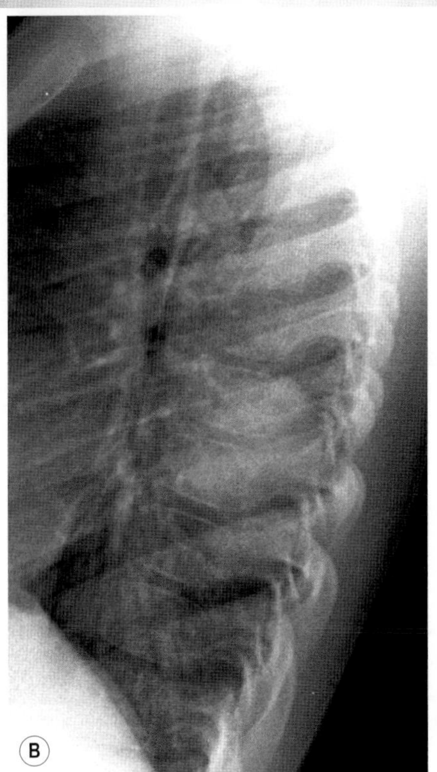

FIGURE 76-25 ■ **Round pneumonia.** This child presented with cough and pyrexia. (A) The CXR shows a rounded opacity behind the left heart adjacent to the mediastinum. (B) The lateral view confirms its position posteriorly within the lung parenchyma. The lesion resolved on a follow-up radiograph following antibiotic treatment.

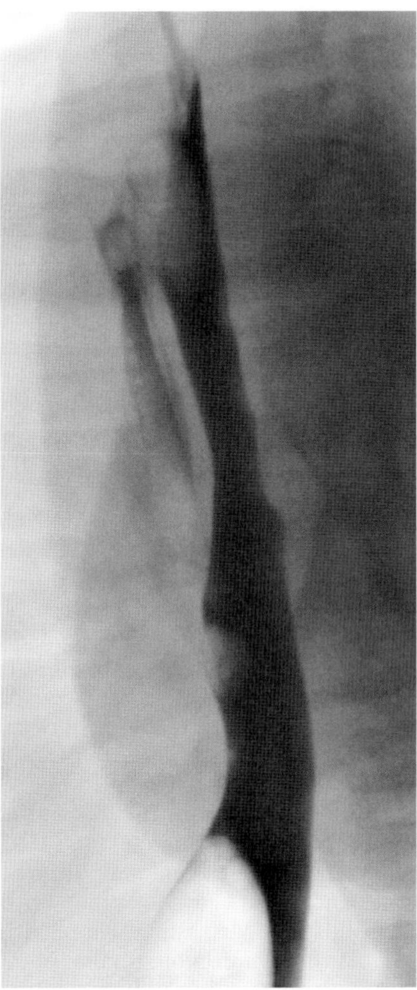

FIGURE 76-26 ■ **H-type fistula.** Tube oesophagram in a child with a history of recurrent unexplained chest infections. There is a mid-oesophageal fistula with abnormal passage of contrast medium into the trachea.

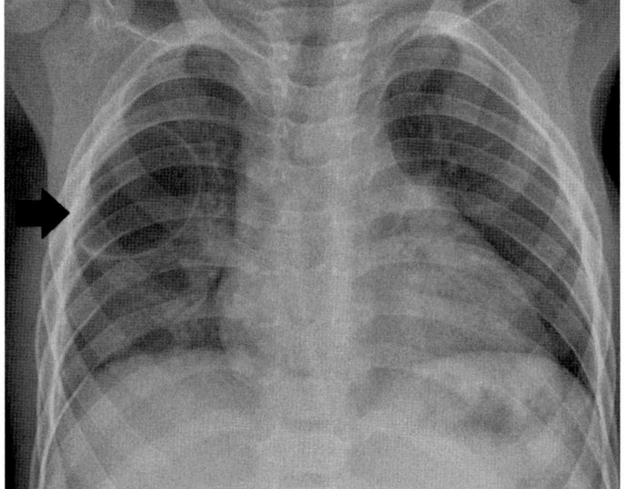

FIGURE 76-27 ■ **Pneumatocele.** Post-severe staphylococcal pneumonia. A thin-walled cyst in the right upper zone is in keeping with a pneumatocele.

increase in world travel, immigration (and in particular the HIV epidemic), infection rates have increased to such an extent that areas of inner city London now have similar TB disease prevalence (according to WHO) as parts of the Third World.

Children, and in particular, infants infected with TB, are at much greater risk of severe (invasive) disease, extrapulmonary dissemination and death, than adults. Many cases of primary TB infection in children do not become symptomatic. Young age (infants are at increased risk) and compromised immune status (HIV, primary immunodeficiency) carry an increased risk.[19,20]

Most cases of paediatric tuberculosis are due to primary infection, and therefore presentation and radiographic appearances are different to the adult-type disease. Early chest X-ray findings are of alveolar consolidation, which has a predilection for the lower lobes. The infection then progresses onto regional and hilar lymph nodes (Fig. 76-28); the combination is referred to as a Ranke complex. The process may spontaneously regress at this point, but can progress onto enlarging and often caeseating lymphadenopathy particularly in those high-risk groups already described. CT is superior to the chest radiograph in the diagnosis and assessment of mediastinal lymphadenopathy.[21] In children the smaller-calibre airways are more easily compressed by enlarged tuberculous lymph nodes and, as a result, lung hyperinflation and air trapping (due to partial airway obstruction and obstructive over-inflation) are commonly seen on CT. Caeseating nodes completely obstruct regional bronchi, causing inflammation and lobar consolidation, with ensuing collapse–consolidation. Mediastinal lymphadenopathy is the hallmark of primary infection.[22] Table 76-2 lists other causes of hilar enlargement in children. Children are also at increased risk of developing disseminated disease; again this is particularly true in infants. Features of disseminated tuberculous disease include multiple lung parenchymal nodules of variable size and distribution, and this has led to the term 'acute disseminated tuberculosis', which is preferred to 'miliary' tuberculosis (Fig. 76-29).[23] The presence of either a sympathetic pleural effusion or cavitations is a rare complication in primary tuberculosis (Fig. 76-30).[24] True tuberculous empyema is exceptionally rare.

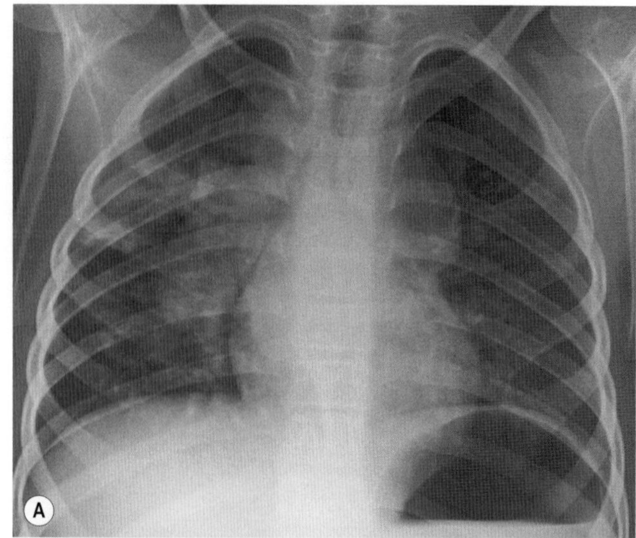

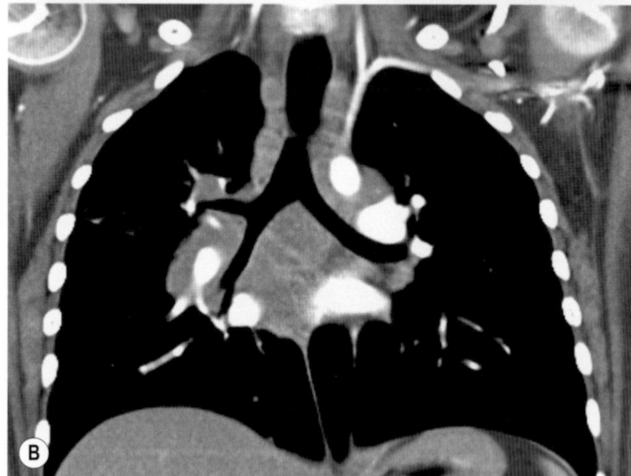

FIGURE 76-28 ■ **Primary tuberculosis.** (A) CXR and (B) coronal CT reformat in a child presenting with tuberculosis infection. Extensive right paratracheal, subcarinal and bilateral hilar adenopathy is demonstrated and is causing tracheal compression.

TABLE 76-2 **Causes of Bilateral Hilar Enlargement**

Bilateral	Unilateral
Lymphadenopathy	
Viral and bacterial infection—common	Tuberculosis
Lymphoma/leukaemia—paratracheal enlargement is frequent	Pulmonary metastases—usually well-defined
Tuberculosis—bilateral involvement is rare	Lymphoma/leukaemia—rarely unilateral
Sarcoidosis—normally presents with extrathoracic symptoms in children	Viral/bacterial/fungal infection—the most common cause
Metastases—lobulated and well-defined	
Vascular Enlargement	
Left–right shunt—ASD/VSD/PDA	Post-stenotic dilatation—enlarged main pulmonary trunk and proximal left pulmonary trunk
Pulmonary hypertension—central enlarged vessels and peripheral pruning	Pulmonary hypertension with absent contralateral pulmonary artery—e.g. in unilateral pulmonary hypoplasia
Cardiac failure—increased vessel calibre with an ill-defined outline	

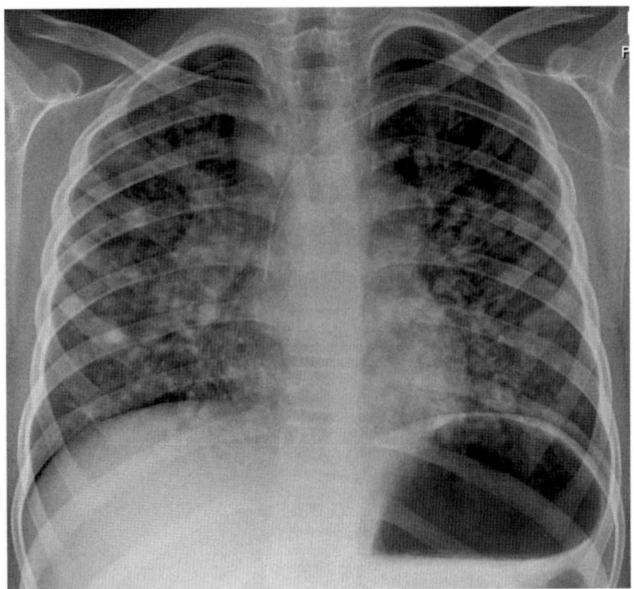

FIGURE 76-29 ■ Acute disseminated (haematogenous/miliary) tuberculosis. Frontal CXR shows widespread ill-defined nodules of varying sizes in a random distribution throughout the lung parenchyma. More confluent areas of consolidation indicate coalescence of the nodules. Appearances of 'miliary' TB in children are more diverse than in adults.

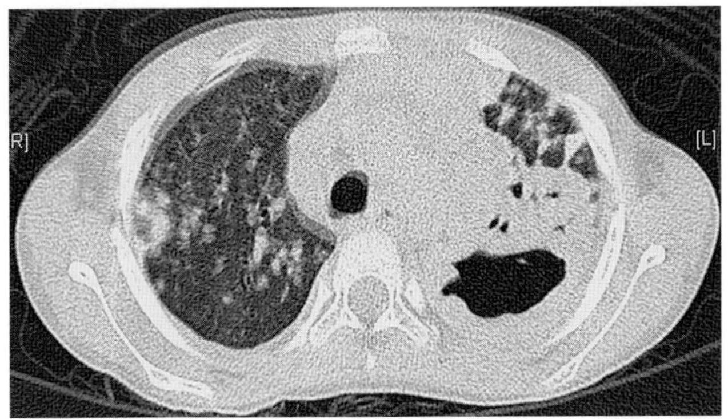

FIGURE 76-30 ■ TB cavitation. Axial CT image shows a large air-filled cavity in an area of consolidation in the left upper lobe. Several nodules throughout the remainder of the lungs are related to endobronchial seeding of TB. Images are degraded due to respiratory motion artefact as the patient was tachypnoeic.

Resolution of radiographic findings is a slow process and may take in excess of 6 months and it is not essential for complete resolution to have occurred prior to cessation of antituberculous therapy.[25]

Mycoplasma pneumoniae

Mycoplasma pneumoniae is a common and important cause of atypical community-acquired pneumonia usually in children of school age. The predominant symptom is often a dry persistent cough. Radiographic findings are non-specific but may range from diffuse interstitial change or perihilar bronchial wall thickening and dilatation through to segmental or lobar consolidation. There is often a discrepancy between the severity of

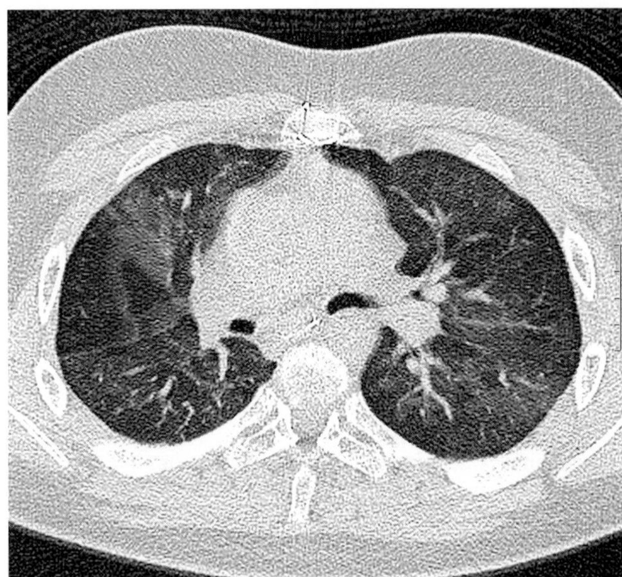

FIGURE 76-31 ■ Constrictive (obliterative) bronchiolitis. Axial expiratory CT slice shows a classic mosaic pattern indicating widespread severe small airways disease.

radiographic findings and the relatively minor clinical picture. Though the majority of cases respond well to medical therapy, *M. pneumoniae* is an important cause of constrictive obliterative bronchiolitis in a minority of those infected, particularly if not treated promptly or effectively.[26]

Late Complications of Infection

The most common chronic complications of pneumonia are bronchiectasis (large airways disease) and constrictive (obliterative) bronchiolitis (i.e. small airways disease), previously known as obliterative bronchiolitis or Swyer–James–Macleod syndrome.

Bronchiectasis is the most frequent chronic complication, and is defined as irreversible dilatation and wall thickening of the bronchi. On high-resolution CT (HRCT) the bronchus is considered dilated if the lumen is larger than the associated adjacent pulmonary artery. Hyperlucent lung, with decreased pulmonary (pruned) vasculature, which persists on expiratory scans, indicates air trapping and is the hallmark of small airways disease (analogous with constrictive obliterative bronchiolitis) (Fig. 76-31), which often coexists with bronchiectasis. Common causative infectious causes include *M. pneumoniae* and adenovirus.[27,28]

Pleural Effusion

There are many causes of pleural effusion in children (Table 76-3) but the most common is due to infection. Parapneumonic effusions are more commonly associated with bacterial infections, usually pneumococcus, but other infections (such as tuberculosis) should be considered, particularly if unresponsive to routine antibacterial therapy. Pleural effusions should be evaluated with US, and can be categorised as low grade (anechoic fluid

TABLE 76-3 **Causes of Pleural Effusion**

Cause	Diagnosis
Infection	• Parapneumonic* • Empyema—commonly secondary to streptococcal or staphylococcal infection • Tuberculosis*—rare in children
Neoplasm	• Common: leukaemia/lymphoma Metastatic—especially Wilms' tumour • Less common—primary lesions such as PNET* or mesothelioma
Inflammatory	• Pancreatitis—small and left-sided
Fluid overload	• Low albumin states • Cardiac failure • Severe sepsis
Trauma	• Haemothorax*—hyperdense on CT (>30 HU)
Congenital	• Diaphragmatic hernia*—opaque hemithorax rather than effusion • Chylothorax—may reflect lymphangiectasia

*Common causes of opaque hemithorax.

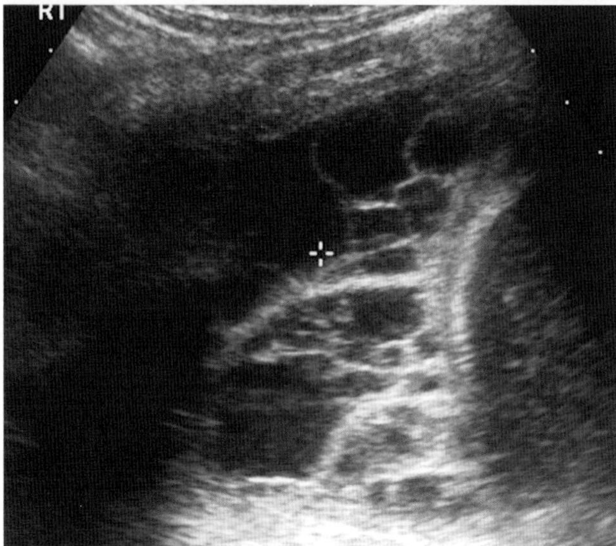

FIGURE 76-32 ■ High-grade parapneumonic effusion. Longitudinal US image shows a complex multiseptated loculated pleural effusion in a child with a known chest infection.

without internal echoes) or high grade (fibropurulent organisation with presence of fronds, septations or loculi) (Fig. 76-32). This is important for further management, as high-grade effusions may require thoracoscopy and surgical debridement, whereas low-grade effusions may be treated more conservatively.[29]

The Acutely Wheezing Child

Asthma[30]

Asthma (reactive airways disease) is a common cause of childhood wheeze, but the diagnosis is clinical and should not normally require radiological intervention unless there are atypical features or complications. However, most children diagnosed with asthma will, at some point in their diagnostic pathway, have a chest radiograph performed. This is useful for excluding other causes of wheeze, such as congenital tracheobronchial/vascular anomalies, lung parenchymal disease or, very importantly, radiographic sequelae of an inhaled foreign body.

In children requiring hospitalisation for an acute asthmatic attack, imaging is useful for assessing complications, such as consolidation related to either mucous plugging or secondary bacterial infection. The chest radiograph commonly shows overinflated lungs, often with peribronchial thickening that is often more marked in the middle lobe. Lobar collapse is frequent, particularly in children with concomitant infections, and is usually due to mucous plugging. Pneumothorax and pneumomediastinum are less frequently observed but important findings.

Inhaled Foreign Bodies

It is important to bear in mind that toddlers are inquisitive and may ingest or inhale foreign bodies, with or without the knowledge of their carer; i.e. the episode may not be witnessed by an adult and may result in acute respiratory distress causing immediate airway compromise, and the need for urgent investigation. Alternatively, the episode may not result in acute symptoms until the child presents at a later stage with a chronic wheeze or recurrent/persistent infections. If there is an unexplained acute respiratory deterioration in a toddler with lung collapse or overinflation, there should be rapid recourse to bronchoscopic assessment, with timely removal of the foreign body to ensure a good short- and long-term prognosis.

A plain radiograph should be the initial investigation of choice in less emergent cases. Findings may include a radio-opaque foreign body (although most are radiolucent, such as nuts and plastic toys), lobar collapse or air trapping. The radiograph should be scrutinised for hypertransradiancy, which may be localised, or diffuse, and occurs due to a ball–valve mechanism in larger airways, causing distal air trapping. A quick fluoroscopic examination using pulsed fluoroscopy can be extremely useful when evaluating differing lung radiolucencies in suspected foreign body aspiration, and in stridor.[31] The obstructed (overinflated) lung will not change in volume with respiration, and the mediastinum will swing contralaterally on expiration.

Certain organic matter, e.g. peanuts, are particularly irritant and cause a severe local inflammatory reaction within the adjacent airway, which may make complete extraction difficult, and they often fragment thence embolise into more distal airways, causing increased consolidation post-bronchoscopy.

Stridor

Stridor may arise secondary to infection in children. Lateral-view fluoroscopy can be useful for dynamic evaluation of tracheomalacia, where the trachea collapses completely during expiration. Barium swallow, with the child in the true lateral position, and good distension of the oesophagus, is still the primary study in patients with a suspected vascular ring or sling. The rings/slings will abnormally indent the contrast column within the

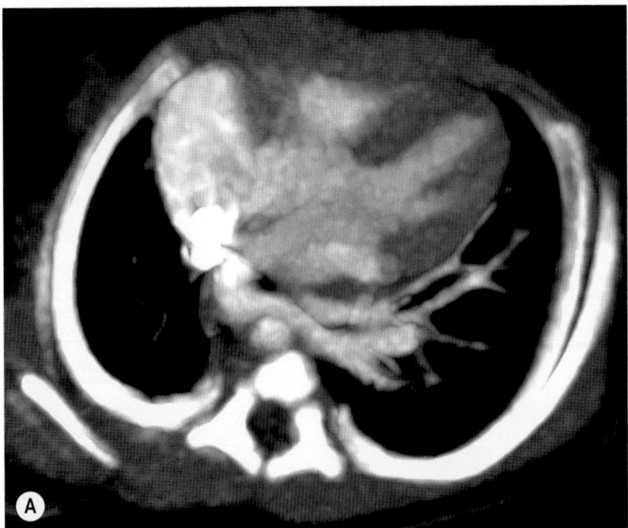

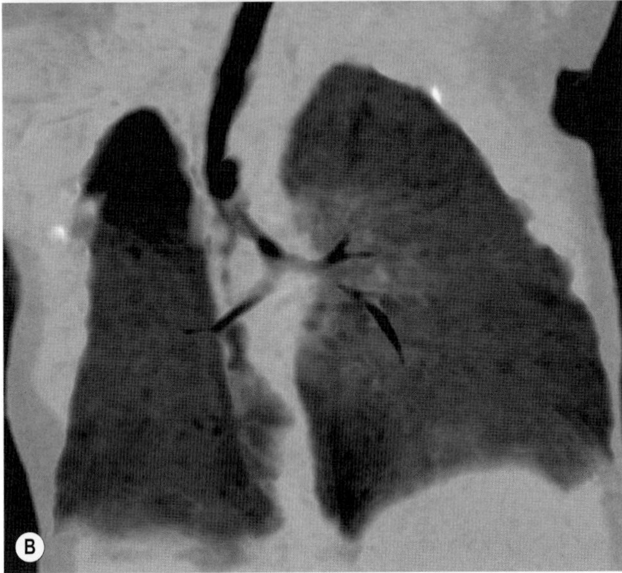

FIGURE 76-33 ■ **Left pulmonary arterial sling.** (A) CTA maximum intensity projection (MIP)—the large left pulmonary artery arises from the right pulmonary artery and passes posterior to the trachea and anterior to the oesophagus. Note the marked narrowing of the trachea at this level. (B) CT minimum intensity projection (MinIP) demonstrates the long-segment tracheal stenosis and wide/splayed carinal angle.

oesophagus. This test may also be valuable for assessing the presence of other extrinsic masses. Thin-section CT with volume rendering and multiplanar reconstruction techniques has almost eliminated the need for contrast bronchography in children being assessed for vascular rings and slings (Fig. 76-33); however, the technique is still used in functional studies for assessing the dynamics of intermittent airway obstruction.

Congenital Chest Abnormalities

Bronchopulmonary Foregut Malformations

Bronchopulmonary foregut malformations (BPFM) are now considered as part of a spectrum of anomalies of lung development ranging from tracheobronchial anomalies such as congenital cystic hamartomatous (adenomatoid) malformations and bronchogenic cysts, to anomalies with abnormal vascularity such as pulmonary sequestration and the hypogenetic lung (or scimitar) syndrome. There is considerable overlap between these groups, with a significant percentage of lesions being of mixed type, i.e. hybrid lesion: for example a 'cystic' malformation with systemic arterial supply (i.e. sequestration). Multidetector CT (MDCT) can offer excellent imaging for this range of anomalies, being able to simultaneously depict detail of lung parenchyma and the systemic arterial vascular supply, and the pattern of venous drainage (either conventional into the pulmonary veins in intralobar types or into the systemic venous systems in extralobar sequestrations).

Congenital Thoracic Cysts

These can occur in the mediastinum (mediastinal bronchogenic cysts, enteric duplication cysts and pleuropericardial cysts) and within lung parenchyma (intrapulmonary bronchogenic cysts). Bronchogenic cysts are more frequently located within the mediastinum (85%), typically in the subcarinal position. Ten to 15% are intrapulmonary, most frequently in the lower lobes, but usually within the proximal third of the lung (Fig. 76-34).[32] Rarely, they can also be located within the diaphragmatic leaflets, or below the diaphragm, and even within the liver or in the neck. These congenital lesions are lined with bronchial epithelium and often communicate with the tracheobronchial tree. The cysts generally contain mucinous or serous fluid, but blood (related to haemorrhage within), or air, can also be contained. Associated congenital malformations include congenital lobar overinflation (emphysema), bronchial atresia and pulmonary (intra- or extralobar) sequestration.[33,34] Mediastinal cysts are often asymptomatic and incidentally found on imaging later in life. They can, however, cause mass effect, resulting in tracheal/bronchial or oesophageal compression, presenting with wheeze, stridor or dysphagia. The cysts can become infected and cause repeated pneumonias. The lesions are often seen as mediastinal masses on plain radiographs, but CT allows better evaluation of the relationships with adjacent structures. The cyst content is usually water attenuation on CT, but may appear iso- or hyperdense due to intracystic haemorrhage or high protein (mucinous) content. MRI, which has a better contrast resolution than CT, can better evaluate the nature of the cyst contents. The cysts are typically hyperintense on T2-weighted spin-echo images. T1-weighted images show different signal intensity, depending on the cyst content.[35] Air within the cyst could be due to infection, instrumentation or communication with the airway or gastrointestinal tract. Surgical treatment is indicated in symptomatic lesions.

The differential diagnosis should include oesophageal duplication (usually located within the posterior mediastinum) and with neurenteric cysts (located in posterior mediastinum and associated with vertebral defects) (Fig. 76-35).

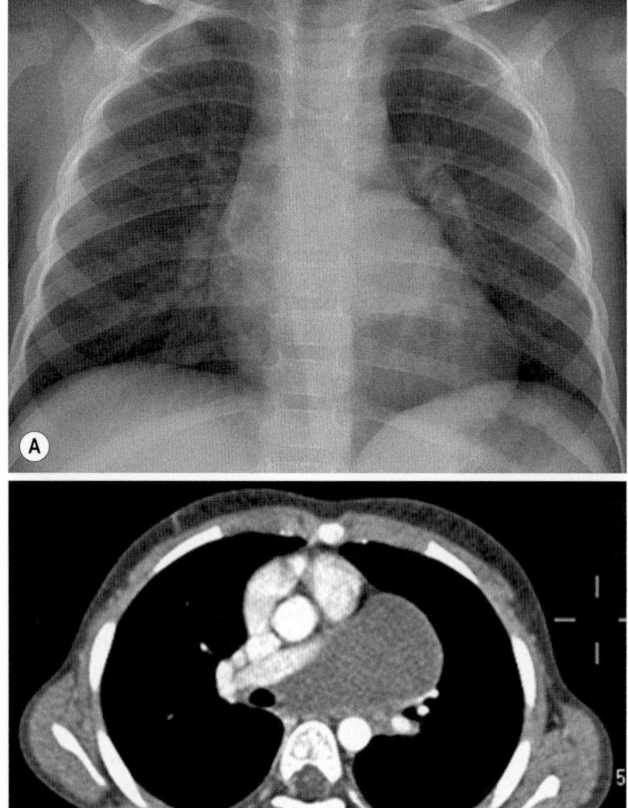

FIGURE 76-34 ■ **Bronchogenic cyst.** (A) CXR in a child showing a smooth round opacity elevating the LMB and splaying the carina. (B) CECT shows an intermediate-density homogeneous mass in a subcarinal position with a classical appearance of a mediastinal bronchogenic cyst.

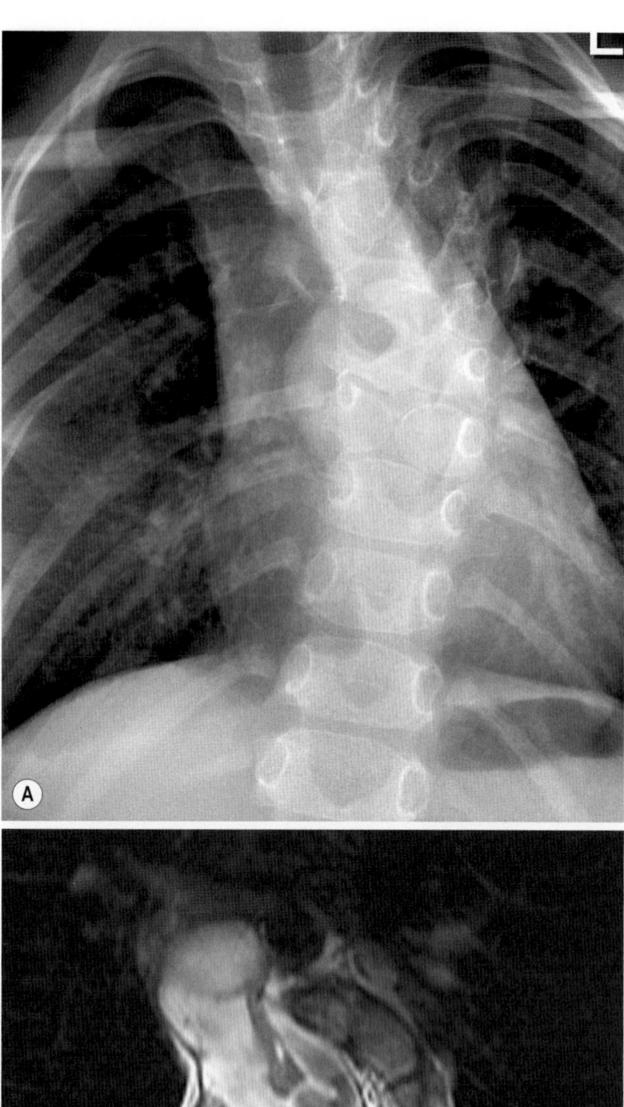

FIGURE 76-35 ■ **Neurenteric cyst.** (A) Thoracic spine radiograph highlights a right-sided paravertebral mass with an associated developmental vertebral anomaly. (B) Axial T2-weighted SE image demonstrates intradural communication.

Congenital Pulmonary Airway Malformations

Congenital pulmonary airway malformations (CPAM) are a group of cystic and non-cystic lung lesions resulting from early airway maldevelopment. It is preferable to use this term instead of the previous nomenclature of congenital cystic adenomatoid malformation (CCAM), as only one type (i.e. type 3) is a true adenomatoid lesion[36] (Table 76-4).[37]

CPAMs can communicate with the airways and are relatively frequently infected (30%).[38] Blood supply is from the pulmonary artery with drainage via pulmonary veins. Hybrid lesions with histological and imaging features of both a CPAM and bronchopulmonary sequestration will have, by definition, a systemic arterial supply.

Fetal US may show an echogenic soft-tissue mass, with multiple variable-size anechoic cysts or a homogeneous echogenic solid mass. Large lesions may cause mediastinal shift, resulting in lung hypoplasia, polyhydramnios and hydrops fetalis.[39,40] Fetal MRI may be carried out to further delineate the mass prior to delivery, and to calculate the overall functional lung volumes. The lesions are hyperintense on T2-weighted sequences and can be uni-/multilocular or solid.[41] Postnatal radiographs demonstrate variable density, depending on the fluid contents of the cysts, and mediastinal shift, depending on the size of the lesion. In the early neonatal period the mass may be completely opaque, as the cysts are still full of fluid. With time, this fluid is gradually replaced with air and prominent air–fluid levels are seen. Approximately 40% of antenatally diagnosed lesions are not detected on plain chest radiography.[37] Spiral CT allows better evaluation, demonstrating a mass made up of multiple cysts of different sizes (Figs. 76-36 and 76-37).[42] Chest

TABLE 76-4 **Modified Stocker CPAM Classification**[37]

Type	Description
0	Incompatible with life
1	Commonest type (>65%) Several large intercommunicating cysts (up to 10 cm) Mediastinal shift is common
2	10–15% of cases Smaller than other types Small evenly sized cysts (up to 2 cm) Often associated with other congenital abnormalities
3	~8% of cases Large solid lesion with small cysts (1.5 cm) Nearly always causes mediastinal shift Poor prognosis
4	10–15% of cases Large cysts (up to 7 cm) May be associated with, or a precursor of, pleuropulmonary blastoma

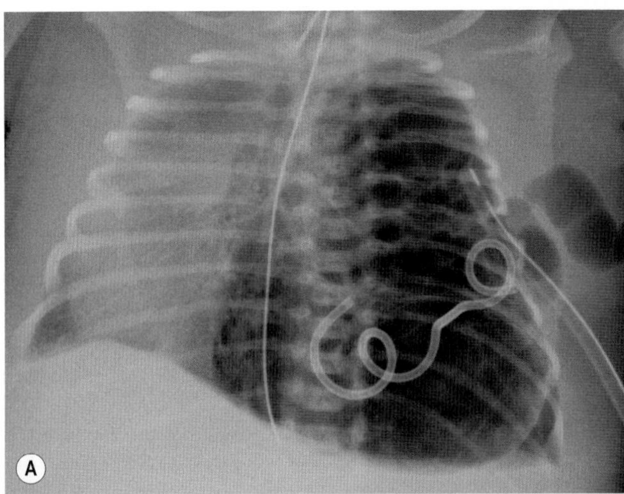

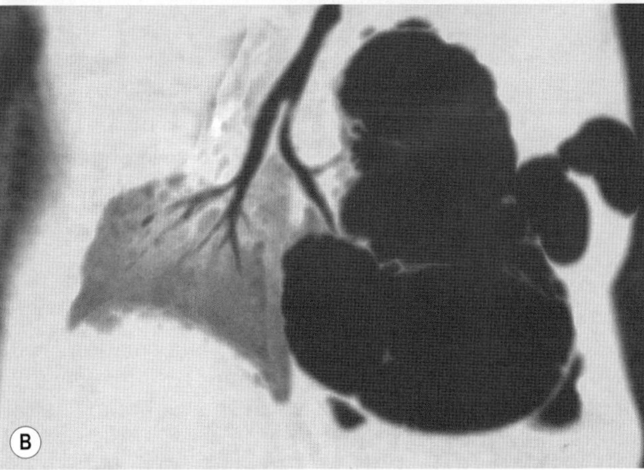

FIGURE 76-36 ■ **Type 1 CPAM.** (A) CXR shows a large air-filled abnormality in the left lung causing marked contralateral mediastinal shift. Attempts have been made to insert intercostal drains. (B) Coronal CT reformat confirms the presence of a large multicystic mass. Note the narrowed and displaced left main bronchus.

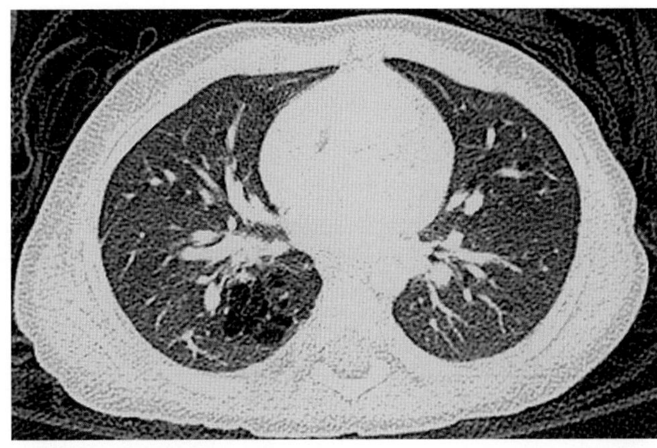

FIGURE 76-37 ■ **Type 2 CPAM.** Axial CT shows a multicystic lesion in the right lower lobe. No significant mediastinal shift is present and the lesion was subsequently excised.

radiography and CT can demonstrate surrounding lung consolidation in cases complicated by infection. Large lesions are usually surgically managed, due to mass effect, but smaller lesions may also be resected owing to frequent infections.

Congenital Diaphragmatic Hernia

One of the differential diagnoses for a large cystic thoracic mass is the congenital diaphragmatic hernia, or Bochdalek hernia, which occurs in approximately 1 in 3000 live births. In 40–50% of cases there are associated congenital abnormalities, most commonly of the central nervous system (CNS). Associated cardiac abnormalities affecting the ventricular outflow tracts (i.e. tetralogy of Fallot and hypoplastic left heart syndrome) are the most important associations, with important impact in terms of prognostic outcome.[43]

In isolated hernias, the most important prognostic factor is the degree of associated lung hypoplasia. The hernia arises from a defect in the posterolateral diaphragmatic leaflet, usually on the left. The lesion is usually detected on antenatal US. These lesions tend to have a worse prognosis owing to associated complications or the degree of lung hypoplasia. Herniation, which occurs later in fetal development, is associated with less severe lung hypoplasia.[44] Fetal MRI can supplement antenatal US, and is particularly useful if prenatal intervention is being considered.[45]

Postnatal chest radiographs are usually sufficient for diagnosis of new presentations, usually demonstrating a large cystic or solid mass, containing bowel loops within the chest (Fig. 76-38). In the minority of cases where there is confusion, contrast studies can demonstrate intrathoracic bowel.

Pulmonary Sequestration

Pulmonary sequestration is a mass of lung tissue, disconnected from the bronchial tree, which derives its blood supply from one or more systemic vessels, commonly the thoracic or abdominal aorta.[46] There are two types, intra- and extralobar sequestration.

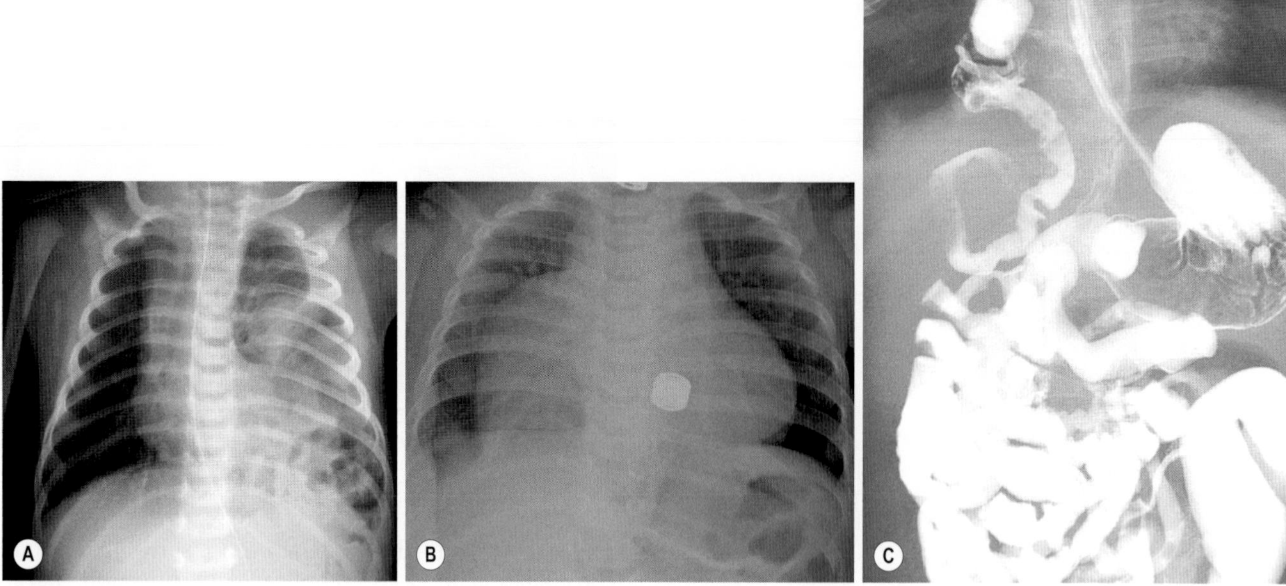

FIGURE 76-38 ■ **Diaphragmatic hernia.** (A) Bochdalek-type hernia with multiple loops of bowel in the left hemithorax. (B) On this frontal CXR, a mass is present at the right cardiophrenic angle in keeping with a Morgagni-type diaphragmatic hernia. These occur through an anterolateral diaphragm defect and typically present later in life. (C) Bowel loops passing into a Morgagni hernia on a contrast study.

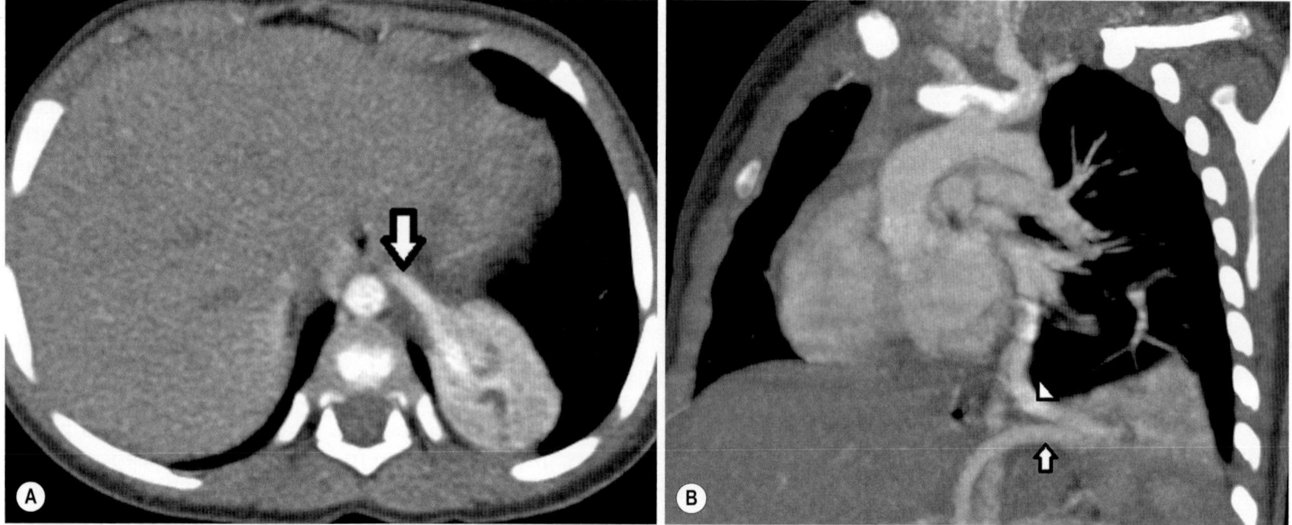

FIGURE 76-39 ■ **Pulmonary sequestration.** (A) Axial CT shows an enhancing mass in the posterior left lower lobe with a large (enhancing) feeding vessel (arrow). (B) Oblique coronal reformat highlights the mass receiving arterial supply from a branch of the coeliac artery (arrow) with venous drainage occurring via a left pulmonary vein (arrowhead).

Intralobar sequestration (ILS) is more common (75%) than extralobar sequestration (ELS) (Fig. 76-39). ILS is surrounded by normal lung, i.e. shares the pleural investment with the surrounding normal lung, and usually drains into the pulmonary venous system. Sixty per cent of the cases are located in the left lower lobe and they relatively frequently become infected.[47] Extralobar sequestration usually has its own pleural covering, and systemic venous drainage to the azygos or portal venous systems.[48] The ELS are usually located at the left base in 77% of cases.[49] Extralobar sequestration can be located below the diaphragm and mimic a neuroblastoma or adrenal haemorrhage.[50] ELS are associated with multiple congenital malformations in 65% of cases, including other types of bronchopulmonary foregut malformation.[51]

A homogeneous opacity at the lung base may be seen on plain chest radiographs. US will show a homogeneous hyperechoic mass, with a systemic feeding artery. CT depicts the feeding artery and the venous drainage, and may show a homogeneous soft-tissue mass, or a mass containing air or fluid cysts. MDCT is more sensitive in detecting small systemic vessels than MRI, due to the superior spatial resolution in CT, especially in small children, and can evaluate lung parenchyma at the same time.

CT is the technique of choice for evaluating pulmonary sequestrations.[52]

MRI demonstrates a solid, well-defined and hyperintense mass on T2-weighted images, with a systemic feeding artery. Hybrid lesions show imaging findings of both sequestration and CPAM.[53] Symptomatic patients require surgical resection.[54]

Congenital Lobar Overinflation[55]

This bronchial abnormality results in a check–valve mechanism, causing progressive hyperinflation of the affected lobe. The left upper lobe is the most frequently affected (42%), followed by the middle lobe (35%). Radiographs in the immediate postnatal period may show a radio-density as the affected lobe is still full of fluid. Later radiographs will demonstrate hyperlucency and overexpansion of the affected lobe with variable degree of mediastinal shift (Fig. 76-40). CT will exclude other causes of secondary lobar overinflation; for example, vascular anomalies, compression of the bronchi or mediastinal masses. In asymptomatic patients, conservative treatment and follow-up can show a reduction in overinflation. Excision of the affected lobe is necessary in symptomatic children.

Bronchial Atresia

Bronchial atresia is a congenital malformation characteristically located within the left upper lobe, characterised by obliteration of a segmental, subsegmental or lobar bronchus. Air enters the affected lobe or segment by collateral channels, producing overinflation and air trapping. Mucous secretions accumulate in the atretic bronchus, forming a mucocele.[56] Chest X-ray (CXR) and CT demonstrate pulmonary overinflation with air trapping during expiration, and a tubular, branched or spherical opacity (mucocele) in a central position (Fig. 76-41). Significant mediastinal shift and collapse of the ipsilateral lobes is more frequent in congenital lobar overinflation. Symptoms may be absent and radiological features may progressively improve. Infection of the unconnected lung is rare.

Lung Agenesis-Hypoplasia Complex

Three categories of pulmonary underdevelopment are grouped under the term of 'agenesis and hypoplasia complex', as they have similar radiologic findings on chest radiograph. Pulmonary agenesis is a complete absence of lung parenchyma, bronchus and pulmonary vasculature; pulmonary aplasia is a blind-ending rudimentary bronchus, without lung parenchyma or pulmonary vasculature; and pulmonary hypoplasia is a rudimentary lung and bronchus, with airways, alveoli and pulmonary vessels decreased in number and size.

They appear on a chest radiograph as a diffuse opacity of one hemithorax, with mediastinal shift and contralateral lung hyperinflation, simulating collapsed lung.[57] Lung agenesis, aplasia and hypoplasia can be differentiated with use of CT or MRI (Fig. 76-42). This lung complex can be associated with other congenital malformations of the cardiovascular, gastrointestinal, genitourinary and skeletal systems.

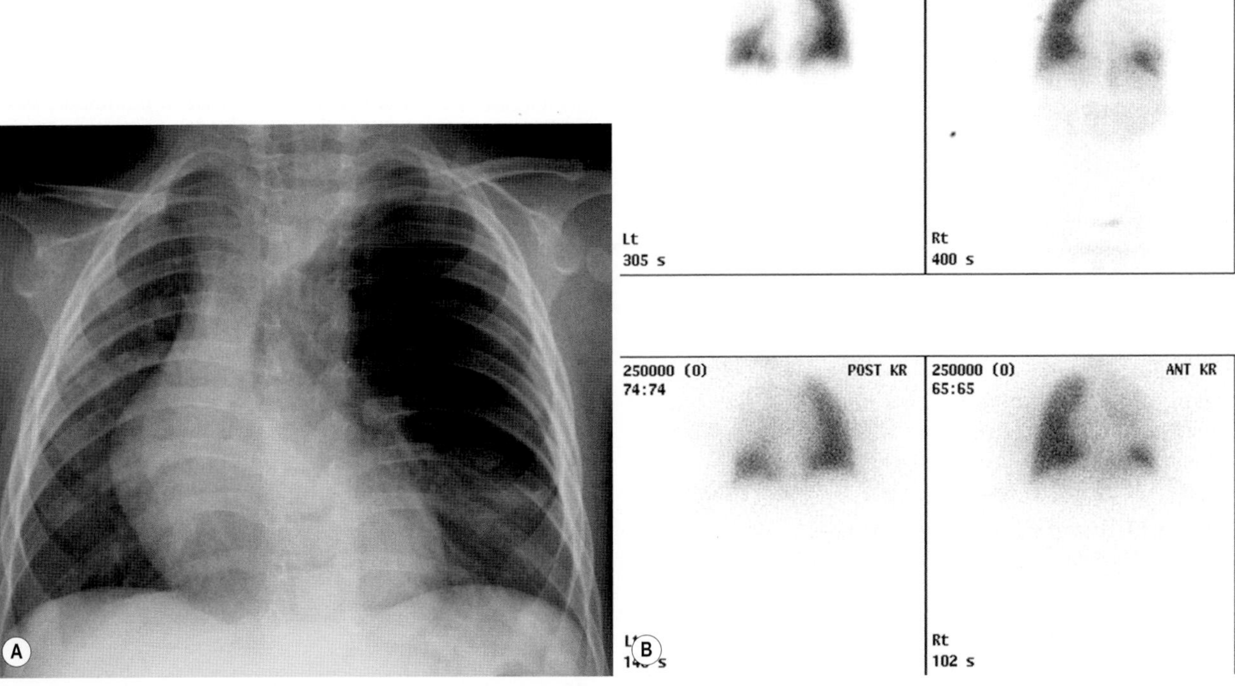

FIGURE 76-40 ■ **Congenital lobar overinflation (emphysema).** (A) CXR shows hyperlucency in the LUL. (B) A V/Q shows limited ventilation but no perfusion within the overinflated segment.

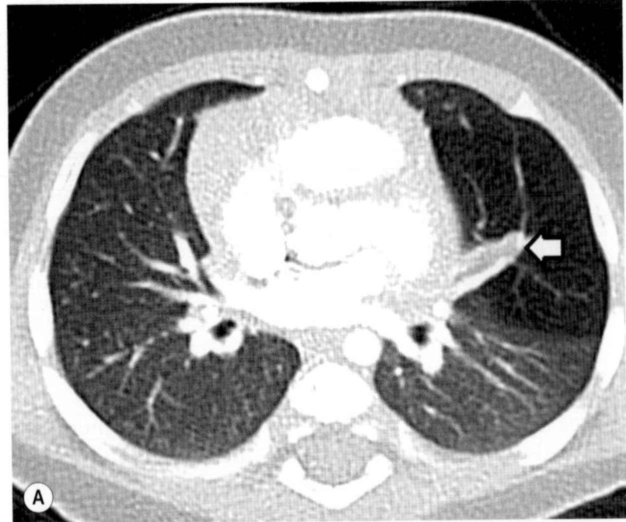

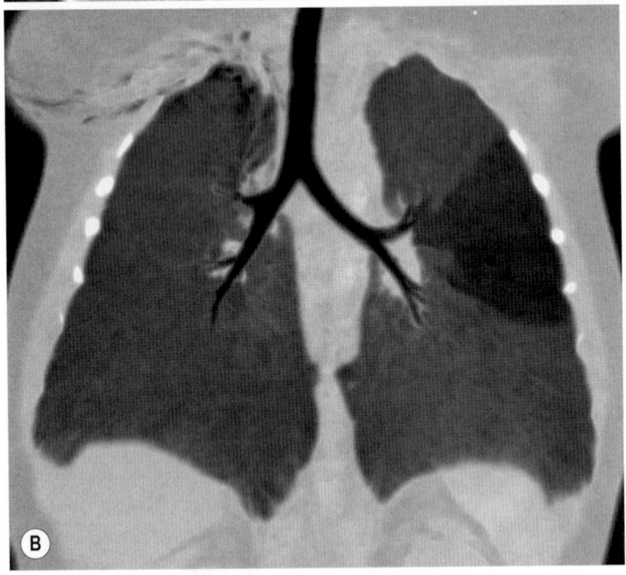

FIGURE 76-41 ■ **Bronchial atresia with mucocele.** (A) Axial CT on lung windows shows segmental hyperlucency in LUL with a soft-tissue density at the left hilum in keeping with an atretic LUL segmental bronchus containing a mucocele. (B) Coronal MinIP confirms the segmental hyperlucency.

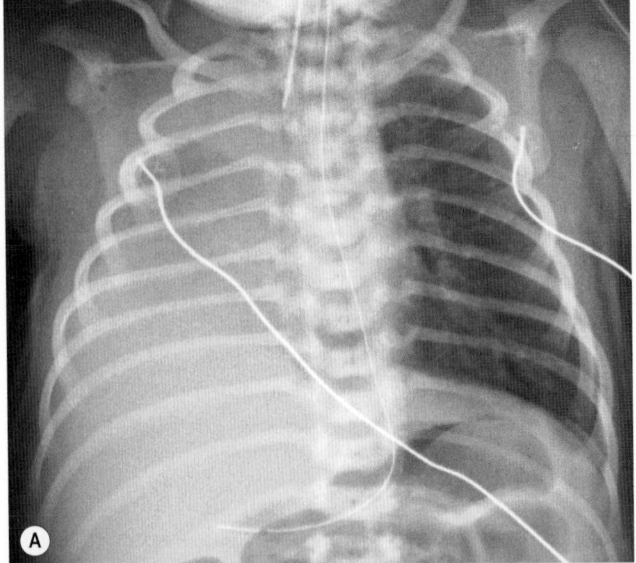

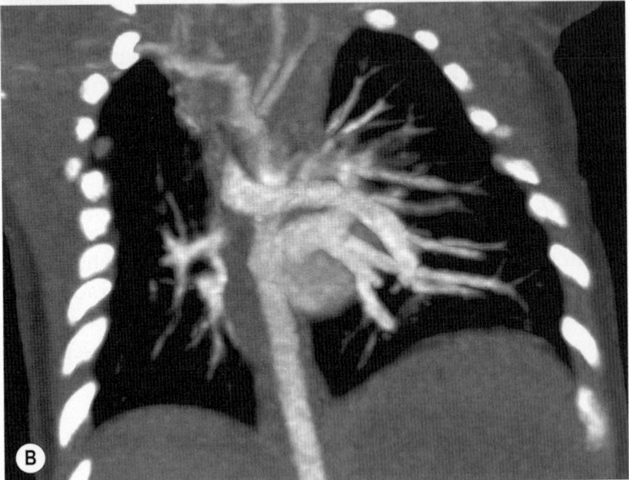

FIGURE 76-42 ■ **Lung hypoplasia.** (A) Right lung hypoplasia in a child with complex congenital cardiac abnormalities. CXR shows complete white-out of the right lung with ipsilateral mediastinal shift. (B) Coronal CT reformat highlights the hypoplastic right pulmonary vein and paucity of pulmonary vessels on the right with a relatively normal left lung.

Pulmonary hypoplasia can also be secondary to lung compression during lung development. The most common intrathoracic cause of hypoplasia is congenital diaphragmatic hernia, but other intrathoracic causes include CPAM and pulmonary sequestration. Extrathoracic causes include severe oligohydramnios secondary to genitourinary anomalies, also known as the Potter sequence, and skeletal dysplasias with a small dysmorphic thoracic cage such as in thanatophoric dysplasia.

Congenital Venolobar Syndrome—Scimitar Syndrome

This is a congenital abnormality comprising lung hypoplasia and ipsilateral anomalous systemic venous drainage. An anomalous pulmonary vein, usually on the right, drains into the inferior vena cava, portal vein, coronary sinus or right atrium. Most patients are asymptomatic but the anomalous venous return constitutes a left-to-right shunt and can lead to pulmonary hypertension.

Radiographic appearances are similar to those of isolated lung hypoplasia. The differential finding is the anomalous (scimitar) vein that may be seen as a tubular shadow, running towards the base of the lung, resembling a curved sword (scimitar), though the vein is not seen in half of the cases on the chest radiograph. CT is the best technique for evaluating the lung, the abnormal vein and to where it drains (Fig. 76-43).

Malignancy

Mediastinal Masses

The mediastinum may be divided into three compartments, anterior, middle and posterior. The most common

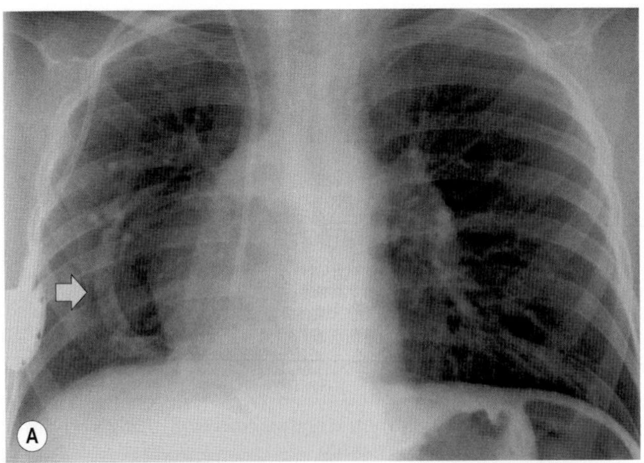

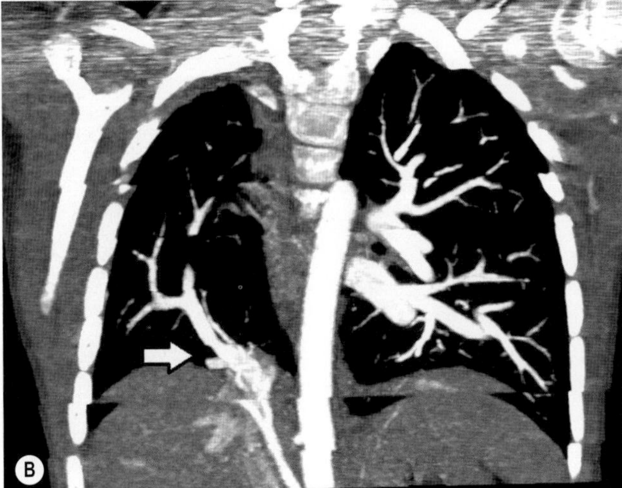

FIGURE 76-43 ■ Congenital venolobar syndrome (scimitar syndrome). (A) CXR showing (1) shift of the heart into the right hemithorax, (2) a small right lung with an abnormal vessel (arrow) paralleling the right heart border and (3) overinflation (compensatory) of left lung. (B) Coronal CT reformat highlights the abnormal 'scimitar vein' (arrow) draining below the diaphragm into the systemic venous system bypassing the pulmonary veins.

anterior mediastinal masses are normal thymus and thymic disorders (abnormalities in thymic size, shape or location), lymphoma or leukaemia (relatively frequent), germ-cell tumours (teratoma, hamartomas, teratocarcinomas, seminomas, dysgerminomas, embryonal cell carcinomas, endodermal sinus tumour, choriocarcinomas) and thymoma. In middle mediastinum, congenital cysts (bronchogenic cyst, duplication, neurenteric cyst) and lymph nodes (infectious and malignant nodes) are usually located. Neurogenic tumours are located in posterior mediastinum (neuroblastomas, ganglioneuromas) (Table 76-5).

The chest radiograph is usually the primary radiologic investigation for a suspected mediastinal mass. US, contrast-enhanced CT or MRI will give further information on the mass itself and its location and anatomical relationships. Bone scintigraphy or PET-CT can be used for staging. Imaging guides the approach for potential biopsy by defining the extent of disease and its relation to major vascular, airway and spinal structures. Involvement of trachea, pericardium, major vessels or spine may necessitate cardiothoracic or neurosurgical input.

Anterior Mediastinum. The most common malignant tumours in children are lymphoma and leukaemia. Abnormal thymic masses appear nodular and lobulated and frequently compress adjacent vascular structures.

Germ-cell tumours are commonly located in the anterior mediastinum (94%). The most common is mature teratoma, with usually well-defined margins, thick walls, some fatty tissue and frequently internal calcification (25%).[58] CT and MRI are superior to US in analysing these anterior mediastinal masses and detecting compression of adjacent structures, tumour extension and invasion of pericardium or pleura.

Middle Mediastinum. The most common mass found in the middle mediastinum is lymphadenopathy, most commonly secondary to infection (TB),[59] but as in the anterior mediastinum, malignancies, in particular, lymphoma and leukaemia, are frequently seen. Other masses encountered in the middle mediastinum are usually congenital, i.e. bronchopulmonary foregut malformations. Middle mediastinal masses, due to their location,

TABLE 76-5 **Mediastinal Masses**

Anterior	Middle	Posterior
Normal thymus	Lymphadenopathy (see Table 76-1)	Neurogenic tumours—neuroblastoma/ ganglioneuroblastoma/ganglioneuroma
Lymphadenopathy (see Table 76-1)	Bronchopulmonary foregut malformations—bronchogenic cyst, oesophageal duplication	Spinal abscess—*Staphylococcus*/TB
Teratoma	Congenital vascular rings	Spinal tumours—PNET/Ewing's
Thymic infiltration—leukaemia/ lymphoma/histiocytosis	Hiatus hernia	Trauma—vertebral haematoma
Thymoma/thymic cyst		Bochdalek hernia
Morgagni hernia		Bronchopulmonary foregut malformations—neurenteric cyst
Cervicomediastinal soft-tissue vascular malformation—lymphangioma/haemangioma		

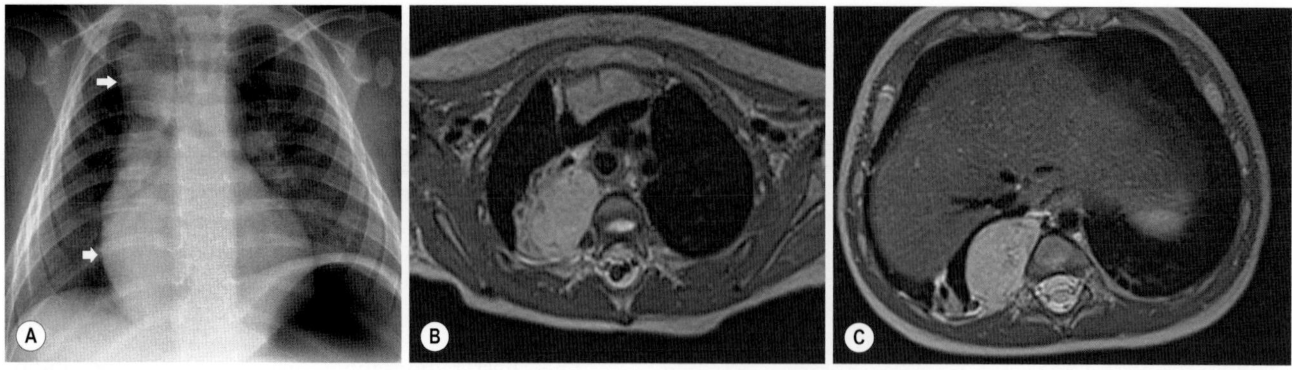

FIGURE 76-44 ■ **Neuroblastoma.** (A) CXR shows two nodular masses in the right posterior mediastinum with mild splaying of the intercostal space at the right 10th and 11th ribs posteriorly. (B, C) Two axial T2-weighted volumetric acquisition MRI studies confirming the presence of the two right-sided thoracic paraspinal masses in keeping with neuroblastoma.

frequently cause airway or oesophageal compression. Contrast-enhanced CT or MRI is the best technique for evaluation.

Posterior Mediastinum. The majority of lesions located in the posterior mediastinum are neurogenic tumours; calcification and extradural spinal extension are commonly demonstrated. Neuroblastoma and ganglioneuroblastoma usually occur in the first decade of life, with the more benign ganglioneuroma seen in older children. Fifteen per cent of neuroblastomas are of a thoracic origin, which is less malignant than a primary abdominal neuroblastoma. They are solid masses which are calcified in up to 40% of cases (Fig. 76-44).

A posterior mediastinal mass is indicated on a chest radiograph, by posterior rib erosion and widening of the intercostal spaces. CT and MRI can both be used for cross-sectional evaluation but MRI is more accurate for detection of extradural mass invasion. Fifty per cent of children with intraspinal extension can be asymptomatic at presentation.[60]

Pulmonary and Endobronchial Tumours

The most common malignant intraparenchymal tumour is pulmonary metastatic disease (Fig. 76-45), usually from an extrapulmonary location, such as Wilms' tumour or osteosarcoma.

In children, particular care and experience with CT imaging techniques are necessary to allow minimisation of the exaggerated dependent atelectasis present, which may mimic or obscure peripheral pulmonary nodules. Prone or decubitus imaging may help to enable detailed scrutiny of problematic cases, helping to aerate lung within the posterobasal segments which may show atelectasis in the conventional (supine) position.

Primary lung malignancies are exceedingly rare in children, with an incidence of approximately 0.05 per 100,000.[61] The most common tumours are pleuropulmonary blastoma, bronchogenic carcinoma and bronchial adenoma.[62]

Pleuropulmonary blastoma usually occurs below 5 years of age. It can be cystic (type I), cystic and solid (type II) and mainly solid (type III).[63] These tumours tend to occur as mixed cystic/solid masses adjacent to the pleura in the lower lobes. They can be confused with the benign lesions, CPAM. Larger lesions often occupy the whole hemithorax and displace mediastinal structures and the contralateral lung.

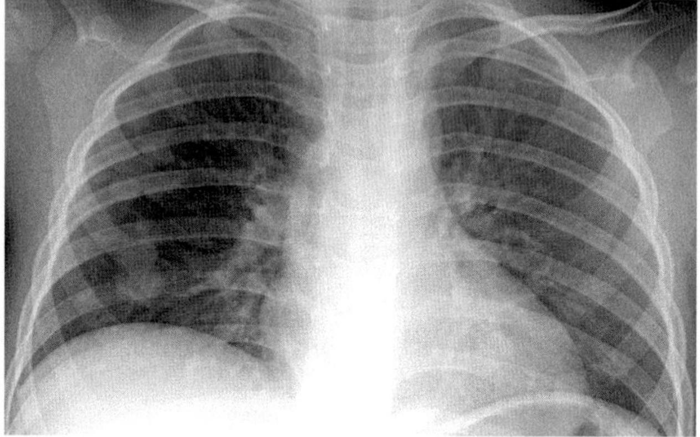

FIGURE 76-45 ■ **Multiple lung metastases.** Child with a primary Wilms' tumour. CXR shows multifocal bilateral soft-tissue density lesions in keeping with metastases.

Bronchogenic carcinoma is very rare in children, representing 17% of primary malignant lung tumours in children. It tends to present in adolescence and is a very aggressive tumour, often with disseminated disease at diagnosis. Radiologically it behaves similarly to the adult tumour.

One-half of all bronchial adenomas, are bronchial carcinoid tumours. Carcinoid syndrome as a cause of Cushing's syndrome (adrenocorticotrophic hormone secretion) is rare in children. Instead, paediatric bronchial carcinoid tumours present with wheezing, lobar collapse or haemoptysis. They usually occur in the central airways, and radiographs may only detect the complications, such as emphysema or collapse. Lung lymphatic metastasis can occur in 5–20% of patients.[64]

Chest Wall Tumours

Chest wall tumours are more frequent than primary lung tumours and they account for 1.8% of all solid tumours in children.[65] The most common are Ewing's sarcoma/primitive neuroectodermal tumours (PNETs), rhabdomyosarcoma and rarely mesothelioma.

PNETs manifest as peripheral chest wall masses, with or without rib destruction and pleural fluid on CXR.[66] Rib destruction is usually the result of a malignant lesion. Rib osteomyelitis, *Aspergillus* or actinomycosis infection can also destroy ribs, but in a different clinical context. US is the first radiological examination in patients where there is complete opacification of the hemithorax, as US can differentiate a solid mass from pleural fluid.

CT or MRI is required for cross-sectional evaluation. CT shows a solid heterogeneous, occasionally calcified mass, lymphadenopathy and pleural fluid. CT is important for determining rib involvement and evaluating the lung parenchyma for metastases. MRI is superior in determining the extent and local invasion of the mass.[67] Bony scintigraphy/PET-CT can be used for detection of distant skeletal metastases.

Rhabdomyosarcoma represents 10% of the solid tumours in paediatrics and it is the most frequent soft-tissue sarcoma in children.[68] Other primary locations of the tumour are more frequent than the thoracic locations. They usually present as a large chest mass with rapid growth. Pleural effusions are relatively uncommon.

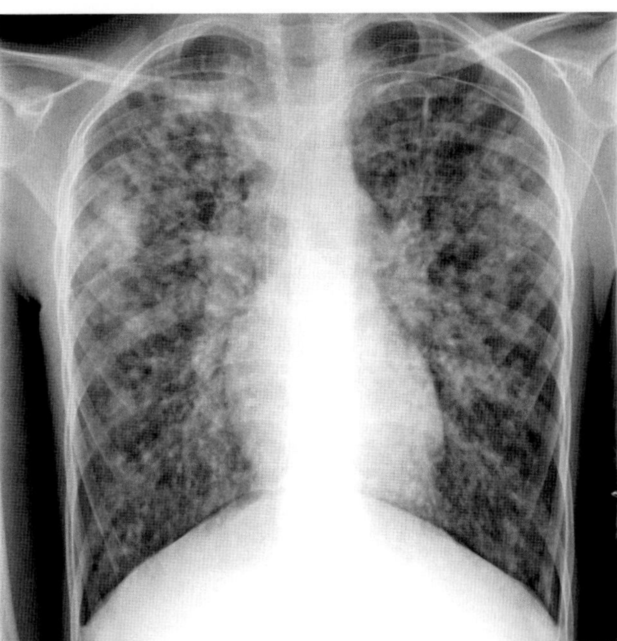

FIGURE 76-46 ■ **Cystic fibrosis.** CXR showing typical features of extensive bilateral bronchial wall thickening in overinflated lungs in a thin patient with advanced bronchiectasis related to CF. There is nodular consolidation in the RUL just above the thickened and elevated (right) horizontal fissure in keeping with an acute infectious exacerbation.

Cystic Fibrosis[69]

Chest radiography is the primary imaging technique and the most widely used diagnostic method for assessing and following progression of cystic fibrosis (CF) lung disease. The current Cystic Fibrosis Trust guidelines recommend annual chest radiographs to assess serial lung parenchymal change in all CF patients.[70]

In children with CF large airways disease, bronchiectasis develops, which is the hallmark feature of established CF. Bronchial wall thickening is universal as the child grows and may precede bronchial dilatation. It is this abnormal wall thickening which allows visualisation of the pathologically thickened airways in the periphery of the lung beyond the level of the segmental bronchi, which are not normally visible.

With further progression of bronchiectasis, large cystic bronchiectatic airways form. Mucoid impaction of the bronchi appears as rounded or band-like opacities of increased density following the course of the dilated bronchi. Lobar and segmental atelectasis may result, most frequently seen in the upper and middle lobes. Interestingly, unlike in the normal host where infection manifests as lobar pneumonia, this pattern is unusual in CF, where patchy nodular areas representing peribronchial consolidation occur (Fig. 76-46).

Immunodeficiency

The immunodeficiency states in children may be subdivided into two major groups: congenital (primary) and acquired (secondary). The spectrum of illness and imaging appearances are similar, regardless of the underlying cause of immunodeficiency. Primary disorders include conditions such as congenital/inherited deficiencies, i.e. SCID (severe combined immunodeficiency). Secondary causes include chemotherapy, bone marrow and solid organ transplantation, and infectious causes such as AIDS. Both primary and secondary immunodeficiency states result in an increased susceptibility to infection, with the respiratory tract being the most common disease site. All immunodeficiency states are also associated with an increased incidence of malignancy, the lymphoproliferative disorders accounting for the majority of tumours.[71]

The low sensitivity of radiographs in detecting incipient pneumonia in these children may promote the use of CT for detection or exclusion of pulmonary infection in an acute clinical deterioration. Multiple agents can cause aggressive infections, in particular fungal (*Aspergillus*, *Candida albicans*, *Pneumocystis jiroveci*) and viral (cytomegalovirus).[72,73]

Human Immunodeficiency Virus (HIV). HIV infection is an important cause of acquired immunodeficiency worldwide. Though it is relatively uncommon in the Western world, in certain groups, particularly those in deprived inner city areas, antenatal testing indicates a prevalence of 1 in 125 to 1 in 200.[74] It is therefore important to be aware of the major complications demonstrated by imaging. Vertical transmission remains the commonest cause of paediatric infection, though the risk is considerably reduced with maternal treatment with antiretroviral therapy. HIV progression is much faster in children than in adults. HIV-associated respiratory disease is the cause of death in 50% of affected children.

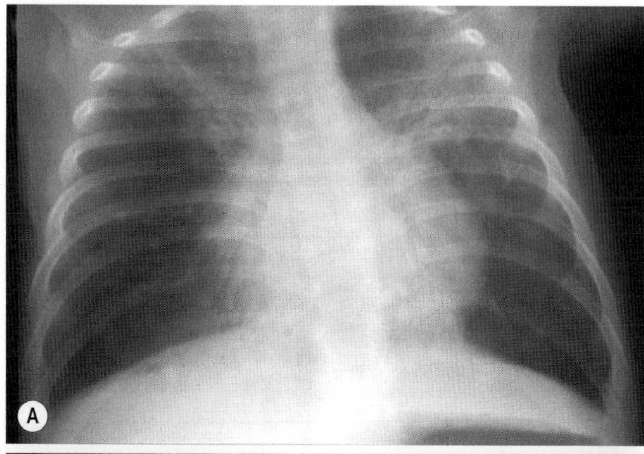

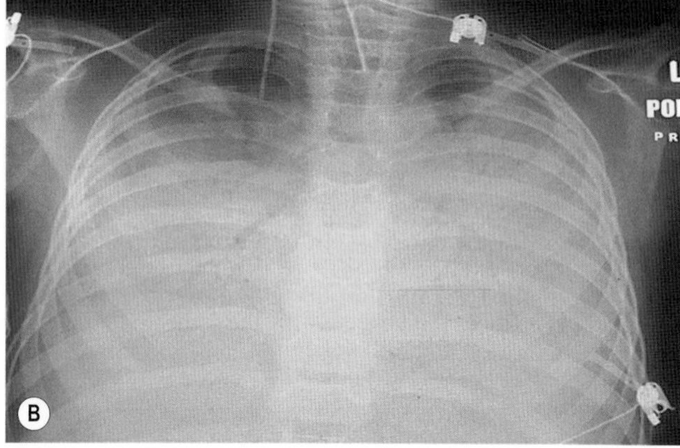

FIGURE 76-47 ■ *Pneumocystis jiroveci (carinii)* pneumonia. (A) CXR shows diffuse perihilar granular shadowing in a non-specific pattern. (B) Severe infection; widespread opacification indicates an ARDS-type pattern.

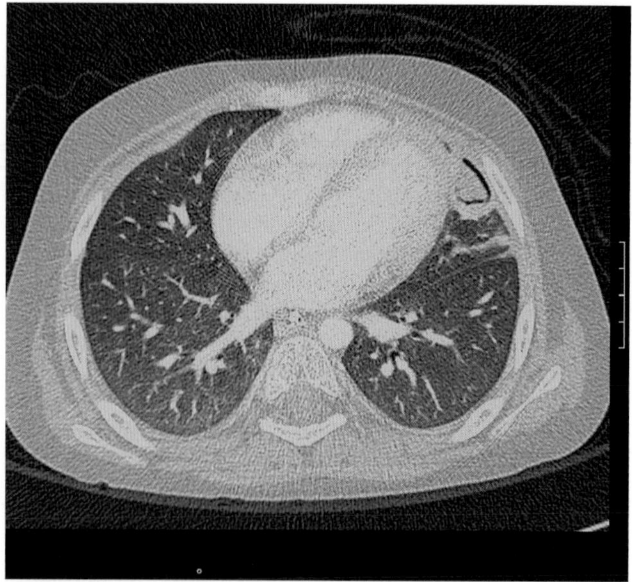

FIGURE 76-48 ■ Air-crescent sign. Axial CT image showing a parenchymal cavity partially filled with a soft-tissue mass and a thin rim of air superiorly.

Infectious Pulmonary Complications of Immunodeficiency

Pneumocystis jiroveci (carinii) Pneumonia. This is an opportunistic infection, common in children with HIV/AIDS, particularly within the first year post-diagnosis. Peak incidence is at 3–6 months of age when the protective effect of transplacental maternal IgG begins to wane.

Classical radiographic appearances include hyperinflation with diffuse bilateral interstitial or nodular infiltrates, which may be subtle initially, progressing rapidly to widespread alveolar shadowing, which may eventually progress to adult respiratory distress syndrome (ARDS) (Fig. 76-47). Following treatment, there may be a significant lag in radiographic resolution compared to the clinical improvement.

Invasive Pulmonary Aspergillosis (IPA). IPA typically manifests as multifocal areas of triangular or nodular parenchymal consolidation caused by haematogenous dissemination of the angioinvasive fungus. Haemorrhagic infarction of the lungs occurs as a result of lung necrosis secondary to vascular obstruction.

Classical radiographic features include either solitary or multiple nodules or masses, with or without cavitation. In some cases, however, the chest radiograph appears normal or may demonstrate a focal infiltrate indistinguishable from a pyogenic pneumonia. Specific HRCT features have been described, probably the most characteristic being a 'halo' of ground-glass attenuation representing perilesional necrosis and haemorrhage, surrounding a central focal fungal nodule or infarct. A second commonly described characteristic feature of IPA is lesional cavitation with the formation of an air crescent (Fig. 76-48). Occasionally IPA may manifest as a necrotising pneumonia with infiltration of local structures or organs. Although these classical features have been described, in many cases, imaging appearances are often non-specific.[75,76]

Non-infectious Pulmonary Complications

Lymphoproliferative Disease (LPD) and Lymphocytic Interstitial Pneumonia (LIP). LPD is the most frequent type of neoplasia in immunodeficiency and may involve the chest, abdomen, CNS and soft tissues. Imaging appearances within the thorax are variable and include focal or diffuse infiltrates, solitary or multiple parenchymal nodules or masses and mediastinal lymphadenopathy, which may be large in volume.[77] LIP is a frequent manifestation of LPD and is characterised by a diffuse interstitial infiltrate of lymphocytes and plasma cells, which may be polyclonal or monoclonal. Radiographic features are variable and include either a predominantly interstitial infiltrate, affecting primarily the perihilar regions and lung bases, or discrete parenchymal nodules and/or patchy ground-glass opacity (Fig. 76-49).[78] Appearances are relatively non-specific and may be indistinguishable from infection with opportunistic organisms.

Diffuse Alveolar Haemorrhage (DAH). DAH occurs in approximately 10% of patients undergoing allogeneic bone marrow transplantation (BMT) and usually occurs at the time of engraftment. DAH is usually associated with other pulmonary complications, particularly (fungal) infection, and is associated with a high mortality.

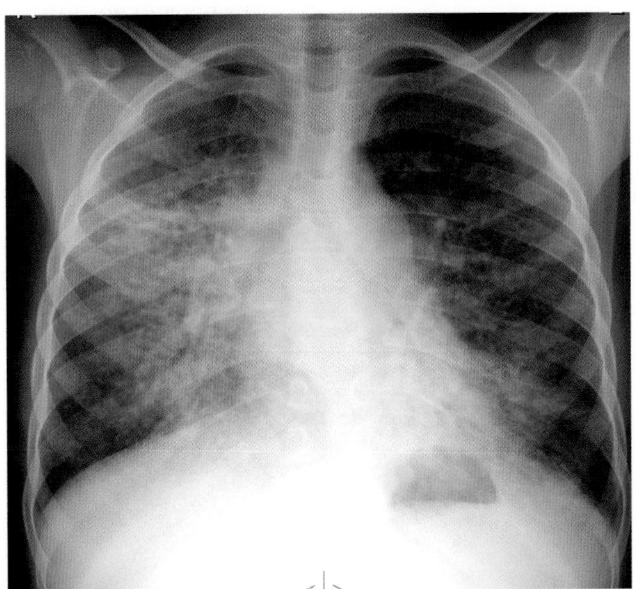

FIGURE 76-49 ■ Lymphocytic interstitial pneumonitis. CXR shows perihilar reticulonodular opacification in a child with known HIV infection. Increased airspace consolidation in the right lower zone indicates an acute infective exacerbation.

Classical radiographic features are those of airspace shadowing, which may be patchy and multifocal or more confluent consolidation with air bronchograms. Cessation of bleeding typically results in rapid clearing over a few days.

Idiopathic Pneumonia Syndrome (IPS). IPS is defined as diffuse lung injury for which no cause has been identified.[79] Both graft-versus-host disease (GVHD) and pre-transplant total body irradiation (TBI) are contributing factors. It usually occurs 6–8 weeks following BMT. Radiographic features are non-specific and variable; they include diffuse airspace shadowing and/or interstitial infiltrates, often with a nodular component. They may be indistinguishable from ARDS.

SUMMARY

In summary chest disease in children is not uncommon. Knowledge of the important categories of disease will help define a diagnostic pathway. Prudent use of chest CT to enable more specific diagnoses may be indicated in selected and complex cases.

For a full list of references, please see ExpertConsult.

FURTHER READING

28. Van Rijn RR, Blickman JG. Differential Diagnosis in Pediatric Imaging. Stuttgart: Thieme; 2011. Chapter 1.

30. Wilmott RW, Boat TF, Bush A, et al. Kendig and Chernick's Disorders of the Respiratory Tract in Children: Expert Consult. 8th ed. New York: Elsevier; 2012. p. 699–735.

55. Castellote A, Enriquez G, Lucaya J. Congenital malformations of the chest beyond the neonatal period. In: Carty H, Brunelle F, Stringer DA, Kao SCS, editors. Imaging Children. Elsevier; 2005. pp. 1049–74.

Hansell DM, Lynch DA, McAdams HP, Bankier AA. Imaging of the Chest. 5th ed. New York: Elsevier; 2010.

Lucaya J, Strife JL. Pediatric Chest Imaging: Chest Imaging in Infants and Children. 2nd ed. Berlin: Springer-Verlag; 2008. pp. 263–87.

Muller NL, Silva CIS. Imaging of the Chest, 2 vols, Expert Radiology series. 1st ed. Philadelphia: Saunders; 2008.

Section 4: Respiratory system in: Coley B. Caffey's Pediatric Diagnostic Imaging. 12th ed. Philadelphia: Saunders; 2013.

CHAPTER 77

Paediatric Abdominal Imaging

Anne Paterson • Øystein E. Olsen • Lil-Sofie Ording Müller

CHAPTER OUTLINE

INTRODUCTION

Paediatric gastrointestinal (GI) radiology is most appropriately thought of according to the age of the patient, and for this reason the chapter has been subdivided into sections; the first details neonatal pathology, the latter relates to older children. The clinical presentation of the conditions remains as before. In this latest edition, newer embryological theories, imaging techniques, management details and updated references have been incorporated. As most children with neonatal GI problems now survive to adolescence or adulthood, data have emerged about adult cohorts and some of the longer-term health problems they face. Information detailing some of these issues has also been included.

THE NEONATE

Visible Abnormalities of the Anterior Abdominal Wall

The ventral wall of the embryo is formed during the fourth week of intrauterine development as the cephalic, caudal and lateral edges of the flat, trilaminar embryonal disc fold in upon themselves and the layers fuse together. The resultant embryo is cylindrical in shape, and protruding centrally from its ventral surface are the remains of the yolk sac connected to the midgut via the omphalomesenteric duct, a structure, which normally regresses in the fifth gestational month.[1,2]

If this complex process is incomplete, then several types of anterior abdominal wall defect may result: ectopia cordis and pentalogy of Cantrell, gastroschisis, bladder and cloacal exstrophy, and omphalocele.

Gastroschisis

In patients with gastroschisis, there is a small defect or split in the ventral abdominal wall, classically to the right side of a normally positioned umbilicus. Gastroschisis typically occurs in the absence of other anomalies and is thought to be due either to a localised intrauterine vascular accident or to asymmetry in the lateral body wall folds with failure of fusion.[1]

The incidence of gastroschisis has increased worldwide over the past two decades and it has been documented to occur in clusters in some geographic regions.[2,3] Mothers under the age of 20 years are at greater risk of having a child with the condition.[4]

Antenatal ultrasound shows bowel loops floating freely in the amniotic fluid, with the diagnosis being possible early in the second trimester. There is no covering membrane. 'Complex gastroschisis' as determined by the presence of intestinal atresia or stenosis, bowel perforation, volvulus or necrosis is found in 10–20% of infants.[3,5,6] Exposure to amniotic fluid causes damage to the bowel; postnatally, this can result in a thick, fibrous 'peel' coating the loops of bowel. Short bowel syndrome, liver disease secondary to intestinal failure and intestinal dysmotility are serious consequences of gastroschisis. Necrotising enterocolitis (NEC) is reported in up to 20% of patients with gastroschisis.[7]

Upper GI contrast studies in infants with repaired gastroschisis will often demonstrate gastro-oesophageal reflux (GOR), malrotation, dilatation of small bowel loops and a markedly prolonged transit time.

Repair of the defect may be possible soon after delivery. If not, the bowel is protected in a silo to prevent fluid loss, and gradually returned to the abdominal cavity.

Omphalocele

An omphalocele (*syn.* exomphalos) is a midline anterior abdominal wall defect through which the solid abdominal viscera and/or bowel may herniate. The extruded abdominal contents are covered in a sac. Larger omphaloceles containing liver tissue may be due to failure of fusion of the lateral body folds. Omphaloceles containing only bowel are thought to arise due to persistence of the physiological herniation of gut after the tenth week of fetal development. The umbilical cord inserts at the tip of the defect. A giant omphalocele is said to be present when the liver is contained within the herniated membranes or when the defect measures more than 5 cm in diameter.[8]

Antenatal ultrasound can detect an omphalocele from the second trimester onwards. The prognosis of the infant is dependent upon associated anomalies. Chromosomal and structural abnormalities are seen in more than 50% of patients.[3] The Beckwith–Wiedemann syndrome has an omphalocele (exomphalos), macroglossia and gigantism as its primary components (the 'EMG' syndrome).

The method of surgical closure of the defect is in part driven by its size. Immediate closure, staged procedures or delayed repair following epithelialisation are all surgical possibities.

Bladder Exstrophy—Epispadias—Cloacal Exstrophy Complex

The terminology of this spectrum of complex disorders is confusing, with many texts using the term OEIS complex (omphalocele, exstrophy, imperforate anus and spinal abnormality) and cloacal exstrophy, interchangeably. In reality, they probably represent different entities of the same spectrum. The epispadias–exstrophy spectrum is rare and complex, extending from epispadias, where males have a urethral meatus opening on the dorsum of the penis, and affected females a cleft urethra, to bladder exstrophy, where the bladder is exposed on the lower abdominal wall and drips urine constantly.

At the far end of the spectrum is cloacal exstrophy, one of the most severe congenital anomalies compatible with life, and which encompasses abnormalities of the genitourinary (GU) and GI tracts, the central nervous and musculoskeletal systems. This condition is thought to arise due to abnormal development of the cloacal membrane[9] and its premature rupture prior to the fifth week of gestation.[10] The cloaca opens onto the lower abdominal wall, where it is seen as an open caecum and prolapsing terminal ileum between two hemibladders. There is an omphalocele of varying size and a blind-ending short gut. The external genitalia are ambiguous. Bilateral inguinal herniae are common to both sexes. There is spinal dysraphism and there is an 'open book' pelvis.[11] Associated renal and lower limb anomalies (club foot and reduction defects) are well described.[9]

Antenatally, the 'elephant's trunk' sign of the prolapsed terminal ileum is said to be pathognomonic for the condition on ultrasound.[9] Non-visualisation of the bladder in association with an omphalocele and myelomeningocele would also be strong predictors of cloacal exstrophy.

Early postnatal imaging includes the extensive use of ultrasound to evaluate the spine and brain, the GU tract and the hips. CT with 3D-VR images is helpful in planning pelvic surgery.[11] Upper GI contrast studies document GI tract anatomy. Magnetic resonance imaging (MRI) of both the pelvis—assessing the genital tract and pelvic floor—and the spine are also required.

Surgery in the immediate postnatal period includes diversion of the faecal stream and colostomy formation, bladder closure ± vesicostomy fashioning, omphalocele reduction and repair, and closure of any open neural tube defects. Genital tract surgeries are often postponed until later in childhood.

Respiratory Distress and Choking

The neonate with disease affecting the proximal GI tract often presents with respiratory symptoms. These symptoms include excess salivation, choking with feeds, coughing, cyanosis and respiratory distress. Conditions that present in this way include oesophageal atresia (OA) with or without tracheo-oesophageal fistula (TOF), laryngeal clefts, swallowing disorders, diaphragmatic hernias, vascular rings and GOR; the latter is by far the most common. The chest radiograph may show airspace disease and atelectasis, should aspiration have already occurred.

Oesophageal Atresia and Tracheo-Oesophageal Fistula

OA with or without a fistulous connection to the trachea is one of the more common congenital anomalies of the GI tract. It is caused by abnormal partitioning of the foregut into separate respiratory (ventral) and GI (dorsal) components early on in the first trimester of fetal life. Five different major anomalies result (Fig. 77-1). The atretic segment of the oesophagus tends to be at the junction of its proximal and middle thirds. Occasionally an isolated TOF occurs without OA; this is the H-type fistula.

Half of all children with OA and TOF have associated congenital anomalies. Features of the VACTERL spectrum (*v*ertebral anomalies, *a*norectal malformation, *c*ardiovascular malformation, *t*racheo-o*e*sophageal fistula with oesophageal atresia, *r*enal anomalies and *l*imb defects) are especially common, with other GI malformations—notably duodenal atresia, small bowel malrotation and volvulus and a more distal congenital oesophageal stenosis often reported.[12]

OA is usually suspected on an antenatal ultrasound. The cardinal findings of maternal polyhydramnios and an absent stomach bubble have a positive predictive value of 50%.[13] A false-negative exam may be as a result of fluid passing via a lower pouch fistula into the stomach. However, OA can be diagnosed with greater certainty by visualising the dilated, blind-ending upper oesophageal pouch and the use of cine-mode fetal MRI.[13,14]

The remaining group of infants present almost immediately in the postnatal period with choking, coughing, cyanosis and drooling, symptoms which are exacerbated during attempts to feed the infant. Patients with an H-type fistula are usually symptomatic from birth.

Postnatally, the diagnosis is usually made on a chest radiograph, which shows an orogastric tube curled in the proximal oesophageal pouch (Fig. 77-2). The lungs may show features of an aspiration pneumonitis. The presence of gas in the abdomen implies a distal fistula. A gasless abdomen is seen with isolated OA or rarely OA with a proximal fistula.

In those infants in whom a primary repair is not possible, the gap between the proximal and distal

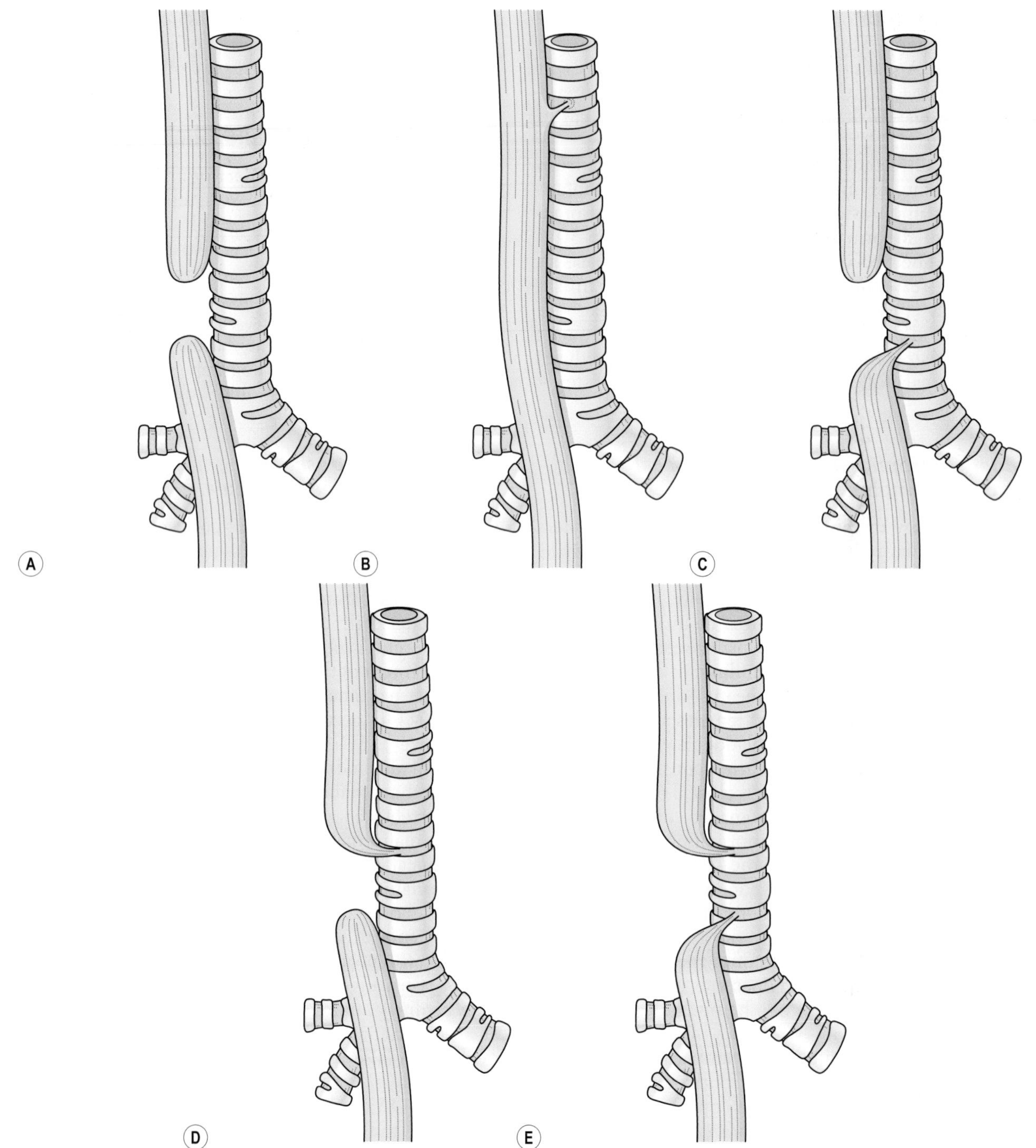

FIGURE 77-1 ■ Oesophageal atresia and tracheo-oesophageal fistula. Diagrammatic representation of (A) isolated OA (9%), (B) H-type fistula (6%), (C) OA with distal TOF (82%), (D) OA with proximal TOF (1%) and (E) OA with TOF from both proximal and distal oesophageal remnants (2%).

oesophageal pouches can be assessed following the formation of a feeding gastrostomy. Under fluoroscopic guidance, a Hegar dilator is inserted though the gastrostomy and passed retrogradely into the distal oesophagus. A Replogle tube is simultaneously used to delineate the superior pouch. As both tubes are radiopaque, the degree of separation between the pouches is easily visualised. Thoracic CT imaging, following simultaneous injection of air into the upper pouch, via the indwelling Replogle tube, and also via the gastrostomy, can alternatively be used.[15,16]

The standard, long-established diagnostic technique for an H-type fistula in most institutions remains the 'withdrawal oesophagram', obtained with the infant in the prone position, with a horizontal X-ray beam (or a steep oblique position with a vertical X-ray beam). The contrast is injected under pressure, via a nasogastric tube (NGT) with its tip in the distal oesophagus, as the tube

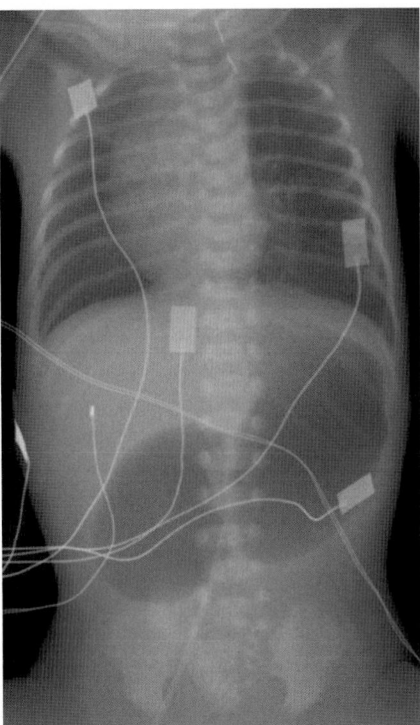

FIGURE 77-2 ■ Oesophageal atresia with distal pouch tracheo-oesophageal fistula and duodenal atresia. Supine chest and abdominal radiograph shows a Replogle tube in the proximal oesophageal pouch, with gas outlining the classical 'double bubble' of duodenal atresia in the abdomen.

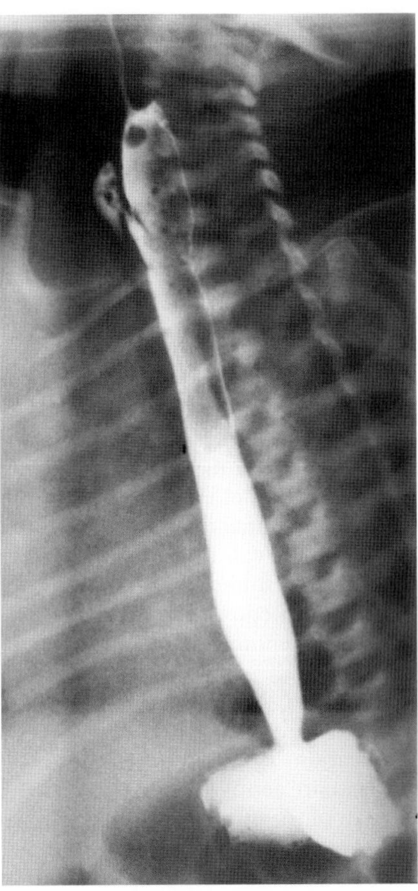

FIGURE 77-3 ■ H-type TOF. Upper GI contrast study shows the fistula running obliquely at the level of the thoracic inlet.

is gradually pulled back under fluoroscopic guidance (Fig. 77-3). Care must be taken not to spill barium via the vocal cords into the trachea, or water-soluble contrast medium can be used. Combined bronchoscopy and oesophagoscopy should be performed if there is a high clinical index of suspicion with negative imaging.

A positive contrast medium injection to outline the proximal oesophageal pouch is rarely necessary, but occasionally required to exclude a proximal pouch fistula. Small quantities (1–2 mL) of isotonic, non-ionic contrast medium should be used under fluoroscopic guidance. A proximal fistula can also be demonstrated if air is injected into the Replogle tube during a multidetector CT (MDCT) imaging.[17]

Given the frequent combination of OA/TOF with VACTERL components, a preoperative work-up should involve assessment of the cardiovascular system and GU tract.

Early Post-Surgical Radiology. The immediate complications following OA and TOF repair are recurrence of the TOF, which occurs in up to 10% of patients, and anastomotic breakdown in a further 10–20% of patients. Major leaks will present early with a tension pneumothorax and require repeat surgery.[18] Presentation of a recurrent fistula may be delayed for months after surgery, and the child can suffer recurrent aspiration pneumonitis and pneumonia. A transanastomotic feeding tube is positioned by most surgeons, who will request a postoperative oesophagram (water-soluble contrast media) prior to the recommencement of enteral feeds.

Anastomotic strictures develop in up to 80% of patients,[19] and are more likely in long gap OA, and in those who have marked postoperative GOR. Oesophageal strictures can easily, safely and repeatedly be treated by balloon catheter dilatation using fluoroscopic guidance.

Longer-Term Problems. As many of the early repair cohorts are now in adulthood, data have emerged regarding the long-term problems patients face following OA/TOF surgery.

Dysphagia of varying degrees is experienced in up to 60%; this can be severe enough to cause food impaction.[19] Almost half of patients report GOR or regurgitation. Biopsy-proven Barrett's oesophagus has been reported in patients' following OA repair.[19]

Respiratory problems lasting into adulthood are common. These are generally mild, but include wheezing and reactive airways disease in 25%, choking sensations in 10% and recurrent infections in up to 30%.[20,21]

Non-bilious Vomiting

Vomiting is a common problem in children of all ages and its presence as a symptom does not necessarily indicate GI disease. Vomiting is common with infections in any body system, in metabolic disease, disorders of the central nervous system, and as a side effect of drugs and poisons. Neonatal non-bilious vomiting due to GI causes implies a lesion proximal to the ampulla of Vater, and is most frequently due to GOR. A full clinical history and physical examination are the most important factors in determining what imaging investigations (if any) are required.

Obstruction of the Stomach

Congenital gastric obstruction is rare. It is usually due to a web or diaphragm in the antrum or pylorus. Occasionally a true atresia is present, with a fibrous cord uniting the two blind ends. Pyloric atresia is associated with epidermolysis bullosa simplex.[22] The diagnosis may be suspected antenatally due to maternal polyhydramnios and a large fetal gastric bubble. Postnatally, non-bilious vomiting and upper abdominal distension are found.

A plain radiograph will show a dilated stomach with no distal air. At ultrasound, webs appear as persistent, linear, echogenic structures arising from the antral or pyloric walls and extending centrally.

Enteric Duplication Cysts

Enteric duplication cysts are uncommon congenital anomalies of obscure aetiology. They can occur anywhere along the length of the gut but are most frequently found in the ileum. Gastric duplications account for less than 5% of cases,[23,24] and are usually found on the greater curve. When located in the antropyloric region they may cause gastric outlet obstruction and present in the neonatal period with non-bilious vomiting and a palpable mass. Confirmation of the diagnosis is by ultrasound. The cysts have a layered wall, with an inner echogenic layer corresponding to the mucosa/submucosa and an outer hypoechoic layer that represents a smooth muscle layer (Fig. 77-4). This appearance is referred to as the 'gut signature'. The contents of the cyst are usually hypoechoic, but debris is seen if there has been haemorrhage or infection has developed. Gastric mucosa takes up ^{99m}Tc-pertechnetate, which is helpful to identify the cysts when children present with GI bleeding (see the section 'Enteric Duplication Cysts' under 'Abdominal Distension').

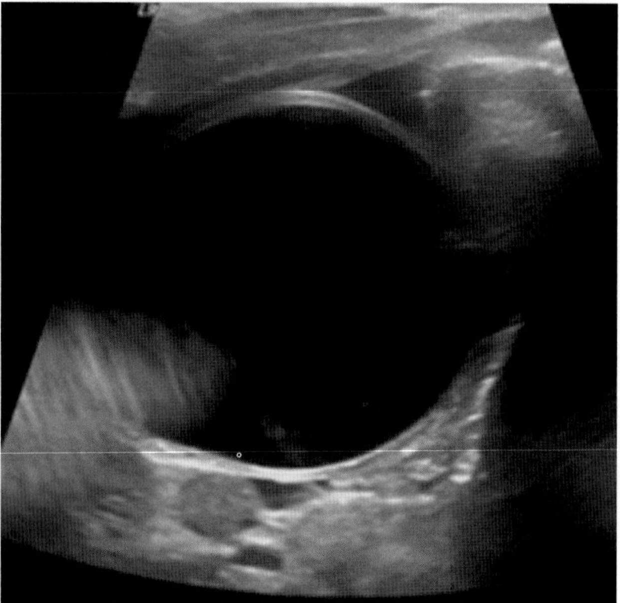

FIGURE 77-4 ■ Ileal duplication cyst. Sonogram showing echogenic mucosal layer and hypoechoic outer muscular layer.

Microgastria

This is a rare abnormality characterised by a small, tubular, midline stomach, severe GOR and a mega-oesophagus. The patients present with recurrent vomiting, failure to thrive, signs of malnutrition and recurrent episodes of aspiration pneumonia. Associated anomalies are found in nearly all cases, and include components of the VACTERL sequence, small bowel malrotation, upper limb reduction defects and asplenia. An upper GI contrast study confirms the diagnosis.

Gastric Perforation

Gastric perforation is uncommon but accounts for a significant proportion of cases of neonatal pneumoperitoneum, and is a life-threatening condition. The underlying cause is unclear, but the rate of enteral feed introduction, ischaemia and increased mechanical pressure have been suggested.[25,26] Iatrogenic gastric perforation is recognised after insertion of orogastric tubes. A massive pneumoperitoneum is seen on a plain radiograph of the abdomen.

Bilious Vomiting

Bilious vomiting in the neonate may be the presenting feature of many different conditions. Sepsis, metabolic upset and gastroenteritis are examples requiring 'medical management', whereas, from a surgical perspective, bilious emesis indicates bowel obstruction distal to the ampulla of Vater. The most urgent of all emergencies in a neonate with bilious vomiting is small bowel malrotation complicated by volvulus.

A plain abdominal radiograph alone will not distinguish between the plethora of underlying conditions causing bilious vomiting. However, a complete high intestinal obstruction (mid-ileal level and above), denoted by a few dilated bowel loops only, requires operative intervention irrespective of the cause, and no further imaging is necessary. If there is a low intestinal obstruction (distal ileum and beyond), as demonstrated by the presence of multiple dilated bowel loops on the plain radiograph, a single-contrast enema will generally be performed prior to any definitive treatment.

Small Bowel Malrotation and Volvulus

Malrotation is a generic term used to describe any variation in the normal position of the intestines. In itself, it is not necessarily symptomatic, but the resultant abnormal position of the duodenojejunal flexure (DJF) ± caecum, mean these two organs lie closer together, shortening the base of the small bowel mesentery (Fig. 77-5). The midgut has a propensity to twist around this

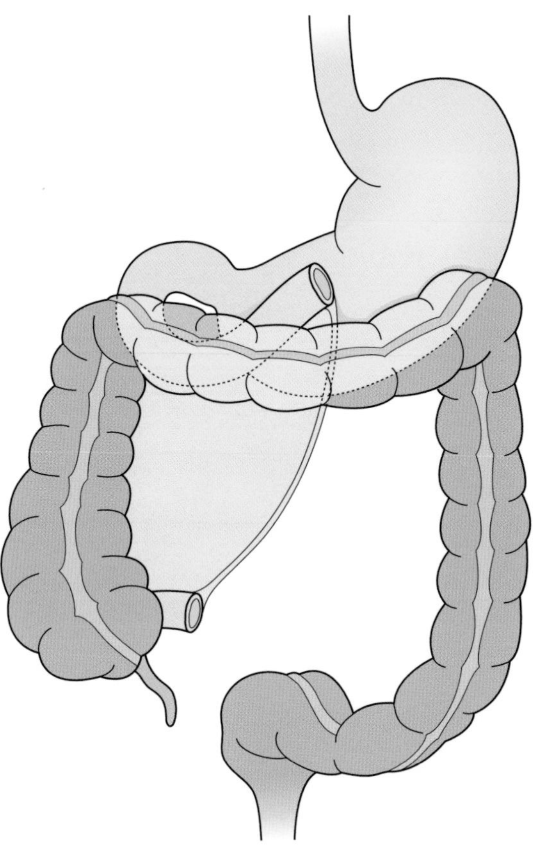

FIGURE 77-5 ■ The base of the normal small bowel mesentery. Diagramatic representation demonstrating the normal small bowel mesentery, which runs from the level of the duodenojejunal flexure (DJF) to the ileocaecal valve.

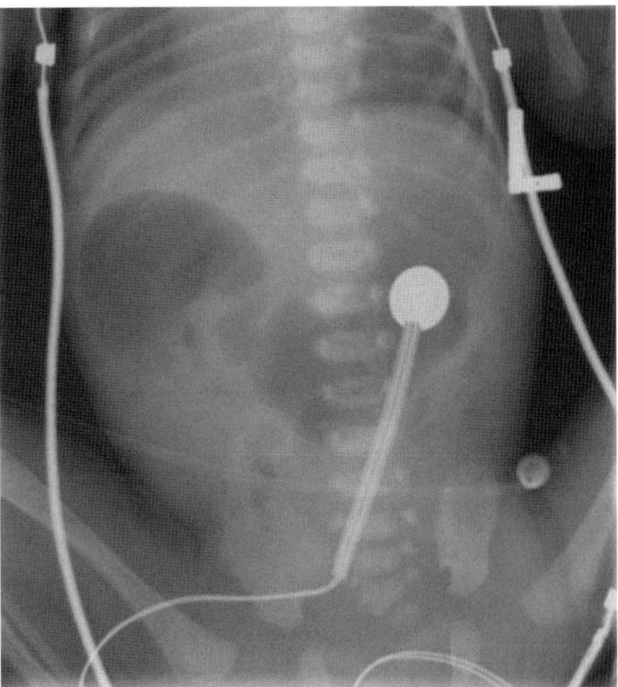

FIGURE 77-6 ■ Surgically proven small bowel malrotation and volvulus. Abdominal radiograph with appearances mimicking the double bubble of duodenal atresia.

narrowed pedicle (volvulus), compromising the arterial inflow and venous drainage of the superior mesenteric vessels, which can lead to ischaemic necrosis of the small bowel. Untreated small bowel volvulus has a high mortality rate.

In fetal life, the gut begins as a straight, midline tube, which, as it elongates and develops, herniates into the base of the umbilical cord. Traditional embryological teaching is based upon the theory that between the sixth and tenth weeks of fetal development, the midgut loop undergoes a complex three-stage anticlockwise rotation process centred around the axis of the superior mesenteric artery (SMA). This is said to explain the position of the DJF in the left upper, and the ileocaecal junction in the right lower quadrants of the abdomen. The mesentery of the small bowel extends between these two fixed points, giving it a broad base. More recent work by Metzger et al.[27] proposes that the anatomical position of the gut relies critically upon localised growth and lengthening of the duodenal loop, which pushes it beneath the mesenteric root.

Should the embryological development of the bowel be interrupted, then a variety of abnormal gut positions can occur; infants with congenital diaphragmatic herniae, gastroschisis and omphalocele by definition all have malrotated, malfixated bowel, although volvulus in these patients is rare after repair of the primary abnormality.[28] In general, small bowel malrotation is an isolated abnormality, though it has been reported in association with pyloric stenosis, duodenal stenosis, web and atresia, preduodenal portal vein, annular pancreas and jejuno-ileal atresias. The heterotaxy syndromes, Hirschsprung's disease and megacystis–microcolon–intestinal hypoperistalsis syndrome are also associated with malrotation and volvulus, as are cloacal exstrophy, prune-belly syndrome and intestinal neuronal dysplasia.

Symptomatic babies with malrotation commonly present within the first month of life, with bilious vomiting. Older children may present with non-specific symptoms of chronic or intermittent abdominal pain, emesis, diarrhoea or failure to thrive. Volvulus, though less common in the older child, still occurs. It is important to suspect malrotation and volvulus in a child of *any* age with bilious vomiting, and to investigate accordingly in an emergent fashion.

There are no specific plain radiographic findings in malrotation, even with volvulus. The radiograph may be completely normal if the volvulus is intermittent or if there is incomplete duodenal obstruction, due to a loose twisting of the bowel. If the volvulus is tight, then complete duodenal obstruction results, with gaseous distension of the stomach and proximal duodenum. The classical picture is of a partial duodenal obstruction, with distension of the stomach and proximal duodenum, with some distal gas (Fig. 77-6).

A pattern of distal small bowel obstruction is seen in a closed loop obstruction and represents a more ominous finding; the small bowel loops may be thick-walled and oedematous, with pneumatosis being evident. These findings represent small bowel necrosis. A gasless abdomen is seen if vomiting has been prolonged, and in both closed loop obstruction with viable small bowel or massive midgut necrosis. In the neonate with bilious vomiting and a complete duodenal obstruction or a seriously ill child with obvious signs of peritonism, radiographic examination should cease after the plain radiograph; and urgent surgery is indicated. In all other children with bilious vomiting and incomplete bowel obstruction, further investigation—usually in the form of an upper GI contrast study—is required. This examination is best performed with barium (single-contrast study).

The intestines in malrotation are malpositioned and the purpose of the upper GI study is to locate the position of the DJF. Meticulous radiological technique is required, and care must be taken not to overfill the stomach with contrast medium, as this can obscure the position of the DJF directly or secondarily by duodenal 'flooding' following rapid emptying of the stomach. The operator should aim to carefully define the position of the DJF on the first pass of contrast medium through the duodenum.

On a supine radiograph, the normal DJF lies to the left of the left-sided vertebral pedicles at the height of the duodenal bulb (Fig. 77-7A). When malrotation is present, the DJF is usually displaced inferiorly and to the right side (Fig. 77-7B). It is important to remember that the DJF can be displaced temporarily by a distended colon or stomach, an enlarged spleen, an indwelling nasoenteric tube or manual palpation.

The 'corkscrew' pattern of the duodenum and jejunum spiralling around the mesenteric vessels is pathognomonic for midgut volvulus on the upper GI study, the calibre of the bowel decreasing distal to the point of partial obstruction (Fig. 77-8). If there is an abrupt cut-off to the flow of contrast in the third part of the duodenum, volvulus cannot be excluded with certainty and these infants too must proceed directly to surgery.

Malfixation of the intestines invariably accompanies malrotation in an attempt to fix the gut in place. Peritoneal (Ladd's) bands stretch from the (sometimes high-lying) caecum and right colon, across the duodenum to the right upper quadrant and retroperitoneum. The Ladd's bands themselves can cause duodenal obstruction.

Ultrasound may demonstrate the dilated, fluid-filled stomach and proximal duodenum when obstruction is present. The relationship of the superior mesenteric vein (SMV) to the superior mesenteric artery (SMA) is abnormal in about two-thirds of patients with malrotation, when the vein lies ventral or to the left of the artery, a finding that is neither sensitive nor specific for malrotation. Ultrasound has also been proposed to confirm the (normal) retromesenteric position of the third part of the duodenum, and has been advocated as a screening tool in neonatal populations.[29] A volvulus may be demonstrated with ultrasound as the 'whirlpool sign'; colour Doppler studies show the SMV spiralling clockwise around the SMA.

Management

The standard operation for small bowel malrotation and volvulus is Ladd's procedure, whereby the bowel is exposed, untwisted and inspected. Any Ladd's bands are divided, and the base of the mesentery is widened. Finally, the bowel is returned to the abdomen, with the duodenum and jejunum to the right side, and the colon to the left; and a prophylactic appendicectomy is often performed.

In those patients with small bowel malrotation diagnosed incidentally on an upper GI contrast study performed for another indication, management is less certain. Many paediatric surgeons will opt to perform an elective Ladd's procedure.

It is important that radiologists understand that a Ladd's procedure does not result in a normal anatomical

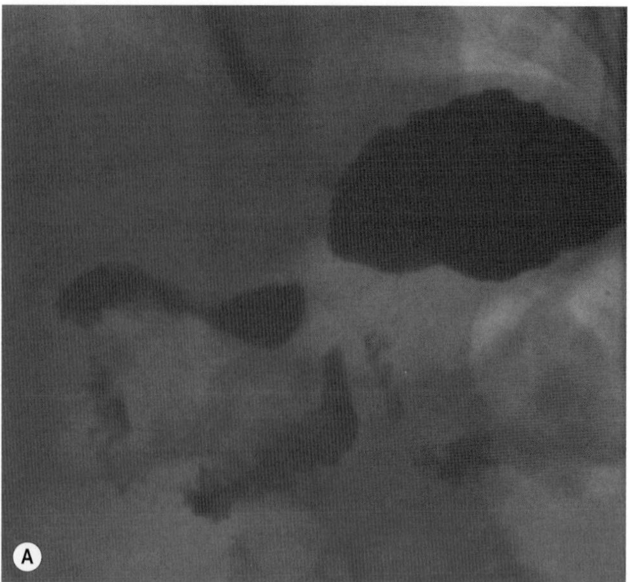

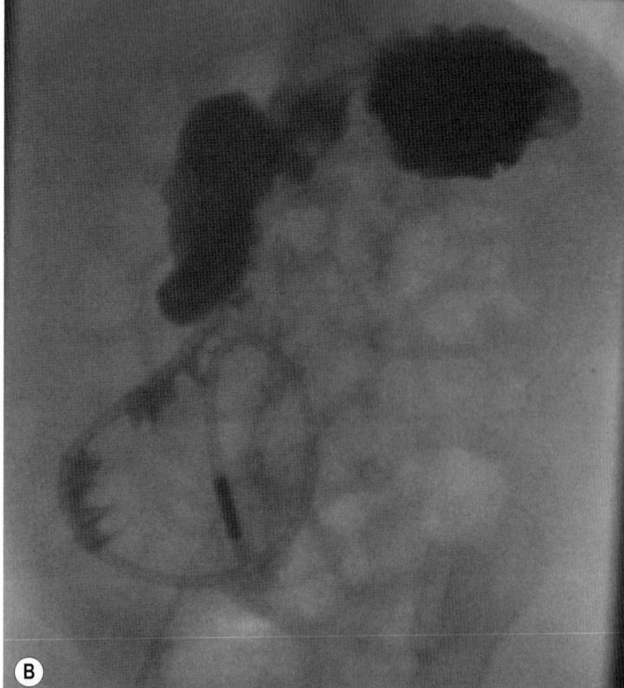

FIGURE 77-7 ■ Demonstration of (A) a normally sited duodenojejunal flexure and (B) a duodenojejunal flexure that is low lying and to the right of the expected position—as shown by the most distal curl of the feeding tube.

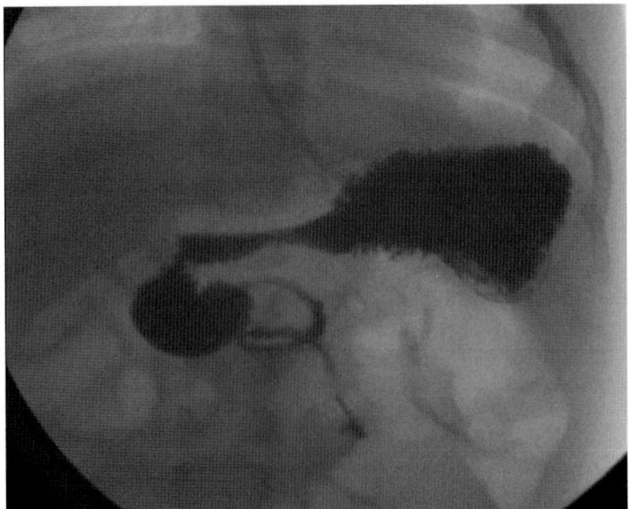

FIGURE 77-8 ■ **Small bowel malrotation and volvulus.** Upper GI contrast study demonstrates the classical 'corkscrew' pattern of the duodenum and jejunum spiralling around the mesenteric vessels. Note the change in bowel calibre at the level of the duodenojejunal flexure.

position of the bowel; the DJF will always be malpositioned in these patients and recurrent volvulus can occur if the mesenteric base is not sufficiently widened at the time of the first surgery.

Duodenal Atresia and Stenosis

Duodenal atresia (DA) is much more common than duodenal stenosis, and both are caused by failure of recanalisation of the duodenal lumen after the sixth week of fetal life. Duodenal obstruction may also be caused by webs or diaphragms. Extrinsic duodenal compression by an annular pancreas or preduodenal portal vein may contribute to the obstruction in some patients. Regardless of the cause, in 80% of cases, the level of the obstruction is just distal to the ampulla of Vater.

Associated anomalies are present in the majority of patients with DA or stenosis. Down's syndrome is present in 30% of patients and congenital heart disease in 20%. Malrotation is present in 20–30% of patients and can only be diagnosed prior to surgery if the duodenal obstruction is partial. Components of the VACTERL association may also be present, with OA coexisting in up to 10% of infants.

DA may be diagnosed antenatally when the dilated stomach and duodenal cap are seen. Fetal growth retardation, maternal polyhydramnios and consequent prematurity are common. Infants otherwise present early in the postnatal period with bilious vomiting and upper abdominal distension. Non-bilious vomiting occurs in those infants with a preampullary obstruction.

Radiographs show a gas-filled 'double bubble' of the stomach and duodenal cap (Fig. 77-9). If the obstruction is partial or in the rare cases of a bifid common bile duct straddling the atretic segment, then distal gas will be present.

In an upper GI study, duodenal stenosis is seen as a narrowed area in the second part of the duodenum, A duodenal web may be seen as a thin, filling defect extending across the duodenal lumen. Ultrasound can also be used to make the diagnosis, the examination made easier if the infant is first given clear fluids orally.

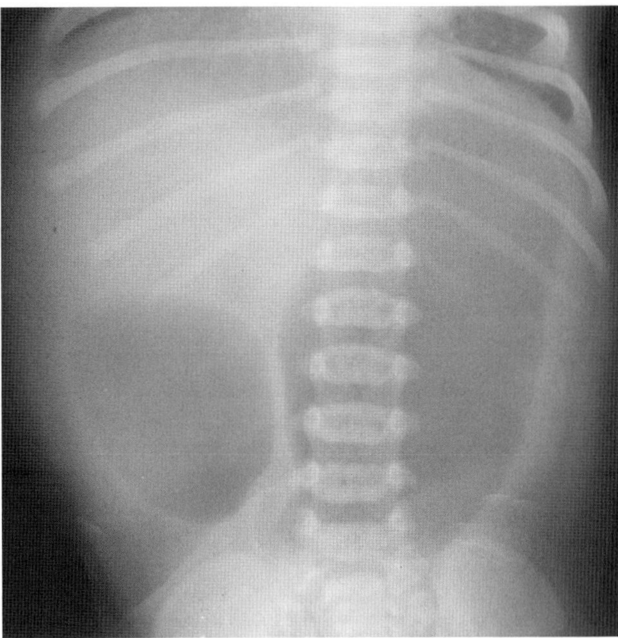

FIGURE 77-9 ■ **Duodenal atresia.** Supine radiograph shows the classical 'double bubble' appearance.

The treatment of both complete and incomplete duodenal obstruction is surgical.

Small Bowel Atresia and Stenosis

Jejunal and ileal atresias have a common aetiology and are thought to be due to an intrauterine vascular accident. The vascular insult may be a primary or secondary event (for example due to antenatal volvulus or intussusception). Jejunoileal atresias have an increased incidence in patients with gastroschisis and meconium ileus.

The 'apple peel' syndrome is thought to follow intrauterine occlusion of the distal SMA. There is a proximal jejunal atresia, with agenesis of the mesentery and absence of the mid-small bowel. The distal ileum spirals around its narrow vascular pedicle, an appearance which gives the syndrome its name. A malrotated microcolon is also usually present. A second, more complex type of intestinal atresia is the syndrome of multiple intestinal atresias with intraluminal calcifications.[30]

The majority of infants with a small bowel atresia present with bilious vomiting in the immediate postnatal period. With more distal atresias, abdominal distension and failure to pass meconium are more commonly recognised clinical features.

On the plain radiograph, there are dilated loops of small bowel down to the level of the atresia. The loop of bowel immediately proximal to the atresia may be disproportionately dilated and have a bulbous contour. A meconium peritonitis with calcification of the peritoneum will be present if an intrauterine perforation has occurred.

Management is surgical, with bowel resection and primary anastomosis if possible. In infants with multiple atresias, the surgeon aims to preserve as much of the bowel length as is feasible.

Abdominal Distension

Abdominal distension in the neonate may be due to mechanical or functional bowel obstruction, an abdominal mass lesion (Table 77-1), ascites or a pneumoperitoneum. A supine abdominal radiograph will show the distribution and calibre of the bowel loops, intra-abdominal calcifications (Table 77-2), the presence of pneumatosis or portal venous gas, any soft-tissue masses and a pneumoperitoneum.

Ultrasound will identify free fluid or the presence of a mass lesion, and is able to confirm the origin of the latter. The majority of neonatal abdominal masses are benign and arise in relation to the GU tract or are of hepatobiliary in origin.

TABLE 77-1 Causes of a Neonatal Intra-abdominal Mass Lesion

- Complicated meconium ileus
- Dilated bowel proximal to an obstruction
- Mesenteric or duplication cyst
- Abscess
- GU causes
  - Hydronephrosis
  - Renal cystic disease
  - Mesoblastic nephroma
  - Wilms' tumour
  - Adrenal haemorrhage
  - Neuroblastoma
  - Retroperitoneal teratoma
  - Ovarian cyst
  - Hydrometrocolpos
- Haemangioendothelioma
- Hepatoblastoma
- Choledochal, hepatic or splenic cysts

TABLE 77-2 Causes of Intra-abdominal Calcifications

- Complicated meconium ileus
- Intraluminal calcifications
  - Low obstruction
  - Anorectal malformations with a fistula to the urinary tract
- Adrenal
  - Haemorrhage
  - Neuroblastoma
  - Wolman's disease
- Hepatobiliary
  - Haemangioendothelioma
  - Hepatoblastoma
  - TORCH infections
- Duplication and mesenteric cysts
- Nephrocalcinosis
- Intravascular thrombus
- Teratomas

Necrotising Enterocolitis (NEC)

NEC is the term used to describe the (often severe) enterocolitis that primarily affects premature infants. The precise aetiology of the condition remains unknown, but a complex interaction of immaturity of the gut mucosa and immune response, impaired gut motility, colonisation of the bowel by pathogenic bacteria and intestinal ischaemia/hypoxia are all in part responsible.[31] There is an inverse relationship between birth weight and gestational age and the development of NEC. The condition is also seen in term infants, particularly those with intrauterine growth retardation, peripartum asphyxia, cyanotic congenital heart disease and gastroschisis.

NEC usually presents in the second week of life, following the commencement of enteral feeds. Initially superficial, the inflammatory process in NEC can extend to become transmural. Diffuse or discrete involvement of the bowel can occur, with the most commonly affected sites being the terminal ileum and colon. The clinical symptoms and signs are non-specific to begin with and include feeding intolerance, lethargy, hypoglycaemia, temperature instability, bradycardia, oxygen desaturation, increased gastric aspirates and gastric distension. Disease progression leads to vomiting, diarrhoea (often with the passage of blood or mucus in the stool) and eventually to shock.

The initial radiographic features of NEC are non-specific. One of the earliest findings is diffuse gaseous distension of both small and large bowel representative of an ileus. Serial radiographs will demonstrate fixed dilatation of one or more bowel loops, and thickening (oedema) and loss of distinction of the bowel walls as the disease progresses.

A more specific sign of NEC on the plain radiograph is intramural gas (pneumatosis intestinalis). Not all infants with pneumatosis will have NEC (Table 77-3). More extensive pneumatosis correlates with an increased severity of NEC. Portal venous gas is seen as branching

TABLE 77-3 Causes of Pneumatosis Intestinalis in the Neonate and the Older Child

- NEC
- Bowel ischaemia, inflammation and obstruction
- Cyanotic congenital heart disease
- Hirschsprung's disease
- Gastroschisis
- Anorectal atresia
- Inflammatory bowel disease
- Lymphoma
- Leukaemia
- CMV and rotavirus gastroenteritis
- Colonoscopy
- Caustic ingestion
- Short bowel syndrome
- Congenital immune deficiency states
- *Clostridium* infection
- Chronic granulomatous disease of childhood
- Chronic steroid use
- Post hepatic, renal or bone marrow transplant
- Collagen vascular disease
- Graft-versus-host disease
- AIDS

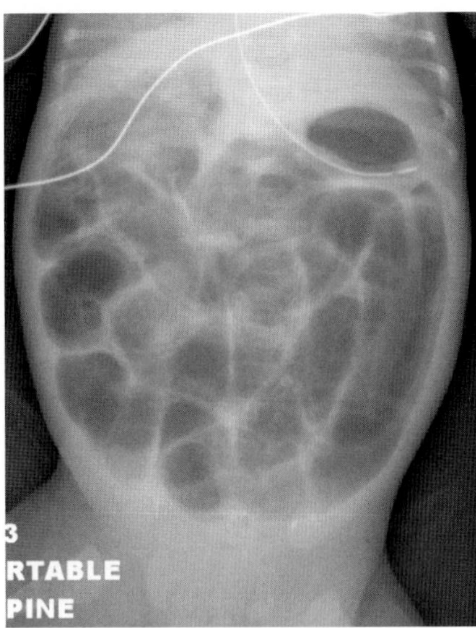

FIGURE 77-10 ■ **Necrotising enterocolitis.** Supine radiograph demonstrates multiple dilated loops of bowel and extensive pneumatosis.

linear lucencies over the liver that radiate from the region of the porta hepatis to the periphery of both lobes. It develops in around 30% of cases and is usually associated with severe NEC, although its presence does not necessarily imply a fatal outcome (Fig. 77-10).[32]

One-third of children with NEC will perforate, most commonly in the ileocaecal region. The supine, cross-table lateral view is useful to detect small amounts of free intraperitoneal air, as there is no need to reposition the infant when the image is taken. Air collects anteriorly, where it is seen as inverted triangles of air. Alternatively, a lateral decubitus radiograph may be used.

Ultrasound can detect signs of NEC before there are plain radiographic abnormalities.[32,33] Thickening of the bowel wall (≥ 2.7 mm), pneumatosis (seen either as echogenic 'dots' or dense echogenic lines within the bowel wall) (Fig. 77-11) and portal venous gas can all be observed. Colour Doppler will show both hyperaemic bowel wall, and the lack of bowel perfusion that accompanies ischaemia and necrosis. Free fluid will be seen clearly; debris within it may represent bowel content or pus, and has been shown to correlate with gangrene or perforation.[34]

Perforation in infants with NEC is not an absolute indication for surgical intervention. Peritoneal drains are used as a temporising measure in these critically ill infants, delaying the need for surgery and allowing time for systemic recovery. Surgery will be required in 20–40% of infants. Necrotic bowel is resected and as much bowel as possible is preserved.

A late complication of NEC is stricture formation, which occurs in up to a third of patients. Contrast studies (with water-soluble contrast media) are indicated to assess the calibre of the gut downstream prior to re-anastomosis of defunctioned bowel.

The overall mortality rate from NEC is approximately 30%, with this figure being even higher in very low birth weight infants.

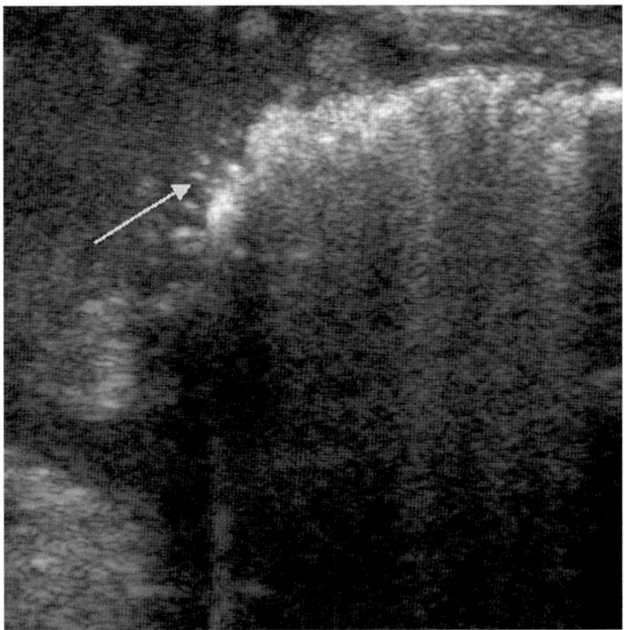

FIGURE 77-11 ■ **The use of ultrasound in the diagnosis of necrotising enterocolitis.** Echogenic dots representing intramural gas bubbles of pneumatosis intestinalis (arrow) in the oedematous bowel wall. (Image reproduced from Imaging in Medicine, August 2011;3(4): 393–410. With the permission of Future Medicine Ltd.)

Colon Atresia

Colon atresia is rare when compared with other intestinal atresias, and colonic stenosis is rarer still. Atresia has long been thought to be due to an in utero vascular accident;[35] however, Baglaj and colleagues have suggested compression of the bowel wall against the closing umbilical ring as an underlying cause.[6]

The affected infant presents after several feeds with abdominal distension, failure to pass meconium and vomiting.

The abdominal radiograph will show the features of a low intestinal obstruction, with the loop immediately proximal to the atretic segment being massively dilated. If multiple atresias are present, then the bowel will be distended only to the level of the most proximal atresia. A contrast enema usually demonstrates a distal microcolon, with obstruction to the retrograde flow of contrast at the point of the atresia.

The management of colon atresia is surgical.

Intra-abdominal Lymphangioma

Intra-abdominal lymphangiomas may be found in the mesentery, omentum or retroperitoneum, which explains the various names that are used to describe them (mesenteric and omental cysts being two of these). The most common location is in the ileal mesentery. These lesions are increasingly being diagnosed by antenatal imaging, meaning asymptomatic infants come for follow-up imaging early in the postnatal period.

Ultrasound will show a thin-walled, multiloculated cystic lesion that may be adherent to adjacent solid organs and bowel. There is no layering of the cyst wall, which helps to differentiate from an enteric duplication cyst. If the fluid within the cyst is chylous, infected or haemorrhagic, then it will be echogenic (see the section 'Mesenteric Cysts').

Megacystis-Microcolon-Intestinal Hypoperistalsis (Berdon's) Syndrome

This syndrome is a rare and severe form of functional intestinal obstruction. The aetiology of the condition remains obscure. The affected infants present with abdominal distension, bilious vomiting and delayed passage of meconium. Antenatal ultrasound shows a massively dilated bladder. Postnatally, an abdominal radiograph will show dilated small bowel with a large soft-tissue mass arising out of the pelvis. The megabladder and the degree of renal upper tract dilatation can be assessed by ultrasound. An upper GI contrast study will confirm malrotation and a short bowel. A contrast enema shows a non-obstructed microcolon. Treatment of this condition is largely unsuccessful—the mortality rate approaches 80%.

Delayed Passage of Meconium

All term infants should pass meconium in the first 24–48 h of life. Delayed or failed passage of the first stool is reported in premature infants, but may also be due to an underlying congenital bowel obstruction (Table 77-4), which will lead to progressive abdominal distension. The more common problems encountered include Hirschsprung's disease, functional immaturity of the colon, meconium plug syndrome, meconium ileus and peritonitis, and distal atresias.

In all cases, a supine abdominal radiograph will show the features of a low intestinal obstruction; there will be multiple, dilated loops of bowel down to the level of the obstruction. Differentiation between small and large bowel to determine the precise level of the obstruction is virtually impossible in the neonate, given that both may be of similar calibre and that the haustra are poorly developed.

Hirschsprung's Disease

Hirschsprung's disease is a neurocristopathy that presents as functional low bowel obstruction. It occurs due to the failure of caudal migration of neuroblasts in the developing bowel during the fifth through twelfth weeks of gestation. Histology reveals an absence of parasympathetic intrinsic ganglion cells in both Auerbach's and Meissner's plexuses in the bowel wall, which is associated with an increase in the number of acetylcholinesterase-positive nerve fibres in the aganglionic portions of the gut. The distal large bowel from the point of neuronal arrest to the anus is aganglionic. In about 75% of cases, the aganglionic segment extends only to the rectosigmoid region (short segment disease). Long segment disease involves a portion of the colon proximal to the sigmoid. Variants of Hirschsprung's disease include total colonic aganglionosis (TCA), which may involve the distal ileum also, and total intestinal Hirschsprung's disease. Ultrashort segment disease is rare and involves only the anus at the level of the internal sphincter. The existence of 'skip lesions' in Hirschsprung's disease is uncommon.[36]

A definitive diagnosis of Hirschsprung's disease is made by a suction or full-thickness rectal biopsy. Current treatment involves resection of the aganglionic bowel segment with a 'pull though' procedure, and anastomosis of the normally innervated gut close to the anal margin. The management of total intestinal Hirschsprung's disease is notoriously difficult and, at the present time, these patients are supported with parenteral nutrition.

Approximately 10% of children with Hirschsprung's disease have Down's syndrome. Other associations with Hirschsprung's disease include ileal, colonic and anorectal atresias, cleft palate, polydactyly, craniofacial anomalies, cardiac septal defects, multiple endocrine neoplasia types 2A and 2B and other neurocristopathies.[37]

Ninety per cent present in the neonatal period, with delayed passage of meconium, abdominal distension and vomiting. Stooling may follow a digital rectal examination or the insertion of a rectal thermometer, before the symptoms recur. Children with longer segment disease and TCA often present later, as their symptoms can paradoxically be milder and their diagnosis missed clinically.[38]

Severe bloody diarrhoea, sepsis and shock are associated with Hirschsprung's enterocolitis, which occurs in up to 30% of patients in both the pre- and postoperative periods. Enterocolitis is the leading cause of death in Hirschsprung's disease and has an increased frequency in long segment disease and those in whom the diagnosis was delayed.

Other postoperative complications of Hirschsprung's disease include anastomotic leaks, fistulae, abscesses and stenoses. Up to 10% of patients will eventually require a permanent colostomy.[37]

The abdominal radiograph will typically show a low bowel obstruction. A contrast enema should be performed. No pre-procedure bowel preparation is given, and there should be an interval of at least 48 hours since the last enema or rectal examination. The catheter tip is placed just inside the rectum. It is important that the catheter balloon is *not* inflated. A catheter balloon can obscure the diagnostic features or, worse, perforate the stiff, aganglionic bowel. The most important film is a lateral (or oblique) view of the rectum during slow filling (Fig. 77-12). In short segment disease the rectum will be

TABLE 77-4 **Delayed Passage of Meconium**

- Ileal atresia
- Meconium ileus
- Functional immaturity of the colon
- Colon atresia
- Anorectal malformations
- Hirschsprung's disease
- Megacystis–microcolon–intestinal hypoperistalsis syndrome
- Extrinsic compression of the distal bowel by a mass lesion
  - Mesenteric cyst
  - Enteric duplication cyst
- Paralytic ileus, sepsis, drugs and metabolic upset

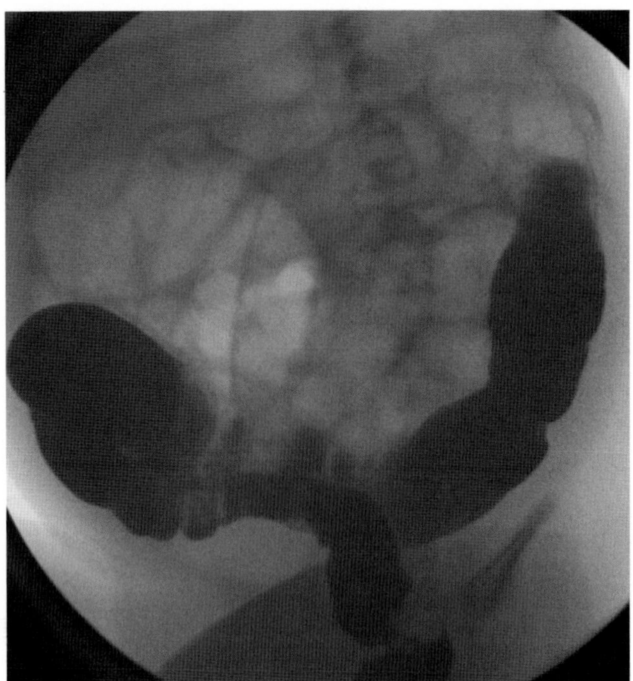

FIGURE 77-12 ■ Rectosigmoid Hirschsprung's disease. Supine oblique view, contrast enema. The cone-shaped transition zone and abnormal rectosigmoid ratio are demonstrated.

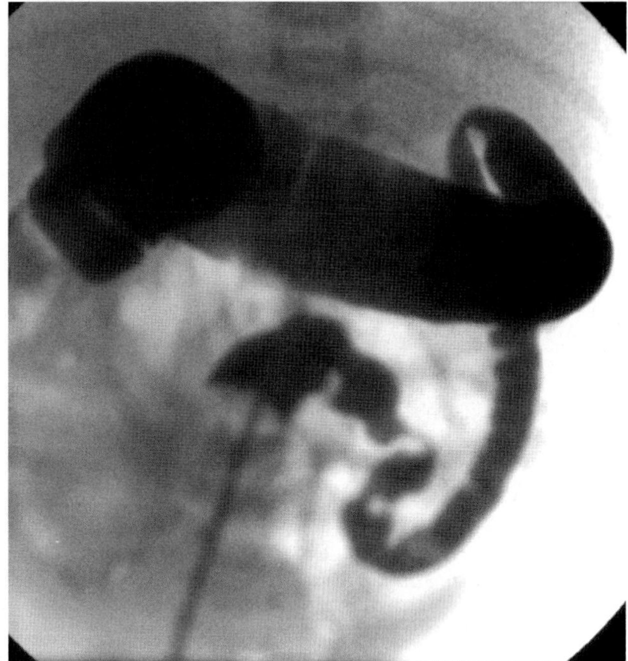

FIGURE 77-13 ■ Small left colon syndrome. Contrast enema shows a microcolon distal to the splenic flexure. The transition point is abrupt.

narrow and there will be a cone-shaped transition zone to the more proximal, dilated, ganglionated bowel. Irregular contractions may be seen in the denervated rectum. A useful calculation is the rectosigmoid ratio; the rectum should always be the most distensible portion of the bowel and have a diameter greater than that of the sigmoid colon (recto: sigmoid ratio > 1). In short segment disease, this ratio is reversed. The radiological features of Hirschsprung's disease may be absent in the neonate as it takes time for the ganglionated bowel to dilate.

Whereas coexistent enterocolitis, mucosal oedema, ulceration and spasm are not infrequently seen, an enema would obviously be absolutely contraindicated in the infant with fulminant colitis. Giant stercoral ulcers may also be seen in older children with a delayed presentation. Overall, the contrast enema has a reported sensitivity of 70% and a specificity of 83%;[39] however, the negative predictive value of a normal contrast enema in patients older than 1 month of age is 98%.[40]

In TCA the contrast enema may be entirely normal. Positive findings include shortening of a normal-calibre colon, with rounding of the contours of the hepatic and splenic flexures.

Functional Immaturity of the Colon and Meconium Plug Syndrome

Immature left colon (*syn.* small left colon) and meconium plug syndrome are relatively common causes of neonatal bowel obstruction. There is overlap in both the clinical features and radiology of the two conditions, and the terms are often used interchangeably in the literature. The former refers to a transient functional obstruction of the colon, which occurs as a result of immaturity of the myenteric plexus. It is common in the infants of diabetic mothers and in those whose mothers have a history of substance abuse. Meconium plug syndrome is a temporary colonic obstruction caused by plugs of meconium. It is associated with both cystic fibrosis and Hirschsprung's disease, both of which should either be confirmed or refuted if a diagnosis of meconium plug syndrome is made.[41] The infants of women who have received magnesium sulphate therapy and premature infants also have an increased incidence of meconium plug syndrome.[42]

In both conditions, the affected infants present with symptoms and signs of bowel obstruction. There is delayed passage of meconium. The plain radiograph shows distension of both small and large bowel loops to the level of the inspissated meconium plugs.

In small left colon syndrome, the contrast enema typically shows a microcolon distal to the splenic flexure, at which point there is an abrupt transition to a mildly dilated proximal colon (Fig. 77-13). The main differential diagnosis is long segment Hirschsprung's disease, and biopsy may be required.

In meconium plug syndrome, the lodged meconium plugs are the cause of the obstruction. The plugs lodge in the region of the splenic flexure, proximal to which there is colonic dilatation. There is no microcolon. The (water-soluble) contrast enema is therapeutic, and once the meconium plugs are passed, the infant recovers.

Meconium Ileus

Meconium ileus is a form of distal intestinal obstruction caused by inspissated pellets of meconium in the terminal ileum. Around 80–90% of infants with meconium ileus have cystic fibrosis and meconium ileus is the

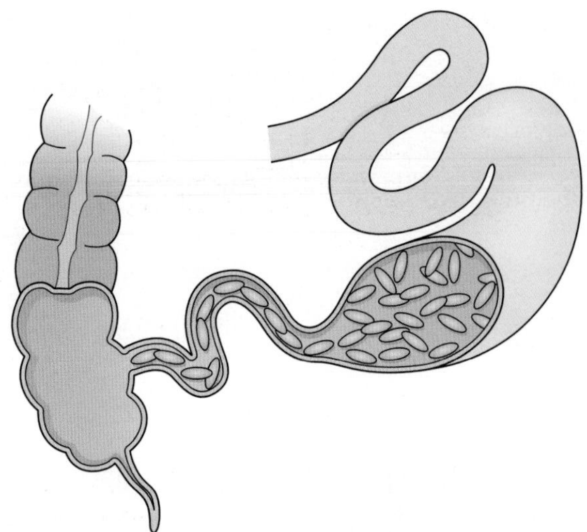

FIGURE 77-14 ■ Diagrammatic representation of meconium ileus. Pellets of desiccated meconium obstruct the terminal ileum, with the more proximal small bowel dilating. The unused colon is extremely narrow in calibre (a microcolon).

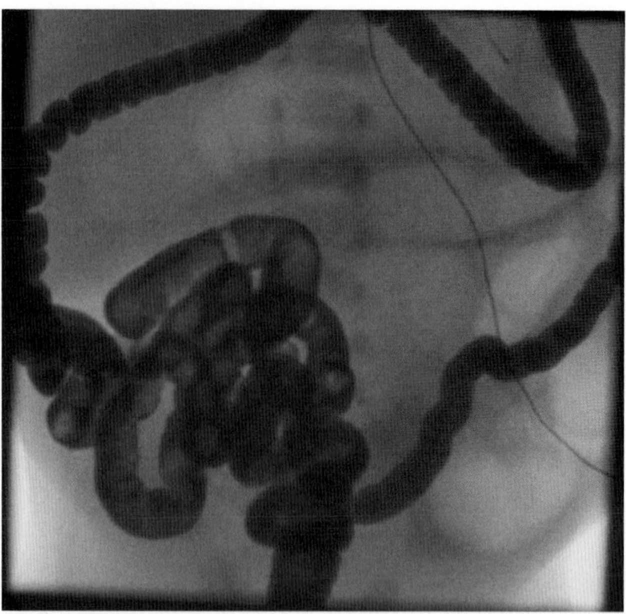

FIGURE 77-15 ■ Meconium ileus. Contrast enema demonstrates the empty microcolon. Contrast medium refluxes into the narrow terminal ileum, where pellets of meconium are outlined.

presenting feature of cystic fibrosis in 10–20% of affected patients. Children with the ΔF508 mutation have an increased incidence of meconium ileus, and those who are homozygous for this mutation have a higher incidence still.[43]

Over half of the affected infants have uncomplicated (or simple) meconium ileus. In utero these babies produce meconium that is thick and tenacious, and which fills and distends the small bowel loops. The meconium desiccates in the distal ileum and becomes impacted, causing a high-grade obstruction (Fig. 77-14). Failure of meconium to pass into the colon results in a functional microcolon, whereas more proximally the small bowel loops are dilated and filled with greenish-black meconium of a toothpaste-like consistency.

Meconium ileus is described as complicated when intrauterine volvulus, intestinal atresias, bowel necrosis, perforation or meconium peritonitis supervene. The presenting clinical symptoms and signs of non-complicated meconium ileus are those of a low bowel obstruction. The plain abdominal radiograph will show dilatation of small bowel loops, which are of varying calibre. Often, there is a 'soap bubble' appearance visible (classically in the right iliac fossa), which is caused by the admixture of meconium with gas.

The contrast enema in meconium ileus demonstrates a virtually empty microcolon. Reflux of contrast medium into the terminal ileum will show that it, too, is small in calibre and numerous pellets of meconium are outlined (Fig. 77-15). More proximal reflux of contrast medium will show the dilated mid-ileal loops. The contrast enema in uncomplicated meconium ileus may be therapeutic as well as diagnostic. Traditionally, 'neat' Gastrografin was the contrast medium of choice, but its hypertonicity led to fluid-balance problems. These days, Gastrografin is diluted to half-strength with saline or water, or another water-soluble contrast medium is substituted. If the infant's clinical condition remains stable, the enema can be repeated as necessary until the obstruction is relieved.

Volvulus of a heavy, meconium-laden loop of bowel occurs in about 50% of patients, and can lead to intestinal stenoses, atresias, necrosis and perforation. Perforation of bowel in utero leads to chemical (sterile) meconium peritonitis. The extruded bowel contents cause an intense inflammatory reaction, with fibrosis and calcification to follow. A meconium pseudocyst is formed when there is vascular compromise in association with an intrauterine volvulus; the ischaemic bowel loops become adherent and necrotic, and a fibrous wall develops around them. The presence of complicated meconium ileus may be suggested by the plain radiographic findings: intra-abdominal or scrotal calcifications, bowel wall calcification, prominent air–fluid levels and soft-tissue masses.

The management of meconium peritonitis is surgical.

Distal Ileal Atresia

Ileal atresia is thought to be due to a prenatal vascular insult. If the atresia is in the distal ileum, then the infant will present with abdominal distension and delayed passage of meconium. The plain radiograph will show a low obstruction with multiple dilated loops of bowel. The contrast enema will outline a microcolon and the contrast medium cannot be refluxed into the dilated small bowel. The condition is managed surgically.

Anorectal and Cloacal Malformations

Anorectal malformations (ARMs) are a not uncommon congenital abnormality of the hindgut. Their precise aetiology is unknown, but the condition results from maldevelopment of the cloacal structure early in the first trimester. The resulting cloacal membrane is too short and the distal cloaca absent, and it is these structures that are necessary for the formation of the lower rectum and anus.[44,45] The abnormality consists of anorectal atresia, with or without a fistulous connection between the atretic anorectum and the GU tract.

Associated congenital anomalies are common. The VACTERL sequence occurs in around 45% of patients, with around 80% of this group having GU tract abnormalities. Musculoskeletal abnormalities are seen in just under half of these VACTERL patients. Cloacal exstrophy and the OEIS complex (omphalocele, exstrophy, imperforate anus and sacral anomalies) are found in up to 5% of patients. Between 2 and 8% of patients have Down's syndrome, with the vast majority of these patients having imperforate anus without fistulae.[46] Currarino's triad is the association between an anorectal malformation, bony sacral anomalies and a presacral mass lesion.

In the past, ARMs were described as either high or low lesions, depending upon where the rectum ended relative to the levator ani muscles. These terms are gradually being replaced by a classification based upon the type of fistula that is present, as this gives information regarding the localisation of the atretic anorectum and has an important bearing upon surgical planning.[46,47] In male patients, the fistula may be to the prostatic or bulbar urethra or bladder neck. In females the fistula may be to the vaginal vestibule, with true posterior vaginal wall fistulae being extremely rare. Perineal fistulae may be present in infants of either sex, as may imperforate anus and rectal atresia or stenosis, the latter groups being without fistulae.

The diagnosis should be made clinically during the baby check immediately following delivery, and if a perineal or anal abnormality is detected, then immediate referral to the local paediatric surgery team is merited.

Should the paediatric surgical team not be able to distinguish between the type of ARM present after a period of 24 h, then the traditional cross-table lateral radiograph, with the infant in the prone position and the buttocks elevated may still have a role. A radiopaque marker is placed over the anal dimple and the distance between the pouch of rectal gas and the marker is measured. A distance of < 1.0 cm implies a more distal atresia. False interpretation of the film is obtained when the film is taken on the first day of life, when there has been insufficient time for gas to reach the rectum or if the infant had not been held prone for sufficient time to allow the gas to reach the tip of the rectal pouch. If the infant is crying or straining, the rectal pouch descends through the levator sling, which will also lead to errors in interpretation. Plain radiographs are useful if they demonstrate intravesical air (implying a rectovesical or rectourethral fistula in a boy). Transperineal ultrasound is also used to measure the distance of the rectal pouch from the perineum but interpretation suffers from similar problems to the radiograph.

Infants who have a perineal fistula usually undergo a posterior sagittal anoplasty within the first 24–48 h of life. All other children with ARMs will have a defunctioning colostomy performed, with the aim of surgery being to separate the GI and GU tracts and stop faecal contamination of the latter. Definitive surgery is postponed until a later stage, when the infant has grown and all other imaging investigations are complete.

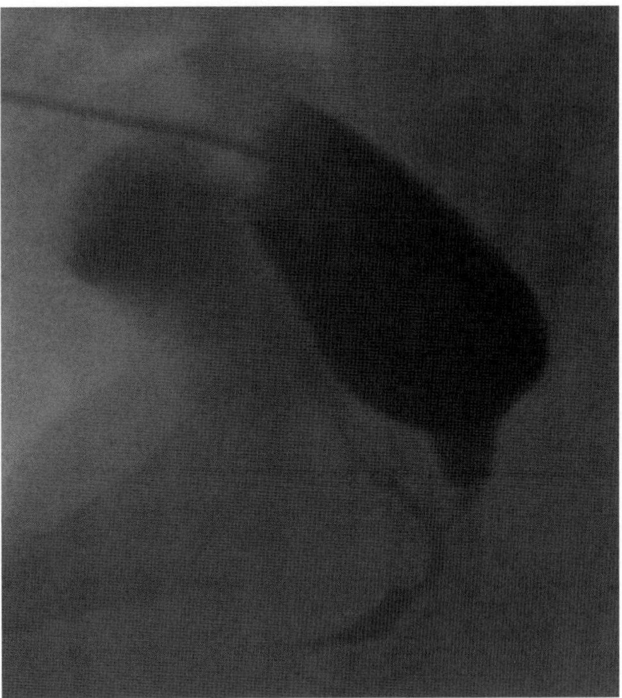

FIGURE 77-16 ■ Rectourethral fistula. Augmented pressure colostogram in a male infant with a high anorectal malformation. Contrast medium is seen passing through the fistula to the posterior urethra, with retrograde flow outlining the bladder.

In terms of defining the precise anatomy of the fistulous tract, the most useful investigation remains the augmented pressure colostogram. A Foley catheter is inserted into the distal segment of the colon and its balloon gently inflated so that it seals the stoma. With the patient in the lateral position, water-soluble contrast medium is hand-injected under mild pressure to distend the distal colon and define the fistulous tract. Interpretation of the images is made easier if there is a bladder catheter in situ, through which some contrast medium has been instilled; this gives anatomical markers for the bladder neck and the course of the urethra (Fig. 77-16).

The cloacal malformation occurs only in female patients. Examination of the perineum reveals a single opening into which the urethra, vagina and rectum drain. Defining the anatomy of these lesions is difficult, but ultrasound, pelvic MRI examinations and contrast studies of the cloaca all play a role. As these girls are all managed with an initial colostomy, then combined fluoroscopic studies of an augmented pressure colostogram, micturating cystourethrogram and 'cloacogram', with images obtained in both the lateral and anteroposterior positions are possible.

Ancillary radiological investigations in infants with ARMs include ultrasound of the GU tract, an echocardiogram along with radiographs of the chest and spine. A tethered spinal cord is seen in almost 50% of patients with ARMs, irrespective of the degree of lesion complexity.[48,49] Ultrasound of the spine is an excellent screening technique in the first few months of life. MRI of the spine and pelvis is extremely helpful to assess not only the spine but also the pelvic organs and pelvic floor muscles.

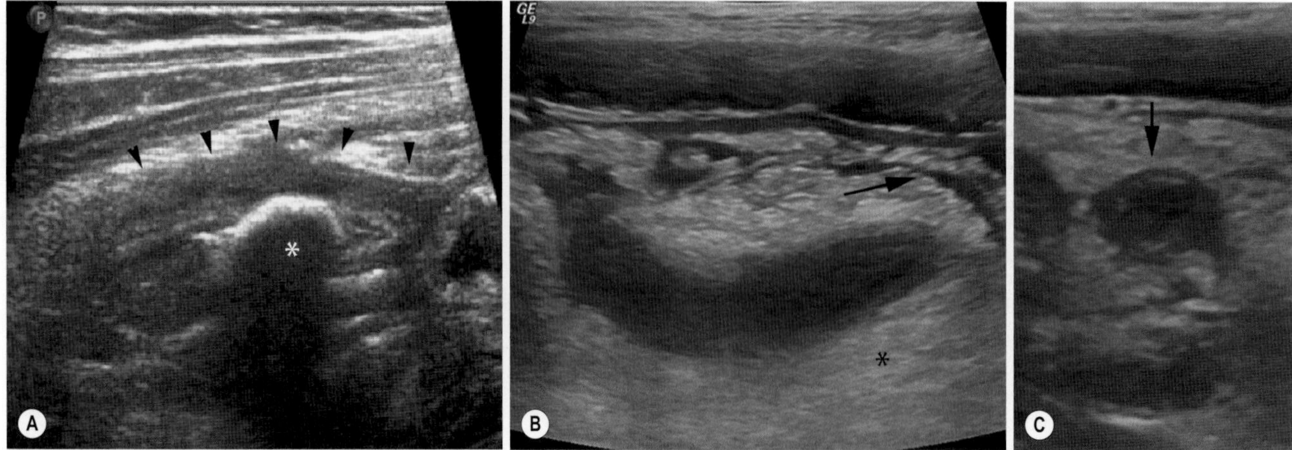

FIGURE 77-17 ■ **Sonographic findings in acute appendicitis.** (A) A longitudinal image showing a thickened appendix (arrowheads) with an appendicolith, casting an acoustic shadow (asterisk). (B, C) Sonographic appearance of a necrotic appendix with surrounding hyperechoic, inflamed mesenteric fat (asterisk) and some free fluid (arrow) suggestive of perforation. The axial view clearly shows a thickened appendix (arrow) with only two remaining layers of the appendix wall due to necrosis.

THE INFANT AND OLDER CHILD

Abdominal Pain

Abdominal pain can have numerous causes, and functional abdominal pain is not uncommon in childhood. However, important entities that may require treatment must be ruled out. One of the challenges in childhood is to accurately define the type, intensity and frequency of pain because children and adolescents have poor ability to recall episodes of abdominal pain, and also to localise and characterise the pain. Therefore the role of radiology is even more important in helping to establish the diagnosis.

The imaging approach will be tailored by the clinical information and the age-specific entities that may cause abdominal pain in childhood. In the majority of cases ultrasound is the primary technique of choice in both chronic and acute abdominal pain. Because of little body fat, children are ideally suited for ultrasound and superb images of excellent quality can be produced. Sonography is therefore a potentially powerful diagnostic tool in children; it is fast, cheap and does not expose the child to radiation. Magnetic resonance imaging (MRI) may be a complementary tool if ultrasound is unable to give sufficient diagnostic information.

The availability of MRI is sometimes limited and, occasionally, abdominal CT imaging may be necessary, especially in acute abdominal pain. However, a restrictive attitude towards the use of CT is important because of the radiation exposure. Plain abdominal radiography after the neonatal period should be reserved for the queries of intestinal obstruction and free intraperitoneal gas (with perforation).

Acute Appendicitis

Appendicitis is the most common cause for acute surgery in childhood. Thirty to 40% of children do not present with the typical findings of appendicitis.[50] Therefore

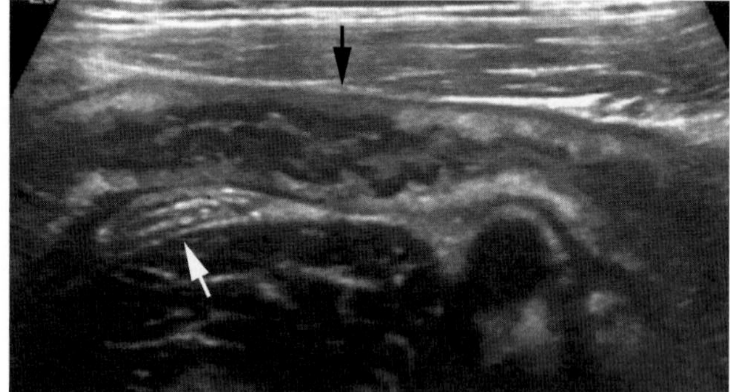

FIGURE 77-18 ■ Sonographic findings in a 12-year-old girl with suspected appendicitis showing a thickened terminal ileum (black arrow) with reduced peristalsis and a normal appendix (white arrow).

imaging is often necessary to confirm or suggest the diagnosis. Use of imaging has reduced the false-positive appendectomy rates from 20–30% to 4–8%.[51] Ultrasound should be the primary imaging technique and performing a comprehensive ultrasound examination will make CT examination redundant in most cases.[52,53] The ultrasound should be performed with a high-frequency linear transducer using a graded compression technique. The primary criteria of acute appendicitis are typically a tubular, blind-ending, non-compressible structure with maximal outer diameter over 6 mm. Other findings include wall hyperaemia or hypoperfusion (depending on the degree of inflammation/necrosis), surrounding hyperechoic mesenteric fat and the presence of an appendicolith (Fig. 77-17).[54]

CT is rarely necessary but may be an important diagnostic tool in difficult cases where ultrasound is unable to clarify and the clinical situation enforce acute surgery. Sonographical mimics of acute appendicitis may be acute salpingitis in teenage girls or terminal ileitis (see below) (Fig. 77-18).

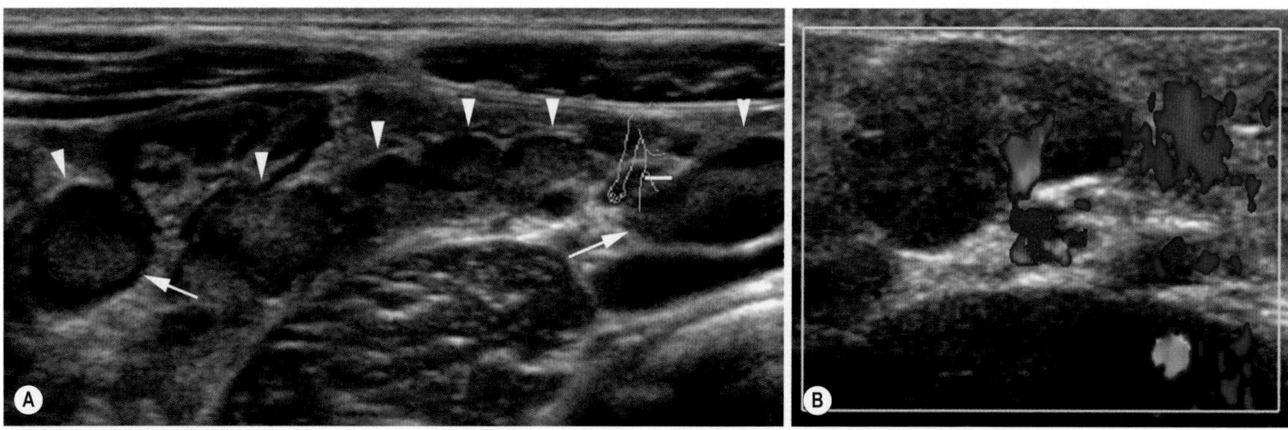

FIGURE 77-19 ■ **Sonographic appearances of mesenteric lymphadenitis.** (A) Multiple, unremarkable mesenteric lymph nodes (arrowheads) with preserved hyperechoic fatty hilum (arrows). (B) Normal hilar flow is seen on Doppler examination.

Mesenteric Lymphadenitis

Mesenteric lymphadenitis is a common cause of abdominal pain in childhood and may present as subacute or acute abdomen. The symptoms are caused by swelling of mesenteric lymph nodes as a reaction to a trivial, often asymptomatic viral infection. On ultrasound, multiple enlarged lymph nodes are seen in the root of the mesentery. The hyperechoic, fatty hilus is preserved and there is normal Doppler signal within the lymph nodes (Fig. 77-19). Mesenteric lymphadenitis is a diagnosis of exclusion and should be established and based on ultrasound findings in the absence of any other plausible explanations for the abdominal pain.[55]

Inflammatory Bowel Disease

The diagnosis of inflammatory bowel disease (IBD) encompasses Crohn's disease, ulcerative colitis and unclassified IBD. IBD is thought to develop as a result of dysregulation of the immune response to gut flora in a genetically susceptible host. The most common symptoms of inflammatory bowel disease are chronic diarrhoea, fever and weight loss but it may also present as acute or subacute abdominal pain. The gold standard for diagnosing IBD is ileocolonoscopy with biopsy. Imaging plays a role in establishing the extent of the disease, to assess possible complications and to select candidates for potential surgery.

Ultrasonography (US). In children ultrasound is the first imaging tool of choice, especially if the diagnosis is unknown. A comprehensive ultrasound to look for bowel wall thickening (BWT) has a strong negative predictive value for IBD. The sensitivity and specificity for BWT on US depends on the threshold used. A small bowel wall thickness greater than 1.5–3 mm and a colonic wall thickness over 2–3 mm is considered to be pathological. Colour Doppler US may reveal hyperaemia of the inflamed bowel and this finding may enhance the diagnosis (Fig. 77-20). Other signs of IBD on US include lack of bowel stratification, altered echogenicity of the bowel wall, hyperechoic mesenteric fat and enlarged lymph nodes. One should always look for complications of the disease, e.g. abscesses and fistula; however, the sensitivity for these features on US is low. US is a quick, radiation-free and easily available technique, but is highly operator dependent and the findings are not necessarily reproducible. The technique also has limited value in obese children and in the presence of gaseous distension of bowel.

Conventional Barium Studies. Conventional barium studies have largely been replaced by other imaging techniques such as MRI and US and play a very limited role in imaging of IBD in children because the techniques are stressful, give a high radiation dose to the patient and are unable to demonstrate extraluminal disease. Small bowel follow through (SBFT) may still play a role in the assessment of bowel obstruction but ultra-low-dose MDCT and capsule endoscopy have replaced SBFT for this indication. Barium enteroclysis should only be performed when the child is unable to undergo an MRI (Fig. 77-21).

Magnetic Resonance Imaging (MRI). The preferred technique for small bowel assessment on MRI is MR enterography. A comprehensive MRI has a high specificity and a sensitivity for bowel inflammation and includes no ionising radiation.[56] This technique is normally well tolerated by children from 6–7 years and older. Sufficient bowel distension is important for a proper assessment of the bowel wall. MR enteroclysis may be an alternative if the child is unable to drink the relatively large amount of fluid required to distend the small bowel. A low-residue diet should be given three days prior to the examination with nil per mouth from 24 h before the imaging.

MRI can estimate the length and localisation of the affected bowel and detect both intra- and extraluminal disease. However, if there is a clinical suspicion of a perianal fistula and/or abscess, dedicated pelvic MR fistulography may be required for detection and delineation of the fistula. A dynamic MRI sequence should be included to find possible bowel strictures, as this may change the treatment approach from medical to surgical. Table 77-5 shows the standard MRI sequences recommended for imaging in IBD. Motion artefacts due to lack of patient cooperation or bowel peristalsis may distort the

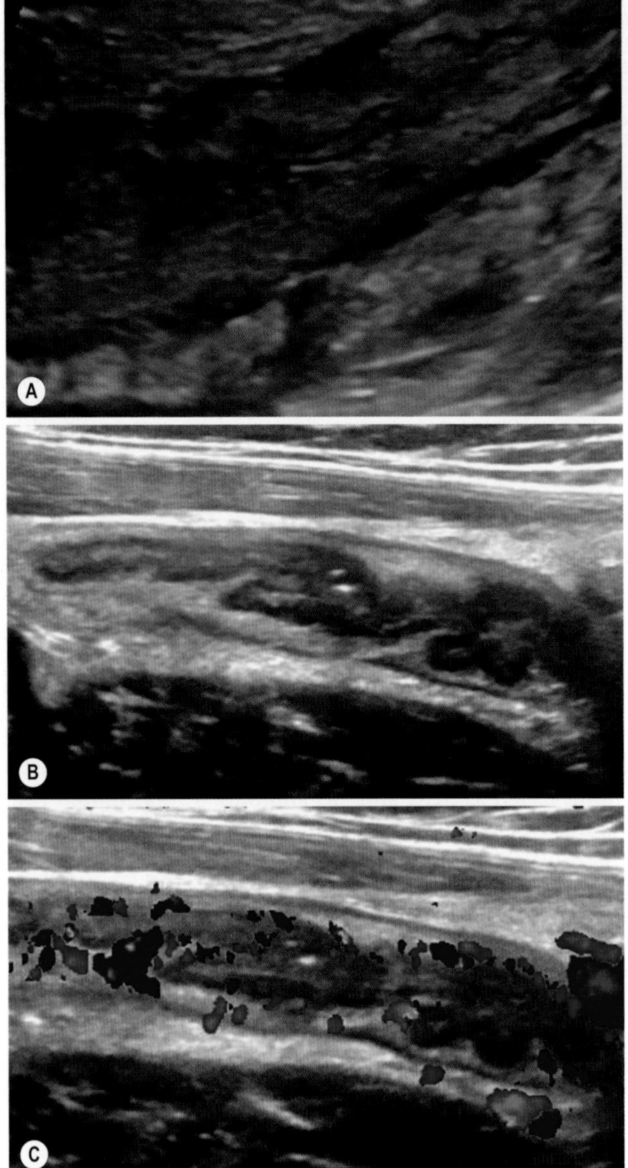

FIGURE 77-20 ■ **Terminal ileitis.** Ultrasound shows marked thickening of the terminal ileum and increased echogenicity of the bowel wall (A). A slightly thickened distal ileum with reduced peristalsis (B). Colour Doppler examination revealed hyperaemic bowel wall in the inflamed bowel segment (C).

images. Controversies exist regarding MRI's ability to determine disease activity, both due to lack of a gold standard and because acute and chronic disease may coexist in the same bowel loop.[57] The development of new imaging techniques such as diffusion-weighted imaging (DWI) have shown to increase the sensitivity and specificity for both intraluminal and extraluminal disease in IBD (Fig. 77-22).[58] MRI signs of IBD are listed in Table 77-6.

Computed Tomography (CT). CT enteroclysis and CT enterography have become widely used techniques

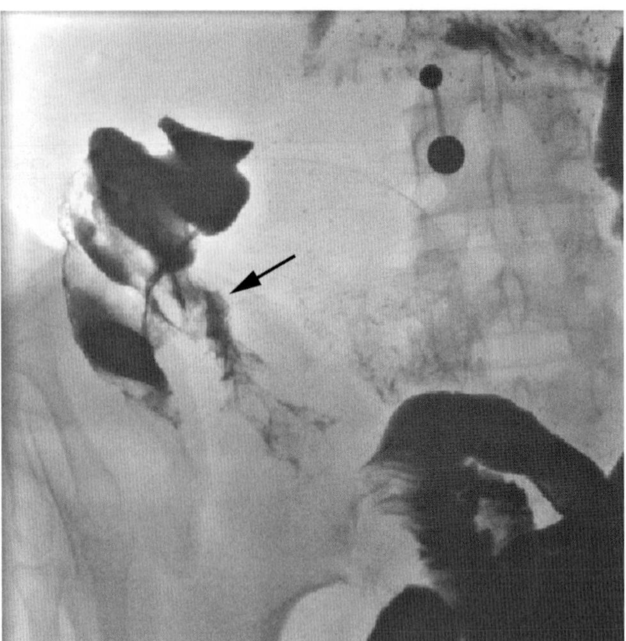

FIGURE 77-21 ■ **Barium follow through (BFT) in terminal ileitis.** BFT shows a narrowed and irregular bowel lumen in terminal ileitis (arrow).

TABLE 77-5 MRI Sequences for Imaging of Inflammatory Bowel Disease

- Hydrographic images: T2-weighted gradient echo (balanced steady-state free precession), in the axial and coronal planes. Alternatively, an ultrafast spin-echo sequence: half-Fourier single-shot turbo spin echo, in the axial and coronal planes
- Dynamic images: cine heavily T2-weighted gradient echo (balanced steady-state free precession) free breathing sequence
- Diffusion-weighted images in the axial plane, b-value >800
- Contrast series: T1W fat-suppressed images in the axial and coronal planes, pre- and post-contrast administration

TABLE 77-6 MRI Signs of Inflammatory Bowel Disease

***Bowel Loop Appearance**
- Fixed
- Dilated
- Pseudo-sacculation appearance
- Strictures

***Bowel Wall**
- Thickness
- Focal lesions (ulceration, pseudo-polyps, mural abscess)
- Enhancement pattern after gadolinium injection (mucosal alone, layered, global, serosal hypervascularity)
- Restricted diffusion
- Extramural signs: fibro-fatty proliferation, distended and enhancing mesenteric vessels fistula, abscess, enlarged lymph nodes

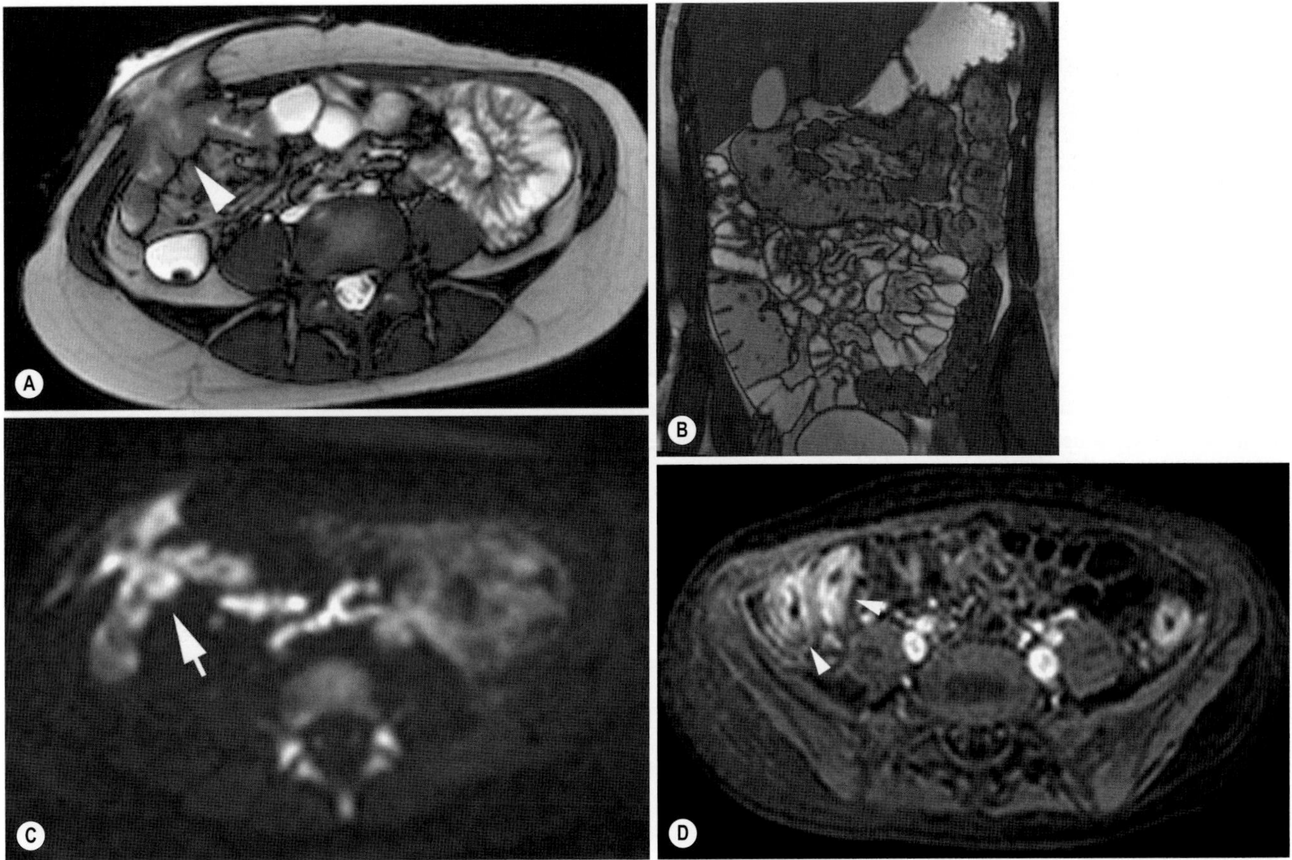

FIGURE 77-22 ■ **Inflammatory bowel disease.** MRI of Crohn's disease. (A) Axial hydrographic sequence showing thickening of the small bowel adjacent to the ileostomy (arrowhead). (B) Diffusion-weighted image of the same bowel segment with high signal suggestive of restricted diffusion. (C) Imaging in IBD should include hydrographic cine images to assess bowel peristalsis. (D) Contrast-enhanced T1W image showing contrast enhancement of thickened bowel loops.

for small bowel investigation in adults. These techniques should be avoided in children due to the high radiation dose. CT should be reserved for investigations of acute complications where US is deemed insufficient, for drainage of complex abscesses, or when the abscess is inaccessible for US-guided drainage.

Intussusception

Intussusception is a common surgical emergency in infants and young children. It is caused by telescoping of a segment of bowel (intussusceptum) into a more distal segment (intussuscipiens). The majority of children are under 1 year of age, with a peak incidence between 5 and 9 months of age; however, it may occur up to school age. Ileocolic intussusceptions are the most common type. Ileoileocolic, ileoileal and colocolic are much less common. Most (over 90%) have no lead point and are due to lymphoid hypertrophy, usually following a viral infection.

Secondary lead points (which include nasojejunal tubes, Meckel's diverticulum, intestinal polyp, duplication cyst and lymphoma) occur in 5–10% of patients. In very young infants or children over 6–7 years of age, intussusception is more likely to be caused by a secondary lead point. The clinical presentation of intussusception varies. The classical clinical signs of colicky abdominal pain, bloody stools and a palpable abdominal mass are present in less than 50% of the children. Intussusception must be treated as a surgical emergency. The clinical situation may deteriorate rapidly, particularly in infants, and may become life-threatening with hypovolaemia and shock. Prolonged symptom duration will reduce the likelihood of successful reduction.[59] Intussusception is diagnosed with ultrasound, with a sensitivity and specificity of 100% in several reported studies, even when performed by inexperienced radiologists, if properly trained.[60,61] The characteristic appearance of intussusception makes its diagnosis or exclusion very easy.

The intussusceptum is usually found just deep to the anterior abdominal wall, most often on the right side of the midline. Sonography must be performed with a high-frequency linear array transducer. The intussusception forms a mass of 3–5 cm in diameter, with a 'target appearance' in the transverse plane and a 'sandwich appearance' in the longitudinal plane. The characteristic 'crescent in doughnut' sign, a hyperechoic semilunar structure caused by the mesenteric fat pulled into the intussceptum, facilitates the differentiation from mimickers of intussusception, like bowel wall thickening, stools and the psoas muscle (Fig. 77-23). Lymph nodes and fluid may be seen between within the intussuceptum and in some studies

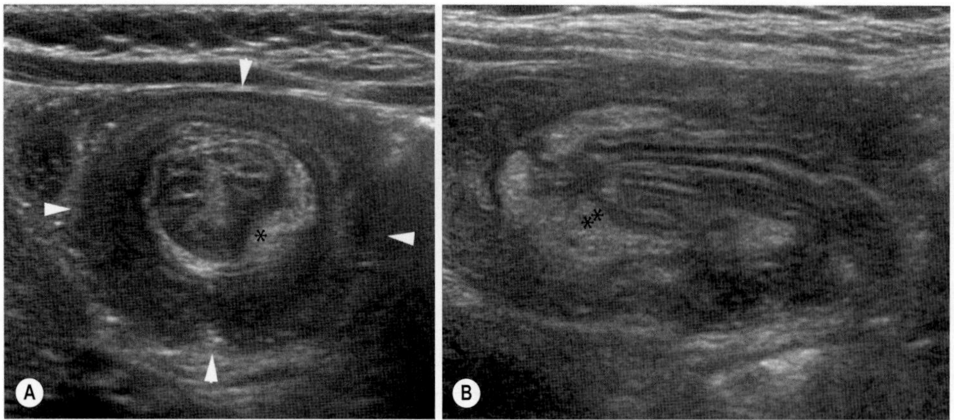

FIGURE 77-23 ■ **Intussusception is easily appreciated on ultrasound.** (A) The axial view shows the 'doughnut'—or 'target sign' (arrowheads)—caused by the multiple layers of bowel and the pathognomonic hyperechoic semilunar appearance of the mesenteric fat within the intussusceptum (asterisk). (B) The longitudinal view reveals the typical 'sandwich' appearance caused by the multiple layers of bowel wall and mesenteric fat (asterisk).

have been found to be associated with decreased hydrostatic reduction rate. Bowel necrosis is difficult to assess by ultrasonography, even with power Doppler examination of the bowel wall. Free intraperitoneal fluid is commonly seen in patients with intussusception and is therefore an unreliable indirect sign of bowel ischaemia. Ultrasonography should not only be performed to establish the diagnosis but also to look for secondary lead points and other intra-abdominal pathology unrelated to the intussusception. However, no sonographic features, including the presence of a secondary lead point, should preclude an attempt at reduction. In a well-hydrated, haemodynamically stable child the only contraindications for hydrostatic or pneumatic reduction are the presence of free intraperitoneal air or frank clinical signs of peritonitis.

The role of plain radiography in the diagnosis of intussusception is controversial. The 'classic' radiographic features of intussusception include a soft-tissue mass contrasting an air-filled bowel loop, the so-called 'meniscus sign' (Fig. 77-24). There may be dilated, gas-filled bowel loops proximal to the intussusceptum, and absence of gas within the caecum may suggest an ileocaecal intussuception. However, the caecum may be difficult to localise in a child, and the sigmoid is located on the left side of the abdomen in almost 50% of children and may be indistinguishable from the caecum on a plain radiograph. Abdominal radiographs should therefore not be routinely used in intussusception. The presence of free intraperitoneal gas is extremely rare in children with intussusception, and may be assessed by a quick fluoroscopic 'frame grab' performed before the fluoroscopically guided reduction.[61]

Image-guided reduction can be performed using a pneumatic technique or by contrast enema, under fluoroscopy or ultrasound guidance. Most centres in the UK use pneumatic reduction under fluoroscopy guidance, but the choice of technique varies across Europe and should be based on experience and expertise of the radiologist who performs the reduction (Fig. 77-25).[62] The use of sedation is also controversial. Animal studies have suggested that the use of sedation may lead to

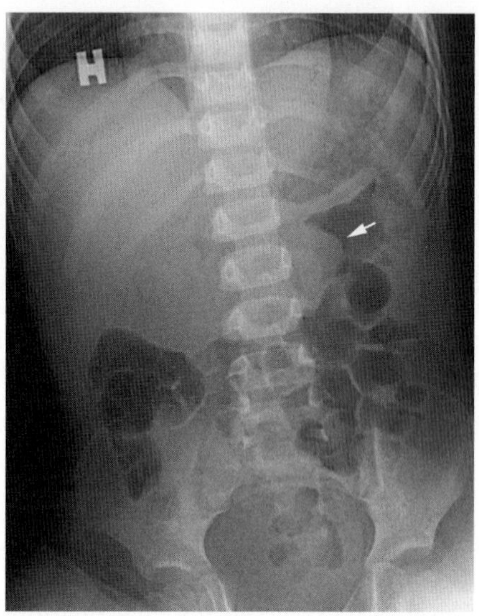

FIGURE 77-24 ■ **Intussusception.** An abdominal radiograph in a child with intussuception may show a soft-tissue mass contrasting an air-filled bowel loop, the so-called 'meniscus sign' (arrow); however, the diagnosis is made by ultrasound and the role of radiography in intussusception is controversial.

increased perforation rates; however, a prospective clinical study found an increased success rate and no difference in complications when using deep sedation with pneumatic reduction of intussusception in children.[63] Regardless of the technique used, one should aim at (and expect) a successful reduction rate over 80%.

Constipation

Constipation is probably the most common gastrointestinal problem in infants and children. Childhood functional constipation has an estimated prevalence of 3% in the Western world. The symptoms are typically infrequent painful defecation, faecal incontinence and abdominal pain.[64] This can lead to encopresis or faecal soiling, and occasionally can cause acute, severe abdominal pain.

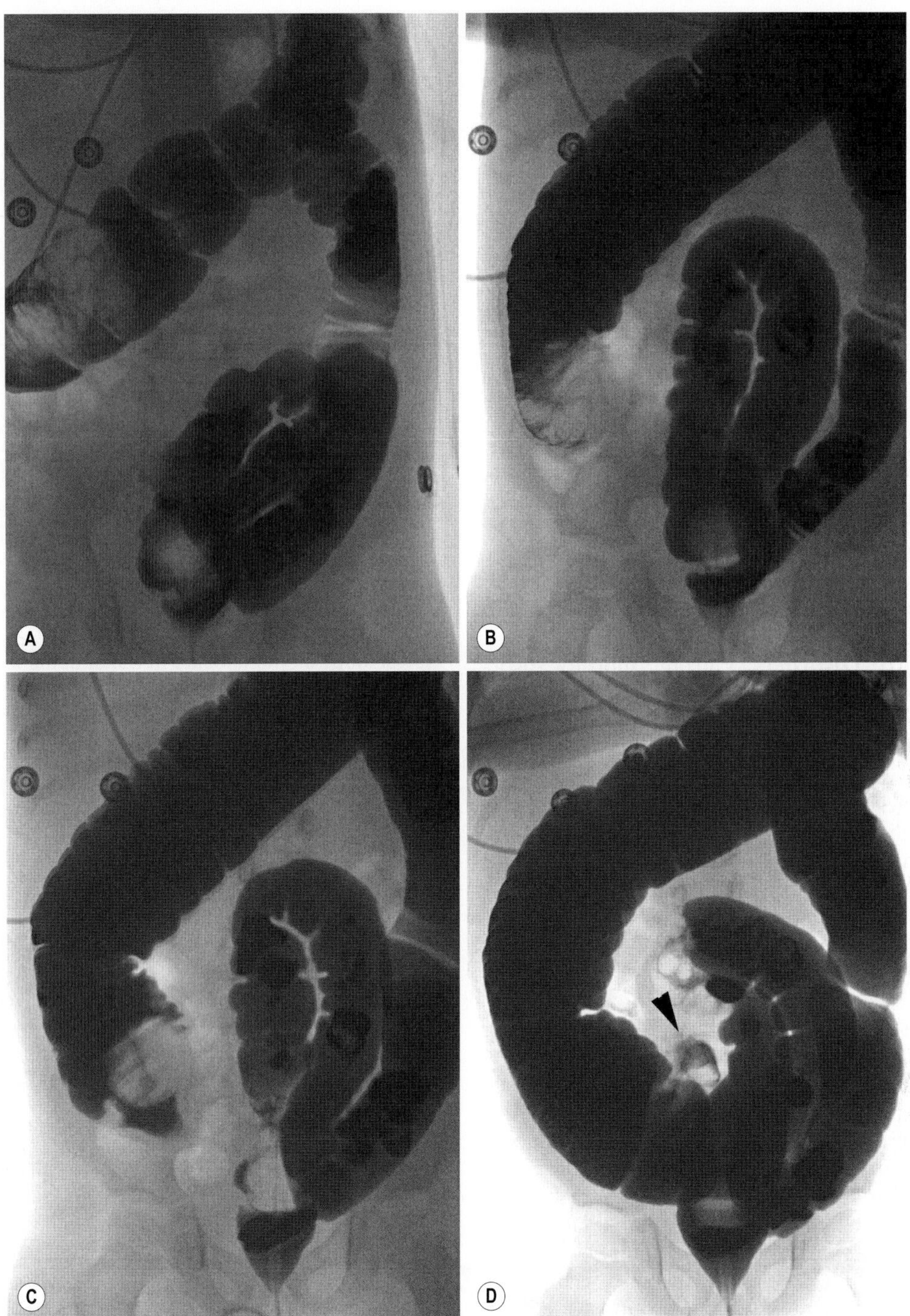

FIGURE 77-25 ■ Hydrographic reduction of intussusception. (A) Contrast defect in the proximal colon transversum due to the intussusceptum. (B) Further reduction of the intussusception into the colon ascendens. (C) Small contrast defect in the caecum. Normally the last part of the reduction is the most difficult due to oedema of the ileocaecal valve. (D) Contrast filling of the terminal ileum (arrowhead) as a sign of successful reduction. Proper filling of proximal small bowel loops is advised to ensure complete reduction.

Less than 5% of children with constipation have an underlying disease. The diagnosis of constipation is essentially clinically and radiological investigations play a very limited role in the work-up of constipation, and should not routinely be performed in children with functional constipation.[65] The plain abdominal radiograph will demonstrate the degree of faecal loading and dilatation of the large bowel; however, the presence of faecal loading on the plain radiograph does not necessarily indicate constipation, and several studies show that plain radiographs have a low sensitivity and specificity for diagnosing constipation.

Radiological investigations should only be performed in a carefully selected group of patients where an underlying cause is suspected. US should be the first imaging tool in chronic abdominal pain when radiological work-up is indicated. US gives a good overview of the bowel and intra-abdominal organs and can help differentiate a faecal mass from a pathological mass. Other imaging techniques described for the evaluation of constipation include the measurement of colonic transit time using radiopaque markers, fluoroscopy and MRI defecography. These are only indicated in highly selected cases.[66]

Intestinal Motility Disorders

'Intestinal motility disorder' is a term used to describe a variety of abnormalities that have, in common, reduced motility of the bowel and no organic occlusion of the bowel lumen. They can be divided into acute and chronic disorders.

Acute Dysmotility. Acute dysmotility includes paralytic ileus in which there is temporary cessation of peristalsis in the gut. This simulates intestinal obstruction, as there is failure of propagation of intestinal contents. Acute gastroenteritis can simulate small bowel obstruction by causing a local paralytic ileus, with dilatation of the affected segment of bowel and multiple fluid levels on an erect plain radiograph of the abdomen.

Chronic Motility Disorders. Chronic motility disorders include primary abnormalities of the bowel—Hirschsprung's disease (aganglionosis), hypoganglionosis which is rare and mimics Hirschsprung's disease, and neuronal intestinal dysplasia, which is a defect of autonomic neurogenesis characterised by an absent or rudimentary sympathetic ganglion innervation of the gut or by hyperplasia of cholinergic nerve fibres and hyperplasia of neuronal bodies in intramural nerve plexuses.

Chronic Intestinal Pseudo-obstruction. Chronic intestinal pseudo-obstruction (CIP) is rare and represents a spectrum of diseases that have in common clinical manifestations consisting of recurrent symptoms mimicking bowel obstruction over weeks or years. The age of presentation varies from the newborn to adulthood. The condition is due to a visceral neuropathy or myopathy, which can be familial or non-familial, resulting in a lack of coordinated intestinal motility. Megacystis–microcolon–intestinal hypoperistalsis syndrome is the most severe form of CIP and is usually fatal in the first year of life. Plain radiographs of the bowel will show loops of bowel with pronounced dilatation (Fig. 77-26). The diagnosis is made by intestinal manometry and biopsy. A contrast medium enema can exclude mechanical obstruction in children with acute symptoms.[67]

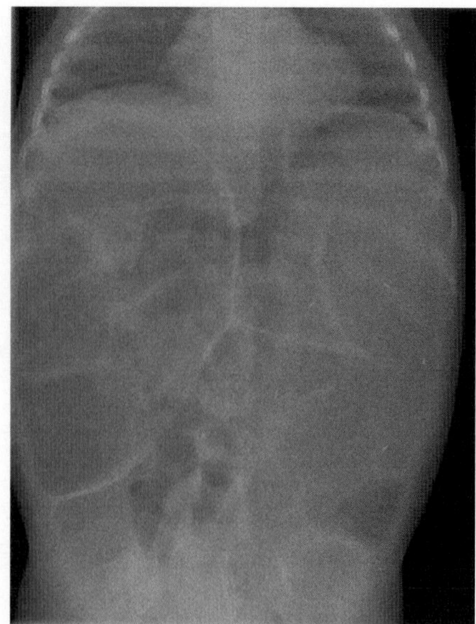

FIGURE 77-26 ■ **Chronic intestinal obstruction.** Multiple, hugely dilated bowel loops throughout the abdomen in a child with chronic intestinal pseudo-obstruction. (Small, dense pellets from intestinal transit time examination are seen within the bowel loops on the left side of the abdomen.)

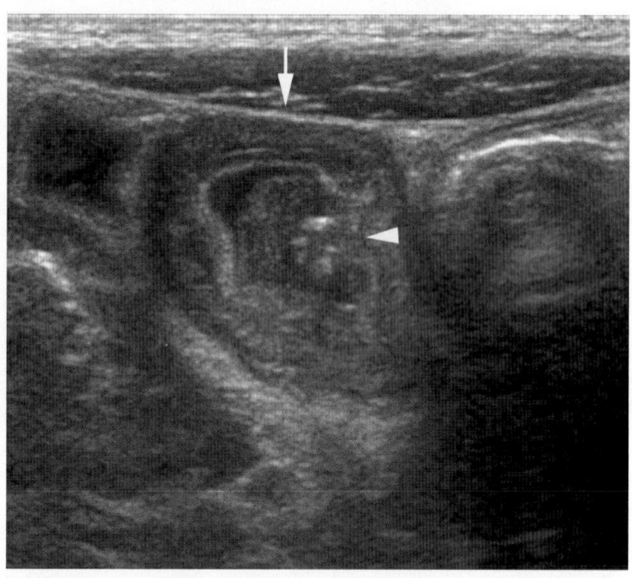

FIGURE 77-27 ■ **Henoch–Schönlein purpura.** Sonographic features of bowel wall thickening (arrow) due to intramural haemorrhage (arrowhead) in a child with Henoch-Schönlein purpura.

Henoch-Schönlein Purpura

Henoch-Schönlein purpura (HSP) is an acute, small vessel vasculitis that occurs almost exclusively in childhood. The manifestations are purpuric skin lesions (without thrombocytopenia), gastrointestinal manifestations, arthritis or nephritis. In most cases the changes of HSP are completely reversible and healing takes place in 3–4 weeks.[68]

Abdominal pain is a common symptom, and the GI involvement is caused by oedema, bleeding, ulceration and intussusception of the intestine. Ultrasound is the imaging technique of choice in HSP and will detect most surgical cases.[69] The sonographic features of HSP are uni- or multifocal thickening of the bowel wall accompanied by reduced peristalsis with normal or slightly dilated bowel loops between the thickened segments (Fig. 77-27).[70] Some patients have a small amount of intraperitoneal free fluid. Intussusception is easily seen on US, with a sensitivity of up to 100%.[61] Intussusceptions in HSP are most often ileoileal, hence not amenable to pneumatic or hydrostatic reduction. However, small bowel intussusception often reduces spontaneously. Ileocoloc intussusception may also occur and should be treated as idiopathic intussusception (see above). Radiographs may show signs of thickened bowel wall (Fig. 77-28) but are less sensitive to these changes than US.

Abdominal Distension

Enteric Duplication Cysts

Enteric duplication cysts are uncommon congenital anomalies and are due to abnormal canalisation of the GI tract. They can occur anywhere along the length of the gut but are most frequent in the ileum where they lie along the mesenteric border and share a common muscle wall blood supply. They have a mucosal lining and 43% contain ectopic gastric mucosa. The majority of duplication cysts do not communicate with the GI tract. Duplication cysts may be diagnosed antenatally. If small and non-obstructing, they may not cause any symptoms.

Clinically they usually present in the first year of life with vomiting or abdominal pain. Infection or haemorrhage into the cyst can cause it to enlarge and suddenly cause pain. A duplication cyst may act as a lead point of intussusception. An abdominal radiograph is useful to assess bowel obstruction or signs of bowel obstruction and may show displacement of bowel loops or even a soft-tissue mass; however, the cyst itself is normally not seen on plain radiographs (Fig. 77-29). US will demonstrate the cyst, which is usually spherical in shape and less often tubular. The cyst is typically anechoic but may have echogenic contents if there has been a bleeding into the cyst. The classical feature of an intestinal duplication cyst is the presence of bowel wall lining the cyst with an inner echogenic mucosal layer and an outer hypoechoic muscular layer (Fig. 77-30).[71] This 'double layer sign' on

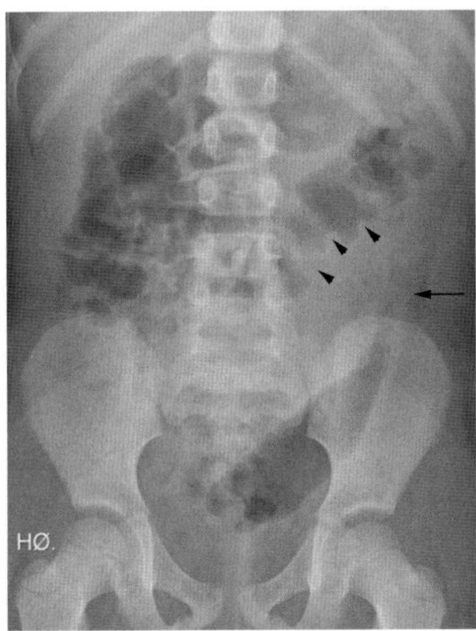

FIGURE 77-28 ■ Radiographic features of bowel wall thickening. 'Thumbprint' appearances of the transverse colon (arrowheads) and narrowing of the lumen (arrow).

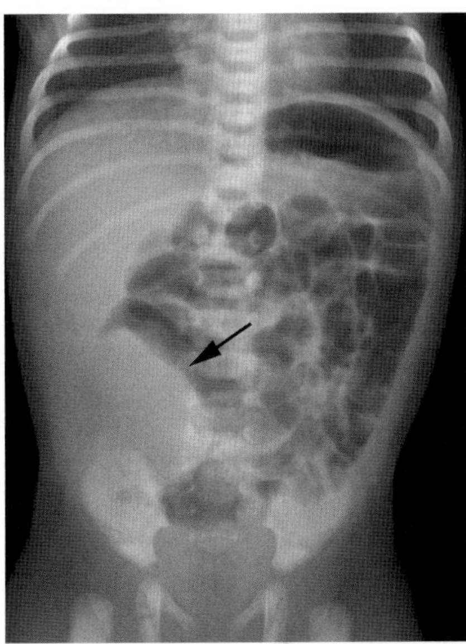

FIGURE 77-29 ■ Intestinal duplication cyst. The initial radiograph in a child with an intestinal duplication cyst showed a round soft-tissue mass on the right side of the abdomen (arrow) and slightly dilated bowel loops. The child presented with abdominal distension and increased regurgitation.

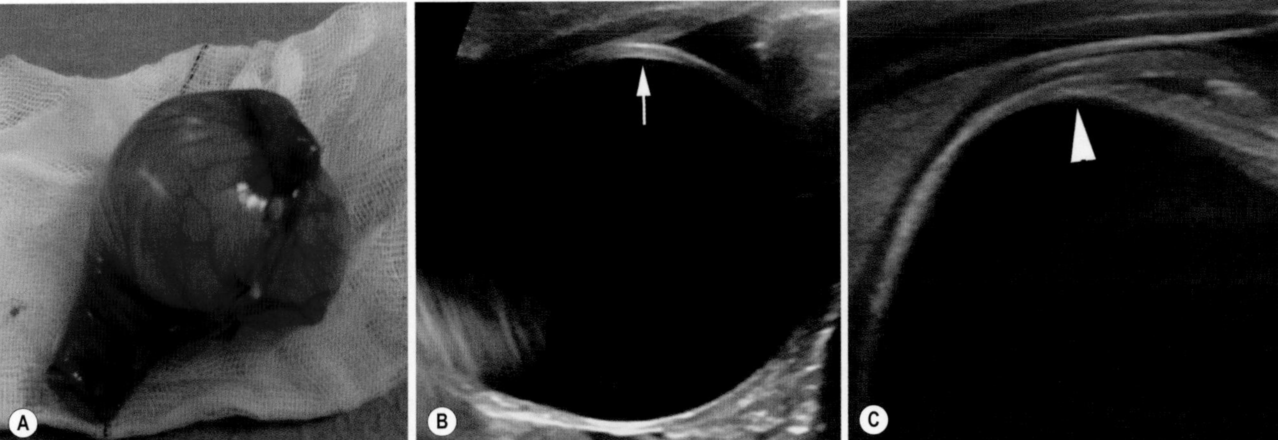

FIGURE 77-30 ■ Intestinal duplication cyst. (A) Pathological specimen of a resected duplication cyst. (B) Sonographic features of the duplication cyst showing an anechoic cyst with a 'double layer' sign of the cyst wall. (C) Magnified image of the cyst wall revealing multiple layers in keeping with an intestinal duplication cyst.

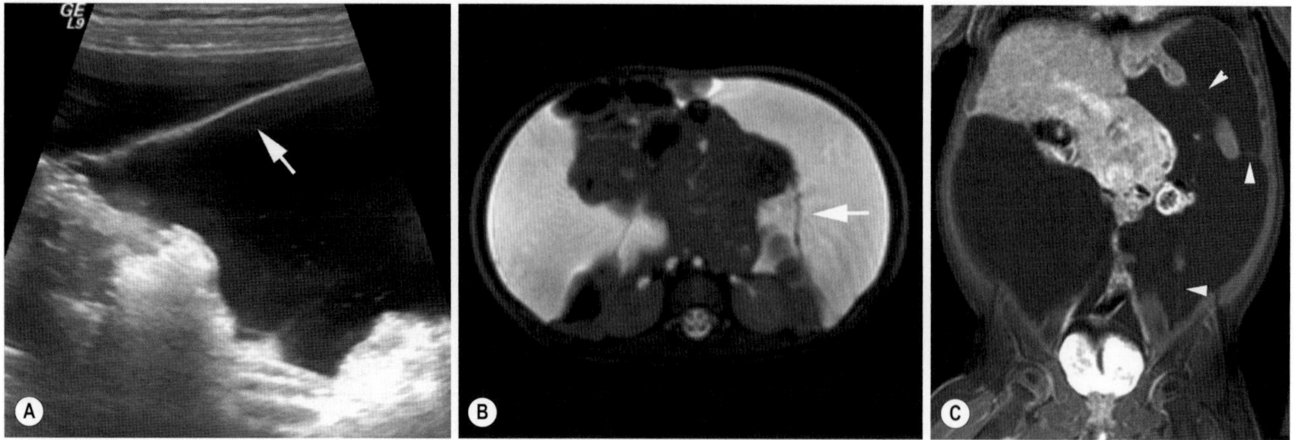

FIGURE 77-31 ■ Imaging characteristics of mesenteric lymphangioma. (A) Ultrasound of the abdomen shows a large, septated fluid-filled structure with debris. (B) T2W MRI shows a large, septated cystic mass, displacing the bowel cranially and towards the mid-abdomen. (C) T1W fat-saturated MRI after administration of intravenous contrast shows subtle enhancement of the intracystic septae.

US is characteristic for intestinal duplication cysts (Figs. 77-4 and 77-30B). However, the sonographic appearance of other intra-abdominal cysts may mimic the double layer sign. Therefore, thorough examination with a high-frequency transducer to identify the split hypoechoic muscularis propria layer (or all five layers of the cyst wall) increases the specificity in making the sonographic diagnosis of a true duplication cyst (Fig. 77-31C).[72] ^{99m}Tc-pertechnetate is taken up by ectopic gastric mucosa and is helpful in diagnosing duplication cysts presenting with gastrointestinal bleeding.[73]

Mesenteric Cysts

Mesenteric cysts (intra-abdominal lymphangioma) have been discussed in 'The Neonate' section. Pathologically there is lack of communication of small bowel or retroperitoneal lymphatic tissue with the main lymphatic vessels, resulting in formation of a cystic mass. They most often present in childhood and children are more likely to present acutely with pain, abdominal distension, fever or anorexia due to haemorrhage into the cyst, infection, or torsion. Large cysts may compress the ureters or lead to bowel obstruction.[74]

Plain abdominal radiographs show a soft-tissue mass, which displaces adjacent bowel loops. Occasionally the cyst wall is calcified. US examination demonstrates a thin-walled, uni- or multilocular cystic mass that may be adherent to the solid organs and bowel. The cyst wall consists of a single layer, which contrasts with the double-layered wall seen with enteric duplication cysts. If the intracystic fluid is chylous, infected, or haemorrhagic, then echogenic debris will be present. MRI or CT can more precisely define the anatomical margins of the cyst, but again, MRI is the preferred imaging method due to radiation protection. MRI can also characterise the cyst content, which will vary according to the cyst content.

Occasionally, large mesenteric lymphangiomas may be misinterpreted as septated ascites; however, the thin septae contain small vessels and may enhance following the administration of intravenous contrast material. Imaging with US, MRI or CT is sensitive to this diagnosis (Fig. 77-31).[75]

Non-bilious Vomiting

Vomiting is not a disease but a symptom that can be caused by numerous conditions, both gastrointestinal and extragastrointestinal (Table 77-7). Vomiting is the forceful ejection of gastric contents from the stomach up the oesophagus, and through the mouth, and is never physiological but the underlying condition may be harmless.

Gastro-oesophageal reflux is the backflow of undigested food from the stomach and up the oesophagus and is common in infants and children and may be normal up to 18 months of age. GOR can occur in healthy children without causing any symptoms. However, GOR may mimic or trigger vomiting. Radiological investigations should be performed when there are warning signals requiring investigation in infants with either GOR or vomiting, to rule out underlying causes that need treatment (Table 77-8).

Gastro-oesophageal Reflux Disease

GORD is present when the reflux of gastric contents causes troublesome symptoms and/or complications. Diagnosing GORD may be difficult, particularly in infants and young children. There is no agreed perfect method for detecting GORD but the diagnosis is usually made on the basis of questionnaires, 24 h pH monitoring and impedance measurements. Both ultrasound and fluoroscopy with contrast medium may show the presence of GOR, but radiological investigations play no role in establishing the diagnosis of GORD.

Barium contrast study of the upper gastrointestinal tract is useful to confirm or rule out anatomical abnormalities of the upper gastrointestinal tract in the presence of GORD, such as malrotation with intermittent volvulus or hiatus hernia (Fig. 77-32).[76]

TABLE 77-7 Causes of Vomiting in Children

***Obstructive Gastrointestinal Causes**
- Pyloric stenosis
- Malrotation with intermittent volvulous
- Intestinal duplication cyst
- Antral or duodenal web
- Severe constipation
- Foreign body
- Incarcerated hernia

***Non-obstructive Gastrointestinal Causes**
- Gastroenteritis
- Achalasia
- Gastroparesis
- Peptic ulcer
- Eosinophilic oesophagitis or gastritis
- Food allergy
- Inflammatory bowel disease
- Appendicitis or pancreatitis

***Neurological Disorders**
- Increased intracranial pressure
- Childhood migraine

***Infections**
- All infections in childhood may cause vomiting, particularly in the younger child

***Metabolic and Endocrine Disorders**

***Renal**
- Obstructive nephropathy
- Renal failure

***Cardiac**
- Heart failure
- Vascular rings

***Others**
- Munchausen syndrome by proxy
- Child neglect or abuse
- Self-induced vomiting
- Cyclic vomiting syndrome

TABLE 77-8 Warning Signals Requiring Investigation in Children with Regurgitation or Vomiting

- Bilious vomiting
- Gastrointestinal bleeding
- Consistently forceful vomiting
- Onset of vomiting after 6 months of life
- Failure to thrive
- Diarrhoea
- Severe constipation
- Fever
- Lethargy
- Hepatosplenomegaly
- Bulging fontanelle
- Macro-or microcephaly
- Seizures
- Abdominal tenderness or distension
- Documented or suspected genetic or metabolic disorder

Organoaxial Torsion and Gastric Volvulus

Sometimes, particularly in younger children, **organoaxial** torsion of the stomach may be the cause of forceful regurgitation or vomiting. The ligaments anchoring the stomach are dynamic to allow expansion. Absence of one or more ligaments and ligamentous laxity increase the risk of gastric volvulus. In **organoaxial** torsion, the stomach flips upward along its long axis and the gastrooesophageal junction and pylorus maintain their normal position. There is no risk of ischaemia; however, there may be full or partial obstruction of the gastric outlet. Gastric distension or gas-filled colon may predispose to this condition. A fluoroscopic barium study will reveal a distended stomach where the greater curvature is positioned superior to and to the right of the lesser curvature (Fig. 77-33). The condition is normal in infancy

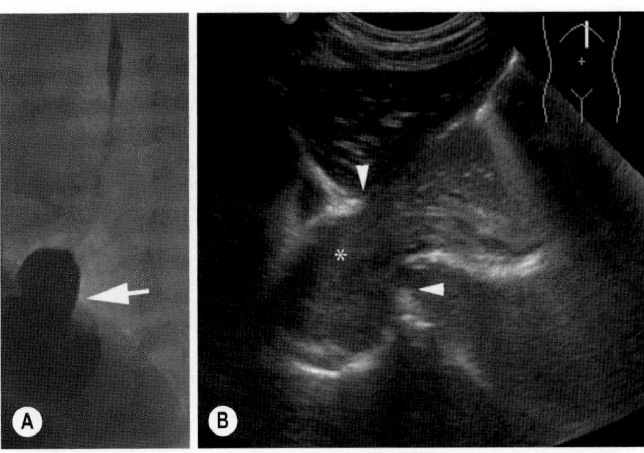

FIGURE 77-32 ■ Hiatus hernia can be diagnosed on ultrasound or an upper gastrointestinal contrast study. (A) Fluoroscopic image of a sliding hiatus hernia (arrow). (B) Sonographic appearance of the hiatus hernia with widening of the oesophageal hiatus (arrowheads) through which the stomach slides to protrude into the thoracic cavity (asterisk).

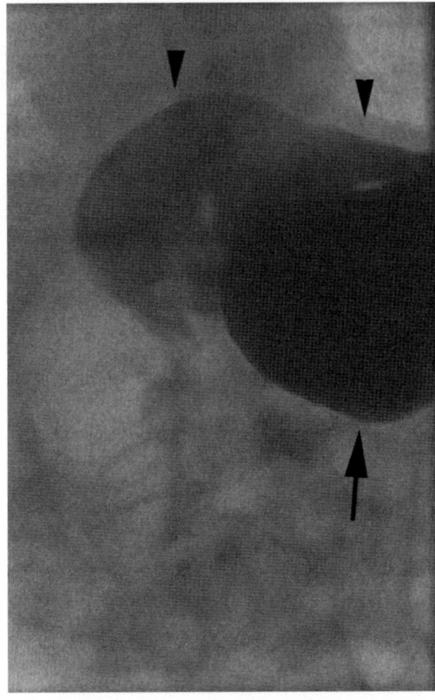

FIGURE 77-33 ■ Organoaxial torsion of the stomach. Fluoroscopic contrast study showing organoaxial torsion of the stomach. The greater curvature is in an inverse position (arrowheads) and the antrum of the stomach is flipped caudally (arrow).

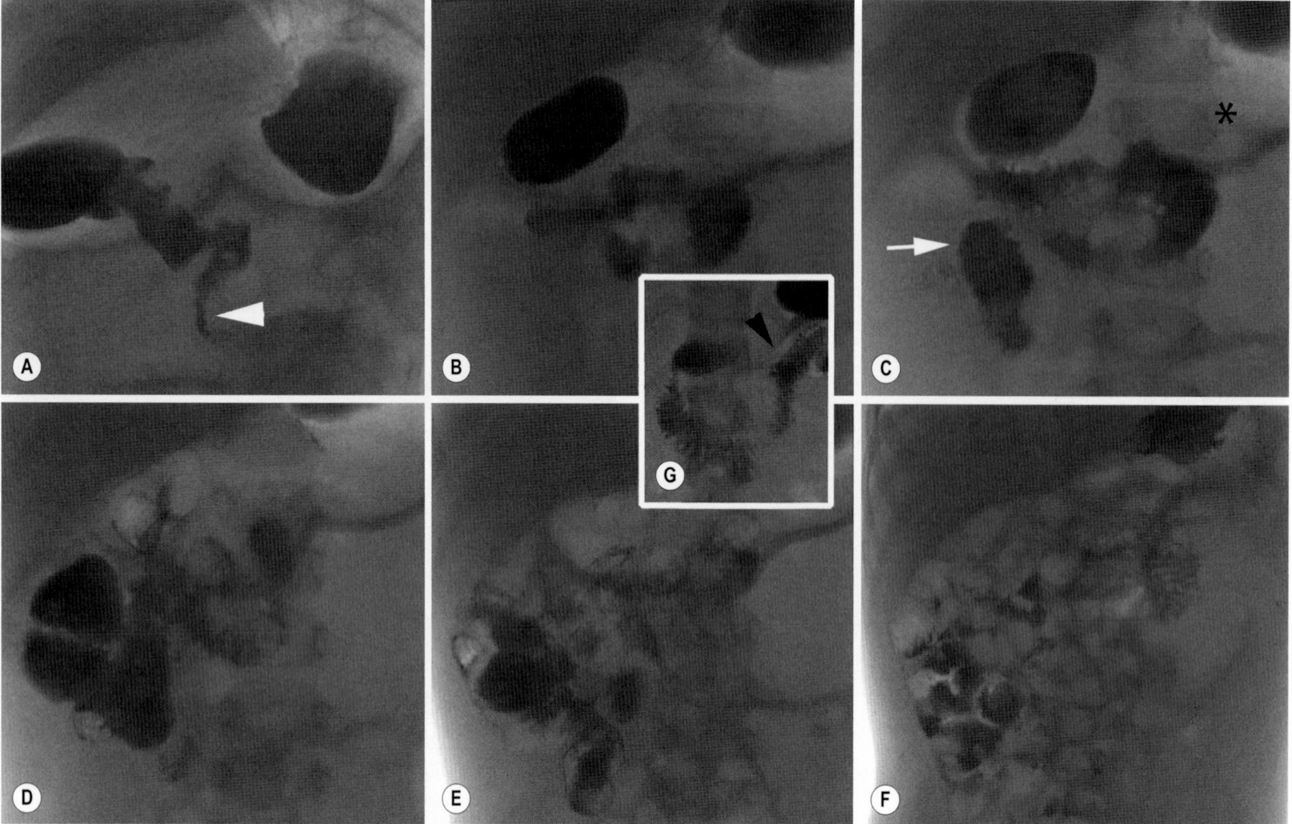

FIGURE 77-34 ■ (A–G) Malrotation without volvulus. An upper gastrointestinal contrast study performed in an 18-month-old girl with intermittent abdominal pain and failure to thrive. The initial, lateral image shows contrast passing to the D2, which turns caudally (arrowhead). Normally the DJF should be placed to the left of the spine, at the level of the duodenal bulb (asterisk). In this patient the duodenum did not have the normal U-shape and the DJF was located low, on the right side of the abdomen. Delayed images show the entire small intestine on the right side of the abdomen. The small image shows a normal, U-shaped duodenum with a normal DJF (arrowhead).

and can be seen as an incidental finding. In symptomatic older children gastropexia may be required.

Mesenteroaxial volulus is a rare entity where the stomach twists transversely around its mesenteric axis, causing close approximation of the gastro-oesophageal junction and pylorus. This is always a surgical emergency, causing gastric obstruction with high risk of ischaemia. The child presents acutely with vomiting and abdominal pain and distension.[77]

Malrotation with Chronic Intestinal Obstruction or Intermittent Volvulus

Malrotation with midgut volvulus is described in detail under 'The Neonate' section. It is, however, important to emphasise that even though symptomatic malrotation most frequently presents in the neonatal period with midgut volvulus, it may also occur in the older child with either acute or chronic symptoms.[78] The chronic presentation is a diagnostic challenge. The most common symptoms are crampy abdominal pain, failure to thrive, recurrent vomiting and signs of malabsorbtion. The symptoms may be non-specific and diagnostic delay is common. Pathophysiology of these chronic symptoms may relate to intestinal obstruction from Ladd's bands or from venous and lymphatic congestion in intermittent volvulus.[79] Surgical treatment is recommended in all patients, even when asymptomatic due to the lifelong risk of complications.[80] The diagnosis can normally be made from an upper gastrointestinal barium examination (Fig. 77-34) but is occasionally seen on cross-sectional imaging investigations for chronic abdominal complaints.

Hypertrophic Pyloric Stenosis

Hypertrophic pyloric stenosis (HPS) is the commonest surgical cause of vomiting in infants. It typically presents with projectile vomiting 2–8 weeks after birth. It is caused by hypertrophy of the pyloric muscle and mucosa with an elongated, narrow pyloric canal that fails to relax, which leads to gastric outlet obstruction. Boys are more frequently affected than girls, and there is a five-fold increased risk with a first-degree relative with this condition. The classic clinical presentation is a dehydrated, cachectic child with a palpable 'olive'-shaped mass in the upper abdomen. However, there has been a change in the epidemiology over the last decades and children are admitted to hospital before they get severe symptoms and so the 'olive' mass is seen in less than 30% of the patients.[81] Ultrasound is the first technique of choice when there is clinical suspicion of HPS, and has replaced barium studies in diagnosing this condition, with a

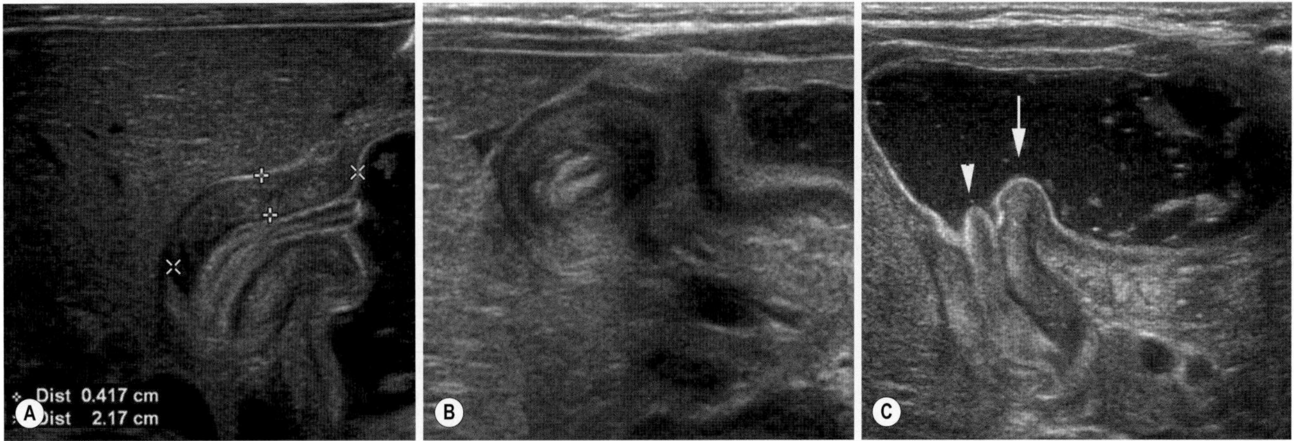

FIGURE 77-35 ■ Hypertrophic pyloric stenosis (HPS). Sonographic appearances diagnostic of HPS with an elongated and thickened pyloric muscle (A, B). A longitudinal image of the pyloric muscle shows the hypertropic mucosa (arrowhead) and the hypertropic muscle (arrow) protruding into the fluid-filled stomach (C).

reported sensitivity and specificity of up to 98 and 100%, respectively.[82] US allows assessment of the pyloric morphology and pyloric movement. The morphological features include a hypoechoic, thickened pyloric muscle, measuring more than 3 mm in transverse diameter and an elongated pyloric canal greater than 12 mm in length (Figs. 77-35A and B). The obstructed pyloric canal is lined with hypertrophic, hyperechoic mucosa. The hypertrophic muscle typically bulges into the antrum of a fluid-filled stomach, creating the so-called 'shoulder sign', and the double-layered hypertrophic mucosa protrudes into the stomach, creating the so-called 'nipple sign' (Fig. 77-35C). The sonographic appearance of the hypertrophied pylorus resembles that of the uterine cervix and is sometimes referred to as the 'cervix sign' (Fig. 77-35C). Abnormal, exaggerated peristaltic waves due to the stomach trying to force its contents past the narrowed pyloric outlet is also seen on real-time US. The treatment is surgical pyloromyotomy most often performed laparoscopically.[83]

Omphalomesenteric (Vitelline) Duct Remnants

The omphalomesenteric (vitelline) duct is a normal fetal structure that connects the midgut to the extraembryonic yolk sac. The omphalomesenteric duct usually involutes in the mid first trimester. Its persistence can give rise to a variety of congenital malformations. The majority of symptomatic omphalomesenteric ducts occur in boys and 60% of patients present before the age of 10. The clinical presentation depends on the exact underlying malformation.

Meckel's diverticulum is the most common end result of the spectrum of omphalomesenteric duct anomalies. Other presentations include umbilicoileal fistula, umbilical sinus and umbilical cyst. There may also be a fibrous cord running from the ileum to the umbilicus. Small bowel obstruction from this cord is the most common cause of ileus in otherwise healthy children and adolescents. Rarely, the entire duct remains patent. The symptoms present in the neonatal period with discharge of faeces from the umbilicus, or the ileum can prolapse onto the anterior abdominal wall.

Meckel's Diverticulum

The most common type of omphalomesenteric duct remnant is the Meckel's diverticulum, which arises on the antimesenteric border of the ileum. This contrasts with the enteric duplication cysts that are located on the mesenteric border of the small bowel. The diverticulum is present in 2–4% of the population. The size of Meckel's diverticula varies, with those greater than 5 cm in length being considered 'giant'. Most are located within 60 cm of the ileocaecal junction. All the layers of the intestine are contained within their walls and frequently contain islands of gastric and/or pancreatic mucosa. The most common presentations are melaena caused by hemorrhage from peptic ulceration, and ileus due to intussusception or volvulus around a Meckel's diverticulum. Meckel's diverticula may also become entrapped within an inguinal hernia, which has become known as Littre's hernia. Patients may present with abdominal pain, and occasionally peritonitis caused by diverticulitis or perforation. The diagnosis of Meckel's diverticulum is difficult to establish preoperatively and the investigations should be tailored by the clinical presentation. The Meckel's diverticula that haemorrhage contain ectopic gastric mucosa in 95% of cases and ^{99m}Tc-pertechnetate scintigraphy can be diagnostic. Plain radiographs can diagnose the presence of ileus and occasionally a soft-tissue mass may be seen (Fig. 77-36); however, the diagnosis is most often made intraoperatively. Occationally, enteroliths may be seen as peripheral calcifications with radiolucent centres. This is the most specific feature for Meckel's diverticulum on plain radiographs. An ultrasound is often performed if the clinical situation allows for further investigation. The diverticulum itself may not be identified on US; however, abscess formation and signs of inflammation with hyperechoic mesenteric fat may be seen in acute diverticulitis. Intussusception caused by a Meckels's diverticulum will also be identified with US. CT is occasionally performed in the evaluation of intestinal obstruction or peritonitis; however, the diverticulum itself is most often difficult to identify. Conventional barium studies may be useful in patients with chronic, persistent symptoms and negative cross-sectional or nuclear imaging. The characteristic feature of a Meckel's diverticulum is a saccular, blind-ending pouch on the antimesenteric border of the ileum with a triradiate fold pattern converging with the ileum. Neoplasms arising in Meckel's diverticula are very rare and do not occur in childhood.[84]

Gastrointestinal Malignancies

Primary gastrointestinal tumours are rare in childhood. Colorectal cancer or gastrointestinal stromal tumours (GIST) may occasionally be seen in children but are most often part of a syndrome. Lymphomas account for 10–15% of all childhood cancers. Extranodal involvement is frequently seen in non-Hodgkin's lymphoma (NHL) and more frequently seen in children compared to adults. The gastrointestinal tract is the most common site of manifestation. The distal ileum, caecum, appendix and ascending colon are most commonly affected and the involvement may be multifocal (Fig. 77-37). There is marked bowel wall thickening with stenosis or dilatation of the affected segment. The lymphomatous infiltrate is hypoechoic on ultrasound and shows soft-tissue attenuation with sparse contrast enhancement on CT or MRI, and diffusion-weighted sequences show restricted diffusion (Fig. 77-38). In contrast to inflammatory causes of bowel wall thickening, loss of stratification appears early in lymphomatous involvement of the bowel wall. Mesenteric and retroperitoneal lymph node involvement may be seen in both Hodgkin's lymphoma (HL) and NHL. Ascites is commonly seen. The spleen is frequently involved in both HL and NHL. Liver involvement rarely occurs without splenic involvement and is most commonly seen in NHL. The imaging findings in diffuse lymphomatous involvement of the liver and spleen are non-specific. On both MRI and US the parenchyma may be normal or show a hazy, salt-and-pepper appearance. There may or may not be hepatosplenomegaly.[85]

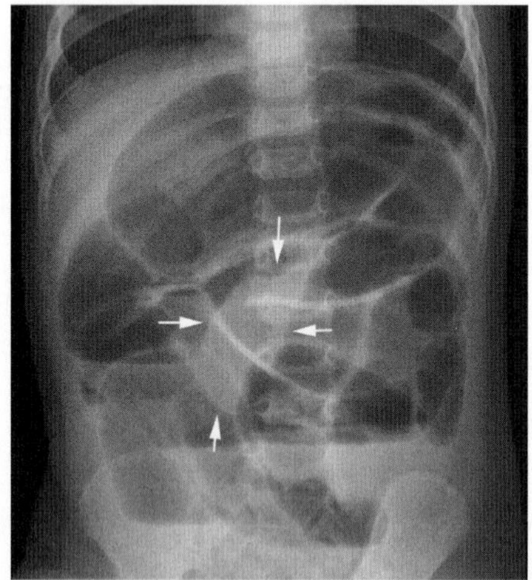

FIGURE 77-36 ■ Meckel's diverticulum. Abdominal radiograph of a 2-year-old boy with acute abdominal pain and clinical signs of peritonitis. The image shows dilated bowel loops and gas–fluid levels suggestive of mechanical ileus. Meckel's diverticulum can be seen as a saccular soft-tissue shadow in the mid-abdomen (arrows).

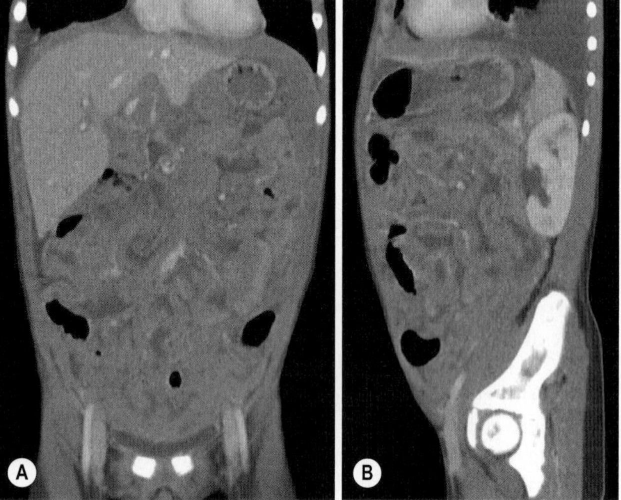

FIGURE 77-37 ■ Small bowel lymphoma (A, B). A coronal and sagittal reformatted contrast-enhanced abdominal CT examination of a 12-year-old boy with non-Hodgkin's lymphoma, presenting with abdominal pain, showing multifocal thickening of the intestinal wall and ascites. Pleural effusion is also present.

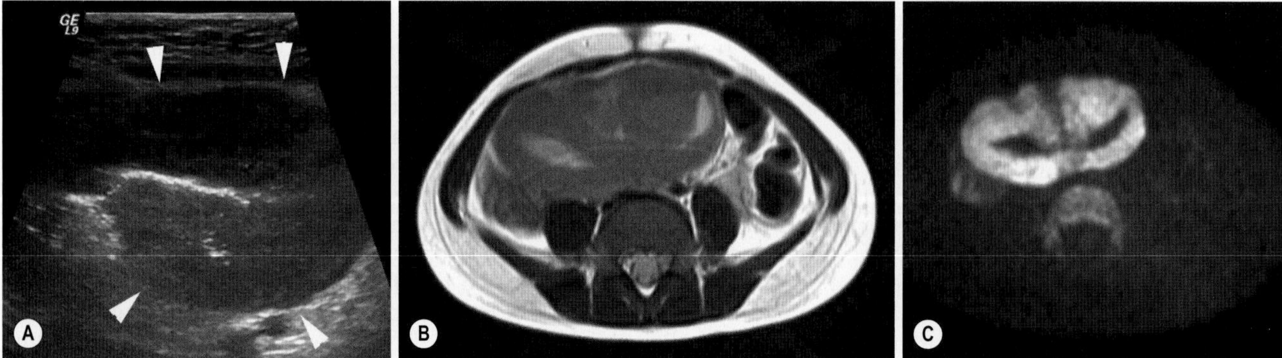

FIGURE 77-38 ■ Focal lymphomatous involvement of the small bowel. (A) Ultrasound revealed a very thick, hypoechoic bowel wall with loss of normal stratification (arrowheads). MRI of the same patient showed a slightly dilated loop of bowel with marked bowel wall thickening, which returned an intermediate signal on a T2W image (B) and a high signal on a diffusion-weighted image in keeping with restricted diffusion (C).

THE IMMUNOCOMPROMISED CHILD

Various abdominal complications can be encountered in young cancer patients following chemotherapy. They often present with diffuse abdominal complaints but may also be asymptomatic. The most common abdominal complications of chemotherapy in childhood are listed in Table 77-9. Some of the entities are rare, and some are specific for children undergoing chemotherapy. It is therefore important to recognise the signs of these complications to improve patient's outcome.

Gallstones, sludge or crystals may be seen as an incidental finding and may be related to the specific drug used or to prolonged illness. The findings may disappear spontaneously. Cholelcystitis may occur as a complication of cholelithiasis; however, acalculous cholecystitis is more commonly seen. The gall bladder is best evaluated with US using the high-frequency linear transducer. Gallstones are freely moving, hyperechoic objects with posterior shadowing within the gall bladder (Fig. 77-39). Sludge is seen as a hyperechoic, liquid material and crystals or sludge balls may resemble gallstones but without posterior shadowing. Acalculous cholecystitis is diagnosed by the presence of a clinically painful gall bladder, and US showing wall oedema with or without overdistension of the gall bladder.

TABLE 77-9 Abdominal Complications of Chemotherapy in Childhood

***Gall bladder**
- Sludge or sludge balls
- Stones
- Acalculous cholecystitis

***Liver**
- Steatosis
- Siderosis
- Veno-occlusive disease

***Typhilitis**

***Pancreatitis**

***Fungal Oesophagitis**

Liver steatosis is a common finding, particularly in children undergoing treatment for acute lymphatic leukaemia. The steatosis may be focal or diffuse. It is important to differentiate liver fatty infiltration from diffuse leukaemic liver infiltration. Focal liver steatosis will follow a typical distribution with hyperechogenic areas on US, due to fat deposition around the main branches of porta hepatis. Steatosis is easily diagnosed on MRI, where there will be loss of signal on the opposed-phase images relative to the in-phase images on proton shift sequences.[86]

Liver fibrosis and siderosis may also occur as a consequence of treatment for childhood malignancies. In both liver fibrosis and siderosis the liver will be hyperechoic relative to the kidney. Siderosis is caused by heamosiderine deposition within the liver, which, due to the ferromagnetic effect of haemosiderin, will return low signal on both T1 and T2 sequences.

Veno-occlusive disease is a rare entity but a severe complication related to chemotherapy with indirect, non-specific findings on imaging. It affects the small hepatic vessels and sinusoids, leading to high resistance within the liver and, importantly, thrombi within the large vessels are not seen. On imaging there may be hepatomegaly, periportal oedema, reversed portal venous flow, high RI within the hepatic artery and ascites. The diagnosis is made by biopsy.

Typhilitis is an opportunistic infection of the bowel caused by the patient's own intestinal flora. It typically occurs in a neutropenic patient and most often affects the terminal ileum and caecum, but may be seen in any part of the bowel. It presents as bowel wall thickening, with or without dilatation of the proximal bowel. Ultrasound is the technique of choice to diagnose and follow up patients with typhilitis but CT may be used in an acute

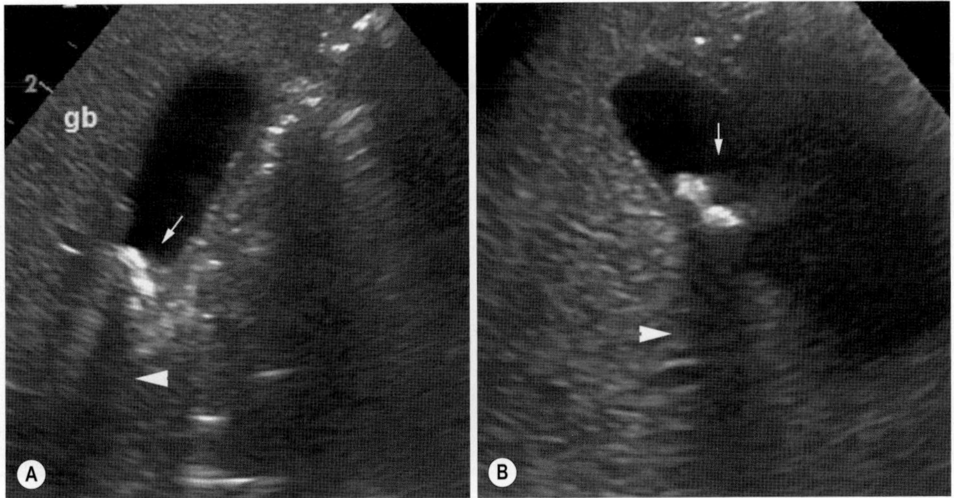

FIGURE 77-39 ■ **Gallstones.** Abdominal ultrasound of a 1-year-old child on chemotherapy for leukaemia, (A) in the supine position and (B) in the decubitus position, revealed two hyperechoic, mobile, round structures (arrows) with posterior shadowing (arrowheads) in keeping with gallstones.

setting to rule out other entities like pneumatosis intestinalis and bowel perforation.[87]

Gastrointestinal Manifestations of Acquired Immune Deficiency Syndrome

Opportunistic infections account for most of the GI tract manifestations of acquired immune deficiency syndrome (AIDS) in children.

Primary lymphoma and Kaposi's sarcoma occur in the adult GI tract but are relatively rare in human immunodeficiency virus (HIV)-infected children. The most common symptoms include acute or chronic diarrhoea, failure to thrive, oesophagitis due to *Candida* invasion, and, less often, cytomegalovirus (CMV) or herpes simplex virus. Imaging is usually not required.[88] Abdominal lymphadenopathy is common in paediatric AIDS and can be idiopathic (where no causative agent is found). Infection, Kaposi's sarcoma and lymphoma also cause lymph node enlargement. Lympadenopathy is the most common finding in intra-abdominal manifestations of tuberculosis in children. US is useful in the evaluation of abdominal lymphadenopathy.[89] Cross-sectional imaging may be required to evaluate the extent of the abdominal disease and potential solid organ involvement.

ABDOMINAL MANIFESTATIONS OF CYSTIC FIBROSIS

The gastrointestinal manifestations of cystic fibrosis (CF) are primarily caused by the abnormal viscous luminal secretions within hollow viscera, and the excretory ducts of solid organs. Abdominal complications of cystic fibrosis can present at any age from neonates to adolescence. The first manifestation of CF may be meconium ileus, which presents in the neonatal period (see 'The Neonate' section). An equivalent to meconium ileus, appearing later in life, is the distal intestinal obstruction syndrome (DIOS). Plain radiographs will reveal faecal impaction in the distal small ileum and right colon with various degrees of proximal small bowel dilatation (Fig. 77-40). Intussusception occurs in 1% of all patients with CF and may manifest as recurrent abdominal pain. Intussusception is diagnosed with US (see above) and is most often ileocolic. Symptomatic small bowel intussusception that necessitates surgery occurs more frequently in children with cystic fibrosis[90] (Fig. 77-41). Fibrosing colonopathy is related to the use of pancreatic enzyme replacement therapy and is also seen more frequently in children with DIOS. A fluoroscopic barium enema study will reveal multiple colonic strictures and irregularities of the colonic mucosa. Enlargement of the appendix is seen in most

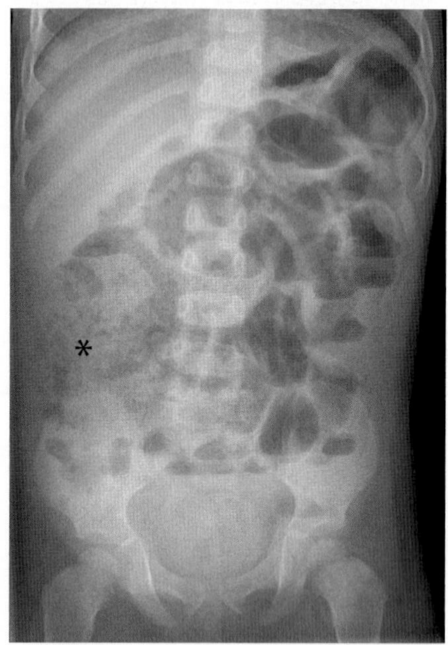

FIGURE 77-40 ■ Distal intestinal obstruction syndrome (DIOS) in a 2-year-old child with cystic fibrosis, presenting with abdominal pain. The plain abdominal radiograph shows faecal impaction (asterisk) in the distal small bowel and proximal colon with dilated small bowel proximal to the obstruction.

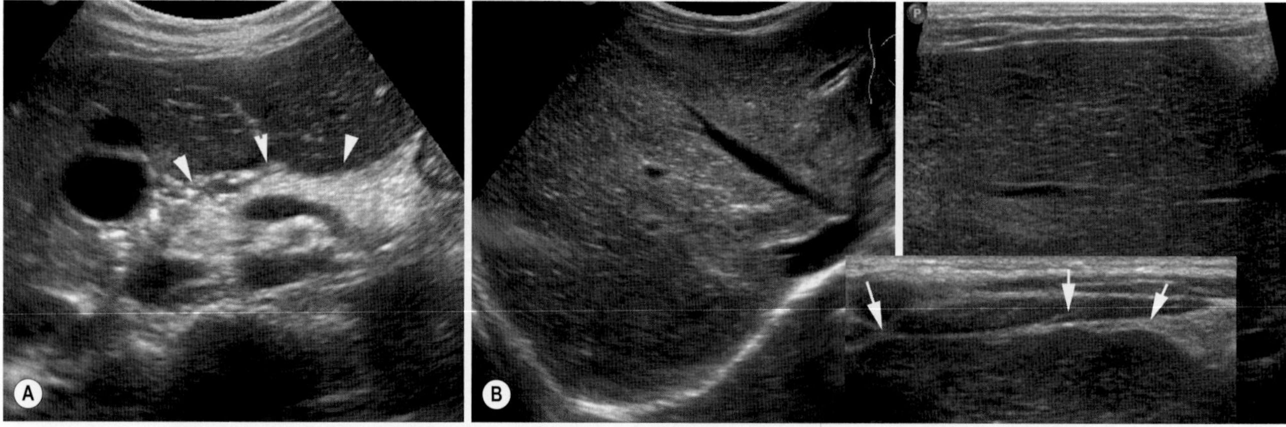

FIGURE 77-41 ■ Sonographic findings in cystic fibrosis. (A) A hyperechoic, small pancreas (arrowheads) is a frequent finding in patients with cystic fibrosis and pancreatic insufficiency. Sonographic findings in cystic fibrosis liver disease include increased echogenicity due to fatty infiltration (B). Careful examination with a high-frequency linear transduser may reveal coarse echogenicity (B) and nodular surface of the liver (small image, arrows) as early signs of cirrhossis.

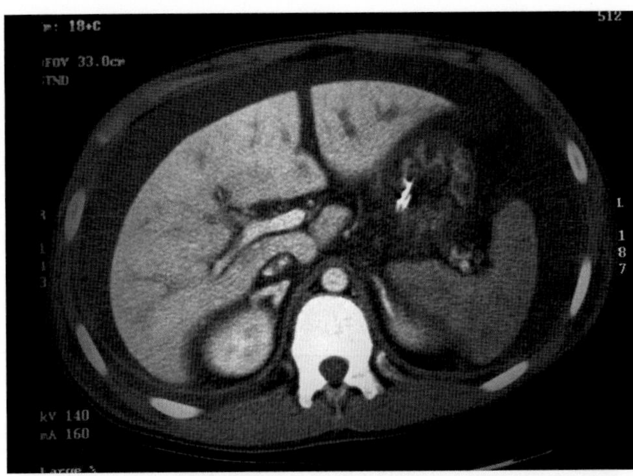

FIGURE 77-42 ■ **Hypoperfusion complex.** Axial CT showing periportal low attenuation, small IVC, diminished and patchy enhancement of the spleen, intense enhancement of the adrenal glands and kidneys and a haemoperitoneum.

asymptomatic patients with CF. This is caused by intraluminal mucus stagnation. US will show an increased diameter of the appendix but without thickening of the appendiceal wall and there is absence of periappendiceal inflammation. Appendicitis occurs less frequently in patients with CF. The symptoms are often misinterpreted as DIOS or masked due to the use of antibiotics. The diagnostic delay leads to increased risk of complications.[91] Exocrine pancreatic insufficiency is seen in up to 95% of children with CF at 1 year of age. The most common findings are fatty replacement or fibrosis; hence the imaging findings vary from a large, lobulated pancreas with fatty infiltration to a small fibrotic panceas. Pancreatic cysts are also a frequent finding as a result of obstructed exocrine ducts. Pancreatic cystosis, where the pancreas is completely replaced by cysts, may be seen. Hepatobiliary involvement is also common in CF and ranges from asymptomatic gallstones to biliary cirrhosis. Hepatosteatosis is the most common abnormality of the liver parenchyma.[92]

ABDOMINAL TRAUMA

Blunt abdominal trauma accounts for 80% of traumatic injuries in childhood. Computed tomography is the imaging method of choice in the evaluation of abdominal and pelvic injury after blunt trauma in haemodynamically stable children. CT classification systems for grading intra-abdominal injuries apply to children as well as adults; however, children are more often treated conservatively. Ultrasound may play a role in follow-up of abdominal trauma, and the application of intravenous ultrasound contrast enhances the sensitivity and specificity of organ injuries and ongoing haemmorhage. Plain radiographs have low sensitivity in detecting intra-abdominal injuries, but may reveal free intraperitoneal gas; however, when bowel perforation is suspected, CT is the technique of choice.

Multi-phase CT should be avoided in children due to the high radiation burden. The morphological characteristics of the paediatric abdomen, abdominal wall and rib cage may lead to different injuries following blunt trauma than normally seen in adults.

The liver is the most commonly affected viscus in blunt trauma in children, followed by splenic injuries. The kidneys are often affected and injuries to the vessels or collecting system typically result from deceleration, because the kidneys in children have greater laxity than in adults.

Bowel injuries and pancreatic injuries are rare in children but can be seen due to compression of the rib cage against the spine. Another mechanism for pancreatic and bowel injury in children is the direct impact from a bicycle handlebar to the abdomen. Associated rib fractures may not always be seen due to the high elasticity of the growing skeleton. Lap-belt ecchymoses represent an important high-risk marker for injury, particularly to the lumbar spine, bowel and bladder.[93] Young children have a relatively high centre of gravity, which produces shearing forces by the seat belt.

The **hypoperfusion complex** or shock bowel is due to poorly compensated hypovolaemic shock, which results in dilated, fluid-filled loops of bowel, and is a more frequent finding in children than adults. On CT there is intense contrast enhancement of the bowel wall mucosa and thickening of the bowel wall. The major abdominal blood vessels and kidneys also show intense enhancement, and the calibre of the aorta and inferior vena cava are reduced. Enhancement of the spleen and pancreas is decreased due to splanchnic vasoconstriction (Fig. 77-42).[94] Always be aware of the possibility of non-accidental injury (NAI) in children with abdominal trauma. NAI is described in Chapter 80, 'Paediatric Musculoskeletal Trauma: The Radiology of Non-accidental and Accidental Injury'.

LIVER

Imaging Techniques

US

Grey-scale US allows detailed assessment of the liver parenchyma provided that every section is imaged systematically[95,96] and a high-frequency linear probe is used. The linear probe is particularly helpful for evaluation of the liver surface (e.g. undulations seen in cirrhosis), small parenchymal focal lesions (e.g. small fungal foci (Fig. 77-43), small or diffuse metastases) and diffuse parenchymal processes (e.g. congenital hepatic fibrosis (Fig. 77-44). A curved or vector probe is helpful for assessing the deeper liver in older children. Lower-frequency probes may be necessary if there is dense hepatic fibrosis.

Colour Doppler is mandatory and is used to assess the hepatic and portal veins and the hepatic artery, the presence of collateral vessels (e.g. cavernoma following extrahepatic portal vein occlusion or recanalisation of fetal veins in portal vein hypertension) and varices. Pulsed-wave Doppler is routinely used to evaluate flow in the portal vein. When traces are difficult to obtain in the moving child, colour Doppler will at least establish

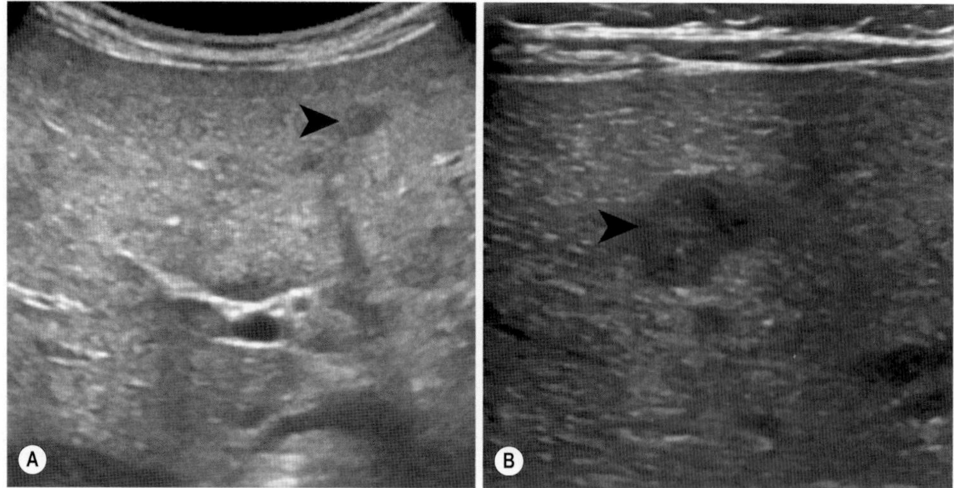

FIGURE 77-43 ■ **US in a neutropenic child with spiking temperature.** (A) The focal fungal lesion (arrowhead) in the liver is easily missed with a low-frequency (5–2 MHz) curvilinear transducer. (B) The lesion (arrowhead) is more conspicuous with a high-frequency (9.5 MHz) linear transducer.

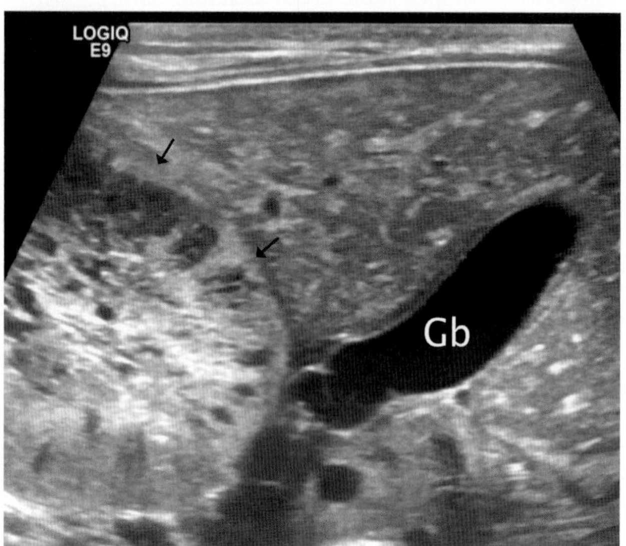

FIGURE 77-44 ■ **US in an infant with congenital hepatic fibrosis shows lace-like hyperechoic bands throughout the liver.** There is associated polycystic kidney disease. Arrows, enlarged polycystic right kidney; Gb, gall bladder.

the flow direction. Twinkling (artefact) seen on colour Doppler is useful to detect calcifications, gallstones and bile duct hamartomas. The sensitivity increases when the focal zone is set deep to the abnormality and with higher colour write priority.[95] Microbubble-based intravenous US contrast media are thought to increase the diagnostic accuracy of US, but are currently only used off-label.[96]

MRI

Provided adequate preparation, MRI allows high-resolution (submillimetre, isotropic) high-contrast imaging of the liver. Respiratory gating is used whenever possible. Useful pulse sequences include short tau inversion recovery (STIR) fast spin-ech, volumetric T2-weighted spin-echo with variable refocusing pulse flip-angle (CUBE, SPACE, VISTA), in-phase and opposed-phase spoiled gradient-echo, diffusion-weighted imaging and T1-weighted gradient-echo before and after intravenous administration of contrast medium (possibly with several post-contrast acquisitions, as in adults to detect, for example, centripetal enhancement in infantile haemangioma and rapid washout in neoplasms).

Non-contrast-enhanced angiographic techniques include selective inversion followed by balanced steady-state free-precession acquisition (NATIVE, TRANCE, FBI). This technique depends on inflow of fresh spins, and may therefore require several acquisitions with varying placement of the inversion volume. The technique is promising for portal venography.

Hepatocyte-specific contrast agents are promising for detection of small lesions and lesion characterisation, and for functional assessment of biliary drainage, but are currently restricted to off-label use (Fig. 77-45).[97,98]

CT

CT should be restricted in children (1) due to its generally poor soft-tissue contrast, (2) because paucity of body-fat in young children hampers identification of tissue planes and (3) for radiation protection. If used, protocols need to be in place to minimise the radiation dose. No pre-contrast run and only one post-contrast run is indicated—with very few exceptions.

Angiography

Angiography is very rarely indicated for diagnosis and, as such, is only performed in specialist centres.

Imaging Anatomy

The neonatal liver is hypoechoic to the kidneys. This reverses during infancy. The umbilical vein and the ductus venosus are patent in the premature and early newborn (< 48 h), and in two-thirds up to 1 week of age.

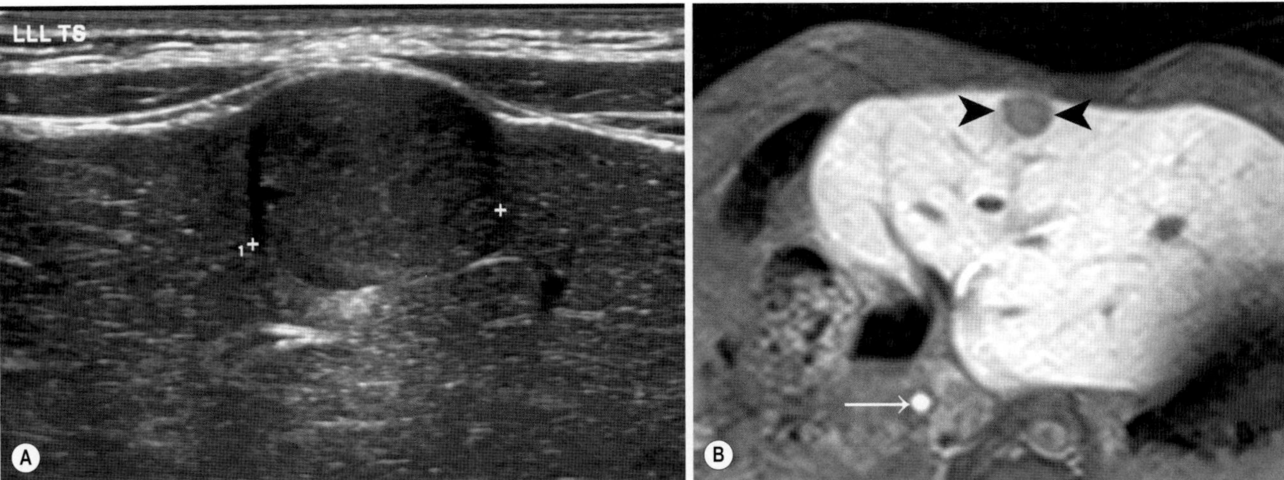

FIGURE 77-45 ■ Imaging in a 3-year-old with Beckwith–Wiedemann syndrome and previously resected hepatoblastoma. (A) During off-treatment surveillance, a 15-mm subcapsular nodule (between markers) is seen with high-frequency US in the left lobe of the liver. (B) Axial spoiled gradient-echo MRI 20 min following intravenous injection of gadoxetic acid (a hepatocyte-specific contrast agent) demonstrates normal enhancement of surrounding liver, but no enhancement in the nodule (arrowheads). Recurrent hepatoblastoma was therefore suspected, and confirmed histopathologically. Note contrast material in the common bile duct (arrow).

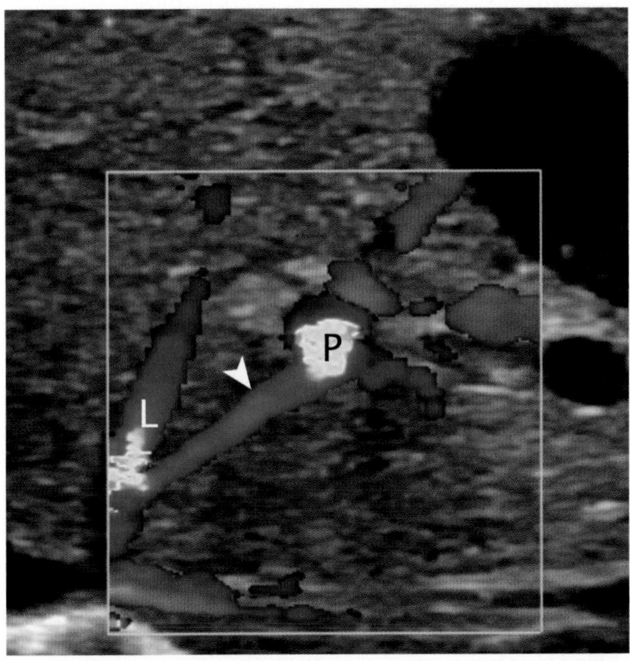

FIGURE 77-46 ■ Duplex Doppler sonography in a neonate demonstrates a patent ductus venosus (arrowhead) between the portal vein (P) and the left hepatic vein (L) just distal to the inferior vena cava. Anatomical variation is common in this fetal umbilicosystemic shunt.

TABLE 77-10 **Suggested Upper Limit of Normal Sonographic Measurement of Liver Size in Children**[83]

Age (months)	Suggested Upper Limit for the Longitudinal Dimension (mm) of the Right Lobe of the Liver in the Midclavicular Sagittal Plane
1–3	90
4–6	95
7–9	100
12–30	105
36–59	115
60–83	125
84–107	130
108–131	135
132–179	140
180–200	145

The limits are based on an ethnically homogeneous material. Considerable intra- and inter-observer variation need to be accounted for.

Patency beyond 2–3 weeks is abnormal. The ductus venosus is seen as a vascular channel between the left portal branch and the left hepatic vein/inferior vena cava (Fig. 77-46). There is considerable variation in the size of normal livers, and measurements are difficult to standardise. Uncritical application of reference measurements is therefore not advised; however, Table 77-10 gives an idea of the upper limit of normal. Portal vein sonographic diameter after 1–3 h of fasting in the supine position was found to range in mm (age group): 3–5 (at birth), 4–8 (1 year), 6–8 (5 years), 6–9 (10 years), 7–11 (15 years).[99] Similar findings were done in a more recent cohort, supine, after at least 2-h fasting, where the 5–95 centiles in mm (age group) were 3.0–6.4 (0–12 months), 4.3–8.3 (1–5 years) and 5.0–10.8 (5–10 years).[100]

Liver Involvement in Congenital Malformation and Infections, Syndromes and Systemic Conditions

Right cardiac isomerisms are associated with two right lobes of the liver, left isomerisms with midline liver and preduodenal portal vein and with biliary and splenic abnormalities (see the sections 'Biliary System' and 'Spleen').[101] Congenital infections (*Toxoplasma*, rubella,

CMV, herpes virus and other) may involve the liver: hepatosplenomegaly, focal calcifications. One differential diagnosis is Aicardi–Goutières syndrome. Periportal hyperechogenicity is non-specific and commonly seen in response to systemic inflammation, and abdominal inflammation in particular.

Non-obstructive Jaundice

Non-obstructive jaundice may be caused by increased production of bilirubin, insufficient conjugation, transport, excretion and/or drainage. All these factors may contribute to physiological jaundice in the neonate with an immature liver. Only prolonged jaundice (beyond 2 weeks) without a clear cause (neonatal hepatitis, haemolytic conditions, sepsis, etc.) requires imaging investigation in the neonate. (Idiopathic) neonatal hepatitis is an increasingly obsolete terms for non-obstructive causes of jaundice,[102] and it follows that the sonographic manifestations are highly variable, e.g. with hyperechoic liver parenchyma and poor visualisation of peripheral portal branches.[103] Severe hepatitis with poor biliary excretion may lead to a small gall bladder and may therefore be confused with biliary atresia (see the section 'Biliary System').

In childhood, the differential is wide and includes metabolic disease (e.g. glycogen storage disorders, Wilson's disease, tyrosinaemia, alpha-1-antitrypsin deficiency) and cystic fibrosis.

The role of imaging is limited in hepatitis: findings are non-specific. However, follow-up to detect and quantify secondary fibrosis (see the section 'Chronic Liver Disease') may be useful.

Infection

Imaging has a more well-defined role in focal infection for detection, image-guided drainage and assessment of treatment response. Estimated globally, liver abscesses in children are most frequently pyogenic (80%; most commonly caused by *Staphylococcus aureus*) and amoebal (most frequently *Entamoeba histolytica*). Fungal causes (often multifocal and involving the spleen) are most likely in the immunocompromised child.[104] US with a high-frequency linear probe is mandatory in febrile neutropaenia since the clinical and laboratory diagnosis is more difficult due to the poor immune response (Fig. 77-43). Repeat US is indicated if the cause remains occult.

In chronic granulomatous disease, the child is susceptible to catalase-positive infections (*Staphylococcus aureus*, fungi and other) and responds with formation of granulomata rather than typical abscesses. It follows that imaging findings are heterogeneous on a spectrum from multilocular to homogeneous, solid (enhancing) lesions, solitary or multifocal, of highly variable size. Calcification is a common sequela post-resolution of acute infection.[105]

Parasitic infections (e.g. *Echinococcus* sp.) are endemic in many parts of the world, and imaging findings are similar to those in adults. Tuberculous infections of the liver are rare.

Chronic Liver Disease

Cirrhosis

Hepatic cirrhosis is advanced fibrosis with anatomical distortion that causes hepatocyte dysfunction. In children, cirrhosis, due to increased intrahepatic vascular resistance, is the leading cause of portal hypertension. As in adults, cirrhosis predisposes for hepatocellular carcinoma. The most common cause of cirrhosis in children is cholestasis, which may be due to biliary anomalies (biliary atresia, persistent intrahepatic cholestasis), cystic fibrosis or long-term total parenteral nutrition.[106–108] Other causes of cirrhosis are necrosis (neonatal, viral and autoimmune hepatitis) and constitutional metabolic disease (e.g. Wilson's disease, alpha-1 antitrypsin deficiency, tyrosinaemia). Non-alcoholic fatty liver disease as a cause of cirrhosis is on the increase in developed countries.[109,110]

Cirrhosis is suggested by typical appearances of a hyperechoic, nodular parenchyma and an undulating surface, atrophy of the right lobe, hypertrophy of the caudate and left lobes, widening of the fissures and of the gall bladder fossa. Doppler investigation of the portal vein is an important part of the investigation (see 'Portal Vein' section).

Imaging is important in surveillance for malignant transformation to hepatocellular carcinoma. US is the primary imaging technique, but is limited to detecting growth of individual nodules, which may be challenging.

MRI has higher, albeit not perfect, accuracy. Regenerative nodules are similar to normal liver on T1- and T2-weighted sequences, opposed-phase sequences and following contrast administration. The steatotic nodule may disclose itself by a high fat concentration, i.e. relatively higher signal intensity on T1- and T2-weighted images, low in opposed phase.

The siderotic nodule has relatively low signal intensity on all sequences due to iron deposition. The hallmark of dysplastic nodules and hepatocellular carcinoma are high signal intensity of T2-weighted images, marked enhancement in the arterial phase following intravenous administration of contrast medium, and rapid washout.[111]

Hepatocyte-specific MRI contrast agents are not licensed for use in children, but there is mounting evidence for their contribution to increasing the diagnostic accuracy for focal lesions, including in cirrhosis (Fig. 77-45).[97,98]

Fibrosis

Non-invasive grading of fibrosis remains difficult. Quantification has been explored by observation of the propagation of mechanical waves (shear-wave velocity) in tissues and subsequent estimation of tissue stiffness (elastography). The feasibility in children has been shown with stand-alone devices and integrated with grey-scale US.[112] Although elastography distinguishes normal and fibrotic liver, there is significant overlap among the intermediate stages of fibrosis.[113] Elastography by MRI has been described in children (using a reduced drive power in children younger than 1 year).[114] However, there are still no normal references for children, so accurate data are not available.

All techniques require standardisation, since several factors other than fibrosis influence liver stiffness, e.g. degree of hydration, postprandial portal flow.

Non-alcoholic Fatty Liver Disease (NAFLD)

In the developed world NAFLD is now one of the most frequent indications for referral for chronic liver disease in children and young people and evidence suggests it is associated with progressive liver disease and cirrhosis.[115] The course from simple steatosis to non-alcoholic steatohepatitis (NASH), possibly via fibrosis to cirrhosis, is poorly understood. Grading of hepatic steatosis is accurate using signal loss in opposed-phase MRI as a severity measurement.[116] The method is also feasible in children, and the range for hepatic fat fraction in obese children without NAFLD was up to 4.7% in one study.[117]

Fibropolycystic Liver Disease

Fibropolycystic liver disease is a spectrum of overlapping phenotypes caused by ductal plate developmental abnormalities. There is variable association with polycystic kidney disease. Secondary cirrhosis is rare. More common complications include portal hypertension, cholangitis and mass effect. Manifestation generally progresses from the peripheral to the central liver. Entities include the following.

Congenital hepatic fibrosis manifests as periportal fibrosis, biliary dysplasia and autosomal recessive polycystic kidney disease (Fig. 77-44). Both the hepatic and renal involvement are variable.[111] US may show mild dilatation of hilar bile ducts. Hepatopetal collateral veins without extrahepatic portal vein occlusion is seen in one-third of affected children.[118] There may be hepatic artery widening and regenerative nodules.

Autosomal dominant polycystic disease was considered 'adult-type' polycystic disease but is now recognised in children, who are often asymptomatic. The liver is usually enlarged and diffusely involved with heterogeneous cysts. Complications are rare in children, but may include infection and rupture of cysts, bleeding and mass effect. Secondary portal hypertension is rare.

Choledochal malformations (see the section 'Biliary System') overlap with fibropolycystic liver disease, in particular in Caroli's syndrome (type 5 choledochal malformation) where there is congenital hepatic fibrosis.

In **hepatoportal sclerosis** US may show a hyperechoic zone (representing fibrosis) surrounding the portal veins with a hypoechoic zone separating it from normal-appearing liver.[119] This entity may have alternative presentation with hepatic nodules.[111]

Biliary hamartomas are uniform cystic lesions < 15 mm in diameter with thin rim enhancement.[120] These may be seen on US and MRI, and are sometimes incidental findings. The entity has not been comprehensively described in children.

Suprahepatic Chronic Liver Disease

Venous stasis is the common denominator for this group, which includes congestive heart failure. Specific entities include the following.

Veno-occlusive disease is associated with antineoplastic therapy and myeloablation. There are no recognised specific imaging findings. However, the severity is correlated with degree of splenomegaly, ascites and flow in the paraumbilical vein and with signs of portal hypertension.[121]

Budd–Chiari syndrome is hepatic venous obstruction due to thrombosis of hepatic veins or of the inferior vena cava. It may be constitutional (primary, associated with myeloproliferative disease) or secondary (hepatic neoplasms and infections). Thrombus is demonstrated on US and Doppler in the acute phase, whereas obliterated veins, reversed flow and collaterals are seen in chronic phase.[111] On CT and MRI there may be heterogeneous arborating enhancement in portal venous phase following contrast medium administration.

Portal Vein

Portosystemic Shunts

Congenital extrahepatic portosystemic shunts, total (type 1) and partial (type 2), are rare.[122] Shunting is to the inferior vena cava, renal vein, iliac veins or azygos system. Establishing the type is important for surgery: total shunts should not be ligated as they represent the sole mesenteric venous return. Several associated congenital anomalies are recognised (e.g. cardiac, gastrointestinal, genitourinary, vascular).[123] Other congenital abnormalities include hypoplasia and atresia, absence of a portal branch and intrahepatic developmental connections between portal and hepatic veins.

Portosystemic shunts are clinically important to recognise since untreated they may cause pulmonary hypertension, hepatopulmonary syndrome and hepatic encephalopathy. US with Doppler is the first technique of choice, with CT or MRI angiography, and catheter portovenography reserved for special cases and for preoperative planning.

Extrahepatic Portal Vein Occlusion

Acquired extrahepatic portal vein occlusion is more common and is, after cirrhosis, the second most common cause of portal hypertension in children. Known causes are umbilical venous catheter, abdominal infection, inflammation, trauma, surgery and neoplasms (hepatoblastoma and hepatocellular carcinoma). The liver is often functionally normal (depending on aetiology), but may be small. The primary finding is cavernous transformation at the porta hepatis and associated signs of portal hypertension.

Portal Hypertension

Slow portal venous flow (< 15–18 mm/s) and loss of respiratory pulsatility suggests portal hypertension, but these findings are unreliable in extrahepatic portal vein occlusion if there is a rich collateral network.[124] US, MRI and CT may all demonstrate varicose veins and aneurysmal dilatations. There is hepatofugal flow with engorged veins in the lesser omentum, at the spleen and gastro-oesophageal junction, recanalised or non-obliterated umbilical vein and/or ductus venosus (Fig. 77-46), and splenomegaly. There is low or absent portovenous flow and high hepatic artery flow.[111] Thickening of the lesser omentum (sagittal sonogram at the level of the coeliac origin) to more that 1.7 times the diameter of the aorta may be seen but it is a non-specific sign.[125]

Portal Venous Gas

US is the most sensitive technique for detecting portal venous gas, seen as hyperechoic dots flowing with the portal blood. When visible on radiographs (or CT) it may be easier to recognise its arborating pattern to within a few centimetres of the hepatic capsule. This is different from biliary gas, which usually collects centrally.[126] The gas may originate from bowel lumen (obstruction), bowel wall (ischaemia or pneumatosis), intra-abdominal abscesses or from gas-forming organisms in the portal venous system itself.

Necrotising enterocolitis is the most common cause in neonates, the gas bubbling from the pneumatotic bowel wall into mesenteric veins. Portal venous gas seen on radiographs is associated with a higher frequency of operative intervention, but not with mortality from necrotising enterocolitis.[127]

Portal venous gas beyond the early stage following liver transplant in children may suggest developing intestinal lymphoproliferative disease.[128]

Preduodenal Portal Vein

There are many case reports of a preduodenal portal vein as an incidental finding or as a cause of duodenal obstruction. It seems associated with other developmental abnormalities, such as the heterotaxia syndromes.

Mass Lesions

Primary liver tumours are rare in children. Before 3 years of age the most common entities are vascular neoplasms, hepatoblastoma, teratoma, rhabdoid tumour and mesenchymal hamartoma; however, primary liver tumours are very rarely malignant in the first few months of life. After 3 years of age the diagnostic distribution becomes increasingly similar to that in adults. Hepatocellular carcinoma occurs, and is associated with cirrhosis. Only lesions that are specific to children are described here.

Imaging Features

Ossification may be seen in teratomas and hepatocellular carcinomas. Fatty content is almost pathognomonic of teratomas. A solid mass with cyst-like low attenuation on CT and/or high signal intensity on T2-weighted MRI suggests undifferentiated sarcoma.[129] Calcification is not a useful discriminator as it is seen in hepatoblastoma, hepatocellular carcinoma, rapidly involuting congenital haemangiona, teratoma and infection.[130]

Hepatoblastoma (Fig. 77-47)

Hepatoblastoma is very uncommon in the first few months of life and after 3 years of age. Known associations include Beckwith–Wiedemann syndrome and biliary atresia. The diagnosis is suggested when there is thrombocytosis and raised serum alpha-fetoprotein (AFP) for age (raised AFP is also associated with the rarer yolk sac tumour). Final diagnosis (tissue) and staging need to be performed in a specialist environment. Staging is based on the number of adjoining liver sections free from tumour, venous encasement/invasion, rupture and metastases.[131] Metastases are most commonly to the lungs, so chest CT is part of the staging procedure.

Vascular Neoplasms

Infantile haemangioma of the liver is similar to those in other locations (e.g. skin) and is associated with multiple skin haemangiomas.[132] Lesions have low vascular resistance and therefore high flow velocities on pulsed-wave

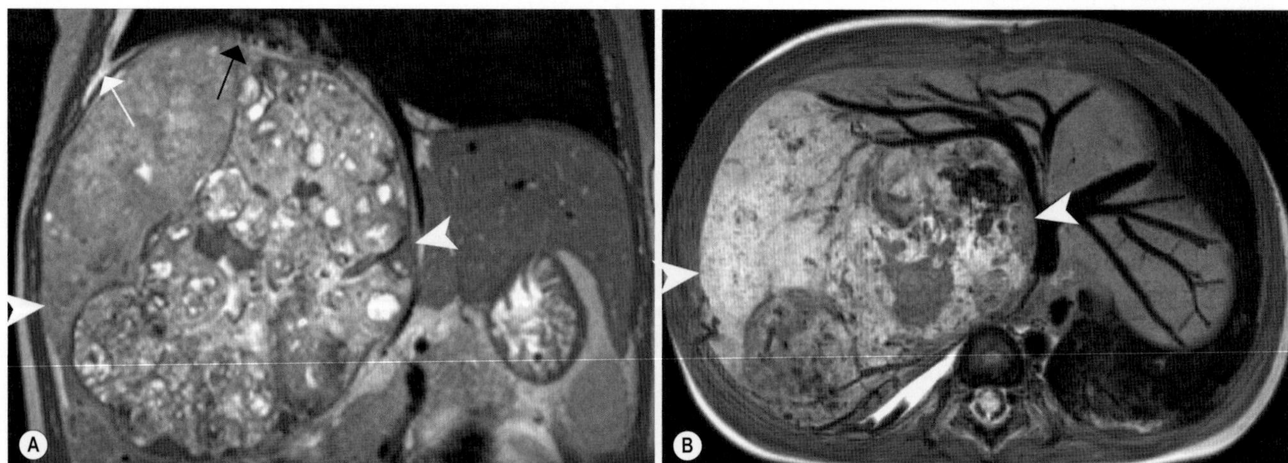

FIGURE 77-47 ■ MRI in a 2-year-old with a hepatoblastoma shows a large, heterogeneous mass (arrowheads) in the right lobe of the liver. (A) Coronal reconstruction of volumetric T2-weighted spin-echo. Note the infiltration of the right hemidiaphragm (black arrow) and the secondary pleural fluid (white arrow). (B) Thick-slab minimum intensity projection in the axial plane of the same sequence demonstrates the relation between tumour and the hepatic veins, the basis for local staging in hepatoblastoma.

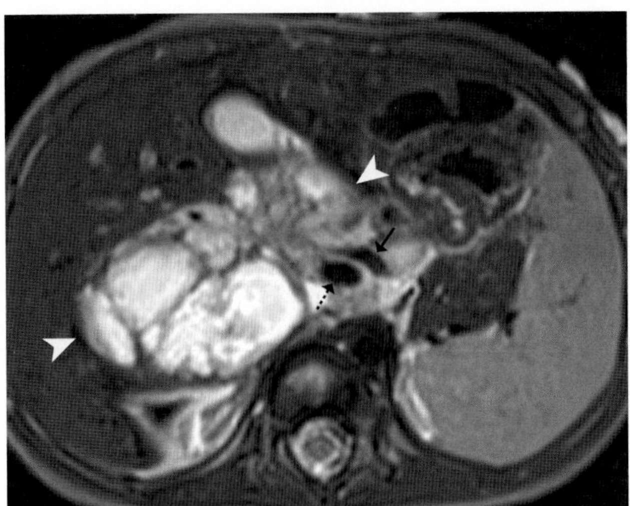

FIGURE 77-48 ■ MRI in a 2-month-old with a partly exophytic liver mass. T2-weighted MRI shows the heterogeneous lesion (arrowheads) with large hyperintense components corresponding to cystic spaces. Tumour encases the inferior vena cava (dashed arrow) and the portal vein (arrow). Mesenchymal hamartoma was established following biopsy. Along with infantile haemangioma and hepatoblastoma, this is one of the top differential diagnoses for a solitary liver tumour in a child younger than 3 years.

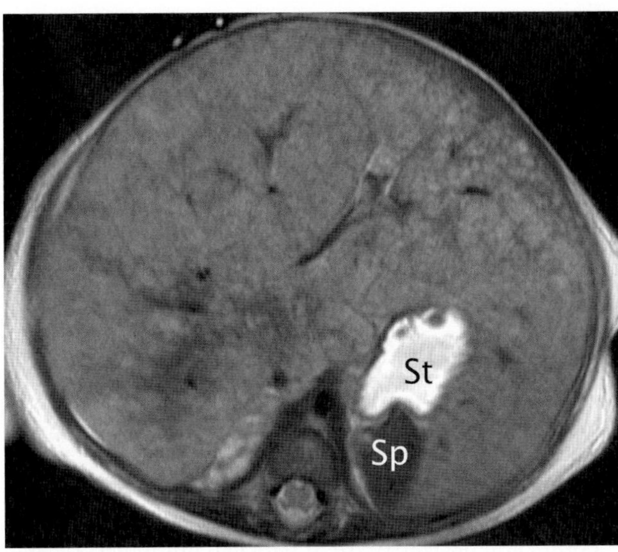

FIGURE 77-49 ■ Axial T2-weighted MRI in an infant with metastatic neuroblastoma shows diffuse infiltration of the liver, which has enlarged to hug the spleen (Sp) and stomach (St).

Doppler,[133] and even arteriovenous shunting. The flow dynamics explain the association with high-output heart failure. On repeated MRI after gadolinium administration there is typically centripetal enhancement. All techniques should demonstrate a non-infiltrating lesion without perilesional oedema.[134]

Congenital haemangiomas are similar on imaging to infantile haemangiomas but may specifically demonstrate vascular aneurysms and thrombosis.[134] The subgroup of rapidly involuting congenital haemangioma (RICH) may present thick, irregular rim enhancement on CT and MRI.[135] These usually involute completely by 14 months of age, as opposed to non-involution congenital haemangioma (NICH).

Mesenchymal Hamartoma (Fig. 77-48)

The majority of children with mesenchymal hamartoma present clinically before the age of 2 years with a palpable mass. Imaging demonstrates variable a mixed cystic/solid mass, which may be very large. Solid may be seen in the youngest. Multifocal variants are known.

Liver Metastases and Other Multifocal Lesions

Liver metastases in children are most frequently from neuroblastoma (Fig. 77-49), lymphoproliferative disease, nephroblastoma and sarcomas. Differentials for multifocal liver lesions include multifocal vascular neoplasm, infection, regenerating nodules, focal nodular hyperplasia, angiomyolipoma, fibropolycystic disease and peliosis hepatis.

Trauma

CT has higher sensitivity than US for liver lacerations.[136] The liver is the most commonly injured organ (particularly the right lobe) in paediatric abdominal trauma due to the soft rib cage. Liver injury accounts for about half of deaths caused by abdominal trauma in children.[137] In children, particularly in the youngest, non-accidental (inflicted) injury needs to be remembered as a possible differential diagnosis. There are no pathognomonic signs. However, the left lobe of the liver is thought most commonly injured due to compression against the spine during a direct impact.[138] (See also the section 'Trauma' under 'Spleen'.)

Transplant

It is important to detect signs of infarction, rejection, post-transplantation lymphoproliferative disorder (PTLD), and vascular and biliary complications.[139] PTLD is frequent in childhood recipients at 9–14%.[140] Apart from typical findings of lymphoproliferation, gas in the portal vein has been suggested a sign of PTLD following liver transplantation.[128] Biliary complications are common (around one-quarter of liver transplantations), and usually present in the first 3 months after transplantation as leakage, stenosis, gallstones, sludge, biloma or infection.

Arterial stenosis or thrombosis occurs in about one-fifth of children. At colour Doppler there is high flow velocity and turbulence across a stenosis, and parvus tardus distally. Portal vein complications are seen in fewer than one-tenth. Significant narrowing may be defined as a reduction of the lumen to less than 50%, but one needs to account for possible differences in vascular calibres due to size mismatch between donor and recipient.

BILIARY SYSTEM

Imaging Techniques

US is the first technique of choice for investigating the biliary system. It may even depict the intrapancreatic portion and the ampulla of Vater. However, for complete biliary anatomy, MR cholangiopancreatography (MRCP) is indicated. Rather than thick-slab multi-direction techniques, volumetric heavily T2-weighted spin-echo images are preferred as they have exquisite resolution and allow multiplanar post-processing. Functional MRI of biliary drainage with a hepatocyte-specific contrast agent has been shown feasible and is promising, e.g. in diagnosis of biliary atresia; however, it is not yet licensed for clinical use in children.[97]

Specific radioisotope imaging in children is performed when there is suspicion of biliary atresia (see 'Jaundice' section), and derivatives of Tc-labelled iminodiacetic acid (IDA) are used. These are actively taken up and excreted by hepatocytes. Infants younger than 2 months with biliary atresia typically have prompt hepatic extraction, no visualisation of a gall bladder, prolonged hepatic tracer retention and no intestinal excretion of tracer.

Imaging Anatomy

The suggested upper limit of normal for the common bile duct diameter is about 2 mm in infants, 4 mm in children and 7 mm in adolescents; the gall bladder length should be at least 1.5 cm in neonates.[141,142]

Jaundice

Jaundice may be caused by increased haemoglobin breakdown (e.g. haemolytic disorders), poor liver function (e.g. immature liver, hepatitis) and/or poor excretion or drainage (e.g. atresia, obstruction). Jaundice is therefore physiological in the newborn due to increased breakdown and an immature liver. However, jaundice beyond 2 weeks is suspicious for liver disease.[143] Of infants with surgical jaundice, about 80% have biliary atresia, and most of the remaining have inspissated bile syndrome or choledochal malformation.[144] Important differential diagnostic imaging findings are summarised in Table 77-11.

Biliary Atresia (Fig. 77-50)

Biliary atresia has an incidence of 1 in 8000–18,000 live births (more common in East and South-East Asia) and is the most common cause of childhood liver transplant.[102] There may be atresia of the common bile duct (type I), common hepatic duct (type II) or intrahepatic ducts (type III), rarely of the cystic duct. A subgroup has an associated cyst at the porta hepatis and may be sonographically similar to choledochal malformation.[145] Importantly, atresia does not cause biliary dilatation or sludge as opposed to choledochal malformations. The main differential diagnoses in a jaundiced infant without biliary dilatation or sludge are neonatal hepatitis and persistent intrahepatic cholestasis. Associated abnormalities (in about one-fifth) include congenital heart disease, preduodenal portal vein, polysplenia, situs inversus and absent

TABLE 77-11 **Important, but not Comprehensive, Imaging Differential Diagnosis in Infantile Jaundice**

Imaging Finding	Biliary Dilatation	Normal Gall Bladder	Hyperechoic Structure at the Porta Hepatis (Triangular Cord)	Biliary Drainage on Radioisotope Scan
Neonatal hepatitis	No	Yes	No	May be detectable
Biliary atresia	No	Rarely	Usually	None
Choledochal malformation	Variable	Usually	No	Usually seen

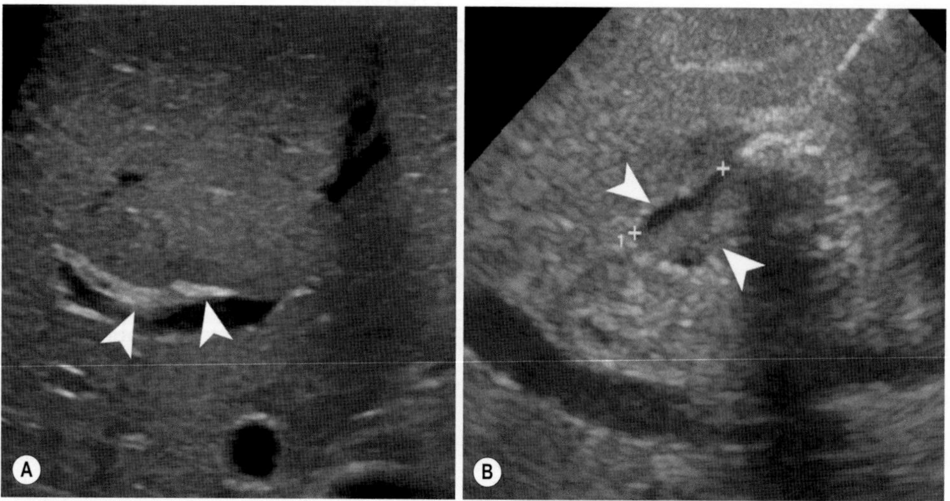

FIGURE 77-50 ■ Typical US findings of biliary atresia in an infant with persistent jaundice. (A) The fibrous atretic plate (arrowheads) is present at the porta hepatis (triangular cord sign). Note that there is no biliary dilatation. (B) A small (about 10 mm) gall bladder (arrowheads) with abnormal wall.

vena cava. The natural history is of progressive fibrosis, cirrhosis and portal hypertension. However, if portoenterostomy (Kasai's procedure) is performed before 8 weeks of age, about half reach adolescence without needing transplant.[146]

The definitive diagnosis is by intraoperative cholangiography. Preoperative percutaneous transhepatic cholecystocholangiography combined with liver biopsy in cholestatic infants has a sensitivity of 100% and a specificity of 93% for diagnosing biliary atresia.[147]

The sonographic signs are (1) absent or abnormal (<1.5 cm fasting and/or no normal wall) gall bladder, (2) a hyperechoic structure ('triangular cord') that represents a fibrous remnant of the extrahepatic bile ducts at the porta hepatis and (3) a wide hepatic artery (diameter > 2 mm at the porta hepatis).[148–153]

In infants up to 3 months of age with conjugated hyperbilirubinaemia, a negative triangular cord sign and normal gall bladder morphology on US has a high negative predictive value (> 90%) for excluding extrahepatic biliary atresia.[154]

Radioisotope studies have high sensitivity but a false-positive rate above 20%. The poor specificity is mostly due to poor biliary excretion/drainage in other conditions, e.g. metabolic disease, infection, persistent intrahepatic cholestasis, total parenteral nutrition and neonatal hepatitis.[155]

Choledochal Malformation (Choledochal Cyst (Fig. 77-51))

Choledochal malformations comprise a spectrum of conditions with overlapping expressions in which there is abnormal widening of the biliary tract without acute obstruction. About 80% manifest clinically during childhood. Malignant transformation in children is not documented.[156] The incidence is 1:100,000–200,000, but as high as 1:1000 in Japan.[157,158]

In infants younger than 3 months with extrahepatic biliary dilatation and conjugated hyperbilirubinaemia, bile duct diameter < 3 mm suggests a non-surgical cause, whereas diameter > 4 mm suggests choledochal malformation. The intermediate cases are often associated with inspissated bile syndrome.[159]

Most commonly there is spherical or fusiform dilatation of the extrahapatic ducts (type 1).[156] A common pancreaticobiliary channel may be seen sonographically[160] and with MRCP, and flux of pancreatic excretions via this into the common bile duct is thought to be a pathogenetic factor. The clinically most important differential diagnosis for a cyst at the porta hepatis is cystic biliary atresia.[145] Other differential diagnoses include duodenal duplication cyst and lymphangioma.

Other variants demonstrate a cystic diverticulum from the common bile duct (type 2), cholodochocele into the duodenum (type 3) or a combination of intra- and extrahepatic dilatation (type 4). Choledochal malformations may be part of the fibropolycystic spectrum (see 'Liver' section). Indeed, Caroli's disease is an association between intrahepatic segmental duct dilatations (type 5 choledochal malformation), (congenital) hepatic fibrosis and cystic kidney disease. Intrahepatic focal biliary dilatation can be recognised by the central dot sign, which represents the encased adjoining portal vein branch. Differential diagnoses to intrahepatic choledochal malformation include sclerosing cholangitis (see later) and recurrent pyogenic cholangitis.[161]

There may be complications like cholangitis (due to stagnant bile), biliary obstruction (calculi), cirrhosis (secondary to obstruction) and cholangiocarcinoma in adults.[162] Surgical treatment is usually hepatoenterostomy.

Inspissated Bile

In infants and young children, obstruction (partial or total) by stagnant-formed bile may be associated with

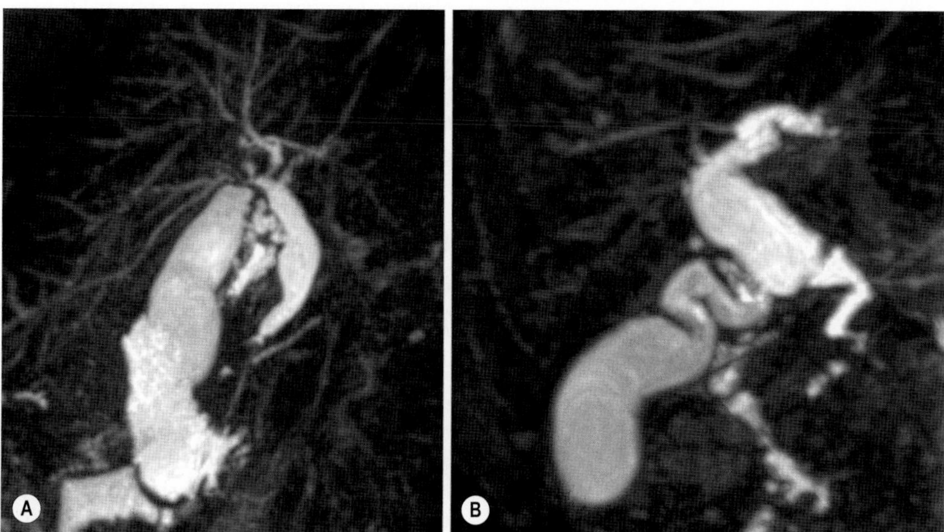

FIGURE 77-51 ■ **Choledochal malformations depicted with thick-slab maximum intensity projections of volumetric heavily T2-weighted fast spin-echo images.** (A) Fusiform widening of the extrahepatic bile ducts (type 1). (B) Widening of the common hepatic duct and central intrahepatic bile ducts (type 4).

prematurity, haemolysis, functional intestinal obstruction (e.g. Hirschsprung's disease), cystic fibrosis and total parenteral nutrition. It is usually idiopathic in infants (inspissated bile syndrome). US demonstrates the (slightly) echogenic bile with no acoustic shadowing, and the secondary biliary dilatation (mainly extrahepatic). There may be increased periportal echogenicity if longstanding. Choledochal malformation is the main differential diagnosis in infants.

Persistent Intrahepatic Cholestasis

This is a spectrum of inherited disorders that need to be considered in infantile jaundice. It includes Alagille syndrome: paucity of intrahepatic bile ducts associated with butterfly vertebrae, congenital heart disease, ocular and/or facial anomalies. There is no documented role for imaging in these conditions; however, this may change with the introduction of hepatocyte-specific contrast agents.[97]

Other causes of biliary obstruction include external compression by cystic (e.g. duplication cysts) or solid (e.g. enlarged lymph nodes) masses. Biliary neoplasms are rare in children (see 'Neoplasia' section).

Sludge and Gallstones

The prevalence of gallstones increases with age; they are rare in children unless there is an underlying cause, such as haemolytic disorders, obesity, cystic fibrosis, small bowel disease, choledochal malformation or total parenteral nutrition. There may not be a developmental continuum from sludge to stone formation.[163]

Spontaneous Perforation of the Bile Ducts

This is a very rare condition. The clinical presentation is increasing ascites, irritability and variable mild jaundice in a young infant. The hepatobiliary radioisotope image demonstrates extrabiliary pooling, and US or MRI may verify coinciding loculated fluid and possibly underlying causes, such as choledochal malformation, gallstone and biliary stenosis.[164]

Cholangitis

Cholangitis in children prompts a search for predisposing conditions. These include anatomical abnormalities (choledochal malformation), congenital hepatic fibrosis, biliary obstruction (gallstone, inspissated bile), congenital immunodeficiency and complications following surgery and transplantation.

Sclerosing Cholangitis

The pathology and imaging findings are similar to those in adults: a beaded appearance of alternating strictures and dilatation of intra- and extrahepatic bile ducts. Primary sclerosing cholangitis is associated with ulcerative colitis in up to 80% (may be metachronous). Conversely, inflammatory bowel disease is found in around half of children with sclerosing cholangitis.[165] Secondary sclerosing cholangitis may be seen in Langerhans cell histiocytosis. Clinical presentation is usually after 2 years of age, but a neonatal form is well known. The differential diagnoses include primary biliary cirrhosis, autoimmune hepatitis, biliary atresia and graft-versus-host disease.

Sclerosing cholangitis leads to progressive cholestasis and cirrhosis. The risk a person with primary sclerosing cholangitis has for developing cholangiocarcinoma is estimated at 0.6–1.5% per year.[166]

Neoplasia

Biliary neoplasms are rare in children. Biliary rhabdomyosarcoma is suspected when there is a mass at the porta hepatis and associated proximal biliary dilatation. It rarely invades the portal vein. Cystic variants are known. Cholangiocarcinoma is an important differential diagnosis in children with sclerosing cholangitis. It is unlikely to arise in childhood from choledochal malformation.

PANCREAS

Imaging Techniques

US usually allows complete depiction of the pancreas in children. The pancreatic tail is seen through a splenic acoustic window. Islet cell neoplasm and other small lesions, however, are not commonly visible, and may also not be seen on MRI. Complete imaging in suspected cases therefore involves radioisotope studies. The pancreatic ducts may be difficult to visualise on MRCP unless the exocrine pancreas is stimulated using intravenous secretin; however, care should be taken in case of recent pancreatitis, which may be exacerbated by secretin.

Imaging Anatomy

Pancreatic size is variable, volumetric references unavailable, and sonographic measurements have unknown reliability. The pancreas may appear large relative to the size of the child. Suggested anteroposterior dimensions on US are (infants–teenagers, cm) 1–2 (head and tail) and 0.6–1.1 (body) with standard deviations of around 0.4 cm.[167] Suggested normal pancreatic duct diameters are 1.1 mm in toddlers to 2.1 mm in late teens, with standard deviations of about 0.2 mm.[168]

Congenital Abnormalities and Associations

Pancreas Divisum (Fig. 77-52)

This is a common, and often uncomplicated, variant. The embryonal ventral and dorsal anlagen have separate ducts that normally connect. This failing, two separate ducts persist. Since the smaller dorsal anlage develops into the larger part (body, tail, part of the head), its duct (of Santorini) may provide inadequate draining capacity through the minor papilla, which may predispose to recurrent acute pancreatitis. However, such an association is disputed (in adults).[169]

Annular Pancreas (Fig. 77-53)

Annular pancreas, i.e. pancreatic tissue encasing the second part of the duodenum, results from erroneous migration of the anlagen. It may result in duodenal obstruction and is a differential diagnosis for the double bubble sign. Associated anomalies are common in children (71%) and differ from those in adults, the most common being trisomy 21, intestinal and cardiac anomalies that often require surgery.[170]

Other

Agenesis of the dorsal anlage is suggested by a short rounded pancreatic head and absence of the body and tail. It is associated with insulin-dependent diabetes mellitus, possibly through a gene mutation.[171] Ectopic pancreatic tissue may exist and is most frequently located in the wall of the stomach, duodenum or jejunum.

Systemic Disorders

Cystic Fibrosis

High-viscosity secretions cause distal obstruction and inevitable destruction of the pancreas in children with cystic fibrosis. The main imaging findings are atrophy and/or fat replacement (Fig. 77-54); however, fibrous tissue and calcifications may be seen.[107] Pancreatitis is a less common complication, occurring in just over 1% of patients with cystic fibrosis.[172]

Other

Diffuse enlargement of the pancreas may be seen in children with Beckwith–Wiedemann syndrome, which also predisposes to pancreatoblastoma, albeit seen very rarely. Both autosomal dominant polycystic kidney disease and von Hippel–Lindau disease may manifest with pancreastic cyst(s).

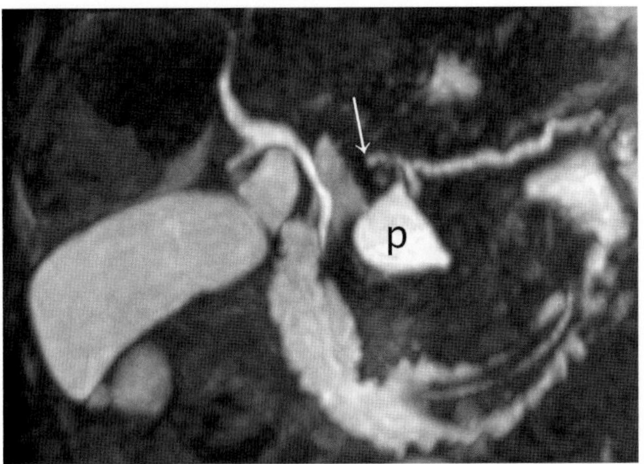

FIGURE 77-52 ■ Thick-slab heavily T2-weighted fast spin-echo in a child following acute pancreatitis. A pseudocyst (p) is seen. The pancreatic duct from the tail, body and proximal head appears to drain exclusively through the duct of Santorini, which narrows abruptly near the minor papilla (arrow).

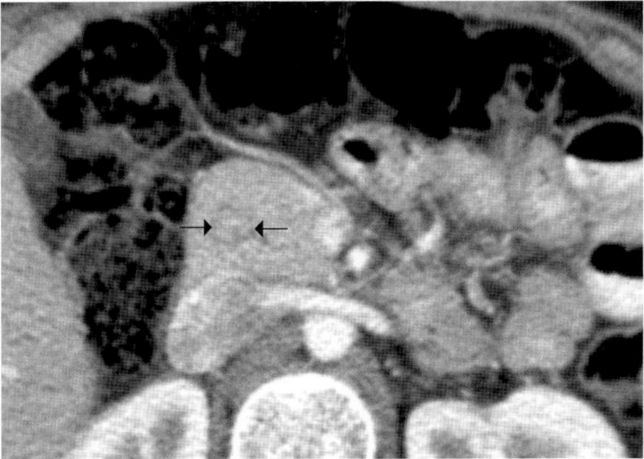

FIGURE 77-53 ■ Contrast-enhanced CT in a toddler with symptoms of partial upper gastrointestinal obstruction demonstrates annular pancreas. The second part of the duodenum (arrows) is completely encircled by pancreatic tissue.

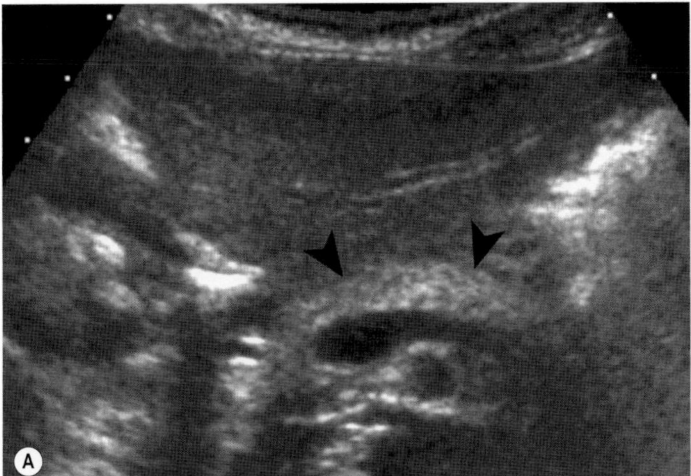

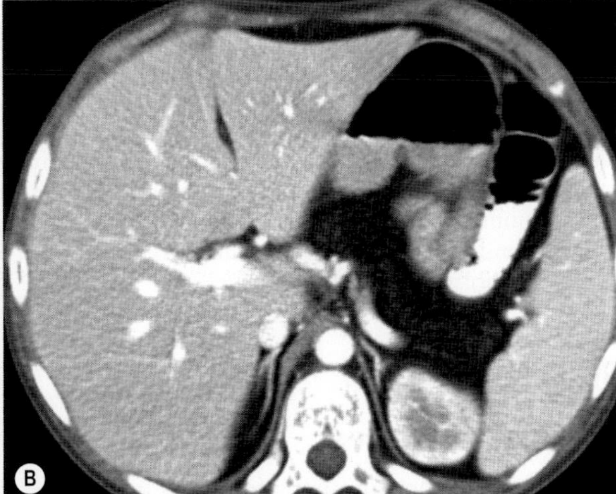

FIGURE 77-54 ■ Fatty replacement of the pancreas in a child with cystic fibrosis. (A) Sonogram demonstrates a small, hyperechoic pancreas (arrowheads). (B) Contrast-enhanced CT shows a fat-attenuated pancreas. Gradual destruction happens during childhood due to stagnant secretions, and may also manifest as fibrosis and calcification.

Pancreatitis

Underlying conditions differ in children. In acute pancreatitis they include congenital biliary abnormalities, viral infections, systemic disease (e.g. Henoch-Schönlein purpura and other vasculitides, metabolic and other hereditary disease) and pancreatic duct abnormalities; however, about one-third are idiopathic.[173] Apart from playing a role in the acute stage (as in adults), imaging in children is directed towards uncovering any underlying anatomical abnormality, for which MRI is used.

Conditions associated with chronic pancreatitis include cystic fibrosis, Shwachman–Diamond syndrome and other hereditary disorders.

Trauma

Children are more prone to pancreatic injury, which may manifest as laceration, transection and/or acute pancreatitis. As with any injury in childhood, non-accidental causes need to be considered, particularly in the youngest.

Congenital Hyperinsulinism

Congenital hyperinsulinism is caused by diffuse or focal inappropriate secretion of insulin. ^{16}F-fluoro-DOPA PET may differentiate the two—important for planning surgical options (partial or complete resection of the pancreas).[174] Co-registration of PET with MRCP images allows assessment of the relation between a focal lesion and the common bile duct.

Neoplasms

Pancreatoblastoma is rare, even in predisposed children with Beckwith–Wiedemann syndrome. Presentation is usually in infants or young children with a heterogeneous solid/cystic mass and variable enhancement.

Solid and papillary epithelial neoplasms (Frantz tumour) is most often seen in adolescent or young adult females. Imaging usually shows a large well-defined mass with cystic-haemorrhagic degeneration, calcifications and low-signal intensity (fibrous) rim on MRI (Fig. 77-55).

Islet cell tumours are associated with multiple endocrine neoplasia type 1 and with von Hippel–Lindau disease. Functioning entities in children are insulinoma (most common; Fig. 77-56), gastrinoma, VIPoma and glucagonoma. These are often small and undetectable on US, CT and MRI, so imaging in suspected cases need to include radioisotope studies.

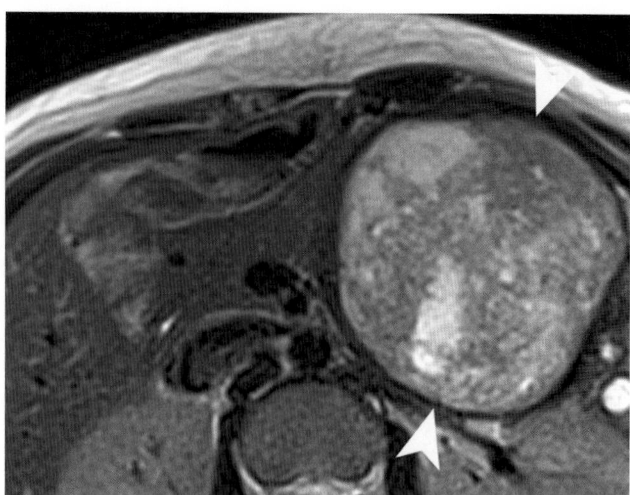

FIGURE 77-55 ■ Solid-cystic and papillary neoplasm (Frantz tumour; arrowheads) in an adolescent girl. Axial T2-weighted fast spin-echo MRI shows a heterogeneous hyperintense mass with a thick hypointense (fibrotic) rim.

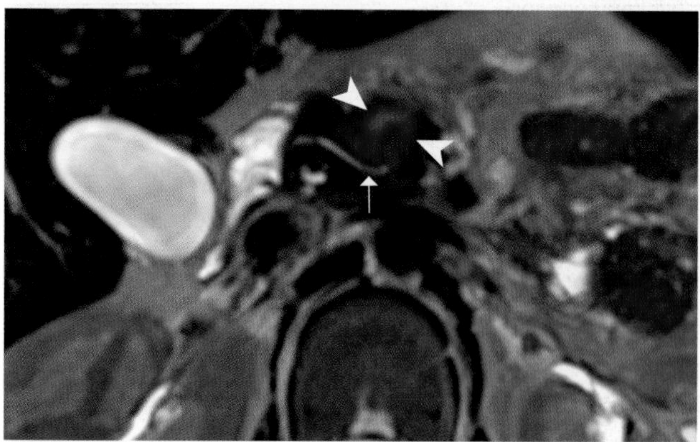

FIGURE 77-56 ■ MRI in a 9-year-old boy with pancreatic insulinoma. Axial T2-weighted MRI (grey scale) with overlay of diffusion-weighted (b, 1000) MRI (red tones) shows the insulinoma (arrowheads) because of its mildly restricted water diffusion. Note also how tumour deflects the main pancreatic duct (arrow) posteriorly.

SPLEEN

Imaging Techniques

US (high-frequency linear transducer) is best for detecting small parenchymal lesions, such as focal fungal infection. MRI is preferred for further investigation of larger (>1 cm) uncertain lesions.

Imaging Anatomy

Accessory spleens are common and of no interest. In the neonate the spleen is hypointense both on T1- and T2-weighted MRI. With increasing white pulp-to-red pulp ratio, its MRI contrast becomes similar to that in adults by 8 months of age. Table 77-12 suggests upper size limits. High-frequency US may demonstrate the spotted appearance of a reactive spleen (Fig. 77-57), which should not be mistaken for multifocal lesions.

Imaging Findings

Splenomegaly

Splenomegaly has a wide differential, as in adults. In children one also needs to consider mononucleosis, depositional disorders (Gaucher's disease, mucopolysacharidosis,

TABLE 77-12 **Suggested Upper Limit of Normal Sonographic Measurement of the Spleen in Children**[177]

Age (months)	Suggested Upper Limit for the Sonographic Longitudinal Diameter (Coronal Orientation) of the Spleen (mm)
1–3	70
4–6	75
7–9	80
12–30	85
36–59	95
60–83	105
84–107	105
108–131	110
132–155	115
156–179	120
180–200	120

The limits are based on an ethnically homogeneous material. Considerable intra- and inter-observer variation need to be accounted for.

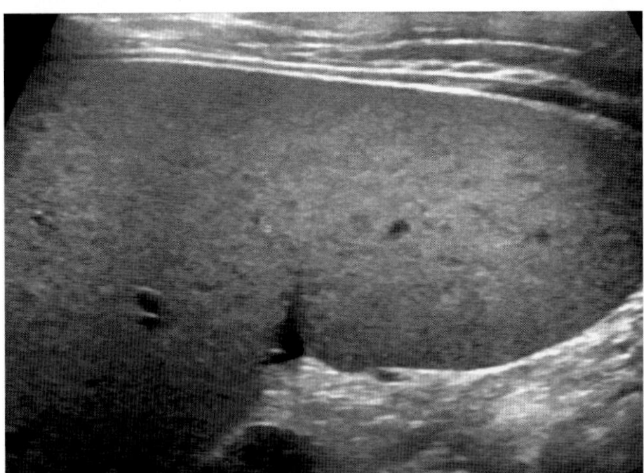

FIGURE 77-57 ■ US in a 10-year-old with falciparum malaria shows an enlarged spleen with a spotted appearance, which is commonly seen in reactive states and should not be mistaken for focal lesions.

Niemann–Pick disease), Langerhans cell histiocytosis and other conditions.

Wandering Spleen

Wandering spleen is associated with prune-belly syndrome, surgery and gastric volvulus, and predisposes to splenic torsion and infarction.

Focal Lesions

Most focal lesions (solitary or multifocal) in the spleen are infectious: abscesses and fungal infection (Fig. 77-58). Granulomata and hydatid cysts often contain calcification. (See also 'Neoplasia' section.)

Lateralisation Disorders (Fig. 77-59)

Both asplenia and polysplenia are associated with congenital heart disease.[101] Asplenia is more commonly associated with immunodeficiency and polysplenia with azygos continuation of IVC, preduodenal portal vein, bilateral left-sidedness of the lungs and biliary atresia. On US the spleen should be located near the greater curvature of the stomach, regardless of its situs. Radioisotope studies can be used to confirm asplenia.

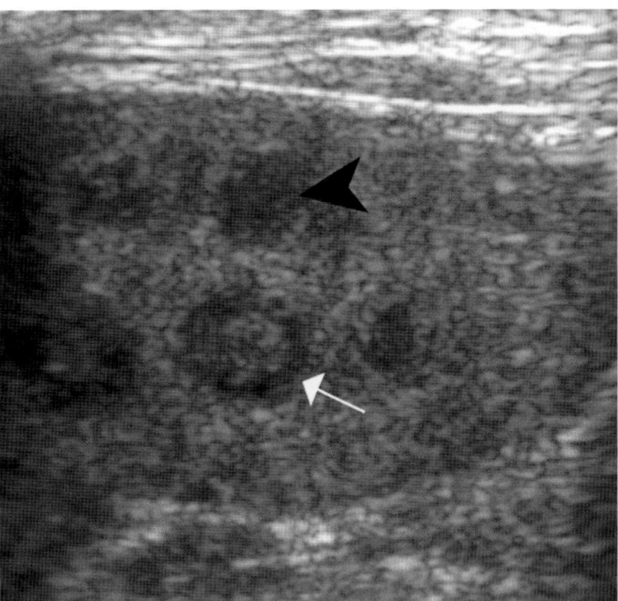

FIGURE 77-58 ■ US with a high-frequency linear transducer in a child with acute lymphoblastic leukaemia and febrile neutropenia shows several hypoechoic (arrowhead) and target lesions (arrow) suggestive of fungal infection.

Infarction

Splenic infarction may occur in disorders with massive sequestration (sickle-cell anaemia), deposition (storage disorders) or infiltration (leukaemia).

Trauma

Trauma epidemiology and mechanisms are different in children than in adults, but imaging is similar. The focused abdominal sonography for trauma (FAST) technique has low (50%) negative predictive value for abdominal injury in haemodynamically stable children post trauma, as compared with CT.[175]

More comprehensive, but still fast (median imaging time 5 min), US, performed by sonographers, in non-selected children post trauma, soon after arrival in an emergency department was reported as highly accurate, but less sensitive, in a prospective study, for any abdominal traumatic injury compared with a combination of CT, peritoneal lavage and laparotomy, with a negative predictive value of 91% for haemoperitoneum.[176]

Non-accidental injury is always an important differential, particularly in the younger age groups.[177] In children with abdominal injury following abuse, the frequency of injury to the spleen has been reported to come third, after small bowel and liver.[138]

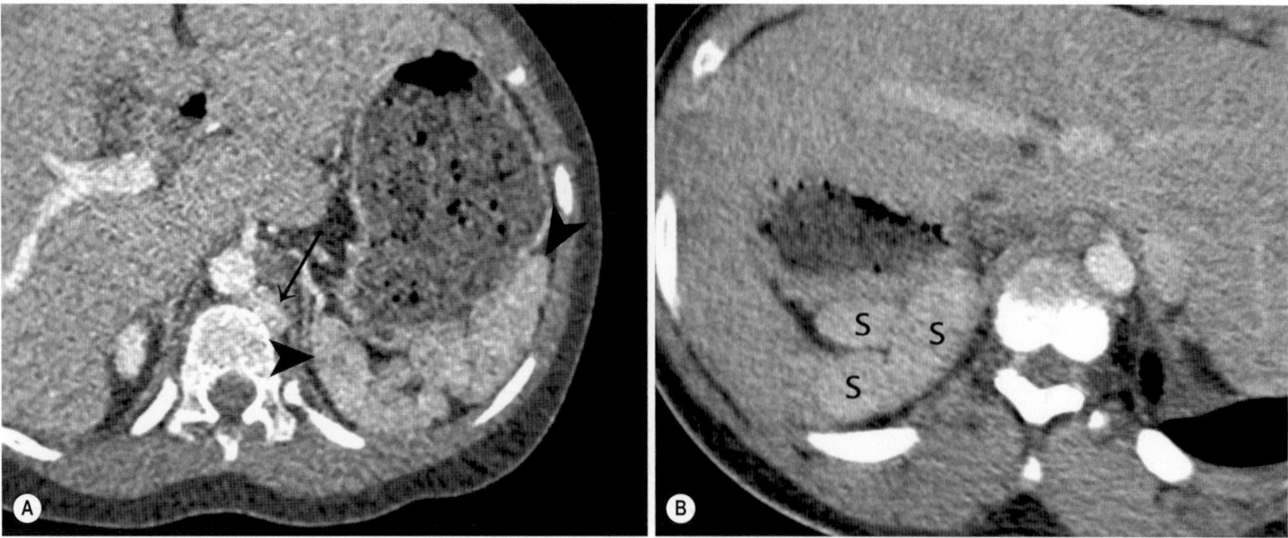

FIGURE 77-59 ■ **Polysplenia on CT.** (A) Multiple spleens (between arrowheads) in this child are associated with minor congenital heart disease and azygos (arrow) continuation of interrupted IVC. (B) Visceral situs inversus, multiple spleens (s) which in this child with primary ciliary dyskinesia was associated with major congenital heart disease and bronchial isomerism (Kartagener's syndrome).

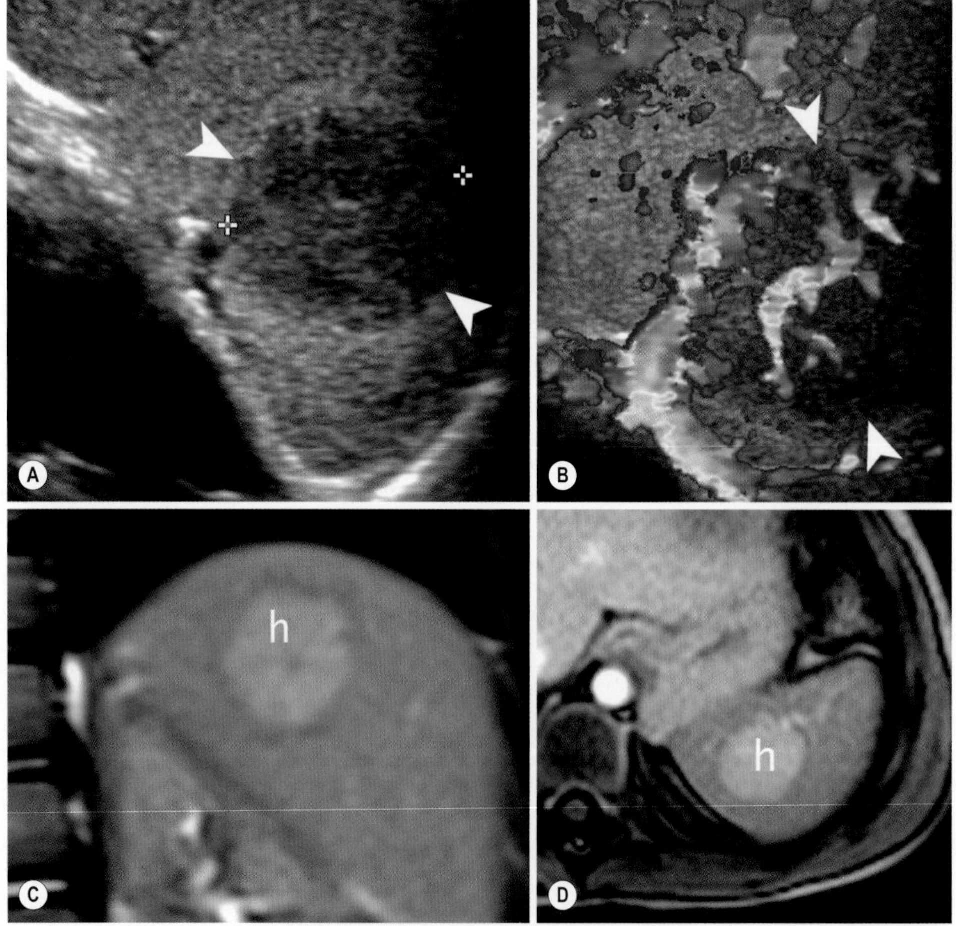

FIGURE 77-60 ■ **Splenic hamartoma as an incidental finding in a child.** Sonogram (A) and duplex Doppler US (B) demonstrate a vascularised well-demarcated, hypoechoic lesion (arrowheads). (C) Coronal T2-weighted MRI shows the lesion (h) as an almost geometrical figure (hexagon) with a fine hypointense perimeter and centre (resembling focal nodular hyperplasia of the liver). (D) There is homogeneous enhancement of the lesion (h) 3 min after intravenous administration of gadoteric acid.

Neoplasia

Most splenic neoplasms are benign. Cystic lesions are usually epidermoid/dermoid cysts, lymphangioma or splenic (epithelial) cysts. Solid lesions include haemangioma and hamartoma (Fig. 77-60). Malignant tumours are most commonly lymphoproliferative disease. Metastases and primary splenic angiosarcoma are rare.

For a full list of references, please see ExpertConsult.

FURTHER READING

Slovis TL, editor. Caffey's Pediatric Diagnostic Imaging. 11th ed. Philadelphia: Mosby Elsevier 2008.

Medina LS, Applegate KE, Blackmore CC, editors. Evidence-Based Imaging in Pediatrics. New York: Springer 2010.

103. Gubernick JA, Rosenberg HK, Ilaslan H, Kessler A. US approach to jaundice in infants and children. Radiographics 2000;20:173–95.
111. Pariente D, Franchi-Abella S. Paediatric chronic liver diseases: How to investigate and follow up? Role of imaging in the diagnosis of fibrosis. Pediatr Radiol 2010;40:906–19.
130. Roebuck D. Focal liver lesion in children. Pediatr Radiol 2008;38(Suppl 3):S518–522.
134. Dubois J, Alison M. Vascular anomalies: What a radiologist needs to know. Pediatr Radiol 2010;40:895–905.
144. Davenport M, Betalli P, D'Antiga L, et al. The spectrum of surgical jaundice in infancy. J Pediatr Surg 2003;38:1471–9.

CHAPTER 78

Imaging of the Kidneys, Urinary Tract and Pelvis in Children

Owen Arthurs • Marina Easty • Michael Riccabona

CHAPTER OUTLINE

OVERVIEW

In this chapter, we cover the important areas of renal, urinary tract and pelvic imaging in children, emphasising the importance of congenital abnormalities and the need for minimising radiation burden and optimising image quality.

Ultrasound (US) is the preferred method for imaging the paediatric population, due to the ease of availability, lack of ionising radiation, reproducibility and because it is usually well tolerated. Modern US is often the only modality required to make a diagnosis, with the high frequency probes and new technology producing exquisite anatomical details in children who are ideal subjects. Alternatively, US can be used to direct other imaging modalities, such as functional assessment of the urinary tract by ^{99m}Tc-MAG3 dynamic imaging.

Intravenous urography (IVU) is now rarely used. Fluoroscopic micturating cystourethrography (MCUG) is essential to exclude bladder outflow obstruction such as in posterior urethral valves and urethral pathology, and to assess for vesicoureteric reflux (VUR). Contrast-enhanced voiding urosonography (ce-VUS) with microbubble contrast is used in some European countries rather than a fluoroscopic examination for VUR assessment, avoiding the radiation burden from conventional MCUG. Direct isotope cystography using ^{99m}Tc-pertechnetate is a low-dose functional study used to assess VUR, particularly in girls, where urethral anatomy is usually normal. Older, continent and cooperative children may benefit from an indirect radionuclide cystogram, IRC, as part of their dynamic ^{99m}Tc-MAG3 renogram, as a non-invasive means of assessing for VUR.

Cross-sectional imaging—computed tomography (CT) and magnetic resonance imaging (MRI)—is crucial in tumour imaging, for disease staging and prognostication as well as for imaging complications. CT is used much less frequently in children than in adults for urolithiasis: indeed, only severe trauma imaging relies on CT in children. The role of MRI is increasing both for anatomical and functional diagnostic information, particularly in cooperative older children, and where nuclear medicine is not available.

Conventional angiography is reserved for specific clinical indications, and is invasive with a high radiation burden. CT and MR angiography (MRA), however, have emerged as replacements for angiography for many diagnostic purposes.

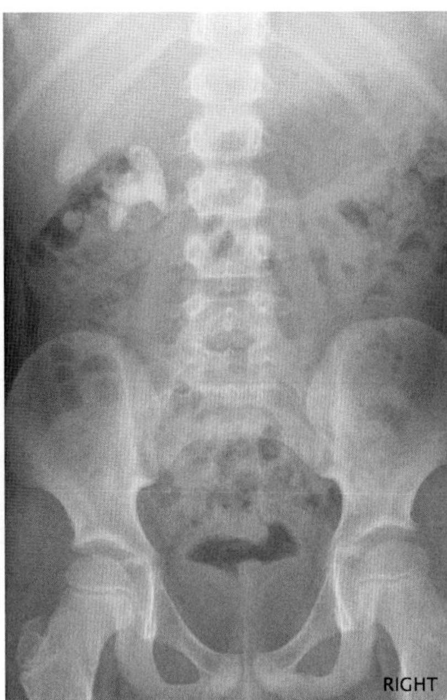

FIGURE 78-1 ■ **Renal calculus.** Plain abdominal radiograph of a large staghorn calculus in the right kidney.

Here we review the relative strengths and weaknesses of these techniques, illustrated using specific pathologies and recommend imaging algorithms.

IMAGING TECHNIQUES

Plain Radiography

Radiographs still have a role to play in babies with congenital renal anomalies, particularly in those cases associated with skeletal anomalies, such as vertebral segmentation anomalies and pubic diastasis (in bladder exstrophy). They may show renal tract calculi (Fig. 78-1) where the exposure should be coned to the kidneys, ureters and bladder (so-called 'KUB film').

Age-appropriate exposure settings and electronic filtering (in digital radiography equipment) are essential.

Ultrasound

Ultrasound is the most useful way of providing anatomical information about the intra-abdominal, pelvic and retroperitoneal structures. The ability to delineate and recognise normal and abnormal findings is directly related to the skill of the ultrasonographer and the equipment used, including high-frequency transducers, and familiarity examining children in a conducive environment, with knowledge of the spectrum of diseases in childhood being paramount. Several European guidelines regarding standard paediatric urinary tract US are available.[1]

Standard Technique

In the young child, ideally a full bladder is necessary, which usually requires at least 30–60 min of encouraged fluid intake to allow adequate hydration. Any US examination of the abdomen should begin by imaging the bladder, to fortuitously attempt to capture a full bladder (as the infant in nappies may void at any time). The distended bladder provides an acoustic window for the lower urinary tract, bladder neck and ureteric orifices (vesicoureteric junction), distal ureters, internal genitalia, retrovesical space, pelvic musculature and vessels (Fig. 78-2).[1]

Well-hydrated patient, full bladder, adequate equipment & transducer, training, etc.

↓

Urinary bladder: size (volume), shape, ostium, wall, bladder neck, include distal ureter & retrovesical space/ internal genitalia

Optional: CDS for urine inflow, perineal US, scrotal US ...

↓

Kidneys: lateral and/or dorsal, longitudinal and axial sections, parenchyma? Pelvicalyceal system?
Standardised measurements in 3 planes & volume calculation.
If dilated: + max. axial pelvis & calyxdiameter, narrowest parenchymal width + ureteropelvic junction

Optional: (a)CDS & duplex Doppler

↓

Post-void evaluation
Bladder: residual volume, bladder neck, shape & configuration
Kidneys: dilatation of pelvicalyceal system/ureter changed?

Optional: ce-VUS, 3DUS ...

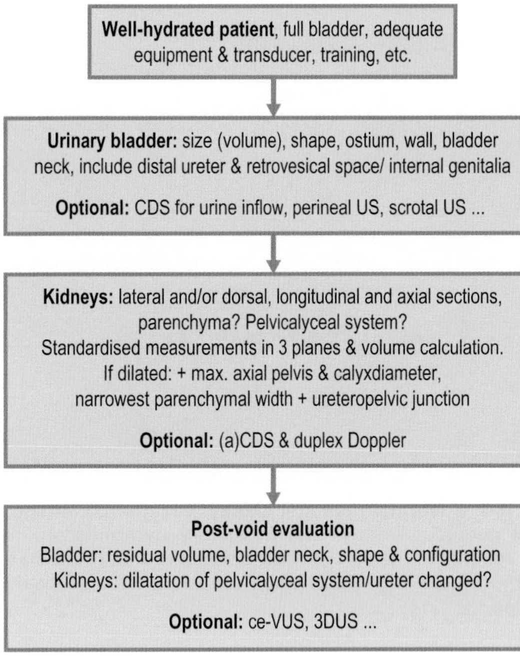

Note: Cursory US of entire abdomen is recommended for first study, and in mismatch of findings and query

FIGURE 78-2 ■ **US of the urinary tract. ESPR imaging recommendations for standard paediatric sonography of the urinary tract.** US = ultrasound, CDS = colour Doppler sonography, ce-VUS = contrast-enhanced voiding urosonography, 3DUS = three-dimensional ultrasound. (Adapted from Riccabona M, Avni F E, Blickman J G, et al 2008 Imaging recommendations in paediatric uroradiology: minutes of the ESPR workgroup session on urinary tract infection, foetal hydronephrosis, urinary tract ultrasonography and voiding cystourethrography, Barcelona, Spain, June 2007. Pediatr Radiol 38(2):138–145.[1])

It is customary to measure pre- and post-micturition bladder volumes, as incomplete voiding may be related to bladder dysfunctions and urinary tract infections, and the presence of pre- and/or post-micturition upper tract dilatation. Normal age-related changes in the kidney must be appreciated. The neonatal kidneys lack renal sinus fat over the first 6 months of life, and the medullary pyramids are typically large and hypoechoic relative to the cortex (the opposite to that found in older children and adults), which may be mistaken for pelvicalyceal dilatation or 'cysts' (Fig. 78-3). The normal neonatal renal cortex is also hyper- to iso-echoic relative to the adjacent normal liver, which again can often be reversed in adults. The neonatal renal pyramids may be echogenic, a transient physiological appearance in up to 5% of newborns, and should not be mistaken for nephrocalcinosis, although it can be seen in older infants with dehydration.[2] The

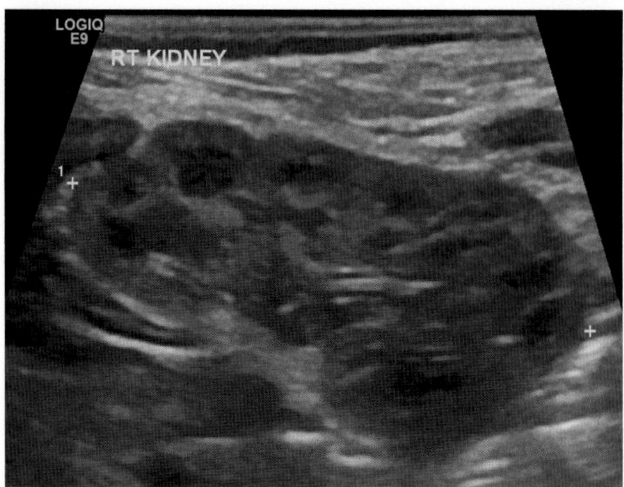

FIGURE 78-3 ■ **Normal neonatal kidney.** Oblique US image of a normal neonatal kidney. The medullary pyramids are hypoechoic relative to the cortex (the opposite to that found in older children and adults), which may be mistaken for pelvicalyceal dilatation.

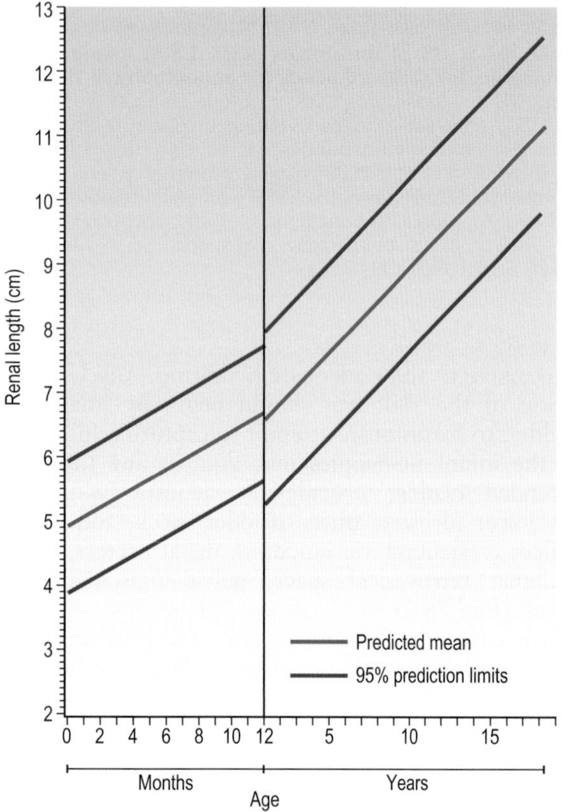

FIGURE 78-4 ■ **Renal growth chart.** Normal reference sizes and 95th centiles given by age of child.

average newborn kidney is approximately 4.5 cm in length, and measurements of bipolar renal lengths can be compared against age/height/weight indexed charts (Fig. 78-4). As the paediatric kidney is more spherical than the ellipsoid adult kidney, renal volumes may be a better assessment using the equation:

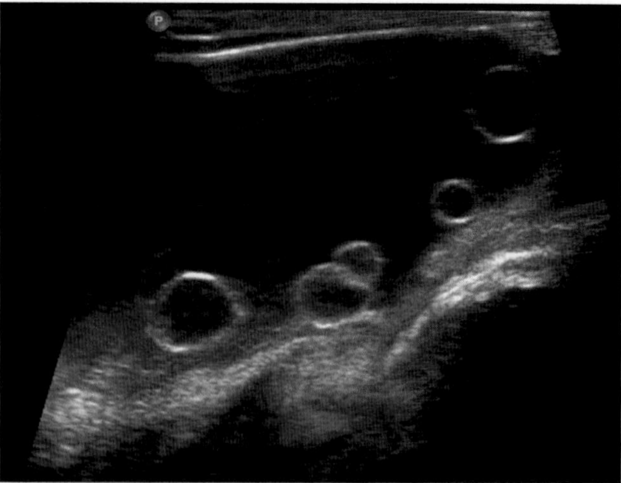

FIGURE 78-5 ■ **Ovarian cysts.** US of a neonatally physiologically large ovarian cyst with daughter cysts.

$$\text{Kidney Volume} = 0.523\ (\pi/6) \times \text{length} \times \text{width} \times \text{depth}$$

Colour Doppler sonography (CDS) of the renal vessels is particularly important in assessing perfusion in a variety of conditions, including infection (segmental perfusion impairment), trauma (hilar vascular injury), biopsy (post-biopsy complications), renal failure, urolithiasis tumours, renal transplants and hypertension, and for the vascular anatomy in hydronephrosis (HN). High-frequency linear transducers yield better images in smaller children, especially in the prone position and should be performed for detailed analysis in all examinations.[1]

Normal Gonadal Imaging in Girls

Normal pelvic structures can be difficult to visualise in children: visualisation of the ovaries by US depends on their location, size and the age of the girl—they are more easily seen in the first few months of life. Ovarian volume is usually under 1 mL in the neonate, and 2–4 mL in the prepubertal child. Ovaries typically look heterogeneous due to the presence of follicles, and larger follicles can appear as small ovarian 'cysts' which are normal at all ages (Fig. 78-5). After puberty, ovarian volumes of 5–15 mL are normal, with normal primordial follicles <10 mm in diameter, and stimulated follicles 10–30 mm in diameter.

The normal uterus also changes dramatically with hormonal changes, and is the most useful guide to pubertal staging. The neonatal uterus is prominent due to circulating maternal oestrogens, typically measuring 2–4.5 cm in length, with thickened and clearly visible endometrial lining (Fig. 78-6A). By 1 year of age it becomes smaller, has changed to the prepubertal tubular appearances: the fundus and cervix are the same size and the endometrium is no longer visible (Fig. 78-6B). At puberty, the fundus starts to enlarge, becomes up to three times the size of the cervix, with a total uterine length of 5–7 cm and the typical adult pear-like shape. The endometrial appearances will clearly vary with the phase of the menstrual cycle.

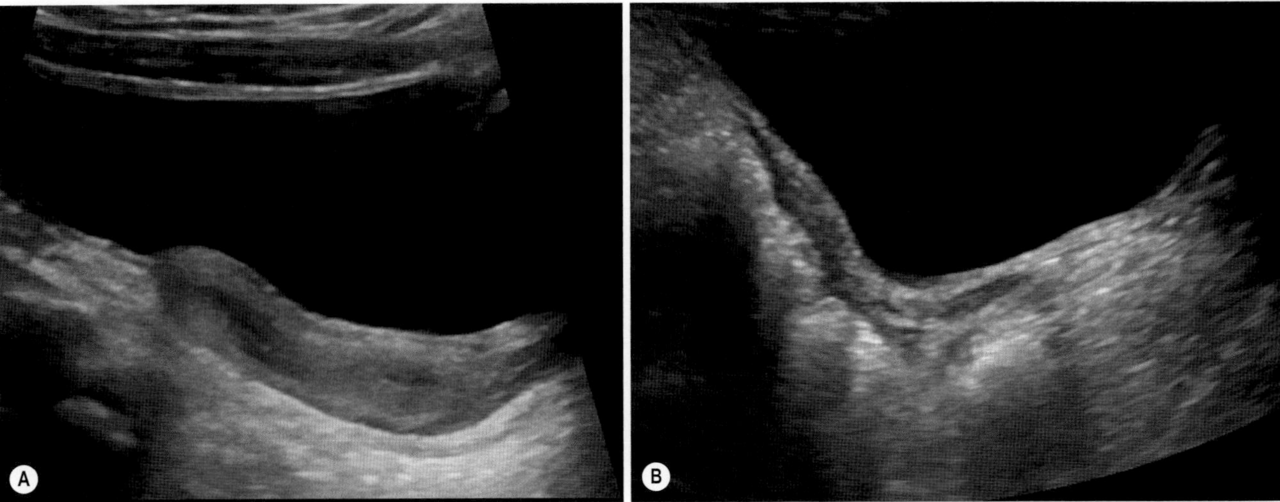

FIGURE 78-6 ■ **Normal uterus.** (A) Sagittal US image of normal neonatal uterus, which is prominent due to circulating maternal oestrogens with a clearly visible endometrial lining. (B) Sagittal US image of the infantile uterus which has a prepubertal tubular appearance: the fundus and cervix are the same size and the endometrium is no longer visible.

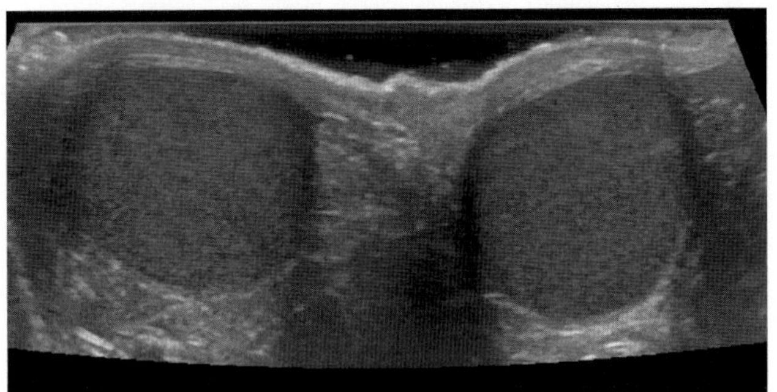

FIGURE 78-7 ■ **Normal testes.** Axial US image of normal prepubertal testes.

The vagina may be visualised by US if airfilled, (shown as a linear bright echo), or if fluid filled. On MRI the vagina is best seen on sagittal T2-weighted spin-echo MRI. As with the uterus, the appearance and the thickness of the vaginal epithelium and the signal from the vaginal wall change with the age and the phases of the menstrual cycle. Ultrasound genitography with saline filling of the vagina, or 3D US can be used for uterine anomalies, and perineal US for vagina and urethral pathology.[3,4]

Normal Gonadal Imaging in Boys

The prostate has an ellipsoid homogeneous appearance, but is difficult to see in newborns, as are the seminal vesicles. As the processus vaginalis remains open for some time after birth (and may never close completely), hydroceles are considered a normal physiological finding in the newborn. Cryptorchidism is discussed later in this chapter.

The normal testis changes in appearance during childhood. It has a homogeneous hypoechoic echotexture and is spherical/oval in shape during the neonatal period, measuring <10 mm in diameter (Fig. 78-7). The epididymis and mediastinum testis are usually not seen at this point, but are clearly identified by puberty. Testicular size in adolescence ranges from 3 to 5 cm in length and from 2 to 3 cm in depth and width (2–4 mL in total). Testicular flow, as measured by Doppler US, also changes with age. The testis in infants shows very low-velocity colour flow, which can be difficult to see despite optimised slow-flow settings, and even normal prepubertal testes may show not exhibit low-velocity flow on power Doppler US. Technically it may be difficult to identify abnormalities in a single testis given the wide range of normal values, and thus a side-by-side comparison can be most useful.

Cystography

There are several ways to visualise the bladder in the paediatric population. The method of choice depends both on the type of pathology suspected and the age of child. All methods, apart from the ^{99m}Tc-MAG3 IRC, require a bladder catheter, which becomes more unpleasant for both child (and the carer who observes) as the child gets older. The modern MCUG, using pulsed fluoroscopy, digital image amplifiers and last image hold, means that high-quality imaging is now available at an acceptably low radiation dose (Table 78-1).

The direct isotope cystogram is useful in the assessment of VUR in young babies (before toilet training), particularly in girls where there is no need to demonstrate the urethral anatomy, or for screening other family members when the index of suspicion for reflux is high.

Micturating (Voiding) Cystogram (MCUG/VCUG)

Indications. If the male baby is found (on US) to have significant bilateral hydronephrosis (HN), a dilated ureter, a pathological urethra or a thick-walled bladder,

TABLE 78-1 **Comparison of Relative Radiation Doses from Urological Examinations**

	DRL (MBq)	Effective Dose (mSv)	Equivalent CXR (0.02 MSv)	Equivalence to NBR (2.6 mSv/year)	Equivalence to a Return Transatlantic Flight (0.1 mSv)
AXR	N/A	0.7	35	3.3 months	7
MCUG in girls	N/A	0.9	45	4.2 months	9
MCUG in boys	N/A	1.5	75	6.9 months	15
DIC	20 MBq	0.3	15	1.4 months	3
DMSA	80 MBq	1.0	50	4.6 months	10
MAG3 renogram	100 MBq	0.7	35	3.3 months	7
MAG3 transplant	200 MBq	1	50	4.6 months	10
DTPA transplant	330 MBq	2	100	9.2 months	20
CT abdomen/pelvis	N/A	10	500	3.85 years	100

CXR = chest radiograph, AXR = abdominal radiograph, DIC = direct radio-isotope cystogram, N/A = not applicable or available. MBq = megabequerel. NBR = national background radiation dose (approximate for UK).

an MCUG is then performed.[5] MCUG is also indicated for VUR assessment, such as after (recurrent or complicated) UTI, or for assessing complex malformations that involve the urinary tract. The MCUG is the only accepted method of lower urinary tract imaging to demonstrate the urethral anatomy clearly, although perineal US performed during voiding also allows assessment of the urethra. It is essential in boys, where urethral pathology is suspected: for example, in boys with suspected posterior urethral valves (Figs. 78-8 and 78-9), cloacal anomaly, or anorectal anomaly and suspected colovesical fistula (Fig. 78-10). The fistula may not be seen on an MCUG. A distal loopogram (i.e. intubating the distal limb of the colostomy and injecting radio-opaque water-soluble iodine-containing contrast under pressure is the best technique to delineate these connections.

MCUG Technique. A sterile narrow feeding tube is used to catheterise the neonatal urethra, secured with tape. A suprapubic catheter may be used in individual cases, or in-dwelling Foley catheter, provided that the balloon is carefully deflated in order to prevent bladder pathology being obscured, or obstruction to bladder emptying increasing the chance of bladder rupture.[1] Warmed water-soluble iodinated contrast is then dripped from a height of no greater than 60 cm (physiological filling pressure of 30–40 cm water). Rapid bladder filling using a syringe may generate high pressures leading to bladder overextension and artificial VUR, as well as altered bladder capacity values. Bladder capacity increases during the first 8 years of life and normal bladder capacity for children 0–8 years can be estimated using the equation (age + 1) × 30 mL.

Early bladder filling views are obtained with the child supine. Tight coning is important to reduce dose. Oblique views are then obtained to assess the vesicoureteric junction and urethra on voiding. In the first few years of life, cyclical filling is advocated, as there is an increased chance of detecting VUR with consecutive voiding cycles.[1] The bladder is refilled and on the second or third void, the catheter is removed so that a well-distended urethral view is obtained. Prophylactic oral or intravesical antibiotics are used, and MCUG is contraindicated in the presence of a urinary tract infection. In a modified

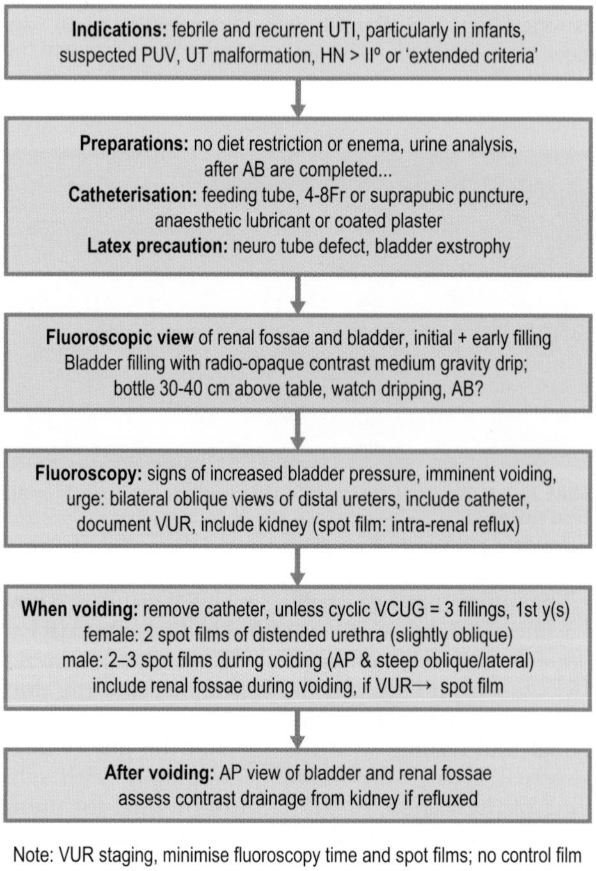

Indications: febrile and recurrent UTI, particularly in infants, suspected PUV, UT malformation, HN > II° or 'extended criteria'

↓

Preparations: no diet restriction or enema, urine analysis, after AB are completed...
Catheterisation: feeding tube, 4-8Fr or suprapubic puncture, anaesthetic lubricant or coated plaster
Latex precaution: neuro tube defect, bladder exstrophy

↓

Fluoroscopic view of renal fossae and bladder, initial + early filling
Bladder filling with radio-opaque contrast medium gravity drip; bottle 30-40 cm above table, watch dripping, AB?

↓

Fluoroscopy: signs of increased bladder pressure, imminent voiding, urge: bilateral oblique views of distal ureters, include catheter, document VUR, include kidney (spot film: intra-renal reflux)

↓

When voiding: remove catheter, unless cyclic VCUG = 3 fillings, 1st y(s)
female: 2 spot films of distended urethra (slightly oblique)
male: 2–3 spot films during voiding (AP & steep oblique/lateral)
include renal fossae during voiding, if VUR→ spot film

↓

After voiding: AP view of bladder and renal fossae
assess contrast drainage from kidney if refluxed

Note: VUR staging, minimise fluoroscopy time and spot films; no control film

FIGURE 78-8 ■ VCUG. ESPR imaging recommendations for voiding cystourethrography (VCUG). AB = antibiotics, HN = hydronephrosis, PUV = posterior urethral valve, UT = urinary tract, UTI = urinary tract infection, VCUG = voiding cystourethrography, VUR = vesicoureteral reflux. (Adapted from Riccabona M, Avni F E, Blickman J G, et al 2008 Imaging recommendations in paediatric uroradiology: minutes of the ESPR workgroup session on urinary tract infection, fetal hydronephrosis, urinary tract ultrasonography and voiding cystourethrography, Barcelona, Spain, June 2007. Pediatr Radiol 38(2):138–145.[1])

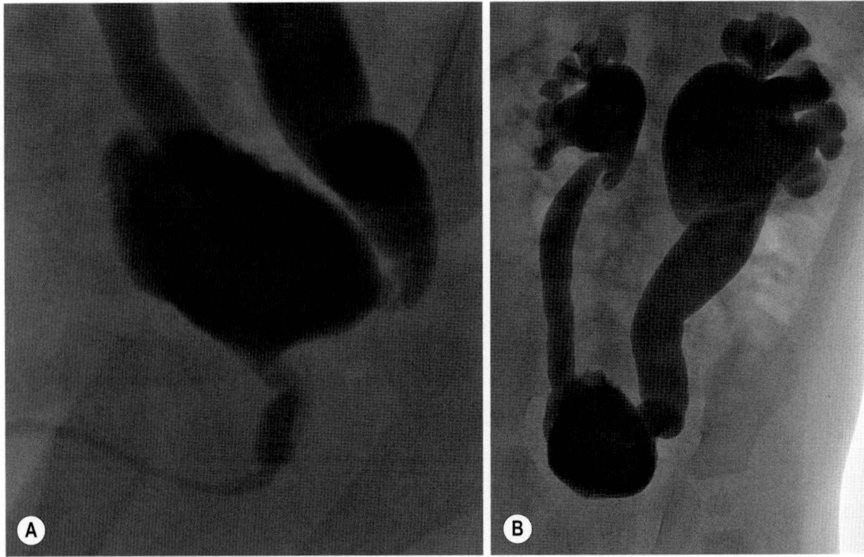

FIGURE 78-9 ■ Posterior urethral valves on MCUG. (A) There is acute calibre change in the posterior urethra caused by posterior urethral valves, with a trabeculated bladder note bilateral gross VUR. (B) Bilateral high-grade reflux is demonstrated.

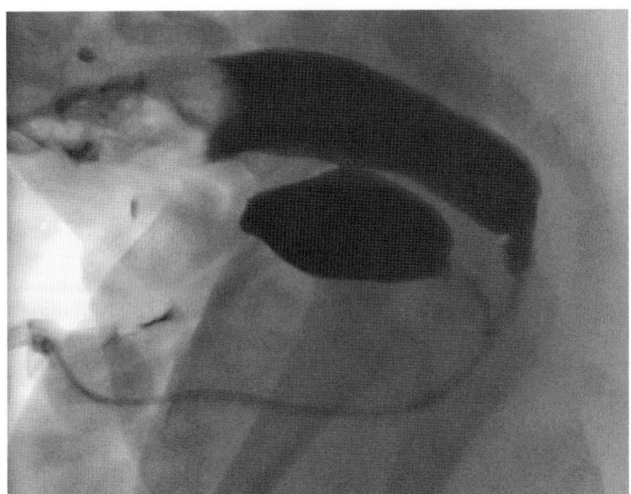

FIGURE 78-10 ■ Colourethral fistula. On micturition in this patient with an anorectal malformation, contrast passed retrogradely into the colon via the fistula.

MCUG, the contrast infusion is monitored for stopping or backflow in drip rate, which may represent dysfunctional sphincter or detrusor contractions, indicating functional disturbances.[6,7]

Contrast-Enhanced Ultrasonography (ce-VUS)

Contrast-enhanced voiding urosonography (ce-VUS) is a non-ionising alternative used throughout Europe, but less commonly used in the UK. Recommended indications for ce-VUS presently include screening populations, in girls, bedside investigations and for follow-up, although none of the ce-VUS contrast agents are currently licensed in children. Study recommendations and VUR grading are available (Fig. 78-11).[1,8]

No diet restriction or enema, urine analysis...
Accepted indications: VUR follow-up, girls, family screening, bedside
Catheterisation: feeding tube, 4–8Fr, or suprapubic puncture
anaesthetic lubricant or coated plaster
Latex precaution: neural tube defect, bladder exstrophy

↓

Standard US of bladder and kidneys (supine, ± prone)
Bladder filling with normal saline (only from plastic containers)

↓

US contrast medium, e.g., SonoVue, 0.2 to 1% of bladder volume,
slow injection, no filters, US monitoring, potentially fractional administration

↓

Peri-/post-contrast US of bladder and kidneys
US techniques: fundamental, HI, CDS, dedicated contrast imaging
alternate scans of right and left side during and after filling

↓

During and after voiding: US of bladder and kidneys supine ± prone,
sitting or standing potentially one cycle for perineal US (Urethra!)

↓

VUR diagnosis: echogenic microbubbles in ureters or renal pelves

FIGURE 78-11 ■ Ce-VUS. ESPR imaging recommendations for contrast-enhanced voiding urosonography (ce-VUS). CDS = colour Doppler sonography, VUR = vesicoureteral reflux. (Adapted from Riccabona M, Avni F E, Blickman J G, et al 2008 Imaging recommendations in paediatric uroradiology: minutes of the ESPR workgroup session on urinary tract infection, fetal hydronephrosis, urinary tract ultrasonography and voiding cystourethrography, Barcelona, Spain, June 2007. Pediatr Radiol 38(2):138–145.[1] and updated in Riccabona M; Vivier HP; Ntoulj A; Darge K, Avni F; Papadopoulou F; Damasio B; Ording-Mueller LS; Blickman J; Lobo ML; Willi U. (2014) ESPR Uroradiology Task Force—Imaging Recommendations in Paediatric Uroradiology—Part VII: Standardized terminology, impact of existing recommendations, and update on contrast-enhanced ultrasound of the paediatric urogenital tract. Report on the mini-symposium at the ESPR meeting in Budapest, June 2013, Pediatr Radiol submit)

Technique. Typically, SonoVue (Bracco/Italy) at 0.2–1.0% of bladder filling volume is given via urinary catheter as for MCUG by saline drip, following standard renal tract US views. Dedicated low-MI contrast imaging of both kidneys and the bladder including the retrovesical space and the urethra during and after filling is performed, with echogenic microbubbles in the ureters or renal pelvis indicating VUR.

Nuclear Medicine

Direct Radio-Isotope Cystogram (DIC)

A DIC is predominantly used to detect the presence of VUR in baby girls, or as VUR follow-up in baby boys.

Technique. Catheterisation using a 6Fr feeding tube can usually be performed with the baby lying on the Gamma camera, wearing a double nappy. Twenty megabequerels of ^{99m}Tc-pertechnetate is introduced into the bladder followed by warmed saline. The baby is restrained with sandbags and Velcro straps, and bladder filling is performed twice. The baby will spontaneously void when the bladder is full and VUR evaluated. The kidneys are kept in the field of view at all times to detect VUR.

Indirect Radio-Isotope Cystogram

This is a useful, well-tolerated and physiological procedure to assess bladder function and for the presence of VUR. It is performed at the end of dynamic renography in cooperative and toilet-trained children who can void on demand. After a non-diuretic stressed dynamic ^{99m}Tc-MAG3 renogram, the gamma camera is turned vertically Children seated on a commode with their backs to the camera. Boys may stand and void. The acquisition is started just before voiding starts and continues for 30 s after voiding, up to approximately 2 min total acquisition time, if required. The study can be repeated if there is still tracer present in the bladder when bladder emptying is incomplete, or when refluxed tracer re-enters the bladder from the upper renal tract. Bladder dysfunction can be assessed and VUR can be seen on the dynamic study. Guidelines are available from the European Association of Nuclear Medicine.[9]

Static Renal Scintigraphy; ^{99m}Tc-DMSA Scans

Dimercaptosuccinic acid (DMSA) is used as a ^{99m}Tc tracer; it is filtered by the glomeruli and reabsorbed, binding to the proximal convoluted tubules to give a static image over several hours. Approximately 10% of the tracer is excreted in the urine. Routinely, three posteriorly acquired views are obtained (posterior, right and left posterior oblique views), with anterior views used in abnormal renal anatomy (transplants, pelvic and ectopic kidneys) or scoliosis. Anterior and posterior views may then be used to estimate the differential renal function (DRF) by the geometric mean. As renal DMSA uptake relies on sufficient glomerular clearance, sufficient renal function is essential for meaningful results, as well as sufficient urinary drainage from the renal pelvis to avoid tracer pooling artefacts.

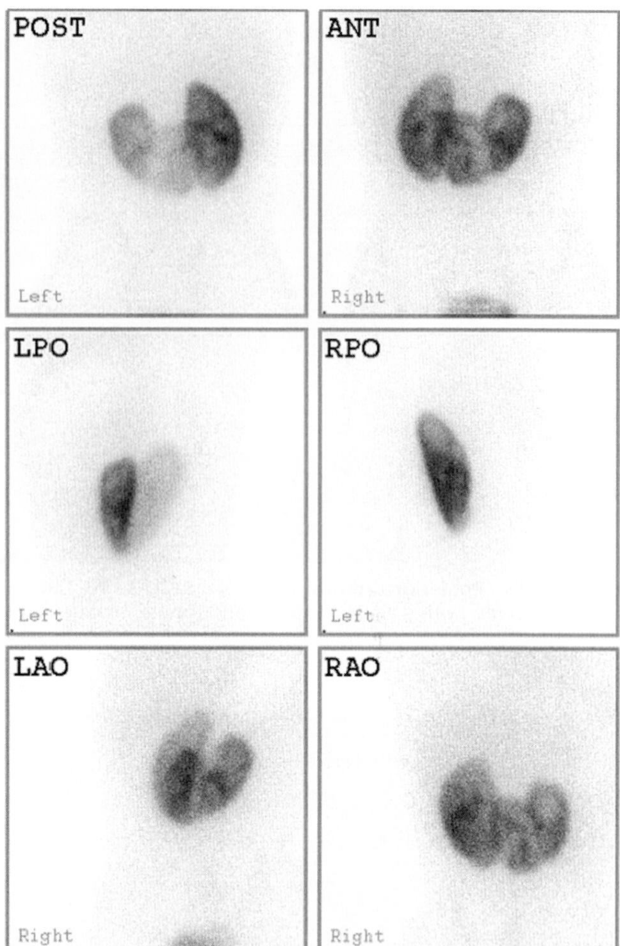

FIGURE 78-12 ■ **Horseshoe kidney.** ^{99m}Tc-DMSA scan of a horseshoe kidney showing fusion at the lower poles in the midline.

The main use of the ^{99m}Tc-DMSA scan is in the assessment of the DRF and cortical abnormalities, such as renal scarring, fusion defects, ectopic or duplex kidneys and in hypertension (e.g. Fig. 78-12). DRF may also be helpful for pre- and post-transplant assessment and in abdominal tumours, where the renal blood supply may be at risk, or where the kidney lies in the radiotherapy field. All indications are given in Table 78-2. There are no contraindications.

Dynamic Renography

Dynamic renography is used to assess split renal function and drainage from the renal collecting systems in suspected obstruction.[10] In Europe, the most common isotope used in paediatric dynamic imaging is ^{99m}Tc-MAG3, which reflects tubular function. ^{99m}Tc-DTPA is also utilised, and uptake reflects glomerular function; thus, it is more commonly is used to calculate the glomerular filtration rate (GFR) and is the least expensive renal imaging agent capable of dynamic assessment. After intravenous administration, about 50% of the ^{99m}Tc-MAG3 in the blood is extracted by the proximal tubules with each pass through the kidneys. The ^{99m}Tc-MAG3 is

TABLE 78-2 **Indications for ^{99m}Tc-DMSA Examination**

- Assessment of differential renal function:
  - e.g. Assessment of functioning renal tissue when renal anatomical variants are encountered, such as duplex kidneys, horseshoe kidneys and cross-fused kidneys, as well as ectopic kidneys
- Assessment for focal parenchymal defects, typically 4–6 months following UTI
- Acute DMSA scans may be performed to confirm pyelonephritis
- Differentiating a multicystic dyplastic kidney from a hydronephrotic kidney
- Assessment of which kidney to biopsy in bilateral disease
- Assessment of function in children with cystic renal disease
- Assessment of focal defects in a hypertensive child, particularly prior to catheter angiography
- Assessment of a transplant kidney in those children with an unfavourable bladder who thus may be prone to reflux and silent infection
- Assessment of functioning renal tissue in children with bilateral Wilms' tumours where renal conserving surgery is being contemplated
- Assessment of DRF in children undergoing abdominal radiotherapy where the kidneys are in the therapy field

TABLE 78-3 **Indications for ^{99m}Tc-MAG3 Dynamic Renography**

- To assess divided renal function and urinary drainage where the collecting system is dilated
- To assess DRF following surgery or procedure, for example post pyeloplasty, or post removal of a double J stent
- Following renal transplant, to assess for urinary leak or possible obstruction

then secreted into the lumen of the tubule. As ^{99m}Tc-DTPA is filtered by the glomerulus, with only 20% extraction fraction, it is not a good agent to use in neonates, children with impaired renal function or in the presence of significant obstruction.

In ^{99m}Tc-MAG3 studies, if there is dilatation of a collecting system, a diuretic is used such as furosemide at a dose of 1 mg/kg (maximum dose 20 mg). Timing of diuretic administration varies widely, but may be given just after the tracer to try to prevent loss of venous access later in the study, in a distressed child. Time activity curves are generated which demonstrate uptake and excretion. Analogue images in the uptake phase may demonstrate renal scarring, albeit less clearly than on the ^{99m}Tc-DMSA static renal scan. Split renal function can also be calculated—being even more accurate than static renography in a significantly obstructed kidney. The indications are given in Table 78-3. Where VUR is suspected, and the child is toilet-trained, cooperative and continent, an IRC may be performed.

Technique. The children are encouraged to drink plenty so that they are well hydrated upon arrival at the department (which is essential for meaningful results). The administered dose is scaled on a body surface area basis, with a maximum dose of 100 MBq of ^{99m}Tc-MAG3. The child empties the bladder, lies supine on the camera face, distracted by television or a film, and is immobilised with sandbags. Ten- to 20-s frames are acquired for 20 min following isotope injection, imaging the heart, kidneys and bladder. The child then voids again before returning to the gamma camera for images following postural change and micturition, at about 40 min post injection.

The DRF estimation is calculated from the renogram between 60 and 120 s from the peak of the vascular curve, expressed as a percentage of the sum total. The recommended methods to evaluate the DRF are the Patlak–Rutland plot and the integral method. Interpretation of the renogram in a dilated kidney, such as pelviureteric junction obstruction (PUJO) needs to be performed carefully. The shape of the time activity curve, response to furosemide and drainage of the collecting system following a change of posture and micturition are evaluated for significant stasis of tracer. There are four classic drainage patterns, described as normal (I), obstructed (II), dilated unobstructed (IIIa) and equivocal (IIIb). Ideally the renogram should be assessed with the US images available so that the degree of HN and the renal parenchyma can be evaluated. Normal kidneys with DRF below 45% should be monitored using US. If dilatation increases, and a ^{99m}Tc-MAG3 demonstrates stepwise fall in function, pyeloplasty may prevent further deterioration in renal function.

TABLE 78-4 **Indications for IVU in Children**

- Suspected ureteral and renal trauma, only if CT is not available
- As a delayed KUB view after contrast-enhanced CT (avoiding a second CT)
- In rare settings where CT is impossible, for instance in intensive care
- Urolithiasis, where USS is inconclusive
- Distinct pelvicalyceal or ureteral pathology (e.g. calyceal diverticula, early stages of medullary sponge kidney, ureteral valves)

Urography (Plain Radiograph and Intravenous Urogram)

With advances of sophisticated US techniques, and availability of cross-sectional imaging, and widespread use of renal scintigraphy, the use of intravenous urography (IVU) has decreased with very few indications remaining (Table 78-4).[11] Except for urolithiasis, an initial 'control' full radiograph is rarely indicated. The radiation exposure should be minimised, using 1–3 properly timed and coned views (KUB film) based on the individual query.

Computed Tomography

CT urography (CTU) may be performed where specialised ultrasound or MR urography is unavailable.[11] Childhood conditions that may require imaging by CT include three main areas: calculi, tumours and trauma (Table 78-5).

TABLE 78-5 Indications for CT of the Renal Tract in Children

- Diagnosis and follow-up of suspected malignant tumour, although MRI is now regarded as equally reliable in assessing abdominal masses
- Major abdominal trauma with suspicion of serious pelvic injury or fracture, or if haematuria is present or bladder rupture is suspected
- Complicated infection, such as suspected abscess if MRI is unavaible and US is inconclusive
- Less common indications may include a suspicion of chronic renal infection or tuberculosis, or of nephrocalcinosis when a US study is inconclusive
- Large calculi or xanthogranulomatous pyelonephritis (XPG) in an older child where surgery may be planned, and where MRI is not available or detailed stone definition is requested
- CT angiography (CTA) may replace conventional angiography in certain circumstances, discussed further in the section 'Hypertension'

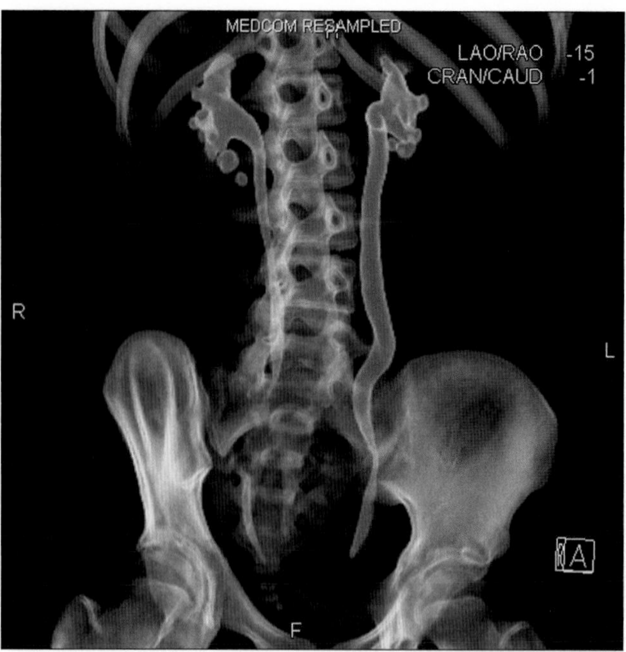

FIGURE 78-13 ■ **CT urography.** This VRT (volume rendered reconstruction) image from a 12 year old shows delineation of the urine within the urinary tract.

Method

Unenhanced CT has almost no role in paediatrics, except for calculi or calcifications,[11] and these are best seen using ultrasound. Thus, standard non-ionic contrast medium (e.g. iohexol 300) is required at an age-adapted dose.[11] Modern imaging techniques using automatic exposure control and low age-adapted kVp and size-based milliampere (mA)s settings will keep the dose to a diagnostic minimum, as will optimal age dependent timing delays and avoiding multiphase acquisitions. In cases of abdominal trauma, topographic delayed imaging after 10–15 min (or a split bolus technique) can be useful in selected cases to detect contrast medium extravasation from the genitourinary tract.[12] Conventional cystography is preferred in suspected urethral injury. Figure 78-13 shows a normal CT urogram.

Magnetic Resonance Imaging

Anatomical MRI is now the imaging modality of choice for abdominal and pelvic masses, as it gives excellent soft-tissue contrast resolution in any imaging plane, decreasing imaging times with modern equipment, improving tissue characterisation without the use of radiation. In most cases, MRI can replace CT, e.g. in the assessment of Wilms' tumour, although thoracic CT may still be required to assess for pulmonary metastases. MRI can also give superior anatomical information to delineate pelvic anatomy, e.g. ambiguous genitalia, or where spinal MRI is needed to evaluate tumoural spread or suspected spinal cord abnormalities (neuropathic bladder). The most common use of MRI/MR urography (MRU) is to evaluate complex urinary tract malformations and urinary tract obstruction, having practically replaced IVU, e.g. Fig. 78-14.[11] MRA is particularly useful to delineate the major renal vessels in preoperative (tumour) imaging, complicated hypertension, or as pre- or post-transplant assessment. The indications are given in Table 78-6.

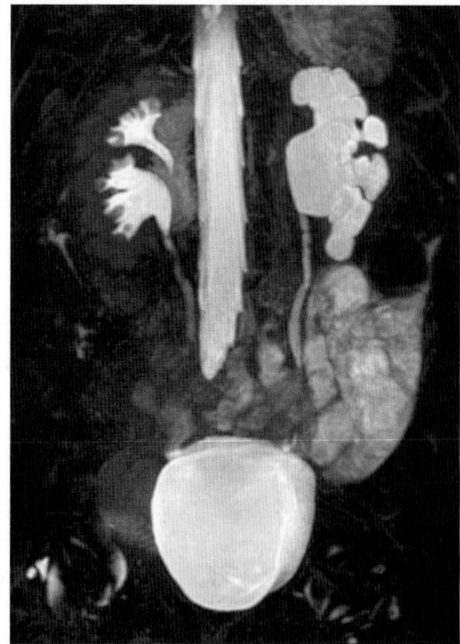

FIGURE 78-14 ■ **MR urography.** Heavily T2-weighted thick-slice coronal MRI image in a 3-year-old girl with right-sided duplex kidney which drains normally, but pelviureteric junction obstruction on the left.

Method

Specific sequences and protocols are now available in most institutions for different clinical scenarios.[13] Axial T1- and T2-weighted imaging are the mainstay of any imaging protocol, and either single-shot coronal heavily T2-weighted imaging or a 3D T2 sequence can give a

TABLE 78-6 Indications for MRI of the Renal Tract in Children

- Diagnosis and follow-up of abdominal or pelvic mass/suspected tumour
- In acute pyelonephritis and its complications, if US inconclusive
- Where spinal imaging is required in children with suspected neuropathic bladder
- Functional MR urography—upper urinary tract obstruction and renal dysplasia
- Contrast-enhanced MRA may have a role in the assessment of hypertension

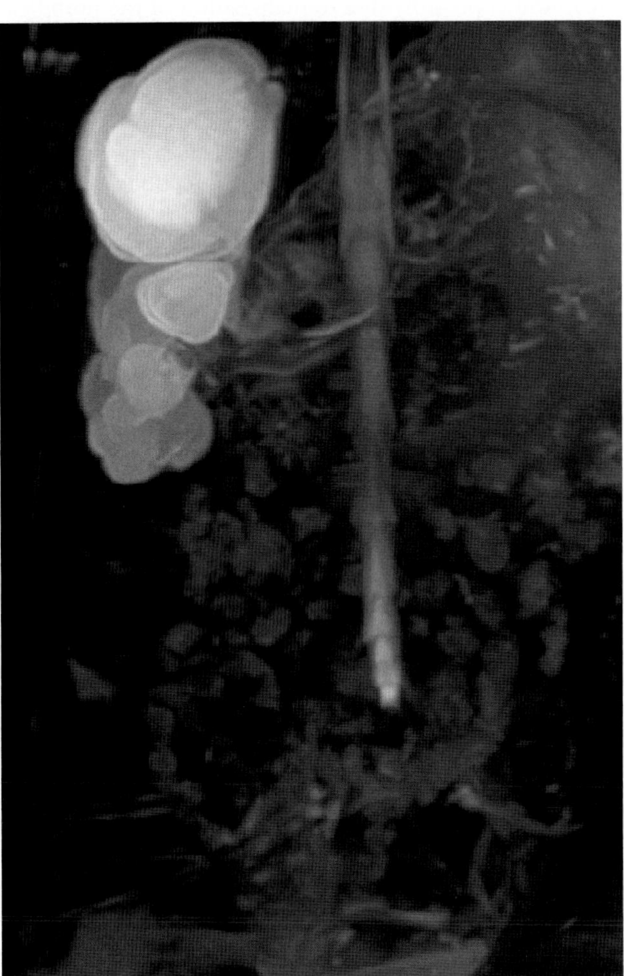

FIGURE 78-15 ■ **MR urography.** Three-dimensional T2 MRU image demonstrates a grossly dilated collecting system of the right kidney CSF is also demonstrated.

'urogram' overview of the entire urinary system (Fig. 78-15). Serial imaging following contrast enhancement is useful to delineate the enhancement of tumours, or arterial enhancement for anatomy. MRU is the only imaging modality to give detailed functional as well as anatomical detail. Full MRU requires a dedicated protocol, including hydration, sedation, catheterisation and diuresis, with prolonged T1 gradient-echo dynamic sequences demonstrating contrast uptake, elimination and drainage similar to radionuclide renograms. Diffusion-weighted MRI (DWI) is rapidly evolving to give an index of tumour cellularity (but does not differentiate benign from malignant tumours), identifying metastases, and in acute pyelonephritis and tumour treatment response. New techniques such as blood oxygen level-dependent (BOLD) MRI are being assessed to demonstrate changes in oxygenation of the kidney during acute obstructive episodes and in transplant imaging.

TABLE 78-7 Indications for Angiography of the Renal Tract in Children

- Hypertension with a high suspicion of renovascular disease, including suspected vasculitis, especially polyarteritis nodosa
- Renal vein sampling for renin values to evaluate which kidney is causing the hypertension
- Before interventional procedures, e.g. embolisation for arteriovenous malformations or balloon dilatation for renal artery stenosis
- Rarely in bilateral Wilms' tumours before surgery
- Testicular vein embolisation for varicocele obliteration

Interventional Procedures

Angiography

Angiography is reserved for specific clinical situations (Table 78-7) by an experienced operator. Selective arteriography with magnification and oblique views is necessary to detect lesions in small renal vessels.

Antegrade Pyelogram

This investigation should be carried out by an experienced operator in the radiology department or in theatre, usually before surgery, to provide anatomical detail of the renal pelvis and/or ureter unavailable from US or IVU. Occasionally antegrade studies are combined with pressure flow measurements with or without urodynamic studies to determine the physiological significance of a dilated upper urinary tract (the 'Whitaker test').

Nephrostomy

The placement of a pigtail or J-J catheter in a dilated renal pelvis or ureter should be undertaken by an experienced operator under US guidance, with similar techniques to adults. US-guided needle placement into an appropriate lower pole calyx with contrast injection gives delineation of the collecting system before insertion of the tube. The complications of placing a nephrostomy tube are generally those of catheter placement, extravasation of contrast medium, and leakage of urine; thus, a combined sonographic–fluoroscopic approach is often recommended.

Retrograde Pyelogram

The instillation of dilute contrast medium into a ureter via a catheter inserted into the distal ureteric orifice is usually undertaken by a urologist in the operating theatre. With modern flexible ureteroscopes, the contrast medium may be instilled into the upper ureter or even the renal pelvis, to outline the ureter and its drainage.

Renal Biopsy

Many disorders affecting the kidney need a biopsy for histological confirmation or diagnosis, particularly glomerular disease, nephrotic syndrome and IgA nephropathy. Surgical exploration or percutaneous US-guided needle biopsy should be considered, with complications such as subcapsular haematoma and AV fistula being fairly rare. Guidelines have recently been formulated for renal biopsy in children.[14,15]

CONGENITAL ANOMALIES

RENAL ANOMALIES

Renal Agenesis

Unilateral agenesis occurs in approximately 1 in 1250 live births. Antenatal diagnosis is uncommon, suggesting that agenesis may be the result of an involuted multicystic dysplastic kidney.

Most functioning kidneys should be identifiable by US wherever they are located, and either ^{99m}Tc-DMSA or MR can be used to detect poorly functioning kidneys. VUR is more common in a non-functioning kidney, and associated ipsilateral abnormalities, including uterine/seminal vesicle or gonadal abnormalities are common, particularly easier to detect in the neonatal period before these structures involute physiologically.

Abnormal Migration and Fusion of the Kidneys

Appreciating renal embryology will assist in the understanding of the various forms of renal malformation and vascular anomalies. The kidney initially forms from an interaction between the mesonephric duct/ureteric bud and the metanephros at around 4 weeks of gestation. The primitive kidney ascends, rotating 90° from horizontal to medial, taking its blood from the aorta and draining via the inferior vena cava. An ectopic kidney may result from excess, incomplete or abnormal ascent. Abnormalities of fusion may occur if the kidneys touch each other in the process of ascending.

Renal Ectopia

Approximately 1 in 1000 kidneys is ectopic, and 10% are bilateral. The commonest is a pelvic kidney, which normally lies anterior to the sacrum just below the bifurcation of the aorta (Fig. 78-16). The true intrathoracic kidney (entering via the foramen of Bochdalek) is rare. Occasionally the kidney may be a superior ectopic kidney lying below a very thin membranous portion of the diaphragm. The adrenal glands are usually normally sited in the presence of renal ectopia, and there are many adrenal anomalies unrelated to renal variation.

Abnormalities of Renal Fusion

The commonest renal fusion abnormality is the horseshoe kidney. The lower poles of the kidneys are fused in the midline, possibly due to malposition of the umbilical arteries causing the developing nephrogenic masses to come together. The isthmus of the horseshoe commonly lies anterior to the aorta and vena cava, at the level of the inferior mesenteric artery, with malrotated collecting systems lying anteriorly, which may lead to pelviureteric junction obstruction and associated infections or calculi. The abnormal axis of the lower poles of the kidneys in a horseshoe should not be missed on US: if bowel gas obscures the anterior view, the loss of the normal medial renal contour and graded compression is useful, and the kidney itself can be used as a window to visualise the parenchymal bridge. The anterior view of a ^{99m}Tc-DMSA may be helpful to assess functioning renal tissue in a horseshoe. MRI also demonstrates abnormalities of renal and (often associated) vascular anatomy and their complications. The horseshoe kidney may become damaged in a road traffic accident because of the position of the lap belt in relation to the kidney. Power Doppler US provides excellent assessment of small traumatic lesions to a horseshoe kidney rather than resorting to CT. There is an increased risk of Wilms' tumour in horseshoe kidneys and the anomaly may be associated with Edwards' syndrome (trisomy 18) and Turner's syndrome.

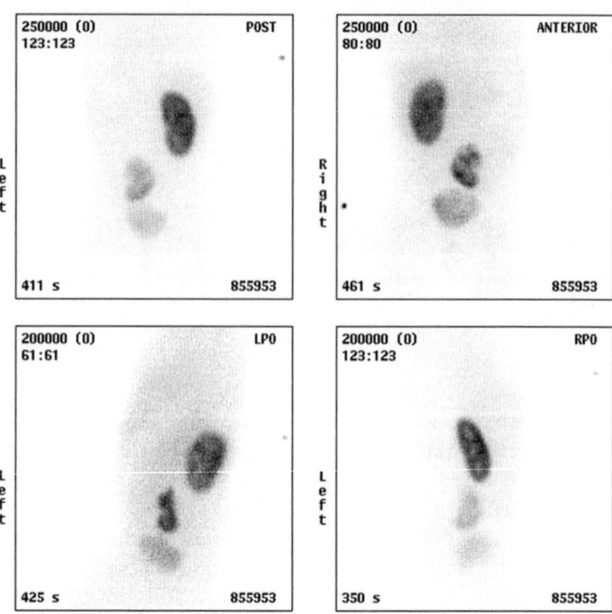

FIGURE 78-16 ■ **Ectopic kidney.** ^{99m}Tc-DMSA scan of a pelvic ectopic kidney which demonstrates scarring from recurrent UTIs.

Cross Fused Renal Ectopia

Crossed fused renal ectopia is seen in 1 in 7000 post mortem examinations. The crossed ectopic kidney lies on the opposite side to its ureteral insertion into the bladder. The left kidney is more commonly the ectopic kidney and the commonest pattern is fusion of the upper pole of the crossed kidney with the lower pole of the normally positioned kidney, in an L shape (Fig. 78-17). Occasionally the crossed kidney remains unfused. Imaging by US demonstrates a unilateral large mass of renal tissue, with contralateral absence of renal tissue. Because of abnormalities in rotation, PUJO is common and a ^{99m}Tc-MAG3 (or dynamic MRU) study is often helpful in assessment of drainage, and VUR is common. Associated anomalies may be seen (for example, VACTERL association).

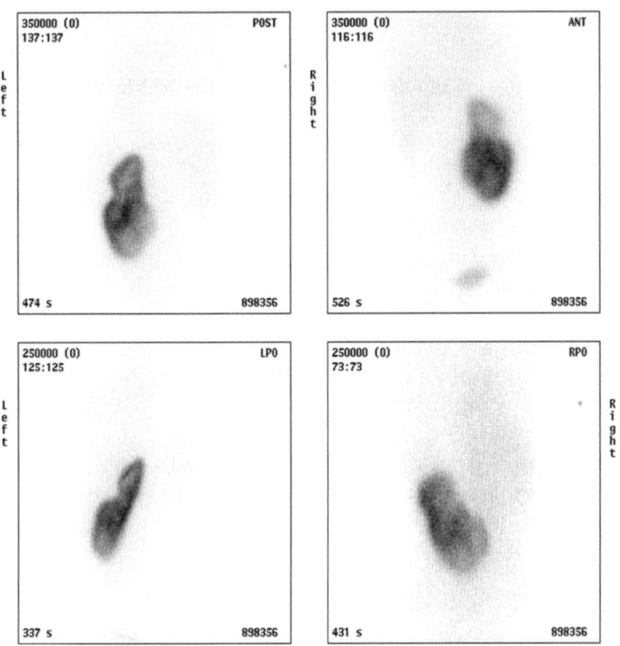

FIGURE 78-17 ■ Crossed fused ectopia. ^{99m}Tc-DMSA scan of crossed fused ectopia.

Duplex Kidneys

The commonest renal anomaly (2% of the population) is an uncomplicated duplex kidney. Complete duplication is caused by two separate ureteral buds presenting onto the mesonephric duct. The ureter draining the lower moiety will come to lie more superior to and lateral to the ureter draining the upper moiety, increasing the VUR risk to the lower moiety. The upper moiety ureteric insertion into the bladder usually is more distally and medially, may even be ectopic, or may be associated with an ureterocele, causing varying degrees of dysplasia and obstruction in the upper moiety (Fig. 78-18). Sometimes the upper moiety is difficult to see and if the upper moiety ureter drains ectopically into the vagina in a girl, continuous wetting or recurrent UTIs result. Careful interrogation by US, complemented by MRI, is essential in order to pick up both echogenic and atrophic upper moieties.

Incomplete ureteric duplication ('incomplete duplication') describes ureteric duplication above the bladder. Yo-yo VUR may be demonstrated by dynamic renography with tracer passing down one ureter and back up the partially duplicated second ureter into the respective renal moiety, but the kidney in these children looks the same as in a complete duplication. A 'septated renal pelvis' is the mildest variant of this condition. An ureterocele prolapsing into the vagina may present as a perineal mass in the newborn, or bladder outlet obstruction due to an ureterocole prolapsing into the posterior urethra (mimicking posterior urethral valves).

Imaging

A duplex kidney may be diagnosed by US, with a larger than normal kidney with two distinct collecting systems being separated by a bridge of renal tissue. The appearances of a duplex kidney vary with the pathology of each moiety. The upper moiety is usually dilated, particularly when associated with a ureterocele or ectopic ureteric insertion, or may be atrophic (Figs. 78-19 and 78-20). (Power) Doppler can estimate the degree of dysplasia and may demonstrate the ectopic ureteric jet. The lower

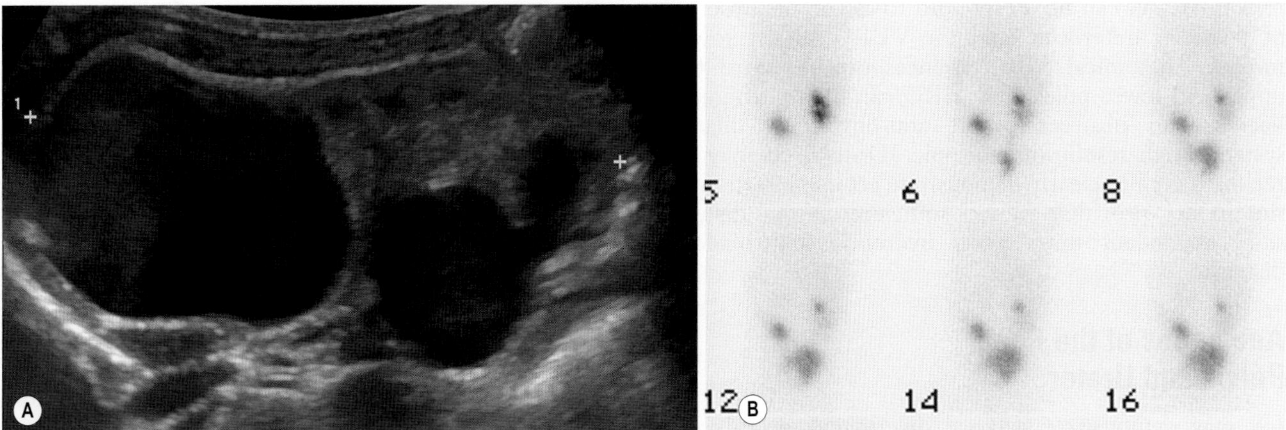

FIGURE 78-18 ■ Duplex kidney. (A) US shows grossly dilated upper moiety of the right kidney, with milder dilatation of the lower moiety. (B) Selected images from the MAG3 shows a duplex left kidney with upper moiety obstruction.

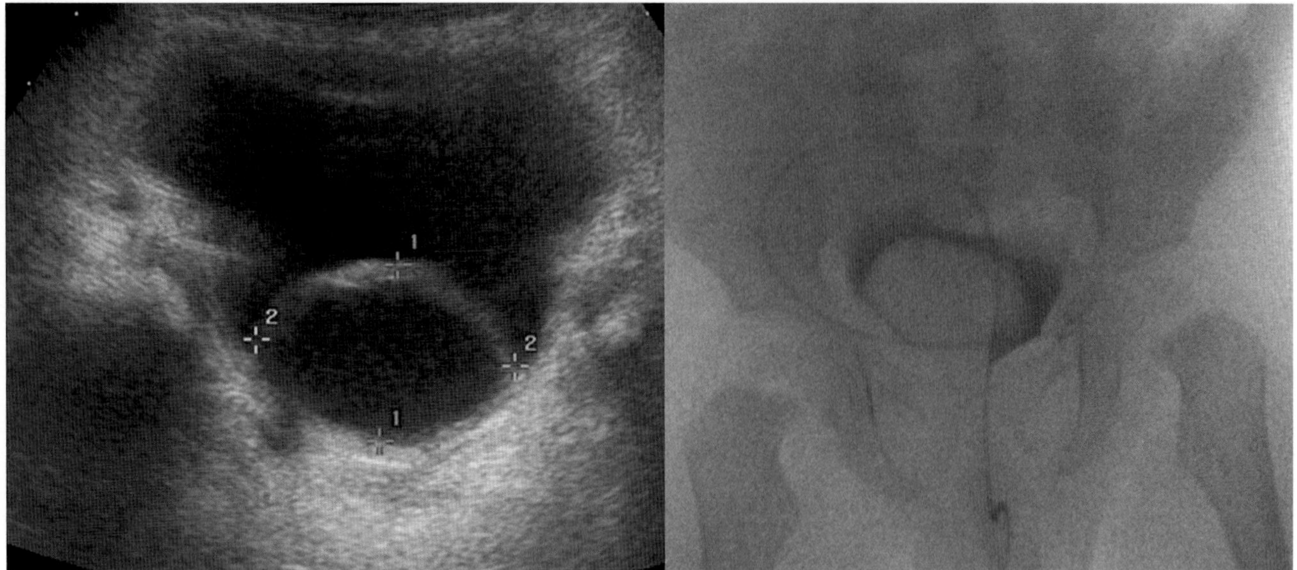

FIGURE 78-19 ■ **Ureterocele.** A large ureterocele is identified on US, clearly visible on the early filling view of the MCUG where contract is seen circumferentially outside the ureterocele within the bladder.

moiety may be dilated in PUJO, or demonstrate scarring and uroepithelial thickening in the collecting system to indicate VUR.

The ^{99m}Tc-MAG3 will be helpful in assessment of renal function, scarring and dysplasia, allowing the relative contribution to function from each moiety to may be calculated. The uncomplicated duplex on a functional study may demonstrate up to 60% DRF compared to a simplex contralateral kidney, giving the false impression of reduced function in the simplex kidney. The axis of the duplex kidney on a DMSA may point towards the ipsilateral shoulder rather than the contralateral shoulder on the image, prompting the radiologist to look carefully on US for the hallmark finding of two separate collecting systems. The ^{99m}Tc-MAG3 renogram is also used to assess function and drainage in a complicated duplex kidney, and an IRC can be used in the toilet-trained child to assess for lower moiety VUR. Correct interpretation and calculations by scintigraphy rely heavily on accurate anatomical knowledge from US or MRI.

An MCUG can be useful both to assess for presence of possible ureterocele and for VUR into the lower moiety. Anatomical MR sequences can delineate the upper and lower poles, and MRU can help distinguish between an obstructed and non-obstructed dilated system. High-resolution isotropic 3D data sets may be reconstructed to clearly demonstrate ectopic insertion of the ureters, provided there is sufficient ureteral distension, dependent upon good hydration and bladder distension.

Anomalies of the Renal Pelvis and Ureter

US may demonstrate calyceal diverticulae or calyceal dilatation due to an infundibular stenosis, either congenital or acquired (secondary to infection or obstruction by calculi). MRI/MRU may further evaluate these appearances. Megacalycosis is a poorly understood condition where the dysplastic calyces are dilated in the absence of obstruction. It is probably due to underdevelopment of the medullary pyramids or maturation defects (resembling the shape of a pelvic kidney), and there may be an association with a megaureter and renal ectopia. Thus ureteric or pelvicaliceal dilatation does not indicate obstruction, and while the condition may predispose to stone formation, corrective surgery for ureteric dilatation is not beneficial.

Pelviureteric Junction Obstruction

PUJO is the commonest cause of renal tract dilatation, comprising up to 40% of cases. Antenatal and then postnatal US of the renal pelvis is useful in suspected PUJO or pseudo-obstruction. Poorly understood, there may be an anatomical abnormality, which can present early with antenatal unilateral HN, or a crossing vessel causing extrinsic compression, which usually presents later with intermittent pain or infection. Abnormal ureteric peristalsis or VUR (with infections) may lead to ureteric kinking, fibrosis or there may be a delayed recanalisation of the fetal ureter. Secondary PUJO may occur due to scarring after UTI and particularly with high-grade VUR, in elongated tortuous megaureters, as well as with obstructing tumours or retroperitoneal fibrosis.

Imaging

Diagnosis of PUJO is important in order to highlight those severe cases which may progress, causing loss of renal function, which may require surgical intervention. The initial US is performed approximately seven days after birth so that the baby is well hydrated and the degree of renal pelvic dilatation is not underestimated.

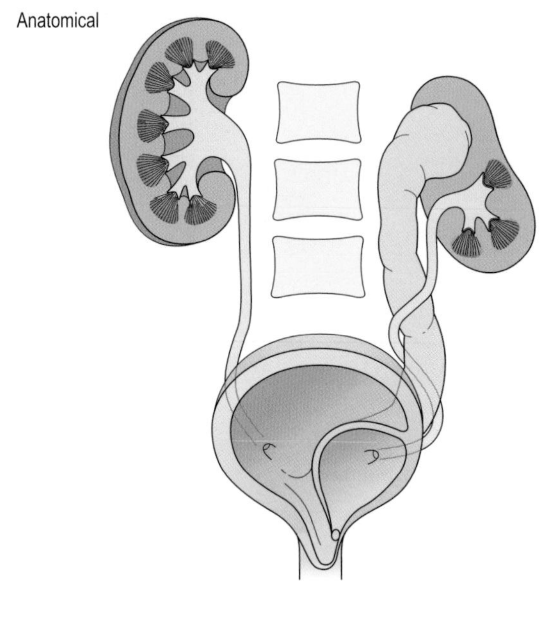

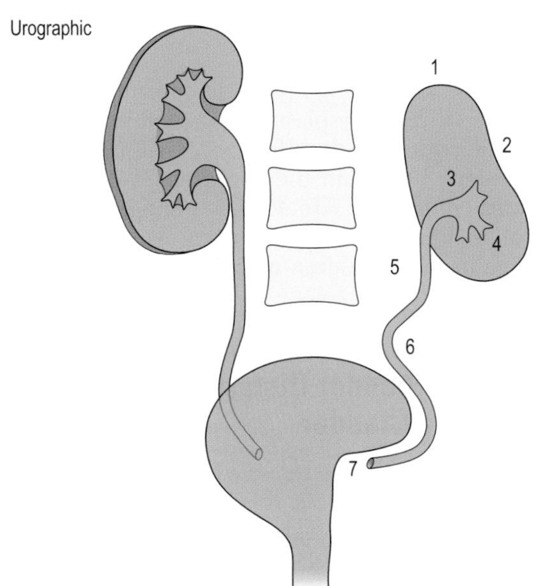

FIGURE 78-20 ■ **Duplex kidney.** Diagrammatic representation of duplex kidneys with an ectopic ureterocele of the left upper moiety without function. Diagnosis depends on recognition of indirect signs: 1 = increased distance from the top of the visualised collecting system to the upper border of the nephrogram; 2 = abnormal axis of the collecting system; 3 = impression upon the upper border of the renal pelvis; 4 = decreased number of calyces compared to the contralateral kidney; 5 = lateral displacement of the kidney and ureter; 6 = lateral course of the visualised ureter; and 7 = filling defect in the bladder.

The prone transverse view of the renal pelvis is used to assess the AP pelvic diameter: between 7 and 10 mm on antenatal US requires follow-up in the newborn period, and greater than 1 cm thereafter; HN can be graded accordingly.[16] Function and drainage is assessed on the diuretic ^{99m}Tc-MAG3 renogram or fMRU (Fig. 78-21). The study is ideally performed when the baby is over 6–8 weeks of age, preferably over 3 months, when there is some renal maturity.

If renal pelvic dilatation is severe and bilateral, and the significantly thinned renal parenchyma is undifferentiated and echogenic, with reduced vascularity on power Doppler, earlier assessment of function is required. Diuretic sonography with serial measurements after furosemide application may help to differentiate dilated from (partially) obstructed kidneys that then require further imaging. In severe bilateral disease, ^{99m}Tc-DMSA may be used as an assessment of the relative contribution of each kidney to total renal function. The study must be performed with careful attention to detail. The baby must be well hydrated and furosemide should be given immediately or soon after the isotope, although a range of timing protocols are in use.

Following the dynamic renogram, a delayed image, following postural change and micturition (if the bladder emptied) should be performed to assess the contribution of gravity to drainage from the dilated upper urinary tract. The degree of urinary stasis cannot be assessed on the supine imaging alone, and a post-micturition/post-catheterisation view is essential. If there is reduced function in the affected kidney and the degree of renal pelvic dilatation on US is changing, urologists may be more inclined to operate. Less than 25% of cases of antenatally diagnosed PUJO undergo surgery.

Megaureter and Hydroureter

In utero, if the fetal ureter is visualised, then it is dilated: it may indicate a primary megaureter, refluxing megaureter, non-refluxing non-obstructive hydroureter or secondary hydroureter (for example, associated with posterior urethral valves and ureterocele).

Imaging

US is used to assess for a ureterocele, or secondary signs of VUR may be evident (e.g. a laterally positioned or gaping ostium, bladder wall trabeculation and thickening, significant post-voiding residual). Bilateral disease is assessed and extrinsic compression leading to secondary hydroureter is readily seen. An MCUG (or ce-VUS) is performed to assess whether ureteric dilatation is caused by VUR, either causing dilatation or coexisting with megaureter. MRU is used to assess anatomy in more complex situations (Fig. 78-22), as the dynamic sequences may demonstrate ureteric peristalsis, and to assess drainage and function.

Bladder Anomalies

Bladder exstrophy–epispadias–cloacal exstrophy complex represents a spectrum of anomalies, with an incidence of around 1 in 20,000 live births, typically male babies. Absence of the normal bladder or the failure to see bladder filling on antenatal US may suggest bladder exstrophy. This results from a failure of closure of the abdominal wall during fetal development, leading to protrusion of the anterior wall of the bladder through the lower abdominal wall defect, and there may be an associated omphalocele. There is an open defect of the anterior abdominal wall or perineal wall and widening of the

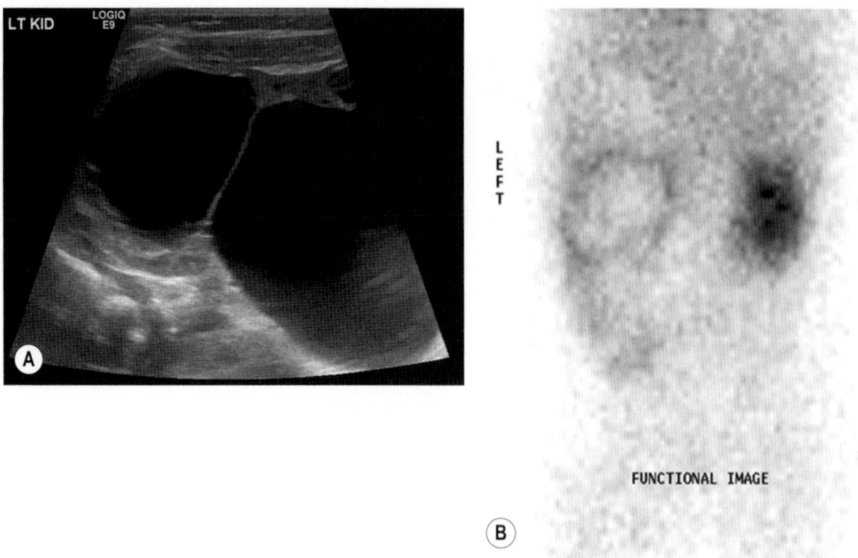

FIGURE 78-21 ■ Pelviureteric junction obstruction. An obstructed left kidney on US (A) with diminished function on MAG3 (B).

pubic symphysis, with epispadias in male babies (dorsal cleft in penis exposing the urethral mucosa). Antenatal diagnosis is difficult and the condition most often presents at birth with the exposed bladder. An estimation of the degree of severity of the condition can be found by measuring the extent of pubic symphysis diastasis on fetal US or plain films (Fig. 78-23). This is normally up to 10 mm, and 10–25 mm suggests epispadias with >25-mm bladder exstrophy. The upper renal tracts are initially normal. Treatment involves staged repair of the bladder and genitalia. Following treatment, careful US and ^{99m}Tc-MAG3 is advised as VUR and obstruction are common following bladder closure.

Prune-Belly Syndrome

The combination of absence/hypoplasia of the abdominal wall musculature, urinary tract dilatation and bilateral undescended testes is known as 'prune-belly syndrome', or abdominal musculature deficiency syndrome. The incidence of prune-belly syndrome is approximately 1 in 40,000 live births, predominantly in male babies; female babies cannot have the complete triad, and the urological manifestations may be less severe. The entire spectrum of prune-belly syndrome is difficult to explain but thought to be either a defect of abdominal wall mesoderm formation early in embryogenesis, or severe bladder outlet obstruction leading to overdistension of the abdominal wall and urinary tract.

Clinical presentation is with a lax abdominal wall with thin wrinkled skin and a protuberant abdomen. US may be challenging but will demonstrate dilated ureters with a large-capacity bladder often with little intrarenal dilatation, as well as absent or hypoplasic abdominal wall muscles. The bladder neck is wide with a dilated proximal posterior urethra and more distal conical narrowing, leading to a poor urinary stream through the anterior urethra ('pseudo-valve'). Prognosis depends on the degree of associated renal dysplasia. These babies are prone to VUR and, consequently, infection. A MCUG is indicated to assess for VUR and the appearances of the urethra. Dynamic diuretic ^{99m}Tc-MAG3 renography may be helpful in long-term follow-up to assess function and drainage in those children without renal compromise.

Functional Bladder Disturbance and Neurogenic Bladder

Children with neurogenic bladder have uncontrolled voiding and incomplete bladder emptying, due to inappropriate detrusor muscle contraction and external sphincter relaxation, e.g. caused by spinal dysraphism, such as a myelomeningocele. Initial spinal US/MRI is essential to rule out spinal abnormality. When no spinal abnormality is found, the term 'non-neurogenic neurogenic bladder' is used: Non-neurogenic voiding disorders or dysfunctional voiding are becoming an increasingly important entity that are identified by modified MCUG or videourodynamics but remain poorly recognised and understood.

Treating neurogenic bladders is aimed towards continence, and preventing deterioration in renal and bladder function. Kidney function deteriorates secondary to poor bladder emptying, leading to HN and VUR, with subsequent complications of infection. Clean intermittent catheterisation, surgical procedures including bladder augmentation, continence procedures and artificial urinary sphincters and medication all have a role in preventing renal damage. Specialised urodynamic clinics are integral in the management of these patients. Regular US of the renal tract with catheterised bladder emptying is necessary to assess renal tract abnormalities. Follow-up dynamic ^{99m}Tc-MAG3 renography with IRC is helpful in

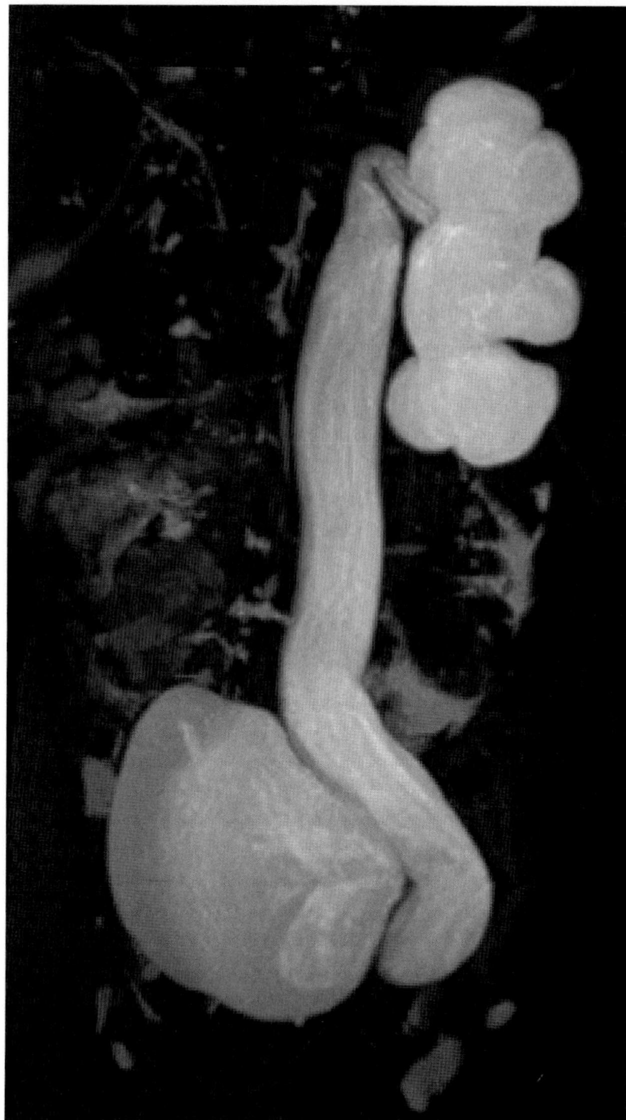

FIGURE 78-22 ■ Megaureter. Three-dimensional T2W MRU image/rotated reconstruction demonstrates a megaureter with an additional kink at the ureteropelvic junction and a markedly dilated collecting system of the kidney.

the assessment of ongoing VUR. MCUG may demonstrate a small-volume trabeculated bladder with diverticula, and VUR into the kidneys; using a modified MCUG protocol or videourodynamic study will give additional functional bladder information. Non-neurogenic bladder and voiding disorders are usually treated by bladder training, often using biofeedback techniques, supported by medications.

URETHRAL ANOMALIES

The urethra is best demonstrated in the oblique lateral projection of the MCUG or by retrograde urethrography. This gives the best view of the bladder neck and posterior urethra, without which an anatomical cause of bladder outlet obstruction cannot be excluded (Fig. 78-9).

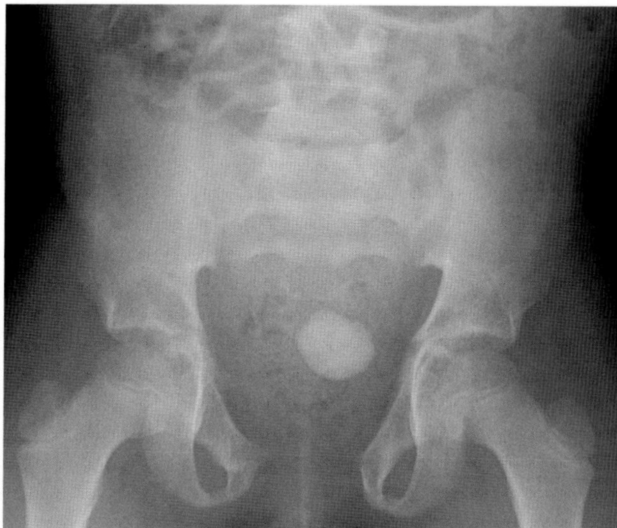

FIGURE 78-23 ■ Bladder exstrophy. Abdominal radiograph showing a radio-opaque calculus in a patient with bladder exstrophy with characteristic diastasis of the pubic symphysis.

Bladder outlet obstruction may be anatomical or functional such as in neurogenic bladder. Anatomical causes of outlet obstruction include posterior urethral valve, ureterocele prolapsing into the posterior urethra causing obstruction, urethral dysplasia, anterior valve/diaphragm/syringocele, meatal stenosis, paraurethral cysts, urethral diverticula or duplication and post-traumatic or infective urethral strictures as well as (severe) hypospadias. Pelvic tumours or urethral polyps can cause obstruction, as can bladder masses such as haemangioma or neurofibroma. These lesions may be demonstrated by (perineal perimicturitional) US, but MRI will be the imaging of choice for assessment and staging of a pelvic mass.

Posterior Urethral Valves (PUV)

Congenital urethral obstruction creates a spectrum of disease, with the timing and severity determining the presenting symptoms. Boys with high-grade obstruction present as neonates with urosepsis, renal insufficiency and pulmonary hypoplasia with severe respiratory distress, detected on antenatal US exhibiting urinary ascites, oligohydramnios, enlarged bladders and renal dilatation. Less severe obstruction may lead to presentation in childhood with UTI. PUV consist of abnormal folds of mucosa between the wall of the urethra and the verumontanum. There are three types, ranging from type I, slit-like orifice between 2 folds at the verumontanum, to type III, valve with eccentric pinpoint aperture causing the valve to balloon forward on micturition ('wind in the sail' appearance on the MCUG). Type III valve is associated with renal dysplasia, even without significant upper tract dilatation. All newborn boys with significant antenatal HN (grade III or higher) and thick bladder wall, ascites or oligohydramnion should be assessed for the presence of PUV. If valves are suspected, the bladder should be drained suprapubically until valves are ablated; with secondary obstruction at the VUJ, a nephrostomy may

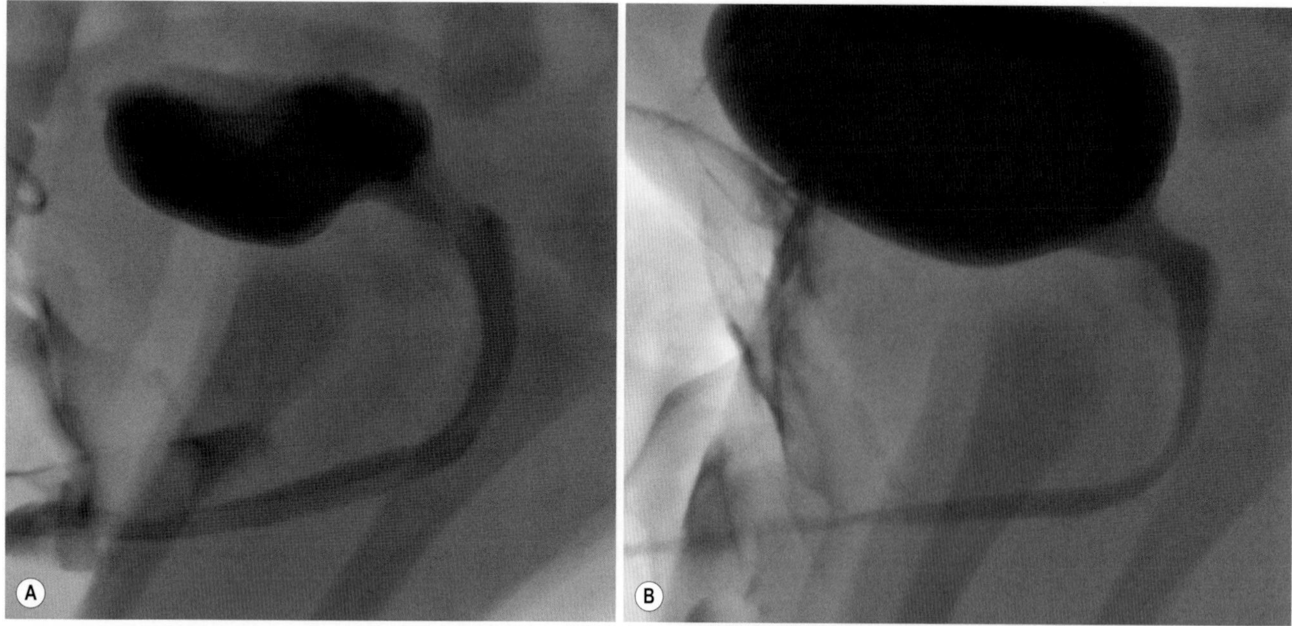

FIGURE 78-24 ■ **Normal urethra.** MCUG demonstrating full-length views of the urethra with a catheter in situ (A) and with the catheter removed (B).

become necessary to ensure sufficient urinary drainage. Note that even with optimal treatment, the associated severe congenital renal dysplasia often still results in renal failure requiring subsequent renal transplantation.

Imaging

In PUV, US may show hydroureteronephrosis, renal dysplasia, or urinomas due to calyceal rupture secondary to increased pressure (the 'pop off' mechanism), and bladder wall thickening with a dilated posterior urethra and hypertrophied bladder neck. If the US is performed before the baby is well hydrated, the degree of hydroureteronephrosis may be underestimated. MCUG is essential (but is contraindicated in acute sepsis). Contrast medium may demonstrate bladder wall trabeculation, a very large (or small) bladder with diverticula, and either unilateral or bilateral VUR, associated with ipsilateral poor renal function. The valve is visualised as an acute-calibre transition on the oblique/lateral urethral projection at micturition. If there is a urethral catheter in situ, a 'catheter out' view when micturating is essential in order to exclude a small valve leaflet compressed by the catheter (Fig. 78-24).

Upper tract drainage by nephrostomy or ureterostomy may be required to preserve renal function. Treatment comprises early cystoscopic valve ablation followed by bladder drainage. A follow-up MCUG after valve ablation may be useful but cystoscopy is required, as remnant valve leaflets may be missed on urethrography. ^{99m}Tc-DMSA is initially used to provide DRF with ^{99m}Tc-MAG3 renography and US follow-up. Antireflux procedures are performed in PUV patients in order to preserve renal function. In boys with severe dysplasia, end-stage renal disease usually occurs in the first 20 years of life.

Anterior Urethral Abnormalities

Anterior urethral valves are around 10 times less common than PUV. The anterior valves may be located anywhere along the anterior urethra, and are often associated with a urethral diverticulum. Severe valves are often diagnosed in the newborn period, but mild valves may present later in childhood. Typical ballooning of the urethra with deviation of the penis may occur during micturition on MCUG. A syringocele is a dilated Cowper's gland or duct that may cause urethral obstruction in the neonate (Figs. 78-25 and 78-26). Sometimes non-specific symptoms of dribbling or haematuria may occur later in childhood. Spontaneous rupture or transurethral incision is curative, but may lead to a urethral stricture.

Urethral Stricture

Strictures may be congenital or acquired and may occur in boys or girls. Seventy-five per cent of male congenital urethral strictures occur in the bulbous urethra (where the embryological proximal urethra merges with the urogenital membrane), and at the urethral meatus in girls. Children with congenital strictures present either as neonates or in the postpubertal period. Early presentation as a neonate may demonstrate significant upper tract dilatation secondary to urethral obstruction. Postpubertal boys present with irritation, urinary dribbling, haematuria and UTI as well as prostatitis or epididymitis. Diagnosis is by MCUG and treatment is usually urethrotomy. Traumatic straddle injuries lead to bulbar strictures. Pelvic trauma and urethral rupture, or catheter induced injuries, tend to cause strictures either at the bladder neck or at the membranous portion of the urethra.

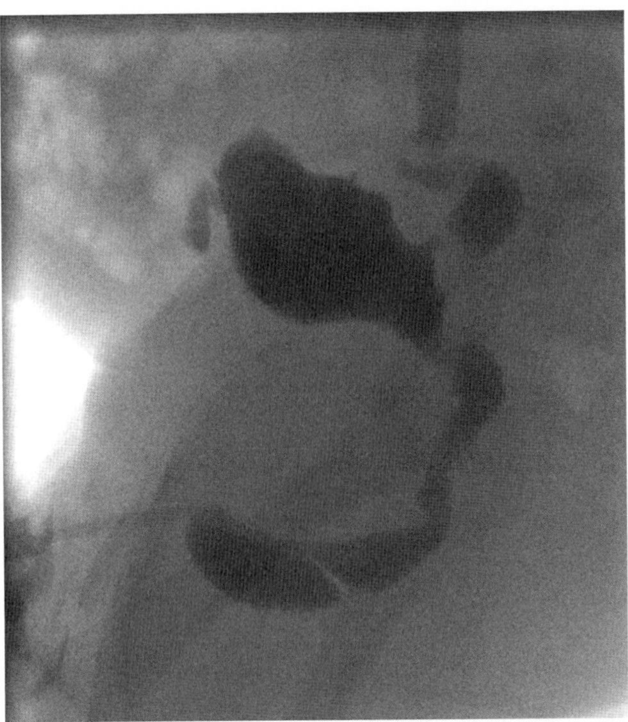

FIGURE 78-25 ■ **Syringocele.** Urethral syringocele demonstrated on MCUG.

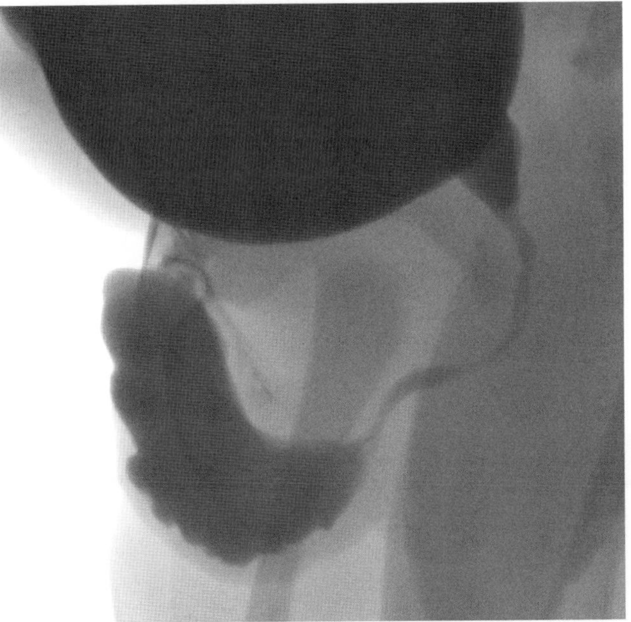

FIGURE 78-26 ■ **Scaphoid congenital megaurethra.** Massive dilatation of the urethra is caused by non-development of the penile erectile tissue, particularly the corpus spongiosum.

Rectourethral Fistula

Rectourethral fistula is usually associated with an imperforate anus and is best demonstrated by a high-pressure loopogram via a distal colostomy which should demonstrate passage of contrast from the bowel to the posterior urethra, or by high-pressure urethrogram/during voiding on a MCUG.

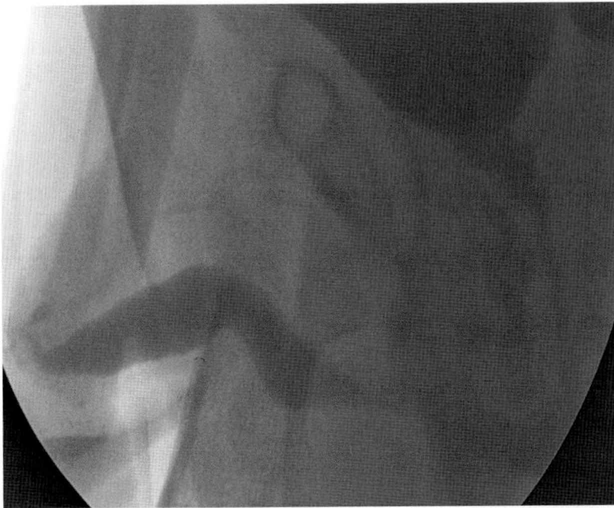

FIGURE 78-27 ■ **Urethal duplication.** There is duplication of the urethra almost from the bladder neck along the whole length of the penis.

Duplication of the Urethra

A rare congenital abnormality usually discovered in childhood with one of the urethras ending as a hypospadias. Duplication of the urethra may be complete and the child presents with a double urinary stream, urinary tract infection, sometimes outflow obstruction and incontinence. The classification of urethral duplication is complex and beyond the scope of this chapter (Fig. 78-27).

UTERUS AND VAGINA

Differentiation of the gonads into ovaries or testes depends on the presence or absence of the Y chromosome. In the absence of hormonal secretion of anti-Müllerian hormone from the fetal testis, the Müllerian ducts meet and differentiate into the uterus, cervix, fallopian tubes and proximal two-thirds of the vagina. The urogenital sinus forms the distal vagina. Uterine development depends on the formation of the Wolffian or mesonephric duct.

Uterovaginal malformations are classified embryologically into either Müllerian agenesis, a developmental defect of the caudal portion of the Müllerian ducts (Mayer–Rokitansky–Küster–Hauser (MRKH) syndrome); disorders of lateral fusion caused by the failure of the two Müllerian ducts to fuse in the midline; and disorders of vertical fusion that are caused by abnormal union between the Müllerian tubercle and urogenital sinus derivatives (leading to disorders of the hymen, cervical agenesis and transverse vaginal septa). Disorders of lateral fusion are heterogeneous and have been classified into six groups. Lateral fusion and vertical fusion abnormalities often coexist and thus congenital vaginal abnormalities can be considered as those with or without obstruction.

Anomalies of the uterus and vagina may present as an abdominal or pelvic mass in the neonatal period. Female genital anomalies are usually suspected on US and diagnosed using MRI, or US genitography using intravaginal saline in centres with experience. Fifty per cent of cases will have an associated renal anomaly and approximately 12% may have associated vertebral segmentation anomalies. Congenital anomalies of the vagina (septation, stenosis, imperforate hymen) often present in pubertal girls with menstrual symptoms but no bleeding due to obstruction (haematometrocolpos; Figs. 78-28, 78-29). Other causes of primary amenorrhoea include Turner's syndrome. MRKH syndrome, which affects 1 in 4000 to 5000 girls, and includes vaginal atresia, uterine anomalies and malformations of the upper urinary tract. Associated renal abnormalities include HN, dysplasia, unilateral ectopia and renal agenesis. Three-dimensional US and MRI are helpful in imaging the spectrum. All girls with genital should have careful US evaluation of the renal tract.

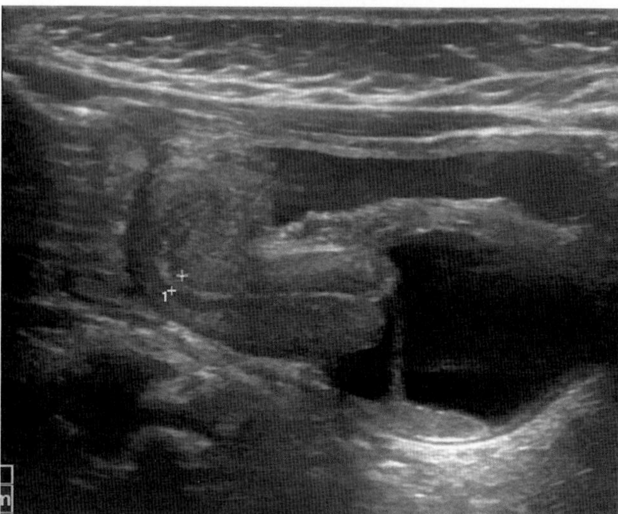

FIGURE 78-28 ■ **Haematocolpos.** Sagittal US image of thickened endometrium with spill of blood into the obstructed, distended vagina lying behind the normal bladder.

UNDESCENDED TESTIS

Cryptorchidism refers to the absence of a testis in the scrotum, affecting 4% of full-term newborns and 30% of preterm newborns, falling to around 0.8% after the first year. It is usually right-sided, but may be bilateral. During embryogenesis, the testes form beside the mesonephric kidneys and descend via the inguinal canal to the scrotum. This normal process may halt anywhere along its descent, causing an undescended testis, or the testis may become ectopic or absent. Early diagnosis and treatment are important to prevent infertility and a risk of malignancy in the undescended testis. Unilateral testicular agenesis is associated with ipsilateral renal agenesis.

There is current debate regarding whether US can confidently localise undescended testes. US has estimated sensitivity and specificity of around 45 and 80%, respectively, in accurately localising non-palpable testes. US is particularly helpful for testicular locations in the inguinal canal or next to the bladder/close to the abdominal wall—deeper positions are more difficult. US can also detect other scrotal pathology, such as hydrocele or cystic dysplasia of the rete testis, which mimics a testicular tumour and is associated with a multicystic dysplastic kidney. MRI is far superior in localising near-normal, non-palable testes, and is preferable in ambiguous genitalia or hypospadias, but small and dysplastic testes may be indistinguishable from non-specific nodules. The testis is typically hypoplastic with low T2 signal. Diagnostic laparoscopy is the definitive investigation and allows for concurrent biopsy or surgical correction.

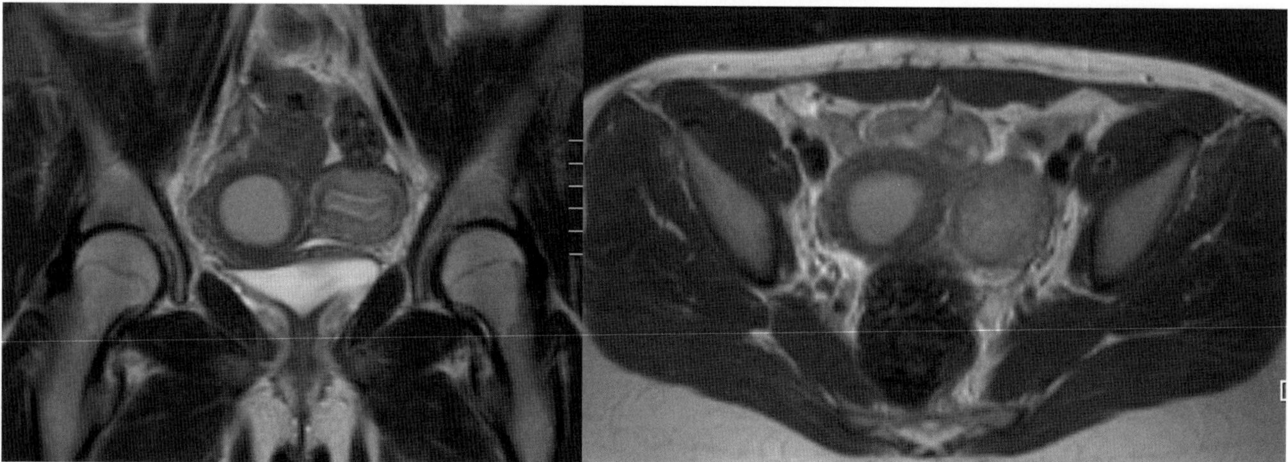

FIGURE 78-29 ■ **Haematometrocolpos.** Only one, i.e. the right of two uterine cavities in this didelphys uterus, demonstrates haematometrocolpos on coronal and axial MRI.

TABLE 78-8 Differential Diagnosis of Prenatal Hydronephrosis

Unilateral Pathology
Renal pelvic dilatation (RPD)
Vesicoureteric reflux (VUR)
Megaureter (with or without reflux)
Multicystic dysplastic kidney
Complicated duplex kidney
Upper moiety dilatation—either ureterocele or ectopic drainage
Lower moiety dilatation—usually VUR but rarely RPD only
Bilateral Pathology
Bilateral renal pelvic dilatation
Bilateral VUR
Bilateral megaureter (with or without reflux)
Bladder pathology, e.g. neurogenic bladder
Bladder outlet pathology (posterior urethral valves)
Bilateral complicated duplex kidneys
Multicystic kidney on one side and cystic dysplastic kidney on opposite side

ANTENATAL DIAGNOSIS OF HYDRONEPHROSIS

Some anatomical renal abnormalities can now be detected antenatally, which begs the question as to what should be done for the child in the immediate postnatal period? The most obvious abnormalities are anatomical disorders, such as renal agenesis and horseshoe kidneys. The next issue is that of HN (pelvicalyceal dilatation) and hydroureter (ureteric dilatation alone). Imaging should try to distinguish between an obstructed and non-obstructed system; the goal of imaging is to direct treatment to preserve renal function and growth potential. There are many imaging algorithms now developed by the European paediatric radiology community, which have been widely publicised.[1]

Prenatal Diagnosis of Renal/Urological Abnormality and Differential Diagnosis

Newborns with a prenatal US diagnosis of a renal tract abnormality do not form a homogeneous group. Transient renal pelvic dilatation (RPD) is thought to be physiological during fetal development, but persistent or enlarging RPD during the antenatal period will typically be referred for postnatal investigation, although most will be determined to be normal. The differential diagnosis is wide (Table 78-8). Bilateral disease must be distinguished from unilateral disease, as unilateral normal kidney and ureter implies that normal function can be achieved. The most important diagnosis to make immediately (US and MCUG within the first 24 h of life) is that of PUV, potentially causing bilateral obstructive HN and renal damage, so that perinatal surgery can be performed for this indication. For those children with less marked abnormalities, repeating US at

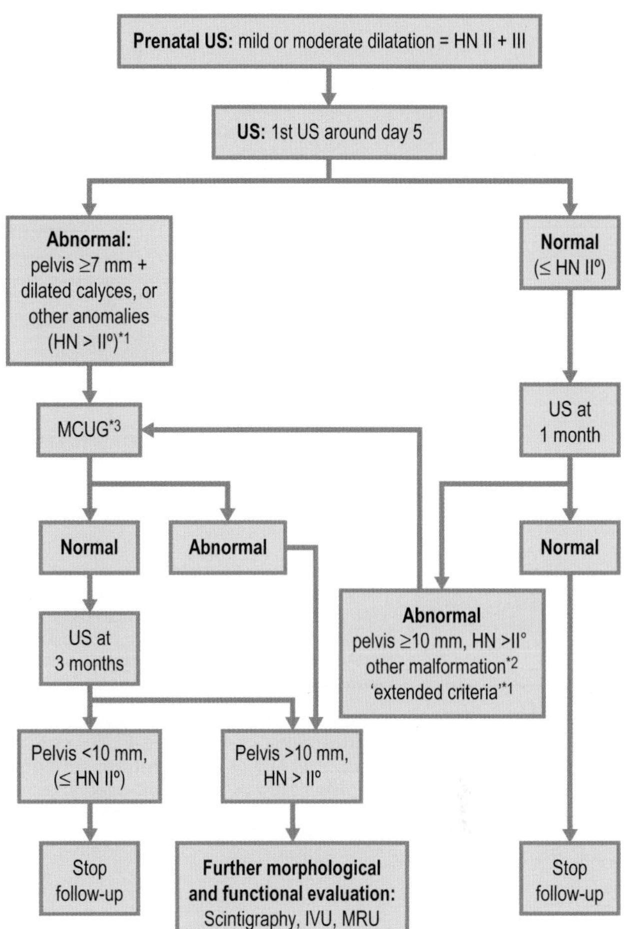

FIGURE 78-30 ■ **Hydronephrosis.** ESPR imaging algorithm for mild or moderate fetal hydronephrosis, IVU = intravenous urography, MCDK = multicystic dysplastic kidney, MRU = magnetic resonance urography. (Adapted from Riccabona M, Avni F E, Blickman J G, et al 2008 Imaging recommendations in paediatric uroradiology: minutes of the ESPR workgroup session on urinary tract infection, fetal hydronephrosis, urinary tract ultrasonography and voiding cystourethrography, Barcelona, Spain, June 2007. Pediatr Radiol 38(2):138–145.[1])

1 and 4–6 weeks of life can often eliminate those in whom the functionally immature system has improved, and no further imaging is required (Fig. 78-30).[1] The urgency of postnatal imaging is heavily dependent on the prenatal US findings and the quality/availability of prenatal US.

Bilateral Renal Pelvic Dilatation

Renal pelvic dilatation (RPD) or hydronephrosis (HN) may be defined as calyceal dilatation plus a renal pelvis of greater than 10–15 mm in its AP diameter with no US evidence of a dilated ureter. This was incorrectly referred to previously as pelviureteric junction (PUJ) obstruction

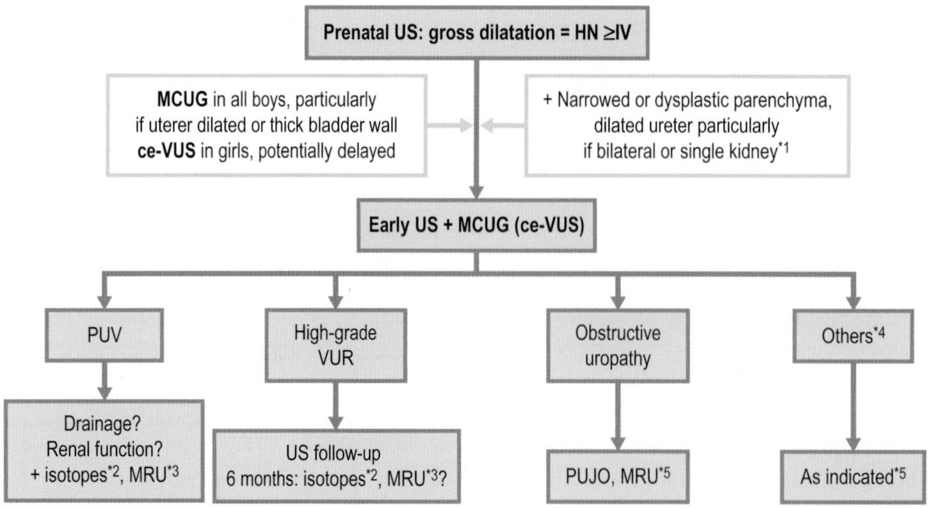

*1 (US) genitography: in patients with single kidney MC1DK, ectopic kidney, suspected genital anomaly
*2 MAG3-better than DMSA in dilated systems and neonates, DMSA usually after 3–6 months, not before 6 weeks;
+ open bladder catheter to avoid VUR-induced errors
*3 MRU-complex anatomy, function, obstructive component, etc.
*4 e.g. MCDK, cystic dysplasia, duplex or horseshoe kidney, other malformations, non-obstructive HN, cysts/cystic tumour, etc.
*5 see relevant algorithm

FIGURE 78-31 ■ Hydronephrosis. ESPR imaging algorithm for postnatally diagnosed severe/high-grade fetal hydronephrosis. MCUG = voiding cystourethrography, ce-VUS = ce-VUS = contrast-enhanced voiding urosonography, PUV = posterior urethral valves, VUR = vesicoureteric reflux, UPUJO = pelviureteric junction obstruction, MRU = MR urography. (Adapted from Riccabona M, Avni F E, Blickman J G, et al; Members of the ESUR paediatric recommendation work group and ESPR paediatric uroradiology work group 2009 Imaging recommendations in paediatric uroradiology, part II: urolithiasis and haematuria in children, paediatric obstructive uropathy, and postnatal work-up of fetally diagnosed high grade hydronephrosis. Minutes of a mini-symposium at the ESPR annual meeting, Edinburgh, June. Pediatr Radiol 39(8):891–898.[17])

or stenosis. The measurement is gestation dependent and equates to approximately 5-mm RPD at 20 weeks' gestation and a 10-mm pelvis in the third trimester. RPD is commonly unilateral but may be bilateral, in which case investigation is essential. Hydronephrosis can be graded according to severity.

High-grade HN or bilateral RPD is frequently associated with severe abnormality, i.e. severe obstructive uropathy and PUV, which may be deteriorate rapidly, and need urgent US and MCUG (Fig. 78-31).[17] The main question in severe HN is whether the child needs early bladder drainage and intervention, after which further imaging work-up may be delayed until physiological maturity of the kidneys occurs.

In mild-to-moderate fetal HN, initial postnatal US is best postponed until after 1 week of age; these US findings should then dictate additional imaging.[1] Treatment and further imaging should then be performed according to the severity of the initial findings (Fig. 78-1). In children with suspected PUJO or ureterovesical junction (VUJ) obstruction (e.g. primary obstructive megaureter, obstructive ureterocele, etc.) a more sophisticated imaging algorithm is proposed (Fig. 78-32),[17] with US findings determining subsequent imaging. MCUG is recommended to differentiate obstructive and refluxing dilatation, and MAG3 renography (increasingly dynamic functional MRU) to assess function and urinary drainage. The exact timing of follow-up will depend on the size of the RPD and DRF: the functionality is much more important than a simple anatomical abnormality which may have no functional consequence. The results should be used as guidance, as satisfactory grading may be difficult, immaturity of renal function may improve, and there is no convincing benefit of early surgical release of obstruction to improve renal function. Those children with functional impairment clearly require closer follow-up than those with an isolated mild RPD alone. Long-term follow-up is recommended until at least 15–20 years of age.

The largest group of children seen with a prenatal diagnosis of HN will have a normal postnatal US, or only mild residual dilatation. Those with persistent significant dilatation require functional and VUR assessment, using both radionuclide investigation of antegrade function and an MCUG, particularly in boys. However, the use of MCUG is falling out of favour, due to the lack of evidence that low-grade VUR has any consequence on the child's outcome or prevention of renal scarring later in life, and the high incidence of VUR resolving spontaneously. It is important to differentiate these children from the group who present later with UTI, on whom much of the data on VUR and renal scarring are acquired. Both VUR and HN may simply be a marker of unilateral renal dysplasia in these children, which results in abnormal renal function and scarring later in life. The use of prophylactic antibiotics in children with unilateral abnormalities detected antenatally is not evidence based, and it is becoming increasingly difficult to justify

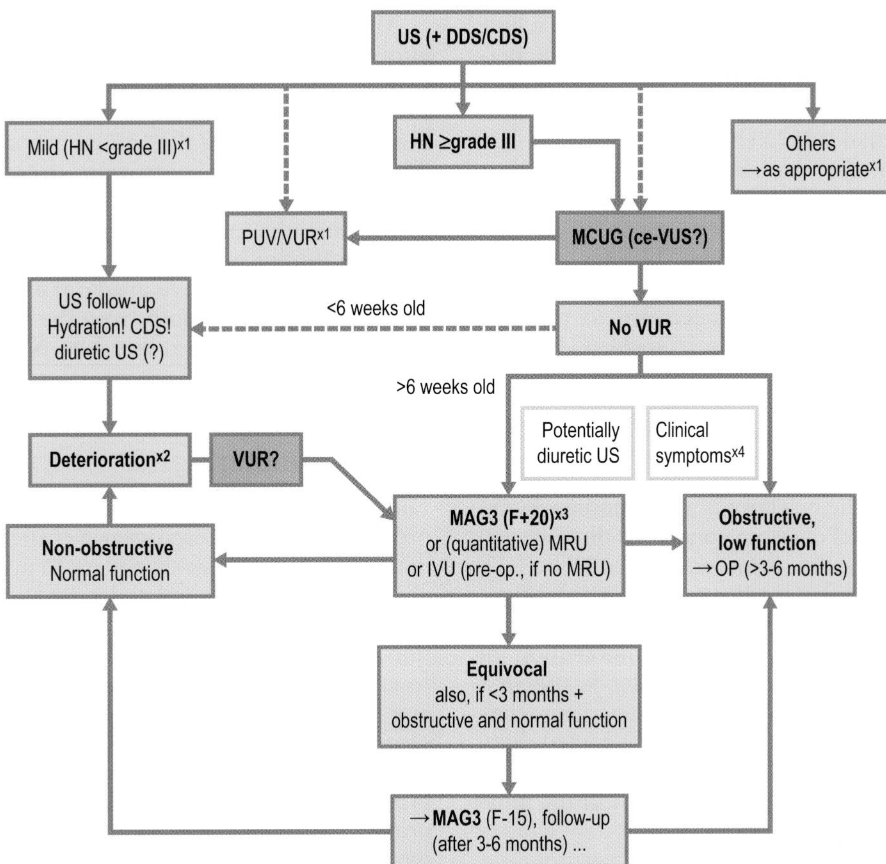

FIGURE 78-32 ■ **Urinary obstruction.** ESPR imaging algorithm for suspected obstructive uropathy. (Adapted from Riccabona M, Avni F E, Blickman J G, et al; Members of the ESUR paediatric recommendation work group and ESPR paediatric uroradiology work group 2009 Imaging recommendations in paediatric uroradiology, part II: urolithiasis and haematuria in children, paediatric obstructive uropathy, and postnatal work-up of fetally diagnosed high grade hydronephrosis. Minutes of a mini-symposium at the ESPR annual meeting, Edinburgh, June. Pediatr Radiol 39(8):891–898.[17])

invasive imaging without being able to offer therapeutic treatment.

There is ongoing uncertainty about the management of bilateral RPD. The investigative protocol in this situation should be as for the unilateral RPD dilatation, but should include an MCUG as well as formal sequential glomerular filtration rate (GFR) estimation.

Unilateral Renal Pelvic Dilatation

The natural history of unilateral RPD is a relatively benign condition which frequently resolves spontaneously. True obstruction will typically lead to parenchymal compression and eventually atrophy. If the child has any of these features, assessment of renal function is imperative, although these changes do not predict progressive renal deterioration. There is no test that will predict which kidney with a prenatal RPD will deteriorate. US assessment within the first 24 h may underestimate RPD due to neonatal dehydration and renal immaturity, and thus US at around 7 days of life should be used to more reliably assess calyceal and pelvic dilatation, measure the transverse diameter of the pelvis and the calyces, assess renal parenchyma and renal volume, and confirm the structural normality of the bladder and opposite kidney.

Megaureter

HN with a dilated ureter is dealt with in the same way as pelvic dilatation above, but suggests that VUR is more likely. The imaging protocol therefore is similar to that of RPD plus a MCUG (ce-VUS) to document or exclude VUR. Careful US of the bladder and VUJ must be performed to exclude a small ureterocele or other bladder abnormality, and ureteric peristalsis. Reimplantation of the ureter into the bladder in a child younger than 1 year of age may result in abnormal bladder function in later life; urodynamics may not be able to clarify this further. In the neonate, a spinal US is useful to exclude spinal cord pathology where a neurogenic bladder may be suspected. Stenting of the ureter or tempory diversion by ureterocutaneostomy may be necessary to preserve renal function, assessed by diuretic ^{99m}Tc-MAG3 drainage studies.

Renal Failure

Acute renal failure in the newborn is a common problem. It may have an antenatal onset, in congenital disease such as renal dysplasia and genetic disorders such as ARPCKD, or hypotensive or hypoxic event at or around delivery, resulting in renal vein thrombosis (RVT), medullary or acute tubular necrosis (ATN), or any combination of these conditions. Ultrasound with Doppler is the first investigation, as all of these disorders result in an echogenic kidney with loss of the normal corticomedullary differentiation. The main task of US is to differentiate between prerenal, intrinsic or postrenal cause of the renal insufficiency.

Renal Vein Thrombosis (RVT)

ATN is typically symmetrical and RVT typically asymmetrical, but can be bilateral. In RVT, swollen echogenic kidneys with prominent interlobular arteries are demonstrated by US. Often no venous flow can be identified at the renal hilum, and echogenic linear streaks of venous thrombi may be seen in the periphery. Seventy-five per cent of RVT is unilateral, starting in the periphery: power Doppler is helpful to depict early stages, around 50% will have IVC involvement, and 10% associated adrenal haemorrhage. Doppler US spectral flow display will show the typical high resistance flow profile with reverse diastolic flow in the affected renal artery. Contrast-enhanced imaging examinations are rarely used in this context; follow-up US (split renal volume assessment) with ^{99m}Tc-DMSA scintigraphy (4–12 months of age) should be performed to assess the long-term effects.

URINARY TRACT INFECTION AND VESICOURETERIC REFLUX

Urinary tract infection (UTI) is a common (bacterial) infection causing illness in infants and children, often with non-specific symptoms. The long-term goal of imaging in UTI is to preserve renal function and growth potential: this is often misinterpreted as (a) identifying VUR on imaging, and (b) minimising future UTIs, although there is limited evidence that these are synonymous.[18]

Many children investigated will be normal; thus, an effort must be made to only image those at high potential clinical risk, and to keep radiation doses to a minimum. Even in those imaged, there is limited evidence to suggest that treatment affects the natural history of renal damage. There is continuing controversy over the significance of VUR in the setting of UTI. In particular, neonatal VUR is now thought to be a transitory condition that, in the majority, diminishes or disappears spontaneously, even in high-grade VUR. There are now in-depth imaging and treatment guidelines both from the ESPR Uroradiology Task Force (Fig. 78-33) and UK National Institute for Clinical Excellence.[1,19]

Clinical Setting

Four per cent of all children under 8 years of age will present with a UTI each year, yet the incidence of children requiring dialysis secondary to pyelonephritis is one child per million age-related population. There is little data to support the belief that hypertension is a complication of mild renal scarring. Most children who respond to antibiotic therapy in the acute setting may not need any imaging. Imaging should be confined to those 'susceptible children' in whom an underlying abnormality may be found. These children may have an atypical UTI presentation, i.e. recurrent infections; clinical signs (poor urinary stream, palpable kidneys, poor response to treatment); unusual organisms (non-*Escherichia coli*) infections; bacteraemia; slow response to antibiotics; or unusual clinical presentation (e.g. older boy).[19] VUR is a radiological sign, not a disease entity (Figs. 78-34 and 78-35) and only 20% of children with VUR show renal damage on DMSA, while scarred kidneys are seen in children where no VUR could be demonstrated by MCUG. Thirty per cent of children with a prenatal diagnosis of HN already have an abnormal kidney at birth; thus VUR may be a marker of dysplasia rather than always reflecting true 'reflux nephropathy'.

Imaging

The aim of imaging is to detect an underlying condition or pyelonephritis. In the acute non-responding UTI, US should be performed to investigate for obstructive uropathy, pyelonephritis and abscess formation in all children. Acute pyelonephritis is best imaged using comprehensive US with power Doppler US, ^{99m}Tc-DMSA or gadolinium-enhanced or inversion recovery (STIR) MRI sequences. European guidelines suggest US imaging in all children following their first upper UTI to exclude anatomical abnormalities which may determine the need for further imaging using MCUG.[1] MCUG is restricted to those younger children with atypical or recurrent upper UTIs, severe infection including pyelonephritis, renal scars or urinary tract anomalies. If there is evidence of obstruction on US then a MAG3 diuretic renogram is required (8 weeks after the UTI). A ^{99m}Tc-DMSA scintigram should be used to detect renal parenchymal defects, not earlier than 4–6 months following the acute infection.

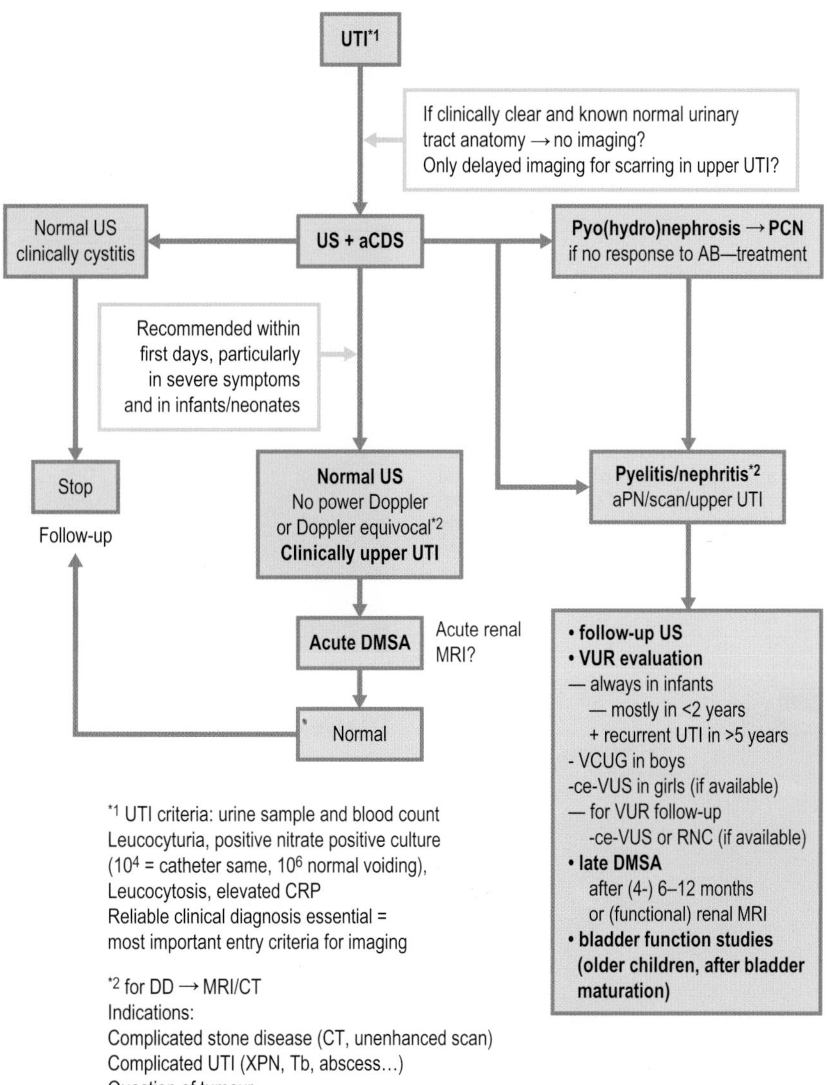

FIGURE 78-33 ■ **Urinary tract infection.** ESPR imaging algorithm for investigation of UTI—aCDS = amplitude-coded colour Doppler sonography, aPN = acute pyelonephritis, CRP = C-reactive protein, DD = differential diagnosis, DMSA = static renal scintigraphy, PCN = percutaneous nephrostomy, RNC = radionuclide cystography, Tb = tuberculosis, XPN = xanthogranulomatous pyelonephritis. (Adapted from Riccabona M, Avni F E, Blickman J G, et al 2008 Imaging recommendations in paediatric uroradiology: minutes of the ESPR workgroup session on urinary tract infection, fetal hydronephrosis, urinary tract ultrasonography and voiding cystourethrography, Barcelona, Spain, June 2007. Pediatr Radiol 38(2):138–145.[1])

In children with recurrent UTI with normal renal appearances on US, the emphasis switches to bladder function: voiding assessment by modified MCUG and (video) urodynamics is more useful than further conventional imaging, allowing assessment of an unstable bladder or destrusor-sphincter dysfunction. The follow-up of children with a damaged kidney and VUR who are on long-term antibiotic prophylaxis is unclear. One approach is to only undertake imaging if it will affect treatment. If surgical intervention has been undertaken to stop VUR, then US and dynamic scintigraphy are essential to exclude obstruction.

Renal Abscess

This complication may follow acute pyelonephritis in a child with a swinging fever with a poor response to antibiotics. Usually the abscess also has a thick wall with heterogeneous internal echogenicity on US. MRI may be helpful, especially if US findings are equivocal or aspiration or drainage is being considered (Fig. 78-36). Lobar nephronia is the term given to focal acute bacterial renal mass without liquefaction, thought to be the stage between acute pyelonephritis and abscess formation, and should not be mistaken for a tumoural mass. Immunodeficient patients may become infected with fungus manifest as 'fungal balls' or fungal abscess formation within the kidney (Fig. 78-37).

Xanthogranulomatous Pyelonephritis

Xanthogranulomatous pyelonephritis (XPN) is a rare chronic inflammatory disease of the kidney in childhood, probably an abnormal inflammatory response to infection

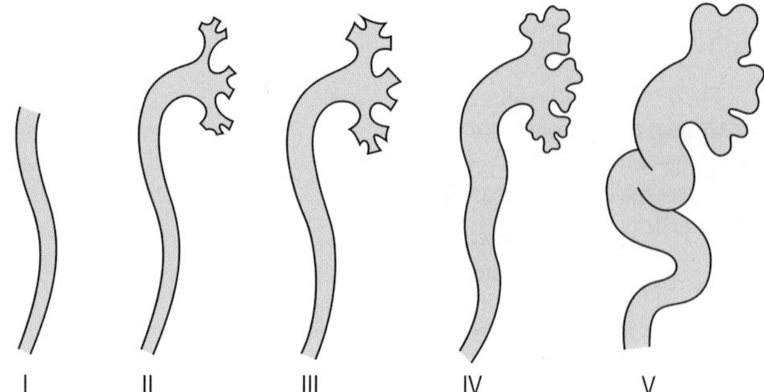

FIGURE 78-34 ■ **Radiographic grading of reflux.** (I) Ureter and upper collecting system without dilatation; (II) mild or (III) moderate dilatation of the ureter and mild or moderate dilatation of the renal pelvis, but minimal blunting of the fornices; (IV) moderate dilatation and/or tortuosity of the ureter with moderate dilatation of the renal pelvis and calyces, and obliteration of the sharp angle of the fornices but maintenance of papillary impression in the majority of calyces; (V) gross dilatation and tortuosity of ureters, renal pelvis, and calyces; papillary impressions are not visible in the majority of calyces. (Reproduced with permission by the American Academy of Pediatrics.)

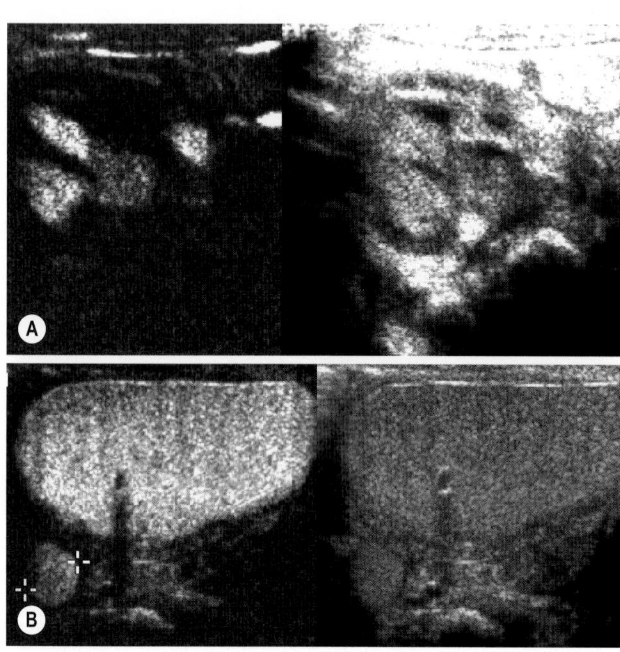

FIGURE 78-35 ■ **VUR using ce-VUS.** (A) Cross-section, upper abdomen/flank during ce-VUS—contrast material depicted in the dilated right renal collecting system in grade IV VUR, easier to see on the dedicated low-MI contrast imaging technique (left image) than on basic US (right image). (B) Cross-section, lower abdomen during ce-VUS—demonstrates contrast material in the dilated distal right ureter retrovesically. VUR is much more conspicuously imaged using a dedicated low-MI contrast imaging technique (left image) than on conventional US (right image).

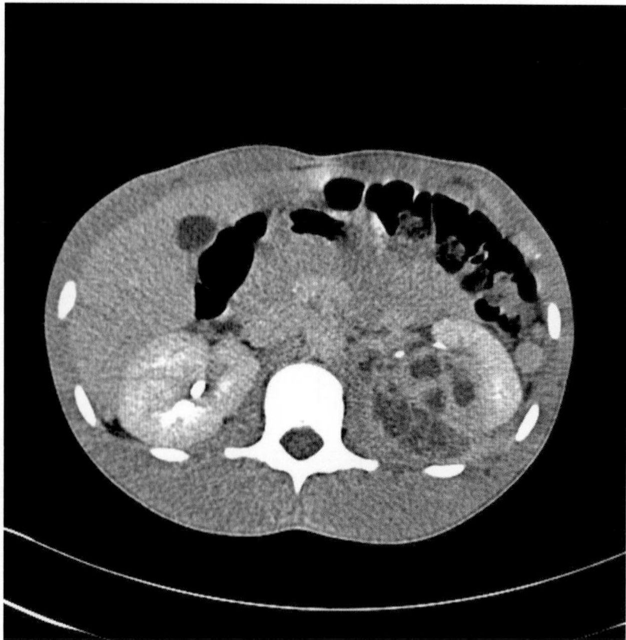

FIGURE 78-36 ■ **Renal abscess.** CT of an adolescent with gross pyelonephritis and abscess cavity formation in the left kidney. This type of image could now be better obtained with MRI.

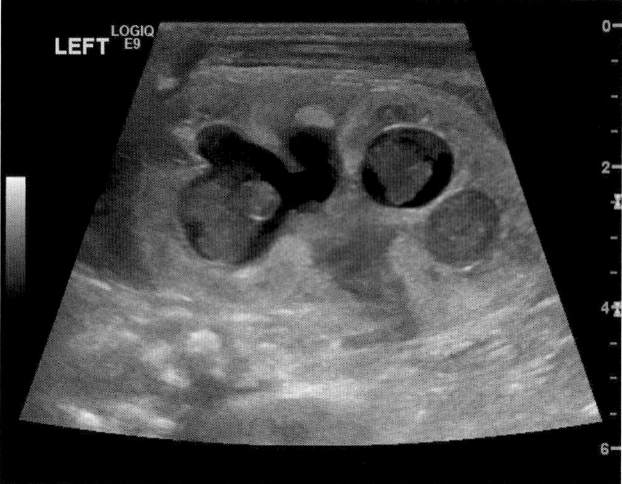

FIGURE 78-37 ■ **Fungal balls within dilated renal calyces.** Longitudinal US of the left kidney in an immunocompromised patient who cultured *Candida* from the urine.

in the presence of a calculus. The clinical presentation is with weight loss, failure to thrive, malaise, anaemia and a renal mass. Urine cultures are positive in 70%, typically for *Proteus* species and *E. coli*. The imaging findings are usually sufficiently characteristic to allow preoperative diagnosis and to avoid confusion with a Wilms' tumour (Fig. 78-38). The diffuse type of XPN, affecting the entire kidney, is more common in childhood, and focal renal involvement is rare.

Focal XPN tends to manifest with a localised intrarenal mass in an otherwise normal kidney. Plain radiographs reveal an abdominal mass with calculi. US demonstrates general renal enlargement in the diffuse form with hypoechoic areas corresponding to inflammatory masses within the kidney. Calcification can be shown, particularly at the contracted renal pelvis, or within the ureter. ^{99m}Tc-DMSA scintigraphy shows a non-functioning kidney or a photon-deficient area. CT after

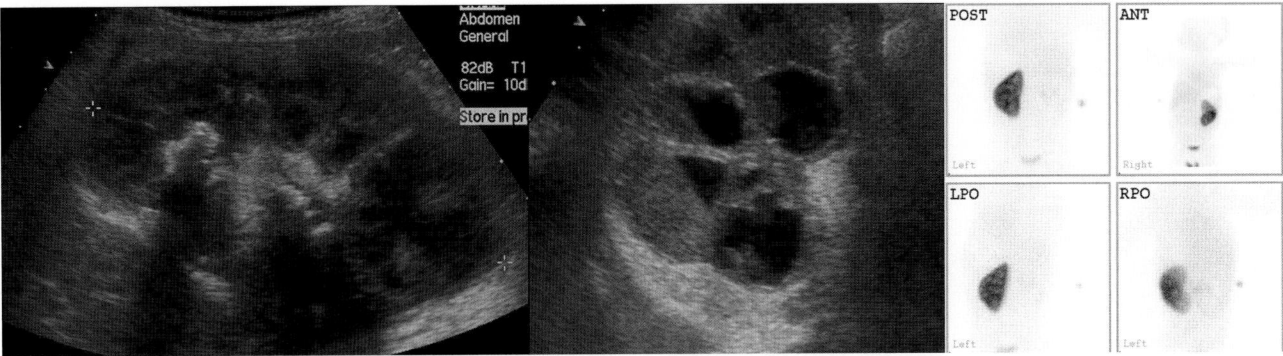

FIGURE 78-38 ■ **Xanthogranulomatous pyelonephritis (XPN).** US demonstrates renal calculi with debris within the right renal collecting system in a hypoechoic, dilated kidney. The DMSA of the same patient shows no function on the right.

intravenous contrast medium characteristically shows global renal enlargement with prominent low-attenuating abscess cavities. The remaining renal parenchyma can often show some rim enhancement due to the perfusion of the inflamed, non-functioning kidney. MRI is preferable, with necrotic areas hyperintense on T2-weighted MRI, with intermediate signal on T1-weighted sequences, which probably represents the high protein content of the cavities. Perinephric extension is common, with hilar or para-aortic adenopathy. The treatment for both types is nephrectomy, but this may be difficult due to the surrounding chronic inflammation. There may be a role for preoperative embolisation to reduce perioperative haemorrhage.

RENAL CYSTIC DISEASE

Antenatal US and fetal MRI have allowed many of the congenital cystic renal diseases to be diagnosed in utero. There is a very wide spectrum of disease with variations in renal involvement both within and between diseases.[20,21] Abnormally large kidneys may be the first indicator of cystic disease prior to the cysts themselves becoming visible: hence the need for accurate age-appropriate renal size assessment. The most widely accepted classification system is based on genetics (Table 78-9); non-genetic cystic renal disease conditions are given in Table 78-10. A careful clinical history must be taken to assess family history of renal disease and a history of diabetes. Consanguinity is a potential risk and evidence of a syndrome should be sought; family members may need to be screened with renal US.

TABLE 78-9 **Genetic Conditions Associated with Renal Cysts**

Autosomal Dominant
- Autosomal dominant polycystic kidney disease
- Tuberous sclerosis
- Medullary cystic disease
- Glomerulocystic disease

Autosomal Recessive
- Autosomal recessive polycystic kidney disease
- Juvenile nephronophthisis

Cysts Associated with Syndromes
- Chromosomal disorders
- Autosomal recessive syndromes, mitochrondrial syndromes
- X-linked syndromes, e.g. Alport's syndrome

TABLE 78-10 **Non-hereditary Conditions Associated with Renal Cysts**

- Cystic dysplasia or dysplasia
- Multicystic dysplastic kidney
- Multilocular cyst
- Multilocular cystic Wilms' tumour
- Localised cystic disease of the kidney
- Parapelvic cyst
- Simple cysts
- Calyceal cyst (calyceal diverticulum)
- Medullary sponge kidney
- Acquired cystic kidney disease (in chronic renal failure)

Cystic Dysplasia

The term 'dysplasia' causes confusion when dealing with abnormal kidneys. Dysplasia is a histological diagnosis based on abnormal metanephric differentiation with persistence of fetal kidney tissue associated with primitive ducts. Many clinicians use the term when US demonstrates a small kidney with increased echogenicity, loss of corticomedullary differentiation with or without cysts (Fig. 78-39). If there is associated VUR, the kidney may demonstrate a dilated collecting system and uroepithelial thickening with a tortuous and dilated ureter, e.g. in boys with dysplastic kidneys secondary to posterior urethral valves or high-grade congenital VUR. The same applies to the so-called 'obstructive dysplasia', probably an early stage of MCDK, with an underlying upper tract obstruction causing the impaired renal development and cyst formation. Care should be taken when interpreting a ^{99m}Tc-DMSA scan in a dysplastic kidney. The appearances of patchy uptake and peripheral photopenic areas may be seen, mimicking renal scarring.

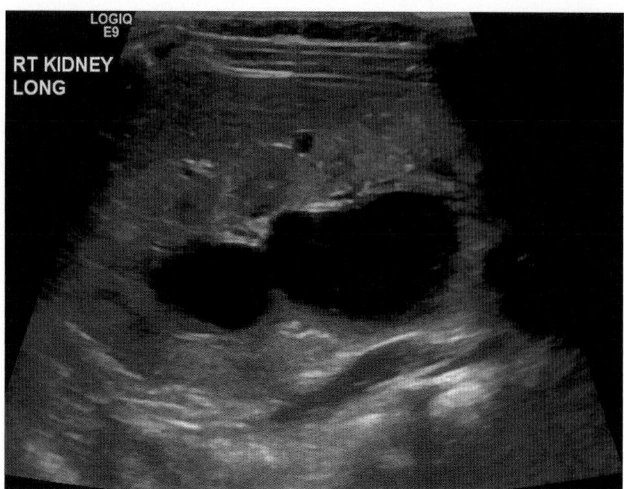

FIGURE 78-39 ■ Cystic dysplastic kidney secondary to chronic obstruction. Dilated PC system hyperechoic renal cortex with tiny peripheral hypoechoic cysts in subcapsular distribution.

Multicystic Dysplastic Kidney (MCDK)

MCDK is a developmental abnormality due to failure of union of renal mesenchyme with the ureteric bud. It is a sporadic condition with an incidence of 1 in 2000–4000 and is twice as common in boys. The MCDK is always non-functioning with an atretic ureter. There is usually contralateral but no ipsilateral VUR. Usually there are multiple anechoic cysts of different sizes, often with a peripheral dominant cyst. The key feature for differentiating a MCDK from a PUJO is the position of the residual parenchyma if present: this tends to be central in MCDK, whereas it is peripheral and rim-like in PUJO; it is always echogenic without differentiation, and may (rarely) exhibit some vascular signal on Doppler US.

Most cases of MCDK are detected antenatally, and typically involute if smaller than 5 cm without demonstrable vasculature. Occasionally, they may increase in size or be large enough to interfere with breathing or feeding; rarely they get infected or cause hypertension. Bilateral MCDK is incompatible with life (formerly called 'Potter syndrome'). There is an association with PUJO or ureteric stenosis in the contralateral kidney in up to 30% of babies and VUR is also associated. A ^{99m}Tc-MAG3 renogram or a MRU is indicated where HN or hydroureter is seen in the contralateral kidney. A ^{99m}Tc-DMSA scintigram will show non-function in the MCDK. This is not normally clinically indicated, and in doubtful cases a MRU is preferred.

Simple Cysts

Simple renal cysts are common incidental findings in adults, but cysts are rare in children and should be considered abnormal at any age, requiring investigation. Cysts are more common in children following abdominal radiotherapy and chemotherapy, and should not be confused with an obstructed upper moiety of a duplex kidney. Calyceal cysts or diverticula are rare findings in children that may be indistinguishable from tertiary calyces or simple cysts, requiring more detailed investigation (Fig. 78-40) and may develop calculi within.

Localised Cystic Disease of the Kidney

This condition, segmental cystic nephroma, is recognised as genetically, radiologically and morphologically distinct from ADPKD. The involved segment of the kidney is usually enlarged, containing multiple, small cysts which gradually merge into normal renal tissue and are not sharply demarcated from the adjacent normal parenchyma. The feature which helps differentiate localised cystic disease of the kidney from the multilocular cystic Wilms' tumour is the absence of a surrounding capsule on imaging and histology. There is no familial trait, there are no cysts in the contralateral kidney and the lesions do not progress in the few cases that have been reported and left in situ. Hypertension has been documented but the natural history is unclear.

Acquired Cystic Renal Disease

Cysts commonly develop in patients undergoing dialysis for renal failure, with 90% of patients developing cysts if on dialysis for over 10 years, without an underlying cystic renal disorder. After renal transplantation, the cysts tend to decrease in size. Complications include renal cell carcinoma, haemorrhage, or infection within the cysts.

Genetic Cystic Disease

Table 78-11 compares some of the findings in the more common cystic renal disorders in children.

Autosomal Dominant Polycystic Kidney Disease (ADPKD)

ADPKD most often presents in the third decade of life; however, there is considerable phenotypic variability in the severity of the renal disease, with some affected individuals presenting in childhood or being detected antenatally. Prevalence is approximately 1 in 1000 with two common genetic loci identified. Ninety per cent of families have the gene located on the short arm of chromosome 16 (*PKD1*). The second gene is on chromosome 4 (*PKD2*). In *PKD1* families, 64% of children <10 and 90% aged <20 years will have cysts. There may be no family history, as spontaneous mutation accounts for approximately half of cases, and phenotypes vary within families.

The extrarenal manifestations of ADPKD include cysts in the liver, pancreas and/or spleen. These are, otherwise, unusual in children and become more common with age. Subarachnoid haemorrhage due to associated intracranial aneurysm is also rare in childhood, but there may be a familial link. Screening for extrarenal manifestations is usually confined to high-risk adults, such as those with strong family history or warning symptoms. Congenital hepatic fibrosis is generally associated with autosomal recessive PKD (ARPKD; see below) and rarely with ADPKD.

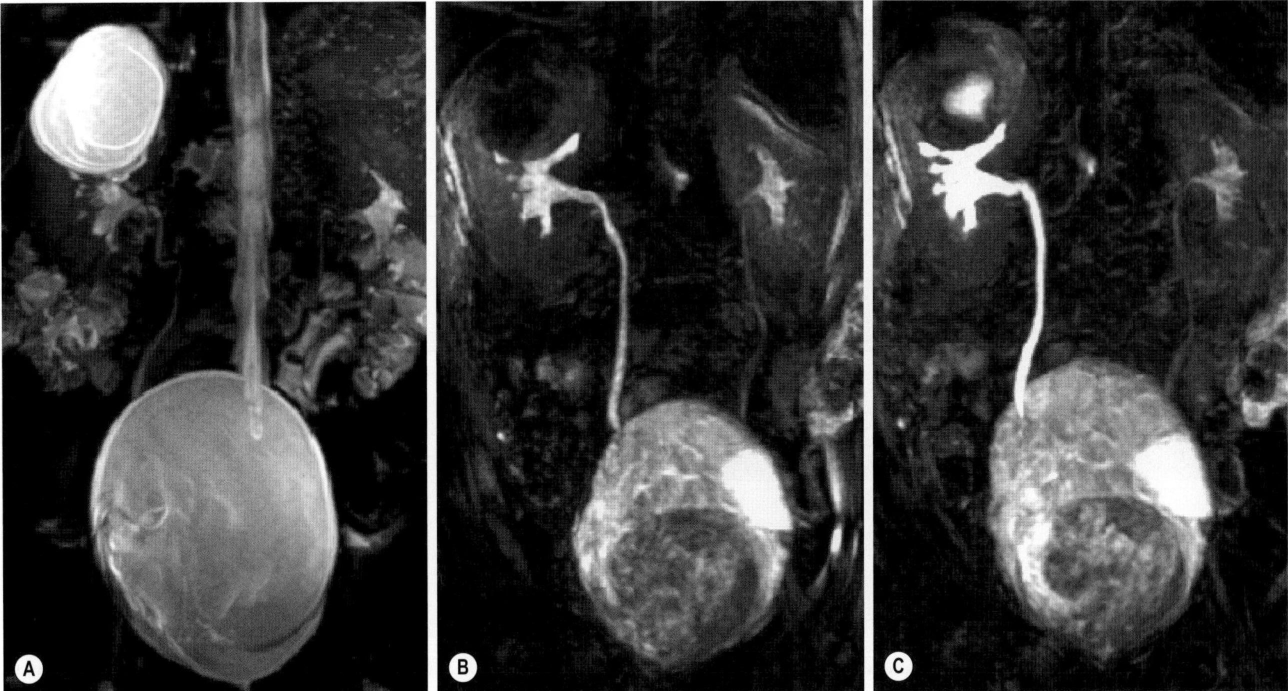

FIGURE 78-40 ■ Diagnostic use of MRU to evaluate a renal cyst. (A) Three-dimensional T2W MRU image demonstrates a large 'cystic' structure on the upper pole of the right kidney; note the disturbance from other fluid-filled structures in this rendered 3D image. (B) Three-dimensional contrast-enhanced T1 GRE MRU in the early excretory phase (10 min, rendered image). Both collecting systems are well visualised; there is no contrast in the 'cyst'. (C) Three-dimensional contrast-enhanced T1 GRE MRU in the delayed excretory phase (45 min, rendered image): this shows obvious contrast influx into the cyst, connecting to the somewhat clubbed and displaced upper calyx, suggesting that this structure is in fact a large calyceal diverticulum.

TABLE 78-11 **Comparison of Features of Renal Cystic Disease**

	ADPKD	Tuberous Sclerosis	ARPKD	MCDK	Simple Cyst
Inheritance	D	D	R	None	None
Uni- or bilateral	Bilateral unequal	Bilateral	Bilateral equal	Uni- or bilateral	Unilateral
Kidney size	Normal or large	Normal or large	Very large > 90th centile	Small or large	Normal
Extrarenal manifestations	Hepatic and pancreatic cysts, cerebral and aortic aneurysms	Cardiac rhabdomyomas, intracranial tubers	Congenital hepatic fibrosis (biliary dysgenesis)	None	None
Age at presentation	Third decade	Often <18 months	Neonate and childhood	Antenatal, rare in childhood	Onset in adult life
Cyst size	Visible cysts of variable size	Similar to ADPKD, ± angiomyolipomas	Generally small, related to collecting ducts	Large then often involute	Variable
Diagnosis	US, genetic	US, cardiac echo, cranial MRI	US, IVU, liver biopsy	US, MAG3	US, IVU
Malignancy risk	No	Yes	No	Rare	No

ADPKD = autosomal dominant polycystic kidney disease; ARPKD = autosomal recessive polycystic kidney disease; D = autosomal dominant; MCDK = multicystic dysplastic kidney; R = autosomal recessive.

Imaging

In the prenatal period, US may demonstrate highly reflective kidneys similar to that in ARPKD. In infancy the US appearances vary, from a normal kidney to a few isolated cysts, to a kidney packed full of cysts (Fig. 78-41). Typically the cysts are scattered throughout both the cortex and medulla with asymmetrical involvement of the two kidneys, which are usually enlarged. The intervening renal parenchyma appears normal. When found in the young child (younger than 5 years of age) with no family history, a diagnosis of tuberous sclerosis (TS) must also be considered and actively excluded. MRI can help, especially to identify fatty tissue in an angiomyolipoma in TS, or for a baseline assessment prior to treatment.

Tuberous Sclerosis

TS is one of the neurocutaneous disorders, an autosomal dominant condition with a prevalence of 1 in 10,000. It is characterised by multiple hamartomas in the brain, skin, heart, kidneys, liver, lung and bone, and cysts are also seen in the kidneys. Two per cent of children with

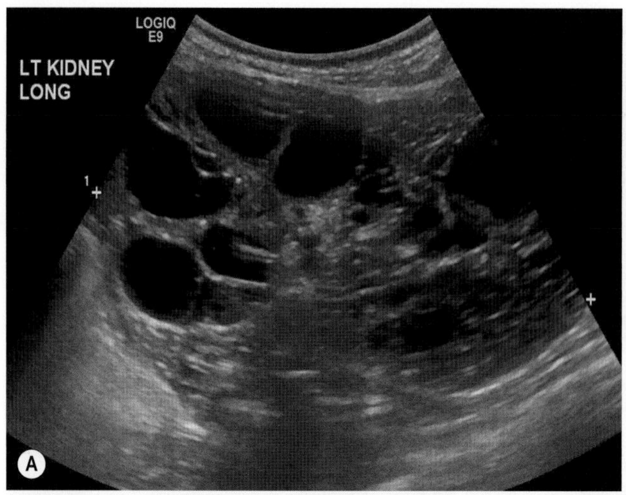

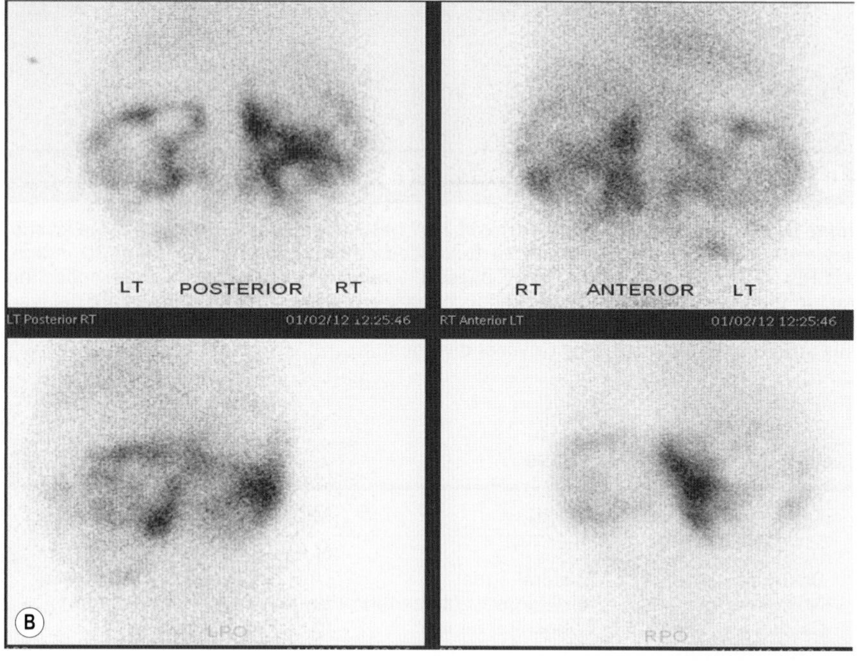

FIGURE 78-41 ■ **ADPKD.** (A) Enlarged kidneys with multiple large cysts in a 3-year-old with no family history of renal disease. (B) ^{99m}Tc-DMSA shows bilateral photopenic areas representing the cysts.

TS have ADPKD, with TS genetically linked to chromosome 9 in about one-third of families, and to chromosome 16 in the same region as the ADPKD1 gene.

Fifty to 75% of TS patients have renal manifestations, most commonly angiomyolipomas, with or without cysts (Fig. 78-42). Renal cysts are found less frequently (20–50%) and occur in younger patients. No imaging modality can currently differentiate cysts in TS from ADPKD. US may demonstrate multiple cysts, or multiple small rounded echogenic foci throughout the renal parenchyma due to multiple angiomyolipomas. Angiomyolipomas greater than 4 cm in diameter are at risk of haemorrhage from abnormal renal vasculature, and some advocate prophylactic embolisation. Renal cell carcinoma may also occur later in life.

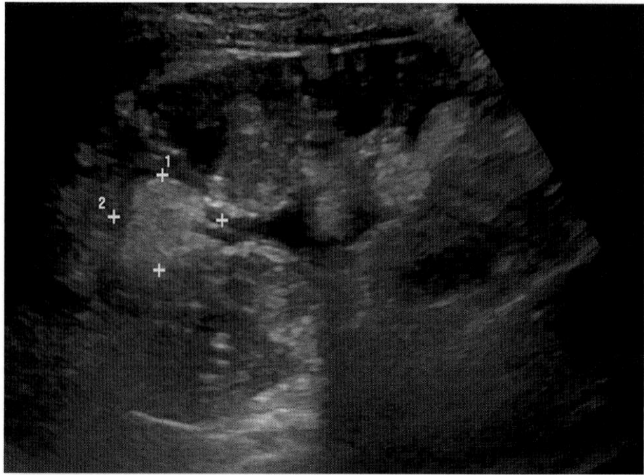

FIGURE 78-42 ■ **Angiomyolipoma.** Oblique US shows hyperechoic mass within the kidney in a patient with known tuberous sclerosis.

Autosomal Recessive Polycystic Kidney Disease

ARPKD is a rare genetic disorder with an incidence of approximately 1 in 55,000 live births. The parents are

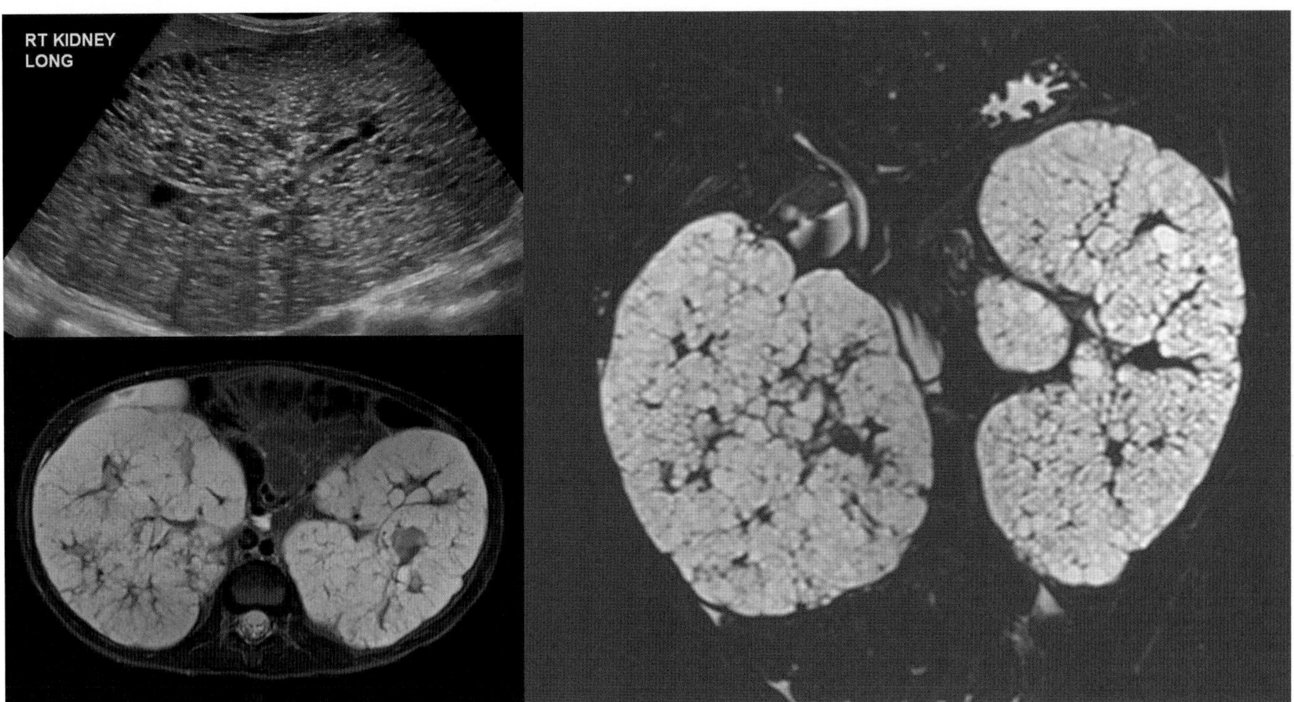

FIGURE 78-43 ■ **ARPKD.** US shows bilateral enlarged hyperechoic kidneys which retain their reniform shape with multiple tiny hypoechoic cysts in a 5-year-old boy, confirmed on axial and coronal T2W MR sequences.

always unaffected. The gene for ARPKD has been located on chromosome 6. All patients with ARPKD have some degree of congenital hepatic fibrosis, the severity of which is usually inversely proportional to the severity of renal disease: early presentation (perinatal/neonatal) has more severe renal involvement, whereas in older children (infantile and juvenile type) the liver disease predominates.

Prenatal diagnosis with US has been reported as early as 14–17 weeks' gestation. However, as bilateral highly reflective kidneys during the fetal period is not specific to ARPKD, caution is necessary before suggesting this diagnosis on prenatal US. Both kidneys are symmetrically involved and markedly enlarged, measuring > 95th centile in early infancy. The characteristic appearance is increased echogenicity in the cortex and medulla, although variations, with the medulla much brighter than the cortex, may be seen (Fig. 78-43). Using high-frequency US probes, 1- to 2-mm cysts may be detected in the medulla ('pepper and salt' kidney). In some cases these may evolve into larger cysts of different sizes with an appearance very similar to ADPKD in older children (Table 78-11).

In the young child (and sometimes even in the neonate) the liver is enlarged with increased periportal echogenicity from bile duct proliferation and fibrosis. Ectatic, dilated and cystic biliary ducts may be indistinguishable from Caroli's disease. A large spleen and evidence of portal hypertension should be excluded in older children. ^{99m}Tc-DMSA scintigraphy can show bilateral focal defects in enlarged kidneys with a high background activity; this combination of US and DMSA appearances is characteristic of ARPKD.

Functional imaging of the liver may be helpful in children with ARPKD. US may fail to show biliary duct dilatation. Children with ARPKD may present in childhood with ascending cholangitis. Liver imaging is performed over the age of 1 year, either using a hepatobiliary agent such as ^{99m}Tc-HIDA, or comprehensive MR evaluation.

Juvenile Nephronophthisis/Medullary Cystic Disease

These are two different terms for conditions that have a different inheritance, different age of onset and different associations, but a similar renal morphology and imaging. Both present with slowly progressive renal failure.

Juvenile nephronophthisis (JN) has an autosomal recessive inheritance, presenting in childhood as chronic renal failure. It is characterised by an early concentrating defect with polyuria and polydipsia, growth retardation, anaemia, and causes end-stage renal disease <25 years of age. Medullary cystic disease (MCD) shows an autosomal dominant inheritance and presents up to the fourth decade of life.

Imaging

The characteristic finding on US is normal or near-normal-sized kidneys with globally increased echogenicity. Corticomedullary cysts are not present until late in the disease. In the early stages of the disease when the tubules are affected to a greater degree than the glomeruli, the ^{99m}Tc-DMSA scintigram may fail to show the kidneys, as the tracer is taken up by the proximal tubules. A ^{99m}Tc-DTPA scintigram may be almost normal as the tracer is filtered by the glomerulus. The diagnosis can only be made on biopsy. Extrarenal manifestations

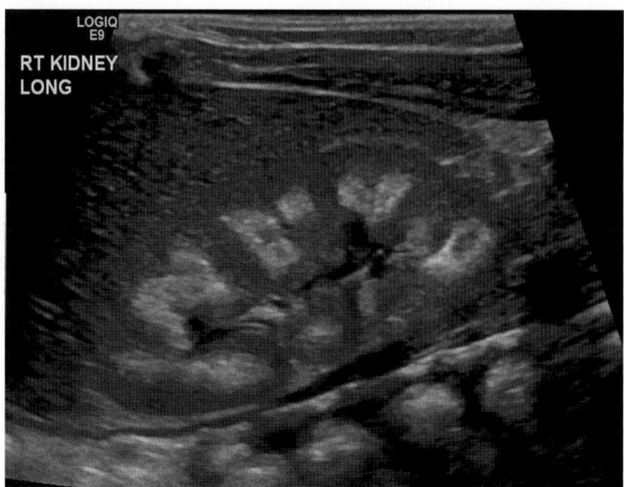

FIGURE 78-44 ■ **Nephrocalcinosis.** Concentric medullary nephrocalcinosis on US consistent with stage II of medullary nephrocalcinosis.

TABLE 78-12 Causes of Increased Medullary Echogenicity in Children

- Nephrocalcinosis (primary hyperoxaluria, cystinuria, xanthinuria)
  - Non-iatrogenic, e.g. idiopathic hypercalcaemia in Williams' syndrome, absorptive hypercalciuria
  - Iatrogenic, e.g. treatment for hypophosphataemic rickets or furosemide for bronchopulmonary dysplasia or cardiac failure in a premature infant
- Tubulopathies, e.g. renal tubular acidosis
- Protein deposits giving transient increased medullary echogenicity in newborns
- Vascular congestion, e.g. sickle cell anaemia
- Infection, e.g. candidiasis and cytomegalovirus
- Metabolic disease, e.g. urate deposits as in Lesch–Nyhan syndrome. Also seen in tyrosinaemia and glycogen storage disease
- Cystic medullary renal disease, e.g. autosomal recessive polycystic kidney disease

reported in JN include skeletal abnormalities, congenital hepatic fibrosis and mental retardation.

No such association has been reported in MCD.

NEPHROCALCINOSIS

Nephrocalcinosis may be a complication of metabolic disorders or genetic diseases, or may be seen in (pre-term) infants following diuretic treatment. Early diagnosis and treatment are essential in order to exclude a progression in nephrocalcinosis, which may lead to deterioration in renal function.

US is much more sensitive in the detection of early calcium deposition in the kidneys than plain radiography of the abdomen. Increased medullary echogenicity of the kidneys in children, while non-specific on US, may be an unexpected finding and indicative of underlying metabolic disease (Fig. 78-44). It always requires a clinical explanation, although there is a wide range of causes (Table 78-12). Iatrogenic nephrocalcinosis (diuretics, vitamin D) is the most common cause in children for an increased echogenicity of the medullary pyramids. Other common causes include idiopathic hypercalciuria and hyperoxaluria, distal tubular acidosis and rare causes include hyperthyroidism and hyperparathyroidism. The differentiation on US among medullary, cortical and global nephrocalcinosis may be important in terms of aetiology, and also to detect complications such as secondary stone formation or papillary necrosis. US can be used for grading medullary nephrocalcinosis, but cannot distinguish between calcium phosphate (nephrocalcinosis) and calcium oxalate (oxalosis) deposition.

RENAL CALCULI

Renal calculi are often asymptomatic in the paediatric population. Older children may present with UTI, pain or haematuria, as in adults, but small children may have non-specific abdominal pain, vomiting or isolated haematuria. Adult standard imaging protocols cannot be directly applied to children because of higher incidence of poorly calcified stones (e.g. cystinuria, infectious stones), and very little fat surrounding a child's small ureter.

US is best used to investigate echogenic foci, dilatation of the ureter and pelvicalyceal system, and increased renal echogenicity and size (Fig. 78-45).[17] An acoustic shadow is not a reliable sign in children, as stones may be too small (<4 mm) or low in calcium content. The twinkling artefact on CDS may enhance the suspicion or diagnosis of urinary calculi. Most stones are found in the pelvicalyceal system or in the proximal (PUJ) and/or the distal (VUJ) ureter, well visualised by US with adequate hydration and bladder distension. In larger patients and with less experienced operators, US may miss mid-ureteral stones (10–20% overall), but as most of these will cause proximal obstruction or frank HN. Stones may also form within ureteroceles or calyceal diverticulae (Fig. 78-46).

A KUB may be necessary for stone localisation prior to lithotripsy, or as a baseline study for follow-up evaluation in selected cases in older children. Ninety per cent of stones contain calcium, and should be visible on an abdominal radiograph. A limited IVU (2–4 images total) is still used by some in the diagnostic imaging of paediatric urolithiasis, especially if CT is not available or access to it is limited. There are very limited data available on the diagnostic accuracy of low-dose CT in children.

One diagnostic algorithm is that if US is negative and there is a low clinical suspicion, a watchful waiting approach may be preferable to further imaging. At present, CT may be complementary in cases with non-diagnostic or equivocal US findings that do not correlate with the clinical findings, or in high suspicion with a negative US examination, or in complex cases. MRI and MR urography for stone imaging needs to be fully evaluated.

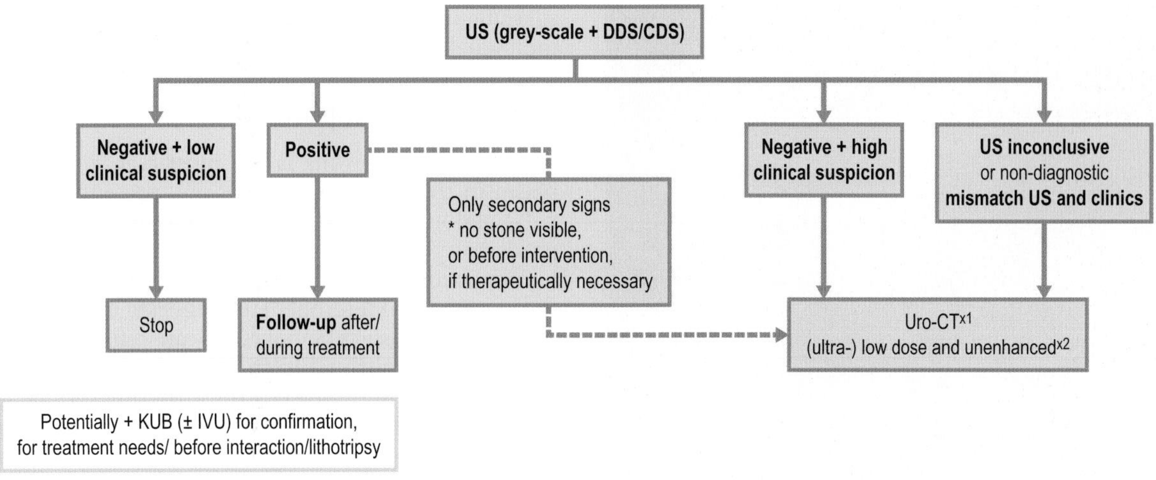

FIGURE 78-45 ■ **Urolithiasis.** ESPR imaging algorithm for suspected urolithiasis. (Adapted from Riccabona M, Avni F E, Blickman J G, et al; Members of the ESUR Paediatric Recommendation Work Group and ESPR Paediatric Uroradiology Work Group 2009 Imaging recommendations in paediatric uroradiology, part II: urolithiasis and haematuria in children, paediatric obstructive uropathy, and postnatal work-up of fetally diagnosed high grade hydronephrosis. Minutes of a mini-symposium at the ESPR annual meeting, Edinburgh, June. Pediatr Radiol 39(8):891–898.[17])

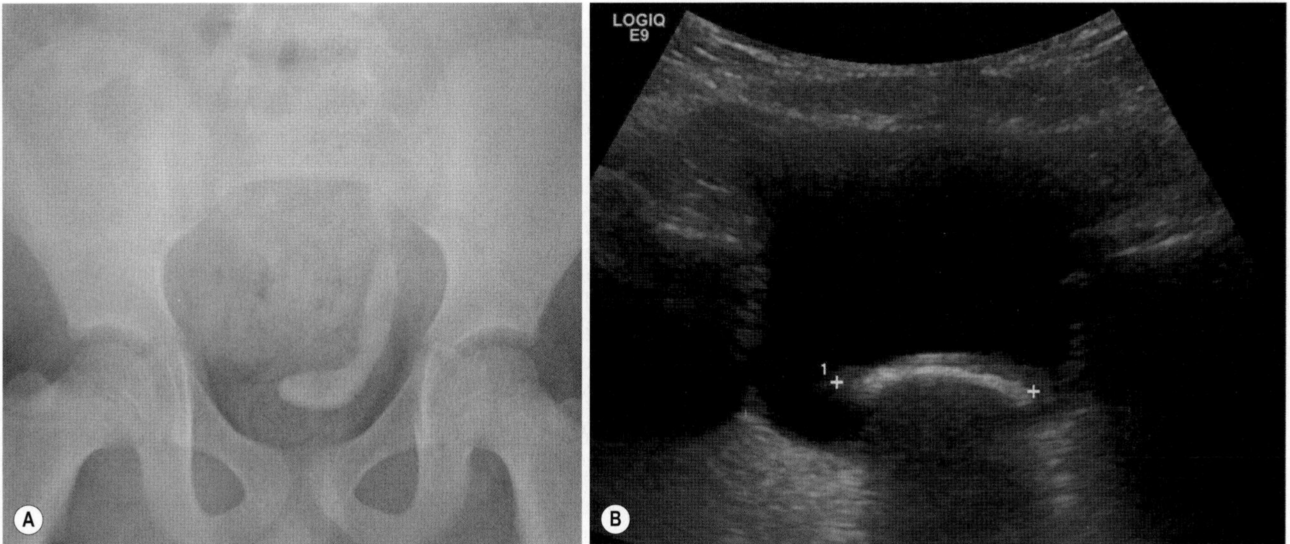

FIGURE 78-46 ■ **Stone in large ureterocele.** Abdominal radiograph of a J-shaped stone (A) which has formed in a large ureterocele, confirmed on US (B) and cystoscopy.

TUMOURS

BENIGN TUMOURS

Nephroblastomatosis

Benign tumours of the paediatric kidney are more common than initially perceived. Nephrogenic rests (NR) are abnormally persistent nephrogenic cells (metanephric blastema, or embryonic renal parenchyma) within the kidney. These may be focal (NR) or diffuse, whence termed 'nephroblastomatosis'. Nephrogenic rests are regarded as precursors of Wilms' tumour (nephroblastoma): nephroblastomatosis occurs in 41% of unilateral Wilms' tumours, 94% of metachronous bilateral Wilms' tumours and 99% of synchronous bilateral Wilms' tumours.[22] They are associated with many syndromes which predispose to Wilms' tumour, such as Beckwith–Wiedemann syndrome, hemihypertrophy and aniridia. However, NR are found in around 1% of tissues at autopsy, and only a minority of nephrogenic rests develop into Wilms' tumour; thus the malignant potential of any individual lesion is uncertain.

Nephroblastomatosis may be unifocal, multifocal or diffuse. Individual foci are usually homogeneous and of low echogenicity on US, although lesions smaller than

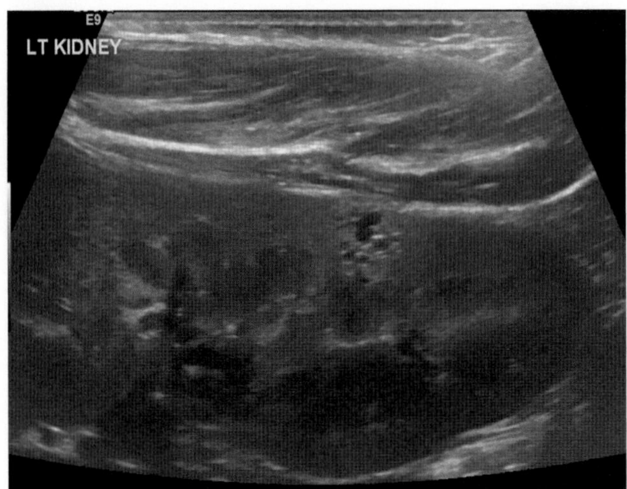

FIGURE 78-47 ■ **Nephrogenic rest.** High-frequency US of this left kidney shows a small echogenic and cystic mass, in a patient with Beckwith–Wiedemann syndrome; difficult to differentiate form a segmental cystic nephroma.

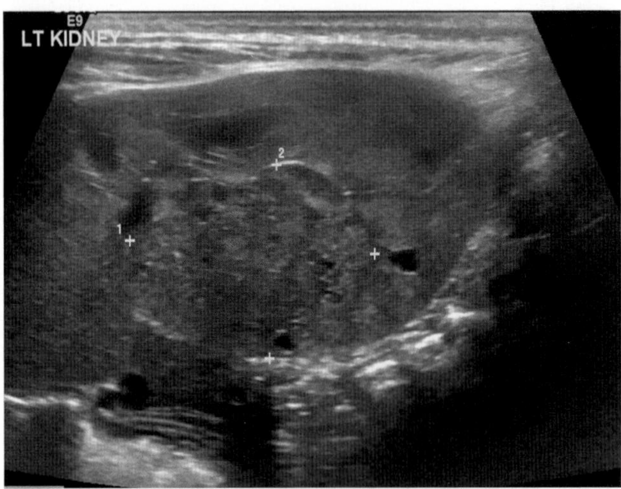

FIGURE 78-48 ■ **Nephrogenic rests.** Larger, more heterogeneous area of nephrogenic rests within the left kidney of a patient who had contralateral Wilms' tumour. Appearances are similar to that of Wilms' tumour.

1 cm may be difficult to depict using US alone; CDS and ce-US, however, improve detection rates (Figs. 78-47 and 78-48). MRI shows homogeneous lesions of low signal intensity; typically they do not enhance with contrast medium due to poorer perfusion than the relatively vascular renal cortex. Diffuse nephroblastomatosis may present as a thick rind of reduced echogenicity on US. Multifocal disease may be difficult to identify as small nephrogenic rests, may resemble normal renal cortex on all modalities, or present as slightly nodular or plaque-like lesions. They are typically identified as small homogeneous lesions in the context of an individual with a Wilms' tumour or genetic predisposition. The differential diagnosis of diffuse nephroblastomatosis on US mainly includes renal lymphoma or leukaemia. Despite the known malignant risk, regular US or MRI surveillance may be chosen in preference to biopsy of individual lesions.

Mesoblastic Nephroma

Mesoblastic nephroma is the most common renal neoplasm in the first 3 months of life, presenting as a neonatal abdominal mass, and accounting for 3–10% of all paediatric renal tumours. The mass is typically solid and homogeneous, with a hypoechoic vascular ring around the periphery. Heterogeneity suggests cystic change or necrosis. Neither US nor CT can reliably distinguish mesoblastic nephroma from Wilms' tumour: the former show uptake of ^{99m}Tc-DMSA. Mesoblastic nephroma does not invade the vascular pedicle, nor does it usually metastasise. Local recurrence may result from incomplete removal or capsular penetration, but complete excision carries an excellent prognosis. US is usually sufficient for diagnosis.

Multilocular Cystic Nephroma (MCN)

Multilocular cystic nephroma is an uncommon cystic renal mass, derived from metanephric blastema, occasionally seen in children. There is a bimodal distribution, seen more commonly in boys under 4 years and in women in the fifth or sixth decade. The child will present with an abdominal mass and US will show a multilocular renal mass with multiple cysts and hyperechoic septations. On cross-sectional imaging, the mass typically has well-defined margins or capsule, multicystic architecture and enhancing septae. It may herniate into the collecting system. Unfortunately, imaging is unable to differentiate the histological spectrum from completely benign (multilocular renal cyst) to malignant (multilocular cystic Wilms' tumour). Typically, the lesion is non-functioning on isotope imaging. (Partial) nephrectomy is curative and is recommended because of the malignant potential.

Angiomyolipoma

Angiomyolipoma (see section above on TS; Fig. 78-42) is rarely encountered as an isolated phenomenon in children but more usually represents one of the renal manifestations of tuberous sclerosis.

MALIGNANT TUMOURS

Wilms' Tumour

Wilms' tumour (nephroblastoma), first described by German surgeon Dr Max Wilms, accounts for up to 12% of all childhood cancers with a peak incidence at around 3 years of age.[23] It commonly presents with an asymptomatic abdominal mass, or haematuria following minor trauma; pain, fever, or hypertension are unusual. Microscopic haematuria is present in 25% of cases. There is equal gender distribution, with the highest incidence being in the black population in the USA and Africa. Around 10% of Wilms' tumours are bilateral, of which two-thirds are synchronous and one-third metachronous.

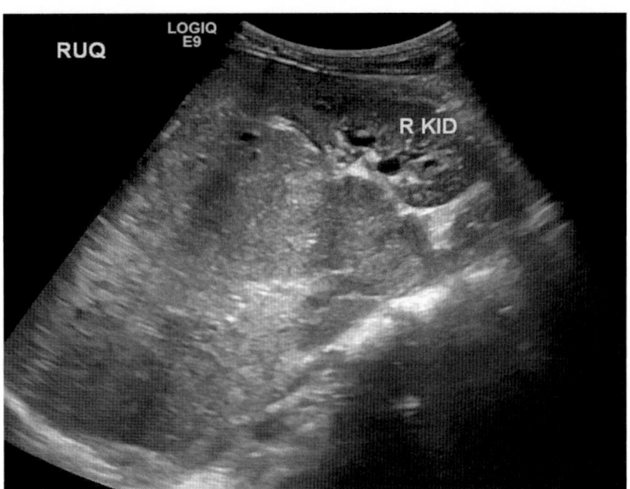

FIGURE 78-49 ■ **Wilms' tumour.** Large heterogeneous mass on US arising from the upper right kidney with inferior displacement of the lower renal pole.

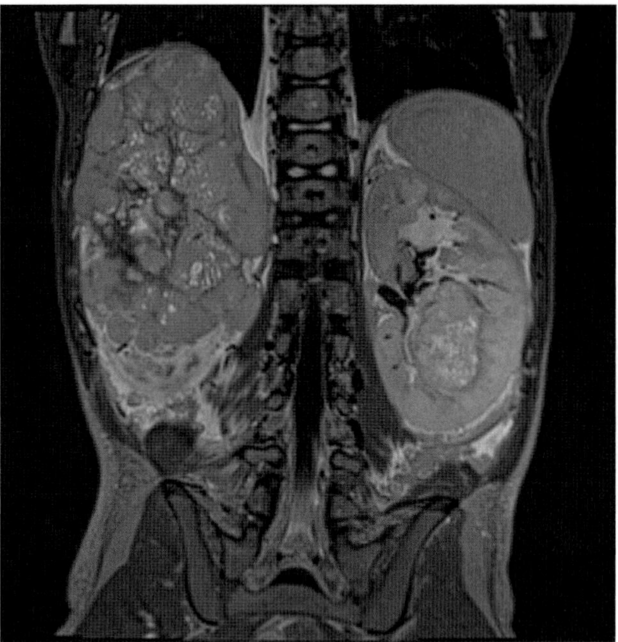

FIGURE 78-50 ■ **Bilateral Wilms' tumour.** MRI is now the gold standard for assessment of bilateral disease. Here, a small mass in the left kidney may be overlooked by the large right-sided mass.

Whereas 75% of Wilms' tumours occur in otherwise normal children, there are associated anomalies in around 15%, including cryptorchidism and horseshoe kidney. Certain syndromes have a predisposition to Wilms' tumour, including aniridia (absence of ophthalmic iris), Beckwith–Wiedemann (macroglossia, exomphalos, gigantism), hemihypertrophy, Denys–Drash (pseudohermaphroditism), Sotos' (cerebral gigantism), Bloom's (immunodeficiency and facial telangiectasia) and Perlman's syndromes. In Denys–Drash syndrome, for example, most but not all patients will develop a Wilms' tumour, the median age at presentation being 18 months, and 20% of cases are bilateral. Routine US screening to detect tumours at an early stage is controversial, because despite 3-monthly US studies large interval tumours may occur (Fig. 78-49).

Wilms' tumours are mostly solid lesions with a fibrous pseudocapsule and variable areas of haemorrhage and necrosis or cysts. The tumour may invade the renal vein and IVC with tumour thrombus extending superiorly, often to the right atrium. Metastases to local para-aortic lymph nodes and haematogenous spread to the lungs, liver or bone are seen.

The (post-surgical) staging of Wilms' tumour according to the North American National Wilms' Tumor Study Group is summarised below:

- Stage I (43%)—tumour confined to the kidney without capsular or vascular invasion.
- Stage II (23%)—tumour extends beyond the renal capsule, vessel infiltration, biopsy performed before resection or intraoperative tumour rupture.
- Stage III (23%)—positive abdominopelvic lymph nodes, peritoneal invasion or residual tumour at surgical margins/unresectable elements.
- Stage IV (10%)—haematogeous spread (typically lung, liver, bone or brain) or metastatic disease outside the abdomen or pelvis.
- Stage V (5%)—bilateral tumours at original diagnosis (Fig. 78-50).

The International Society of Paediatric Oncology (SIOP) in Europe generally uses the same staging system with the exception of masses that have been biopsied regarded as Stage I disease when later excised.

As with all abdominal masses, US must be the first radiological method of assessment. The tumour typically is large, with a mixture of solid hyperechoic masses and relatively cystic areas; often the cystic components predominate. Normal native renal tissue can be difficult to detect and may be stretched at the periphery of the lesion (Fig. 78-49). The renal vein, IVC, liver, contralateral kidney and lymph nodes should be carefully assessed for spread of disease.

US is the best way to assess renal vein and IVC tumour invasion/thrombus, and movement of the mass separate from adjacent organs such as the liver (suggesting a lack of direct invasion).

Contrast-enhanced CT or MRI is necessary for further delineation of tumour extent. Although MRI is the imaging modality of choice, as it can be easily repeated and does not involve ionising radiation, chest CT may still be needed to exclude pulmonary metastases. Wilms' tumours are typically heterogeneous with areas of low attenuation. Calcification is unusual (<10%) and the lesions enhance less than normal renal parenchyma. A 'claw' or 'beak' of normal renal tissue may be seen to stretch around the periphery. Cross-sectional imaging helps to assess the contralateral kidney, and to exclude localised lymphadenopathy, peritoneal or liver lesions, and bone metastases. Small superficial or intrarenal nephroblastomatosis lesions are often not identified, even with high-resolution CT images. Wilms' masses on MRI are generally hypointense on T1, variably hyperintense on

T2, and enhance heterogeneously, and often poorly, with gadolinium contrast administration. Gadolinium is required to assess the contralateral kidney for nephroblastomatosis or another Wilms' mass, and to guide biopsy.

The value of chest CT at initial diagnosis remains controversial, as the commonly used staging systems are based on chest radiographs alone. The presence of (small) metastases on chest CT which are not apparent on chest radiographs is currently of uncertain prognostic significance.

The typical North American treatment practice is initial surgical removal followed by adjuvant chemotherapy as dictated by the staging at surgery. European oncologists favour initial chemotherapy after biopsy confirmation with later resection. It is not surprising, therefore, as tumour response to chemotherapy is often dramatic, that preoperative chemotherapy increases the percentage of Stage I and II patients. The prognosis for Wilms' tumour patients is excellent, irrespective of approach taken. The 4-year overall survival (presumed cure) rate ranges between 86 and 96% for Stages I–III disease, 83% for Stage IV and 70% for Stage V (bilateral) disease. Patients with the diffuse anaplastic Wilms' tumours have a much poorer outcome, with 4-year survival rates of 45% for Stage III and only 7% for Stage IV disease.

Clear Cell Sarcoma of the Kidney

Clear cell sarcoma of the kidney is a rare tumour with marked male preponderance, but perhaps one of the most common with an 'unfavourable' histology (Fig. 78-51). There are no known genetic associations and no reports of bilateral tumours; it does not have an association with nephrogenic rests. The peak age of incidence is similar to that of Wilms' tumour. There are no specific radiological features to help distinguish clear cell sarcoma of the kidney from a Wilms' tumour; the distinction is purely histological. Only 5% of patients present with metastases, but metastases to bone first: hence, the alternative name was 'bone metastasising renal tumour BMRT'. ^{99m}Tc-MDP bone scintigraphy is used for staging. The presence of bone lesions but absence of lung lesions with a presumed Wilms' tumour should raise the possibility of a clear cell sarcoma.

Rhabdoid Tumour of the Kidney

Rhabdoid tumour of the kidney is the most aggressive malignant renal tumour in childhood and accounts for 2% of paediatric renal neoplasms. They are characterised by early metastases and resistance to chemotherapy, with survival rates of only 20–25%. Most cases are diagnosed in the first year of life, but indistinguishable from Wilms' tumour on imaging. Metastases to the lungs, liver and brain have been reported. There is also an association with synchronous primitive neuroectodermal tumours, usually in the posterior fossa. Hypercalcaemia is a recognised finding in rhabdoid tumour but it is not specific, found occasionally in mesoblastic nephroma.

Renal Cell Carcinoma

Renal cell carcinoma (RCC) rarely presents in the first two decades of life, with less than 1% of all cases in children, with mean paediatric presentation age 9 years. Abdominal mass or flank pain is more common than haematuria at presentation. A typically solid intrarenal mass cannot be distinguished from a Wilms' tumour; the age of the patient is a better discriminating factor. Histologically RCCs are characteristically high-grade, high-stage, papillary tumours with numerous ring-like calcifications. Metastases to the lungs, liver, skeleton or brain are present in 20% of patients at diagnosis. A third of RCCs are associated with other diseases, such as tuberous sclerosis, neuroblastoma, Saethre-Chotzen syndrome, chronic renal failure or inherited disorders.

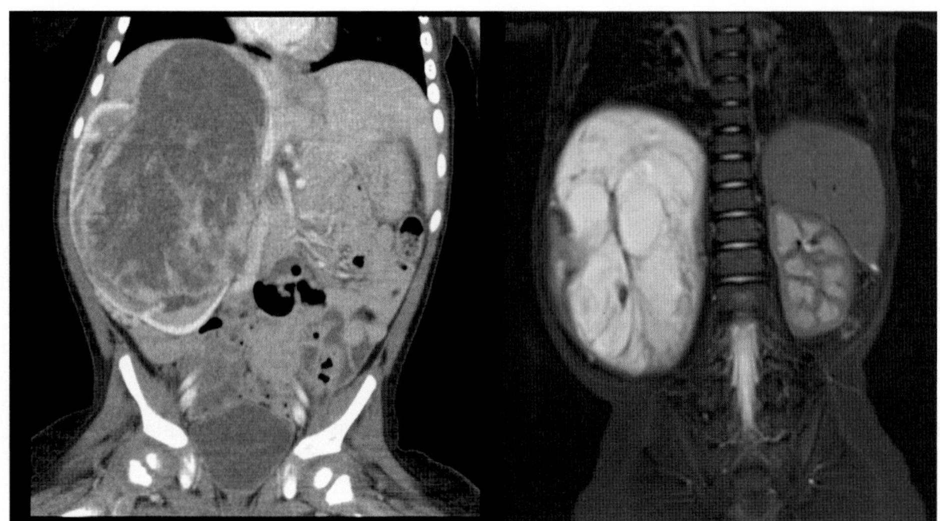

FIGURE 78-51 ■ **Clear cell sarcoma.** Coronal CT and MRI STIR sequences show a large heterogeneous mass arising from the right kidney.

Lymphoma and Leukaemia

Renal involvement with or without retroperitoneal adenopathy is seen in 12% of children with non-Hodgkin's lymphoma, most commonly B-cell Burkitt's lymphoma. Multiple, usually bilateral, nodules are typical, although diffuse renal infiltration may be seen. There is generally widespread disease elsewhere. Renal enlargement on US with altered echo texture is characteristic of both renal lymphoma and leukaemia. The changes in the kidneys can be quite subtle on CT and may be more conspicuous on contrast-enhanced MRI. US is recommended in all children with leukaemia/lymphoma before starting chemotherapy to detect tumour infiltration or calyceal dilatation. Before and during initial chemotherapy, a large fluid load is administered, which, in addition to the excretion of tumour metabolites, may result in renal obstruction or uric acid nephropathy.

Rhabdomyosarcoma

Rhabdomyosarcoma is the most common malignant neoplasm of the pelvis in children. The genitourinary tract is the second most common site of rhabdomyosarcoma in children after head and neck locations. Although the term suggests a mesenchymal tumour derived from striated muscle, the tumour frequently arises in sites lacking striated muscle. The two major cell types are embryonal (commoner, better prognosis) and alveolar. Five per cent are a botryoid subtype of embryonal rhabdomyosarcoma, characterised macroscopically by the presence of grape-like polypoid masses which classically occur in the vagina, rarely metastasise and have a good prognosis.

In general, pelvic tumours may be very large at presentation and present as abdominal masses. Prostate tumours may cause urinary obstruction and manifest with marked bladder distension or acute retention. The mass is typically solid but heterogeneous on US, with variable vascularity. Regional lymph nodes must be evaluated.

MRI is recommended in general for all pelvic tumours. Coronal or sagittal T1-weighted imaging without contrast can often be the most useful sequences for follow-up. Staging includes chest CT (10% of rhabdomyosarcomas have pulmonary metastases) and ^{99m}Tc-MDP skeletal scintigraphy.

Rhabdomyosarcomas in favourable sites such as the vagina have up to 94% 3-year survival (Fig. 78-52). Prostatic tumours commonly infiltrate locally into the perivesical tissues and bladder base, and have a worse prognosis with a 3-year survival of approximately 70%. The goal of therapy for bladder or bladder/prostate tumours (as it is frequently very difficult to tell the exact organ of origin) is survival with an intact bladder.

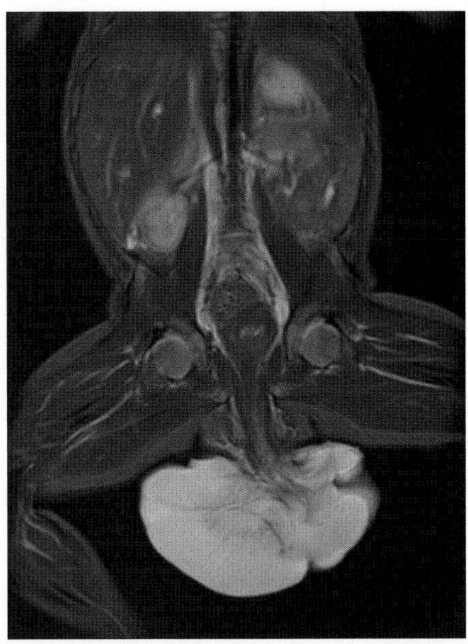

FIGURE 78-52 ■ **Rhabdomyosarcoma.** Coronal MRI shows an exophytic vaginal mass, subsequently found to be a vaginal rhabdomyosarcoma.

INFLAMMATORY DISEASES OF THE SCROTUM

The more common causes of acute pain and/or swelling in the scrotum include testicular torsion, torsion of the testicular appendages, epididymitis with or without orchitis, trauma, acute hydrocele, incarcerated hernia and acute scrotal oedema. US is the imaging modality of choice, although Doppler examination in the very young child may be limited as even modern high-resolution linear array transducers may be not reliably detect very slow flow in small testes.

Testicular torsion is a surgical emergency; if suspected clinically, the scrotum should be explored without delay. Torsion shows ipsilateral increased echogenicity with absence of intratesticular flow (always perform spectral analysis and compare to contralateral side—any asymmetry is suspicious, e.g. for partial or intermittent torsion), occasionally with surrounding fluid. Following the vessels into the inguinal canal may reveal a corkscrew-like appearance, proving torsion. The main differential is epididymitis or orchitis, where there is normal or increased testicular colour flow. The other entity is torsion of testicular appendices, where the testis is normal with a swollen appendix, with scrotal fluid. Acute scrotal oedema presents clinically with abrupt onset of a swollen, painful, red scrotal sac, with normal underlying structures on US. In children with recurrent epididymitis, always consider an associated urinary tract anomaly.

SCROTAL MASSES

Intratesticular benign and malignant tumours are relatively common neoplasms in children. Primary testicular neoplasms include germ cell tumours (teratomas, most common and often with calcification), endodermal sinus tumour and embryonal carcinoma. The testes are also secondary sites of disease in children with leukaemia, lymphoma and neuroblastoma, although much less frequently than in adults.

Paratesticular rhabdomyosarcoma includes tumours arising in the spermatic cord, testis, epididymis and penis.

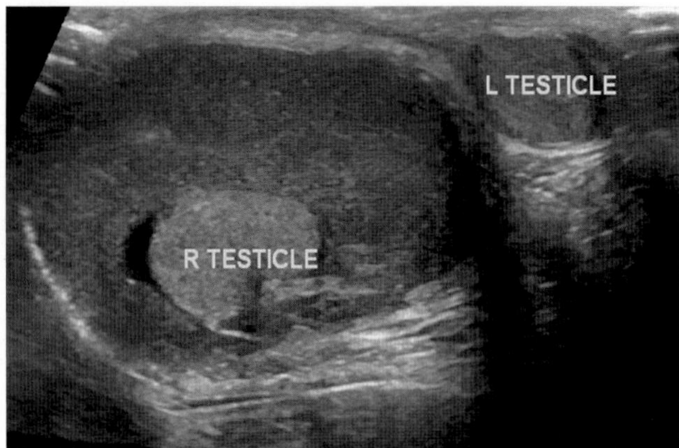

FIGURE 78-53 ■ Paratesticular rhabdomyosarcoma. US confirms a large homogeneous mass surrounding the right testis, which is lying centrally and appears normal otherwise.

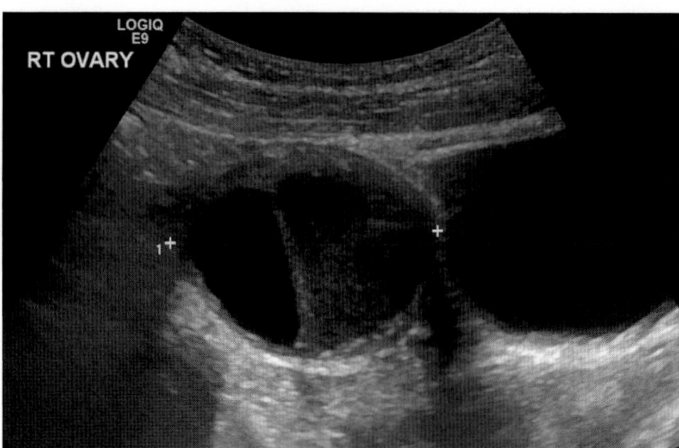

FIGURE 78-55 ■ Haemorrhagic ovarian cyst. The medial aspect of the cyst demonstrates a blood/fluid level on US.

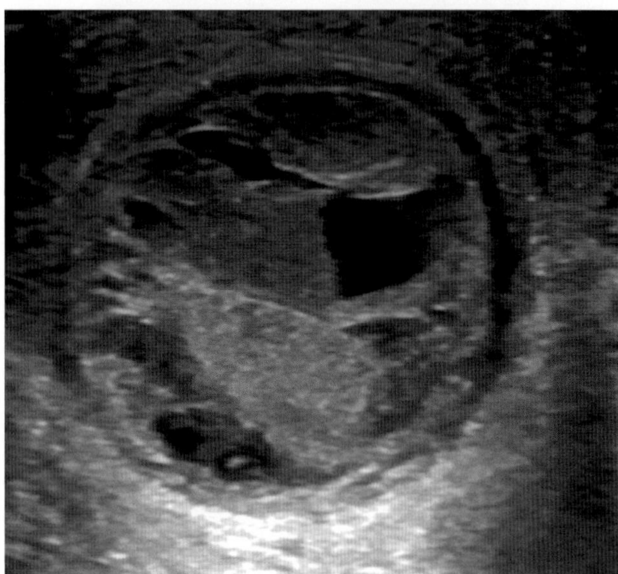

FIGURE 78-54 ■ Paratesticular haematoma. Following localised trauma during a football match, this US confirms a multiseptated hypoechoic mass surrounding a testis with patchy appearances. This patient made a full recover with integrity of vascular supply to the testis.

US is the first-line examination to evaluate scrotal disease (Figs. 78-53 and 78-54). A heterogeneous appearance within the testis with increased flow on Doppler may mimic infection, but may have presented with a palpable mass rather than infection. Cross-sectional imaging (CT or MRI) is essential to assess for lymphatic spread to the para-aortic nodes, as retroperitoneal lymph node dissection may be necessary. Paratesticular rhabdomyosarcoma has a good prognosis in young children, with a >90% 5-year survival.

OVARIAN MASSES

Ovarian Cysts

Simple ovarian cysts are large follicles and represent the majority of ovarian masses. In the neonate they usually present as abdominal masses, and the differential may include mesenteric cysts, intestinal duplication and urachal cysts. In pubertal girls, ovarian cysts result from continuous growth of a follicle after failed ovulation, or when it does not involute after ovulation. Most follicular cysts are 3–10 cm in size and contain clear fluid. Corpus luteal cysts contain serous or haemorrhagic fluid, and, as with follicular cysts, usually involute spontaneously. Most ovarian cysts are asymptomatic, but when complications such as haemorrhage (Fig. 78-55), torsion, or rupture occur, patients present with acute abdominal pain, nausea, vomiting and leucocytosis. Torsion of the ovaries and Fallopian tubes results from partial or complete rotation of the ovary on its vascular pedicle. US can demonstrate a fluid–debris level or septa, which can indicate haemorrhage or infarction. A more specific sign of torsion is the presence of multiple follicles in the cortical portion of a unilaterally enlarged and hyperechoic ovary. As there is dual blood supply to the ovary, a lack of Doppler signal is a much less reliable sign than in testicular torsion. Physiological or pathological cysts may be found coincidentally in patients with lower abdominal or pelvic pain. Repeating the US study at a different phase of the menstrual cycle is useful, and may detect more adult-type pathology such as endometriosis.

Ovarian Tumours

Ovarian neoplasms account for 10% of all childhood tumours, and 10–30% of these are malignant, commonly malignant germ cell tumours. Tumours include dysgerminoma, immature teratoma, embryonal carcinoma, endodermal sinus tumour and choriocarcinoma. The differentiation between tumour and ovarian torsion may be difficult, requiring MRI and serum markers. Tumours can occur at any age, but typically present as abdominal pain or mass after puberty. Mature teratomas and dermoid cysts account for two-thirds of paediatric ovarian tumours and have a wide spectrum of imaging characteristics (Fig. 78-56). Usually, US shows a low reflectivity mass with an echogenic mural nodule, with fat–fluid levels and calcification. Cystadenomas represent 20% of ovarian tumours in children and are of epithelial origin; they are

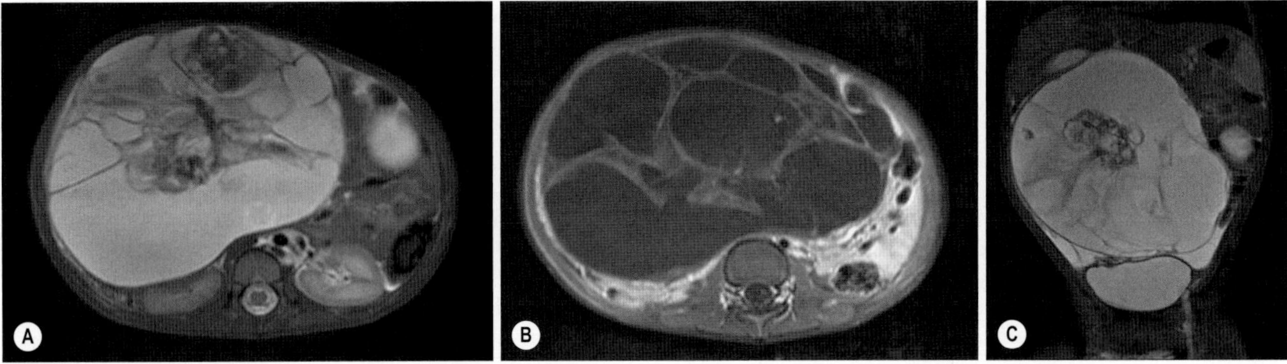

FIGURE 78-56 ■ **Ovarian teratoma.** (A) Axial STIR, (B) axial contrast-enhanced and (C) coronal STIR MRI show a multiseptated mass arising from the pelvis with peripheral enhancement.

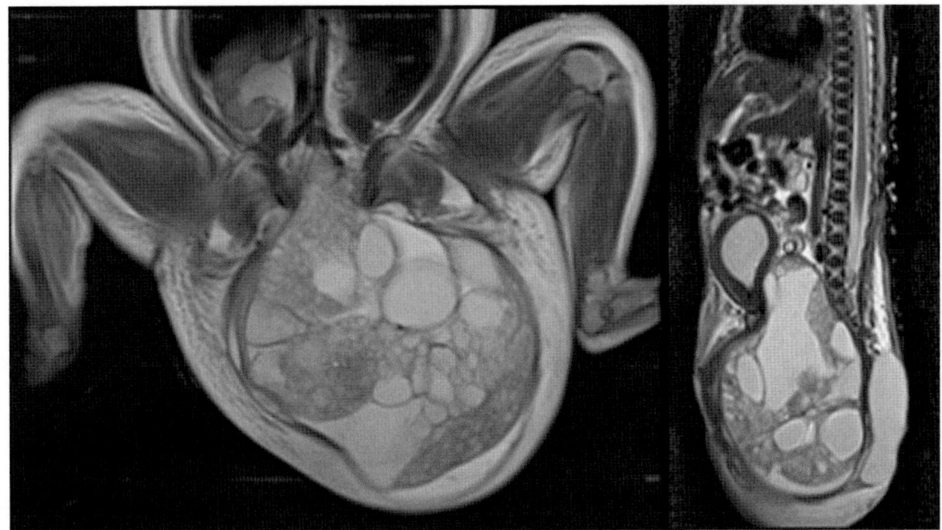

FIGURE 78-57 ■ **Sacrococcygeal teratoma.** Coronal and sagittal MRI show the large presacral mass which protrudes outside the perineum. These masses are sometimes large enough to obstruct vaginal delivery of the baby. Normal appearances to the spinal cord.

large tumours, with loculations. Imaging cannot differentiate between malignant and benign cystadenomas. Leukaemia, lymphoma and neuroblastoma are among the primary tumours that metastasise to the ovaries in children.

PRESACRAL MASSES

Sacrococcygeal germ cell teratomas are the most common presacral tumour and the most common solid tumour in neonates. These lesions occur more frequently in girls, are mostly non-familial, and are classified according to the degree of intrapelvic or extrapelvic involvement.[24] Sacrococcygeal teratomas have solid components, and are attached to the sacrum, with the internal component best depicted on sagittal MRI sequences (Fig. 78-57), allowing differentiation from an anterior sacral meningocele. Benign teratomas are usually cystic, with calcification and fat. Malignant teratomas are predominantly solid and may invade adjacent structures. All sacrococcygeal teratomas are removed due to the potential for malignant transformation. Other presacral lesions include anterior myelomeningocele and neuroenteric cyst, and forms of spinal dysraphism associated with a sacral defect. Neuroblastoma, ganglioneuroma and lymphoma in the pelvis are less common.

HYPERTENSION

Renovascular hypertension is rare in children. However, unlike in adults, renovascular is more common than idiopathic hypertension: renal disease is the cause of hypertension in over 90% of children after 1 year of age. The more severe the hypertension and the younger the child, the more likely it is to be secondary hypertension. Any abnormal kidney may produce renin and so generate hypertension. Renal scarring and glomerular disease are the most common causes, and occasionally PUJ obstruction, neuroblastoma, or Wilms' tumours present with hypertension.

Renovascular disease accounts for approximately 10% of cases, with fibromuscular dysplasia being the most common cause. Other associations are neurofibromatosis, idiopathic hypercalcaemia of infancy, an arteritic illness or middle aortic syndrome. Phaeochromocytomas, albeit uncommon in childhood, are seen and are often both multiple and extra-adrenal in origin. Essential hypertension is usually encountered in milder cases, often with a positive family history of hypertension.

Optimal imaging and managing children with suspected renovascular hypertension remains controversial (Fig. 78-58).[12] Angiography with vascular intervention offers the highest diagnostic accuracy, with the option of simultaneous treatment. MRA is feasible in older children and is relatively sensitive for significant stenoses of the main renal artery, but less sensitive in smaller children and for the more peripheral interlobar and arcuate arteries due to the lower temporal and spatial resolution. The use of non-invasive CT angiography (CTA) is particularly controversial.

US may demonstrate a small kidney, a severely scarred kidney, significant HN, and both renal and most adrenal tumours. Doppler US of the aorta and intrarenal arteries may reveal aortic narrowing or renal artery stenosis. However, Doppler findings and flow parameters have not been widely or adequately evaluated for diagnostic

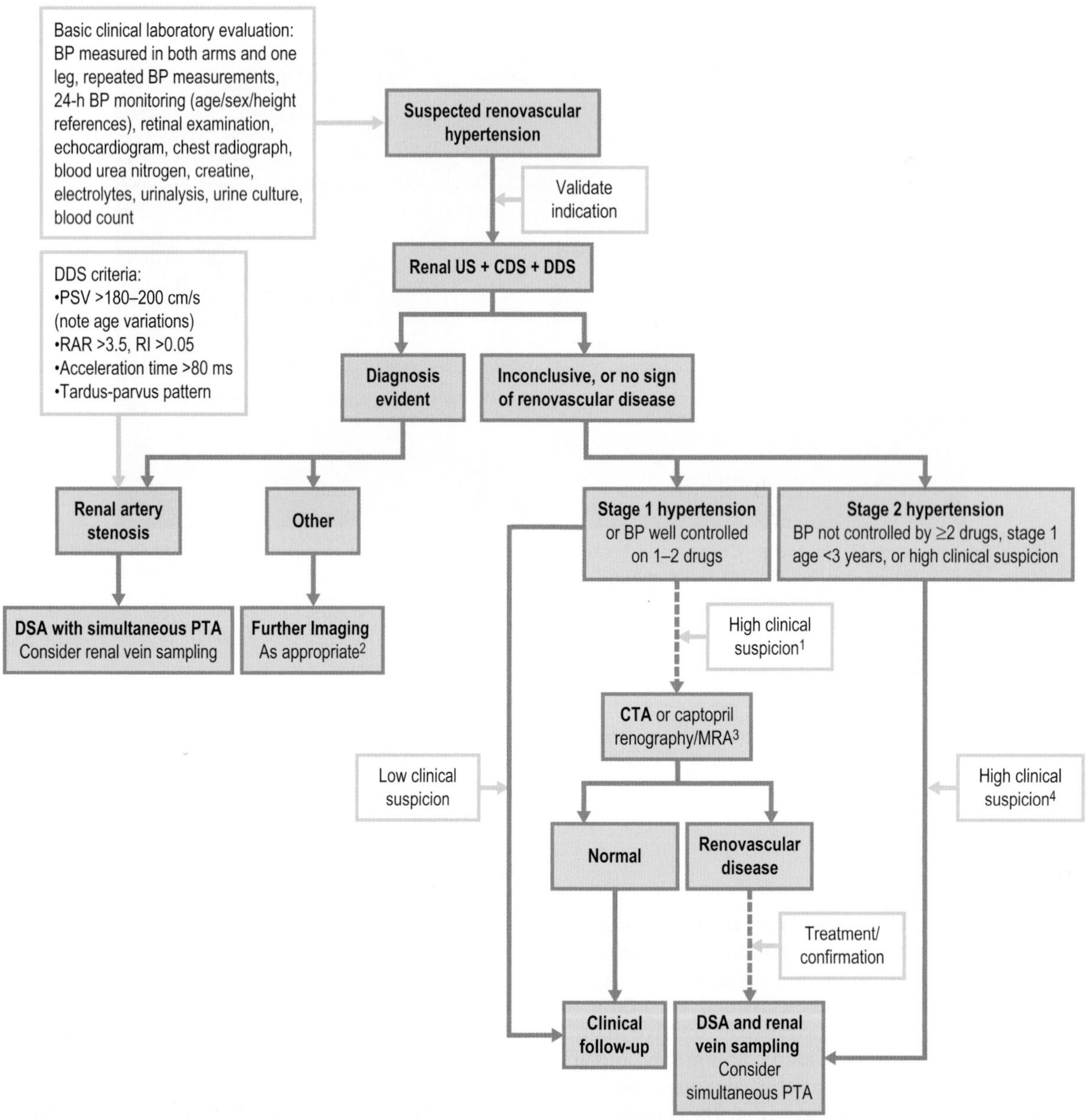

FIGURE 78-58 ■ ESPR imaging algorithm for suspected renovascular hypertension. BP = blood pressure, CDS = colour Doppler sonography, CTA = computed tomography angiography, DDS = spectral duplex Doppler, DSA = digital subtraction angiography, PSV = peak systolic velocity, RAR = renal-aortic ratio, δ-RI = resistive index difference. (Adapted from Riccabona M, Lobo M L, Papadopoulou F, et al 2011 ESPR uroradiology task force and ESUR paediatric working group: imaging recommendations in paediatric uroradiology, part IV: Minutes of the ESPR uroradiology task force mini-symposium on imaging in childhood renal hypertension and imaging of renal trauma in children. Pediatr Radiol 41(7):939–944.[12])

performance in childhood renal arterial stenosis (RAS). It is unclear whether adult criteria (e.g. a peak systolic velocity >180–200 cm/s) are applicable to children. Only the typical distal pulsus tardus and parvus waveforms, and the direct visualisation of the stenosis on CDS (turbulent flow at increased velocity causing aliasing) are reliable predictors for childhood RAS. The current recommendation, although not evidence based, is that children with a high pre-test probability of renovascular disease and positive Doppler US findings should be referred for catheter angiography with renal vein sampling, potentially with simultaneous endovascular treatment (Fig. 78-59).[25] Further non-invasive imaging by CTA or MRA currently has no significant benefit in these children as it cannot demonstrate intrarenal vasculature stenoses adequately, but this may improve in the future.

TRAUMA

Children have a higher risk of renal damage from trauma than adults following blunt abdominal trauma. This is due to increased organ mobility and less body fat protection of the kidneys. Haematuria is common, but the degree of haematuria does not necessarily correlate with the presence or severity of possible renal injury; therefore, every child with haematuria after abdominal trauma should undergo renal imaging.

CT is considered the imaging modality of choice in severe abdominal trauma; its use at first-line evaluation is unequivocally accepted in haemodynamically stable children, especially in suspected spinal or pelvic trauma, and suspected rupture of the urinary bladder. CT is the safest, most reliable and most widely available method to exclude significant urinary tract injuries. However, CT encompasses transporting an injured patient to the scanner, a significant radiation dose and the need for intravenous iodinated contrast medium. Some authors feel that a comprehensive US examination, including power, colour and spectral Doppler analysis, may be sufficient to reliably exclude major renal injury when performed by an experienced examiner. US will undoubtedly miss some subtle lesions that will be identified by CT, although the clinical significance of this is limited. US is therefore the imaging modality of choice in minor or moderate paediatric trauma, and CT should be considered where the US is limited, inconclusive, discordant with worsening clinical findings, or warrants further investigation. There is no role for following up renal lesions or severe urinary tract trauma with CT, even if initially evaluated by CT. US should be used, and MRI used wherever possible, if further cross-sectional imaging is needed (Fig. 78-60).[12]

RENAL TRANSPLANTATION

In the UK in 2009 the prevalence of patients (both adult and child) receiving renal replacement therapy was 794 per million population. It is well recognised that mortality is much higher in dialysed children than in those who have received a transplant, and that results are better in those transplanted before dialysis. Unlike adults, the majority of children with chronic renal failure are suitable candidates for renal transplantation. Live donation is increasingly being used in the paediatric population, with better outcomes than with cadaveric transplants. ABO-incompatible kidney transplantation is now possible following desensitisation by using plasmapheresis and immunoabsorption. The three most common causes of end-stage renal disease leading to transplantation are renal dysplasia, glomerular disease and pyelonephritis.

Pre-Transplantation

Ultrasound of the kidneys and abdominal vessels is essential in prerenal transplantation assessment. US of the abdominal, pelvic and femoral vessels is all that may be needed if the child has not had previous venous access; otherwise an MR venogram and MR angiogram are warranted. Intravenous gadolinium is contraindicated in patients with renal failure, and therefore non-enhanced ‘time of flight’ or ‘fresh blood techniques’ are used. Patients needing to undergo haemodialysis may require arm venography or vascular US pre-fistula formation. Follow-up US for fistula complications such as stenosis or thrombus in the fistula circuit may be required. Donor imaging of adult patients is not covered in this chapter.

Post-Transplantation

Following transplantation, an initial US scan in theatre or in the recovery area is advised, particularly using CDS to assess renal perfusion. This may be particularly helpful if there were several renal arteries to anastomose or if any renal vessels were sacrificed (Fig. 78-61). Collections may also be assessed (Fig. 78-62). Regular follow-up US are performed, or when complications such as haemorrhage following biopsy may occur (Fig. 78-63).

If the child has an unfavourable bladder (unused, or thick walled and non-compliant), the chance of pyelonephritis is high, with additional VUR up the short transplant ureter. An early ^{99m}Tc-DMSA scan is performed at 4–6 weeks following surgery to give baseline imaging in case scarring develops. ^{99m}Tc-DTPA or ^{99m}Tc-MAG3 studies are no longer routinely used in post-transplant imaging unless obstruction or urinary leak is suspected. As no single technique allows specific diagnosis of graft dysfunction, often a direct biopsy is required. The role of MRI in post-transplant assessment is being developed.

Complications of immunosuppressive therapy after transplant include post-transplant lymphoproliferative disorder. A diagnosis of PTLD is made by having a high index of suspicion in the appropriate clinical setting; histopathological evidence of lymphoproliferation on tissue biopsy; and the presence of EBV DNA, RNA or protein in tissue. Most cases of PTLD are observed in the first post-transplant year. The more intense the immunosuppression used, the higher the incidence of PTLD and the earlier it occurs. Successful treatment of PTLD involves reduction or withdrawal of immunosuppression, which

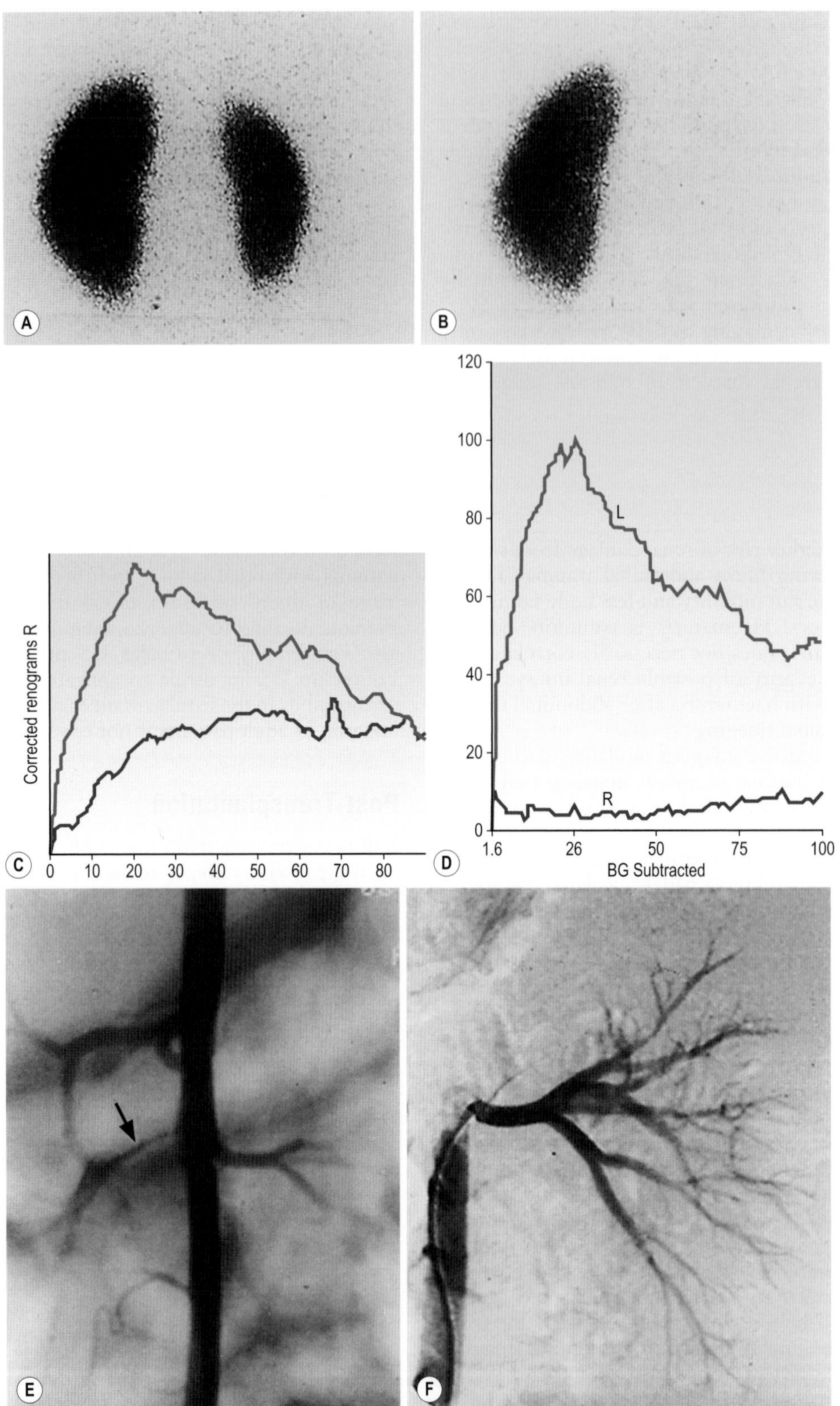

FIGURE 78-59 ■ **Hypertension.** A 7-year-old boy presented with left facial nerve palsy, a well-recognised presenting feature of hypertension in paediatrics. (A) A ^{99m}Tc-DMSA scintigram at outset shows a smaller unscarred right kidney contributing only 31% to overall function. US was unremarkable. (B) Repeat ^{99m}Tc-DMSA scintigraphy 1 month later following oral captopril ingestion shows absent function in the right kidney while the left kidney remains normal. (C) The ^{99m}Tc-DTPA renogram curves after background subtraction show a normal left kidney (L); the right kidney (R) shows a decreased uptake of radionuclide with a poor renogram. (D) Following oral captopril the ^{99m}Tc-DTPA renal curves reveal no change on the left, and a very abnormal right curve. (E) Free-flush aortic angiogram. The aorta is normal; the right renal artery shows narrowing from its origin all the way to the renal hilum (arrow). The left renal artery looks normal apart from narrowing at the origin of the artery inferiorly. (F) Selective left renal arteriogram reveals a normal intra-arterial supply within the left kidney.

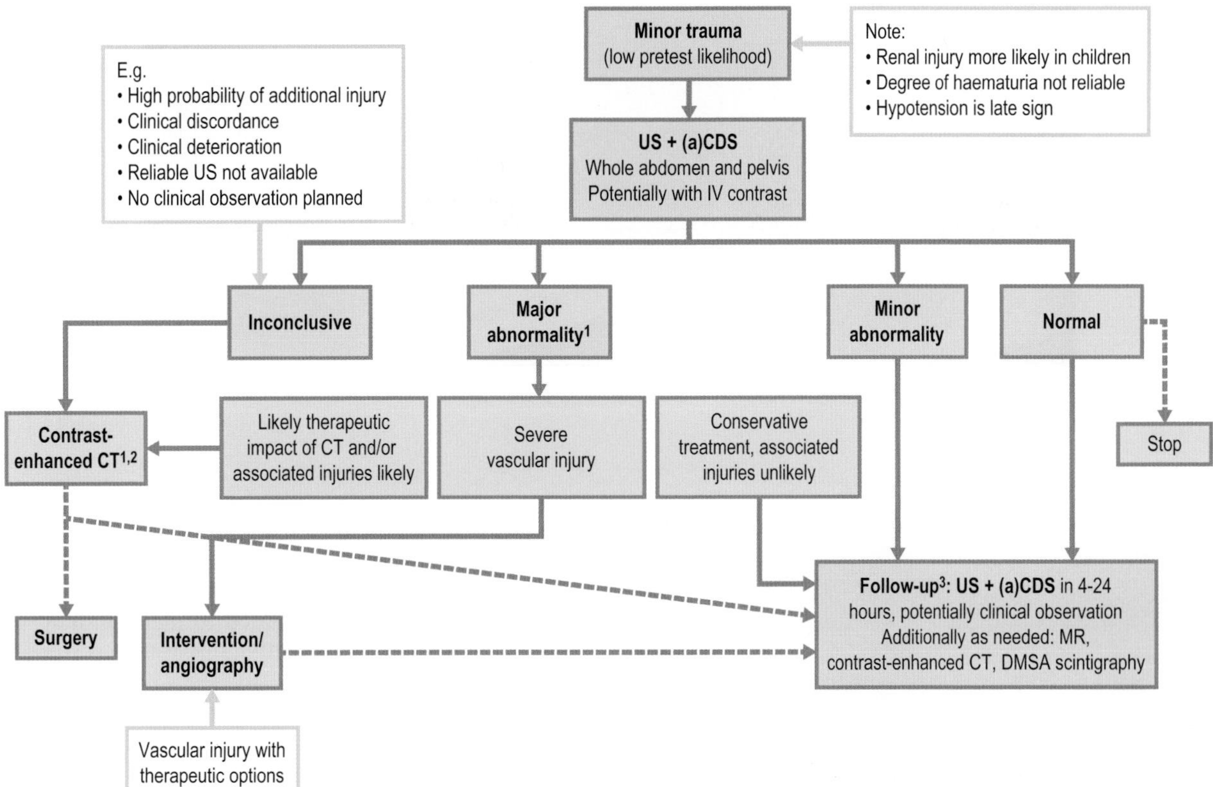

FIGURE 78-60 ■ **Trauma.** ESPR imaging algorithm for mild paediatric urinary tract trauma. DMSA = Dimercaptosuccinic acid static renal scintigraphy, CT = computed tomography, MRI = magnetic resonance imaging, US = ultrasound. (Adapted from Riccabona M, Lobo M L, Papadopoulou F, et al 2011 ESPR uroradiology task force and ESUR paediatric working group: imaging recommendations in paediatric uroradiology, part IV: Minutes of the ESPR uroradiology task force mini-symposium on imaging in childhood renal hypertension and imaging of renal trauma in children. Pediatr Radiol 41(7):939–944.[12])

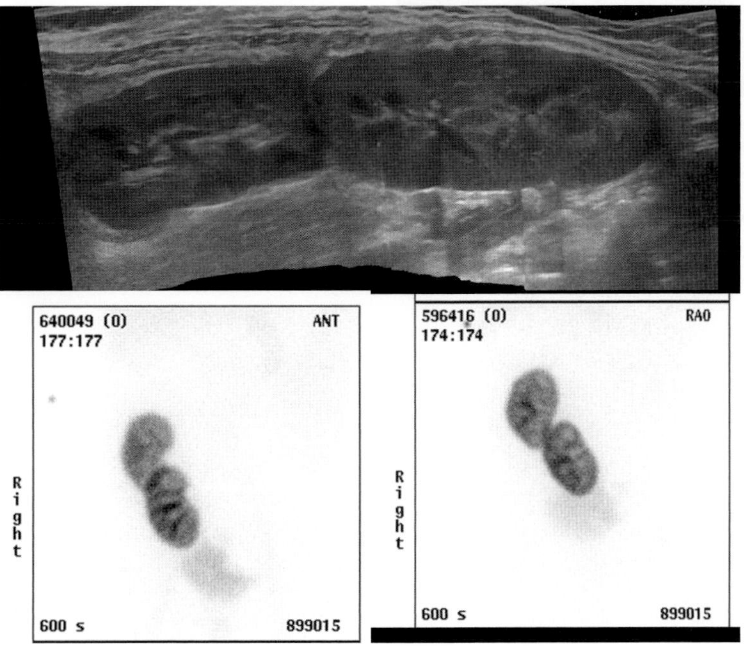

FIGURE 78-61 ■ **En bloc renal transplant.** Often from very young donors, both (paired) kidneys will be transplanted in the recipient. Normal appearances on US and DMSA.

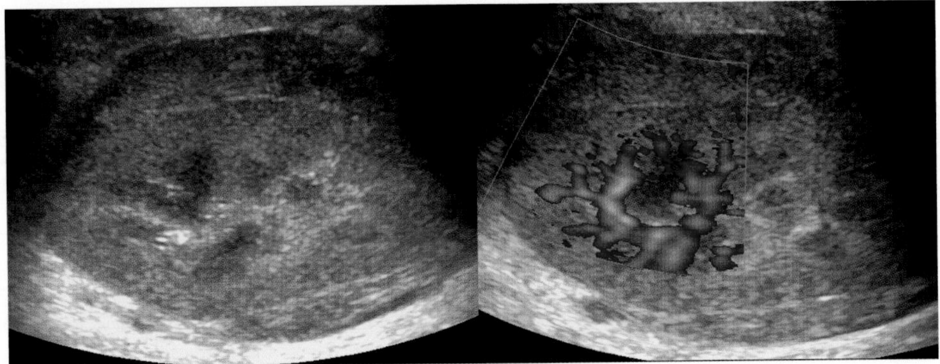

FIGURE 78-62 ■ There is a non-vascular subcapsular haematoma which may be easily overlooked, but can cause significant compression of the kidney.

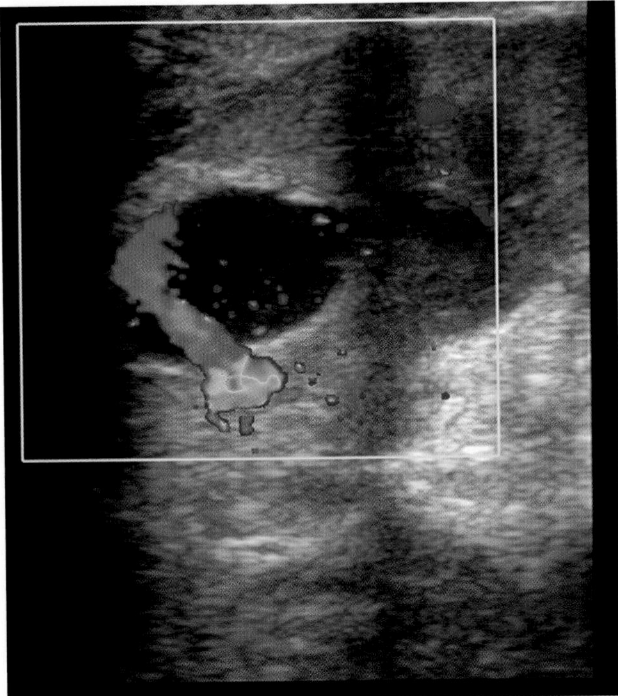

FIGURE 78-63 ■ **Arteriovenous fistula.** US shows high-flow AV fistula following biopsy of a renal transplant for suspected rejection.

inherently carries the risk of allograft dysfunction or loss. US imaging is useful in the search for lymphadenopathy or solid organ infiltration, and cross-sectional imaging with CT or MRI may be needed to plan the biopsy and to stage the lymphoproliferative disease.

For a full list of references, please see ExpertConsult.

FURTHER READING

Carty H, Brunelle F, Stringer DA, Kao SCS, editors. Imaging Children. 2nd ed. Edinburgh: Churchill Livingstone; 2005.

Fotter R, editor. Paediatric Uroradiology. 2nd ed. Springer; 2008.

Gearhart JP, Garrett RA, Rink R, Mouriquant P. Pediatric urology. Philadelphia: WB Saunders; 2001.

Hogg R, editor. Kidney Disorders in Children and Adolescents. London: Taylor & Francis; 2006.

CHAPTER 79

Skeletal Radiology in Children: Non-traumatic and Non-malignant

Amaka C. Offiah

CHAPTER OUTLINE

CONSITUTIONAL DISORDERS OF BONE

Nomenclature

The constitutional disorders of bone include osteochondrodysplasias and dysostoses.

Osteochondrodysplasias consist of dysplasias (abnormalities of bone and/or cartilage growth) and osteodystrophies (abnormalities of bone and/or cartilage texture). Abnormalities in the osteochondrodysplasias are intrinsic to bone and cartilage,[1] and because of gene expression will continue to evolve throughout the life span of the individual.

Dysostoses occur as a result of altered blastogenesis in the first 6 weeks of intrauterine life. In contrast to the osteochondrodysplasias, the phenotype is fixed, and previously normal bones will remain so. However, more than one bone may be involved.

Inevitably there is some overlap and, from the radiological point of view, when establishing a diagnosis it is useful to consider them together. Most are genetically determined but some malformation syndromes are the result of environmental effects. In addition to making a diagnosis, radiologists are required to identify complications of the condition itself and complications of medical (see Fig. 79-1) and/or surgical intervention.

The 2011 international nosology and classification of genetic skeletal disorders[1] includes 456 different conditions subdivided into 40 groups defined by molecular, biochemical and/or radiographic findings. Of these 456 conditions, 316 are associated with one or more of 226 different genes. Major conditions are summarised in Table 79-1.

While the international classification lists only those conditions with a proven genetic basis, there are currently over 2000 malformation syndromes, many of which are associated with skeletal abnormalities. In this chapter, only an approach to diagnosis can be given and only the more common conditions are used as illustrative examples.

Prevalence

Although individually rare, collectively malformation syndromes and skeletal dysplasias form a large group, which is expensive in both medical resources and human care and commitment. The prevalence of affected patients is difficult to ascertain. As a rough estimate, approximately 1% of live births have clinically apparent skeletal abnormalities. This figure does not take into account the large numbers of spontaneous abortions or elective terminations, many of which have significant skeletal abnormalities. Nor does it include those dysplasias presenting only in childhood, or those relatively common conditions that may never present for diagnosis because they are mild, e.g. hypochondroplasia and dyschondrosteosis, both of which merge with normality in individual cases. At orthopaedic skeletal dysplasia clinics in England and Scotland, approximately 10,000 patients are seen; 6000 of whom will require repeated hospitalisation for surgical procedures and some will require more prolonged admissions.

Diagnosis

Arriving at an accurate diagnosis requires a multidisciplinary approach with combined clinical, paediatric, genetic, biochemical, radiological and pathological (molecular, cellular and histopathological) input.

Rapid advances are being made in the field of gene mapping, with many conditions being localised to abnormalities at specific loci on individual chromosomes. Identification of genetic mutations allows 'families' of conditions to be recognised, with some common clinical and radiological features. One example of this is the recently described TRPV4 group of disorders, consisting of autosomal dominant brachyolmia, spondylometaphyseal dysplasia-type Kozlowski and metatropic dysplasia. Although classification based on genetic mutations is of value in determining an underlying causative defect, this diagnostic approach does not necessarily arrive at a precise clinical diagnosis, with prediction of natural history, morbidity and mortality, and in individual cases may be conflicting and indeterminate.

The international classification of skeletal dysplasias recognises the radiological features as being paramount in accurate diagnosis. Whilst clinical features, such as cleft palate, deafness and myopia, are of diagnostic

Text continued on p. 1899

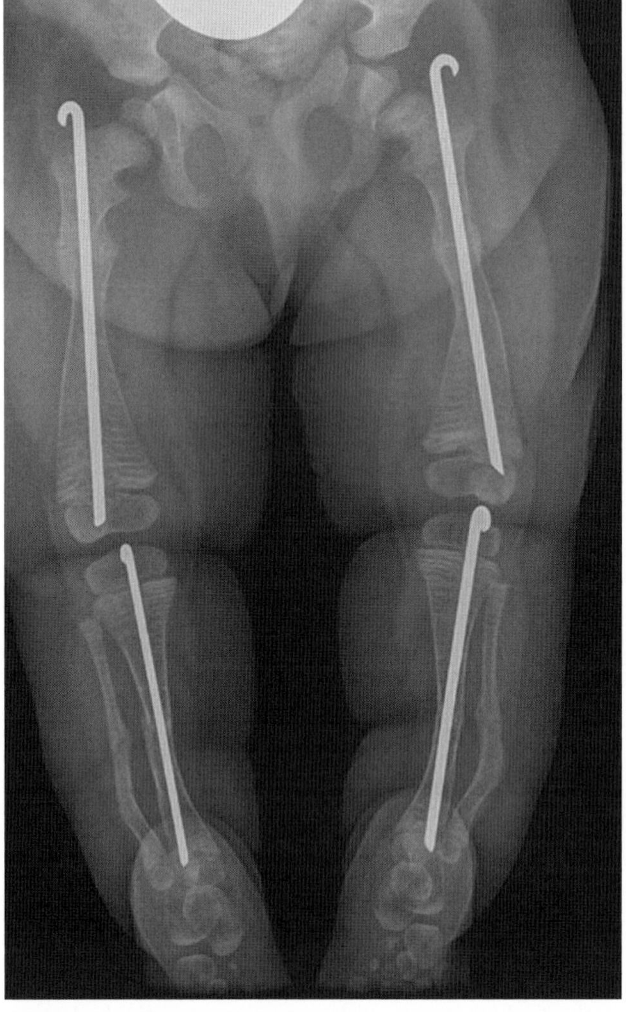

FIGURE 79-1 ■ **Osteogenesis imperfecta.** Bilateral femoral and tibial intramedullary nails. Note multiple bisphosphonate lines (see also Fig. 79-17F).

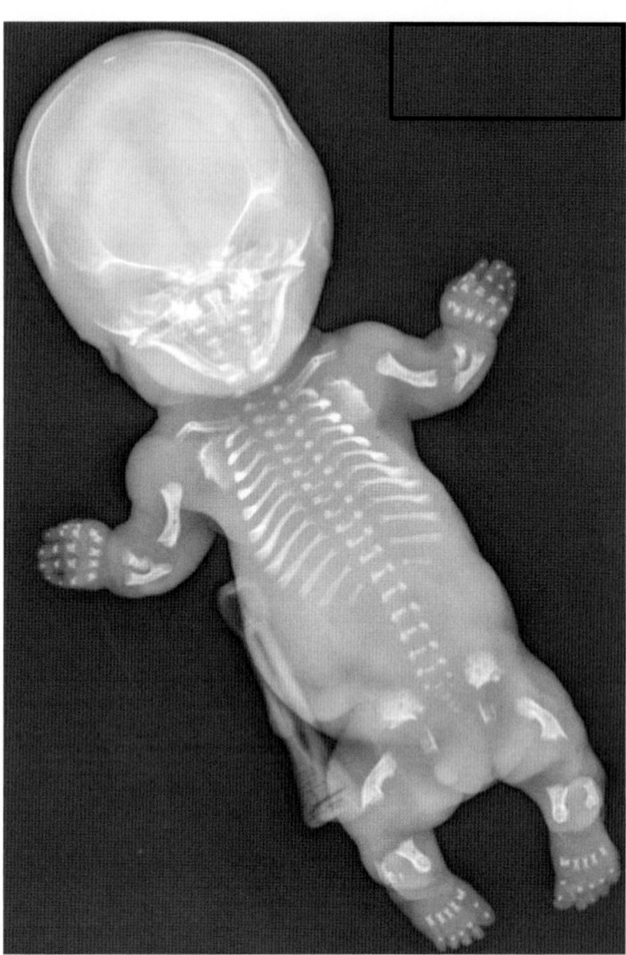

FIGURE 79-2 ■ **Thanatophoric dysplasia type 1.** Micromelia with bowed femora and metaphyseal spurs. Short ribs with a small thorax. Platyspondyly. Trident acetabula.

TABLE 79-1 **Clinical and Radiographic Features of Selected Osteochondrodysplasias and Dysostoses**

	Clinical Features	Radiological Features
Group 1 (FGFR3 Chondrodysplasia Group)		
Thanatophoric dysplasia (Fig. 79-2)	Most common lethal neonatal skeletal dysplasia Short markedly curved limbs Respiratory distress, small thoracic cage Inheritance: Sporadic AD mutation Gene: *FGFR3*	Short ribs with wide costochondral junctions Severe platyspondyly 'Trident acetabula': horizontal roofs with medial spikes Marked shortness and bowing of the long bones ('telephone receiver femora') Irregular metaphyses Short broad tubular bones of the hands and feet Small scapulae Type 1—Normal skull Type 2—'Clover leaf' skull

TABLE 79-1 **Clinical and Radiographic Features of Selected Osteochondrodysplasias and Dysostoses (Continued)**

	Clinical Features	Radiological Features
Achondroplasia (Fig. 79-3)	Common Short limbs, short trunk Narrow thorax with respiratory distress in infancy Bowed legs Prominent forehead with depressed nasal bridge Hydrocephalus and brainstem and spinal cord compression Inheritance: AD Gene: *FGFR3*	'Bullet-shaped' vertebral bodies Decrease of the interpedicular distance of lumbar spine caudally (in older child and adult) Short vertebral pedicles Posterior vertebral body scalloping (in older child and adult) Squared iliac wings with small sciatic notch Flat acetabular roofs Short ribs Short wide tubular bones Relative overgrowth of fibula Large skull vault, relatively short base Small foramen magnum Dilatation of lateral cerebral ventricles V-shaped notches In growth plates ('chevron deformity') 'Trident' hands
Hypochondroplasia	Variable short stature Prominent forehead Inheritance: AD Gene: *FGFR3*	Absence of normal widening of the interpedicular distance of the lumbar spine caudally Short, relatively broad long bones Elongation of the distal fibula and of the ulnar styloid process Variable brachydactyly
Group 2 (Type 2 Collagen Group)		
Spondyloepiphyseal dysplasia congenita (Fig. 79-4)	Short stature with short trunk at birth Cleft palate Myopia Maxillary hypoplasia Thoracic kyphosis and lumbar lordosis Barrel-shaped chest Inheritance: AD Gene: *COL2A1*	Oval, 'pear-shaped' vertebral bodies Irregular-sized vertebral bodies with L5 smaller than L1 in infancy, 'anisospondyly' Odontoid hypoplasia and cervical spine instability Short long bones Absent ossification of epiphyses of knees, shoulders, talus and calcaneus at birth Pubic and ischial hypoplasia at birth Severe coxa vara developing in early childhood Horizontal acetabulum Relatively normal hands
Group 8 (TRPV4 Group)		
Metatropic dysplasia (Fig. 79-5)	Short limbs Relatively narrow chest Small appendage in coccygeal region ('tail') Progressive kyphoscoliosis Progressive change from relatively short limbs to relatively short trunk (hence name, 'metatropic') Inheritance: AD Gene: *TRPV4*	Short long bones with marked metaphyseal widening ('dumb-bell') Platyspondyly with relatively wide intervertebral disc spaces Flat acetabular roofs Short iliac bones Short ribs with anterior widening Progressive kyphoscoliosis Hypoplastic odontoid peg
Group 9 (Short Rib Dysplasias (with or without Polydactyly) Group)		
Ellis–van Creveld (Fig. 79-6)	Short stature Short limbs, more marked distally Polydactyly Hypoplasia of the nails and teeth Ectodermal dysplasia with sparse hair Congenital cardiac defects (ASD, single atrium) Fusion of upper lip and gum Inheritance: AR Gene: *EVC1, EVC2*	Short ribs (in infancy) Short iliac wings; horizontal 'trident' acetabula (pelvis becomes more normal in childhood) Premature ossification of proximal femoral epiphyses Laterally sloping proximal tibial and humeral epiphyses Polysyndactyly; carpal fusions (90% cases) Cone-shaped epiphyses of middle phalanges Exostosis of upper medial tibial shaft
Asphyxiating thoracic dysplasia—Jeune (Fig. 79-7)	Often lethal Respiratory problems with long narrow thorax Short hands and feet Nephronophthisis in later life in survivors Inheritance: AR Gene: *IFT80, DYNC2H1*	Small thorax with short ribs, horizontally orientated Widened costochondral junctions High clavicles Short iliac bones Trident acetabula Premature ossification of proximal femoral epiphyses Cone-shaped epiphyses of phalanges Polydactyly (10% cases)

Continued on following page

TABLE 79-1 **Clinical and Radiographic Features of Selected Osteochondrodysplasias and Dysostoses (Continued)**

	Clinical Features	Radiological Features
Group 10 (Multiple Epiphyseal Dysplasia and Pseudoachondroplasia Group)		
Pseudoachondroplasia (Fig. 79-8)	Short limbs with normal head and face Accentuated lumbar lordosis Genu valgum or varum Joint hypermobility <u>Inheritance</u>: AD <u>Gene</u>: *COMP*	Platyspondyly with 'tongue-like' anterior protrusion of the vertebral bodies Biconvex upper and lower vertebral end plates Atlantoaxial dislocation Small proximal femoral epiphyses Short iliac bones Wide triradiate cartilage Irregular acetabulum Small pubis and ischium Pointed bases of the metacarpals Short tubular bones with expanded, markedly irregular metaphyses Small irregular epiphyses with delayed bone age Wide costovertebral joints Relatively long distal fibula
Multiple epiphyseal dysplasia (Fig. 79-9)	Joint stiffness ± limp Early osteoarthritis Mild limb shortening <u>Inheritance</u>: AD <u>Gene</u>: *COMP, MATN3, COL11, COL9A1, COL9A2, COL9A3*	Delayed ossification and irregularity of the epiphyses of the tubular bones Delayed bone age of carpus and tarsus Short tubular bones of the hands and feet Only mild irregularity of the vertebral bodies Mild acetabular hypoplasia Early osteoarthritis *Multilayered patella only seen in autosomal recessive MED due to mutations in the *DTDST* gene (Group 4, sulphation disorders)
Group 11 (Metaphyseal Dysplasias)		
Metaphyseal chondrodysplasia type Schmid (Fig. 79-10)	Short limbs, short stature presenting in early childhood Waddling gait Genu varum <u>Inheritance</u>: AD <u>Gene</u>: *COL10A1*	Metaphyseal flaring Irregular widened growth plates, most marked at hips Increased density and irregularity of metaphyses, especially of hips and knees Large proximal femoral epiphyses Coxa vara; femoral bowing Anterior cupping of ribs Normal spine
Group 18 (Bent Bone Dysplasias)		
Campomelic dysplasia (Fig. 79-11)	*Neonatal* Respiratory distress Cleft palate Prenatal onset of bowed lower limbs Pretibial dimpling *Survivors* Short stature Learning difficulties Recurrent respiratory infections Kyphoscoliosis <u>Inheritance</u>: AD (sex reversal) <u>Gene</u>: *SOX9*	11 pairs of ribs Hypoplastic scapulae Angulation of femora (junction of proximal third and distal two-thirds) Angulation of tibiae (junction of proximal two-thirds and distal third) Short fibulae Progressive kyphoscoliosis Dislocated hips Deficient ossification of the ischium and pubis Hypoplastic patellae
Group 21 (Chondrodysplasia (CDP) Group)		
Chondrodysplasia punctata (Fig. 79-12)	Flat nasal bridge, high arched palate Cutaneous lesions, e.g. ichthyosis Asymmetrical or symmetrical shortening of long bones Joint contractures Cataracts <u>Inheritance</u>: XLD, XLR, AR, AD <u>Gene</u>: XLD—*EPP, NHDSL* XLR—*ARSE* AR—*LBR, AGPS, DHPAT, PEX2* AD—Unknown (also some AR types)	Stippled calcification in cartilage, particularly around joints and in laryngeal and tracheal cartilages. Disappears later on in life Shortening, symmetrical or asymmetrical of the long bones Short digits in some types Coronal cleft vertebral bodies Punctate calcification is also seen in some chromosomal disorders, fetal alcohol syndrome, mucolipidoses (Fig. 79-20), neonates of mothers with autoimmune disorders, Pacman dysplasia, warfarin embryopathy and Zellweger syndrome

TABLE 79-1 **Clinical and Radiographic Features of Selected Osteochondrodysplasias and Dysostoses (Continued)**

	Clinical Features	Radiological Features
Group 22 (Neonatal Osteosclerotic Dysplasias)		
Caffey disease (infantile cortical hyperostosis)	Usually present in the first 5 months of life Hyperirritability Soft-tissue swelling Inheritance: AD, AR Gene: AD—*COL1A1* AR—Unknown	Commonly affects mandible, clavicle, ulna May be asymmetrical Periosteal new bone and cortical thickening Abnormality limited to diaphyses of tubular bones Proximal pointing of 2nd to 5th metacarpals
Group 23 (Increased Bone Density without Modification of Bone Shape)		
Osteopetrosis (Fig. 79-13)	Several types Enlargement of liver and spleen Bone fragility with fractures Cranial nerve palsies Blindness Osteomyelitis Anaemia Inheritance: Severe types—AR Milder/delayed types—AD Gene: AR—*TCIRG1, CLCN7, RANK, RANKL* AD—*LRP5, CLCN7*	Generalised increase in bone density Abnormal modelling of the metaphyses, which are wide with alternating bands of radiolucency and sclerosis 'Bone-within-bone' appearance Rickets Basal ganglia calcification (in the recessive form associated with carbonic anhydrase deficiency)
Pyknodysostosis (Fig. 79-14)	Short limbs with a propensity to fracture Respiratory problems Irregular dentition Inheritance: AR Gene: *CTSK*	Multiple Wormian bones Delayed closure of fontanelles Generalised increase in bone density Straight mandible (reduced mandibular angle) Prognathism Deficient ossification of terminal phalanges Re-absorption of lateral clavicles Pathological fractures
Osteopoikilosis (Fig. 79-15)	Often asymptomatic May be associated with skin nodules (Buschke-Ollendorff syndrome) Inheritance: AD Gene: *LEMD3*	Sclerotic foci/bone islands, particularly around pelvis and metaphyses
Melorheostosis (Fig. 79-16)	Sclerodermatous skin lesions over affected bones Asymmetry of affected limbs Vascular anomalies Abnormal pigmentation Muscle wasting and contractures Inheritance: Sporadic	Dense cortical hyperostosis of affected bones with 'dripping candle wax' appearance Long bones most commonly affected
Group 24 (Increased Bone Density Group with Metaphyseal and/or Diaphyseal Involvement)		
Diaphyseal dysplasia (Camurati–Englemann disease)	Muscle weakness Pain in the extremities Gait abnormalities Exophthalmos Inheritance: AD Gene: *TGFβ*	Sclerotic skull base Progressive endosteal and periosteal diaphyseal sclerosis Narrowing of medullary cavity of tubular bones Isotope bone scan: Increased uptake
Group 25 (Osteogenesis Imperfecta and Decreased Bone Density Group)		
Osteogenesis imperfecta (Fig. 79-17)	See Table 79-5 Inheritance: Types I & V—AD Types II, III and IV—AD, AR Genes: Type I—*COL1A1, COL1A2* Type II—*COL1A1, COL1A2, CRTAP, LEPRE1, PPIB* Type III—As for type II plus *FKBP10, SERPINH1* Type IV—*COL1A1, COL1A2, CRTAP, PKBP10, SP7* Type V—Unknown	See Table 79-5

Continued on following page

TABLE 79-1 **Clinical and Radiographic Features of Selected Osteochondrodysplasias and Dysostoses (Continued)**

	Clinical Features	Radiological Features
Group 27 (Lysosomal Storage Diseases with Skeletal Involvement (Dysostosis Multiplex Group))		
Mucopolysaccharidoses (Figs. 79-18 and 79-19) This group of conditions is characterised by an abnormality of mucopolysaccharide and glycoprotein metabolism. Differentiation between the types is dependent upon laboratory analysis (of urine, leucocytes and fibroblastic cultures)	Typically present in early childhood Variable clinical manifestations Short stature Distinctive coarse facies Intellectual impairment (in some) Corneal opacities (in some) Joint contractures Hepatosplenomegaly Cardiovascular complications Inheritance: AR, except for MPS type 2 which is XLR Gene: Hurler/Scheie (type 1H/1S)—*IDA* Hunter (type 2)—*IDS* Sanfilippo (type 3)—*HSS, NAGLU, HSGNAT, GNS* Maroteaux–Lamy (type 6)—*ARSβ* Sly (type 7)—*GUSβ*	Macrocephaly Thick skull vault with 'ground-glass' opacification Elongated 'j-shaped' sella turcica Wide ribs, short wide clavicles, poorly modelled scapulae Ovoid, hook-shaped vertebral bodies with hypoplastic vertebral body(ies) and gibbus at thoracolumbar junction Odontoid hypoplasia Flared iliac wings with constricted bases of iliac bones Small irregular proximal femoral epiphyses Coxa valga Poorly modelled long bones with thin cortices Coarse trabecular pattern Short wide phalanges with characteristic proximal pointing of 2nd to 5th metacarpals Neurological changes include hydrocephalus, leptomeningeal cysts and a variety of abnormalities best demonstrated by MRI
Morquio syndrome (MPS type 4) (Fig. 79-19)	Normal intelligence Joint laxity Knock knees Short stature Corneal opacities Inheritance: AR Gene: *GALNS, GLβ1*	Hypoplastic/absent odontoid peg (cervical instability may lead to cord compression) Platyspondyly with posterior scalloping of vertebral bodies Anterior 'beak' or 'tongue' of vertebral bodies Flared iliac wings with constricted bases of the iliac bones Progressive disappearance of the femoral heads Coxa valga and genu valgum Irregular ossification of metaphyses of long bones Small irregular epiphyses Proximal pointing of 2nd to 5th metacarpals
Mucolipidoses type II (I-cell disease) (Fig. 79-20)	Symptoms may be apparent in neonatal period Craniofacial dysmorphism Gingival hyperplasia Joint stiffness Inheritance: AR Gene: *GNPTα/GNPTβ*	Osteopenia with coarse trabeculae Periosteal cloaking Pathological fractures Stippled/punctate calcification Metaphyseal irregularity Flared iliac wings Broad ribs Ovoid vertebral bodies
Group 29 (Disorganised Development of Skeletal Components Group)		
Multiple cartilaginous exostoses (Fig. 79-21)	Multiple bony prominences, particularly at the ends of long bones, ribs, scapulae and iliac bones Secondary deformity and limitation of joint movement Ulnar deviation of wrist Inheritance: AD Gene: Type 1—*EXT1* Type 2—*EXT2* Type 3—Unknown	Multiple flat/protuberant, polypoid/sessile exostoses Secondary joint deformities Reverse Madelung deformity (short distal ulna) Iliac crest and scapulae may be involved Vertebral bodies rarely involved Skull vault spared
Enchondromatosis (Ollier) (Fig. 79-22)	Asymmetrical limb shortening Expansion of affected bones Occasional pathological fracture Absence of vascular malformation (Ollier) Presence of vascular malformation (Maffucci) Malignancy rare in Ollier Malignancy relatively common in Maffucci (at least 15%) Inheritance: Non-genetic Gene: Non-genetic (*PTHR1* and *PTPN11* mutations found in a few patients—significance unknown)	Typically asymmetrical Shortening of affected long bones Rounded/streaky radiolucencies, particularly in metaphyses Expansion of bone with cortical thinning Areas of calcification within lesions Pathological fractures Joint deformity Reverse Madelung deformity (short distal ulna) Calcified phleboliths within vascular malformations (in Maffucci, but not usually seen until adolescence)

TABLE 79-1 **Clinical and Radiographic Features of Selected Osteochondrodysplasias and Dysostoses (Continued)**

	Clinical Features	Radiological Features
Fibrous dysplasia (Fig. 79-23)	Pain and deformity of involved bones Monostotic—only one bone involved Polyostotic—multiple bones involved McCune–Albright syndrome consists of polyostotic fibrous dysplasia, patchy café au lait skin pigmentation and precocious puberty (usually in girls) Inheritance: Sporadic Gene: *GNAS1* (polyostotic)	Asymmetrical thickening of skull vault, with sclerosis of the base; multiple rounded opacities Obliteration of the paranasal air sinuses Marked facial deformity ('leontiasis ossea') 'Ground glass' or radiolucent areas of trabecular alteration in the long bones associated with patchy sclerosis and expansion, with cortical thinning and endosteal scalloping Pathological fractures and deformities due to bone softening e.g. 'shepherd's crook' femoral necks Localised or asymmetrical overgrowth Secondary spinal stenosis
Neurofibromatosis type 1 (Fig. 79-24)	See Table 79-6 Inheritance: AD Gene: *NF1*	See Table 79-6
Group 32 (Cleidocranial Dysplasia and Isolated Cranial Ossification Defects Group)		
Cleidocranial dysplasia (Fig. 79-25)	Macrocephaly Large fontanelle with delay in closure Multiple supernumerary teeth Excessive shoulder mobility Narrow chest Inheritance: AD Gene: *RUNX2*	Frontal bossing Wide sutures of the skull with persistently open anterior fontanelle Multiple Wormian bones Prominent jaw with supernumerary teeth Variable hypoplasia/pseudoarthrosis of the clavicle Small scapulae Absent or delayed pubic ossification
Group 33 (Craniosynostosis Syndromes)		
Pfeiffer syndrome (Figs. 79-26A and 79-26B)	Craniofacial dysmorphism Broad, medially deviated thumbs and 1st toes Soft-tissue syndactyly of fingers and toes Inheritance: AD Gene: *FGFR1, FGFR2*	Sagittal/coronal craniosynostosis Squamous temporal craniosynostosis ('clover leaf skull') Dysplastic proximal phalanges of 1st toes Medial deviation of thumbs and 1st toes Hypoplastic or absent middle phalanges ⅔ and/or ¾ soft-tissue syndactyly of fingers and toes Carpal fusions
Apert syndrome (Fig. 79-26C)	Craniofacial dysmorphism present from birth Proptosis High arched/cleft palate Bifid uvula 'Mitten/sock deformity' of hands/feet Inheritance: AD Gene: *FGFR2*	Coronal craniosynostosis Bony and soft-tissue syndactyly of hands and feet Progressive carpal and tarsal fusions Progressive symphalangism Progressive fusion of cervical spine (commonly C5/C6) Progressive fusion of large joints Hypoplastic glenoid fossae Dislocated radial heads
Group 35 (Dysostosis with Predominant Vertebral with or without Costal Involvement)		
Spondylocostal dysostosis	Short thorax with respiratory distress More or less symmetrical chest Protuberant abdomen Kyphoscoliosis (mild, non-progressive) Inheritance: Types 1 to 4—AR Type 5—AD Others—AD/AR Gene: Type 1—*DLL3* Type 2—*MESP2* Type 3—*LFNG* Type 4—*HES7* Type 5 and others—Unknown	Vertebral segmentation defects affecting 10 or more contiguous vertebral bodies 'Pebble beach' appearance of vertebrae in early childhood Kyphoscoliosis Intrinsic rib anomalies (malalignment, broadening, intercostal fusions, bifid ribs, missing ribs)
Spondylothoracic dysostosis	Short thorax with respiratory distress (≥50% infant mortality) Symmetrical chest Protuberant abdomen Kyphoscoliosis (mild or absent) Inheritance: AD Gene: *MESP2*	Vertebral segmentation defects affecting 10 or more contiguous vertebral bodies 'Tramline' appearance (on AP projection) of prominent vertebral pedicles in early childhood 'Sickle cell' appearance of vertebral bodies on lateral projection Ribs regularly aligned Posterior fusion of ribs at their costovertebral origins, fanning out in a 'crab-like' appearance No intercostal fusions

AD = autosomal dominant; AR = autosomal recessive; XLD = X-linked dominant; XLR = X-linked recessive.

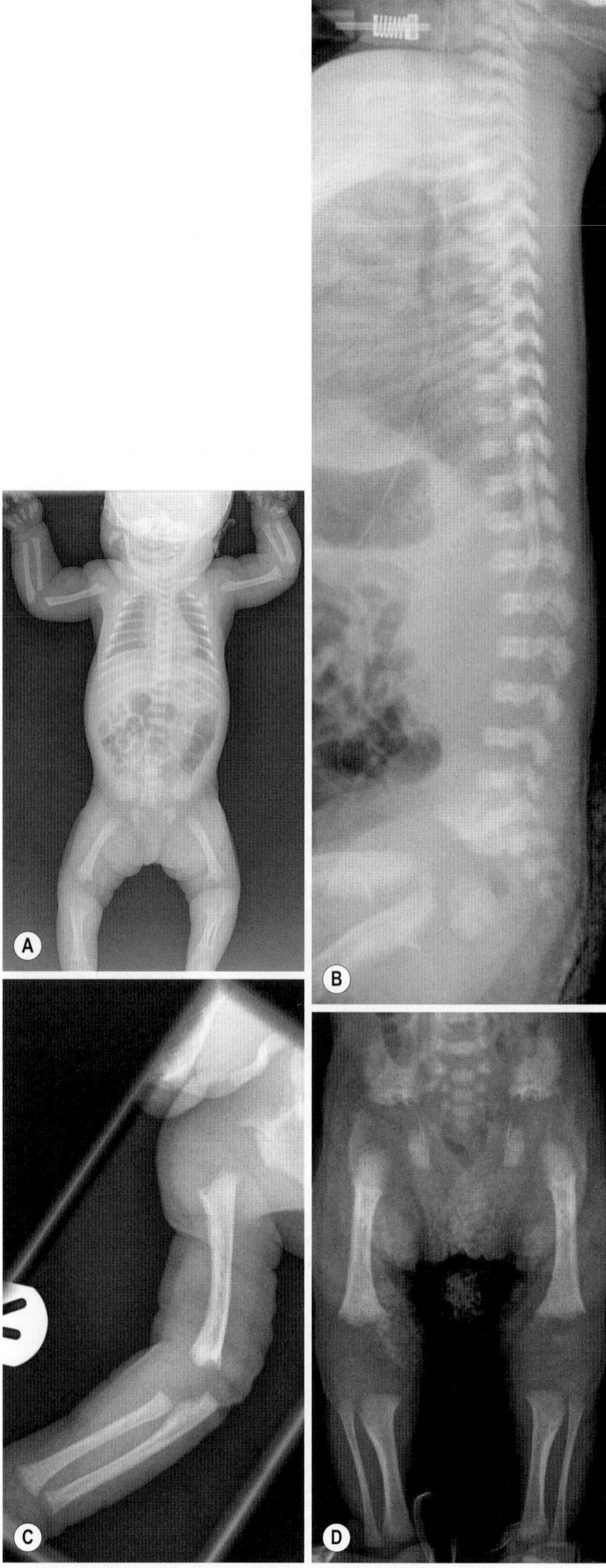

FIGURE 79-3 ■ Achondroplasia in a neonate. Narrow interpedicular distances of the lumbar spine and posterior scalloping of the vertebral bodies develop with age. (A) Micromelia, short ribs with a small thorax, sloping metaphyses. (B) Platyspondyly and bullet-shaped vertebral bodies. (C) Sloping metaphyses of proximal and distal humerus. (D) Small square iliac wings, short sacrosciatic notches, horizontal trident acetabula, sloping metaphyses, relatively long fibula.

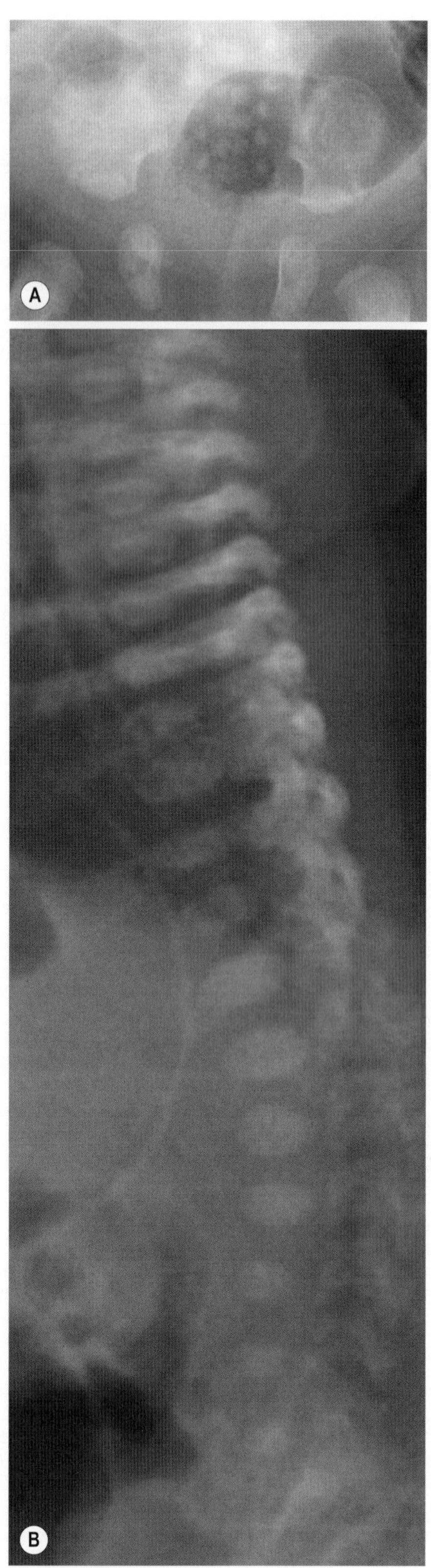

FIGURE 79-4 ■ Spondyloepiphyseal dysplasia congenita in a 3-week-old infant. (A) Hypoplastic superior pubic rami. (B) Anisospondyly (varying shape and size of the vertebral bodies). L5 is smaller than L1 (may be more subtle than in this example).

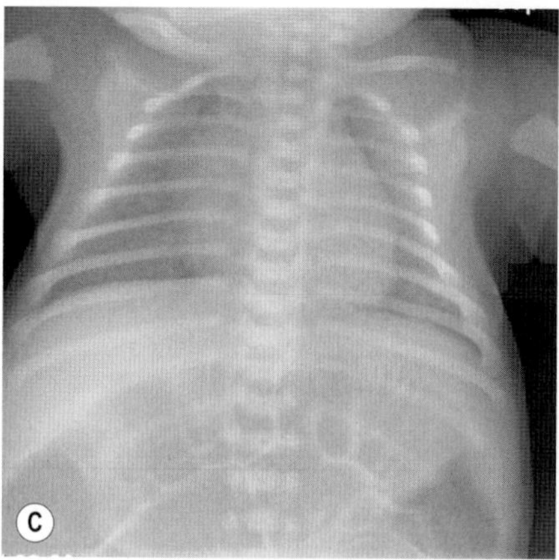

FIGURE 79-4, Continued ■ (C) Small chest with delayed appearance of the proximal humeral epiphyses.

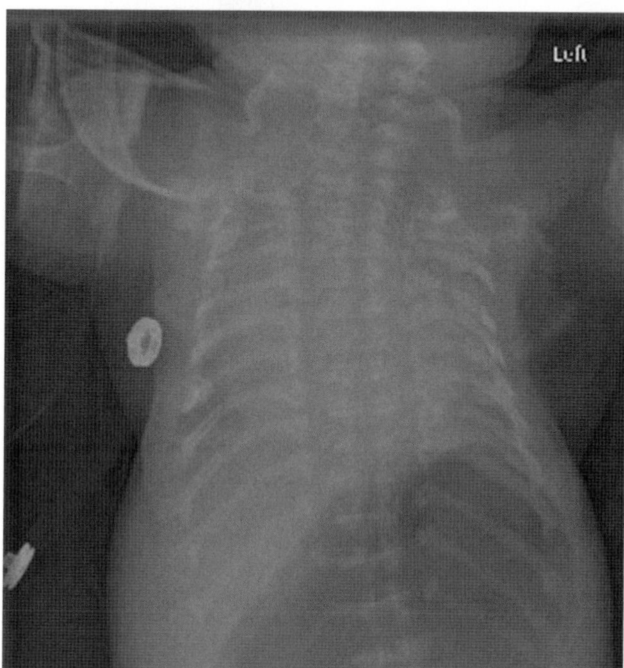

FIGURE 79-5 ■ **Metatropic dysplasia.** Narrow thorax, short ribs with prominent anterior ends and marked platyspondyly. Expanded metaphyses (seen here of the right proximal humerus) with narrow diaphyses gives rise to the so-called 'dumb-bell' appearance of the long bones.

importance, the onus is still on the radiologist to evaluate the wealth of findings on the radiographic skeletal survey by careful observation and accurate interpretation, and thereby arrive at an accurate diagnosis. An approach to the radiological interpretation of skeletal surveys performed in the context of suspected dysplasia is available.[2]

Because of the large number of relatively rare conditions, it is difficult or impossible for an individual radiologist to be familiar with every feature of every disorder. In addition, many of these conditions may have

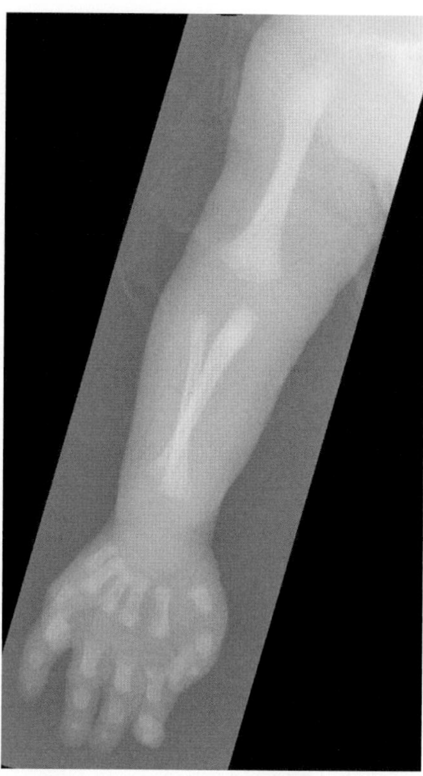

FIGURE 79-6 ■ **Ellis–van Creveld syndrome.** Postaxial polydactyly, short middle and terminal phalanges, cupped metaphyses (the epiphyses will be cone-shaped when they ossify) and sloping of the proximal humeral metaphysis.

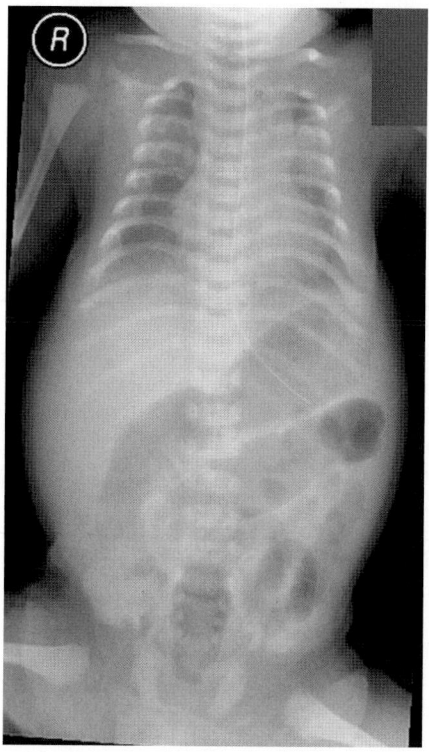

FIGURE 79-7 ■ **Jeune asphyxiating thoracic dystrophy.** Short ribs, trident acetabula. No platyspondyly.

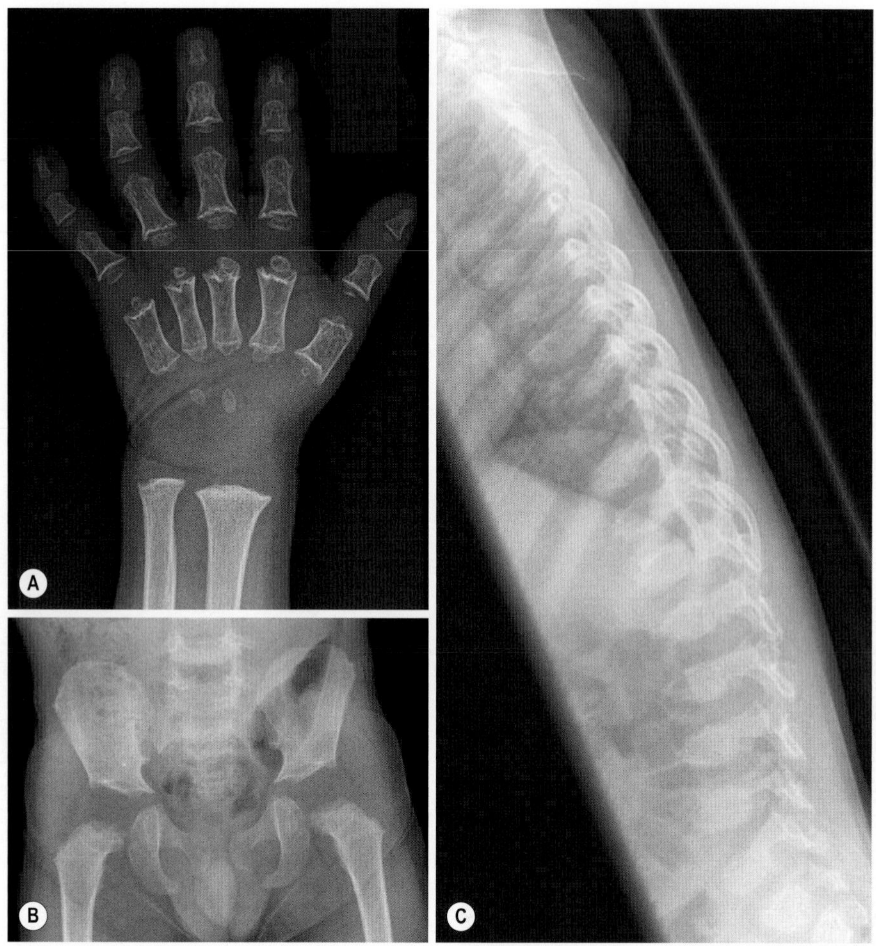

FIGURE 79-8 ■ Pseudoachondroplasia in a 3 year old. (A) Short tubular bones of the hand, small epiphyses with delayed bone age, pointed bases of the metacarpals with pseudoepiphyses, irregular metaphyses, flared metaphyses of distal radius and ulna. (B) Irregularity of acetabula and proximal femoral metaphyses, delayed ossification of femoral heads with short femoral necks, wide triradiate cartilages. (C) Mild platyspondyly with anterior protrusions of the vertebral bodies.

age-dependent features such that the radiological findings evolve or even resolve with time.

Examples of this temporal change include:

1. Spondyloepiphyseal dysplasia congenita (SEDC). Radiological features in the neonate (Fig. 79-4) include absent ossification of the pubic rami and short femoral necks. However, by the age of 10 to 12 years, the pubic rami will have ossified and there will usually be some degree of coxa vara.
2. Morquio disease (mucopolysaccharidosis, MPS type 4) in which the capital femoral epiphyses are well ossified at the age of 2 years, but at 8 years are small and flattened, and by 10 years have typically disappeared (see Fig. 79-19D).

Each radiologist's personal experience of the individual conditions will be limited because of the vast numbers of conditions involved. Textbooks are also of limited value because of the necessarily restricted number of illustrations and obsolescence. For these reasons, skeletal dysplasias and malformation syndromes as a group lend themselves to computer and web-based applications.

Computer assistance may take the form of menu-driven databases of clinical and radiological features. A number of findings in a particular case can be matched and a group of conditions selected from the database for further consideration before arriving at a diagnosis, e.g. the Winter Baraitser Dysmorphology Database.[3] This approach is really an automated method for cross-referencing gamuts. An alternative method is by means of a knowledge-based expert system in which experts in the field lead the user (the general radiologist) with a series of questions through a differentiation strategy to arrive at a diagnosis. Either system can be linked to a computerised image database capable of illustrating many thousands of images. Web-based resources include those that allow individuals to refer cases to a group of experts, e.g. the European Skeletal Dysplasia Network (ESDN)[4] or those that allow individuals to attempt to make a diagnosis themselves, e.g. the digital Radiological Electronic Atlas of Malformation Syndromes (dREAMS).[5]

A specific diagnostic label should only be attached to a patient when it is secure. An inaccurate diagnosis may have a profound effect upon the family in terms of genetic counselling, and upon the patient in terms of management and outcome. There may be a need to monitor and re-evaluate the evolution of radiological findings over

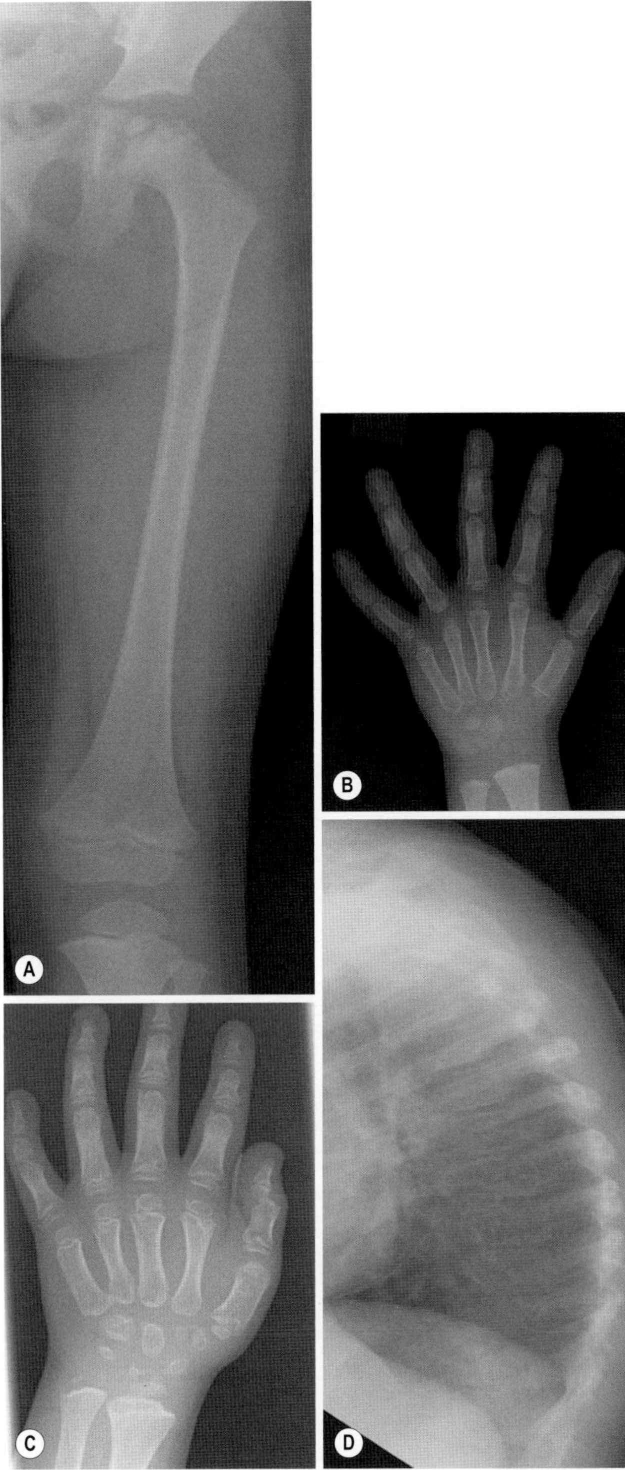

FIGURE 79-9 ■ **Multiple epiphyseal dysplasia.** (A) Small proximal femoral epiphysis with irregularity of the metaphysis. Flattened epiphyses of the knee. (B) Delayed bone age (chronological age of 4 years) with small carpal bones. (C, D) Another child with proven *COMP* mutation. Small irregular carpal bones, metaphyseal irregularity, cone-shaped epiphyses (C). Mild irregularity of vertebral end plates and narrow intervertebral disc spaces (D). Relative sparing of the spine differentiates this from pseudoachondroplasia (Fig. 79-8).

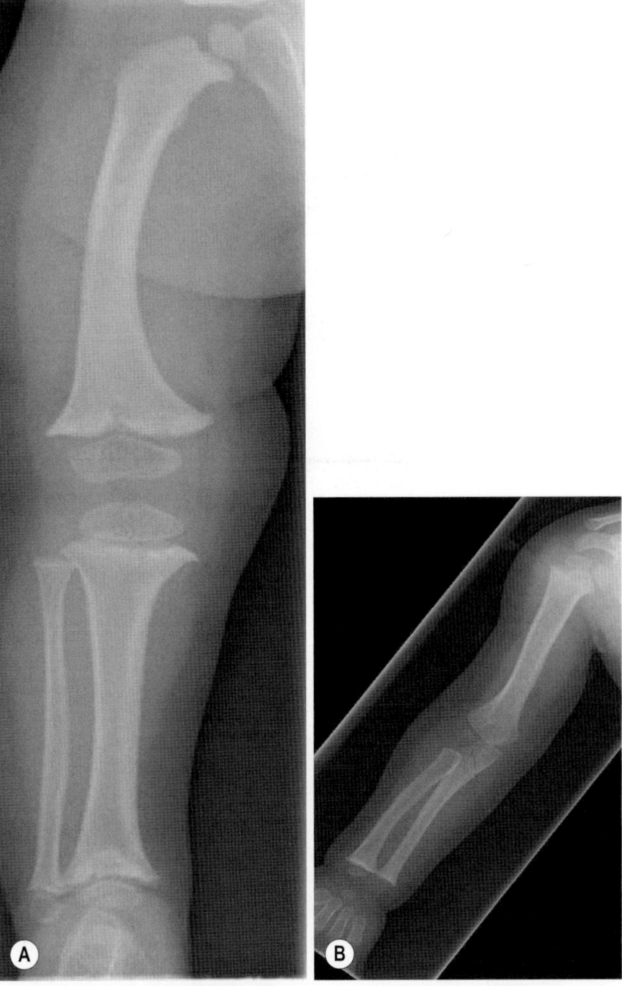

FIGURE 79-10 ■ **Metaphyseal chondrodysplasia type Schmid.** Bowed femur and coxa vara (A) and irregular cupped metaphyses of upper (B) and lower (A) limbs are shown. Bone density is normal.

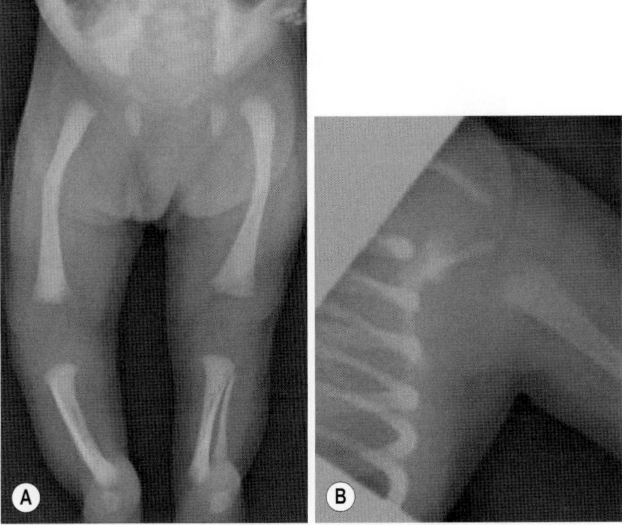

FIGURE 79-11 ■ **Campomelic dysplasia.** (A) Narrow iliac wings, flared iliac bones, mesomelic shortening and characteristic angulation of the femora (although usually affected, the tibiae in this child are not angulated). (B) Hypoplastic scapula.

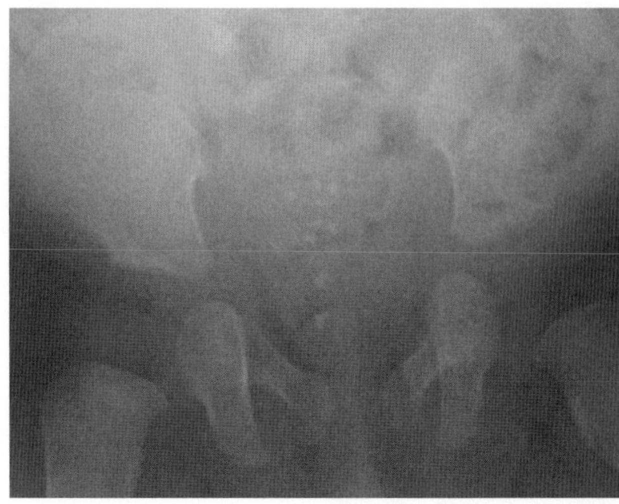

FIGURE 79-12 ■ **Chondrodysplasia punctata.** Punctate stippling of sacrum and coccyx.

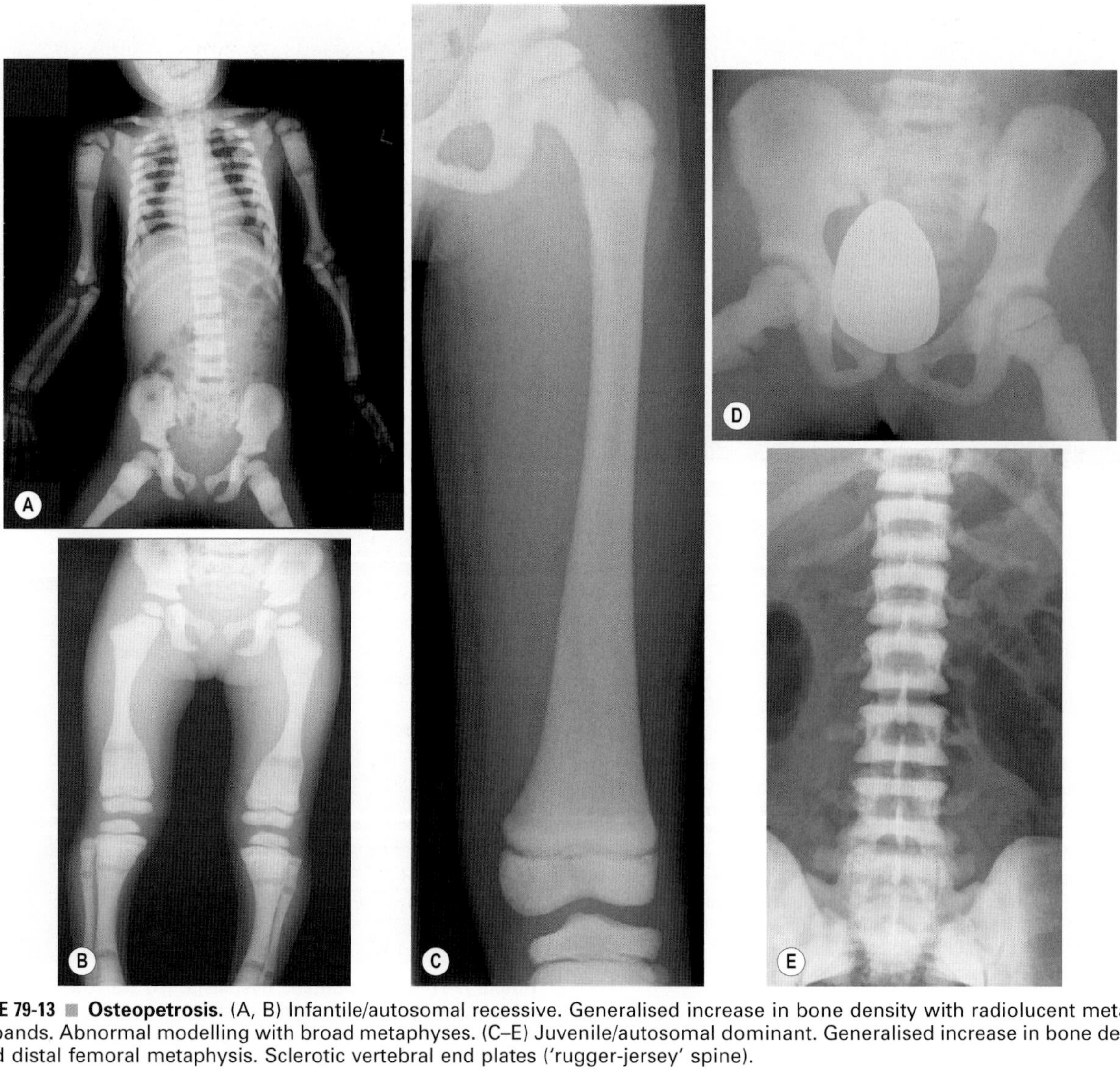

FIGURE 79-13 ■ **Osteopetrosis.** (A, B) Infantile/autosomal recessive. Generalised increase in bone density with radiolucent metaphyseal bands. Abnormal modelling with broad metaphyses. (C–E) Juvenile/autosomal dominant. Generalised increase in bone density. Broad distal femoral metaphysis. Sclerotic vertebral end plates ('rugger-jersey' spine).

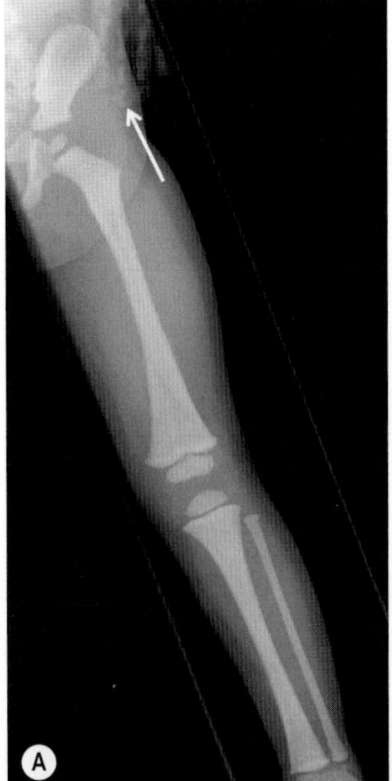

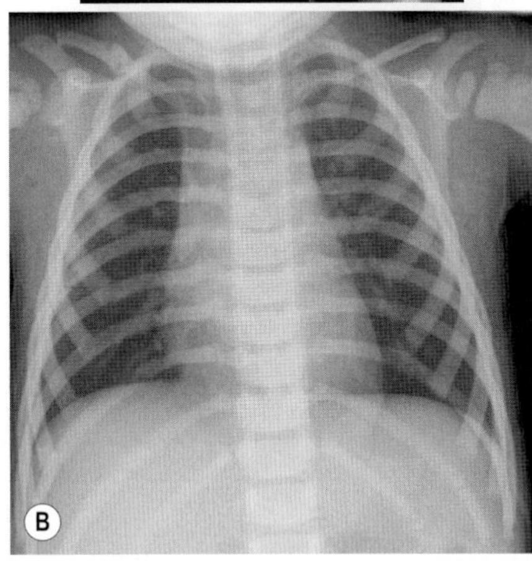

FIGURE 79-14 ■ **Pyknodysostosis.** (A) Generalised increase in bone density. Slender overmodelled long bones. Hypoplastic terminal phalanges of the left hand can just be appreciated on the edge of the radiograph (arrow). (B) Increased bone density. Fracture of the right clavicle. Mild narrowing of the thorax.

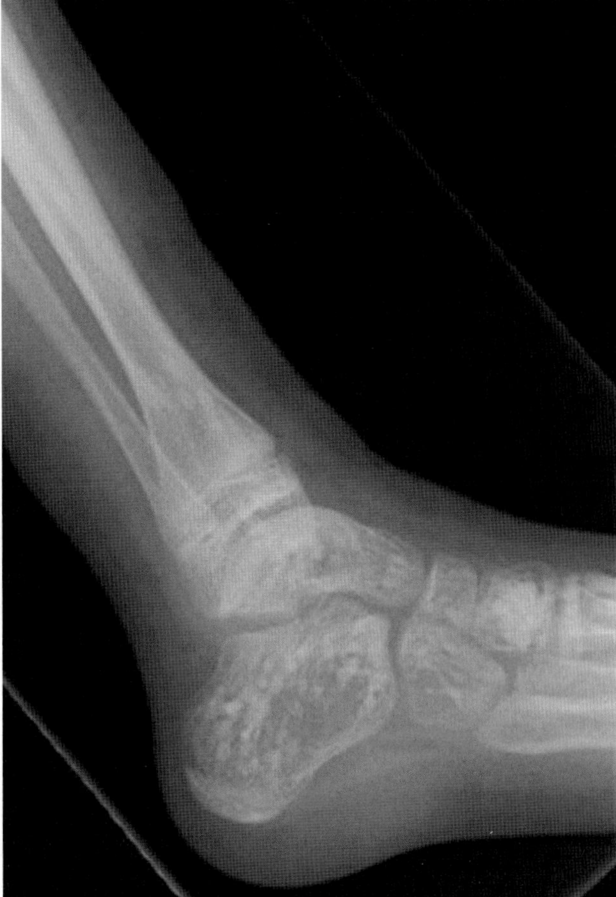

FIGURE 79-15 ■ **Osteopoikilosis.** Multiple sclerotic bone islands.

time before establishing a diagnosis. A significant proportion of cases (approximately 30%) are unclassifiable because the combination of findings does not conform to any recognised condition. It is important that data, both clinical (Table 79-2) and radiological, and specimens, such as bone, tissue and blood, are stored and that the information can be widely disseminated. Only in this way will it be possible to 'match' conditions and to establish the natural history of a disorder.

TABLE 79-2 **Clinical Data Used in the Diagnosis of Skeletal Dysplasias and Malformation Syndromes**

Stature—proportionate, disproportionate, asymmetry
Abnormal body proportion—short trunk, short limbs, macrocephaly, microcephaly
Abnormal limb segments—rhizomelic, mesomelic, acromelic
Local anomalies and deformities—cleft palate, polydactyly
Facies—dysmorphology
Other—hearing, sight, learning difficulties
Temporal changes
Pedigree

Prenatal Diagnosis

In the UK, almost all pregnant women now undergo prenatal US screening at between 14 and 18 weeks' gestation. All neonatally lethal skeletal dysplasias may be diagnosed at this stage by demonstrating short limbs, bowed limbs (Fig. 79-2), or a narrow thorax. Where there has been a previously affected sibling, specific malformations such as polydactyly, polycystic kidneys, or micrognathia may be assessed. Skeletal US findings are highly significant but are not very specific, and in general it is unwise to offer a precise diagnosis on the basis of US findings alone. Pregnancy terminations offered on the grounds of such US findings should subsequently have radiological and histopathological evaluation to determine the precise diagnosis, and before genetic counselling is offered.

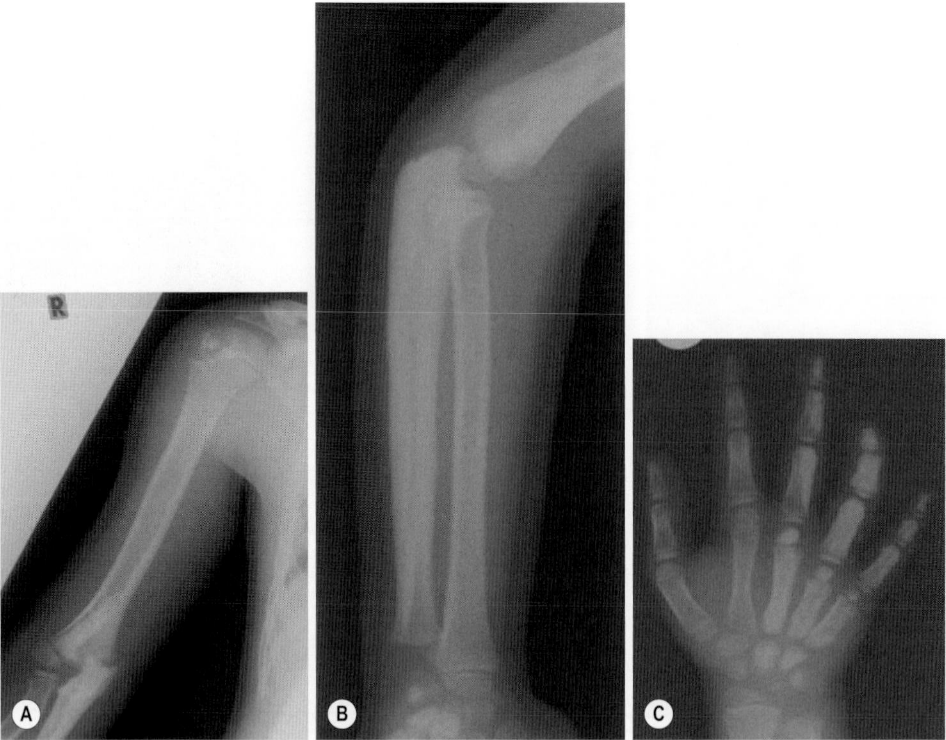

FIGURE 79-16 ■ **Melorheostosis (same patient as in Fig. 79-15).** Dense cortical bone ('dripping candle wax') in a ray distribution affecting (A) the right humerus, (B) the ulna and (C) the medial three digits and their associated carpal bones.

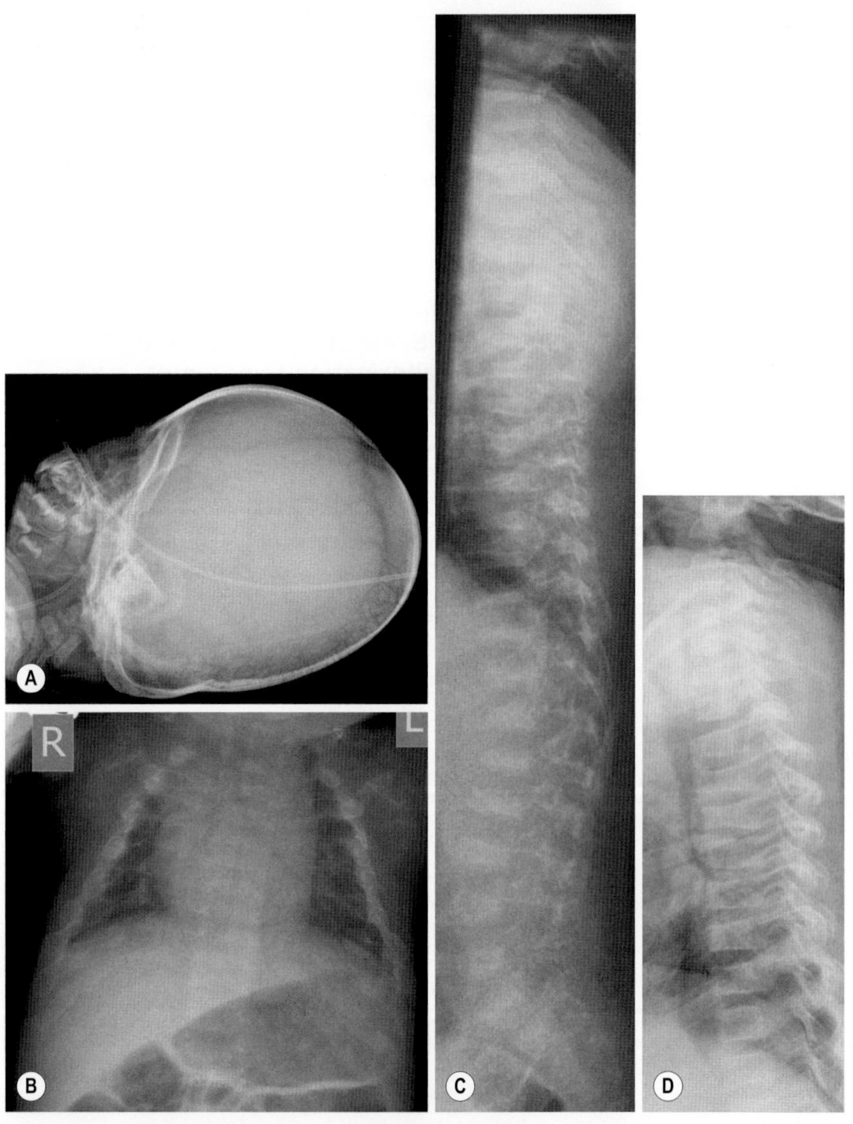

FIGURE 79-17 ■ **Osteogenesis imperfecta (OI).** (A) OI type III. Turricephaly, platybasia (but no basilar invagination) and multiple Wormian bones. (B, C) OI type III 4-week-old child: (B) reduced bone density, broad ribs with multiple healing fractures, platyspondyly; and (C) multiple vertebral compression fractures with reduced bone density. (D) OI type III aged 4 years and 7 months (same child as depicted in (B, C)). Improved bone density on bisphosphonate therapy. Multiple vertebral wedge fractures.

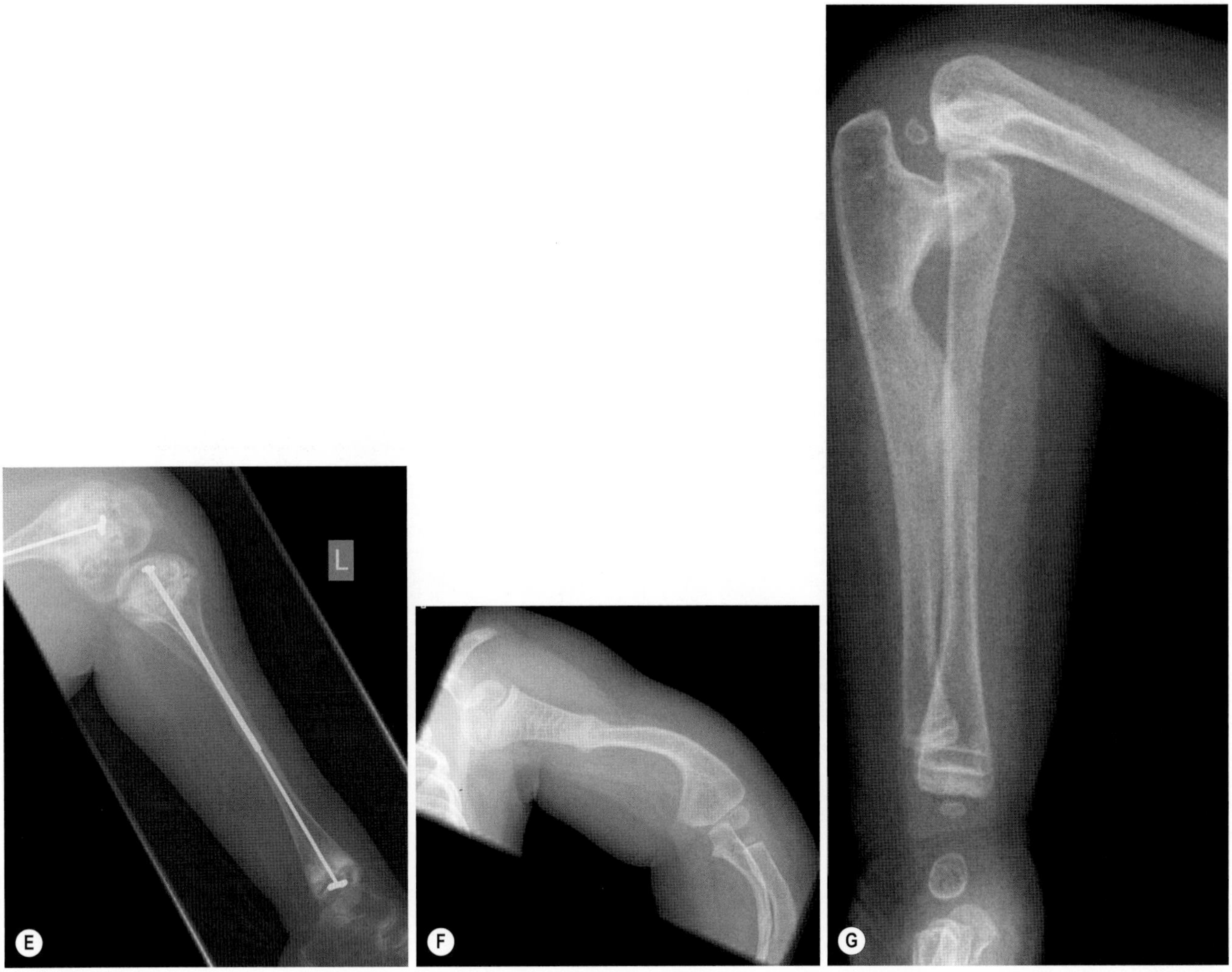

FIGURE 79-17, Continued ■ (E) OI type III. Reduced bone density. 'Popcorn' calcification of the metaphyses. Intramedullary rodding of femur and tibia. (F) OI type III. Bowing deformity of the bones. Healing shaft fractures of the humerus and ulna. Multiple bisphosphonate lines of the proximal humerus. See also Fig. 79-1. (G) OI type V. Ossification of the interosseous membrane. Dislocated radial head.

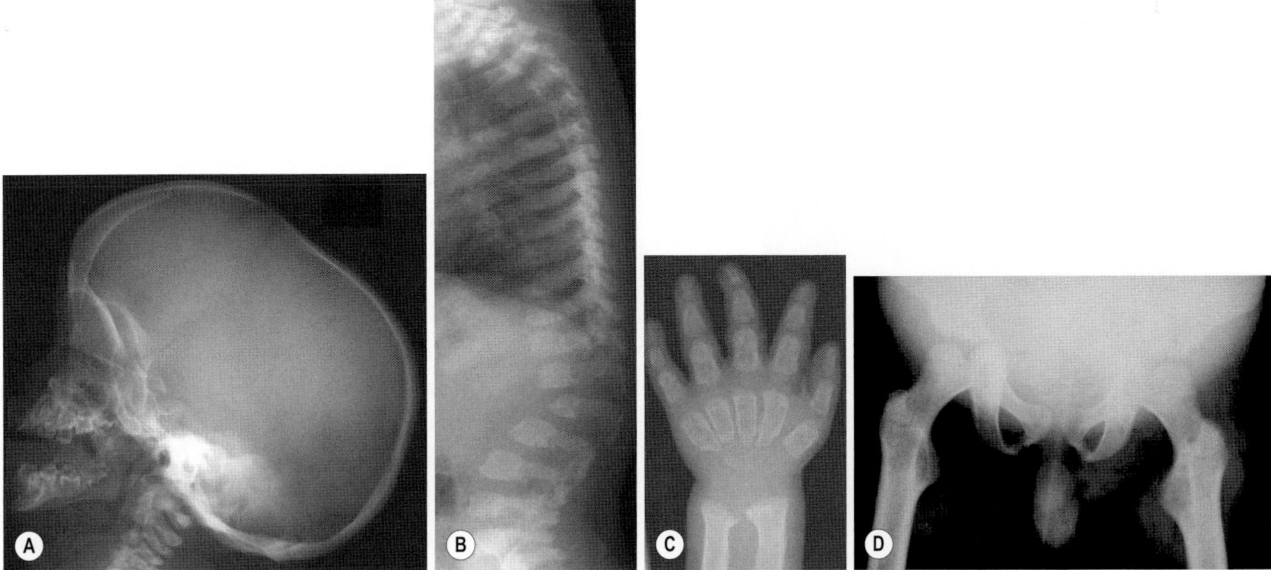

FIGURE 79-18 ■ **Mucopolysaccharidosis type 1H/1S (Hurler/Scheie).** (A) Macrocephaly, ground-glass appearance, elongated 'j-shaped' sella turcica. Mild hypoplasia of the odontoid peg. (B) Hypoplastic L2 vertebral body with a kyphosis at this level. Anterior beaking of vertebral bodies. Mild posterior scalloping of the upper lumbar vertebral bodies. Broad ribs. (C) Undermodelled tubular bones of the hand with proximal pointing of the second to fifth metacarpals. Short terminal phalanges. Undermodelling of the distal radius and ulna with a reduced carpal angle. (D) Flared iliac wings, elongated femoral necks with small proximal femoral epiphyses.

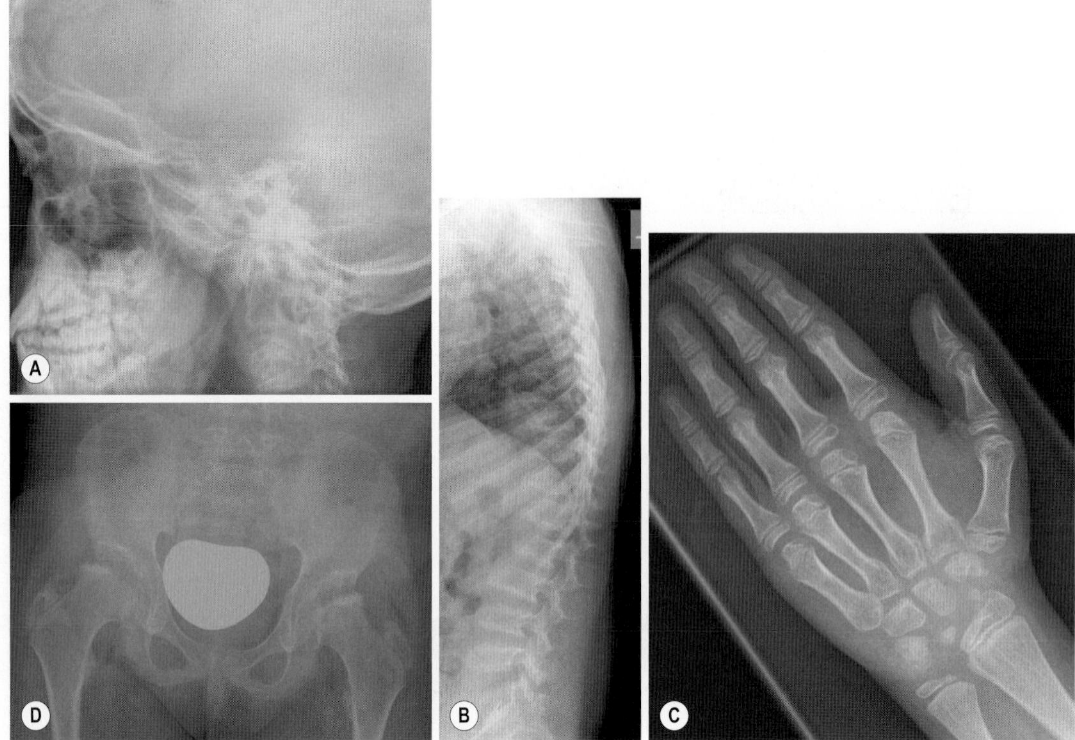

FIGURE 79-19 ■ Mucopolysaccharidosis type 4 (Morquio) in a girl aged 10 years and 8 months with corneal clouding and normal intelligence. (A) Hypoplastic odontoid peg. (B) Platyspondyly, anterior beaking and posterior scalloping of the vertebral bodies. (C) Flattened metacarpal heads and irregular carpal bones. (D) Small (nearly absent) and sclerotic femoral heads (progressive fragmentation over the preceding few years), irregular acetabula.

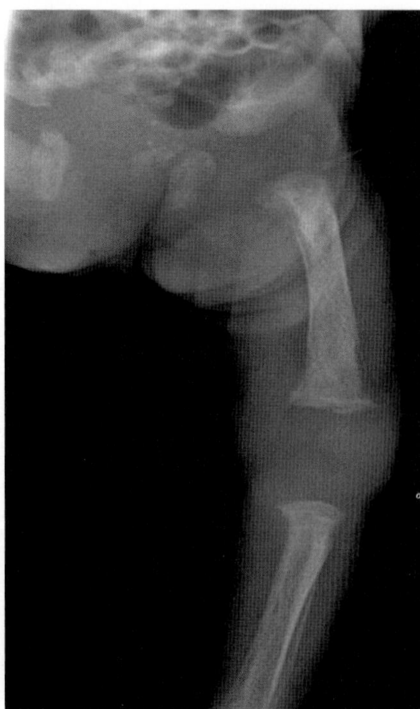

FIGURE 79-20 ■ Mucolipidosis type II (I-cell disease). Coarse trabeculation and periosteal cloaking of the long bones. Stippling of the lower spine and at the knee.

Many non-lethal conditions which may present at birth can also be ascertained on prenatal US. Fetal anomaly US examinations are offered to parents of previous babies who have had congenital dysplasias or malformation syndromes, and to at-risk parents with high maternal or paternal ages, or with specific environmental exposures (including certain medications).

Occasionally, other imaging techniques may help to confirm a suspected prenatal diagnosis. Maternal abdominal radiographs are now almost obsolete; the poor diagnostic quality does not justify the radiation risk to either fetus or mother, particularly as the fetus may be normal or have the potential to survive with a good quality of life.

Low-dose prenatal CT is being successfully performed in some centres for the evaluation of skeletal anomalies.[6]

Magnetic resonance imaging (MRI) is increasingly used for in utero evaluation of specific anomalies, particularly of the central nervous system but more recently of other systems including the musculoskeletal[7] and for the assessment of lung volumes.[8]

Chorionic villus sampling can be used for biochemical evaluation of fetuses at risk from storage disorders when a previous pregnancy has been affected. Fetal chromosomal analysis from skin biopsy can be assessed when a sibling or carrier parent is affected.

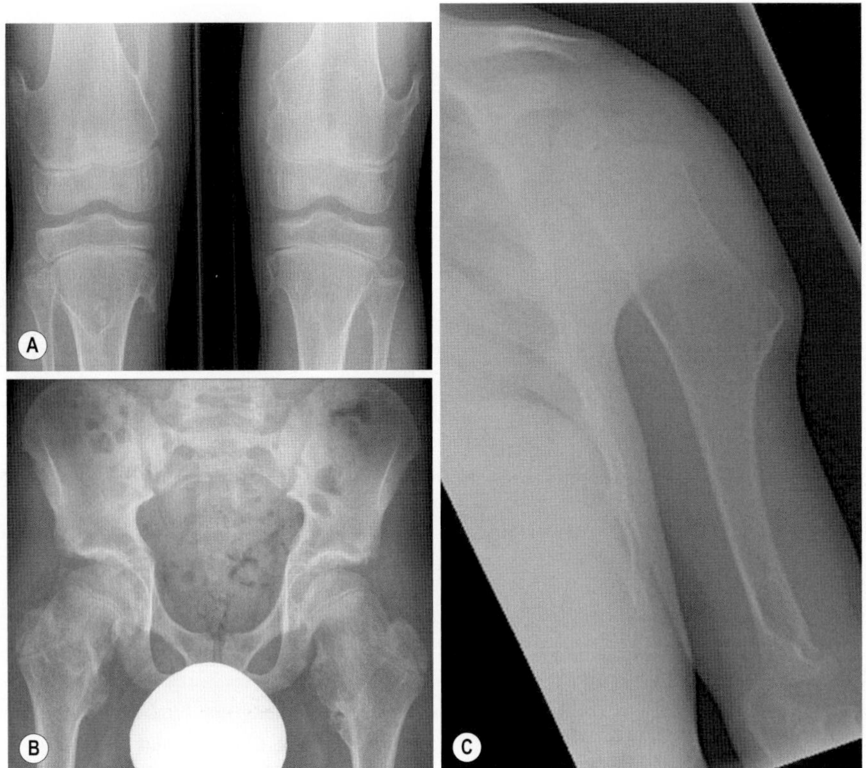

FIGURE 79-21 ■ **Multiple cartilaginous exostoses.** (A) Multiple exostoses around the knee. Note that they point away from the growth plates. (B) Exostoses causing broadening of the femoral necks. (C) A large sessile exostosis of the proximal humerus—again pointing away from the nearest growth plate.

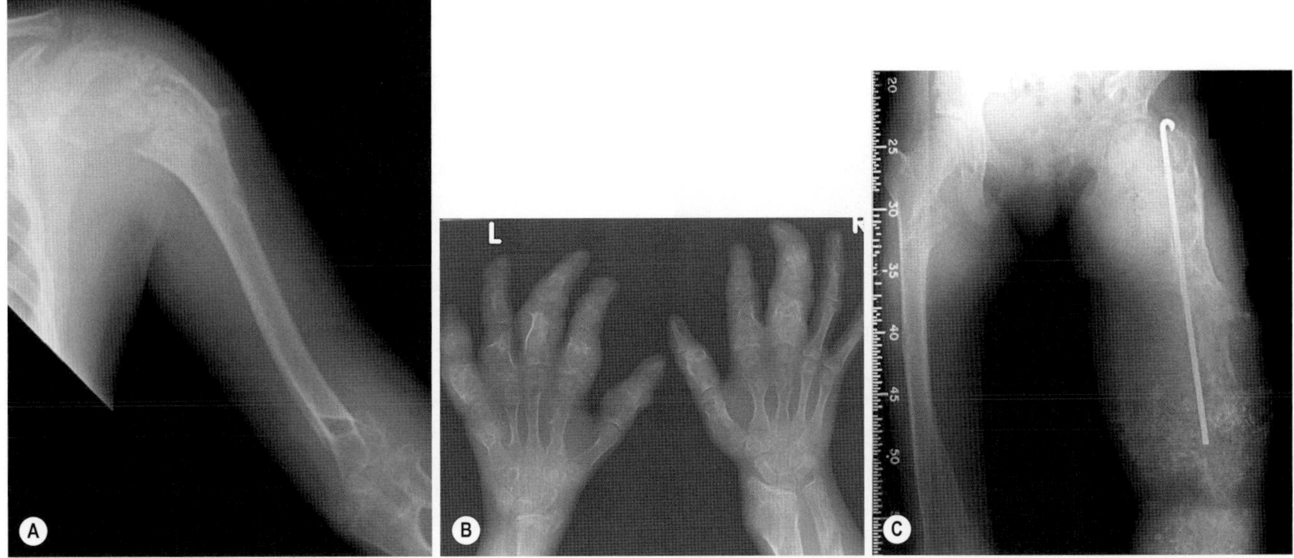

FIGURE 79-22 ■ **Multiple enchondromatosis (Ollier's disease).** (A) Enchondromata of the proximal humerus appear as metaphyseal striations and stippled calcification. Bowing deformity of proximal humerus. (B) Multiple expansile lytic lesions with associated soft-tissue swelling of some fingers. Short left distal ulna (reverse Madelung deformity). (C) Characteristic asymmetrical involvement with severe involvement of the left femur and tibia and milder involvement of the right femur.

Imaging

Making the Diagnosis

In addition to prenatal US, a skeletal survey should be performed on any pregnancy termination resulting from a US diagnosis of short-limbed dwarfism or significant malformation. Also, a skeletal survey should be performed on any stillbirth. Although this may involve anteroposterior (AP) and lateral 'babygrams' of the entire infant, ideally additional views of the extremities should

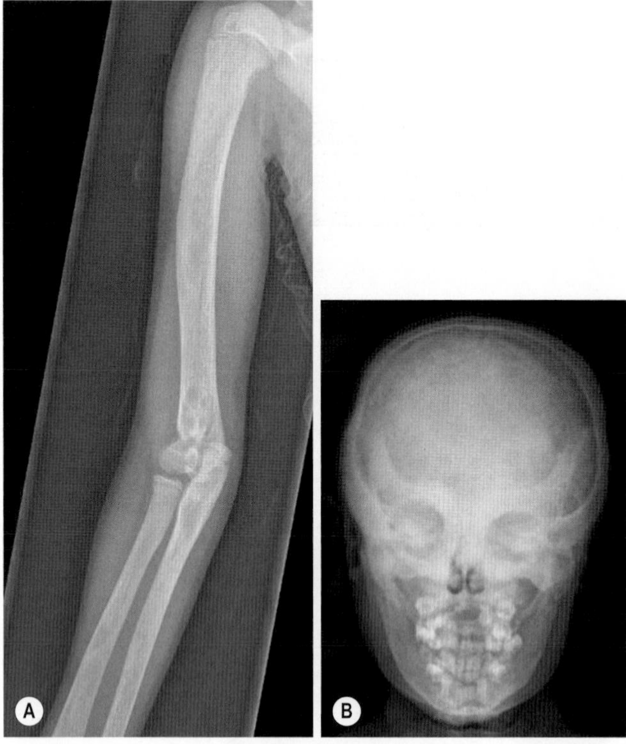

FIGURE 79-23 ■ **Fibrous dysplasia.** (A) Expansile radiolucent lesions, some with a sclerotic margin ('rind' appearance). Some cortical scalloping. (B) Patchy sclerosis of the skull vault and facial bones.

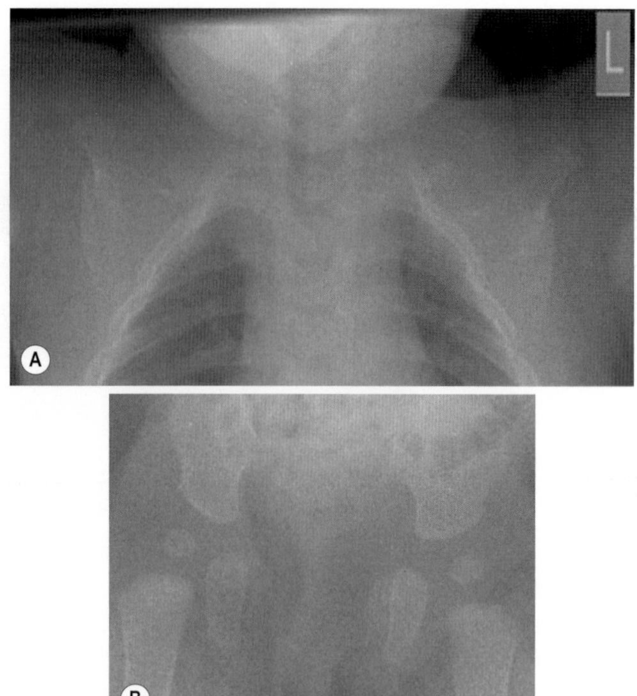

FIGURE 79-25 ■ **Cleidocranial dysplasia.** (A) Hypoplastic lateral ends of the clavicles. (B) Hypoplastic pubic rami. Bilateral coxa valga.

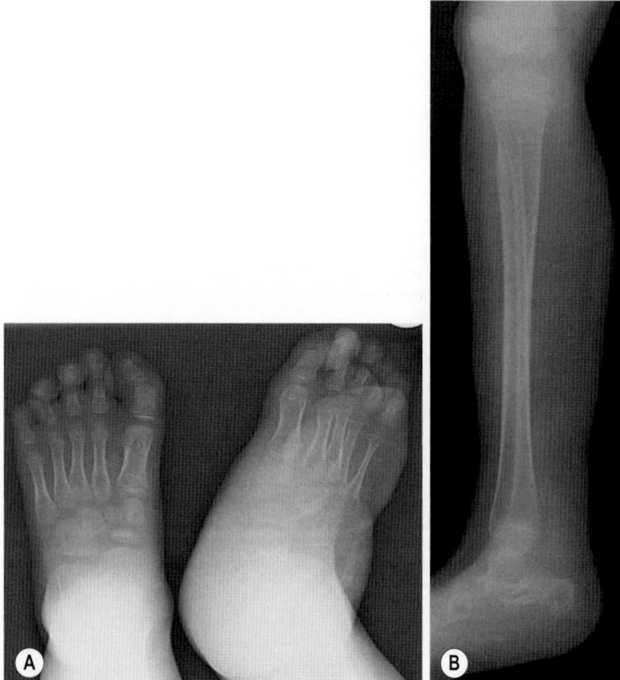

FIGURE 79-24 ■ **Neurofibromatosis.** (A) Soft-tissue and bony overgrowth of the right foot. (B) Soft-tissue overgrowth of the right leg. Thickened heel pad with characteristic erosion of the calcaneum.

be performed. Spontaneous abortions should also have a radiographic skeletal survey. However, this can rarely be achieved.

After birth, a standard full skeletal survey is indicated when attempting to establish a diagnosis for short stature or for a dysmorphic syndrome. This should include:

- AP and lateral skull (to include the atlas and axis)
- AP chest (to include the clavicles)
- AP pelvis (to include the lumbar spine and symphysis pubis)
- lateral thoracolumbar spine
- AP one lower limb
- AP one upper limb
- posteroanterior (PA) one hand (usually the left; allows bone age assessment).

Occasionally, additional views will be required, particularly with specific clinical abnormalities, and these may include views of the feet, e.g. if polydactyly is present, or views of the cervical spine if cervical instability is suspected with specific diagnoses, or both upper and lower limbs if asymmetry or deformity is a clinical feature.

If a diagnosis cannot be established, then (limited) follow-up imaging is indicated (e.g. at 1 and 3 years), to evaluate progression and evolution of radiographic appearances.

Occasionally a technetium radionuclide skeletal scintigram showing the photon-deficient area of avascular necrosis (AVN) may be of value in differentiating bilateral Perthes disease from the small fragmented capital femoral epiphyses of multiple epiphyseal dysplasia. In this regard, contrast-enhanced MRI is also useful.

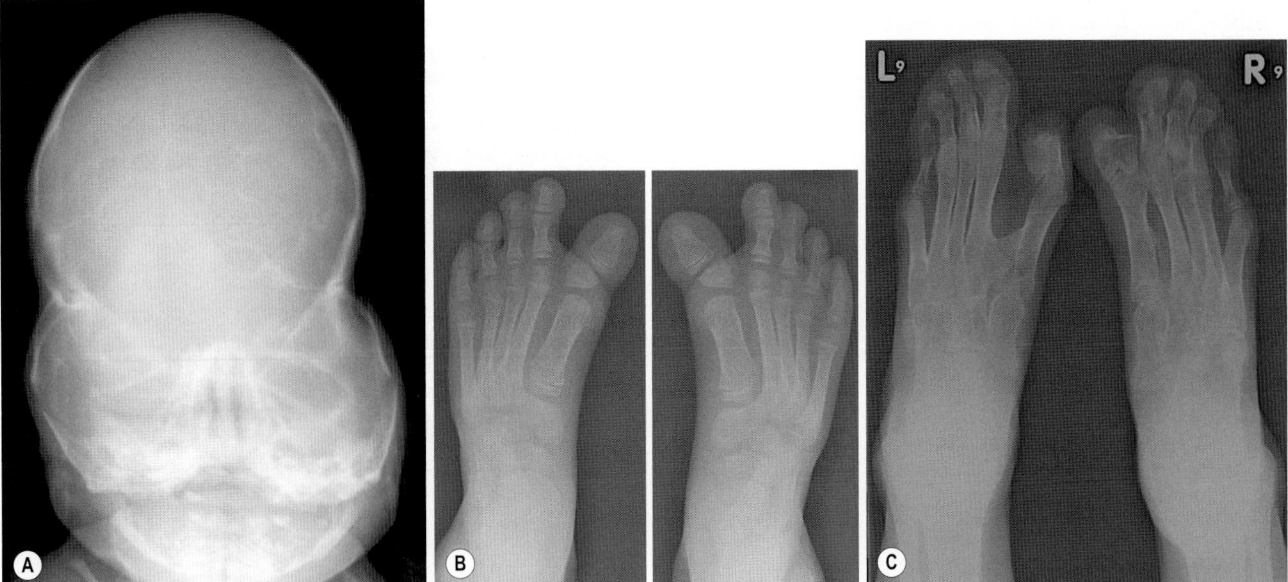

FIGURE 79-26 ■ **Acrocephalosyndactyly syndromes.** (A) Pfeiffer syndrome. Craniosynostosis with a clover-leaf skull. Prominent sutural markings and wide anterior fontanelle. (B) Pfeiffer syndrome. Characteristic hypoplastic trapezoid proximal phalanges of broadened great toes, which are medially deviated. Significant hypoplasia of all middle phalanges, bilateral two-thirds soft-tissue syndactyly. (C) Apert syndrome. Single dysplastic phalanx of broadened great toes and only two phalanges for second to fifth toes. Fusion of the metatarsophalangeal joints of second to fourth toes. Fusion of metatarsal bases. Bony bar between first and second metatarsals bilaterally (left more prominent). Soft-tissue syndactyly of second to fifth toes ('sock foot').

Conditions with decreased bone density may be assessed and monitored by means of dual-energy X-ray absorptiometry (DEXA).

Assessing Complications

When a confident diagnosis is established, further imaging is essential to monitor the progress of potential complications. Complications may result as part of the natural evolution of the condition, but may also be iatrogenic.

Radiography and MRI of the cervical spine in flexion and extension will monitor instability; AP and lateral views of the spine will monitor kyphosis and scoliosis. Long limb radiographic views or (increasingly) computed tomography (CT) scannograms will help to assess asymmetry, genu varum and genu valgum, and to monitor progression of limb length discrepancy. CT or MRI may monitor the development of hydrocephalus or the presence of neuronal migration defects and structural defects, such as the absence of the corpus callosum. CT may also demonstrate encroachment on the cranial nerve foramina and both CT and MRI are of value in assessing spinal cord compression.

US can demonstrate associated organ anomalies, e.g. cystic disease of the kidneys or hepatosplenomegaly, and echocardiography may reveal associated intracardiac abnormalities.

Arthrography, US, CT and MRI are of value in the assessment of joint problems, particularly when surgical intervention is proposed or following surgery.

Technetium skeletal scintigrams are occasionally used to determine the extent of bony involvement in specific disorders, e.g. asymptomatic lesions identified in chronic recurrent multifocal osteomyelitis. However, in patchy disorders such as fibrous dysplasia, radiographically affected areas may not demonstrate abnormal uptake of radionuclide.

Postoperative Imaging

US has a place in assessing the development of new bone formation following osteotomies and limb-lengthening procedures and plain radiography and CT in confirming the correct alignment in this situation. CT is also of value for the assessment of hip reduction in developmental hip dysplasia (see Fig. 79-30F). All imaging investigations are brought into play in the assessment of a patient following bone marrow transplantation.

Management

Only when an accurate diagnosis has been established can the prognosis and natural history be given. For example, myopia can be corrected and retinal detachment prevented in Stickler syndrome (hereditary arthro-ophthalmopathy); cord compression can be prevented in conditions with instability of the cervical spine (Table 79-3) or with progressive thoracolumbar kyphosis and spinal stenosis, as in achondroplasia. Various imaging techniques have a role in evaluating the cervical spine.[9]

In some conditions, cure may be achieved, e.g. in the severe form of osteopetrosis (which is lethal in childhood unless treated), by means of a compatible bone marrow transplant in the first 6 months of life. Not only do the radiographic changes revert to normal but also the

TABLE 79-3 Disorders with Instability in the Cervical Spine

Cervical Spine Instability with Odontoid Peg Absence or Hypoplasia
Achondroplasia
Chondrodysplasia punctata
Diastrophic dysplasia
Dyggve–Melchior–Clausen disease
Hypochondrogenesis
Infantile hypophosphatasia
Kniest dysplasia
Metaphyseal chondrodysplasia, type McKusick
Metatropic dysplasia
Morquio disease (MPS type 4) and other mucopolysaccharidoses (MPS)
Mucolipidoses (MLS)
Multiple epiphyseal dysplasia
Neurofibromatosis type 1
Opsismodysplasia
Pseudoachondroplasia
Pseudodiastrophic dysplasia
Spondyloepiphyseal dysplasia congenita
Trisomy 21
Cervical Spine Instability with Cervical Kyphosis (C2/C3)
Diastrophic dysplasia
Spondyloepiphyseal dysplasia congenital
Lethal
Atelosteogenesis
Campomelic dysplasia

TABLE 79-4 Asymmetric Shortening or Overgrowth

Beckwith–Wiedemann syndrome
Chondrodysplasia punctata (Conradi–Hünermann)
Dysplasia epiphysealis hemimelica
Epidermoid nevus syndrome
Hereditary multiple exostoses
Hypomelanosis of Ito
Klippel–Trénaunay syndrome
Maffucci syndrome
McCune–Albright syndrome
Melorheostosis
Neurofibromatosis
Ollier's disease (multiple enchondromatosis)
Polyostotic fibrous dysplasia
Silver–Russell syndrome
Sturge–Weber syndrome

predisposition to fractures resolves, cranial nerve compression is arrested and life expectancy improved.

Bone marrow transplantation has also been used with some success in treating selected patients with mucopolysaccharidoses. Although this treatment has resulted in iatrogenic manipulation of the natural history of the mucopolysaccharidoses (skeletal abnormalities persist), with the associated improved quality of life and increased life expectancy, later complications, often the result of spinal cord compression, are now being recognised.

In many conditions, orthopaedic procedures are invaluable in maintaining or improving mobility. For example, osteotomies prevent or correct dislocations or long bone bowing deformities. Patients with osteogenesis imperfecta may require multiple osteotomies to correct severe deformities, as well as intramedullary rodding to reduce fractures, maintain alignment and provide support and stability (see Fig. 79-1). These patients suffer from basilar invagination, resulting in compression of the brainstem. Surgical intervention may prevent severe neurological impairment. Spinal deformities, kyphosis and scoliosis are common in the constitutional disorders of bone. Prevention and treatment consists of spinal bracing and timely arthrodeses or laminectomies for cord compression. Joint replacements may be necessary, especially in those dysplasias, such as multiple epiphyseal dysplasia, in which major involvement of the epiphyses may result in premature osteoarthritis. In some conditions, limb-lengthening procedures may be appropriate to improve mobility. This is usually offered in disorders with asymmetric shortening (Table 79-4), but is sometimes offered to selected patients with achondroplasia (Fig. 79-3) or other short-limbed dysplasias for cosmetic reasons. Achondroplasia has proved particularly amenable to limb-lengthening procedures because redundant soft tissues are a feature of this dysplasia and insufficient soft tissue has proved to be a limiting factor in lengthening procedures in other conditions. An increase of approximately 30% in the length of the long bones may be achieved in achondroplasia, compared with 15% in other disorders.

Only with an accurate diagnosis in those conditions presenting at birth can those that are likely to be lethal be predicted. The diagnosis of a lethal dysplasia can prevent unnecessary and distressing prolongation of life, help to reduce parental expectations and anguish and help save on economic resources.

Termination of pregnancy may be offered with prenatally diagnosed lethal conditions, or where there is intrauterine evidence of short limbs. When a sibling has suffered from a disabling condition associated with particular malformations, these may be specifically looked for prenatally in subsequent pregnancies. This practice is leading to a change in the incidence of certain conditions formerly presenting at birth.

With the identification and localisation of specific chromosomal abnormalities associated with particular disorders, the development of gene therapy for clinical use poses many challenges and offers great potential for the future.

Growth hormone therapy is used in selected disorders to influence final height. Growth hormone stimulates Type I collagen production and is being used, in particular, to augment growth rate in children with osteogenesis imperfecta (see Table 79-5).

Bisphosphonates are pyrophosphate analogues that inhibit osteoclast function. They have been used in osteogenesis imperfecta to improve bone density, and have also been used to treat bone pain and osteopenia in a variety of rheumatological and dermatological conditions. The radiological hallmark of bisphosphonate therapy, so-called 'bisphosphonate lines', are now well recognised (see Figs. 79-1 and 79-17F).

TABLE 79-5 **Osteogenesis Imperfecta Clinical (Based on the Sillence Classification) and Radiological Findings**

	I	II	III	IV	V[a]
Clinical Findings					
Incidence	1:30,000	1:30,000	Rare	Unknown (rare)	Unknown (rare)
Severity	Mild	Lethal	Severe	Mild/moderately severe	Moderate
Death	Old age	Stillborn	By 30 years	Old age	Old age
Sclerae	Blue	Blue	Blue, then grey	White	White
Hearing impairment	Frequent	—	Rare	Rare	Rare
Teeth	IA normal	—	DI[b]	IVA normal	Normal
	IB DI	—		IVB DI	
Stature	Normal	—	Short	Normal/mildly short	Normal/mildly short
Radiological Findings					
Fractures at birth	<10%	Multiple	Frequent	Rare	Rare
Osseous fragility	Moderate/mild	Severe	Moderate/severe	Moderate/mild	Moderate
Deformity	Mild	—	Severe	Variable	Moderate/severe

[a]Other radiological findings in type V OI include dense metaphyses in the paediatric age range, healing of fractures with hyperplastic callus formation, ossification of the interosseous membrane and dislocated radial head.
[b]DI = dentinogenesis imperfecta.

TABLE 79-6 **Clinical and Radiographic Features of Neurofibromatosis**[28,29]

Clinical Features	Radiographic Features
Focal gigantism (soft-tissue overgrowth or plexiform neurofibroma)—Fig. 79-24	Neuromas and/or fibromas (with enlarged cranial foramina[30]), schwannomas and neurofibrosarcomas[29]
Macrocrania	Aplasia/hypoplasia of the sphenoid wings (empty orbit)
Axillary freckling	Dumb-bell neurofibromas/lateral meningoceles
Multiple café au lait macules	Hypoplasia of posterosuperior orbital wall (pulsatile exophthalmos)
Molluscum fibrosum	Mesodermal dysplasia (calvarial defects)
Anteromedial bowing of tibia	Angular kyphoscoliosis
	Posterior scalloping of the vertebral bodies (dural ectasia)
	'Ribbon' ribs (mesodermal dysplasia), rib notching
	Pseudoarthroses of the tibia, fibula or clavicle
	Fibrous cortical defects (multiple and large)
	Intraosseous cysts

Genetic Counselling

When an accurate diagnosis has been made, meaningful genetic counselling can be given, both to the parents and to the affected individual. Most conditions are inherited in an autosomal dominant (AD) or autosomal recessive (AR) manner. In conditions with an AD inheritance, the affected individual has a one in two chance of passing the same abnormality on to his/her offspring. However, many of these conditions arise as a spontaneous mutation, which means that the parents of the affected individual, who are themselves normal, have an extremely low risk of having another affected child. In AR conditions, both the parents are carriers of the disorder, but are not affected, and they have a one in four chance of having another affected child.

Other important, although uncommon, modes of inheritance are the result of somatic or gonadal mosaicism or uniparental disomy. Mosaicism is the presence of at least two cell lines in a single individual or tissue that derive from a single zygote. Somatic mosaicism for AD conditions results in asymmetric or patchy disorders (Table 79-4). It is thought that when not a mosaic, these disorders are lethal. Clinical evidence of somatic mosaicism includes asymmetry, localised overgrowth, pigmentation and haemangiomas. In uniparental disomy, both copies of a chromosome or part of a chromosome are inherited from one parent, e.g. paternal uniparental disomy 14 (patUPD14). Imprinting refers to the situation where a gene's expression depends on the parent of origin: hence, paternal UPD15 leads to Angelman syndrome, while maternal UPD15 causes Prader–Willi syndrome.

Osteochondrodysplasias

The clinical and radiographic features of selected osteochondrodysplasias and dysostoses are described in Tables 79-1, 79-5 and 79-6.

Chromosomal Disorders

Trisomy 21 (Down's Syndrome)

Craniofacial abnormalities include brachycephaly, microcephaly, hypertelorism and relatively small facial bones. The iliac wings are flared with relatively sloping acetabula. Frequently there are 11 pairs of ribs and the ribs themselves are gracile. There are often two ossification

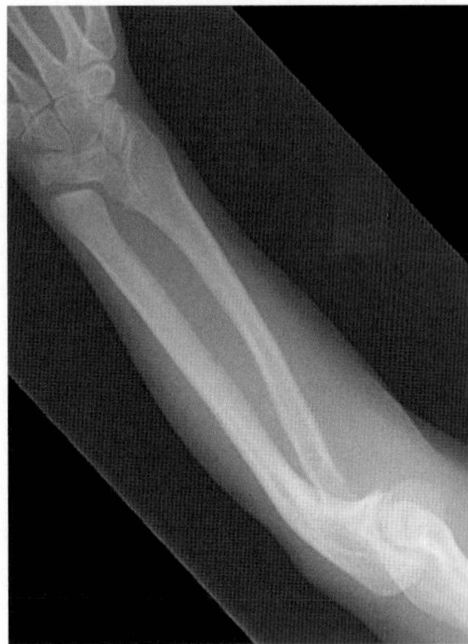

FIGURE 79-27 ■ **Dyschondrosteosis (Léri–Weill syndrome).** Premature fusion of the ulnar half of the distal radial epiphysis with sloping of the distal radius and reduced carpal angle. Dislocation of the radial head.

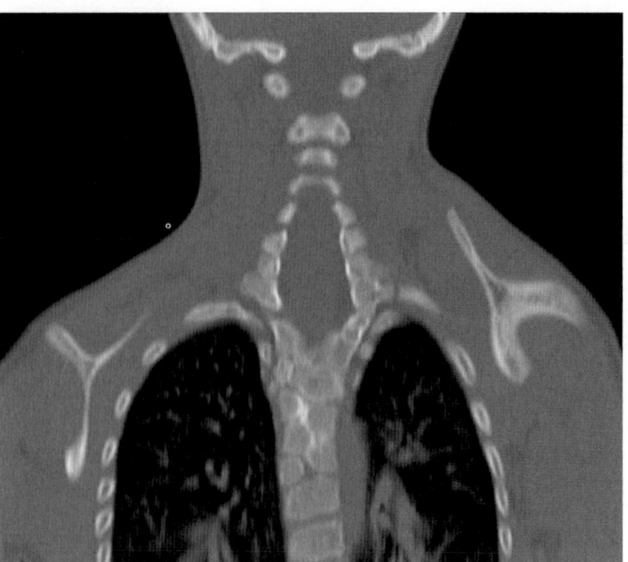

FIGURE 79-28 ■ **Klippel–Feil syndrome.** Coronal CT of the thorax on bone windows showing a high-riding left scapula and segmentation defects of the upper thoracic spine.

centres in the manubrium sterni. Atlantoaxial subluxation and instability with hypoplasia of the odontoid process are a frequent cause of myelopathy. There is generalised joint laxity. The vertebral bodies are relatively tall. The hands are short, with fifth finger clinodactyly due to a hypoplastic middle phalanx. Congenital heart lesions include endocardial cushion defects and intra- and extracardiac shunts. Duodenal atresia, duodenal stenosis, Hirschsprung's disease and anorectal anomalies are associated.

45XO (Turner's Syndrome)

Short stature and lymphoedema may be clinically obvious. Important radiological findings include short fourth metacarpals, a reduced angle between the distal radial and ulnar metaphyses similar to that seen in dyschondrosteosis (Madelung deformity; Fig. 79-27; see also Fig. 79-29 below), flattening of the medial tibial condyle with a transitory exostosis, osteoporosis, scoliosis, coarctation of the aorta, and increased occurrence of urinary tract anomalies, such as horseshoe kidneys.

LOCALISED DISORDERS OF THE SKELETON

Sprengel Deformity (Congenital Elevation of the Scapula)

This is the most common congenital abnormality of the shoulder. There is failure of the normal descent of the scapula from its initial mid-cervical to its final mid-thoracic position. This descent should occur between the sixth and eighth weeks of gestation. Males and females are affected equally. It may affect one or both sides. When unilateral, the left shoulder is more often involved. It may occur in isolation or in association with fusions of the cervical spine (Klippel–Feil syndrome). The scapula is elevated and rotated with the inferior edge of the glenoid pointing towards the spine. The superomedial angle is high and prominent, and the affected scapula is larger than the normal one. An autosomal dominant inheritance has been suggested.

An omovertebral bone (bony or fibrous connection between the superomedial angle of the scapula and the spinous process, lamina or transverse process of a vertebral body between C4 and C7) occurs in approximately 50% of cases. Both MRI[10] and CT (Fig. 79-28) are useful for depicting the deformity, associated vertebral segmentation defects and the omovertebral bone (when present).

Madelung Deformity

This condition results from abnormality (premature fusion) of the medial half of the distal radial epiphysis. The radii are short and bowed. There is reduction of the carpal angle, with wedging of the carpal bones between the distal radius and ulna. Madelung deformity may be inherited when it occurs as an autosomal dominant mesomelic dysplasia (dyschondrosteosis) or it may present as an isolated disorder, for example following trauma or infection (Fig. 79-29A).

In reverse Madelung deformity, there is bowing of the forearm bones, in association with a short (abnormal) ulna. Causes of reverse Madelung include trauma, multiple cartilaginous exostoses and multiple enchondromatosis (Fig. 79-29B).

Developmental Dysplasia of the Hip

This may occur as an isolated disorder (increased female incidence, breech presentation, first-born children, oligohydramnios, and when there is a positive family history) or in association with other conditions (e.g. sternomastoid tumour, torticollis, talipes calcaneovalgus, arthrogryposis multiplex and trisomy 21). The incidence in the UK approaches 1 in 400 live births, while in the USA it is 3–4 in 1000.

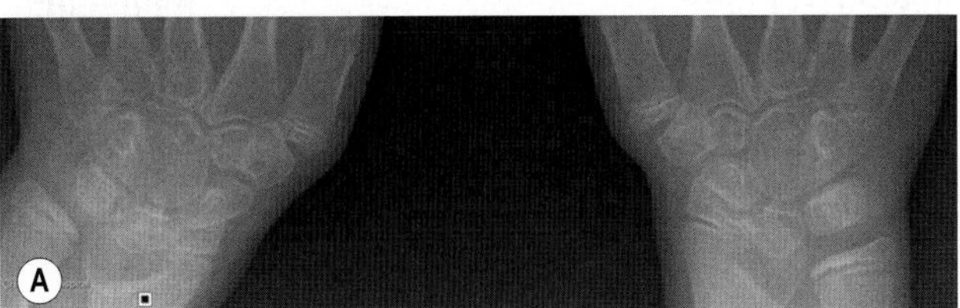

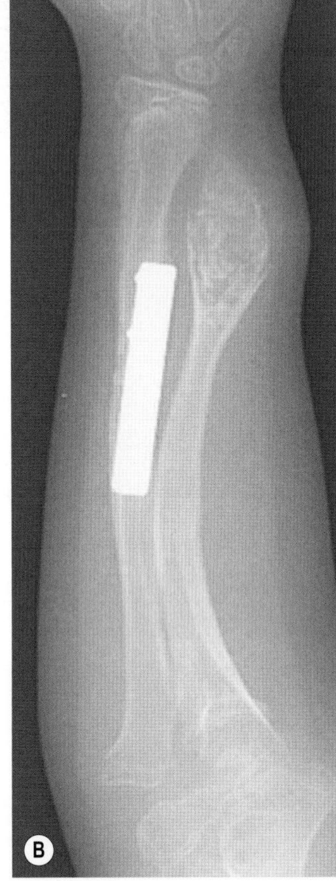

FIGURE 79-29 ■ Compare the bilateral Madelung deformity (long ulna) in dyschondrosteosis (A) with the reverse Madelung deformity (short ulna) in a patient with multiple enchondromatosis (B).

Although guidelines may vary slightly, both in the UK and the USA, static and dynamic US examination is performed on all newborn infants with a positive Ortolani and/or Barlow test, breech presentation, or positive family history. US should usually be performed when the infant is about 6 weeks old. A high-frequency linear probe is used to obtain a coronal view of the hip joint. Measurements and their interpretation are summarised in Figs. 79-30A, B and in Table 79-7. The various imaging appearances of developmental dysplasia of the hip (DDH) are illustrated in Figs. 79-30C–G.

When ossification of the proximal femoral epiphysis renders US examination difficult, then radiographs are useful for follow-up and monitoring the response to treatment. CT is useful for assessing the position of the femoral head following operative reduction (Fig. 79-30F). Screening programmes[11] for at-risk infants have led to earlier detection and treatment, and cases such as those with bilateral dislocation and formation of pseudoacetabulae are now less common. When it occurs, osteonecrosis secondary to surgical treatment for DDH is a relatively benign complication, not significantly affecting general physical function or quality of life.[12]

Femoral Dysplasia (Idiopathic Coxa Vara/Proximal Focal Femoral Deficiency Spectrum)

The spectrum of femoral dysplasia encompasses all conditions from the mild idiopathic coxa vara, through moderate forms with deficiency of the proximal femur (Fig. 79-31), to severe forms in which only the distal femoral condyles develop.

Idiopathic Coxa Vara

In this condition, there is coxa vara (reduction of femoral neck/shaft angle). A separate fragment of bone (Fairbank's triangle)—from the inferior portion of the femoral neck—is characteristic. If the neck/shaft angle is less than 100°, then without surgical intervention the varus deformity will progress.

Proximal Focal Femoral Deficiency

Proximal focal femoral deficiency (PFFD) is bilateral in only 10% of cases. Varying degrees of agenesis of the

TABLE 79-7 **Graf Angles**

Type	α Angle (°)	β Angle (°)	Bony Roof	Ossific Rim	Cartilage Roof	Interpretation
Ia	>60	<55	Good	Sharp	Covers femoral head	Mature
Ib	>60	>55	Good	Usually blunt	Covers head	Mature
IIa	50–59	>55	Deficient	Rounded	Covers head	Physiological ossification delay
IIb	50–59	>55	Deficient	Rounded	Covers head	
IIc	43–49	<77	Deficient	Rounded/flat	Covers head	
IId	43–49	>77	Severely deficient	Rounded/flat	Compressed	On point of dislocation
IIIa	<43	>77	Poor	Flat	Displaced up Echo poor	Dislocated
IIIb	<43	>77	Poor	Flat	Displaced up Reflective	Dislocated
IV	<43	>77	Poor	Flat	Interposed	Dislocated

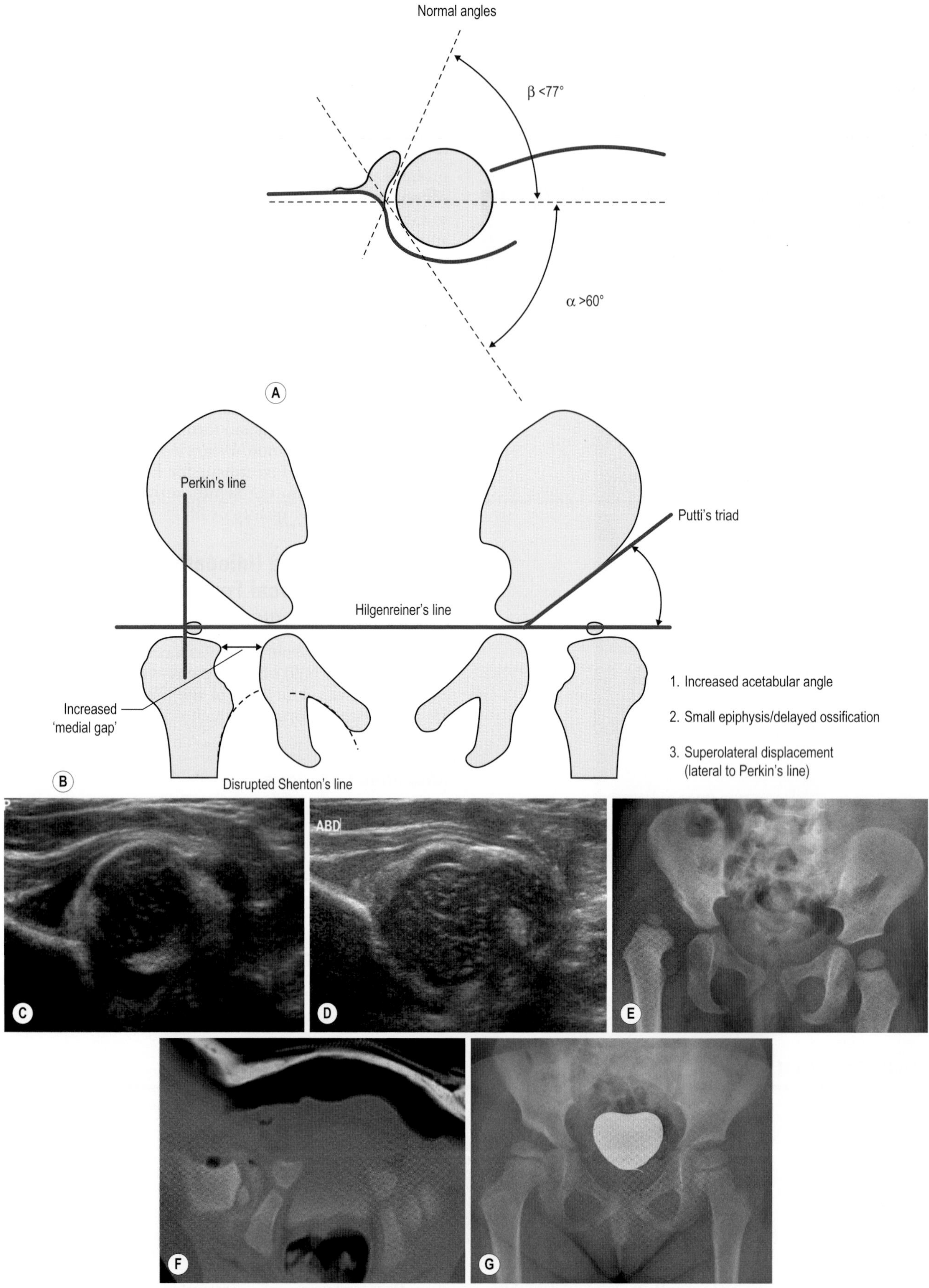

FIGURE 79-30 ■ **Developmental dysplasia of the hip.** (A) Graf α and β angles. (B) Putti's triad. (C, D) Ultrasound in a 2-week-old neonate showing dislocation of the left hip. The dislocated left hip reduces in abduction (D). (E) Dysplastic right acetabulum with dislocated femoral head at 1 year and 5 months. (F) Same patient at 1 year and 7 months. Postoperative axial CT images confirm satisfactory reduction of the femoral head. (G) Same patient at 3 years and 11 months. Shallow right acetabulum with bony fragments beneath the acetabular roof. Flattening of the femoral head. Mild coxa magna.

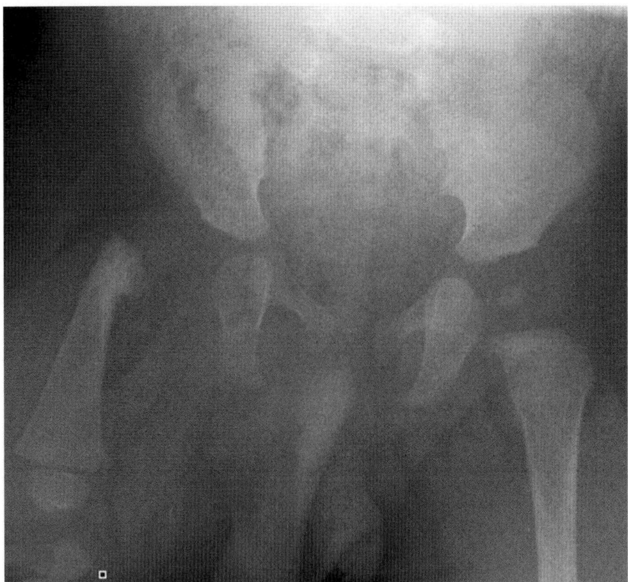

FIGURE 79-31 ■ Proximal focal femoral deficiency. Hypoplastic proximal right femur. Absent ossification of the femoral head with a normal acetabulum.

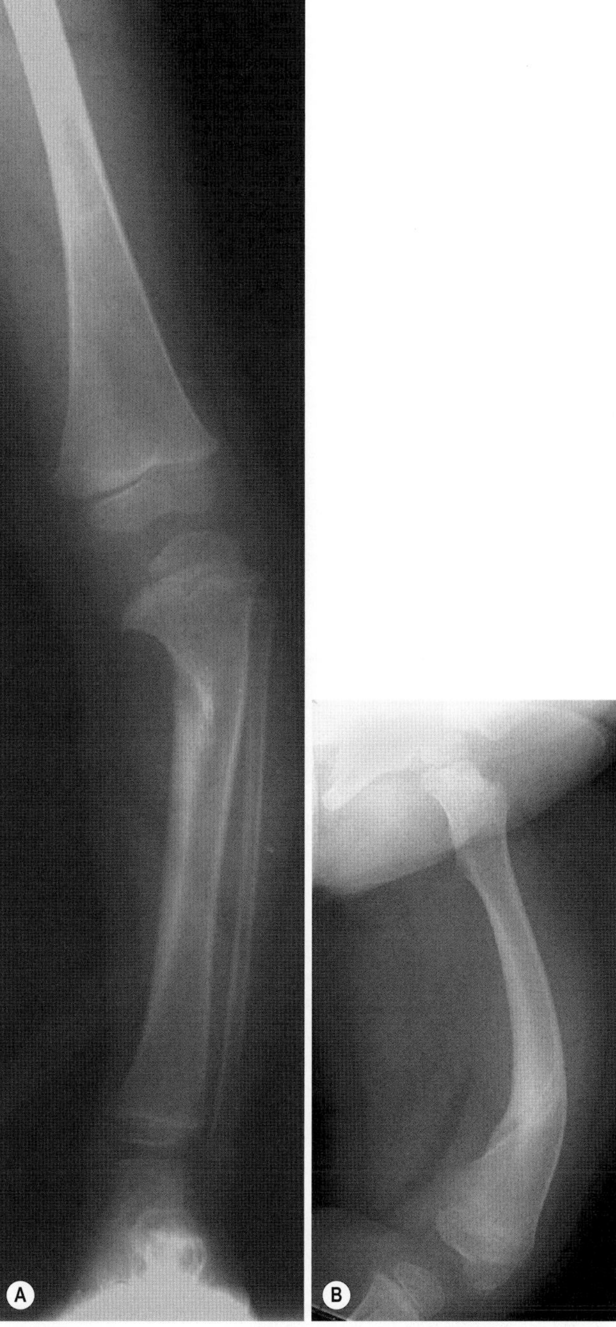

FIGURE 79-32 ■ Focal fibrocartilaginous dysplasia (FFCD). (A) Pathognomonic appearance of the proximal tibia with bowing deformity and a cortical radiolucent band. This condition is usually self-resolving and should be managed conservatively. The proximal tibia is the commonest site to be affected. (B) FFCD of the distal femur.

proximal femur occur (Fig. 79-31); there is an association between severity of femoral dysplasia and severity of acetabular dysplasia. Based on the presence or absence of the femoral head and the morphology of the acetabulum and shortened femur, Aitken classified PFFD into four groups of increasing severity from A to D. In addition to the femoral shortening, the lower leg may also be short, and the fibula absent or hypoplastic.

Radiography demonstrates the degree of aplasia and, particularly in younger children, MRI[13] and/or arthrography is useful for the visualisation of unossified cartilage. Because PFFD is associated with absence or deficiency of the cruciate ligaments, MRI also has a role in imaging the knee(s) of affected patients.

Tibia Vara

This refers to unilateral or bilateral bowing of the legs.[14] Bowing may occur at the level of the knee joint or proximal tibia. Causes include physiological bowing (bilateral and self-resolving), rickets, trauma, infection, neurofibromatosis, Ollier's disease, Maffucci syndrome, fibrous dysplasia, focal fibrocartilaginous dysplasia (Fig. 79-32) and Blount's disease (Fig. 79-33).

Focal fibrocartilaginous dysplasia[15] (Fig. 79-32) characteristically affects the proximal tibia, appearing as a linear radiolucency extending inferolaterally from the proximal tibial metadiaphysis. It causes bowing of the affected bone, but is benign and usually self-resolving. Surgery is required in those children with severe bowing or in whom the bowing does not resolve with time.

Blount's disease (Fig. 79-33) affects the medial aspects of the proximal tibial epiphyses. It is unilateral in 40%. There are infantile and adolescent presentations. The infantile form of the disease occurs between the ages of 1 and 3 years. Adolescent Blount's disease has a higher post-surgical recurrence rate than the infantile form. Tibial bowing occurs below the level of the knee. Initial beaking of the medial proximal tibial metaphysis progresses to irregularity, fragmentation and premature fusion of the medial aspect of the proximal tibial growth plate.

Talipes

Talipes equinovarus (congenital clubfoot) consists of varus (inversion) and equinus (fixed plantar flexion) of the

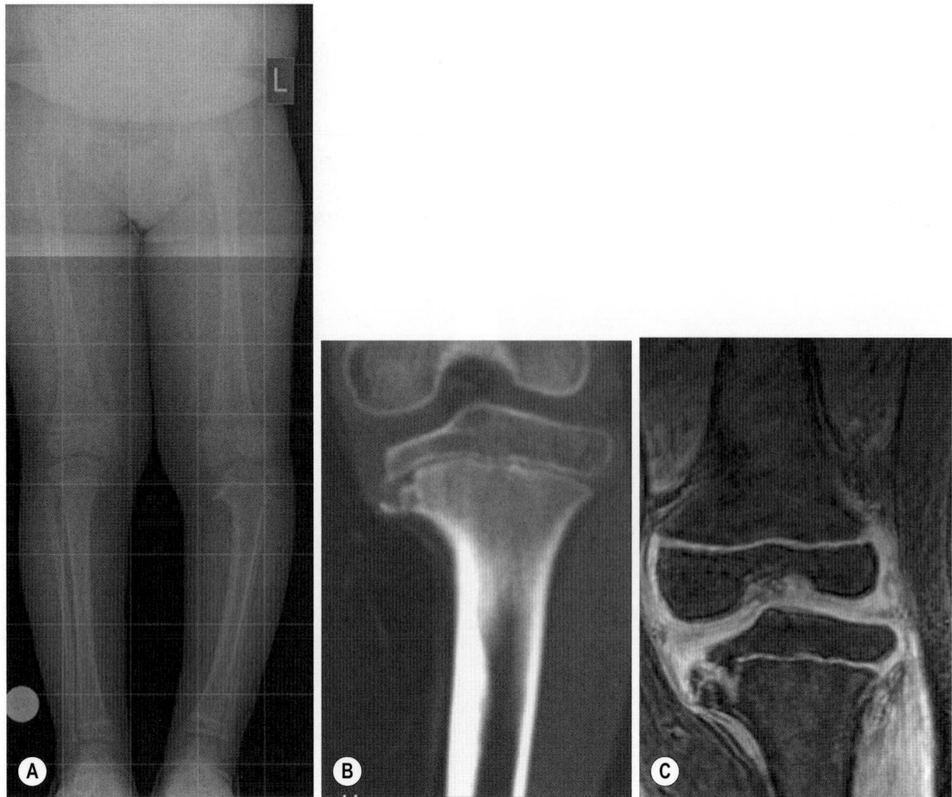

FIGURE 79-33 ■ **Blount's disease.** Fragmentation of the medial half of the left proximal tibial epiphysis. (A) Radiograph showing varus angulation. (B) CT appearance in a different patient with no varus angulation. (C) MRI appearance in the same patient in (B).

TABLE 79-8 **Diagnosis of Talipes**

Deformity	DP Radiograph	Lateral Radiograph
Hind foot varus	Talocalcaneal angle: <15° Midtalar line lateral to first metatarsal base	Talocalcaneal angle: <25°
Hind foot valgus	Talocalcaneal angle: >50° in newborns; >40° in older children Midtalar angle medial to first metatarsal base	Talocalcaneal angle: >50° in newborns; >45° in older children
Hind foot equines	—	Calcaneotibial angle: >90° plantar flexion of calcaneus
Hind foot calcaneus	—	Calcaneotibial angle: <60° dorsiflexion of calcaneus
Forefoot varus	Narrow with increased overlap of metatarsal bases	Fifth metatarsal most plantar (normal); first metatarsal most dorsal
Forefoot valgus	Broad with reduced overlap of metatarsal bases	First metatarsal most plantar

hindfoot, and varus of the forefoot. It results from abnormal development around the ninth week of gestation. Aetiological considerations include genetic factors and early amniocentesis (before 11 weeks), with recent work providing tentative evidence for aetiologically distinct subtypes.[16] It occurs two to three times more commonly in boys. Useful measurements are summarised in Table 79-8.

Idiopathic Avascular Necrosis of the Femoral Head (Perthes Disease)

Osteonecrosis of the femoral head usually presents with pain or limping between 5 and 8 years of age. It is most often unilateral, but when bilateral (approximately 15%) is asymmetrical, helping to distinguish it from an epiphyseal dysplasia. There are four stages of disease: devascularisation; collapse and fragmentation; re-ossification; and finally the stage of remodelling.

The earliest radiographic feature is that of a radiolucent subchondral fissure—the crescent sign (Fig. 79-34A). Disease progresses with loss of height, fragmentation and sclerosis of the femoral head (Figs. 79-34B, C). A coxa magna deformity may ensue, with lateral uncovering of the capital femoral epiphysis. There may be associated irregularity of the acetabular margin. The extent of subchondral fracture is said to be a good predictor of the final outcome.[17] Several radiological classification systems have been developed and shown to be reliable when used by an experienced observer.[18]

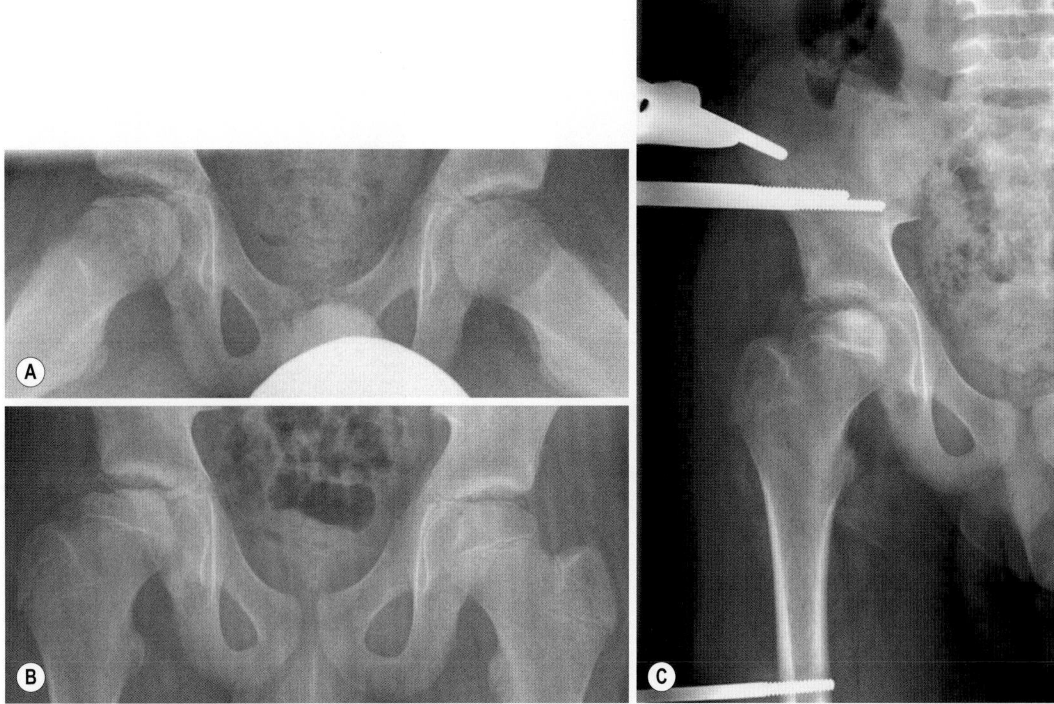

FIGURE 79-34 ■ Idiopathic avascular necrosis (AVN) of the femoral head (Perthes disease). (A) Frog lateral on day of presentation showing the characteristic crescent sign of early AVN of the right capital femoral epiphysis. (B) Ten days after (A): rapid progression with irregularity, loss of height and sclerosis of the femoral head. (C) Nine months after (A) and a month following hip distraction.

US may reveal capsular distension from a hip effusion, which if persisting for longer than 6 weeks may be associated with the development of Perthes disease. Additionally, irregularity/fragmentation of the capital femoral epiphysis and poor coverage of the femoral head may be demonstrated.

While skeletal scintigraphy is highly sensitive and specific for detecting AVN, MRI has now largely replaced it (see Fig. 79-41C below). Six patterns of signal abnormality have been described.[19] T1-weighted images show low signal intensity, compared to high signal on T2-weighted, fat-suppressed/inversion recovery (STIR) sequences. In those with normal signal intensity or complete loss of signal on both sequences (dead bone), intravenous enhancement is not necessary. In those with normal/low T1- and high T2-weighted signal, intravenous contrast medium will identify areas of viable bone. Dynamic contrast and DWI MRI have an increasing role in the diagnosis of Perthes disease.[20,21]

Slipped Capital Femoral Epiphysis (SCFE)

This is the commonest hip disorder of adolescence. Anterolateral and rotational forces of the hip muscles on the femoral shaft result in anterosuperior translation of the proximal femoral metaphysis relative to the epiphysis. By definition, a slip occurs through the non-rachitic physis.[22]

It is more common in boys, in Afro-Americans and in the obese. The age range for girls is 11–12 years and for boys 12–14 years. It most commonly occurs at the time of the pubertal growth spurt at Risser grade 0 (see Fig. 79-37 below), and is rarely seen in girls after menarche or in boys after Tanner stage 4. Bilateral slips occur in about 25% of Caucasian and up to 50% of Afro-American children. When unilateral, the left side is more often involved (65%). Endocrine disorders associated with SCFE include hypothyroidism, growth hormone deficiency, hypogonadism and panhypopituitarism.

Clinically, SCFE may be classified based either on duration of symptoms—acute (symptoms for less than 3 weeks); chronic (symptoms for more than 3 weeks); or acute on chronic (symptoms for more than 3 weeks with an acute exacerbation). A second system based on patient mobility classifies SCFE as either stable (patient able to walk with or without crutches) or unstable (patient unable to walk with or without crutches). The condition is most commonly of chronic onset.

Radiography remains the investigation of choice. Klein's line is drawn on the AP projection (Fig. 79-35A) and the slip angle measured on frog lateral radiographs (Fig. 79-35B). Based on the slip angle obtained, SCFE can be classified as mild (≤30°), moderate (31°–50°) or severe (≥51°). It is important to ensure adequate patient positioning if measurements are to be accurate and reliable.[23]

Complications of SCFE include chondrolysis (narrowing of the joint space), AVN and osteoarthritis.

Scoliosis

Scoliosis (a lateral curvature of the spine greater than 10°) may be congenital or idiopathic. In contrast to idiopathic scoliosis, congenital scoliosis is related to a developmental abnormality of the spine. Based on the age of the

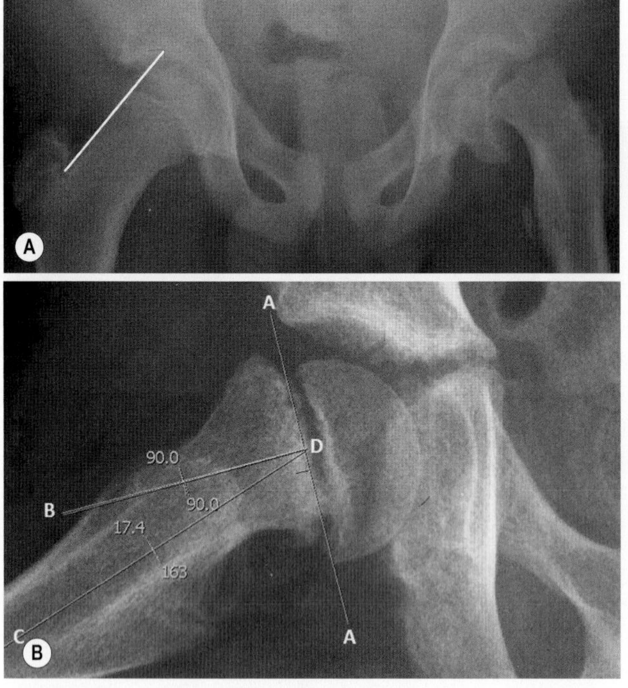

FIGURE 79-35 ■ Slipped capital femoral epiphysis. (A) Left slipped capital femoral epiphysis. Klein's line is shown on the right. This line should normally intersect approximately the lateral sixth of the capital femoral epiphysis in the AP projection. (B) The slip angle—between (1) a line [BD] perpendicular to the plane of the growth plate [AA] and (2) a line [CD] parallel to the longitudinal axis of the femoral shaft in the frog lateral projection—is 17.4°.

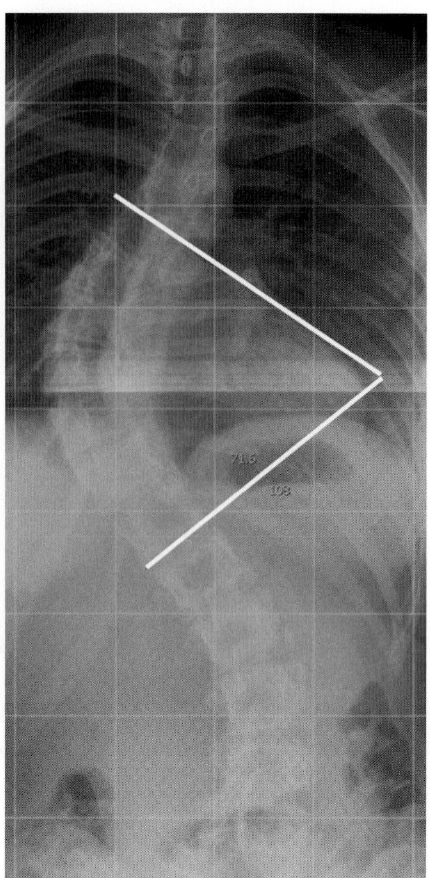

FIGURE 79-36 ■ Scoliosis concave to the left. The Cobb angle between the superior end plate of D6 and the inferior end plate of D12 is 71.6°.

patient at diagnosis, idiopathic scoliosis may be further subdivided into infantile (onset before 3 years of age), juvenile (between 3 and 10 years of age) and adolescent (from 10 years to skeletal maturity). The majority of children who present with idiopathic scoliosis do so in the adolescent period.[24] There is a strong hereditary component to idiopathic scoliosis and candidate regions on chromosomes 6, 9, 10 and 16 have been identified.[25,26]

Congenital scoliosis is associated with such vertebral anomalies as hemivertebrae, block vertebrae and butterfly vertebrae. It may be associated with syndromes such as Alagille, spondylocostal and spondylothoracic dysostoses, VACTERL, Goldenhar and Klippel–Feil. Other conditions associated with a scoliosis include connective tissue disorders (Marfan's, Ehlers–Danlos and homocystinuria), neurological conditions (cerebral palsy, tethered cord, neurofibromatosis), and any cause of a leg length discrepancy.

The risk of curve progression depends on the patient's gender (worse in girls), the severity of the curve and the child's growth potential. The latter two may be determined radiographically.

The magnitude of the curve is determined by measuring the Cobb angle (Fig. 79-36). An estimation of growth potential can be made by an assessment of the Tanner stage (clinical) and the Risser grade (radiological; Fig. 79-37). The Risser grade is based on the degree of maturation of the iliac crest apophysis, and gives an estimation of how much growth remains. It correlates directly with the risk of curve progression.

Cross-sectional imaging (CT and MRI) is useful for the exclusion of underlying vertebral and spinal cord anomalies; indications for cross-sectional imaging include a left thoracic curve, pain, abnormal neurological examination, or other unexpected findings in order to exclude underlying causes such as tumour, syringomyelia or spondylolisthesis.[27]

NEUROCUTANEOUS SYNDROMES

Neurofibromatosis

See Tables 79-1 and 79-6.

Tuberous Sclerosis

Clinical and radiographic features are listed in Table 79-9.

Juvenile Idiopathic Arthritis (JIA)

The 1997 International League of Associations for Rheumatology (ILAR) initial criteria for classification into various JIA subtypes was revised in 2001.[32] JIA is arthritis

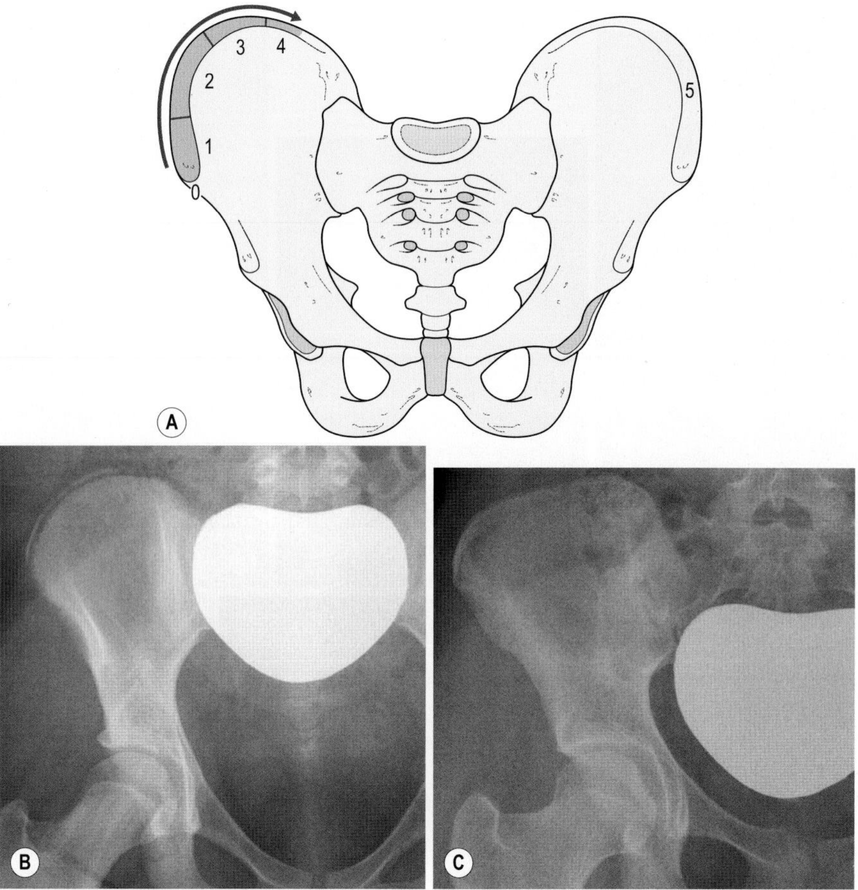

FIGURE 79-37 ■ **Risser grades of maturation of the iliac apophysis.** (A) Grade 0—no ossification. Grades 1 to 4 correspond to sequential 25% increments in ossification. Grade 5 indicates skeletal maturity. (B) Grade 3 in a 12-year-old girl. (C) Grade 4 (very close to complete fusion i.e. grade 5) in a 15-year-old girl.

TABLE 79-9 **Clinical and Radiographic Features of Tuberous Sclerosis**[30,31]

Clinical Features	Radiographic Features
Adenoma sebaceum	Renal angiomyofibromas[30]
Leukoderma	Cardiac myomas
Shagreen patches	Cyst-like phalangeal lesions
Subungual fibromas	Irregular undulating periosteal reaction along metacarpals and other tubular bones
Café au lait spots	Bone islands in the vertebral bodies and pedicles

of unknown aetiology occurring before the age of 16 years. It is subdivided to include: 'oligoarthritis' (one to four joints affected in the first 6 months of the disease); 'polyarthritis' (more than four joints affected within the first 6 months); 'systemic arthritis' (arthritis accompanied by systemic illness); 'psoriatic arthritis'; 'enthesitis-related arthritis' (often HLA B-27 positive); and 'other arthritis' (disease that does not fall into the listed groups).

The wrist is affected in 61% of patients with polyarticular JIA, being second only to the knee as the most frequently affected joint. The hip and wrist are the most vulnerable joints to radiographically visible destruction. In some children, isolated involvement of the hips with bilateral protrusio acetabuli has been documented. It has been suggested that this isolated inflammatory coxitis may represent a separate subtype of oligoarthritic JIA.[33]

Joint involvement is characterised by synovial inflammation progressing to synovial hyperplasia and pannus formation. Pannus erodes cartilage and bone and leads to articular destruction and ankylosis. Affected joints are swollen, stiff with reduced motion, painful, erythematous and warm.

The best predictors of poor outcome are severity and extent of joint involvement at onset of disease; early hip and/or wrist involvement; positive rheumatoid factor; and prolonged active disease.[34]

Radiography (Fig. 79-38), dual-energy X-ray absorptiometry (DEXA), ultrasound, CT and MRI are all employed, both for the initial evaluation and diagnosis of patients with JIA and for monitoring response to and complications of therapy.

Radiography allows the assessment of soft-tissue swelling, osteoporosis, erosions, joint destruction and ankylosis. Early in the course of the disease, the presence of effusions causes the joint spaces to appear widened. As disease progresses in severity, the joint spaces are narrowed (seen in the wrist as loss of height of the carpus) until finally there may be bony ankylosis. Inflammation

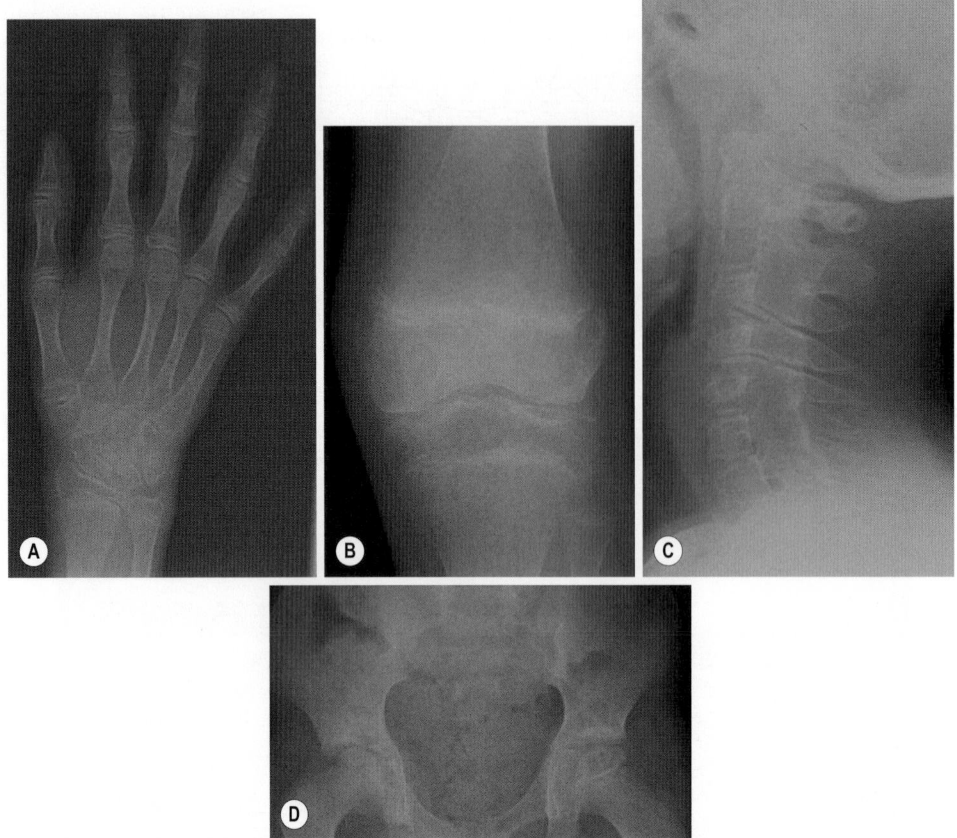

FIGURE 79-38 ■ **Juvenile idiopathic arthritis.** (A) Periarticular osteoporosis, soft-tissue swelling around proximal interphalangeal joints of second to fourth fingers, erosions of carpal bones with loss of joint space of intercarpal and wrist joints. (B) Wide intercondylar notch, reduced bone density, loss of joint space and erosion of the lateral femoral condyle. (C) Ankylosis of the cervical spine. (D) Erosions of both femoral heads, loss of joint spaces and irregular acetabula.

causes hyperaemia with osteopenia, relative overgrowth of the femoral condyles and patella and premature fusion of the epiphyses. The pressure from the hypertrophied synovium causes widening of the intercondylar notch. Evaluation of bone density from digital radiographs has poor sensitivity and interobserver reliability.[35] Other disadvantages of radiography include its low sensitivity for the detection of joint effusions, synovial thickening and differentiation of active from quiescent disease.

MRI has the advantage of not exposing the child to radiation. Furthermore, it allows improved demonstration of articular cartilage, joint effusions, synovial hypertrophy, fibrocartilaginous structures and muscles. Although a recent systematic review concluded that Doppler ultrasound has a higher sensitivity for the identification of synovitis than clinical examination,[36] contrast-enhanced MRI allows assessment of the perfusion of cartilage, synovium and bone and is the most sensitive method for determining whether an arthritic condition is present.[37] Enhancement of thickened synovium suggests active disease and differentiates it from fluid.

AVN is a recognised complication of both JIA and of steroid therapy. The presence of AVN may be determined using either radiography or MRI. Although it is more sensitive than radiography for the detection of early AVN, MRI is said to be less sensitive for the detection of osteochondral fractures[38]. MRI is also useful for imaging the sacroiliac joints (Fig. 79-39).

Juvenile Dermatomyositis

Juvenile dermatomyositis (JDM) is a multisystem disease defined as affecting those under 18 years of age, although it more commonly affects children aged 2–15 years. It is of unknown aetiology, but both genetic and infectious agents have been implicated. The disease is characterised by a non-suppurative inflammation of skin and skeletal muscle and is associated with a typical (pathognomonic) rash.[39]

Diagnostic criteria include this rash and any three of the following: symmetrical proximal muscle weakness, elevated muscle enzymes, diagnostic histopathology findings and characteristic features on electromyogram (EMG). The latter two are invasive procedures and with the advent of MRI the diagnosis is often based on clinical, laboratory and MRI findings. Indeed, the development of new diagnostic criteria that include MRI findings has been advocated.[40]

Disease activity and response to therapy may be monitored by documenting muscle strength and function, serum muscle enzyme levels, range of joint movement, physician's global assessment and MRI. The Paediatric

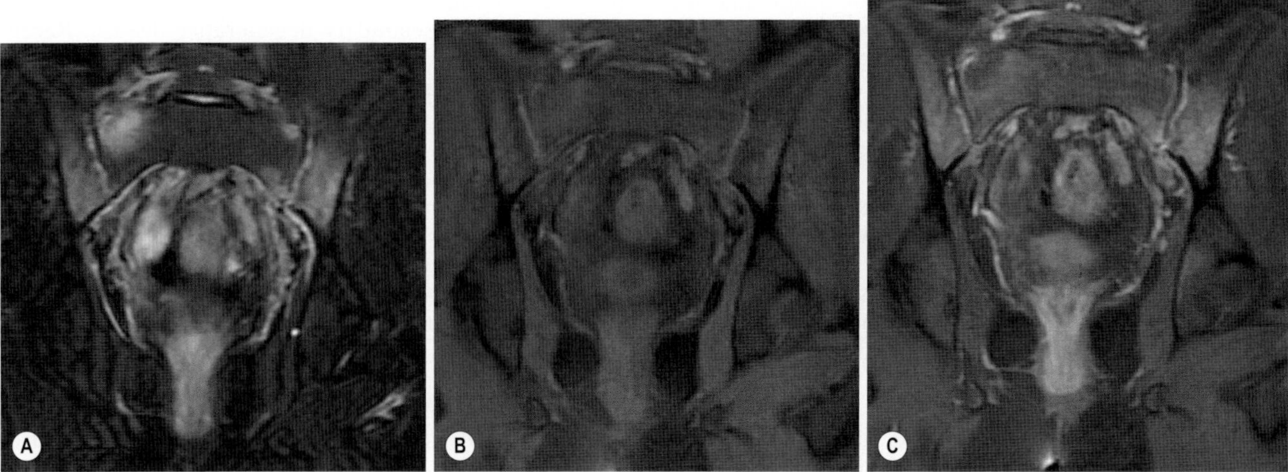

FIGURE 79-39 ■ Sacroiliitis in a girl with ulcerative colitis. Coronal fat-saturated T2 (A), coronal T1 (B) and coronal T1 post-gadolinium (C) images show oedema and enhancement of sacroiliac joints and surrounding bones.

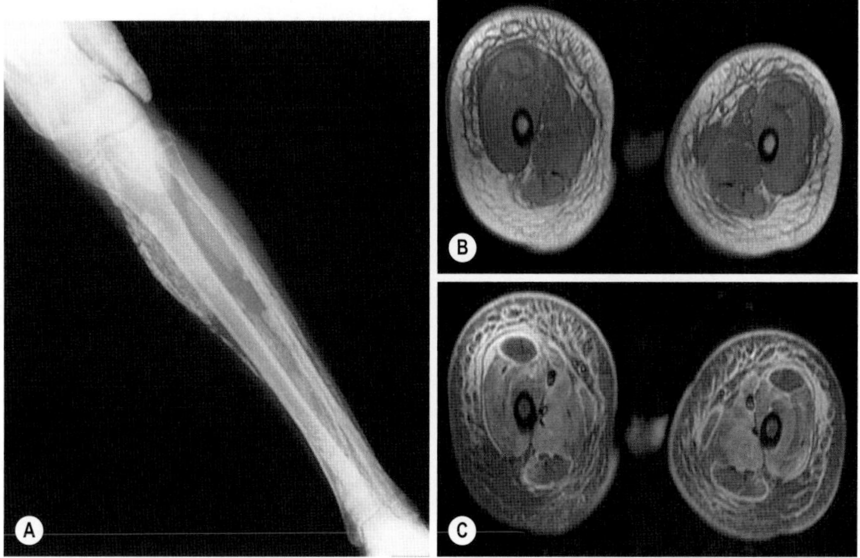

FIGURE 79-40 ■ Juvenile dermatomyositis. (A) Significant soft-tissue calcification. (B) T1 axial of both thighs. Marked soft-tissue oedema. (C) Axial STIR image of same patient in (B) more clearly illustrates soft-tissue and muscle oedema and perifascicular fluid.

Rheumatology International Trials Organisation and the Pediatric Rheumatology Collaborative Study Group have recently validated core sets of measures for disease activity and damage assessment in JDM, which bring together several of the tools listed above. However, they include neither ultrasound (because it has not been sufficiently validated), nor MRI (as it is relatively expensive and not universally available).[41]

Abnormal radiographic findings include loss of muscle bulk, disuse osteopenia and soft-tissue calcification (Fig. 79-40A).

Ultrasound will demonstrate oedema of affected muscles, with Doppler highlighting areas of increased vascularity.[42]

The MRI features of active dermatomyositis are best illustrated on axial T1 (Fig. 79-40B) and T2-weighted or inversion recovery (Fig. 79-40C) sequences. Features include increased signal intensity, perimuscular oedema, enhanced chemical-shift artefact and increased signal intensity in subcutaneous fat. More recently it has been shown that the T2 relaxation time can be used as a quantitative measure of muscle inflammation in JDM.[43] Furthermore, a new MRI scoring system has been trialed, is being further developed and may prove useful, particularly as a non-invasive biomarker of response to therapy.[44]

MRI will also demonstrate loss of muscle bulk with relative and absolute increases in subcutaneous fat, fatty infiltration of muscles, and occasionally soft-tissue calcification. The resolution and relapse of signal abnormality during the course of JDM has been documented using serial MRI. However, there have been no controlled studies. Currently there are no recommendations for the timing of MRI in JDM, and it is not known how soon the abnormal signal intensity begins to respond to therapy or when it normalises.

The bisphosphonates are a group of drugs that are pyrophosphate analogues. They act by reducing bone resorption through an inhibitory effect on osteoclast function. Although not yet licensed for children, they are increasingly used in this age group, most commonly to increase bone mass in osteogenesis imperfecta. However, other indications include improvement of bone pain and density in rheumatological conditions such as JIA, JDM and SAPHO (synovitis, acne, palmoplantar pustulosis, hyperostosis and osteitis) syndrome. The radiographic hallmark of bisphosphonate therapy is the presence of dense metaphyseal bands (treatment pulses) alternating with bone of normal density (periods off treatment) (Figs. 79-1 and 79-17F).

NON-INFLAMMATORY DISORDERS

Haemophilia

In this X-linked recessive disorder, a defect in blood coagulation leads to an increased tendency to haemorrhage. Depending on the severity of the disease (and compliance with therapy), bleeding may be spontaneous or occur following relatively mild trauma. Sites of bleeding include the brain, joints, abdomen and retroperitoneal cavity.

Bleeding into the joints is common and usually involves the large joints of the knee (Fig. 79-41A), elbow, ankle (Fig. 79-41B), hip (Fig. 79-41C) and shoulder. Haemarthrosis begins in the first two decades of life, but the number of affected joints stabilises by the age of 20.

Recurrent episodes of intra-articular bleeding cause villous synovial hypertrophy with accumulation of haemosiderin within macrophages. The arthropathy may progress to cause significant and irreversible cartilage destruction with secondary degenerative disease. Rarely (1–2% of patients), recurrent subperiosteal haemorrhage may become encapsulated and cause bony erosion, giving rise to the so-called haemophilic pseudotumour. This is more common in adult patients.[45]

Based on radiography, five stages of disease may be recognised; however, in any given patient, the chronology may not necessarily follow the stages, nor is progression to the final stages inevitable in all affected joints. The stages are:

- Stage I—soft-tissue swelling and/or joint effusion—normal joint surfaces.
- Stage II—stage I plus periarticular osteoporosis—epiphyseal overgrowth.
- Stage III—erosions, sclerosis and subchondral cysts—joint spaces preserved.
- Stage IV—stage III plus focal/diffuse joint space narrowing.
- Stage V—stiff contracted joint with significant degenerative change.

Although CT and US may be used in the assessment of haemophilic arthropathy, MRI (with its ability to demonstrate early disease, including synovial abnormality, ligamentous tears, periarticular bleeding, cartilaginous and osseous bruising, erosions and joint space narrowing) is the investigation of choice and classification systems based on MRI findings have been developed.[46–48] Intra-articular haemorrhage will usually be evident as a joint effusion; fluid–fluid levels may be demonstrated. Gradient-echo sequences will more readily demonstrate deposits of haemosiderin compared to spin-echo sequences (due to magnetic susceptibility artefact). Three-dimensional spoiled gradient-echo and fast spin-echo sequences allow early identification of focal cartilage defects and thinning.

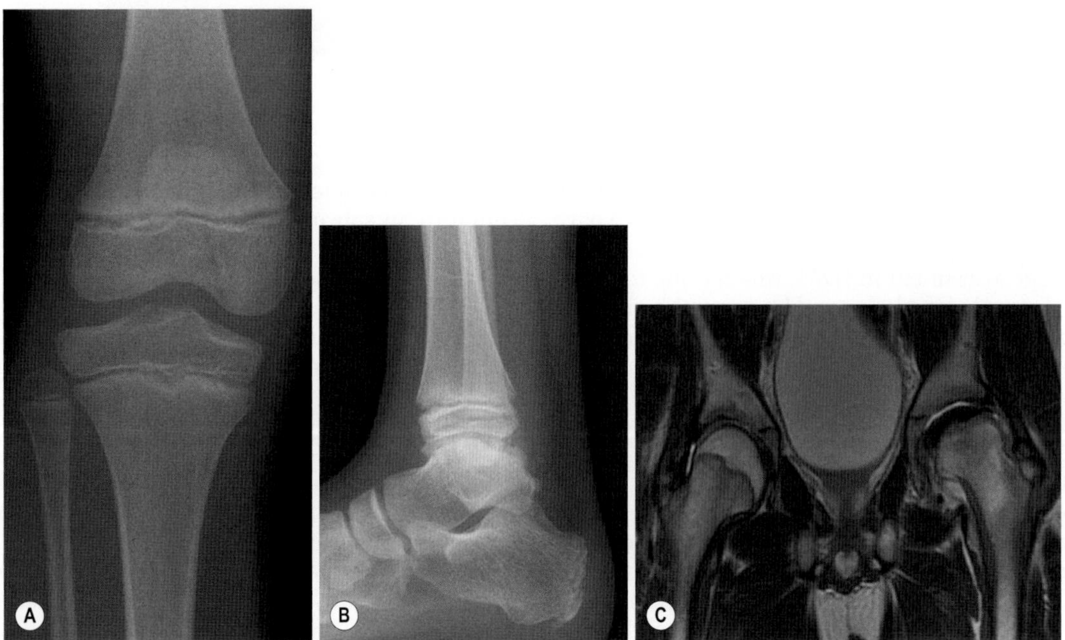

FIGURE 79-41 ■ **Haemophilia.** (A) Wide intercondylar notch. (B) Destructive change secondary to bleeding into the ankle joint. (C) Avascular necrosis of the left capital femoral epiphysis in another patient.

Pigmented Villonodular Synovitis

Pigmented villonodular synovitis (PVNS) refers to benign villous or nodular proliferation of synovium of uncertain aetiology. It most commonly affects a single joint, with the knee being involved in 80%. Although most patients present in the third and fourth decades of life, the disease may also present in childhood. Synovial joints, tendon sheaths, or bursae may be involved.

Presentation is with a slow-growing painless mass that may be tender to palpation. In long-standing cases there may be destruction of cartilage, secondary degenerative change and pain.

Radiographic findings include soft-tissue swelling, joint space narrowing and bony erosion (particularly in the hip where subchondral cysts with sclerotic rims are typical). Calcification is rare.

Non-enhanced CT will show high attenuation due to haemosiderin within the mass. The synovial proliferation enhances following administration of contrast medium.

Diagnostic MRI features include a nodular lesion with areas of haemosiderin (low signal on all sequences) and haemorrhage. Joint effusions and bony erosions are well demonstrated. As with CT, contrast enhancement is typical.

The differential diagnosis includes haemophilia and synovial haemangioma (rare, phleboliths in soft tissue).[49]

Synovial Osteochondromatosis

This benign condition is characterised by synovial membrane proliferation and metaplasia. Fragments of proliferated synovium detach from the synovial surface into the joint, where, nourished by synovial fluid, the fragments may grow, calcify or ossify. The intra-articular fragments may vary in size from a few millimetres to a few centimetres. The extent of calcification seen on radiographs (Fig. 79-42) is variable, and may underestimate the degree of intra-articular bodies. The calcified bodies are well depicted by CT and ultrasound. Although the fragments will appear as foci of reduced signal on MRI (not well seen on gradient-echo sequences),[50] the condition may be confused with PVNS if radiographs or CT is not available. Other features include synovial hypertrophy, joint effusions and changes of osteoarthritis.

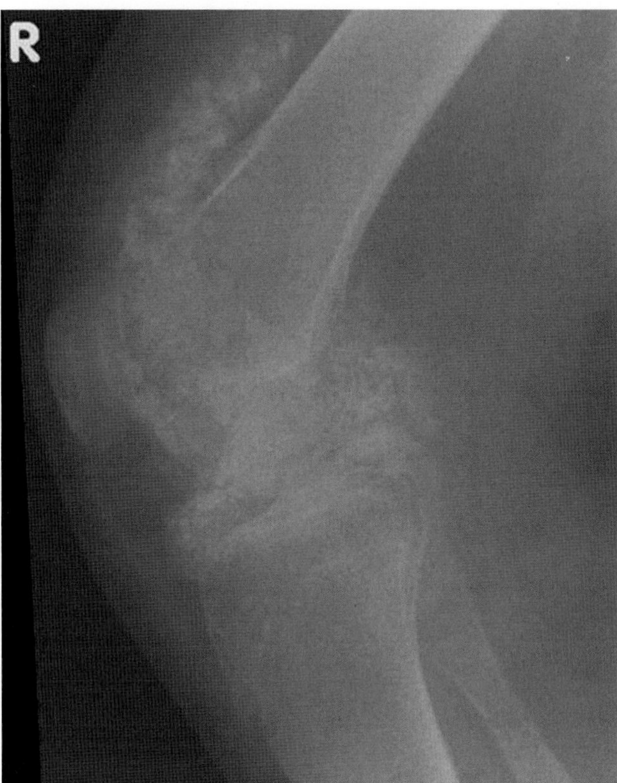

FIGURE 79-42 ■ **Synovial osteochondromatosis.** Multiple calcified intra-articular loose bodies.

METABOLIC AND ENDOCRINE DISORDERS

Metabolic Disorders

Rickets

Rickets is osteomalacia in children. There is an excess of unmineralised osteoid. The serum alkaline phosphatase is elevated, while serum and urinary calcium and phosphate levels are low. Serum levels of calcium and phosphate are controlled in part by vitamin D.

The active form of vitamin D (cholecalciferol) is 1,25-dihydroxy-D_3. Hydroxylation of D_3 occurs first in the liver at the 25-position, and then in the kidney (regulated by parathyroid hormone) at the 1-position. It acts (with parathyroid hormone) on bone to stimulate the release of calcium and phosphate from osteoclasts; it stimulates intestinal absorption of calcium and phosphate; it inhibits secretion of parathyroid hormone; and, finally, it stimulates renal tubular re-absorption of phosphate.

The radiographic features of rickets are best seen at sites of rapid growth (metaphyses and epiphyses of the distal radius, ulna and femur and proximal humerus and tibia (Fig. 79-43)). Features include widening and cupping of the metaphyses, which have irregular, frayed margins. There is apparent widening of the physis (due to the unossified zone of provisional calcification). The epiphyses have indistinct margins and are relatively osteopenic. Looser zones may be seen, particularly at the pubic rami, medial margins of the proximal femora, posterior aspects of the proximal ulnae, axillary margins of the scapulae and the ribs. The 'rachitic rosary' occurs as a result of expansion of the costochondral junctions.

Complications include bowing of the long bones (bone softening, especially of the lower limbs), irregular vertebral end plates and fractures. It should be noted that, in a recent study, fractures in children with rickets were only present in those with radiographic evidence of rickets.[51]

Renal Osteodystrophy

Chronic renal failure causes rickets as a result of failure of hydroxylation of inactive 1-hydroxy-D_3 to the active 1,25-dihydroxy-D_3 within the renal glomeruli. In chronic renal failure there is retention of phosphate and hypocalcaemia, which leads to parathyroid hyperplasia and

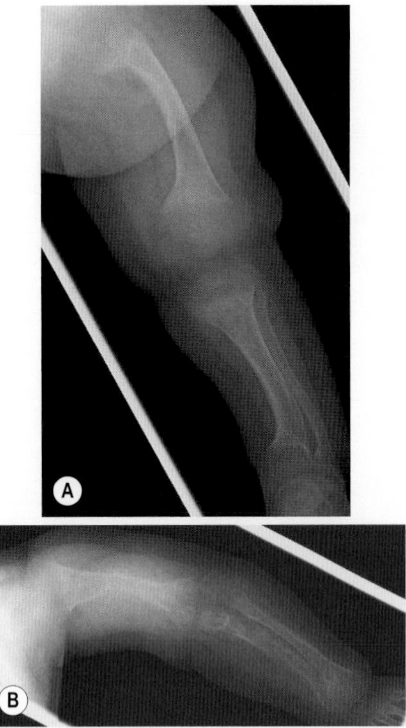

FIGURE 79-43 ■ Severe nutritional rickets. Marked reduction in bone density with bowing deformity. Cupped frayed metaphyses with wide growth plates. Pathological fractures of the humerus and ulna.

secondary hyperparathyroidism. In addition there is reduced gastrointestinal absorption of calcium and end-organ resistance to parathyroid hormone. Serum phosphate and alkaline phosphatase are elevated, while serum calcium is normal or low.

Radiologically, in addition to features of rickets, those of secondary hyperparathyroidism (osteosclerosis, acro-osteolysis and subperiosteal bone resorption) are also present.

Vitamin D-Dependent Rickets

In these autosomal recessive conditions, vitamin D levels are not reduced. Type I is due to a defect in 1-α-hydroxylase, while in Type II vitamin D-dependent rickets there is end-organ resistance to 1,25-dihydroxy-D_3. Patients may have alopecia and abnormal dentition.

Vitamin D-Resistant Rickets

In these disorders renal tubular re-absorption of phosphate is defective. Renal excretion of calcium and phosphate is increased. Serum vitamin D levels are normal or even elevated. X-linked hypophosphatasia, vitamin D-resistant rickets with glycosuria (defective glucose and phosphate resorption), Fanconi's syndrome and acquired hypophosphataemic syndrome are the four conditions in which vitamin D-resistant or -refractory rickets may be seen.

Tumour Rickets

Certain tumours are thought to secrete a phosphaturic substance with consequent elevation in urine phosphate and alkaline phosphatase. Serum calcium is normal. Implicated tumours include haemangiopericytoma, linear sebaceous naevus syndrome, non-ossifying fibroma, giant cell tumour, osteoblastoma, fibrous dysplasia and mixed sclerosing dysplasia. Resection of the tumour leads to resolution of the rickets.

Neonatal Rickets

Radiographic features of neonatal rickets are not usually seen before 6 months of age. Rickets may develop in the neonate because dietary levels of calcium, phosphate and vitamin D cannot meet the needs of a rapidly growing skeleton. Rickets occurring in preterm infants on parenteral nutrition is now relatively uncommon as a result of supplements in feeds.

Scurvy

In this condition there is deficiency (usually dietary) of vitamin C (ascorbic acid). Infants typically present between 6 and 9 months of age. There is defective osteoid production by osteoblasts with reduced endochondral bone ossification.

The bones are osteopenic with relatively dense margins (white lines of scurvy) where mineralisation of osteoid continues. In the epiphyses this pencil outline is termed the 'Wimberger' sign. Other features include metaphyseal (pelcan) spurs, which may fracture, exuberant periosteal reaction (recurrent subperiosteal bleeding), lucent metaphyseal bands and increased density of the end of the metaphyses (white line of Fraenk).

MRI may show broad bands of abnormal metaphyseal signal (low on T1- and high on T2-weighted sequences),[52] or more diffuse marrow signal abnormality. Marrow change may be isolated or coexistent with subperiosteal collections and muscle signal abnormality.

Gaucher's Disease

This autosomal recessive storage disorder occurs most frequently in Ashkenazi Jews. The deficient enzyme is glucocerebrosidase. Glucocerebroside accumulates in the reticuloendothelial system and the bone marrow is infiltrated by lipid-laden Gaucher cells. Infantile and juvenile forms are associated with mental retardation and early death. A milder adolescent form presents in childhood or early adulthood.

Radiological features include osteopenia, bone infarcts, AVN (particularly of the femoral head), flattening of the vertebral bodies, which may be significant (vertebra plana), Erlenmeyer flask deformity of the femora and localised lytic bone lesions (focal deposition of Gaucher cells).

Radiology helps to estimate disease burden, detect skeletal complications and monitor response to treatment. In children, physiological conversion of red to yellow marrow may cause confusion when interpreting MRIs. Radiologists should be aware of the patterns of conversion of low-signal red marrow to high-signal fatty marrow.[53,54]

Endocrine Disorders

Hyperparathyroidism

In hyperthyroidism serum phosphate is decreased, serum calcium and alkaline phosphatase increased, and urine calcium and phosphate increased.

Primary hyperthyroidism is due to a parathyroid adenoma or may occur in multiple endocrine neoplasia and is rare in children. Secondary hyperthyroidism is seen in chronic renal failure and tertiary hyperthyroidism occurs when the parathyroid glands become resistant to the regulatory effects of serum calcium (usually in patients on haemodialysis).

Radiographs reveal features either of bone resorption and/or bone formation. Sites of bone resorption include:

- subperiosteal (radial sides of phalanges)
- subchondral (sacroiliac joints, acromioclavicular joints, with resorption of the acromial ends of the clavicle and symphysis pubis)
- subligamentous (calcaneum at the site of insertion of the Achilles tendon)
- trabecular (diploic space causing a 'salt and pepper' skull)
- intracortical (intracortical tunnelling/striations)
- endosteal.

Additional findings include osteosclerosis (localised or diffuse), rugger-jersey spine, brown tumours, chondrocalcinosis and soft-tissue and vascular calcification.

Neonatal hyperparathyroidism (Fig. 79-44) may occur as a primary disorder or as a result of poorly controlled maternal hypoparathyroidism, pseudohypoparathyroidism, hypocalcaemia, vitamin D deficiency, chronic renal failure and renal tubular acidosis. Radiological features in these infants with failure to thrive include severe osteopenia with an increased tendency to fracture, coarse trabeculae, metaphyseal cupping, metaphyseal spurs and subperiosteal resorption. It may be associated with severe respiratory distress and death. Intrauterine fractures may rarely occur.

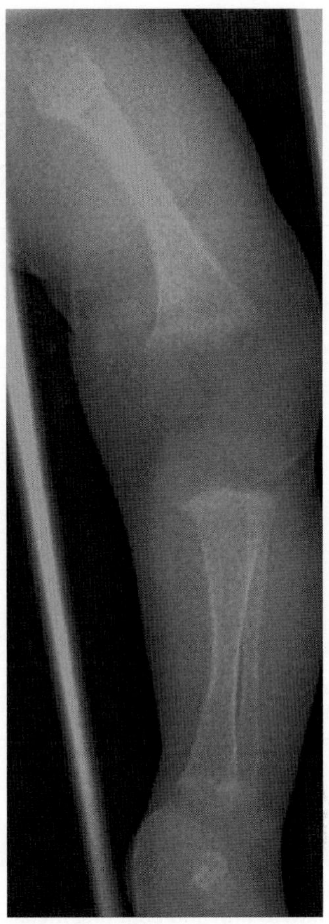

FIGURE 79-44 ■ **Neonatal hyperparathyroidism.** Reduced bone density and metaphyseal spurs.

Hypoparathyroidism

A reduced level of parathyroid hormone causes hypocalcaemia, hypophosphataemia and neuromuscular malfunction. It may be idiopathic or occur after surgical removal, disease, or trauma.

Radiographs demonstrate osteosclerosis, skull vault thickening, soft-tissue calcification, calcification of the basal ganglia, hypoplastic dentition and thickened lamina dura. Less commonly, osteoporosis, dense metaphyseal bands, dense vertebral end plates, premature fusion of the growth plates, vertebral hyperostosis and enthesopathy may occur.

Pseudohypoparathyroidism and Pseudo-Pseudohypoparathyroidismm

Features in common with hypoparathyroidism include osteosclerosis, dense metaphyseal bands and calcification of the soft tissues and basal ganglia. Secondary hyperparathyroidism may be seen in 10% of patients with pseudo-hypoparathyroidism (PHP), but is never seen in pseudo-pseudohypoparathyroidism (PPHP).

Both PHP and PPHP are caused by epigenetic (imprinting) mutations in GNAS.[55]

1. PHP type 1a: Albright's hereditary osteodystrophy (AHO). This is caused by specific loss of function mutations inherited from the mother. There is end-organ resistance to normal or increased serum levels of parathyroid and other hormones. Clinically there is obesity, short stature and a rounded facies. Hypocalcaemia results in muscular tetany. Radiological features include exostoses and brachydactyly (short fourth (and fifth) fingers and toes (Fig. 79-45)) with a positive metacarpal sign (a line joining the heads of the little and middle fingers fails to intersect the head of the fourth metacarpal).
2. Inheritance of the same GNAS mutations from the father gives rise to PPHP. These patients have the skeletal phenotype of PHP; however, serum calcium and phosphate levels are normal. Cone-shaped epiphyses of the tubular bones of the hands and feet fuse prematurely, causing brachydactyly.
3. PHP type 1b is due to a different GNAS mutation, and has no skeletal manifestations. Patients have end-organ resistance to parathyroid hormone.

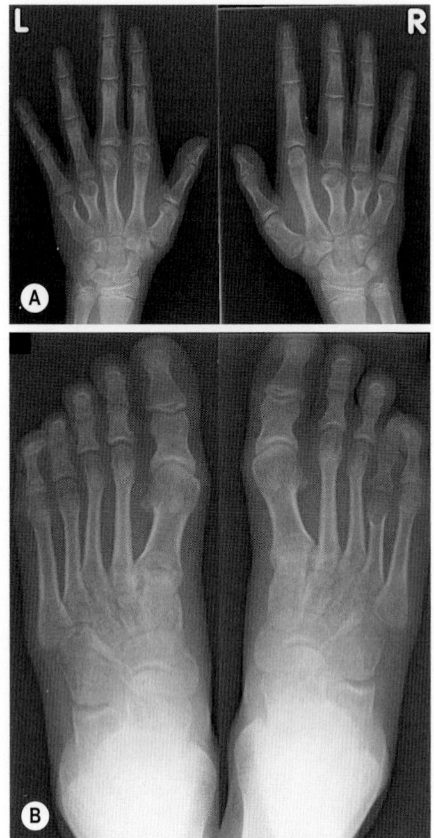

FIGURE 79-45 ■ Pseudohypoparathyroidism. (A) Short left fourth and fifth, right third to fifth and both first metacarpals. (B) Short right fourth metatarsal.

Hypothyroidism

In all types of hypothyroidism (infantile, juvenile and adult) there is either deficiency, or failure, of end-organ response to thyroxine. A mutation in the thyroid hormone receptor alpha gene causing end-organ resistance to thyroxine and presenting with recognised radiographic features of hypothyroidism has recently been identified.[56]

Radiological features in the paediatric age group include delayed bone age, delay in appearance of secondary ossification centres, epiphyseal fragmentation, stippling and short stature. Additional findings include osteoporosis, multiple Wormian bones, delay in closure of the sutures and fontanelles, delayed dentition, dense metaphyseal bands, shortened long bones, increased atlantoaxial distance, kyphosis at the thoracolumbar junction and an increased incidence of slipped capital femoral epiphysis.

TOXIC DISORDERS

Fluorosis

Radiologically, fluorosis manifests as a generalised increase in bone density, particularly of the axial skeleton. There is periosteal proliferation, ligamentous calcification, degenerative enthesopathy and fractures. In children, exposure before the age of 8 years causes patchy opaque areas of the enamel of permanent teeth.

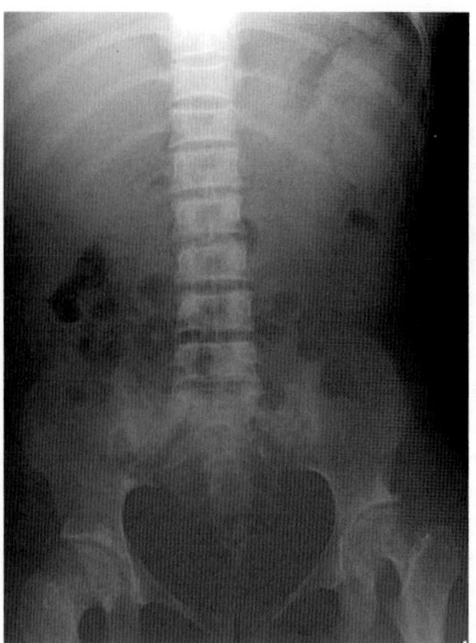

FIGURE 79-46 ■ Sickle cell anaemia. Cod fish vertebrae and bilateral avascular necrosis of the femoral heads.

Lead Poisoning

This manifests radiologically as dense metaphyseal bands. Other features include widened sutures (raised intracranial pressure) and radio-opacities on abdominal radiographs (ingested lead).

HAEMOGLOBINOPATHIES

Sickle Cell Disease

Bone pain is the most common reason for hospital admission of patients with sickle cell disease. Thromboembolic infarcts and haemolysis (with chronic anaemia and secondary marrow expansion) is the underlying pathophysiology of the skeletal complications that occur.

Acute bony involvement includes bone infarcts, osteomyelitis, stress fractures, vertebral collapse, bone marrow necrosis, orbital compression (infarction of the orbital bone) and dental complications (caries, mandibular osteomyelitis). Chronic complications include osteoporosis (secondary to marrow hyperplasia), AVN, chronic arthritis and growth failure.[57]

Bone infarcts of the small bones of the hands and feet will lead to dactylitis; of the vertebral end plates to the so-called 'cod fish' or 'H-shaped' vertebrae (Fig. 79-46); of the epiphyses will lead to joint effusions and AVN. Osteomyelitis is common, with *Salmonella* species being isolated in up to 70%. The infection most commonly involves the diaphysis of the humerus, femur and tibia (Fig. 79-47A).

The diagnostic challenge is to differentiate acute osteomyelitis from vaso-occlusive disease. Imaging findings may be very similar. The presence of a collection or

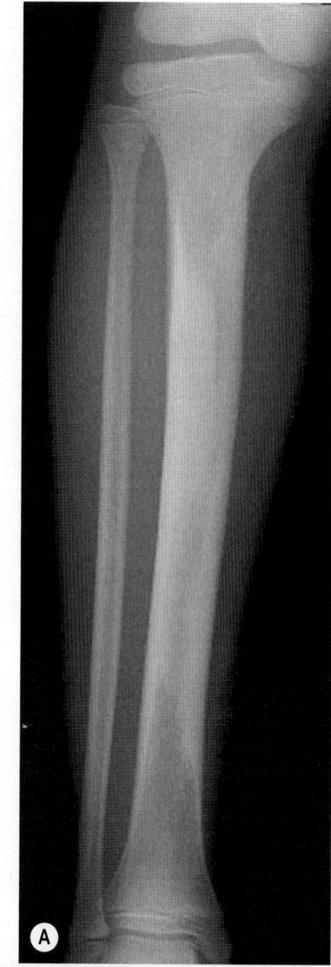

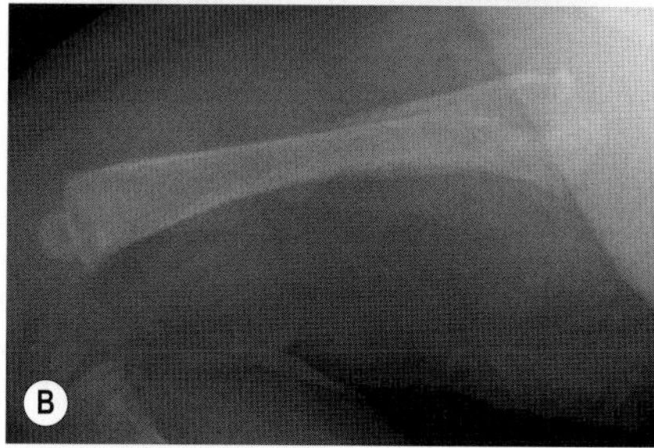

FIGURE 79-47 ■ **Osteomyelitis.** (A) Low-grade infection in a child with sickle cell anaemia showing sclerosis of the tibia. (B) Radiolucency of the proximal femoral metaphysis and periosteal reaction along the proximal femoral shaft in an infant with acute osteomyelitis.

of a break in the cortex makes infection more likely than simple infarction.

Thalassaemia

Skeletal changes in thalassaemia arise from the chronic anaemia associated with the condition.

In the skull, there is widening of the diploic spaces (low signal on all MRI sequences), with thinning of the outer table of the skull vault. The trabecular markings are oriented perpendicular to the inner and outer tables and on plain radiographs give rise to the 'hair-on-end' appearance. There is frontal bossing and overgrowth of the facial bones with reduced pneumatisation of the paranasal sinuses. The so-called 'rodent facies' arises from marrow hyperplasia in the maxillae, causing lateral displacement of the orbits and ventral displacement of the central incisors.

In the spine there may be marked osteoporosis and cortical thinning, resulting in fractures of the vertebral bodies and platyspondyly. Imaging may reveal paraspinal masses (as a result of extramedullary haematopoiesis). Cord compression can result if these masses extend into the extradural space. MRI findings are secondary to blood transfusion and chelation therapy.

There may be expansion of the head and neck of the ribs and osteoporosis. A rib within a rib appearance may result. Extramedullary haematopoiesis can cause erosions of the inner cortex of the ribs or manifest as a posterior mediastinal soft-tissue mass.

Premature fusion of the growth plates (particularly of the proximal humerus and distal femur) is a recognised feature. Irregular sclerosis at the metaphyses and anterior rib ends is a recognised complication of treatment with desferrioxamine.[58]

INFECTION OF THE BONES AND JOINTS

Osteomyelitis

Infection may reach the bone through the bloodstream (haematogenous), from direct implantation (e.g. penetrating injury, surgery), or from infection elsewhere adjacent to bone (e.g. soft tissues). Because of the rich blood supply, osteomyelitis of the long bones in children most commonly affects the metaphyses. In infants, metaphyseal vessels penetrate the growth plate, and therefore in this age group there is a higher incidence of epiphyseal and joint involvement.

Infection of the bones may be acute, subacute (Brodie's abscess) or chronic.

Acute osteomyelitis is most commonly seen in infants (*Staphylococcus aureus*, *Escherichia coli*) and young children (*S. aureus*, *Streptococcus pyogenes*, *Haemophilus influenzae*). Patients with sickle cell disease are more disposed to *Salmonella* infection. Subacute and chronic osteomyelitis result from incomplete eradication of infection following acute osteomyelitis, or from infection by less virulent organisms. Mycobacterial osteomyelitis occurs from haematogenous spread in a patient with primary tuberculosis. Fungal causes include coccidioidomycosis, blastomycosis and cryptococcosis.

In acute disease there is oedema, vascular congestion and thrombosis of small vessels. Clinical features include fever, irritability, lethargy and local signs including swelling, erythema and warmth (inflammation). If not treated promptly (or aggressively), the vascular compromise leads to areas of dead bone (sequestra), which are the hallmark of chronic infection.[59,60] Periosteal new bone formation is another feature of chronic osteomyelitis. This new bone (involucrum) encases areas of live bone. Pus may track from the medullary cavity through gaps in the involucrum into the soft tissues. These tracks may eventually penetrate the skin surface (sinus tracts).

Radiographic changes (Fig. 79-47B) may not be apparent for up to 2 weeks after the onset of disease, and therefore radiographs may appear entirely normal. More specific signs include soft-tissue swelling, cortical irregularity (bony destruction) and periosteal reaction. A Brodie's abscess may be seen as a well-defined lytic lesion with a sclerotic rim. In chronic infection, sequestra appear as dense foci, and soft-tissue wasting and sinus tracts may be appreciated. Even on appropriate therapy, radiographic signs of improvement may lag behind clinical recovery. Spina ventosa implies tuberculous dactylitis. Radiographically there are cyst-like cavities associated with diaphyseal expansion. It more commonly affects the bones of the hands than the feet.[61]

High-resolution US provides a simple and non-invasive assessment of infants and children with osteomyelitis. US helps to localise the site and extent of disease, and to confirm the presence and degree of the fluid component of the abscess, and provides guidance for interventional procedures. Chau and Griffith provide a useful review of the US appearances of musculoskeletal infection.[62]

Skeletal scintigraphy is useful if multifocal infection is suspected.

CT helps to define the extent of cortical destruction and to exclude the presence of sequestra.

MRI has the highest sensitivity and specificity for detecting osteomyelitis in children. In subacute infection a characteristic penumbra sign may be recognised.[63] This consists of a peripheral relatively high-signal ring (granulation tissue) surrounding a low-signal central zone (abscess cavity). Enhanced fat-suppressed sequences show avid enhancement of the granulation tissue. Contrast medium also helps to identify soft-tissue abscesses. On T2-weighted sequences the high signal of reactive oedema may exaggerate the extent of infection.

Complications include joint destruction, damage to growth plates and resorption of bone (Fig. 79-48), resulting in limb-length discrepancies, angular deformity and premature osteoarthritis.

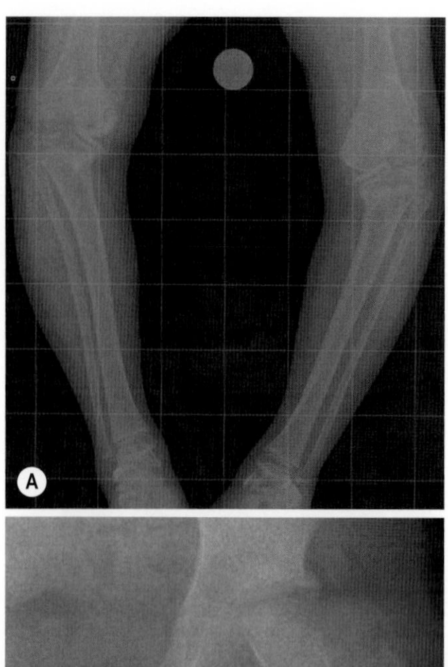

FIGURE 79-48 ■ **Complications of infection.** (A) Premature fusion of the distal femoral and proximal tibial growth plates with genu varum following meningococcal septicaemia (bilateral knee and ankle arthrograms were performed prior to obtaining this image). (B) Almost complete resorption of the femoral head following infective arthritis.

Chronic Recurrent Multifocal Osteomyelitis

This is a condition of unknown aetiology characterised by a fluctuating clinical course of relapses and remissions. It affects multiple sites (synchronous or metachronous) and most commonly involves the long bones, clavicle, spine and pelvis. The ribs and sternum may also be affected. No causative agent is found. When associated with acne and palmoplanter pustulosis it is termed SAPHO syndrome.

Radiographic features (Fig. 79-49) suggest subacute or chronic osteomyelitis; however, abscess formation, involucra and sinus tracts are not a feature. In the tubular bones lytic metaphyseal lesions sometimes extending to the diaphysis are typical. Quiescent periods are characterised by bony expansion and sclerosis. In the clavicle, lytic medullary lesions are a feature of active disease, with expansion and sclerosis again being features of a quiescent phase. Chronic recurrent multifocal osteomyelitis (CRMO) manifests in the spine as loss of height of the affected vertebral bodies and is a differential diagnosis of vertebra plana.

Bone scintigraphy is useful for the detection of asymptomatic lesions. MRI, by failing to demonstrate abscesses and sinus tracts, excludes chronic osteomyelitis. Active disease is confirmed by the presence of high signal marrow on T2/STIR sequences.

Infective Arthritis

As with osteomyelitis, infection may spread to joints via the bloodstream, direct inoculation, or spread from a contiguous site. The most common organism is *S. aureus*. Imaging features (Fig. 79-50) include soft-tissue swelling, oedema and joint effusion. In infants, effusions may lead to dislocation (particularly in the hip joint). Other findings include metaphyseal irregularity, destruction and avascular necrosis. Septic arthritis in children is a clinical emergency, and early drainage is required to prevent severe bony destruction with resultant shortening and deformity. In this regard US is helpful, both to exclude

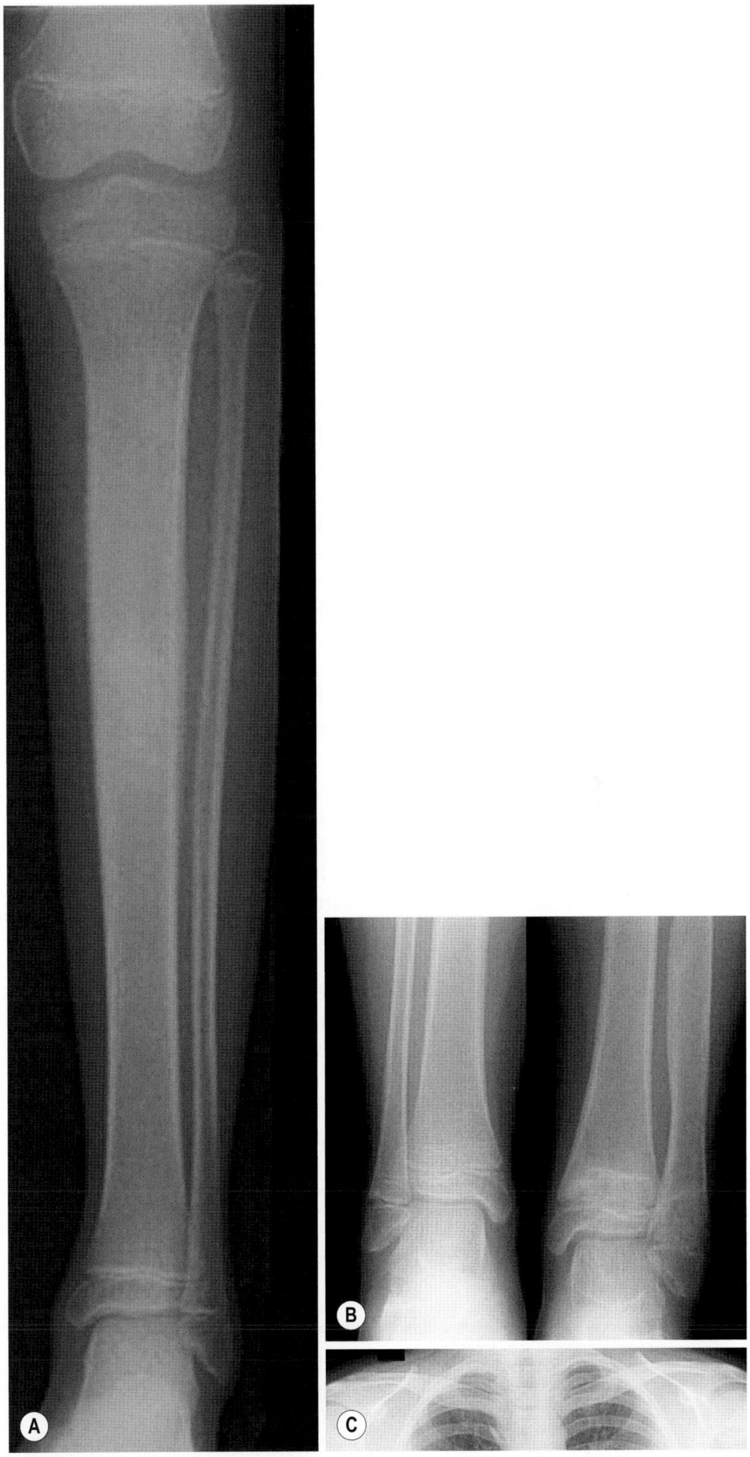

FIGURE 79-49 ■ Chronic recurrent multifocal osteomyelitis. (A) Periosteal reaction with sclerosis of the mid-tibial shaft. (B) Lucent lesions with a permeative appearance adjacent to the growth plates of the left distal tibia and fibula. Broad left distal fibula with cortical thickening. (C) Broad medial ends of the clavicles (right more than left).

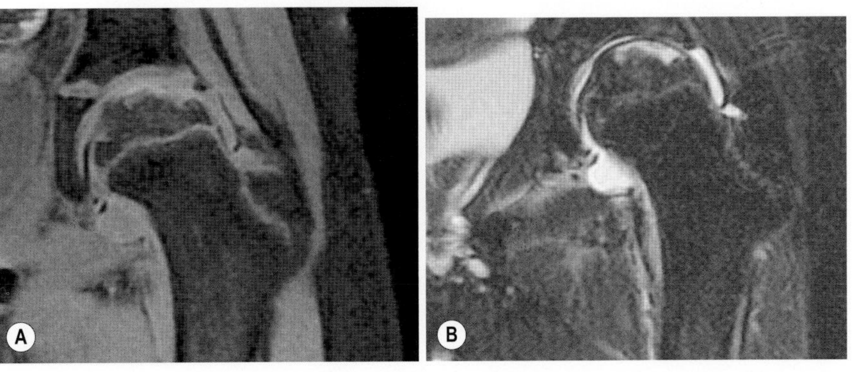

FIGURE 79-50 ■ Infective arthritis in a child with thalassaemia. Coronal fat-saturated T1 (A) and T2 (B) images show a joint effusion and avascular necrosis of the femoral head.

the presence of an effusion (a difference of 1–2 mm between the two sides is suggestive) and to assist in its drainage.

Infection of the Spine (Discitis and Osteomyelitis)

Discitis refers to infection of the intervertebral disc space, whereas osteomyelitis of the spine implies pyogenic destruction of the vertebral body, which may then spread to involve the disc. Differentiation of the two is important, as management may differ. Discitis can involve any spinal level, but most commonly affects the lumbar region in children younger than 5 years of age.[64] Generally children with discitis are younger, and clinically less toxic than those with osteomyelitis.[64] Children with either condition will present with back pain, refusal to mobilise, or irritability depending on age at presentation. Although there is much debate as to the aetiology of discitis, a low-grade infection has been postulated. In 70% of cases, the causative organism is not identified. When an organism is cultured, it is most commonly *S. aureus*. In discitis, radiological changes are confined to the disc and adjacent vertebral end plates, in comparison to osteomyelitis, in which the disease begins in and destroys the vertebral body. Infection may then spread to an adjacent vertebral body either via the intervertebral disc or via the subligamentous spread of pus (e.g. in spinal tuberculosis).

In discitis, radiographs/CT of the spine show characteristic features, including loss of disc height and irregularity of the adjacent vertebral end plates. Vertebral body height is preserved. It has been suggested that in the clinical context of suspected discitis, further imaging is not required if the radiographs demonstrate characteristic findings. However, if radiographs are normal or equivocal, or the child is toxic (suggesting spinal osteomyelitis), then further imaging is indicated.[65]

MRI can exclude intraspinal or other soft-tissue (e.g. psoas) collections. T1 sagittal and axial and T2 sagittal views are often sufficient. In equivocal cases, intravenous administration of contrast medium may be helpful. The pattern of enhancement may aid in differentiating tuberculous spondylitis (avid, heterogeneous rim enhancement, involving several vertebral bodies) from vertebral osteomyelitis. However, regardless of the pattern of enhancement, tissue should be obtained for microbiological examination, usually by CT-guided biopsy.

For a full list of references, please see ExpertConsult.

FURTHER READING

1. Warman ML, Cormier-Daire V, Hall C, et al. Nosology and classification of genetic skeletal disorders: 2010 revision. Am J Med Genet A 2011;155A:943–68.
2. Offiah AC, Hall CM. Radiological diagnosis of the constitutional disorders of bone. As easy as A, B, C? Pediatr Radiol 2003;33:153–61.
22. Loder RT. Unstable slipped capital femoral epiphyses. J Pediatr Orthop 2001;21:694–9.
29. Jacquemin C, Bosley TM, Liu D, et al. Reassessment of sphenoid dysplasia associated with neurofibromatosis type 1. Am J Neuroradiol 2002;23:644–8.
32. Petty RE, Southwood TR, Manners P, et al; (International League of Associations for Rheumatology). International League of Associations for Rheumatology classification of juvenile idiopathic arthritis: second revision, Edmonton, 2001. J Rheumatol 2004;31:390–2.
36. Collado P, Jousse-Joulin S, Alcalde M, et al. Is ultrasound a validated imaging tool for the diagnosis and management of synovitis in juvenile idiopathic arthritis? A systematic literature review. Arthritis Care Res 2012;64(7):1011–19.
39. Martin N, Krol P, Smith S, et al; Juvenile Dermatomyositis Research Group. A national registry for juvenile dermatomyositis and other paediatric idiopathic inflammatory myopathies: 10 years' experience; the Juvenile Dermatomyositis National (UK and Ireland) Cohort Biomarker Study and Repository for Idiopathic Inflammatory Myopathies. Rheumatology 2011;50:137–45.
48. Doria AS, Lundin B, Kilcoyne RF, et al. Reliability of progressive and additive MRI scoring systems for evaluation of haemophilic arthropathy in children: expert MRI Working Group of the International Prophylaxis Study Group. Haemophilia 2005;11:245–53.
51. Chapman T, Sugar N, Done S, et al. Fractures in infants and toddlers with rickets. Pediatr Radiol 2010;40:1184–9.
60. Offiah AC. Acute osteomyelitis, septic arthritis and discitis: differences between neonates and older children. Eur J Radiol 2006;60:221–32.
62. Chau CLF, Griffith JF. Musculoskeletal infections: ultrasound appearances. Clin Radiol 2005;60:149–59.
64. Early SD, Kay RM, Tolo VT. Childhood diskitis. J Am Acad Orthop Surg 2003;11:413–20.

CHAPTER 80

Paediatric Musculoskeletal Trauma and the Radiology of Non-accidental Injury and Paediatric Factures

Karen Rosendahl • Jean-François Chateil • Karl Johnson

CHAPTER OUTLINE

Fractures account for up to 25% of all injuries in children, being commoner in boys.[1] The type and distribution of injuries varies between different age groups in children and adults because of the physiology of the developing skeleton. A child's bones are more elastic than those of an adult. When a force is applied to a bone, it will generate stresses within that bone, which may be compressive, tensile or shearing. These stresses will result in deformity of the bone, which will progress as the stress increases. When the force is removed, the bone may eventually return to normal. However, at some point, namely the yield stress, the bone enters a phase of plastic deformity, resulting in microscopic fractures on the tensile side of the bone.[2] This bone may initially be radiographically normal, but follow-up radiographs may show evidence of a healing periosteal reaction in response to these microfractures. With further increases in the deforming force, the bone's ultimate stress point will be reached and the bone then fractures.

In adults, the yield point and ultimate stress points are very close together, so plastic deformity is rare. In the younger child, the greater degree of elasticity of the bone means that there can be a significant difference between the yield point and ultimate point, with a greater propensity for plastic deformity. Cortical bone will tolerate compressive stresses better than tensile or shearing forces. Consequently, childhood fractures may be complete or partial (incomplete). A complete fracture occurs when there is complete discontinuity between two or more bone fragments. An incomplete fracture involves trauma and damage to the bone, but a portion of the cortex remains intact due to the increased elasticity of the bone.

Greenstick, buckle and plastic bowing fall into the category of incomplete fractures (Fig. 80-1). Stress injuries can occur due to repeated forces acting upon the bone, which are less than the force needed to fracture the bone (Fig. 80-2). Fractures may also be classified with regards to the fracture line; a simple fracture is where there is only a single fracture line. These fractures can be further described as transverse, oblique or spiral, depending on the appearances of the fracture line with respect to the bone's long axis. A comminuted fracture is where there are several fracture lines and these include segmental fractures and those with butterfly fragments (Fig. 80-3). Open or compound fractures occur when a wound extends from the skin surface to the fracture. Displacement refers to when there is a space and altered alignment between the fracture fragments.

For the majority of injuries, a good-quality anteroposterior and lateral radiograph is the only imaging which will be required. From these projections, the fracture pattern, along with any shortening or angulation, can be determined. Rotation is best assessed from the relative position of the joints above and below the fracture, which should be included on the radiograph as standard practice. Careful inspection of a fracture may allow the mechanism of injury to be determined, which may have implications as to the stability and hence help determine management.

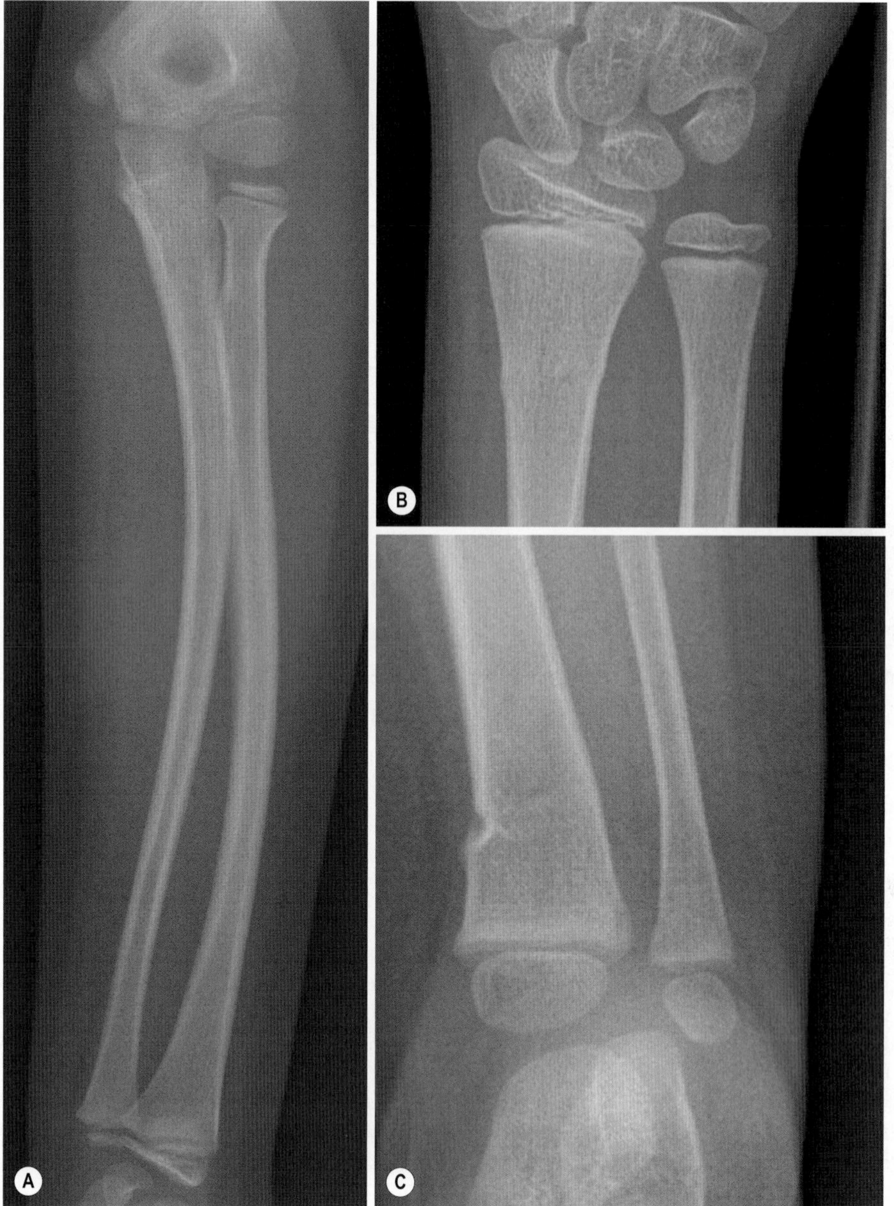

FIGURE 80-1 ■ (A) Fracture of the left radius and ulna. (B) Torus fracture of the distal right radius. (C) Greenstick fracture of the distal left tibia.

PHYSEAL INJURIES

A cartilaginous physis (growth plate) occurs between a bone and its epiphysis or apophysis. An epiphysis contributes to longitudinal growth while an apophysis does not. In early childhood, not all the epiphysis or apophysis will be ossified and so will not be visible on a radiograph. The transitional zone between the physeal cartilage and the metaphyseal portion of the bone, 'the zone of provisional calcification', is the weakest point in the growing skeleton. The physeal cartilage is weaker than bone, which, in turn, is weaker than the surrounding ligaments.

Injuries which may result in a ligamental tear or joint dislocation in an adult are more likely to cause a physeal injury in a child.[3] Up to 15% of fractures of the tubular bones in children affect the growth plate and the majority of physeal fractures are due to shearing or avulsion stresses. The classification of physeal injuries typically uses the system of Salter and Harris, which separates fractures into five main types (Figs. 80-4 and 80-5).[4] Other fracture types and other categories of injury have been proposed since the original classification.[5,6] The importance of the classification system is that for higher grades of injuries, there is an increased likelihood that the growth plate will be damaged, which will result in long-term complications such as malunion, premature fusion (resulting in growth impairment) and avascular necrosis (Fig. 80-6). The latter is most likely to occur in fractures of the femoral or radial neck. Whilst

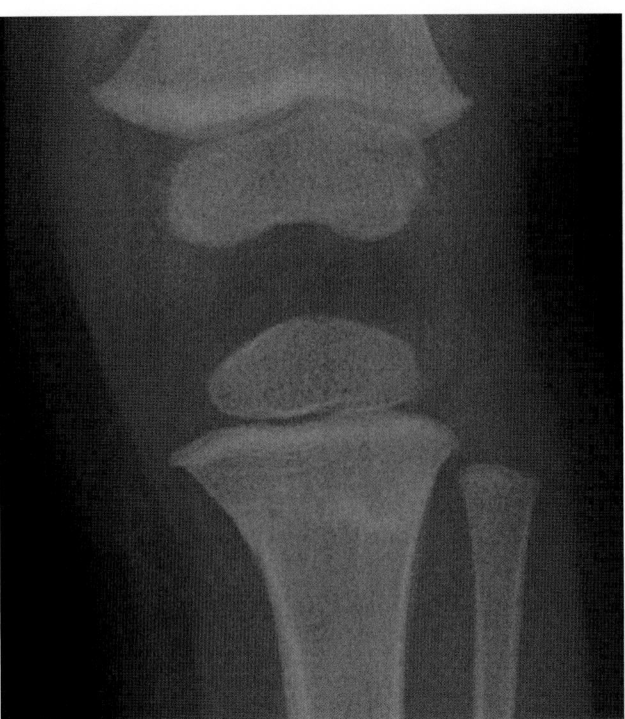

FIGURE 80-2 ■ Healing stress fracture of the proximal tibia.

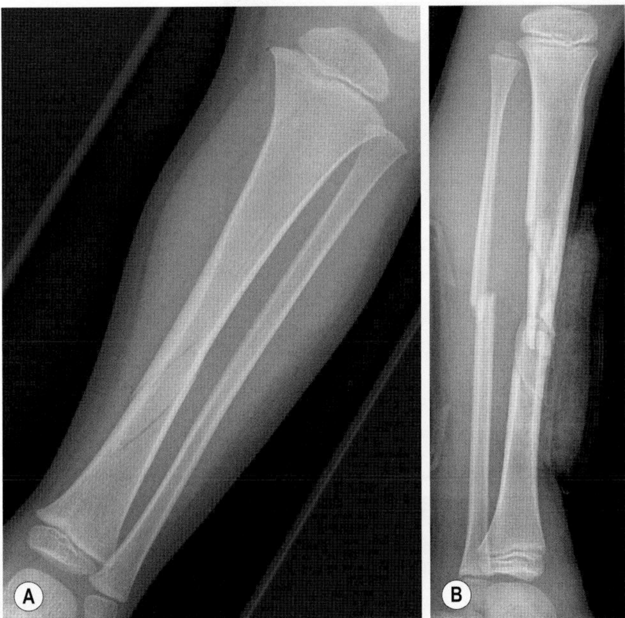

FIGURE 80-3 ■ (A) Spiral fracture of the left tibia. (B) Comminuted fracture of the right tibia with associated fracture of the fibula.

the majority of injuries are clearly shown on standard radiographs, magnetic resonance imaging (MRI) can be used to better visualise the physeal cartilage and the non-ossified portion of the epiphysis (Fig. 80-7).[7]

The other site of potential physeal damage is at the musculotendinous insertion into an apophysis,

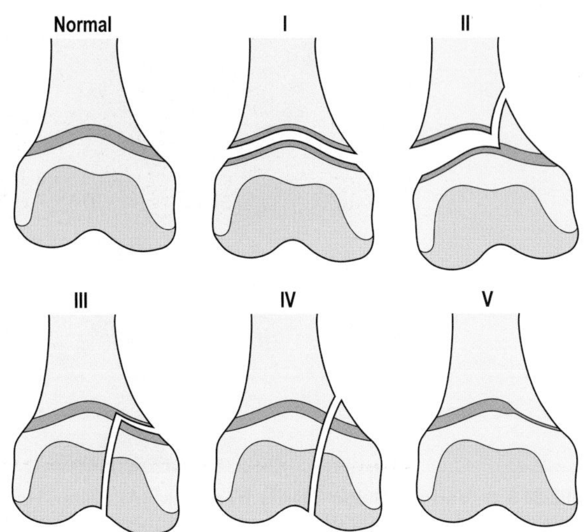

FIGURE 80-4 ■ Illustration of the Salter–Harris classification of fractures. (Type I) The fracture is isolated to the growth plate and causes epiphyseal separation, without adjacent bone fracture. The fracture line passes through the hypertrophic layer of the physis. (Type II) This is the most common growth plate fracture and is usually seen in children between the ages of 10 and 16. As a result of shearing or avulsive force, the fracture splits the growth plate and then passes into the metaphysis, separating a small fragment of bone. (Type III) The fracture line passes through the epiphysis, and then horizontally across the growth plate. This is most commonly seen at the distal tibia in children aged 10–15. (Type IV) This is a vertically orientated fracture, involving both the epiphysis and metaphysis, and crossing the growth plate. This is most commonly seen in the distal humerus and tibia. (Type V) This fracture, results from a compressive force, crushing the growth plate. Damage to the growth plate can cause subsequent deformity. The diagnosis is often made retrospectively when growth arrest is discovered at a later date.

particularly following an avulsion injury. In children, the apophyseal physis is the weakest point of the bone, tendon and muscle interface and, consequently, severe traction on the muscle will result in avulsion of a bone or cartilaginous fragment. Avulsion injuries are common sports injuries and most usually seen around the pelvis and elbow (Figs. 80-8 and 80-9).

Low-energy repetitive traction forces can result in microtrauma, causing a chronic apophysitis. Around the medial epicondyle of the humerus, this is eponymously called 'little leaguer's elbow'. Radiographs are usually sufficient to diagnose acute avulsion injuries, providing the avulsed fragment is ossified. MR imaging or ultrasound can be helpful in demonstrating soft-tissue swelling, effusion and marrow oedema in the more chronic presentations.

THE UPPER LIMB

Shoulder/Humerus

Fractures of the clavicle can occur from either a direct blow or a fall onto the shoulder or outstretched arm. Typically, they occur in the middle third and there is a

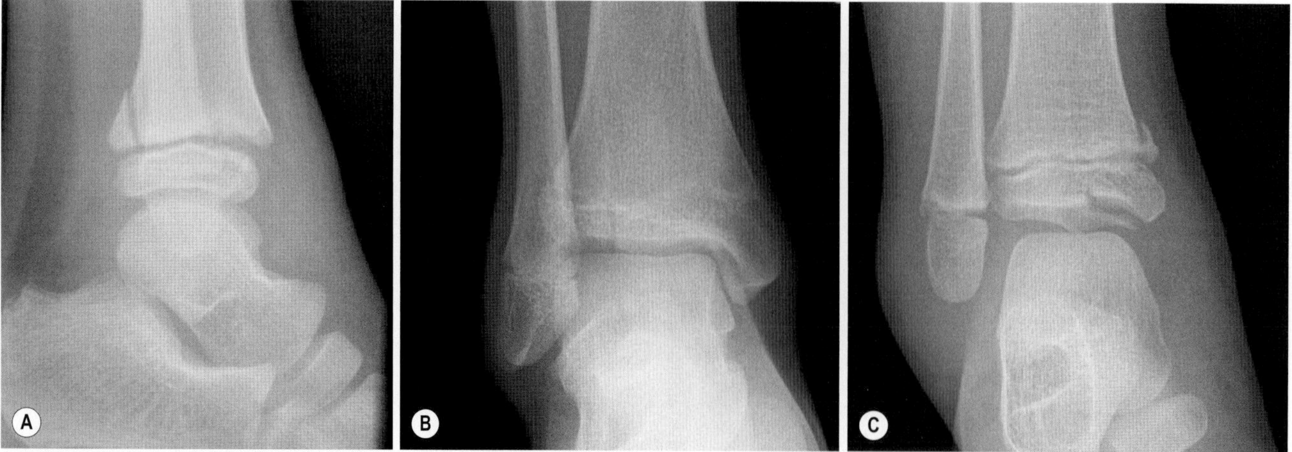

FIGURE 80-5 ■ Various Salter–Harris fractures. (A) Salter–Harris II fracture of the distal left tibia. (B) Salter–Harris III fracture of the distal right tibia. (C) Salter–Harris fracture of the distal left tibia.

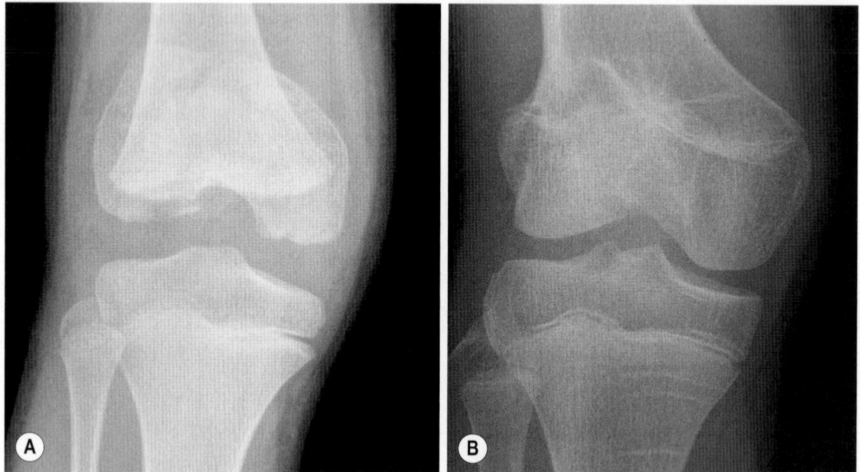

FIGURE 80-6 ■ (A) Fracture through the growth plate of the distal right femur with significant displacement and distortion of the epiphysis. (B) Follow-up radiographs after surgical correction show premature fusion of the lateral aspect of the distal femoral physis, resulting in abnormal remodelling and development.

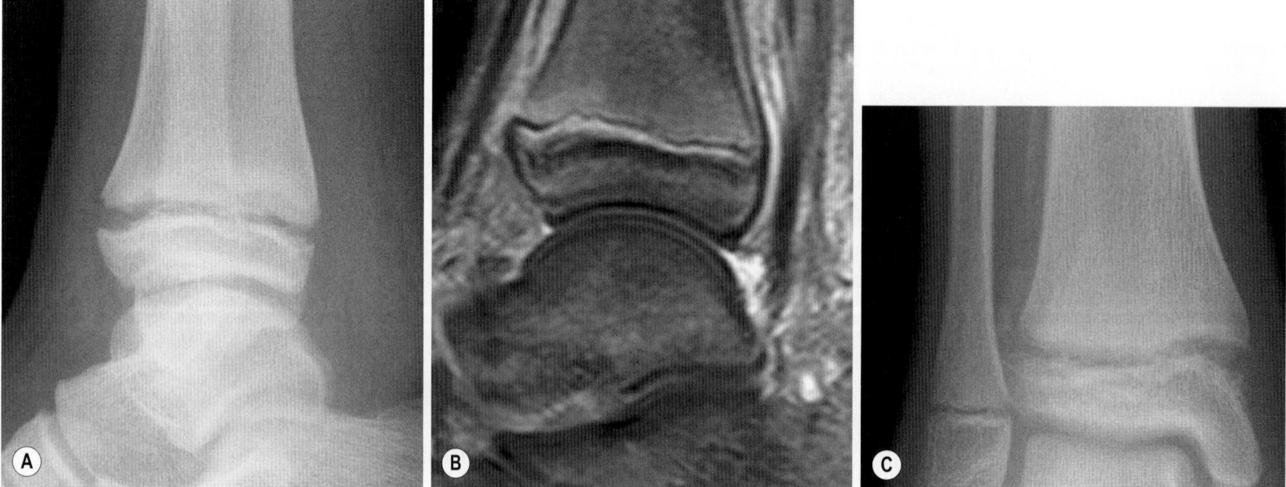

FIGURE 80-7 ■ (A) Salter–Harris I fracture of the distal right tibia. Note widening of the growth plate. (B) MRI of the same patient showing abnormal increased signal on the T2-weighted sequences through the growth plate. (C) Follow-up films in the same patient as (A) show subperiosteal new bone formation around the fracture site confirming the injury.

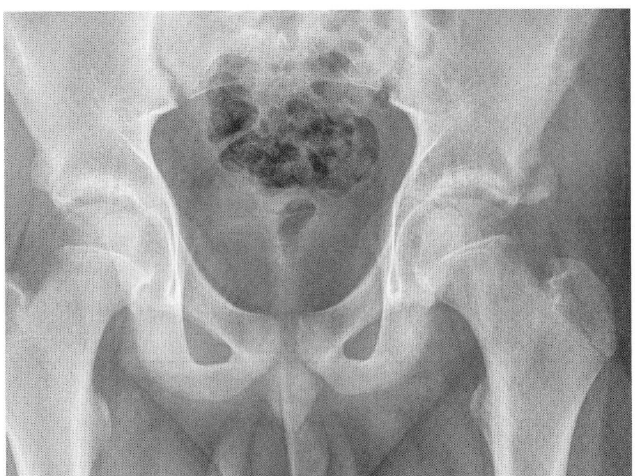

FIGURE 80-8 ■ Avulsion fracture of the left anterior inferior iliac spine.

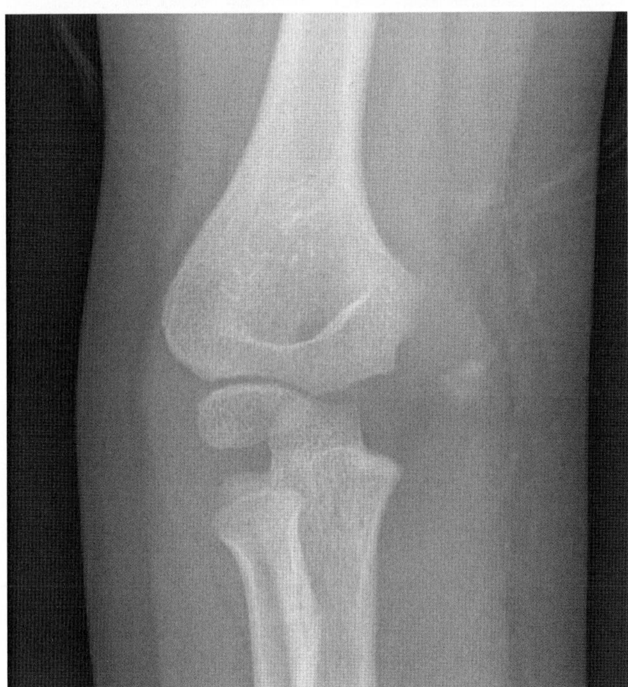

FIGURE 80-9 ■ Avulsion of the medial epicondyle of the distal humerus.

high propensity for greenstick injuries due to the plastic nature of the periosteum.[8] The clavicle is the commonest site of birth-related fracture and is associated with shoulder dystocia and obstetric brachial plexus palsy. This may cause the neonate to present with reduced arm movement, the differential diagnosis of which includes septic arthritis, osteomyelitis, shoulder dislocation and non-accidental injury (NAI).[9]

Shoulder dislocation is uncommon under 10 years of age, the presence of the humeral physis appearing to be in some way protective. Displacement is typically anteriorly and the humeral head lies under the coracoid process on the AP radiograph. On the axial view, the humeral

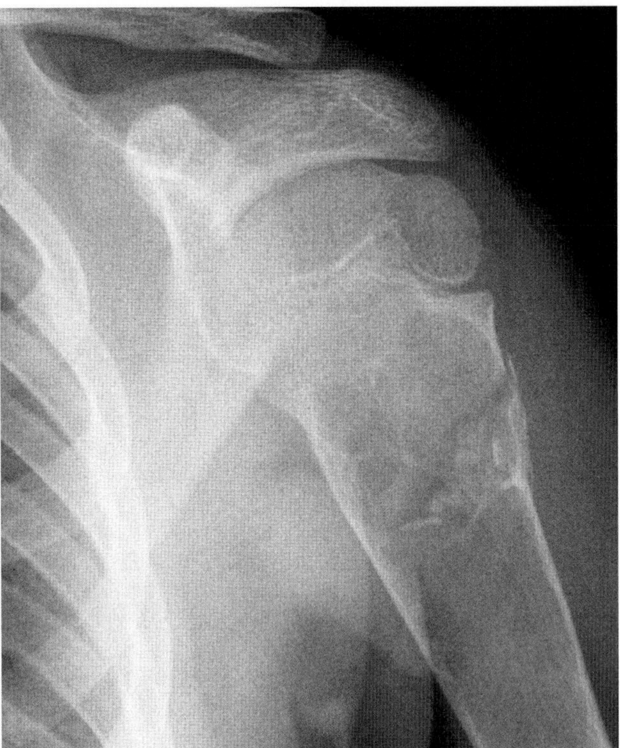

FIGURE 80-10 ■ Pathological fracture of the proximal left humerus through a simple bone cyst. There is a small bony fragment within the cystic cavity.

head is displaced anteriorly and no longer covers the glenoid.

Proximal humeral fractures are uncommon, with those involving the physis representing just 3% of such injuries. However, the consequences of fractures here may be significant as the physis accounts for 80% of longitudinal growth of the humerus. Care must be taken in reviewing the proximal humerus, as the normal growth plate has an irregular contour which should not be mistaken for a fracture.[10]

Under 10 years of age, the fractures are typically metaphyseal, whilst in adolescents, they are usually a Salter–Harris type II fracture. Conversely, the proximal humerus is a relatively common site for pathological fractures, typically through a simple bone cyst, creating the 'fallen fragment sign', due to a piece of cortical bone lying within the fluid-filled cavity (Fig. 80-10).[11]

Elbow

There are six separate ossification centres around the elbow joint which appear and fuse in a relatively predictable temporal sequence. These are shown in Table 80-1. Recognition of this sequence is important in determining the presence and type of any injury. While some variation in the appearances can be seen, the internal apophysis should always appear before that of the trochlea, and any deviation from this, with a history of trauma, is suspicious for an avulsed or malpositioned internal apophysis (Fig. 80-11).[12]

TABLE 80-1 **The Ossification Centres around the Elbow Joint**

	Age Range at Which The Ossification Centre Becomes Visible Radiographically (Years)	Age Range at Which They Fuse (Years)
Capitellum	0–2	13–16
Radial head	3–6	13–17
Internal (medial) epicondyle	3–9	Up to 20
Trochlea	7–13	13–16
Olecranon	8–10	13–16
Lateral (external) epicondyle	8–12	13–16

The age at which they appear and then subsequently fuse. In general it occurs earlier in girls than in boys.

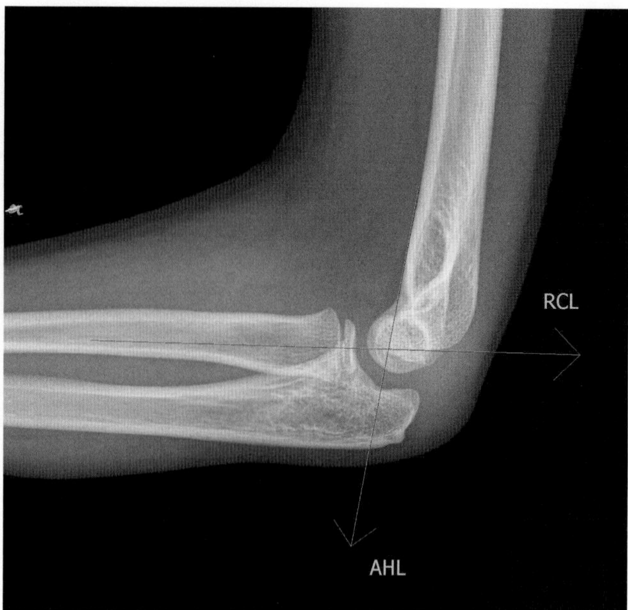

FIGURE 80-12 ■ Normal lateral film of the elbow. The two lines drawn on the radiograph are used to assess the elbow joint. Anterior humeral line (AHL): one-third of the capitellum should lie anterior to this line. In the young child where there is only partial ossification of the capitellum, this measurement is less valid. RCL—on a lateral film, a line drawn along the shaft of the proximal radius should pass through the capitellum.

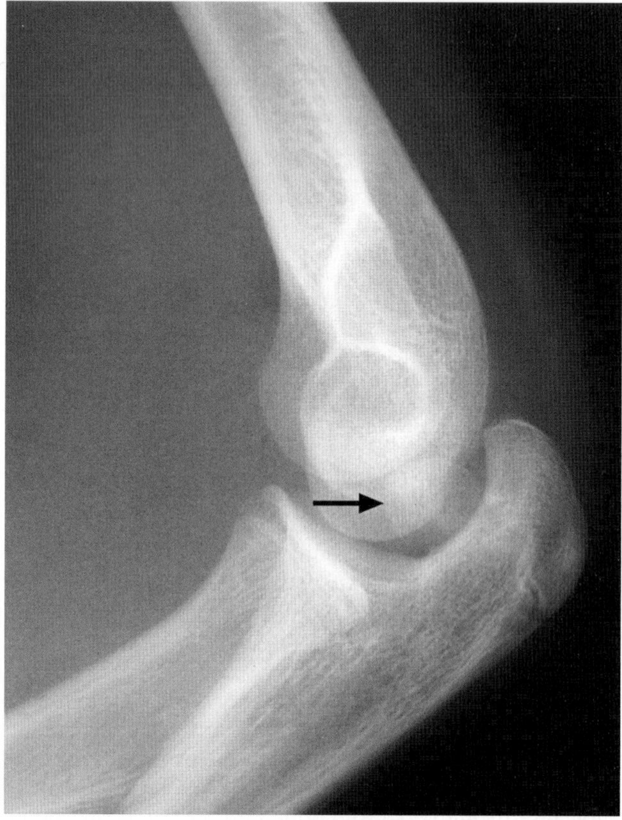

FIGURE 80-11 ■ Medial epicondyle epiphysis (arrow) trapped within the elbow joint following avulsion.

A good-quality AP and lateral radiograph is essential for evaluating the elbow joint following trauma, for the important assessment of crucial anatomical landmarks (Figs. 80-12 and 80-13). Fracture, haematoma or effusion into the elbow joint will cause capsular distension and elevation of the fat pads overlying it. A visible posterior fat pad should be regarded as abnormal due to a potential occult injury, particularly a fracture/dislocation of the radial head or undisplaced supracondylar fracture.

A visible anterior fat pad may be a normal finding. The absence of any visible fat pad does not exclude the presence of a fracture. The medial and lateral epicondyles are extracapsular and so are not associated with capsular distension.

Supracondylar fractures are the commonest fractures under the age of 7 years. The majority are the extension type, with posterior displacement of the distal fracture fragment, typically due to a fall on an outstretched arm. Flexion-type fractures with anterior displacement are due to a direct blow on a flexed elbow and are often unstable (Fig. 80-14).[13]

Complications include nerve entrapment, malunion (leading to either cubitus valgus or varus) and vascular compromise. The absence of the radial pulse may be an indication for arteriography prior to surgical exploration.

Lateral condylar fractures are due to a varus force on an extended elbow. It is important to realise that this fracture may extend through the unossified portion of the capitellum into the joint space (Salter–Harris type IV).[14]

Forearm/Wrist/Hand

Radial and ulnar fractures can occur together or in isolation, the radius being the commoner single injury site. Forearm fractures may also occur with dislocation at either the elbow or wrist joint, the so-called Monteggia and Galeazzi fractures. To avoid missing a dislocation, it is vital the joints above and below a forearm fracture are visualised properly (Fig. 80-15).

Incomplete fractures of the distal forearm metadiaphysis are common, the mechanism of injury typically being a fall on an outstretched hand. The peak incidence

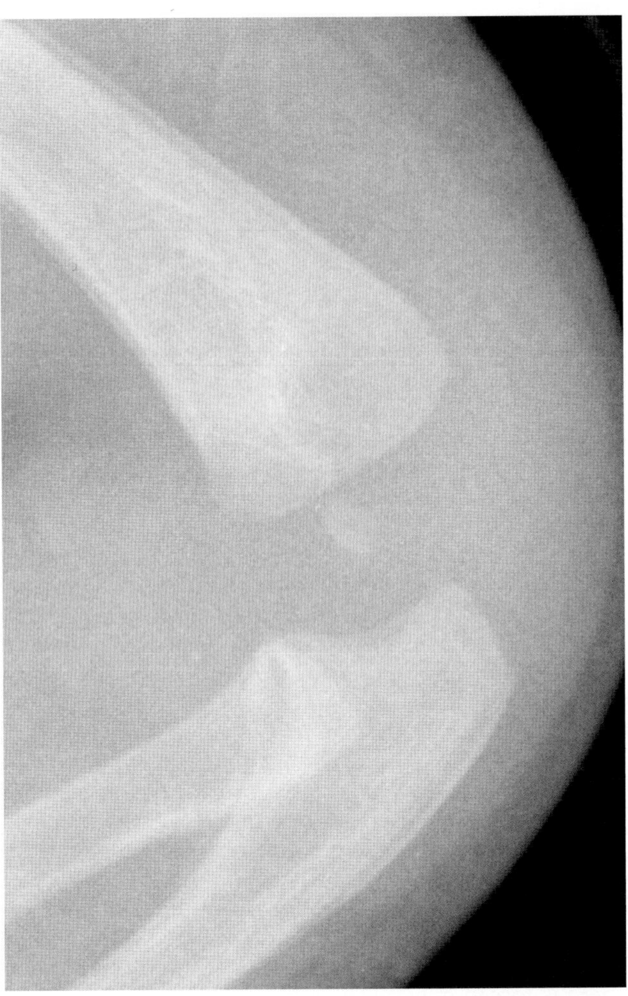

FIGURE 80-13 ■ Dislocated radial head. Note a line along the proximal radius does not pass through the capitellum.

in boys is between 12 and 14 and in girls 10 and 12 years.[15] This corresponds to the adolescent growth spurt and relative weakness of the metadiaphysis (Fig. 80-1).

Carpal injuries in childhood are infrequent, the commonest being the scaphoid, which more typically occurs in adolescence. The site of injury is more likely to be the distal third of the scaphoid, compared with the waist in adults, and so the risk of vascular compromise is lower in children. Scaphoid fractures may be radiographically occult, and MR imaging is useful in confirming the diagnosis and expediting appropriate management (Fig. 80-16).[16]

Metacarpal fractures have an increased incidence in older schoolchildren where the mechanism is usually punching or contact sports. The metacarpal of the little finger is most often injured, with the commonest type of fracture being a Salter–Harris type II.[17]

The phalanges may fracture from direct trauma or as a result of avulsion forces. Crush injuries of the phalanges are typically seen in the preschool child. It is important that all the ossified phalangeal epiphyses are reviewed, as any avulsed fragments may travel a significant distance proximally.

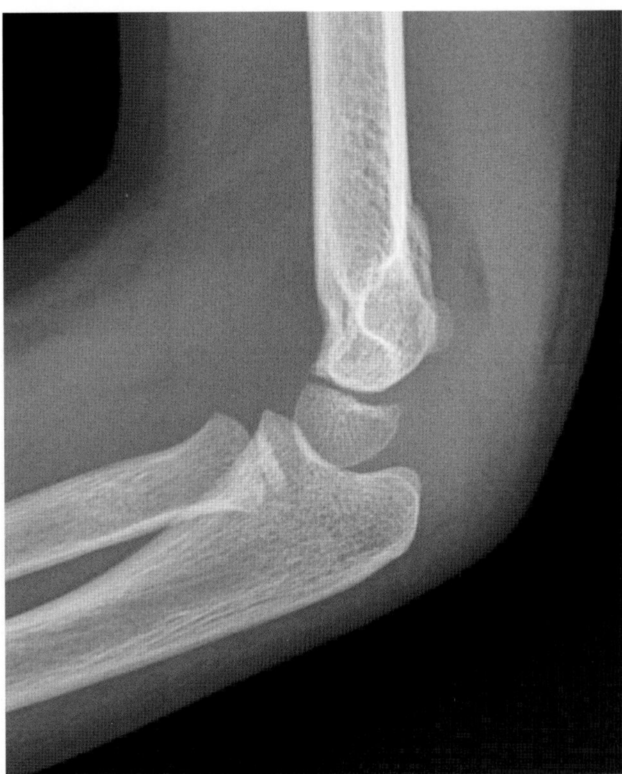

FIGURE 80-14 ■ Left supracondylar fracture with posterior displacement and a large elbow effusion.

THE LOWER LIMB

Pelvis

A number of classifications of pelvic fractures have been proposed, with the general aim being to predict the degree of morbidity associated with the injury and to try to assess the mechanism and force vectors involved in the causation. An improved understanding of causation helps plan treatment. In principle, the classification systems all detail the type of fracture and the anatomical sites within the pelvis. Unsurprisingly, the more severe injuries which result in significant disruption of the pelvis are associated with greater long-term morbidity. They are generally associated with high-velocity impacts and often occur with injuries in other anatomical areas, particularly the brain.[18–21]

The least severe fractures are avulsion injuries, which are common in adolescence and are typically the result of athletic activity. These can occur at a number of sites related to muscle attachments.

Standard AP radiographs are usually the initial investigation and are useful in assessing for avulsion injuries. For higher-grade injuries, CT is a more sensitive investigation and in most circumstances is part of a more general screening of a child following high energy/impact trauma.

Acetabular, Hip and Femur

Acetabular fractures are an uncommon, but significant, injury in childhood, because if the triradiate cartilage is

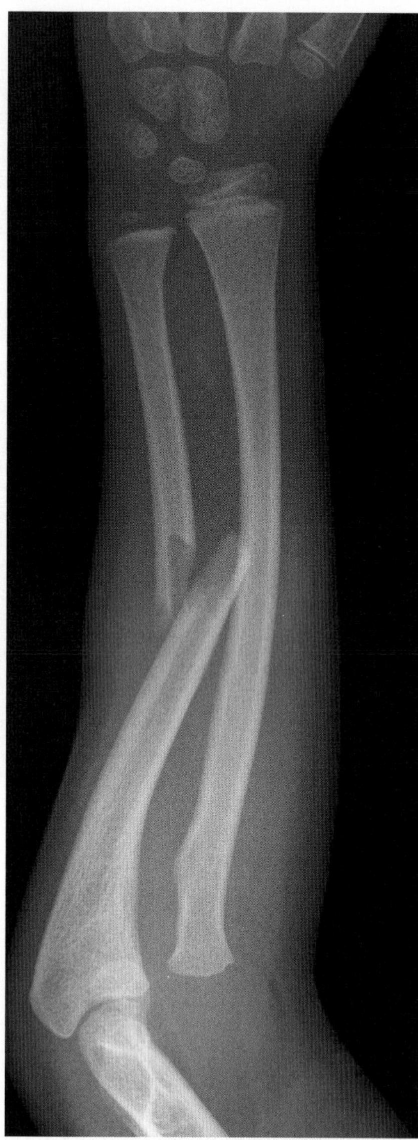

FIGURE 80-15 ■ Monteggia fracture of the left radius and ulna (fractured ulna dislocated radial head).

involved, growth and acetabular development may be affected.

Posterior dislocation of the hip is commoner than anterior, and while dislocation in children is less likely to result in acetabular injury, avascular necrosis of the femoral capital epiphysis is a serious potential complication if the femur remains unreduced for over 24 hours. With dislocations, proper assessment of the acetabular margins is vital to exclude occult fractures and this will be improved with CT or MR imaging (Fig. 80-17).[22,23]

Femoral head and neck fractures are relatively uncommon and may be associated with femoral head dislocation. They are classified with reference to their location along the femoral neck: namely, transepiphyseal, transcervical, cervicotrochanteric and intratrochanteric. Complications include osteonecrosis (the occurrence of which is increased the more significant the fracture displacement), premature physeal fusion, varus deformity and non-union.[24]

Femoral diaphyseal fractures may be associated with significant displacement if the fracture line means that there is unopposed muscle traction of the bone fragment. It is vital to check for rotation, as this will not be corrected without manipulation.

Knee

Acute knee trauma is a common childhood symptom. Studies which have been validated in paediatrics have devised rules to determine the need for radiographs within this cohort of patients. Radiographs are only indicated when there is isolated tenderness of the patella and head of the fibula, an inability to flex the knee to 90° or if the patient cannot weight bear. AP and lateral radiographs are standard and the use of the skyline view is arbitrary.[25]

An effusion within the knee joint will outline the suprapatellar region and obliterate fat planes. A horizontal beam lateral film will show a lipohaemarthrosis due to the different densities of fat and blood within the joint. The presence of a lipohaemarthrosis is suspicious of an intra-articular injury.

Outside of acute trauma, MR imaging is the modality of choice when assessing for pathological conditions of the knee, as it will obviously provide an assessment of ligaments, menisci and cartilage. CT is valuable for detecting intra-articular fracture displacement and detached bony fragments.

In contrast to adults, anterior tibial spine fractures are more likely to occur in childhood compared with anterior cruciate ligament (ACL) ruptures. This occurs when there is forced hyperextension and rotation of the knee. In children, the tensile strength of the ACL is greater than that of the bone, causing avulsion of the tibial spine. The detached bony fragment may be seen on radiographs within the knee joint. Both CT and MRI are more sensitive in assessing the degree of displacement and rotation (Fig. 80-18).

Osteochondral fractures are associated with traumatic lateral dislocation of the patella or axial compressive loading on the femur. Typical sites for injury are the lateral femoral condyle or patella. The fracture is through the subchondral bone and there may be a small bony (loose) fragment within the knee joint.

Osteochondritis dissecans is a defect within the subchondral region of the distal femur, typically occurring on the posterolateral aspect of the medial femoral condyle. Other anatomical sites are the talar dome and capitellum. The full aetiology is unknown, but there is necrosis of the subchondral bone which may be the result of repetitive overloading. On radiographs, there is an oval lucency adjacent to the articular margin.[26]

The patella is infrequently fractured in children, the commonest types being the comminuted and transverse. Sleeve fractures are avulsion injuries of the inferior pole of the patella with a small amount of detached ossified periosteum, but a large amount of unossified cartilage and retinaculum. This may be difficult to detect on standard radiographs as there is only a small of flake of detached bone, but it is well shown on MR imaging.

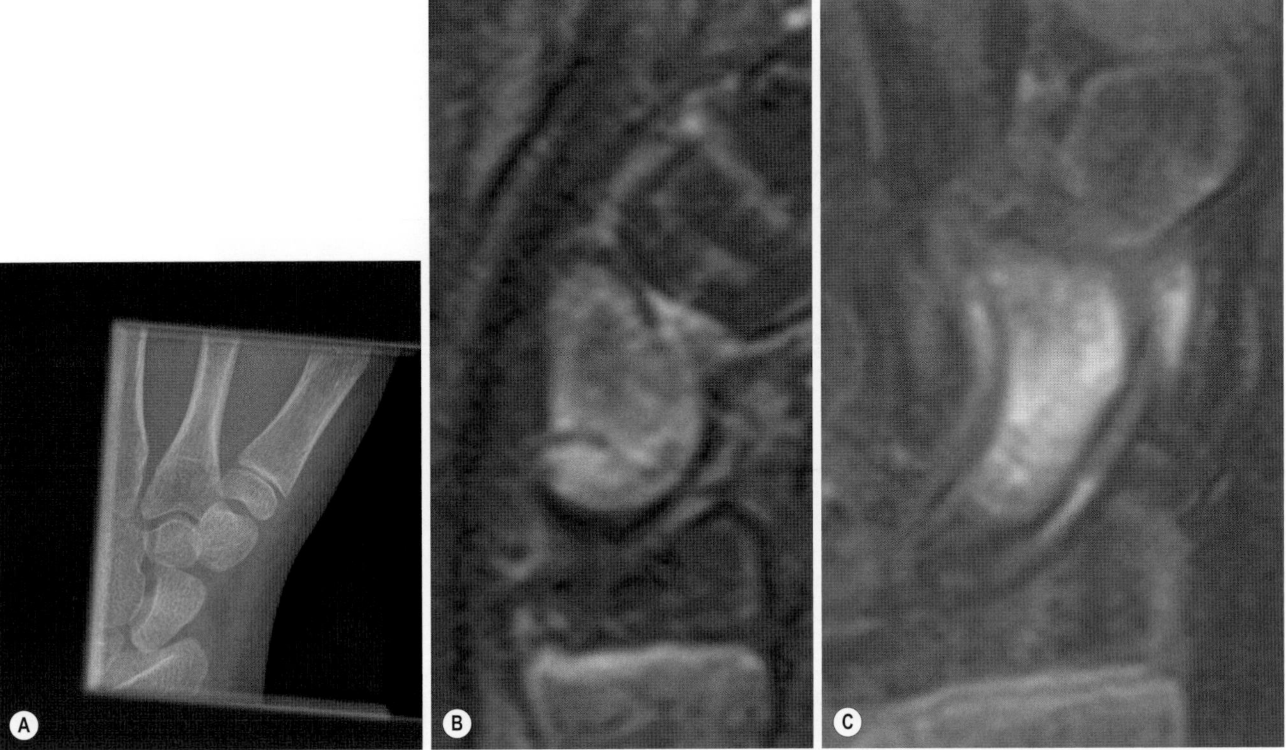

FIGURE 80-16 ■ (A) Normal radiographs of the left scaphoid. (B, C) MR images in the same patient demonstrate extensive marrow oedema within the scaphoid and a fracture line.

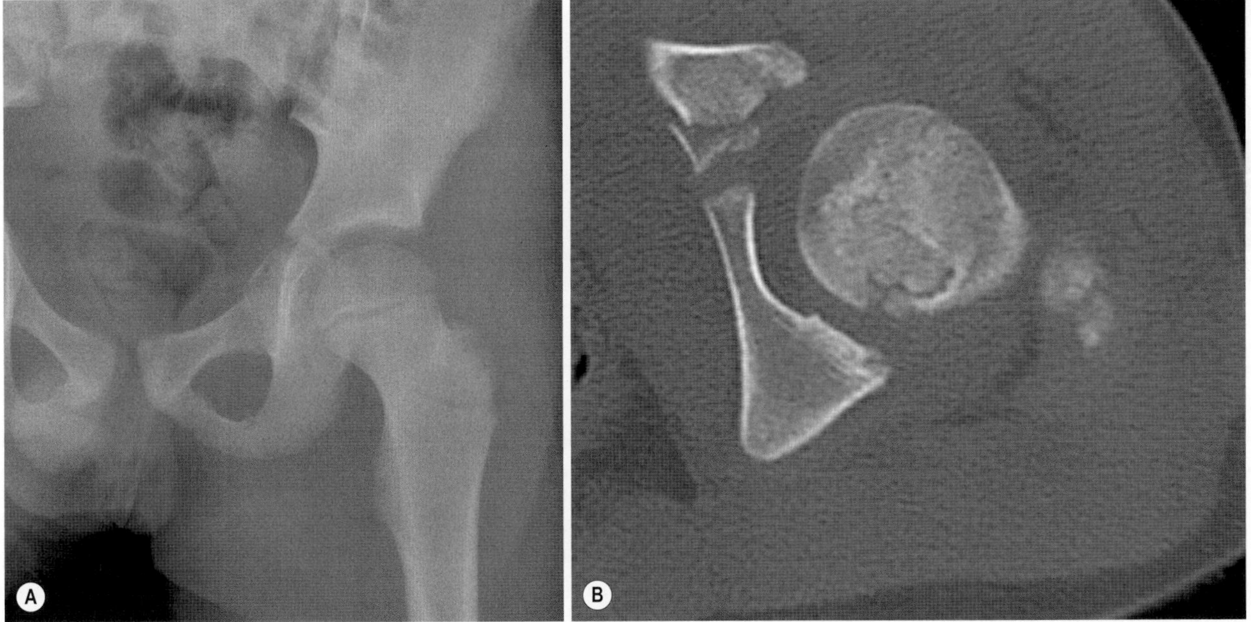

FIGURE 80-17 ■ (A) AP radiograph of the pelvis demonstrates a fracture of the left acetabulum and left inferior pubic ramus. (B) Axial CT confirms the presence of the acetabular fracture and demonstrates involvement of the triradiate cartilage.

Tibia/Ankle/Foot

Tibia

The classical toddler's fracture is an undisplaced fracture of the middle/distal tibial diaphysis, which may not be initially visible on the convential AP and lateral radiograph (being more discernible on oblique views). The toddler's fracture is a cause for a child to be non-weight bearing. If there are no other clinical concerns, follow-up imaging is not routinely indicated, due to radiation dose considerations. However, if repeat imaging

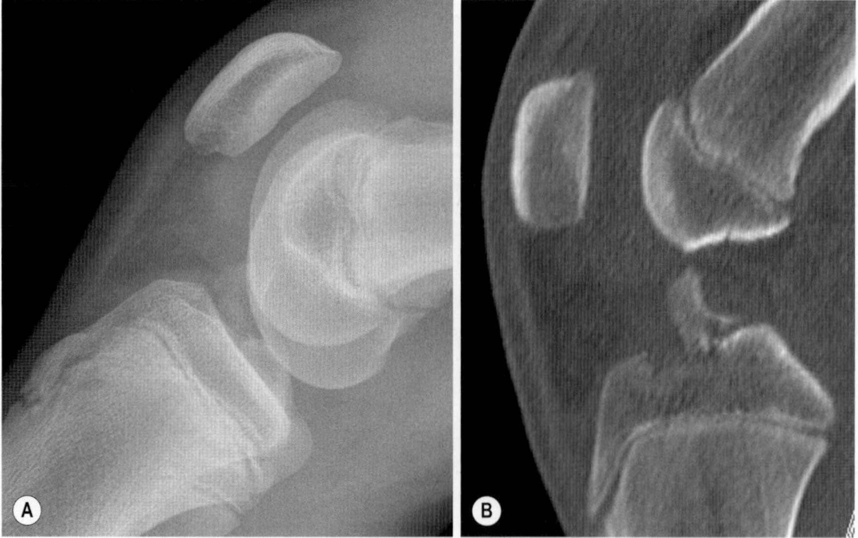

FIGURE 80-18 ■ (A) Lateral radiograph of the right knee demonstrates a bony fragment within the knee joint due to an avulsed tibial spine. (B) Avulsed tibial fragment clearly shown on sagittal reformatted CT image.

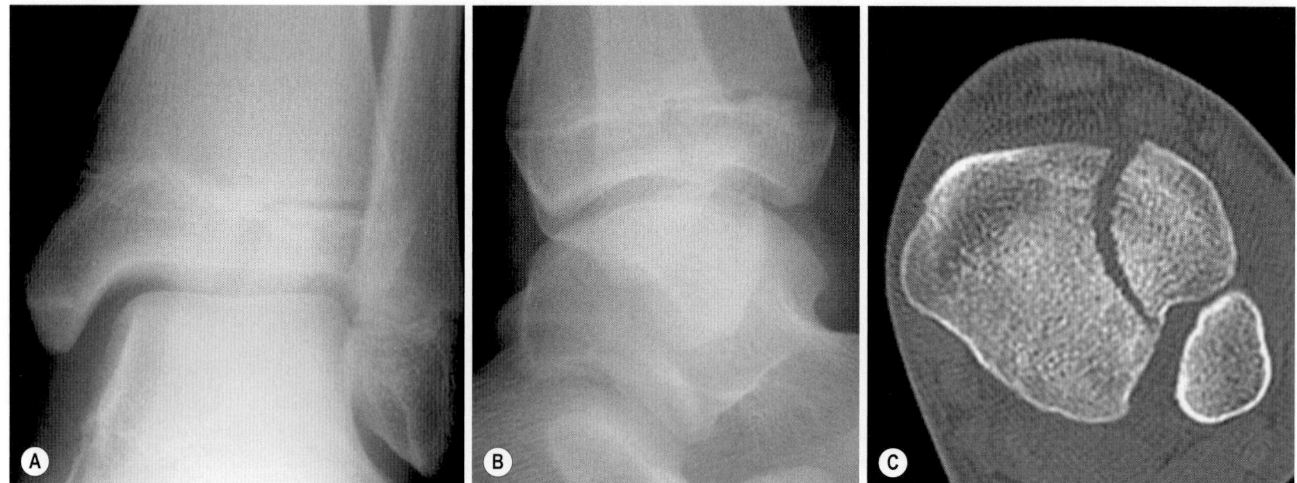

FIGURE 80-19 ■ **(A–C) Tillaux fracture of the distal tibial epiphysis.**

is performed, periosteal reaction and sclerosis along the fracture line may become visible after about a week (Fig. 80-3).

Stress fractures of the tibia are generally located in the upper third in children aged around 10–15 years and are associated with excessive or continuous physical exercise (Fig. 80-2). Approximately 70% of tibial shaft fractures are isolated, with the remainder also involving the fibula. The tibia shows a reduced tendency to remodel and there may be a risk of varus angulation due to the pull of the long flexors and an intact fibula. Isolated fibular fractures are rare and usually occur from a direct blow.[27]

Ankle

Most ankle fractures are adequately assessed with standard radiographs (i.e. AP, lateral ± mortice view). Some confusion can occur from the numerous accessory ossification centres which may be visible, particularly adjacent to the malleoli.

Epiphyseal, avulsion and Salter–Harris type I and II fractures of the distal tibia account for the majority of injuries. Injuries are usually caused by indirect trauma with the foot being fixed and forced either into dorsiflexion, plantar flexion, eversion, inversion or rotation (external or internal). The physes of the distal tibia and fibula fuse at the same time, initially centrally followed by medially and then laterally. If only one physis is visible, the suspicion of an epiphyseal injury is raised.

Transitional fractures (triplane and juvenile tillaux) occur in adolescence, as the name implies, as the skeleton becomes more mature (Figs. 80-19 and 80-20). Triplane injuries are fractures caused by external rotation which causes the fracture to extend in the axial, sagittal and

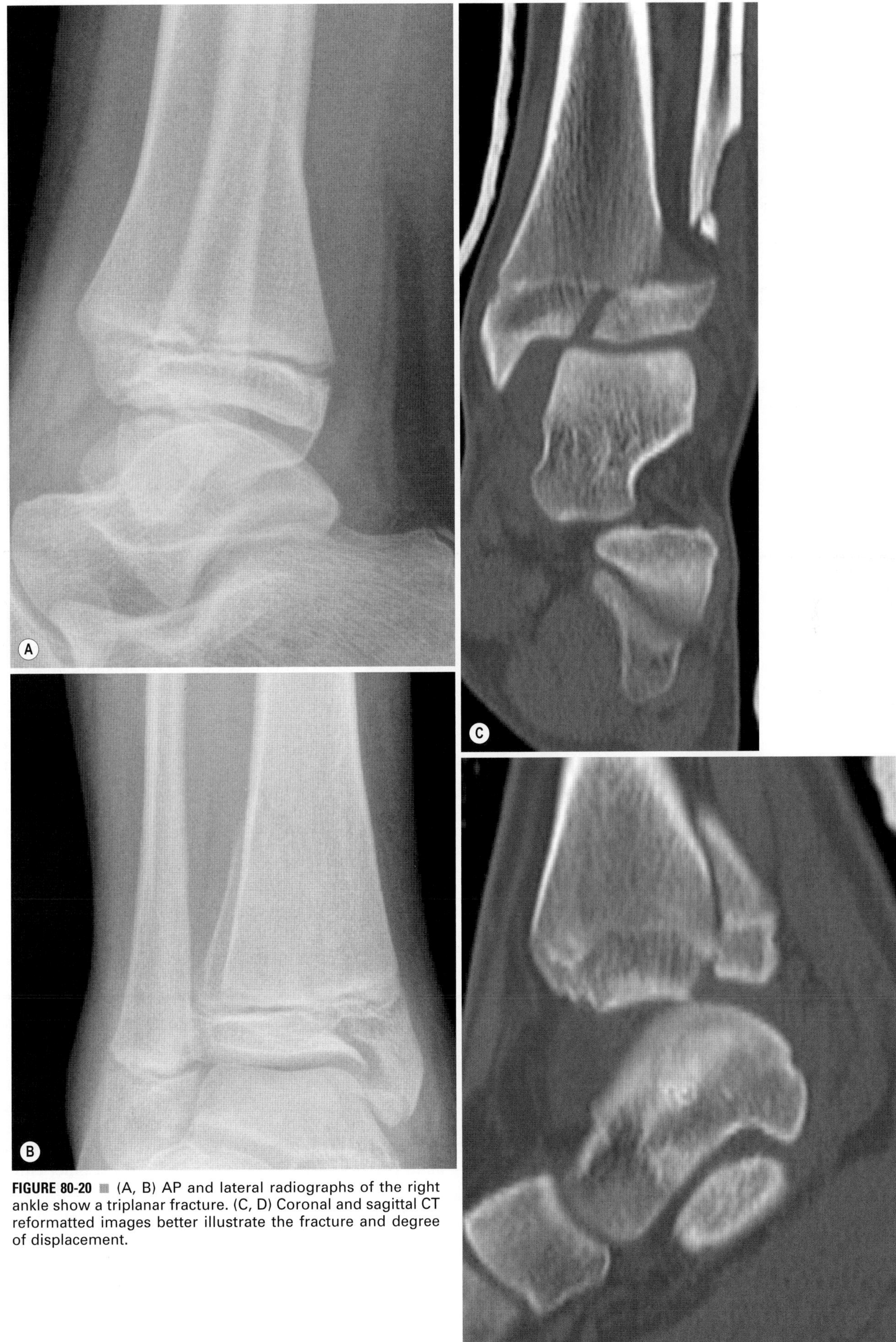

FIGURE 80-20 ■ (A, B) AP and lateral radiographs of the right ankle show a triplanar fracture. (C, D) Coronal and sagittal CT reformatted images better illustrate the fracture and degree of displacement.

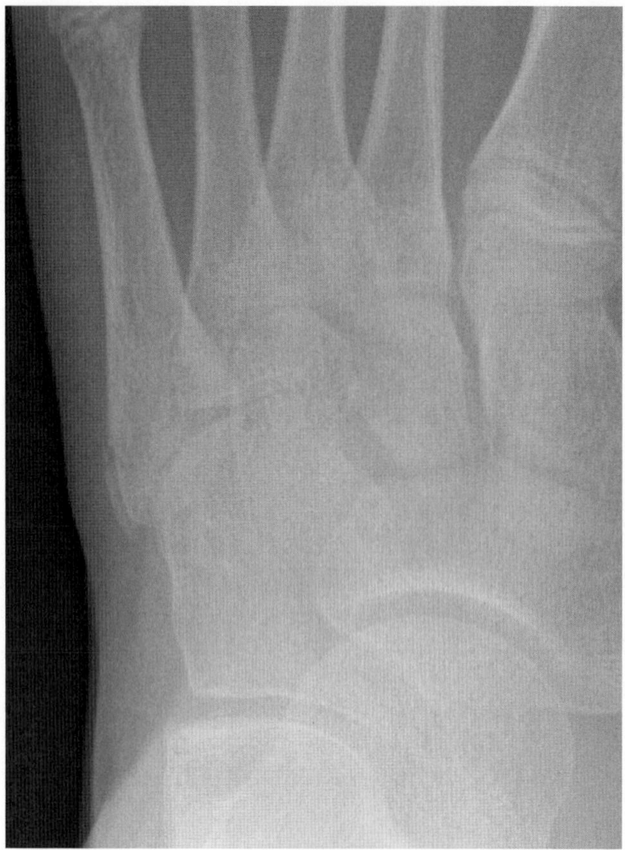

FIGURE 80-21 ■ The normal apophysis of the fifth metatarsal, which runs in a longitudinal direction parallel to the metatarsal. Fractures are typically transverse.

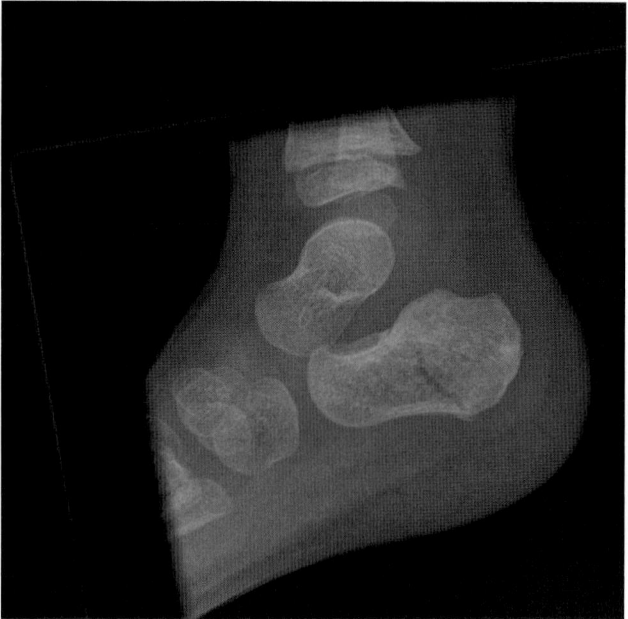

FIGURE 80-22 ■ Fracture of the calcaneum.

coronal planes. If the fibula is also fractured, it suggests a more severe rotational force. The lateral radiograph may suggest a Salter–Harris type II fracture while the AP view demonstrates a type II injury.[28]

Tillaux fractures are Salter–Harris type III fractures of the epiphysis and the unfused anterolateral portion of the distal tibial physis, due to avulsion of the anterior tibiofibular ligament. The lack of a fracture component in the coronal plane distinguishes it from a triplane fracture.[29,30]

In all Salter–Harris type III and IV fractures, there will be intra-articular extension of the fracture line and any degree of displacement should be properly evaluated with CT. Displacement greater than 2 mm often requires precise surgical reduction and fixation.

Foot

Foot fractures account for less than 10% of paediatric fractures,[31] the majority of which occur in the metatarsals and phalanges, particularly the fifth metatarsal. However, children under 5 years have a higher proportion of first metatarsal fractures, of which greenstick and torus are the commonest types. It is important not to confuse the apophysis of the fifth metatarsal with a fracture (Fig. 80-21).

The calcaneum is the commonest tarsal bone to be fractured, classically as a result of a fall from a height (Fig. 80-22). An extra-articular fracture which involves the tuberosity and avoids the posterior facet is commoner in the immature skeleton. There is an association with other injuries to the limb. Bohler's angle is unreliable under the age of 10 years and a normal Bohler's angle does not exclude a fracture.[32] CT is the imaging modality of choice for all suspected tarsal injuries.

Talar fractures are uncommon, as it is believed that the high cartilage to bone ratio in the young child is protective. Displaced fractures of the talar neck carry the risk of avascular necrosis. Isolated fractures of the cuboid, navicular and cuneiforms are rare and tend to be simple avulsions.

Stress fractures in the athletic child may occur in any tarsal bone.

CERVICAL SPINAL INJURIES

Paediatric spinal trauma is uncommon, with childhood injuries accounting for less than 10% of reported spinal injuries. Spinal fractures account for no more than 2% of all paediatric fractures,[33] the majority of which are the result of road traffic accidents.

Due to the disproportionate size of a young child's head and underdeveloped neck musculature, injuries under the age of 12 typically affect the first and second cervical bodies. Younger children are more likely to suffer distraction and subluxation injuries compared with the adult pattern of fractures which occur in the older child.

In children, the spinal column has significantly more flexibility than the spinal cord. Consequently, severe flexion extension injuries may not result in a fracture or ligamental disruption, but will cause significant spinal cord injury. The term 'spinal cord injury without radiographic abnormality' (SCIWORA) was described.[34] The increased use of MR imaging has been able to demonstrate abnormal cord findings in these patients. However,

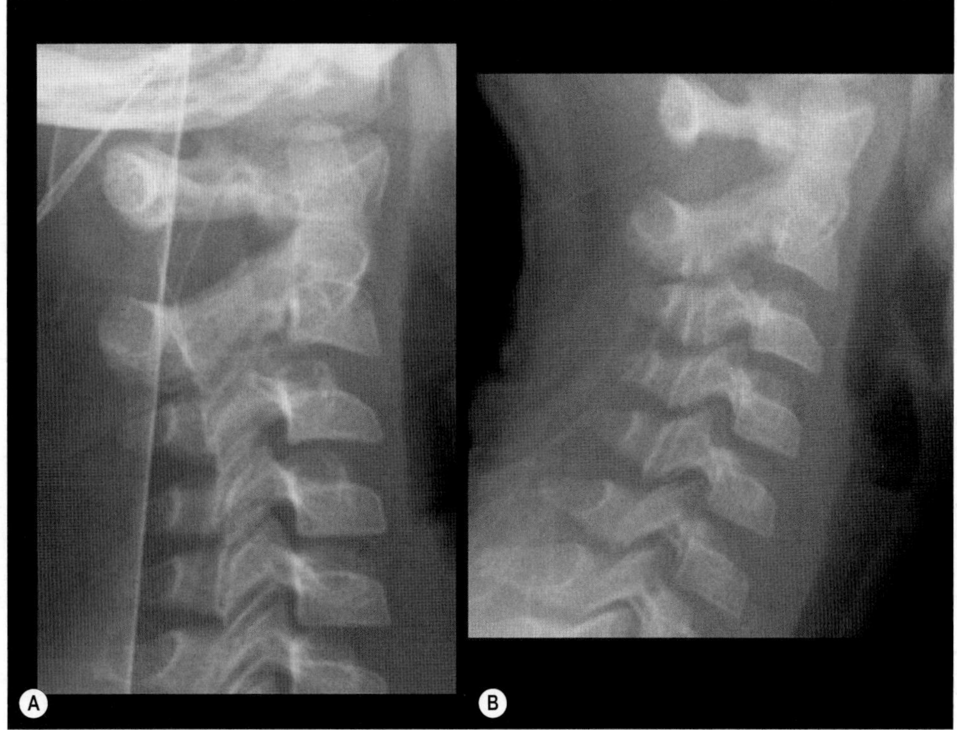

FIGURE 80-23 ■ **(A, B) A Pseudosubluxation of C2 upon C3.** In the same patient, extension view shows normal anterior alignment.

there is a small group of patients where even the MR imaging is normal despite clinical evidence of cord injury and damage.

It is important that normal anatomical variations are not misinterpreted as possible injuries. The commonest variant is pseudosubluxation at the C2/3 and C3/4 levels. Pseudosubluxation of up to 4 mm is acceptable. A line connecting the anterior aspects of the spinous processes (spinolaminar junction) of C1–C3 should pass within 2 mm of the spinolaminar junction of C2 (Fig. 80-23).

When the C2 spinolaminar junction lies 2 mm or more behind this line then the possibility of a fracture or true subluxation is raised. On an open mouth view, a pseudo-Jefferson fracture may be observed due to ossification of the lateral mass of C1 exceeding that of C2, so that they appear to overhang the axis by up to 6 mm. Pseudo anterior wedging of the vertebral bodies of up to 3 mm can be a normal variation and is particularly common at the C3 level.

Unfused apophyses and ossification centres may cause some confusion with fractures.

Atlantoaxial rotatory fixation (AARF) may or may not follow trauma in children and is a commoner occurrence than in adults.

Four types have been described and CT is the imaging modality of choice. An axial CT is performed in a neutral position, followed by repeat imaging in voluntary, maximal, ipsilateral and contralateral head rotation. In patients with fixation, no rotation of the atlas on the axis is observed while with transient torticollis, a reverse or reduction of rotation occurs.

Thoracic and lumbar injuries are typically the result of hyperflexion, which will result in stable anterior wedge compression fractures, and are commoner in children more than 8 years of age.

Flexion distraction forces causing bone and ligament disruption to the lumbar spine can occur with lap seatbelt restraint. Multilevel injuries are common and warrant imaging evaluation of the entire spinal column. The prognosis for neurological recovery is related to the initial severity of the injury. Some children with significant spinal cord injuries can recover substantial neurological function. Associated injuries within the thorax and abdomen are not uncommon.

NON-ACCIDENTAL INJURY

The incidence of physical abuse, a subset of child abuse, varies according to age, ethnicity and the specific definition used, and is both under-reported and under-recorded. Common to all definitions is the presence of an injury that the child sustains at the hands of his (or her) caregiver(s) (<http://www.yesican.org/definitions/CAPTA.html>, <http://www.yesican.org/definitions/WHO.html>, <http://www.yesican.org/articles.html>). These injuries are also referred to as inflicted or non-accidental injuries, battered child syndrome[35] or shaken baby syndrome.[36] When first described in 1946, the shaken baby syndrome included subdural and retinal haemorrhages in conjunction with fractures; however, during the past decade this term has been more and more linked to the abusive head injuries sustained by shaking.

During the past decades, efforts have been made to systematically register the occurrence and nature of child abuse. In the USA, the National Child Abuse and Neglect

Data System (NCANDS) has reported annually since 1990 (<http://www.acf.hhs.gov>). For 2010, the unique victim rate was 9.2 per 1000 children in the total population, increasing to around 20 per 1000 for those below 1 year of age. Victimisation was split between the sexes, with boys accounting for 48.5%. As in prior years, the greatest percentage of children was neglected while 17.6% suffered physical abuse. The overall rate of child fatalities was 2.1 deaths per 100,000 children, with nearly 80% being younger than 4 years old. Boys had a higher child fatality rate than girls; 2.5 versus 1.7 per 100,000. Around one-third of child fatalities were attributed exclusively to neglect, while around 40% were caused by multiple maltreatment types, i.e. neglect, physical abuse, psychological maltreatment and/or sexual abuse. More than 80% of duplicate perpetrators of child maltreatment were parents, and another 6% were other relatives of the victim. Of the perpetrators who were parents, more than 80% were the biological parent of the victim. In the USA, child abuse is responsible for approximately 1400 deaths per year[37] (<http://www.childwelfare.gov/pubs/factsheets/fatality.cfm>).

The UK does not publish statistics on the number of substantiated child abuse cases recorded every year; however, as at March 2010, there were 46,700 children on child protection registers or the subject of child protection plans, i.e. at risk of abuse (National Society for the Prevention of Cruelty to Children, NSPCC, <http://www.nspcc.org.uk/Inform/research/statistics/statistics_wda48748.html>). A UK-wide study of child maltreatment carried out by the NSPCC in 2009 suggested that one in 14 children (6.9%) aged 11–17 have experienced severe physical violence at the hands of an adult.[38]

Further, in England, the Department for Education and the Office for National Statistics have collected and reported statistics on children being looked after every year since 1989 (<http://www.education.gov.uk/rsgateway/DB/SFR>). At 31 March 2011, there were 65,520 looked after children in England, an increase of 9% since 2007. Overall, the main reason why social services first engaged with these looked after children was because of abuse or neglect (54%).

In Australia, the 13th annual comprehensive child protection report *(Child Protection Australia 2008–09)* showed that the number of children subject to a notification of child abuse or neglect increased by 47% from 4.8 to 7.0 per 1000 children over the past 5 years.[39]

Taken together, the rate of physical child abuse is fairly high in industrialised countries. Infants and young children are at greatest risk, with up to 80% of cases being younger than 5 years and up to half being infants (< 1 year of age).

CLINICAL PRESENTATION AND THE ROLE OF THE RADIOLOGIST

The clinical presentation takes many forms, but the physically abused child typically presents with an obvious injury such as soft-tissue swelling, haematomas, bruises, burns and/or fractures. Fractures are seen in a high proportion of physically abused children and more often in infants.[40,41] It is not uncommon, however, for the abused child to present with symptoms of occult injury, particularly in cases of head and abdominal trauma.

Infants with head injuries may present with nonspecific symptoms, such as lethargy, irritability, persistent, unexplained vomiting, apnoea, coma or seizures. Abusive head injury is the most common cause of NAI-related death.[42] Similar to head injury, severe abdominal trauma may present without visible external signs or history to suggest such an injury.

As radiologists, we have important medical and legal roles in the diagnosis of cases of child abuse. We may be the first to raise a question of abuse, if characteristic or unexplained findings are encountered during imaging. The possibility of physical abuse when the parent or another adult caregiver offers conflicting, unconvincing, or indeed no explanation for the child's injury, should always be considered. Immediate and direct communication with the referring physician and also a named and designated child protection colleague (if available) is imperative in all such cases. If there is any doubt as to the presence or significance of a lesion, a second opinion should be sought from a paediatric radiologist experienced in NAI cases, as both a missed, and also an incorrect, diagnosis may be devastating for the child and the family.

INJURY PATTERNS

Our current understanding of injuries and injury patterns in physical abuse is the result of early observations by neurosurgeons, identifying an association between trauma-induced subdural haemorrhages (SDHs) and retinal haemorrhages.[43] Subsequently, in the 1940s, radiologists noticed SDHs in conjunction with skeletal injuries.[36] Physicians' recognition of abuse as the cause of these injuries emerged in the 1950s.[35,44] Observational studies of accidental versus non-accidental injuries are summarised in a recent review,[45] large epidemiological series on fractures in children,[46,47] cadaver and animal studies,[48] and more recently, biomechanical studies.[49]

Physical abuse can produce various injuries and injury patterns in children, of which none are pathognomonic for non-accidental injury.[45] In various clinical series, fractures are observed in approximately 30% of the children and more often in infants,[44] burns are observed in 10%, bruises are common and are present in approximately 40% of maltreated children, and inflicted CNS injury is observed in around a quarter of children treated for head injury.[50] Abdominal trauma is rare, with a reported incidence of 1% of abused children, and is more predominantly seen after the child is able to move around freely.[51]

Shaken Baby Syndrome

The description of findings referred to as the 'shaken baby syndrome' (SBS) has been widely ascribed to the paediatric radiologist John Caffey, who, in 1946, observed and published case reports on six infants suffering chronic subdural haematoma.[36] These six patients also had fractures of long bones, without evidence of an underlying, predisposing skeletal disorder or a history of trauma. During subsequent years he continued to collect data, and in 1974, he published his sentinel paper in which he linked violent manual shaking of an infant to brain damage, retinal haemorrhage and residual mental retardation.[52,53]

Since then our understanding of this syndrome has been modified as a result of new medical research and multiple legal challenges. Biomechanical studies have repeatedly failed to show that shaking alone can generate the triad of subdural haemorrhage, retinal haemorrhage and encephalopathy, in the absence of significant neck injury.[49] Moreover, the importance of a concomitant impact has been recognised, i.e. 'shaken baby—impact syndrome'. More recently, an even wider term, namely 'abusive head trauma', has been introduced to cover the whole spectrum of CNS pathology sustained by violent shaking.[54] Controversy still exists, however, as to the cause and mechanisms of the observed head and spinal injuries. The majority of all cases of abusive head injury are limited to children under 2–3 years of age, and most often seen in infants younger than 6 months.[55] Small children and infants are at a high risk due to their small size in comparison to their adult perpetrators.

GENERAL IMAGING STRATEGIES

The appropriate imaging of children being evaluated for suspected physical child abuse depends on the age of the child and the presence of neurological, thoracic or abdominal signs and symptoms. Several referral and imaging guidelines exist, of which the American College of Radiology (ACR) Appropriateness Criteria,[56] recommendations by the Royal College of Radiologists/the Royal College of Paediatrics and Child Health (RCR-RCPCH)[57] and referral guidelines from the Royal College of Radiologists (RCR)[58] have been widely adopted.

Both the ACR and the RCR recommend a skeletal survey in all children younger than 2 years of age in whom there is suspicion of abuse. As for the use of additional imaging, there are minor differences between the two, and the radiologist should be familiar with the local policy.

The RCR referral guidelines include:

- Skeletal survey, including skull radiographs, as these are essential to demonstrate skull fractures even when CT of the brain is performed.
- Brain CT, indicated for:
  - any infant (< 1 year) where there is evidence of physical abuse[57]
  - any child who presents with evidence of physical abuse with encephalopathic features, focal and neurological signs or haemorrhagic retinopathy.
- Brain MRI is helpful if CT shows evidence of subdural haemorrhage or brain injury, or if there is neurological deficit.
- Consider including the cervical spine.[59]
- Bone scintigraphy, of value if the skeletal survey is equivocal or if there are ongoing clinical concerns despite a normal survey. It should, however, only be performed in departments which have expertise in bone scanning in infants.

For the older children, 2–5 years of age, a skeletal survey is of less value, but should be considered for each specific case, individually. Alternatively, the radiographs may be tailored to the area(s) of suspected injury.[56]

Furthermore, all children with suspected injury to the chest or abdomen should have an enhanced CT scan, following per-oral contrast if possible. Children suffering sudden infant death should have a skeletal survey before an autopsy is undertaken.

SKELETAL INJURY

The role of skeletal imaging in cases of suspected child abuse is to accurately detect, and possibly date, any injuries, to exclude normal variants of growth (which may mimic injuries or fractures) and possibly to diagnose any underlying metabolic or genetic disorders of bone, which may predispose a child to pathological fractures.[60]

The Skeletal Survey

The skeletal survey should be performed by experienced radiographers, under the supervision of a consultant radiologist. High-quality images of each anatomical site, and not a whole-body radiograph ('babygram'), should be performed, and all images should be appropriately labelled and stored. The following views are advised:[57]

- Skull (anteroposterior (AP) and lateral; additional Townes view if there is a suspected occipital fracture).
- Spine (lateral views of cervical, thoracic and lumbar spine); if the whole of the spine is not included on the chest and abdominal radiographs then additional views will be required.
- Chest (AP, including the clavicles, and oblique views of both sets of ribs).
- Abdomen, including pelvis and hips (AP).
- Long bones (AP views of both humeri, both forearms, both femora and both tibiae and fibulae).
- Hands (PA).
- Feet (DP).

When an abnormality is suspected, these views should be supplemented with:

- Lateral views of any suspected shaft fracture.
- AP and lateral coned views of the elbows, wrist, knees and ankles, when a fracture is suspected at these sites—as directed by the supervising consultant radiologist. These may demonstrate metaphyseal injuries in greater detail than AP views of the limb alone.[57]

Follow-up radiographs have been shown to be of value in improving the detection of rib and metaphyseal fractures.[61,62] Repeat radiographs after 11–14 days should be considered if there are questionable areas or areas of persistent clinical concern, particularly to rule out rib fractures. This is pertinent as up to two-thirds of acute fractures may be missed.[63] In cases of suspected metaphyseal injury, a repeat radiograph after 2 weeks may show ongoing healing, while a repeat radiograph after 5–6 weeks may clarify whether a metaphyseal irregularity represents a normal variant, as most fractures will have healed at this stage.

Bone Scintigraphy

The role of bone scintigraphy in diagnosing child abuse is controversial, and the technique is not routinely used in large parts of Europe.[64] According to the guidelines (as published by the ACR and RCR-RCPCH), bone scintigraphy may be considered in cases with a normal radiographic skeletal survey, but with a high clinical index of suspicion of child abuse. To increase sensitivity, the bone scan should include the use of pinhole collimators and differential counts of the metaphysis. A bone scan is especially good for detecting periosteal trauma, and rib, scapular, spinal, diaphyseal, pelvic and acromial fractures, whilst the sensitivity is lower for fractures of flat bones, old healed fractures and metaphyseal injuries.[65] Scintigraphy becomes positive within hours of an injury.[66] Familiarity with the normal scintigraphic appearances in children is crucial, in particular the normal high metaphyseal uptake, which should not be mistaken for a metaphyseal injury.

Magnetic Resonance Imaging (MRI)

MRI is not routinely used for the assessment of bony injury in infants with suspected NAI, and the literature is sparse as to its validation. One study demonstrated a low sensitivity for both metaphyseal and rib fractures.[67] Others have shown that more than half of healthy children aged 5–15 years have findings consistent with bone oedema in at least one of the carpal bones, reflecting a wide normal variation of the MRI appearances within paediatric bones.[68,69]

Ultrasound

Ultrasound may be a useful supplementary technique in selected cases of bony injury; however, its use in NAI has not been validated, and it cannot be advocated as a primary tool for the investigation of bone injury. Of note is the mild periosteal 'elevation' close to the growth plate, which can be seen as a normal feature, and thus should not be mistaken for injury (Fig. 80-24).

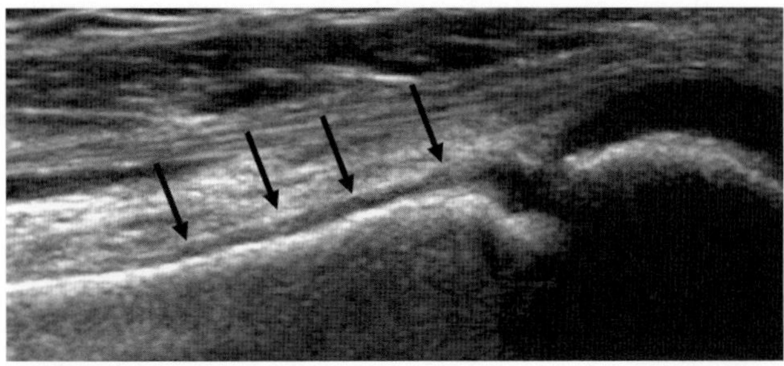

FIGURE 80-24 ■ Ultrasound of the distal femur in a 6-month-old female, showing a normal, diaphyseal elevated periosteum, not to be mistaken for an injury.

Fracture Patterns in Accidental vs Non-Accidental Injury

Fractures are a common problem in childhood, with approximately one-third of girls and boys sustaining at least one fracture before 16–17 years of age.[46,70] Rates are higher among boys than girls, with peak incidences at 14 and 10–11 years of age, respectively.[70,71] The most common site affected in both sexes is the radius/ulna, although the type and location varies considerably at different stages of the child's age and development.[46,72] In toddlers, fractures to the tibia and fibula predominate (Fig. 80-25), while fractures of the clavicle and skull are more common in infants.[71] Multiple fractures are uncommon, and seen in only 16% of non-abused versus 74% of abused children.[41]

In various clinical series of non-accidental injury, skeletal fractures are diagnosed in up to a third of the children, and more often in those under the age of 2.[41,50] Any bone can be involved, but some locations are more frequent than others.

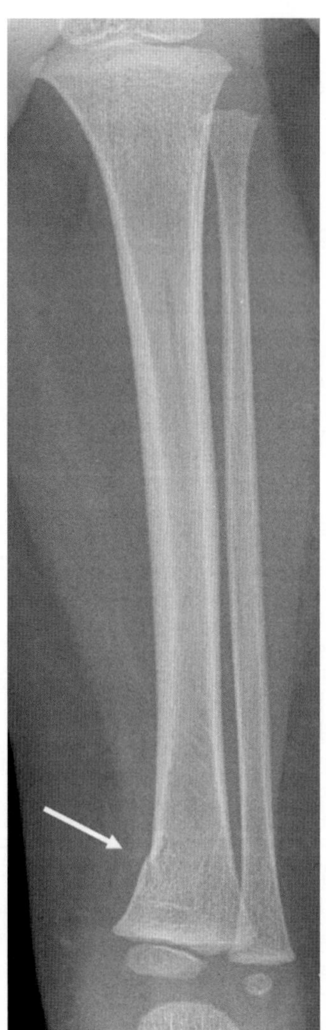

FIGURE 80-25 ■ Buckle fracture (arrow) of the distal metaphysis in a toddler.

TABLE 80-2 **Specificity of Skeletal Injuries in Child Abuse; Highest Specificity Applies in Infants**[75]

Specificity	Type of Fracture/Skeletal Lesion
High specificity	Classic metaphyseal lesion
	Rib fractures, especially posterior
	Scapular fractures
	Spinous process fractures
	Sternal fractures
Moderate specificity	Multiple fractures, specifically bilateral
	Fractures of different ages
	Epiphyseal separation
	Vertebral body fractures and subluxations
	Digital fractures
	Complex skull fractures
Common but low specificity	Subperiosteal ne-bone formation
	Clavicular fractures
	Long bone shaft fractures
	Linear skull fractures

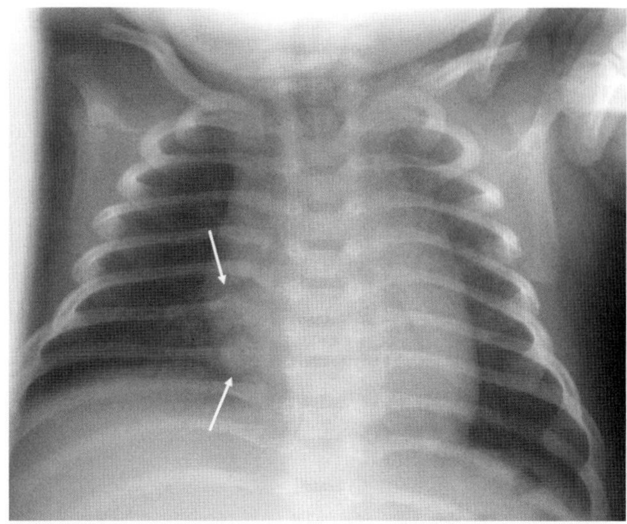

FIGURE 80-26 ■ Healing fractures to the posterior right seventh and eighth ribs (arrows). Also note a healing fracture to the left clavicle.

Overall, long tubular bones are affected in about one-third of cases, metaphyses in a quarter, ribs in a quarter and skull fractures in approximately 15%.[73] No fracture is considered pathognomonic for physical abuse on its own, although fractures to the ribs, particularly to the posterior aspects and to the long bone metaphysis, should raise particular concern.[45] In a recent systematic review on fracture patterns in child abuse, the authors conclude that physical abuse should be considered in the differential diagnosis when a child (under 18 months of age) presents with a fracture, in the absence of an overt history of important trauma or a known medical condition that predisposes to bone fragility. The authors present several features associated with possible child abuse[45] such as multiple fractures, rib fractures—(regardless of type), for example femoral fractures—in particular in children who are not yet walking and humeral fractures (in particular affecting the mid-shaft) and skull fractures.

Additional features found to be associated with abuse are metaphyseal injuries,[74] uncommon fractures for example at the scapula, especially at the spinous process, the sternum, and any fracture with a delayed presentation (Table 80-2).[41,75]

Careful correlation of the observed radiological findings with the proposed mechanism of injury, with the child's age and clinical status, is crucial in the evaluation, knowing that a missed diagnosis could lead to a second and potentially fatal abusive injury.

Rib Fractures

Because of the relative elasticity of the thoracic cage, rib fractures in otherwise healthy infants and young children are rare. Any such injury should be regarded with suspicion if no plausible explanation, such as an underlying diseases leading to bone fragility, a motor vehicle accident or violent trauma, is offered.[45,76]

A child with rib fractures has a 7 in 10 chance of having been abused.[45] Most rib fractures are clinically occult, in contrast to around 60% of extremity fractures, and are discovered incidentally during imaging.[77] They are not usually associated with bruising of the chest wall, although finger marks may be an accompanying clinical sign. Abusive rib fractures can occur at any point along the rib, from the costovertebral articulations to the costochondral junctions, but fractures to the posterior rib arches are believed to be particularly associated with NAI[78–80] (Figs. 80-26–80-29). A recent literature review has, however, challenged this assumption, as findings of posterior rib fractures were variable.[45] While Barsness and colleagues found that posterior rib fractures were significantly more common in abuse than in non-abuse,[80] their findings were not supported by others.[81,82]

Abusive rib fractures are typically multiple, positioned immediately above each other in a line, are unilateral in up to 50%, but may also be solitary.[76] In up to 29% of cases, one or more rib fractures are the only skeletal finding in an abused child, underscoring the importance of high-quality radiographs and a keen eye for detail.[80]

The mechanism of rib fractures is believed to be thoracic compression by adult hands, causing fractures along the rib arches, including the posterior aspects, when the posterior end of the rib is levered over the transverse process[48] (Fig. 80-30). Most posterior rib fractures occur near the costovertebral articulations, but can also involve the rib head and neck.[76] Mid-posterior fractures are typically seen in conjunction with fractures to the rib neck in adjacent ribs, whilst lateral and anterior fractures can have the appearances of greenstick or buckle fractures. Injuries to the costochondral junction mirror the classic metaphyseal lesion (CML) due to similar anatomy, with a growth plate present between the osseous anterior rib end and the costal cartilage (Fig. 80-31). As opposed to the others, and similar to the CMLs, these fractures appear to heal by a process of consolidation without callus formation. They can also be associated with abdominal visceral injury.

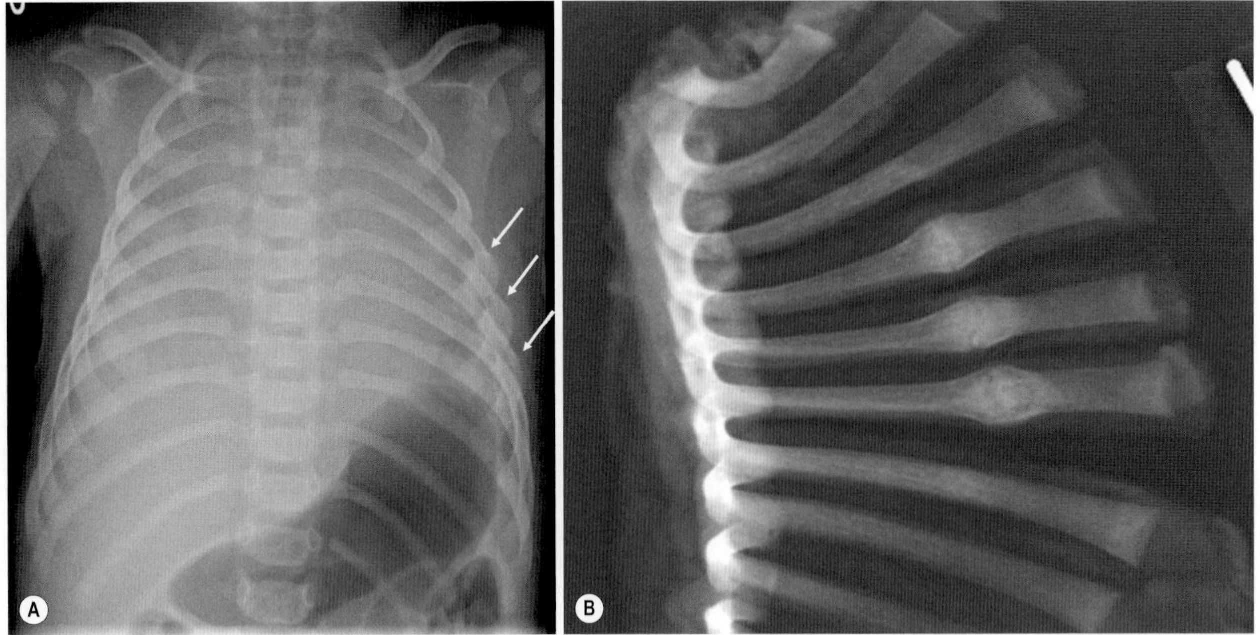

FIGURE 80-27 ■ **Healing fractures to the lateral left fourth through sixth ribs (arrows) in a 3-month-old infant.** (A) Pre- and (B) postautopsy.

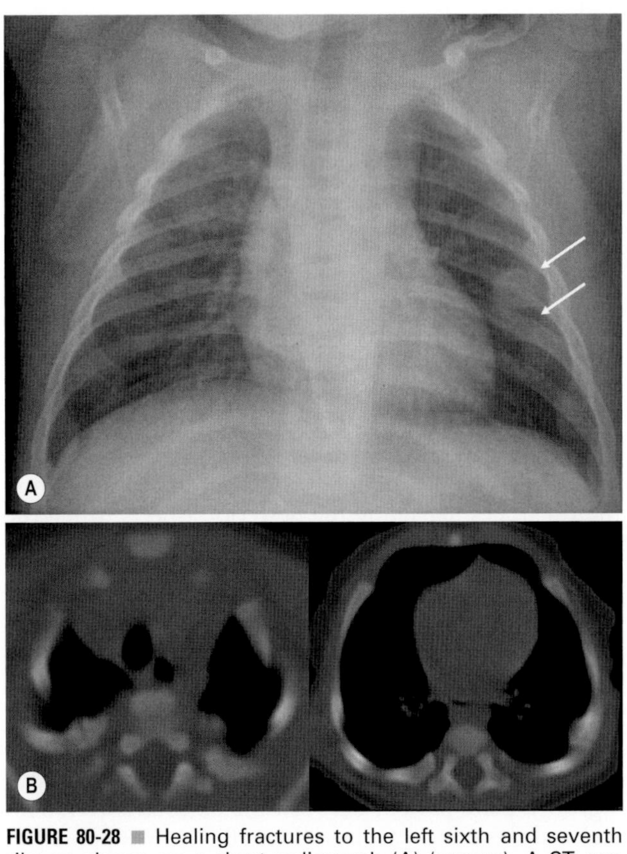

FIGURE 80-28 ■ Healing fractures to the left sixth and seventh ribs as shown on a chest radiograph (A) (arrows). A CT performed 4 days later also demonstrated healing fractures to the second through fifth right ribs, and to the second left rib, all of which had been missed on the initial, slightly suboptimal radiograph (B).

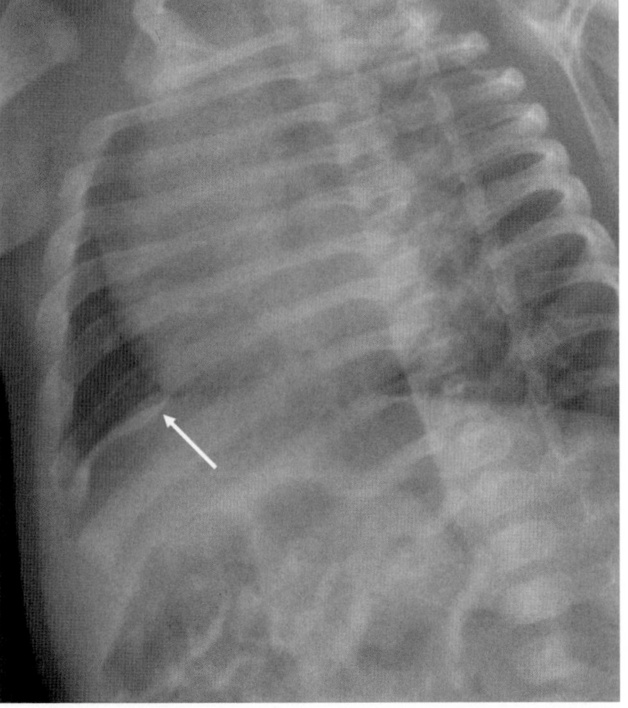

FIGURE 80-29 ■ **Old fracture to the right seventh rib (arrow).**

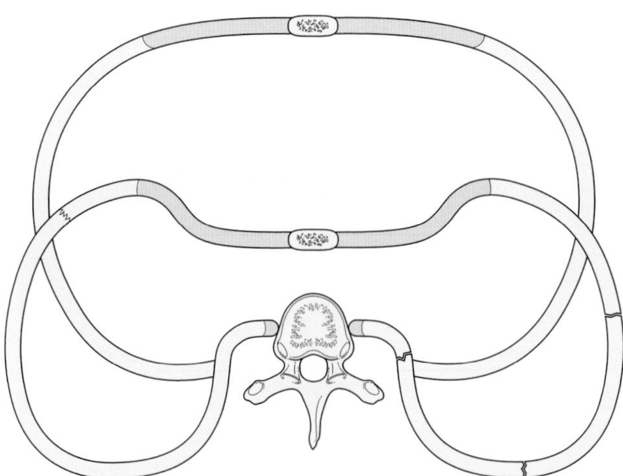

FIGURE 80-30 ■ During violent shaking, the perpetrator's hands wrap around the child's chest, exerting a bidirectional force. The vertebrae act as a fulcrum, resulting in posterior rib fractures. Lateral and anterior fractures may also occur. (Illustration courtesy of E M Hoff, Department of Photo and Drawing, University of Bergen.)

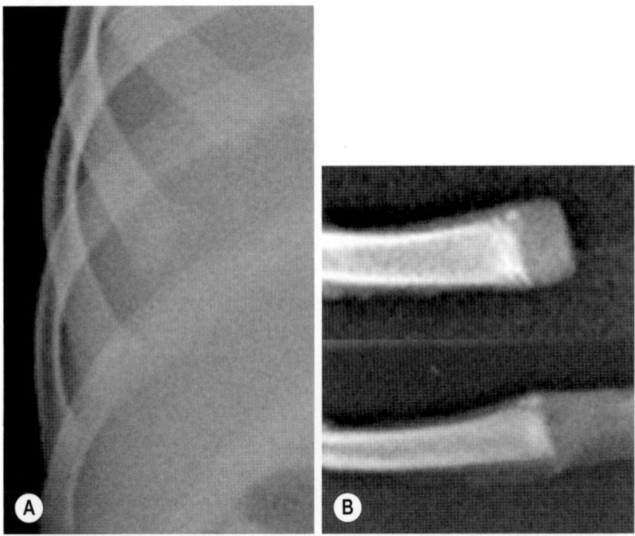

FIGURE 80-31 ■ Fracture to the costochondral junction, mimicking a classic metaphyseal lesion. (A) Pre- and (B) postautopsy.

Rib fractures can also be seen after blunt trauma to the chest wall. Unlike in the adult skeleton, rib fractures due to cardiopulmonary resuscitation are uncommon, and if present, involve the lateral or anterior arches of the ribs.[83,84] Recently, however, there have been some reports on rib fractures, posterior, anterior and lateral, after two-handed CPR delivered by trained medical personnel.[85] Similarly, fractures caused by physiotherapy in children treated for bronchiolitis have been reported.[86] However, fractures to the first rib are rare.

Metaphyseal Injury

Metaphyseal injury, or classic metaphyseal lesions (CMLs), are seen in a high proportion of physically abused infants, most commonly in non-mobile infants under the age of 12 months.[87] CMLs have been perceived as strong predictors of abuse,[76] although the literature is inconclusive.[45,74] Histologically, the CML is a series of microfractures across the entire width of, or part thereof the metaphysis, through the immature portion of the primary spongiosa.[88] The injury is a result of 'shearing forces' sustained during violent shaking or handling of the infant, outside those forces associated with daily care. The CMLs are usually asymptomatic and not evident clinically. They are most frequently seen in the distal femur, the tibia and the proximal humerus, but also occur in the elbow and wrist. They may be uni- or bilateral.

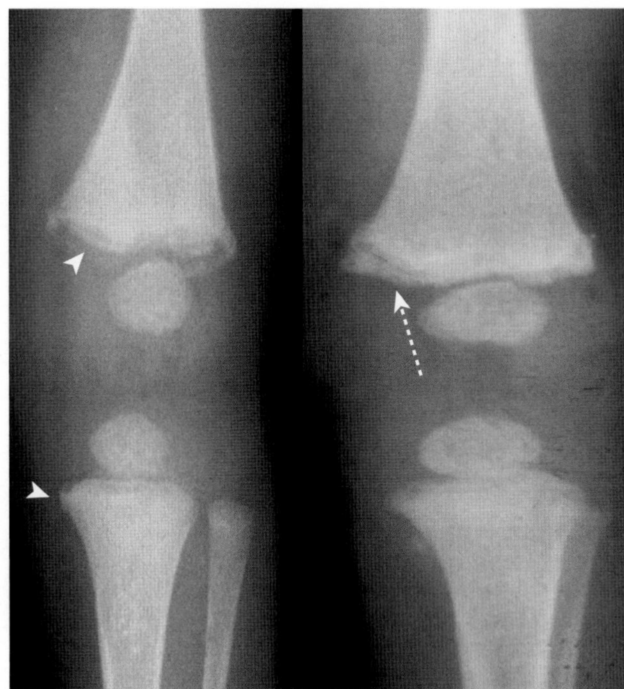

FIGURE 80-32 ■ Classic metaphyseal lesions with different appearances. 'Corner fracture' (a thick rim only, arrowhead), 'bucket handle' (a thick rim projected away from the shaft, arrow) and a thin disk with a thick rim (stippled arrow).

Radiographically, the CML appears as:

1. a thin wafer of bone separated from the metaphysis, thicker at the periphery ('bucket handle fracture');
2. a thick rim only ('corner fracture'); or
3. a thin disk with a thick rim (Fig. 80-32).

Small CMLs tend to heal without callus formation, by gradual bone consolidation, within 4–8 weeks.[76] When the adjacent periosteum is injured, or stripped by the shearing forces, a subperiosteal haemorrhage occurs, which, during the healing process, is evident as a periosteal reaction. Occasionally the fracture heals with a local disturbance of growth.

CMLs must be differentiated from normal growth variations, which may take the form of subtle irregularities, 'step-off' (also termed a metaphyseal collar) (Fig. 80-33) or even mimic a bucket handle fracture (Fig. 80-34). In children over the age of 15 months, metaphyseal fragmentation can be seen in bow-legs due to abnormal stresses associated with early weight bearing.[89]

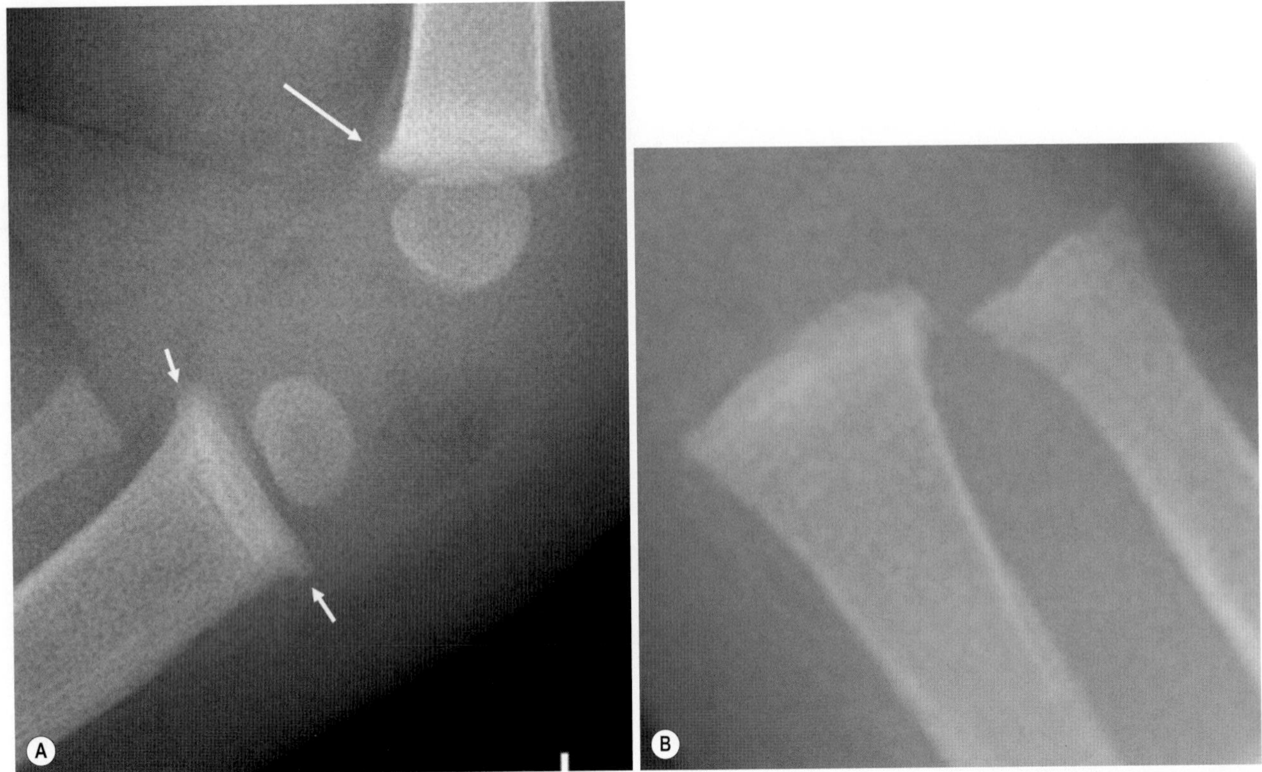

FIGURE 80-33 ■ **Normal metaphyseal irregularities in the distal femur (A) and in the distal radius (B) in an 8-month-old boy who had a skeletal survey after presenting with a head injury suspect of abuse.**

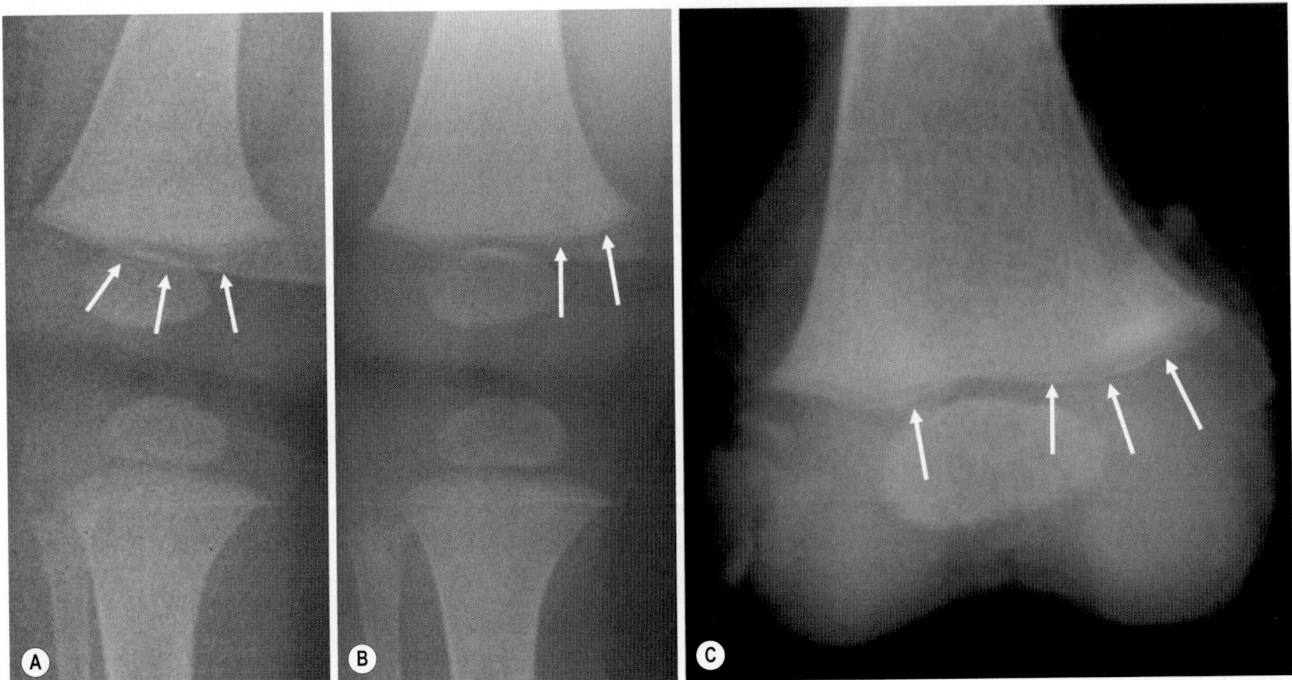

FIGURE 80-34 ■ **Lucent line through the distal right femur metaphysis (arrows), mimicking a CML (bucket handle fracture) in a 3-month-old boy who died from abusive head injury.** (A, B) Initial radiographs and (C) post-mortem specimen. No fracture was found at autopsy.

FIGURE 80-35 ■ Avulsion fracture to the proximal left humerus (white arrows) in a 3-month-old boy who died from abusive head trauma. (A) Initial radiograph and (B) radiograph of the specimen at autopsy. Note the normal, flanged appearances of the posterolateral ribs, not to be mistaken for periosteal reaction (short, black arrows).

Long Bone Fractures

Fractures to the long tubular bones are seen in about one-third of physically abused children, most commonly involving the femur, humerus and tibia (Fig. 80-35).

There is no specific fracture pattern or type specific to NAI.[45] The type of fracture may suggest a possible mechanism that, again, can assist the clinician in attempting to assess the truthfulness of the explanation given by the carers.

In general, a spiral fracture indicates a twisting force; an oblique fracture may result from levering, for instance by lifting a child by a limb; and a transverse fracture may be the result of a direct impact. A greenstick or buckle fracture, commonly seen in toddlers, will be caused by compression in relation to a fall.

Overall, a child with a femoral fracture has approximately a 1 in 3 chance of having being abused, and femoral fractures resulting from abuse are more commonly seen in children who are not yet walking.[45] Similarly, a child under the age of 3 years with a humeral fracture has a 1 in 2 chance of having been abused. Midshaft diaphyseal fractures are more common in abuse than non-abuse, whereas supracondylar fractures are more likely to have non-abusive causes.[45]

The significance of long bone fractures increases when they are multiple (Fig. 80-36), particularly when of different ages, when bilateral, and when associated with clinical findings suggestive of physical abuse.

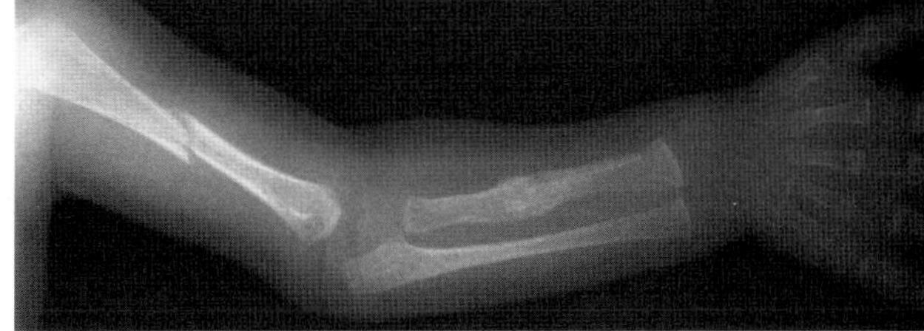

FIGURE 80-36 ■ A recent fracture to the midshaft of the left humerus, and an old, healing fracture to the mid-radius in a 6-week-old girl, highly suggestive of abuse.

Periosteal new bone formation along the shaft of the long bones is a normal feature in up to 35% of infants between the ages of 1 and 3–4 months of age, and should be differentiated from subperiosteal new bone formation (SPNBF) as a result of an occult fracture, or a gripping injury (Fig. 80-37).[90] SPNBF is usually bilateral but can also be unilateral, and most commonly involves the femur or tibia, and less commonly the humerus or forearm.[76] It is confined to the diaphysis and never extends to the metaphysis.

Unusual Fractures

Fractures to the spine, scapula (most commonly the acromion), sternum, pelvis, fingers and toes, in a

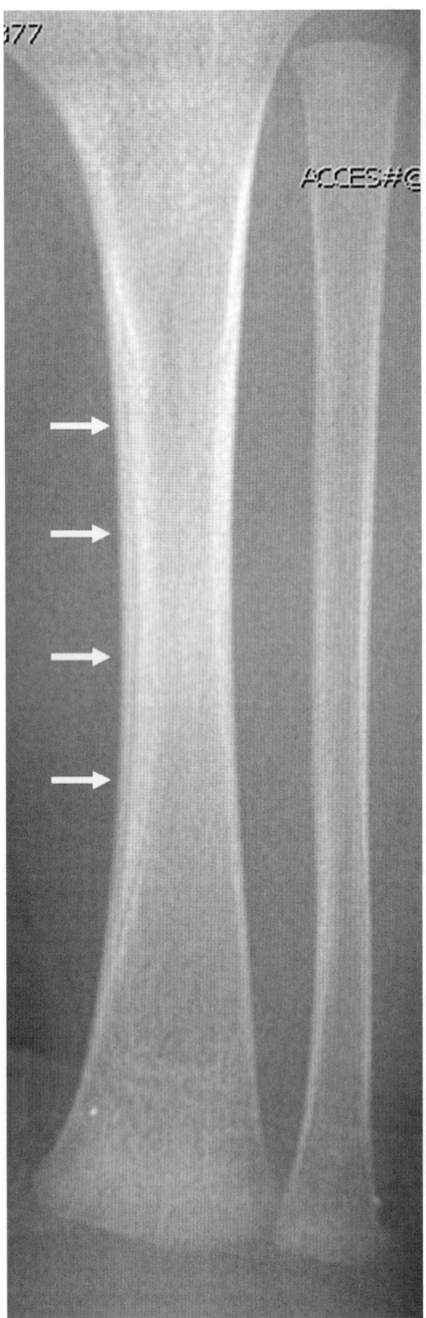

FIGURE 80-37 ■ A smooth band of mineralised density separate from the underlying cortex, not exceeding 2-mm thickness, along the tibial shaft in a 4-week-old, healthy boy, consistent with physiological SPNBF.

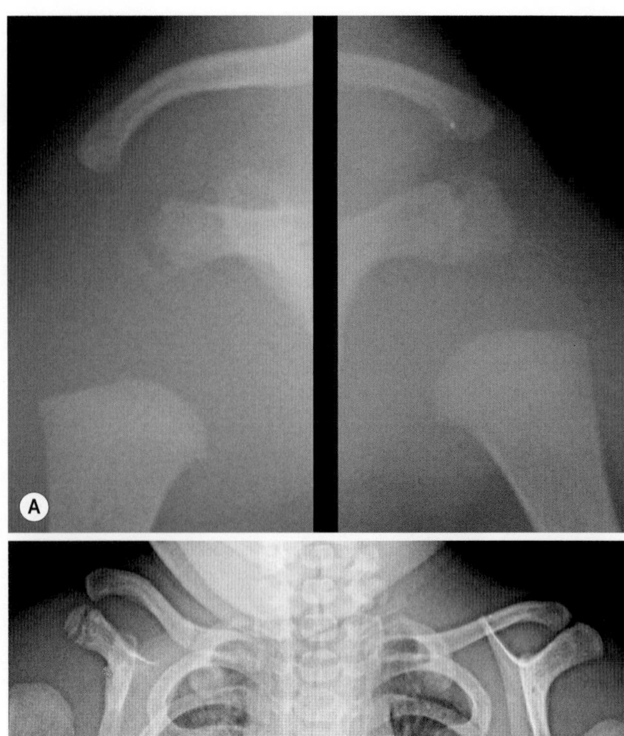

FIGURE 80-38 ■ Lucent, irregular lines with surrounding sclerosis through both acromions in a 3-month-old boy having a skeletal survey for suspected abuse. (A) Initial radiographs and (B) follow-up radiograph after 6 weeks, showing healing of the left, but not the right, suggestive of a healing, left-sided fracture from unrecognised trauma.

non-ambulant child are rare, and should raise concern when no plausible explanation can be provided.

Acromial fractures, which tend to be clinically overt, must be differentiated from normal variations in acromial ossification[76,91] (Fig. 80-38). In acromial fractures, the radiolucent defect appears to be initially smooth or slightly irregular but then, probably within a month, the margins become quite irregular and sclerotic, indicating early healing.[88] More advanced or complete healing of the fracture is usual thereafter. In the developmental anomaly, the margins of the defect remain smooth and corticated for more than a year, becoming thickened and slightly irregular thereafter. The defect becomes progressively narrow and remains visible for 3 years or more. Both injury and ossification defects can be bilateral, but can also be unilateral. Fractures are thought to be the result of indirect forces, and have also been observed in severe neonatal tetanus.

Vertebral compression fractures, particularly to the thoracolumbar region, very occasionally occur during violent shaking.

Fracture Healing

Radiological dating of fractures is of medicolegal importance, but unfortunately the evidence base for current methods of dating is sparse.

Most radiologists date fractures based on their own clinical experience, and guidance offered by textbooks (Table 80-3).[76,92,93] The radiological features of bone healing are a continuum with considerable overlap,[94] and depend on age of the child, fracture site and mobility. A systematic review of the international, scientific literature from 2005 concluded that:[94]

- Radiologists can clearly differentiate recent from old fractures.

TABLE 80-3 **Chronology (in Days) of Radiographic Changes during Fracture Healing[75]**

	Early	Peak	Late
Appearance of SPBNF	4–10	10–14	14–21
Loss of fracture line definition owing to formation of soft callus	10–14	14–21	
Appearance of hard callus (formation of lamellar bone)	14–21	21–42	42–90

- Periosteal reaction is seen as early as 4 days and is present in at least 50% of the cases by 2 weeks after the injury.
- Remodelling peaks 8 weeks after the injury and, moreover, bone scintigraphy has no place in fracture dating, as fractures show increased uptake for as long as a year.

A recent study, addressing the timetable for the radiographic features of fracture healing, concluded that fractures in young children may be dated as acute (< 1 week), recent (8–35 days), or old (≥ 36 days) on the basis of six key radiological features; soft-tissue swelling, periosteal reaction, soft callus, hard callus, bridging and remodelling.[95]

Differential Diagnosis

The differential diagnoses include accidental injury, including birth trauma, and generalised bone disease.

Birth Trauma

Birth trauma most commonly involves the clavicle, femur or humerus, but classical metaphyseal lesions have also been reported.[96] Clavicular fractures typically affect the middle third, and when left sided, must be differentiated from congenital pseudarthrosis. The fracture may be noted during birth, or later when a carer palpates the forming callus. The absence of callus 11 days or more after birth excludes a birth-related injury.

Accidental Injury

The most common explanation offered for a fracture and its plausibility will rest on relating the fracture morphology to the mechanism of injury, radiological age to temporal history of events, and personal and published data on common injuries at different ages. Numerous registries on paediatric injuries and fractures have been established worldwide during the 20 years.

Generalised Bone Disease

Differential considerations for bone injury include metabolic disorders such as rickets; copper deficiency, particularly Menkes syndrome; metaphyseal chondrodysplasia of the Schmid type; spondylometaphyseal dysplasia; corner fractures; and the occasional fragmentation occurring in osteogenesis imperfecta.

BRAIN INJURIES

Brain injuries are a major cause of morbidity and mortality in abused children under 2 years of age.[97] The clinical presentation may be hyperacute (respiratory failure, cerebral oedema), acute or subacute. Again, lack of a plausible explanation to the child's symptoms and clinical findings should raise concern. The clinical signs may be non-specific, such as changes in the mental status, vomiting, pallor, apathy, cyanosis, seizures, and even shock or severe respiratory distress. Children with hypoxic-ischaemic injury often present with apnoea and loss of consciousness. Notably, an interval of several hours to days may exist between the initial trauma and the first neurological manifestations, underscoring the importance of a meticulous medical history.

Differentiation between accidental and non-accidental head injury (NAHI) is of major legal importance, but remains difficult.[98] In one retrospective study, cases in which a perpetrator confessed to violence toward the child were compared with cases in which there was no confession. There was no significant difference between the two groups for any of the variables studied: gender, mortality, fractures, retinal haemorrhage, ecchymosis, symptoms and SDH pattern. In cases with confession, shaking was described as extremely violent (100%) and was repeated (55%) from 2 to 30 times (mean, 10) because it stopped the infant's crying (62.5%). Impact was reported in around a quarter of the cases. No correlation was found between repeated shaking and SDH densities on CT.[99] There is reason to believe that some of the NAHI cases remain undiagnosed, and the converse that is some 'unexplained sudden infant deaths' may represent NAHI.[100]

Pathophysiology of Skull, Brain and Spinal Canal Lesions

From a pathophysiological point of view, NAHI, or abusive head trauma,[54] may be caused by direct trauma with skull fractures and underlying brain damage, repeated trauma, shaking, or even strangulation. These mechanisms could lead to subdural/subarachnoid haemorrhage, contusion and intraparenchymal haemorrhage as well as other injuries such as diffuse axonal (shear) injuries and hypoxic-ischaemic damage.[101–103] The overall prognosis of intracranial lesions in this context is generally relatively pejorative compared to isolated head injuries.

Shaking injuries to the head and neck usually occur in infants younger than 1 year of age, but can be seen up to 2 years. Infants this age have relatively large heads compared to body size, and their neck muscles are weak, providing little head support.[99] Thus, repeat whiplash movements can result in ruptured cortical veins at their influx to the fixed sagittal sinus, with subarachnoid and/or subdural haemorrhage, often bilateral.[55,104,105] Further, axonal injuries can occur in the brain parenchyma due to differences in density between white and grey matter, and also in the midbrain, due to the limited mobility of the upper brainstem (set by the tentorium).

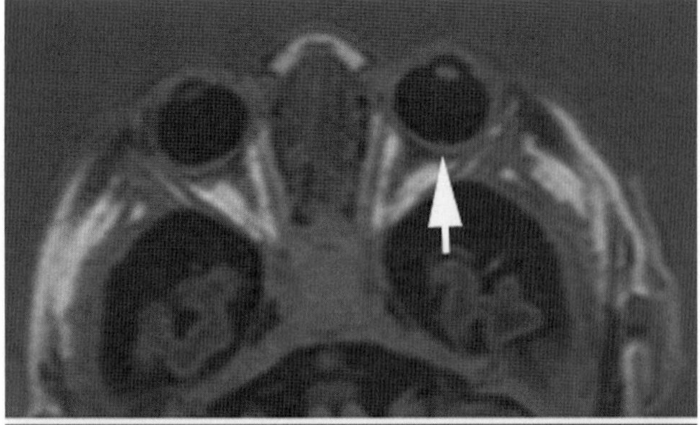

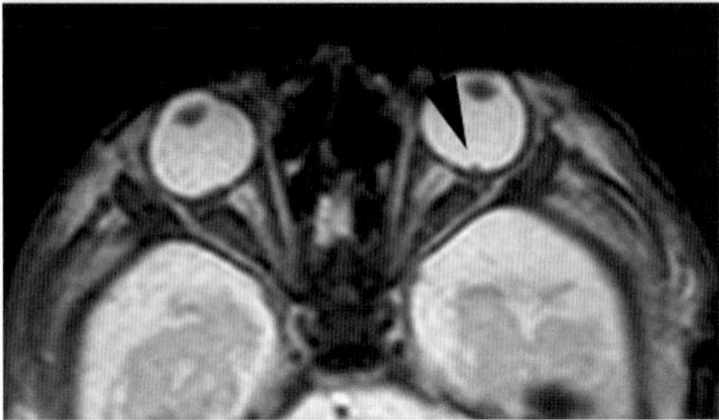

FIGURE 80-39 ■ Axial T1- and T2*-weighted images showing left retinal haemorrhages in a 3-month-old girl with a subdural haematoma. The findings were also demonstrated on fundoscopy.

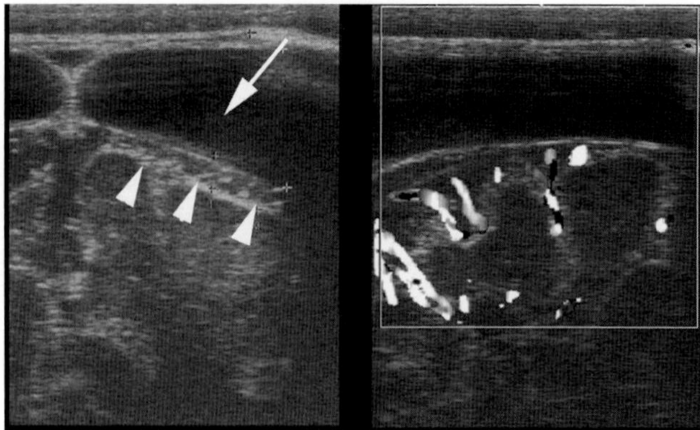

FIGURE 80-40 ■ A 9-month-old boy presenting with hypotonia and macrocrania. Cranial ultrasound demonstrates a bilateral subdural chronic haematoma (arrow) with compressed subarachnoid space (arrowhead) containing vessels between subdural spaces and brain.

Shaking also causes retinal haemorrhages, which must be systematically searched for ophthalmoscopically, and described in detail as to location, severity, extent and bilaterality.[106,107] Notably, both retinal and vitreous haemorrhages can also be seen on MRI (Fig. 80-39).[108,109]

Spinal injuries can be associated with NAHI. Parenchymal cord injury, meningeal haemorrhage (epidural/subdural), nerve root avulsion or ganglion haemorrhages have been reported in post-mortem examinations. They usually occur without evidence of muscular or ligamentous damage, or of bone dislocation or fracture.[110] A recent study demonstrated that 60% of children with abusive head trauma also suffered spinal canal subdural bleeding. The two proposed mechanisms regarding the origin of spinal subdural hemorrhage are mainly tracking of intracranial subdural haemorrhage[104] or, more uncommonly as a consequence of, direct injury to vessels in or around the spinal cord, but within the dural compartment.[111]

Imaging in NAHI

Skull radiographs, including AP and lateral views, are mandatory to demonstrate skull vault fractures. An additional Townes view may help diagnose occipital fractures, as well as the presence and number of Wormian bones, which may be of value for the differential diagnoses, such as osteogenesis imperfecta and Menkes' disease.

The value of head ultrasound is limited in the diagnosis of NAHI; however, it may add useful information when the initial presentation is misleading (macrocrania, stupor).[112] Pericerebral spaces are well seen with high-frequency probes. A subdural haematoma is visible outside the subarachnoid space, as a peripheral anechoic collection limited by a deep echoic thin line separating the two spaces, causing a compression more or less marked on the adjacent cortical sulci (Fig. 80-40). Parenchymal contusions, when located in an area accessible to the probe, at the convexity, can be found with hypoechoic, hypoechoic or cystic lesions, particularly at the junction of grey matter and white matter.

CT is the initial examination in suspected head trauma,[113] and should include thin, contiguous slices of the entire skull and of the craniocervical junction. Parenchymal algorithm reconstructions should be completed by specific bony reconstruction with VRT projections.

MRI is indicated when CT is equivocal or discordant with clinical signs, or to give more details about pericerebral spaces or parenchymal lesions.[114] In most cases sedation or general anaesthesia is required. The examination should include T1-weighted images (two orthogonal planes), T2-weighted (axial or coronal) or gradient-echo T2* to better detect degradation products of haemoglobin; susceptibility-weighted imaging (SWI) is more sensitive for small haemorrhages and is considered as the best tool to depict a bleed. FLAIR can be difficult to analyse during the first months of life, but is also useful for demonstrating an extra-axial, acute bleed.[59]

Diffusion-weighted imaging (DWI) is now mandatory, especially in the initial phase of trauma, to look for hypoxic-ischaemic changes and axonal injuries.[112]

Additional, alternative sequences include MR angiography and MR spectroscopy. Sagittal T1- and T2-weighted images of the spine are useful to detect intraspinal haemorrhage, and should be supplemented with axial scans in cases of equivocal or positive findings.

In most cases, the use of contrast medium, both in CT and MRI, is unnecessary;[112] it may in some cases be useful to confirm the presence of a subdural haematoma.[53,73,115]

Skull Fractures

Most skull fractures, both accidental and abusive, are linear. The presence of bilateral, stellar or depressed fractures or fractures through the midline, increase the clinical suspicion of abuse, in particular when there is a history of a mild trauma or no trauma (fall from a couch).[116] Dating is difficult, as skull fractures heal without any callus formation, within 6 months.

Loss of fracture-line definition can be seen after around 2 weeks' interval. A growing fracture with leptomeningeal cyst formation is more commonly seen in NAHI than in accidental injury. With CT, some parallel linear fractures in the plane of slices may be missed, highlighting the need for conventional radiographs. CT with thin sections and 3D volume reconstruction and VRT views are useful to demonstrate these fractures[53] (Fig. 80-41). Bone scintigraphy, on the other hand, may fail to visualise skull fractures due to low osteoblastic activity during fracture repair.

Extra-Axial Haemorrhages

Acute extradural haemorrhage is rare, and can be found in both abusive and accidental head injury.[113]

Subarachnoid haemorrhage (SAH) is better seen in the initial phase with CT than with conventional T1 and T2 WSE MRI,[117] but FLAIR (hyperintensity) and SWI (hypointensity) are still sensitive. In young infants, the diagnosis may be overdiagnosed on CT since the difference in density between the dura and parenchyma is higher than in the older child.

Subdural haematoma (SDH) is the most frequent haemorrhage encountered in NAHI. It is caused by the primary trauma, and not secondary hypoxia or brain swelling.[101,118] At the time of presentation, SDHs can be acute, subacute or chronic and seen as a hyper-, iso- or hypodense collection, respectively, on CT.[109]

In the context of abuse, SDHs are frequently bilateral, closely related to the falx, layering over the tentorium and then highly suggestive of abuse, especially if they are accompanied by cerebral oedema[116] (Figs. 80-42A-C). Haemorrhages can also occur within the falx itself.[119,120] In accidental trauma, SDHs are mainly localised over the cerebral convexities, while involvement of the posterior fossa is more common in abusive trauma.

MRI is more sensitive than CT for detecting small collections, and is also useful in the differentiation between CSF in the subarachnoidal space and chronic SDHs in cases where the CT scan shows low-attenuation extra-axial fluid[116] (Figs. 80-42B, 80-43A, B and 80-44A, B). Dating of haemorrhages is inaccurate on both CT and MRI.[101,121] After the acute phase, several concentric compartments can be seen within the SDH, with different signal regarding the weighted sequences. Is appears very difficult to affirm that they correspond to repetitive trauma, or to give a specific calendar of these bleedings, because in case of SDH, new spontaneous bleedings can occur within the first one.

Moreover, in terms of differential diagnosis, it should be remembered that a subdural collection is not necessarily related to abuse, but may also occur in children with 'benign macrocrania', with enlarged transitional subarachnoid spaces and tensioning of the cortical veins. Searching for an association between a sudden increase in head circumference and intraparenchymal lesions is therefore important in order to avoid overdiagnosis of NAHI.[104,109,122,123]

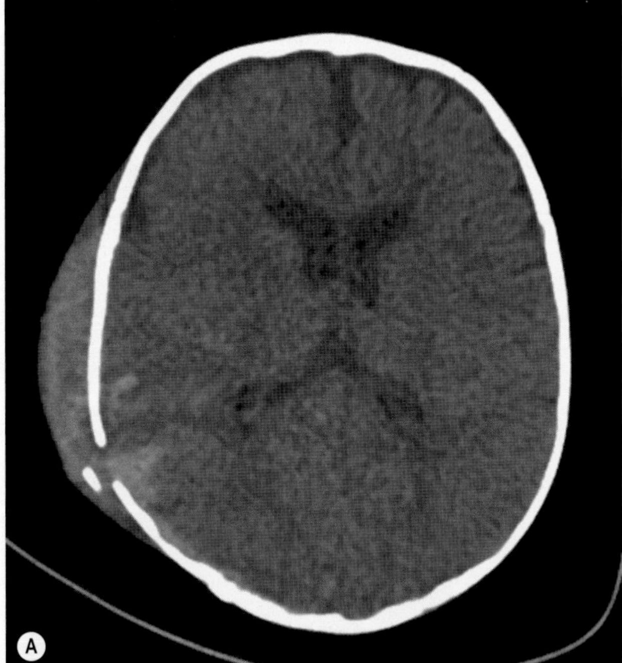

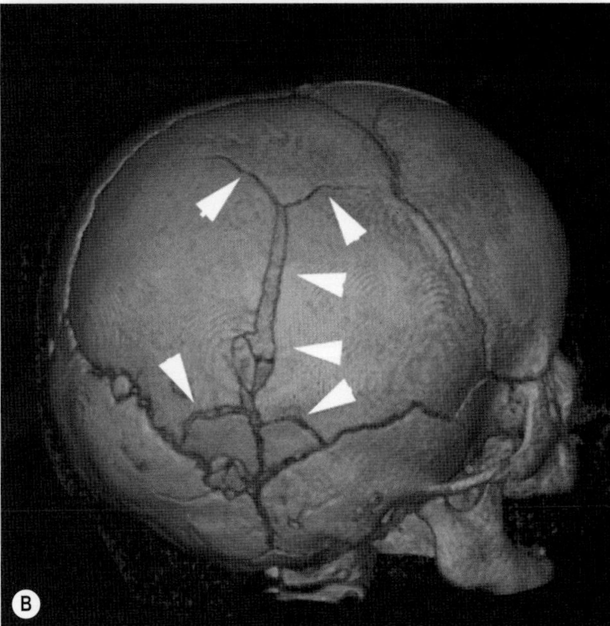

FIGURE 80-41 ■ (A) Cerebral CT in a 6-month-old boy, showing a soft-tissue swelling in the right parietal region with an underlying skull fracture and haemorrhagic brain contusions. The baby had been thrown to the floor. (B) A 3D reconstruction of the skull, demonstrating a stellar parietal fracture.

It remains difficult, without previous imaging studies demonstrating a 'benign' enlargement of subarachnoid spaces, to affirm that an acute or subacute SDH is present only in relation to this pre-existent situation.[53,124] Other

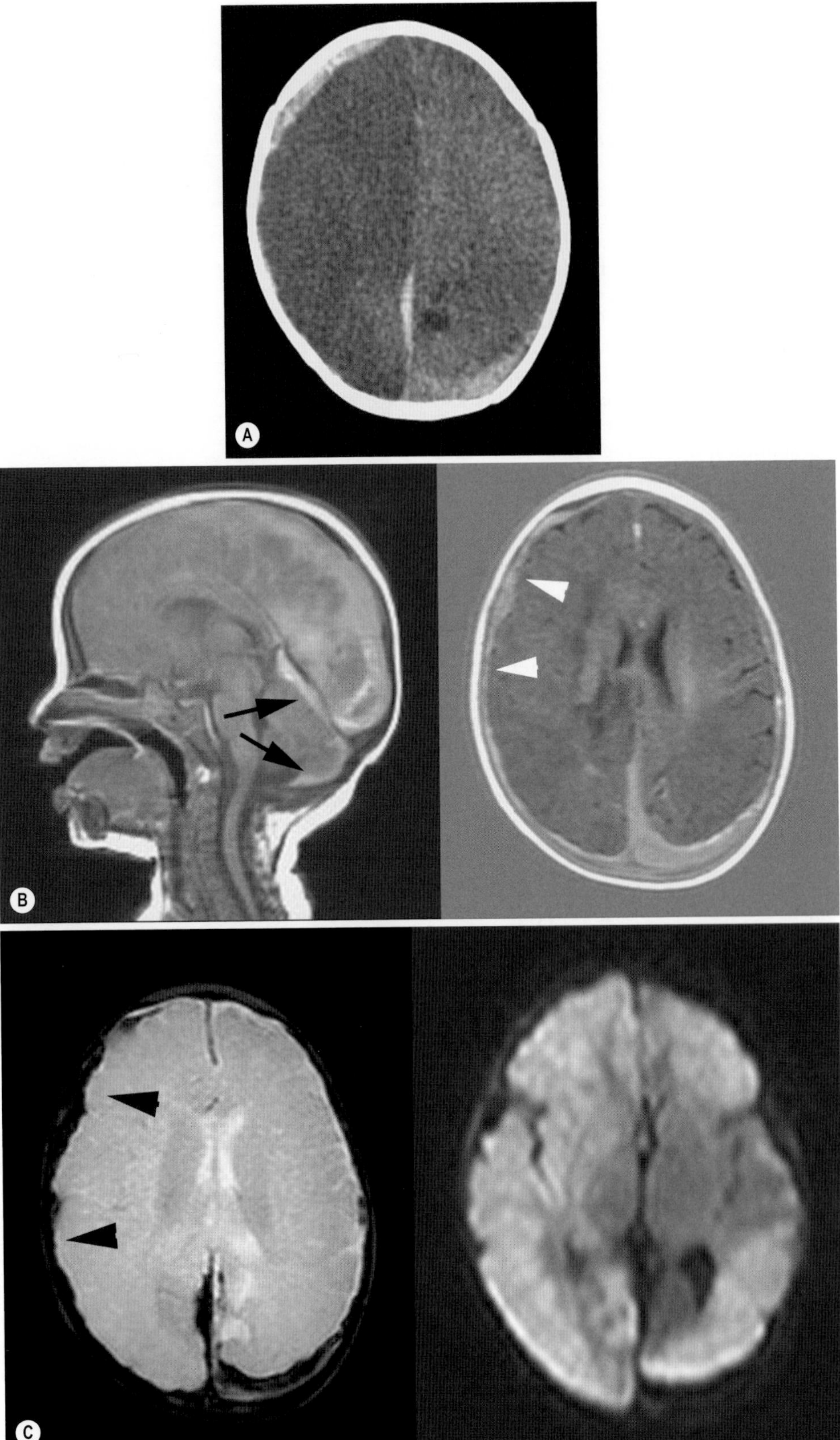

FIGURE 80-42 ■ (A) A 4-month-old girl presenting with apnoea and loss of consciousness. The initial CT demonstrated acute, subdural haematomas in the right frontal and left parietal regions, a haemorrhage within the posterior part of the falx and oedema of the right hemisphere with loss of grey–white matter differentiation. (B) Continuing, sagittal and axial T1-weighted MR images confirmed the hemispheric subdural acute haematoma (arrowheads). Note also a subdural bleeding within the posterior fossa (arrows). (C) Continuing, an axial T2*-weighted MR image shows hypointensity in relation to blood. Diffusion-weighted image confirms restriction of water diffusion within the right hemisphere, but also in the left frontal and parietal lobes.

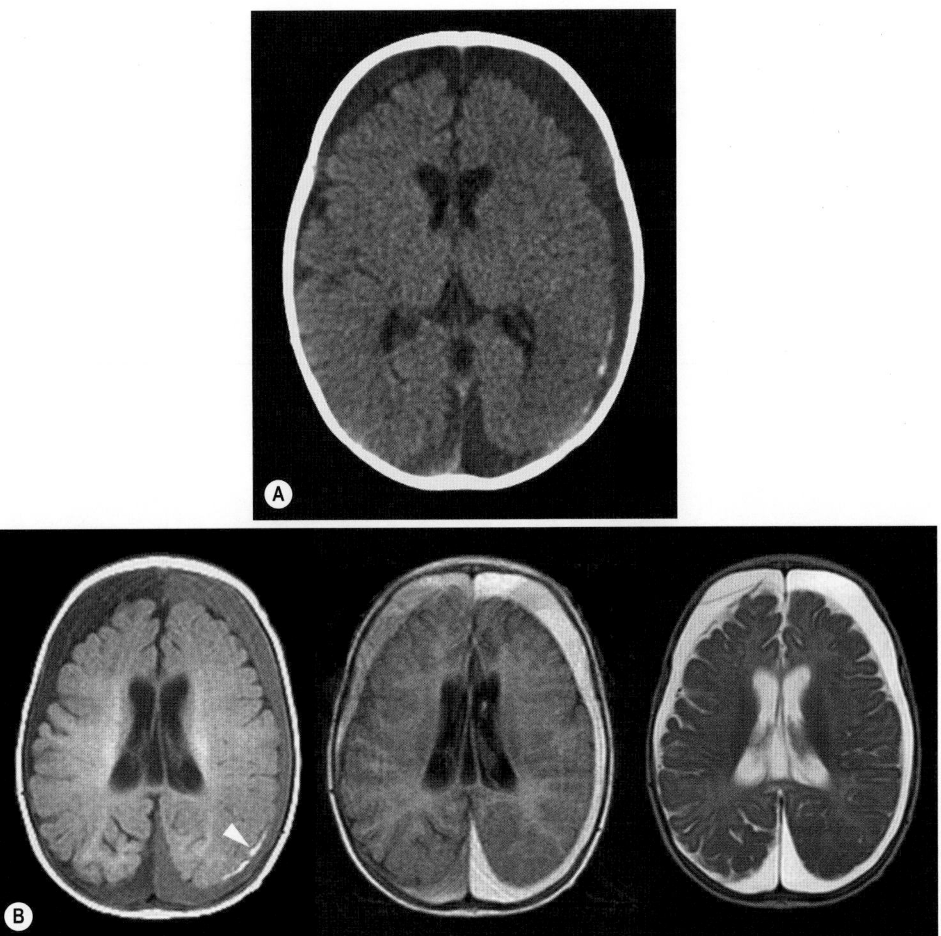

FIGURE 80-43 ■ (A) A 4-month-old boy, somnolent, presenting with a right periorbital haematoma. CT demonstrated subacute, subdural collections bilaterally, with recent bleeding on the left side. (B) Continuing, MRI performed 3 days later. Axial T1, flair and T2-weighted images. Right and left subdural collections exhibit different signal intensities, maybe in relation to different bleeding but also to blood concentration in each collection. Note also subarachnoid bleeding on the left side, better seen on T1 (arrowhead). Skeletal survey revealed multiple rib fractures.

options to be considered would be coagulopathies, subdural collections after acute dehydratation or meningitis, or in relation to congenital metabolic diseases, such as glutaric aciduria type I or Menke's disease.

Intraventricular haemorrhage may occur in the 'shaken baby' in connection with a subependymal venous injury, and is easily detected on CT in the acute phase. On MRI, changes on T2*-weighted or SWI sequences will remain for a while. Secondary, obstructive hydrocephalus may be seen.

Parenchymal Brain Injuries

Focal or generalised brain injury can be related to the severity of the trauma itself, or to hypoxic-ischaemic change. CT is useful for detecting focal haemorrhages in the acute phase, while MRI is more sensitive for their recognition at any stage.

Intraparenchymal haemorrhagic contusions, visible at the white matter and cortex junction, are spontaneously hyperdense on CT in the acute phase and become hypodense after a few days. They are also secondarily better seen with MRI, due to the presence of degradation products of haemoglobin, with increased signal intensity on T1, at the intermediate phase, then a low signal on T2*, SWI in the late phase (Fig. 80-44C). It may, however, be difficult, once again, to precisely date the haemorrhage.[73] Non-haemorrhagic lesions are well depicted by MRI. Multiple subcortical lesions affect the neurodevelopmental outcome and prognosis.[125]

Shearing lesions (diffuse axonal lesions) are sought in the subcortical region, but also at the centrum ovale, in the corpus callosum and the cerebral peduncles. They can be haemorrhagic, and then initially visible on CT, or in most of cases non-haemorrhagic: MRI (FLAIR, T2 and DWI) is then essential to demonstrate them.[126] DWI is useful to look for changes in regional brain anisotropy and fibre tracking helps to characterise axonal lesions, although this is not routine clinical practice.

Diffuse Hypoxic-Ischaemic Lesions

The association of focal ischaemic lesions, in multiple locations, either in the MCA territory, with a subarachnoid haemorrhage is highly suggestive of abuse. Ischaemic lesions preferentially involve the basal ganglia. Moreover, the lesions are more diffuse, preserving only the posterior fossa (especially in lesions resulting from

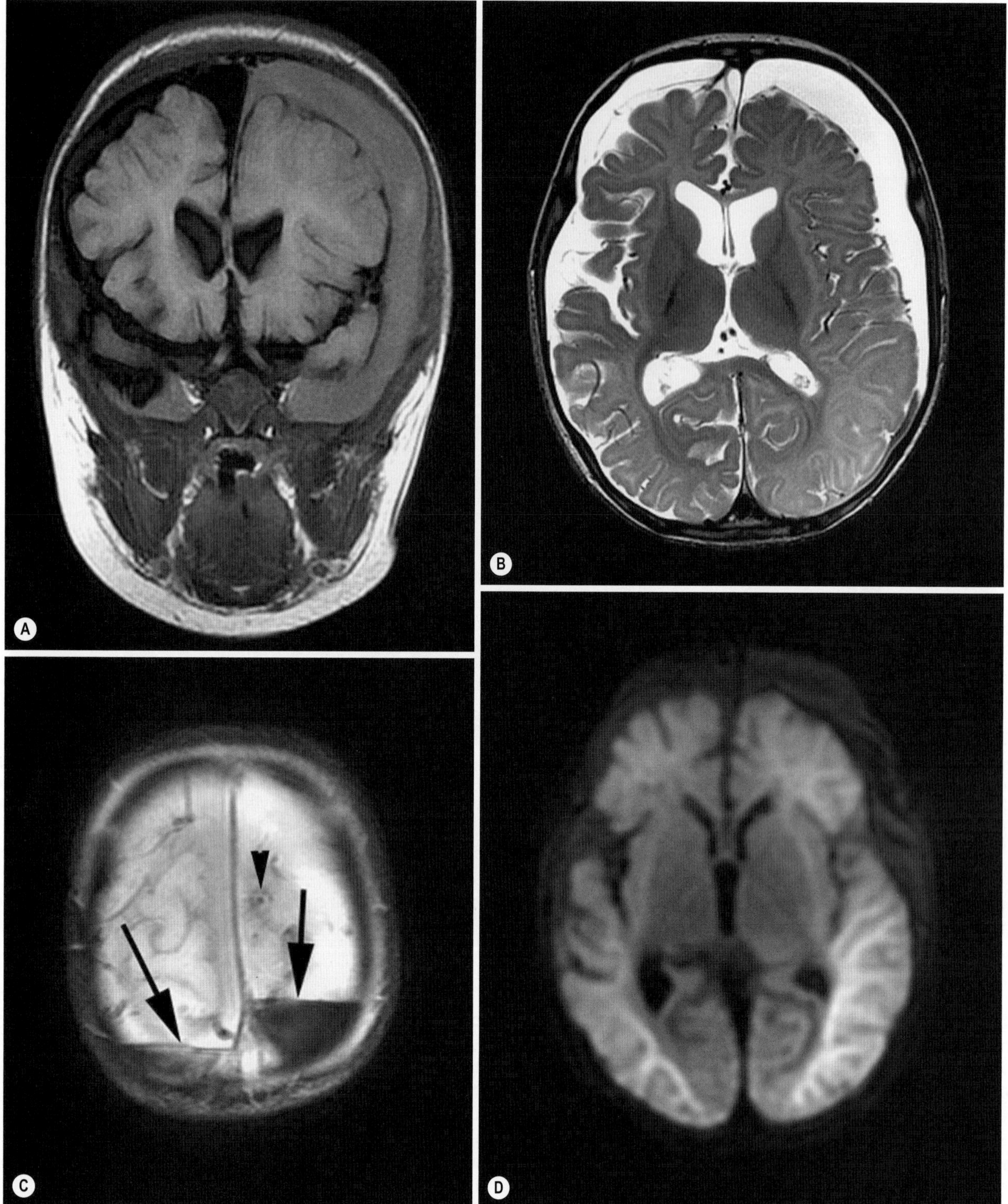

FIGURE 80-44 ■ (A) A 4-month-old boy. Macrocrania, malaise. Coronal FLAIR image demonstrates circumferential bilateral subdural collections. (B) Continuing, T2 axial slice confirms subdural collections, with hyperintensity of the posterior regions of the brain. (C) Continuing, susceptibity-weighted image shows punctiform parenchyma bleeding (arrowhead) and fluid–fluid levels within the surrounding subdural collections. (D) Continuing, diffusion-weighted image better demonstrates bilateral cortico-subcortical ischaemic lesions.

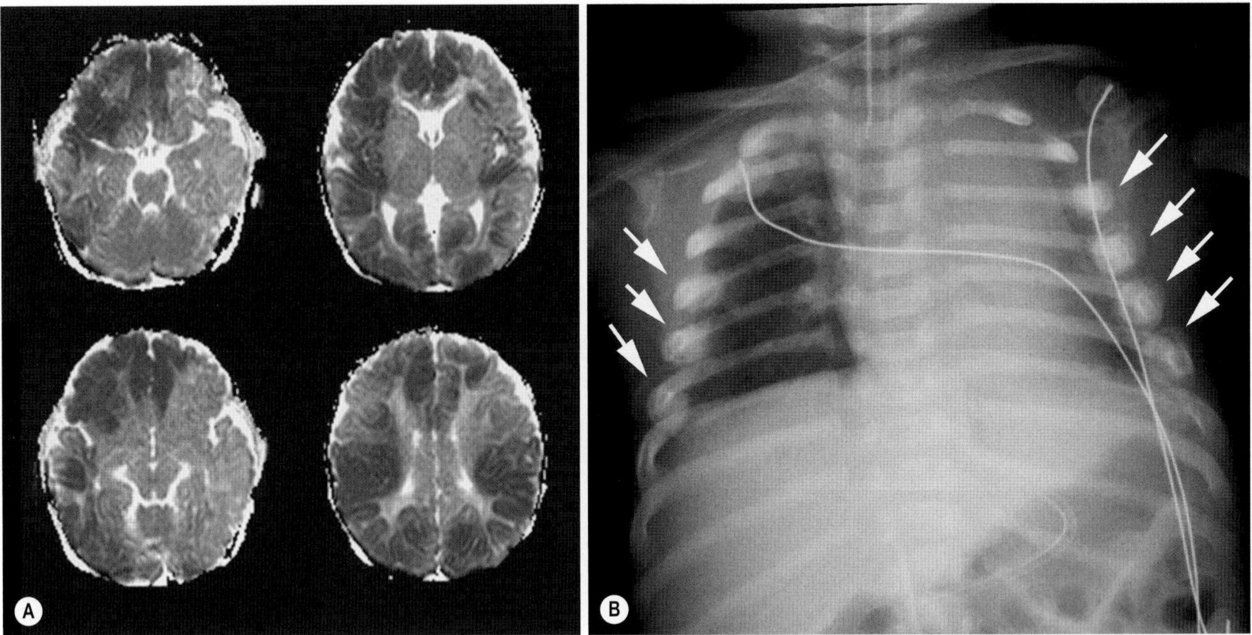

FIGURE 80-45 ■ (A) A 3-month-old girl. Sudden pallor, loss of consciousness, then seizures; blood found with lumbar puncture. DWI with ADC maps reveals multiple ischaemic lesions. (B) Continuing, chest radiographs after resuscitation in the intensive care unit: multiple rib fractures with callus (arrows). Shaken baby.

strangulation), sometimes associated with specific signs of shock.

CT may show parenchymal hypoattenuation or loss of grey–white matter differentiation, and the 'reversal sign', where the cerebellum is of higher attenuation than the cerebral hemispheres. MRI with DWI is very sensitive in demonstrating early hypoxic-ischaemic changes, by demonstrating cytotoxic oedema with restriction of water diffusion (Figs. 80-42C, 80-42D and 80-45). MR spectroscopy adds some prognostic information when a high relative concentration of lactate, compared to creatine and *N*-acetylaspartate (NAA), is obvious[53,109] (Fig. 80-46). CT or MRI will secondarily depict late outcome with brain atrophy or multicystic encephalomalacia.[127]

Intraspinal Lesions

Spinal injuries in NAHI are believed to be underdiagnosed,[110,128] and additional MRI series covering the whole spine are therefore recommended by some authors.[111] Signal abnormality of the cord may suggest contusion or infarction. Haemorrhage in the epidural or subdural spaces is suspected when there is a nodular or smooth dural thickening, a mass effect upon the cord and/or effacement of the subarachnoid space. Recognition of the normal epidural fat allows for distinction between epidural or subdural location.[111] Spinal ultrasound represents a valuable alternative to demonstrate a spinal subdural haematoma.[129]

Strategy and Prognosis

In summary, the initial work-up of children having sustained a head injury should include skull radiographs, an unenhanced head CT and an ophthalmic examination.

In the majority of cases, MRI is indicated to better depict the parenchymal lesions and is particularly useful for follow-up. The MRI should include T1-weighted series, T2, T2* or SWI and DWI. The assessment and report should preferably be done by a neuroradiologist or a paediatric radiologist with experience in NAHI cases, and should include a thorough description of the nature and the extent of the lesions, possible mechanisms and possible differential diagnoses. Dating intracranial lesions should be performed with caution.[113] The evaluation of head injuries in infants requires a high level of awareness and thorough and systematic examination by a trained multidisciplinary team.[57,98]

Overall, prognosis is worse in NAHI than in accidental trauma. Parenchymal haemorrhages and cerebral contusions, better seen on MRI with SWI and DWI, correlate with poor clinical outcome.[130] Preventative efforts must be focused within the child welfare system, assisting parents and caregivers as well as child welfare professionals to facilitate early identification of abusive head injury.[54,131,132]

ABDOMINAL AND CHEST INJURIES

Non-accidental skeletal and cerebral trauma are features of the non-ambulant child, whilst visceral injuries are common after the child is mobile, with an average age of 2 years.[51] The incidence of these injuries is lower than that reported for skeletal and head injury, but the mortality rate is as high as 50%.

This could be related to the vague clinical history at presentation and consequent delayed diagnosis.[76] The clinical presentation can be acute, with symptoms

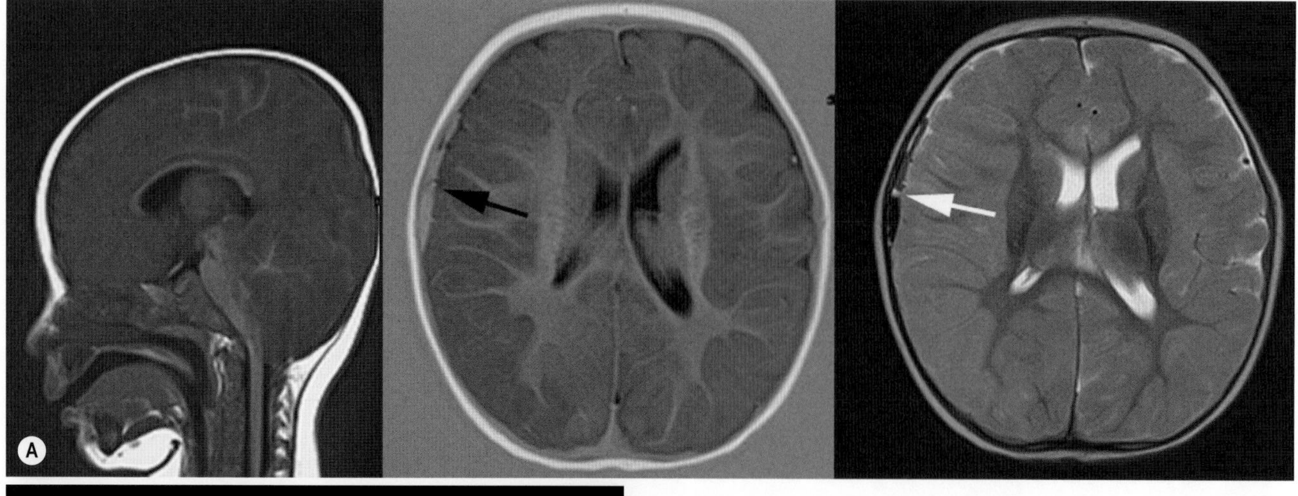

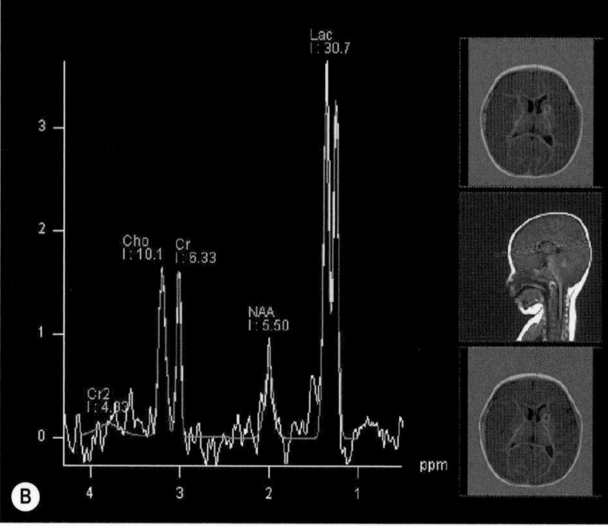

FIGURE 80-46 ■ (A) A 4-month-old boy. Acute respiratory distress, admitted for near-miss syndrome. Sagittal and axial T1-weighted images, axial T2-weighted slice demonstrate massive brain oedema without visibility of cerebral cisterns. Note also subdural bleeding on the right side (arrows). (B) Continiuing, MR spectroscopy demonstrates a low *N*-acetylaspartate (NAA) peak and a very high concentration of lactate. Post-mortem pathological confirmation of an acute subdural haematoma with rupture of bridging veins.

suggestive of perforation, obstruction or bleeding, such as vomiting, severe pain, tenderness, shock or sepsis.

Others may present with more ill-defined, chronic symptoms like weight loss, malaise or non-specific abdominal pain. The radiologist should be familiar with the different scenarios, and also be aware that incidental findings, e.g. rib fractures on an abdominal radiograph, may represent markers for abuse. The most common abdominal injuries involve the duodenum, pancreas and mesentery, but injuries to the liver, kidney and spleen also occur. Injuries to the chest are rare, and include pneumothorax/pneumomediastinum, haemothorax, chylothorax, contusions to the lung and heart, as well as injuries to the oesophagus.

Imaging

In unstable patients, a focused assessment with sonography (FAST) ultrasound, which has now become an extension of the physical examination of the trauma patient, should be considered. Performed in the trauma room by properly trained and credentialed staff, it allows the timely diagnosis of potentially life-threatening haemorrhage and is a decision-making tool to help determine the need for transfer to the operating room, CT scanner or angiography suite.

CT scans of the chest, abdomen and/or the pelvis are indicated if there are signs and symptoms of abuse or if abnormal findings are seen on conventional radiography, particularly if there is a discrepancy with clinical history.[56]

The chest scan should generally be performed with intravenous contrast to detect vascular injuries, while CT scans for suspected intra-abdominal injury should include contrast-enhanced images of both the abdomen and pelvis, as well as oral contrast where possible.

For a full list of references, please see ExpertConsult.

CHAPTER 81

Bone Tumours and Neuroblastoma in Children

Paul Humphries • Claudio Granata

CHAPTER OUTLINE

This chapter should be read in conjunction with the descriptions of bone tumours in adults (see Chapters 47 and 48).

BONE TUMOURS

The most common presenting symptom of bone neoplasms is skeletal pain. Plain radiography remains the first diagnostic step. Lesion location, appearance and patient age may help suggest a diagnosis. Magnetic resonance imaging (MRI) defines soft tissue, intramedullary extent, joint involvement and relationship to muscular compartments and neurovascular structures. If a malignant lesion is suspected, computed tomography (CT) of the chest and bone scintigraphy are used to evaluate distant metastatic disease.

In the paediatric population, unusual clinical presentation, suspected metastatic spread from an unknown primary, adult-type neoplasms, chemo- and radiotherapy-induced malignancies and tumours associated with genetic syndromes may lead to diagnostic dilemmas. Imaging must be closely coordinated with clinical assessment and histology. It is essential that all potentially malignant lesions in children be referred to an expert centre with an appropriate multidisciplinary team so that discussion about potential biopsy is discussed with the surgeon and oncologists who will be responsible for future care. A biopsy should be obtained through tissue planes related to subsequent surgery to avoid the risk of tumour seeding, and this may avoid contamination of uninvolved muscle compartments.[1]

The aim of initial tumour assessment is to differentiate aggressive from chronic disease and to distinguish benign from malignant lesions (Table 81-1).[2]

MALIGNANT BONE TUMOURS

Primary bone tumours have a peak incidence between 10 and 20 years, with Ewing's sarcoma family of tumours most commonly occurring before 9 years and osteosarcoma most common between 10 and 29 years.[3]

Osteosarcoma

Osteogenic sarcoma (OS) is the most common primary malignant tumour of bone in children and accounts for 55% of all bone tumours seen in adolescence. The aetiology is unknown but there are recognised associations with previous retinoblastoma, prior alkylating agent treatment, prior radiotherapy and some genetic syndromes, such as Rothmund–Thomson syndrome. Often, patients have a history of trauma, which brings the problem to clinical attention.

Radiographically, OS is variable but most frequently appears as a destructive metaphyseal long bone lesion, with poorly demarcated margins, osteoid production, aggressive periosteal reaction and a soft-tissue mass (Fig. 81-1). The lesion may cross the growth plate. Locoregional staging is performed using MRI and pulmonary metastatic disease using CT. Distant bony metastases are usually assessed using scintigraphy.

MRI staging should include wide field-of-view T1-weighted sequences to assess the entire bone involved,

TABLE 81-1 Types of Bone Tumours Seen in Children

Type of Tumour	Benign	Malignant
Bone forming	Osteoid osteoma, osteoblastoma, enostosis	Osteosarcoma
Fibro-osseous	Non-ossifying fibroma, fibrous dysplasia, osteofibrous dysplasia	Fibrosarcoma, malignant fibrous histiocytoma
Cartilage forming	Enchondroma, chondroblastoma, chondromyxoid fibroma, osteochondroma	Chondrosarcoma
Vascular/connective tissue	Haemangioma, lymphangioma, myofibrosis, Gorham's disease	Haemangiopericytoma
Cystic	Simple bone cyst, aneurysmal bone cyst	
Small round cells		Ewing's sarcoma family of tumours, lymphoma
Other	Langerhans cell histiocytosis	

Modified from Wootton-Gorges S L 2009 MR imaging of primary bone tumors and tumor-like conditions in children. Magn Reson Imaging Clin N Am 17(3):469–487.[2]

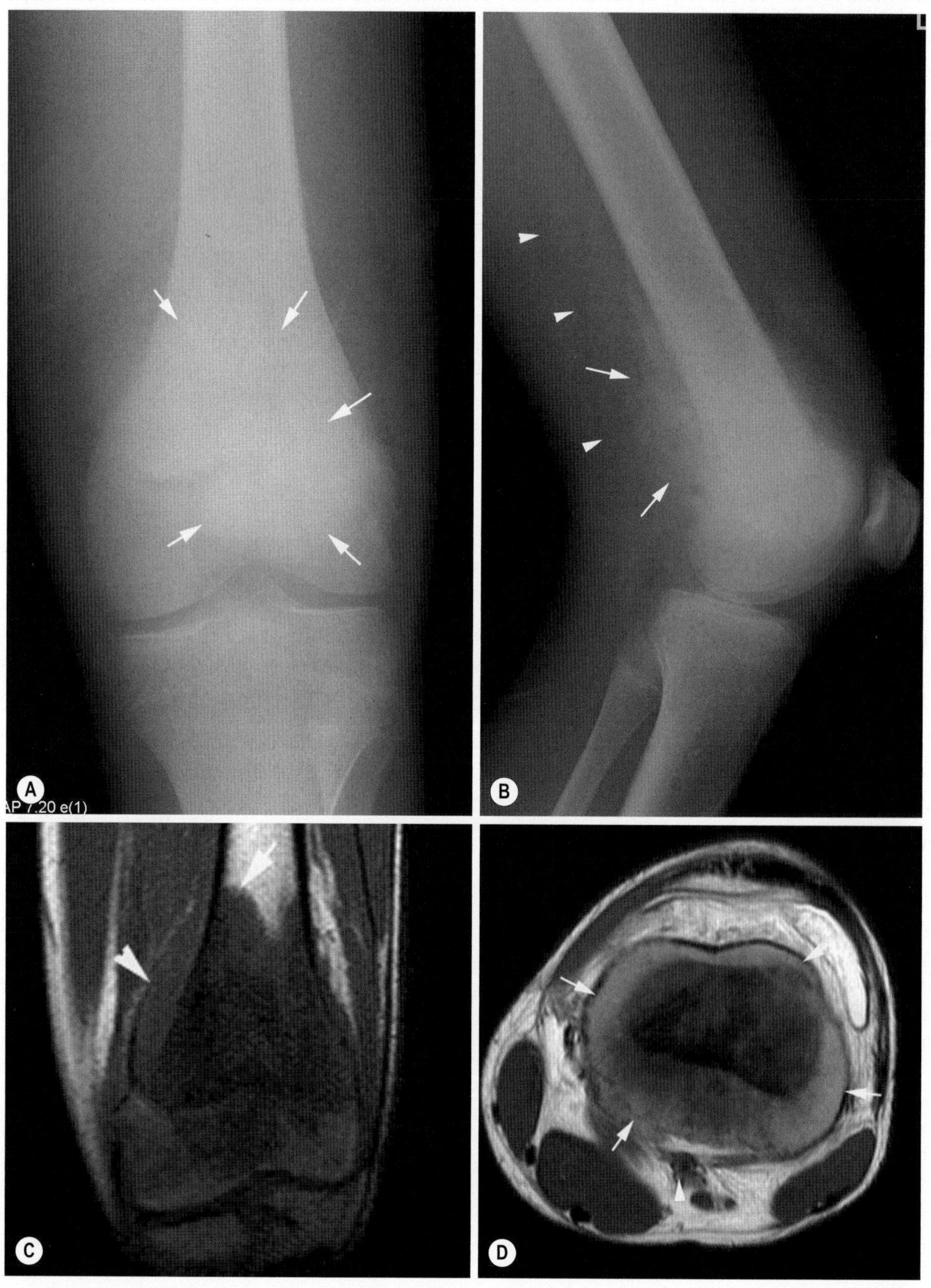

FIGURE 81-1 ■ Osteosarcoma. AP radiograph (A) showing a poorly defined dense lesion within the distal left femoral metaphysis, crossing the growth plate into the epiphysis (short arrows). Lateral radiograph (B) demonstrating new bone formation (short arrows) and displacement of surrounding fat planes by an extraosseous mass. Coronal T1-weighted MRI (C) showing both the intramedullary tumour (arrow) and extraosseous soft-tissue mass (arrowhead). Axial PD-weighted MRI (D) demonstrating the circumferential nature of the extraosseous soft-tissue mass (arrows) and the relationship to the popliteal neurovascular bundle (arrowhead).

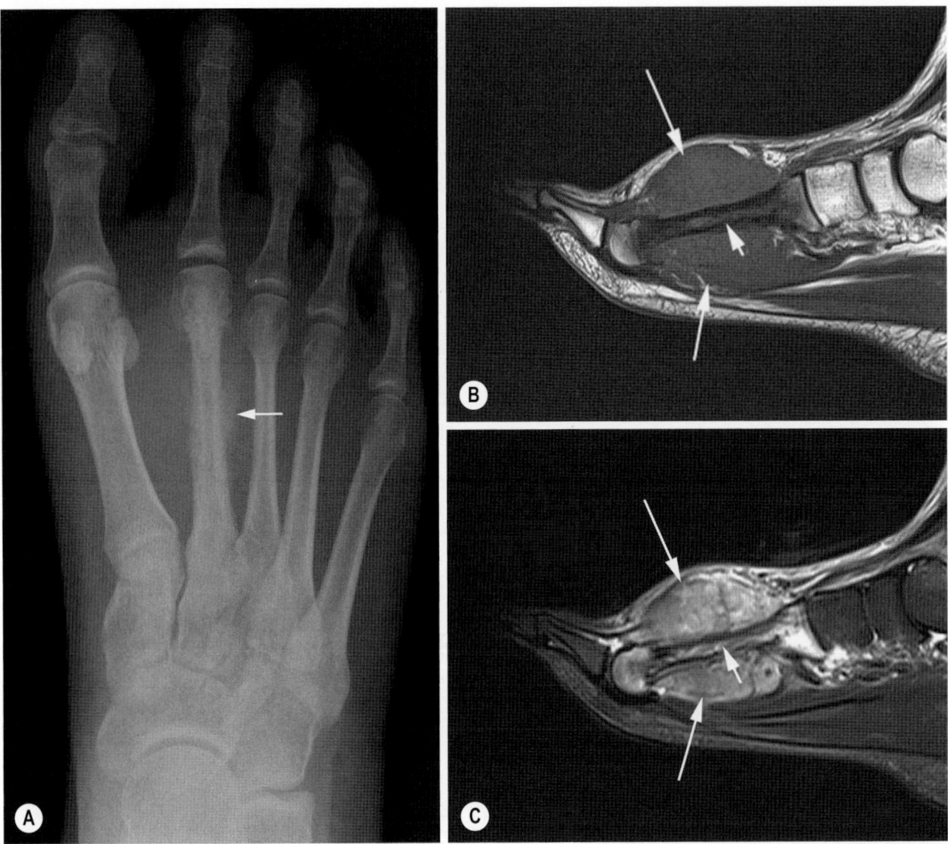

FIGURE 81-2 ■ **Ewing's sarcoma.** DP radiograph (A) demonstrating a periosteal reaction of the second metatarsal. Sagittal T1- (B) and STIR-weighted MRI (C) showing a surrounding soft-tissue mass (long arrows) and bone marrow replacement (short arrows).

and the contralateral side to look for skip and synchronous contralateral lesions.

Paediatric OS variants include telangiectatic OS characterised by dilated blood-filled cavities, periosteal OS arising from the deep periosteal layer and high-grade surface OS involving the bone surface.

Treatment with chemotherapy may lead to a decrease in tumour volume, haemorrhagic signal change and organisation of periosteal reaction. Diffusion-weighted imaging, dynamic MRI contrast imaging and positron emission tomography are all said to assess tumour response and necrosis fraction, an important prognostic indicator, but these are currently research tools.[4–6]

Ewing's Sarcoma Family of Tumours (ESFTs)

ESFTs are the second most common bone tumour in adolescents and children. The pathogenesis of ESFT is unknown. ESFT occurs more commonly in adolescents but a peak of incidence in very young children is well recognised. Classically, flat bone involvement (such as ribs or iliac crest) is seen in ESFT, but any bone may be involved, with 50% arising in the femur or pelvis.

The clinical presentation is non-specific: local pain, fever and swelling can mimic an acute osteomyelitis, delaying the diagnosis. Children with a chest wall tumour usually present with pain. The destructive rib lesion is often initially overlooked and by the time of diagnosis, a pleural effusion is usually present. Metastatic spread is haematogenous, and metastases occur to the lungs, bones and bone marrow. Lymph node, liver and skip metastases are rare. Radiographic features include a permeative appearance, with an 'onion skin' periosteal reaction. There is often a large associated soft-tissue mass (Fig. 81-2), which in the case of pelvic origin tumours may not be clinically apparent and radiographically may be difficult to interpret, possibly delaying diagnosis. ESFT staging is as for OS; however, PET may have some advantages over scintigraphy in evaluating bone metastases in ESFT.[7]

Bone Metastases

Bone metastases are not as common in children when compared to adults. Metastases as the first manifestation of a primary tumour are unusual, as the primary tumour is usually evident initially. Metastatic bone disease in children is most frequently due to leukaemia and neuroblastoma, but lymphoma, ESFT, rhabdomyosarcoma and medulloblastoma may metastasise to bone (Figs. 81-3 and 81-4).

Lytic appearances ± periosteal reaction are the most common radiographic characteristics in metastatic locations, but sclerotic lesions are also reported, particularly in medulloblastoma and leukaemia. Metaphyseal radiolucent lines are typically described in leukaemia and, less commonly, neuroblastoma. Bone scintigraphy, MRI or

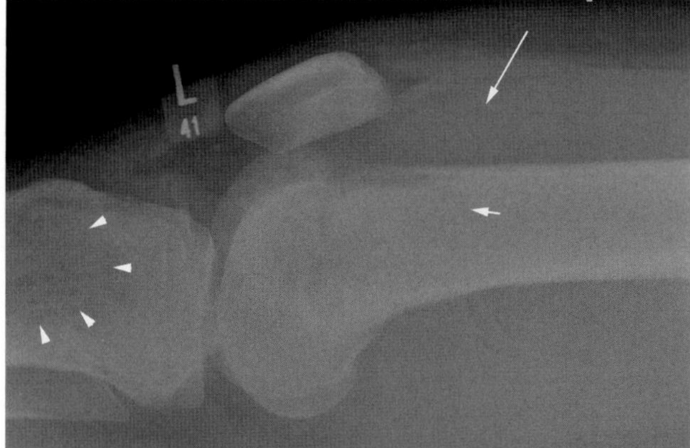

FIGURE 81-3 ■ **Leukaemic infiltration.** Lateral knee radiograph showing an ill-defined permeative osteolytic lesion within the tibia (arrowheads), further permeative lesion within the distal femur (short arrow) and an associated joint effusion (long arrow).

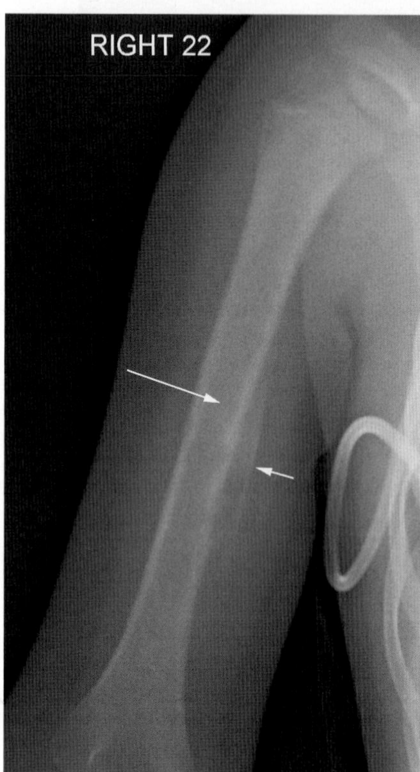

FIGURE 81-4 ■ **Neuroblastoma metastases.** AP humeral radiograph demonstrating an ill-defined permeative appearance of the right humerus (long arrow), with an associated periosteal reaction (short arrow). Note the similarity to the lesions in Fig. 81-3.

metaiodobenzylguanidine (mIBG) studies may be utilised, depending on the clinical scenario.

Rare Malignant Bone Tumours in Children

- Chondrosarcoma
- Primary malignant lymphoma of bone
- Haemangiosarcoma of bone.

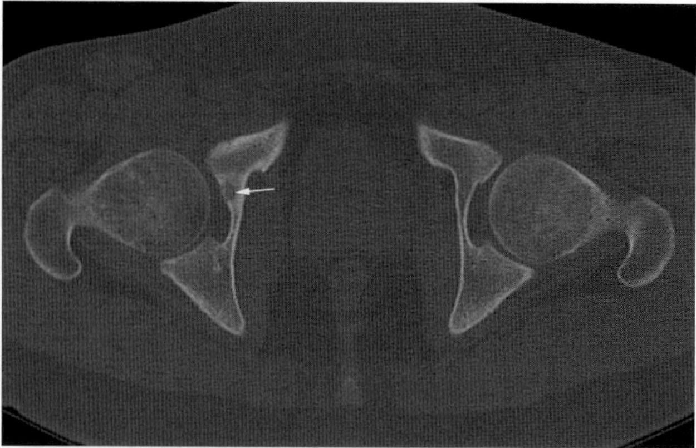

FIGURE 81-5 ■ **Pelvic osteoid osteoma.** Axial CT section depicting a central nidus within the right iliac bone (arrow), with surrounding bony sclerosis.

BENIGN BONE TUMOURS

Bone-Forming Tumours

- Enostosis (bone island)
- Osteoid osteoma
- Osteoblastoma.

Osteoid Osteoma

This painful lesion composed of woven bone and osteiod occurs in children and adolescents but more than 80% of cases occur in the second decade of life.[8] The pain is typically worse at night, relieved by aspirin. Classically, lesions occur in tubular bones but they may also affect the vertebral appendages, presenting clinically with painful scoliosis, seen as a dense pedicle, or are identified following positive scintigraphy. Osteoid osteoma may be polyostotic.

Plain radiographs, supplemented by CT with direct visualisation of a central nidus and surrounding sclerotic reaction, provide the diagnosis (Fig. 81-5). Sometimes, the nidus may contain calcification. On MRI, cortical thickening returns low signal on all sequences. The nidus has a variable appearance depending on the site and relative amounts of osteoid and matrix.[9] There may be prominent soft-tissue or bone marrow oedema, which may lead to diagnostic confusion (Fig. 81-6).

A typical tumour pattern on three-phase skeletal scintigrams is described, characterised by focal hypervascularity and high uptake.[10] A negative scintigram excludes the presence of osteoid osteoma. Scintigraphy can confirm recurrence or incomplete removal if pain persists following surgery. Historically, surgical treatment has been the mainstay; however, image-guided ablation therapy, for example using radiofrequency, is now possible.[11]

Osteoblastoma

Osteoblastoma is rare and difficult to differentiate histologically from osteoid osteoma, whilst, radiographically, it is distinct, with a nidus measuring greater than 1.5–2 cm in diameter.[12] The main site is the posterior elements of the spine. Radiographically, osteoblastoma is expansile, and may be either lucent or sclerotic, with a sclerotic rim (Figs. 81-7 and 81-8). The cortex may occasionally be broken. There is usually surrounding oedema (Fig. 81-9).

Tumours of Fibrous Tissue Origin

- Non-ossifying fibroma (NOF)
- Metaphyseal fibrous cortical defects
- Fibrous bone dysplasia (Jaffe–Lichtenstein) (FBD)
- Osteofibrous bone dysplasia (Campanacci) (OBD)

Non-Ossifying Fibroma and Metaphyseal Fibrous Cortical Defects (Synonyms: Fibroxanthoma, Benign Fibrous Histiocytoma)

Although histologically different, these two lesions appear radiologically similar, NOF being greater than 2 cm in

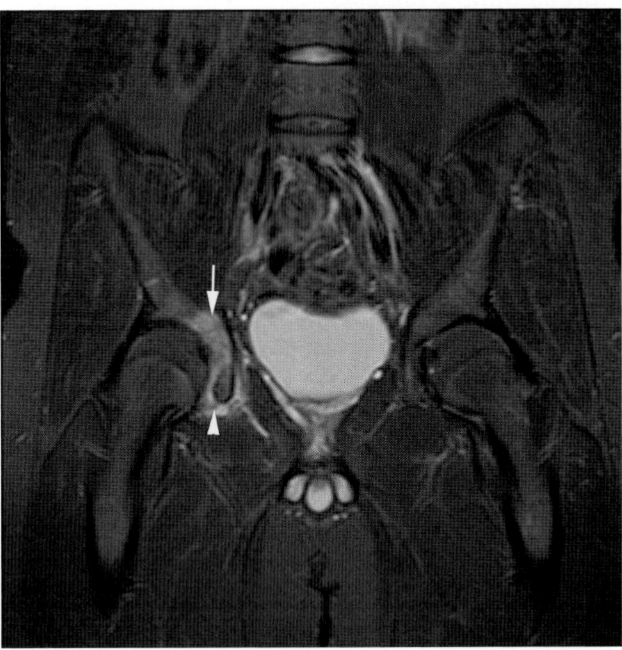

FIGURE 81-6 ■ **Pelvic osteoid osteoma.** Coronal STIR MRI demonstrating marked bone marrow oedema (arrow) and adjacent soft-tissue oedema (arrowhead).

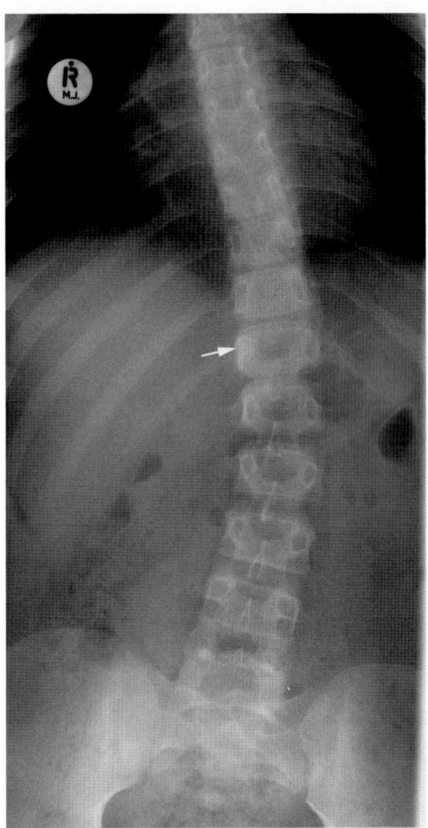

FIGURE 81-7 ■ **Spinal osteoblastoma.** AP spinal radiograph demonstrating a left convex thoracolumbar scoliosis, with a sclerotic right T12 pedicle at the apex of the curve.

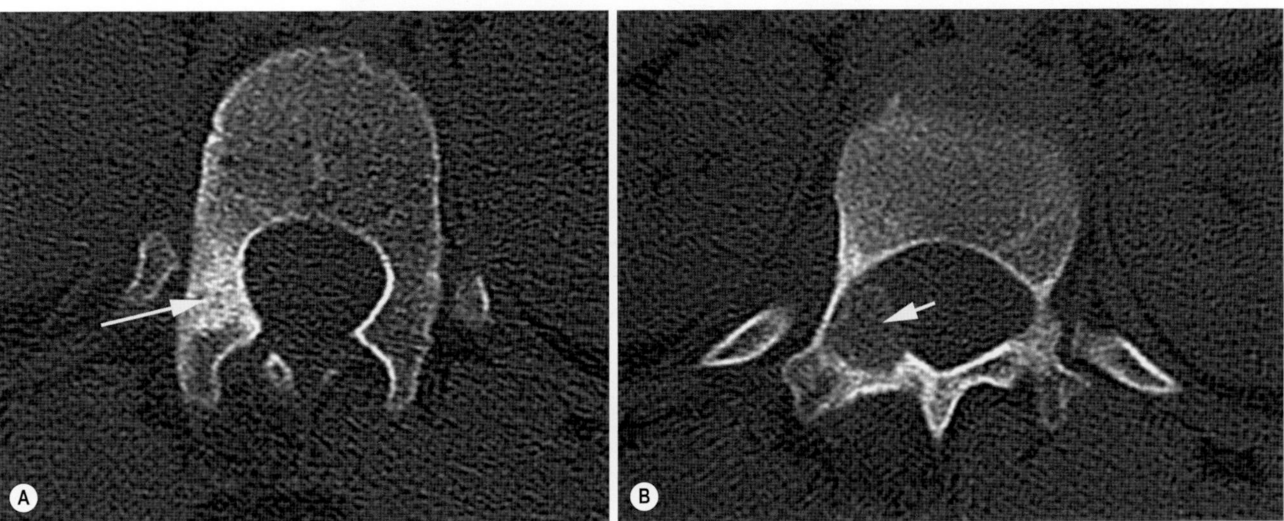

FIGURE 81-8 ■ **Spinal osteoblastoma.** Axial CT sections demonstrating a sclerotic right vertebral pedicle (arrow, panel A), with an adjacent expansile, lytic lesion (short arrow, panel B). The cortex is thinned but intact.

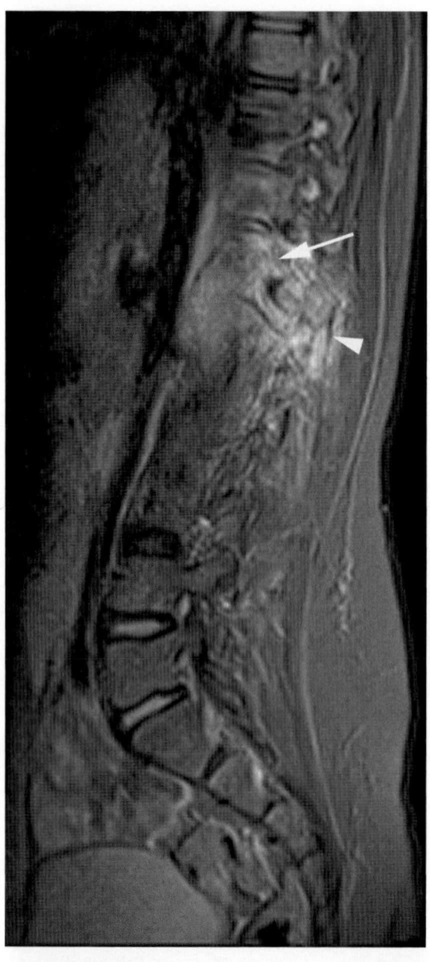

FIGURE 81-9 ■ **Spinal osteoblastoma.** Sagittal STIR MRI depicting both extensive bone marrow (arrow) and adjacent soft-tissue oedema (arrowhead).

size. NOF is the most common benign tumour in children and is typically incidentally encountered during childhood and adolescence, appearing as a well-defined multilocular osteolytic defect in the metaphysis of a long bone, with marginal sclerosis. The most frequent sites are the tibia and proximal femur.[13] Although MRI is not routinely indicated for simple cases of NOF, T1-weighted MRI shows low signal intensity within the lesion compared with the skeletal muscle. T2-weighted signal intensity is variable. The lesion usually enhances avidly (Fig. 81-10).

Fibrous Bone Dysplasia

FBD is a common developmental anomaly in which the bone is centrally replaced by fibrous tissue.[14] Local bending or pathological fractures may occur. Radiologically the appearance is typically of a widened medullary cavity, bony expansion and a ground-glass appearance (Fig. 81-11). A rare condition, McCune–Albright syndrome, consists of unilateral polyostotic FBD associated with precocious puberty. The most frequent locations for FBD are the ribs, proximal femur, skull, scapula and pelvis.

Osteofibrous Bone Dysplasia

This occurs in the shaft of long tubular bones, classically the tibia. It is a cortically based multicystic lesion surrounded by sclerosis with intact cortex and no periosteal reaction (Fig. 81-12). It may be multifocal. Moth-eaten margins and complete involvement of the

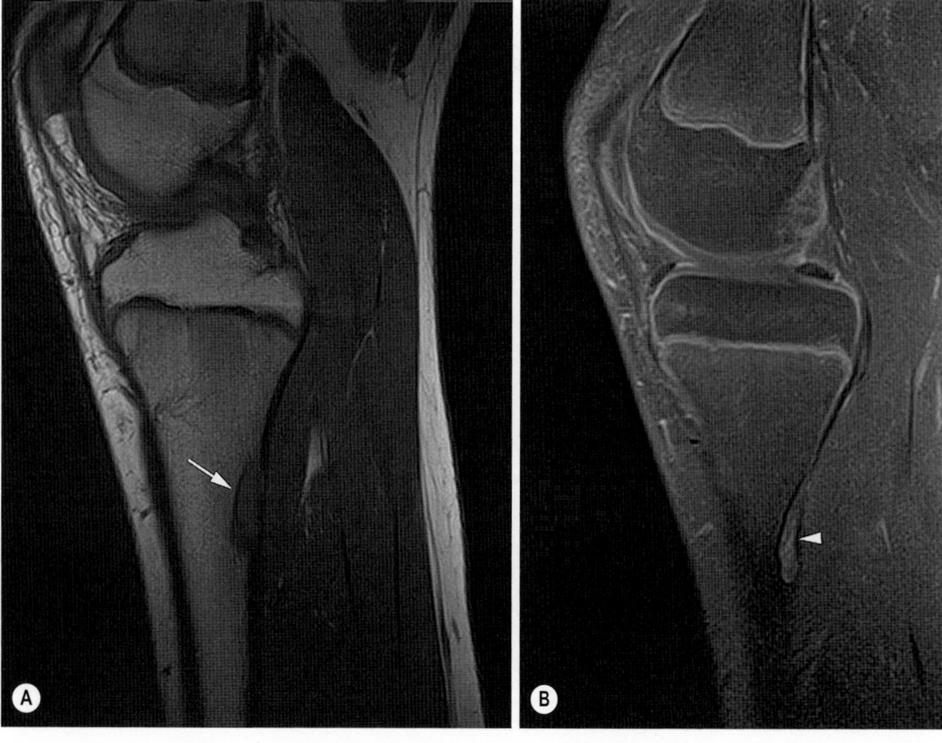

FIGURE 81-10 ■ **Non-ossifying fibroma: MRI.** Sagittal pre- (A) and (B) post-gadolinium T1-weighted MRI with fat saturation, depicting a well-defined cortical lesion with a sclerotic low signal rim (arrow) (A). The lesion avidly enhances following contrast administration (arrowhead) (B).

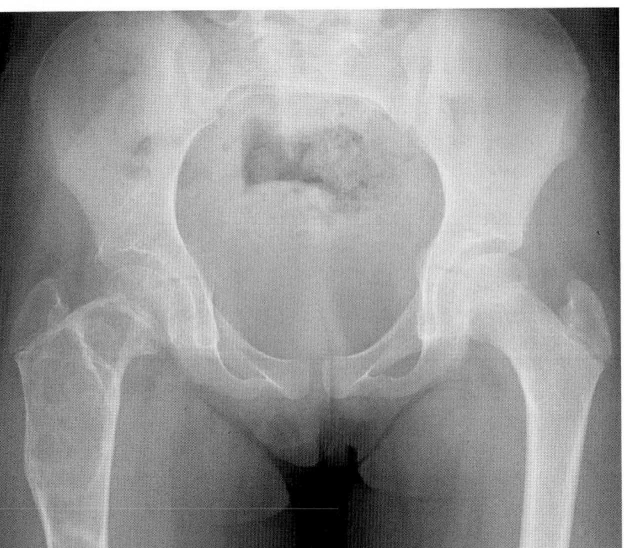

FIGURE 81-11 ■ **Fibrous dysplasia.** AP pelvic radiograph showing an expansile lytic lesion of the right proximal femur, extending to the growth plate. The internal aspect of the lesion demonstrates ground-glass appearance.

medullary cavity suggest adamantinoma rather than OFD.[15]

Cartilage-Forming Tumours

- Chondroma (enchondroma)
- Osteochondroma
- Chondroblastoma.

Osteochondroma (Exostosis)

Osteochondromas are developmental anomalies resulting from physeal cartilage displaced to the metaphyseal region, the knee being the most common site.[16] Osteochondromas are covered by a cartilaginous cap from which growth occurs. Osteochondromas may be pedunculated (Fig. 81-13) or sessile (Fig. 81-14), solitary or multiple, as seen in the autosomal dominant condition multiple hereditary exostoses (MHE). Local pressure effects on adjacent structures, deformity and shortening may result, particularly in MHE.

Plain radiography is usually diagnostic. On MRI T2-weighted sequences the hyaline cartilage appears hyperintense with a good visualisation of its structural layers. MRI demonstrates the thickness of the cartilaginous cap of the tumour. In children and adolescents, the cap may be as thick as 3 cm. Growth may continue until skeletal maturity. Growth after maturity suggests malignant degeneration, which occurs in 1% of solitary exostoses and between 3 and 5% in MHE. Persistent pain is also a worrying feature, which should prompt investigation to exclude malignant degeneration.

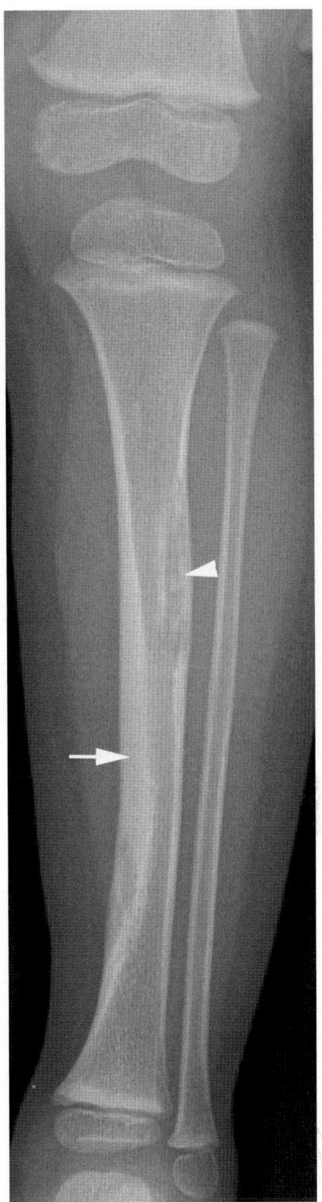

FIGURE 81-12 ■ **Osteofibrous dysplasia.** Frontal left tibial radiograph showing multifocal cortically based lesions with both sclerosis (arrow) and lucency (arrowhead). There is no periosteal reaction or cortical destruction.

Chondroblastoma

This is a rare benign cartilaginous tumour found in the epiphysis or epiphyseal equivalents. It is a monostotic lesion with chondroid matrix, calcification, a sclerotic rim and commonly a periosteal reaction. Aggressive features may rarely be seen. The most common sites are the femur (proximal > distal) and proximal tibia.

The radiographic appearance is that of a well-defined radiolucent lesion. Calcified matrix may be more apparent on CT. MRI shows low (reflecting haemosiderin) to intermediate heterogeneous signal on T2 with a lobulated pattern. Bone marrow oedema may be present and ABC components may be seen.

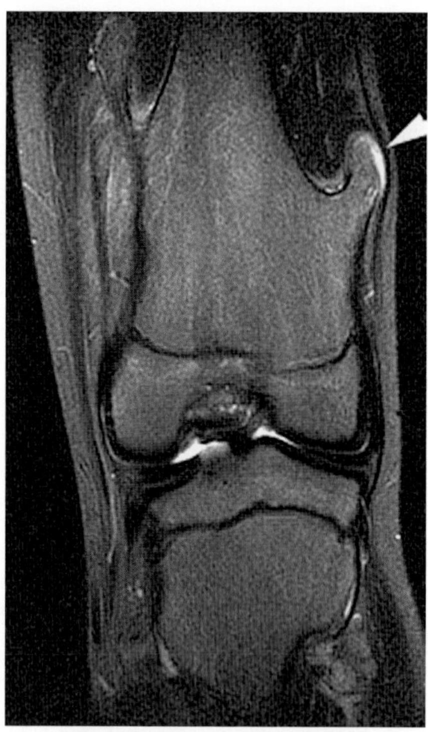

FIGURE 81-13 ■ Pedunculated osteochondroma. Coronal proton density MRI depicting two pedunculated osteochondromas. Note the bony medullary continuity. A thin cartilage cap is shown (arrowhead).

Vascular and Other Connective Tissue Tumours

- Bone haemangioma
- Bone lymphangioma
- Massive osteolysis (Gorham's disease)
- Myofibromatosis
- Lipoma of bone.

Myofibromatosis

Myofibromatosis presents most often in infancy, but can occur even in adults. The solitary or multiple lesions involve skin, subcutaneous tissues, muscles, bones and viscera (particularly lung, heart, gastrointestinal tract and dura). The skeletal lesions appear lytic and sharply defined, sparing the periphyseal area. Sclerotic margins appear later.[17]

Gorham's Disease

A rare disorder of unknown aetiology, typically arising in childhood, Gorham's disease presents as osteolysis, which may be dramatic ('vanishing bone disease') (Fig. 81-15). Pathologically characterised by lymphovascular proliferation, both bone and multisystem involvement can be seen.[18] The most commonly afflicted sites are the

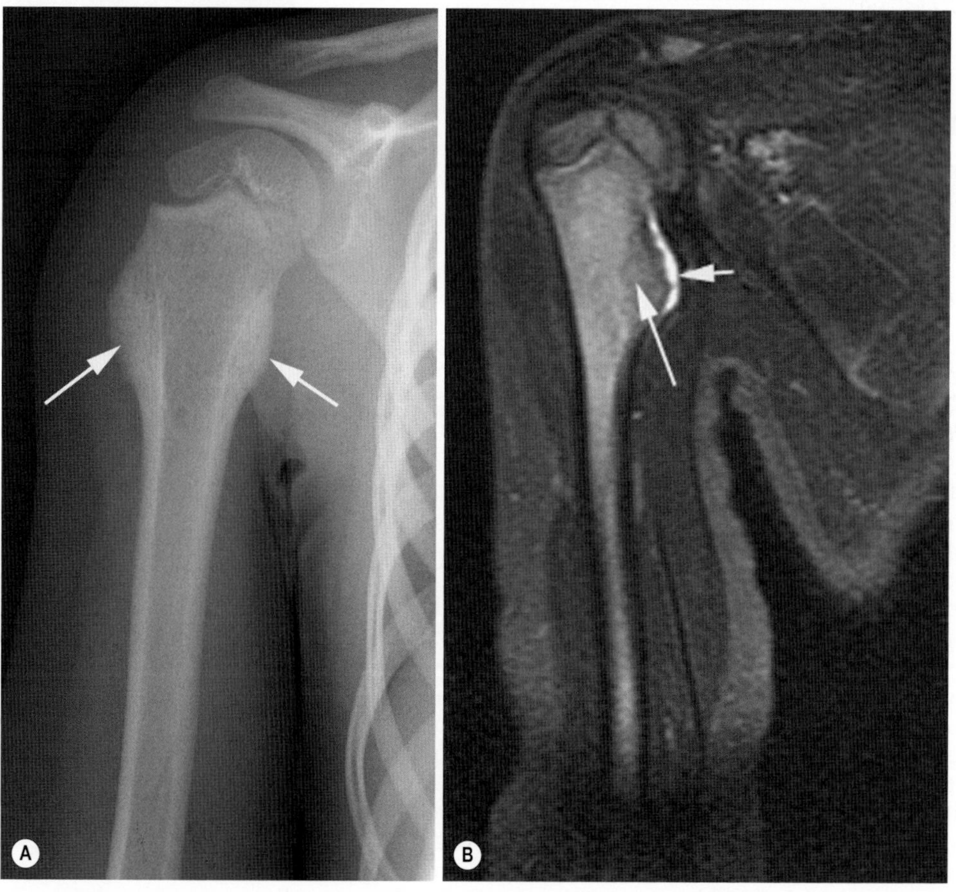

FIGURE 81-14 ■ Sessile osteochondroma. AP right humeral radiograph (A) and coronal STIR MRI (B) depicting sessile osteochondromas (arrows). Note the thin cartilage cap (short arrow, B).

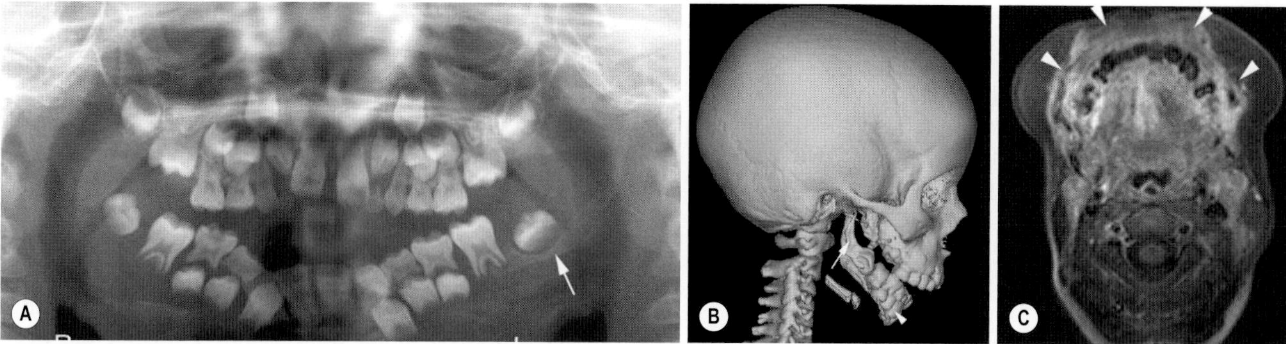

FIGURE 81-15 ■ **Gorham's disease.** Orthopantomogram (A) showing almost complete absence of the mandible, with a small remnant demonstrated (arrow). 3D surface-shaded display CT of the face (B) depicting the mandibular remnant (arrow) and 'floating teeth' (arrowhead). Post-gadolinium T1-weighted fat-saturated MRI (C) demonstrating enhancing lymphovascular soft tissue replacing the mandible.

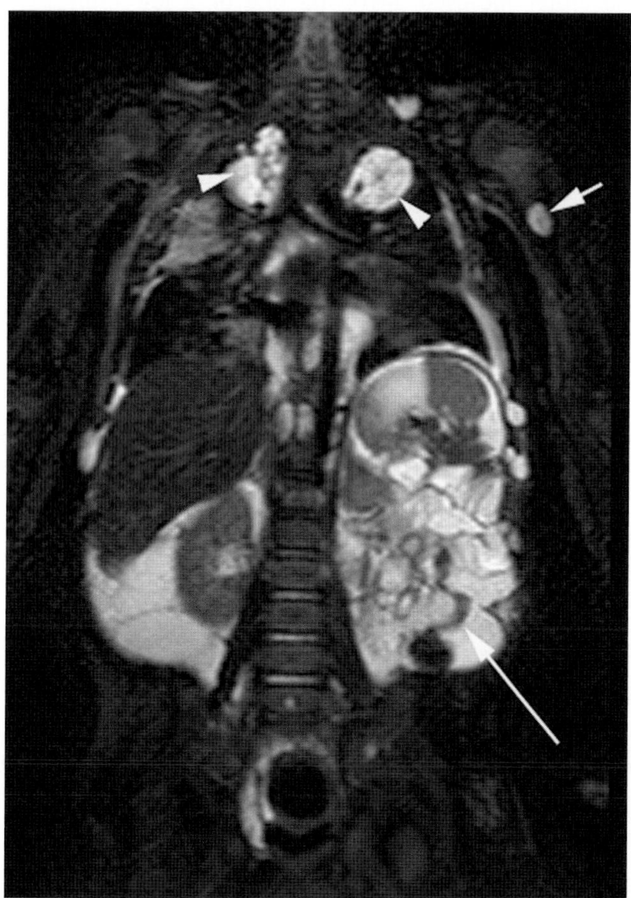

FIGURE 81-16 ■ **Multisystem lymphangiomatosis.** Coronal STIR MRI demonstrating abdominal (long arrow), left humeral (short arrow) and thoracic (arrowheads) lymphangiomatosis.

shoulder, face, spine and pelvis. There is no standard therapy, with interferon alpha being used successfully in some cases. Bone involvement may also be observed with diffuse multisystem lymphatic malformations (Fig. 81-16).

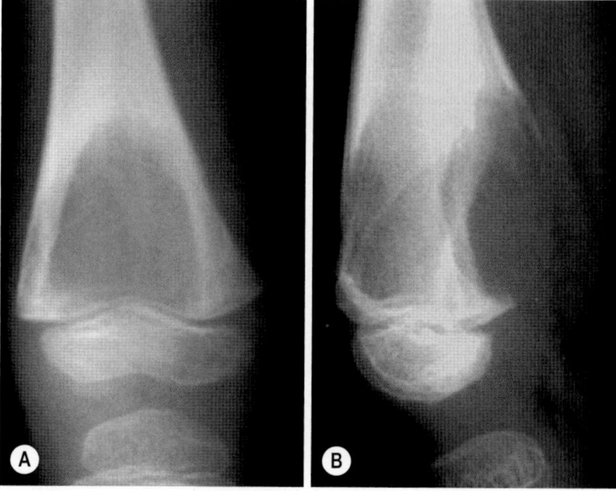

FIGURE 81-17 ■ **Chondromyxoid fibroma of the distal femoral metaphysis.** (A, B) Large osteolytic defect bulging outward.

Locally Aggressive Tumours

- Desmoplastic bone fibroma
- Chondromyxoid fibroma
- Haemangiopericytoma
- Osteoclastoma (giant cell tumour).

Chondromyxoid Fibroma

This is a rare bone tumour that accounts for only 0.5% of all bone tumours. It is mainly seen in the second decade of life, but cases have been described in the first decade. Typically, chondromyxoid fibromas are located in the metaphyseal region of the long tubular bones, near the growth plate, and can cross into the epiphysis. The lesion is well circumscribed, with an eccentric osteolytic lobulated aspect that bulges outward, thinning the cortex (Fig. 81-17). It is usually benign in character but may cause local invasion with a high recurrence rate if incompletely removed.

Tumour-Like Lesions

- Simple juvenile bone cyst
- Aneurysmal bone cyst (ABC)
- Fibrous cortical defect: see fibrous tissue tumours
- Fibrous bone dysplasia (Jaffe–Lichtenstein) (FBD)
- Osteofibrous bone dysplasia (Kempson, Campanacci) (OBD)
- Eosinophilic granuloma (Langerhans cell histiocytosis).

Simple Bone Cyst (Synonyms: Juvenile, Solitary or Unicameral Bone Cyst)

SBC is a benign lesion that develops in the centre of the metaphysis, usually of the proximal femur or humerus adjacent to the epiphyseal plate (Fig. 81-18). Most patients present with a pathological fracture, but SBC may be an incidental finding. There is cortical thinning with mild expansion. With maturity, the cyst migrates down the shaft of the bone. Following fracture, fluid–fluid levels and solid areas may be seen.

Aneurysmal Bone Cyst

This is a cystic expansile lesion, often containing haemorrhage, which occurs in the vertebral appendages, the flat bones, and most frequently in the metaphysis of the long bones in the femur, tibia and humerus (Fig. 81-19). The lesion develops eccentrically without crossing the growth plate. The lesion is frequently multilocular and may cause subtle cortical thinning. Within the vertebral column, a destructive expansile lesion is seen in the appendages and may encroach into the spinal canal. ABC can be primary or secondary to other bone tumours in up to 30% of cases. Telangiectatic OS is a mimic of ABC.

Full evaluation of ABCs requires cross-sectional imaging and biopsy. MRI demonstrates the architecture and fluid–fluid levels within the lesion, which may be haemorrhagic (Fig. 81-20). In selected cases percutaneous sclerotherapy under fluoroscopic guidance has been used with successful clinical results.[19]

Langerhans Cell Histiocytosis (LCH)

LCH is uncommon, accounting for less than 1% of bone biopsy specimens. This disorder, involving proliferation of Langerhans cell histiocytes and their precursors, may be either localised, involving one or a few bony sites (70%), or multifocal, affecting bone and extraskeletal sites. Solitary lesions (eosinophilic granuloma) frequently involve flat bones (skull, mandible, ribs and pelvis being most common) and typically appear as a geographic lytic lesion, with a variable degree of surrounding sclerosis, depending on the degree of healing (Fig. 81-21). Vertebra plana, classically, is seen within the spine; however, LCH may have variable appearances and is a great mimic of other lesions.[20]

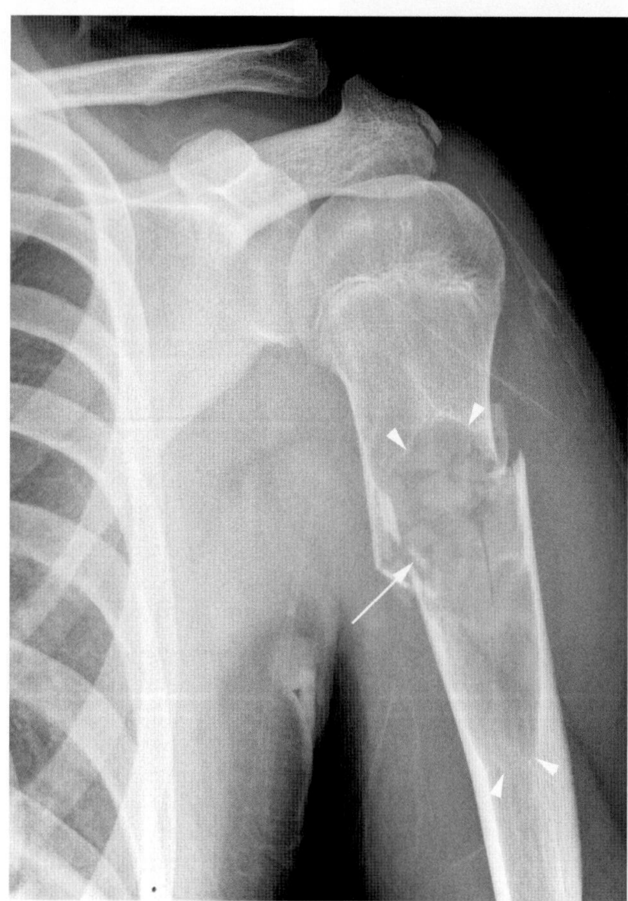

FIGURE 81-18 ■ Simple bone cyst. AP left humerus demonstrating a well-defined osteolytic lesion within the diaphysis (arrowheads), with a pathological fracture and internal fragments (arrow).

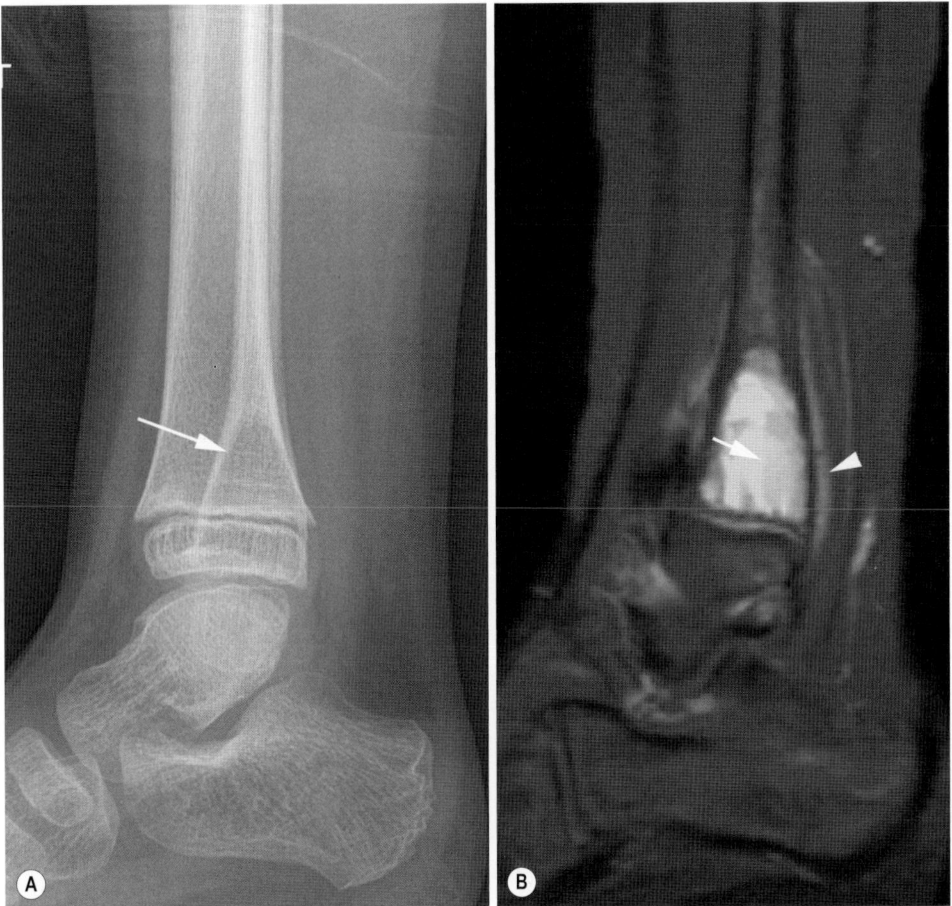

FIGURE 81-19 ■ **Aneurysmal bone cyst.** Lateral radiograph of the ankle (A) showing an expansile lytic lesion of the fibula (arrow). Sagittal STIR MRI (B) demonstrates multiple fluid–fluid levels (short arrow), with some adjacent soft-tissue oedema (arrowhead), which can be seen in association with an ABC.

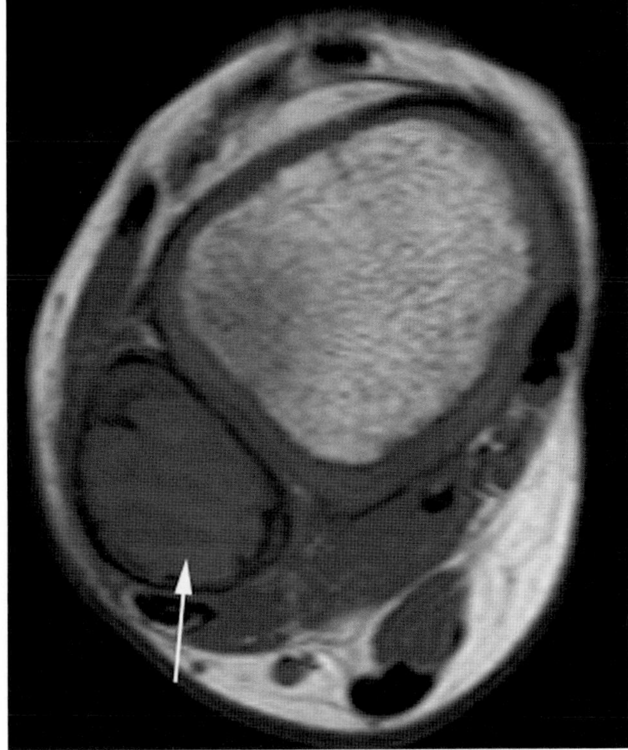

FIGURE 81-20 ■ **Axial T1-weighted MRI demonstrating the haemorrhagic nature of the fluid–fluid levels, with subtle T1 shortening observed (arrow).**

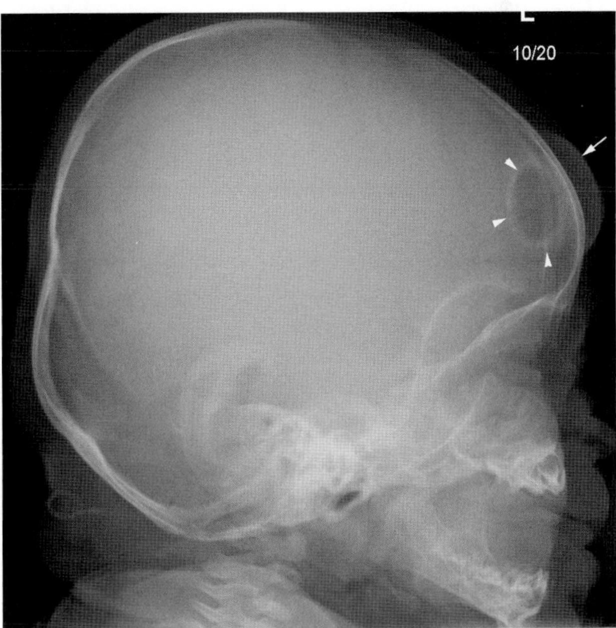

FIGURE 81-21 ■ **Langerhans cell histiocytosis.** Lateral skull radiograph showing a well-defined lytic frontal bone lesion with sclerotic margins (arrowheads) and an associated soft-tissue mass (short arrow).

NEUROBLASTOMA

Neuroblastomas (NBs)—with the less common, but more differentiated and mature ganglioneuroblastoma and ganglioneuroma (GN)—are neoplasms arising from the primordial neural crest cells. Neuroblastic tumours represent the most common extracranial solid neoplasms occurring in children, with median age at diagnosis of 2 years, and 90% of cases occurring under the age of 5 years. Overall, NBs account for 8–10% of all childhood cancers. NBs are also seen in newborns and may be detected in the fetus by antenatal imaging, most often associated with favourable prognostic features.[21] Common sites for primary NB are the adrenal glands (48%), extra-adrenal retroperitoneum (25%), chest (16%), neck (3%) and pelvis (3%). About 50% of patients have metastatic disease at diagnosis.

The signs and symptoms of NB reflect the tumour site and extent of disease. The tumours may manifest as an incidental mass, or may cause abdominal pain. Because metastases are frequently present (skeleton, bone marrow, lymph nodes, liver and, rarely, lung and brain), the clinical symptoms are often due to metastatic disease. Children may have bone and joint pain, proptosis from orbital metastases, anaemia, weight loss and fever. Horner's syndrome may be the presenting feature of cervical or thoracic NB involving the stellate ganglion. Children may also present with the effects of production of hormones such as catecholamines (hypertension) and VIP (intractable watery diarrhoea). Another paraneoplastic syndrome associated with NB is myoclonic encephalopathy of infancy (MEI). The precise pathogenesis of MEI is unknown.

NBs in infants younger than 1 year of age are often associated with extensive hepatic metastases. Hepatomegaly may be massive despite a small, sometimes not evident, primary lesion. These infants usually have bone marrow lesions and palpable subcutaneous nodules. In infants, this type of NB has a better prognosis and has a tendency to spontaneous regression, although the very young patients are at high risk because of severe respiratory complications, occurring as a result of massive hepatomegaly.

Extradural extension (dumb-bell syndrome) with possible compression of the spinal cord is relatively common with thoracic NB, but rare in abdominal tumours.

Approximately 90% of patients with NB have elevated levels of catecholamines (vanillylmandelic acid, homovanillic acid, noradrenaline, dopamine) in the urine. However, no more than 60% of newborns with NB have elevated levels of urinary catecholamines.[21] The combination of a positive bone marrow aspirate and an increase of urinary catecholamine metabolites are sufficient to confirm the diagnosis.

NB shows a broad spectrum of clinical behaviour, as in some cases it may spontaneously regress or mature, whereas in other cases it may progress despite intensive multimodality treatment. Its outcome appears to correlate with a series of well-known clinical, histological and biological features, which can be used for risk group stratification and treatment assignment, according to current treatment protocols.

GN often occurs in the posterior mediastinum and, unlike NB, does not contain neuroblastic cells. In comparison with NB, GN occurs in older patients, as the median age at diagnosis is approximately 7 years. GN often manifests as an asymptomatic mass discovered on a routine radiographic study, such as a chest radiograph. The imaging features of GN are similar to those of ganglioneuroblastoma (GNB) and NB; hence, they most often cannot be discriminated with imaging in isolation.

IMAGING

The initial diagnosis of an abdominal NB is made most frequently by ultrasound or by chest-X-ray in the case of a thoracic mass. The evaluation of the primary tumour includes CT or MRI, whereas ^{123}metaiodobenzylguanidine (^{123}I-mIBG) scintigraphy and ^{99m}Tc-MDP bone scintigraphy are required for the detection of metastases.

Radiographs

Radiographs may show a calcified mass in the thorax and/or in the abdomen. Erosion of vertebral pedicles may suggest an intraspinal extension. Radiographs of the long bones with metastases may be normal or may show ill-defined areas of bone destruction. A solitary lesion may appear as a lytic, moth-eaten or a permeative destructive area, interspersed with sclerotic trabeculae. New periosteal bone formation, often parallel to the shaft, may be present. The radiographic features indicate malignant growth but are not specific. The most common skeletal sites are the skull and metaphyses of long bones (humerus and femur).

Ultrasound

Ultrasound, performed to confirm the presence of an abdominal mass, often suggests the diagnosis of NB. Typical features are a retroperitoneal location, varying echogenicity with hyperechoic foci representing calcification, and usually rich vascularisation on colour Doppler. The retroperitoneal location of the mass can be confirmed by demonstration of anterior displacement of the aorta and inferior vena cava (Fig. 81-22). Hypoechoic areas secondary to haemorrhage and necrosis are frequent. Completely cystic NB has been described, especially in newborns.

Computed Tomography and Magnetic Resonance Imaging

CT of the chest, abdomen and pelvis requires a bolus intravenous administration of contrast medium. Examinations of the chest should extend from the lung apices to the lower edge of the liver during relatively early contrast enhancement; the abdominal study should cover the

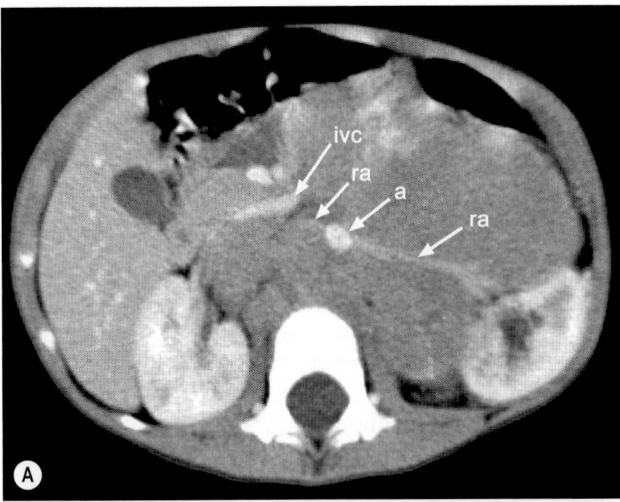

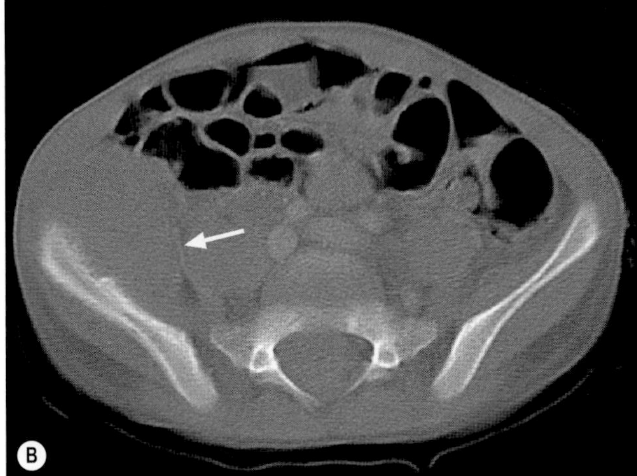

FIGURE 81-22 ■ **Abdominal neuroblastoma.** Contrast-enhanced CT. (A) A prevertebral tumour extends across the midline in the retroperitoneum, displaces and encases the aorta (a) anteriorly and encases the renal arteries (ra). The inferior vena cava (ivc), partially encased, is displaced anterolaterally and compressed by the tumour and nodes. The mass extends to the renal hila. (B) Infiltrative lesion to the right iliac bone with a large soft-tissue component (arrow) that projects inward as a space-occupying mass.

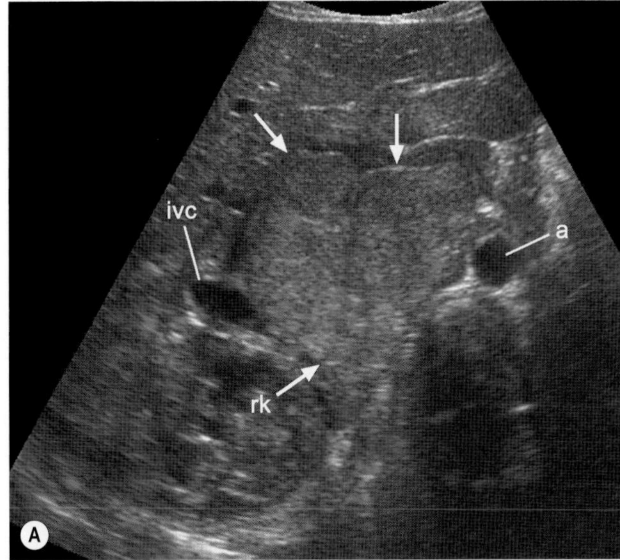

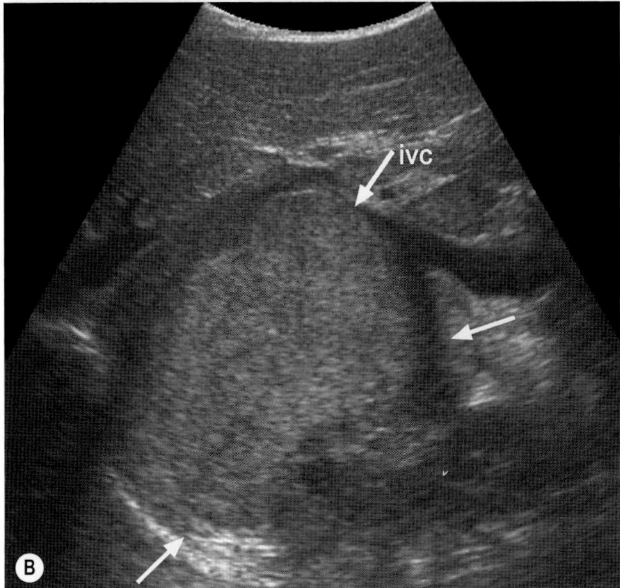

FIGURE 81-23 ■ **Abdominal neuroblastoma.** (A) Transverse ultrasound through the right abdomen shows a solid paraspinal mass (arrows) anterior to the right kidney (rk). The aorta (a) and inferior vena cava (ivc) are displaced by the mass. (B) Longitudinal image through the right flank shows the mass (arrows) and the stretched inferior vena cava (ivc).

liver in the portal phase and extend down to the pubic symphysis. Multiple pre- and post-contrast phases usually do not add useful information for diagnosis and staging and thus should be avoided.[22] On CT, NB appears as a large and heterogeneous mass; calcifications are detected in up to 85% of cases. Low-attenuation areas represent regions of necrosis or haemorrhage. NB usually shows mild heterogeneous enhancement, reflecting areas of vascularity alternating with areas of necrosis, haemorrhage and cystic change.

Using MRI the patient must be imaged in at least two planes by T1-weighted spin-echo (SE) and fat-saturated T2-weighted fast SE sequences, and with transverse T1-weighted gradient-echo angiographic sequences. The T1-weighted SE sequence must be repeated with fat suppression after intravenous injection of gadolinium. On MRI, NB has prolonged T1 and T2 signal. High signal intensity on T1-weighted images represents haemorrhage. After administration of gadolinium the tumour enhancement is usually heterogeneous. MRI may also show bone marrow involvement with areas of abnormal signal intensity (low on T1- and high on T2-weighted images).

As separation of the primary tumour from adjacent enlarged lymph nodes is usually not possible, measurement must include the entire mass. The tumour may invade the spinal canal, kidney, or liver. Although intraspinal extension may be suspected at CT, it cannot be thoroughly evaluated: MRI should be performed on any paraspinal mass suspected of extending into the extradural space (Fig. 81-23).

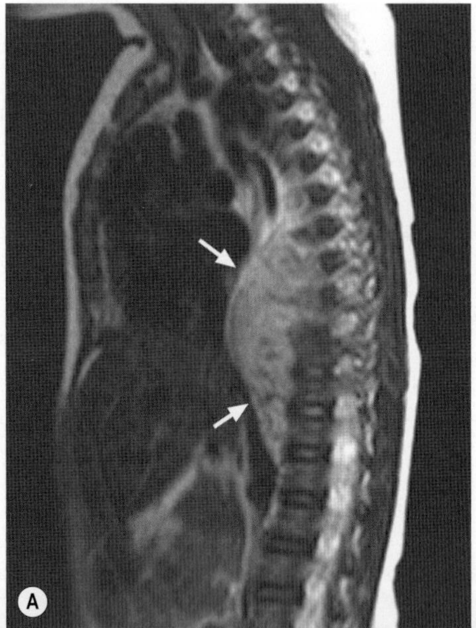

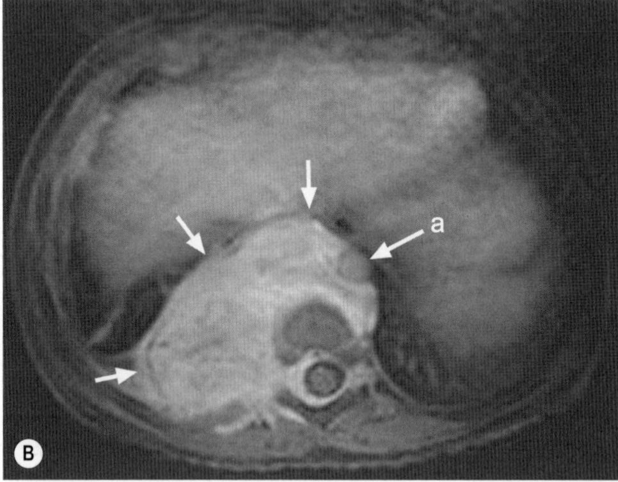

FIGURE 81-24 ■ (A) Sagittal T1-weighted images with Gd-DOTA enhancement. (B) Axial T2-weighted image. Large posterior mediastinal mass (arrows) with anterior and lateral displacement of the aorta (a), which is encased. There is massive tumour extension into the canal through the right neural foramina to displace the spinal cord to the left. Extension into the right paraspinal soft tissues is evident.

Hepatic metastases and renal atrophy (due to ischaemia secondary to encasement or compression of the renal vessels) may be seen. Indeed, NB often has an invasive pattern of growth encasing the vessels (Fig. 81-24). Therefore, with imaging it is crucial to define the extent of the tumour and its relationships to adjacent vessels, according to standardised criteria (see the section below on 'NB Staging') in order to define feasibility of a complete resection.

CT or MRI may allow the evaluation of skull and iliac bone metastases. Usually, skull metastases are located in the spheno-orbital region. They appear as an infiltrating mass causing permeative bone destruction and spiculated bony changes, which may extend into the soft tissue of the scalp or push through the inner table of the skull.

Radionuclide Radiology

^{123}I-mIBG scintigraphy has a pivotal role in the diagnosis of NB: i.e. characterisation of the mass, localisation of the primary tumour in patients with MEI and evaluation of metastatic disease and in follow-up; i.e. new areas of uptake generally indicate new active disease. mIBG is a guanethidine derivative and an analogue of noradrenaline, which is specifically taken up and stored in those tumours derived from the cells of the sympathetic nervous system. In children such uptake is usually specific for NB (both primary tumour and metastases). Unfortunately, about 20% of primary lesions do not take up mIBG, and in other rare cases the uptake may stop despite the presence of persistent demonstrable disease. Furthermore, mIBG cannot differentiate bone marrow uptake from cortical bone uptake.[23] Therefore, ^{99m}Tc-MDP bone scintigraphy should be performed in all patients, as two-thirds of patients have metastatic bone disease at diagnosis.

NBs which cannot be resected at diagnosis, because of their size and/or infiltration into adjacent structures, require chemotherapy. With chemotherapy, a NB mass tends to regress in size, but the regression is frequently incomplete, leaving a small, often calcified residual mass. Determining whether this residual mass is just fibrosis or a viable tumour usually requires ^{123}I-mIBG scintigraphy.

Emerging Imaging Techniques

Recently, fluorodeoxyglucose(^{18}F) positron emission tomography (FDG-PET) coupled with computed tomography (^{18}F-FDG PET/CT) has gained a major role in the treatment of adult cancer, whereas the reported experience with childhood tumours is still limited. Preliminary reports suggest that ^{18}F-FDG-PET/CT may be useful in evaluating neuroblastoma (Fig. 81-25), contributing to disease management and even providing opportunity for modification and minimisation of treatment effect (such as in radiation treatment planning) when utilised at diagnosis for disease staging, during therapy to assess response and during follow-up after completion of therapy.[24] However, ^{18}F-FDG-PET/CT is an imaging technique carrying a high radiation exposure, which causes concern in children because of their sensitivity to ionising radiation, and especially in children with cancer, as repeated studies with ionising radiation are expected during the course of the disease.

Whole-body MRI (WBMRI) is an emerging imaging technique with great potential in paediatric oncology. Usually, T1-weighetd and short T1 inversion recovery (STIR) sequences in coronal and sagittal planes are used to image the whole body. Experience with WBMRI in NB is still limited, although preliminary studies show that WBMRI may play a role as a result of the excellent sensitivity in detecting both local disease and metastases, with no radiation burden (Fig. 81-26). However, low specificity is the main downside of WBMRI. Further studies are required to confirm the potential of WBMRI in children with NB.[25]

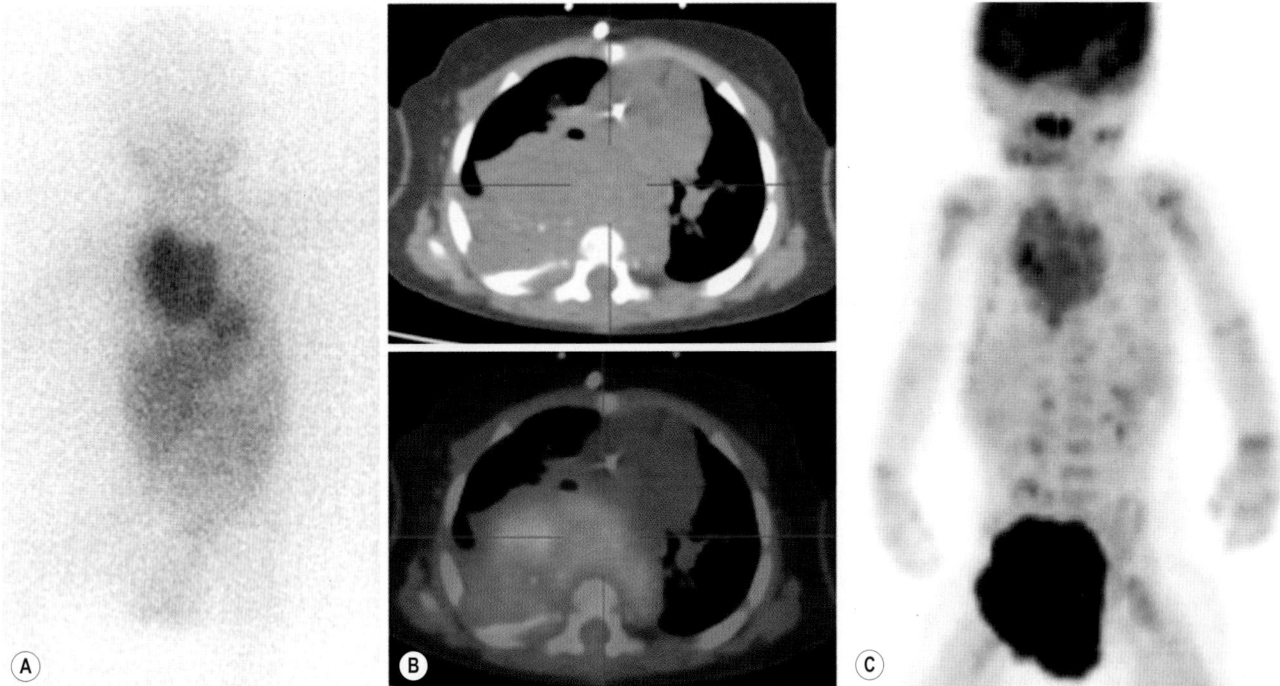

FIGURE 81-25 ■ Infant with thoracic neuroblastoma. ^{123}I-mIBG scintigraphy (A) shows avid uptake in the mediastinum and right hemithorax. There is no uptake within the bones. ^{18}F-FDG-PET (B) shows a similar pattern of uptake in the mediastinum and right hemithorax. Bone/bone marrow uptake is weak and diffuse, not specific for disease infiltration. (C) CT and ^{18}F-FDG-PET/CT. CT (upper image) shows a large mass in the posterior mediastinum with calcific spots, crossing the midline and spreading into the right hemithorax. ^{18}F-FDG-PET/CT (lower image) shows avid uptake in the mass. (Images courtesy of Arnoldo Piccardo, MD, Service of Nuclear Medicine, Galliera Hospital, Genoa, Italy.)

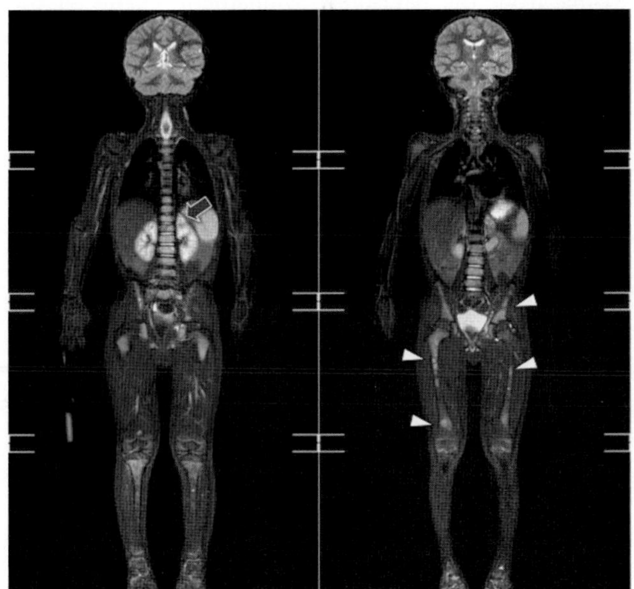

FIGURE 81-26 ■ Two-year-old boy with left adrenal neuroblastoma. Whole-body MRI. STIR images. Left image shows an enlarged left adrenal gland (arrow). Right image shows metastatic infiltration in both femora and left iliac bone (arrowheads).

NB STAGING

Disease staging at diagnosis relies on diagnostic imaging, which is of paramount importance for prognosis, risk group stratification and treatment, being the most statistically significant prognostic factor. Until very recently, the only staging system for NB was the International Neuroblastoma Staging System (INSS) (Table 81-2).[26] This staging system is largely based on the extent of surgical excision of the NB mass and lymph node sampling at surgery. However, some issues are evident with INSS. For example, with INSS the same tumour can be either stage 1 or 3, depending on the extent of surgical excision. Lymph node sampling is subject to the diligence of the individual surgeon. Infants with localised disease, who are just observed because tumour regression is anticipated, cannot be properly staged.[27] These difficulties can make direct comparison of clinical trials based on INSS very difficult.

Furthermore, this staging system does not address the issue of a safe and complete excision of the mass, leaving this decision to the personal evaluation of the individual surgeon. The increased awareness of this issue led the International Society of Paediatric Oncology Europe Neuroblastoma Group (SIOPEN) to classify locoregional tumors as resectable or unresectable on the basis of the presence, or absence of a series of 'image-defined risk factors' (IDRFs) detected with diagnostic imaging. This led to the new International

TABLE 81-2 International Neuroblastoma Staging System[26]

Stage	
1	Localised tumour confined to the area of origin; complete gross resection with or without microscopic residual disease; identifiable ipsilateral and contralateral lymph nodes negative macroscopically
2A	Localised tumour with incomplete gross excision; identifiable ipsilateral and contralateral lymph nodes negative microscopically
2B	Unilateral tumour with complete or incomplete gross resection with positive ipsilateral regional lymph nodes; contralateral lymph nodes negative microscopically
3	Tumour infiltrating across the midline with or without regional lymph node involvement; unilateral tumour with contralateral regional lymph node involvement; midline tumour with bilateral lymph node involvement
4	Dissemination of tumour to bone, bone marrow, liver, distant lymph nodes or other organs
4s	Limited to infants < 1 year of age. Localised primary tumour as defined for stage 1 or 2A or 2B with dissemination limited to liver, skin and/or bone marrow

TABLE 81-3 International Neuroblastoma Risk Group Staging System

Stage	
L1	Localised tumour not involving vital structures as defined by the list of image-defined risk factors and confined to one body compartment
L2	Locoregional tumour with presence of one or more image-defined risk factors
M	Distant metastatic disease (except stage MS)
MS	Metastatic disease in children younger than 18 months with metastases confined to skin, liver and/or bone marrow

Adapted from Monclair et al.[27]

Neuroblastoma Risk Group Staging System (INRGSS) (Table 81-3),[27] which now add to INSS. IDRFs and can be defined as features detected on imaging that make safe and complete tumour excision impracticable at the time of diagnosis, thus suggesting a need for preoperative chemotherapy. In INRGSS, staging of local disease—at variance with INSS—is based on imaging, as stage assignment is determined by IDRFs absence (stage L1) or presence (stage L2).[27]

A detailed description of INRGSS and IDRFs is beyond the scope of this chapter, and can be found in two recent articles by Cohn et al[28] and Monclair et al.[27] In this chapter our description will be limited to the basic principles and guidelines.

CT and/or MRI are the best-suited imaging modalities to assess the presence of IDRFs. The primary tumour should be measured with three-dimensional orthogonal measurements and the presence or absence of each individual IDRF should be systematically verified according to tumour site. Measurement of the tumour volume is crucial for prognosis and follow-up. By definition, if the mass crosses the contralateral aspect of the vertebral body, it has crossed the midline: this determination is important for INSS staging, but not for INRGSS.

The majority of IDRFs pertain to abdominal NBs, due to their usual close relationship with major abdominal vessels. Therefore, aorta, celiac axis, mesenteric arteries, renal pedicles, inferior vena cava, iliac vessels and portal vein should be accurately assessed. Specific terms should be used to describe the relationship observed between the mass and adjacent vital structures, i.e. structures that cannot be sacrificed without impairment of normal function.[22]

- *Separation*: the interposition of a layer between the tumour and any neighbouring structure.
- *Contact*: no visible layer is present between the tumour and the adjacent structure, without obvious invasion. Contact is not an IDRF, with the exception of renal vessels as their dissection from a mass is very risky and may lead to nephrectomy or renal infarction.
- *Encasement*: a neighbouring structure is surrounded by the mass, an IDRF. With reference to a vessel, more than 50% of its circumference should be in contact with the mass.
- *Compression*: a tumour is in contact with the airway and reduces its short axis, thus representing an IDRF.
- *Infiltration*: a structure other than vessel shows ill-defined margins with the tumour, and it is an IDRF.

IDRFs are specific according to tumour site. NB arising from the paraspinal sympathetic chains in the mediastinum and abdomen may extend into the foraminal spaces, causing intraspinal involvement (the so-called 'dumb-bell' tumors) with possible cord compression. On imaging, finding invasion of more than one-third of the spinal canal diameter or loss of leptomeningeal fluid spaces is considered an IDRF. These imaging features, however, are better assessed with MRI. Intraspinal tumour extension below L2 causes radicular involvement and it does not represent a contraindication for excision of the extraspinal tumour component.[22]

A mediastinal tumour involving the costovertebral junction between T9 and T12 may cause spinal cord ischaemia during surgical excision of the mass, because of injury to the Adamkiewicz artery, which originates between T9 and T12. This should be considered an IDRF, although abundant collateral vessels are usually present due to the usual slow growth of NB located at this site. Therefore, angiography is not mandatory, although this issue is still controversial.

DIFFERENTIAL DIAGNOSIS

The differential diagnosis encompasses all paediatric abdominal masses, particularly Wilms' tumour (see Chapter 78) and neonatal adrenal haemorrhage. Concerning Wilms' tumour (WT), the mean age at onset is 3 years (for NB it is younger than 2 years). WT tends to displace the vessels, whilst NB surrounds vessels; WT may invade the renal vein and inferior vena cava and arises from the kidney with the typical 'claw sign', whereas NB classically displaces the kidney without distorting the renal collecting system. Calcifications are uncommon in NBs. In WT, lung metastases are present in 20% of cases, whereas they are very uncommon in NBs.

The diagnosis of neonatal adrenal haemorrhage is usually made by ultrasound, which identifies the mass and shows in sequential examinations, progressive decrease in size and cystic evolution. Colour Doppler is useful for showing absence of vascularisation. MRI may show the classic signal intensity pattern of ageing blood products, but diagnostic difficulties can occur because of bleeds of different ages. Other paediatric adrenal tumours, such as phaeochromocytoma and adrenal carcinoma, are much less common.

In the neck, firm/hard masses can be cysts, ectopic thymus, abscesses, inflammatory or neoplastic adenopathies, benign and malignant tumours or parotid and thyroid lesions. The most common cancers are lymphomas, thyroid cancers, rhabdomyosarcomas and NBs. In the mediastinum, NB is located in the posterior mediastinum. Other abnormalities encountered are neurofibroma, neurenteric cyst, meningocele and paraspinal inflammation due to vertebral osteomyelitis.

For a full list of references, please see ExpertConsult.

FURTHER READING

2. Wootton-Gorges SL. MR imaging of primary bone tumors and tumor-like conditions in children. Magn Reson Imaging Clin N Am 2009;17(3):469–87.

Charron M. Contemporary approach to diagnosis and treatment of neuroblastoma. Q J Nucl Med Mol Imaging 2013;57(1):40–52.

Gains J, Mandeville H, Cork N, et al. Ten challenges in the management of neuroblastoma. Future Oncol 2012;8(7):839–58.

Sharp SE, Parisi MT, Gelfand MJ, et al. Functional-metabolic imaging of neuroblastoma. Q J Nucl Med Mol Imaging 2013; 57(1):6–20.

CHAPTER 82

Paediatric Neuroradiology

Maria I. Argyropoulou • Andrea Rossi • Roxana S. Gunny • W.K. 'Kling' Chong

CHAPTER OUTLINE

NORMAL BRAIN MATURATION

Brain maturation is assessed by observing tissue characteristics related to myelination, as well as variations in morphology. Most of the changes associated with myelination occur in the first 2 years of life and gyral and sulcal development mainly occurs in utero or in the premature brain, while other morphological changes are observable later in life.

Normal Myelination

Myelination is the process by which brain oligodendrocytes produce layers of myelin that wrap around the neuronal axons and act as a layer of insulation for the transmission of electric action potentials down the neuronal axon. Axonal transmission is facilitated at the junctions between these myelin sheaths or nodes of Ranvier by a process known as saltatory conduction. The extent of myelination of the infant brain can be assessed by magnetic resonance imaging (MRI) according to specific milestones which are analogous to the normal milestones of clinical development. During earliest brain development none of the brain is myelinated. By term, key structures such as the ventrolateral thalami, dorsolateral putamina, posterior limb of the internal capsule, inferior colliculi, medial longitudinal fasciculus and dorsal brainstem nuclei are already myelinated. As the brain matures, there is progressive T_1 and T_2 shortening of the white matter due to an increase in the lipid content and reduced water content of developing myelin and packing of myelinated white matter tracts.[1] This follows a centrifugal posterior-to-anterior and caudal-to-cranial pattern and is virtually complete by the age of 2 years (Fig. 82-1). Advanced MRI techniques show progressive reduction in free water diffusion, increased fractional anisotropy (assessed by diffusion tensor imaging) and increased magnetisation transfer.[2–4] Brain myelination is detected in grey matter earlier on T_2-weighted fast spin-echo (FSE) and in the white matter tracts earlier on T_1-weighted spin-echo (SE) or inversion recovery (STIR) sequences. Most myelination occurs post-term in the first 8 months of life, although the final parts of this process may extend into adulthood. The brain should appear virtually fully myelinated on T_2-weighted sequences by 2 years, with almost an adult appearance on T_1-weighted sequences by 10 months (Fig. 82-2).

The newborn has limited motor function but a well-developed sensory system. Thus the myelination pattern seen at birth at full term is primarily in the sensory tracts. During the first 6 months of life the process of myelination is easiest to follow on T_1-weighted images, where the myelinated areas appear bright. T_2-weighted images are less sensitive and it takes much more myelin to produce a hypointense signal within the white matter. During this period T_2-weighted images show only subtle myelination.

At full term, T_1-weighted images should show high signal in the dorsal medulla and brainstem, the cerebellar peduncles, a small part of the cerebral peduncles, about a third of the posterior limb of the internal capsule, the central corona radiata, and the deep white matter in the region of the pre- and post-central gyrus.[5] Progression of myelination is seen in the optic radiations during the first

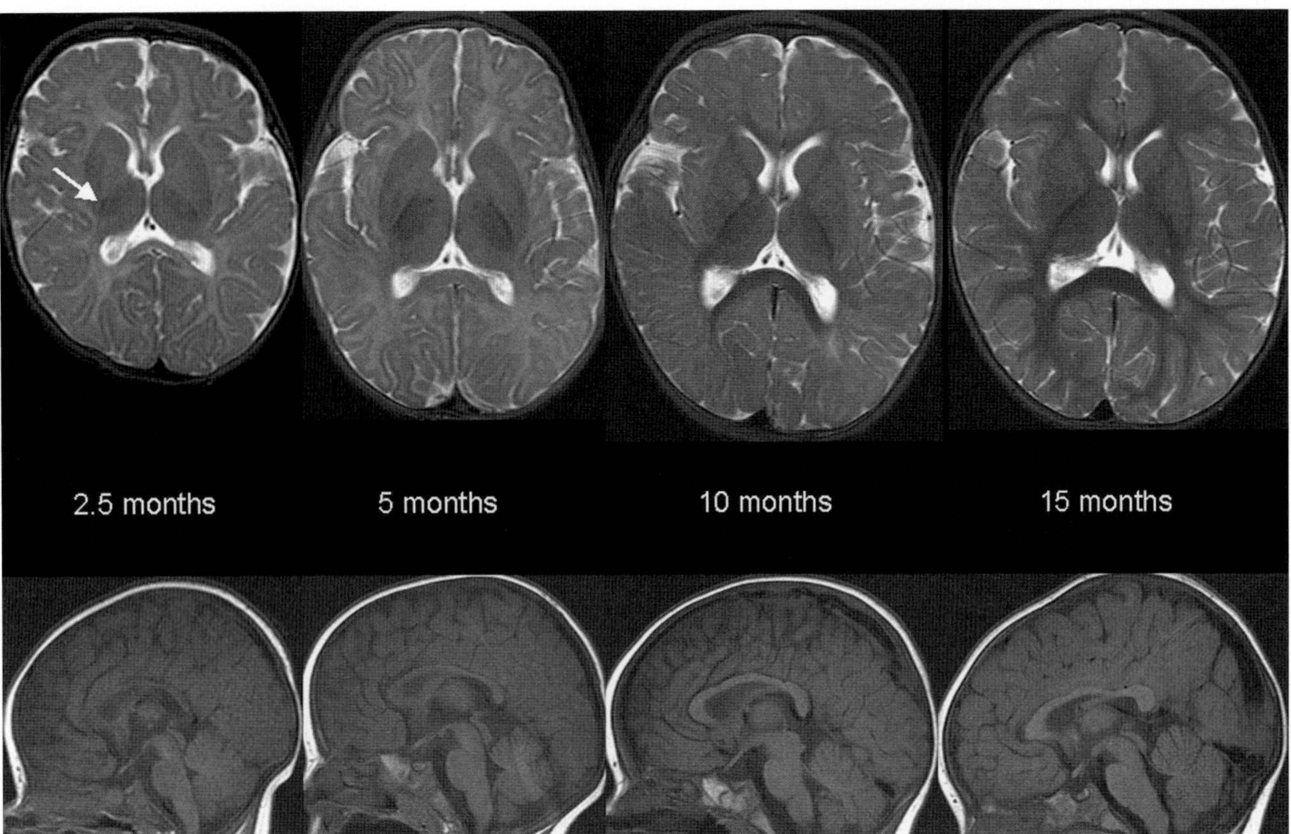

FIGURE 82-1 ■ Normal brain development with age seen on T_2- (top row) and T_1-weighted (bottom row) MRI. On T_2-weighted images myelination at term and at 2.5 months is seen centrally as signal hypointensity within the posterior limbs of the internal capsules. This progresses from posterior to anterior with age, as does myelination of the corpus callosum. Myelination also progresses centrally to peripherally. The sagittal T_1-weighted image shows progressive bulking up of the corpus callosum. By 6 months the corpus callosum should reach approximately its normal childhood size. The splenium is slightly enlarged with respect to the genu.

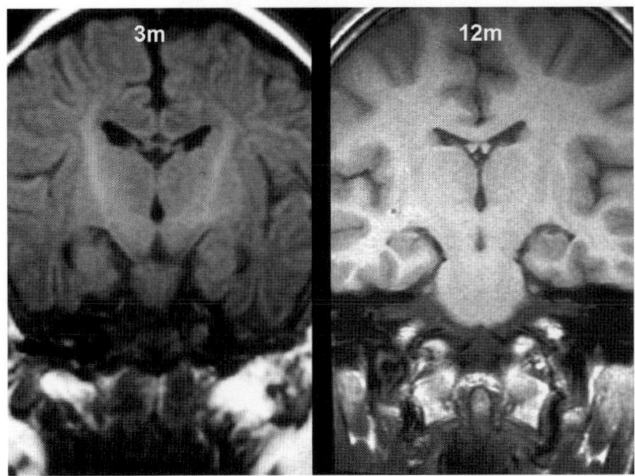

FIGURE 82-2 ■ Normal brain myelination at 3 and 12 months. On T_1-weighted MRI at term, T_1 shortening is seen within the posterior limb of the internal capsule. This progresses posteriorly to anteriorly and centrally to peripherally until by 12 months the brain appears fully myelinated.

months of life. The internal capsule will demonstrate T_1 shortening within the anterior limb by 3 months, while on T_2-weighted images the hypointensity due to myelin is not seen until about 8 months of age. The splenium of the corpus callosum on T_2-weighted images becomes hypointense at 3 months of age. The hypointense signal extends anteriorly along the body and genu, and the complete corpus callosum is myelinated at 6 months.[6]

After 6 months the signal pattern on T_1-weighted images becomes less precise, and after 10 months the brain is fully myelinated by T_1 criteria. T_2-weighted images are then used to assess the myelination from 6 months to 24 months of age, when the signal pattern generally is fully mature and has a completely adult pattern, though the milestones of myelination are much more imprecise than during the first 6 months of life.

On T_2-weighted images the first signs of mature subcortical white matter are found around the calcarine fissure at 4 months and in the pre- and post-central gyri at 8 months. By 10 months the occipital subcortical white matter appears isointense with the overlying grey matter and finally shows mature hypointense signal around 1 year of age. This process proceeds anteriorly and by 18 months has finally reached the most frontal parts and the frontal poles of the temporal lobes.

Regions of persistent hyperintensity on T_2-weighted sequences known as the 'terminal myelination zones'[7] may be seen within the peritrigonal areas well into adulthood. They can be distinguished from white matter disease by the presence of a rim of normal myelinated brain between these areas and the ventricular margin, and no evidence of white matter volume loss such as ventricular enlargement or irregularity of the ventricular margins. Other areas may also persist as regions of signal hyperintensity beyond 2 years, e.g. in the frontotemporal subcortical white matter and peritrigonal white matter, and should not be mistaken for disease (Fig. 82-3).

Normal Gyral Development

Gyration is the process by which the individual gyri and sulci of the cerebral hemispheres form (Fig. 82-4). The MRI appearances lag behind the extent of gyral formation seen at the same age at post-mortem. The surface of the cerebral hemispheres is initially smooth, with the interhemispheric fissure and Sylvian fissures having already formed by 16 weeks' gestation. Other primary sulci, such as the callosal sulcus and parieto-occipital fissure, are recognisable at 22 weeks' gestation, followed by the cingular and calcarine sulci. The central sulcus is seen in most infants by 27 weeks. Gyration then continues into the post-term period in a standardised and

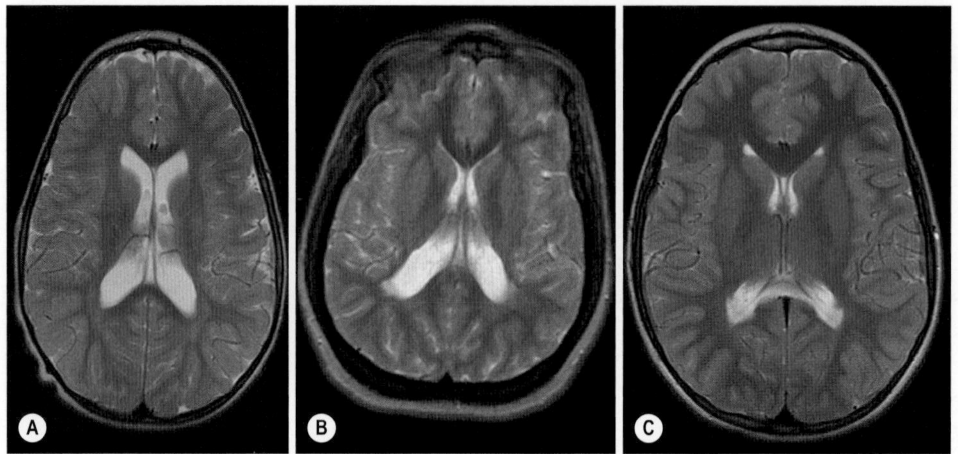

FIGURE 82-3 ■ Normal terminal myelination zones compared to pathological states. (A) T_2-weighted MRI shows signal hyperintensity adjacent to the trigones of the lateral ventricles but with a rim of darker signal between this and the ventricular margins. This is the normal appearance of the terminal myelination zones. (B) Periventricular signal hyperintensity extending down to the ventricular margin. The ventricles are dilated posteriorly and there is irregular scalloping of the ventricular margins in keeping with white matter volume loss. These are the typical features of periventricular leukomalacia due to hypoxic ischaemia. (C) Peritrigonal and splenial signal abnormality. The ventricles are not dilated. This is the typical pattern of adrenoleukodystrophy.

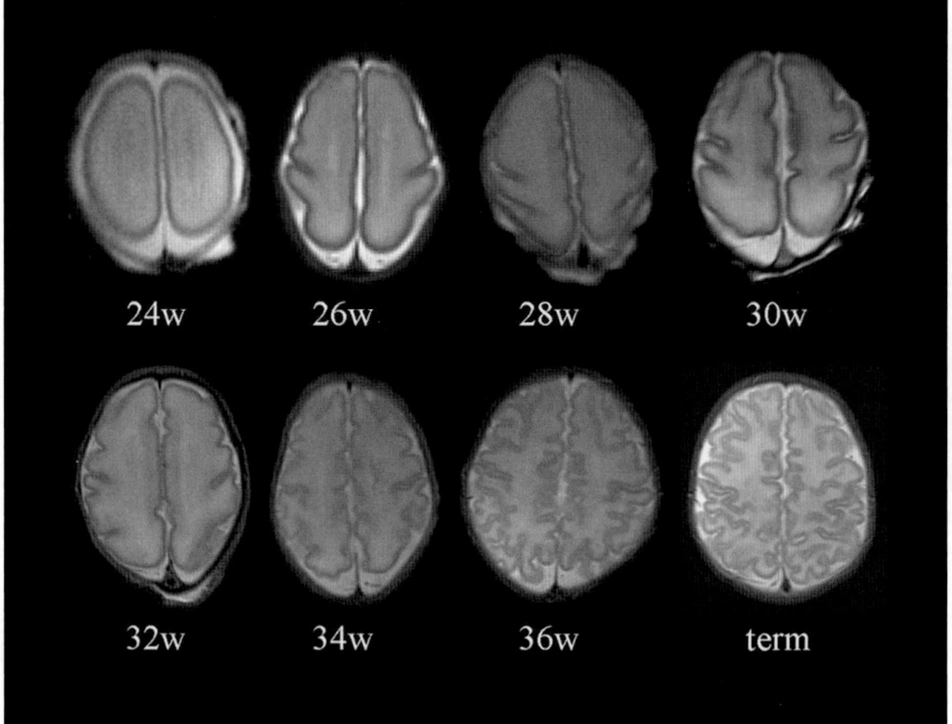

FIGURE 82-4 ■ Normal gyral development in the fetal period seen from 24 weeks' gestational age until term on MRI. Further sulcal development and cortical folding occurs to reach the adult gyral pattern by term. Postnatally, the sulci continue to deepen. Images are a combination of in utero fetal MRI and postnatal MRI. (Acknowledgements: Dr Cornelia Hagmann and University College Hospital, London.)

consistent sequence, beginning with the sensorimotor regions and visual pathways, areas that are also myelinating at the same time. The slowest regions of gyration are also those with the slowest myelination, such as the frontal and temporal poles. By term the gyral pattern is nearly the same as the appearance in adults, with further deepening of the sulci occurring post-term. The Sylvian fissures are also wider and vertically oriented and these continue to mature post-term.[8,9]

Other Postnatal Maturational Changes

Development of the corpus callosum begins with the posterior genu, body and splenium, and then the anterior genu and rostrum. All these components are present by 20 weeks' gestation; however, it continues to grow in length and thickness through the rest of the fetal period and post-term. The adult appearance with full thickness of the corpus callosum is achieved by 8–10 months of age, and bulking up of the splenium as the visual pathways mature occurs by 4–6 months.[10]

In the adult there are several regions where there is relative T_2 hypointensity, considered to be due to the normal deposition of iron; these are the basal ganglia, particularly the globus pallidus, substantia nigra, and red nucleus. In the infant the basal ganglia begin to appear relatively T_2 hypointense to cortex by about 6 months of age due to myelination, but the putamen and globus pallidus are isointense to each other and the internal capsule. They then become relatively bright with respect to white matter as this begins to myelinate. By 9 or 10 years there is a second stage of T_2 shortening in the globus pallidus, substantia nigra and red nucleus, which reduces further during the second decade.[11] The dentate nuclei show similar though less marked changes by about age 15 years. This phase is due to iron deposition, which continues throughout adult life.

In normal infants up to the age of 2 months the anterior pituitary gland has a convex upper border and is of relatively high T_1-weighted signal.[12] From 2 months the pituitary gland has a flat surface and is isointense with grey matter. It slowly grows during childhood and ranges from 2 to 6 mm in vertical diameter until puberty, when it enlarges again.

BRAIN MALFORMATIONS AND DEVELOPMENTAL ABNORMALITIES

Posterior Fossa Abnormalites

Cerebellar Hypoplasia

The cerebellum may be small due to lack of formation or due to cerebellar atrophy. Cerebellar hypoplasia may be due to an acquired brain injury, such as infection (especially congenital cytomegalovirus (CMV)), infarction or preterm ischaemic insult, toxins or a paraneoplastic condition, or the hypoplasia may be due to a genetic, neurometabolic or neurodegenerative condition, or a malformation. In many children (up to 50% in our series), despite extensive testing the cause remains unknown. It has been suggested that the timing of onset is the key feature which determines whether the cerebellum is involved in isolation or whether the pons is also involved. This imaging finding may indicate an earlier disease onset with early neuronal injury to the cerebellum causing pontine hypoplasia by affecting the development of synaptic connections from the hypoplastic cerebellum or supratentorial white matter.

The inherited neurometabolic or neurodegenerative conditions causing cerebellar hypoplasia comprise an extremely wide range of aetiologies. Most are autosomal recessive, but autososomal dominant (often seen in adults), X-linked or maternally inherited forms are recognised. Clinically the child may present with progressive or intermittent hypotonia or ataxia, although there is often no clear correlation between the severity of the imaging findings and the clinical presentation. Among common causes are Friedreich's ataxia, oculomotor apraxia types 1 and 2, ataxia telangiectasia, infantile onset spinocerebellar ataxia, congenital disorders of gylycosylation and infantile neuroaxonal dystrophy (Fig. 82-5). The imaging findings in this large group of conditions are abnormal but are non-specific and include: symmetrical atrophy of the cerebellar folia with widened cerebellar fissures; progressive cerebellar atrophy on sequential images; and variable cerebellar signal changes (less common). The vermis is more frequently affected but the atrophy may be diffuse and bilateral. In most cases there are no additional imaging changes pointing to a specific imaging diagnosis. However, unilateral cerebellar atrophy is more likely to be due to an acquired insult, including

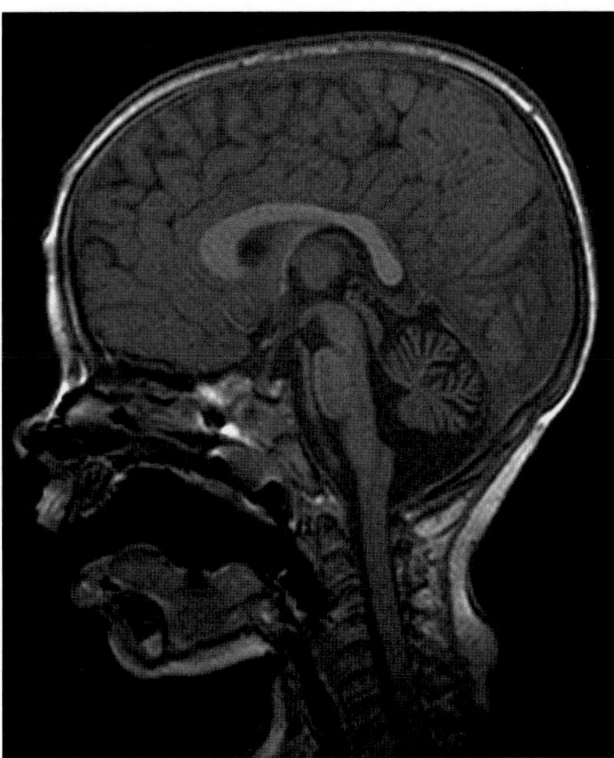

FIGURE 82-5 ■ Child with infantile neuroaxonal dystrophy. The cerebellar folia are underformed and the fissures are widened. The brainstem is also small.

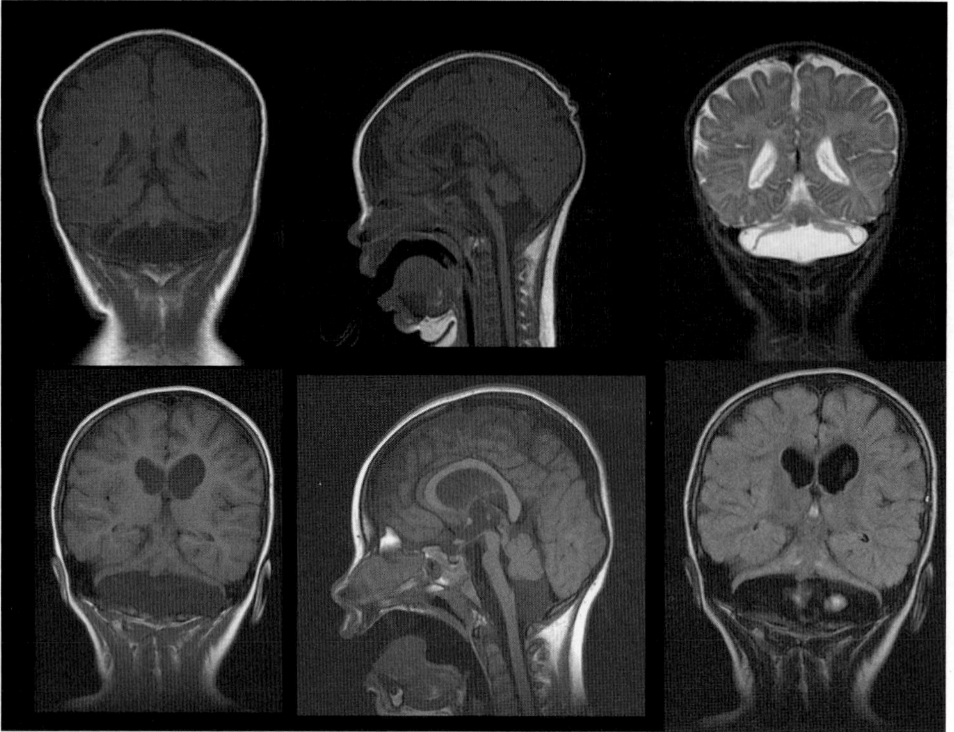

FIGURE 82-6 ■ (Top row) MRI brain images (coronal, sagittal T1W and coronal T2) at 3 months of age. (Bottow row) MRI brain images at age 4 in a child with pontocerebellar hypoplasia and confirmed TSEN54 mutation. The pons is small and there is a 'dragonfly' cerebellum with cerebellar hemisphere hypoplasia and relative sparing of the vermis. There are bilateral cerebellar hemisphere cysts.

in utero infection, stroke or germinal matrix haemorrhage. Many cases of genetic degenerative cerebellar hypoplasia are not associated with significant brainstem hypoplasia. Cerebellar white matter changes are seen in infantile Refsum's disease, adrenomyeloneuropathy and cerebrotendinosis xanthomatosis. Cerebellar grey matter signal abnormality is uncommon but may suggest diagnoses such as infantile neuroaxonal dystrophy, late infantile neuronal ceroid lipofuscinosis, mitochondrial disorders or Marinesco Sjögren's syndrome.

There is also a specific group of conditions in which the pons is more severely affected along with the cerebellum. These are known as the pontocerebellar hypoplasias (PCH) and there are six types (PCH1–6). Some are associated with a typical clinical phenotype, and others with both a classical clinical and imaging phenotype. PCH1 is associated with muscle hypotonia, joint contractures, microcephaly and breathing difficulties from birth with loss of spinal cord motor neurons. Most affected children do not survive infancy. In children with PCH2 there is lack of voluntary movements, dysphagia and absent speech as well as clonus, muscle spasms and classically dystonia, though some children may present purely with spasticity. PCH4 has a similar phenotype but is more severe. PCH3 is associated with optic atrophy. PCH6 is characterised by hypotonia, poor feeding in infancy, progressive developmental delay and seizures; typically a rapidly progressive neonatal or early infancy epileptic encephalopathy with intractabale seizures is seen.

The pontocerebellar hypoplasias may be associated with mutations in specific genes related to neuronal development and survival. Some cases of PCH1 have a specific genetic mutation, VRK1. PCH2 is associated with three related genetic mutations: TSEN54 (the commonest), TSEN2 and TSEN34. PCH4 is also associated with TSEN54 mutation. RARS2 may be seen in PCH6, while specific genetic mutations for PCH3 and PCH5 are not yet known.

All have varying degrees of pontocerebellar hypoplasia on brain MRI. A 'dragonfly' appearances of the cerebellum is recognised typically in PCH2 commonly with TSEN54 mutations; there is marked cerebellar hemisphere atrophy with relative vermian sparing. Cerebral hemisphere cortical atrophy and cerebellar hemisphere cysts may also be seen (Fig. 82-6). In other mutations or unknown genetic mutations a more non-specific 'butterfly' appearance may be seen when there is equal involvement of the cerebellar hemispheres and vermis. Another group of conditions which can present with both cerebellar and pontine hypoplasia are the congenital disorders of glycosylation type IA.

The cerebellum may also be involved in acute presentations of neurometabolic disease or with supratentorial abnormalities and will be discussed in the context of neurometabolic disease later in the chapter.

Dandy–Walker Malformation and Its Variants

This describes a spectrum of cystic posterior fossa malformations ranging from the complete Dandy–Walker malformation to a persistent Blake's pouch and mega

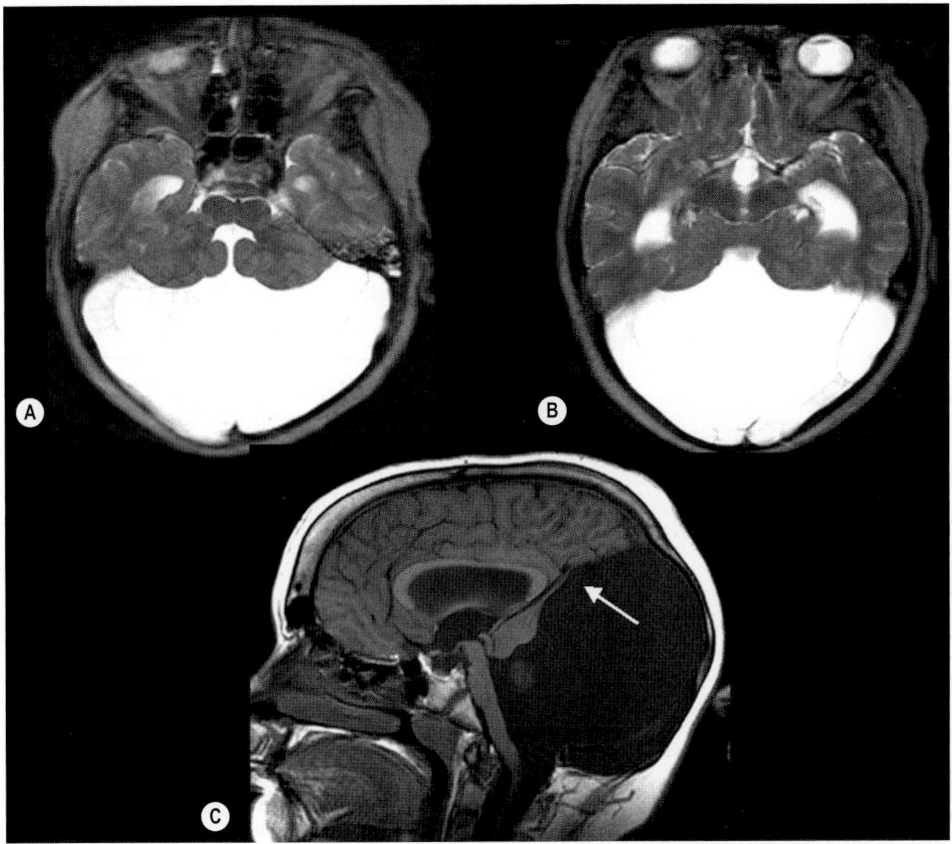

FIGURE 82-7 ■ **Dandy–Walker malformation.** (A, B) The fourth ventricle opens into a large posterior fossa cyst. There is associated hydrocephalus. (C) The cerebellum is hypoplastic and a thin rim of cerebellar tissue is seen forming the wall of the posterior fossa cyst (arrow). The vein of Galen, straight sinus and venous confluence are elevated above the level of the lambdoid suture.

cisterna magna, all of which have in common a focal extra-axial cerebrospinal fluid (CSF) collection continuous with the fourth ventricle, and variable cerebellar hypoplasia.[13] The classical Dandy–Walker malformation is the most severe posterior fossa malformation in this spectrum. It is characterised by cystic dilatation of the fourth ventricle, an enlarged posterior fossa, often with elevation of the venous confluence of the torcula above the lambdoid suture, which may be seen on plain radiography, computed tomography (CT) and MRI, and elevation of the tentorium. There is aplasia or hypoplasia of the cerebellar vermis, with vermian rotation (Fig. 82-7).[14] The Dandy–Walker malformation is associated with hydrocephalus and other midline anomalies, and can be an indicator for underlying clinical syndromes and chromosomal abnormalities. Children with any of these developmental anomalies may present as incidental findings or with developmental delay, seizures and hydrocephalus.

At the mildest end of the spectrum, the mega cisterna magna is seen as an incidental finding of no clinical significance and consists of an infracerebellar CSF collection (or normal cisternal space), with a normal cerebellum and fourth ventricle. The presence of crossing vessels and falx cerebelli favours the mega cisterna magna over a posterior fossa arachnoid cyst. Unlike the mega cisterna magna, posterior fossa arachnoid cysts are not in continuity with the fourth ventricle. They may be associated with mass effect on the adjacent cerebellum and enlargement of the posterior fossa. Mainly these are clinically incidental findings but, like suprasellar arachnoid cysts, may occasionally increase in size in the neonatal period or infancy and cause obstructive hydrocephalus requiring surgical intervention. Arachnoid cysts do not communicate with the fourth ventricle.

Joubert's Syndrome and Related Disorders (JSRD)

These are a group of recessive congenital ataxia disorders in which typically there is neonatal hypotonia, tachypnoea, abnormal eye movements and mental retardation[15] associated with a particular pattern of cerebellar dysgenesis with a molar tooth-type malformation and vermis hypoplasia. The typical imaging findings may be seen in children without the full triad of clinical features. Cilia are found as projections from the neuron and ependyma; to date three known causative genes have been identified in primary ciliary protein genes and JSRD is, therefore, considered to be a cilopathy. Several syndromes with additional features such as renal cysts, ocular abnormalities, liver fibrosis, hypothalamic hamartoma and polymicrogyria have been classified with this anomaly, so that detection of the typical midbrain changes should prompt additional investigation for these. The cardinal feature of the Joubert malformation is the presence of a 'molar tooth' sign which is created by a combination of midbrain hypoplasia with an abnormally deep interpeduncular fossa and a failure of the superior cerebellar peduncles to decussate across the midline (Fig. 82-8). On axial imaging the fourth ventricle is abnormally shaped with a 'batwing appearance', there is cerebellar hypoplasia and there is a midline vermian cleft and dysplastic small vermis. The midbrain is small.[16]

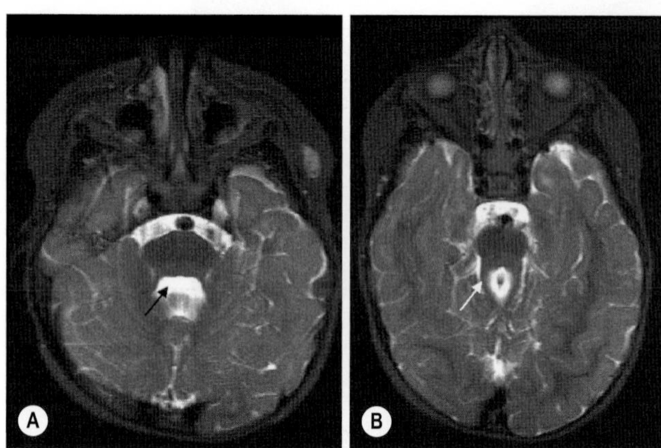

FIGURE 82-8 ■ Child with Joubert's syndrome. (A) Typical batwing appearance to the fourth ventricle (arrow) and (B) prominent superior cerebellar peduncles with failure of the normal midline decussation (arrow). This gives the typical 'molar tooth' appearance. The midbrain is hypoplastic in this condition.

Other Posterior Fossa Malformations or Developmental Disorders

Rhombencephalosynapsis. Rhombencephalosynapsis is a very rare cerebellar malformation in which the cerebellar hemispheres, deep cerebellar nuclei and superior cerebellar peduncles are fused across the midline and there is hypoplasia or aplasia of the vermis (Fig. 82-9).[17] It may be associated with hydrocephalus typically due to aqueduct stenosis, as well as fusion of midbrain colliculi and other midline supratentorial anomalies such as absence of the septum pellucidum, and corpus callosum.

Pontine Tegmental Cap Dysplasia. The diagnosis of pontine tegmental cap dysplasia is made on the basis of characteristic imaging findings in children presenting with multiple cranial neuropathies and evidence of cerebellar dysfunction. There is a characteristic 'cap' or projection on the dorsal surface of the pons which projects into the fourth ventricle. This is continuous with the middle cerebellar peduncles and diffusion tensor imaging studies suggest this is caused by failure of decussation and abnormal axonal pathways at this level. There is also a 'molar tooth' appearances of the superior cerebellar peduncles which fail to decussate. The cerebellar vermis and hemispheres are all small as well as the pons distal to the dorsal pontine 'cap'. The vestibulocochear nerves are absent, there is a cochlea dysplasia and there is a duplicated internal auditory canal for the facial nerve (Fig. 82-10).

Lhermitte-Duclos or Dysplastic Cerebellar Gangliocytoma. Lhermitte-Duclos or dysplastic cerebellar

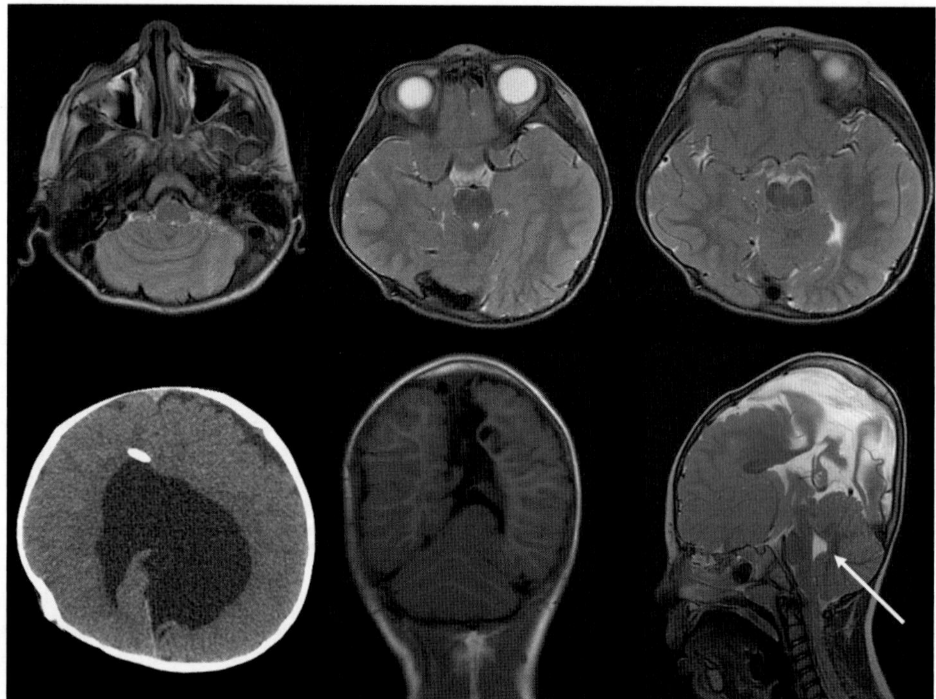

FIGURE 82-9 ■ Child with rhombencephalosynapsis, absent septum pellucidum, initial hydrocephalus and porencephalic cyst. Note the complete fusion across the midline of the cerebellum which herniates cranially thorugh the tentorial hiatus, absent vermis and resulting abnormal configuration of the fastigial point (arrow).

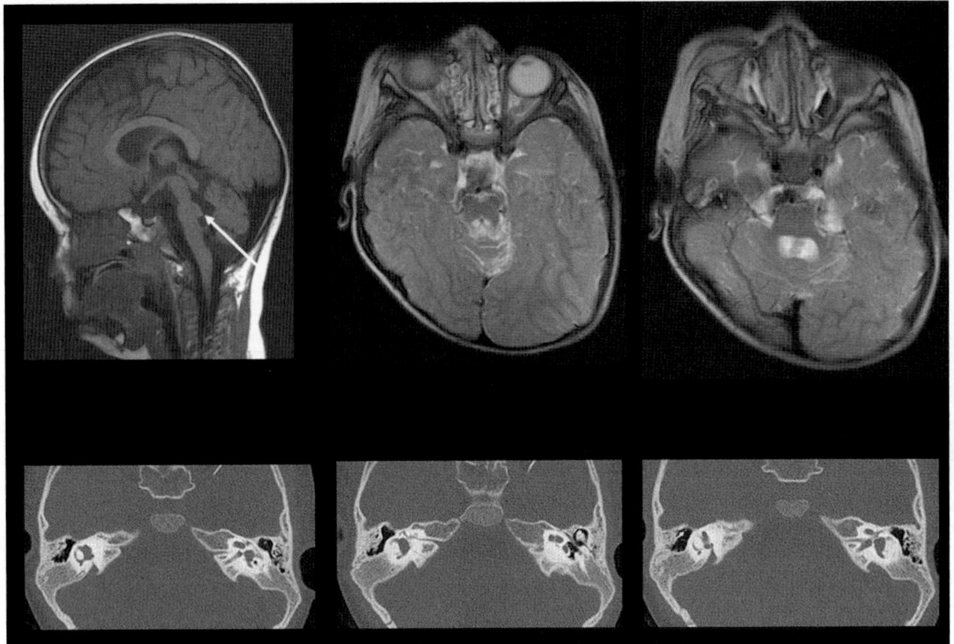

FIGURE 82-10 ■ MRI brain images in this 3-year-old with congenital sensorineural deafness as well as congenital paresis of IV, V and VII, hypotonia, vertical pendular nystagmus and developmental delay show flattened ventral pons, pontine 'cap' projecting into the fourth ventricle (arrow), very thin middle cerebellar peduncles in keeping with pontine tegmental cap dysplasia. CT petrous bones show widened bilateral vestibular aqueducts and dysplasia, small IAM on the right, which is the bony canal for the right facial nerve and on the left two bony canals instead of a single normal-sized IAM, with absence of the VIII nerves.

gangliocytoma is a developmental lesion with a distinctive radiological appearance in which there is enlargement of the cerebellar cortex, usually affecting one hemisphere. On MRI there is a non-enhancing mass with diffusely enlarged cerebellar folia.[18] Pial enhancement may be demonstrated.

There are many other forms of non-specific cerebellar dysgenesis for which as yet there are no universally accepted classification systems.

The Chiari malformations are discussed separately as they represent separate entities.

Chiari II Malformation

This is a true hindbrain malformation which is clinically, radiologically and embryologically distinct from the Chiari I malformation described below. The Chiari II malformation is aetiologically and epidemiologically intimately related to the myelomeningocele with an association that is close to 100%. It is therefore part of a spectrum of consequences of open spinal dysraphism or other failures of closure of the neural tube during fetal development. The clinical presentation is usually at birth or by earlier in utero detection of a lumbosacral meningocele. This entity is discussed in more detail in the 'Disorders of Dorsal Induction' section.

Chiari I Malformation

This may be considered a form of hindbrain deformation rather than a true malformation and is characterised by cerebellar tonsillar descent through a normal-sized foramen magnum. It may be an acquired condition and has occasionally been observed either to improve or worsen over time without intervention. Clinical symptoms are more likely when there is greater than 5 mm descent below the foramen magnum, and therefore descent below this level is considered to be clinically significant. However, neuroimaging does not reliably predict those who are symptomatic. Children between 5 and 15 years have greater tonsillar descent up to 6 mm as a normal finding compared to children under 5 years or adults. There may be an associated syringomyelia. Symptoms including cough-induced headache, lower cranial nerve palsies and disassociated peripheral anaesthesia have been described.

Supratentorial Abnormalities

The earliest malformations to appear relate to the formation of the neural tube, and are described as abnormalities of dorsal induction or cranial dysraphism (occurring at 3–4 weeks' gestation). Anencephaly, cephaloceles and Chiari II (Arnold–Chiari) malformation are generally considered to be consequences of abnormalities of dorsal induction. The events which follow the formation of the neural tube are known as ventral induction, when the two separate cerebral hemispheres are formed (5–8 weeks). The holoprosencephalies are all abnormalities of ventral induction. The structures in the posterior fossa are also formed during this period. Neurons form and proliferate in the subependymal layer of the lateral ventricles known as the germinal matrix and subventricular zone from around 7 weeks' gestation. The neurons subsequently migrate peripherally along radially oriented microglia to form the layers of the cerebral

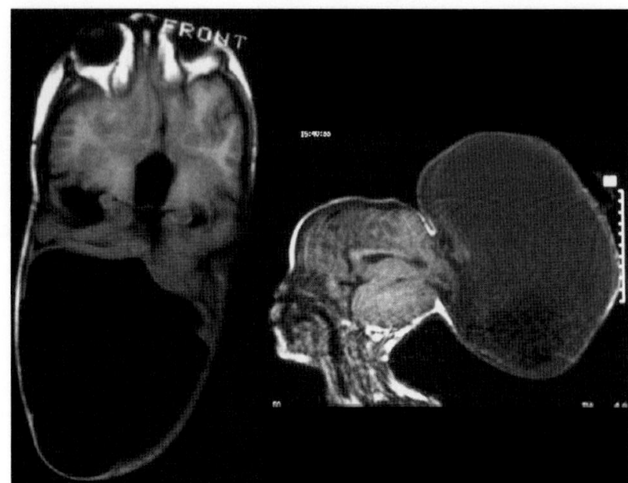

FIGURE 82-11 ■ Parieto-occipital cephalocele with herniation of the brain and meninges through a calvarial defect. Most of the herniated component is in the form of a cerebrospinal fluid-containing meningocele.

cortex from 2 to 5 months' gestation, the deeper layers forming first.

Disorders of Dorsal Induction

Anencephaly. Anencephaly is the most common cerebral malformation in the fetus and is incompatible with life. Most anencephalics are stillborn, but a few survive for a few days.

Cephalocele. A cephalocele is an extracranial protrusion of intracranial structures through a congenital defect of the skull and dura mater (Fig. 82-11). Some authors consider this to be a failure of neurulation or ventral induction (or primary neural tube closure) while others consider this as a post-neurulation event in which brain tissue herniates through a mesenchymal defect in the future dura and cranium.

The cephalocele may be clinically palpable. Unlike myelomeningoceles in the spine, there is usually no skin defect. When the cephalocele contains only leptomeninges and CSF it is a meningocele, and when it also contains neural tissue, typically abnormal and non-functioning with areas of necrosis, calcification and cerebral malformation, it is an encephalocele. The herniation may also include part of the ventricle when it is known as an encephalocystocele. These congenital cephaloceles mainly occur in the midline and at predictable and consistent points, assumed to be multiple closure points of the neural tube to produce frontonasal, parietal, occipital or cervico-occipital cephaloceles. As expected, the bigger the extent of herniating brain, the more microcephalic the affected child is and the more cognitive impairment is present. Occipital cephaloceles are often syndromic.

Cephaloceles are named by the bones which border the bone defect. In nasofrontal cephaloceles the bone defect lies between the frontal and the nasal bones at the level of the 'fonticulus frontalis', a small developmental communication that usually regresses during the fetal period. These lesions can be midline or just off the midline and can be associated with other midline defects such as callosal agenesis and callosal lipomas. If the communicating channel persists, there may be a cephalocele. If the more proximal part eventually obliterates, there may be a dermoid or ectopic brain tissue along the residual track but without intracranial communication. Frontoethmoidal ('sincipital'), nasoethmoidal, naso-orbital, transethmoidal, sphenoethmoidal and sphenonasopharyngeal cephaloceles are also seen, although they are less common.

The primary role of imaging is to establish the presence of neural tissue, other intracranial malformations and hydrocephalus as well as the bone defect. This requires a combination of MRI and CT. Small meningoceles that do not have an intracranial connection may not require surgery, since their size may decrease with time, producing the appearance of an 'atretic meningocele'. As well as the detection of persistent intracranial connection, the detection and localisation of vascular structures is important before any neurosurgical intervention.

Chiari II Malformation (Arnold–Chiari). This is discussed here as a congenital malformation of the hindbrain that is almost always associated with a neural tube defect, usually a lumbosacral myelomeningocele (open neural tube defect). Affected children may have hydrocephalus at birth (25%) but if not most (80%) will develop hydrocephalus following closure and repair of the lumbar myelomeningocele after birth. Other symptoms of complications of the malformation include upper airway problems, such as apnoea and stridor, and feeding problems, such as dysphagia due to brainstem compression or underdevelopment and which occur in about a third of patients. Patients can be developmentally normal or may have delay or seizures. Urinary retention may occur as well as congenital hip dislocations and feet deformities.

The Chiari II malformation is characterised by a small posterior fossa and downward displacement of the cerebellum, pons, medulla oblongata and cervical cord through an enlarged foramen magnum. Associated features include medullary kinking, an inferiorly displaced, elongated and slit-like fourth ventricle, beaking of the tectum of the midbrain, flattening of the ventral pons and low attachment of the tentorium.[19,20] The tentorial incisura is enlarged and the cerebellum herniates superiorly into the supratentorial space. The falx is partially absent or fenestrated, resulting in interdigitation of gyri across the midline, and the massa intermedia of the thalami is enlarged. The foramen magnum is enlarged and 'shield-shaped' (Fig. 82-12).

Other malformations that may be associated with the Chiari II malformation but are less consistent include a lacunar skull dysraphism (luckenschadel), disorders of neuronal migration, malformation of the corpus callosum, dorsal midline cyst and absence of the septum pellucidum.

The diagnosis can be readily made with CT by identifying the wide tentorial incisura, typical configuration of the wide foramen magnum and the small fourth ventricle and posterior fossa. Interdigitation of the cerebral hemispheres may be also identified. MRI is the

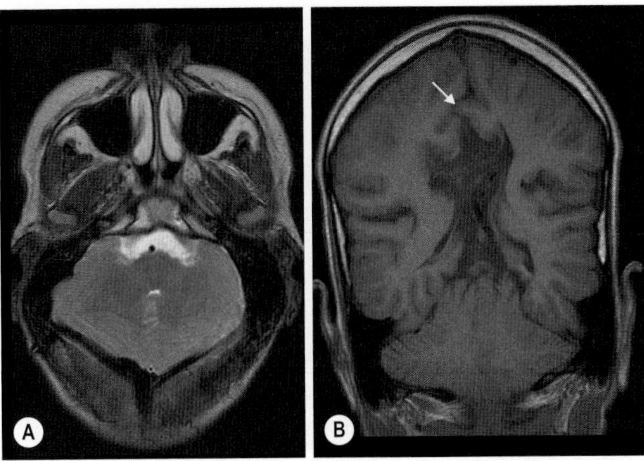

FIGURE 82-12 ■ Chiari II malformation. (A) The posterior fossa is enlarged and 'shield-shaped'. The fourth ventricle is small and slit-like. (B) The cerebellum towers superiorly through the tentorium and there is interdigitation of a cerebral gyrus through the fenestrated falx (arrow).

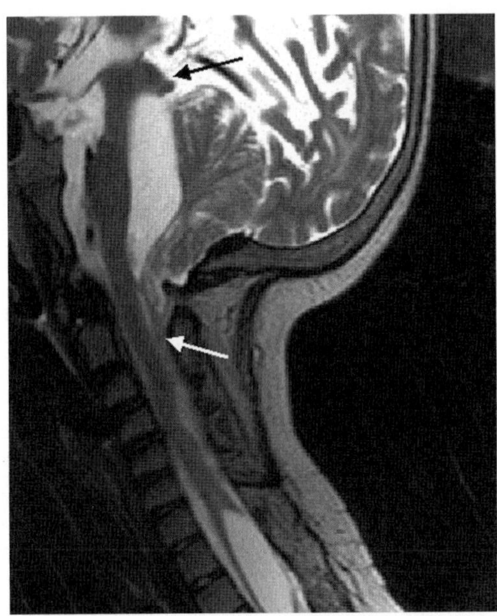

FIGURE 82-13 ■ Chiari II malformation. The fourth ventricle, which should normally be small and slit-like in this condition, is enlarged, indicating hydrocephalus. There is cascading tonsillar tissue herniating through the foramen magnum (white arrow). Beaking of the tectal plate is also seen (black arrow), as well as a cervical spinal cord syringomyelic cavity.

best investigation to show complications, which include hydrocephalus, an isolated fourth ventricle, hydrosyringomyelia and compression of the craniocervical junction. The fourth ventricle in Chiari II malformation should be slit-like: a normal or enlarged ventricle suggests hydrocephalus or that the ventricle may be isolated (Fig. 82-13). A spinal cord syrinx may be present.

The term 'Chiari III' malformation has been used by some authors to describe the association of the brain anomalies commonly seen in Chiari II malformation (inferior cerebellar, medulla and spinal cord displacement, medullary kinking and tectal beaking, etc.) plus an

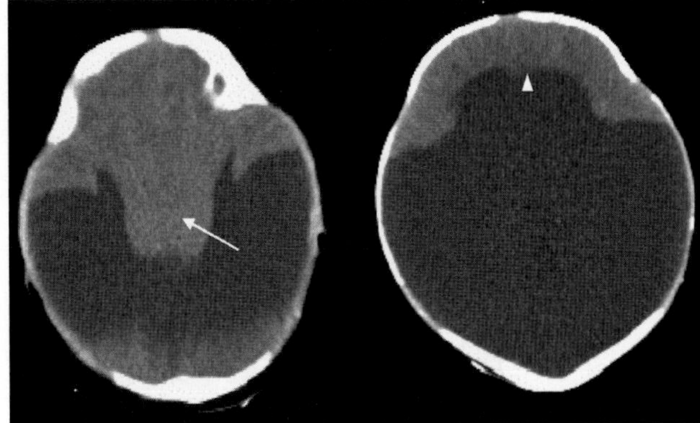

FIGURE 82-14 ■ CT brain of this infant shows that the cerebral hemispheres have failed to form and there is no interhemispheric fissure or corpus callosum. Instead there is a thin pancake of cerebral tissue crossing the midline anteriorly (arrowhead) and a single holoventricle continuous with a large dorsal cyst. The midbrain and deep grey structures are fused into a single indiscriminate mass (arrow).

occipital or cervical encephalocele with occipital bone defect.

Disorders of Ventral Induction

Holoprosencephaly. Holoprosencephaly is a relatively common structural abnormality of the human forebrain, occurring in up to 1 in 10,000 live and stillbirths. It results from a disturbance in the usual signalling pathways required for separation of the embryonic prosencephalon into two separate cerebral hemispheres. Holoprosencephaly is found in association with chromosomal abnormalities, and various teratogenic factors including maternal diabetes. At least 13 different holoprosencephaly loci on chromosomal regions, nine of which are on known holoprosencephaly genes such as sonic hedgehog, ZIC2 and TGIF are recognised. The primary pathway involved in midline developmental anomalies is the sonic hedgehog pathway. This malformation is seen in trisomy 13, 18 and in triploidy. Other abnormalities of midline development are frequently also found.

Classification of holoprosencephaly is based on the degree of separation of the cerebral hemispheres and it appears this is a continuous spectrum of failure of separation. The most severe form is alobar holoprosencephaly in which there is complete or nearly complete failure of separation of the cerebral hemispheres. Many infants are either stillborn or do not survive until term, while infants who do survive are very abnormal with abnormal reflexes, tone and seizures in the neonatal period as well as severe midline facial deformities. The facial deformities can include cyclops or a single eye on a stalk, midline clefts and hypotelorism. Only a minority of patients survive beyond the first year. The medial and ventral parts of the brain have not formed in these patients and the septum pellucidum is absent. On imaging there is a crescent-shaped holoventricle continuous with a large dorsal cyst and the cerebrum consists of a pancake-like mass of tissue with no interhemispheric fissure, corpus callosum or falx cerebri (Fig. 82-14). The hypothalamic and basal ganglia

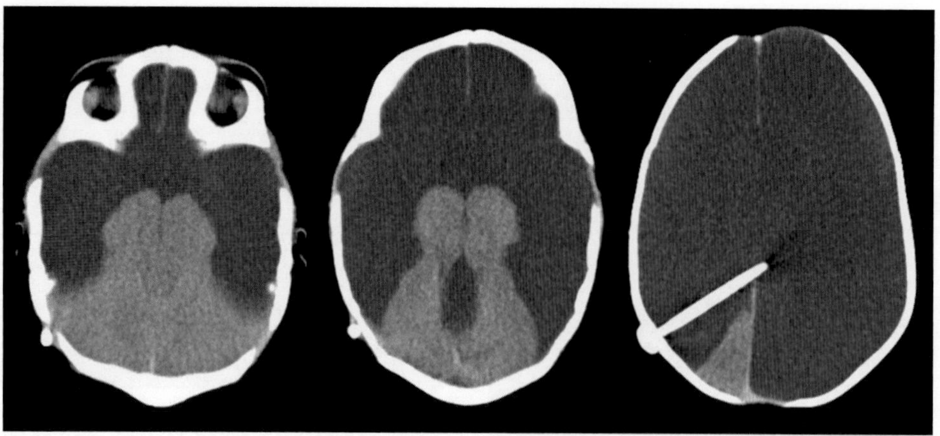

FIGURE 82-15 ■ Child with hydranencephaly in which the cerebral hemispheres are absent with the exception of some of the parieto-occipital lobes, and preservation of the thalami and posterior fossa structures.

are fused. There is no normal circle of Willis and the arterial supply comes directly from the internal carotid and basilar arteries without normal anterior, middle and posterior cerebral arteries. Despite the underlying microcephaly, hydrocephalus often develops and CSF diversion with a shunt may be required as a palliative procedure to help manage head size for nursing. Holoprosencephaly should be distinguished from gross hydrocephalus in which there is a very thin, barely visible cerebral cortical mantle and from hydranencephaly caused by a global early in utero insult (thought to be ischaemic) in which much of the cerebral hemisphere parenchyma is destroyed, leaving a fluid-filled cavity but with relative preservation of mesial temporal occipital lobes, deep grey matter and brainstem (Fig. 82-15). Semilobar holoprosencephaly is less severe; although posteriorly the interhemispheric fissure is partially formed, anteriorly the hemispheres fail to separate. As the brain is less dysmorphic, the midline facial abnormalities are also mild or absent. These children present later with developmental delay or concerns over reduced or increasing head size due to hydrocephalus. The frontal lobes are fused, but the thalami are partially separated. There is still a single ventricle instead of the two lateral ventricles seen normally but the failure of separation of the hypothalami, thalami and basal ganglia is less severe compared to the alobar form and there may be an indication of a third ventricle. The posterior corpus callosum is partially formed. The temporal horns are rudimentary and the hippocampi are underdeveloped.

Lobar holoprosencephaly is associated with mild (or absent) facial malformations and intellectual abilities that range from mild impairment to normal. They may have endocrine disturbance of the hypothalamic–pituitary axis. The brain is generally of normal volume and shows almost complete separation into two hemispheres, though in the depth of the frontal lobes there is continuous cerebral cortex between the two lobes.

Finally there is the interhemispheric variant of holoprosencephaly, also known as syntelencephaly, which has a mild clinical presentation with mild learning and visual impariments. In this condition the interhemispheric fissure is formed anteriorly at the level of the anteroir frontal lobes, and posteriorly at the level of the occipital lobes but in the middle the posterior frontal and parietal lobes are fused and there is no interhemispheric fissure, falx and corpus callosum (Fig. 82-16). This results in an unusual callosal malformation in which the genu and splenium are present but the body is absent

Malformations of Commissural and Related Structures

Agenesis of the Septum Pellucidum. Absence of the septum pellucidum is not a severe malformation, but should be recognised as an indicator of other cerebral malformations. Associated malformations include septo-optic dysplasia, agenesis of the corpus callosum, holoprosencephaly, Chiari II malformation, schizencephaly and other migration disorders. Septo-optic dysplasia or de Morsier's syndrome describes the triad of hypopituitarism, hypoplasia of the optic nerves and absence of the septum pellucidum (Fig. 82-17). Less than 1% are associated with mutations in the HESX1 gene. However, the the clinical manifestations are quite variable. Neuroimaging may show absence of the septum pellucidum with a typical box-like configuration of the frontal horns, small optic nerves and chiasm, small anterior pituitary gland and ectopic 'bright spot' of the posterior pituitary gland on T1W imaging. Isolated absence of the septum pellucidum may also occur and it is important to look for other associated brain anomalies such as callosal agenesis, holoprosencephaly, cobblestone cortical malformations and bilateral polymicrogyria. The septum pellucidum may also be absent as an acquired lesion in the context of hydrocephalus.

Commissural Agenesis or Dysgenesis. The major interhemispheric commissural connections are the corpus callosum and anterior and hippocampal commissures. The corpus callosum consists of the rostrum, genu, body and splenium with the isthmus defining a normal point of narrowing between the body and the splenium of the corpus callosum. The corpus callosum may be partially

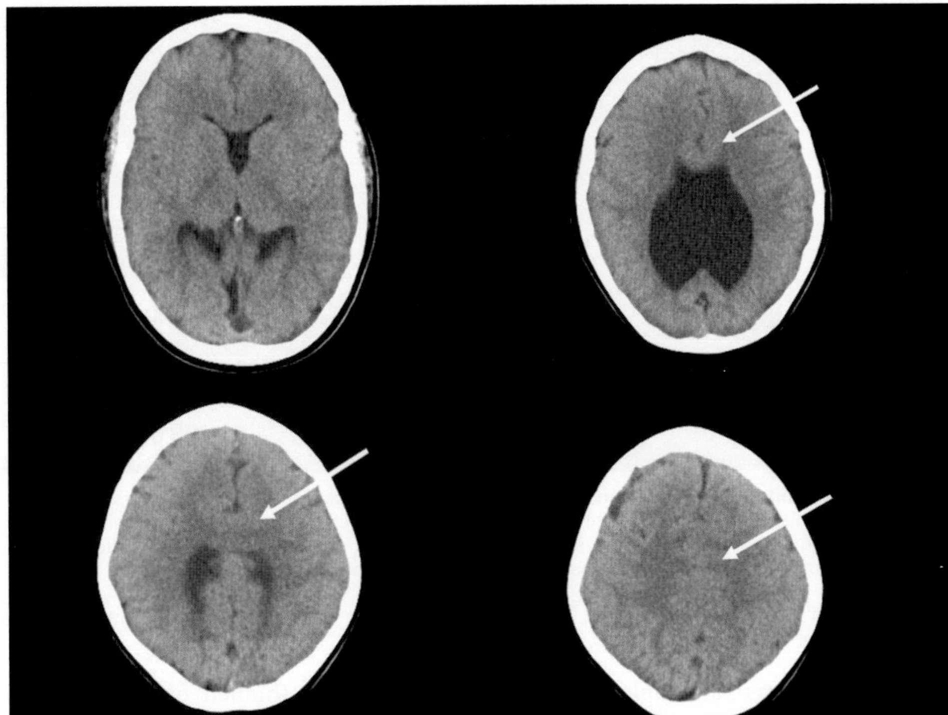

FIGURE 82-16 ■ Syntelencephaly or 'middle interhemispheric' variant of holoprosencephaly in which the anterior interhemispheric fissure is present and frontal lobes and occipital lobes are separate, but the posterior frontal and parietal lobes have failed to separate (arrows).

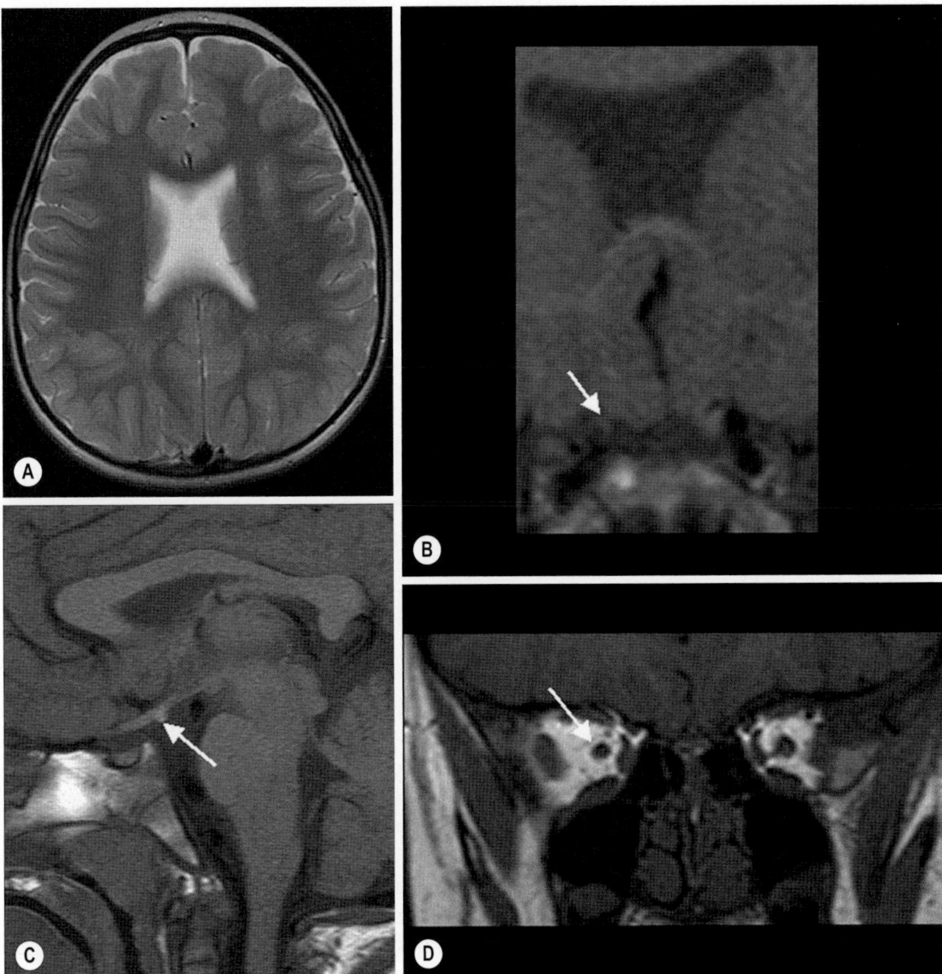

FIGURE 82-17 ■ **Septo-optic dysplasia in a child with HESX1 gene mutation.** (A) The septum pellucidum is absent and the frontal horns have a typical box-like configuration. (B) The posterior pituitary gland is ectopic (arrow). (C, D) The right optic nerve is small (arrows).

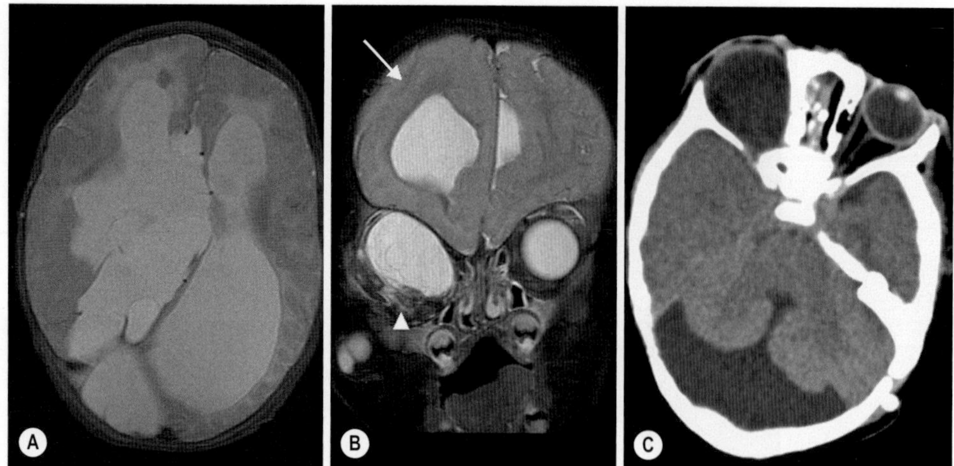

FIGURE 82-18 ■ **Child with skin lesions and right orbital cyst in oculocerebrocutaneous syndrome.** (A) There is callosal agenesis with dorsal interhemispheric cysts. (B) The right cerebral hemisphere is dysplastic with thickening of the cortex and an indistinct grey–white matter junction (arrow). There is a cyst expanding the orbit with a small calcified globe seen inferiorly (arrowhead). (C) An associated Dandy–Walker posterior fossa malformation is also present.

formed (dysgenesis) or completely absent (agenesis). The anterior part (posterior genu and anterior body) is formed before the posterior part (posterior body and splenium). Hence a small or absent genu or body, with an intact splenium and rostrum, is more likely to suggest secondary destruction rather than abnormal development. The structure develops between about 7 and 20 weeks' gestation, which parallels the development of the rest of the cerebrum and the cerebellum; abnormalities of the corpus callosum are therefore commonly associated with other congenital malformations of the brain, such as Chiari II malformation, Dandy–Walker malformation, lipoma, abnormalities of neuronal migration and organisation, dysraphic anomalies, encephaloceles, septo-optic dysplasia, ocular anomalies and other midline facial anomalies.[21]

There are many well-defined syndromes in which callosal abnormalities feature, including Aicardi's syndrome which is X-linked dominant occurring in females and characterised by seizures, intellectual impairment, chorioretinal lacunae seen at fundoscopy examination and brain malformations such as polymicrogyria, ectopic grey matter and cortical dysplasias. Callosal agenesis is a feature of oculocerebrocutaneous syndrome or Delleman's syndrome (Fig. 82-18), Alport's syndrome, orofacial-digital syndrome and many other syndromes. Dysgenesis of the corpus callosum is also frequently seen in fetal alcohol syndrome.

Agenesis of the Corpus Callosum. On axial imaging the lateral ventricles have a parallel orientation and a typical posterior dilatation known as colpocephaly. The third ventricle extends more superiorly than normal within the interhemispheric fissure between the bodies of the lateral ventricles and the normal convergence of the bodies of the ventricles towards the midline is absent. On sagittal imaging, partial or complete absence of the corpus callosum must be distinguished from a generally thinned one (which is more likely to be an acquired abnormality). In callosal agenesis the vertically oriented sulci extend right down to the ventricle without formation of the cingulate gyri which normally run parallel to the corpus callosum and there is no horizontally running cingulate sulcus. On coronal imaging the corpus callosum is absent in the midline, the third ventricle is high-riding and there is a characteristic indentation on the medial aspect of the lateral ventricles caused by the bundles of Probst, which are the white matter tracts that are no longer able to cross the midline in the corpus callosum (Fig. 82-19). Presence of one midline anomaly, such as callosal agenesis, should prompt the reporting radiologist to look carefully for other midline anomalies that are frequently associated, such as midline lipomas and cephaloceles.

Agenesis of the Corpus Callosum with Interhemispheric Cyst. In some cases the interhemispheric cyst frequently seen with this malformation originates from the herniated third ventricle and is in continuity with it and the rest of the ventricular system, while in others continuity between the cyst and the third ventricle is lost. In both cases progressive increase in head circumference with hydrocephalus may occur in the neonate and infant, requiring shunting/drainage.

Malformations of Cortical Development—Histogenesis, Neuronal Migration and Cortical Organisation

Abnormalities of the cerebral cortex are a common finding in children with developmental delay and children with partial epilepsy. After neurulation, the process by which the neural tube is formed, has occurred, an important stage in the development of the brain is the formation of the cortex. The cortex is formed from neuroblasts that are generated in the germinal matrix,

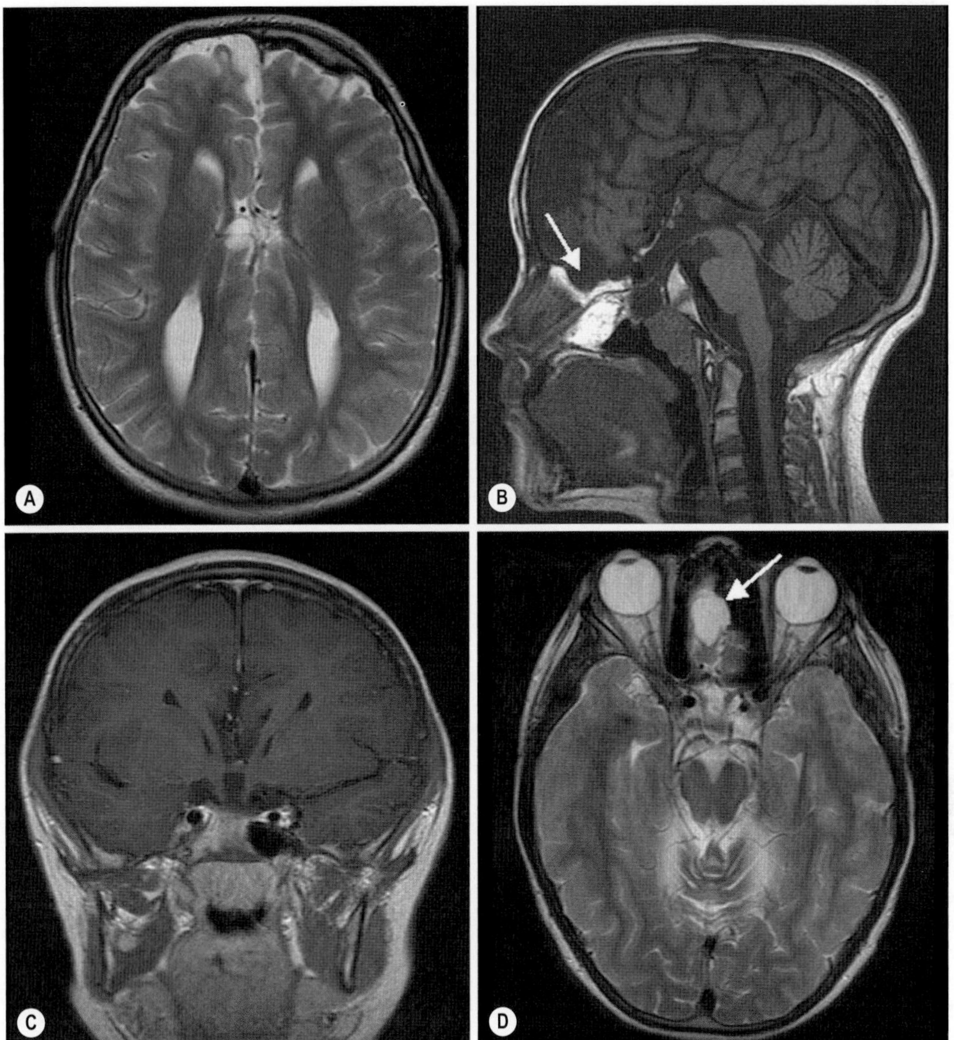

FIGURE 82-19 ■ **Callosal agenesis.** (A) Axial T_2-weighted MRI shows separated ventricles with parallel orientation. The superior part of the third ventricle is just seen. (B) Sagittal T_1-weighted MRI through the midline confirms callosal agenesis. There is no cingulate sulcus and the vertically oriented cerebral sulci extend right down to the third ventricle. This finding is associated with other midline anomalies such as a frontoethmoidal cephalocele (arrow), seen also on the axial T_2-weighted MRI (arrow, C). (D) The optic chiasm is absent.

located at the ependymal border of the ventricular wall. There is a migration of excitatory glutaminergic neurons by radial migration from the ventricular zone at the ependymal surface. These neuroblasts migrate to the surface of the brain along radially oriented glia, passing neurons previously laid down to form the layers of cortex. Thus the six layers of the cortex are formed, with the youngest neurons on the surface and the oldest ones adjacent to the subcortical white matter. The migration of the neuroblasts starts at about week 7 of gestation, is most intense during weeks 15–17 and is largely complete by weeks 23–24. In parallel with this, another process of tangential migration occurs involving inhibitory GABA-ergic interneurons which migrate from the ganglionic eminences. There organise in a precise manner with the radially migrating neurons described earlier.

Malformations of cortical development result from disorders of cell proliferation (or histogenesis), cell migration or cell organisation. Based on this neuroembryology, it is convenient to attempt to classify malformations of cortical development broadly according to these embryological principles.[22] For the purposes of this chapter, these malformations will be described by radiological pattern, starting with disorders of neuronal organisation, then migration, then histogenesis.

Polymicrogyria

This is considered to be a disorder of neuronal organisation, occurring after neuronal migration. The extent of polymicrogyric cortex may vary from small, isolated, unilateral areas to larger areas of bilateral disease (Fig. 82-20). The key pathological feature to identify on

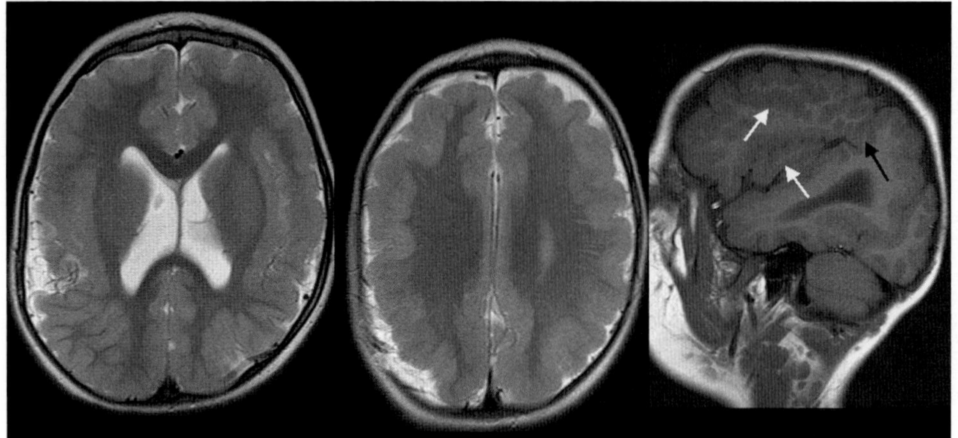

FIGURE 82-20 ■ **Extensive bilateral cerebral hemisphere polymicrogyria.** Virtually no normal cortex is seen. At first glance the cortex appears thickened, but closer inspection reveals an overconvoluted gyral pattern and a 'lumpy bumpy' grey–white matter interface (including regions marked by white arrows). The Sylvian fissure is abnormally oriented with a parietal cleft that extends posteriorly (black arrow).

imaging is an overconvoluted and fused cortex of normal thickness. The appearances on imaging may vary from apparently broad, thickened gyri mimicking pachygyria (particularly when examined with relatively thick imaging slices), to clearly overconvoluted multiple gyri with irregular outer and inner cortical surfaces.

The identification of polymicrogyria assists with genetic counselling. There are recessive and dominant forms that are often bilateral and symmetrical, as well as disease believed to be acquired from intrauterine infection such as CMV infection or an underlying neurometabolic disorder, which may often be asymmetrical in distribution. There may be associated dystrophic calcification in these lesions, which typically may only be visible on CT.

Schizencephaly

Schizencephaly is a defect that involves the complete cerebral mantle and connects the calvarium and the outer surface of the brain with the lateral ventricles. The defect is a cleft lined by grey matter and leptomeninges, which differentiates it from a transmantle infarction in which the defect is lined by white matter. The schizencephaly may have an 'open lip' with a wide open defect (Fig. 82-21), or a 'closed lip' when the cleft is closed but lined with grey matter entirely into the ventricle. The convolutional pattern of the cortex adjacent to the clefts is abnormal and consists of polymicrogyria.

The clinical features are variable, depending on the size and location of the lesion. Severe seizures are quite common, as is spasticity. Children with bilateral clefts have severe mental and psychomotor developmental delay. Wide clefts usually correlate with moderate-to-severe developmental delay, while children with narrow or closed-lipped lesions may only have hemiplegia and/or seizures. The location of the lesion is typically central, involving the pre- and post-central gyri. However, the clefts may also be found in parasagittal, frontal or occipital sites when the clinical manifestations are often mild.

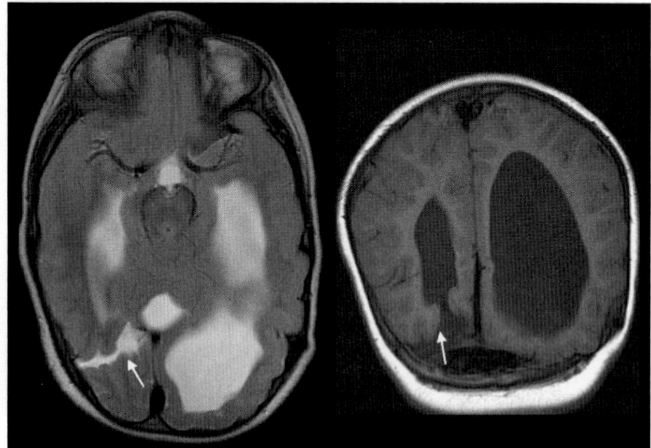

FIGURE 82-21 ■ Schizencephaly with a grey matter-lined cleft (arrows) extending from the leptomeningeal surface through the brain parenchyma to the ventricular margin.

In most cases the diagnosis can be made with CT, but this may not detect all cases of closed lip schizencephaly, which are best detected using coronal T_1-weighted MRI, preferably a three-dimensional (3D) volume acquisition. MRI also shows the abnormal appearance of the cortical mantle along the cleft and the cortex appearing thicker than normal owing to the presence of polymicrogyria. The contralateral hemisphere may also have developmental abnormalities, such as polymicrogyria and subependymal heterotopia. CT may show subependymal or parenchymal calcification in many cases, which suggests that one cause of schizencephaly may be intrauterine infection such as CMV infection.

Lissencephaly–Agyria–Pachygyria

The lissencephaly–agyria–pachygyria group includes the severest forms of abnormal neuronal migration. Lissencephaly literally means 'smooth brain'. The classical or

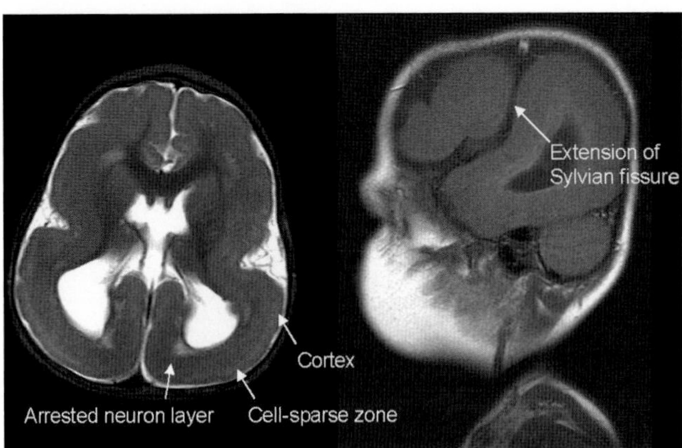

FIGURE 82-22 ■ Classical with lissencephaly. This child was 'floppy' at birth and then had developmental delay, seizures and strabismus. MRI shows a smooth gyral pattern which is slightly more developed frontally in keeping with classical lissencephaly (*LIS1* mutation). The cerebral cortex is generally thin and there is a band of arrested neurons deep to the 'cell-sparse zone'. The Sylvian fissures are vertically oriented and extend into a vertical cleft.

type 1 Lissencephaly will be discussed first. The cortex is thickened and the brain has very few or no gyri, opercularisation (development of the Sylvian fissures) is abnormal, and the Sylvian fissures are shallow and wide. Other associated features are agenesis or hypoplasia of the corpus callosum or septum pellucidum. Agyria refers to the total or almost total absence of a convolutional pattern, i.e. there are no gyri or sulci, and is synonymous with 'complete lissencephaly'. In pachygyria, the gyri are relatively few and are unusually broad and flat. The entire brain is not affected and therefore it is sometimes referred to as 'incomplete lissencephaly'. Macroscopically and on standard thick-slice MRI, the thickened cortex of pachygyria may be difficult to differentiate from the overconvoluted, fused and normal-thickness cortex of polymicrogyria, but the latter may be distinguished more easily on higher-resolution imaging, e.g. with volumetric T_1-weighted imaging (e.g. MPRAGE, SPGR, FLASH).

In complete lissencephaly the brain surface is smooth and the Sylvian fissures are wide and vertically orientated. The posterior fossa structures are typically spared and appear normal. The cortex has a thin outer layer, an underlying 'cell-sparse zone' and a thicker broad band of grey matter, the 'arrested neurons' that have failed to migrate to the cortex, deep to it (Fig. 82-22). The gyral pattern of the brain resembles the appearance of the 23- to 24-week normal fetal brain. The implication of this is that lissencephaly is unlikely to be reliably diagnosed on early fetal MRI (before 24 weeks), though there may be clues to the diagnosis before this, such as the immature appearance of the Sylvian fissures, cell-sparse zone and the broad band of arrested neurons.

With incomplete lissencephaly there is an anteroposterior gradation of disease severity. In the *LIS1* mutation (chromosome 17) the frontotemporal gyri are more developed than the parieto-occipital gyri and in the X-linked form (*DCX* a.k.a. *XLIS* mutation) the posterior gyri are more developed. Subcortical band heterotopia is a feature of these mutations and is therefore discussed here. On imaging, band heterotopia appears as a homogeneous band of grey matter between the lateral ventricle and the cerebral cortex, separated from both by a layer of white matter. The overlying cortex is usually of normal thickness but has shallow sulci. *DCX* mutations result in subcortical band heterotopia or 'double cortex' that is predominantly seen in girls (> 90%), as boys with these mutations usually develop lissencephaly. Impairment to neuronal migration is more severe anteriorly, so the band heterotopia is typically seen symmetrically in the frontal regions. Although the imaging appearances may be severe, the degree of developmental delay may be quite variable. Some children may even be normal except for a relatively mild seizure disorder.

Variants of classical lissencephaly are now increasingly recognised. They account for a minority of cases and may demonstrate additional findings on imaging. These include X-linked lissencephaly with abnormal genitalia (XLAG) demonstrating agenesis of the corpus callosum and associated with *ARX* mutations, lissencephaly with cerebellar hypoplasia (LCH) associated with *RELN* or *VLDLR* mutations and tubulin mutations such as *TUBA1A* which result in a per-Sylvian pachygyria, absent anterior limbs or the internal capsules and dysplastic basal ganglia (Fig. 82-23).

Type 2 or Cobblestone lissencephaly is distinct from the above, the result of overmigration of neurons and is characterised by thick meninges adherent to the smooth cortical surface. There is disordered lamination of the cortex on histological examination. Extensive subcortical heterotopia are a feature and delay in myelination is frequently present. The posterior fossa structures are usually abnormal with the appearance of dysplasia with microcysts of the cerebellar hemispheres, a flattened shape of the pons in the AP dimension with a midline cleft or with a Z-shaped brainstem in the sagittal plane. The congenital muscular dystrophies (CMDs) are a heterogeneous group characterised clinically by hypotonia at birth, muscle weakness and joint contractures, developmental delay and seizures. The cobblestone lissencephaly in these cases may range from the severe clinical phenotype of the Walker–Warburg syndrome with coexistent ocular abnormalities to the milder phenotype of Fukuyama CMD with relatively normal eyes. In parallel with these clinical phenotypes, several genes have been identified with these clinical syndromes, including *POMT1*, *POMT2*, *FKRP*, *POMGnT1* and *LARGE*.

Grey Matter Heterotopia

Grey matter heterotopia refers to the occurrence of grey matter in an abnormal position anywhere from the subependymal layer to the cortical surface, but the term is usually reserved for ectopic neurons in locations other than the cortex. Its most common clinical presentation is as a seizure disorder. However, small isolated areas of heterotopia may be seen occasionally as incidental findings in normal patients.

Heterotopia can be subependymal, focal subcortical or band formed, or parallel to the ventricular wall (double cortex). They are isointense with cortical grey matter on

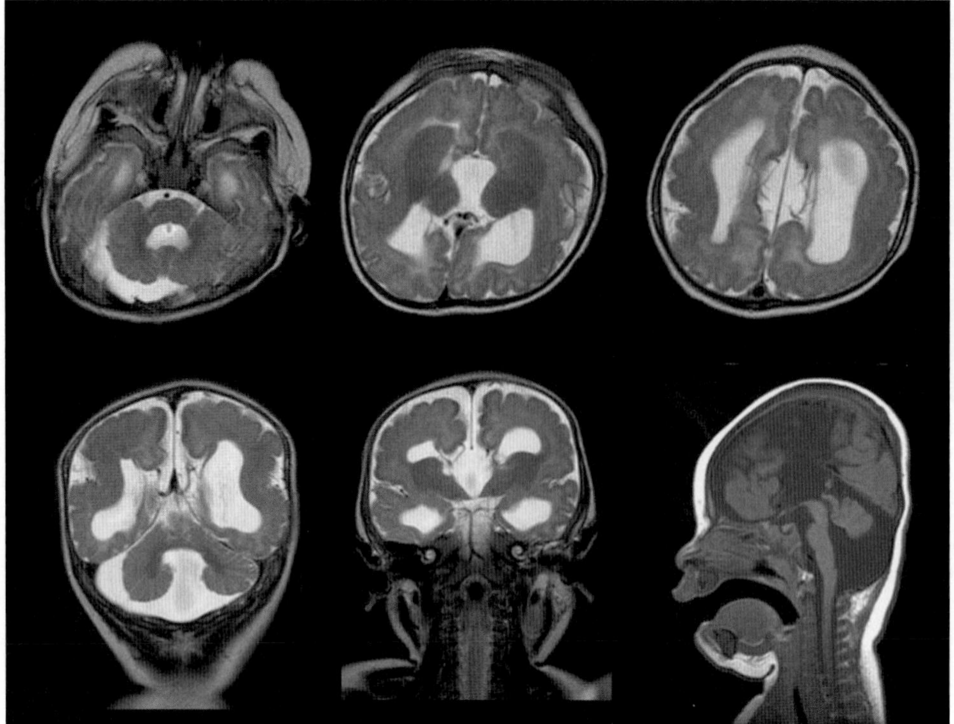

FIGURE 82-23 ■ MRI brain of a child with confirmed *TUBA1A* mutation shows frontal and peri-Sylvian pachygyria with more normal gyral differentiation anteriorly and posteriorly, absent corpus callosum, cerebellar vermian hypoplasia and rotation, small pons and absent anterior limb of internal capsule.

all imaging sequences and do not enhance after the intravenous infusion of paramagnetic contrast agents. Subcortical band heterotopia has already been discussed with classical lissencephaly.

Subependymal heterotopia are smooth and ovoid, with their long axis typically parallel to the ventricular wall, quite different from subependymal hamartomas in tuberous sclerosis which are irregular and have their long axis perpendicular to the ventricular wall (Fig. 82-24). In contrast, hamartomas seen in tuberous sclerosis are more heterogeneous depending on the presence of calcification, gliois, etc., and do not have signal characteristics of grey matter. They may also enhance after the intravenous infusion of a paramagnetic contrast agent.

Focal subcortical heterotopia produces variable motor and intellectual impairment, depending on the size and location of the lesions. The overlying cortex is thin with shallow sulci. The foci may be isolated or may coexist with other malformations such as schizencephaly, microcephaly, polymicrogyria, dysgenesis of the corpus callosum, or absence of the septum pellucidum.

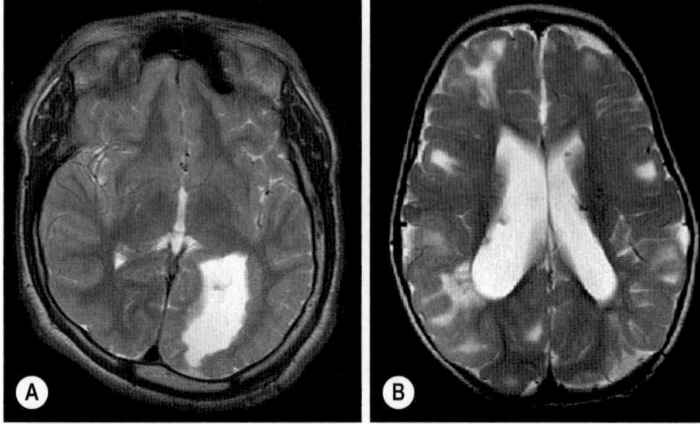

FIGURE 82-24 ■ **Subependymal grey matter heterotopia (A) and subependymal hamartomas of tuberous sclerosis (B).** (A) Multiple subependymal continuous 'nodules' running along the ventricular margin with signal intensity isointense to grey matter. (B) Scattered nodules which project into the ventricles and with variable signal intensity. Some are markedly hypointense in keeping with calcification. Note also the multiple regions of cortical and subcortical white matter abnormality with slight mass effect in keeping with cortical tubers.

Hemimegalencephaly

This is a structural malformation due to defective neuronal proliferation, migration and organisation, leading to hamartomatous overgrowth of all or part of one hemisphere. It may occur in isolation or in association with syndromes such as Proteus, epidermal naevus and Klippel–Trénaunay–Weber syndromes, neurofibromatosis type 1 (NF1) and tuberous sclerosis. The affected hemisphere contains regions of pachygyria, polymicrogyria, heterotopia, as well as dysmyelination and gliosis. Usually (but not always) the hemisphere is enlarged, there is diffuse cortical thickening, white matter signal abnormality and there may be calcification. The ipsilateral lateral ventricle is enlarged and there is a very characteristic configuration of the

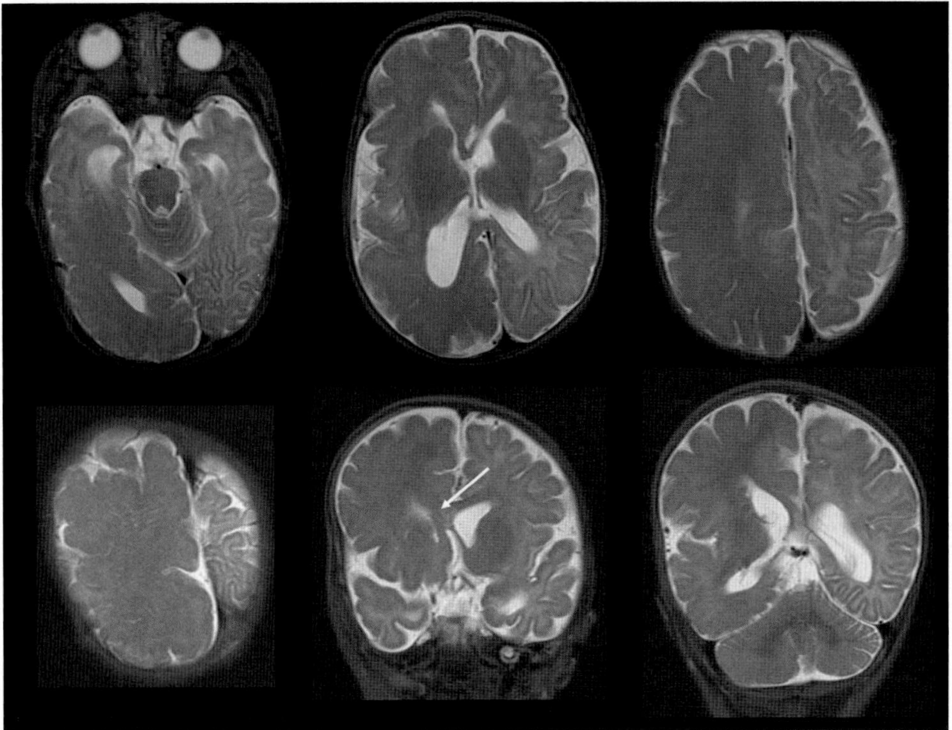

FIGURE 82-25 ■ Enlargement of the right cerebral hemisphere in keeping with hemimegalencephaly. There is thickening of the cortex with broad, thickened gyri, underdeveloped sulci and extensive white matter signal abnormality. Note the straightening of the right frontal horn and thickening of the genu of the corpus callosum and right anterior fornix (arrow).

frontal horn which is straight and pointed (Fig. 82-25) and associated thickening of the septum pellucidum. Occasionally this may be the only imaging clue to an underlying malformation.

Focal Cortical Dysplasia (FCD)

These are localised regions of malformed cerebral cortex and are frequently associated with epilepsy in children and adults. They are the commonest lesion found in paediatric epilepsy surgical series and were first described by Taylor et al. in 1971. This term is now used for a wide spectrum of lesions including cortical dyslamination, cytoarchitectural lesions and underlying abnormalities of white matter. Classification may be imaging-based[22] or pathologically based and the challenge remains to identify discriminating imaging features to differentiate the different histopathological subtypes of FCD. A recent classification produced by the ILAE describes FCD I (a–c), II (a, b), both isolated, and III (associated with a principal lesion such as hippocampal sclerosis, glioneuronal tumour, vascular malformation or adjacent to an early acquired insult).[23] Overall they can be located in any part of the cortex, have variable size and location and can affect more than one lobe. If seizures become resistant to medical treatment, patients with these lesions may be considered for epilepsy surgery and lesion resection. Neuroimaging is a crucial part of the clinical assessment of these children in order to identify and localise lesions which may be resectable.

FCD type IIB is a particular subtype of FCD that is characterised by the presence of balloon cells. On imaging there are features which are commonly seen with these lesions: subcortical white matter signal abnormality, blurring of the grey-white matter junction, well-defined margins, single lobe involvement, abnormal gyration/sulcation, 'transmantle sign', in decreasing order of frequency (Fig. 82-26). The key point about these lesions is that they may be a group associated with a better seizure-free outcome as they are often small, well-defined and more frequently completely resectable than other FCDS.

Imaging is ideally performed in the epilepsy surgical centre and focuses on multiplanar, multisequence imaging, including thin-section volumetric T_1- and T_2-weighted imaging. Some centres obtain surface views of the cortex to detect abnormal gyral patterning, though this can often be seen without using this technique. There is a correlation between abnormal venous drainage and dysplastic cortex, so it can be useful to look for large cortical vessels on MRI in the search for the abnormal area of cortex. The lesion may sometimes be calcified and this may be detected more easily on CT. The detection of FCDs depends largely on the conspicuity of the lesion and relative differences in signal intensity between the FCD and adjacent brain. FCDs may appear different or may be easier to detect at different ages—for example, it can be easier to detect the lesion by the presence of signal change suggesting accelerated myelination in the unmyelinated brain (so the lesion will appear dark on T_2, bright

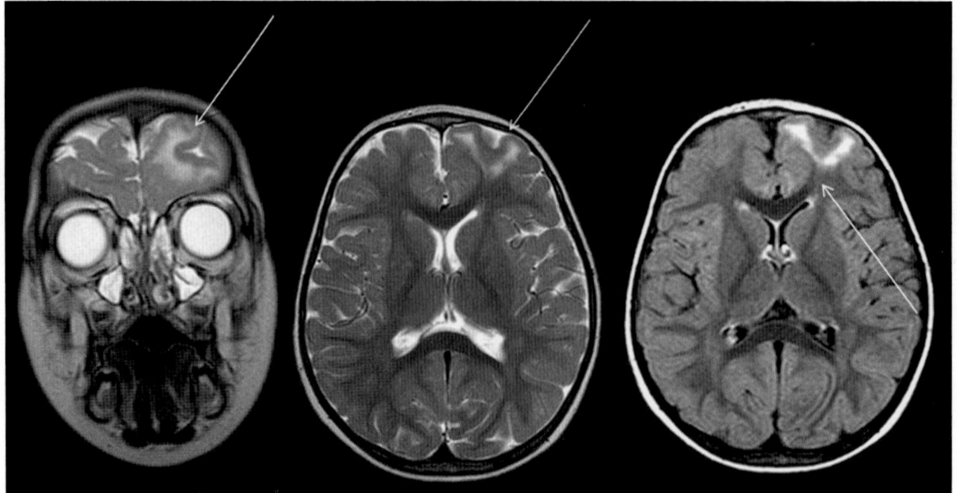

FIGURE 82-26 ■ Child with focal epilepsy and type 2B focal cortical dysplasia. There is abnormal gyral patterning, apparent cortical thickening and abnormal subcortical signal change extending towards the lateral ventricle ('transmantle' sign—arrow).

on T_1 images compared to the adjacent white matter). Sometimes the lesion may be very difficult to see on later imaging acquired when the brain is completely myelinated as the signal contrast between the lesion and the adjacent brain tissue is much less, giving rise to the so-called 'disappearing' lesion. Therefore when reviewing the imaging as part of the epilepsy surgery assessment, it is important to review all imaging acquired at different ages and to have a low threshold for repeating the imaging, using different sequences and tissue contrasts, optimising sedation/anaesthesia and considering higher field strength imaging.

NEUROCUTANEOUS SYNDROMES

The neurocutaneous syndromes or phakomatoses are congenital malformations affecting particularly structures of ectodermal origin, i.e. the nervous system, skin and eye. The most frequently seen are NF1, tuberous sclerosis, neurofibromatosis type 2 (NF2), von Hippel–Lindau disease and Sturge–Weber syndrome.[24,25]

Neurofibromatosis Type 1

The most common neurocutaneous syndrome is NF1, with an incidence of 1 in 3000–4000 births. As well as being one of the most common inherited central nervous system (CNS) disorders, it is the most common autosomal dominant condition, due to a mutation on chromosome 17 which encodes for the tumour suppressor gene product neurofibromin, and the most common inherited tumour syndrome. Half of children affected have new mutations. The diagnosis is made on the basis of at least two major criteria (Table 82-1).[26] Minor criteria are supportive of the diagnosis.

CNS tumours in NF1 include visual pathway gliomas, plexiform neurofibromas and cranial and peripheral nerve gliomas. These may be diagnosed radiologically without recourse to biopsy and the diagnostic criteria allow the diagnosis of NF1 to be made purely on neuroimaging or as an adjunct to clinical findings. Visual/optic pathway gliomas (OPGs) are usually WHO Grade I pilocytic astrocytomas and are the most common brain abnormality in NF1, occurring in up to 15% of patients. Most of these are diagnosed in childhood but only half are symptomatic. OPGs in NF1 are more likely to affect the optic nerves rather than the chiasm and post-chiasmatic pathways, as opposed to non-NF1 OPGs, and are also associated with a better prognosis. Once the tumour involves the chiasm and hypothalamus there is a risk of precocious puberty and a greater risk of visual deterioration.[27] They have a wide spectrum of biological behaviours, ranging from static or minimal growth in most to rapidly increasing size in a minority.

Fusiform expansion of the optic nerve and widening of the optic foramen may be detected on CT, along with the very characteristic sphenoid wing dysplasia and

TABLE 82-1 Diagnostic Criteria for Neurofibromatosis Type 1

Major Criteria	Minor Criteria
Café-au-lait spots	Small stature
Freckling in the inguinal or axillary areas	Macrocephaly
One plexiform neurofibroma or two neurofibromas of any type*	Scoliosis*
Visual pathway glioma*	Pectus excavatus*
Two or more Lisch nodules of iris	'Hamartomatous lesions' of NF1*
Distinctive osseous lesion, e.g. sphenoid dysplasia or thinning of cortex*	Neuropsychological abnormalities
First-degree relative with neurofibromatosis type 1 (NF1)	

*Radiologically detectable features.

plexiform neurofibroma which are frequently associated. Although CT can detect the intraorbital involvement of OPG, this involves irradiating the eye and is less sensitive than MRI for delineating tumour within the chiasm and intracranial extension. Other orbital features seen in NF1 include dilatation of the optic nerve sheaths due to dural ectasia and intraorbital extension of plexiform neurofibroma. Variable extension into the chiasm, the lateral geniculate bodies or optic radiations is best detected on MRI. A suggested NF1 imaging protocol includes orbital MRI with axial and coronal dual-echo STIR, coronal and T_1-weighted pre- and fat-saturation post-gadolinium images, all with a slice thickness of 3 mm or less. Images obtained with a fat-saturation pulse allow elimination of chemical shift artefact at the interface of the optic nerve sheath complex and intraorbital fat, making assessment easier, and contrast medium improves visualisation of the normal intraorbital optic nerves.

The whole of the optic nerve may be expanded or there may be subarachnoid extension of tumour around a normal-sized nerve. Tumour infiltration within the nerve is detected as expansion of the nerve within the optic nerve sheath, often but not always with enhancement following a paramagnetic contrast agent, whereas if the tumour is predominantly subarachnoid, a rim of tumour around a minimally enhancing nerve is sometimes detected. It is important to identify the expanded nerve within the optic nerve sheath in order to distinguish it from NF1-associated dural ectasia in which the optic nerve sheath is expanded by CSF rather than tumour. Generally these optic pathway tumours are kept under observation unless symptomatic or progressive (≤ 5%). Spontaneous involution of tumour is also well recognised.

There is an increased risk of other CNS tumours in NF1 with OPG. These are usually WHO Grade I pilocytic astrocyomas occurring in 1–3% of patients, particularly within the cerebellum and brainstem, although other low-grade and higher-grade tumours also occur. In the brainstem they are usually less aggressive than non-NF1 brainstem astrocytomas and are more likely to be seen in the medulla and midbrain (e.g. tectal plate gliomas) than the pons. A tectal plate tumour may cause aqueduct stenosis and hence hydrocephalus. These brainstem NF1 tumours are often biologically benign and may regress spontaneously, and therefore clinical management is generally not aggressive unless clinical/radiological tumour progression is seen.

Another characteristic lesion of NF1 is the so-called 'hamartomatous' changes of NF1, also known as 'unidentified bright objects (UBOs)', 'neurofibromatosis bright objects (NBOs)' or areas of myelin vacuolation. These are seen in 60–80% of NF1 cases, depending on the age at which the child is imaged, and in 95% of children with NF1 and OPG, and may have an impact on cognitive function.[28] They are few in number before the age of 4 years, increase in number and volume between 4 and 10 years and then decrease in the second decade, being rare over the age of 20. Therefore, they are rarely seen in the adult NF1 population. Multiple hyperintense lesions are seen on T2W images. They have normal signal on T_1-weighted images, apart from lesions in the basal ganglia which are often slightly hyperintense on T1W images. They have minimal mass effect and no contrast enhancement and occur in typical sites such as the pons, cerebellar white matter, internal capsules, basal ganglia, thalami and hippocampi (Fig. 82-27). Their lack of growth, eventual regression and lack of contrast enhancement distinguish them from gliomas. Astrocytomas, however, may develop in the areas involved by UBOs and radiologically it can be difficult to distinguish them without serial imaging. Enhancement and increasing mass effect are suspicious for tumour development, in which case the involved areas should be kept under regular imaging review. Other non-CNS neoplasia recognised in NF1 include phaeochromocytoma, carcinoid, rhabdomyosarcoma and childhood chronic myeloid leukaemia.

Plexiform neurofibromas are one of the main diagnostic criteria of NF1. These are multinodular lesions formed when tumour involves either multiple trunks or

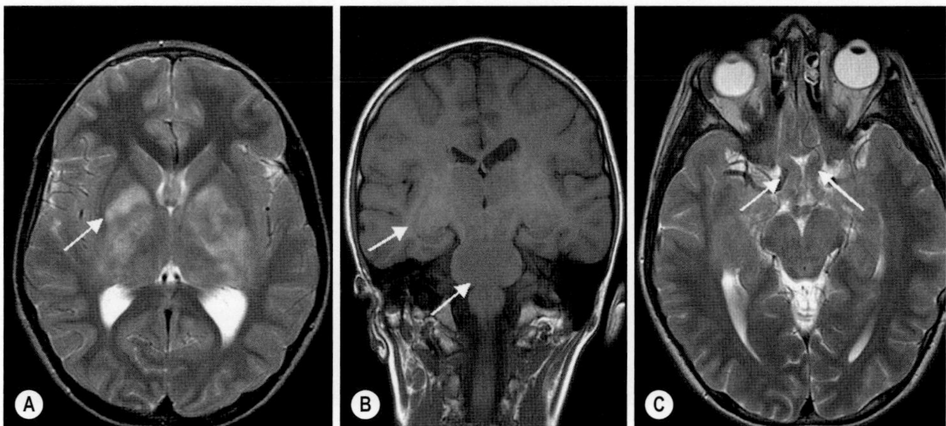

FIGURE 82-27 ■ Child with neurofibromatosis type 1 (NF1). (A, B) There are very characteristic lesions within the lentiform nuclei, brainstem and midbrain, the so-called 'hamartomatous' lesions or 'unidentified bright objects' of NF1 (arrows). They are hyperintense on T_2-weighted imaging, with minimal mass effect. Basal ganglia lesions may demonstrate some T_1 shortening, as in this case, or are hypointense on T_1-weighted imaging. (C) There are also bilateral optic nerve gliomas extending into the optic chiasm (arrows).

multiple fascicles of a large nerve. A typical location is the orbit where the tumour grows along the ophthalmic division of the trigeminal nerve in association with sphenoid wing dysplasia. They are hypodense on CT and generally do not enhance with contrast agents. On MRI they have a more heterogeneous appearance, of low signal intensity on T_1 images and hyperintensity on T_2 images, with variable contrast enhancement, although at least part of the tumour normally enhances. Extension occurs along the nerve pathways into the pterygomaxillary fissure, orbital apex/superior orbital fissure and cavernous sinus (Fig. 82-28). Other characteristic sites include the lumbosacral and brachial plexi. There is a malignant potential with transformation to fibrosarcoma quoted at between 2 and 12%, though probably within the lower range. Neurofibromas are more homogeneous and well-defined lesions which cause diffuse expansion of nerves. It may be possible to distinguish plexiform from other types of neurofibroma radiologically, as the former are more diffuse lesions. Neurofibromas appear on MRI as nodules seen along the spinal nerves of the cauda equina and, as they enlarge, they extend out through the neural exit foramina, enlarging them. They may have a central region of hypointensity on T_2 images, producing a target appearance. NF1 is associated with some characteristic bone dysplasias, including lambdoid sutural dysplasia, thinning of long bone cortices and kyphoscoliosis with a high thoracic acute curve. One of the most common is sphenoid wing dysplasia marked by a bone defect which allows herniation of the temporal lobe through the orbit. On plain radiography this produces the 'empty' or 'bare' orbit (Fig. 82-28A). Clinically there may be pulsatile exophthalmos due to transmission of CSF pulsations. The globe may also be affected with proptosis or enlargement.

As well as kyphoscoliosis due to a primary skeletal dysostosis, there may be dural ectasia with vertebral scalloping and lateral meningoceles containing CSF. Scoliosis may be seen in association with an intrinsic spinal cord tumour or peripheral nerve neurofibroma.

Tuberous Sclerosis

Tuberous sclerosis (TS) is a multisystem genetic neurocutaneous syndrome characterised by hamartomas, cortical tubers and benign neoplastic lesions (giant cell astrocytomas), with an incidence of around 1 in 5800 live births. The most frequently affected organs are the skin,

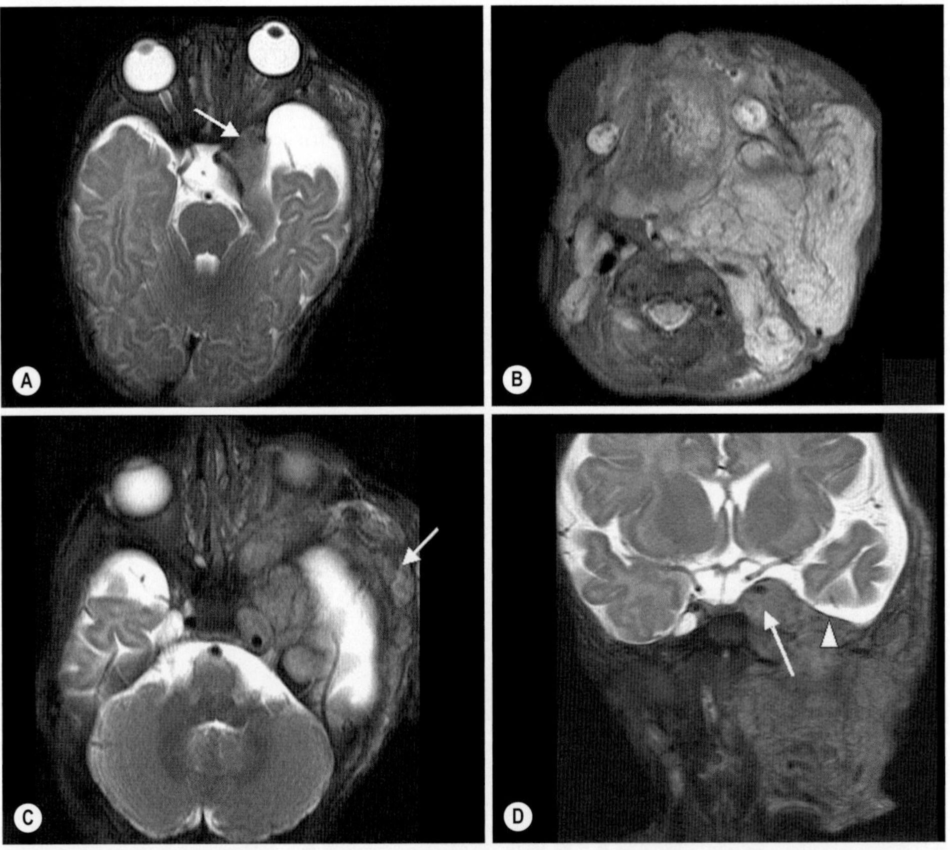

FIGURE 82-28 ■ Infant with neurofibromatosis type 1. The diagnosis was made from these images. (A) There is sphenoid wing dysplasia causing expansion of the middle cranial fossa (arrow) and absence of the lateral orbital wall, which causes the 'bare orbit' sign (arrow) on AP plain radiographs. (B) There is an associated extensive plexiform neurofibroma involving the deep and superficial fascial spaces of the neck, tongue and orbit. (C, D) This is almost indistinguishable on imaging from multiple cranial nerve fibromas involving the left cavernous sinus (arrows) and middle cranial fossa. Note the neurofibroma has extended through the foramen ovale and is elevating the dura, seen as a black line (arrowhead).

brain, retina, lungs, heart, skeleton and kidneys, but the few manifestations that are associated with the reduced life expectancy seen in this condition are, in order of highest to lowest frequency, neurological disease (seizures and subependymal giant cell tumour), renal disease (angiomyolipoma and renal cell carcinoma), pulmonary disease (lymphangioleiomyomatosis and bronchopneumonia) and cardiovascular disease (rhabdomyosarcoma and aneurysm). TS is autosomal dominant with a high level of penetrance and variable phenotypic expression; 60–70% of cases are sporadic and two gene mutations have been identified, TSC1 and TSC2, encoding protein products with a tumour suppressor function.

The classical clinical presentation of TS is the triad of intellectual impairment, epilepsy and adenoma sebaceum, but there is a wide phenotypic range. There are a large number of diagnostic primary, secondary and tertiary criteria for TS, some of which are radiological and which categorise TS as 'definite', 'probable' or 'possible'. Radiological primary criteria are the presence of calcified subependymal nodules, while non-calcified subependymal nodules and tubers, cardiac rhabdomyoma and renal angiomyolipoma are secondary criteria.[29,30] In 80% of patients with TS, infantile spasms or myoclonic seizures are the presenting symptom. Conversely, 10% of children with infantile spasms will have evidence of TS, so structural MR neuroimaging is indicated in these children.

Ocular manifestations of TS include retinal hamartomas seen near the optic disc in 15% and are often bilateral and multiple. On CT they appear as nodular masses originating from the retina and when calcified may be difficult to distinguish from retinoblastomas unless there are also calcified subependymal nodules. Subretinal effusions may also be detected. Micro-ophthalmia and leukocoria are other features.

The intracranial manifestations include subependymal hamartomas or nodules (SENs), subependymal giant cell astrocytomas (GCAs), radially oriented linear bands and cortical tubers (Fig. 82-29). SENs are the most common lesion and are seen in 88–95% of individuals with TS. They may be calcified, which is a useful diagnostic feature on CT or T_2* MRI; calcification increases with age and

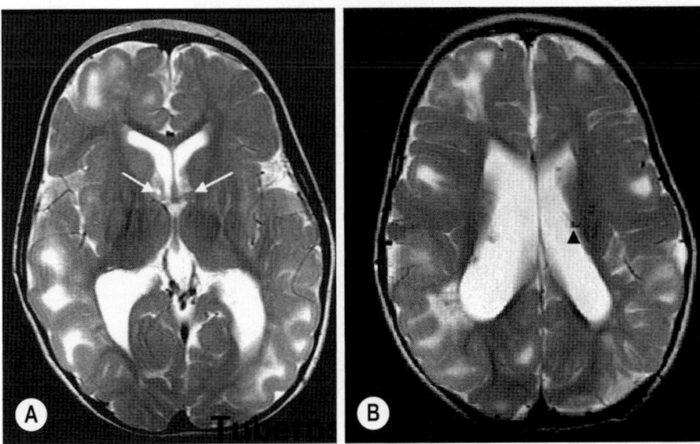

FIGURE 82-29 ■ **Intracranial manifestations of tuberous sclerosis.** (A) Multiple tubers involving the cortex and subcortical white matter. Bilateral lesions are seen at the foramina of Monro, in keeping with giant cell astrocytomas (arrows). (B) Subependymal nodules project into the ventricles, some of which are markedly hypointense, in keeping with calcification (arrowhead).

is rarely detected under the age of 1 year.[30] Histologically, they are indistinguishable from GCAs. The latter are determined by location in the caudothalamic groove adjacent to the foramen of Monro, progressive growth on serial imaging and the presence of hydrocephalus. Contrast enhancement may be seen in both SENs and GCAs. The lack of myelination in infants helps to identify white matter anomalies, which become less visible as myelination progresses.[31] SENs and linear parenchymal tuberous sclerosis lesions in infants under 3 months old are hyperintense on T_1-weighted images and hypointense on T_2-weighted images as opposed to the reverse pattern of signal intensity in older children and adults.

Sturge–Weber Syndrome

Sturge–Weber syndrome is a congenital syndrome characterised by a port-wine naevus on the face and ipsilateral leptomeningeal angiomas with a primarily parieto-occipital distribution.[32] Bilateral involvement may occasionally occur. The clinical manifestations include the onset of focal seizures, appearing during the first year of life, and developmental delay with progressive hemiparesis, hemianopsia and intellectual impairment. The seizures progressively become refractory to medication.

The leptomeningeal angiomas cause abnormal venous drainage with chronic ischaemia, leading ultimately to cortical atrophy and calcification, the latter feature being usually very prominent. By 2 years of age, skull radiographs may reveal 'tramline calcifications' within the cortices.

In early imaging the brain may look normal on CT as well as on MRI even with intravenous contrast enhancement as the pial angioma may not be conspicuous until after 2 years of life. The involved hemisphere progressively becomes atrophied and the pial angioma is seen as diffuse pial enhancement of variable thickness (Fig. 82-30).[33] The ipsilateral white matter appears hypointense on T_1-weighted images and hyperintense on T_2-weighted images. Other findings include enlargement of the ipsilateral choroid plexus and dilatation of transparenchymal veins that communicate between the superficial and deep cerebral venous systems. In 'burnt out' cases the pial angioma may no longer be detected after contrast enhancement, leaving only a chronically shrunken and calcified hemisphere.

Neurofibromatosis Type 2

This is located to an abnormality on chromosome 22 and occurs in 1 in 50,000 live births. Nearly all have bilateral vestibular schwannomas, other tumours such as meningiomas and other cranial and peripheral nerve schwannomas and ependymomas, including spinal tumours (Fig. 82-31). While in adults hearing loss is a common presentation, seizures and facial nerve palsy are more common in children.

Other Neurocutaneous Syndromes

These include hypomelanosis of Ito in which hypomelanotic skin lesions are associated with polymicrogyria,

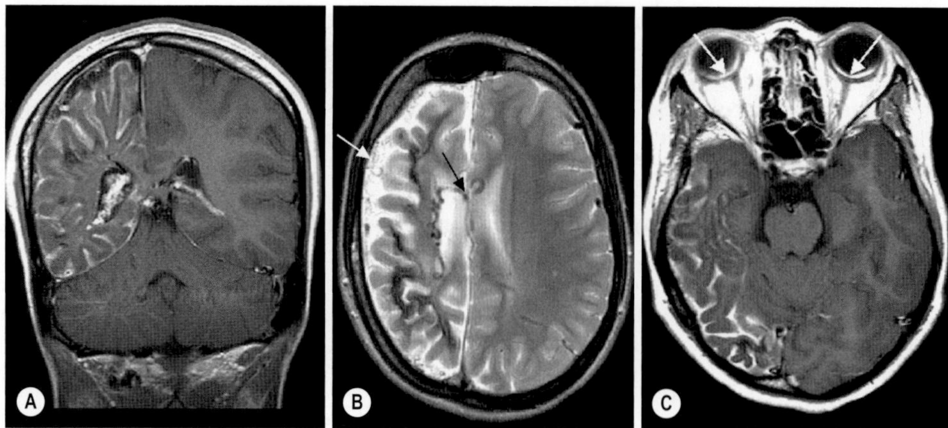

FIGURE 82-30 ■ Sturge–Weber syndrome. (A) Coronal T_1 post-contrast image shows an enhancing pial angioma overlying the right cerebral hemisphere which is atrophic. The right choroid plexus is enlarged. Foci of signal hypointensity within the gyri and adjacent white matter are due to calcification. (B) Axial T_2-weighted image shows in addition prominent superficial cortical veins and ependymal veins (arrows). (C) Axial post-contrast T_1-weighted image shows bilateral choroidal angiomas (arrows) in addition to the pial angioma.

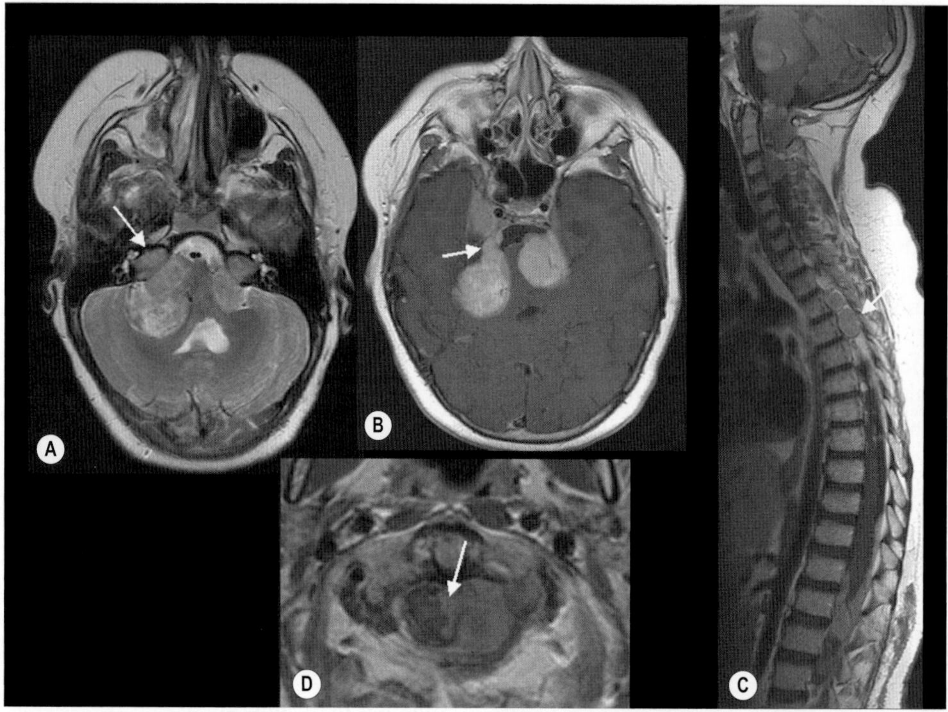

FIGURE 82-31 ■ Neurofibromatosis type 2 (NF2). (A) Bilateral cerebellopontine angle masses extending into the internal auditory meati and causing expansion (arrow) in a child with NF2 and bilateral acoustic neuromas. (B) Trigeminal schwannomas extending into the cavernous sinus on the right. The arrow indicates the cisternal segment of the right trigeminal nerve. (C) Sagittal T_1-weighted images show expansion of the neural exit foramina by enhancing nerve or nerve sheath tumours (arrow). (D) Axial image shows a mainly dural mass extending out through the neural foramen with a small intradural component (arrow).

heterotopias and callosal dysgenesis, basal cell naevus syndrome and PHACES (posterior fossa malformations, facial haemangiomas, arterial anomalies, cardiac and eye anomalies and sternal cleft) syndromes. Neurocutaneous melanosis is a rare syndrome in which giant congenital melanocytic naevi on the skin are associated with intracranial melanosis (Fig. 82-32). Neuroimaging detects the clusters of melanocytes by the melanin that they are associated with, therefore appearing as regions of T_1 shortening on MRI in characteristic locations: the anterior and mesial temporal lobe, cerebellum and pons. CT may detect areas of increased density but these are much more difficult to appreciate. Diffuse melanosis with intracranial and intraspinal leptomeningeal spread may occur and therefore hydrocephalus. Degeneration into malignant melanoma is rare.

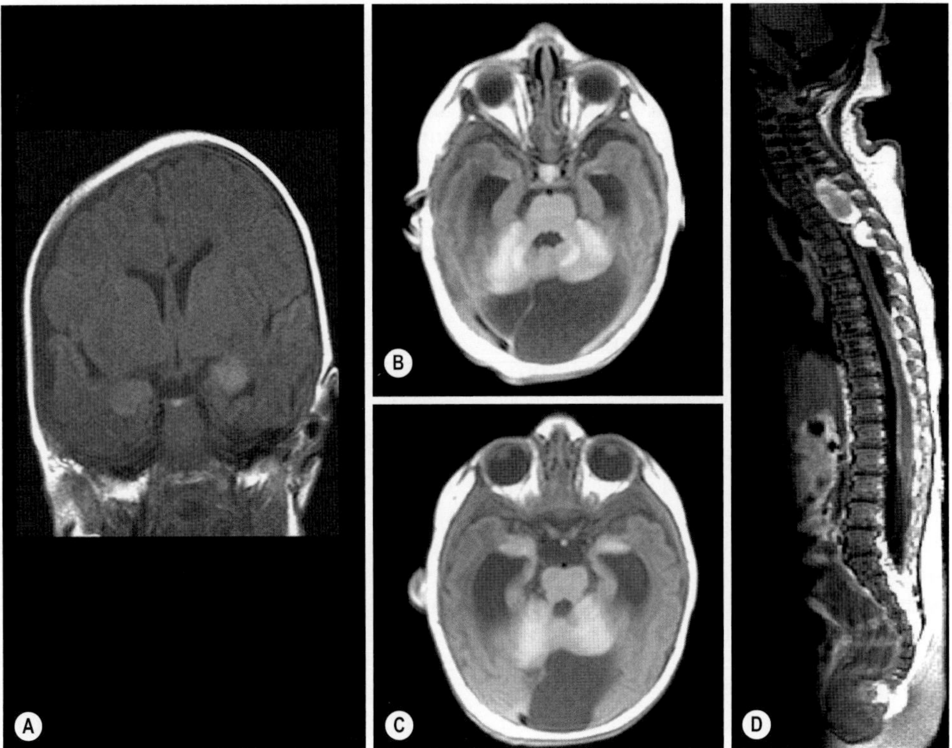

FIGURE 82-32 ■ Child with giant pigmented naevus and neurocutaneous melanosis. (A) Initial coronal T_1-weighted MRI shows the typical regions of T_1 shortening within the amygdalae of the mesial temporal lobes. (B, C) Axial T_1-weighted MRI obtained 2 years later shows hydrocephalus in addition to the regions of melanin deposition within the mesial temporal lobes and cerebellum. These do not show any enhancement. There is a posterior fossa arachnoid cyst, a described association. (D) Within the spine there is diffuse pial enhancement over the spinal cord in addition to focal haemorrhagic and partly enhancing extramedullary lesions, indicating malignant melanoma, which was subsequently confirmed histologically.

SPINAL MALFORMATIONS

Normal Development

The spinal cord forms during three embryological stages known as gastrulation (at 2–3 weeks of gestation), primary neurulation (3–4 weeks) and secondary neurulation (5–6 weeks). During gastrulation the embryonic bilaminar disc consisting of epiblast and hypoblast is converted to a trilaminar disc by migration of cells from the epiblast through Hensen's node, a focal region of thickening occurring at the cranial end of the midline 'primitive streak' of the disc. This results in the midline notochord and a layer that will form the future mesoderm. During primary neurulation the notochord induces the overlying ectoderm to become neurectoderm and form the neural plate. Subsequent folding and bending occurs until the margins unite to form the neural tube. The cranial end closes at day 25, while the caudal end closes a couple of days later. Finally the caudal cell mass arises from the primitive streak and undergoes retrogressive differentiation with cavitation. This is the origin of the foetal neural tissue and vertebrae distal to S2, and will become the conus medullaris. A focal expansion of the fetal canal known as the terminal ventricle occurs as a result of incomplete retrogressive differentiation. This may be seen as a normal asymptomatic finding in young children and may persist in a small minority into adulthood. It is seen on all post-mortem studies but is bigger in those detectable on MRI. Spinal dysraphisms can result from abnormalities occurring during any of these periods.[34–36]

Definitions

Spinal dysraphisms may be open, in which case nervous tissue is exposed, or closed, in which case the defect is covered by skin, although a cutaneous lesion such as a dimple, sinus, hairy naevus or haemangioma may be seen as a marker of an underlying defect in 50% of these cases.[35,36] Spina bifida refers to the failure of fusion of the posterior spinal bony elements. The neural placode is a flat segment of un-neurulated nervous tissue that may be seen at the end of the spinal cord or at an intermediate position along its course.

The normal level of the spinal cord termination has a normal or Gaussian distribution. It is a popular misconception that the spinal cord lies lower in the neonate and continues to rise as the vertebral column grows during childhood. In fact most authors agree that it has already reached its adult position by term, and in 98% lies above L2/3, the majority lying between T11/12 and L1/2.[37,38] The spinal cord termination should be considered unequivocally abnormal if seen at or below L3. Tethered cord syndrome is a clinical diagnosis of progressive neurological deterioration (usually leg weakness, deformities such as scoliosis or foot abnormalities, loss of bladder and bowel function), presumed to be due to traction damage on the tethered cord. Although there may be some suggestive features such as a low positioned conus and associated spinal cord syrinx, this is not a diagnosis made radiologically; and the position of the conus or neural placode following successful surgical 'untethering' typically remains unchanged.

Open Spinal Dysraphism

Most open spinal dysraphisms (OSDs) are myelomeningoceles and these are virtually always associated with Chiari II malformation The neural placode protrudes beyond the level of the skin and there is an expanded CSF-containing sac lined by meninges.[35,36] A small proportion of OSDs are myeloceles where the placode is flush with the surface and there is no meningocele component. Both disorders result from defective closure of the primary neural tube and persistence of un-neurulated nervous tissue in the form of the neural placode, usually at the lumbosacral level at the spinal cord termination. Nerve roots arising from the everted ventral surface of the placode cross the widely dilated subarachnoid spaces of the meningocele to enter the neural exit foraminae. The posterior elements of the vertebral column and any other mesenchymal derivatives, such as the paravertebral muscles, remain everted. Hemimyelomeningoceles and hemimyeloceles may occur with diastematomyelia (split cord syndrome) and may be associated with an asymmetric skin abnormality and clinical presentation. These can be hypothesised to occur as the result of an embryological failure of primary neurulation of one hemicord in addition to a gastrulation abnormality.

Myelomeningoceles are operated on soon after birth; if untreated, the exposed neural tissue is prone to ulceration and infection. In some centres, in utero repair has been correlated with subsequent failure to develop the typical hindbrain malformation of Chiari II, although other abnormalities such as the enlarged massa intermedia and falx fenestration persist. The advocates of this technique suggest that hydrocephalus and the need for surgical drainage may also be delayed and even reduced in these children Hydrocephalus usually develops 2–3 days post-neonatal repair of the myelomeningocele but may occur preoperatively. Other causes of postoperative deterioration include re-tethering of the spinal cord and the development of a syrinx, which may, later, be associated with scoliosis.[39] The Chiari II malformation is described in more detail with brain malformations in the 'Disorders of Dorsal Induction' section.

Closed Spinal Dysraphism

Closed spinal dysraphisms (CSDs) are often associated with midline cutaneous stigmata or a mass.[40,41] This may be a subcutaneous lipomatous mass overlying the spinal defect, as in lipomyeloceles and lipomyelomeningoceles. In these conditions there is an intraspinal lipoma. In a lipomyelocele the junction between the placode and the lipoma lies within the spinal canal (Fig. 82-33), while in lipomyelomeningoceles it lies outside. Typically the placode is rotated to one side while the lipoma rotates on the other. McClone's hypothesis is that during primary neurulation there is premature disjunction of the cutaneous ectoderm from the adjacent neuroectoderm, allowing mesenchymal elements to come into contact with the open neural tube and then differentiate into fat. These lipomas may be dorsal, with a normal conus below, or transitional where the lipoma extends caudally along the conus. In both these situations the lipoma–placode junction is dorsal, well-defined and complete removal of the lipoma at surgery is feasible. A third form exists, known

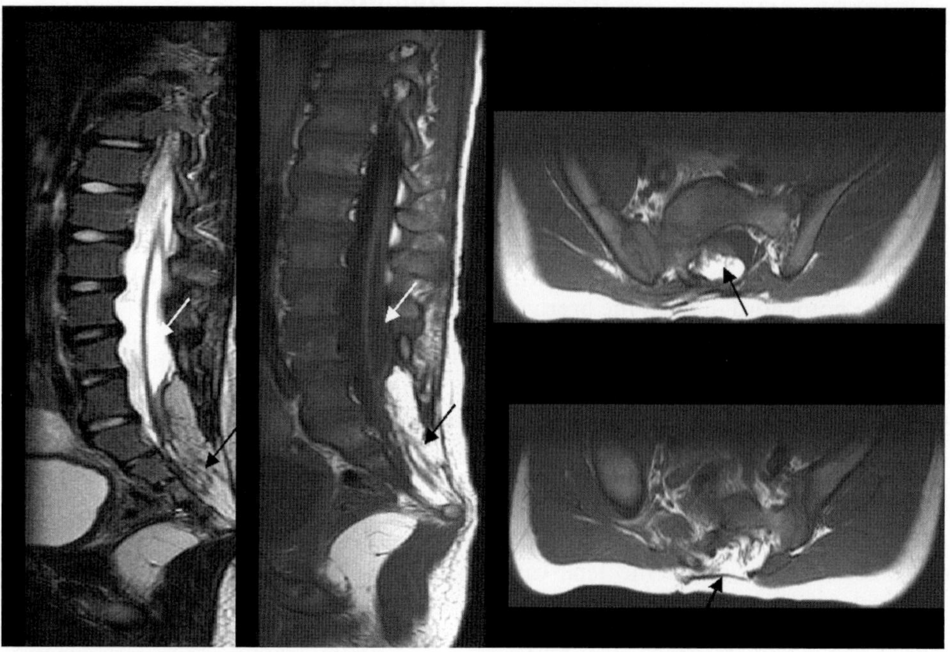

FIGURE 82-33 ■ **Closed spinal dysraphism.** The spinal cord is too low and the neural placode terminates at the lumbosacral junction in a lipomyelocele (black arrows). There is an associated spinal cord syringomyelic cavity (white arrows). The posterior elements are deficient and everted.

as 'chaotic' where the lipoma extends ventrally around the neural placode and the lipoma is much more difficult to resect.[42] These are less common conditions but are more commonly seen with sacral agenesis. It is harder to explain these by the premature disjunction theory, given the ventral fat, and it may be that these are disorders of caudal cell mass development. The terminal lipoma and filum terminale lipoma are also considered to arise from a disturbance of caudal regression. Other examples of these are described in a separate section below.

A posterior meningocele consists of herniation of a CSF sac lined by dura and arachnoid through a posterior spinal defect, resulting in a clinically apparent mass covered by skin. These are mainly lumbosacral but may be seen at any level. Anterior meningoceles are typically presacral, are seen with caudal agenesis and are present in older children and adults with low back pain and bladder/bowel disturbance. The terminal myelocystocele is a rare condition associated with syndromes such as VACTERL in which the central canal is dilated by a hydromyelic cavity that herniates into a posterior meningocele through the posterior spinal bony defect. Sometimes it can be difficult to see the communication with the central canal of the spinal cord which is the key finding of the terminal cystocele cavity. The cystocele cavity is seen at the most caudal aspect of the spinal canal, with a myelomeningocele seen ventrally and posteriorly around the neural placode, giving rise on MRI to two fluid-filled sacs (Fig. 82-34).

CSDs without a mass include simple intramedullary and intradural lipomas. These typically occur along the posterior midline in a subpial juxtamedullary location at the cervicothoracic level. Embryologically they are also the result of premature disjunction and the lipoma fills in the gap between the unopposed folds of the neural placode. On MRI they have the signal characteristics of fat, including signal suppression on STIR sequences.

Fatty change within the filum terminale is detected on MRI, and may be more easily seen on axial T_1-weighted sequences extending caudally from the conus. This is estimated to occur in 1.5–5% of the normal adult population and may be considered a normal variant in the absence of the clinical tethered cord syndrome. The 'tight' filum terminale, also due to abnormal retrogressive differentiation, is a short, thick filum greater than 2 mm in diameter associated with clinical tethering and a low-lying spinal cord.

Dorsal Dermal Sinus

A dermal sinus is an epithelial-lined opening on the skin with variable fistulous extension to the dural surface, typically seen in the lumbosacral region and often associated with cutaneous stigmata, such as hairy naevus and capillary haemangioma.[40,41] Embryologically it arises from a failure of disjunction of neuroectoderm from cutaneous ectoderm. Dermal openings seen at the sacrococcygeal level are directed inferiorly below the thecal sac and are known as sacrococcygeal pits. They do not require further imaging unless there are neurological features to suggest additional spinal dysraphism, as there should be no risk of CNS infection in the absence of a

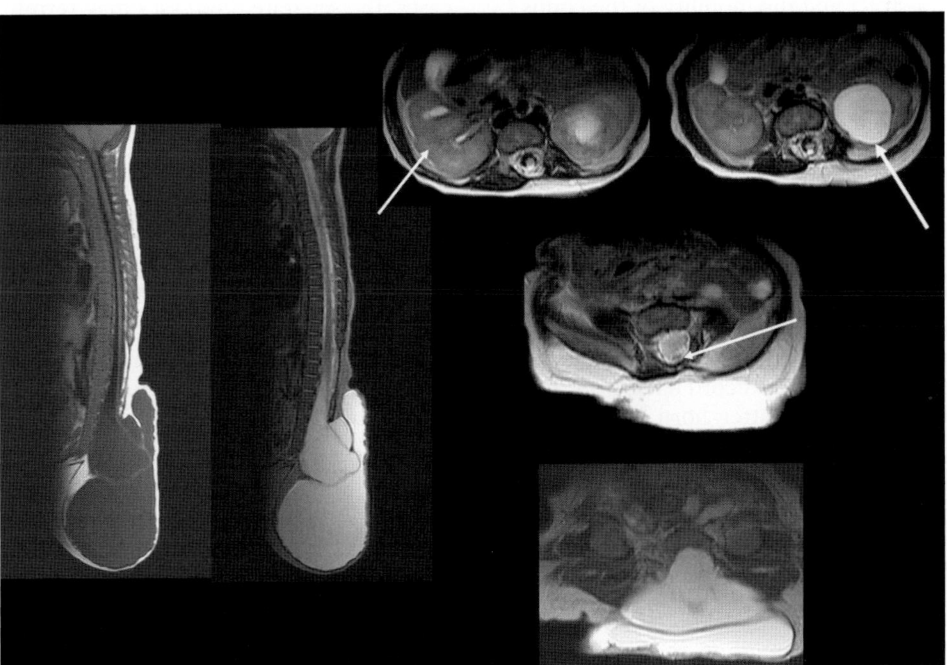

FIGURE 82-34 ■ There is a right duplex kidney and dilated left pelvicalyceal system (axial top images). The termination of the spinal cord is very low and the neural placode is seen at the sacrum. The distal bony lumbosacral spine is deficient. The placode splits in two, forming a disatemyelia (middle axial image) and two cystic structures are identified. At surgery there was an inner sac (myelomeningocele) with nerve roots seen within it and an outer sac (the cystocele cavity), into which the neural placode opened.

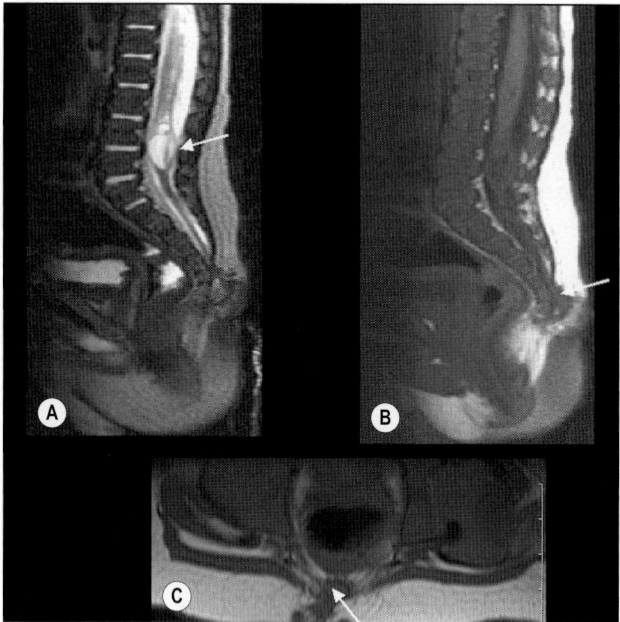

FIGURE 82-35 ■ Dorsal dermal sinus. (A) The termination of the spinal cord is very low and there is a syringomyelic cavity with internal septations. In addition there is a more focal cyst within the conus confirmed at surgical untethering to be a dermoid cyst (arrow). (B, C) There is an associated dermal sinus track (arrows).

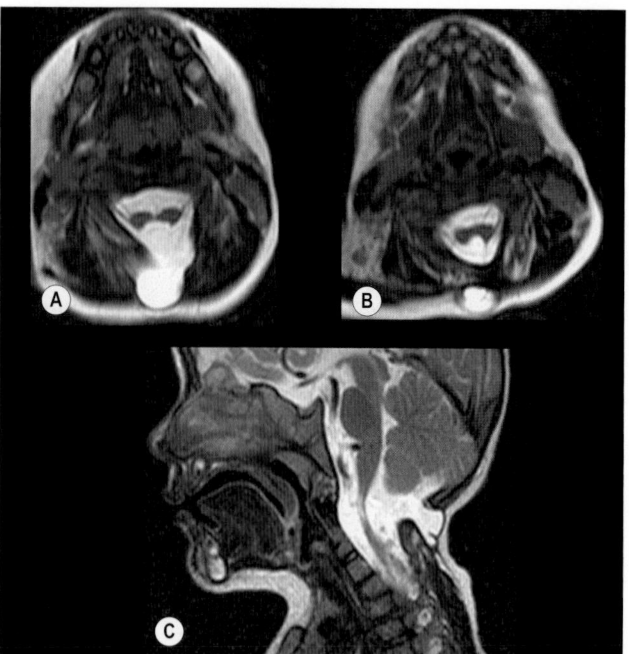

FIGURE 82-36 ■ Cervical spinal cord diastematomyelia type II with associated craniocervical meningocele. (A) Sagittal T_2-weighted MRI appears to show signal abnormality and thinning of the spinal cord, and is the clue to the diastematomyelia seen on the axial images. (B, C) Axial T_2-weighted MRI shows that the cord has split into two hemicords. The apparent signal abnormality is in fact normal cerebrospinal fluid interspersed between the two hemicords. These reunite inferiorly. The meningocele is seen herniating through a bony defect in the vertebral posterior elements.

connection with the thecal sac. Those seen above the natal cleft have a more cranial direction and may form a fistulous connection with the dural sac and warrant further investigation as they may need to be resected to prevent future CNS infection. Ultrasound (US) may provide useful information about the intradural extension of the dermal sinus tract and the mobility of the conus.[43] MRI is more sensitive for additional intraspinal findings such as spinal cord syrinx and intraspinal dermoid. On MRI the dermal sinus is seen as a thin linear strip of tissue hypointense to adjacent fat but MRI is not particularly reliable for determining whether there is continuity with the thecal sac and surgical exploration may be required (Fig. 82-35).

Diastematomyelia

The split notochord syndromes are disorders of notochord midline integration. In diastematomyelia the spinal cord is split in two, with each hemicord having one anterior and one posterior grey matter horn.[44,45] In type I diastematomyelia there are two complete dural sacs. There is a craniocaudal gradient of division, ranging from partial clefting cranially to two complete dural sacs separated by an osteocartilaginous spur inferiorly. There may be plain radiographic features, including scoliosis or hemivertebrae or bifid/fused vertebrae at the level of the bony spur. The bony spur in type I diastematomyelia is completely extradural, usually midline, though it may be seen coursing obliquely from the posterior vertebrae to the laminae, and may be complete or incomplete. It is seen at the caudal end of the split and the hemicords fuse tightly just below it. On MRI marrow signal may be detected within it and this distinguishes it from a simple fibrous band. Above it the split is much longer. In rare cases, the separate dural sacs may terminate distally with different fates, one as an OSD and the other as a CSD. In diastematomyelia type II (Fig. 82-36) there is a single dural sac in which the two hemicords lie, and a fibrous septum, seen as a band of hypointensity, may be seen passing intradurally between the two hemicords. There may be no septum or there may only be partial clefting of the cord. The conus is often low and there may be a tight or fatty filum. Both forms of diastematomyelia may be associated with hydromyelia within the spinal cord.

Neurenteric Cysts

The severest and rarest form of notochordal midline integration anomaly occurs with dorsal enteric fistulas and neurenteric cysts.[46] The cysts are usually seen intradurally anterior to the spinal cord and are derived from endodermal remnants trapped between a split notochord. They have signal characteristics of CSF or of proteinaceous fluid with T shortening (Fig. 82-37). The commoner variants of these involve cysts that extend through a ventral bony defect through abnormally formed verterbral bodies, called the canal of Kovalevsky (Fig. 82-38). Rarer cases demonstrate the neurenteric cyst extending between a split cord malformation. It is possible for such a fistula to connect the dorsal skin with bowel across duplicated spinal elements.

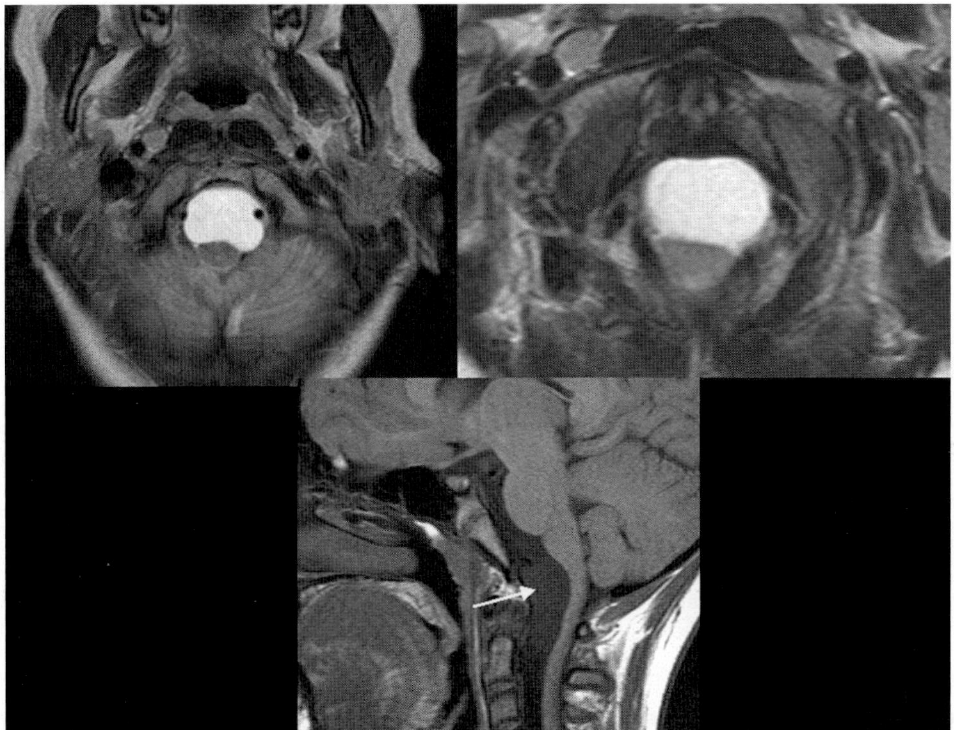

FIGURE 82-37 ■ Neurenteric cyst ventral to the medulla and upper cervical spinal cord, displacing them posteriorly, and with the vertebral arteries displaced around it. The cyst is hyperintense on the T_2-weighted images and there is also some mild T_1 shortening (arrow).

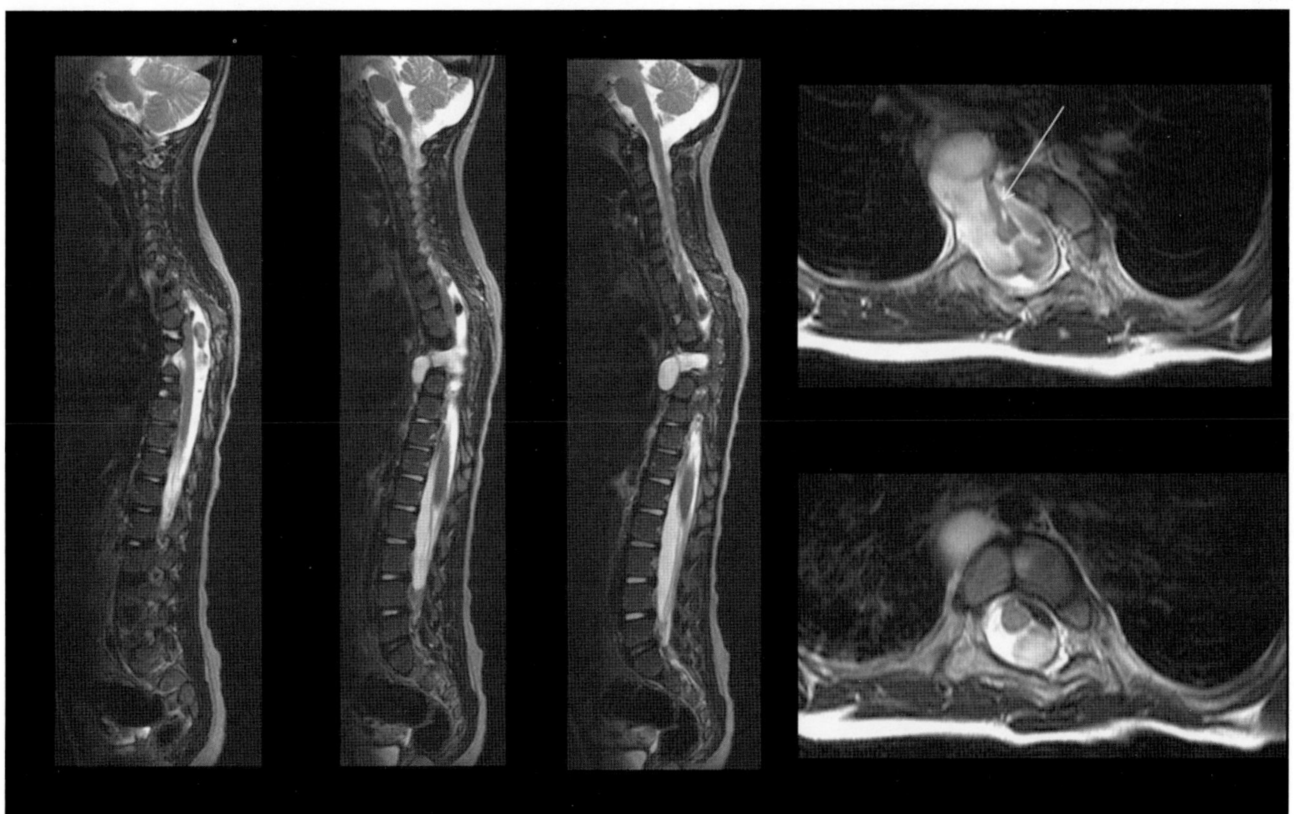

FIGURE 82-38 ■ Sagittal and axial T2W images show ventral herniation of a sac through a thoracic bony defect (the canal of Kovalevsky) at the level of a vertebral segmentation anomaly. The spinal cord appears stretched and a ventral component extends into the sac (arrow). There is a small syrinx cavity within it.

Disorders of the Caudal Cell Mass/ Caudal Regression Syndrome

The last group of developmental spinal abnormalities affects development of the caudal cell mass.[47] Caudal agenesis and the rarer condition of segmental spinal dysgenesis are considered to occur as a result of apoptosis of notochordal cells which have not formed in their correct craniocaudal position. In caudal agenesis there is a severe abnormality which results in absence of the vertebral column at the affected level, as well as a truncated spinal cord, imperforate anus and genital anomalies. It may be seen with OEIS (omphalocele, exstrophy, imperforate anus, spinal defects), VACTERL and the Currarino triad in which there is partial sacral agenesis (or sometimes a 'scimitar'-shaped sacrum), anorectal malformation and a presacral mass which may be a teratoma or anterior meningocele[48–50] (Fig. 82-39). In type I caudal agenesis, which affects secondary neurulation and formation of the caudal cell mass, there is a high (often at T12) abrupt spinal cord termination with a characteristic wedge-shaped configuration and variable coccygeal to lower thoracic vertebral aplasia (Fig. 82-40). Clinically the neurological deficit due to absence of the distal spinal cord is stable. In type II caudal agenesis the true notochord is not affected and only the caudal cell mass is involved. The vertebral aplasia is less extensive, with up to S4 present as the last vertebra. It may be difficult to detect partial agenesis of the conus because it is stretched and tethered to a fatty filum terminale, lipoma, lipomyelomeningocele, or anterior sacral meningocele.

Segmental Spinal Dysgenesis

These represent a segmental abnormality affecting the spinal cord, segmental nerve roots and vertebrae, and are associated with a congenital paraparesis and lower limb deformities. A short segment of the spinal column is deficient and the spinal canal may be obliterated. On imaging there may be an acute angle kyphus, and the spine and spinal cord in the most severe cases may appear 'severed', but with functioning spinal cord neural tissue anatomically present above and below the affected segment. In less severe cases the cord is focally

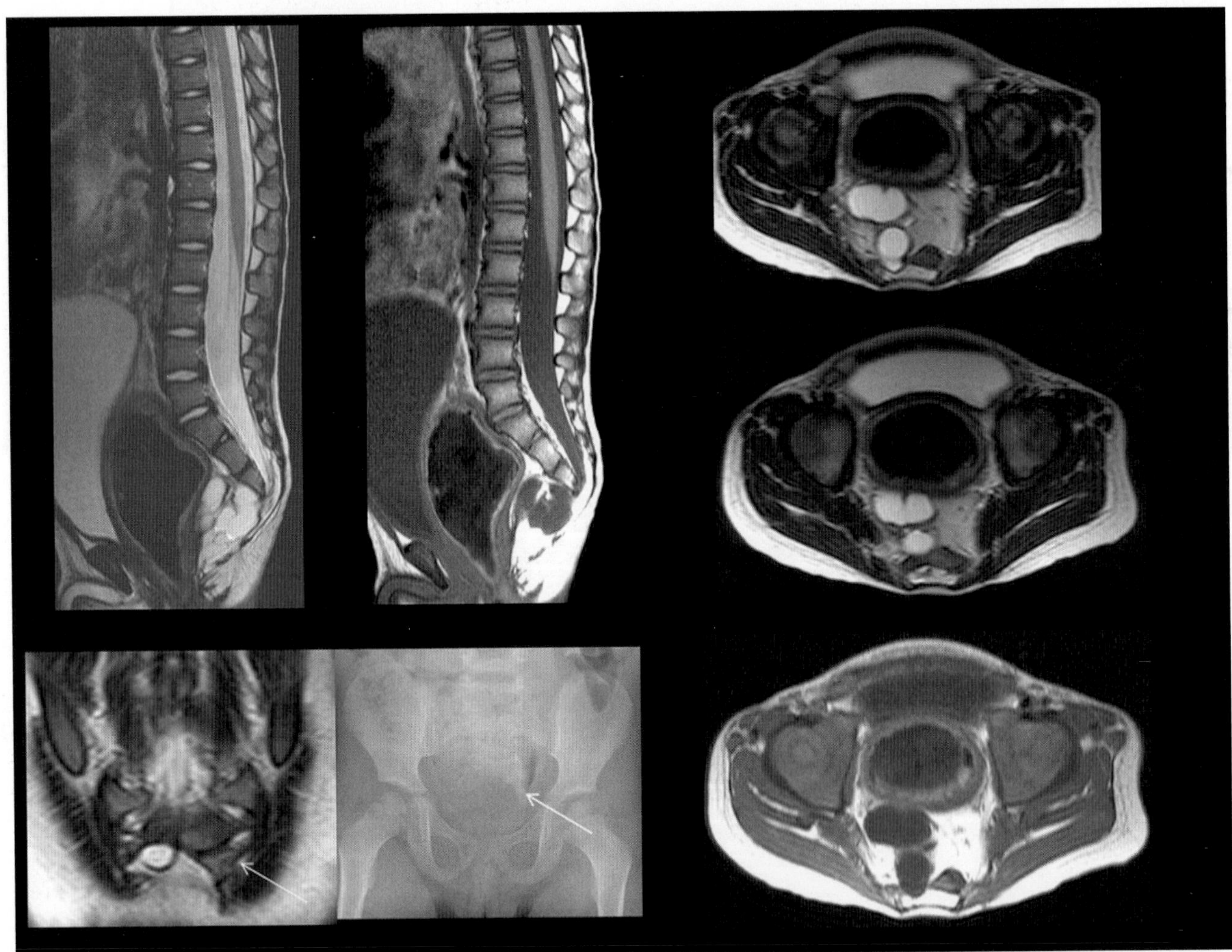

FIGURE 82-39 ■ **There is a presacral cystic lesion in continuity with the thecal sac at the level of the sacrum.** A small solid component is seen in keeping with a benign teratoma with associated meningocele. The conus is seen at the L2/3 level and the spinal cord was untethered at surgery. The left side of the sacrum has a scimitar configuration, with the meningocele seen on the right. These are the features of the Currarino triad.

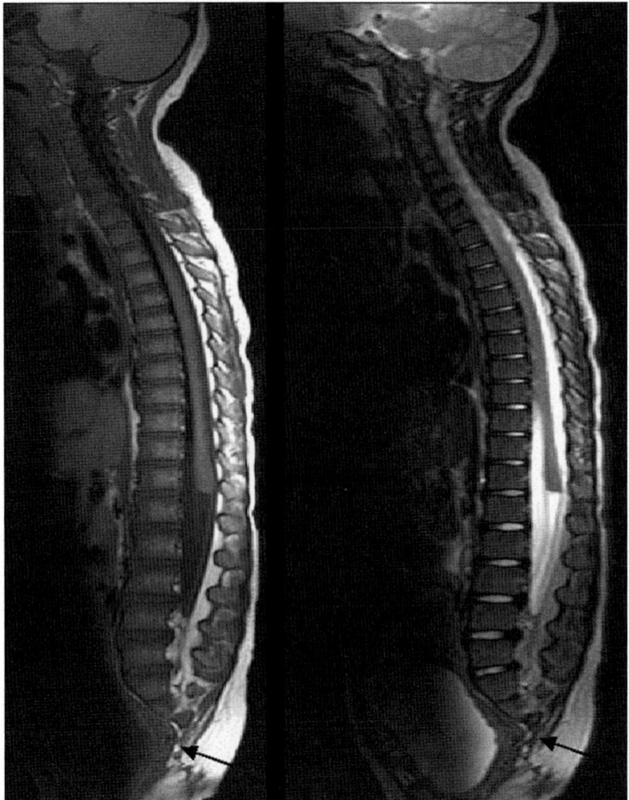

FIGURE 82-40 ■ **Caudal regression syndrome.** The spinal cord is truncated with a typical blunt edge seen at the inferior margin of T12. The thecal sac terminates at the superior margin of L4. The sacrum distal to S2 is agenetic (arrows).

hypoplastic. These anomalies may be a result of a post-neurulation insult.

INBORN METABOLIC BRAIN DISORDERS

Metabolic disorders may be inborn or acquired. Inborn errors of metabolism may result from an enzyme deficiency leading to the build-up of a directly toxic metabolite, or have an indirect toxic effect by activation or inhibition of another metabolic pathway, leading to increased levels of a different toxic metabolite.

The inborn errors of metabolism may be subdivided according to a number of different classification systems, one of which is radiological. One system classifies them by cellular organelle involvement into mitochondrial (usually meaning disorders of mitochondrial energy metabolism), lysosomal and peroxisomal disorders. Another scheme classifies them by the biochemical enzyme pathway affected, e.g. the organic acidaemias, aminoacidopathies or disorders of heavy metal metabolism. In the radiological approach, neuroimaging can be used to help classify them according to white or grey matter involvement, by anatomical distribution of disease, contrast enhancement and other radiological features, mostly by MRI characteristics. Interested readers can also refer to Van der Knaap and Valk[51] and Patay.[52] With each of these methods, advances in molecular genetics and genetic classifications are leading to a deeper understanding of specific gene defects in the manifestation of disease.

There are some general principles that may be helpful in detecting and characterising the radiological features. The abnormalities of metabolic disease are characteristically bilateral and symmetrical. Assessment on MRI should include analysis of the selective involvement and/or sparing of deep grey, cortical grey and white matter structures. When describing white matter abnormalities it is helpful to describe them in terms of general location (lobar involvement, centripetal/centrifugal distribution and AP gradient), juxtacortical U-fibre involvement, involvement of deep white matter structures such as the internal capsule, corpus callosum and white matter tracts such as the pyramidal tracts as they descend from the motor strip (pre-central gyrus) through the posterior limbs of the internal capsules and cerebral peduncles to the decussation within the medulla and then into the spinal cord.

Assessment of the grey matter should include analysis of the cerebral and cerebellar cortex and basal ganglia and thalami for signal abnormality, swelling and volume loss. Signal changes include T_2 and T_1 prolongation, but faint T_1 shortening within the basal ganglia may be seen also when there is calcification. Other deep grey matter structures include the red nuclei, and subthalamic and dentate nuclei. Calcification is much better assessed on CT. Macrocephaly is a useful clinical pointer to diseases such as megalencephalic leukodystrophy with subcortical cysts (MLC), Canavan's and Alexander's leukoencephalopathies, glutaric aciduria type I, GM2 gangliosidosis and L-2-hydroxyglutaric aciduria.

An assessment of the degree of myelination is useful as delay or hypomyelination is frequently seen in metabolic disorders. Although often non-specific, it is a helpful clue to an underlying neurometabolic condition. Myelination requires active energy-dependent metabolism and therefore may also be seen with cardiorespiratory illness. However, hypomyelination may also be seen as a general marker of developmental delay and correlates well with clinical developmental milestones. In premature infants the appropriate MRI markers for corrected age should be assessed before deciding that myelination is immature. There are also specific inherited hypomyelination disorders that may be detected on MRI as a myelination pattern which is immature for the child's age. These include Pelizaeus–Merzbacher disease, in which T_2-weighted imaging often shows more severe hypomyelination compared to T_1-weighted imaging (Fig. 82-41).

Serial imaging should be assessed for progressive cerebral atrophy. This may involve white matter, shown as ventricular enlargement and thinning of the corpus callosum, cortical grey matter, shown as sulcal widening, or deep grey matter with atrophy of the specific basal ganglia and thalamic structures.

Pathognomonic imaging patterns are seen in X-linked adrenoleukodystrophy (ALD), Alexander's disease, glutaric aciduria type I, Canavan's disease, L-2-hydroxyglutaricaciduria, neonatal maple syrup urine disease and MLCs.

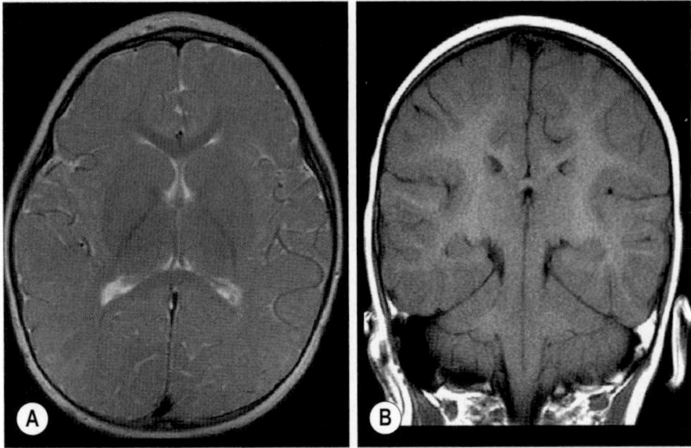

FIGURE 82-41 ■ Pelizaeus–Merzbacher disease in a 2-year-old child with nystagmus and developmental delay. (A) Axial T_2-weighted image shows dark regions of myelination in the posterior limbs of the internal capsules, splenium and genu of the corpus callosum, and within the parieto-occipital lobe white matter. The rest of the cerebral hemispheres are not myelinated (the white matter is too bright). This pattern is severely delayed and equivalent approximately to an age of 6 months. (B) Paradoxically coronal T_1-weighted MRI shows much more advanced myelination, which appears virtually complete, with T_1 shortening extending right out into the subcortical white matter.

Classic X-linked adrenoleukodystrophy is the most common leukodystrophy of children and affects 1 in 20,000 boys. It is due to a defect in a peroxisomal membrane protein leading to defective incorporation of fatty acids into myelin. Screening of family members of affected cases for the specific gene defect should be considered. Clinically, boys present between the ages of 5 and 10 years with learning difficulties, behavioural problems, deteriorating gait and impaired visuospatial perception. Adrenal insufficiency may precede the CNS presentation or may be absent. Without bone marrow transplantation (which replaces the defective gene), the disease progresses to spastic paraparesis, blindness and deafness. Lorenzo's oil may also delay disease progression. Imaging features are of low attenuation on CT and hyperintensity on T2W images in the posterior central white matter, specifically the splenium and peritrigonal white matter progressing to the corticospinal tracts and visual and auditory pathways. The regions of T_2 signal abnormality show increased diffusion. The leading edge of the demyelination enhances where there is active inflammation and disruption of the blood–brain barrier (Fig. 82-42). MR spectroscopy may detect early changes

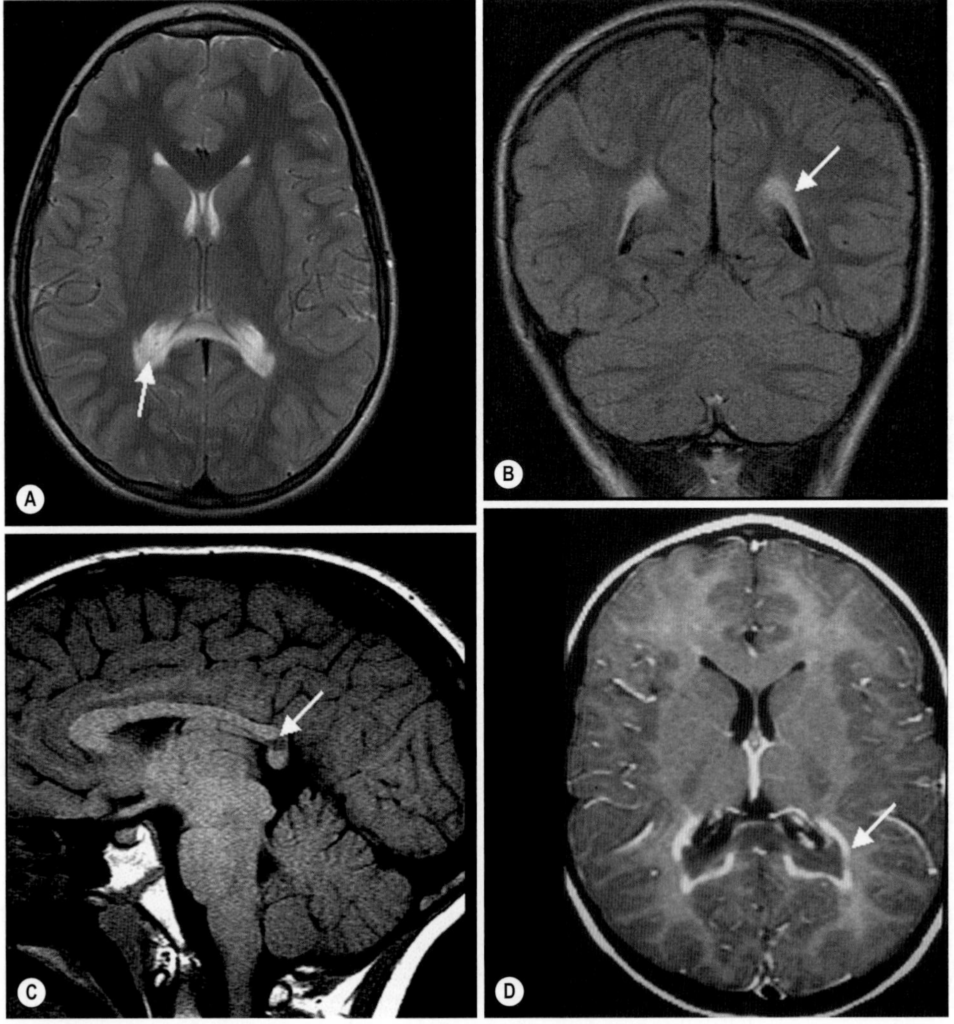

FIGURE 82-42 ■ Adrenoleukodystrophy. MRI of a 6-year-old boy with increasing gait disturbance and impaired vision demonstrates peritrigonal and splenial signal abnormality (increased signal on T_2-weighted images and low signal on T_1-weighted images), and (A–C, arrows) marginal enhancement at the leading edges where there is active inflammation, typical of adrenoleukodystrophy (D, arrow).

and may, in the future, guide early bone marrow transplantation before overt and irreversible changes in the white matter have occurred. Adrenomyeloneuropathy is a variation on ALD which presents in young adults or adolescents, usually boys, with progressive paraparesis and cerebellar signs. It has a less specific radiological pattern causing diffuse disease of the white matter, and it more commonly involves the cerebellum and less frequently the cerebral hemispheres.

In **Alexander's disease**, which has a neonatal, juvenile and adult form, imaging shows extensive white matter abnormality beginning in the frontal and periventricular white matter (Fig. 82-43). Large cystic cavities are seen within the frontal and temporal regions. The basal ganglia may also be involved. Contrast enhancement or garland appearance may be seen along the ventricular ependyma. Less typical forms can show symmetrical or nodular lesions in the brainstem (Fig. 82-44).

L-2-Hydroxyglutaricaciduria is a slowly progressive disorder which is usually discovered in childhood or early adulthood, although it is likely to have started earlier than this. The clinical presentation is non-specific with learning difficulties, epilepsy and pyramidal and cerebellar signs. The MRI findings show white matter involvement with peripheral involvement, particularly of the subcortical U fibres, internal, external and extreme capsules, sparing of the periventricular white matter and corpus callosum, and with a slight frontal predominance. There is macrocephaly. There is also grey matter involvement affecting the basal ganglia, especially the globus pallidi, and sparing the thalami (Fig. 82-45).

Maple syrup urine disease (MSUD) is an autosomal recessive disorder presenting in the neonate in which an enzyme deficiency leads to an accumulation of amino acids (leucine, isoleucine and valine) and their metabolites. A characteristic feature at acute presentation is marked swelling and oedema of the white matter tracts and brainstem often best appreciated in the corticospinal tracts as they course through the internal capsules (Fig. 82-46).

Megalencephaly with leukoencephalopathy and cysts (MLC) is a recently identified autosomal recessive

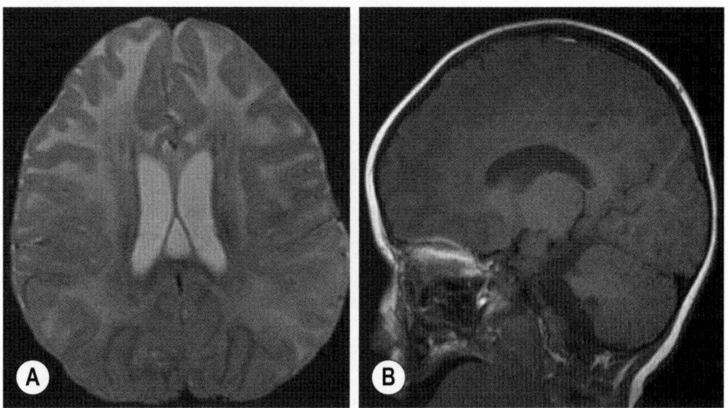

FIGURE 82-43 ■ **Child with Alexander's disease.** Head circumference charts showed the child had macrocephaly. (A) Axial T_2-weighted MRI shows extensive bilateral symmetrical deep and subcortical white matter signal hyperintensity with a frontal predominance and mild swelling. (B) Sagittal T_1-weighted MRI shows corresponding low signal in the affected areas without evidence of cavitation but in keeping with oedema.

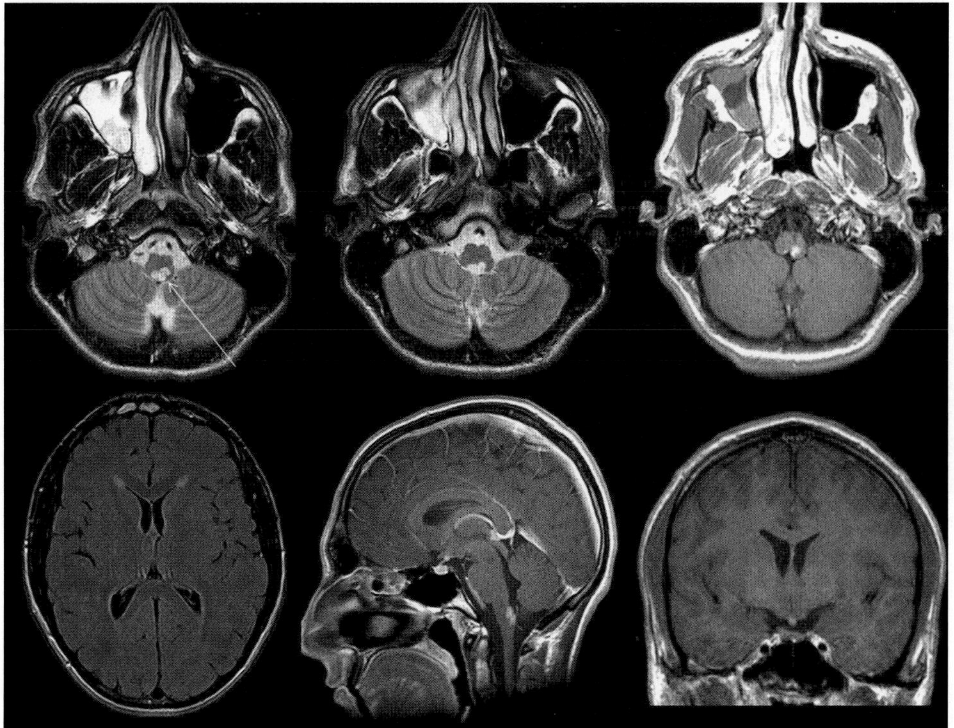

FIGURE 82-44 ■ **A 15-year-old with a 3-year history of progressively worsening nausea, vomiting and hiccups, triggered by exercise.** The MRI images show asymmetrical enhancing nodular lesions in the dorsal medulla and pituitary infundibulum. Very subtle periventricular white matter changes were seen. A de novo GFAP mutation for Alexander's disease was confirmed.

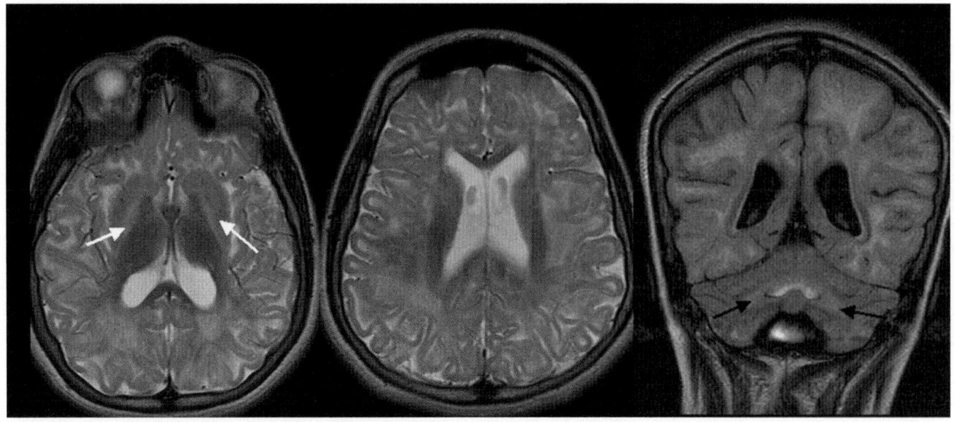

FIGURE 82-45 ■ L-2-Hydroxyglutaricaciduria axial T_2-weighted MRI. Coronal FLAIR images show extensive white matter signal hyperintensity involving mainly deep and subcortical white matter but with relative sparing of the periventricular white matter, and bilateral pallidal involvement. The dentate nuclei are also abnormal.

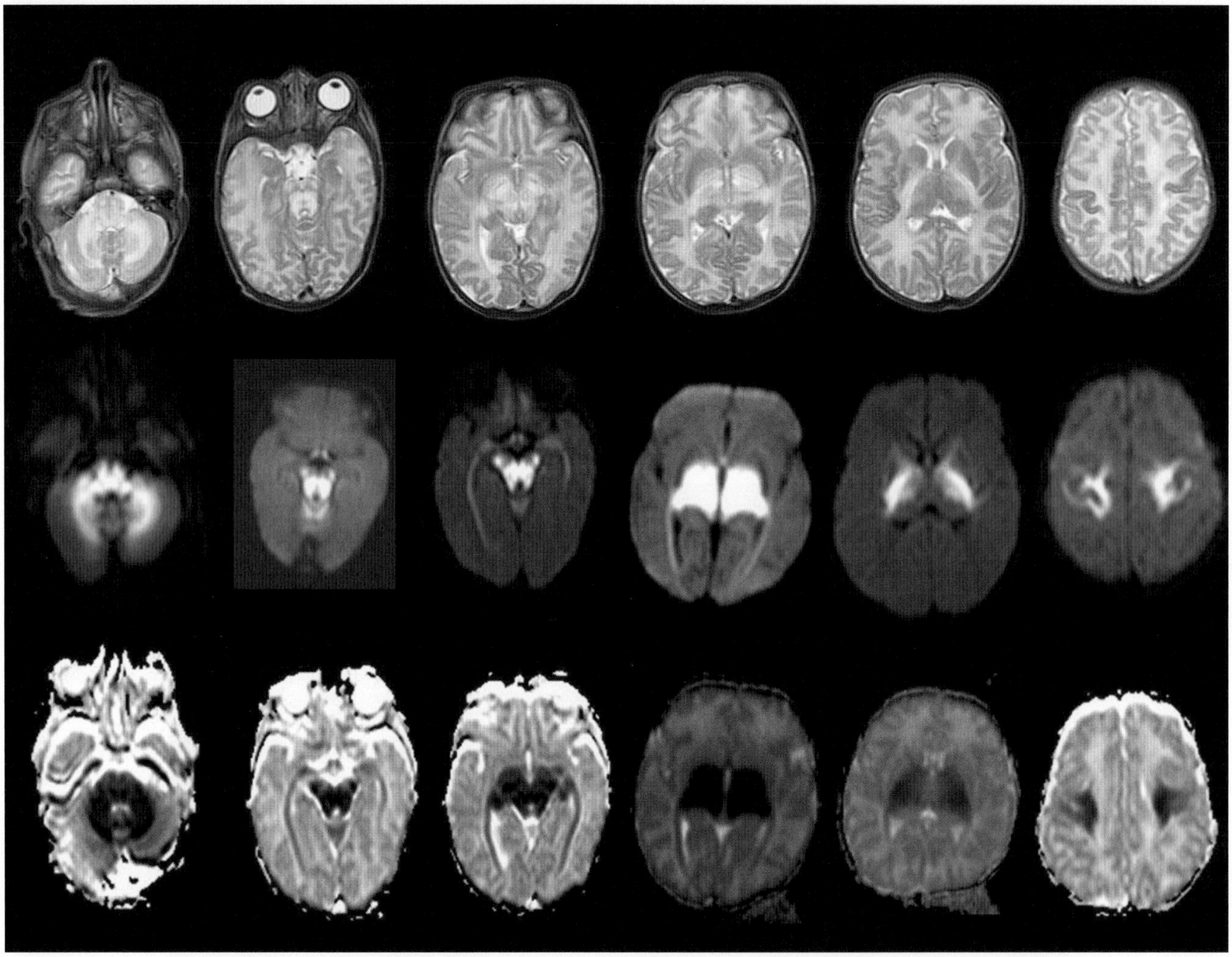

FIGURE 82-46 ■ Neonate presenting with acute encephalopathy on day 5 of life. There is global cerebral swelling and oedema within the white matter. There is also oedema and swelling with restricted diffusion (bright on diffusion-weighted images and dark on ADC maps) within the basal ganglia, thalami, internal capsules and perirolandic cortex/white matter along the course of the corticospinal tracts as well as the midbrain, pons and both cerebellar hemispheres.

leukodystrophy with macrocephaly. A characteristic feature is the relatively mild clinical course despite very abnormal findings of extensive signal change and rarefaction of white matter, particularly in the parietal and anterior temporal lobe regions.

Suggestive MRI patterns include methylmalonicacidaemia in which there is bilateral symmetrical involvement of the globus pallidus with sparing of the thalami and the rest of the basal ganglia (Fig. 82-47). The cerebral cortex is also normal. In the acute stage there is swelling

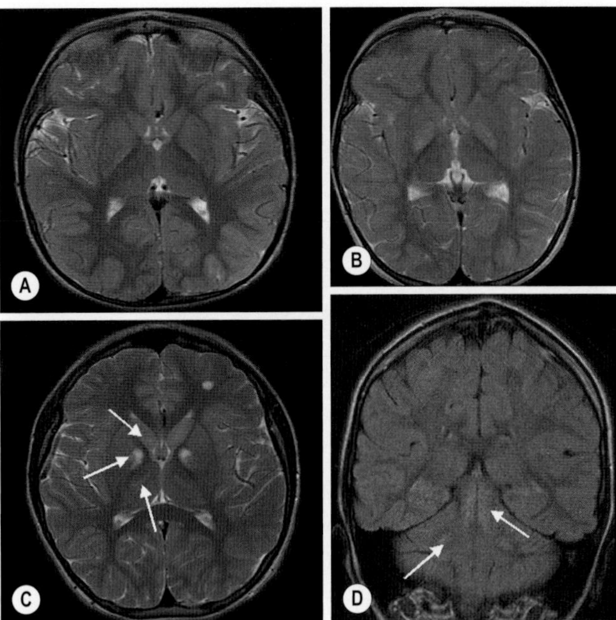

FIGURE 82-47 ■ Examples of signal abnormality affecting both globus pallidi. (A) Kernicterus. (B) Methylmalonicacidaemia. (C) Kearns–Sayre syndrome. This child also has hyperintense signal in both caudate nuclei and thalami, left frontal white matter and (D) dorsal midbrain and cerebellar dentate nuclei (arrows).

and oedema of these structures, while in the chronic phase there is imaging evidence of atrophy and gliosis. Bilateral pallidal involvement is also seen in other rarer inborn errors of metabolism, such as GAMT (guanidinoacetate methyltransferase deficiency), Kearns–Sayre syndrome and some acquired and toxic disorders, such as kernicterus and carbon monoxide poisoning (Fig. 82-47).

Disorders of heavy metal metabolism include Wilson's and Menkes' diseases, both disorders of copper metabolism, molybdenum cofactor deficiency and disorders of magnesium and manganese metabolism. **Wilson's disease** results from defective extracellular copper transport and leads to multiorgan copper deposition. Hyperintensities on T_2-weighted MRI are seen in the basal ganglia, midbrain and pons, thalami and claustra, and there is T_1 shortening in the basal ganglia and thalami, as in other hepatic encephalopathies. **Menkes' disease** is X-linked and affects transcellular copper metabolism at the level of the cell membrane. There is a systemic failure of copper-requiring enzymes, particularly those of the cytochrome-*c* oxidase system. Affected children have connective tissue defects with 'kinky hair', inguinal herniae, hyperflexible joints and bladder diverticula. In the brain there is progressive cerebral atrophy, which may allow subdural collections of CSF or subdural haematomas (and therefore this is a mimic of non-accidental head injury). The basal ganglia may also show T_1 shortening. Children develop a severe cerebral vasculopathy in which vessels are tortuous and prone to dissection.

Another cause of neonatal encephalopathy is **molybdenum cofactor deficiency** in which acutely there is global cerebral swelling and oedema with many features similar to the brain infarction seen in hypoxic-ischaemic injury, but in addition focal symmetrical, selective changes within the globus pallidi and subthalamic nuclei (mocod paper).

Disorders of cellular organelle function include mitochondrial, lysosomal and peroxisomal disorders. Mitochondria are involved in energy metabolism; lysosomes in the degradation of macromolecules, e.g. those involved in the maintenance of cell membrane integrity such as lipids and lipoproteins; and peroxisomes have a role in both catabolic and anabolic metabolism. Mitochondrial disorders include those of mitochondrial energy metabolism affecting oxidative phosphorylation, fatty acid oxidation and ketone metabolism. Respiratory chain disorders affect the respiratory chain, an enzyme pathway mostly located on complex proteins on the inner membrane of the mitochondria. This has an integral role in oxidative phosphorylation and these disorders tend to be multisystem or organ diseases. In the brain they may result in multiple cerebral infarcts in non-vascular territories.

Leigh's disease is not one single entity and can be caused not only by respiratory chain defects but also by enzyme disorders such as those of pyruvate and tricarboxylic acid metabolism. It is characterised by a typical radiological pattern. Bilateral, typically symmetrical, signal change is seen within the brainstem, deep cerebellar grey matter, subthalamic nuclei and basal ganglia (Fig. 82-48). The midbrain changes have been described as a 'panda face' with involvement of the substantia nigra and tegmentum, and the medulla is frequently involved and may account for the apnoeic episodes often seen clinically. Cerebral grey matter infarction may also be seen. MELAS (mitochondrial encephalomyopathy with lactic acidosis and stroke-like episodes) is another mitochondrial disease, typically occurring between the ages of 4 and 15 years but which can occur at any age. Acute metabolic decompensation may be provoked by any insult which causes increased metabolic demand, e.g. febrile illness. Patients may also have a cardiomyopathy and endocrinopathies. Imaging features are those of cerebral infarcts in non-vascular territories and symmetrical basal ganglia calcification.

Lysosomal disorders include Krabbe's disease and metachromatic leukodystrophy. Imaging features which might suggest Krabbe's disease are white matter changes, more severely posteriorly and centrally; basal ganglia and thalamic involvement, specifically dark signal in the thalami on T2W images; cerebellar white matter abnormality, sparing the dentate nuclei; and involvement of the pyramidal tracts within the brainstem. Peroxisomal disorders include Zellweger's syndrome and X-linked ALD. Imaging features of Zellweger's syndrome include severely delayed myelination, periventricular germinolytic cysts, peri-Sylvian polymicrogyria and grey matter heterotopias. When this combination is seen in the clinical context of severe hypotonia with visual and hearing deficits, seizures, hepatomegaly and jaundice, the pattern may be considered pathognomonic.

CRANIOSYNOSTOSIS[53]

Craniosynostosis is a disorder of growth, one of the manifestations of which is premature closure of one or more

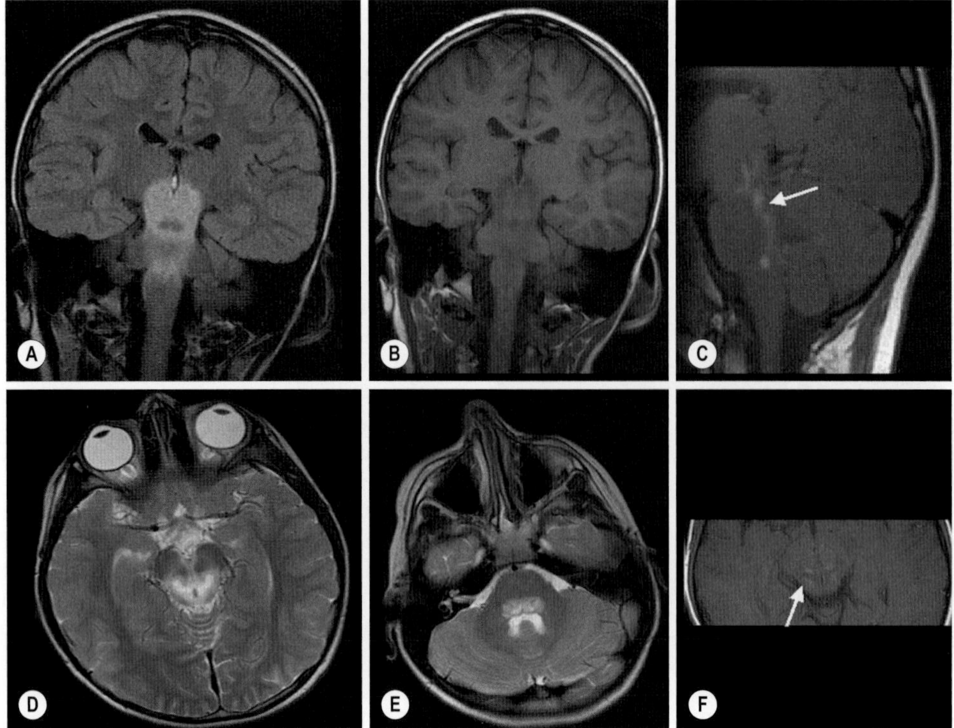

FIGURE 82-48 ■ **Leigh's disease.** There is bilateral symmetrical signal hyperintensity on the coronal FLAIR (A) and axial T_2 images (D, E) matched by hypointensity on the coronal T_1-weighted MRI (B) affecting the midbrain, pons and medulla. Symmetrical contrast enhancement (C, F) indicates breakdown of the blood–brain barrier in keeping with active disease.

calvarial or skull base sutures. The three broad categories of craniosynostosis are the simple non-syndromic type, usually involving one suture; complex syndromic forms involving many sutures; and secondary craniosynostosis due to disrupted growth caused by a wide range of insults such as drugs and metabolic bone disease or secondary to an underlying small brain, as in chronic, treated hydrocephalus or any other cause of microcephaly. The most common type of primary craniosynostosis is simple sagittal synostosis.

The diagnosis is made initially by clinical assessment of the skull shape. Imaging provides confirmatory evidence and information regarding the skull base and orbits, and is important in the assessment of intracranial complications of craniosynostosis, such as hydrocephalus and visual failure. Standard radiographs will allow assessment of the coronal, sagittal, lambdoid and metopic sutures on the AP view; lambdoid and sagittal sutures on the Towne's view; and coronal and lambdoid sutures on the lateral view in addition to assessment of the skull shape, foramen magnum and fontanelles. The affected suture may be absent, indistinct, show bridging sclerosis or a heaped-up or beaked appearance, but also may appear normal if the synostosis is fibrotic not bony. Skull growth decreases perpendicular to the suture and increases parallel to it. Therefore, greater weight is given to the skull shape than the radiological evidence of direct sutural involvement on plain film or CT. Conversely, if the sutures are not clearly visualised but the skull shape is normal, then primary craniosynostosis is unlikely.

Sagittal synostosis produces an elongated head shape called scaphocephaly (Fig. 82-49). Bicoronal synostosis causes brachycephaly or foreshortening in the AP direction, which is accompanied by lateral elevation of the sphenoid wings producing the characteristic 'harlequin' deformity, upward slanting of the petrous apices and hypertelorism. Unicoronal synostosis causes anterior plagiocephaly or asymmetrical skull deformity and may be associated with compensatory growth on the unaffected side, resulting in frontoparietal bossing (Fig. 82-50). Metopic synostosis causes trigonocephaly or 'keel deformity' and an AP view may show parallel, vertically oriented medial orbital walls. True unilateral lambdoid

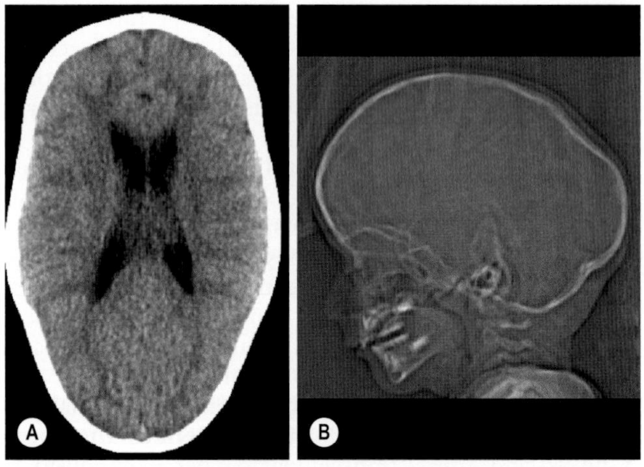

FIGURE 82-49 ■ **Sagittal synostosis.** (A) Brain CT and (B) lateral scout view showing the typical 'boat-shaped' skull or scaphocephaly of sagittal synostosis.

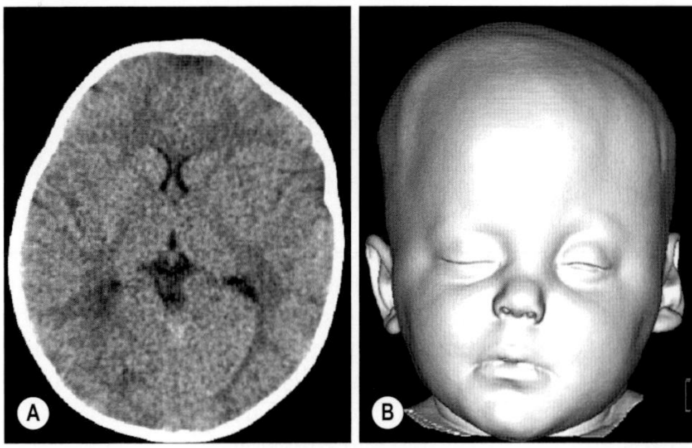

FIGURE 82-50 ■ Unicoronal synostosis. (A) Axial CT and (B) 3D surface-shaded reformat show the asymmetrical head shape of left frontal plagiocephaly due to unicoronal craniosynostosis, with bossing seen on the right side.

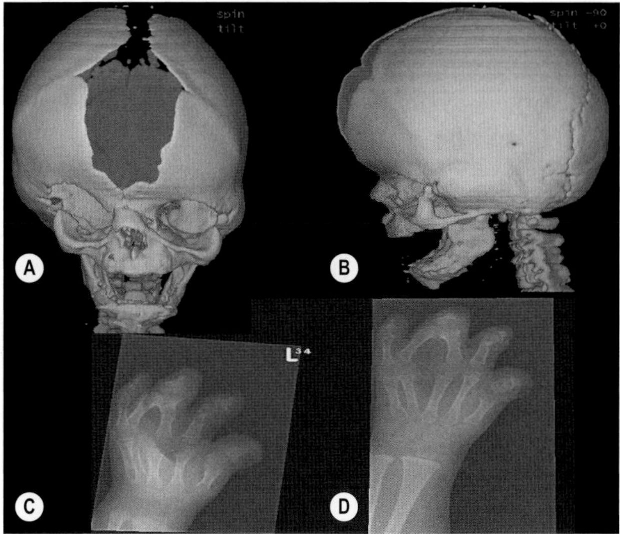

FIGURE 82-51 ■ Apert's syndrome. (A, B) 3D CT surface-shaded display shows the wide open defect of the sagittal suture and brachycephaly with bicoronal synostosis typical of Apert's syndrome. The coronal sutures appear fused and are ridged. (C, D) Plain radiographs of the hands show the 'mitten' hand appearance with syndactyly and shortened metacarpals.

synostosis, the rarest form of monosutural synostosis, causes posterior plagiocephaly. This should be distinguished from the much more common positional or deformational plagiocephaly in which the suture is normal, and which is seen more often since the 1992 recommendation of the American Academy of Pediatrics to place newborns supine rather than prone in their cots to reduce the incidence of sudden infant death. In this case the skull deformity is caused by the child lying on one side in preference to the other, and may also be seen in children with torticollis or developmental delay. On plain radiographs and CT the lambdoid sutures appear open. Imaging of the spine may reveal segmentation anomalies, e.g. C5 and C6 in Apert's syndrome, and atlanto-occipital assimilation and basilar invagination in Apert's and Crouzon's syndromes.

CT is more sensitive and specific than plain radiographs for detecting radiological evidence of craniosynostosis, such as sclerosis and bony bridging, and CT venography may be helpful to assess the jugular foramina, variations in venous anatomy and patency of the venous sinuses. Three-dimensional CT surface-shaded bone and soft-tissue reconstructions or maximum intensity projections (MIPs) with a low milliampere technique may also be acquired, preferably in the craniofacial unit where treatment is being considered. The sutures should be assessed on both the axial 2D CT and 3D CT as either technique may miss relevant diagnostic features. There is also increasing prenatal diagnosis of craniosynostosis, particularly the syndromic forms, by ultrasound and fetal MRI.

In Apert's syndrome there are features of brachycephaly due to bicoronal synostosis, a wide open midline calvarial defect from the root of the nose to the posterior fontanelle in what would normally be the sagittal and metopic sutures and anterior fontanelle (Fig. 82-51). The sutures never form properly and, instead, bone islands appear within the defect, eventually coalescing to bony fusion by about 36 months. There is also hypertelorism with shallow anterior cranial fossae, depressed cribriform plate, as well as maxillary hypoplasia causing midface retrusion with exorbitism. Indeed, the globe may actually sublux onto the cheek. The hand and feet deformities distinguish this condition from most other syndromic craniosynostoses and include syndactyly, phalangeal fusion and a short radially deviated thumb producing the 'mitten' or more severe 'hoof' hand. Children with Crouzon's syndrome demonstrate a more complex syndromic synostosis involving the coronal, sagittal, metopic and squamosal sutures, with early rather than late fontanelle closure. There is no midline calvarial defect but there is maxillary hypoplasia, hypertelorism, exorbitism and dental malocclusion. The limbs are usually clinically normal.

CT will detect any underlying structural brain abnormality. Although the brain usually appears structurally normal, midline anomalies such as callosal and septum pellucidum agenesis, limbic system abnormalities in Apert's, ventriculomegaly or distortion of the posterior fossa and skull base causing Chiari I malformations (tonsillar descent) may be detected. Tonsillar herniation is more frequently seen in Crouzon's syndrome, probably because there is more frequent skull base sutural synostosis in these conditions compared to Apert's.

Predicting raised intracranial pressure is known to be difficult by imaging, and correlation with clinical assessment is extremely important. Sometimes, however, direct invasive intracranial pressure (ICP) monitoring will be required. Hydrocephalus, seen in 4–25% of craniosynostosis and more commonly in the syndromic forms, may be multifactorial; possible aetiologies include tonsillar herniation and altered craniocervical junction CSF dynamics and venous hypertension due to venous foraminal narrowing, such as the jugular foramina, which ultimately may lead to venous occlusion and the development of venous collateral pathways such as enlargement of the stylomastoid emissary veins. Hydrocephalus is the most sensitive radiological indicator (see below) but only detects 40% of these children with raised ICP.

Finally CT may also be useful to assess the airway. Midface hypoplasia, small maxilla with dental overcrowding and basilar kyphosis may contribute to nasopharyngeal obstruction. Deviation of the nasal septum and choanal atresia may also be detected.

NEONATAL NASAL OBSTRUCTION: NASAL CAVITY STENOSIS/ATRESIA

The most common cause of neonatal nasal obstruction is mucosal oedema, followed by choanal atresia, skeletal dysplasias and congenital dacrocystocele due to distal nasolacrimal duct obstruction.

Choanal Atresia and Pyriform Stenosis

Choanal atresia/stenosis, a congenital malformation of the anterior skull base characterised by failure of canalisation of the posterior choanae, is the most common form of nasal cavity stenosis. It may be bony and/or fibrous in nature, unilateral presenting in later childhood with chronic nasal discharge and bilateral presenting in newborns with respiratory distress, particularly during feeding and which is a surgical emergency. Bilateral forms are more likely to be syndromic (50%) than unilateral forms and common associations are Crouzon's, Treacher Collins, CHARGE and Pierre Robin syndromes. The CHARGE syndrome describes the association of colobomas of the eye, heart defects, atresia of the choanae, retardation of growth and development, genitourinary anomalies and ear anomalies. The atresia is best evaluated on CT by direct axial and direct coronal imaging on a bone algorithm after administration of a nasal decongestant. The nasal cavity appears funnel shaped with a fluid level proximal to the obstruction. The posterior vomer is thickened and the nasal septum is deviated to the side of the stenosis. A bony, fibrous or membranous bridging bar across the posterior choana is seen (Fig. 82-52). There is also congenital nasal pyriform aperture stenosis in which there is focal stenosis of the nasal aperture anteriorly caused by medial displacement of the nasal process of the maxilla assessed on axial bone CT at the level of the inferior meatus, often associated with a single central maxillary incisor (Fig. 82-53).

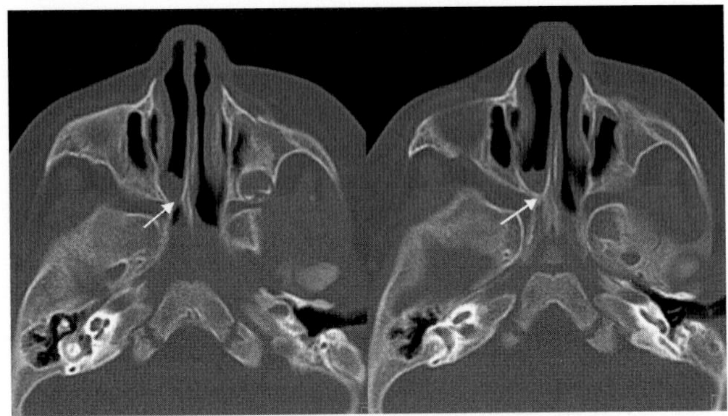

FIGURE 82-52 ■ **Choanal atresia.** Axial skull base CT in a child with chronic nasal discharge shows right-sided choanal atresia. There is bony narrowing of the funnel-shaped posterior right choana down to a bony bridging bar (arrows) and pooling of secretions proximally.

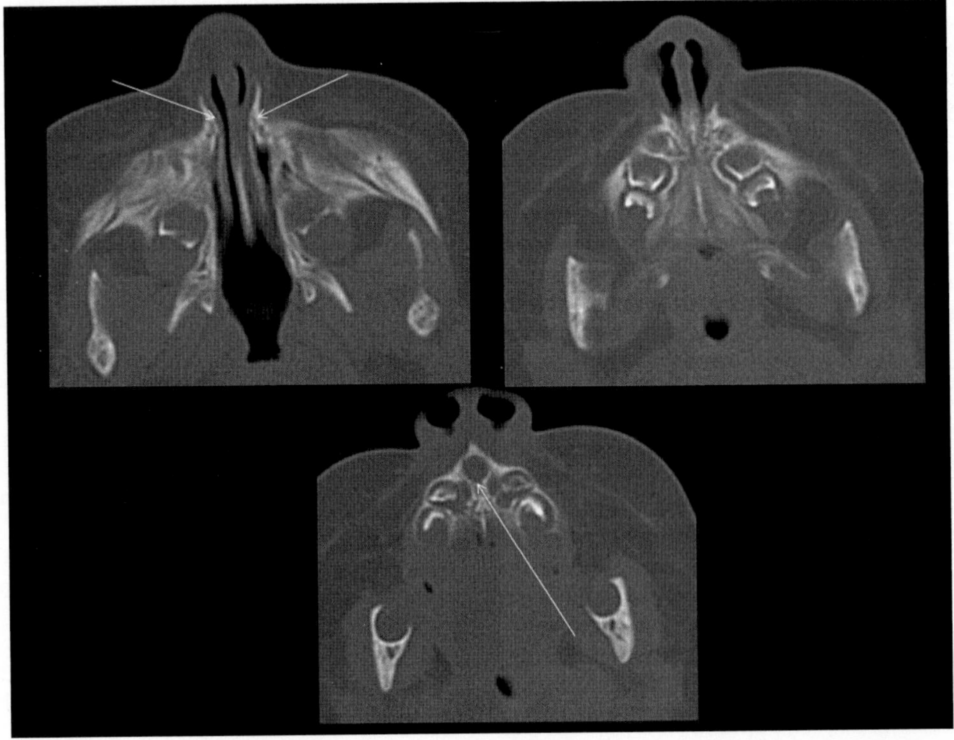

FIGURE 82-53 ■ **Pyriform stenosis and single central incisor.**

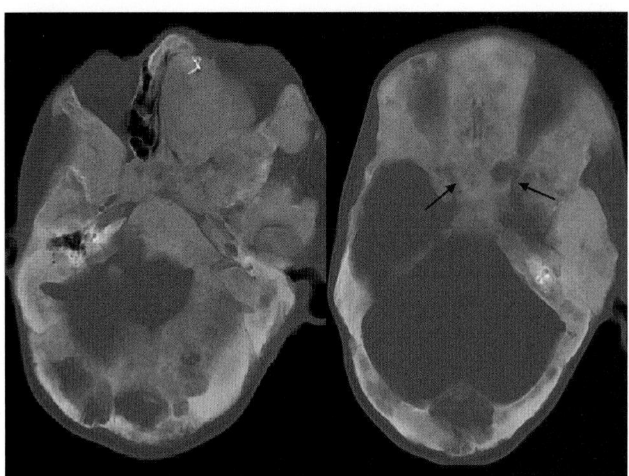

FIGURE 82-54 ■ Polyostotic fibrous dysplasia with diffuse calvarial expansion, mixed lytic lesions and sclerosis. The optic nerve canals are markedly narrowed (arrows).

Skeletal Dysplasias

Fibrous dysplasia is a benign congenital disorder in which bone is gradually replaced by fibrous tissue. McCune–Albright syndrome is a subtype of polyostotic fibrous dysplasia in which there is pituitary hypersecretion (hence precocious puberty but also Cushing's syndrome, etc.) and café-au-lait spots. Cherubism refers to fibrous dysplasia of the mandible and maxilla, and unlike the other forms of fibrous dysplasia is an inheritable condition. Typically the mandibular condyles are spared. The teeth may be displaced, impacted, resorbed or appear to be floating.

Clinical symptoms other than cosmetic deformity relate to the site of bony involvement; hence, cranial nerve impingement caused by narrowing of the skull base foramina, exophthalmos and optic foraminal narrowing caused by orbital involvement are all seen. On CT the typical lesion is a region of bony expansion with a 'ground-glass' appearance, but lesions may be lytic or sclerotic, or a combination of all three (Fig. 82-54).

BRAIN TUMOURS[54]

The Children's Cancer and Leukaemia Group (CCLG) Guidelines[55]

At initial presentation all paediatric brain tumours should have brain and whole-spine MRI, including contrast-enhanced images. A suggested protocol includes T_2-weighted FSE axial coronal FLAIR, T_1-weighted SE pre- and post-contrast imaging in three orthogonal planes for the brain (axial, coronal, sagittal), diffusion-weighted imaging and post-contrast imaging of the whole spine. Ideally spine imaging should be performed at the outset, but if the need for surgery is immediate, then postoperative spinal imaging (pre- and post-contrast T_1-weighted MRI to allow exclusion of T_1 shortening due to post-surgical blood products) should be performed. The immediate postoperative MRI should be performed within 48 h (or 72 h maximum, according to the CCLG guidelines), the rationale being that post-surgical nodular enhancement which mimics tumour will not be seen before then. Post-surgical linear enhancement may be seen within this time period and, indeed, intraoperatively, and should therefore be interpreted with caution. The management strategy and frequency of subsequent surveillance imaging is determined by the tumour histology and presence of residual or recurrent tumour.[56–58] There remain regional differences in outcome in the UK, emphasising the importance of managing children with these tumours in a paediatric neuro-oncology centre with multidisciplinary support of neurosurgery, radiology and pathological condition.

Posterior Fossa Tumours

The most common intra-axial cerebellar tumours in children are medulloblastoma (generically known as infratentorial primitive neuroectodermal tumour or PNET), pilocytic astrocytoma, ependymoma and atypical teratoid/rhabdoid tumour, of which medulloblastoma and astrocytoma are the most common. Cerebellar haemangioblastoma may be seen in the context of von Hippel–Lindau disease but otherwise is an unusual tumour in the paediatric age group. Other posterior fossa tumours include brainstem gliomas and extra-axial tumours, such as dermoid and epidermoid cysts, schwannoma, neurofibroma, meningioma and skull base lesions, such as Langerhans' cell histiocytosis, Ewing's sarcoma and glomus tumours.

Clinically all of these tumours may present as a 'posterior fossa' syndrome with lethargy, headache and vomiting due to hydrocephalus and/or direct involvement of the brainstem emetic centre. Before the fontanelles have closed, infants may present with macrocephaly and sunsetting eyes. Truncal and gait ataxia is seen more often in older children and adults.

Infratentorial PNET (medulloblastomas) are highly malignant small, round cell tumours. They are slightly more common than pilocytic astrocytomas in most pathological series, are more common in boys, and account for 30–40% of posterior fossa tumours. They are also associated with some rare oncogenetic disorders such as Li–Fraumeni syndrome, Gorlin's or basal cell naevus syndrome (with falcine calcification), Turcot's and Cowden's syndromes. They are aggressive, high-grade tumours (WHO Grade IV) and tend to have a shorter onset of symptoms, typically shorter than 1 month, compared to other cerebellar tumours. The peak age of presentation is 7 years but they have a wide age range and may be seen from the neonatal period to late adulthood. There is a second peak in young adults presenting with the 'desmoplastic', less-aggressive type of medulloblastoma, which is seen more frequently in the cerebellar hemisphere than the vermis. Closely related to this is the medulloblastoma with extensive nodularity found in young children and also with a better prognosis than standard medulloblastoma (Fig. 82-55). Occasionally there may be symptoms and signs or imaging evidence of intracranial or intraspinal leptomeningeal metastatic disease at presentation, a

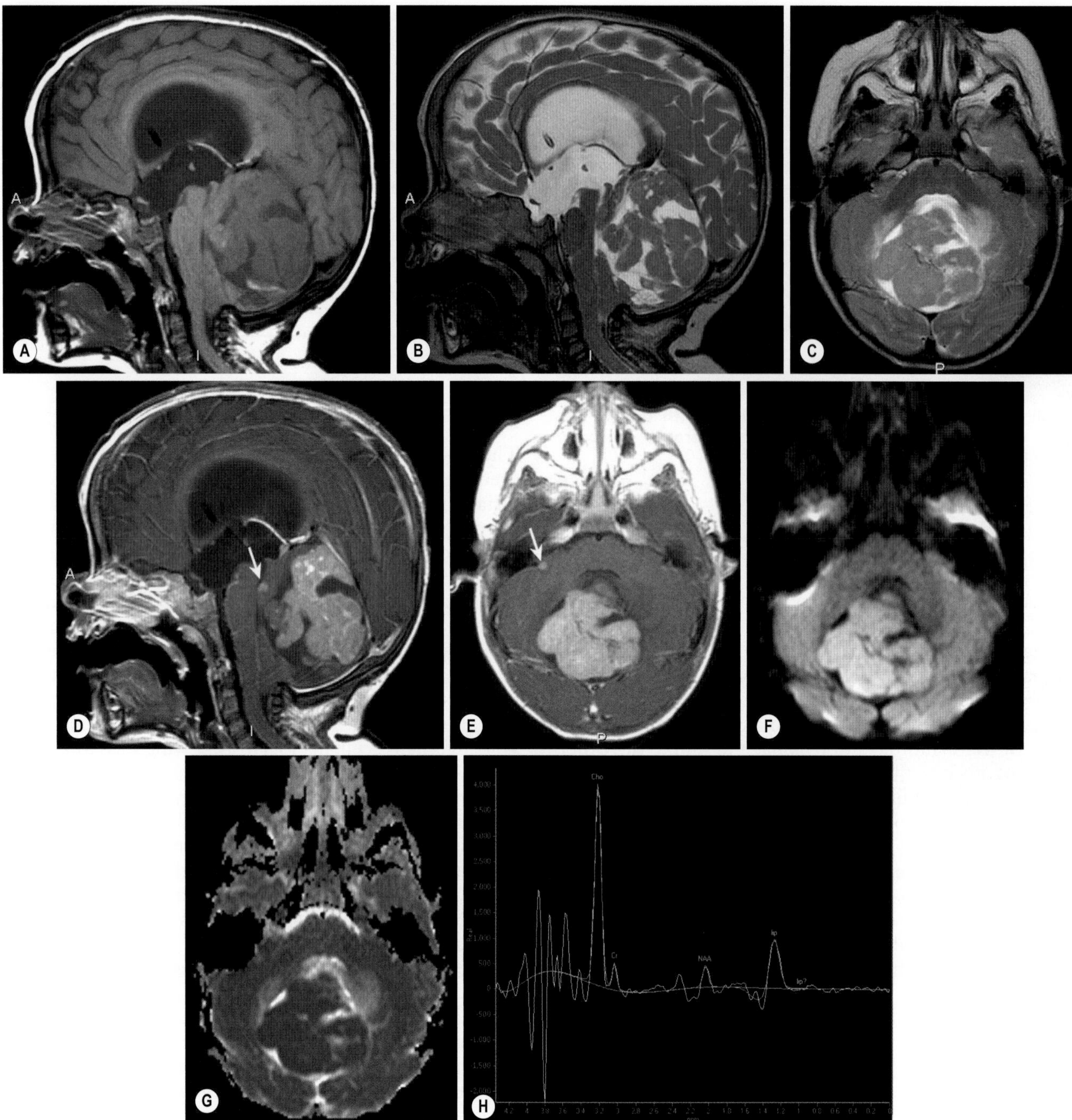

FIGURE 82-55 ■ Medulloblastoma with extensive nodularity (MB-EN). (A) Sagittal T1-weighted image and (B, C) sagittal and axial T2-weighted images show a large, cerebellar mass predominantly involving the vermis, composed of a macronodular conglomerate. There is marked supratentorial hydrocephalus. (D, E) Post contrast T1-weighted images show enhancement of the macronodules as well as secondary lesions in the cerebral acqueduct and right cerebellopontine cistern (arrows). Note the mass is superficially located in the cerebellar vermis and abuts the pial surface posteriorly, whereas the fourth ventricle is compressed. (F, G) Diffusion-weighted image and corresponding ADC map show restricted diffusion consistent with hypercellularity. (H) MR spectroscopy (PRESS, TE 144 ms) shows markedly elevated choline, reduced creatine and NAA, and an abnormal lipid peak, consistent with a high-grade lesion.

feature observed more commonly than with other posterior fossa tumours.

The typical appearance of the childhood medulloblastoma on CT is of a hyperdense midline vermian mass abutting the roof of the fourth ventricle, with perilesional oedema, variable patchy enhancement and hydrocephalus. The brainstem is usually displaced anteriorly rather than directly invaded. Cystic change, haemorrhage and calcification are frequently seen. On MRI, the mass is hypointense or isointense compared to grey matter. The CT finding of hyperdensity and MRI finding of T_2 hypointensity, supported by the presence of restricted diffusion on diffusion-weighted imaging, are the most reliable observations in prospectively differentiating

TABLE 82-2 **Differential Diagnosis of Posterior Fossa Tumour with CT Hyperdensity and T_2 Hypointensity**

- Infratentorial PNET (medulloblastoma) or atypical teratoid/rhabdoid tumour
- Choroid plexus carcinoma
- Ewing's sarcoma
- Chondrosarcoma
- Chordoma
- Lymphoma
- Langerhans' cell histiocytosis

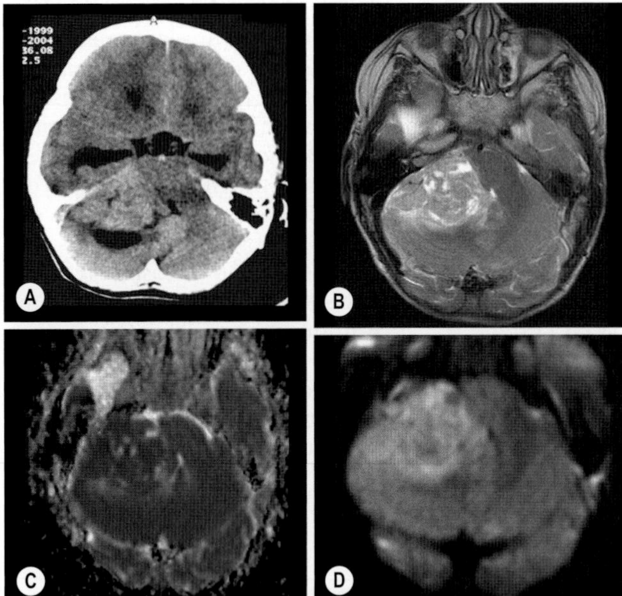

FIGURE 82-56 ■ **Medulloblastoma.** (A) CT and (B–D) axial T_2, ADC and diffusion MRI show a mixed solid and cystic mass within the right cerebellopontine angle encroaching on the pons and fourth ventricle and causing hydrocephalus. The solid component is hyperdense on CT, is hypointense on the T_2-weighted sequence and demonstrates restricted diffusion in keeping with a cellular tumour. Despite some less typical features, such as lateral site (more usually seen in older patients and associated with the desmoplastic variant) and cystic components, on the basis of the signal characteristics this was correctly diagnosed as a medulloblastoma.

medulloblastoma (and atypical rhabdoid tumour which on imaging appears identical to medulloblastoma) from ependymoma or other posterior fossa tumours (Fig. 82-56, Table 82-2).[59] Both the CT hyperdensity and MRI T_2 signal hypointensity reflect the increased nuclear-to-cytoplasmic ratio and densely packed cells of the tumour, and are particularly useful in differentiating medulloblastomas with 'atypical' features, such as a lateral site involving the foramen of Luschka or extrusion through the foramen of Magendie, which are more commonly seen with ependymomas. Medulloblastomas demonstrate restricted diffusion and reduced *N*-acetyl asparatate (NAA) peak with an increased choline-to-creatine ratio, and occasionally lactate and lipid peaks on MR spectroscopy.

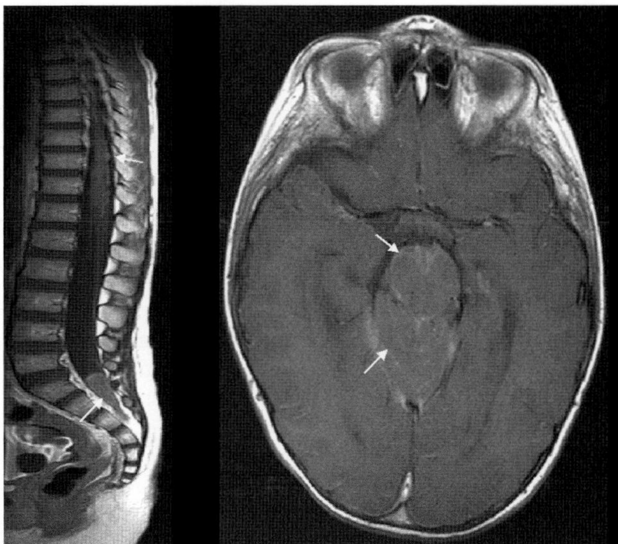

FIGURE 82-57 ■ **Medulloblastoma.** Same patient as described in the legend to Fig. 82-56, with posterior fossa medulloblastoma, has evidence of disseminated metastatic disease. There is nodular enhancement over the conus medullaris and a mass within the thecal sac in addition to pial enhancement over the midbrain and cerebellar folia (arrows).

In medulloblastoma, both intracranial and intraspinal subarachnoid dissemination should be actively looked for, and is seen in a third of cases at presentation, most often occurring as irregular, nodular leptomeningeal enhancement (Fig. 82-57). Imaging is reported as being more sensitive than CSF cytology and false positives can be avoided by preoperative imaging of the brain and spine. Occasionally, enhancement may not always be detected or may be very mild, making the detection of both disseminated disease and residual or recurrent tumour on surveillance imaging more difficult. Other features of leptomeningeal disease include sulcal and cisternal effacement and communicating hydrocephalus; thickening, nodularity and clumping of nerve roots; and pial 'drop' metastases along the surface of the spinal cord.

Standard treatment for infratentorial primitive neuroectodermal tumour (PNET) (medulloblastoma) is by surgical resection, with adjuvant craniospinal radiotherapy for those over 3 years of age (as the infant brain is more susceptible to radiation effects) and chemotherapy. The 5-year survival varies from 50% to 80%. Favourable prognostic factors include complete surgical resection, lack of CSF dissemination at presentation, onset in the second decade, female gender and lateral location within the cerebellar hemisphere, while poor prognostic factors include specific oncogene expression. Surveillance imaging detects recurrences earlier than clinical presentation, allows earlier therapeutic intervention and correlates with increased survival.

Atypical teratoid/rhabdoid tumours are unusual malignant tumours with a poor prognosis. For practical purposes, the imaging features are indistinguishable from medulloblastoma/PNET. They are more aggressive tumours, are often large at the time of presentation and occur in slightly younger children, typically under the age of 2 years.

The next most common cerebellar tumour in children after medulloblastoma, and accounting for 30–40%, is the cerebellar low-grade astrocytoma (CLGA), which in most cases (85%) is a pilocytic tumour (WHO Grade I) and in up to 15% is a more diffuse fibrillary type with a higher histological grade. The 5-year survival for cerebellar pilocytic astrocytoma is in excess of 95% in most reported series, including the original description by Cushing in 1931. The CLGA is a well-circumscribed, slowly growing lesion of children and young adults, though it is occasionally seen in older people. There is an association with NF1, as there is for other neuro-axis pilocytic astrocytomas. The duration of symptom onset is more insidious than that of medulloblastomas, typically being intermittent over several months.

On CT and MRI the tumour is typically a cerebellar vermian or hemispheric tumour which is cystic with an enhancing mural nodule. The solid component is hypointense to isodense on CT, hyperintense on T_2-weighted FSE and hypointense on T_1-weighted sequences reflecting the hypocellular and loosely arranged tumoural architecture.[60] The solid component is highly vascular with a deficient blood–brain barrier and therefore enhances avidly and homogeneously (Fig. 82-58).

Occasionally the pilocytic astrocytoma may present with diffuse nodular enhancement of the leptomeninges, indicating intracranial or intraspinal pial dissemination. This is typically seen with WHO Grade I tumours, does not imply a higher-grade tumour and, like the tumour primary, tends to grow slowly.

Ependymomas (WHO Grade II) account for approximately 10% of paediatric posterior fossa tumours and the posterior fossa is the most common site for ependymomas in children. Their mean age at presentation is 6.4 years, with a range of 2 months to 16 years. They are well-defined tumours which typically originate from the floor or the roof of the fourth ventricle, extend into the cerebellopontine angle and extrude through the foramina of Luschka and Magendie (Fig. 82-59). Perivascular pseudorosettes and ependymal rosettes are the cardinal histopathological features. They are more cellular than CLGAs but usually demonstrate CT and MRI features consistent with a greater water content than medulloblastomas. Therefore they are still hypodense or isodense on CT, hypointense on T_1 and isodense to hyperintense on MRI. Foci of microcystic change, haemorrhage and calcification are common features. They can also disseminate throughout the neuro-axis by leptomeningeal spread, although this is much less common than for medulloblastoma, and tends to occur later in the disease rather than at initial presentation. Incomplete resection, age under 3 years and anaplastic histopathological features correlate with a worse prognosis. The 5-year progression-free survival is 50% but worse under the age of 2 years.

Children with von Hippel–Lindau disease may occasionally present with cerebellar haemangioblastoma (WHO Grade I), which in the sporadic form is usually a tumour of adults. It consists of a rich capillary network in addition to large vacuolated stromal cells. On imaging, haemangioblastomas may mimic a CLGA with an intensely enhancing mural nodule and a cystic component. The tumour abuts the pial surface, but unlike the CLGA it may be associated with prominent vascular flow

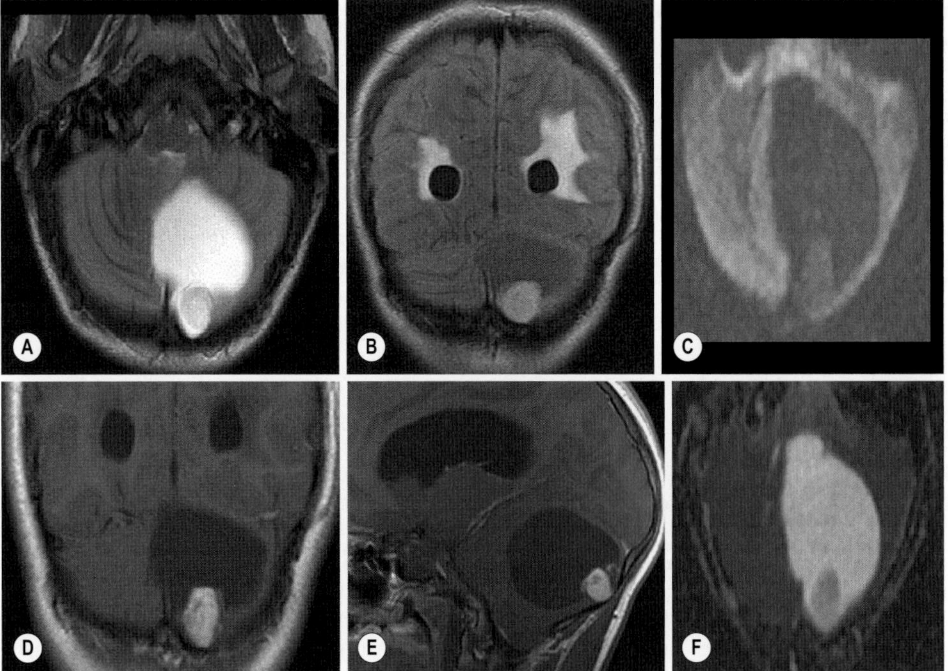

FIGURE 82-58 ■ Cerebellar hemispheric tumour in a child with a history of ataxia, nausea and vomiting over several months. (A, B, D, E) Axial T_2, coronal FLAIR, coronal and sagittal T_1-enhanced MRI show a left cerebellar hemispheric tumour with a large cystic component and solid homogeneously enhancing component which is bright on T_2-weighted sequences (compare with the images of posterior fossa medulloblastoma, Figs. 82-56 and 82-57). The solid component is not restricted on the diffusion-weighted image (C) and ADC map (F) compared to medulloblastoma and there is free diffusion in the cystic component.

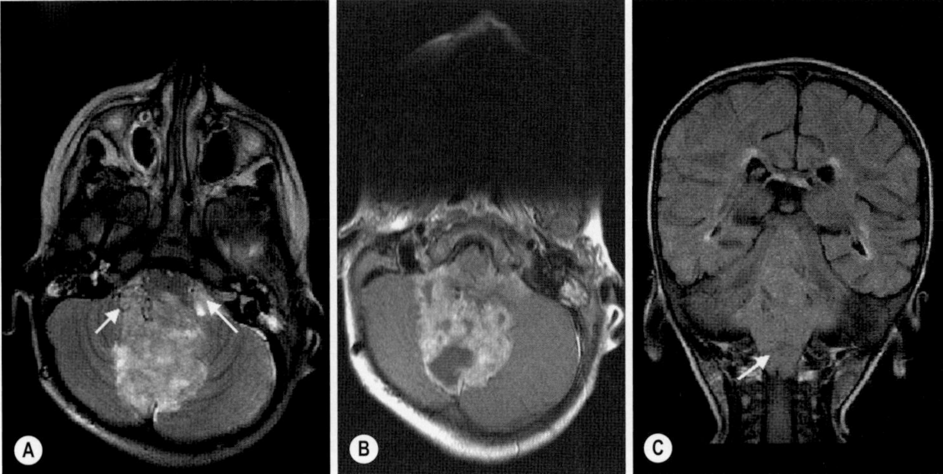

FIGURE 82-59 ■ **Ependymoma.** (A–C) Axial T_2, enhanced T_1 and coronal FLAIR images showing a solid and microcystic fourth ventricular tumour extending out through the foramina of Luschka, Magendie and the foramen magnum (arrows), the typical features of an ependymoma.

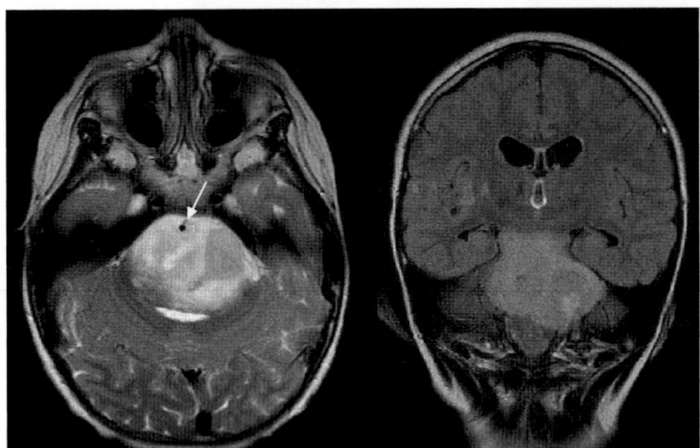

FIGURE 82-60 ■ **Diffuse brainstem astrocytoma.** Note the mass effect within the pons distorting the fourth ventricle and the encasement of the basilar artery (arrow).

voids. Haemorrhage and frank necrosis may occur but are less common.

Most brainstem tumours in children are astrocytomas. Medullary tumours may present with symptoms and signs of raised intracranial pressure and cranial nerve dysfunction. The two major groups are diffuse tumours and focally exophytic tumours.[61] Diffuse tumours extend up and down the brainstem and are seen best as ill-defined signal hyperintensity on T_2-weighted (including FLAIR) images in association with expansion of the brainstem. Their enhancement if present is usually minimal unless the tumour has been irradiated (Fig. 82-60). Focal exophytic tumours are usually dorsally exophytic, well-defined tumours, which do not extend along white matter tracts in the same ways as diffuse astrocytomas (hence their exophytic growth), but often enhance. They are usually Grade I pilocytic or Grade II astrocytomas and are associated with a better prognosis than diffuse astrocytomas, particularly focal tumours within the midbrain tectum.[62] Occasionally, however, anaplastic gangliogliomas or PNET tumours may appear like this.

TABLE 82-3 **Differential of Enhancing Infundibular Lesions**

- Germinoma
- Langerhans' cell histiocytosis
- Lymphocytic hypophysitis
- Granuloma (tuberculosis, sarcoid)

Suprasellar Tumours

Some knowledge of the typical clinical presentation of certain suprasellar tumours can be very helpful in differentiating them even before imaging. For example, hypopituitarism is more likely to be seen with craniopharyngioma, delayed puberty with hypothalamic astrocytoma or Langerhans' cell histiocytosis and occasionally pituitary adenoma, precocious puberty due to hypothalamic infundibular lesions, such as Langerhans' cell histiocytosis, germinoma, craniopharyngioma, hamartoma and non-neoplastic granulomatous disease, such as sarcoidosis and tuberculosis (Table 82-3). Large suprasellar mass lesions have the ability to produce hydrocephalus by obstruction at the foramen of Monro, and visual field defects by compression or involvement of the optic chiasm.

Craniopharyngioma

Although histologically benign (WHO Grade I), this tumour is associated with significant morbidity and mortality because of its site and often large size at presentation. It is the most common suprasellar tumour in children, accounting for 1–3% of intracranial tumours of all ages, but usually occurring from age 5 to 15 years. Most craniopharyngiomas have a suprasellar mass and a smaller intrasellar component. In 5% of cases it is purely intrasellar and may be difficult to distinguish from a Rathke's cleft cyst. Classically it appears as a calcified, mixed cystic and solid tumour with enhancement of the solid component and the cyst wall (Fig. 82-61). Large

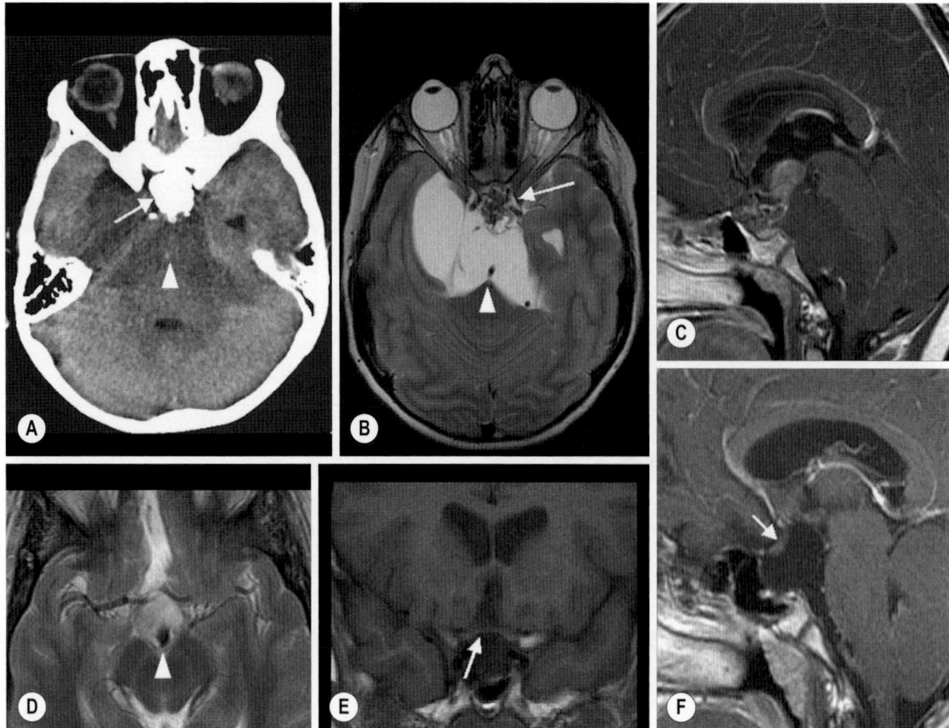

FIGURE 82-61 ■ **Craniopharyngiomas in two children.** (A–C) The first child has a large suprasellar, pre-pontine and middle cranial fossa tumour which is causing considerable mass effect on the brainstem and is encasing the basilar artery (arrowheads). There are solid enhancing and calcified components (arrows). The cystic components are of higher density on CT and there is T_1 shortening on MRI in keeping with proteinaceous contents. (D–F) The second child has a smaller suprasellar lesion, which is also calcified (arrowhead). The optic chiasm is clearly separate from the lesion and is draped over the top (E, F).

tumours may cause hydrocephalus and compression and distortion of the optic chiasm. The cystic components may extend behind the clivus and into any of the cranial fossae. On T_1-weighted sequences the cyst may demonstrate T_1 shortening due to proteinacaeous components, which have been described macroscopically as appearing like 'machine oil'. The cystic components are of increased signal on T_2-weighted FSE. MR spectroscopy demonstrates high lipid peaks. Surgical resection is often incomplete (in > 20%) because of the close adherence of the tumour to the optic chiasm; despite this, long-term survival is good (> 90% in children). Partial surgical resection with adjuvant radiotherapy with preservation of the hypothalamic–pituitary axis is a considered treatment strategy which aims to maximise outcome and reduce long-term endricological morbidity. This is advocated in the UK, while more aggressive surgical resection may be the strategy pursued in other centres.

Hypothalamic–Optic Pathway Glioma

Astrocytomas of the optic chiasm and hypothalamus account for 10–15% of supratentorial tumours in children. Optic chiasm tumours often extend into the hypothalamus and vice versa; hence they are discussed here together. Optic nerve tumours are usually pilocytic astrocytomas with a very indolent course, while hypothalamic/chiasmatic tumours may be of slightly higher histological grade (for example, WHO Grade II tumours) and more aggressive biological behaviour.

CT and MRI both define involvement of the optic nerves. CT can detect expansion of the optic canal. However, MRI is the best technique for delineating expansion of the chiasm and hypothalamus and involvement of the posterior visual pathways (Fig. 82-62). Tumour appears isointense to hypointense on T_1weighted imaging and hyperintense on T_2-weighted imaging. There may be diffuse fusiform expansion of the nerve from subarachnoid dissemination of tumour around the optic nerve. Enhancement is variable. The main differential diagnosis is from craniopharyngioma, which tends to present later, is usually calcified and is adherent to the chiasm rather than arising from it and causing expansion.

Infundibular Tumours

These include germinomas and Langerhans' cell histiocytosis, both of which cause expansion and enhancement of the pituitary infundibulum (Fig. 82-63). Onset of diabetes insipidus appears to correlate with absence of high T_1 signal in the posterior pituitary gland. The hypothalamic hamartoma (by definition a hypothalamic mass rather than a tumour) presents either with precocious puberty or with gelastic seizures. These may be sessile or pedunculated and are well-defined lesions arising from the floor of the third ventricle and extending inferiorly into the suprasellar or interpeduncular cistern. They are typically isointense to grey matter on T_1- and T_2-weighted MRI and do not enhance (Fig. 82-64).

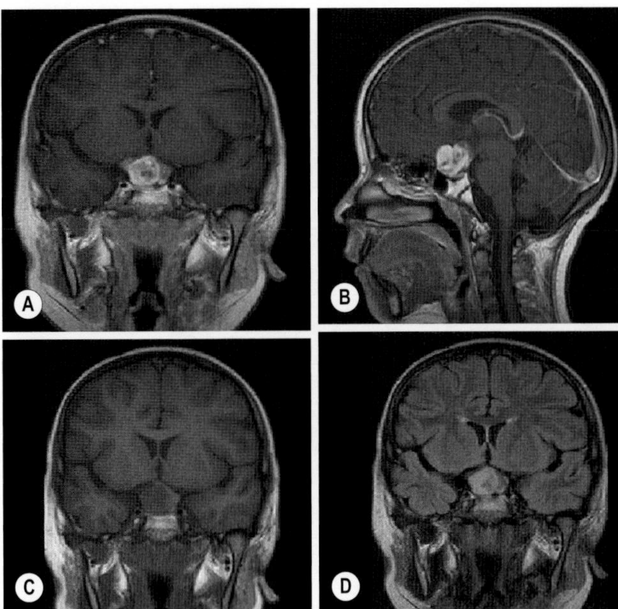

FIGURE 82-62 ■ **Hypothalamic–optic pathway glioma.** (A) Coronal T_1-weighted, (B) sagittal and (C) coronal enhanced T_1-weighted MRI and (D) coronal FLAIR show an optic chiasm glioma. The chiasm is not identified separately from the tumour.

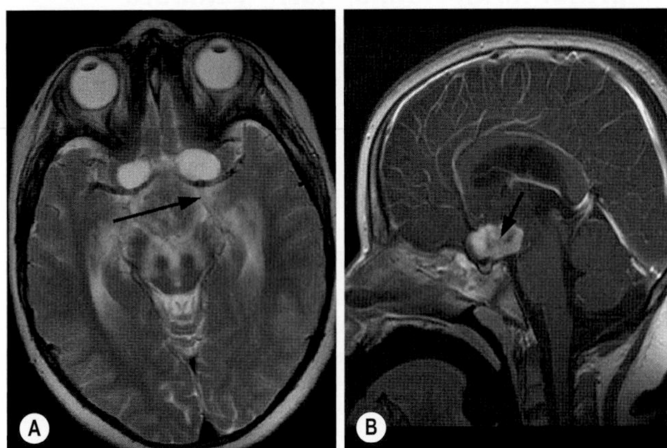

FIGURE 82-63 ■ **Langerhans' cell histiocytosis.** (A) Axial T_2-weighted image. (B) Sagittal T_1-weighted post-contrast image. Suprasellar T_2 hypointense and enhancing mass (arrows) with associated oedema extending superiorly along white matter tracts in a child with multisystem Langerhans' cell histiocytosis.

Pituitary Tumours

Pituitary adenomas are uncommon in children but may present in adolescents, and account for 2% of all pituitary adenomas. The most common functional tumours are prolactinomas and corticotrophin- and growth hormone-secreting tumours. A quarter of paediatric pituitary tumours are non-functioning. The imaging appearances are the same as in adults. Rathke's cleft cysts are also rare in children.

Pineal Region Tumours

The pineal region is a descriptive term and encompasses the posterior third ventricle and its contents, including

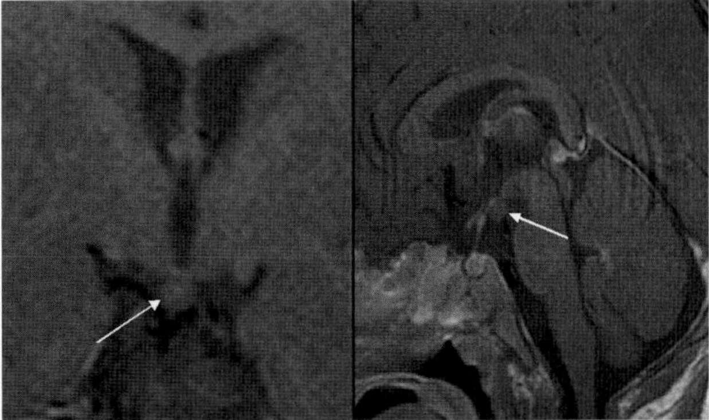

FIGURE 82-64 ■ **Hypothalamic hamartoma.** Coronal T_1 and sagittal T_1-weighted post-contrast MRI shows a non-enhancing lesion arising from the floor of the third ventricle posterior to the pituitary infundibulum and projecting inferiorly into the suprasellar cistern (arrows).

the pineal gland itself, the tectal plate and aqueduct, the posterior septum pellucidum, corpus callosum and thalami, internal cerebral veins in addition to the quadrigeminal cistern containing the posterior cerebral arteries, vein of Galen and straight sinus. Lesions may arise from any of these components and therefore the differential diagnosis of a pineal region tumour is wide. The most common lesions are germ cell tumours (GCTs), followed by primary pineal gland masses. Gliomas are also relatively common lesions at this site, usually derived from adjacent brain parenchyma. Pineal region tumours can cause hydrocephalus by obstruction of the cerebral aqueduct. Direct compression or invasion of the tectal plate, specifically the colliculi, may cause failure of upward gaze and convergence (Parinaud's syndrome). They may also cause precocious puberty.

Central Nervous System Germ Cell Tumours

CNS GCTs are primarily tumours of the young, over 90% occurring in the under-20 age group and with a peak incidence from age 10 to 12 years. They are more common in Asia but in the West account for 1% of intracranial neoplasms in children. Germinoma is the most common type of CNS GCT, followed by non-secreting teratoma. Other GCTs include rarer secreting forms such as yolk sac, embryonal and choriocarcinoma, and may be of mixed cellular types, the latter associated with the worst prognosis.

Germinomas are characteristically found in the midline, in the pineal or suprasellar regions. A minority of lesions may be found in the basal ganglia, thalami, or cerebellum. Pineal and suprasellar lesions may be synchronous, and when so, are pathognomonic. Most pineal region GCTs occur in boys and suprasellar GCTs in girls. Pathologically the tumour is solid and consists of large, glycogen-rich germ line cells with variable desmoplastic stroma and lymphocytic infiltrate. Necrosis and haemorrhage are unusual, with the exception of lesions seen in the basal ganglia.

Germinomas are classified as malignant tumours but respond extremely well to radiotherapy and may melt away over just a few days of treatment. Overall they are

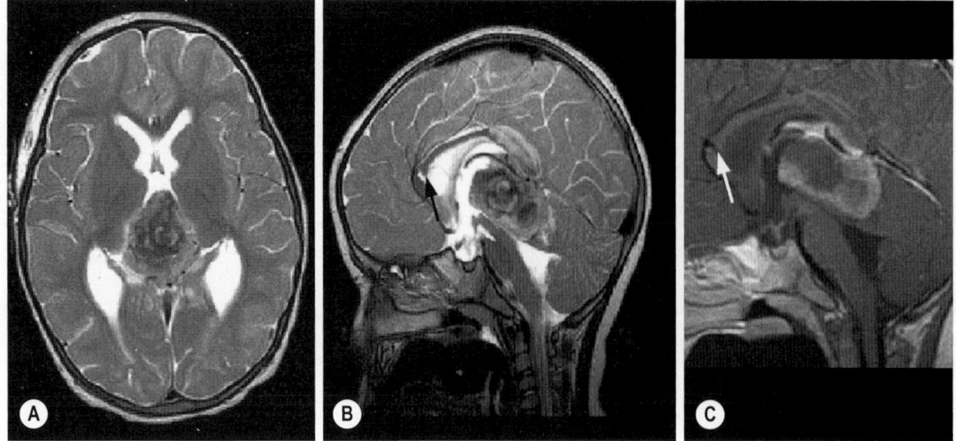

FIGURE 82-65 ■ **Pineoblastoma.** (A) Axial, (B) sagittal T_2-weighted fast spin-echo and (C) enhanced sagittal T_1-weighted MRI in a 2-year-old girl show a pineal region tumour effacing the tectal plate. The hydrocephalus is treated by a frontal extraventricular drain (track through the genu of the corpus callosum marked by the arrows). The tumour is hypointense on the T_2-weighted images with rings of lower signal consistent with calcification and haemorrhagic products, and peripheral rim enhancement, and was confirmed as a pineoblastoma.

more common in young adolescent males. On CT they appear as a hyperdense, solid mass within the posterior third ventricle and enhance avidly and homogeneously. They tend to engulf the pineal gland, which may be calcified. Occasionally this may be difficult to differentiate from intrinsic tumoural calcification more suggestive of a teratoma or primary pineal gland tumour, such as a pineoblastoma, although both of these lesions are typically more heterogeneous with haemorrhage and cyst formation. On MRI the cellularity of the tumour is reflected by T_2 hypointensity relative to grey matter. The tumour may be less homogeneous than on CT and cystic change may be detected, although enhancement remains a marked feature. Germinomas demonstrate restricted diffusion. Synchronous germinomas in typical midline sites, such as the suprasellar region, and evidence of early CSF dissemination should be actively looked for.

Benign teratomas are very heterogeneous, mixed cystic, solid and well-defined masses characterised by calcification and fat. Enhancement is not usually seen unless there are areas of malignant degeneration. Other GCTs are also heterogeneous in appearance and do not contain fat, but the individual tumour types are not distinguishable radiologically.

Primary Pineal Tumours: Pineoblastoma and Pineocytoma

Pineoblastomas are malignant (WHO Grade IV), small, round cell tumours which histologically are similar to medulloblastomas and share similar imaging characteristics in terms of hyperdensity on CT and are hypointense to isointense signal on T_2-weighted FSE relative to grey matter. They may contain areas of calcification and rarely haemorrhage. The solid parts of the tumour enhance intensely. They may be distinguished from Grade II pineocytomas by the age at presentation, as they occur most frequently in the first two decades of life compared to pineocytomas, which are tumours of young adults; by their size (> 3 cm); and by their relative T_2-weighted hypointensity (Fig. 82-65).

Supratentorial Hemispheric Tumours

Overall, supratentorial tumours occur as frequently as posterior fossa tumours in the paediatric age group but are more common under the age of 2 and over the age of 10, while posterior fossa tumours are more common from the ages of 2 to 10. The presenting symptoms are due to a large mass-occupying lesion and include headaches and vomiting. In the under 2-year-old age group the tumour may be very large at the time of presentation; the fontanelles are open so that infants present with increasing head size as often as they do with hydrocephalus. Seizures are seen more particularly with temporal and frontal cortex lesions.

Astrocytomas

The most common paediatric cerebral hemispheric tumour is the astrocytoma, accounting for 30% of supratentorial brain tumours in children. In children under 2 years, other diagnoses should be considered; teratomas and desmoplastic infantile gangliogliomas are seen in neonates and PNET, atypical teratoid/rhabdoid tumours, and ependymomas are seen in slightly older infants. Some children who present with a longer history and refractory epilepsy may have low-grade, indolent glioneuronal tumours, including the dysembryoplastic neuroepithelial tumour.

As with cerebellar astrocytomas, hemispheric astrocytomas may be cystic with an enhancing mural nodule, entirely solid with variable enhancement or solid with a necrotic centre. On CT the solid part of the hemispheric astrocytoma is isodense or hypodense and on MRI T_2-weighted sequences it is hyperintense, helping to distinguish these tumours from small, round cell tumours such as supratentorial PNET. They may rarely be multicentric. The histological grade cannot be reliably determined by the radiological features. Contrast enhancement can be seen in both low- and high-grade tumours. A simple cyst with non-enhancing walls, minimal surrounding oedema and a single enhancing mural nodule is more likely to be a pilocytic astrocytoma. Lesions containing haemorrhage and associated with marked adjacent oedema are more likely to be of higher grade. Glioblastoma is seen in children and in children is associated with a better prognosis than in adults. The pleomorphic xanthoastrocytoma is an uncommon astrocytoma of children and young adults. It is usually a WHO Grade II lesion, though it may have anaplastic features. Typically it has a superficial location within the temporal lobe and consists of a cyst and enhancing mural nodule with minimal adjacent oedema. Radiologically it is often indistinguishable from ganglioglioma and some other glioneuronal tumour subtypes.

Ependymomas

Supratentorial ependymomas occur more commonly in boys, with a peak incidence between the ages of 1 and 5 years, and again are similar to the posterior fossa ependymoma. However, they are more usually extraventricular in site and therefore CSF dissemination is less common than with their posterior fossa equivalent. They are isodense to hyperdense, well-defined lesions on CT with variable enhancement of the solid component. Tumour heterogeneity with cystic areas and foci of calcification are common (Fig. 82-66). Haemorrhage may also be seen.

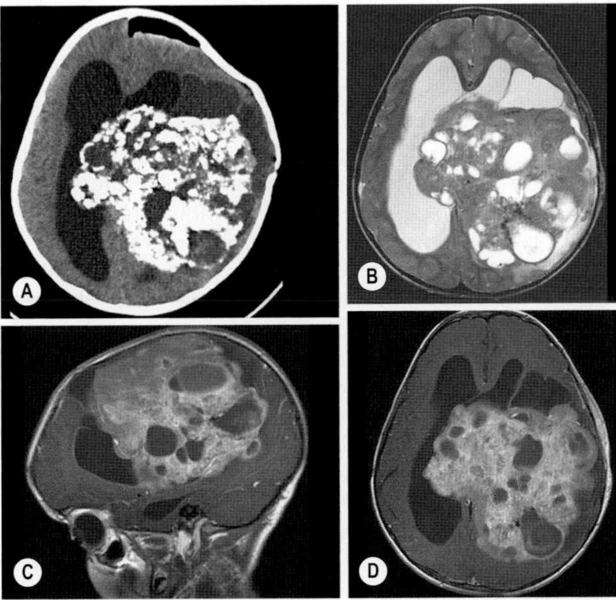

FIGURE 82-66 ■ **Supratentorial Grade II ependymoma.** The left cerebral hemisphere tumour extends across the midline into the right ventricle. (A) CT (post partial debulking) shows it is heavily calcified and (B–D) MRI (axial T_2-enhanced, sagittal T_1 and axial T_1-weighted MRI) show a mixed cystic and solid heterogeneously enhancing tumour. There is associated hydrocephalus.

Supratentorial Primitive Neuroectodermal Tumours

PNET (WHO Grade IV) is a cellular tumour of primitive cell types and may be seen in children as young as 4 weeks to 10 years, with a mean age of 5.5 years. A rare subtype that includes more neuronal cells is known as cerebral neuroblastoma. PNET is found more frequently in the posterior fossa (where it is also known as medulloblastoma) than in the supratentorial compartment. Poor prognostic factors for PNET include age under 2 years and a supratentorial location. The 5-year survival drops from 85% for tumours in the posterior fossa to 34% for supratentorial tumours. They are frequently haemorrhagic, necrotic and have foci of calcification. The solid parts of the tumour are hyperdense on CT and hypointense on T_2-weighted FSE. There is always some enhancement, although the degree is variable. Although the tumour may appear well-defined radiologically, tumour cells are likely to extend beyond the apparent margins. Widespread dissemination of tumour, both through the CSF space and to the lungs, liver and spleen, is not infrequent.

Medulloepithelioma is a rare, highly malignant tumour usually affecting children between the ages of 6 months and 5 years. Solid components are hypercellular; therefore, the density and signal characteristics may be similar to PNET. They are large at the time of presentation with extensive areas of haemorrhage and necrosis but may be distinguished from other tumours, including PNET, by their lack of contrast enhancement.

Desmoplastic Infantile Gangliomas

These typically present as a massive cyst with an enhancing cortically based mural nodule in an infant with increased head size and bulging fontanelle. Adjacent dural enhancement may also be seen. The cyst, which is hypointense on T_1, hyperintense on T_2 and may contain septations, usually does not enhance.

Choroid Plexus Tumours

These are 'cauliflower-like' tumours arising from the epithelium of the choroid plexus and are more frequently benign (papilloma) than malignant (carcinoma). Both types may disseminate within the CSF space. They are the most common brain tumour in children under 1 year and present with hydrocephalus, possibly due to CSF hypersecretion or obstructive hydrocephalus due to haemorrhage, arachnoiditis or carcinomatosis in carcinomas. For papillomas the 5-year survival approaches 100%, while for carcinomas it ranges from 25 to 40%, with a higher survival if the tumour is completely resected.

On CT they are seen as hyperdense or isodense, lobulated 'frond-like', avidly and homogeneously enhancing masses with punctate calcifications, occasionally with haemorrhage and with hydrocephalus. The typical site is the trigone of the lateral ventricle, while in older children the cerebellopontine angle or fourth ventricle

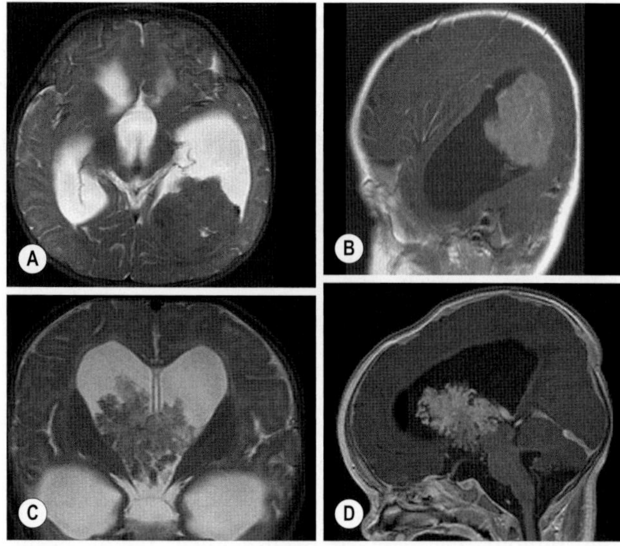

FIGURE 82-67 ■ Choroid plexus tumours. (A, B) Axial T_2, enhanced sagittal T_1-weighted MRI in a boy aged 6 months demonstrate a lobulated homogeneously enhancing intraventricular tumour with relative T_2 hypointensity, in keeping with a highly cellular tumour closely related to the choroid plexus. The ependyma is enhancing and the interface between tumour and adjacent brain is indistinct. Histology confirmed the tumour to be a choroid plexus carcinoma and this was subsequently embolised before surgery. There is a communicating hydrocephalus which may be due to increased cerebrospinal fluid production or to proteinaceous/haemorrhagic exudate. (C, D) A different child with choroid plexus papilloma. Choroid plexus tumours, although commonly seen within the trigone of the lateral ventricle, may arise from anywhere within the ventricular system. This child has a frondy choroid plexus papilloma arising within the third ventricle and extending superiorly through the foramina of Monro. In this case the hydrocephalus was obstructive.

may be involved (Fig. 82-67). On MRI the papillary appearance is more readily appreciated: they are more mottled and isointense or hypointense on T_1-weighted imaging with intense enhancement. Vascular flow voids, usually from choroidal arteries, are often seen in association, and arterial embolisation may be considered before surgery in an attempt to reduce the vascularity of the tumour. Haemorrhage and localised vasogenic oedema are suggestive of carcinoma with invasion but the two histological types cannot be reliably distinguished on imaging.

Other intraventricular tumours include meningiomas, which are rare in children outside NF2 and ependymomas.

Dysembryoplastic Neuroepithelial Tumours

Dysembryoplastic neuroepithelial tumour (DNT) is a WHO Grade I benign tumour which classically presents with complex partial seizures in children and young adults under the age of 20. It is a cortically based lesion which may have associated foci of cortical dysplasia.

On imaging it appears as a well-defined cortically based lesion with a characteristic 'bubbly' internal structure, minimal mass effect and no associated vasogenic oedema (Fig. 82-68). There may be some adjacent bony scalloping consistent with a long-standing lesion and a third of lesions demonstrate calcification. On MRI they are hypointense on T_1 and have a hyperintense rim on FLAIR or proton density-weighted imaging. Most tumours do not enhance and, if present, enhancement is faint and patchy.

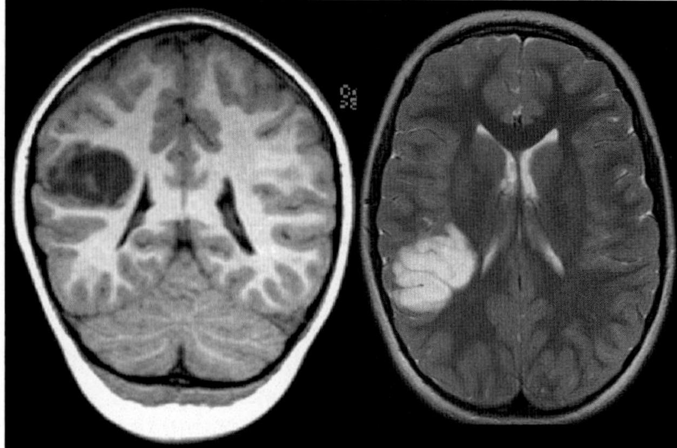

FIGURE 82-68 ■ Dysembryoplastic neuroepithelial tumour (DNT) in a child with long-standing refractory focal epilepsy referred to the epilepsy surgical programme. Several MRI examinations over 3 years had shown no change in the appearances of this right inferior parietal lobe lesion. The lesion is well-defined and cortically based, extends towards the ventricular margin and has the typical lobulated internal architecture of DNT.

CEREBROVASCULAR DISEASE AND STROKE

Stroke is an important paediatric illness, with an incidence of around 2 cases per 100,000 children per annum. The aetiology of paediatric stroke is significantly different from adult stroke, as large artery atherosclerosis, cardio-embolic and small vessel disease combined account for only 10% of cases in children.[63]

There have been several misconceptions regarding stroke in children. Paediatric stroke was said to be idiopathic, associated with a good prognosis with low recurrence rates and good recovery of motor function and school performance, and was minimally investigated on the assumption that this would not affect management. Recent work has shown that there are many different aetiologies associated with stroke in children and a single episode may be multifactorial. Associated factors, some of which may be amenable to treatment, include congenital heart disease, anaemias, prothrombotic disorders such as protein C and S deficiencies, hyperhomocystinaemia, lipid abnormalities, recent infections and respiratory chain disorders (Fig. 82-69). Equally, long-term follow-up has shown a poor outcome with some degree of dependency in 60% of affected children. Although difficult to quantify due to selection bias, the risk of recurrence for ischaemic stroke ranges from 5 to 20%. Children who have a stroke at a young age have a worse physical and intellectual outcome and behavioural problems may be significant. Hence children with acute stroke should be referred to, or have their management discussed with, a paediatric neurologist, and thoroughly investigated on

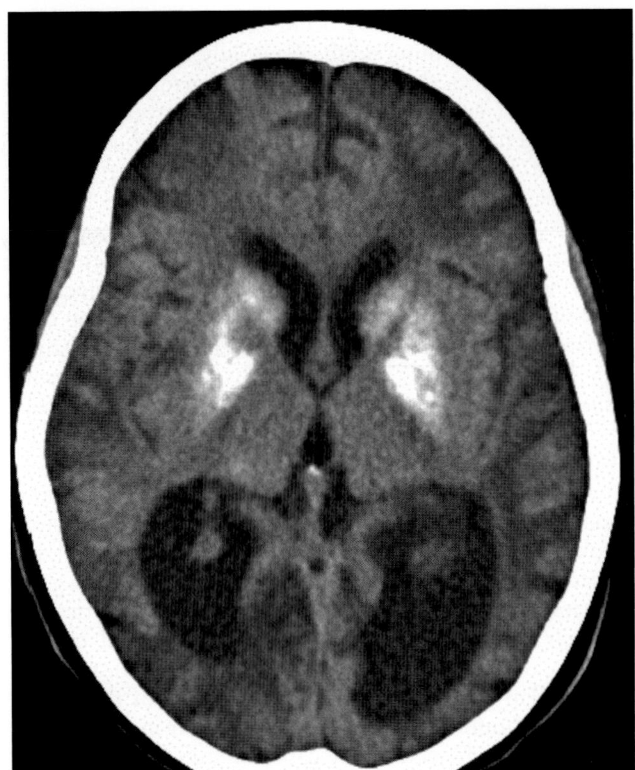

FIGURE 82-69 ■ **Strokes occurring in mitochondrial cytopathy.** Bilateral symmetrical lentiform and caudate calcification and extensive cerebral infarction crossing arterial territories in a child with a mitochondrial disorder (MELAS).

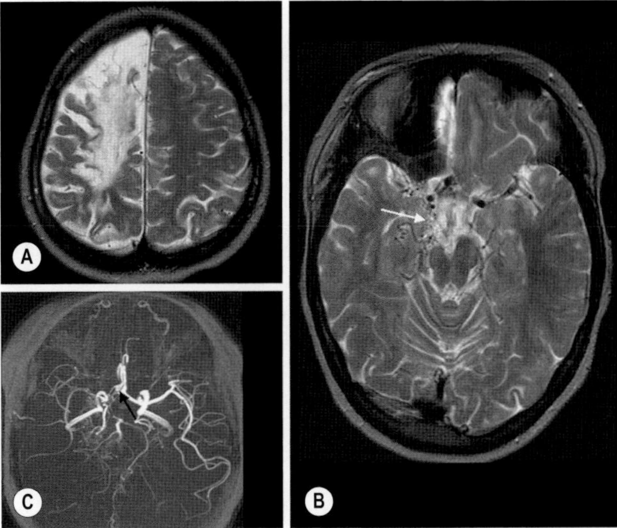

FIGURE 82-70 ■ **Sickle cell disease and moya moya syndrome.** Child with extensive frontal, deep and posterior watershed infarction (A). (B) Extensive perimesencephalic 'moya moya' collaterals (arrow) and attenuated right middle cerebral artery (MCA) flow voids. (C) Compressed maximum intensity projection image shows narrowed terminal internal carotid artery (ICA), reduced filling of right MCA, and A1 segment of the anterior cerebral artery. There is an aneurysm at the A1/anterior communicating artery (ACOM) junction (arrow).

each occasion to detect all potential risk factors. Cross-sectional brain imaging is mandatory in children presenting with clinical stroke. Brain MRI is recommended and should be performed as soon as possible after presentation. If MRI is not available within 48 h, CT is an acceptable initial alternative. Imaging should be undertaken urgently in those who have a depressed conscious level or whose clinical status is deteriorating.[64]

The purpose of neuroimaging is to confirm the diagnosis and exclude alternative treatable lesions, as well as to help understand the underlying cause, guide treatment and monitor progression of the disease. The radiological findings of brain parenchymal involvement in stroke are not significantly different from findings in adults. There is, however, some evidence that restricted diffusion may occur for a shorter time in younger children and pseudonormalisation may occur earlier than in adults. Vascular abnormalities in paediatric ischaemic stroke are common.[65] These are more frequently intracranial than extracranial, involve the anterior rather than posterior circulation and typically consist of occlusion of proximal large arteries, i.e. middle cerebral artery (MCA), anterior cerebral artery (ACA) and terminal internal carotid artery (ICA).

Sickle cell disease, a chronic haemolytic anaemia in which abnormal haemoglobin (HbS) forms with a tendency to cause red blood cells to distort and block small blood vessels, is the most common cause of ischaemic stroke in children worldwide. Even within this single disease entity there are several factors that contribute to stroke. These include a cerebral vasculopathy known as moya moya disease, an underlying predilection to infection, tissue hypoxia and precipitation of sickling vaso-occlusive crisis resulting from chronic anaemia, high white cell count, adenotonsillar hyperplasia causing obstructive sleep apnoea, cardiomegaly and a generalised procoagulant state.

Stroke in sickle cell disease is clinically apparent in 9% of children with sickle cell disease under the age of 20 years, but silent infarction occurs in as many as 25%. The imaging pattern of infarction is typically of arterial watershed infarction between the major cerebral arterial territories. A fifth of strokes in sickle cell disease may be haemorrhagic. The diploic space of the calvarium may be diffusely thickened due to increased haematopoiesis in order to compensate for the chronic haemolytic anaemia.

The brain MRI and circle of Willis MR angiogram (MRA) may show evidence of a cerebral vasculopathy known as moya moya syndrome. In this there is typically progressive stenosis of the terminal ICA and proximal segments of the major intracranial arteries (Fig. 82-70). There is a predilection for the anterior circulation. As the stenosis progresses, increased flow occurs through proximal collateral vessels, particularly the lenticulostriate and thalamoperforator arteries, resulting in the 'puff of smoke' appearance to which moya moya refers. These are seen as multiple small flow voids within the basal ganglia. Prominent transmedullary veins and pial enhancement may also be seen. Other acquired vascular abnormalities include aneurysms and small arteriovenous malformations.

Referral to a neurosurgical paediatric centre for consideration of external-to-internal carotid (EC–IC) bypass may be indicated. At this point cerebral perfusion imaging to detect 'diffusion–perfusion mismatch' may be helpful in order to assess for critical ischaemia or to select which hemisphere should be revascularised first. This involves a bolus of intravenous contrast medium for MRI perfusion studies and it is important that the child with sickle cell disease is well hydrated for this. Surgical EC–IC bypass may be performed indirectly by mobilisation of part of the temporalis muscle with its blood supply, the superficial temporal artery (STA), and laying it onto the pial surface of the brain, or by direct end-to-side anastomosis between the STA and distal MCA branch. Some centres use multiple calvarial burr holes alone to promote superficial angiogenesis and collateral revascularisation. Postoperative MRA and perfusion imaging after successful EC–IC bypass should show flow through the STA and increased collateral flow within the distal MCA branches. Perfusion imaging will show increased cerebral blood volume and flow to the revascularised hemisphere.

Moya moya accounts for up to 30% of cerebral vasculopathy in paediatric stroke but it is not unique to sickle cell disease, being also idiopathic, secondary to NF1, cranial irradiation, Down's syndrome, human immunodeficiency virus (HIV) and even tuberculous meningitis. Postinfective angiitis associated with varicella zoster, in which the terminal ICA and proximal MCA are usually affected and there is infarction of the basal ganglia, is relatively common (Fig. 82-71). MRA in the majority (but not all) shows evidence of stabilisation or remodelling and improvement of the angiographic appearances at 6-month follow-up.

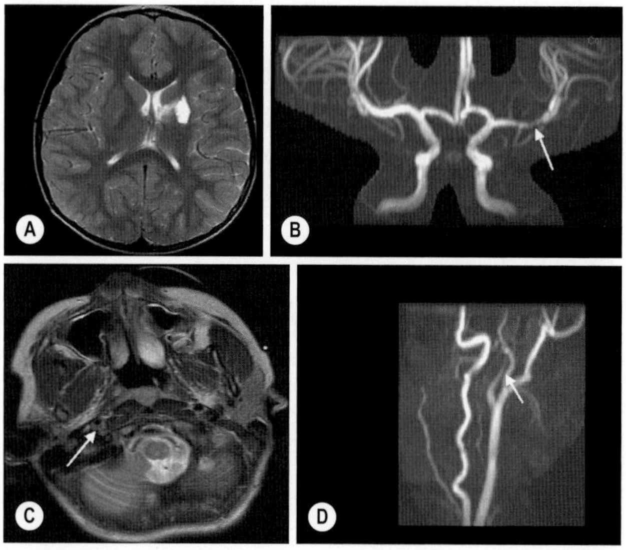

FIGURE 82-71 ■ **Vasculitis.** (A, B) In a child with chicken pox vasculitis, axial T_2 and maximum intensity projection (MIP) image of time-of-flight (TOF) circle of Willis MRA show a mature proximal left middle cerebral artery branch infarct with reduced and turbulent flow (arrow) and reduced distal filling. **Arterial dissection.** (C, D) In a 14-year-old girl with acute-onset left hemiplegia, large right middle cerebral artery territory infarct, and internal carotid artery (ICA) dissection is seen. On the axial T_2-weighted image there is an eccentric filling defect within the lumen of the right internal carotid artery which is narrowed, confirming the presence of dissection (arrow). The MIP image of the TOF MRA shows a typical rat's tail appearance of a tapering stenosis distal to the right ICA bifurcation (arrow).

Arterial dissection may occur intracranially but is also seen, as it is in young adults especially, not infrequently within the cervical arteries. Vertebral arterial dissection occurs most commonly as the vertebral artery exits the transverse foramen of C2 before passing posterolaterally over the lateral masses of C1 to enter the foramen magnum, and ICA dissection occurs above the bifurcation (Fig. 82-71). Dissections may involve intracranial and extracranial arteries. There may be other rarer causes of cervical arterial disease with more diffuse involvement proximal to the bifurcation, e.g. that seen with the connective tissue disorders such as Marfan's, Ehlers–Danlos type IV, osteogenesis imperfecta type I, autosomal dominant polycystic kidney disease, fibromuscular dysplasia, or other causes of cystic medial necrosis and Menkes' disease. Cervical arterial dissection may occur without an antecedent history of trauma. As this is a potentially treatable cause of stroke,[66] we advocate in all paediatric stroke non-invasive imaging by MRA not only of the intracranial circle of Willis but also of the entire great arteries of the neck from their origins at the aortic arch to their intracranial terminations. Radiological criteria for the diagnosis of dissection are visualisation of an intimal flap or a double lumen in the wall of the artery. These pathognomonic signs are detected in fewer than 10% of adult dissections by catheter angiography, which remains the gold standard for diagnosis. However, tapering arterial occlusion, the 'string sign' or 'rat's tail' appearance (Fig. 82-71), aneurysmal dilatation of the artery and eccentric mural thrombus are other less specific signs. Non-invasive angiographic techniques, CTA and MRA, are less sensitive and less specific than the gold standard of the more invasive DSA. The differences are more marked with the calibre of the vessel under consideration. It may be prudent to consider childhood posterior circulation strokes as caused by vertebral dissection until proven otherwise or cleared by DSA.

Vein of Galen aneurysmal malformations (VGAMs) are a rare cause of paediatric stroke but have a wide range of clinical presentations and account for 30% of vascular malformations in children. Their recognition is important as there is increasing evidence that appropriate endovascular treatment by neuroradiologists with specialist skill in dealing with paediatric high flow AV shunts in a multidisciplinary setting with access to neonatologists, anaesthetists and neurologists is associated with improved outcome. VGAMs are unique congenital malformations of the intracranial circulation characterised by an enlarged midline venous structure, a persistent embryological remnant, with multiple arteriovenous communications leading to aneurysmal dilatation, presumably secondary to high arteriovenous flow. Neonates may present with severe cardiac failure. In infants and children who present with VGAMs the degree of shunting is much smaller and they may have evidence of hydrocephalus with cerebral atrophy. Older children may have headaches and seizures, and also are more likely to develop intracerebral or subarachnoid haemorrhage.

MRI will demonstrate the dilated venous sac, location of fistulous connections and the arteries involved, venous drainage and any evidence of thrombus within the venous sac (Fig. 82-72). MRI can determine the extent of parenchymal damage, including focal infarctions and

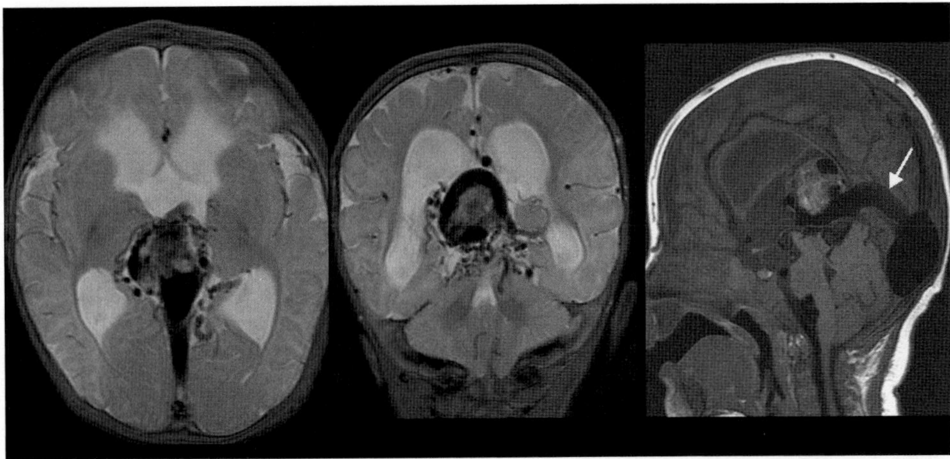

FIGURE 82-72 ■ Vein of Galen malformation (partly occluded by embolisation glue) showing residual flow through the promesencephalic vein, containing a combination of glue and thrombus, via the falcine sinus (arrow) towards the venous confluence. Arterial supply is via a number of choroidal vessels.

generalised cerebral atrophy, although CT is more sensitive for the parenchymal calcification which accompanies chronic venous hypertension. Angiography is the gold standard of diagnosis and ideally should be performed at the time of endovascular treatment. In imaging follow-up, evidence of significant arteriovenous shunting, progressive cerebral damage/atrophy and jugular vein occlusion as a chronic effect of venous hypertension should be sought.

HYPOXIC–ISCHAEMIC INJURY IN THE DEVELOPING BRAIN

Introduction

In the neonatal period brain injury due to hypoxia–ischaemia depends on the degree of brain maturation and on the severity of the event. Babies born preterm (gestational age at birth ≤ 36 weeks) react to hypoxia–ischaemia differently than full-term babies.[1,2] White matter injury is predominant in preterm babies, while grey matter is mostly injured in full-term babies.[3–5] Imaging plays an important role in the diagnostic work-up of these patients, with brain US being the first-line examination performed at bedside, followed by brain MRI. State-of-the-art brain US should be performed using sectorial and high-frequency linear transducers through the anterior, posterior and posterolateral fontanelles.[1,5] The MRI protocols consist of T_2 and T_1 conventional sequences, while diffusion imaging is increasingly becoming part of the routine. Special equipment for monitoring the vital signs, ventilators and, for very premature babies, MR-compatible incubators are necessary for safe and state-of-the-art brain MRI.

Encephalopathy of Premature Neonate—Patterns of Injury

Periventricular leukomalacia and brain haemorrhagic disease are the two main patterns of brain injury associated with hypoxia–ischaemia in the premature neonate.

Periventricular Leukomalacia

There are two forms of periventricular leukomalacia (PVL), the focal form (fPVL) and the diffuse form (dPVL). The pathological substrate of fPVL is necrosis of all cell elements of the brain tissue surrounding the lateral ventricles and that of dPVL is injury of the premyelinating oligodendrocytes (pre-OLs) associated with astrocytosis and microgliosis.[2,6] Long and short penetrating arteries with underdeveloped distal parts vascularise the immature brain.[2] Brain tissue between and at the end of these arteries represents watershed areas that receive deficient blood supply under conditions of hypoxia–ischaemia.[2] fPVL represents a watershed infarct in the periventricular white matter giving rise to micro- and macrocysts.[1] In dPVL, injury of pre-OLs results in decreased numbers of mature oligodendrocytes responsible for myelination and is characterised by hypomyelination and microstructural changes in brain connectivity.[2,7] In fPVL, brain US initially demonstrates hyperechogenic periventricular white matter which progressively (8–25 days) gives rise to the development of coalescent macro- or microcysts[1,5] (Figs. 82-73A, B). On brain MRI areas of impending fPVL appear with restricted diffusion and those with cystic components with increased diffusion.[8] Areas of established PVL are characterised by ventriculomegaly, irregular (in the case of fPVL) or regular (in dPVL) outline of the body of lateral ventricles, thinning of the periventricular white matter and signal abnormalities of the white matter in the peritriginal regions[9] (Figs. 82-73C, D). Cystic lesions of PVL appear with low signal intensity on T_1- and high signal on T_2-weighted sequences.[10] After corrected age of 1 month, the presence of abnormal signal intensity (low on T_1 and high on T_2) in the posterior limb of the internal capsule predicts a poor motor outcome.[5] Brain US is usually normal at the initial stages of dPVL. On brain MRI, dPVL is characterised by ventriculomegaly with regular outlines of the lateral ventricles (Fig. 82-74).

Brain Haemorrhagic Disease

Brain haemorrhagic disease consists of germinal matrix haemorrhage (GMH), intraventricular haemorrhage

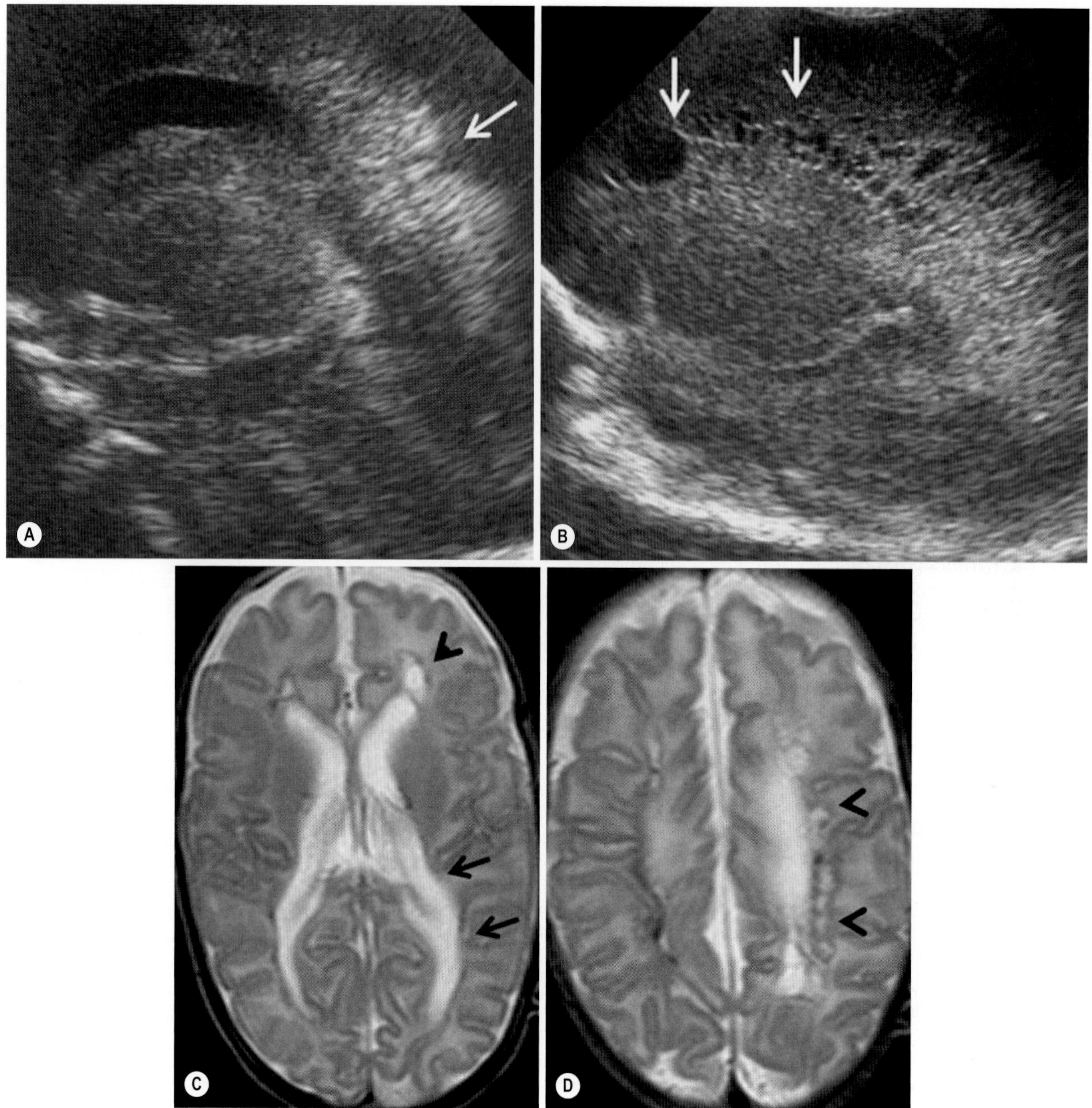

FIGURE 82-73 ■ Prematurity, history of birth at 32 weeks' gestational age due to placental abruption. (A, B) Brain ultrasound. Day 10 of life: sagittal (A) image demonstrating increased heterogeneous echogenicity of the periventricular white matter (arrow). Day 25 of life: sagittal (B) images demonstrating multiple cysts of the periventricular white matter (arrows). (C, D) Brain MRI. Chronological age 2.5 months: T_2-weighted axial images (C, D) demonstrating thinning of the periventricular white matter, irregular outline of the lateral ventricles (arrows) and periventricular cysts (arrowheads).

(IVH) and paraventricular haemorrhagic infarct (PHI). GMH may appear 24 h after birth and starts from the germinal matrix, a highly vascular collection of neuroglial precurcor cells located under the ventricular ependymal.[1,5] Regression of the germinal matrix starts at 12–16 gestational weeks and disappears at term. Around 24 gestational weeks, germinal matrix is only present under the frontal horns of the lateral ventricles. Increased vessel fragility and immature autoregulation of the cerebral blood flow are responsible for germinal matrix haemorrhage in premature babies.[5] Haemorrhage may be limited at the germinal matrix or extend into the ventricle with or without associated ventricular dilatation. Brain US shows an ovoid lesion located anterior to the caudothalamic groove, initially homogeneously hyperechogenic, then heterogeneously hyperechogenic and finally cystic[5] (Figs. 82-75A, B). IVH may result from rupture of GMH into the ventricles or from bleeding at the level of choroid plexuses. Brain US shows echogenic material into the lateral ventricles, sometimes extending into the third ventricle[1] (Fig. 82-76). MRI demonstrates a variety of signal intensities, depending on the age of haemorrhage, with high signal at the subacute stage and signal void at the chronic stage.[5] Post-haemorrhagic hydrocephalus may appear as complication of large IVH. Paraventricular haemorrhagic infarct (PHI) is almost always associated with IVH and results from compression and obstruction of terminal veins lying under the germinal matrix.[5] Brain US shows a frontoparietal hyperechogenic triangular lesion pointing towards the lateral ventricle. A liquefaction and sometimes communication of the lesion with the lateral ventricle is observed at the latter stages[1] (Fig. 82-77). Lesions lying proximal to the ventricular trigones carry a better neurological outcome.[11] Early MRI demonstrates a haemorrhagic paraventricular lesion associated with IVH; late MRI shows a cystic lesion surrounded by gliosis and communicating with the lateral ventricle.

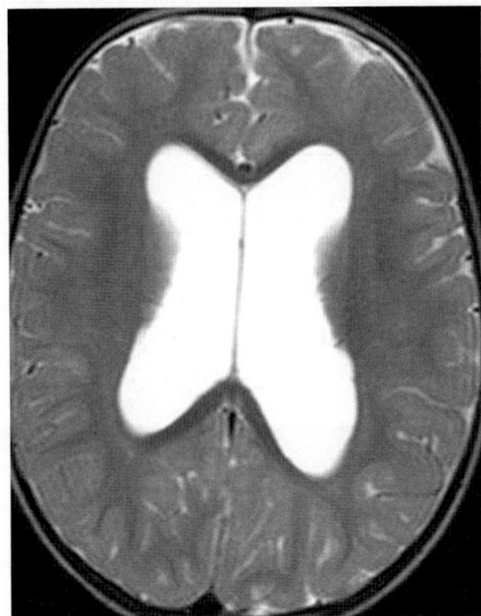

FIGURE 82-74 ■ Prematurity, history of birth at 30 weeks' gestational age. Brain MRI. Chronological age 2.5 months: T_2-weighted axial image demonstrating thinning of the periventricular white matter with regular outline of the lateral ventricles.

Encephalopathy of Term Neonate—Patterns of Injury

Depending on the severity of hypoxia–ischaemia, three main types of lesions have been described:[4,12]

1. Parasagittal lesions represent watershed infarcts affecting the cortex and the subcortical white matter at the territories between anterior and middle and posterior and middle cerebral arteries.[3,4] Decreased brain perfusion is the underlying cause. Brain US shows subcortical leukomalacia, initially hyperchogenic and then multicystic. In older children brain atrophy is observed in the affected areas.[13,14] Brain MRI reveals T_1 and T_2 prolongation of the affected areas.[12]
2. Diffuse lesions affecting the cortex, the basal ganglia and the white matter are due to partial prolonged asphyxia (1–3 h). Brain US shows initially increased echogenicity of the cortex and the basal ganglia and later macrocystic encephalomalacia.[4,13,14] Brain MRI reveals heterogeneous signal

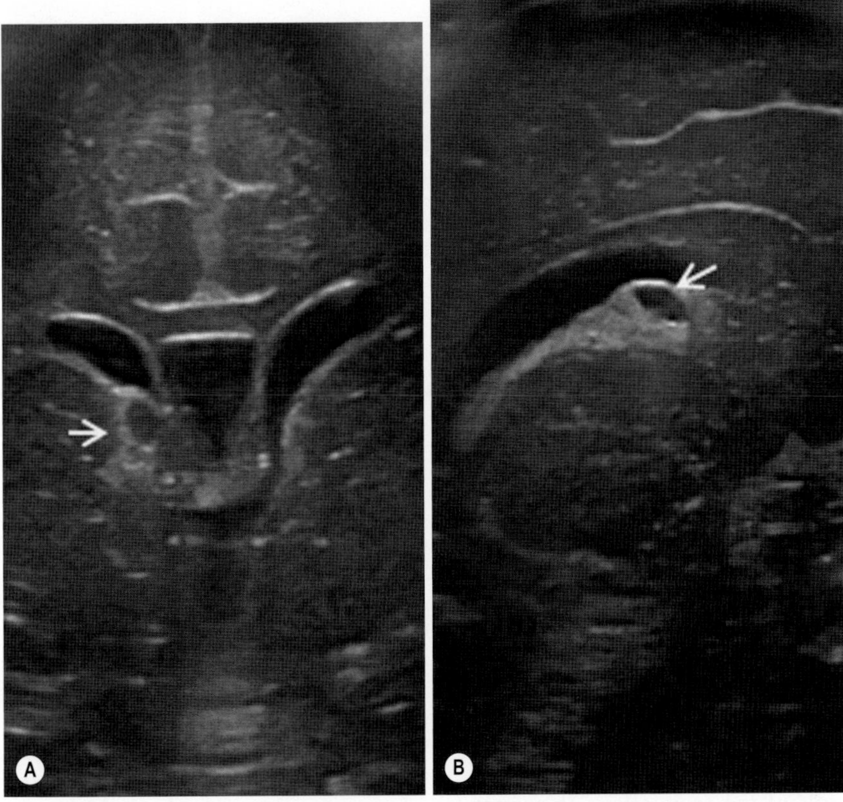

FIGURE 82-75 ■ Prematurity, history of birth at 31 weeks' gestational age. Brain ultrasound. Day 7 of life: coronal (A) and sagittal (B) images demonstrating a centrally cystic ovoid lesion located at the right lateral ventricle, anterior to the caudothalamic groove (arrows).

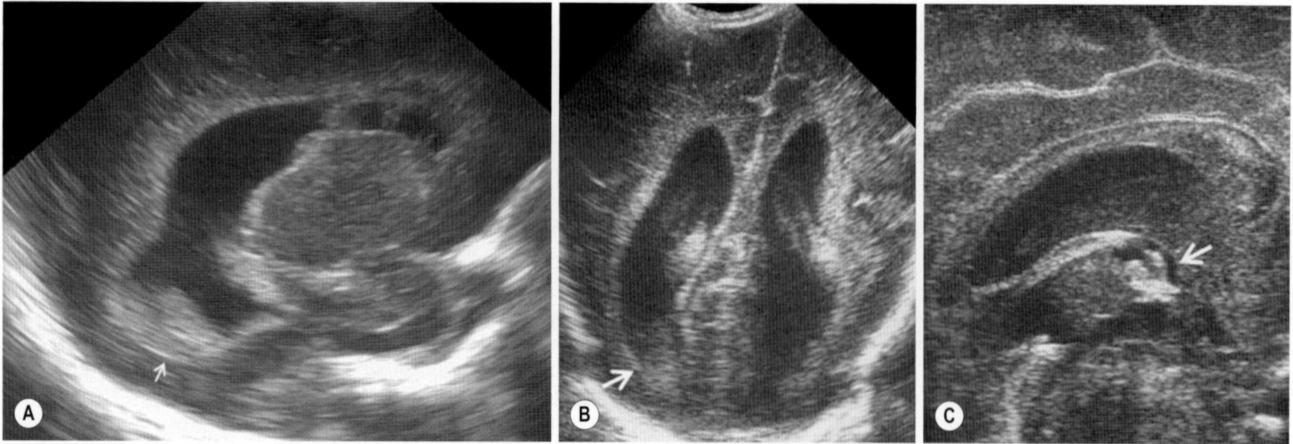

FIGURE 82-76 ■ Prematurity, history of birth at 29 weeks' gestational age. Brain ultrasound. Day 8 of life: sagittal (A) and coronal (B) images demonstrating echogenic material into the right lateral ventricle (arrows) compatible with blood. Midline sagittal (C) image demonstrates echogenic clot pending from the foramen of Monro into the third ventricle (arrow).

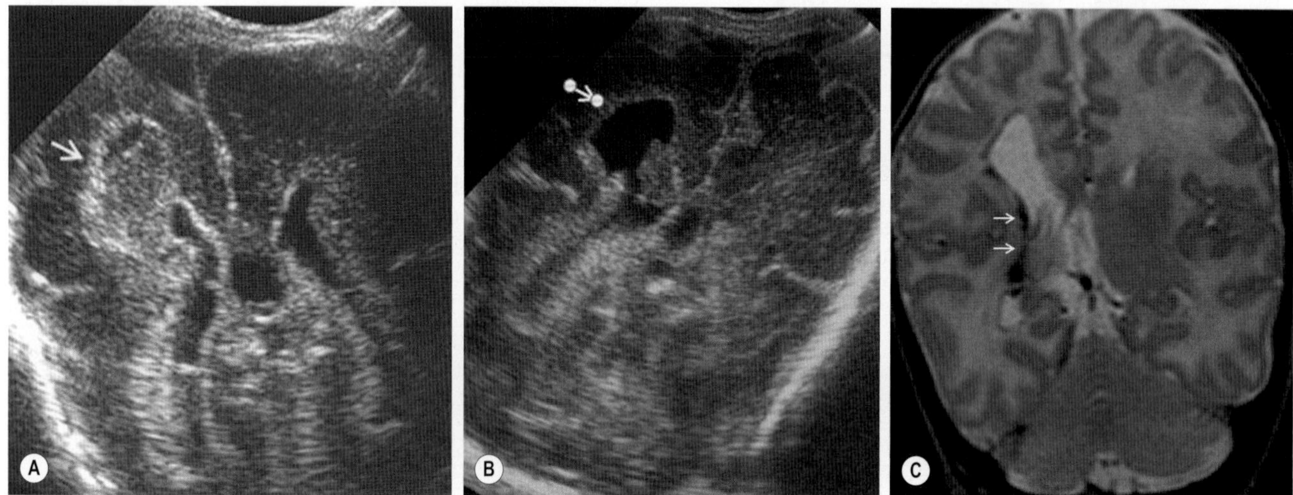

FIGURE 82-77 ■ Prematurity, history of birth at 25 weeks' gestational age. Brain ultrasound. Day 10 of life: (A) coronal image demonstrating echogenic venous infarct adjacent to right lateral ventricle (arrow). Day 20 of life: (B) coronal image demonstrating liquefaction of the lesion and the formation of a cavity communicating with the lateral ventricle (arrow). Brain MRI. Day 21 of life: (C) coronal T_2-weighted image shows the cystic infarct communicating with the right lateral ventricle. Signal void at the lateral wall of the ventricle (arrows) represents haemosiderin.

intensity of the white matter and focal loss of the grey–white matter differentiation ('missing cortex' sign). Follow-up MRI demonstrates macrocystic encephalomalacia[3,4] (Fig. 82-78).

3. Lesions of the basal ganglia, the perirolandic cortex and the brainstem may occur after acute total asphyxia (10–15 min).[12–14] Brain US reveals hyperechogenicity of the affected areas, and brain MRI shows heterogeneous increased signal intensity (Fig. 82-79). At later stages, atrophy develops.

MISCELLANEOUS ACQUIRED TOXIC OR METABOLIC DISEASE

Kernicterus is the result of the toxic effect of neonatal unconjugated hyperbilirubinaemia on the brain. The brain regions that have selective susceptibility include the globus pallidi, subthalamic nuclei and hippocampi, as well as cranial nerves VIII, VII and III. Neonates with bilirubin encephalopathy have a depressed conscious level, hypotonia and seizures with opisthotonus. Delayed effects include extrapyramidal signs (athetosis), deafness, gaze palsies and developmental delay. In the acute stage there is signal abnormality with bilateral symmetrical T_2 prolongation and swelling of the globus pallidi. There may be T_1 shortening also. Eventually the pallidal changes will progress to atrophy with variable persistent gliotic change. US and CT are initially normal, although later there may be evidence of calcification.

Hypoglycaemia may also present with a non-specific encephalopathy, subsequently leading to seizures. This is a problem particularly with neonates who have immature enzyme pathways and relatively poor glycogen reserves, particularly in the context of increased requirements due to sepsis or associated hypoxia–ischaemia but may also be

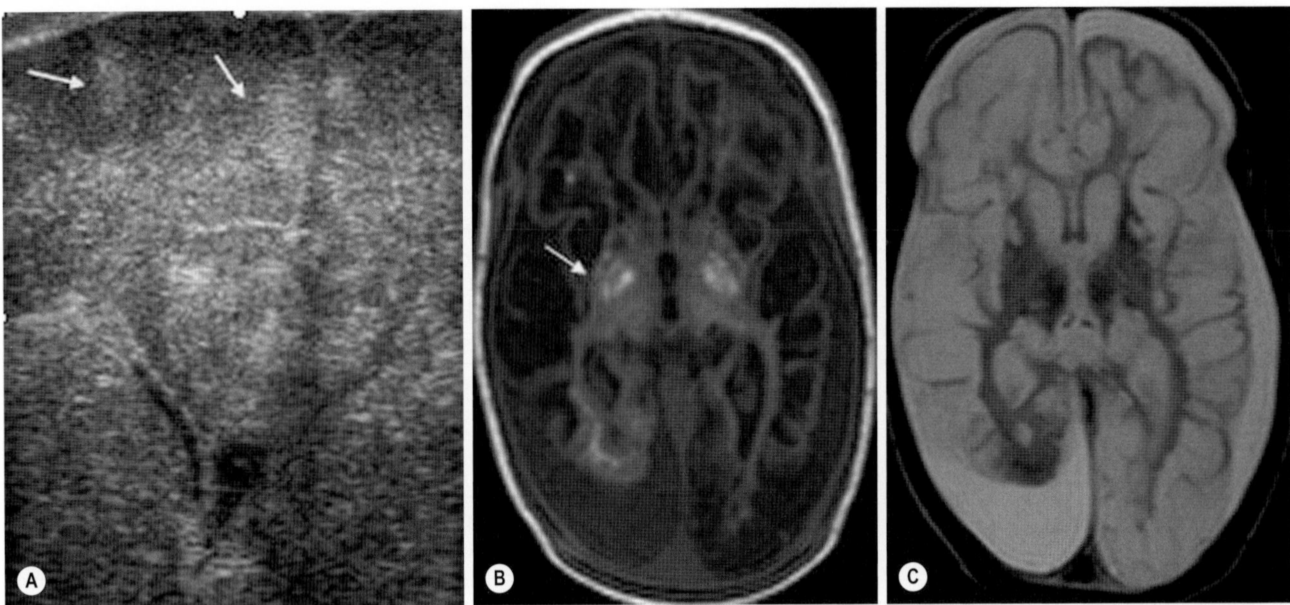

FIGURE 82-78 ■ Full term, 37 weeks' gestational age severe prolonged perinatal asphyxia. (A) Brain US. Day 3: coronal image demonstrating, heterogeneity of brain echostructure and increased echogenicity of the cortex (arrows). (B, C) Brain MRI. Day 20: axial T_1- and T_2-weighted images demonstrate extensive macrocystic encephalomalacia in the white matter and hypersignal of the putamen the pallidum (arrows).

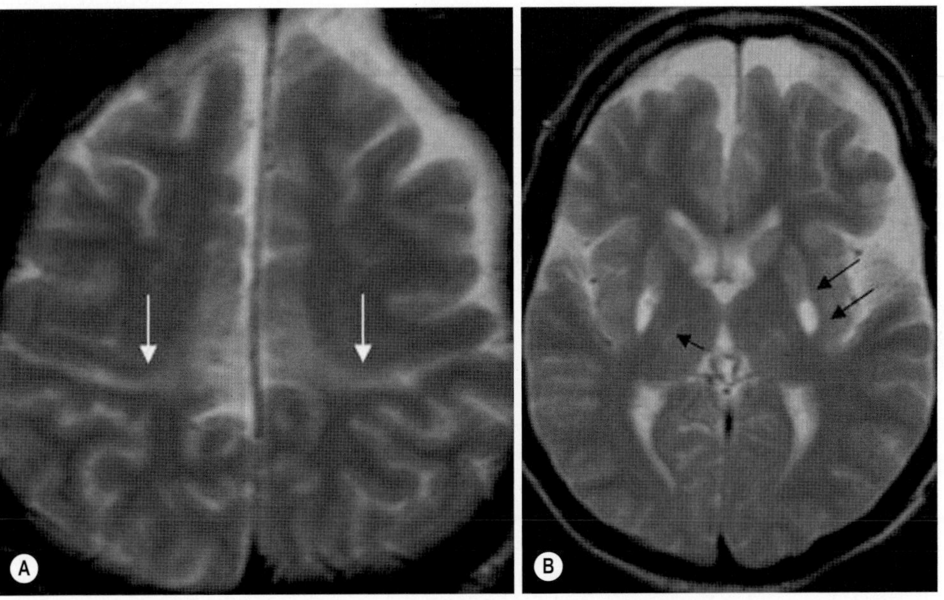

FIGURE 82-79 ■ Full term, 38 weeks' gestational age severe perinatal asphyxia. Dyskinetic cerebral palsy epilepsy, mental retardation. Brain MRI. 30 years: (A, B) axial T_2-weighted images demonstrating atrophy of the lentiform nuclei (arrowhead), signal abnormalities in the thalami (black arrows) and abnormal signal intensity in the perirolandic cortex (white arrows).

the end result of some inborn errors of metabolism or hyperinsulinism. Imaging studies may show evidence of a diffuse encephalopathy with brain swelling and oedema, but the findings are typically most severe in the parieto-occipital regions and thalami. There is T_1 and T_2 prolongation with swelling affecting the cortex and subcortical white matter with variable restricted diffusion (Fig. 82-80), progressing to the chronic sequelae of cerebral infarction with evidence of gliosis, cavitation and atrophy. Pallidal damage may also occur.

Hypernatraemia is most commonly seen in premature infants, particularly if there is additional dehydration, e.g. due to diarrhoea. Affected infants have a depressed conscious level and irritability. There is an osmotic water shift from the intracellular to the extracellular space, resulting in interstitial oedema, manifest by T_1 and T_2

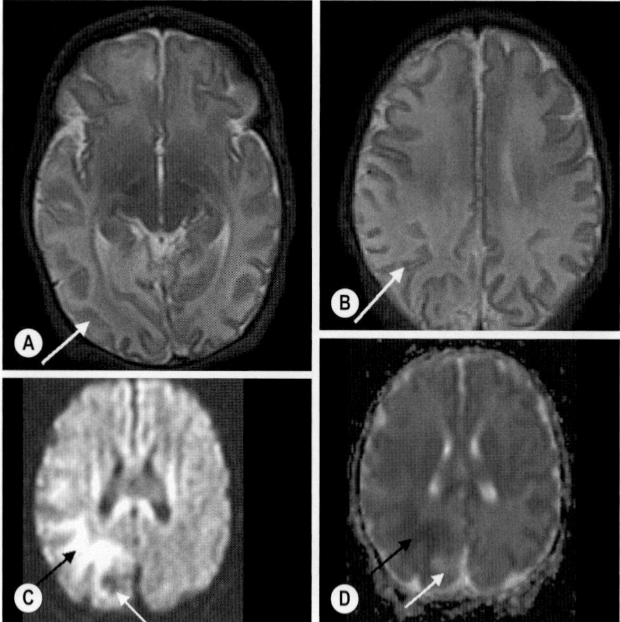

FIGURE 82-80 ■ Neonate with seizures and hypoglycaemia shows (A, B) increased signal within the parieto-occipital cortex and white matter, with patchy loss of the normal cortical low signal (arrows). (C) Diffusion-weighted image and (D) ADC map show that the diffusion changes are a mixture of restricted (black arrows) and increased diffusion (white arrows). *All* of these changes, including the T_2 and restricted areas of diffusion, completely resolved on follow-up.

prolongation with increased diffusion, but also in parenchymal haemorrhage as the brain shrinks and bridging dural veins are torn as they are pulled away from the calvarium.

Toxic exposure should be considered in children, particularly adolescents, with acute neurological symptoms and bilateral symmetrical grey matter involvement. Toxins include toluene or other organic solvents, cyanide and carbon monoxide poisoning, the latter also associated with bilateral symmetrical pallidal signal changes.

INTRACRANIAL AND INTRASPINAL INFECTIONS

Congenital Infections (TORCH)

These infections are acquired in utero or during passage through the birth canal; bacterial infections spread from the cervix to the amniotic fluid while toxoplasmosis, rubella, cytomegalovirus (CMV), syphilis and human immunodeficiency virus (HIV) spread via the transplacental route, and herpes simplex virus (HSV) is acquired from direct exposure to maternal type II herpetic genital lesions during delivery. The stage of brain development judged by the gestational age is more important than the actual organism in determining the pattern of CNS injury. Therefore in utero infections acquired before 16–18 weeks, when neurons are forming within the germinal matrix and migrating to form the cerebral cortex, produce lissencephaly and a small cerebellum. Spontaneous abortion is also a frequent outcome during this time. Between 18 and 24 weeks, when the cortical neurons are organising but the immature brain is unable to mount an inflammatory response, the infective insult may produce localised dysplastic cortex, polymicrogyria and porencephaly. This is seen as a smooth-walled cavity isointense to CSF on all sequences in continuity with the ventricular system and without evidence of gliosis. From the third trimester onwards the insult results in asymmetrical cerebral damage with gliosis, cystic change and calcification.

CMV is the most common cause of serious viral infection in fetuses and neonates in the West, occurring in up to 1% of all births. It is acquired transplacentally and the vertical transmission rate is 30–40%. The classical manifestations of CMV disease at birth include hepatosplenomegaly, petechiae, thrombocytopenia, microcephaly, chorioretinitis and sensorineural deafness occurring in up to 10% of CMV infection, but there is also an increased risk of developing deafness and other neurological deficits up to 2 years after exposure. The mechanism of injury may be due to a direct insult to the germinal matrix cells leading to periventricular calcification, cortical malformations with microcephaly and cerebellar hypoplasia, or due to the virus causing a vascular insult.

Transfontanelle cranial US may demonstrate branching curvilinear hyperechogenicity in the basal ganglia, or 'lenticulostriate vasculopathy', which may also be seen with other congenital infections, hypoxia–ischaemia and trisomy 13 and 21. Infants affected in the second trimester have lissencephaly with a thin cortex, hypoplastic cerebellum, ventriculomegaly and periventricular calcification, which is more reliably detected on CT than MRI. Those injured later, probably during the period of cortical organisation in the second trimester, have polymicrogyria, with less ventricular dilatation and cerebellar hypoplasia, and later infection produces parenchymal damage, large ventricles, calcification and haemorrhage without an underlying structural brain malformation. Temporal pole cysts are also a feature.

Toxoplasmosis is a protozoan infection caused by ingestion by the mother of *Toxoplasma gondii* oocytes in undercooked meat. The transmission rate is high and increases from 30% at 6 months' gestation to approaching 100% at term. The incidence of congenital infection is approximately 1 in 1000 to 1 in 3400 but it accounts for 1% of all stillbirths. When the CNS is involved the infection may cause a granulomatous meningitis or diffuse encephalitis. Most infants at birth are asymptomatic, although sequelae such as seizures, hydrocephalus and chorioretinitis may appear later. Imaging features of microcephaly and parenchymal calcification are similar to CMV infection, although cerebellar hypoplasia and polymicrogyria are not seen, and the ventriculomegaly may be due to an active ependymitis causing obstructive hydrocephalus rather than diffuse cerebral damage (Fig. 82-81). The severity of brain involvement correlates with earlier maternal infection.

The CNS involvement in HSV is a rapidly disseminating diffuse encephalitis, unlike the pattern of involvement in children or adults in which disease starts within the mesial temporal lobes and spreads within the limbic

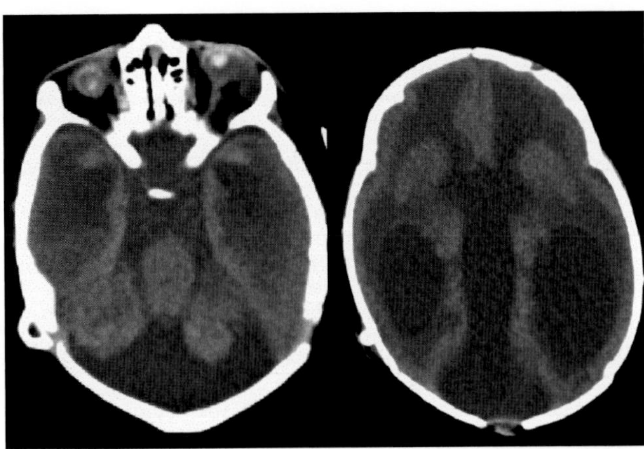

FIGURE 82-81 ■ CT of a neonate with congenital TORCH infection. Both the globes are small and calcified (phthisis bulbi). There is a Dandy–Walker malformation and hydrocephalus with transependymal oedema.

system. CT and MRI of neonatal infection show widespread asymmetrical regions of hypodensity or T_2 hyperintensity mainly in the white matter. As the disease progresses there is increasing swelling and cortical involvement (CT cortical hyperdensity and T_1/T_2 shortening on MRI) and meningeal enhancement. Subsequent loss of brain parenchyma occurs early on, often as early as the second week, eventually resulting in profound cerebral atrophy, cystic encephalomalacia and calcification.

Congenital rubella is now very rare in the West following the introduction of mass immunisation programmes, but immigrant populations remain at risk as do populations where uptake of the MMR vaccine is low. In the first 8 weeks, cataracts, glaucoma and cardiac malformations occur, while in the third trimester infection may be asymptomatic. Brain imaging appearances demonstrate similar changes to other congenital infections depending on the timing of the insult.

It is estimated that over 60 million people worldwide are infected with HIV. Almost half are women and vertical transmission of HIV accounts for 90% of newly diagnosed cases. Children with congenitally acquired AIDS usually present between the ages of 2 months and 8 years with non-specific signs such as hepatosplenomegaly and failure to thrive. Neonatal presentation is unusual. Affected children may develop a progressive HIV encephalopathy in which dementia, spasticity and increasing head size occur. A more static form is also seen in which cognitive and motor developmental delay predominate. Global atrophy and bilateral basal ganglia calcification are the most common imaging findings. Diffuse symmetrical periventricular and deep white matter abnormalities are seen in almost half of children with HIV encephalopathy and are usually associated with mild atrophy. HIV may also cause corticospinal tract degeneration.

Meningitis

Meningitis is the most common infection in childhood. The diagnosis is made not on imaging but on the presence of clinical symptoms and signs and the results of lumbar puncture. Indeed, in uncomplicated meningitis, the imaging is usually normal, and the role of neuroimaging is to detect the complications of meningitis. Neuroimaging is indicated when the diagnosis is unclear, if the meningitis is associated with persistent seizures or focal neurological deficits, if symptoms or signs suggest raised intracranial pressure, or when recovery is unduly slow.

Pathophysiology

Organisms reach the meninges by five main routes: direct spread from an adjacent infection, especially otitis media and sinusitis; haematogenous spread; rupture of a superficial cortical abscess; passage through the choroid plexus; or from direct penetrating trauma. Cerebral infarction (venous and arterial) is seen in 30% of neonates with bacterial meningitis. Infection spreads along the adventitia of penetrating cortical vessels within the periventricular spaces. Arterial thrombosis may arise from the resulting arterial wall inflammation and necrosis, or from a similar process affecting the arteries that traverse basal meningitic exudates. Venous thrombosis and subsequent infarction is particularly common in the presence of subdural empyemas due to veins becoming thrombosed as they traverse the infected subdural space. Extension of the infection through thrombosed vessels into the brain parenchyma can result in cerebritis and abscess formation. Fibropurulent exudates in the basal cisterns, ventricular outlet foramina or over the brain convexity result in hydrocephalus due either to the obstruction of CSF flow or failure of resorption. Ventriculitis occurs in about 30% of children with meningitis and is particularly common in neonates with ependymal changes seen in severe or prolonged meningitis. Later on, ventricular enlargement may persist due to damage to the adjacent periventricular white matter and parenchymal loss.

Neonatal meningitis has two distinct clinical presentations. The first presents in the first few days of life with overwhelming generalised sepsis, often in association with complicated labour, such as premature rupture of membranes. The second develops after the first week, with milder systemic sepsis but with more meningitic features.

In older infants and children acute bacterial meningitis has a mortality of 5% in the developed world, which rises to between 12% and 50% in developing countries where there is a high incidence of permanent neurological sequelae.

Uncomplicated Meningitis

Although neuroimaging is not performed for this indication alone and is usually normal, occasionally meningeal enhancement may be seen on CT or MRI. MRI is more sensitive than CT, but the sensitivity of either/both is insufficient to warrant imaging as a diagnostic test for meningitis. Imaging findings are more useful for chronic and granulomatous meningitides where dense enhancing basal exudates may be seen within the cisternal spaces. Recurrent meningitis is unusual and full neuro-axis imaging is often applied to identify underlying risk factors (see below).

Imaging of Complications (Table 82-4)

Hydrocephalus may be detected on CT or MRI and may reflect a combination of obstructed CSF flow and impaired absorption. Ependymitis may cause debris/haemorrhage within the ventricular system, resulting in obstructive hydrocephalus at the foramen of Monro, cerebral aqueduct and fourth ventricular outlet foramina. Purulent exudates may impair CSF absorption within the subarachnoid space, resulting in communicating hydrocephalus.

Sterile subdural effusions are often seen as a complication of meningitis, particularly in neonates with *Streptococcus pneumoniae* or *Haemophilus influenzae*. They are not empyemas, do not need to be surgically treated and will regress as the meningitis is treated. On imaging, the subdural collections have density and signal characteristics similar to CSF on CT and MRI, though they may be slightly hyperintense to CSF on MRI. Enhancement is not usually seen; however, leptomeningeal (pial) enhancement, to be distinguished from pachymeningeal (dural) enhancement, may be seen as a result of underlying brain infarction or due to leptomeningeal inflammation.

Subdural empyemas may require urgent surgical drainage to prevent further cerebritis and cerebral infarction. These appear as more proteinaceous subdural collections (increased density on CT, intermediate T_1 signal intensity relative to CSF, T_2 hyperintensity) with pachymeningeal (dural) and leptomeningeal enhancement (Fig. 82-82).

Imaging evidence for ventriculitis, usually spread via the choroid plexus, comes from the finding of debris layered posteriorly within the ventricular system and ependyma which are hyperdense on CT. Hydrocephalus may be seen and there may be isolation of various components of the ventricular system, resulting in some parts draining adequately while others remain dilated as debris obstructs the CSF outlet foramina. Infection may extend directly into the adjacent brain parenchyma, causing cerebritis.

Thrombosis of deep venous sinuses and cortical veins may occur, particularly in children with dehydration (Fig. 82-83). The symptoms of deep venous sinus thrombosis, such as headache, impaired consciousness and prolonged fitting, cannot be distinguished from the symptoms of the underlying meningitis and neuroimaging is required for confirmation. Cavernous sinus thrombosis is uncommon, is more commonly seen with paranasal sinus, dental or orbital infection, and tends to present with ophthalmoplegia due to involvement of the cranial nerves II, IV and VI as they pass through the cavernous sinus. Direct involvement of the cavernous carotid artery by infection may produce a mycotic aneurysm. In generalised sepsis, the sagittal and transverse sinuses are most commonly involved.

Deep venous sinus thrombosis may be seen as a hyperdense expanded sinus on unenhanced CT. As the thrombus becomes less dense, intravenous enhancement may demonstrate the 'empty delta' sign as a filling defect within the sinus lumen. A dense cortical vein may also be seen on CT, but neither CT nor MRI can reliably detect cortical vein thrombosis.

The diagnosis of deep venous sinus thrombosis may be missed in up to 40% of patients at CT; MRI with MR venography (MRV) is more sensitive. In the subacute phase thrombus is seen as T_1 shortening within an expanded sinus and this finding may be sufficient to make the diagnosis. In the acute phase when the thrombus is isointense on T_1-weighted imaging and hypointense on T_2-weighted imaging, it can be mistaken for flowing blood, although the sinus, in the latter, should not be expanded. MRV is useful to confirm absence of flow in the thrombosed sinus.

Venous infarction may occur in up to 40% of children with deep venous sinus thrombosis. Venous infarcts are often bilateral, do not conform to an arterial territory but to the territory of venous drainage, and are frequently haemorrhagic. They are parasagittal when the superior sagittal sinus is involved, thalamic when the internal cerebral veins or straight sinus/vein of Galen is involved and temporal lobe when the transverse or sigmoid sinus or vein of Labbé (one of the deep superficial venous system anastomoses connecting the middle cerebral vein to the transverse sinus) are involved. On diffusion imaging, there is a mixture of restricted and free diffusion even when non-haemorrhagic.

Arterial infarction may be seen as wedge-shaped cortical and white matter hypodensity conforming to a major

TABLE 82-4 Intracranial Complications of Meningitis in Infants

Pathology	Imaging
Cerebritis	Diffuse hypodensity (CT), hyperintensity (T_2-weighted MRI) involving cortex and white matter, gyral swelling, ill-defined enhancement
Abscess formation	Peripheral rim enhancement surrounding central necrotic cavity, adjacent oedema
Subdural effusion	Cerebrospinal fluid density/signal subdural collection, no pathological enhancement
Empyema	Higher density (CT), restricted diffusion (MRI) subdural collection with pachymeningeal/dural enhancement
Deep venous thrombosis	Hyperdense expanded venous sinus (CT), lack of T_2 flow void, expanded sinus (MRI), variable haemorrhagic venous infarction
Cavernous sinus thrombosis	Expanded cavernous sinus, filling defects on CTV, signal drop off MRV
Arterial thrombosis	Large arterial territory infarct, basal ganglia/thalamic small perforating arterial territory infarcts
Ventriculitis	Debris within ventricular system, hyperdense ependyma (pre-contrast), ependymal contrast enhancement, ventricular isolation
Hydrocephalus	Obstructive intraventricular (foramen of Monro, cerebral aqueduct), obstructive extraventricular, communicating
Deafness	CT/MRI evidence of labyrinthitis ossificans

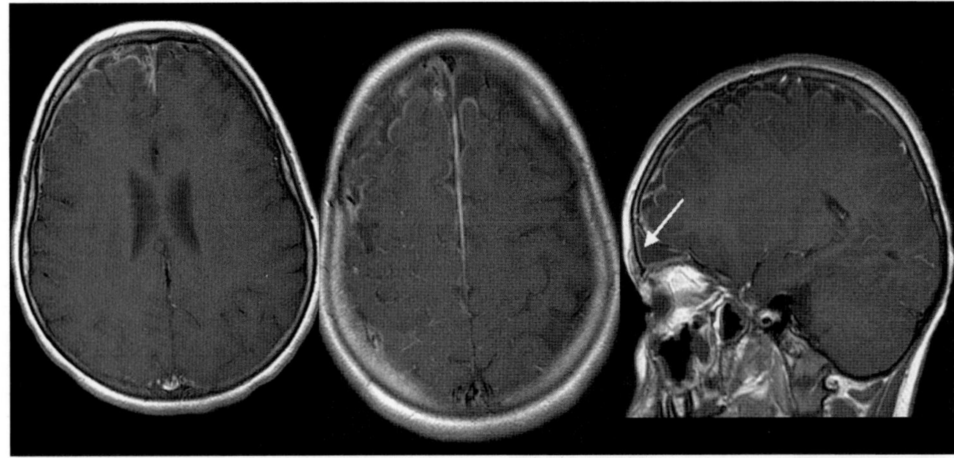

FIGURE 82-82 ■ **Bilateral subdural empyemas.** There is leptomeningeal and pachymeningeal enhancement (arrows) most marked over the right cerebral convexity and extending back to the vertex (on the sagittal view). There is enhancing debris within the subdural space and the signal is slightly increased compared to cerebrospinal fluid. The source of infection was from the frontal sinus (arrow).

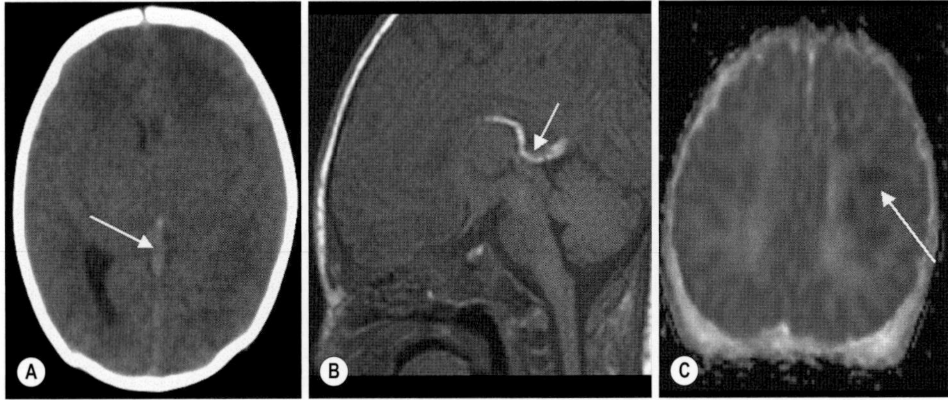

FIGURE 82-83 ■ **Venous sinus thrombosis in a child with recent history of nausea and vomiting.** (A) CT shows hyperdense thrombus within the vein of Galen just reaching the internal cerebral veins (arrow). There is diffuse cerebral swelling with more hypodense change and swelling affecting the left hemisphere and thalami. (B) Sagittal T_1-weighted MRI confirms the diagnosis with T_1 shortening in keeping with methaemoglobin in the internal cerebral veins and vein of Galen (arrow). (C) The ADC map shows patchy restricted diffusion (low signal) (arrow) within the deep white matter in keeping with infarction.

arterial territory on CT or as T_2 hyperintensity and T_1 hypointensity with cortical highlighting on MRI. The basal meningitis may occlude small perforating branches from the circle of Willis, causing small infarcts in the region of the deep grey nuclei (basal ganglia and thalami).

Labyrinthitis ossificans, the most common cause of acquired deafness in childhood, is one of the sequelae of bacterial meningitis resulting from direct spread of infection from the meninges into the inner ear. Faint enhancement of the membranous labyrinth may be seen on enhanced T_1-weighted images in acute infection. In some children inflammation persists; fibrosis and ossification subsequently develop and may be detected on high-resolution CT of the temporal bone, as increased density within the membranous labyrinth. High-resolution T_2-weighted MRI (e.g. performed with 3DFT-CISS imaging) may be more sensitive than CT to the changes of labyrinthitis ossificans, and T_2 signal drop-off may detect the fibrous stage before ossification when children are still suitable for cochlear implantation. Once the typical appearances of diffuse labyrinthitis ossificans develop, cochlear implantation is much more difficult (Fig. 82-84).

Tuberculous Infection

Tuberculosis (TB) has risen in incidence recently, and while it remains a serious problem in children, there does not appear to have been an increase in tuberculous meningitis in children as yet, possibly due to targeted immunisation of at-risk immigrant populations. TB may cause meningitis, cerebritis and abscess formation (tuberculomas). With leptomeningeal disease, which may be seen without evidence of miliary TB elsewhere, thick enhancing purulent soft-tissue exudates may be seen in the subarachnoid space, particularly in the basal cisterns, and associated with hydrocephalus, basal ganglia and thalamic infarcts. Larger major arterial branch cortical infarcts are seen less frequently. Tuberculomas are seen as solid or ring-enhancing lesions, particularly at the grey–white matter junction.

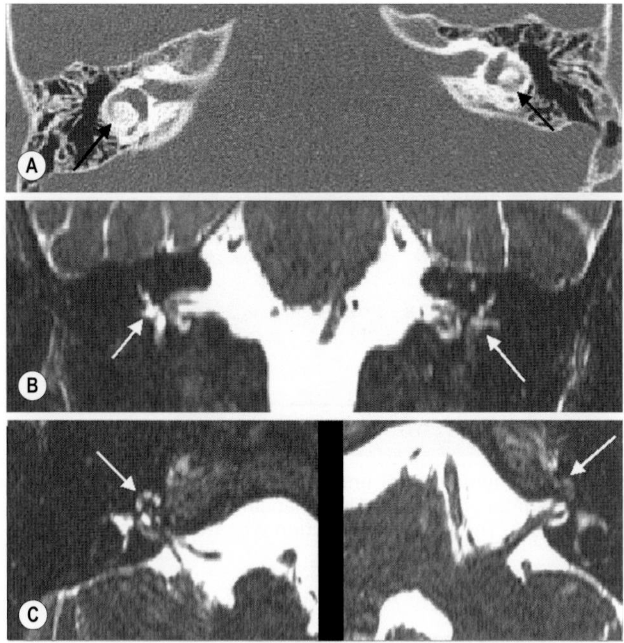

FIGURE 82-84 ■ Child with recent meningitis and new sensorineural deafness. (A) High-resolution axial CT through the petrous bones shows increased density in keeping with calcification within the lateral semicircular canals (arrows). (B) Coronal and (C) axial CISS MRI show reduced T_2 signal within all the semicircular canals (arrows), particularly the left, confirmed on the oblique axial views (C). There is reduced signal within the cochlea, again worse on the left (arrows). These are typical features of labyrinthitis ossificans.

Bacterial Infection: Cerebritis and Abscess Formation

Cerebritis is the earliest stage of purulent brain infection, may be focal or multifocal, and may resolve or evolve into frank abscess formation. Predisposing conditions include middle ear, dental and paranasal sinus infection, penetrating injury, postoperative complication or dermal sinus, immune deficiency, and any cause of arteriovenous shunting (e.g. cyanotic congenital heart disease). Fungal infection may also cause brain abscesses, particularly in immunocompromised children, but in this case the lesion may not be able to encapsulate because this requires the ability to mount an adequate immune response. Radiological differentiation between cerebritis and abscess formation is important because cerebritis may respond to antibiotics while an abscess may require surgical drainage as an adjunct. During the cerebritis stage CT and MRI show an ill-defined area of oedema with swelling with or without variable ill-defined enhancement and haemorrhagic transformation. As the infection becomes more established, focal areas may become walled-off and abscess formation occurs. On imaging this appears as a space-occupying lesion with a central region of pus manifest as low density on CT, or T_2 hyperintensity on MRI, surrounded by an enhancing wall. The wall of the cavity may demonstrate T_1/T_2 shortening. Typically there is surrounding oedema. The central region of pus shows restricted diffusion and this may help to differentiate abscesses from necrotic or cystic tumours which usually demonstrate central areas of increased diffusion. Imaging can be used to monitor response to treatment although there may be a lag time between the resolution of imaging findings and clinical response.

Neurocysticercosis

Cysticercosis occurs from ingestion of the encysted form of *Taenia solium* (porcine tapeworm). Humans act as the intermediate host and neurological disease occurs as the host mounts an inflammatory response and the parasites die. In children a typical presentation is with parenchymal cysts associated with seizures, headache and focal neurological deficits. These may occur anywhere within the brain but typically at the grey–white matter interface. Calcification may occur and may be punctate within the solid component or may occur within the wall of the cyst. Perilesional oedema is the result of the inflammatory response to the dying larva. Lesions at various stages of development may be seen. Therefore active lesions seen as regions of oedema may coexist with ring or solid enhancing lesions with or without oedema, and with foci of calcification without oedema or enhancement which are burnt-out lesions following the death of the parasite.

There are also leptomeningeal, intraventricular and racemose forms of neurocysticercosis. Leptomeningeal disease is demonstrated on CT or MRI by soft tissue filling the basal cisterns with marked contrast enhancement. Granulomata with variable calcification may be seen within the subarachnoid space. Hydrocephalus and brain infarcts are also complications. Intraventricular cysticerci are important to detect because of the risk of acute-onset hydrocephalus and sudden death. MRI is more sensitive than CT at identifying the cysts with their scolex. In the racemose form there are multilobular cysts without a scolex within the subarachnoid space, typically in the cerebellopontine angles, suprasellar region and basal cisterns and Sylvian fissures. They may demonstrate enhancement and may coexist with leptomeningitis.

Viral Encephalitis

The typical pattern of viral encephalitis is that of patchy and asymmetrical disease with a predeliction for grey matter. The anterior temporal and inferior frontal cortical regions are a classical location for herpes encephalitis. Another characteristic herpes virus pattern is the involvement of the hippocampi and cingulate gyrus as a limbic encephalitis. More widespread hemispheric involvement is seen with a variety of enteroviruses, echovirus and Coxsackie virus in particular.

A more unusual pattern of deep grey matter and upper brainstem disease is seen with rare types of viral encephalitis. Patchy enhancement with oedema has been seen with Epstein–Barr virus infection and may also be mimicked by mycoplasma infection. Thalamic and upper brainstem involvement, occasionally with haemorrhagic change, is a feature of Japanese encephalitis and the related West Nile virus.

Acute cerebellitis presents infrequently in children with sudden onset of truncal ataxia, dysarthria, involuntary eye movements due to a swollen cerebellum, and nausea, headache and vomiting due to resulting hydrocephalus. Fever and meningism may also be present. The many causes of a swollen cerebellum include infectious (e.g. pertussis), post-infectious (e.g. acute disseminated encephalomyelitis [ADEM]), toxic, such as lead poisoning, and vasculitis. Imaging shows effacement of the cerebellar fissures, enlarged cerebellum, signal abnormality affecting the cortex and white matter, and variable hydrocephalus. Although the cerebellar swelling may resolve spontaneously, surgical CSF diversion may be necessary as a temporary measure.

Infection in Immunocompromised Children

Children with primary, acquired or iatrogenic immunodeficiencies are vulnerable to opportunistic and unusual organisms. Examples include fungal infections such as aspergillosis, actinomyces and unusual bacterial infections such as atypical mycobacteria. The host's ability to develop an inflammatory response may be limited and the interpretation of images should be considered in this context. Contrast enhancement remains a useful hallmark. A diffuse pattern of nodular leptomeningeal and parenchymal disease may be seen. Conversely, focal large parenchymal abscesses or mycetomas may develop.

Spinal Infections

The patterns of discitis and spondylitis in children are similar to those of young adults and do not need to be discussed in detail in this chapter. However, special mention should be made of congenital spinal abnormalities that may harbour or increase the risk of spinal infection. These children may present with recurrent meningitis. Spinal imaging may reveal a dorsal dermal sinus tract or an intraspinal dermoid.

Brain and Cord Inflammation

Children may develop CNS disease known as acute disseminated encephalomyelitis (ADEM) following an infection, usually viral, or vaccination. This is assumed to be a post-infectious inflammatory immune-mediated phenomenon. Affected children present with focal neurological deficits, headache, fever and altered consciousness following a recent infection. Classically, ADEM is a monophasic disease occurring at multiple sites within the brain and spinal cord. Most children recover completely, although 10–30% will have a permanent neurological deficit. Occasionally ADEM may present with relapses occurring within a few months of the original presentation, but these are still considered as part of a monophasic inflammatory process. When relapses occur that are more disseminated in time or place, the diagnosis of multiple sclerosis (MS) may be made. On follow-up imaging, children with ADEM have no new lesions and complete or partial resolution of the majority of old lesions, while in MS there are new lesions which may or may not be symptomatic.

On MRI, multiple asymmetrical areas of demyelination seen as increased signal intensity on T_2-weighted imaging with swelling occur within the subcortical white matter of both hemispheres and may also involve the cerebellum and spinal cord. Cortical and deep grey matter may also be involved but to a lesser extent (Fig. 82-85). Diffusion-weighted imaging shows increased free diffusion within the lesions. Occasionally, a fulminant haemorrhagic form may develop. Periventricular and callosal lesions (such as Dawson's fingers) are more in keeping with MS lesions, while cortical abnormality is not seen with MS and deep grey matter involvement, though seen in both, is more frequent in ADEM. Other differentials include viral encephalitis, which typically is more cortically based, and vasculitis (the lesions should also show restricted diffusion).

TRAUMA

Birth Trauma

Extracranial haemorrhage may be seen as a consequence of birth trauma and more often with instrumental

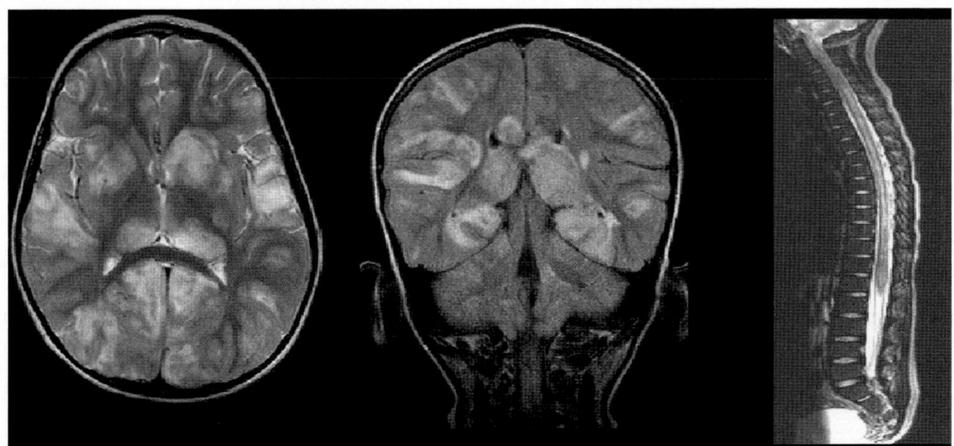

FIGURE 82-85 ■ Acute disseminated encephalomyelitis in an 11-year-old boy with recent viral illness and acute impaired consciousness. MRI shows bilateral, asymmetrical, mainly subcortical, cerebral hemisphere white matter lesions but also involving the cortex and deep grey matter. The cerebellum and spinal cord are also involved. There is focal swelling of the involved regions. The imaging features are typical of acute disseminated encephalomyelitis. The child made a full recovery.

delivery. It does not usually require imaging but may be detected on images done for intracranial assessment. Subgaleal haemorrhage may occur deep to the scalp aponeurosis. As there is a large potential space, the extent of haemorrhage may occasionally be severe, requiring transfusion. Cephalhaematoma is a traumatic subperiosteal haemorrhage between the vault and the outer layer of periosteum and is therefore confined by the sutures. It may calcify peripherally where the periosteum calcifies. Very rarely, forceps may cause skull fractures. These may be linear, depressed or 'ping pong' (depressed without a fracture line, but to be distinguished from an asymptomatic parietal depression which is a normal variant) with a cephalhaematoma overlying them. Caput succedaneum is due to diffuse oedema and bleeding under the scalp and is more commonly seen with prolonged vaginal or ventouse delivery.

Birth trauma can result in a subdural haematoma, which may be seen even without instrumental delivery. Most are small, clinically silent and infratentorial, although they may extend above the tentorium cerebelli, and resolve spontaneously within 4 weeks. Occasionally they are large and associated with extensive intracranial haemorrhage and hydrocephalus. However, small posterior fossa subdural bleeds are common incidental findings on MRI when newborn infants are imaged for clinical CNS illness.

The spinal cord may be injured by distraction during a difficult delivery, usually a breech delivery, typically affecting the lower cervical and upper thoracic regions. The cord can be transected while the soft and compliant spine remains undamaged. A more common birth-related neurological injury is brachial plexus damage secondary to traction of the shoulder during a breech delivery of the head. Brachial plexus MRI may show CSF signal pseudomeningoceles around the avulsed nerve roots.

Growing Skull Fractures

Growing skull fractures are seen when there is a dural tear deep to the fracture and usually also when there is localised brain parenchymal damage, which may be associated with a focal neurological deficit or seizures (Fig. 82-86). CSF pulsation may keep the tear open, preventing healing of both the dura and the fracture. The fracture margins become progressively widened on serial radiographs and are bevelled and sclerotic. It usually occurs in children under 1 year with 90% occurring under the age of 3. A leptomeningeal cyst with arachnoid adhesions can cause further pressure erosion.

Spinal Trauma

The investigation of spinal trauma in children requires knowledge of the normal appearances of the developing spine on plain radiographs. The distance between the anterior arch of C1 and the dens can be up to 5 mm in normal children, and there is increased mobility not only between C1 and C2 but also between C3 and C4. The prevertebral soft tissues should not exceed two-thirds of the width of the C2 vertebral body. Increased mobility in many children allows anterior 'pseudoluxation' of C2 on

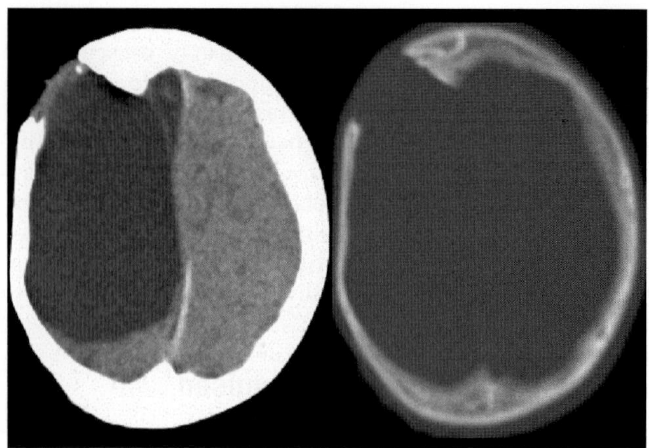

FIGURE 82-86 ■ Large cerebral parenchymal defect in association with frontal bone defect which increased in size following a frontal bone linear fracture. Note the well-corticated margins of the fracture.

C3 by up to 4 mm but the posterior elements should always remain correctly aligned and the distance should reduce in extension.

There is generalised ligamentous laxity of the immature spine. This may allow significant injury to the spinal cord in the absence of detectable bony injury causing SCIWORA (spinal cord injury without radiographic abnormality). In the appropriate clinical setting a proper evaluation may therefore require carefully performed flexion and extension views, and MRI to look for soft tissue and cord injury.

Atlanto-Axial Rotatory Fixation

This entity is discussed in this section for convenience, although there is often little or no history of trauma in these cases. Torticollis is common in children. Most cases are acute and the symptoms disappear without treatment within a week. Rarely it may be caused by rotatory fixation between C1 and C2, and with variable degrees of subluxation, and may occur within a normal range of movement and without subluxation. Atlanto-axial rotatory fixation should be suspected if the symptoms of torticollis persist for more than 2 weeks. The diagnostic test (CT is best) must prove that there is a fixed relationship between C1 and C2 in all positions, and in particular, on turning the head to the opposite side of the clinical presentation. Atlanto-axial rotatory fixation is present if there is rotation between C1 and C2 which remains constant throughout all positions. The treatment is aggressive with traction; if it is unsuccessful, the atlanto-axial rotatory fixation will result in a permanent rotatory malalignment requiring surgery. Secondary degenerative changes and eventually fusion may occur.

Non-Accidental Head Injury

Imaging of the brain is particularly important for the diagnosis of the so-called 'shaken baby syndrome' (see also Chapter 80). The triad of retinal haemorrhages, subdural haemorrhages and encephalopathy is accepted as a useful marker for this condition. The mechanism for injury is thought to be that of vigorous or violent shaking or such shaking followed by an impact injury. The emphasis is on rapid and alternating forces of acceleration and deceleration acting on an unsupported head. The strength of force required to cause these injuries is unknown and not easy to study scientifically. However, experienced workers would agree that such injuries cannot occur from the normal handling of an infant or young child. Subarachnoid haemorrhage, cerebral contusions, lacerations or 'splits' in the brain parenchyma and diffuse cerebral oedema with little evidence of external impact injury are supportive hallmarks of the shaken baby syndrome.

During shaking, the brain also comes into contact with the inner surface of the skull, and there may also be a final impact, and cerebral contusions are seen. The mechanism behind the repeated trauma also causes shearing injuries in the brain, often located in the subcortical region at the junction of white and grey matter. MRI detects these injuries more frequently than CT. Brain oedema is a very important feature of the shaken baby syndrome, the mechanism of which is hypothesised to be due to hypoxic–ischaemic injury. The oedema is usually massive, with reduced or absent grey–white matter differentiation, and is worst in the parieto-occipital regions. The basal ganglia, brainstem and cerebellum are, in turn, relatively preserved. The outcome of brain injury caused by shaking when severe brain oedema is present is usually grim. There is rapid destruction of brain tissue and significant atrophy becomes obvious after 2–3 weeks. In severe cases the end result is multicystic encephalomalacia, and microcephaly with marked mental and motor disability (Fig. 82-87).

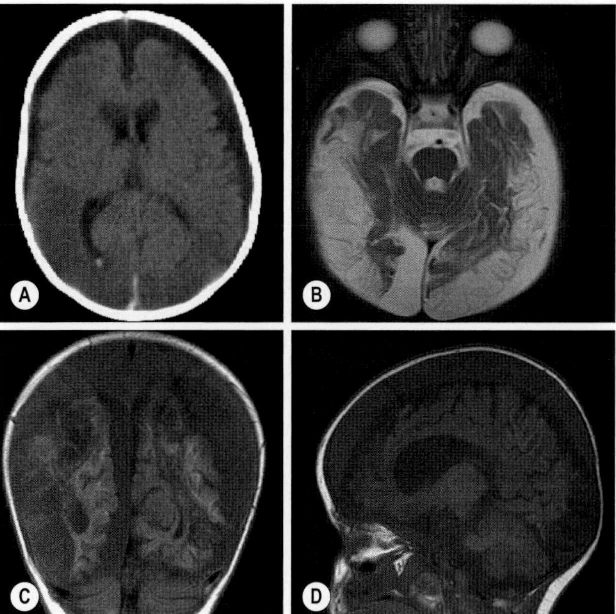

FIGURE 82-87 ■ Brain injury in 'shaken baby syndrome'. (A) The initial CT shows posterior interhemispheric subdural and intraventricular blood. There are bilateral hypodense subdural collections overlying both hemispheres. Extensive bilateral hypodense parenchymal lesions consistent with contusions or infarction are seen. (B) Follow-up MRI shows evolution of the parenchymal damage with marked atrophy and large chronic subdural collections. (C) Coronal and (D) sagittal T_1-weighted sequence shows the subdural collections have signal slightly greater than cerebrospinal fluid in keeping with proteinaceous contents from previous haemorrhage. There is cortical T_1 shortening suggesting the parenchymal lesions are regions of cerebral infarction.

HYDROCEPHALUS

The term 'hydrocephalus', literally 'water on the brain', is unfortunately a non-specific term which refers to any condition in which the ventricles are enlarged, including cerebral atrophy. The clinical and radiological challenge is to identify those forms that are likely to benefit from intervention. Some qualifying terms have been used to distinguish some of these entities. The terms communicating and non-communicating hydrocephalus are used to indicate extraventricular obstructive hydrocephalus and intraventricular obstructive hydrocephalus, respectively. These need to be distinguished from ventriculomegaly due to underlying lack of brain parenchyma, through atrophy or primary lack of brain development; some authors have suggested avoiding the use of the term hydrocephalus altogether for these cases. The concepts fail to hold true in a sizeable minority of cases, where the changes following intervention may not appear to follow expectations. For these, an appreciation of the complexities of CSF physiology may be helpful. Although it is generally accepted that those forms of hydrocephalus that are likely to benefit from interventions are caused by an imbalance between CSF production and absorption, the exact pathophysiology of these mechanisms remains incompletely understood. CSF is produced by the choroid plexuses and is mostly absorbed through the brain and cord with a lesser contribution from the arachnoid granulations. There is a net flow of CSF through the ventricular system, from lateral to third to fourth ventricles, which is influenced by cerebrovascular pulsations.

Post-haemorrhagic and post-infective hydrocephalus account for a significant proportion of hydrocephalus presenting in neonates and infants. Apart from these, congenital causes include aqueductal stenosis/gliosis, Chiari II malformation (usually occurring after repair of the associated lumbosacral myelomeningocele) and other malformations such as the Dandy–Walker malformation. Rarer causes include congenital midline tumours and vascular (e.g. vein of Galen) malformations. Before closure of the fontanelles (i.e. up to 2 years), the most reliable clinical sign is progressive macrocephaly documented by serial head circumference measurements. Caution should be exercised in the case of an asymmetrical skull or preferential growth in one direction due to craniosynostosis, which may give a spuriously enlarged head circumference without hydrocephalus. Alongside an increasingly disproportionate head circumference which crosses centiles on growth charts, other features of hydrocephalus in this age group include frontal bossing, calvarial thinning, presence of a tense, bulging anterior fontanelle, sutural diastasis and enlargement of scalp veins. Sunsetting eyes with failure of upward gaze, lateral rectus palsies and leg spasticity due to stretching of the corticospinal tracts as they descend from the motor strip around the ventricles are also seen.

In older children posterior fossa neoplasms and aqueduct stenosis are the most common causes of hydrocephalus. Early morning headache, nausea, vomiting, papilloedema, leg spasticity, cranial palsies and alterations in conscious level are the dominant clinical features as the skull is rigid. The fontanelles have fused and the sutures are fusing, and therefore increasing head circumference, fontanelle bulging and sutural diastasis are not features.

Imaging indicators of intraventricular obstructive (non-communicating) hydrocephalus include dilatation of the temporal horns disproportionate to lateral ventricular dilatation, enlargement of the anterior and posterior recesses of the third ventricle with inferior convexity of the floor of the third ventricle, transependymal (periventricular interstitial) oedema and bulging of fontanelles The sulcal spaces, major fissures and basal cisterns are small or obliterated. A careful survey of the regional ventricular dilatation may reveal the location as well as the cause of obstruction. Other features, such as changes in the configuration of the frontal horns of the lateral ventricles, specifically widening of the radius of the frontal horn, and a decrease in the angle it makes with the midline plane, are less useful. Further features classically described in chronic hydrocephalus, such as erosion of the dorsum sellae and copper-beaten skull, are even less reliable.

Extraventricular obstructive (communicating) hydrocephalus, however, may reveal a range of findings from ventricular and sulcal prominence to 'normal' CT/MRI appearances. It may have a variety of causes, ranging from haemorrhage and proteinaceous cellular debris with infection and disseminated malignancy to venous hypertension from impaired venous drainage to impaired arterial compliance from diffuse arteriopathies. In some cases, a combination of both forms of obstructive hydrocephalus would be expected.

Assessment of the cortical sulci for effacement disproportionate to ventricular size in children can be difficult and it requires some knowledge of the normal appearances for age; in normal younger children, under 2, the ventricles and subarachnoid spaces are more prominent, and should not be misinterpreted as 'atrophic' or due to hydrocephalus. Knowledge of the head size is important in making this distinction, being large in hydrocephalus and benign enlargement of the subarachnoid spaces, or small if there is cerebral atrophy. Again it may not be possible to be certain about the findings in the absence of serial measurements documenting trends. In benign enlargement of the subarachnoid spaces, there is believed to be a mismatch between the rate of skull growth and rate of growth of the developing brain. The child is neurologically normal. There is rapid skull growth, often to above the 95th centile by the time of presentation, but this then stabilises and both the size of the subarachnoid spaces and head size have usually normalised by age 2 years. The extra space anterior to the cerebral convexities is distinguishable from subdural collections by lack of mass effect on the adjacent brain and the presence of crossing veins within the subarachnoid space. The importance of its recognition is to indicate that no intervention is required, with the expectation that the situation will normalise with age.

In the second decade the hemispheric cortical sulci become much less conspicuous and the ventricles less prominent, which should equally not be misinterpreted as due to cerebral oedema or the presence of a 'tight' brain. In this case in the normal child the basal cisterns should not be effaced.

An attempt should be made to identify a structural cause for the hydrocephalus. The narrowest parts of the ventricular system are the most susceptible to mechanical obstruction, i.e. the foramina of Monro, cerebral aqueduct and fourth ventricular outflow foramina. Masses causing obstructive hydrocephalus at the foramina of Monro include superior extension of suprasellar tumours and arachnoid cysts, colloid cysts, which may cause sudden acute and life-threatening hydrocephalus, and giant cell astrocytomas in tuberous sclerosis. Masses effacing the cerebral aqueduct include tectal plate gliomas, superior extension of midline posterior fossa tumours and brainstem diffuse astrocytomas and inferior extension of pineal region tumours. Atrial diverticula from dilated lateral ventricles may herniate into the quadrigeminal and supracerebellar cisterns and may also compress the tectum. These may be distinguished from large arachnoid cysts using multiplanar MRI to confirm continuity with the ventricular system.

More diffuse patterns of obstruction, including isolation of pockets of CSF, may be caused by haemorrhage, infection, disseminated tumour and reparative fibrosis. Clues to the underlying cause include evidence of haemosiderin staining or superficial siderosis in previous haemorrhage; focal atrophy or porencephaly from previous haematomas; the presence of hyperdense exudates in the basal cisterns, subarachnoid space and pial enhancement with infection or pial neoplastic dissemination.

Aqueduct stenosis is one of the most common causes of hydrocephalus in children but may present at any time from birth to adulthood. It may be developmental or acquired gliosis secondary to infection or intraventricular haemorrhage. Classically, the lateral and third ventricles are dilated and the fourth ventricle is of normal size, and there is no evidence of a tectal plate tumour. On sagittal MRI there is focal narrowing of the cerebral aqueduct, normally proximally at the level of the superior colliculi or at the intercollicular sulcus with posterior displacement of the tectal plate. Proximal to this, the aqueduct is dilated. Occasionally a congenital web may be seen as a very thin sheet of tissue across the distal aqueduct.

Overproduction of CSF is a very rare cause of hydrocephalus, most often seen with choroid plexus papillomas. These tumours may cause hydrocephalus by other mechanisms, e.g. obstructive hydrocephalus of the lateral ventricle due to mass effect at the body/trigone or foramen of Monro of the lateral ventricle, and haemorrhage within the ventricular system. A highly proteinaceous exudate produced by the tumour can cause communicating hydrocephalus due to impaired extraventricular drainage of CSF. Spinal cord tumours may be associated with hydrocephalus due to proteinaceous exudates or pial dissemination of disease, both causing impaired absorption of CSF. Indeed, in the cases of unexplained hydrocephalus, spinal imaging is recommended to exclude a possible occult intraspinal lesion.

Chiari II malformation is a common cause of hydrocephalus presenting early in life. The underlying aetiology is disputed; it may not be due to simple craniocervical junction obstruction but due to the displacement of the fourth ventricular outlet foramina within the spinal canal inferior to the foramen magnum, i.e. within the spinal canal, where the capacity for CSF absorption is reduced. Some specific features should be looked for when assessing these children for hydrocephalus or shunt malfunction. Children with occipital headaches at night probably have some degree of shunt malfunction which may present with potentially fatal signs of brainstem compression and apnoeic attacks. Also, the fourth ventricle should be slit-like, so the presence of a normal-sized or enlarged fourth ventricle suggests a shunt malfunction or isolation of the fourth ventricle requiring diversion.

Finally, hydrocephalus may be seen as a consequence of raised intracranial venous pressure. Examples include syndromic skull base abnormalities in craniosynostosis(es) and leading to stenosis of the jugular outflow foramina. Vascular causes include venous thrombosis, the vein of Galen aneurysmal malformation and dural arteriovenous shunts. Persistent untreated raised intraventricular pressure may result in secondary parenchymal damage affecting adjacent white matter and resulting in impaired cognitive function, permanent spasticity and blindness.

As well as by removing the obstructive lesion, hydrocephalus can be treated by CSF diversion. This can be performed initially by external ventricular drainage, or more permanently by ventriculoperitoneal, ventriculoatrial shunting, or third ventriculostomy. Here a surgical defect is made in the floor of the third ventricle, allowing CSF drainage into the suprasellar cistern.

Shunt malfunction from obstruction of the shunt by choroid plexus or glial tissue and subsequent ventricular dilatation is best assessed by comparison with baseline or previous imaging. In addition to a recurrence of the signs of hydrocephalus, there may be the appearance of fluid tracking along the length of the shunt tubing. Assessment of shunt tubing integrity may be made by plain radiograph imaging of the tube from the skull to the abdomen/pelvis. The scout view of a brain CT may also be useful to pick up disrupted shunt tubing or disconnection of the valve. As well as separation of the fragments, calcification may be seen at either end of the shunt disruption due to inflammation and fibrotic change where the shunt has become tethered and then distracted. Knowledge of the type of shunt inserted, or discussion with the neurosurgeon who inserted it, should allow distinction of the normal radiolucent components of the shunt (often as it exits the calvarium) from shunt distraction.

Patency of a third ventriculostomy can be inferred on MRI by visualising the surgical defect and detecting rapid CSF flow through it into the suprasellar cistern, manifest as large hypointense flow voids on T_2-weighted imaging. This may be aided by imaging without any flow compensation.

The incidence of shunt infection has declined over the years and in most neurosurgical centres runs at around 1–5%, being slightly higher in infants. Imaging may detect evidence of ventriculitis: enlarged ventricles with hyperdense ependyma on CT, ependymal enhancement and debris within the ventricular system. This may progress to cerebritis with devastating consequences for the developing brain parenchyma. Other shunt complications include the development of abdominal ascites, pseudocyst formation and perforated abdominal viscus. Rarely, shunted hydrocephalic patients may become symptomatic without ventricular dilatation and develop the 'slit ventricle' syndrome. This has a number of potential causes which include overdrainage of CSF, stiff, poorly compliant ventricles which allow raised intraventricular pressure without ventricular dilatation, intermittent shunt malfunction and headaches unrelated to the shunt.

SUMMARY

Paediatric neuroradiology is a subspecialist field drawing from knowledge and expertise in neuroimaging, neuropathology, paediatrics, embryology and genetics. Some skill is required in adapting neuroimaging techniques to suit the paediatric population, especially in terms of sedation/general anaesthesia and image optimisation. The range of conditions encountered is very different from that seen in adults. The management aims and options are also often different from adult cases.

For a full list of references, please see ExpertConsult.

FURTHER READING

22. Barkovich AJ, Kuzniecki RI, Jackson GD, et al. Developmental and genetic classification for malformations of cortical development. Neurology 2005;65:1873–87.
23. Blumcke I, Thom M, Aronica E, et al. The clinicopathological spectrum of focal cortical dysplasias: a consensus classification proposed by an ad hoc Task Force of the ILAE Diagnostic Methods Commission. Epilepsia 2010;52(1):158–74.
42. Pang D, Zovickian J, Oviedo A. Long-term outcome of total and near-total spinal cord lipomas and radical reconstruction of the neural placode: part 1—surgical technique. Neurosurgery 2009;65:511–29.

Barth PG, Majoie CB, Caan MW, et al. Pontine tegmental cap dysplasia: a novel brain malformation with a defect in axonal guidance. Brain 2007;130(Pt 9):2258–66.

Desai NK, Young L, Miranda MA, et al. Pontine tegmental cap dysplasia: the neurotologic perspective. Otolaryngol Head Neck Surg 2011;145(6):992–8.

Namavar Y, Barth PG, Kasher PR, et al. Clinical, neuroradiological and genetic findings in pontocerebellar hypoplasia. Brain 2011;134(Pt 1):143–56.

Vedolin L, Gonzalez G, Souza CF, et al. Inherited cerebellar ataxia in childhood: a pattern-recognition approach using brain MRI. Am J Neuroradiol 2013;34(5):925–34.

Vijayakumar K, Gunny R, Grunewald S, et al. Clinical neuroimaging features in molybdenum cofactor deficiency. Pediatr Neurol 2011;45(4):246–52.

SECTION I

INTERVENTIONAL RADIOLOGY

Section Editors: Anna-Maria Belli • Michael J. Lee • Andreas Adam

CHAPTER 83

BASIC CLINICAL REQUIREMENTS OF INTERVENTIONAL RADIOLOGY

Jim Reekers

CHAPTER OUTLINE

IR

Interventional radiology (IR) is a recognised subspecialty of radiology both within the Union of European Medical Specialties (UEMS) and the European Society of Radiology (ESR). IR is unique and distinct from all other surgical, radiological and medical subspecialties and specialties.

IR is performed by trained IR specialists who have expertise in interpreting diagnostic imaging as well as expertise in image-guided minimally invasive procedures and techniques as applied to various diseases and organs. There are a huge variety of therapeutic procedures performed by IR. They can be divided into broad categories of vascular, non-vascular and oncological interventions. For a more detailed description of IR and what interventional radiologists do, please read the Global Statement on IR.[1]

TRAINING

Training in IR should be under an accredited training programme and the minimum length of training is 2 years. In several countries there are special training curricula for IR and there is also a European IR training curriculum which can be viewed at <http://www.cirse.org>.

There is a European IR examination which can be taken by every interventional radiologist after the completion of training. This examination is called the European Board of Interventional Radiology (EBIR) and is held under the auspices of an independent European Board. Maintenance of IR skills by performing an adequate number and range of procedures and demonstration of continuous medical education by CME certification is an essential requirement.

CLINICAL INVOLVEMENT

Interventional radiology involves interaction with patients and their families, taking decisions and judging outcome and risks. Most important is the clinical evaluation and management of patients with diseases or conditions amenable to image-guided interventions. The IR as a clinician should keep the following questions in mind when entering into a patient consultation: Is the proposed procedure necessary? Is the patient suitable or fit for the procedure? What is the potential for harm? Are there better alternatives for the patient?

For these reasons an IR should be clinically trained. Clinical involvement may include seeing patients in consultation particularly for complex treatments (see the next section), but this is not always feasible and for more routine work it is often not necessary. It is becoming more common for IRs to have their own clinics and beds. Access to day case and inpatient beds is necessary to optimise provision of an IR service. An on-call service should also be provided on a 24/7 basis, which means having an adequate number of IRs available or providing an on-call service through formation of a network of IRs from adjacent hospitals.

INFORMED CONSENT

Informed consent is an essential requirement in contemporary medicine, especially in cases where there is clinical equipoise, as is sometimes the case in IR treatments. Informed consent should be based on an ethical assessment of the clinical situation, including the invasiveness of the procedure, the clinical indications and not simply on practical issues. Focusing on the whole decision-making process, effective communication and an individualised approach to consent is essential, also because it will reduce much of the patient's anxiety for the procedure to follow. A combination of information both written and verbal is often the best approach. Informed consent should ideally be obtained by the operator performing the procedure or, if this is not possible, the task can be delegated to a suitably trained doctor. Informed consent should also be obtained at least 24 h before any procedure so that the patient has time to digest the information and make an informed decision. The risks, intended benefits and alternatives should be discussed with the patient and any follow-up care that is planned should be itemised. Informed consent is a prerequisite for good clinical IR practice as IR is increasingly the first line of treatment and the interventional radiologist the primary clinician.[1]

IR CHECKLIST

In 2009, Haynes et al. published the results of a study which implemented a 19-item surgical safety checklist to determine whether this checklist could reduce complications and deaths associated with surgery.[2] A significant reduction in the rate of death and complications occurred after the introduction of the surgical safety checklist. The death rate fell from 1.5% before the introduction of the checklist to 0.8% afterwards. The complication rate fell from 11 to 7%. Although complications in IR are significantly fewer than with surgery, patient contact before IR procedures is often quite short, and sometimes it is difficult for the interventionalist to gather all the necessary clinical information in a timely manner. This increases the risk of complications. A standarised checklist has the advantage of ensuring that human error, in terms of forgetting key steps in patient preparation, intraprocedural care and postoperative care are not overlooked.[3] This checklist can be downloaded and modified through <http://www.cirse.org/files/files/Profession/IR_Checklist_new.pdf>.

However, the patient safety checklist is only one part of a comprehensive patient safety strategy. Regular morbidity and mortality meetings, reporting of errors, participation in hospital risk management committees and a culture of patient safety are all important items in the overall strategy for patient safety. In an ideal world, competence should match performance but this is not always the case. Performance may be hindered by both system and individual influences. Individual influences on performance can be aided by a lifelong commitment to learning, while system influences may be difficult to deal with and may involve not peforming some procedures if the necessary support is not available locally.

COAGULATION

Management of coagulation status and haemostasis risk in percutaneous image-guided interventions is very important. Haemorrhage is a major complication of IR procedures and guidelines for the management of coagulation status and haemostasis risk are available.[4] IR procedures can be divided into two categories: those with low and those with moderate risk of bleeding. For each category special attention should be given to the clotting status of the patient. In elective treatments, the coagulation status should be optimised unless there are other important contraindications to stopping anticoagulation. General rules for haemostasis management are given in Table 83-1.

TABLE 83-1 **IR Procedure Categories: Haemorrhagic Risk**

Low Risk of Haemorrhage		
Vascular • Dialysis access interventions • Venography • Central line removal • IVC filter placement • PICC line placement **Non-Vascular** • Drainage catheter exchange • Superficial abscess drainage	• INR: Routinely recommended for patients receiving warfarin anticoagulation or with known or suspected liver disease • Activated PTT: Routinely recommended for patients receiving intravenous unfractionated heparin	• INR > 2.0: Threshold for treatment (i.e., FFP, vitamin K) • PTT: No consensus • Platelets: Transfusion recommended for counts < 50,000/µL
Moderate Risk of Haemorrhage		
Vascular • Angiography, arterial and venous intervention with access size up to 7Fr **Non-Vascular** • Intra-abdominal, chest wall or retroperitoneal abscess drainage or biopsy • Lung biopsy • Transabdominal liver biopsy (core needle) • Percutaneous cholecystostomy • Gastrostomy tube: initial placement • Radiofrequency ablation: straightforward • Spine procedures (vertebroplasty, kyphoplasty, lumbar puncture, epidural injection, facet block)	• INR: Routinely recommended for patients receiving warfarin anticoagulation or with known or suspected liver disease • Activated PTT: Routinely recommended for patients receiving intravenous unfractionated heparin	• INR: Correct above 1.5. • Activated PTT: No consensus (trend toward correcting for values _1.5 times control, 73%) • Platelets: Transfusion recommended for counts > 50,000/µL • Hematocrit: No recommended threshold for transfusion • Plavix (clopidogrel): Withhold for 5 days before procedure • Aspirin: Do not withhold • Low-molecular-weight heparin (therapeutic dose): Withhold one dose before procedure

CONTRAST MEDIUM ALLERGY

Contrast medium carries a risk for allergic reactions, but this has been reduced to a very low level since the advent of low-osmolar contrast media. A treatment protocol for anaphylaxis and allergy should be available in the interventional suite. Patients with known previous allergic reactions to contrast media should be pretreated with steroids. An oral regimen often used is dose 1, prednisone 50 mg 13 h prior; dose 2, prednisone 50 mg 7 h prior; and dose 3 (final dose), prednisone 50 mg 1 h prior to the intervention. If oral prednisone is not an option for the patient one of the following equivalent alternatives should be considered: 8 mg Decadron (dexamethasone) IV × 3 doses starting 13 h prior to intervention or 200 mg Solu-Cortef (hydrocortisone) × 3 doses starting 13 h prior to the procedure.

KIDNEY FUNCTION

Low-osmolar contrast medium has a small but definite benefit over high-osmolar contrast media for patients with pre-existing renal impairment.[5] Pre-procedural hydration may have a protective effect in high-risk patients and some newer drugs may also have a role in protection from contrast medium-induced nephrotoxicity (CIN). For the purposes of this standard, CIN as a major complication is clinically defined as an elevation of serum creatinine requiring care which delays discharge or results in unexpected admission, readmission or permanent impairment of renal function. This definition focuses on the outcome of renal impairment, which is the central issue in any monitoring programme. The threshold chosen is 0.2% and is based on consensus and a review of the pertinent literature. Three factors have been associated with an increased risk of contrast-induced nephropathy: pre-existing renal insufficiency (such as creatinine clearance <60 mL/min (1.00 mL/s)), pre-existing diabetes and reduced intravascular volume.

Adenosine antagonists such as the methylxanthines theophylline and aminophylline may help, although studies have produced conflicting results. Administration of sodium bicarbonate 3 mL/kg/h for 1 h before, followed by 1 mL/kg/h for 6 h after administration of contrast medium was found superior to plain saline in one randomised controlled trial of patients with a creatinine level of at least 1.1 mg/dL (97.2 µmol/L).[6]

A randomised controlled trial involving patients with a creatinine over 1.6 mg/dL (140 µmol/L) or creatinine clearance below 60 mL/min studied the use of 1 mL/kg of 0.45% saline per hour for 6–12 h before and after the administration of contrast medium[7] and suggested that *N*-acetylcysteine (NAC) 600 mg orally twice a day, on the day before the procedure, *may* reduce nephropathy, but the results are inconclusive.

SEDATION AND PAIN MANAGEMENT

Sedation and pain management during IR procedures are becoming more important as many complex percutaneous procedures are performed without general anaesthesia. Sedation should, however, only be performed in those circumstances when adequate resuscitative equipment and organisational support are available. For more complex cases in ill patients and in instances where deep sedation is desired, the assistance of a dedicated anaesthetist is mandatory. Conscious sedation is often used in interventional procedures to minimise discomfort. There are three main categories: benzodiazepines, opioids and intravenous anaesthetics. The most common side effects of conscious sedation are described in Table 83-2.

TABLE 83-2 **Common Side Effects of Conscious Sedation**

Hypotension	• Volume replacement therapy by crystalloids or colloids • Sympathomimetic agents such as ephedrine (5–10 mg boluses) or phenylephrine (100 µg boluses)
Respiratory depression	• Reversal of narcotics by naloxone (0.1–0.3 mg IV every 30–60 s, with no specific maximum dose) • Reversal of benzodiazepines by flumazenil (0.2 mg IV every 60 s, usually up to 1 mg) • Respiratory support
Nausea	• Reversal with antiemetic agents
Prolonged sedation	• Reversal with naloxone or flumazenil

Benzodiazepines

These drugs are reasonably safe to use during IR procedures, as their cardiorespiratory suppressive effects are minimal. However, even commonly used doses of benzodiazepines can cause apnoea. Therefore, it is important to adequately monitor patients receiving benzodiazepines. The most commonly used benzodiazepines include midazolam and lorazepam. Midazolam has a rapid onset and short duration of action, which makes it an ideal drug for most interventional procedures.

In patients where a benzodiazepine overdose occurs, **flumazenil** (0.2 mg IV every 60 s, usually up to 1 mg) should be administered.

Opioids

For most interventional radiological procedures, and especially for elderly patients, shorter-acting narcotics like fentanyl and alfentanil are preferred. The regular dose for fentanyl is 25–50 µg IV. Duration of effect becomes longer with higher doses/infusions

In case of opioid overdose, **naloxone** (0.1–0.3 mg IV every 30–60 s, with no specific maximum dose) should be administered.

Intravenous Anaesthetics

Ketamine and propofol can be used for conscious sedation in IR procedures. These drugs should, however, only be reserved for situations in which all necessary provisions for administration of general anaesthesia are available, which includes the participation of an anaesthetist.

COMPLICATIONS REGISTER

The periprocedural management of patients undergoing image-guided interventional procedures is continually evolving. Local factors such as procedure types and patient selection will influence management. In addition, advances in technology and image guidance may have a significant effect on periprocedural management. The use of arterial closure devices, smaller-gauge catheters and biopsy devices, adjunctive haemostatic measures such as postbiopsy tract plugging/embolisation and colour flow ultrasonography or computed tomographic fluoroscopy can affect the incidence of periprocedural haemorrhagic complications. One of the most effective methods of improving the safety of IR procedures is to maintain a local complication register and to hold a regular complication meeting. This should lead to improved local procedural guidelines, protocols for interventional radiological procedures and training.

THE INTERVENTIONAL RADIOLOGY SUITE

Common medications used during arterial interventions and their doses are indicated in Table 83-3.

TABLE 83-3 **Doses of Common Medications Used during Arterial Interventions**

Medication	Dose	Use
Glyceryl trinitrate (nitroglycerin)	0.1 mg/mL/dose IA, repeated up to 3 times	Treatment of vasospasm
Heparin	75–100 IU/kg IV	Prevent arterial thrombosis
Protamine	10 mg IV per 1000 IU heparin	Heparin reversal
Papaverine	1 mg/kg IA	Treatment of vasospasm
Lidocaine	0.5 mL/kg (5 mg/kg) 1% (without adrenaline)	Local anaesthesia

INVENTORY

An inventory of interventional radiological devices, catheters and guidewires should be available. Also the essential materials to deal with complications, such as covered stents, in case of an arterial rupture after angioplasty, should be part of the inventory. In general it is recommended to keep the stock small, as technology changes rapidly and most devices have a limited period of sterility. No specific recommendations can be given here and local practice will dictate how sufficient stock and stock control is achieved. In many European countries separate storage of interventional equipment outside the interventional room is required by hospital infection committees.[8]

For a full list of references, please see ExpertConsult.

CHAPTER 84

Angiography: Principles, Techniques and Complications

James E. Jackson • James F.M. Meaney

CHAPTER OUTLINE

INTRODUCTION

The non-invasive imaging of blood vessels continues to evolve and there have been significant new developments in cross-sectional imaging techniques since the 5th edition. As discussed in the previous edition of this textbook these have made many diagnostic catheter angiographic techniques almost obsolete; this is a welcome change as they are clearly less invasive and, therefore, safer and will in many instances give more diagnostic information than could be obtained by conventional catheter arteriography because of the concurrent visualisation of surrounding tissues and the ability to reconstruct the data in any plane.[1] A good understanding of the basic principles and techniques of catheter angiography remains essential, however, for those intending to become interventional radiologists and this information is still included in this chapter. The newer cross-sectional techniques for imaging blood vessels will, however, be discussed first as these will, quite rightly, be requested before (and often instead of) conventional catheter angiography.

Ultrasound plays a key role in a few areas, notably evaluation of the carotid bifurcation and follow-up of peripheral bypass grafts for patency, but it falls to CT and MR to provide detailed information of the vasculature for most other territories. The major advance in CT has been the introduction of multiple rows of detectors, which, in combination with a continuously rotating X-ray source and continuous table movement, allows rapid imaging of a large region of interest during first pass of an intravenously injected bolus. For MR, the key development has been the progressive increase in gradient speed, which, when coupled with parallel imaging that greatly increases acquisition speed, also allows rapid imaging of a large region of interest during first pass of an intravenously injected bolus. MR has the additional advantage that for some indications intravenous contrast injection is not necessary.

MULTIDETECTOR CT ANGIOGRAPHY (MDCTA) TECHNIQUES

The development of CT equipment combining a fan-shaped X-ray source, multiple detector rows and continuous table movement has led to the ability to acquire image data from a large tissue volume in a short time period.[1] Two major advantages result from rapid CTA acquisition times: firstly, blood vessels of the thorax and abdomen can be imaged during breath-holding; and secondly, it is possible to capture the relatively short 'arterial' phase following injection of contrast medium intravenously. Optimal imaging of the vessels during the first arterial passage of contrast material requires both a relatively rapid IV injection of iodinated contrast medium (usually 3–5 mL/s) to ensure adequate arterial opacification, and data acquisition at the appropriate time of vascular enhancement. The latter can be estimated based upon the 'expected' time of arrival of the contrast medium within the organ being imaged, but as this varies between patients it can be inaccurate and may result in poor-quality studies. These have been replaced by automated contrast bolus detection techniques in which the 'arrival' of contrast medium within a large vessel is measured on images obtained at a single level and data acquisition is initiated when a certain increase in density within the region of interest has been reached. 'Tight' boluses of contrast medium using a chaser of normal saline may be useful not only to improve vascular opacification but also to reduce the total volume of contrast medium required.

Rapid acquisition of images results in large data sets; for example, comprehensive evaluation of the peripheral vasculature from the level of the renal arteries to the feet with an acquired slice thickness of 0.8 mm will generate approximately 1500 images. Whilst all the diagnostic information is available in this data set, evaluation of the source images is not only extremely time-consuming but also confusing and is helped considerably by reconstruction of the data in axial, coronal and oblique planes without loss of resolution, so-called multiplanar reconstruction (MPR). Tortuous vessels can be 'straightened' by curved MPR to aid in the assessment of luminal narrowing caused by, for example, atheromatous disease or encasement by tumour. Maximum intensity projection (MIP) and volume rendering (VR) techniques are additional tools that help greatly in the assessment of blood vessels.[2] Each of these reconstruction techniques has its advantages and disadvantages:

1. *MPR* is very useful for the rapid review of blood vessels in any plane, including the relationship to surrounding bone and soft tissues. It also allows the assessment of vessel walls that might be obscured in MIP and VR techniques by, for example, calcification or endoluminal stents. Each image, however, gives only one 'slice' of information and multiple separate images are often required to demonstrate the vessel in its entirety.
2. *MIP techniques* produce a planar image from a volume of data within which the pixel values are determined by the highest voxel value in a ray projected along the data set in a specified direction. The images format mimics a conventional arteriogram but a disadvantage of this technique is that any tissue of high density (such as bone, fresh haematoma or vascular calcification) will be reprojected in the final image and may misrepresent the blood vessel. This is a common cause of overestimation of vascular stenoses.
3. *Volume-rendering techniques* assess the entire volume of data with an attenuation threshold for display and produce a three-dimensional image. Typically, tissues are assigned a colour that is dependent upon their attenuation values, facilitating the differentiation of structures of differing density. The final images can be rotated in real time to find the best projection to display anatomy and pathology and this is the most important feature of this technique. Vascular stenoses can be overestimated, however, and small vessels may not be clearly visualised.

It should be remembered that, whilst these post-processing techniques are very helpful for diagnostic assessment and for display in multidisciplinary team meetings, the axial source images are essential and allow the operator to distinguish between artefact and disease when an abnormality is suggested on reformatted views.

MAGNETIC RESONANCE ANGIOGRAPHY (MRA) TECHNIQUES

Magnetic resonance angiography is a method for generating images of blood vessels with magnetic resonance imaging (MRI). With improved understanding of the nature of the signals emanating from blood vessels on MR images, it became evident that rather than simply contributing a source of artefacts on MR images, flow phenomena could be harnessed to generate diagnostic 'angiograms'.[3] Although MR angiograms can be generated without use of contrast medium, non-contrast techniques suffer from frequent artefacts and are time inefficient. Contrast-enhanced techniques, which can be completed within seconds rather than the several minutes of earlier methods, have revolutionised clinical practice over the last decade and extended the reach of MRA into all vascular territories with the exception of the coronary arteries.[3]

Contrast Mechanisms

Unenhanced Time-of-Flight (TOF) MRA

TOF angiography relies on the fact that the blood enters the volume under consideration with relatively high velocity and traverses it rapidly, so that it receives very few radio frequency (RF) pulses.[3] In order to maximise inflow effect, protons within the imaging volume must be replenished between successive repetition times (TRs), although maximal inflow may not be necessary in clinical practice and some trade-offs can be accepted. Oblique course of the blood vessel being imaged in relation to the slice orientation and short TRs adversely affect signal-to-noise ratios (SNR) as a result of protons under these circumstances experiencing more RF pulses whilst in the imaging slice. The severity and length of stenoses also tend to be overestimated on TOF MRA images because of intravoxel dephasing secondary to turbulent, slow or pulsatile flow.[3]

As a result of these limitations, TOF MRA has failed to offer a viable non-invasive screening alternative to conventional arteriography, and has not had a major impact on clinical practice outside the brain, where it remains the primary approach for evaluation of the intracranial arteries.

Phase-Contrast MRA

Phase-contrast angiography (PCA) is now seldom used in clinical MRA. The methodology underpinning the technique is somewhat complex and, like TOF MRA, images are prone to artefacts and data acquisition is lengthy.[4]

Contrast-Enhanced MRA (CEMRA)

Because of their unmatched high contrast-to-noise ratios, high spatial resolution, rapid speed of acquisition and relative freedom from artefacts, contrast-enhanced techniques have almost universally replaced non-contrast techniques in clinical practice.[5–9] Unlike TOF and PCA techniques, where the intravascular signal is dependent on inherent properties of flow and is, therefore, at the mercy of alterations in flow rate secondary to vascular disease, intravascular signal for contrast-enhanced MRA (CEMRA) depends on a T1 shortening effect induced by the injection of a paramagnetic contrast agent (usually gadolinium based). Images can, therefore, be acquired in any plane, including coronal, which affords the best anatomical coverage for virtually all vascular territories outside the brain.[5] In addition, the ability to exploit ultrafast 3D acquisitions (by using the shortest TRs possible and parallel imaging), allows rapid image acquisition that can easily be accommodated within a single breath-hold, an important factor when imaging in the chest and abdomen. In order to generate 'selective' arteriograms, images are acquired during the first arterial passage of the contrast agent before its arrival within the veins. The synchronisation of data acquisition with the peak arterial bolus is one of the major challenges of CEMRA, as the rate of transit of contrast medium from the peripheral vein injection site to the vessel of interest is affected by a number of factors, including heart rate, stroke volume and the presence or absence of proximal steno-occlusive lesions. Although the circulation time can be measured using a test bolus, or can be inferred by making some assumptions about the patient's cardiovascular status, the process is now automated by employing an MR fluoroscopic approach—a technique that demonstrates contrast medium arrival in real time on the display monitor, thus signalling the appropriate time for data acquisition.[7,8]

The unique nature of k-space (the array of data from which the final image is generated), whereby the central lines determine image contrast and the peripheral lines determine image resolution, can be uniquely exploited to generate CEMRA images with unrivalled signal-to-noise ratios. In situations where breath-holding is not required (e.g. vascular territories which do not move with respiration such as the peripheral arteries and carotid arteries), assuming acquisition of the contrast-defining central lines of k-space is completed during the arterial peak, the continued collection of resolution-defining peripheral lines of k-space during venous enhancement does not result in venous contamination of the images. CEMRA is now the standard of reference for MRA against which all new techniques must be measured.

New Non-Contrast Techniques

Because of concerns regarding nephrogenic systemic fibrosis,[10] there has been renewed interest in non-contrast techniques for body (extracranial) imaging where TOF and PCA techniques are limited.[11,12] A new family of 'balanced' techniques, where image contrast reflects the ratio of T1/T2, have been developed which portray the vessels as high signal structures. Background tissues are suppressed and either arteries or veins can be highlighted. In many instances the information provided allows contrast injection to be avoided.[11,12]

CLINICAL APPLICATIONS OF CTA AND MRA

Although CT and MR generate broadly similar angiographic images, the former is still favoured in many instances for a number of reasons: MR remains less widely available than CT especially out-of-hours and requires more expertise and operator input; although the time required for acquisition of first pass contrast-enhanced MRA and CTA is similar, the set-up time for MRA is greater; and it is more difficult to monitor unstable patients in the MR environment.[1]

It is clear, however, that the role of MRA has markedly increased since the last edition of this book, particularly in elective studies of thoracic and abdominal vessels, and it remains important in patients in whom contrast medium is contraindicated.

Thorax

Thoracic Aorta and Great Arteries

Because of the relatively large size of these vessels, conditions such as aneurysms, stenoses, aberrant anatomy and the relationship between blood vessels and adjacent tumours are equally well demonstrated with both CTA or MRA (Figs. 84-1 and 84-2).[13,14] With improvements in spatial resolution, the blood supply to the thoracic cord can be delineated with either technique, information that is useful to the surgeon and helps prevent spinal cord infarction in patients undergoing repair of thoracic aortic aneurysms.

Pulmonary Arteries

CTA (CTPA – CT pulmonary angiography) has been the technique of choice for detection of pulmonary embolism for at least the last decade (Fig. 84-3).[15,16] Advantages include high accuracy compared to catheter angiography in a wide range of reported studies, wide availability (including out of hours), short total examination time, ease of patient monitoring during the study and a high degree of clinician confidence in the test. Although several studies have established high accuracy for MRA compared with pulmonary angiography for the evaluation of suspected pulmonary embolism, it is not widely used clinically[17,18] (Fig. 84-4). Reasons for this include a reluctance to refer potentially unstable patients to MRI and the availability of CT pulmonary angiography.

Improvements in spatial resolution for MRA and additional techniques, such as MR perfusion and ventilation (mirroring the ventilation and perfusion components of nuclear medicine studies albeit at much higher resolution), offer additional functionality to determine the location and distribution of small emboli and may improve the acceptability of MR for PE.[17,18]

Abdomen

Abdominal Aorta and Abdominal Veins

Assessment of the abdomen in virtually all patients with suspected acute vascular emergencies such as abdominal aortic aneurysm rupture and acute mesenteric ischaemia is performed with CTA but the elective assessment of vascular pathology within the abdomen can be performed with either CTA or MRA.[5–7,19,20] Abdominal aortic aneurysm morphology can be equally well assessed by CTA and MRA (external dimensions, tortuosity and relationship to visceral arteries) but calcium within the wall is

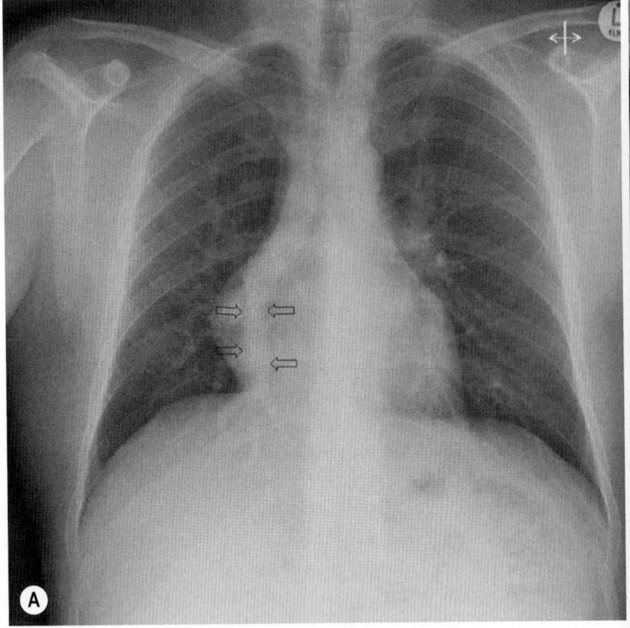

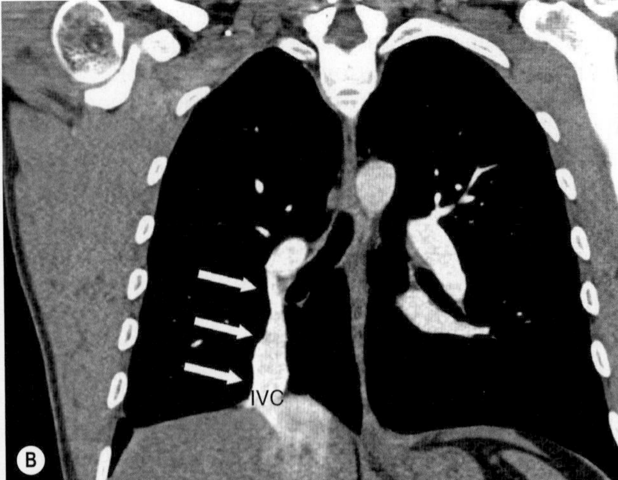

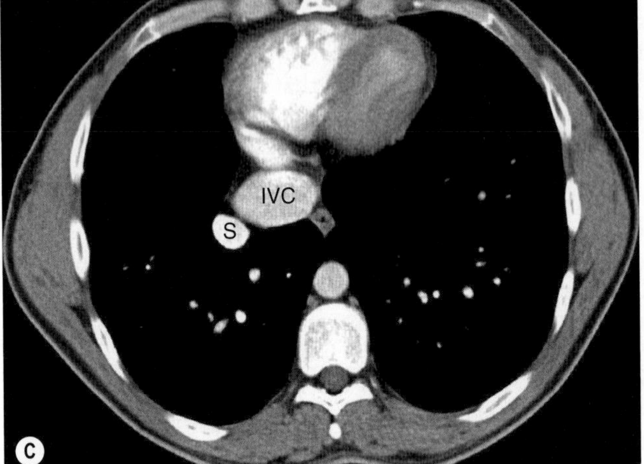

FIGURE 84-1 ■ **Asymptomatic patient undergoing routine preoperative assessment.** CXR (A) shows an unusual tubular structure (arrows) projected behind the right heart border. Coronal reformat (B) from CTA demonstrates an abnormal vein (arrows) draining from the right lung into the IVC. The axial source image (C) demonstrates the vein (S) just before it joins the IVC. The appearance is that of a Scimitar syndrome, a variant or anomalous pulmonary venous drainage in which part or all of the right lower lobe drains into the inferior vena cava.

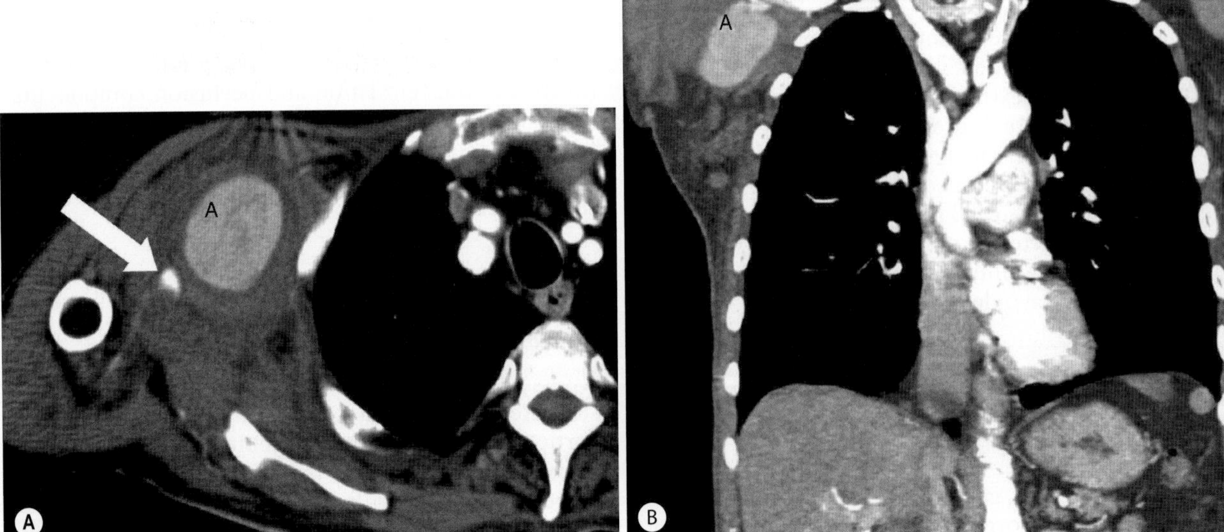

FIGURE 84-2 ■ **Patient with embolic episode to right arm.** CTA in axial (A), coronal (B), sagittal (C) reformat demonstrates a large pseudoaneurysm arising from the subclavian artery (denoted by the arrow). The arrow denotes the subclavian artery and A, the aneurysm sac in all 3 parts.

Continued on following page

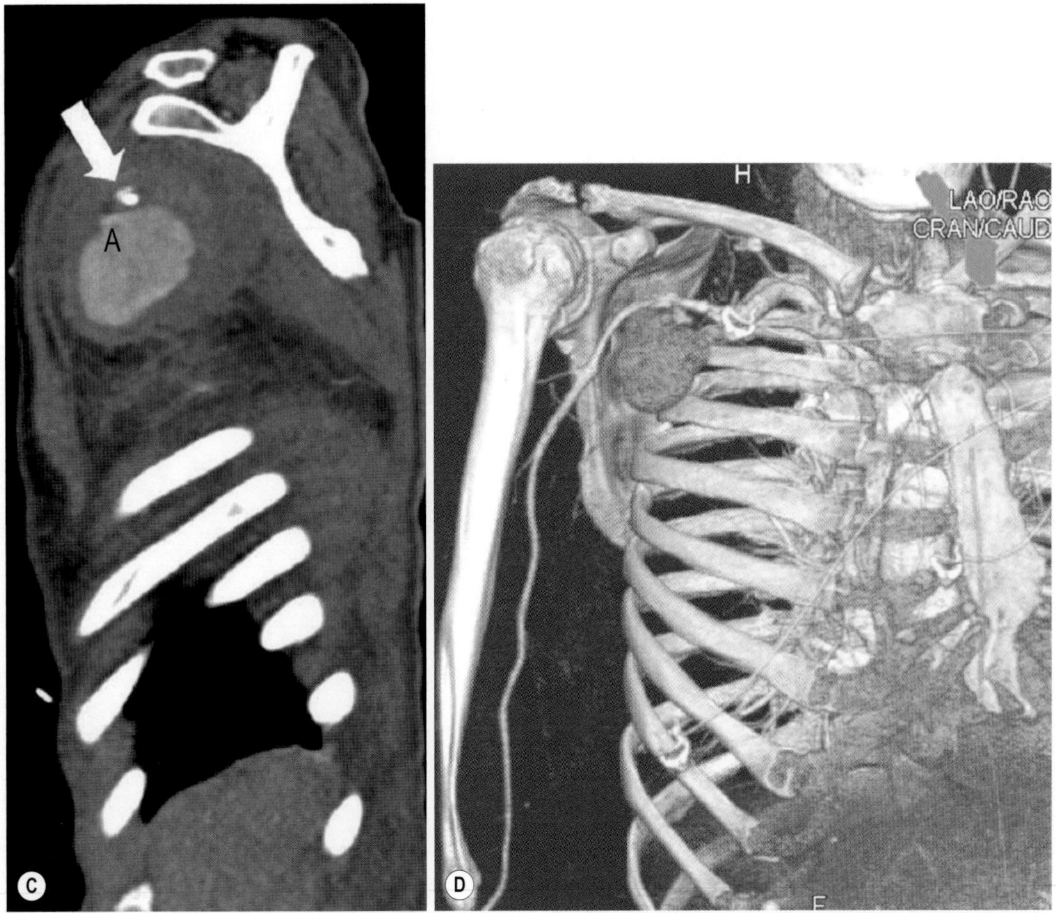

FIGURE 84-2, Continued ■ Surface shaded display (D) shows the relationship of the aneurysm to the parent artery and the status of the distal run-off arteries.

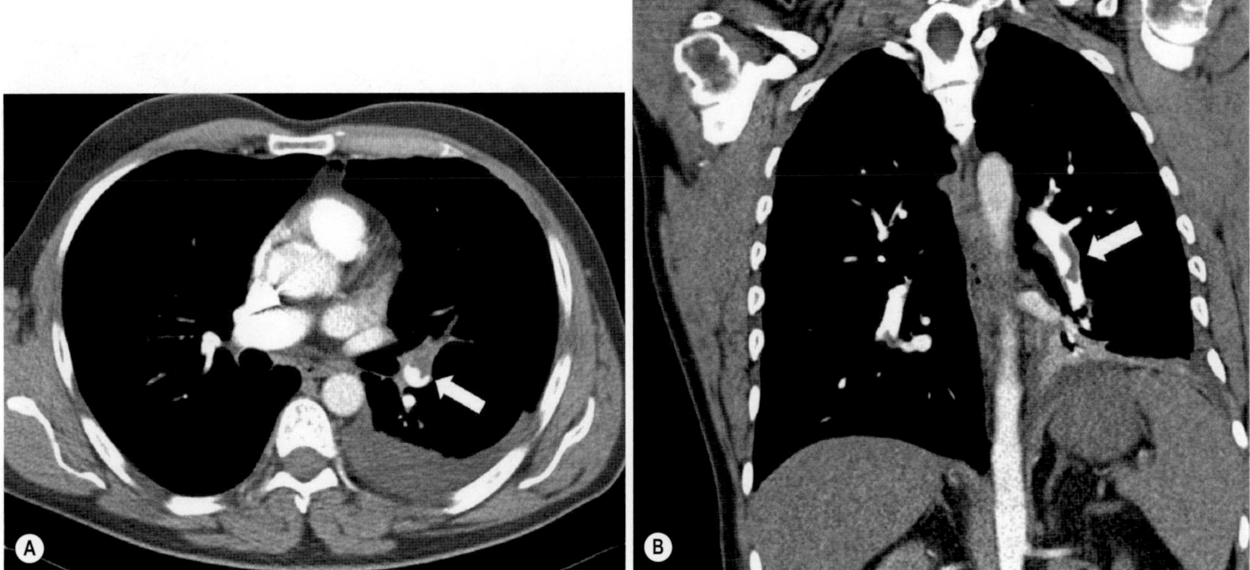

FIGURE 84-3 ■ **CTPA in a patient presenting with left pleuritic chest pain and shortness of breath.** (A) There is a large filling defect within the left lower lobe pulmonary artery (arrow) consistent with acute pulmonary embolism. Coronal reformat (B) confirms the extensive clot (arrow).

Continued on following page

better demonstrated by CTA; for this reason aneurysm assessment before and after endovascular stenting is usually performed with CTA.[19]

Thrombosis of the spleno-portal system or IVC is usually detected by performing delayed imaging after acquisition of the arterial phase for CTA or MRA (Fig. 84-5). An advantage of MRA is that venographic images can also be acquired using a non-contrast technique.

Renal, Mesenteric and Hepatic Arteries

The assessment of native and transplant renal arteries and the staging of hepatopancreaticobiliary neoplasm is well performed with both CTA and MRA, supplemented by additional standard imaging of the parenchyma as indicated.[19,20] CEMRA, however, has many advantages for imaging the renal arteries and proximal mesenteric arteries.[10] (Fig. 84-6). Numerous studies and meta-analyses attest to the accuracy of MRA in the assessment of significant visceral artery stenotic disease.[8] An additional significant benefit of MRA lies in its ability to measure

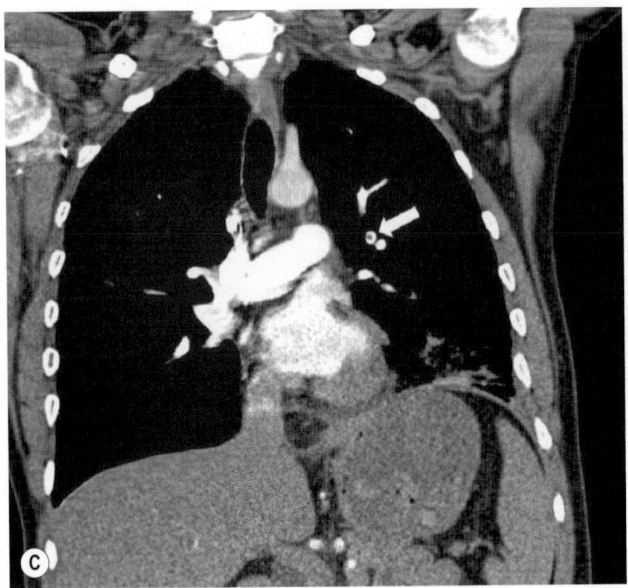

FIGURE 84-3, Continued ■ (C) A more anterior image confirms further embolism to the upper lobe pulmonary artery (Arrow points to filling defect of embolus within the artery).

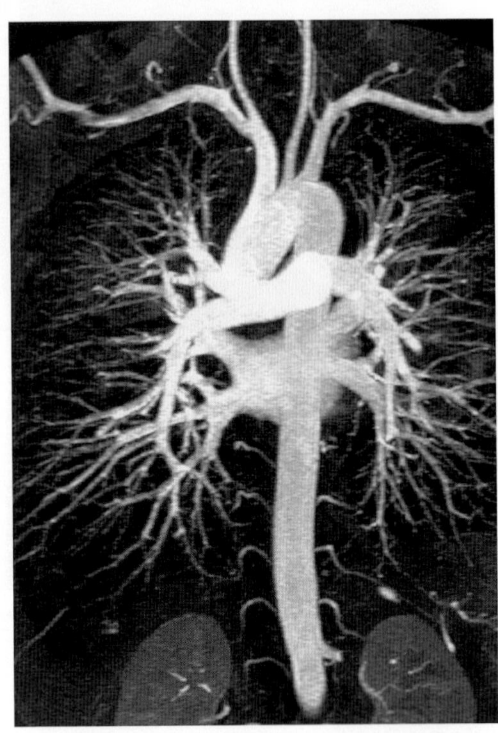

FIGURE 84-4 ■ Normal pulmonary MRA.

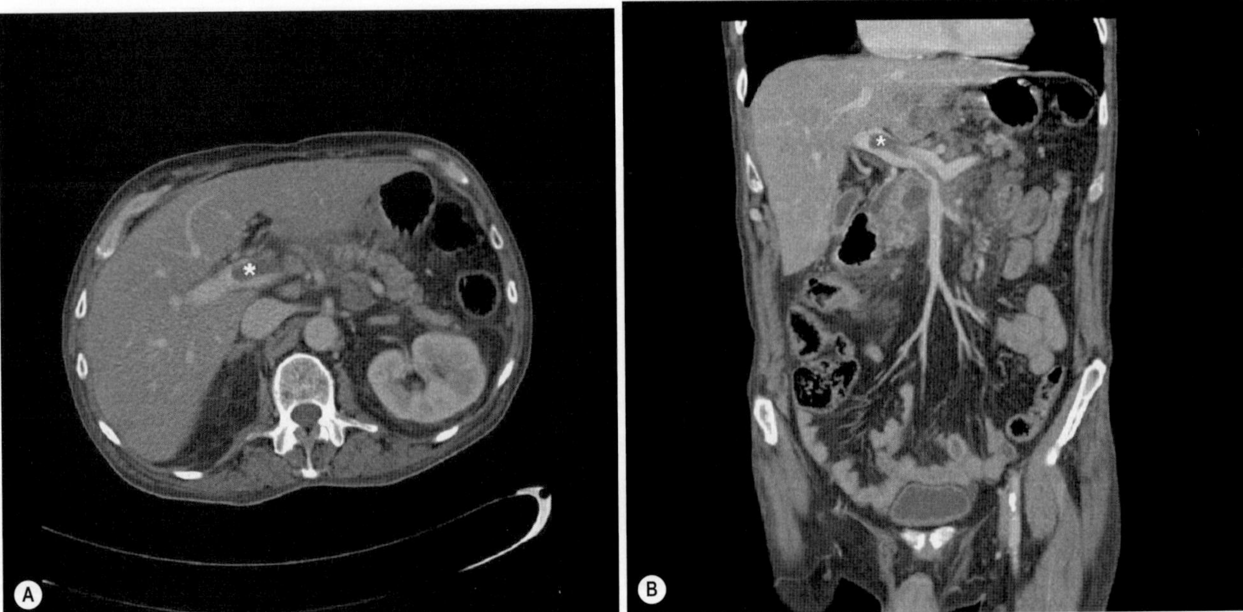

FIGURE 84-5 ■ CT venogram of the portal veins demonstrates acute thrombus (*) within the main portal vein on axial image (A) and coronal reformat (B).

directly the flow rate to each kidney using a two-dimensional (2D) cardiac-triggered, phase-contrast approach, which facilitates both the assessment of end-organ damage and the likelihood of success of transluminal angioplasty.[1]

As mentioned above, renewed interest in non-contrast techniques has led to the development of reasonably robust techniques which benefit the patient in avoiding the risks of contrast agents in patients with renal impairment or other contraindication to gadolinium contrast agents.[11,12]

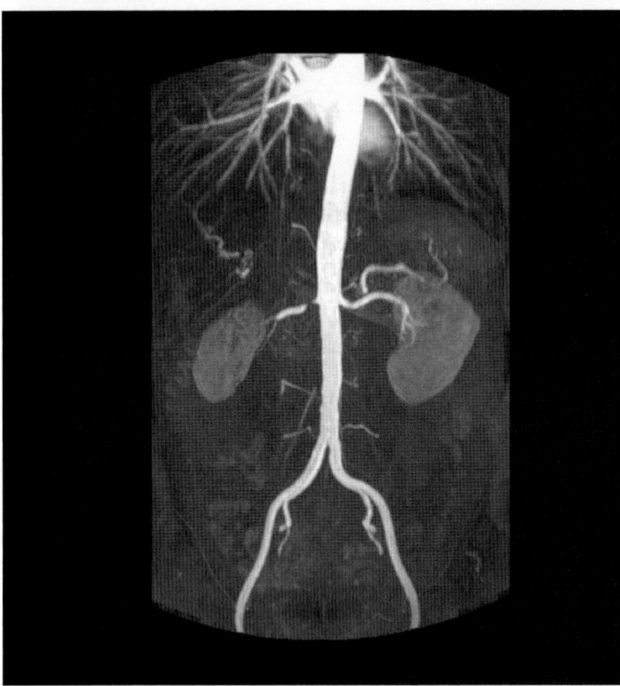

FIGURE 84-6 ■ Patient with severe hypertension refractory to treatment. CEMRA demonstrates severe proximal right renal artery stenosis with reduced size of the right kidney.

Carotid and Vertebral Arteries and Intracranial Arteries

TOF MRA remains the technique of choice for depiction of the intracranial arteries (Figs. 84-7 to 84-10).[1,3] Because of the requirement accurately to differentiate stenoses at a 70% cut-off within a relatively small (internal carotid) artery, there are stringent spatial resolution requirements for carotid evaluation[9] (Fig. 84-9). For CTA, excellent quality is achieved but the presence of intramural calcification (calcified plaque) at the bifurcation may interfere with accurate stenosis grading, whereas the signal void of calcium on MR does not interfere with image interpretation.[1]

A further advantage of MRA lies in the assessment of patients with suspected subclavian steal syndrome. Although both CTA and MRA are equal in their ability to detect subclavian stenosis, the reversed flow within the vertebral artery that confirms the diagnosis can only be made with MRA.[1]

A particular situation exists in the imaging of carotid and vertebral artery dissections where imaging of the lumen alone with CTA or MRA simply demonstrates narrowing indistinguishable from other causes.[1,9] In all cases of suspected carotid or vertebral dissection, therefore, pre-contrast T1- and T2-weighted fat-saturation MR images should be performed, as these will demonstrate the bright appearance of an intramural haematoma, which is typically crescent-shaped. Failure to do so results in the identification of a focal stenosis only, and robs the patient of the opportunity to receive anticoagulation therapy, the treatment of choice for dissection.

Peripheral Arteries

For assessment of the peripheral arteries, both CTA and MRA are well validated.[7,21,22] In the peripheral arteries, as in most other areas, TOF MRA has been superseded by CEMRA.[7,23] Although the spatial coverage offered by single-field-of-view imaging is insufficient to address all of the relevant anatomy, the introduction of moving-table

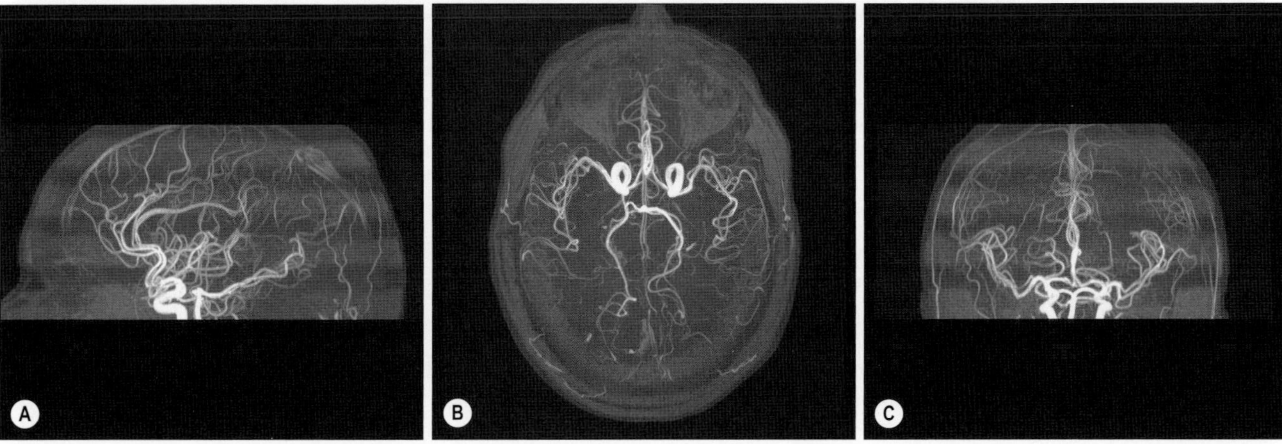

FIGURE 84-7 ■ Normal time-of-flight MRA performed at 3.0 tesla. Note excellent detail of the intracranial arteries on lateral (A), basal (B) and anteroposterior (C) MIPs.

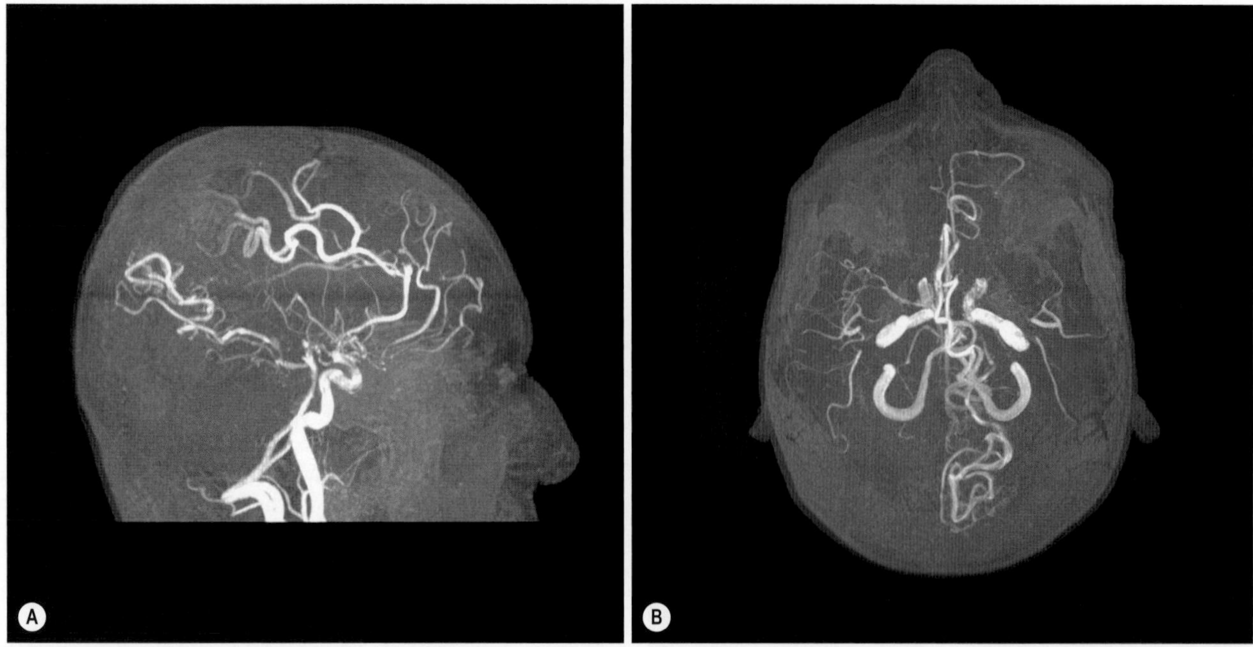

FIGURE 84-8 ■ Patient with left cortical blindness. Lateral (A) and basal (B) projections from TOF MRA demonstrate a large left occipital arteriovenous malformation.

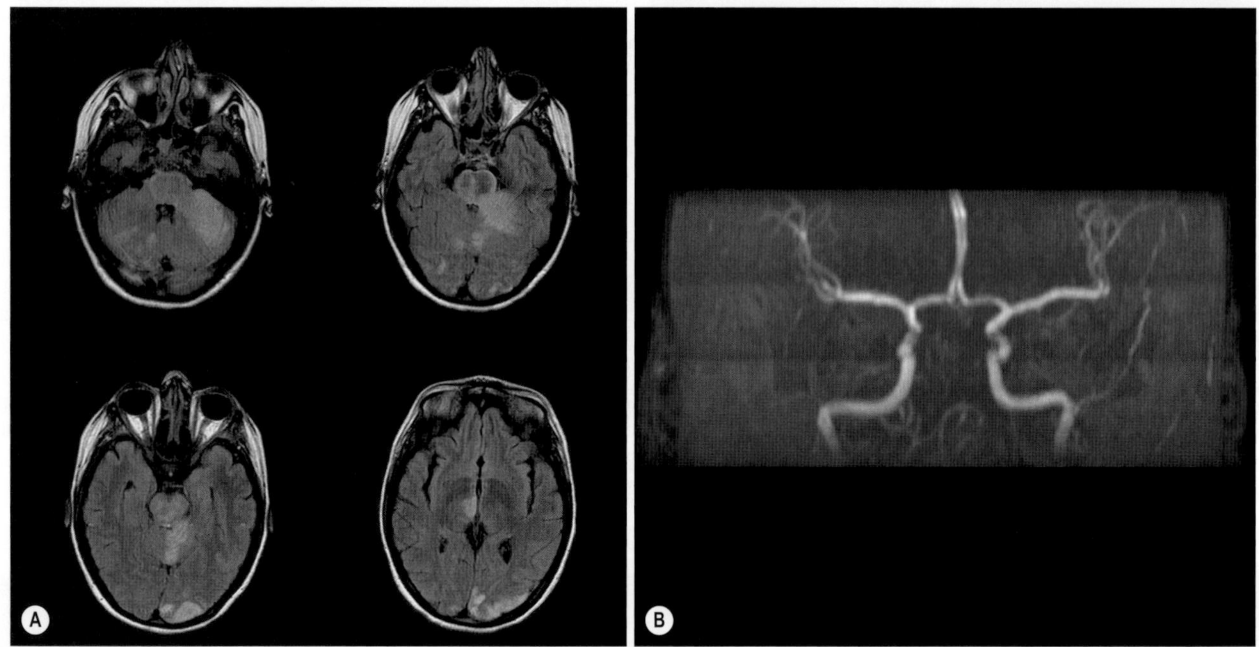

FIGURE 84-9 ■ Patient admitted unconscious and unresponsive. FLAIR images (A) demonstrate widespread bilateral parenchymal abnormality affecting both cerebellar hemispheres, pons, midbrain, right thalamus and left occipital lobes. TOF MRA in anteroposterior (B) and basal (C) projections demonstrates absence of the basilar artery, indicating thrombosis.

Continued on following page

MRA has opened the way for routine non-invasive MRA of the entire run-off arteries in a short timeframe (<20-min examination)[23] (Figs. 84-11 and Fig. 84-12). The major limitation of moving-table MRA is venous contamination in the legs. Methods to eliminate this include the use of tourniquets inflated to subsystolic pressures to delay onset of venous enhancement, careful attention to detail in setting up the examination (to avoid any redundancy in anatomical coverage), the use of high parallel-imaging factors and the exploitation of ultra-short TR imaging.[23]

FUTURE DIRECTIONS

Following the breathtaking developments in both CT and MR technology over the last two decades, clinicians now have at their fingertips readily available, reproducible

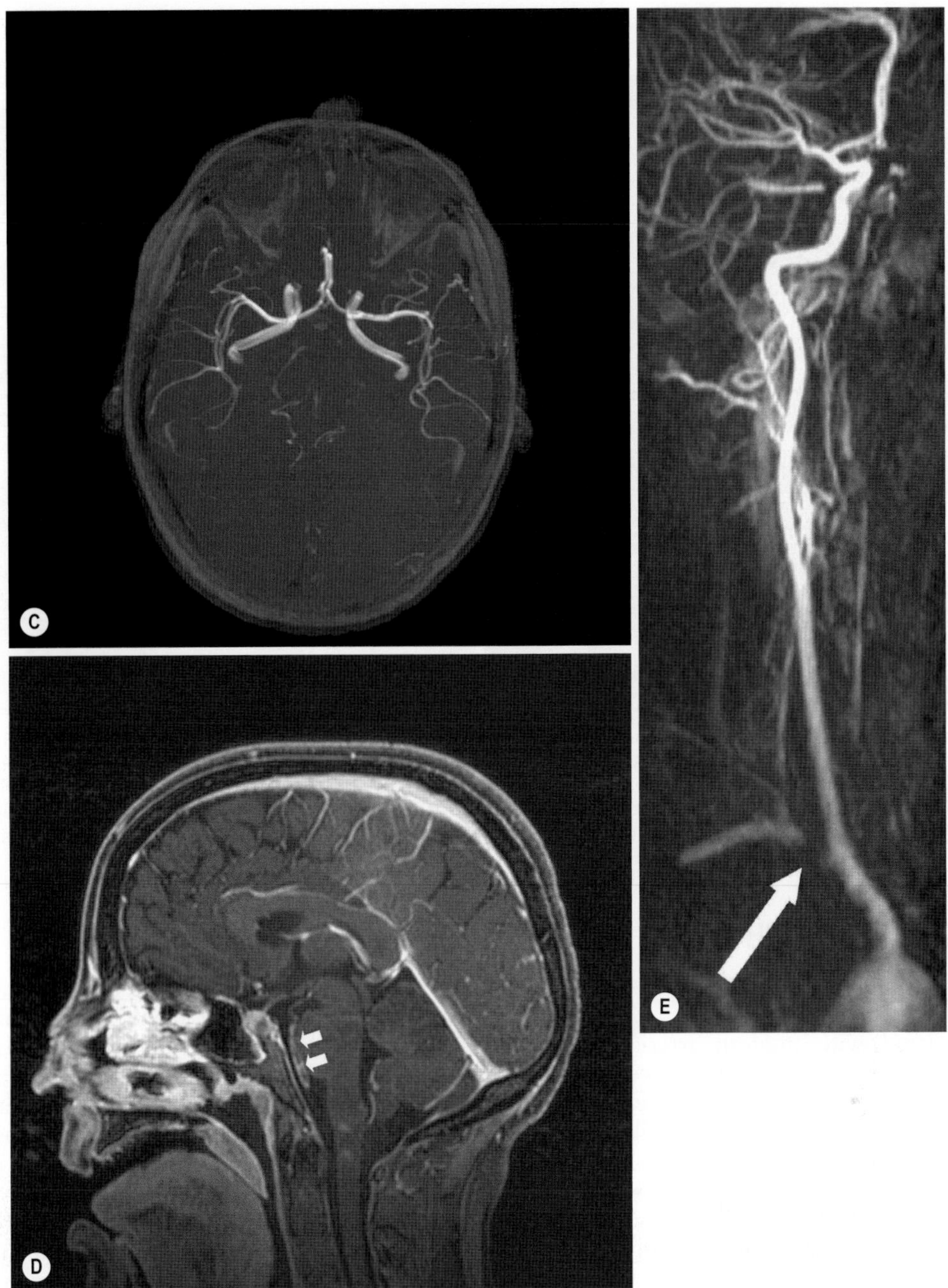

FIGURE 84-9, Continued ■ This is confirmed on the post-contrast sagittal midline image (D), which demonstrates intravascular thrombus within the basilar artery (arrows). Contrast-enhanced MRA of the neck vessels (E) demonstrates a tight stenosis at the origin of the right subclavian artery (arrow), thought to be the source of embolism. Note also irregularity of the right vertebral artery consistent with atheroma.

and accurate modalities in both CTA and MRA for non-invasive assessment of virtually all vascular territories. CTA offers ease of use, rapid performance, wide availability and ease of interpretation. MRA offers virtually identical, or, in some cases, improved 'road-mapping' potential and, in addition to the widely implemented contrast-enhanced techniques, a number of non-contrast techniques that offer truly non-invasive vascular imaging. Additionally, it allows assessment of functional aspects of flow and the ability to perform follow-up studies without risk to the patient. Further improvements in spatial resolution can be expected in CTA but this is likely to result in only modest diagnostic benefit given the excellent image quality already achievable. Improvements in spatial resolution are also likely in MRA, together with greatly improved temporal resolution facilitated by better coil efficiency and new parallel imaging methods that increase acquisition speed and/or spatial resolution by a factor of 2–16. 3-Tesla imaging (3T imaging),[24] new targeted contrast agents and the potential for routine functional imaging of end-organ damage offer exciting prospects for the future.

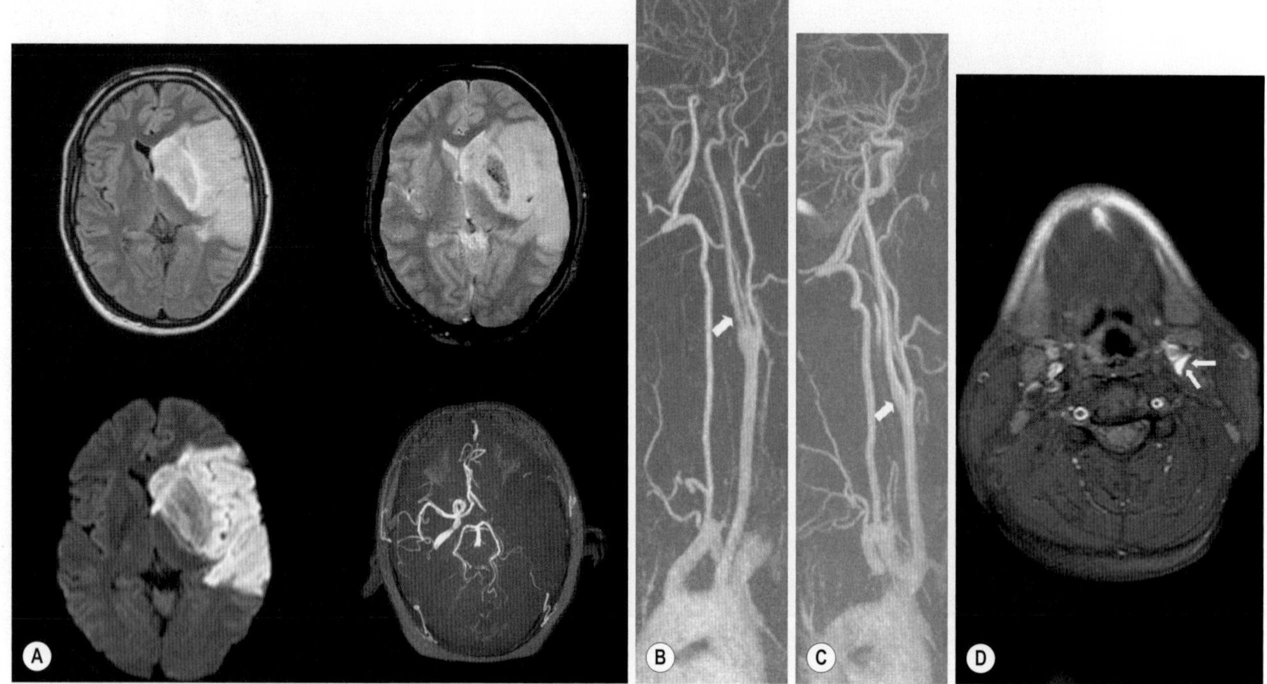

FIGURE 84-10 ■ Patient admitted with sudden-onset dense right hemiplegia. (A) Panel of 4 images (top left FLAIR, top left GRE T2, bottom left DWI, bottom right TOF MRA) demonstrates widespread acute left middle cerebral artery infarction with some haemorrhage and mass effect secondary to left middle cerebral artery occlusion. CEMRA (B) demonstrates diffuse narrowing of the internal carotid artery at the bulb (arrow). The normal right side is shown for comparison (arrow denotes normal carotid bulb) (C). Axial fat-saturation image (D) through the area of narrowing shown on (B) demonstrates crescentic high signal intensity (arrows), confirming the presence of acute carotid artery dissection.

CATHETER ARTERIOGRAPHY

Technique

The risks associated with modern arteriography are extremely small. Arteriography is still, nevertheless, an 'invasive' procedure and it should never be undertaken unless the radiologist is satisfied that the likely benefits justify the potential risks. An arteriogram should never be carried out simply because it has been scheduled or 'routinely requested' by a clinical team; mistakes inevitably occur and the radiologist responsible for the procedure should be satisfied in every case that proper indications exist for the particular study requested.

Preparation of the Patient

Informed consent should be obtained for arteriography. A doctor, preferably the responsible radiologist or a member of the radiology department, should see the patient before the procedure to explain what is to be done, check that no contraindications to the study exist, check the appropriate pulses and ensure that adequate premedication is arranged. The groin should be shaved if a femoral approach is to be used. It is generally recommended to ask the patient to stop solid foods for a few hours before the procedure but to permit free oral fluids unless general anaesthesia or heavy premedication is being used. Dehydration should be avoided and adequate measures should be taken to avoid this during the procedure and the recovery period.

Contraindications

There are very few absolute contraindications to arteriography but there are many factors that considerably increase the hazards of the technique. Always check that a patient is not pregnant before arteriography, as the radiation dose may be considerable. If arteriography is essential in a pregnant patient, the dose to the fetus should be minimised by protection, field collimation and careful choice of filming sequences. Caution should be exercised in patients on anticoagulant therapy or with other bleeding diatheses. Arteriography should be avoided if possible in such cases; if it is essential, then all possible steps should be taken to correct or improve the coagulation defect before and during the procedure if this is clinically acceptable. Other factors that increase the risk of bleeding from an arterial puncture site include systemic hypertension and disorders predisposing to increased fragility of the vessel wall such as Cushing's syndrome, prolonged steroid treatment and rare connective tissue disorders such as certain Ehlers–Danlos subtypes (especially type IV).

Arteriography may be necessary in a patient with a suspected or known previous adverse reaction to contrast medium and this problem is discussed in Chapter 2. Arteriography can require larger doses of contrast medium than any other radiological procedure and particular care must be exercised in infants and in dehydrated or shocked patients, patients with serious cardiac or respiratory disease, patients in hepatic or renal failure, and other patients with serious metabolic abnormalities.

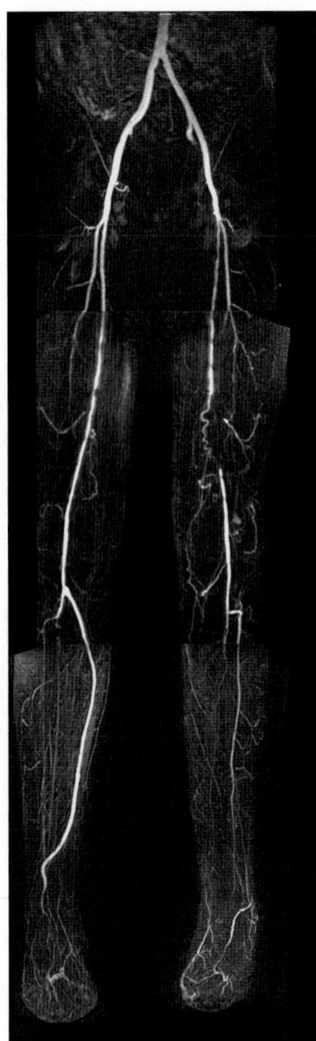

FIGURE 84-11 ■ Peripheral MRA performed using a three-station, moving-table approach. The study demonstrates excellent visualisation of the entire run-off arteries from the mid-abdominal aorta to the level of the pedal arch. Note extensive vascular stenoses and occlusions and a bypass graft from the right popliteal artery to the right anterior tibial artery.

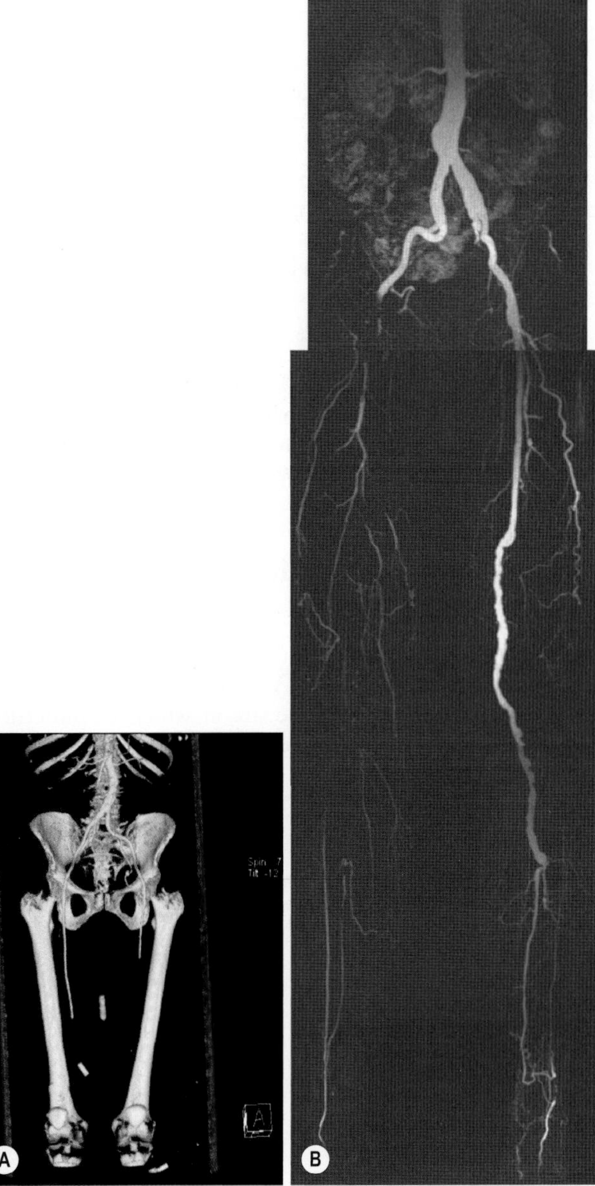

FIGURE 84-12 ■ (A) Patient with acute onset of rest pain in both lower legs. Peripheral CTA using a surface-rendered reformat demonstrates acute cut-off of the superficial femoral arteries on both sides consistent with bilateral acute embolism. (B) Patient with long-standing claudication right leg: peripheral MRA demonstrates occlusion of the right common femoral, superficial femoral and popliteal arteries with reconstitution of flow via collaterals.

Anaesthesia

Most arteriography is performed under local anaesthesia, though general anaesthesia is necessary for babies and young children, for confused, difficult or very nervous patients, and in some complex procedures. Although general anaesthesia can be more pleasant for the patient than local anaesthesia and reduces motion artefact on the radiographs, it nevertheless adds to the risks of arteriography. This is not only because of the (small) risks inherent in general anaesthesia but also because it masks the patient's subjective symptoms and reactions. These may provide the radiologist with immediate warning of a mishap such as the subintimal injection of contrast medium or the inadvertent wedging of the catheter tip in a small artery: a warning that may well prevent more serious injury.

Arterial Puncture

It is often said that the most important part of an angiographic procedure is the initial vessel puncture and there is no doubt that a good technique is likely to make the subsequent angiogram not only more comfortable for the patient but also easier for the angiographer. It should go without saying that the most suitable route of access in order to achieve the aims of the study should have been chosen before the patient enters the angiographic suite; this decision will often depend upon a number of factors, including previous imaging studies, operation notes and clinical examination.

The most common vessel punctured for diagnostic and therapeutic angiography is the common femoral artery. Axillary, brachial or radial approaches can be used, but these routes are usually reserved for those patients in whom a femoral approach is not possible due to iliac occlusive disease. A popliteal artery puncture may be useful in certain instances such as angioplasty of the superficial femoral artery when it is not possible to catheterise this vessel via an antegrade approach.

The technique of arterial puncture and catheterisation of the common femoral artery will be described. Access via other less commonly used vessels such as the brachial, radial and popliteal arteries will not be discussed further in this chapter. Interested readers are referred to previous editions of this textbook or specialist interventional radiology texts.

Retrograde Femoral Artery Puncture (Fig. 84-13)

The artery is palpated to select the site of puncture before local anaesthetic is injected. Various anatomical descriptions are given regarding the site at which to puncture, but the aim should be to enter the common femoral artery a short distance below the inguinal ligament. This is best achieved by puncturing the vessel where it can be most easily palpated, irrespective of the relationship of this point to the inguinal skin crease. Since this is the point where the artery crosses the femoral head, it is also the easiest point at which to achieve haemostasis afterwards. Ultrasound is also recommended to help select the most appropriate site of puncture, avoiding atherosclerotic plaques, and is also used to guide needle entry.

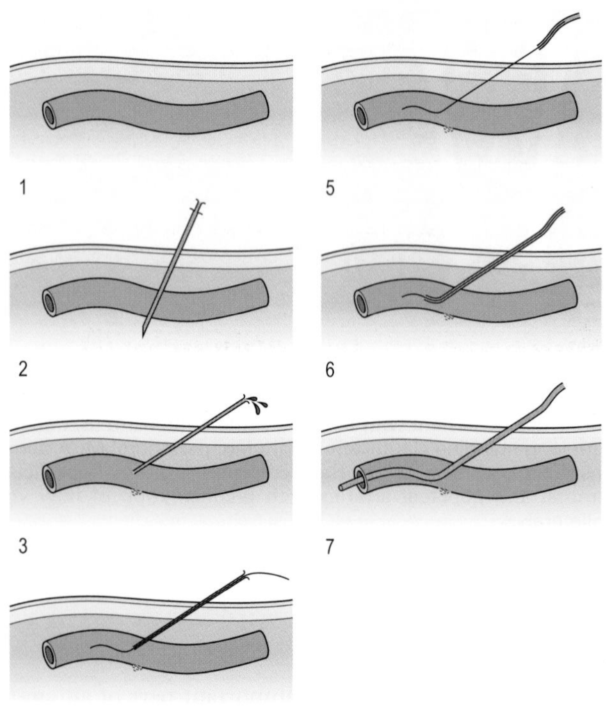

FIGURE 84-13 ■ Percutaneous catheterisation. One of the commonly used techniques of percutaneous arterial catheterisation. The artery (1) is transfixed (2). The needle is partially withdrawn and re-angled (3). A guidewire is passed into the needle during free backflow of blood (3, 4), the needle is removed and a catheter or introducer is inserted over the wire (5, 6). When the catheter is safely within the arterial lumen, the wire is withdrawn (7).

It is important that the arterial puncture site should be adequately anaesthetised. After cleansing the skin with a suitable preparation, 5–10 mL of 0.5–1% lidocaine is infiltrated around the artery. It is important to inject the local anaesthetic agent posterior to the artery as well as anterior to it, even if a single-wall puncture of the vessel is subsequently made, as it makes the arterial puncture and subsequent catheter manipulation much more comfortable for the patient. In addition, if the puncture site is inadequately anaesthetised arterial spasm is more likely, which may make selective catheterisation very difficult because of the lack of free catheter movement.

After local anaesthesia, a small scalpel incision is made in the skin (large enough to accommodate the anticipated catheter), the skin being temporarily drawn laterally during the incision to avert the risk of a scalpel injury to the arterial wall. A pair of fine artery forceps is inserted into the incision and used to create a tunnel through the subcutaneous tissues down to the artery. This manoeuvre is particularly important in large or obese patients, for it not only facilitates catheterisation but also reduces the risk of a postoperative haematoma: any escaping blood emerges through the incision and is immediately apparent, instead of collecting subcutaneously.

The technique employed for puncturing the artery is a matter of personal preference. A reliable way is to feel the artery with the middle and index fingers of the left hand and insert the needle (held in the right hand) between the two palpating fingers. The needle is held angled forwards and passed through the anterior wall alone or right through the artery, depending upon the angiographer's preference. A single-wall puncture technique is most commonly performed with a one-part needle, in which case free pulsatile blood flow will occur as soon as the needle enters the vessel lumen. When a double-wall puncture technique is performed a two-part needle is used; after passing through the vessel, the central stylet is removed, the needle angled slightly more towards the horizontal and then withdrawn at an even rate, assisted by gentle rotatory movements to avoid any sudden jerking. When the tip of the needle is safely in the arterial lumen there will be a free, spurting backflow of blood from the hub. While the needle is held steady with one hand, the soft tip of a guidewire is threaded through the needle into the artery. When a sufficient length of wire is inside, the needle is removed and firm manual pressure maintained on the puncture site until the needle has been exchanged for a catheter or dilator. The guidewire is removed when the tip of the catheter is in a satisfactory position and the catheter is then flushed free of blood with heparinised saline. At the end of a correctly conducted insertion procedure there should be no bleeding around the catheter, which will move freely and painlessly through the puncture site when manipulated.

There are arguments in favour of both single- and double-wall arterial punctures; some radiologists prefer to puncture only the anterior wall of the artery to minimise the trauma to the vessel, although puncture to both vessel walls does not increase the risk of complications as these are usually caused by the subsequent manipulations with guidewires and catheters. Proponents of a double-wall puncture technique maintain that this method is safer, particularly when first learning angiography, with a lesser risk of intimal dissection when introducing the guidewire through the needle when compared with a single-wall technique. Whichever method is employed, if a guidewire does not pass freely into the arterial lumen it should not be forced; this technique is never successful and usually causes an intimal dissection. If there is good backflow of blood the reason for failure of the wire to pass freely may be either that the needle is angled sharply towards one wall of the blood vessel or that the wire is passing into a small branch vessel such as the deep circumflex iliac artery. A number of manoeuvres may help, including fluoroscopy, cautious repositioning of the angle of the needle or changing to a J-wire. A gentle injection of contrast medium is possible to help ascertain the nature of the problem but only if good backflow is present. If there is poor backflow then the needle may be positioned near an atheromatous plaque or a stenosis, may be only partially in the lumen, or may have caused an intimal dissection. In these circumstances discretion is advised and it is wise to start again with a fresh puncture. In difficult cases remember that there is usually a patent femoral artery in the opposite leg! Better two groin punctures than a dissection or a large haematoma.

The catheter is flushed with a heparinised saline solution throughout the procedure to prevent clotting. It is almost always preferable to give a firm hand flush intermittently, rather than maintain a continuous slow flush infusion. This technique not only leaves the proximal end of the catheter free for manipulation but also is more effective, since a slow infusion may only clear the proximal holes of a catheter with multiple side-ports; clot forms in the end-port and the more distal side-ports, and is then blown out into the vascular system when a pressure contrast injection is performed.

Antegrade Femoral Artery Puncture

The most common indication for an antegrade puncture of the femoral artery is when performing ipsilateral superficial femoral, popliteal or infragenicular artery angioplasty. Once again, the aim should be to puncture the common femoral artery just below the inguinal ligament. The most common problem associated with this procedure is catheterisation of the profunda femoris and many methods have been described in order to manipulate the catheter out of this vessel into the superficial femoral artery when this has happened. With a good technique and ultrasound guidance, however, this complication should rarely occur.

Preparation of the patient is important; obese patients may have an abdominal 'apron' that hangs over the groin and this should be lifted superiorly and strapped out of the way with heavy-duty tape. It is well worthwhile when performing an antegrade femoral puncture to screen over the femoral head to determine the correct site for vessel puncture, as this is often considerably higher than anticipated when using palpation alone. The fovea of the femoral head is a useful landmark for the correct site of arterial access and this can be marked on the skin before local anaesthetic is infiltrated in the same way as for a retrograde puncture. A skin incision is made with a scalpel blade and blunt dissection is again performed of the soft tissues over the femoral artery. The vessel is then punctured with the needle angled slightly towards the feet. The best wire to use is a wide-angled J-wire with a curvature of radius 7.5 mm. This should be introduced through the needle with the tip of the curve directed anteriorly, so that, as it exits the needle tip within the vessel lumen, it is directed into the superficial femoral artery rather than the profunda femoris. A straight guidewire is much more likely to pass directly into the latter vessel because of the posterolateral orientation of this artery.

Selective Catheterisation

By manipulating a catheter under fluoroscopic control it is possible to insert the catheter selectively into various branches of the vascular system such as the renal artery, coeliac axis, axillary artery, etc. Different catheter shapes are available, each of which is suitable for a particular manoeuvre or for catheterising certain arterial branches. Superselective catheterisation (also known as subselective embolisation) is the term used for the catheterisation of small subsidiary arteries that themselves arise from named branch arteries and is most frequently performed during embolisation procedures. A coaxial catheter (one that passes through the lumen of a diagnostic or guiding catheter) is often used for the catheterisation of these small vessels.

DIGITAL SUBTRACTION ANGIOGRAPHY

With any DSA examination, particular attention must be paid to the elimination of movement artefact. Respiratory motion needs to be controlled (a nose-clip is often helpful) and in the case of abdominal and pelvic examinations the effects of bowel movement can be minimised by the use of paralytic agents. Multiple mask acquisition is a simple and much neglected technique for counteracting the effect of inevitable movement such as, say, the artefacts produced in pulmonary arteriograms by cardiac motion. If several pre-contrast images are taken so as to embrace all the different phases of the cardiac cycle, then appropriate mask selection will subsequently permit virtually any contrast-filled image to be presented free of artefact. The same technique can be used in those individuals who are unable to hold their breath for any length of time. Such patients should be asked to breathe normally throughout the run and multiple images are obtained *before* the injection of contrast medium so that a suitable mask for subtraction is available for every phase

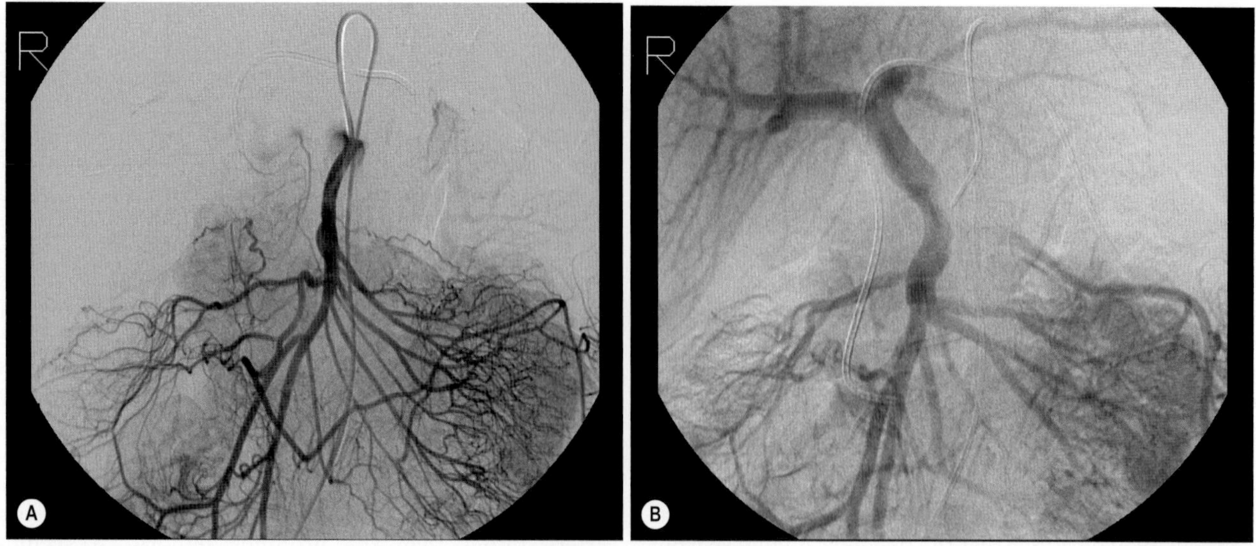

FIGURE 84-14 ■ Example of use of breathing technique during visceral angiography. Arterial (A) and venous (B) images from a superior mesenteric arteriogram acquired during patient respiration. Intestinal peristalsis has been obliterated with hyoscine butylbromide. The arterial and venous images were acquired at different phases of respiration but the use of different masks (mask 2 for the arterial image and mask 10 for the venous image), acquired before the injection of contrast medium, has resulted in excellent-quality images.

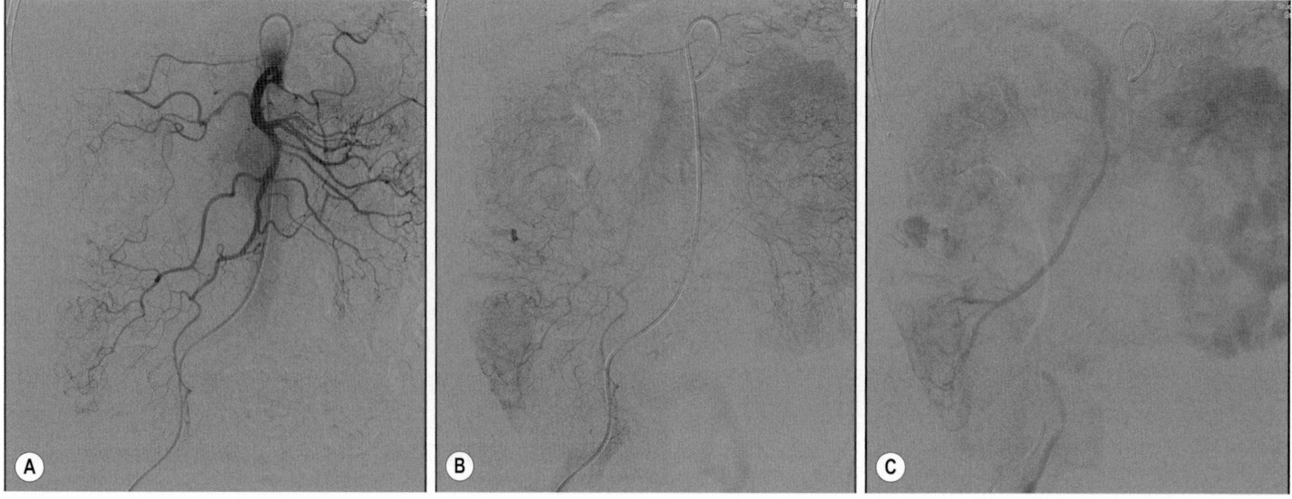

FIGURE 84-15 ■ Superior mesenteric artery angiogram in a 79-year-old patient with acute gastrointestinal haemorrhage. Images were obtained with the patient breathing throughout the acquisition using the technique described in the text. (A) Arterial phase image demonstrates normal arterial anatomy. (B) Late arterial/early capillary phase image demonstrates an area of active contrast medium extravasation into a proximal ascending colon diverticulum. (C) Delayed image demonstrates that extravasated contrast medium has spilled into the colonic lumen. Normal venous drainage is seen from the caecum.

of respiration. This technique is particularly suited to visceral angiography (Fig. 84-14) and allows the acquisition of images during arterial and late venous phases that are often of much better quality than those obtained in patients who are asked to hold their breath (Fig. 84-15).

AFTERCARE

When an arteriographic study is completed, the catheter is withdrawn and firm manual pressure applied to the puncture site for 5–10 minutes. The radiologist should be absolutely satisfied that bleeding has stopped before the patient leaves the angiography suite. The wound site is then checked at regular intervals by the nursing staff, who should also record pulse and blood pressure observations for a reasonable period following the procedure and check that distal pulses remain palpable. Pressure pads, sand bags and other accoutrements are generally a waste of time. It is much better to be able to see the puncture site than to cover it up. If bleeding does not stop from a puncture site, press for longer! Almost all post-catheterisation bleeding can ultimately be controlled by local pressure unless the artery has been torn or there is a coagulation abnormality. Several devices are now available that are used to seal the puncture point in the vessel wall at the time of catheter withdrawal in order to allow rapid mobilisation and discharge of the patient, often within 1–2 h.[25–27] These have become popular in many centres following cardiac catheterisation and are being utilised more commonly in peripheral angiography. A description of the various devices that are currently available and a discussion of the arguments for and against their use lie outside the scope of this chapter and the interested reader is referred to specialist texts.

An adequate record of the procedure should be entered in the patient's case notes. This should include:

- date
- name of the operator
- puncture site
- catheter size
- studies performed
- names and doses of anaesthetic agents
- volumes and concentrations of contrast medium and other drugs administered
- preliminary findings
- any complications during the procedure
- integrity or otherwise of the pulses peripheral to the puncture site at the end of the procedure
- post-procedural nursing instructions.

These notes are important not only for patient care but also as a medico-legal record and they should be comprehensive and accurate.

COMPLICATIONS

Contrast Medium Reactions

The many possible adverse effects of contrast media, together with details of their prevention and treatment, are discussed in OldChapter 2.

Puncture Site Complications

Haemorrhage

Haemorrhage may occur from the puncture site and may cause external blood loss or a subcutaneous haematoma, which can result in extensive bruising. Retroperitoneal bleeding is uncommon but may occur if the arterial puncture is performed above the inguinal ligament. Perhaps the commonest reason for this is the introduction of the needle during retrograde femoral artery catheterisation at too acute an angle so that it passes through the back wall of the external iliac artery above the inguinal ligament. It is less well recognised, however, that this complication may also occur when the femoral artery is correctly punctured; this is probably due to a downward extension of the pelvic and abdominal wall fascial layers around the femoral artery and vein, the so-called femoral sheath. If this sheath is transgressed at the time of vessel puncture, and bleeding subsequently occurs from the puncture site after catheter or sheath removal for any reason, then blood may spread along the fascial planes continuous with the femoral sheath into the retroperitoneum or, indeed, into the anterior abdominal wall.

Four types of haematoma may occur after femoral artery puncture: (A) abdominal wall, (B) retroperitoneal, (C) groin and thigh and (D) intraperitoneal. The first three may all result from puncture of the common femoral artery (i.e. below the inguinal ligament), with (A) and (B) resulting when there is bleeding into the femoral sheath and (C), the commonest, when there is spread into the femoral triangle. Intraperitoneal haemorrhage is even less frequent than retroperitoneal bleeding and generally requires transgression of the peritoneum itself, which is more likely to occur if vessel puncture is performed above the level of the inguinal ligament. Some intraperitoneal bleeding has also been described, however, when the arterial puncture is below the inguinal ligament; it has been postulated that this may be due to the presence of defects in the parietal peritoneum.

Excessive bleeding is usually the result of bad technique. Particular caution is necessary in patients with a bleeding diathesis or hypertension and following the use of balloon catheters in transluminal angioplasty. If inexplicable bleeding continues, check that inadvertent overheparinisation has not occurred. This can be corrected if necessary by the administration of protamine sulphate (10 mg of which counteracts the effects of approximately 1000 IU heparin).

Intramural and Perivascular Contrast Medium Injection

Contrast medium may be inadvertently injected into the wall of a vessel or outside the vessel (perivascular). In most cases little harm (apart from pain) results from a perivascular injection but it is possible to dissect and occlude an artery with a subintimal injection of contrast medium. Never inject into a needle or catheter that does not exhibit free backflow.

Vascular thrombosis can result from severe trauma to the vessel at the puncture site or from a subintimal contrast injection. It is also possible that thrombus wiped off the outside of the arterial catheter during its extraction forms a nidus for thrombus at the puncture site. Vascular trauma at the puncture site can be minimised by good technique. Never use force to introduce a wire into a vessel; if it does not pass easily something is wrong! It is often better for the inexperienced operator to start again with a fresh needle puncture and/or call for help than to persist with one that is causing problems. A 10-minute delay with a successful outcome is always preferable to a dissection and/or a groin haematoma.

Peripheral embolisation from the puncture site probably occurs to a minor degree in many cases but clinically obvious embolisation is rare.

Local vascular complications such as false aneurysm (pseudoaneurysm) or AV fistula formation and late stenosis or occlusion can all result from arterial procedures. Good technique is the best preventative measure. Femoral artery pseudoaneurysms are usually caused by a combination of a low puncture—the superficial femoral or profunda femoris arteries have often been cannulated instead of the common femoral artery when this complication occurs—and inadequate compression of the vessel at the end of the procedure.

Local sepsis may occur following an arterial puncture (although it is extremely rare) and this factor is particularly important if early surgery is contemplated. The utmost care should be taken to observe sterile precautions and when a study is performed in a patient with local skin contamination (e.g. open wound, ileostomy, etc.) a protective adhesive sheet helps to keep the operative field uncontaminated.

Injury to local structures such as nerves, joints and bones is rarely of clinical significance. Occasionally damage to branches of the femoral nerve gives rise to areas of cutaneous anaesthesia or paraesthesia in the thigh.[28] These normally recover completely, although this may take several months in some instances.

Catheter-Related and General Complications

1. *Thrombi* can form in or on a catheter and be ejected into the vascular system. This is always undesirable and in areas such as the cerebral or coronary circulation is extremely dangerous. Catheters should be flushed assiduously during all arteriographic procedures to prevent thrombus formation. Other types of embolism that may occur are air embolism (sometimes from incorrectly loaded pressure injectors) and thread embolism from fragments of gauze swab.
2. *Vascular injuries* distant from the puncture site may be produced by the catheter or guidewire, or by the intramural injection of contrast medium or saline. If there is ever any doubt about whether a needle or catheter tip is in a satisfactory position, contrast medium should always be injected in preference to saline. Under fluoroscopic control, it is then possible to stop the injection immediately if any extravasation or other mishap is apparent. The most common injury is dissection of the tunica intima from the tunica media and this complication is far more likely to occur in previously diseased vessels than in normal vessels. The intima forms a raised flap that may completely occlude the vessel. It is also possible to perforate vessels with a guidewire or to rupture them when a forced injection is made through a catheter wedged into a vessel of the same calibre.
3. *Injuries to organs* are normally caused by ischaemia during arteriographic procedures (other than those related to the effects of contrast medium). This may occur through wedging of the catheter so that the normal flow to an organ is obstructed; dissection of the feeding artery; spasm, thrombosis or rupture of the feeding artery; or embolism. The ischaemia resulting from one or more of the earlier mentioned events may have no observable clinical sequelae, may result in temporary or permanent functional abnormalities in the affected organ or system, or may cause infarction of the organ. The clinical importance of these accidents depends very much on the vascular territory in which they occur; complete occlusion of a carotid, coronary or renal artery is likely to have disastrous consequences whereas occlusion of, say, a hepatic artery may not necessarily produce any adverse effects.
4. *Guidewire fracture*. Occasionally fragments of guidewire or catheter may become detached within the vascular system. Catheters may also become knotted during overenthusiastic manipulation procedures. With good technique these complications should not occur.
5. *Injection accidents*. Tragedies have occurred when toxic substances have been inadvertently injected into blood vessels. Skin-cleansing fluids should always be removed from the instrument trolley immediately after the puncture site has been prepared. Drugs should always be double-checked before injection through a catheter.
6. *Vasovagal reactions*. Vagally mediated reactions may occur during arteriography in response either to the injection of contrast medium or to the discomfort and psychological effects of the procedure. Bradycardia is a prominent feature of such reactions, which must be distinguished from acute allergic responses to the contrast medium or local anaesthetic. The incidence of vasovagal reactions is considerably reduced if proper premedication is employed.

For a full list of references, please see ExpertConsult.

FURTHER READING

6. Zhang HL, Schoenberg SO, Resnick LM, Prince MR. Diagnosis of renal artery stenosis: combining gadolinium-enhanced three-dimensional magnetic resonance angiography with functional magnetic resonance pulse sequences. Am J Hypertens 2003;16:1079–82.
7. Nelemans PJ, Leiner T, de Vet HC, van Engelshoven JM. Peripheral arterial disease: meta-analysis of the diagnostic performance of MR angiography. Radiology 2000;217:105–14.
8. Meaney JF, Prince MR, Nostrant TT, Stanley JC. Gadolinium-enhanced MR angiography of visceral arteries in patients with suspected chronic mesenteric ischemia. J Magn Reson Imaging 1997;7:171–6.
9. Remonda L, Heid O, Schroth G. Carotid artery stenosis, occlusion, and pseudo-occlusion: first-pass, gadolinium-enhanced, three-dimensional MR angiography—preliminary study. Radiology 1998;209:95–102.
10. Kaewlai R, Abujudeh H. Nephrogenic systemic fibrosis. Am J Roentgenol 2012;199(1):W17–23.
11. Khoo MM, Deeab D, Gedroyc WM, et al. Renal artery stenosis: comparative assessment by unenhanced renal artery MRA versus contrast-enhanced MRA. Eur Radiol 2011;21(7):1470–6.
12. Miyazaki M, Akahane M. Non-contrast enhanced MR angiography: established techniques. J Magn Reson Imaging 2012;35(1):1–19.

CHAPTER 85

Aortic Intervention

Christopher J. Hammond • Anthony A. Nicholson

CHAPTER OUTLINE

INTRODUCTION

Open surgical treatment of aortic pathology is often technically demanding for the surgeon and invasive for the patient, being associated with a significant physiological insult. Surgery for the thoracic aorta requires thoracotomy or median sternotomy, aortic cross-clamping, often single lung ventilation and sometimes cardiopulmonary bypass or circulatory arrest. Surgery for the abdominal aorta requires laparotomy, or extensive retroperitoneal dissection, medial visceral rotation and aortic cross-clamping. The aortic tissue is usually diseased and may be friable (especially in the case of dissection and intramural haematoma (IMH)) or calcified and brittle. In either situation, working with, dissecting and suturing the aorta is challenging.

The cohort of patients requiring aortic intervention is usually that least able to withstand it. In most cases, aortic pathology is associated with generalised cardiovascular disease, including ischaemic heart disease, cerebrovascular, renovascular and peripheral vascular disease as well as other comorbidites such as respiratory impairment. Mortality rates for elective open surgery for thoracic and abdominal aneurysms are in the region of 8 and 5%, respectively,[1,2] and morbidity is significant.

These considerations have driven the development of minimally invasive endovascular therapies for aortic disease. Endovascular repair of the aorta using covered stents (stent-grafts) was first described in 1991[3] and is generally associated with a smaller physiological insult and lower mortality than open surgical repair.[2,4] However, there are a number of unique limitations (particularly relating to anatomy) and complications. Although the current generation of stent-grafts is easier to insert and performs better in the long term than their predecessors, they are by no means a panacea for all aortic pathology. A multidisciplinary approach to aortic disease is vital and should include cardiothoracic and vascular surgeons, interventional radiologists, vascular anaesthetists and device specialists (e.g. company representatives). This multidisciplinary approach should ensure that the patient receives the most appropriate treatment, be it open surgery, endovascular repair or medical management.

This chapter will discuss the endovascular management of aortic pathology and in particular the indications, anatomical and technical considerations and complications of the technique.

STENT-GRAFTS AND BASIC PRINCIPLES OF STENT-GRAFTING

A stent-graft (Fig. 85-1) is composed of a fabric tube, usually woven polyester or expanded polytetrafluoroethylene (Gore-Tex). Circular or crown-shaped metal struts ('ring stents'), usually made of nitinol or Elgiloy, are attached to the tube by either suturing or gluing. The exact design of the ring stent varies from manufacturer to manufacturer, but in all cases serves to provide support for the fabric and provide firm apposition of the stent-graft to the wall of the aorta. Some devices have uncovered stents at one end to provide additional support and anchorage above or below the covered portion of the device. The stent-graft is held in place by the radial force of the ring stents, which produce friction against the aortic wall and prevent distal device migration. Additionally, some devices have small hooks (usually at the top end of the fabric or on an uncovered stent) which engage with the aortic wall to prevent migration (Fig. 85-1B). Most manufacturers make a range of stent-graft

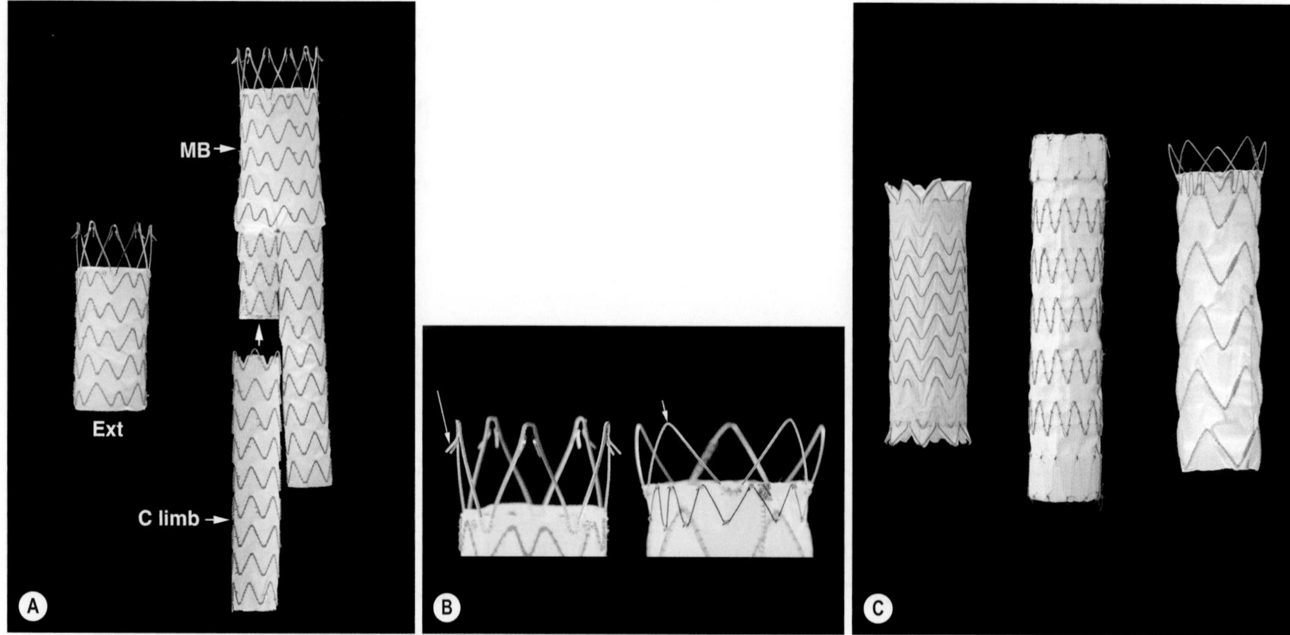

FIGURE 85-1 ■ Stent-grafts. (A) Typical bifurcated stent-graft, consisting of a main body (MB) with a short and a long limb, a contralateral limb (C limb), which is docked into the short limb stump (short arrow) during deployment inside the aneurysm sac, and a proximal extension cuff (Ext), which can be deployed within the main body to extend the seal cephalad if necessary. Note the ring stents (zig-zag lines) which are sutured to the fabric and the proximal bare metal (uncovered) stent which acts to increase device fixation. (B) Types of proximal bare stent. The device on the left has a bare metal proximal stent to which small hooks have been soldered (long arrow). The device on the right has a bare metal proximal stent (short arrow) but no hooks. (C) Three thoracic stent-grafts. Gore-TAG (left), Cook TX2 (middle) and Medtronic Talent (right). Note the differences in ring stent design, fabric and presence (or absence) of hooks.

diameters and lengths to allow 'off the shelf' device selection. Complex devices (such as fenestrated or branched devices or devices in sizes outside the normally manufactured ranges) can be ordered but are expensive and there is a lead-time associated with their manufacture. Currently (July 2013), the approximate cost of a typical single thoracic aortic stent-graft (Fig. 85-1C) is £10k. A bifurcated abdominal aortic device costs about £6k and a custom-made device can cost £15k or more.

Good quality high-resolution imaging is required to choose the correct stent-graft for a particular aneurysm. This is usually achieved with thin-section contrast-enhanced arterial phase computed tomography (CT) to include the whole of the diseased section of the aorta and the access vessels (see below) in a volumetric acquisition. Magnetic resonance (MR) angiography is sometimes utilised. Multiplanar reformatting software is essential to allow measurement of true axial diameters and vessel length. Expert systems are available to automate this process, though many clinicians prefer to do it by hand.

To achieve a good 'seal' between the device and the aortic wall, the stent-graft is usually oversized relative to the aorta by 10–20%. The aorta at the point of seal (sometimes called the 'neck') should be relatively disease free and straight-sided. Most stent-grafts require a neck length of 8–15 mm to achieve a seal. Shorter necks (Fig. 85-2A) and diseased necks (e.g. those containing marked atheroma or thrombus, Fig. 85-2B) risk a suboptimal seal and leakage between the device and the aortic wall. A neck which is sharply angulated relative to the more distal aorta (Fig. 85-2C) risks the stent-graft not deploying truly perpendicular to the aortic wall. This can increase the risk of suboptimal apposition and leak, though modern devices are designed to accept a greater degree of neck angulation than earlier designs, and some devices are specifically marketed for greater neck angulation. This requires specific design features to prevent graft lumen collapse. Finally, markedly barrel or conical shaped necks (Fig. 85-2D) increase the risk of poor seal as the degree of oversize needed to achieve a seal at the narrower portion of the neck may not be sufficient to achieve seal at the wider portion. The considerations outlined above for the 'neck' apply equally to the distal sealing point, often called the 'landing zone'.

Approximately 40% of abdominal aortic aneurysms are unsuitable for conventional (as opposed to fenestrated or branched) endovascular repair because of adverse morphology.[5] A description of the degree to which an operator can compromise on an 'ideal' neck (minimal angulation, straight-sided, long and disease free) is beyond the scope of this chapter though there are many reports of operators deploying devices in 'off-label' morphologies (where the characteristics of the aorta are outwith the published 'indications for use' (IFU) limits of the device) with satisfactory results.[6,7]

Stent-grafts are supplied preloaded on a deployment system. They are usually constrained within a sheath, which, at deployment, is gradually withdrawn, allowing the stent to expand under its own radial force. Many delivery systems have mechanisms to allow partial

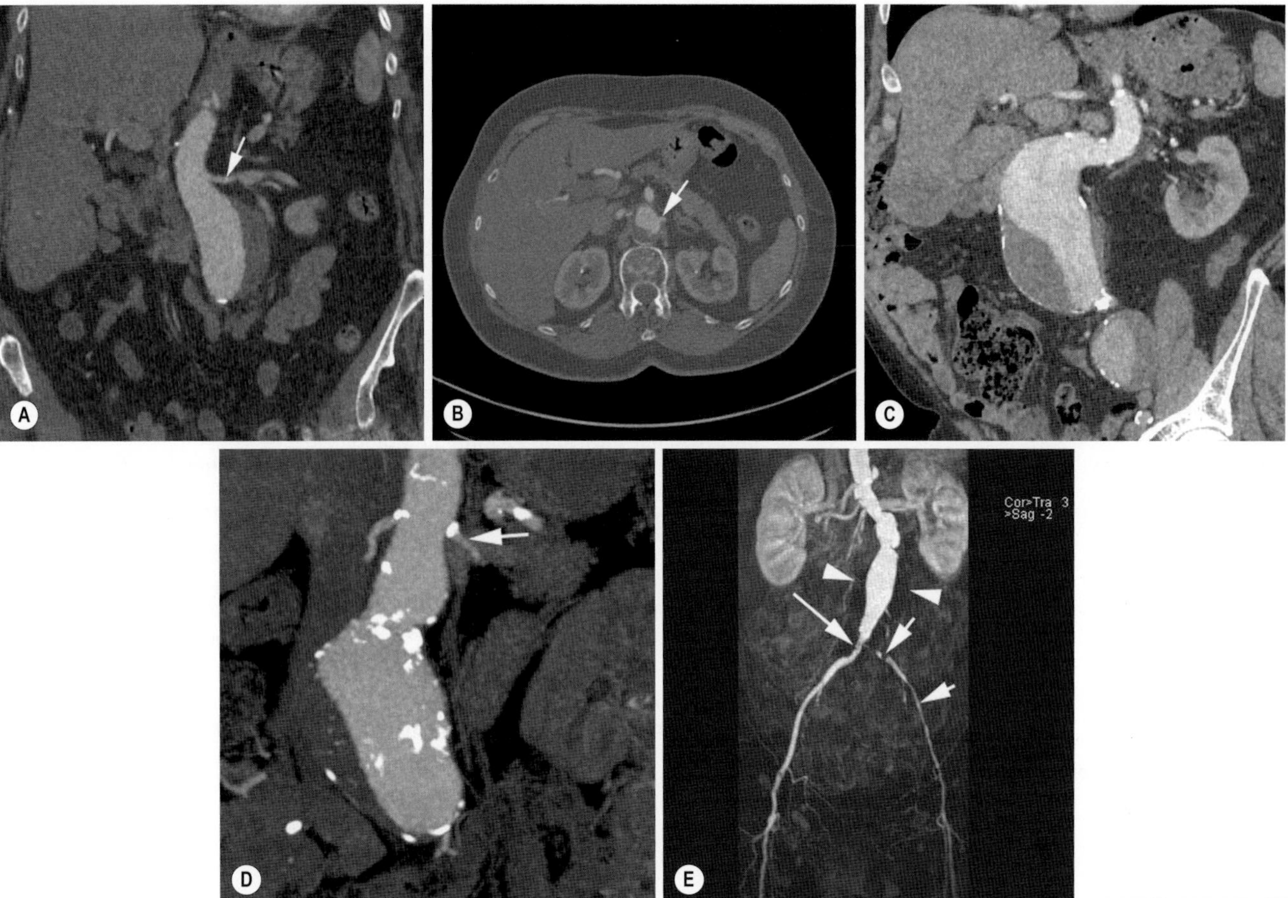

FIGURE 85-2 ■ **Adverse anatomy for EVAR.** (A) Short neck between the renal artery (short arrow) and the aneurysm. (B) Significant atheroma/thrombus in the aneurysm neck (posteriorly) at the level of the renal artery (short arrow). (C) Markedly angulated neck with 90° bends between the suprarenal aorta and the neck (which runs horizontally in the image) and between the neck and the aneurysm itself. (D) Conical neck below the renal artery (short arrow). (E) Stenosed access vessels precluding passage of a device delivery system. There is a right common iliac artery origin stenosis (long arrow) and multifocal left iliac stenoses (short arrows). The true diameter of the AAA (between the arrowheads) is discernible from the dark bands of thrombus outwith the flowing lumen.

deployment and repositioning before final release. The 'windsock' effect of systolic pressure during the cardiac cycle forcing a partially deployed device distally from its intended deployment position is occasionally problematic, though usually only in the proximal thoracic aorta. Some thoracic delivery systems have mechanisms to constrain the proximal portion of the stent-graft until the remainder of the device is fully deployed to minimise this windsock effect. Where the proximal positioning of a thoracic stent-graft is critical (e.g. in short or angulated necks) overdrive cardiac pacing or pharmacological manipulation to lower blood pressure may be used as the device is deployed.

Once completely released, a device cannot be retrieved or repositioned without open surgery.

Deployment systems vary in diameter between 14 and 25Fr (approximately 4–9 mm). Patients in whom the access vessels (usually the common femoral and iliac arteries) are narrower than the diameter of the delivery system required (Fig. 85-2E) cannot undergo endovascular repair without adjunctive procedures such as previous angioplasty or stenting of the stenosed segment or the placement of a temporary surgical conduit to allow the device to be inserted from above any stenosis. Heavily calcified or tortuous access vessels may also preclude endovascular repair as they will not straighten sufficiently to allow passage of the delivery system. Attempts to force a large delivery system through suboptimal access can result in access vessel rupture or avulsion with potentially disastrous consequences.

Table 85-1 summarises the absolute and relative contraindications to endovascular repair of aortic pathology with conventional stent-grafts. The characteristics of some currently manufactured stent-grafts are summarised in Table 85-2.

SURVEILLANCE IMAGING AND COMPLICATIONS

Endovascular repair of aortic pathology is associated with a number of novel complications that may occur months or years following the procedure. For this reason, patients undergoing endovascular repair undergo a programme of surveillance imaging over a number of years (and sometimes indefinitely) following the procedure. The exact

TABLE 85-1 **Absolute and Relative Contraindications to Endovascular Repair of Aortic Pathology**

Contraindication	Comment
Absolute	
Patient preference for open surgical repair	
Limited life expectancy	Where the risks of intervention outweigh the benefits
Poor cardiopulmonary reserve or other comorbid condition	Where the risks of intervention outweigh the benefits
Significant (>50%) or circumferential thrombus at seal zone	
Unstable patients	Where they are deemed unable to withstand the small delay associated with imaging of the pathology
Ascending aortic pathology	Unless there is absolutely no surgical alternative
Relative	
Contrast allergy	Procedures can be performed with carbon dioxide angiography or intravascular ultrasound as imaging guidance
Renal insufficiency	Procedures can be performed with carbon dioxide angiography or intravascular ultrasound as imaging guidance
Suboptimal proximal seal zone ('neck') • Angulation • Length • Shape	Proceed accepting an increased risk of endoleak, or use fenestrated or branched device
Poor access vessels • Stenosis • Tortuosity • Calcification	Can be mitigated with angioplasty or proximal surgical conduit
Children	Where physiological growth may result in loss of seal and device dislocation
Young patients	As long-term durability of endovascular repair has not yet been established
Not Contraindications	
Rupture	
Malignancy	
Mycotic aneurysms	

details of the surveillance vary from institution to institution though most will involve cross-sectional imaging initially (arterial phase CT or MR angiography at 1 or 3 months, or both) and regularly (at least annually) thereafter for a number of years. Plain radiographs of the device are also obtained to assess for ring stent fracture, device dislocation and migration. Ultrasound (US) and contrast-enhanced US may be used to detect sac expansion and endoleak. Some authors have advocated replacing CT with US as early as 1 year post-abdominal EVAR (within certain strict criteria) to minimise radiation, dose of iodinated contrast agent, cost and inconvenience to the patient.[8] Such programmes of less intensive surveillance will evolve as device performance improves with successive stent-graft generations.

The novel complications of endovascular repair are endoleak, device migration and dislocation, kinking and occlusion (Fig. 85-3).

Endoleak

This is defined as continuing flow of blood into the diseased segment of aorta outside the lumen of the stent-graft. There are five types of endoleak described.

Type 1 Endoleak (Fig. 83-3A)

Poor sealing between the device and the aortic wall, at both the proximal and distal seals (the neck and distal 'landing zone'), can result in leakage of blood between the aortic wall and the device and incomplete exclusion of the treated segment of the aorta from the circulation. This is a type 1 endoleak. It is often associated with adverse neck morphology[9,10] and sometimes with device migration over time. Errors in device sizing can also be a cause. Type 1 endoleak is associated with poor long-term outcome, with ongoing sac pressurisation, expansion and rupture.[11] It typically requires treatment. Therapeutic options include insertion of proximal or distal extension cuffs, balloon moulding or restenting of the seal zones, open surgical buttressing, device explantation and repair or attempts at transcatheter embolisation of the endoleak.

Type 2 Endoleak (Figs. 85-3B and C)

Small side branches of the aorta (e.g. the intercostal, lumbar or inferior mesenteric arteries) are not usually occluded during endovascular repair. This allows the possibility of retrograde flow of blood into the diseased segment of aorta via these side branches—a type 2 endoleak. These endoleaks often cease spontaneously. They do not require treatment in the absence of aneurysm sac or false lumen expansion.[11] Such expansion is uncommon, but, if it occurs, it can cause alteration in the morphology of the proximal or distal stent-graft seal zones with eventual loss of seal and type 1 endoleak (which would require treatment). Therefore type 2

TABLE 85-2 **Summary of Characteristics of Some Currently Manufactured Aortic Stent-Grafts**

Name	Endurant AAA	Excluder C3	Anaconda	AorFix	Zenith LP	Zenith Flex	Valiant Thoracic	TAG Conformable	TX2
Manufacturer	Medtronic	Gore	VascuTek Terumo	Lombard Medical	Cook	Cook	Medtronic	Gore	Cook
Date to Market	2012 (2nd gen)	2010	2007	1999	2010	1999	2009	2009	2009
Intended Deployment Site	Abdominal	Abdominal	Abdominal	Abdominal	Abdominal	Abdominal	Thoracic	Thoracic	Thoracic
Fabric	Polyester	ePTFE	Polyester	Polyester	Polyester	Polyester	Polyester	ePTFE	Polyester
Stent Material	Nitinol	Nitinol	Nitinol	Nitinol	Nitinol	Stainless steel	Nitinol	Nitinol	Stainless steel
Bare Stent—Distal	No	No	No	No	No	No	Yes (on some components)	No	Yes (distal components only)
Bare Stent—Proximal	Yes	No	No	No	Yes	Yes	Yes (on some components)	Yes (partially uncovered)	No
Hooks	On proximal bare stent	On proximal ring stent	On proximal ring stent	On proximal ring stent	On proximal bare stent	On proximal bare stent	No	No	On proximal ring stent and distal bare stent
IFU(*)									
Minimum Neck Length (mm)	10	15	15	20	15	15	15	20	20
Maximum Neck Angulation (°)	60	60	Not defined. Used up to 90	90	60	60	Not defined	Not defined	Not defined
Delivery System Diameter (Fr)**	18–20	18–20	20–23	22	16	18–22	22–25	18–24	20–22
Device Size Range (mm)	23–36	23–31	21–34	24–31	22–36	22–36	22–46	21–45	22–42
Comments			'Fish mouth' deployment system with marked repositionability. Magnet system for cannulation of contralateral limb	CE marked for 90° necks	Low profile version of Flex		Tip capture delivery system		Two-piece system (proximal and distal components). Trifold delivery system

*IFU = Indications for use.
**Diameter (mm) = French size /π.

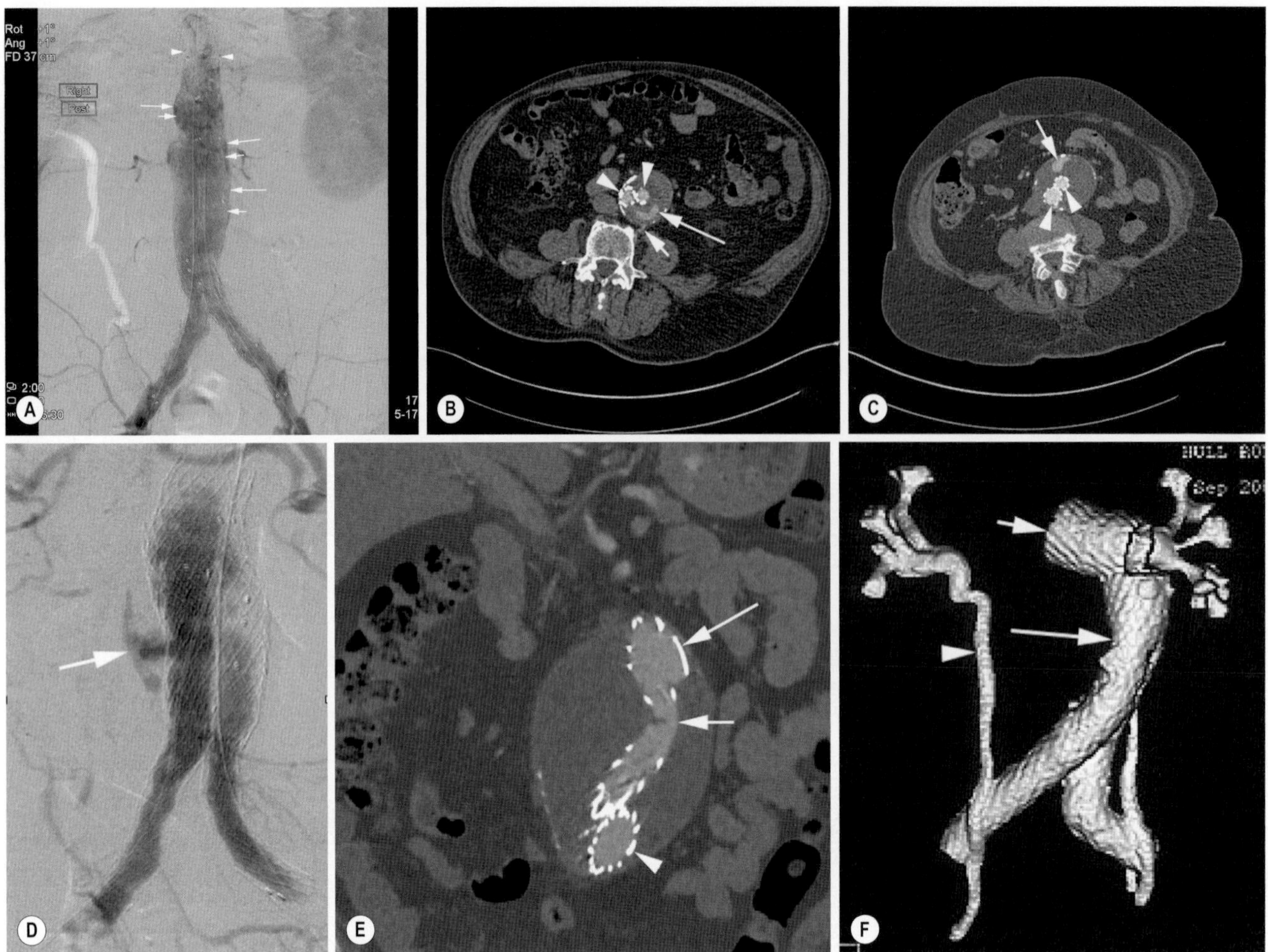

FIGURE 85-3 ■ **Complications of EVAR.** (A) Type 1 endoleak. Pigtail aortogram immediately following stent-graft deployment. The outer margins of the stent-graft are indicated by the lateral edges of the ring stents (short arrows). Contrast can be seen outside the stent-graft in the aneurysm sac and neck (long arrows). The lumbar vessels were filling antegradely, indicating this was not a type 2 leak. The proximal markers on the stent-graft fabric (arrowheads) are evident just below the proximal bare metal stent. (B) Type 2 endoleak from a lumbar vessel. A pool of contrast (long arrow) is evident posteriorly in the aneurysm sac outside the stent-graft limbs (arrowheads). It lies in close association with a prominent lumbar vessel (short arrow). (C) Type 2 endoleak from the inferior mesenteric artery. A pool of contrast (arrow) is evident anteriorly in the aneurysm sac outside the stent-graft limbs (arrowheads). It lies in close association with the inferior mesenteric artery (not shown). (D) Type 3 endoleak. A defect in the graft fabric has resulted in leakage of contrast from the graft lumen into the aneurysm sac (arrow). (E) Limb kinking. A fold of stent-graft fabric (short arrow), causing significant stenosis in one of the limbs of a bifurcated device (reformatted oblique image), is evident. The other limb (arrowhead) and proximal main body (long arrow) are unremarkable as they course through the image plane. (F) Device dislocation. Morphological changes in the aneurysm post EVAR have resulted in marked dislocation of a proximal extension cuff (short arrow) out of the main body (long arrow) of this bifurcated device. The renal collecting systems have been opacified by iodinated contrast media at the time of scan (arrowhead).

endoleaks with ongoing expansion are treated, usually with embolisation. Routine embolisation of prominent side branches before stent-graft deployment is time-consuming and has not been shown to alter rates of subsequent sac expansion.[12] The exceptions to this are the left subclavian artery and the internal iliac artery, both of which are moderately large vessels with prominent collateral circulation and, untreated, are a source of significant type 2 endoleak.

Type 3 Endoleak (Fig. 85-3D)

Graft defects and fabric tears are rare with modern devices but for modular devices (such as bifurcated abdominal aortic stent-grafts, or long segment thoracic aortic devices) the seal between components can be incomplete or dislocation of one component from another can occur. The associated type 3 endoleak causes repressurisation of the diseased segment of aorta and (for aneurysmal disease) sac expansion and rupture. It requires treatment, usually by balloon moulding any joints, relining defects with a secondary device or operative repair.

Types 4 and 5 Endoleak

Type 4 endoleak refers to transient graft 'porosity'—equivalent to the 'sweating' sometimes seen with knitted open surgical grafts. It is rare with modern stent-graft fabric and does not require treatment. Type 5 endoleak refers to ongoing aneurysm sac expansion in the absence of any other demonstrable endoleak. It may be due to unidentified very low volume or intermittent endoleak, osmotic effects of dissolving atheroma and thrombus or low-grade infection. Treatment, if required (e.g. if the proximal or distal seal is threatened), can be difficult and complex.

Device Migration, Dislocation, Kinking and Occlusion

Each cardiac cycle produces a force estimated to be approximately 10 N (equivalent to 1 kg) tending to push the graft distally in the aorta. This can result in graft migration over time, especially where the proximal seal zone is short or diseased when device apposition to the wall of the aorta is suboptimal. Device migration can result in limb kinking (Fig. 85-3E), which predisposes to occlusion or thrombus formation and distal embolisation. Migration can also result in type 1 or 3 endoleak (if the device migrates out of the neck, or the migration results in a change in device geometry and dislocation of modular components—Fig. 85-3F). Longer-term morphological changes in the treated aortic segment can alter device geometry and cause kinking and dislocation in the absence of migration.

Device kinking and migration are rare with modern devices, occurring in approximately 1 and 2% of patients, respectively.[5] If there is little risk of complication associated with the migration or kinking (e.g. a small amount of migration in a long neck or a minor kink unlikely to cause haemodynamically significant stenosis), no treatment is required. However, if needed, treatment can be complex. Options include extension stent-grafting, device reinforcement with stent-grafts or uncovered stents, surgical buttressing of the neck or device explantation and open repair.

INFRASTRUCTURE AND STAFFING[13]

The management of patients with aortic disease is complex and should not be undertaken without adequate supportive infrastructure, staffing, processes and governance. The decision on how (and whether) to treat relies on detailed anatomical, physiological and clinical information. Electively, patients should undergo a formal assessment of their general cardiovascular fitness (such as a cardiopulmonary exercise test (CPX)) with treatment and optimisation, where possible, of any underlying pathology. Once clinical information and data on aortic morphology and cardiovascular fitness are available, the patient should be discussed at a multidisciplinary team meeting and a plan for treatment constructed. Written information should be provided to the patient about their aortic pathology and the proposed treatment. In an emergency such detailed work-up is clearly impossible, though there is occasionally time to optimise the patient's physiology to an extent.

Endovascular aortic repair should be carried out by experienced staff in a sterile environment of theatre standard with optimal imaging facilities and equipment to convert rapidly to open repair in an emergency. The ideal is an angiography theatre with fixed C-arm image intensification and theatre-grade air change and lighting, anaesthetic and surgical equipment, piped gases and suction and facilities for rapid (level 1) infusion and cell salvage.

Postoperative care in an intensive-care or high-dependency unit should be available if needed with facilities for invasive ventilation and renal support. Vascular surgical, anaesthetic and radiological support should be available on a 24/7 basis. Written protocols for accelerated postoperative recovery, mobilisation and discharge are desirable. Data should be submitted to national or international registries (such as the National Vascular Database (NVD) in the UK).

There is evidence of improved outcomes for open abdominal aortic aneurysm (AAA) repair at centres that undertake a greater volume of work.[14] This is almost certainly as much to do with pre- and post-procedural process as it is to do with individual surgical competence. There is likely to be a similar relationship for endovascular repair of all aortic lesions.[15] Centralisation of services for aortic repair is being undertaken currently in the UK.

THORACIC AORTIC INTERVENTION

Anatomical Considerations

For the purposes of endovascular repair, thoracic aortic pathology is best classified according to its location relative to the left subclavian artery (the Stanford classification, described originally for thoracic aortic dissection— see Fig. 85-4). Pathology affecting the aortic root and ascending aorta (Stanford A disease) is generally unsuitable for endovascular repair due to the frequent

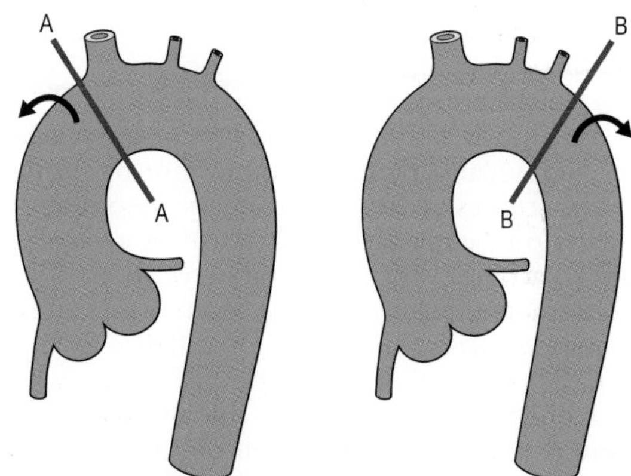

FIGURE 85-4 ■ **Stanford classification of aortic dissection.** Dissection is classified according to the site of the primary entry tear (curved arrows). If the tear lies proximal to the brachiocephalic artery, it is type A. If it lies distal to the left subclavian artery it is type B.

involvement of the aortic valve (which may also need repair) and close association of critical branch vessels (the coronary arteries and great vessels). There are occasional situations where endovascular intervention is preferable, though at present these must be considered experimental.[16]

Disease affecting the aorta distal to the left subclavian artery (Stanford B disease) is amenable to endovascular repair, assuming there is enough disease-free aorta proximally to achieve a seal (usually 15–20 mm). The left subclavian artery can be covered by the device to increase the available useable neck proximal to the diseased aorta without significant morbidity[17] and an even more proximal seal can be achieved with prior carotid–carotid bypass (which allows a seal proximal to the left common carotid origin) or complete arch debranching (with all the great vessels transposed onto the more proximal ascending aorta—Fig. 85-5), which allows coverage around the entire arch, distal to the reimplanted innominate artery. These techniques make distal- and mid-arch disease amenable to endovascular repair, though they increase the invasiveness and complexity of the intervention. Carotid–carotid bypass can be performed via incisions in the neck but complete arch debranching requires median sternotomy (though not cardiopulmonary bypass).

Angulation is a particular problem in the aortic arch and proximal descending thoracic aorta where the arch is not a smooth curve (like a Norman arch) but rather is peaked with an apex (like a Gothic arch; Fig. 85-6). This can lead to type 1 endoleak, particularly around the inner curve of the aorta. If there is a marked 'stand-off' between the device and the inner curve of the aorta the stent-graft can be folded in on itself by the action of blood flowing around the stent-graft rather than through it. Device placement such that the seal zone is (where possible) in a straight segment of aorta a few centimetres either proximal or distal to the point of angulation will avoid issues of poor seal and stand-off, but frequently such placement is impossible and a compromise must be struck between neck length and angulation. Modern devices conform to angled aortic morphology more readily than their predecessors but marked angulation remains a problem which can preclude thoracic aortic endovascular repair.

The blood supply to the spinal cord arises from the anterior spinal artery, a branch of the vertebral artery which usually arises from the first part of the subclavian artery. Additionally there is supply directly from the intercostal arteries as they arise from the descending thoracic aorta and enter the spinal canal as radicular (or medullary) arteries with the dorsal nerve roots. There is frequently a dominant radicular artery—the artery of Adamkiewicz—arising between T8 and L1, usually on the left. Repair of thoracic aortic pathology (whether open or endovascular) carries a risk of coverage (and therefore occlusion) of some or all of this spinal supply with resultant spinal cord ischaemia and diplegia. Open repair offers the possibility of intercostal vessel reimplantation but endovascular repair does not. The overall risk of diplegia with endovascular repair of thoracic aortic aneurysm is in the region of 3%.[18] The risks are higher if the left subclavian is covered, if longer lengths of the thoracic aorta are covered and if there has been prior abdominal aortic repair.[19] Cerebrospinal fluid drainage preserves spinal cord blood flow during aortic cross-clamping and minimises rebound hyperaemia thereafter in animal models.[20] A prophylactic lumbar cerebrospinal fluid drain is protective during open and endovascular repair of thoracic aortic aneurysm (TAA) where the risks of cord ischaemia are thought to be high.[21,22]

THORACIC AORTIC ANEURYSM

The incidence of TAA is approximately 10 per 100,000 people per year,[23] with the incidence increasing as the population ages. Most (70%) involve the ascending aorta. They present frequently as incidental findings on chest X-rays (CXRs) or other imaging, or may cause hoarseness, stridor, dypnoea, dysphagia or pain due to local mass effects. Rupture presents with chest pain and shock and patients with rupture rarely survive to hospital.

The risk of rupture of a TAA is determined by size, site, rate of growth and association with genetic syndromes such as Marfan's. Untreated, most TAAs will eventually rupture[24] but the annual risk of rupture is difficult to accurately quantify. A retrospective review of outcomes of patients with TAA demonstrated annual rupture risk to be 0.3% for TAAs 4–4.9 cm in diameter, 1.7% for TAAs 5–5.9 cm in diameter and 3.6% for TAAs 6 cm or above. Similar annual risks of dissection in TAAs were noted.[25] These estimates are compound risks for all TAAs (ascending, arch and descending aortic sites). Descending thoracic aortic site was an additional (independent) predictor of rupture and descending thoracic aortic aneurysms were larger at presentation.

Repair should be considered when the risks of rupture exceed the risks of intervention. Guidelines from a joint US task force suggest that endovascular repair be considered when an asymptomatic descending aortic TAA reaches 5.5 cm.[26] A higher threshold (6 cm) is suggested for open repair given its greater risks.[26] There have been no clinical trials to demonstrate that observation only is safe up to a given aortic diameter for TAA (unlike the UK small aneurysm trial[27] for abdominal aortic aneurysm (AAA)—see below).

Rapidly expanding aneurysms or symptomatic aneurysms usually require treatment whatever their size. Pseudoaneurysms, saccular aneurysms and mycotic aneurysms are perceived to be at a greater risk of rupture than fusiform degenerative aneurysms and generally require early intervention.

Outcomes of Endovascular Repair and Comparison with Surgery

The aims of endovascular repair of a TAA are a proximal and distal seal in disease-free segments of the aorta and complete exclusion of the aneurysm sac from the circulation. Frequently the length of the aneurysm may require

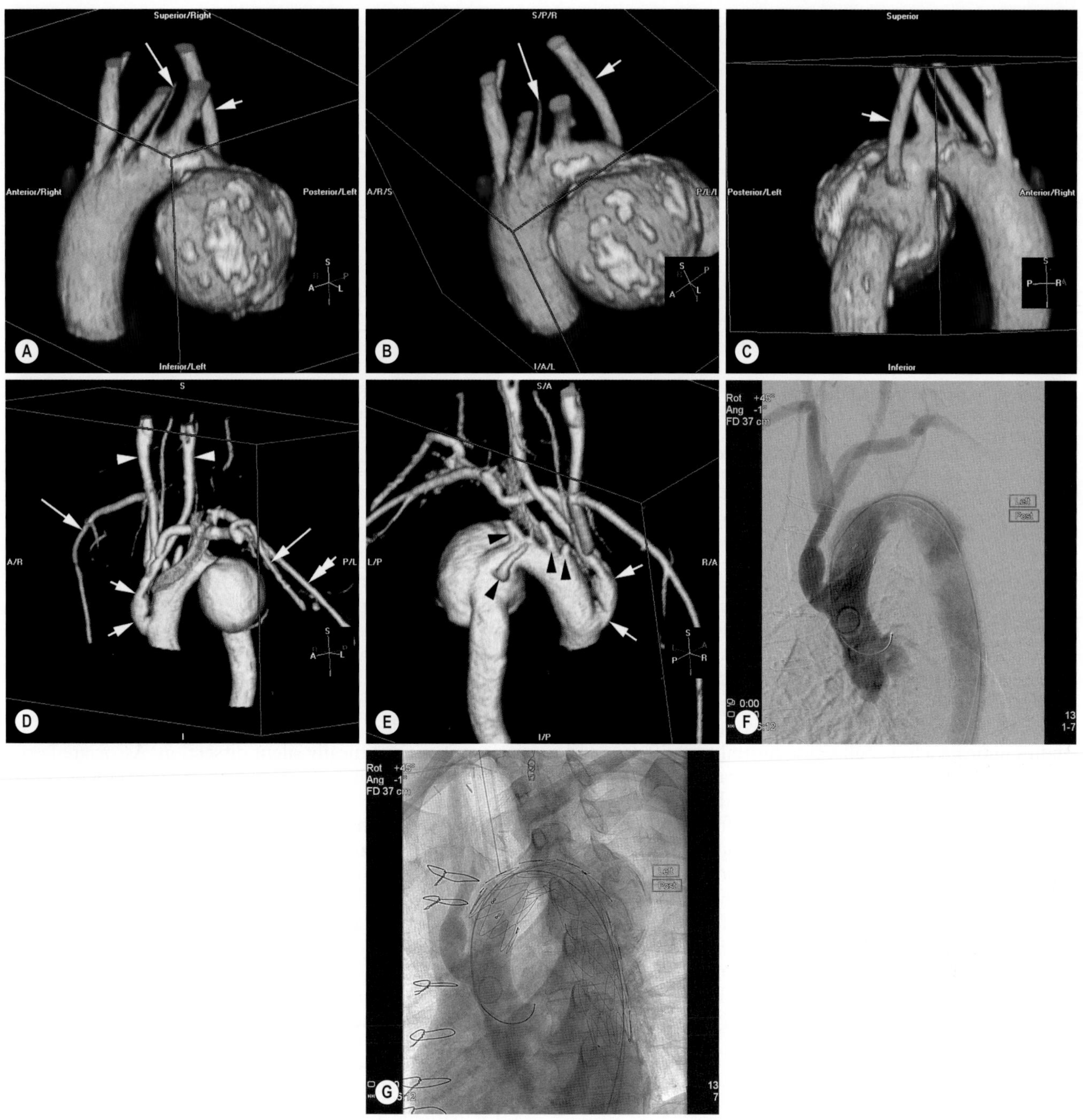

FIGURE 85-5 ■ Proximal arch aneurysm treated with complete aortic debranching and stent-grafting. (A–C) Surface-shaded volumetric CT reconstruction of the aortic arch in left anterior oblique (A), left superior anterior oblique (B) and right posterior oblique (C) projections. The great vessels can be seen arising from the superior surface of the arch. Additionally there is an aberrant left vertebral artery arising directly from the arch (long arrow) and an aberrant right subclavian arising from the aneurysmal proximal descending thoracic aorta (short arrow). (D, E) Surface-shaded volumetric MRA reconstruction following arch debranching in left anterior oblique (D) and right superior posterior oblique projections (E). A 'Y' graft (short arrows) has been constructed between the ascending aorta and the distal great vessels (arrowheads: common carotid arteries; long arrows: subclavian arteries). Gadolinium has been injected into the left arm, resulting in dense opacification of the left subclavian vein (double arrowhead). The ligated stumps of the great vessels (black arrowheads) are evident on the posterior view (E). Subtracted (F) and unsubtracted (G) angiographic images following stent-graft placement over the origins of the ligated great vessels, to the origin of the bypass graft.

several devices to be 'telescoped' one into the other to provide coverage. This may require considerable overlap of components to prevent subsequent dislocation and type 3 endoleak.

Registry data indicate that the overall 30-day mortality for endovascular repair of TAA is in the region of 2–5%.[28–30] Complications include stroke (4–7%), spinal cord ischaemia (2–4%), access vessel damage (2–5%), myocardial infarction (2–4%) and respiratory failure (5%). Endoleaks usually occur early and are seen in 10–20%, and device migration occurs in approximately 3%, though the requirement for secondary intervention

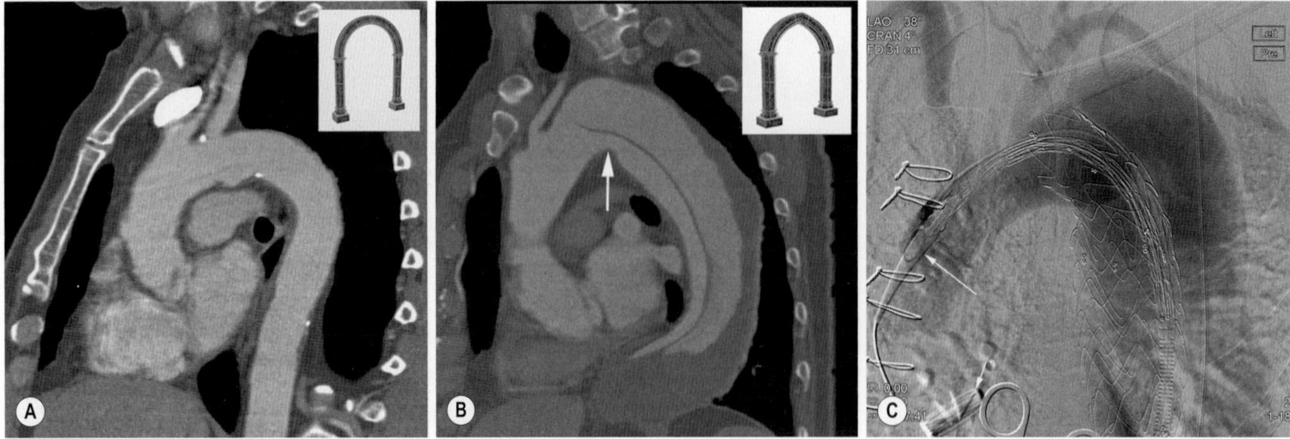

FIGURE 85-6 ■ **Aortic arch configurations for thoracic EVAR.** (A) Norman arch configuration with a shallow ulcer on the inner curve at its apex. Note the smooth curve around the arch without a focal angle (inset: architectural drawing of a Norman arch). (B) Gothic arch configuration with an aortic dissection. Note the angle (arrow) at the apex of the arch (inset: architectural drawing of a Gothic arch). (C) Complication of stent-grafting into a short neck around the apex of a Gothic arch. The device has dislocated out of the short neck at the point of arch angulation, resulting in a significant type 1 endoleak. A new device is being deployed (arrow: delivery system nosecone), extending the stent-graft more proximally in the arch (covering the left subclavian artery) to seal the leak. (Architectural images courtesy of Redwood Stone, West Horrington, Well, UK.)

to treat these problems is low (6–8%).[1] Aneurysm-related mortality by 1 year following endovascular repair of TAA is low (2%). Overall 1-year survival is 80%.[28]

Elective surgical mortality is approximately 10%,[31] dependent on the type of the repair necessary. There are no randomised studies comparing open surgical and endovascular repair of TAAs. Data from non-randomised studies indicate a lower all-cause mortality at 30 days and lower aneurysm-related (but not all-cause) mortality at 12 months for patients treated with endovascular repair.[1] The long-term durability of stent-grafts in the management of thoracic aortic disease is unknown, but 15 years of worldwide experience gives no reason to doubt their structural integrity in the lifespan of the patient. Newer generations of stent-graft might perform better long term than their predecessors, but this is unproven. In the UK, the National Institute for Health and Clinical Excellence (NICE) recommendation is that endovascular repair of TAA is a suitable alternative to surgery in appropriately selected patients.[32]

ACUTE AORTIC SYNDROME

Acute aortic syndrome is a general term used to encompass three aortic lesions with similar presentation: aortic dissection, intramural haematoma (IMH) and penetrating atherosclerotic ulcer (PAU). The exact pathological relationship between these entities is unclear. In aortic dissection, intimal disruption that allows blood to track through a dissection plane in the media can be identified. However, the initiating event for this may be a direct tear in the intima (due to shear stresses on the aortic wall) or intramural haemorrhage (from vasa vasorum) weakening the intima at the site of the tear. Thrombosis of the false lumen of a dissection may give rise to appearances identical to IMH or IMH may be due to microscopic dissection-like intimal tears. Bleeding at the base of a PAU could give rise to IMH or act as a focus for dissection.

Clinical presentation of acute aortic syndromes is usually with abrupt onset of severe chest pain. The classical description is of 'tearing interscapular' pain but pain may be anterior, abdominal or migratory. The symptom complex overlaps with many other potential diagnoses (e.g. myocardial infarction) and diagnosis relies significantly on index of suspicion. A small proportion of patients have a clinically silent dissection. Associated presenting features may be cerebrovascular accident, renal failure and acutely ischaemic bowel or limbs (due to branch vessel occlusion), myocardial infarction and acute aortic regurgitation (due to involvement of the aortic root or coronary ostia), pericardial tamponade, massive haemothorax and profound shock (due to rupture) or progression to aneurysm formation. These complicating features are more common with dissection than with IMH.[33]

Definitive diagnosis is usually made by cross-sectional imaging or transoesophageal ultrasound. A normal CXR does not exclude aortic dissection, IMH or PAU, although it may confirm an alternative diagnosis in patients with low clinical risk.

Of patients presenting with acute aortic syndrome, three-quarters have dissection, with 10–20% having IMH and a small proportion having PAU. Dissection involves the ascending aorta and arch in three-quarters of cases. IMH involves the descending thoracic aorta more frequently and tends to occur in older patients. PAU usually occurs in markedly atheromatous aortic segments, usually the descending thoracic aorta. Whatever the exact pathological relationship between these entities, the principles of management are broadly similar.

THORACIC AORTIC DISSECTION

The incidence of thoracic aortic dissection is about 5–10 per 100,000 people per year and is increasing with an ageing population. Dissection is associated with hypertension (especially if uncontrolled), inherited disorders of elastin such as Marfan's syndrome and certain vasculitides. TAA is a risk factor for dissection and vice versa.

Classification of dissection is important for management. It is classified according to its age (acute: less than 14 days old; subacute: 14 days–2 months; chronic: older than 2 months), the presence of associated complications and location (Stanford A or B).

Untreated, the prognosis of aortic dissection is poor, with an approximately 1% mortality per hour for the first 48 h after presentation. The mortality for type A dissection is worse than that for type B: uncomplicated type B dissection is associated with a 30-day mortality of 10%, though complications occur in 30% and are associated with significantly higher mortality (20% by 48 h, 30% by 30 days).[34]

Management

All patients with aortic dissection should be managed in a high-dependency environment with invasive monitoring. They should have aggressive management of heart rate (HR) and blood pressure to reduce aortic wall stress (HR <60 bpm, sBP <120 mmHg)[35]—though this can sometimes be difficult, requiring a combination of agents. Intravenous β-blockade and nitrates are commonly titrated to an adequate response. Pain control is essential.

As discussed above, disease affecting the ascending aorta is generally unsuitable for endovascular repair and definitive management should be surgical.

For Stanford type B dissections (involving the descending aorta, beyond the left subclavian artery) close clinical observation and serial imaging is mandatory as the requirement for definitive management is determined by the development of complications. A recent randomised trial demonstrated no additional benefit of endovascular repair of uncomplicated Stanford type B dissection over best medical therapy[36] and prophylactic surgical or endovascular repair in the absence of complications is not indicated.

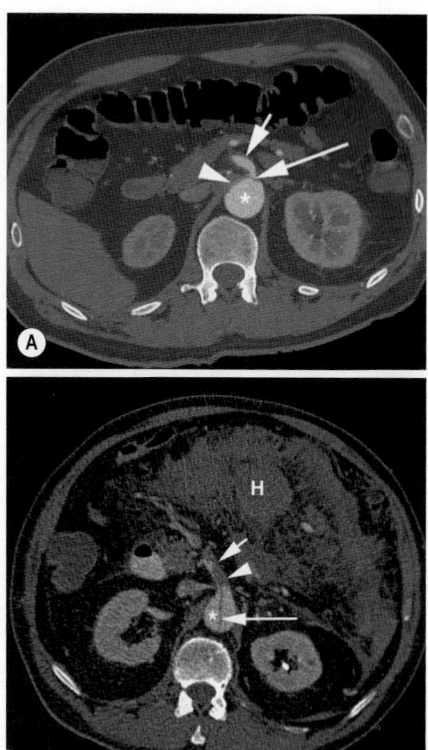

FIGURE 85-7 ■ Static and dynamic branch vessel occlusion. (A) Dynamic branch vessel occlusion. The true lumen (arrowhead) is markedly compressed by the false lumen (asterisk). The dissection flap (long arrow) is seen to prolapse across the ostium of the superior mesenteric artery (SMA) (short arrow), compromising its inflow (though the SMA is still filling). The patient had abdominal pain, rising lactate and thickening of small bowel loops (not shown) consistent with small bowel ischaemia. (B) Static vessel occlusion. The dissection flap (long arrow) has extended into the SMA (short arrow) and there has been thrombosis of the false lumen in the SMA (arrowhead). The true lumen (asterisk) is obliterated distally in the SMA by the combination of the dissection and the thrombus. A large intraperitoneal haematoma is evident (H) due to bleeding from infarcted bowl.

Complicated Type B Dissection

The aim of endovascular management of complicated type B dissection is to treat the complications of the pathology (branch vessel occlusion and end-organ ischaemia) and prevent aneurysm formation and rupture.

Restoration of branch vessel flow is achieved by closure (i.e. coverage with a stent-graft) of the dissection entry tear with the aim of depressurising the false lumen and allowing true lumen re-expansion. Where branch vessels have been occluded dynamically (where the dissection flap has prolapsed across their aortic true lumen ostium—Fig. 85-7A), depressurisation of the false lumen allows the flap to move away from the ostium, with restoration of flow. Where the dissection has extended into a branch vessel (static occlusion—Fig. 85-7B) or where dynamic obstruction is not adequately relieved, additional branch vessel stenting or the deliberate formation of holes in the flap ('fenestration') may be needed.

Not infrequently there are several tears ('fenestrations') in the dissection flap. Coverage of all these fenestrations necessitates stent-grafting a longer length of aorta with increased risk of diplegia, though (theoretically at least) with a greater chance of false lumen collapse. Whether all fenestrations or just the 'primary' entry tear should be covered is debatable. If the dissection extends below the diaphragm there are often fenestrations at the level of the renal arteries or in the infrarenal aorta. Stent-graft placement from the thorax into the abdominal aorta is clearly impossible, as it would necessitate splanchnic and renal artery coverage. In this situation the proximal entry tear (or tears) in the thoracic aorta only are covered in the hope that this will alter the haemodynamics enough to allow abdominal true lumen re-expansion.

Ideally the false lumen should collapse entirely (and be obliterated) or should at least thrombose (Fig. 85-8). False lumen thrombosis protects against rupture and aneurysm formation and is associated with good

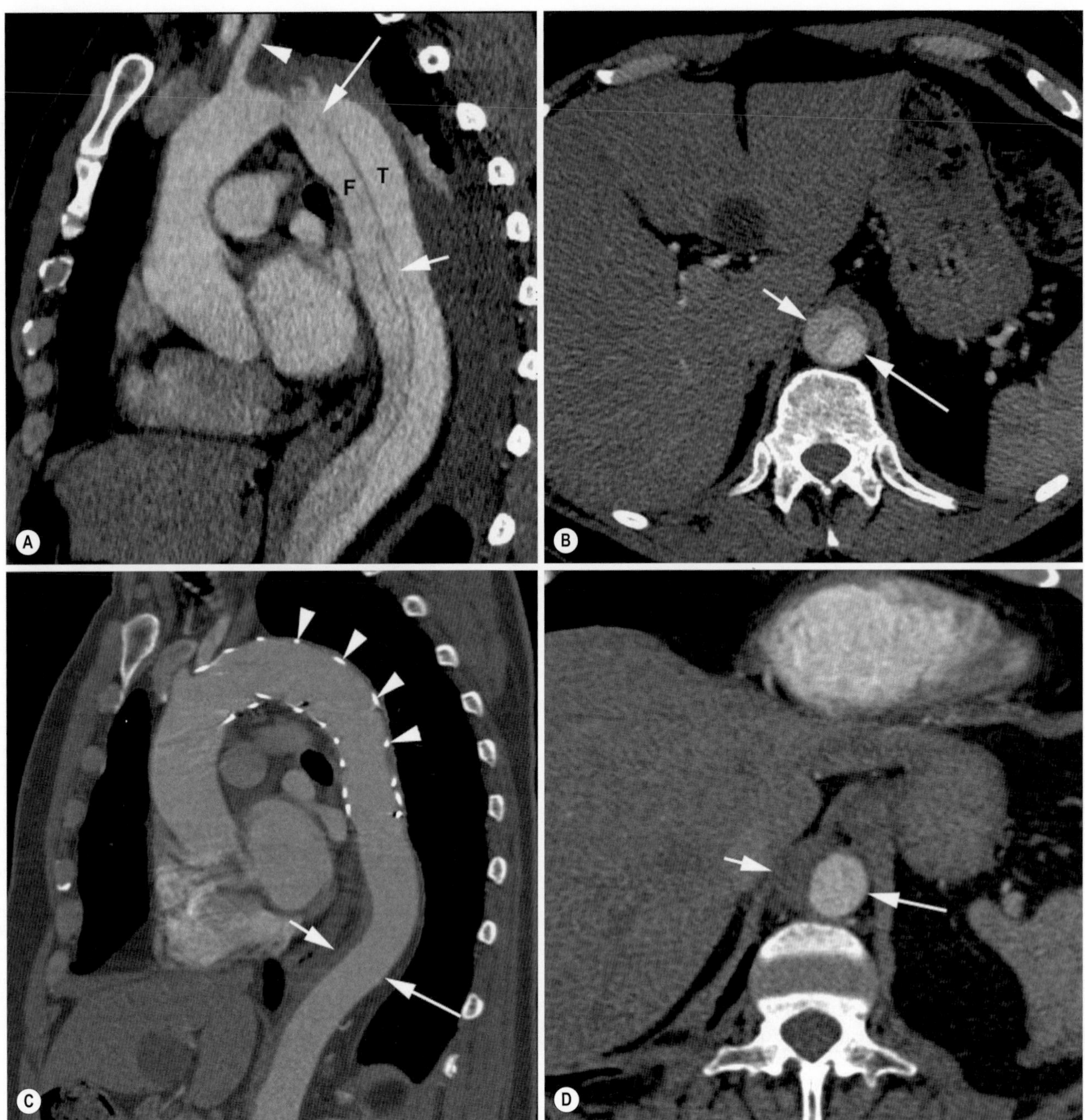

FIGURE 85-8 ■ Coverage of proximal entry tear of a dissection with false lumen thrombosis and collapse. (A) Acute type B dissection. The entry tear (long arrow), a more distal fenestration (short arrow) and the dissection flap are clearly visualised. Arrowhead: left common carotid artery; F: false lumen; T: true lumen. (B) Representative aortic cross-section at the level of the diaphragmatic crura. The true lumen (long arrow) and false lumen (short arrow) both opacify with contrast, indicating patency. (C) Following stent-graft (arrowheads) placement in the true lumen, covering (and sealing) the proximal entry tear. The false lumen (short arrow) has thrombosed and partially collapsed. The true lumen (long arrow) remains patent. (D) Representative aortic cross-section (same level as B), demonstrating thrombosis of the false lumen (short arrow) and retained patency of the true lumen (long arrow).

long-term outcome.[37] Ongoing false lumen perfusion after stent-graft coverage of the entry tear (Fig. 85-9) can occur via uncovered fenestrations, retrogradely from the distal end of the dissection or via backbleeding from branch vessels.

Other techniques to eradicate the false lumen include scissoring or 'cheese-wiring' the flap or using large uncovered stents to pin it back in place. Often a combination of techniques is used.

Stent-grafts for treating acute dissection should not be oversized relative to the vessel to be treated (in contrast to sizing for TAA) as the vessel wall is extremely friable. Aggressive oversizing and the use of balloon moulding can result in aortic rupture or proximal or distal extension

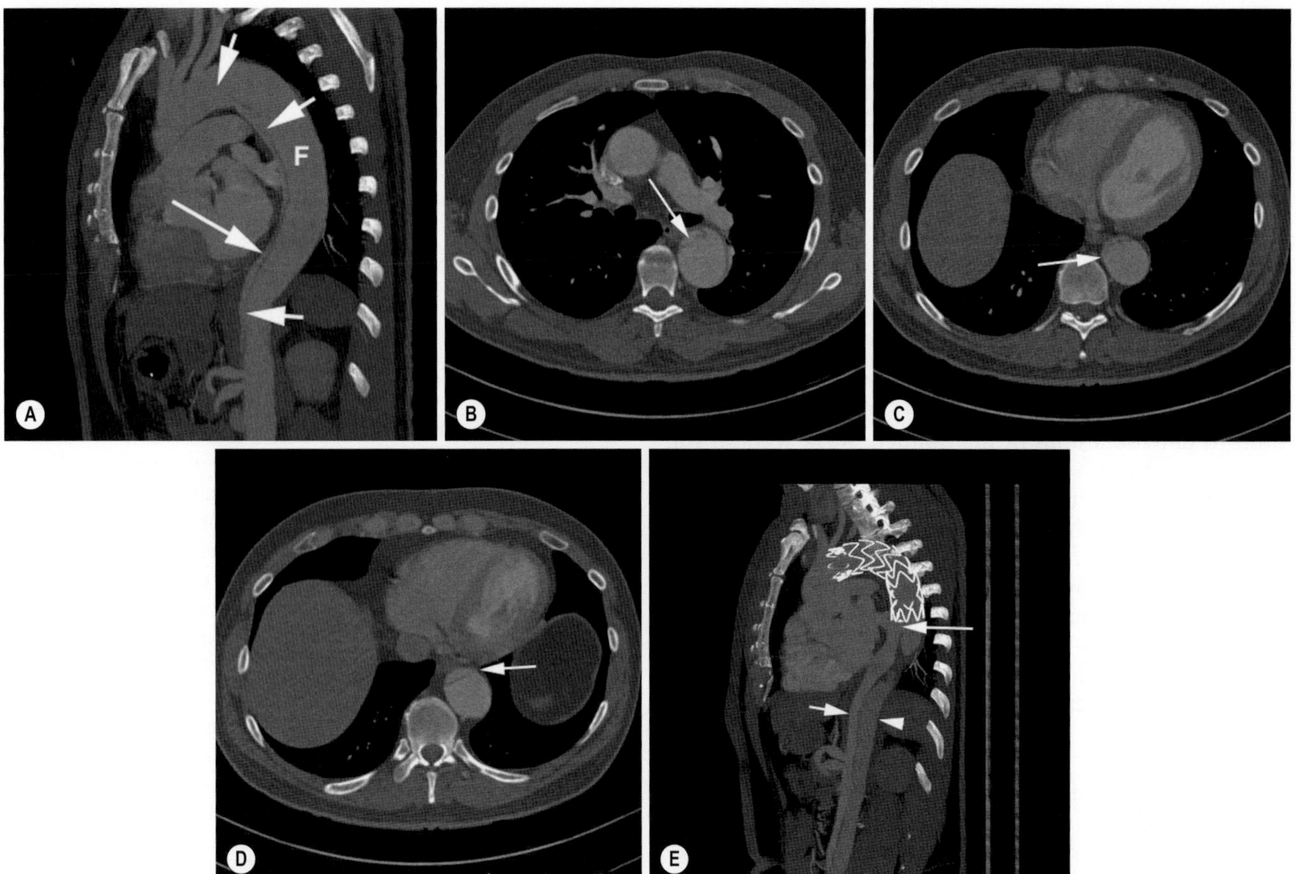

FIGURE 85-9 ■ Coverage of proximal entry tear of a dissection with failure of false lumen thrombosis and ongoing perfusion. (A) Acute type B dissection. The true lumen (long arrow) is significantly compromised by the false lumen (F). In addition to the proximal entry tear, several other fenestrations (short arrows) are evident in the dissection flap. (B–D) Representative aortic cross-sections in the mid (B) and distal (C, D) thoracic aorta demonstrating the fenestrations (arrows) in the flap. The true lumen is compromised by the false lumen. (E) Following stent-graft placement in the true lumen covering (and sealing) the proximal entry tear. The false lumen persists due to ongoing perfusion via a large fenestration just distal to the stent-graft (long arrow), and the other smaller fenestrations demonstrated on the pre-EVAR CT (A–D). Short arrow: true lumen; arrowhead: false lumen.

of the dissection, potentially converting a type B dissection into a type A.[38]

Chronic Dissection and Aneurysmal Development

Thoracic aortic dissection may be associated with aneurysmal development of the aorta at presentation, or it may develop over time following acute dissection. Dissection may also occur de novo in a pre-existing TAA. Management (as for TAA) requires exclusion of the aneurysmal segment of aorta from the circulation by obtaining a proximal and distal seal above and below the aneurysmal segment. This is difficult if the aneurysm is extensive (and especially if it extends below the diaphragm). Moreover, with time, the dissection flap becomes stiffer and fibrous, and is more difficult to displace. It may prevent a stent-graft from opening fully. Not infrequently there has been previous placement of stent-grafts in the aorta (e.g. as treatment for the acute phase of the dissection), which can make subsequent device placement challenging as multiple layers of metalwork and device markers can become confusing.

Outcomes of Endovascular Repair and Comparison with Surgery

A recent meta-analysis of 609 patients undergoing endovascular repair of type B aortic dissection indicated rates of 30-day mortality of 5%, in-hospital major complication of 11% and aortic rupture (during mean follow-up of 20 months) of 2%. False lumen thrombosis was seen in 75% of patients.[39] For studies with follow-up to 2 years, the overall survival was 90%. This compares favourably with surgical outcomes (in-hospital mortality: 34%; in-hospital major complication: 40%).[40] NICE recommendations are that endovascular repair of thoracic aortic dissection is a suitable alternative to surgery in appropriately selected patients.[32]

ACUTE INTRAMURAL HAEMATOMA AND PENETRATING ULCER

The management of these lesions is broadly similar to that of acute aortic dissection. Aggressive medical management should be instituted. Type A lesions require surgery. Complicated type B PAU (with or without associated IMH) should be treated similarly to aortic dissection, with the PAU being considered the 'entry tear'. Complicated type B IMH without an identifiable intimal defect represents a therapeutic challenge as there is no 'target' for limited stent-graft coverage even though the IMH itself may be extensive. It may be necessary to cover the entire involved aorta.

TRAUMATIC LESIONS OF THE THORACIC AORTA

Blunt traumatic lesions of the thoracic aorta account for approximately 15% of road traffic accident fatalities in the UK.[41] The most common site of blunt injury is at the aortic isthmus, at the site of the ligamentum arteriosum, probably because of differential torsional and shear forces acting on the relatively mobile arch and the less mobile descending thoracic aorta during sudden deceleration or acceleration. Other mechanisms such as osseous pinch or hydrostatic injury have been proposed.

A range of appearances is seen on imaging for traumatic aortic injury from minor flaps of intima to traumatic dissection, intramural haematoma or abrupt (sometimes circumferential) changes in aortic contour[42] (Fig. 85-10). Mediastinal haematoma may be evident, though it is unlikely to be aortic in origin (arising instead from damaged mediastinal vessels). A full-thickness tear in the aorta, with high-pressure bleeding into the loose connective tissue of the mediastinum, is unlikely to seal spontaneously and will result in exsanguination and death, usually at-scene. It follows therefore that most patients who survive to imaging will have some form of incomplete aortic injury (IAI), with at least one layer of the aortic wall (often the adventitia) intact.

Untreated, the prognosis of patients with IAI is very poor, with an approximately 30% mortality within 6 h and 50% mortality at 24 h.[43] There are invariably significant associated injuries and prognosis reflects the compound effects of diffuse and significant trauma to multiple organs and organ systems, rather than being due to the aortic injury alone.

The observation that early mortality in patients with IAI was high led to a doctrine of early aortic repair as paramount whatever the priorities for management of associated injuries. More recently, extrapolating from medical management of type B aortic dissection, several studies have demonstrated that immediate aggressive blood pressure control (mBP<80 mmHg) markedly reduces the risks of rupture,[44,45] allowing time for treatment of other life-threatening injuries and control of haemorrhage, sepsis, hypothermia and acidosis. Control of blood pressure in this manner may allow definitive aortic repair to be safely delayed by days or weeks.[44,45] Sometimes blood pressure control may be incompatible with requirements for treatment of other injuries (especially the maintenance of cerebral perfusion pressure in head injury), in which case earlier definitive repair is indicated. Senior clinical consultation is essential in these complex cases[46] to ensure sequencing of therapeutic interventions is optimised and timely.

The mortality associated with endovascular repair of IAI is significantly less than that for open surgical repair (7 vs 15%).[47] Rates of significant morbidity are also lower (diplegia: 0 and 6%; stroke 1 and 5%, respectively) with identical rates of technical success.[47] However, the long-term performance of stent-grafts in these (often young) patients is unknown. American College of Cardiology guidelines on management of thoracic aortic disease[26] state that endovascular repair of IAI 'be considered'. There are currently no guidelines in the UK.

Penetrating Injury to the Thoracic Aorta

Full-thickness penetrating injury to the thoracic aorta usually results in death at-scene. IAI is uncommon but if it occurs, it can be managed similarly to blunt injury.

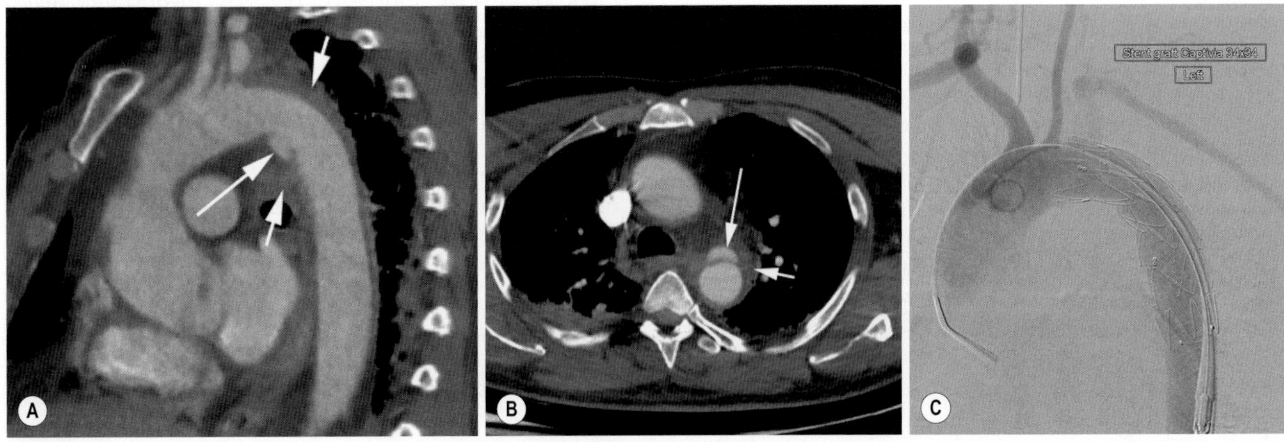

FIGURE 85-10 ■ **Aortic trauma.** (A, B) Typical appearances of blunt traumatic incomplete aortic injury with irregularity of the external aortic contour in the region of the ligamentum arteriosum (long arrow) and periaortic blood (short arrow) from damage to vasa-vasorum and mediastinal vessels. (C) Stent-graft repair with coverage of the site of aortic injury with a short device.

Iatrogenic injury (usually the result of misplaced attempts at central venous cannulation) is survivable if recognised immediately and ideally before the device is removed.

AORTIC COARCTATION

Most cases of aortic coarctation are diagnosed in childhood and early repair is associated with improved outcome and rates of complication.[48] Endovascular treatment of coarctation in childhood is problematic as access vessels are small and stent deployment can interfere with the later growth of the treated aortic segment, leading to recoarctation despite initial technical success. Angioplasty (without stenting) is possible, though it cannot deal with elastic vessel recoil. In general, endovascular management of coarctation is therefore reserved for older children and adults.

Outcomes after endovascular repair for coarctation (Fig. 85-11) are good with technical success rates in excess of 90%.[49] Peri-procedural mortality is low (2–3%) for both endovascular and open-surgical repair.[50,51] Rates of restenosis are approximately 10% following primary surgical repair and 5% following stent placement.[50,51] Redo surgery is complex and in this situation endovascular repair may be preferable.

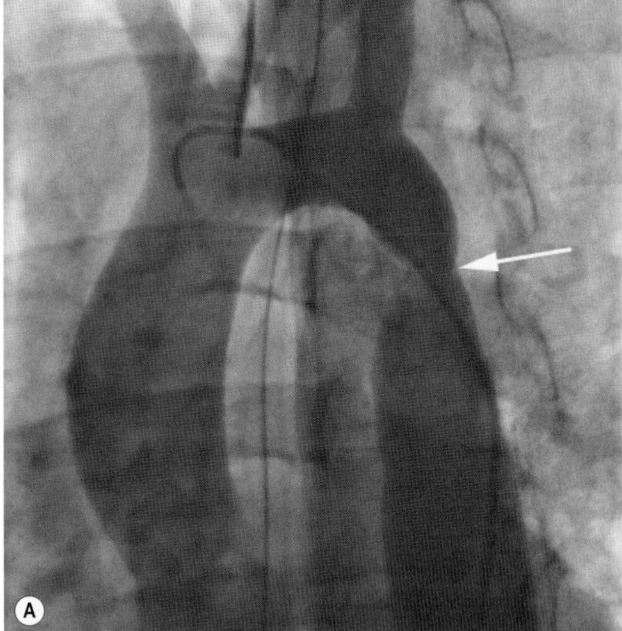

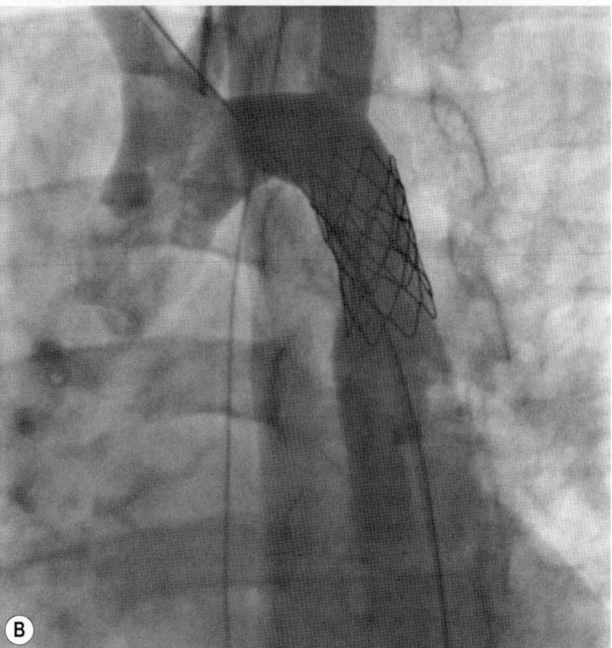

FIGURE 85-11 ■ Aortic coarctation. (A) Aortic coarctation (arrow). Note the hypertrophied great vessels (particularly the left subclavian) which supply collateral pathways (e.g. via the internal thoracic artery and intercostals) to beyond the coarctation. (B) Coarctation (same patient as A) treated with a balloon mounted stent.

ABDOMINAL AORTIC ANEURYSM

Abdominal aortic aneurysm (AAA) is a disease of the elderly with a prevalence of 8% in the over 60s. The male : female ratio is 7 : 1. AAA is six times more common than TAA. Most are occult and are only diagnosed incidentally during investigation of other disorders or when they rupture. Occasionally, AAAs present with symptoms other than rupture—usually abdominal or back pain.

The risk of AAA rupture is a function of size: a 5.5-cm AAA has an annual risk of rupture of about 6%, but for an 8-cm AAA the risk it is 25%.[52,53] Symptomatic AAAs are at greater risk of rupture and usually require urgent intervention.

The aetiology of AAA is unclear. There is a strong familial tendency, and most patients are smokers or ex-smokers. Patients often have atherosclerotic disease elsewhere. An inflammatory infiltrate is seen in the walls of large AAAs though whether this arises in response to atheromatous deposits or merely as a response to common risk factors is unknown. In a small proportion of AAAs (5–10%) the inflammatory infiltrate is marked. These patients tend to be younger, and are more often symptomatic, though the risks of rupture for a given size are lower. Unlike 'atherosclerotic' AAA there is often elevation of serum inflammatory markers and a cuff of periaortic 'haziness' on CT.

Anatomical Considerations in AAA repair

Most AAA stent-graft systems comprise a main body with a long limb on one side and a short limb (or 'gate') on the other (see Fig. 85-1). Once the main body is deployed, the short limb is catheterised from the opposite side. A second limb is then inserted over a wire into the short limb of the main body, sealing inside the main body at a flow divider. Innovative single-piece stent-graft designs are available (for example, with limbs that are pulled into place) though these have, as yet, not been widely adopted.

As stated earlier, the anatomy of the proximal 'neck' is critical for the efficacy of any endovascular repair. For AAA the 'neck' refers to the segment of aorta between the lowest renal artery and the aneurysm. Short, angled or thrombus-filled necks increase the risk of endoleak and device failure. Proximal bare stents can be deployed across the renal arteries to achieve a more secure fixation in short necks.

The distal 'landing zone' in AAA repair is usually the common iliac artery. However, where this vessel is also aneurysmal, or is short, extension to the external iliac artery is necessary, usually with previous proximal embolisation of the internal iliac artery (IIA) to prevent a significant type 2 endoleak via back-filling. Embolisation of the IIA on one side is associated with buttock claudication in up to 31% and erectile dysfunction in up to 17%.[54] Risks of buttock claudication are higher if the IIA embolisation is necessary bilaterally. Iliac branched devices which preserve IIA patency are available.

Risks and Timing of Repair

Scheduling intervention to aortic aneurysms is a balance between the risks of intervention (be it open surgery or EVAR) and the risks of rupture. The patient's overall fitness needs to be carefully considered as this affects both the risks of intervention and the likelihood of the patient surviving long enough beyond the intervention to see the benefit of it. The UK Small Aneurysm Study[27] demonstrated that surgical treatment of AAAs smaller than 5.5 cm (on US) was associated with a greater overall mortality than conservative management and this has underpinned the practice of 'watchful waiting' with serial imaging of AAAs smaller than 5.5 cm. Intuitively, any new method of treating AAA with an improved perioperative mortality over that of open surgery (6%)[2,4] would alter the balance of risks between watching and intervening, so that treatment could be offered safely for smaller AAAs. Endovascular repair of AAA is associated with a 30-day mortality approximately one-third that of open repair (2%),[2,4] though whether this means smaller aneurysms should be treated with EVAR remains unproven. A recent randomised trial to test this hypothesis in AAAs 4–5 cm in diameter demonstrated equal mortality for EVAR and surveillance groups though the study was probably underpowered to detect a difference.[55]

Outcomes of Endovascular Repair and Comparison with Surgery

There are two randomised trials that compared EVAR with open surgical repair of AAA: the UK EVAR 1 trial and the Dutch DREAM Trial.[2,4] Both these trials demonstrated a threefold reduction in 30-day mortality with EVAR (2 vs 6% for open repair). At 4 years aneurysm-based mortality was also reduced in patients randomised to EVAR though all-cause mortality (principally due to non-aneurysm-related cardiovascular death) was the same in both EVAR and open repair groups.[5]

Critics of endovascular repair note that there is an increased rate of secondary interventions in the EVAR group (20 vs 6% for open surgery by 4 years, mostly for type 1 or 2 endoleak), that not all patients are anatomically suitable for EVAR, that an economic analysis of the EVAR 1 trial's data suggests that by 4 years EVAR is more expensive than open repair (£13,257 vs £9946) and that the durability of EVAR in the medium-to-long term is unknown. However, both of the randomised trials of EVAR versus open surgery were carried out relatively early in the development of endovascular aneurysm repair (EVAR 1 recruited from 1999 to 2003). Since they reported, rates of secondary intervention have fallen[56] due to the improved performance of newer generations of devices and a greater awareness of what is and is not suitable anatomy for EVAR. More conformable, fenestrated and scalloped devices increase the applicability of an endovascular approach in challenging anatomy, meaning more patients are treatable with EVAR. Device costs are falling and, as less intensive follow-up protocols are advocated,[8] the cost of follow-up (a significant proportion of the cost of EVAR) is decreasing. Finally, though long-term durability of EVAR remains unproven, the significant cumulative cardiovascular mortality of the cohort of patients with large AAA[57] renders this consideration rather moot.

ENDOVASCULAR REPAIR OF RUPTURED AAA

The mortality of ruptured AAA (rAAA) exceeds 85%. About half of patients with ruptured aneurysms die in the community and of those arriving alive in hospital only a quarter will survive to discharge. These figures have changed little over the past 50 years.[58] The incidence of rAAA is increasing.[59]

Emergency endovascular repair (eEVAR) of rAAA (Fig. 85-12) necessitates taking a haemodynamically compromised patient to CT (to allow device sizing and procedural planning) before the point of definitive care, introducing a small delay with potential adverse effects on mortality. About half of all patients with rAAA have aneurysm morphology suitable for endovascular repair.[60] On the other hand, the theoretical benefit of a minimally invasive repair over open surgery is enhanced in a critically ill patient. The trade-off between these three factors (delay, suitability and invasiveness) is fundamental in determining the possible role of eEVAR in rAAA. In practice, logistical issues (such as availability of skilled staff) will also be critical, especially out-of-hours.

Meta-analyses of pooled data from numerous small studies of eEVAR have demonstrated in-hospital mortality of about 20%.[60,61] Open repair of rAAA is associated with 30-day mortality of about 40%.[58,62] The transfusion requirements, intensive care and hospital stay and cost of eEVAR also appear to be lower.[61,63,64] Some of the improved outcomes seen with eEVAR may be accounted for by publication[61] and selection bias (more stable patients being transferred to CT for EVAR work-up, whilst the less stable ones are taken immediately to open surgery). There is, as yet, no level 1 evidence comparing eEVAR with open repair for rAAA, though a multicentre randomised controlled trial (IMPROVE)[65] is due to report in November 2013 and it would not be surprising if eEVAR became the treatment of choice for rAAA once the results of this trial are known.

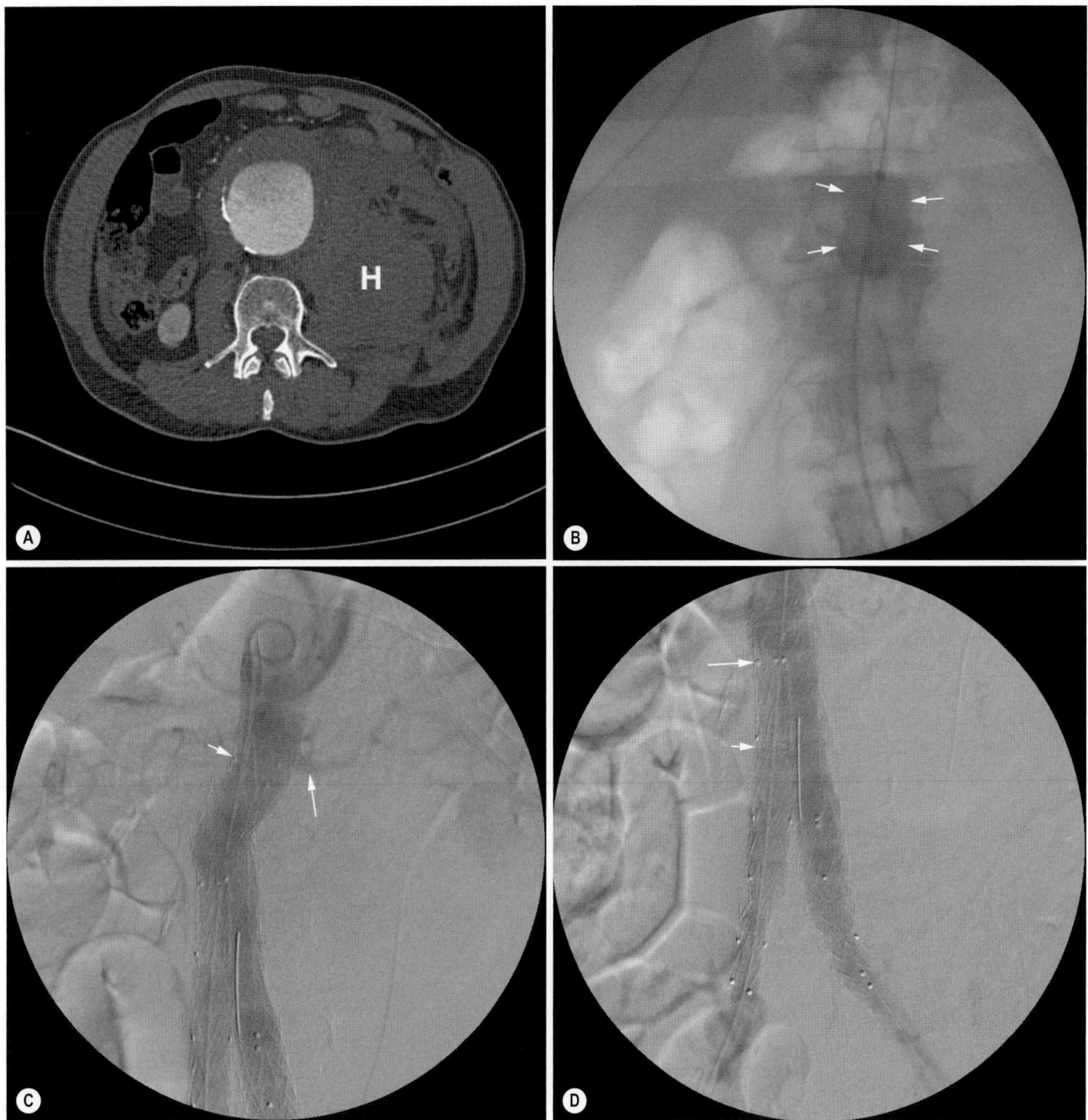

FIGURE 85-12 ■ **Emergency EVAR for ruptured AAA.** (A) Typical appearances of a ruptured AAA with a sizable left retroperitoneal haematoma (H) and a 7-cm AAA. (B) Suprarenal aortic occlusion balloon (arrows) has been placed (percutaneously) via a common femoral artery approach as a temporising measure to prevent further bleeding while the patient is prepared and the stent-grafts chosen and readied. (C, D) Completion angiograms following emergency stent-graft repair demonstrating complete exclusion of the AAA from the circulation and good flow into the common iliac arteries bilaterally. (C) Long arrow: left renal artery; short arrow: marker on upper edge of stent-graft fabric. (D) Long arrow: upper markers of contralateral limb aligned with flow divider of the main body; short arrow: ring marking lower extent of contralateral limb stump or 'gate'. The patient was discharged 3 days later.

THORACO-ABDOMINAL ANEURYSMS

So far this chapter has dealt specifically with aneurysms arising solely above or below the renal and mesenteric arteries. Thoraco-abdominal aneurysms cross these anatomical arterial boundaries and present very significant challenges for both open and endovascular repair. Thoraco-abdominal aneurysms are classified into four types depending on their anatomical location and extent. They are invariably fatal when they rupture but (as with TAA) there are no studies to guide timing of intervention.

The peri-procedural mortality of open repair is around 19%.[66] This usually involves replacement of the affected portions of the aorta with a synthetic graft, with reimplantation of branch vessels either individually or as

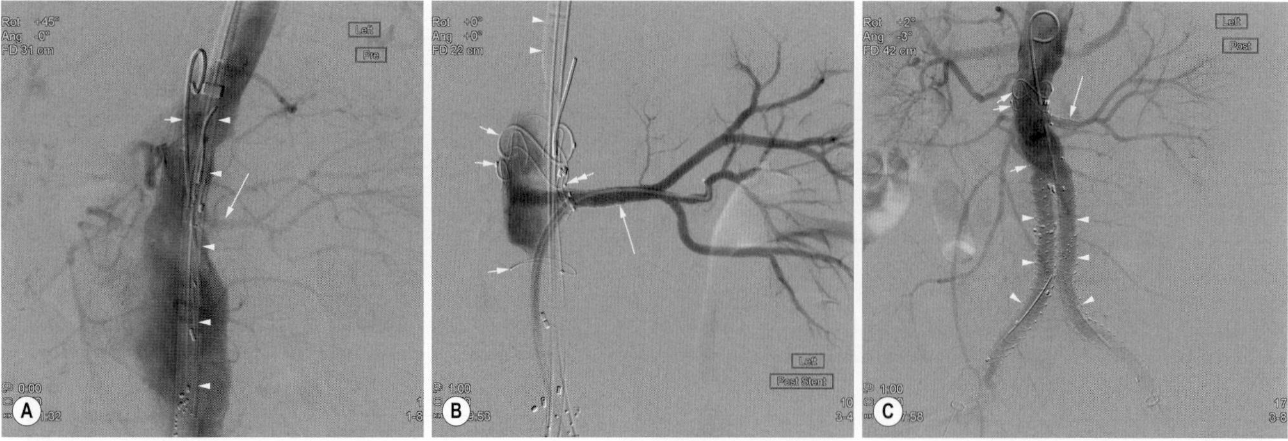

FIGURE 85-13 ■ **Branched stent-graft repair.** AAA with a short conical neck, unsuitable for repair with a conventional device, being repaired with a custom-built branched device (same patient as in Fig. 85-2A). (A) Main body of the device about to be deployed. Long arrow: left renal artery; short arrow: pigtail catheter; arrowheads: delivery system sheath within which the constrained main body is evident. (B) Angiogram following main body and branch vessel stent-graft deployment. The main body (short arrows) has been deployed above the left renal artery. A ring of high-density markers can be seen in the main body wall (double arrowhead) surrounding a custom-made fenestration (hole). A short covered stent (long arrow) has been placed through this into the left renal artery, preserving flow into it. Arrowheads: main body delivery system nose cone. (C) Completion angiogram following branched stent-graft repair. The proximal seal is above the left renal artery but below the right. Flow into the left renal artery is preserved via the fenestration and covered stent (long arrow). There is good flow into the common iliac arteries via iliac extensions (arrowheads). The aneurysm is completely excluded from the circulation. Short arrows: main body.

'islands' of native aorta from which several vessels arise. Cardiopulmonary bypass is sometimes necessary. A 'hybrid' repair involves insertion of a stent-graft to exclude the aneurysm, with the mesenteric and renal arteries then surgically reimplanted onto a conduit from the iliac arteries. The peri-procedural mortality of hybrid repair is in the region of 15–20%.[66]

Endovascular grafts that have a means of preserving flow into the visceral vessels have been developed, principally to allow treatment of complex juxtarenal AAAs. Such devices have fenestrations (holes) or branches to allow aortic side branch perfusion (Fig. 85-13). Series of fenestrated stent-grafts to treat thoraco-abdominal aneurysms have been published with encouraging intermediate-term mortality (about 5%),[66] though these results are predominantly from three institutions (worldwide) with expertise in the technique and may not be generalisable more widely.[67]

AORTIC STENOSES AND OCCLUSIONS

Haemodynamically significant stenoses of the infrarenal aorta are rare. Surgical options include localised aortic endarterectomy or bypass. Endovascular options include 'kissing balloon' angioplasty, 'kissing' aortic to common iliac artery stents or primary aortic stenting (first described in 1985[68]). These procedures are significantly less invasive than open aortic surgery, usually requiring a single night's stay in hospital. In some institutions they are performed as day cases. Primary stenting has 5-year patency rates of 80–100% for aortic stenosis and 60% for stenoses extending into the iliac ateries.[69,70] Complications are uncommon.[69]

SUMMARY AND CONCLUSION

Management of aortic disease is complex, requiring the involvement of vascular radiologists, vascular surgeons and anaesthetists skilled in the management of vascular patients. Stent-grafts offer a minimally invasive option for aortic repair though they are associated with some novel complications and clinical and imaging follow-up is essential. The evidence suggests that, in general, endovascular repair is associated with lower procedural mortality, though at the expense of greater rates of secondary interventions over time, than open surgical repair. There remains a cohort of patients who are unsuitable for endovascular repair, principally because of morphological constraints. Emergency EVAR for aortic trauma and spontaneous rupture is promising, with particularly low mortality relative to open surgery.

As stent-graft technology develops, the results and applicability of endovascular repair of aortic pathology would be expected to improve further. Branched and fenestrated technologies are particularly exciting developments. It is possible that, in the near future, the majority of aortic pathology is treated with an endovascular technique, with open surgery being the exception rather than the rule.

For a full list of references, please see ExpertConsult.

FURTHER READING

5. EVAR trial participants. Endovascular aneurysm repair versus open repair in patients with abdominal aortic aneurysm (EVAR trial 1): randomised controlled trial. Lancet 2005;365:2179–86.
27. Hiratzka LF, Bakris GL, Beckman JA, et al. ACCF/AHA/AATS/ACR/ASA/SCA/SCAI/SIR/STS/SVM Guidelines for the diagnosis

and management of patients with thoracic aortic disease. A Report of the American College of Cardiology Foundation/American Heart Association Task Force on Practice Guidelines, American Association for Thoracic Surgery, American College of Radiology, American Stroke Association, Society of Cardiovascular Anesthesiologists, Society for Cardiovascular Angiography and Interventions, Society of Interventional Radiology, Society of Thoracic Surgeons, and Society for Vascular Medicine. J Am Coll Cardiol 2010;55:e27–129.

39. Eggebrecht H, Nienaber CA, Neuhäuser M, et al. Endovascular stent-graft placement in aortic dissection: a meta-analysis. Eur Heart J 2006;27:489–98.
42. McPherson SJ. Thoracic aortic and great vessel trauma and its management. Semin Intervent Radiol 2007;24:180–96.
64. Cochrane Database of Systematic Reviews. Endovascular treatment for ruptured abdominal aortic aneurysm. 1996. Available at: <http://dx.doi.org/10.1002/14651858.CD005261.pub2>. Accessed 7 April 2012.

CHAPTER 86

Peripheral Vascular Disease Intervention

Robert A. Morgan • Anna-Maria Belli • Joo-Young Chun

CHAPTER OUTLINE

Since the first edition of this textbook, vascular radiology has changed beyond recognition. It was only 30 years ago that the role of radiology in the vascular system was mainly to provide diagnostic images using invasive angiography. Since the development of interventional techniques in the late 1980s, interventional radiologists have assumed a major role not only in the diagnosis of vascular disorders but also in their treatment.

The other main advance in vascular radiology has been the development of non-invasive imaging such as duplex ultrasound, multidetector computed tomographic angiography (MDCTA) and magnetic resonance angiography (MRA). The current range of diagnostic and interventional techniques is too extensive to be described fully in a general textbook of radiology. The aim of this chapter is to provide a brief overview of salient features of diagnostic angiography and to describe the role of the main interventional techniques in the vascular system. A description of non-invasive angiographic imaging is described in Chapter 84 and a discussion of aortic and renal arterial disease is covered in Chapter 85 and Chapter 90.

INTERVENTIONAL RADIOLOGY TECHNIQUES

The following are brief descriptions of the main therapeutic procedures used by vascular interventional radiologists.

Angioplasty

Percutaneous transluminal angioplasty (PTA) refers to treatment of a vascular stenosis or occlusion with a balloon catheter, which is introduced into the blood vessel and advanced to the site of the lesion. The balloon is inflated for a short period of time. After deflating the balloon, a check angiogram is performed to assess the success of the procedure (Fig. 86-1).

Stenting

This refers to the placement of a metallic mesh tube across a vascular stenosis or occlusion. There are two main types of stent: balloon expandable stents are mounted on a balloon catheter and deployed by inflating the balloon; self-expanding stents are compressed on a delivery catheter and released by withdrawing an outer sheath, allowing them to expand by their own radial force (Fig. 86-2).

Stents may be used as the primary method of treatment or may be reserved for use if PTA is unsuccessful, depending on the location and type of lesion.

Embolisation

Embolisation refers to the occlusion of a blood vessel by delivery of embolic material through a catheter. Embolisation has a wide range of applications, including the treatment of haemorrhage, aneurysms, vascular malformations and the treatment and palliation of cancer, particularly primary and secondary hepatic malignancy.

There are a large variety of embolic agents, including metallic springs (coils), particulate matter, gelatin sponge, glue and liquids such as absolute alcohol. The choice depends on the anatomical site, the nature of the lesion and the personal preference of the operator.

Some embolic agents, such as gelatin sponge, are considered temporary, and can be used to control

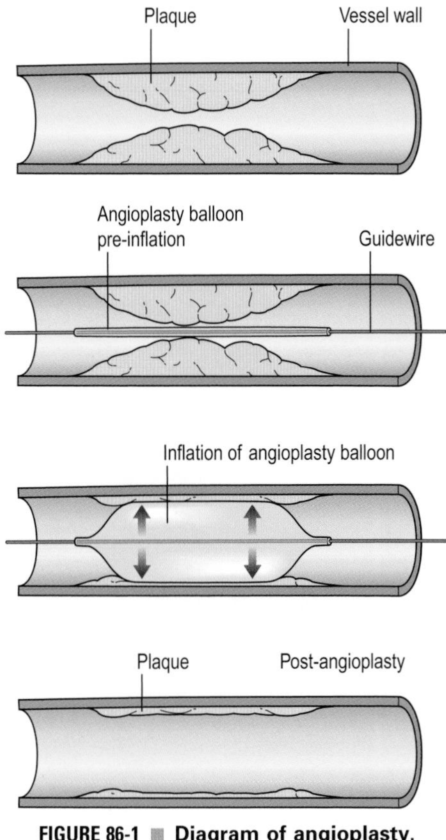

FIGURE 86-1 ■ **Diagram of angioplasty.**

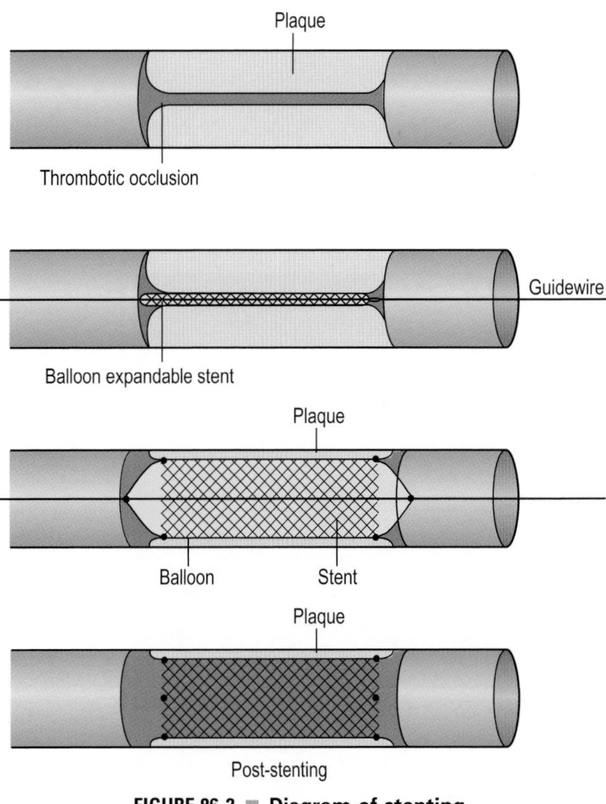

FIGURE 86-2 ■ **Diagram of stenting.**

haemorrhage when recanalisation of the parent vessel may be desirable once the 'acute' lesion has healed, e.g. traumatic injury to the internal iliac artery following pelvic trauma. Permanent particulate emboli are made from various agents, but polyvinyl alcohol (PVA) is the best known example. These agents are not radio-opaque and must be suspended in contrast medium. They cause occlusion by 'silting up' the blood supply. The level of occlusion depends on the size and type of particles chosen. Particulate emboli are used in the treatment of benign and malignant tumours, such as uterine leiomyoma and renal angiomyolipoma (Fig. 86-3). They may be used in combination with chemotherapeutic agents (drug-eluting beads) in hepatic chemoembolisation. Coils are used in situations analogous to tying of a vessel surgically, but knowledge of vascular anatomy is important for avoiding retrograde filling of a lesion from collateral vessels. They are used widely in the embolisation of haemorrhage (Fig. 86-4) and the exclusion of aneurysms and pseudoaneurysms.

Liquid embolic agents include sclerosants such as absolute alcohol, sodium tetradecyl sulphate (STD), glue (e.g. n-butyl-2-cyanoacylate) and newer agents such as Onyx. Sclerosants are useful in venous embolisation, e.g. varicoceles and low-flow vascular malformations. Glue and Onyx are particularly useful in dealing with high-flow arteriovenous malformations and visceral artery aneurysms.

Thrombolysis

This refers to the dissolution of blood clots within an artery or vein by the injection or infusion of a thrombolytic (clot-dissolving) drug directly into the thrombus through a catheter, which has been advanced directly into the thrombus. Although successful thrombolysis may be achieved within a short time, it is not uncommon for the lytic agent to be infused over 24–48 h. Patients undergo periodic check angiography to assess the progress of the treatment. In most cases, successful clearance of the thrombus reveals an underlying causative lesion, which should be treated by angioplasty or stenting during the same procedure. Thrombolysis was a very popular technique for the treatment of acute lower limb ischaemia about 10–15 years ago. It is less often used now but it is still performed in selected cases.

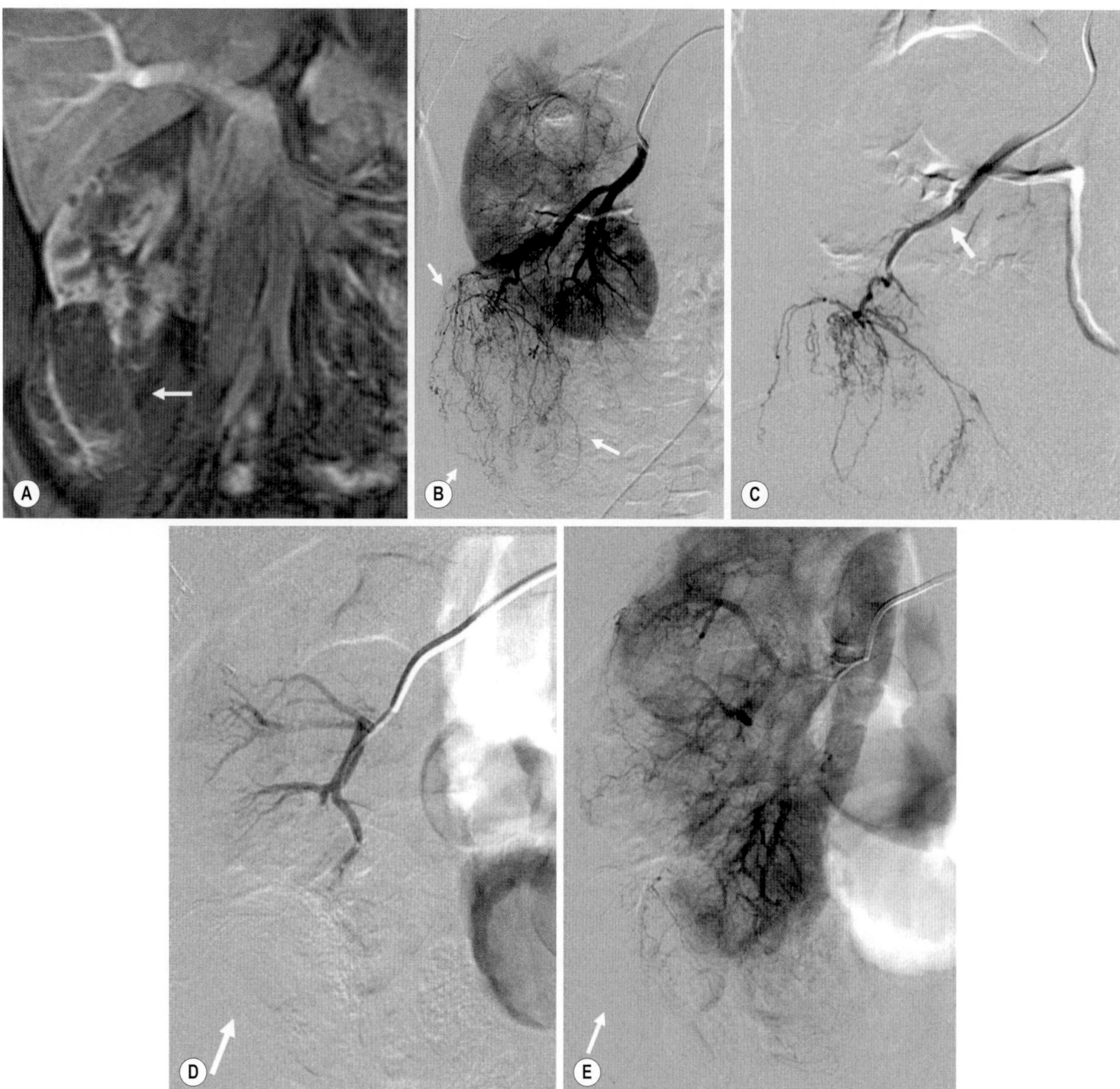

FIGURE 86-3 ■ **Embolisation of angiomyolipoma (AML).** (A) Large AML in the lower pole of right kidney in a patient with tuberous sclerosis (arrow). (B) Right renal angiogram demonstrating tumour vascularity within the AML (arrows). (C) Super-selective catheterisation of an interpolar segmental artery that supplies the AML with a coaxial microcatheter (arrow). (D, E) Angiograms after embolisation with PVA demonstrating devascularisation of the AML (arrows).

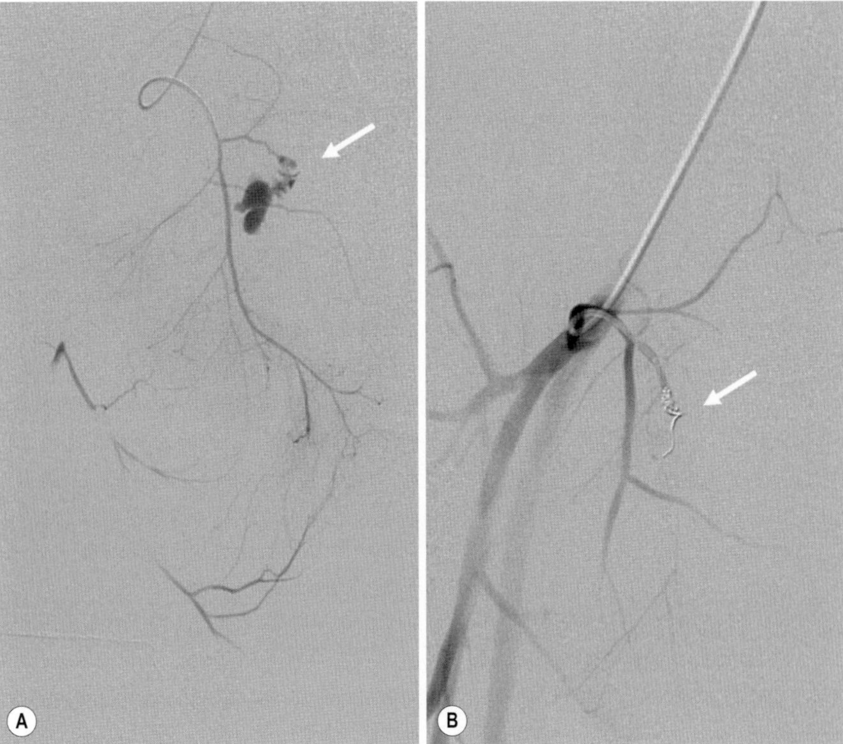

FIGURE 86-4 ■ Embolisation of bleeding lower limb artery. (A) Femoral angiogram in a patient who incurred penetrating traumatic arterial injury to the upper thigh. There is active extravasation of contrast medium from a branch of the profunda femoris artery (arrow). (B) The bleeding has ceased after selective embolisation with metal coils (arrow).

ARTERIAL SYSTEM

PELVIC AND LOWER EXTREMITY ARTERIES

Angiographic Anatomy (Fig. 86-5)

At the level of L4, the aorta divides into the common iliac arteries, which pass in front of the iliac veins and give off no major branches. At the level of the mid sacrum, they divide into the external and internal iliac arteries. The internal iliac arteries supply the pelvis and surrounding musculature. They divide into anterior divisions, which supply the viscera, and posterior divisions, which mainly supply the musculature. The external iliac artery has no major branches, although it gives rise to the inferior epigastric artery at the junction with the common femoral artery. At the level of the inguinal ligament, the external iliac artery becomes the common femoral artery—a short vessel that gives rise to the profunda femoris (or deep femoral artery), which supplies the muscles of the thigh; and the superficial femoral artery (SFA), which has no major branches and passes distally. At the level of the adductor canal, the SFA becomes the popliteal artery, which gives rise to the vessels of the calf, which are the anterior and posterior tibial arteries and the peroneal artery. At the level of the ankle, the anterior tibial artery becomes the dorsalis pedis artery and the posterior tibial artery becomes the medial and lateral plantar arteries. The anterior tibial artery is the most lateral calf vessel, whereas the posterior tibial artery is the most medial. In the forefoot, the plantar arch is formed by the lateral plantar branch of the posterior tibial artery and the dorsalis pedis artery. Anatomical variations of the lower extremity arteries are outside the scope of this chapter.

Arterial Disease Affecting the Lower Extremity

The most common condition affecting the arteries of the lower extremity is tissue ischaemia due to occlusive disease. Occlusive disease may be acute, acute-on-chronic (where acute occlusion occurs in the presence of a previous chronic stenosis or occlusion) or chronic occlusion. Most patients present with symptoms of chronic occlusive disease, usually caused by atherosclerosis. Less common causes include thromboembolism, acute thrombotic occlusion, microembolism, entrapment syndromes, cystic adventitial disease, trauma and vasculitis, including vasospastic disorders and Buerger's disease.

The clinical presentation varies, depending on the type, location and number of the arterial lesions. Patients may be asymptomatic, may suffer from pain on walking (intermittent claudication), pain while at rest, or tissue loss in the form of either ulceration or gangrene. In general, patients with intermittent claudication are not treated with invasive procedures unless their claudication distance is very short or their symptoms substantially limit their lifestyle. Patients with rest pain and tissue loss

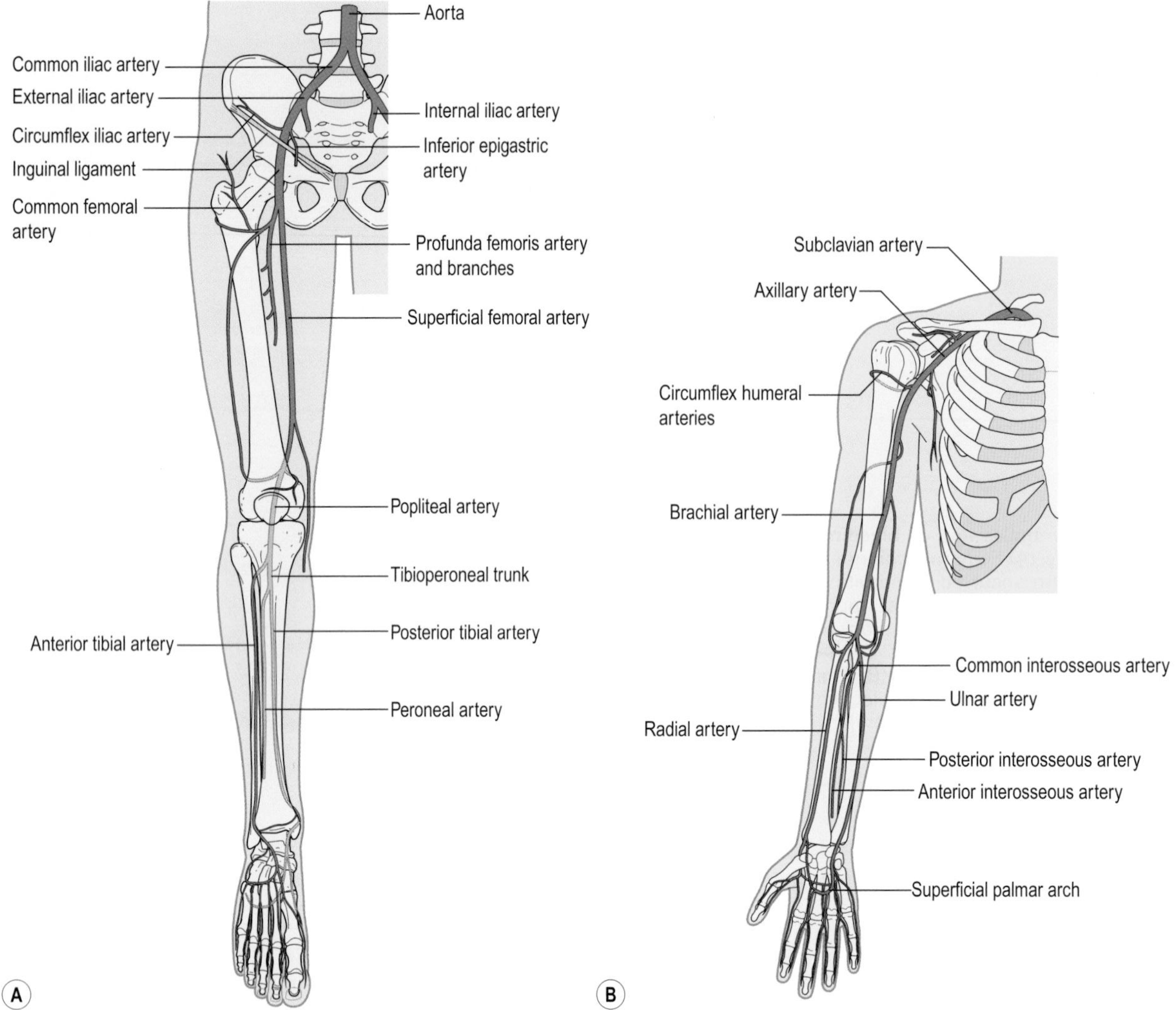

FIGURE 86-5 ■ **Diagram of (A) lower and (B) upper limb anatomy.**

are at risk of limb loss and must be treated by angioplasty, stenting or surgery.

Angiographic Diagnosis

Most pathological processes affecting the lower extremity arteries cause stenosis, occlusion or dilatation, i.e. aneurysm formation. Atherosclerosis may affect the arteries at any level, from the iliac arteries to the small vessels of the foot. While it is true that a stenosis or occlusion is almost always due to atherosclerosis, it is important to consider other possible causes. The clinical history may often be of help in this respect. For example, a patient who develops acute severe pain in the lower leg with no previous history or symptoms has probably sustained an acute embolus in the femoral or popliteal arteries, rather than a long-standing atherosclerotic occlusion. Patients with diabetes develop arterial occlusive disease, which involves mainly the distal vessels of the calf and feet. Patients with a history of radiotherapy to the pelvis for the treatment of carcinoma of the cervix may develop occlusive lesions of the common and external iliac arteries due to ischaemic vasculitis induced by the radiation.

Treatment of Chronic Limb Ischaemia

Iliac Artery Disease

Stenosis. In the treatment of stenotic lesions, PTA has a technical success rate approximating 100% (Fig. 86-6). Stents are used when PTA is immediately unsuccessful or when lesions recur soon after a previous angioplasty. There is no evidence that primary stenting is better than a policy of angioplasty with selective stenting for PTA failure.[1,2] Five-year patency rates are around 64–75%,[3] which, although lower than those of surgical aortobifemoral bypass, are acceptable considering the minimally invasive nature of this treatment.

Patients with diffusely stenosed iliac arteries respond less well to PTA. These patients are often treated with stents, although there is no definite evidence to support this policy.

Occlusions. Occlusions of the iliac artery are usually amenable to endovascular treatment, with a technical success rate of recanalisation of around 80% (Fig. 86-7). Most operators favour primary stent insertion because angioplasty carries a 7–24% risk of significant distal

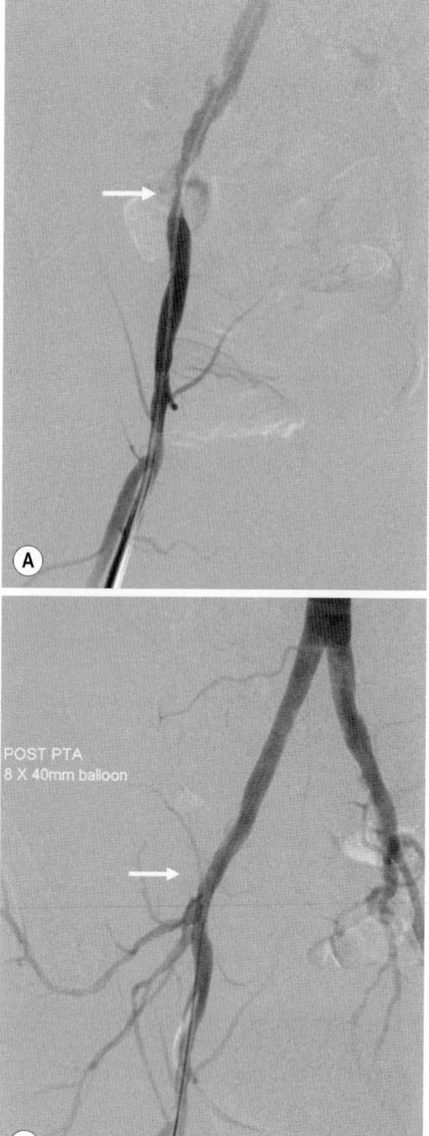

FIGURE 86-6 ■ Iliac angioplasty. (A) Flush angiogram from the distal aorta shows a tight stenosis at the right iliac bifurcation (arrow). (B) Improved lumen following 8-mm balloon angioplasty (arrow).

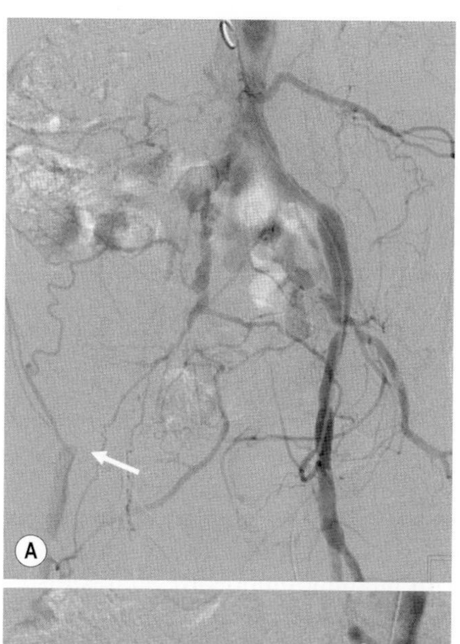

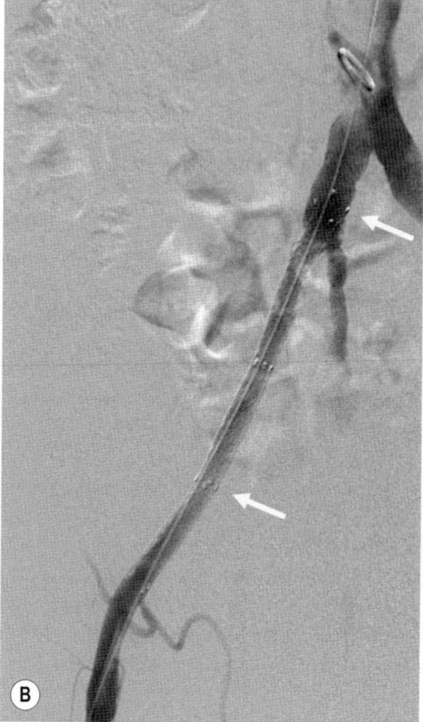

FIGURE 86-7 ■ Iliac stenting. (A) A pelvic angiogram showing occlusion of the external iliac artery with reconstitution distally via collateral vessels (arrow). (B) A guidewire has been passed retrograde through the occlusion from the right and two 8-mm self-expanding stents deployed. This has resulted in successful recanalisation of the occluded segment. The proximal and distal extents of the stents are indicated (arrows).

embolisation.[4] The durability of endovascular treatment of iliac artery occlusion is similar to that for iliac artery stenosis.

Common Femoral Artery and Profunda Femoris

Stenoses of the common femoral artery are amenable to PTA. Access to these lesions is usually gained from the contralateral groin involving catheter and guidewire manipulation across the aortic bifurcation. However, common femoral endarterectomy is a straightforward procedure and may be performed under local anaesthesia. Surgery is considered a better option than PTA at this site when lesions are calcified and eccentric. If the SFA is patent or salvageable by intervention, PTA of a stenosis in the profunda artery is usually not carried out. However, if the SFA is occluded, then any stenosis of the main profunda trunk should be treated by PTA or at the time of endarterectomy. The success and durability rates of PTA are similar to those for the SFA (see below).

Occlusions of the common femoral artery and profunda femoris are generally treated surgically.

Superficial Femoral Artery

Stenosis. Angioplasty is the first-line treatment for stenosis of the superficial femoral artery. Patency is around 55% at 5 years,[3] which is lower than for surgical bypass using vein grafts. However, most patients are treated by PTA because of the lower rate of complications compared with surgery. Angioplasty can be repeated if lesions recur. An additional advantage of angioplasty is that it spares the long saphenous vein, which is commonly used for femoropopliteal bypass, but which is also used for coronary artery bypass. The results of angioplasty are less satisfactory if the vessel is diffusely stenosed or if the number of calf run-off vessels is reduced. The technical success of stenting is higher than for angioplasty, but studies have found no convincing long-term benefit for stents versus PTA. More recently, drug-eluting balloons and stents have been introduced. These devices are coated with immunosuppressive and anti-proliferative drugs (e.g. sirolimus and paclitaxel) that have been shown to limit neointimal hyperplasia, and therefore inhibit vessel restenosis. Early evidence suggests improved patency of femoropopliteal lesions after treatment using either of these devices when compared with standard PTA balloons and bare metal stents.[5–7]

Occlusions. SFA occlusions are usually treated by PTA (Fig. 86-8) followed by selective stent placement in cases where angioplasty is unsuccessful. Many radiologists use a technique called subintimal angioplasty in which a catheter and guidewire are manipulated outside the lumen of the vessel underneath the intima and into the subintimal space. Unless the vessel is heavily calcified, it is usually easy to advance the catheter and guidewire down the occluded vessel via the subintimal space. When the guidewire reaches the level of the patent vessel below the occlusion, it re-enters the lumen. After replacing the catheter with a balloon catheter, the subintimal space is dilated in the usual manner. Overall, the results for endovascular management of SFA occlusions are lower than for stenoses.[3] Although there is no conclusive evidence, primary stenting is often preferred for the treatment of occlusions. Drug-eluting balloons and stents may be used for these lesions if the long-term outcomes of these devices replicate early published data. In general, endovascular treatment is favoured over surgery in view of its lower morbidity and repeatability.

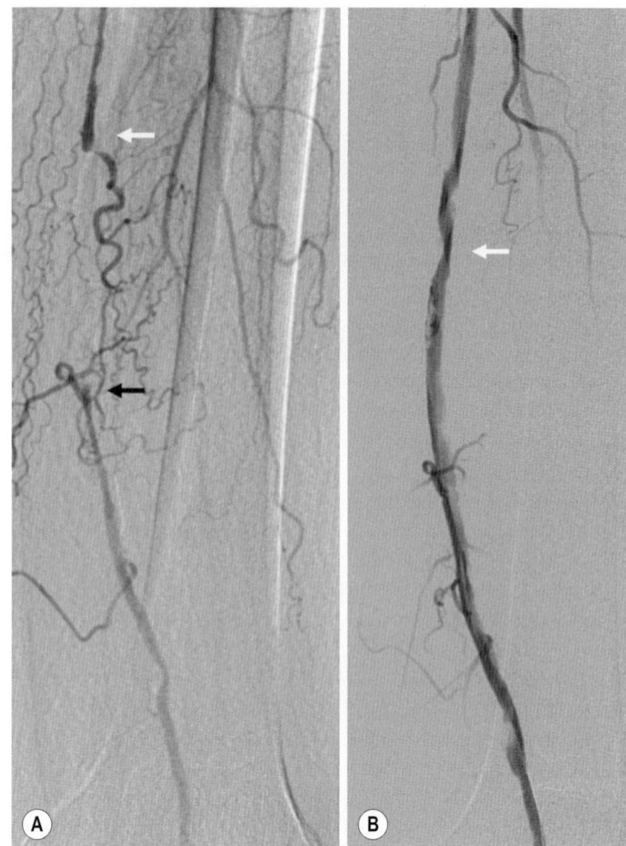

FIGURE 86-8 ■ **Subintimal angioplasty.** (A) Occlusion of the SFA (white arrow). There is reconstitution of the distal SFA via collaterals (black arrow). (B) The occlusion has been crossed subintimally with a hydrophilic guidewire and a 5-mm PTA performed (white arrow), restoring flow.

Popliteal Artery

The principles of treatment, results and durability are similar to those in the SFA. In general, the more distal the lesion, the more likely it is to produce symptoms of critical limb ischaemia. If treatment of these lesions fails, the limb may be lost. In general, lesions in the popliteal artery are only treated if the patient has critical limb ischaemia or very short distance claudication.

Calf Vessels

Angioplasty has become the main method of treatment for focal or diffuse lesions (stenosis or occlusions) of the tibial and peroneal arteries (Fig. 86-9). In view of the size of these vessels, it is necessary to use small-calibre catheters and guidewires. Interventions in the calf vessels are performed in the setting of critical limb ischaemia, i.e. rest pain or tissue loss. The primary patency and limb salvage rates are 49 and 82% at 3 years, respectively.[8] More recently, bare metal stents, drug-eluting stents and drug-eluting balloons have been introduced to the market for use in the tibial arteries.[9] The data regarding their efficacy remain limited and studies are ongoing. Endovascular intervention in the pedal circulation is now being performed more frequently, with reasonable outcomes, but limited data.

Treatment of Acute Lower Limb Ischaemia

Patients with acute limb ischaemia usually present with severe rest pain. In many cases, the limb is threatened and patients may develop paraesthesia or motor dysfunction. In such circumstances urgent treatment is required to prevent limb loss. In the 1990s, this condition was often treated by intra-arterial thrombolysis. However,

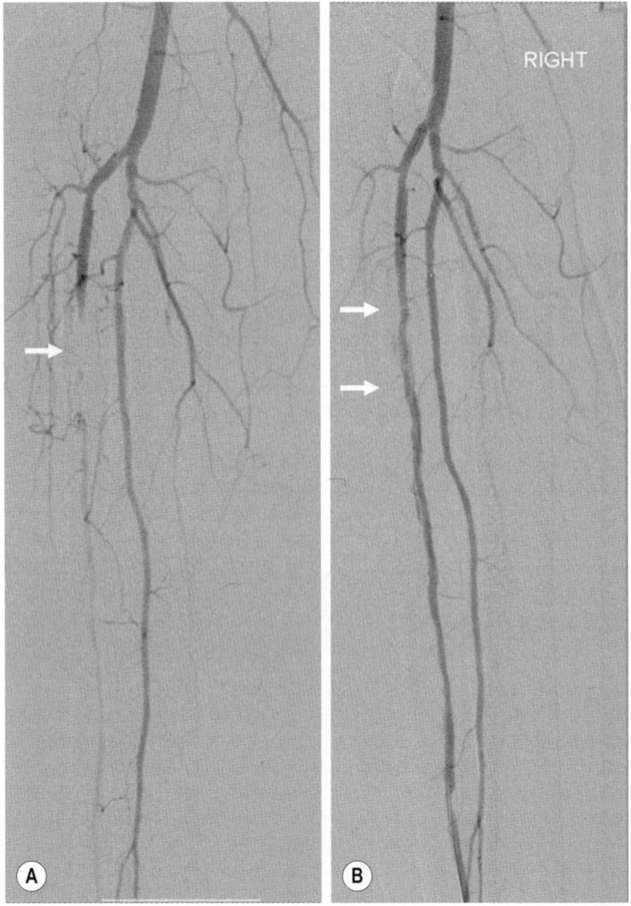

FIGURE 86-9 ■ **Tibial artery angioplasty.** (A) Angiogram of the tibial vessels in a patient with critical limb ischaemia. There is occlusion of the proximal anterior tibial artery (arrow) with reconstitution via collaterals. The posterior tibial artery is occluded. (B) Appearance after angioplasty with a 2.5-mm balloon with improved distal flow (arrows).

because of the overall lack of data showing a benefit for thrombolysis compared with surgery and a high rate of haemorrhagic complication, the technique is now used less frequently, although it is still employed on a selected patient basis.[10,11]

Some patients presenting with acute limb ischaemia have emboli lodged in the popliteal artery. They can be treated by percutaneous aspiration of the thrombus using wide-bore catheters placed directly into the thrombus via the femoral artery. A variety of mechanical thrombectomy devices for fragmenting thrombus either as an adjunct or instead of thrombolysis in patients with a large thrombus load are also available.

UPPER EXTREMITY ARTERIES

Anatomy

The subclavian artery extends to the lateral border of the first rib and continues as the axillary artery. The axillary artery extends to the lower border of the Teres major muscle, where it becomes the brachial artery. At the elbow, the brachial artery gives rise to the radial artery and ulnar arteries. At the wrist, the radial artery gives rise to the deep carpal arch that anastomoses with branches of the ulnar artery. The ulnar artery gives rise to the superficial carpal arch. The digital arteries originate from both arches.

Pathology

Most lesions involving the arteries of the upper limb are caused by atherosclerosis. However, other processes form a greater proportion of lesions compared with the legs, including Takayasu's arteritis, giant cell arteritis, thoracic outlet syndrome and thromboembolism.

Endovascular Treatment

Stenoses and occlusions of the subclavian artery (Fig. 86-10) usually occur at the origin, and are amenable to angioplasty and/or stent insertion with technical success

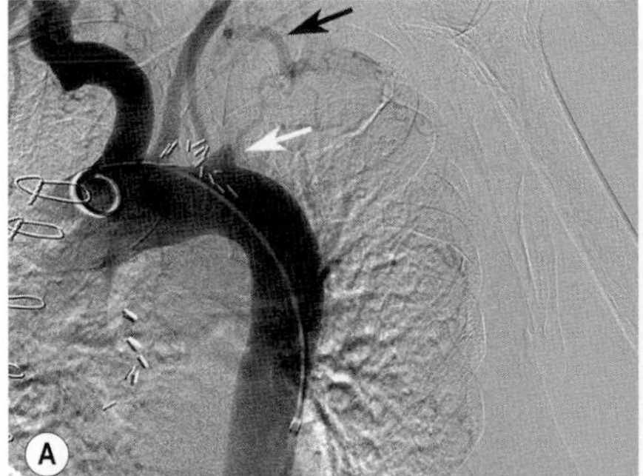

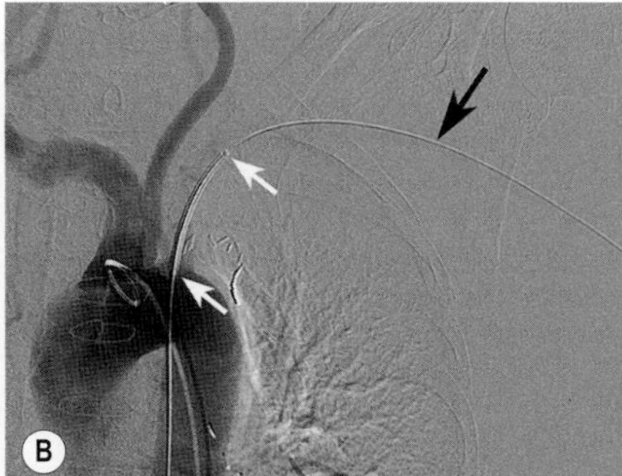

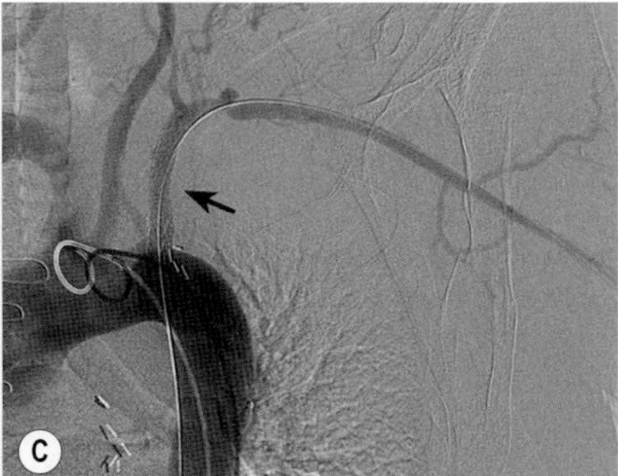

FIGURE 86-10 ■ **Subclavian artery occlusion.** (A) Left anterior oblique projection flush aortogram performed via a pigtail catheter in the ascending aorta. There is left subclavian artery occlusion in this patient who presented with arm claudication. Note that the left vertebral artery (the third vessel from the right) arises directly from the aortic arch, rather than off the left subclavian. The stump of the left subclavian is marked (white arrow). There is reconstitution of the distal left subclavian artery (black arrow). (B) A guidewire (black arrow) has been placed across the occlusion from the left brachial artery. A balloon expandable stent (white arrows) is seen in position ready for deployment. (C) After deployment of a 7-mm stent (arrow). Continuous flow has been restored.

rates of around 95% (less for occlusions). There are no convincing data on the superiority of stents versus angioplasty (although most interventionalists treat these lesions with stents).

Thromboembolism is a common cause of acute upper extremity ischaemia that is almost always treated surgically. Thrombolysis is rarely performed, because of significant haemorrhagic and embolic stroke complications.

The role of angioplasty or stenting in the treatment of stenotic or occlusive lesions distal to the subclavian arteries is very limited, with very little evidence for it.

GASTROINTESTINAL SYSTEM

The coeliac axis and the superior mesenteric artery (SMA) usually arise at the level of T12 and L1, respectively. The inferior mesenteric artery (IMA) arises at the level of L3. The coeliac axis and SMA anastomose with each other via the pancreaticoduodenal arcades, while the superior and inferior mesenteric arteries anastomose via the middle colic branch of the SMA and left colic branch of the IMA, just proximal to the splenic flexure.

Angiography (Fig. 86-11)

The main problems affecting the gastrointestinal circulation are haemorrhage, occlusive disease and aneurysms.

Mesenteric Haemorrhage

Upper gastrointestinal (GI) haemorrhage is defined as bleeding proximal to the duodenojejunal flexure. It is

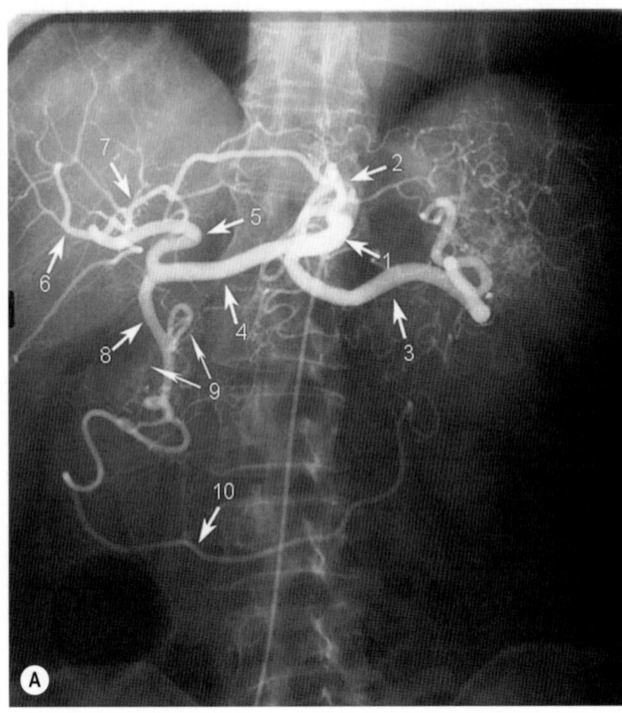

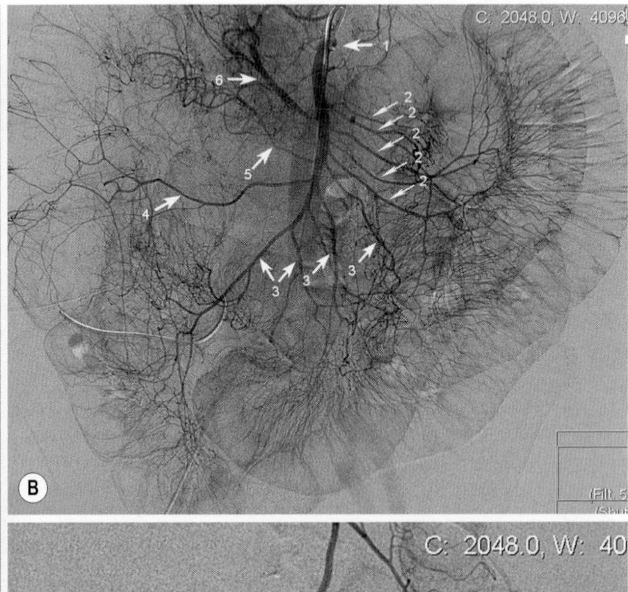

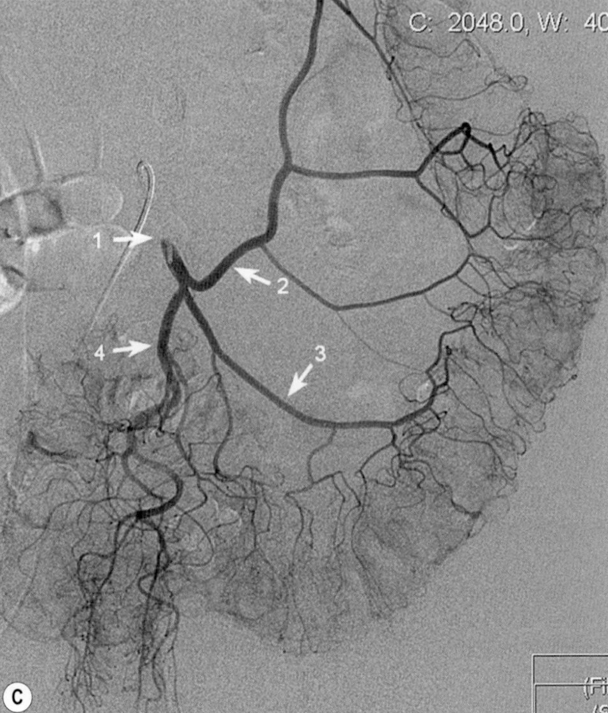

FIGURE 86-11 ■ **Mesenteric anatomy.** (A) Coeliac artery: 1 = coeliac axis, 2 = left gastric artery, 3 = splenic artery, 4 = common hepatic artery, 5 = proper hepatic artery, 6 = right hepatic artery, 7 = left hepatic artery, 8 = gastroduodenal artery, 9 = superior pancreaticoduodenal arteries, 10 = right gastroepiploic arteries. (B) Superior mesenteric artery: 1 = sidewinder catheter in the superior mesenteric artery, 2 = jejunal arteries, 3 = ileal arteries, 4 = ileocolic artery, 5 = right colic artery, 6 = middle colic artery. (C) Inferior mesenteric artery: 1 = catheter in the inferior mesenteric artery, 2 = left colic artery, 3 = sigmoid artery, 4 = superior rectal artery.

commonly caused by peptic ulceration, inflammatory disease such as pancreatitis, or as a complication of endoscopic, surgical or percutaneous biliary procedures. Lower GI haemorrhage is less common and is usually due to angiodysplasia, diverticular disease, neoplasms or haemorrhoids.

MDCTA has transformed the diagnostic algorithm for acute GI hemorrhage as it allows fast, accurate and non-invasive detection and localisation of bleeding. MDCTA may be performed as the first-line investigation or after a negative endoscopy. MDCTA has a high sensitivity for detecting active arterial bleeding, with a threshold bleeding rate of approximately 0.35 mL/min.[12] A triphasic scan protocol that includes unenhanced, arterial and portal-venous phase imaging should be used (Figs. 86-12A, B). Active bleeding is diagnosed when extravasated contrast material is seen within the bowel lumen during the arterial phase, which increases or pools during the portal-venous phase. Unenhanced images ensure that high-attenuation materials such as clips, suture material and faecoliths are not mistaken for acute bleeding. CTA may detect the cause of bleeding even when there is no active haemorrhage at the time of the scan, by identifying underlying pathology such as pseudoaneurysms. The information from the MDCTA allows the interventional radiologist to plan arterial embolisation by identifying the source branch. This enables faster selective catheterisation of the target vessels, reducing radiation exposure and contrast volume during the procedure.

Catheter angiography can detect active bleeding at a rate of 0.5 mL/min. If there is no active haemorrhage but the site of bleeding is known or clinically suspected because of associated pathology or recent intervention, prophylactic embolisation may be successful. This is easier in the upper GI than the lower GI tract, where collateral supply is less good and precise identification of the bleeding site is required to avoid bowel ischaemia or infarction.

The only direct sign of haemorrhage is contrast medium extravasation into the bowel lumen (Figs. 86-12C–E), but this may not be visible if the bleeding is intermittent or if the rate is too low. Indirect signs indicating the source of haemorrhage include the presence of a pseudoaneurysm, vessel truncation, early venous return, vascular lakes or tumour circulation and irregularity of the vessel wall.

Once the source of haemorrhage is identified, embolisation can be therapeutic, or enable stabilisation of the patient's condition before surgery. Consideration of the anatomical site will dictate the type of agent used and the extent of the embolisation required to avoid tissue

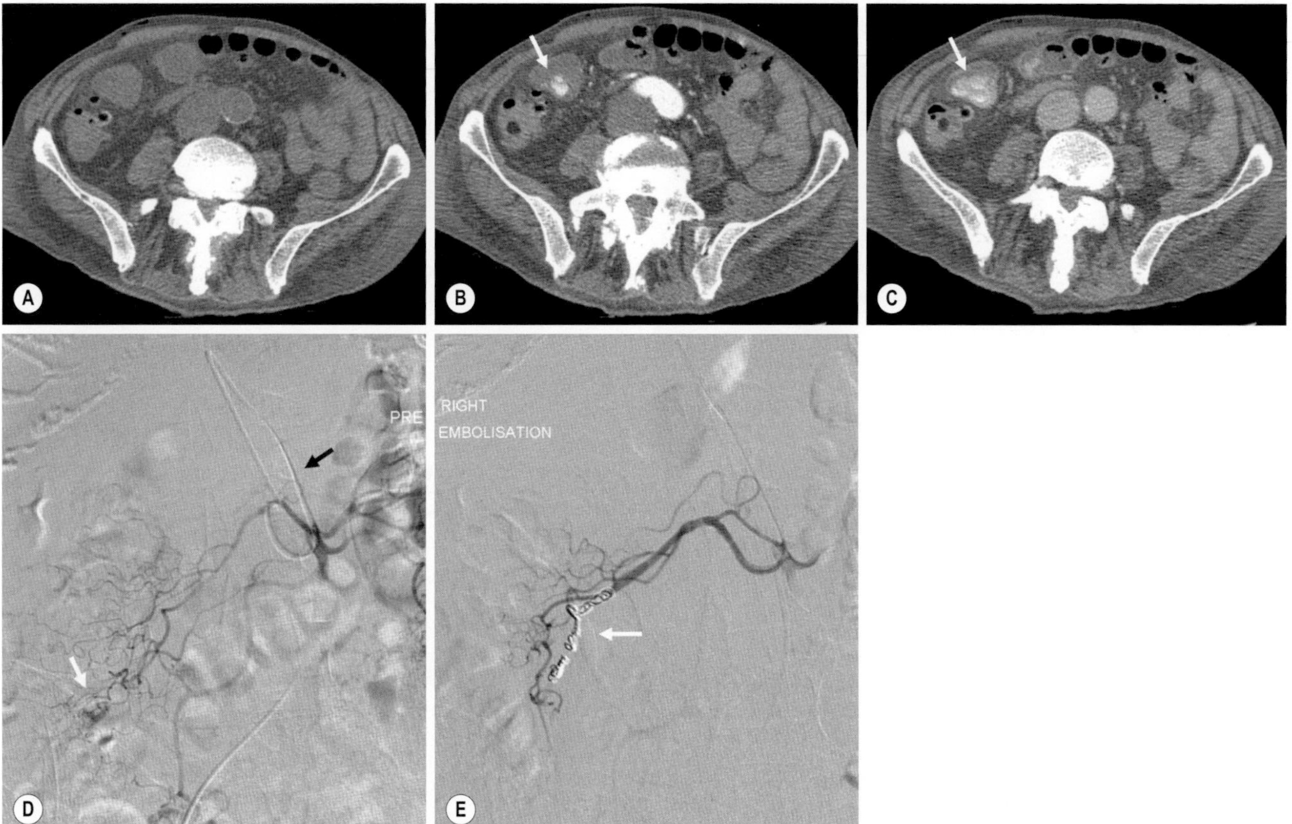

FIGURE 86-12 ■ Acute lower gastrointestinal haemorrhage on MDCTA and catheter embolisation. (A) Unenhanced axial CT image shows no evidence of high attenuation in relation to the bowel wall or lumen. (B) Arterial phase shows contrast material extravasation into the lumen of the ascending colon. (C) There is pooling of contrast in the bowel lumen on portal-venous phase. (D) Superselective angiogram performed via a coaxial microcatheter (black arrow). Contrast extravasation is seen from a right colic branch (white arrow). (E) After embolisation with microcoils (white arrow), there is no further bleeding.

ischaemia or infarction. For example, consideration should be given as to whether the vessel is an end artery (when the risk of infarction is greater) or whether there is significant collateral supply. The embolic agent is selected, depending on the anatomy and presence of collateral supply. As a very general rule, particulate emboli are used in the upper GI tract where there is good collateral supply, and coils are placed very distally in the branches of the lower GI tract where the collateral supply is poor.[13,14]

Visceral Artery Aneurysms

These are uncommon. The splenic artery is the vessel most frequently involved, followed by the hepatic artery and SMA. The aneurysms may be found incidentally on imaging, or present due to symptoms or actual rupture. Visceral artery aneurysms (VAA) may be true or pseudoaneurysms and occur as a result of atherosclerosis, arteritis, collagen vascular disorders (true aneurysms), or trauma and infection (pseudoaneurysms) (Fig. 86-13).

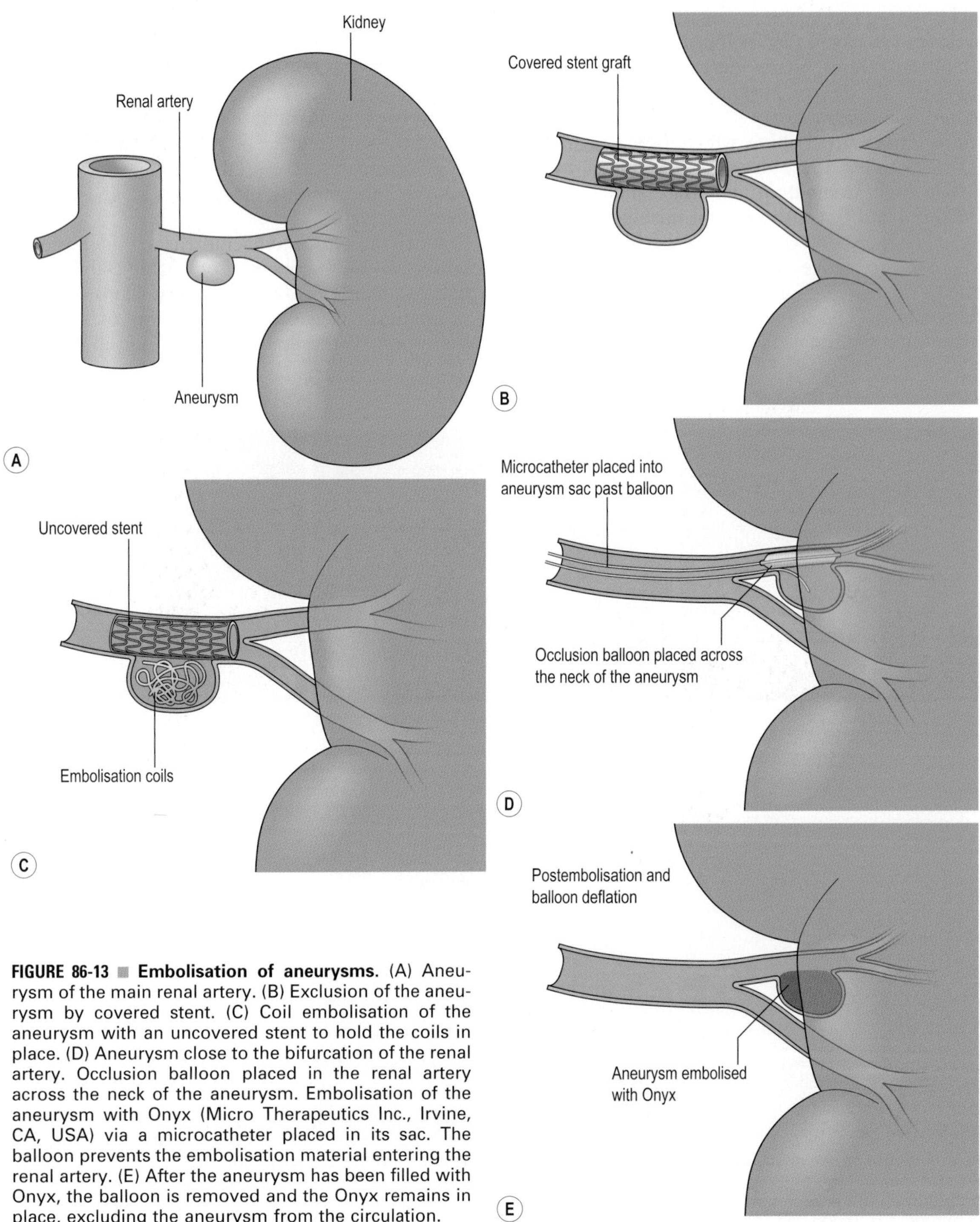

FIGURE 86-13 ■ Embolisation of aneurysms. (A) Aneurysm of the main renal artery. (B) Exclusion of the aneurysm by covered stent. (C) Coil embolisation of the aneurysm with an uncovered stent to hold the coils in place. (D) Aneurysm close to the bifurcation of the renal artery. Occlusion balloon placed in the renal artery across the neck of the aneurysm. Embolisation of the aneurysm with Onyx (Micro Therapeutics Inc., Irvine, CA, USA) via a microcatheter placed in its sac. The balloon prevents the embolisation material entering the renal artery. (E) After the aneurysm has been filled with Onyx, the balloon is removed and the Onyx remains in place, excluding the aneurysm from the circulation.

Continued on following page

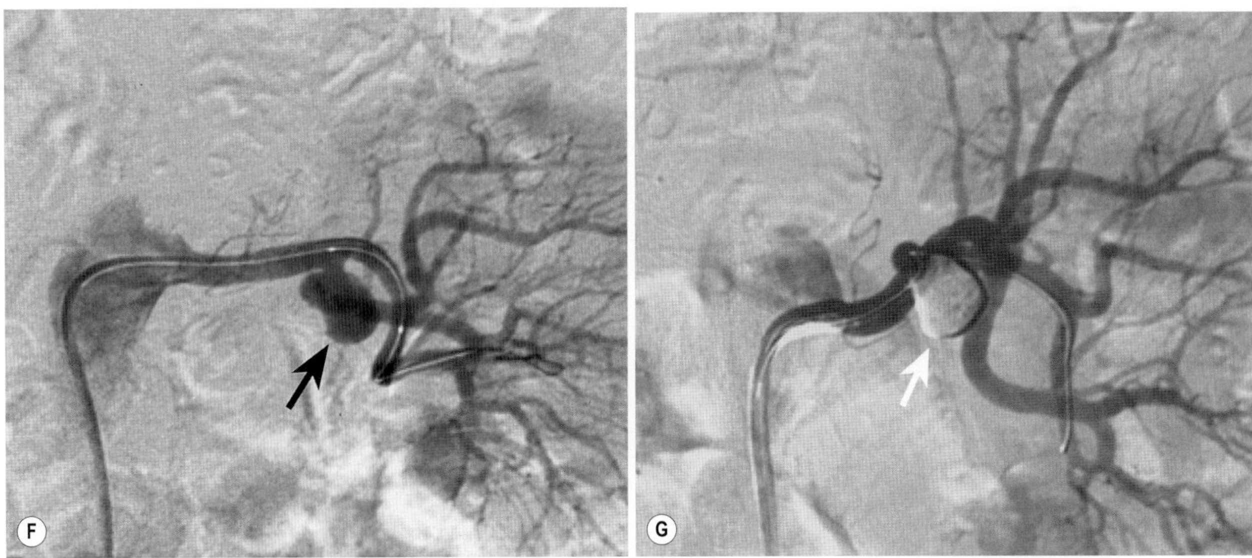

FIGURE 86-13, Continued ■ (F) Angiogram demonstrating a saccular aneurysm (arrow) of the anterior division of the left renal artery. (G) Appearance after embolisation with Onyx (arrow). Both anterior and posterior divisions remain patent.

Depending on the vascular anatomy, endovascular treatment may involve embolisation (with coils, glue or Onyx), insertion of stent grafts or a combination of these methods.[15] A new type of stent called a flow diverting stent which occludes the neck of the aneurysm whilst maintaining patency of side branches has been developed, but early experience is very limited.

Occlusive Mesenteric Vascular Disease

Nowadays, acute mesenteric ischaemia (AMI) is more frequently diagnosed on CT than at laparotomy. If suspected, and the bowel is deemed viable, targeted thrombolysis is a potential treatment option, although the evidence for this treatment is limited to small case series and reports.

Chronic mesenteric ischaemia (CMI) presents with post-prandial abdominal pain and weight loss. Autopsy series quote mesenteric vessel atherosclerosis in 35–70% of unselected patients.[11] However, clinical symptoms are rare because of the excellent collateral vessels between mesenteric arteries. At least two of the three mesenteric arteries must be significantly stenosed for symptoms to occur.

The main therapeutic options for CMI are surgery and arterial stenting (Fig. 86-14). The diagnosis may be made non-invasively by Doppler ultrasound, CT or MRI. Catheter angiography is reserved for confirmation at the time of intervention. Lateral aortography is the best way to assess the anatomy before intervention. It is important to exclude extrinsic compression of the coeliac axis by the median arcuate ligament of the diaphragm (MALC) as this requires surgery. MALC causes a non-ostial asymmetric narrowing on the superior aspect of the coeliac axis, accentuated on expiratory angiography.

Angioplasty of the mesenteric vessels may be performed using a femoral or brachial approach. Most lesions occur at the vessel origins, and are treated by primary stenting. In general, treatment of one vessel will relieve symptoms, although treating more than one vessel, if technically feasible, might improve long-term outcomes. Technical success is 80–100% in most series.[16]

Bronchial Artery Embolisation

Haemoptysis can be a life-threatening respiratory emergency. Massive haemoptysis is defined as more than 300 mL of blood loss over 24 h and moderate haemoptysis is more than three episodes of 100 mL/day within 1 week. The aetiology is variable and includes tuberculosis, cystic fibrosis, malignancy, bronchiectasis, aspergilloma and lobar pneumonia.

The bronchial arteries are the most common source of bleeding in haemoptysis. They arise anterolaterally from the descending thoracic aorta at the level of the fifth or sixth thoracic vertebrae. Their anatomy is highly variable; the most common configuration is of an intercostobronchial trunk (ICBT) on the right and two bronchial arteries on the left, although other variations are almost as common.

Bronchoscopy can localise the side of haemorrhage when there is bilateral pulmonary disease but care must be taken in interpreting its findings as they may be misleading. MDCTA can identify the source of bleeding and the underlying disease process as well as providing a roadmap of the thoracic vasculature. The images should be carefully reviewed to search for not only abnormal bronchial arteries but also non-bronchial collaterals that can arise from branches of the subclavian artery in upper lobe disease and infradiaphragmatic branches in lower lobe disease.

Bronchial artery embolisation (BAE) is an effective and safe treatment for massive and recurrent haemoptysis. Bronchial arteries are selectively catheterised with

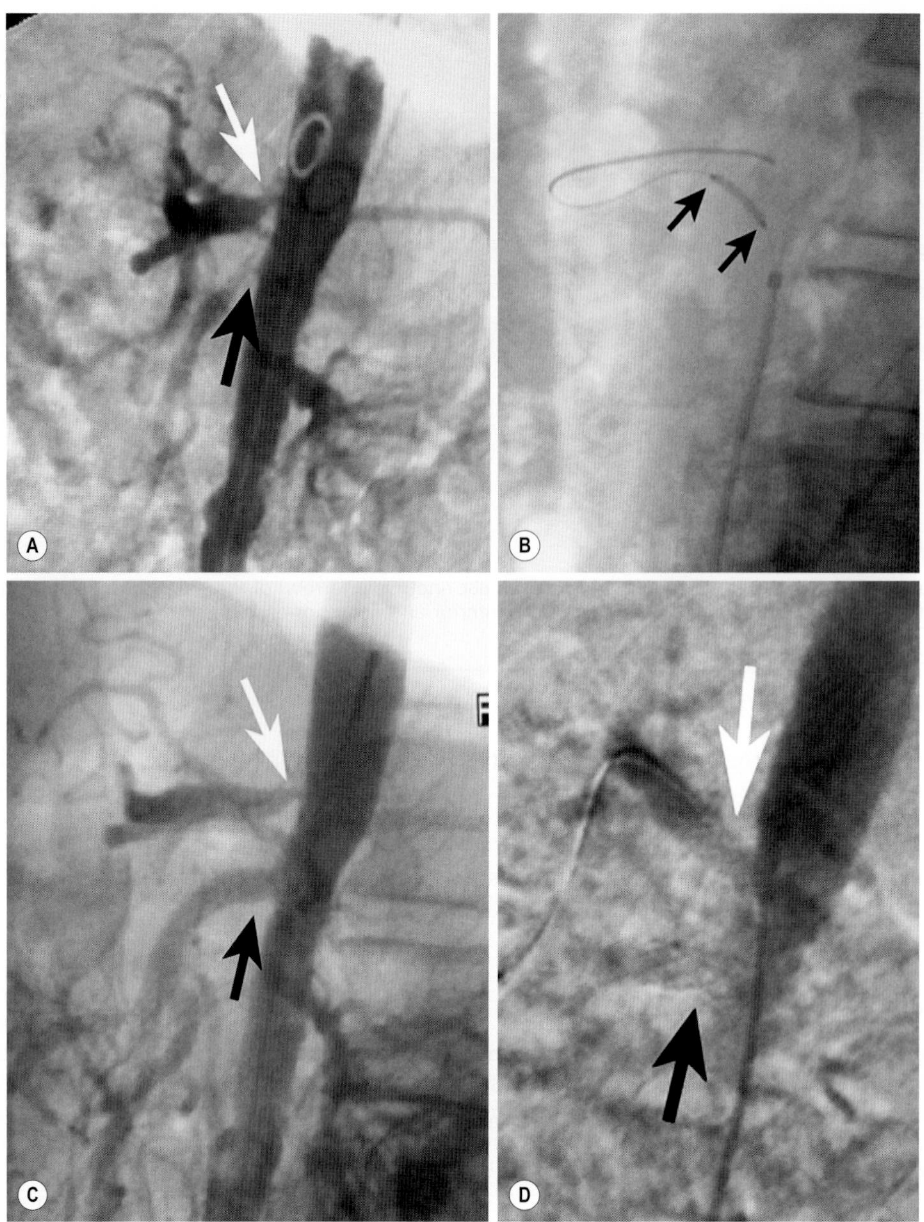

FIGURE 86-14 ■ **Mesenteric revascularisation.** (A) Lateral flush aortogram in a patient who had significant weight loss and post-prandial pain. There are critical stenoses of the coeliac axis (white arrow) and superior mesenteric artery (SMA) (black arrow). The inferior mesenteric artery (IMA) was occluded. (B) Image demonstrating a guidewire in the SMA and a 6-mm balloon expandable stent ready for deployment. The proximal and distal markers of the stent are indicated (arrows). (C) Appearance of the SMA after stent insertion (black arrow). Angioplasty of the coeliac axis had been attempted. The vessel exhibits considerable elastic recoil and continued stenosis at its origin (white arrow). (D) Final angiogram after insertion of stents in the coeliac axis (white arrow) and SMA (black arrow).

pre-shaped catheters, such as cobra and sidewinder. Signs of abnormality include hypertrophy, areas of hypervascularity or neovascularity, shunting of blood into the pulmonary artery or vein, aneurysm and contrast extravasation (Fig. 86-15). Coaxial microcatheters may be used to obtain a super-selective position to avoid any reflux of embolic material into the aorta or into important side branches, such as the anterior medullary artery that can arise from the right ICBT in 5–10% of cases. Embolisation is usually performed using PVA. It is prudent to check for non-bronchial collaterals which may arise from the subclavian, axillary and internal mammary arteries in upper lobe disease or from branches of the coeliac axis or inferior phrenic artery in lower lobe disease.

BAE provides immediate relief of symptoms in 73–99% of cases.[17] If bleeding does not stop immediately, repeat angiography and embolisation should be performed. The source of haemorrhage lies in the bronchial arteries in 85–90% and in non-bronchial arteries in 10–15% of cases. The pulmonary arteries are rarely the cause of massive haemoptysis. It is important to note that BAE does not address the underlying disease process and

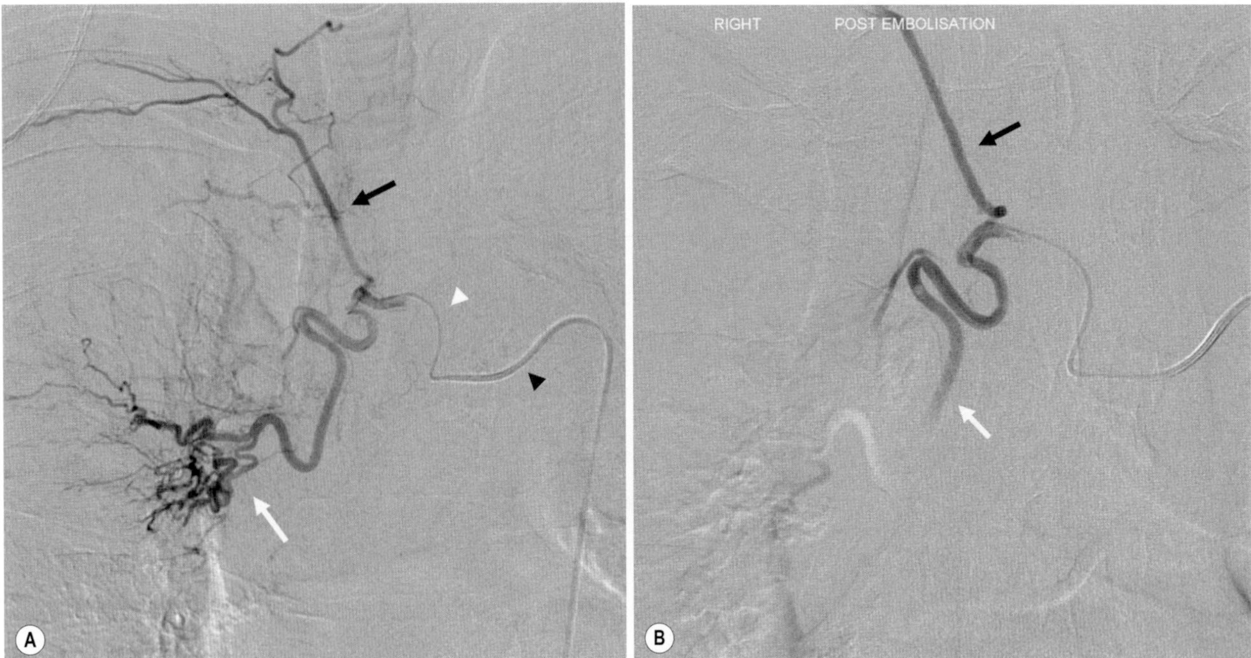

FIGURE 86-15 ■ **Bronchial artery embolisation.** (A) Right bronchial angiogram in a patient with lower lobe bronchiectasis who presented with haemoptysis. The right intercostobronchial trunk has been selectively catheterised with a cobra catheter (black arrow head) and a more stable position achieved with a coaxial microcatheter (white arrow head). An enlarged tortuous right bronchial branch is seen to supply an abnormal hypervascular area of lung corresponding to the bronchiectatic area (white arrow). The intercostal branch is unremarkable (black arrow). (B) Angiogram after superselective embolisation of the right bronchial branch with polyvinyl alcohol particles. The abnormal bronchial branch has been successfully embolised (white arrow) while the intercostal branch remains patent (black arrow).

re-bleeding is likely if the cause of hemoptysis is not treated effectively. Complications of bronchial embolisation include chest pain, dysphagia, broncho-oesophageal fistula, spinal cord ischaemia and stroke.

THE CAROTID ARTERIES

Internal carotid artery stenosis is an important cause of ischaemic stroke and transient ischaemic attack (TIA) (Fig. 86-16). Patients with symptomatic carotid stenosis are at a higher risk of developing further ischaemic cerebral events than patients with asymptomatic stenosis. Standard non-medical treatment is surgical carotid endarterectomy, although carotid stenting is an alternative to surgery.

Two trials (European Carotid Surgery Trial (ECST) and the North American Symptomatic Carotid Endarterectomy Trial (NASCET)) showed benefit in surgically treating patients with 70–99% stenosis. The criteria for treating patients by stenting are the same as for surgery. There remains controversy regarding the management of asymptomatic significant carotid artery disease.

Imaging

The standard imaging methods for delineating the carotid arteries are duplex ultrasound, MDCTA and MRA. Catheter angiography has little place in the diagnosis of carotid disease except as a problem-solving tool when the non-invasive methods are discordant.

Angiography

Selective carotid angiography is associated with a risk of stroke in 1% of procedures.[18] Selective angiography is performed using one of a variety of pre-shaped catheters, such as the sidewinder, the Berenstein, Headhunter or Mani.

Endovascular Treatment of Carotid Artery Stenosis

The stenting technique differs slightly from procedures at other sites in that cerebral protection devices are usually used to prevent distal emboli, and predilatation is generally performed before stenting.

An overview of the available evidence suggests that stenting is associated with more minor strokes, especially in the elderly, and surgery with more myocardial infarction.[19] The decision to treat symptomatic and asymptomatic carotid stenosis should be made by a multidisciplinary team, which should include an interventional radiologist/neuroradiologist, a vascular surgeon and a physician with a special interest in stroke.

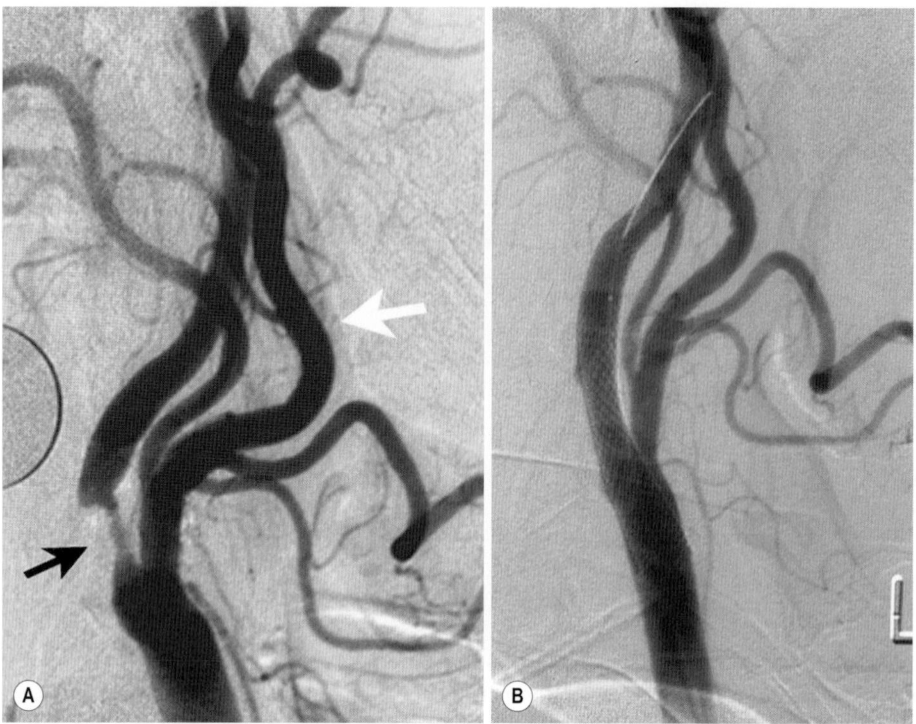

FIGURE 86-16 ■ **Carotid stenting.** (A) Lateral projection angiogram following selective injection into the common carotid artery. There is a tight stenosis at the origin of the internal carotid artery (black arrow). The external carotid artery is marked (white arrow). (B) Angiogram following self-expanding stent deployment.

VENOUS SYSTEM

LOWER EXTREMITY VENOUS SYSTEM

The main pathology affecting the lower extremity venous system is thrombosis. This may be due to factors causing procoagulation such as patient immobility, dehydration and thrombocythaemia; or due to an underlying stenosis/occlusion in the iliac veins. Although some interventionalists advocate catheter-directed thrombolysis as first-line treatment for patients with acute lower limb venous thrombosis, this technique has not yet been widely adopted. Thrombolysis is occasionally performed for patients with limb-threatening ischaemia as a result of acute venous occlusion in the condition of phlegmasia caerulea dolens.

Occasionally, an underlying stenosis or occlusion of the common iliac vein is the underlying cause of thrombosis, which can be treated by stenting. Left lower limb vein thrombosis or oedema due to compression by the right common iliac artery is called May–Thurner syndrome.

UPPER EXTREMITY VENOUS OBSTRUCTION

The main causes of upper limb venous occlusion are thoracic outlet syndrome (Paget–Schroetter syndrome) and occlusive disease related to the presence of dialysis fistulae.

Paget–Schroetter syndrome refers to acute subclavian or axillary vein thrombosis caused by underlying venous obstruction due to muscles or bony structures of the thoracic outlet. Patients presenting with subclavian or axillary vein thrombosis due to thoracic outlet syndrome are usually treated first by thrombolysis. If the thrombus can be cleared by this method, the first rib should be resected to create space for the vein, followed by angioplasty of any residual stenosis.

Patients with high pressure in the upper extremity veins resulting from the presence of dialysis fistulae are prone to develop venous stenoses and occlusions. These can be treated by angioplasty or stenting with high technical success rates. However, recurrence is frequent and long-term durability is very uncommon.

INFERIOR VENA CAVA FILTERS

Inferior vena cava (IVC) filters are placed to prevent fatal pulmonary embolism (PE) in patients with a documented PE, or IVC, iliac or femoropopliteal DVT who cannot be treated with anticoagulants, or in whom anticoagulants have failed to prevent further PE or progression of thrombus.

Other possible indications for IVC filters include protection against PE in pregnant women with proven DVT during Caesarean section or childbirth; in patients

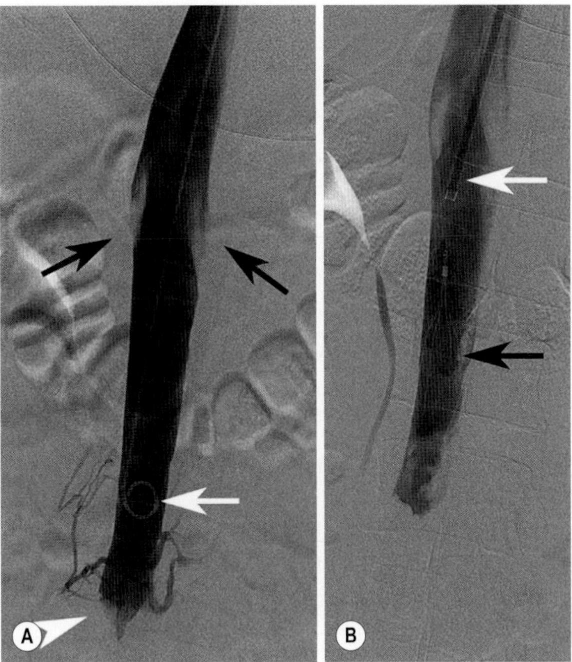

FIGURE 86-17 ■ Inferior vena cava filter. (A) Cavogram performed with a pigtail catheter (white arrow) placed from the right internal jugular vein. Unopacified blood from the renal veins creates a void (black arrows) in the column of contrast medium and thus delineates their position. Thrombus is seen as a filling defect distally (white arrowhead). (B) Post-filter (black arrow) deployment. The delivery catheter is marked (white arrow).

post-severe trauma; and preoperatively in patients with iliofemoral DVT when anticoagulation is contraindicated or pelvic manipulation is expected.

IVC filters may be permanent or optional, meaning they can be retrieved after a period of time, which varies with the individual filter, or left in permanently.

Before placing a filter, the IVC should be assessed by inferior vena cavography, the diameter of the IVC measured to ensure the filter will not migrate and the position of the renal veins documented (Fig. 86-17). The ideal position for the IVC filter is in the infrarenal IVC with the apex of the filter at or just below the level of the renal veins. Filters can be inserted via the femoral or jugular venous route depending on the site and extent of the thrombus. Retrieval is via the jugular route, the right jugular vein being the ideal choice.

Suprarenal positioning of the filter may be necessary when IVC thrombosis extends above the renal veins or there is renal vein thrombosis. Other indications include thrombus above a previously placed filter, pregnant women in whom there will be compression of the infrarenal vena cava, PE following gonadal vein thrombosis and anatomical variants (double IVC).

COMPLICATIONS OF ENDOVASCULAR PROCEDURES

Complications occurring after endovascular procedures are divided into major and minor. Major complications include death and those complications where intervention is required, while minor complications are usually self-limiting and do not require treatment.

Death occurring after angioplasty or stenting procedures occurs in less than 1% of cases and is usually related to comorbidity rather than to the procedure itself. Other major complications of angioplasty or stenting include vessel rupture, access vessel pseudoaneurysm formation, haemorrhage, distal embolisation and vessel dissection, stent migration and severe reactions to intravascular contrast medium. Major complications occur in around 1% of procedures.[3]

Minor complications of these procedures are self-limiting haematoma, dissection not requiring treatment, minor contrast medium reactions, self-limiting fever and nausea. Thrombolysis is associated with haemorrhage, mainly at the access site, in up to 30% of cases.[20]

For a full list of references, please see ExpertConsult.

FURTHER READING

2. Klein WM, van der Graaf Y, Seegers J, et al. Dutch iliac stent trial: long-term results in patients randomized for primary or selective stent placement. Radiology 2006;238:734–44.
3. Norgren L, Hiatt WR, Dormandy JA, et al. Inter-society consensus for the management of peripheral arterial disease (TASC II). Eur J Vasc Endovasc Surg 2007;33:S1–S75.
7. Dake MD, Ansel GM, Jaff MR, et al. Paclitaxel-eluting stents show superiority to balloon angioplasty and bare metal stents in femoropopliteal disease: twelve-month Zilver PTX randomized study results. Circ Cardiovasc Interv 2011;4:495–504.
8. Romiti M, Albers M, Brochado-Neto FC, et al. Meta-analysis of infrapopliteal angioplasty for chronic critical limb ischemia. J Vasc Surg 2008;47:975–81.
9. Siablis D, Karnabatidis D, Katsanos K, et al. Infrapopliteal application of sirolimus-eluting versus bare metal stents for critical limb ischemia: analysis of long-term angiographic and clinical outcome. J Vasc Interv Radiol 2009;20:1141–50.
12. Roy-Choudhury SH, Karandikar S. Multidetector CT of acute gastrointestinal bleeding. Radiology 2008;246:336.
13. Weldon DT, Burke SJ, Sun S, et al. Interventional management of lower gastrointestinal bleeding. Eur Radiol 2008;18:857–67.
14. Schenker MP, Duszak R Jr, Soulen MC, et al. Upper gastrointestinal hemorrhage and transcatheter embolotherapy: clinical and technical factors impacting success and survival. J Vasc Interv Radiol 2001;12:1263–71.
16. Cognet F, Ben Salem D, Dranssart M, et al. Chronic mesenteric ischaemia: imaging and percutaneous treatment. Radiographics 2002;22:863–79.
17. Chun J-Y, Morgan R, Belli A-M. Radiological management of hemoptysis: a comprehensive review of diagnostic imaging and bronchial artery embolization. Cardiovasc Intervent Radiol 2010; 33:240–50.
19. Macdonald S. Carotid artery stenting trials: conduct, results, critique, and current recommendations. Cardiovasc Intervent Radiol 2012;35:15–29.

CHAPTER 87

Image-Guided Biopsy and Ablation Techniques

David J. Breen • Elizabeth E. Rutherford • Beth Shepherd

CHAPTER OUTLINE

IMAGE-GUIDED BIOPSY

INTRODUCTION

There is an increasing role for imaging in the planning and performing of biopsy procedures. It is becoming unacceptable in modern practice to perform 'blind' liver or renal biopsies when imaging can provide real-time monitoring of needle position and hence reduce complication rates.[1,2] Ongoing technological advances are providing us with new and improved imaging modalities to aid biopsy and there are a number of modality fusion techniques which promise to further improve lesion targeting in the future.

PRINCIPLES OF IMAGE-GUIDED BIOPSY

Percutaneous image-guided needle biopsy is now a standard technique for the diagnosis of most tumours throughout the body and also has a role in the diagnosis of certain infective and inflammatory conditions. It is particularly helpful in the staging of cancer, most notably when the definitive treatment may not involve surgical intervention. Advances in imaging techniques have led to greater precision in the targeting of lesions. Advantages of percutaneous biopsy over surgical excision biopsy include time and cost savings and reduced morbidity. The complication rates associated with percutaneous biopsy vary according to the organ studied, but are generally lower than 0.1%.[3]

CASE SELECTION

Most image-guided biopsies can be performed using local anaesthesia and sedation. General anaesthesia may be preferable in some patients, including children. Pertinent patient history includes bleeding diatheses and anticoagulant usage. Contraindications to biopsy include an uncorrected coagulopathy and lack of a safe needle approach route. The benefits of confirming a suspected diagnosis need to be evaluated against the inherent procedural morbidity.

PRE-PROCEDURAL ASSESSMENT

Pre-procedural assessment aims to reduce complication rates by optimising the patient's physiology and identifying contraindications in a timely fashion. It is also useful in alleviating patient anxiety and discussing post-procedural care to enable the patient to plan time off work, etc. The pre-procedural assessment is also a good time to obtain patients' written consent.

Careful questioning can determine whether a day case procedure is appropriate, taking into account the patient's clinical status and home circumstances. Any language, cultural or religious barriers can also be identified. Regularly updated and referenced departmental patient information leaflets should be available for all common procedures and include links to web-based information and relevant telephone numbers for further advice. These help inform the consent process and provide post-procedural advice as it is well documented that patients retain little of any verbal information they are given.[4]

Another role of pre-procedural assessment is to highlight potential problems related to patient co-morbidity or the nature of the biopsy target. If the patient is on anticoagulants or has a coagulopathy, the timing of the biopsy procedure should be carefully planned around the cessation of anticoagulant medication or admission for correction of coagulation disorders. These patients have an increased risk of post-procedural haemorrhage and may require an extended period of observation. The nature of the target lesion also needs consideration as vascular lesions are at increased risk of bleeding; it may be necessary to establish peripheral venous access and ensure the availability of cross-matched blood. Wherever possible, an obstructed organ should be decompressed prior to biopsy using techniques such as biliary drainage or percutaneous nephrostomy.

Patients should be told how and when they will receive biopsy results and a follow-up outpatient clinic appointment booked prior to discharge.

CORE BIOPSY VS FINE NEEDLE ASPIRATION

Fine needle aspiration (FNA) utilises a small calibre needle (20 to 25G) to obtain a sample of cells from a target organ/lesion for cytological analysis. Core biopsy involves larger calibre needles (14 to 19G) and reveals more structural information, which is often necessary for histological diagnosis (Table 87-1).[5,6] Each method has its own advantages and disadvantages and the decision as to which one to use depends on many factors:

FNA with a small calibre needle may be employed in situations where a structure (e.g. bowel loop) needs to be transgressed as it is interposed between the target lesion and skin. Similarly, where a deep lesion lies in close proximity to critical vascular structures (e.g. a central liver lesion abutting the vena cava), core biopsy may be deemed too hazardous.

TABLE 87-1 **Needle Gauge and Calibre**

Needle Gauge	Diameter (mm)
22	0.72
21	0.82
19	1.10
18	1.26
16	1.67
14	2.13

Aside from the reduced risk of iatrogenic injury, FNA can be useful in frail or unwell patients who cannot tolerate a prolonged procedure. A further advantage is that cytological slides can be examined immediately to check for adequacy and formal pathology reports can be issued rapidly if required.

The degree of confidence in cytological diagnosis will vary according to the indication; the diagnosis of recurrent malignancy can be more easily made on a cytological sample if previous tumour tissue is available for comparison. For a new diagnosis of malignancy, however, a larger sample of tissue is usually required and hence core biopsy is generally preferred over cytology. This is particularly important where different subtypes of malignancy exist (e.g. lymphoma), and accurate histological typing is necessary to plan treatment.[7–9] Other pathologies requiring histological confirmation include diffuse disease such as cirrhosis and renal parenchymal disease (e.g. glomerulonephritis).

BIOPSY NEEDLES

Needles vary in calibre, tip design, length and mechanism of action and there are a wide range of different products on the market. Needle choice depends on a number of factors including the lesion to be targeted, the number of cores required, the modality chosen for image guidance, personal preference, cost and local availability. They can be broadly classified as follows.

Fine Needle Aspiration Cytology Needles

Cytological samples are usually taken with small calibre needles (20–25G). Different lengths of small calibre needle are available and the needle should be carefully selected according to the depth and size of lesion to be sampled. For abdominal FNA, the target will often be deep and a spinal or other stylet needle is often used. The presence of a needle stylet helps to avoid luminal contamination with tissue before it reaches its target. When using very fine needles, a stylet also aids insertion by stiffening the needle to prevent it deviating from its course.

Core Biopsy Needles

For core biopsy, larger calibre cutting needles are employed (usually 16–18G for abdominal biopsies). The size of biopsy needle chosen depends on the organ being targeted and may also vary according to the number of samples being obtained. For a routine 'background' liver biopsy, a single pass is usually sufficient and so a larger (e.g. 16G) biopsy needle may be chosen. If the operator anticipates that several cores will need to be obtained, e.g. in the case of multiple lesions, then an 18G needle may be more appropriate to reduce the risk of bleeding following multiple liver capsule punctures.

The shape of the tissue core obtained varies according to the design of the chamber within the biopsy needle; various manufacturers have designed biopsy instruments

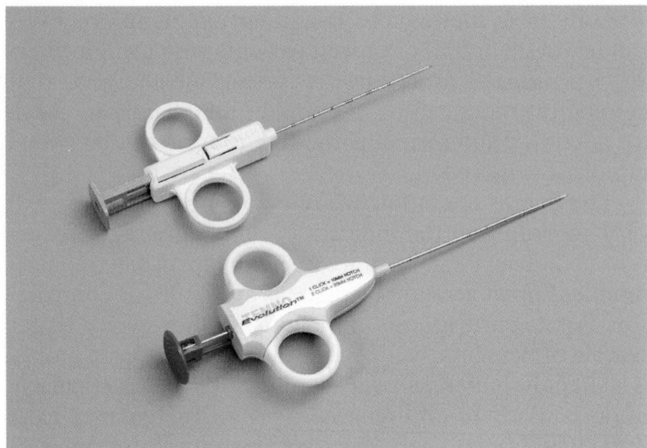

FIGURE 87-1 ■ Examples of semi-automatic core biopsy instruments. These allow placement of the central notch at the exact position required with the cutting sheath subsequently fired over the stylet. There is therefore no additional forward excursion of the needle upon firing, so minimising the risk of damage to adjacent structures.

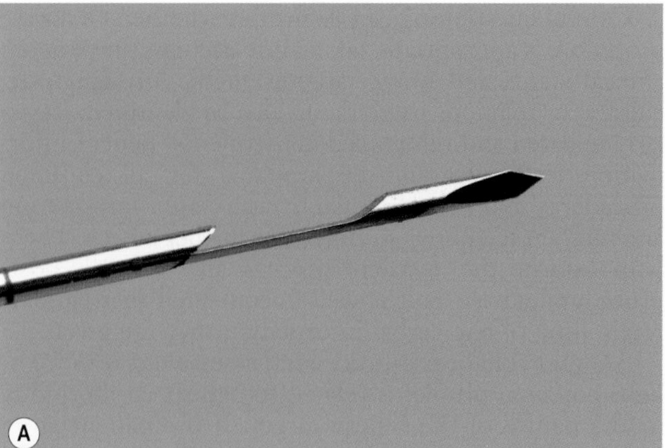

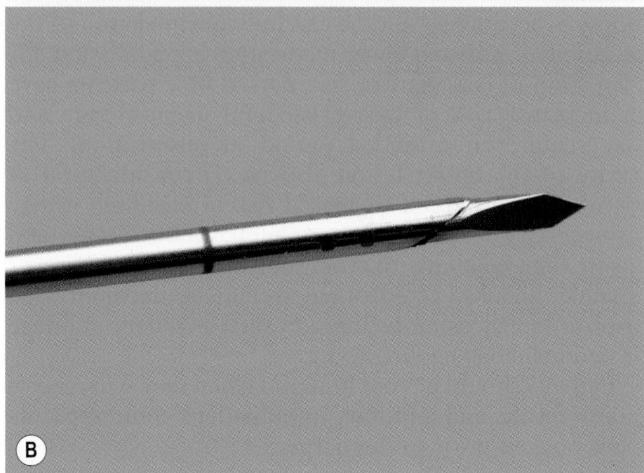

FIGURE 87-2 ■ The mechanism of a semi-automatic biopsy instrument. (A) The central notched stylet is advanced to the point required. (B) The cutting sheath is then fired over the stylet with the cored sample of tissue residing in the notch of the stylet.

which optimise the volume of tissue obtained for a given needle gauge[10] as there is evidence that increasing needle calibre is related to increased risk of haemorrhage.[11]

Menghini Technique Biopsy Needles, e.g. Surecut

These operate using a suction mechanism but are no longer in common use. They are based on the Menghini principle in which the needle, stylet and syringe form a single unit.

Sheathed Biopsy Needles

Manual, e.g. Tru-Cut

These needles consist of a biopsy chamber that can be opened and closed. After insertion to the correct depth, the needle is opened by manually advancing the inner portion so that the surrounding tissue falls into the biopsy notch. As the outer part of the needle is then advanced, the tissue in the chamber is cut by its leading edge. This requires two hands to operate and so is impractical for ultrasound-guided procedures.

Semi-Sutomatic, e.g. Temno, SuperCore (Fig. 87-1)

Some biopsy instruments allow placement of the central notch at the exact position required and then fire the cutting sheath over the stylet (Fig. 87-2). There is therefore no additional forward excursion of the needle upon firing the cutting part of the needle, so minimising the risk of damage to adjacent structures. This is useful in the case of small lesions or those adjacent to critical structures such as large veins. When the target tissue is fibrous or very firm in texture it can, however, be difficult to manually advance the cutting needle through the lesion without displacing it. This is often overcome by the use of spring-loaded fully automated devices that exert more forward force to advance the needle into the target.

Fully Automatic, e.g. Biopty gun, Achieve, Biopince, Bard Max-Core (Fig. 87-3)

These can take the form of metal biopsy guns, which are designed for use with disposable biopsy needles of different gauges, or fully disposable integrated plastic biopsy devices, which have a similar mechanism of action. Whilst the disposable devices are more expensive, they avoid the difficulties associated with sterilisation of the metal biopsy guns and have generally been adopted as the biopsy instrument of choice in many radiology departments. Fully automatic biopsy instruments fire both a central stylet and cutting sheath in a rapid forward motion such that the tissue core is obtained at a preset distance or 'throw' (e.g. 2 cm) ahead of the visualised needle tip. Many of the instruments offer a choice of throw (usually 1 or 2 cm) depending on the size of target lesion or organ. This mechanism of action means that the operator needs to be aware of the size of the lesion to be sampled relative to the throw of the biopsy needle. Often the

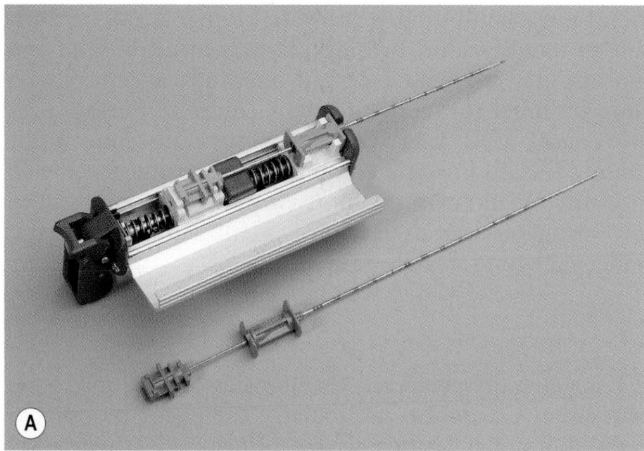

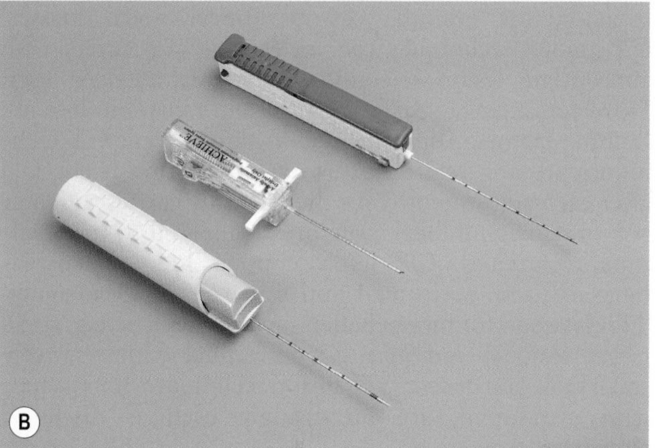

FIGURE 87-3 ■ Examples of fully automatic core biopsy instruments. Fully automatic biopsy instruments fire both a central stylet and cutting sheath in a rapid forward motion such that the tissue core is obtained at a preset distance or 'throw' (e.g. 2 cm) ahead of the visualised needle tip. (A) Non-disposbale metal biopsy guns, which are designed for use with disposable biopsy needles of different gauges. (B) Fully disposable integrated plastic biopsy devices, which have a similar mechanism of action.

needle tip can be positioned at the superficial margin of the target lesion to avoid injury to adjacent structures.

COAXIAL TECHNIQUE

Most biopsies are performed by making one or more passes into an organ or mass with a single biopsy needle. Occasionally it may be helpful to employ a system whereby a coaxial needle is radiologically guided into the lesion/mass, the central stylet is removed and then a smaller calibre biopsy needle can be inserted through the coaxial system to obtain multiple cores (Fig. 87-4). This has the advantage of allowing several samples to be taken without re-puncturing the superficial soft tissues or organ capsule, which theoretically reduces the risk of haemorrhage and time taken to target the lesion,[12] although studies have not demonstrated any significant difference in complication rates between coaxial and non-coaxial techniques.[13] The coaxial needle can be angled between samples to increase the volume of tissue sampled. This technique is commonly employed during CT-guided biopsy, particularly for lung lesions where minimising the number of passes through the pleura, reduces the risk of pneumothorax (Fig. 87-5). It is also used for biopsy of deep abdominal/pelvic masses, as it reduces the radiation dose and trauma involved in re-positioning biopsy needles for each core. There is also a theoretical advantage that coaxial systems reduce the risk of track seeding. A disadvantage is that the calibre of the coaxial needle must be larger than that of the biopsy needle, increasing the overall size of the needle track, with a possible increased risk of damage to adjacent tissues.

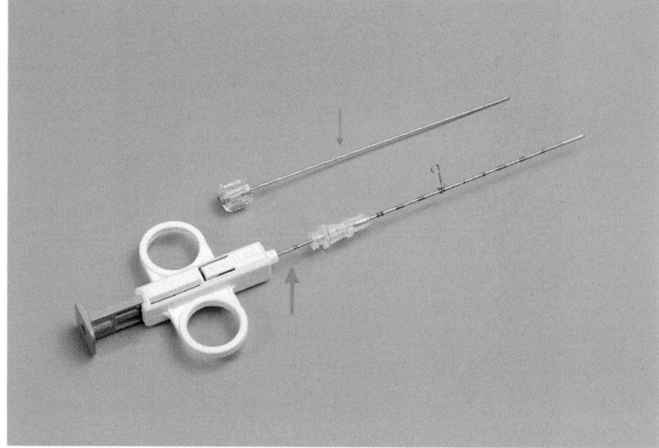

FIGURE 87-4 ■ Example of a coaxial biopsy system. The coaxial needle is radiologically guided into the lesion then the central stylet (thin arrow) is removed; a smaller calibre biopsy needle (thick arrow) can then be inserted through the coaxial system to obtain multiple cores.

IMAGING MODALITIES FOR BIOPSY

Choice of modality for biopsy varies according to the size, location and visibility of the lesion. Most intra-abdominal lesions can be approached using either ultrasound or CT imaging. Modern technology is increasingly allowing a combination of modalities to be used during biopsy procedures (fusion imaging) to aid targeting of lesions. Previously, this required time-consuming manual registration of imaging but newer automated registration/fusion software is considerably reducing the time taken for co-registration of different modalities and it is likely that this technique will become commonplace in the future.

Ultrasound

Ultrasound-guided biopsy is considered an accurate, safe, widely accessible and relatively cheap technique. It has the advantage of real-time visualisation of the needle (particularly important for biopsy of organs such as the liver where the time the biopsy needle remains within liver parenchyma should be limited to minimise haemorrhagic complications). In addition, it allows a multiplanar angled approach that may be more challenging at CT or MR imaging. Ultrasound-guided biopsy procedures have

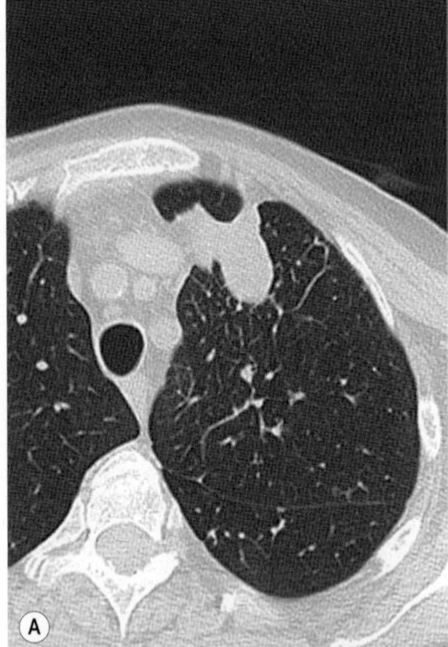

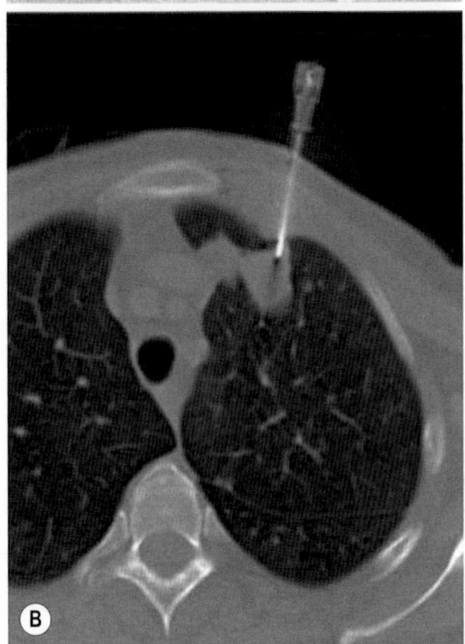

FIGURE 87-5 ■ A coaxial system has been utilised so there is only one pass through the pleura during lung biopsy. (A) CT images of the lesion prior to biopsy. (B) A coaxial needle has been placed under CT guidance (seen here on bone windows) through which a biopsy needle can be passed to obtain multiple biopsies.

the advantages of portability and lack of ionising radiation. However, ultrasound-guided biopsies are more operator-dependent than procedures guided by other imaging modalities. Ultrasound platforms and software are becoming increasingly advanced, enabling the operator to benefit from additional information to aid lesion targeting. Intravenous ultrasound contrast agents and elastography data are being used with increasing frequency.

Technology which enables co-registration of real-time ultrasound imaging with CT/MRI studies is becoming more accessible.[14] One example of this is using MRI data to aid ultrasound-guided prostate biopsy. It can be difficult to identify focal prostatic lesions at ultrasound and cancers may be missed despite methods which allow a large number of cores to be acquired. Fusing pre-procedural MRI data with real-time transrectal ultrasound (TRUS) imaging combines the advantages of each modality by allowing the biopsy needle to be introduced into suspicious lesions previously identified with MRI but under real-time TRUS guidance.[15]

CT

CT is generally preferred for biopsies of the lung, bone and spine. CT is also particularly useful for biopsies of deep abdominal lesions where ultrasound visualisation is poor, for example retroperitoneal nodal masses. CT-guided techniques can be extremely accurate with appropriate lesion selection and an experienced user. However, access to scanning time and radiation dose are limiting factors. Additionally non-fluoroscopic CT techniques are not 'real time', as needle position is checked after each adjustment. This theoretically carries a greater risk of damaging local structures compared to true real-time techniques. CT fluoroscopy technology enables biopsies to be performed under real-time CT imaging. This is useful for more challenging procedures (e.g. small target lesions) and may be performed with relatively small radiation doses.[16] CT fusion techniques, for instance with ultrasound, are increasingly used as discussed elsewhere.

MRI

Recent advances in MRI have made it increasingly useful, particularly where an oblique approach is required, e.g. for subdiaphragmatic liver and adrenal masses.[17,18] MRI also provides improved soft tissue detail when imaging certain organs and structures compared with CT or ultrasound and hence can be invaluable in targeting lesions in areas such as the prostate which are difficult to visualise with ultrasound or certain liver lesions which cannot be appreciated on unenhanced CT imaging.[19,20]

MRI-guided breast biopsies are also performed, particularly for lesions that are difficult to localise with mammography or ultrasound. Within the field of musculoskeletal imaging, MRI-guided biopsy is useful for lesions in the bone marrow that cannot be identified with CT. The use of MRI guidance is likely to increase as the technology improves.

The main disadvantage of MRI-guided biopsies is the magnetic environment, which limits equipment usage, making some procedures more complex. This in turn can lead to increased procedural times which may be an issue where MRI capacity is limited. There are also increased costs to consider, and patients may find MRI-guided procedures more uncomfortable due to positioning constraints. Open magnets allow direct access to the patient during the entire procedure, enabling real-time monitoring of needle insertion. A further problem with MRI-guided biopsy is the need for motion correction during the biopsy procedure. In addition, patients may not be able to tolerate MRI due to claustrophobia or have other contraindications such as pacemakers. MRI-safe biopsy equipment is now mass-produced but is expensive and the range is limited.

PET CT

The mechanism by which PET images are obtained is an intrinsic barrier to their use in biopsy, in that images are obtained over a period of time and proximity to the patient during acquisition results in radiation safety issues. However, novel fusion techniques that combine real-time CT with pre-procedural PET/CT to identify lesions that are not easily visualised on conventional CT and are only identified due to their differential FDG uptake have been described.[21]

Fluoroscopy

Plain fluoroscopic biopsy techniques are most frequently used for musculoskeletal lesions, as bony landmarks are easily identified. Fusion techniques are being increasingly developed, for example the use of pre-procedural MRI and CT overlaid on real-time fluoroscopic images; this is useful for sampling multiple targets, including head and neck lesions.[22]

Fluoroscopy is also utilised in transvascular biopsy techniques, where intravascular contrast is used to guide access, e.g. transvenous liver biopsy via the jugular or femoral vein,[23] which is usually performed when liver biopsy is essential but contraindicated percutaneously.

Stereotactic

This technique is mainly limited to the biopsy of breast lesions that are seen on mammography but cannot be visualised with ultrasound. They are performed most commonly for microcalcification and architectural distortion. This technique relies on computer software to interpret angled mammography views to give a three-dimensional location of the lesion.

Endoscopy/Endoscopic Ultrasound (EUS) and Bronchoscopy/Bronchoscopic Ultrasound

More often performed by appropriately trained clinicians than radiologists, direct visualisation biopsies and endoscopic/bronchoscopic ultrasound-guided aspiration or biopsy procedures have an important role in obtaining tissue from areas which are difficult to access percutaneously. EUS can also be combined with elastography to aid lesion identification and biopsy.[24]

TIPS AND TRICKS

'Look Before you Leap'—Procedural Set Up

As with any procedure, time spent reviewing pre-procedural imaging and planning biopsy approach and modality is very well spent. Particularly when performing ultrasound-guided procedures, the operator should try and ensure that the patient's bed is at an appropriate height. Small changes to patient position and room setup can increase or decrease significantly the difficulty of performing the biopsy.

Avoiding Inadequate Samples

In centrally necrotic tumours, it is important to plan a needle trajectory through the periphery of the lesion to obtain useful tissue for histological analysis. Obtaining fibrous or gelatinous material can often result in failure to secure a histological diagnosis. Therefore it is advantageous to identify and subsequently avoid these areas. Often it is possible to assess the likelihood of a diagnosis being reached by visually assessing the sample (e.g. white tissue which sinks in formalin) but if there is doubt, urgent cytological/histological assessment can help to decide whether the biopsy should be repeated.

Improving Needle Tip Visualisation in Ultrasound-Guided Biopsy

This can be technically difficult, particularly when sampling anatomically deep structures or tissues which are particularly echogenic. Accurate needle/transducer alignment is also crucial to good visualisation. The conspicuity of the needle is increased by turning the bevel upwards. 'Jiggling' the needle gently, injecting a tiny volume of air or local anaesthetic, optimising ultrasound platform settings (focal zone, depth, etc.) and use of needle guides can also help to increase needle conspicuity. Many biopsy needles are manufactured with a roughened tip or polymer coating to aid ultrasound scatter/beam reflection.

POST-PROCEDURAL CARE

Good post-procedural care reduces the morbidity associated with percutaneous biopsy by prompt recognition of complications and subsequent instigation of appropriate management. Immediate post-procedural imaging to identify problems can be helpful (e.g. in looking for pneumothorax following lung biopsy) but overall it has a low sensitivity and specificity for identifying complications, the majority of which become evident during the early post-procedural period. Patients should therefore be closely observed to a standard protocol in a dedicated unit with appropriately trained staff. Within the radiology departmental setting, in the initial post-procedural period, patients are best observed in a radiology day case unit. Post-procedural pain is common and usually responds to simple non-steroidal analgesia and reassurance. If opiate analgesia is required, the patient should be clinically assessed for early evidence of complications such as haemorrhage. Standard procedure-specific post-biopsy observation sheets which highlight the management of suspected complications should be used. These are particularly beneficial when patients return to their wards where staff may not have any specialist knowledge of the procedure and its associated risks.

SPECIMEN HANDLING

All core biopsy samples obtained should be very carefully handled to avoid tissue disruption or 'lost samples'. The operator should ensure that clear clinical information is provided on the request form. Specimen handling is aided by the presence of an assistant. Following core biopsy, the needle gate should be opened carefully to reveal the specimen which can be then placed in formalin. The cores obtained should be inspected to make an initial assessment of adequacy: soft tissue generally sinks in the formalin while fat floats to the surface.

COMPLICATIONS AND SAFETY ISSUES

Day case biopsy procedures should be scheduled on morning lists in order to enable an appropriate period of post-biopsy observation. This allows complications to be identified and managed during normal working hours. Higher risk biopsy procedures should be performed in a unit where any associated complications can be managed definitively, in order to avoid the need for emergency patient transfer. For the purposes of clinical governance, those performing biopsy or drainage procedures should audit their complication rates against published standards and monitor their success rate in terms of the percentage of adequate samples for histological evaluation obtained.

Complications are specific to the organ/lesion undergoing biopsy but are more likely to occur in patients who have co-morbidity or abnormal coagulation.

Haemorrhage is the most common major complication after biopsy procedures. If there is clinical suspicion regarding haemorrhage, ultrasound examination can be used to look for free fluid but false negative scans are not unusual and CT imaging is often necessary. The other major general complication of image-guided biopsy is infection (wound infection, deeper abscess formation, septicaemia or peritonitis). Minor complications include post-procedural pain and vasovagal reactions. Procedure-specific complications include haematuria after prostate biopsy and pneumothorax following lung biopsy.

Track Seeding

Seeding the needle track with malignant tumour cells when performing percutaneous needle biopsy is rare and must be differentiated from local tumour recurrence. It has been reported from a number of different tumour sites but certain tumours, such as hepatocellular carcinoma, soft tissue sarcomas, colorectal liver metastases and primary pleural malignancy, have been associated with a higher risk of track seeding.[25] Multidisciplinary team discussion is often appropriate in these cases. Careful consideration should be given to the proposed course of the needle to limit the tissues traversed. Knowledge of proposed surgical/radiotherapy treatment is helpful, particularly in the case of sarcoma biopsy where the needle track should be limited to the same compartment as the target lesion.

CONCLUSION

Image-guided biopsies are increasingly performed as an alternative to open biopsy or resection. Radiologists have a vital role in providing a safe and reliable biopsy service that enables clinicians to make an accurate diagnosis. Although ultrasound and CT are the commonest modalities utilised, the principles of safe biopsy technique can be applied across the modalities. As with all procedures, patient selection and preparation are key considerations and a firm understanding of the benefits and associated risks is essential in the selection and counseling of patients.

Technological advances include the use of MRI and multi-modality fusion imaging. These emerging techniques are enabling biopsies to be undertaken in more challenging patient groups, facilitating the biopsy of lesions that are difficult to identify with conventional imaging and providing more accurate guidance in the biopsy of smaller target lesions.

IMAGE-GUIDED TUMOUR ABLATION

THE CASE FOR TUMOUR ABLATION

Advances in diagnostic imaging have led to ever more frequent identification of small malignant tumours in different organs. It is becoming increasingly difficult to justify traditional, major surgical resection for such small volume disease. An additional consideration is that these tumours are often found in elderly patients who are less likely to tolerate the morbidity of traditional surgical techniques.

Although modern combination chemotherapy is yielding increasingly better results and has improved survival in a number of common cancers, it does not eradicate the disease in the 'surgical' sense. This consideration has stimulated the development of minimally invasive techniques for the treatment of small volume disease. In some cases this is a replacement for surgical resection, as in image-guided ablation of renal tumours, which is increasingly yielding outcomes equivalent to those of partial nephrectomy. In other situations, such as metastatic colorectal disease in the liver, ablation is more likely to be seen as a minimally invasive adjunct to systemic chemotherapy.

This section will set out to discuss the principles of effective tumour ablation and the ablative energies involved. Sound oncological outcomes also require a clear understanding of image guidance as it influences procedural planning and execution, intraprocedural monitoring and perhaps most importantly radiological follow-up of this inherently 'in situ' surgical technique.

THE PRINCIPLES OF TUMOUR ABLATION

Tumour ablation is used mainly in the treatment of small tumours. Image-guided ablation (IGA) sets out to reduce the morbidity of invasive surgery and spare background functioning parenchyma. It has inherent physical limitations but treatment efficacy can be improved by the use of adjunctive techniques such as hydrodissection, (chemo)embolisation and modulation by systemic chemotherapy.

ABLATIVE ENERGIES

The operator must have a firm understanding of the ablative energies currently used and their relative limitations and merits in different environments. Most ablative technologies employ thermal energy to achieve coagulative tissue necrosis through both the target tumour and a surrounding margin of organ parenchyma, in order to reduce the risk of local recurrence. This process of localised thermal destruction is modified in vivo by local tissue interactions, which affect how well the thermal energy is propagated through adjacent tissue. The degree to which the tumour is heated can be modified by heat loss as a result of perfusion-mediated tissue cooling and 'heat-sumping' arising from the cooling effect of blood flow in adjacent vessels of > 3 mm in diameter.[26,27]

The operator must address the shape of the target tumour and aim to incorporate it within a contiguous ablation zone along with an adequate 'resection' margin in the surgical sense. The energy applied must be sufficient not only to denature tumour but also to achieve effective ablation of adjacent normal tissue. An adequate margin is necessary because adjacent parenchyma may harbor microsatellites of disease or small foci of microvascular invasive disease. The aim should be to obtain tissue lethal temperatures in a consistent margin around the tumour without causing thermal injury to adjacent structures.

Radiofrequency Ablation

Radiofrequency ablation (RFA) has evolved rapidly since its first application to tumour ablation in the early 1990s into the most commonly utilised ablative device to date.[26] Monopolar radiofrequency ablation involves the application of high-frequency (460–500 kHz) alternating current to the target tissue using a needle-like applicator. Water molecules, which are inherently polarised, are agitated within the alternating electric field. Large, dispersive grounding pads are attached to the patient's trunk or thighs but the resultant current flux density around the uninsulated probe tip causes 'radiofrequency' agitation of

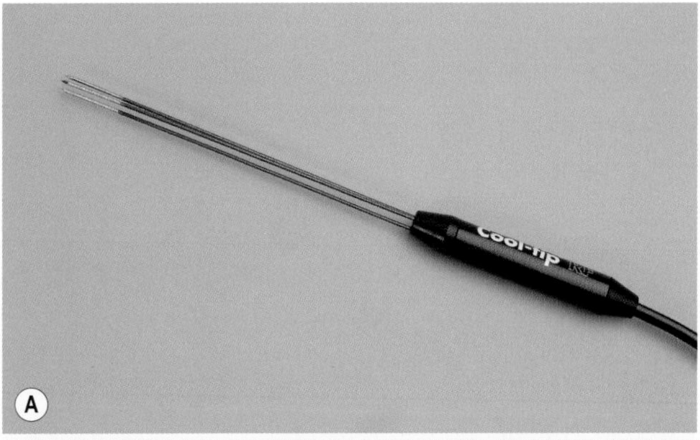

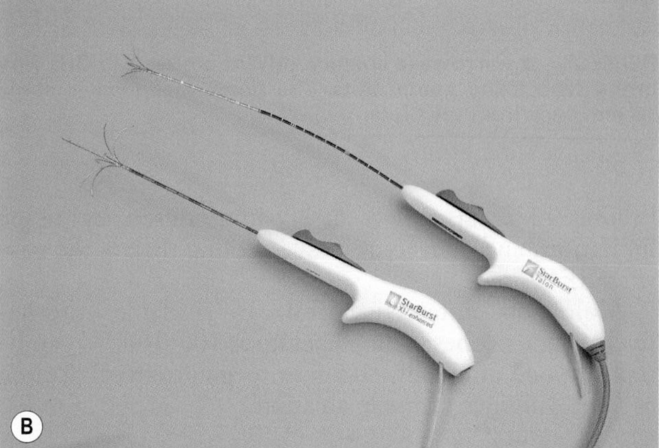

FIGURE 87-6 ■ **Radiofrequency ablation (RFA) devices.** The manufacturers have developed clustered (A) or expandable probe arrays (B) to overcome the limitations of single-probe RFA.

water molecules and local frictional heating within a few millimetres of the tip of the electrode.

Coagulative necrosis results if the target tissue can be maintained at temperatures above 45°C. RFA can induce temperatures of 100–110°C within a few millimetres of the probe but beyond this zone it relies on conductive heating to raise the temperature of the target tumour. The temperature of the tissue near the edge of the tumour may not be high enough for effective ablation leading to marginal recurrences.

Modern needle applicators can achieve reproducible 3–5 cm spheres of contiguous tissue destruction within 15–20 minutes. Larger ablation volumes can be achieved by 'clustering' needles on a single-hand piece, using expandable multi-tined devices or through multipolar arrays (Fig. 87-6).

Microwave Ablation

Microwave ablation (MWA) employs needle-like probes harbouring a microwave broadcast antenna within the 'feedpoint' towards the tip of the device (Fig. 87-7). These are tuned to interact with soft tissue in the range of 900–2400 MHz. Water molecules oscillate when subjected to microwave (electromagnetic) radiation. There is an inherent physical inefficiency to this process—'lossy dielectrics'—which results in localised tissue heating, often to very high temperatures. This results in effective

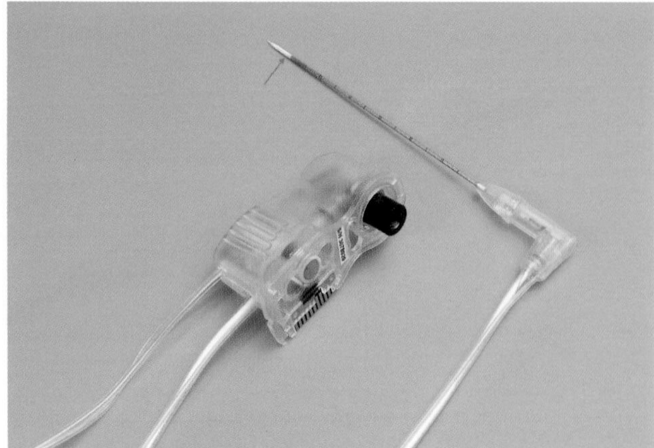

FIGURE 87-7 ■ **Microwave ablation (MWA) probe, 2.45 GHz MW probe with inline pump units.** The probe feedpoint is some 16 mm back from the tip (arrow).

heating of local tissues, less compromised by tissue limitations and convective tissue cooling than is the case with RFA.[28]

Multiprobe, interactive arrays are available. Alternatively single probes, which operate at 100–180 W, can be repositioned after only 3–5 min to good effect, leading to large volumes of tissue ablation.

Cryoablation

This form of thermal energy has been in variable use for some decades but only in the past few years has there been renewed interest due to the introduction of narrow guage (17G) argon cryoprobes, which have made percutaneous cryoablation (CRA) a practical proposition (Fig. 87-8).[29] In practice several parallel probes (usually 3–4) are placed under image guidance into the tumour, approximately 10 mm from the edge and 15–20 mm apart. The phase change of liquid to gaseous argon can induce temperatures as low as –150 to –170°C in the immediate vicinity of the probes. The cell lethal isotherm lies at –20 to –30°C and is ensured in practice by a double freeze–thaw cycle.[30]

The mechanism of cell injury is multifactorial but intracellular ice formation disrupts cellular organelles whilst extracellular ice formation and osmotic dehydration also aids in achieving cellular disruption. These mechanisms are compounded by microvascular endothelial injury.[29]

The outstanding feature of cryoablation is the physical iceball created through the tissues during the treatment cycle. The evolution of the iceball is more predictable and the phase change to ice is clearly visualised by current ultrasound, CT and MR imaging modalities. This provides a readily visualised 'therapeutic' ovoid iceball.

Focused Ultrasound

Focused ultrasound does not require placement of an invasive probe. Small focal areas of tissue destruction are achieved by focusing sound energy in the 1-MHz range, using an extracorporeal acoustic lens. This has the clear

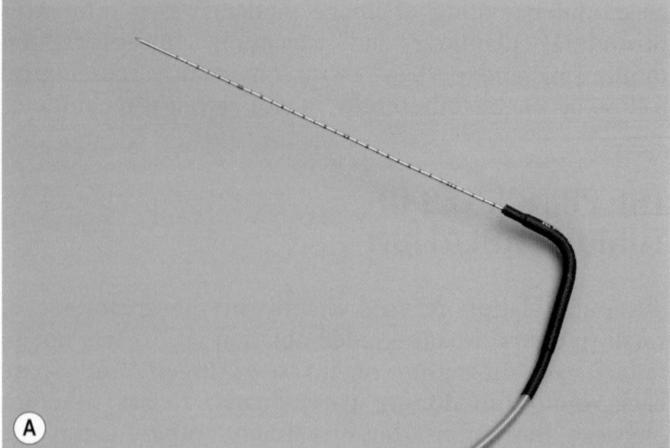

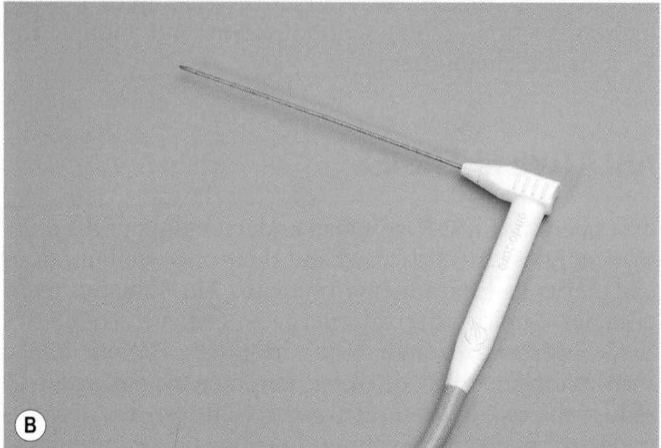

FIGURE 87-8 ■ **Cryoablation (CRA) probes.** Two examples of standard organ cryoprobes.

advantage of avoiding breach of the body wall but the sound energy can be severely attenuated by intervening structures such as bone or gas. The focused energy results in small ovoids of tissue destruction usually of about rice grain size, i.e. 12 × 3 mm.[31] These areas are stacked together contiguously to create larger ablation zones. This process requires complex motion correction and respiratory gating in organs such as the liver and kidney, and this explains why to date applications have centred on stationary organs such as the prostate or the uterus.

Irreversible Electroporation

Irreversible electroporation (IRE) is a non-thermal ablative technique that acts by the application of millisecond pulses of direct current between monopolar probes or using a single bipolar probe. These bursts of current can temporarily disrupt the electrical potential of the cell membrane and thereby perforate—or 'porate'—the cell membrane. A reversible form of electroporation has been used for some in the laboratory to permit genetic transfection of cells through temporary cell wall permeability. By applying the direct current for slightly longer the cells can be permanently porated—irreversible electroporation—resulting in controlled cell death.[32]

The major disadvantage associated with IRE is the severe muscle contractions induced by the application of direct current pulses. This necessitates the use of a general anaesthetic and muscle relaxants. On occasion cardiac dysrhythmias have been induced by the direct current pulses and as a result the technology is now ECG-synchronised in order to avoid these.[33] Clinical experience with IRE remains in its infancy.

Interstitial Laser Photocoagulation

Interstitial laser photocoagulation (ILP) is known by a number of synonyms including laser interstitial thermotherapy and laser thermal ablation. Laser fibres are coupled to an energy source, commonly neodymium:yttrium aluminium garnet (Nd-YAG), and the fibres emit low energy laser light which interact with chromophobes in the tissue, producing heat. This slow heating can induce useful small zones of tissue destruction over a range of about 10 mm. In practice multiple fibres must be placed using a beam splitter to yield clinically useful volumes of tissue destruction. The unwieldy nature of this device has limited its utilisation in clinical practice although a few centres have produced promising results.[34]

Chemical Ablation

This form of tumour ablation involves the instillation of chemical agents that denature tissue; the main ones are absolute alcohol and acetic acid. Ethanol ablation has been used widely to treat small nodular hepatomas.[35] Excellent results have been achieved in small homogeneous hepatomas. However, in the treatment of larger tumours multiple sessions of ethanol instillation are required because of inhomogeneous distribution of alcohol through the lesion. In recent years multi-tined alcohol infusion needles have been developed and have been advocated by some groups in the treatment of smaller hepatomas, especially in countries with very limited health care budgets.[36]

IMAGE GUIDANCE

This is of defining importance in terms of safety and the achievement of good clinical outcomes. The ablation device must be placed accurately to achieve the desired effect and avoid injury to adjacent structures. In many cases, repositioning of the device is necessary in order to achieve the desired effect. The aim is to destroy the tumour whilst avoiding injury to transgressed or threatened intervening organs.

Pre-Procedural Planning

Ablative techniques are largely aimed at smaller tumours (generally ≤ 5 cm) with the best results obtained in most organ systems for tumours smaller than 3 cm. The aim is to treat the tumour in its entirety without injury to adjacent structures. Injury to structures such as the bowel can be avoided by physical displacement through the use of injected 5% dextrose (Fig. 87-9). The addition of 2% iodinated contrast medium to this fluid can enhance its visualisation. Carbon-dioxide gas insufflation within the retroperitoneum can also be used to displace adjacent bowel for the purpose of renal tumour ablation.[37]

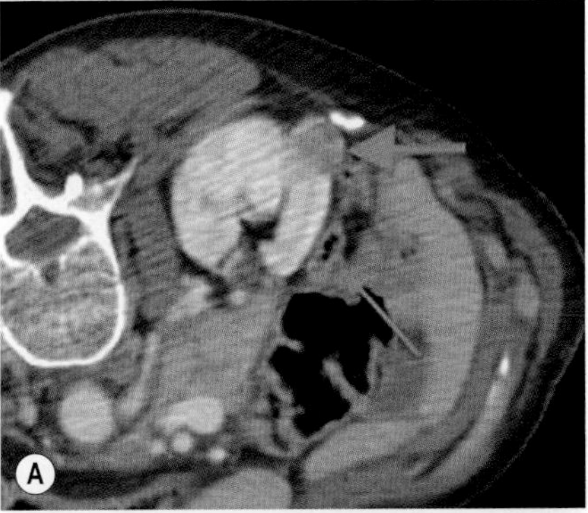

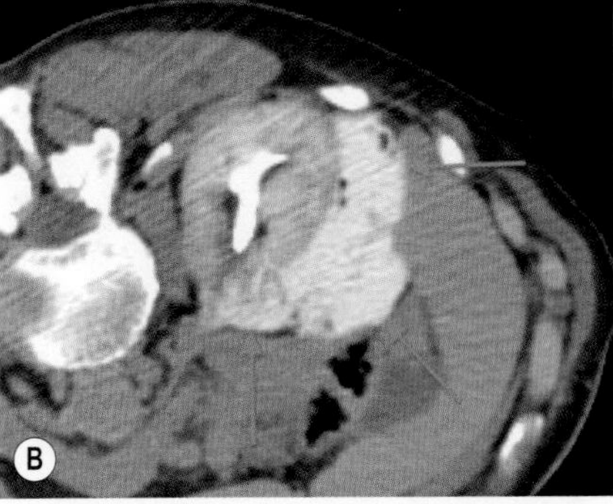

FIGURE 87-9 ■ **Sequence demonstrating the need for hydrodissection during cryoablation of a renal tumour (thick arrow).** (A) Portal venous phase CT; directly adjacent loops of small bowel (thin arrow) that would be at risk if incorporated in the ablation zone. (B) A hydrodissection needle is placed to the interposed retroperitoneum and contrast-tinted saline injected (arrowed), displacing adjacent at risk structures.

Good positioning of the patient can increase the likelihood of a successful ablation. For example, placing a patient with an adrenal tumour in a lateral decubitus position with the target adrenal lowermost can often help to displace the intervening lung in the deep costodiaphragmatic recess and any adjacent bowel away from the treatment volume.

Procedural Targetting

With current ablative technologies most appropriate tumour targets are in the range of 10–40 mm in diameter. Smaller tumours can be difficult to visualise; for example, small hepatomas clearly visible in the late arterial phase CT within a cirrhotic liver can be very difficult to target using ultrasound guidance. Sound outcomes from IGA require a clear visualisation of the tumour and adjacent structures, ideally in real time. Ultrasound provides real-time imaging but may not be able to demonstrate clearly adjacent threatened bowel. Many operators use a combination of ultrasound and CT. It is possible to combine volumetric CT and ultrasound data on a single display platform, allowing display of real-time ultrasound image and 'cold' CT data in any plane. MR guidance can provide image guidance in multiplanar formats with excellent soft-tissue contrast and is under evaluation with regard to resolution and image feedback speed.[38]

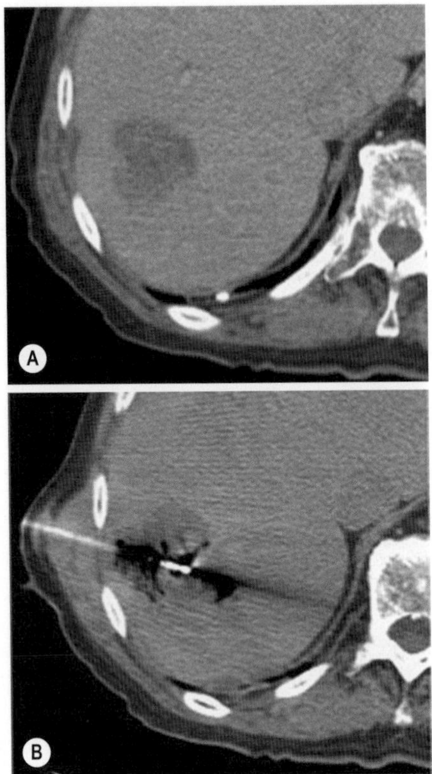

FIGURE 87-10 ■ **Example demonstrating the problem of outgassing following RFA or MWA.** (A) Colorectal metastases in segment 7 for microwave ablation. (B) At initial probe placement and treatment there is considerable 'outgassing' obscuring the target tumour and rendering probe repositioning and treatment dosimetry difficult.

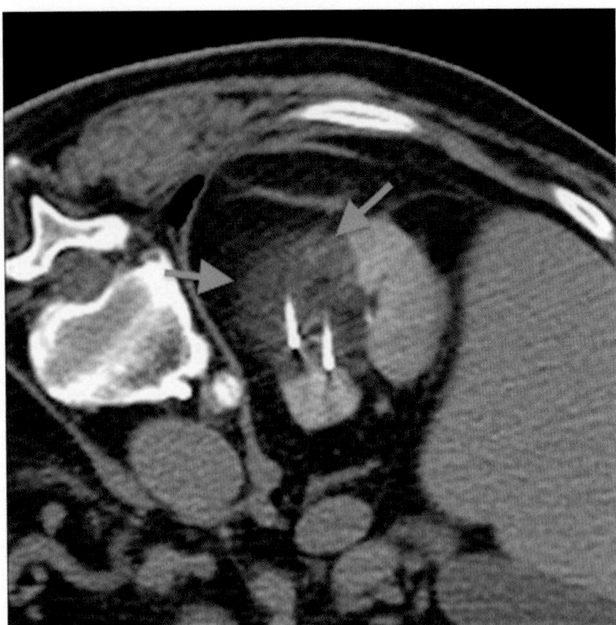

FIGURE 87-11 ■ **Two cryoprobes in a renal tumour demonstrating the formation of the clearly defined low attenuation iceball during the freeze cycle of CRA.**

Peri-Procedural Monitoring

Intraprocedural confirmation of treatment adequacy remains an issue for almost all of the ablation modalities. Visualisation of RFA and MWA procedures is severely compromised by 'outgassing' of the treated lesion (Fig. 87-10), which obscures the target tumour and can impede accurate re-positioning of the probe. Several studies have suggested that contrast-enhanced ultrasound[39] and MR thermometry[38] can guide tumour treatment but each have their limitations in terms of robustness and accuracy.

Cryoablation has the considerable merit of inducing a well-defined and perceivable iceball which can be readily visualised by a number of imaging modalities during the treatment procedure (Fig. 87-11). This feature permits assessment of the effect of treatment with the lethal isotherm of –30°C deemed to reside 5 mm deep to the advancing margin of the iceball.

Post-Procedural Imaging

IGA must assess a 360° global resection margin to confirm treatment adequacy. There is broad acceptance that non-enhancement on CT or MRI during injection of intravenous contrast medium is a surrogate marker of tumour ablation.[40] In some organs such as the kidney and lung other surrogates of complete tumour ablation have been utilised, such as the 'post-treatment' halo artefact seen in the perirenal fat around completely ablated renal tumours[41] and the contiguous ground-glass opacification seen around completely denatured lung tumours.[42]

Follow-up imaging can be delayed for 1–2 weeks after the primary treatment as the ablation zone matures and becomes better defined with immediate post-treatment phenomena such as irregular penumbral arterialisation steadily resolving (though often this can take up to 3 months) and thereby facilitating post-procedural assessment. Degraded blood products within the treatment zone should not be mistaken for residual, viable enhancing tissue. In this respect, subtraction imaging, particularly subtraction T1 volumetric imaging at MR, can help to confirm tumour ablation.

Over time the ablation zone should slowly involute become darker on CT with an increasingly well-defined and sharp margin (Fig. 87-12). In the case of renal tumours and hepatocellular carcinoma, late arterial phase imaging helps to illustrate residual or recurrent disease, which tends to adopt a marginal nodular or crescenteric pattern. Recurrent colorectal metastatic disease can declare itself as an expanding ablation zone with softening of the margins—coined a 'halo' recurrence (Fig. 87-13).

The post-treatment follow-up protocol will clearly be determined by the natural history of the treated tumour. Ablated renal tumours can be indolent and, rarely, recurrent disease can declare itself 2–4 years after the initial treatment. Most local recurrences of colorectal metastases and hepatocellular tumours will be apparent at follow-up within 10 months. As a result most authors advocate follow-up at 3-monthly intervals within the first year, 6-monthly to 2 years and annually out to 5 years.

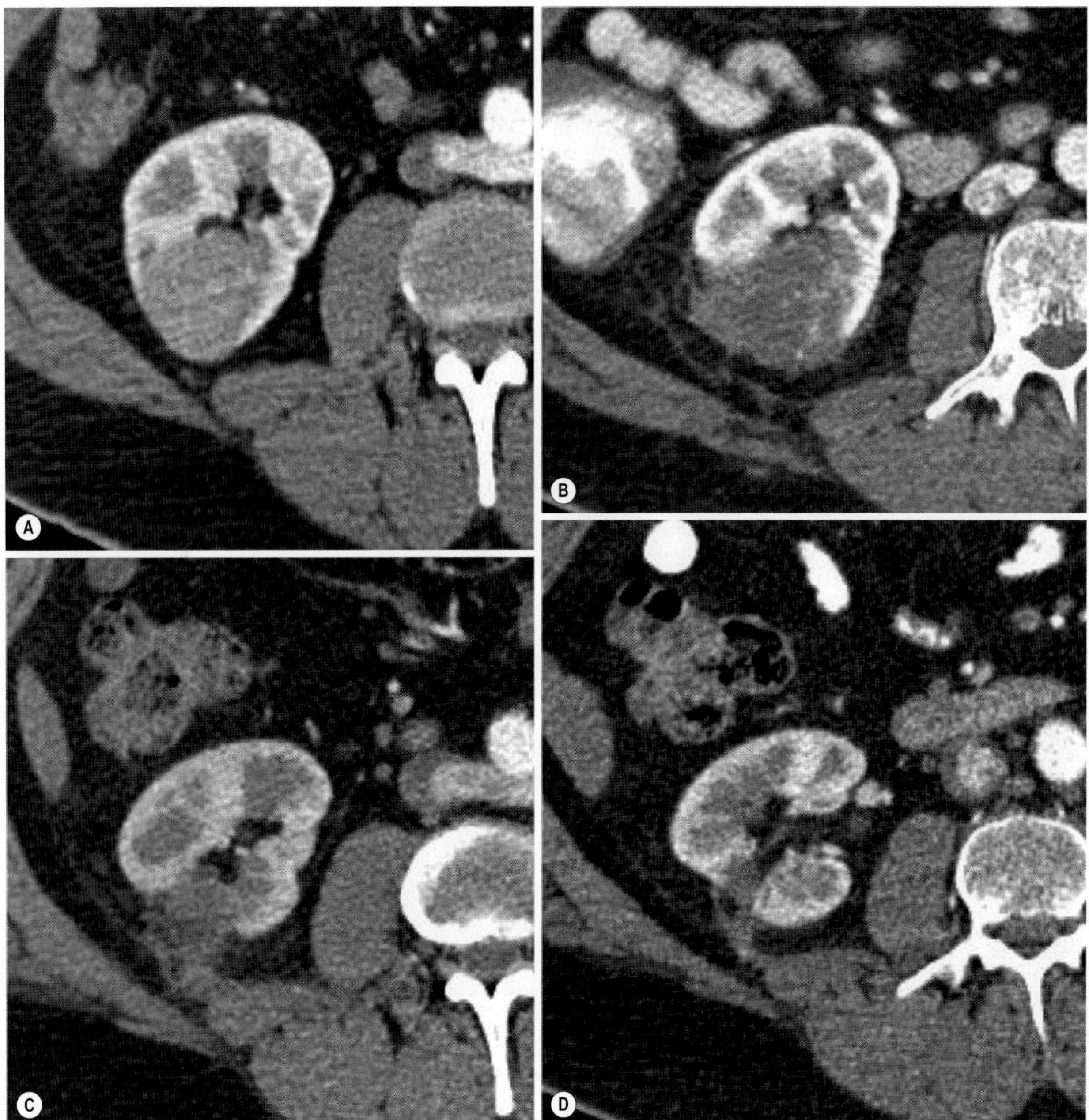

FIGURE 87-12 ■ Sequential images showing involution of a successfully cryoablated 44-mm renal cell carcinoma on late arterial phase CT. (A) Pre-treatment. (B) One month post-treatment. (C) Six months post-treatment. (D) Sixteen months post-treatment.

As we become better able to predict treatment success it may be possible to reduce the intensity of follow-up protocols.

Lung tumours are uniquely problematic in that straightforward imaging markers of treatment success are not readily to hand. A circumferential ground-glass opacification after treatment has been advocated as a marker of completion[42] but it is a very indirect surrogate in that it only represents adjacent airspace injury or haemorrhage. Functional imaging such as FDG PET/CT seems set to play a significant role in confirming the absence of tumour metabolism.[43]

UNDERSTANDING AND MODIFYING TUMOUR PATHOPHYSIOLOGY

During RFA, perfusion-mediated tissue cooling, particularly in the adjacent normal parenchyma, can compromise the zone of thermal injury. Similarly 'heat-sumping', in relation to adjacent blood vessels of ≥ 3 mm, can limit the achievement of tissue-lethal temperatures and result in perivascular tumour sparing.

These problems may be overcome through various techniques such as hypotensive anaesthesia, adjacent temporary vessel occlusion and pre-embolisation. Some

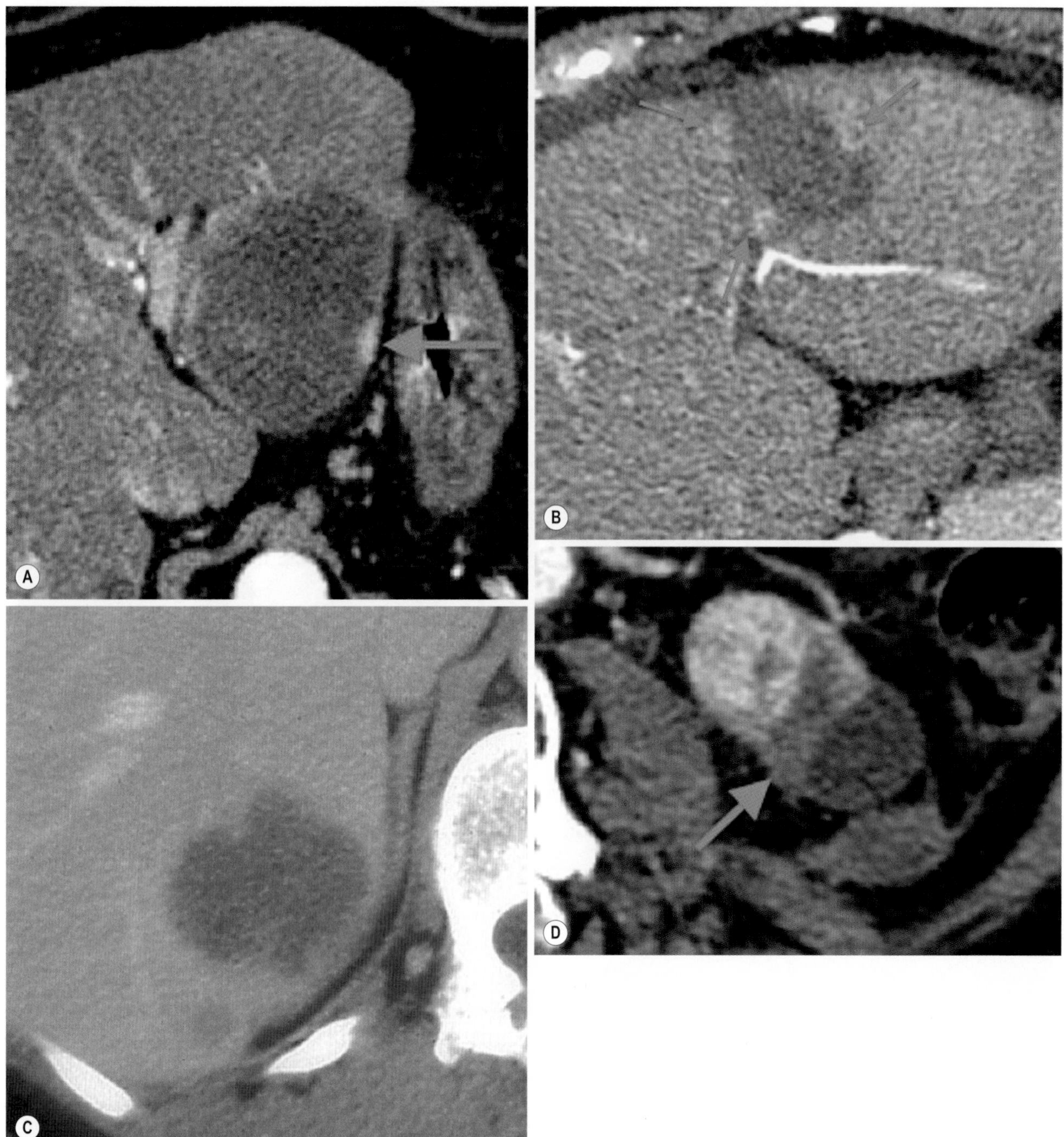

FIGURE 87-13 ■ Patterns of local recurrence can vary according mainly to tumour type. Examples of local recurrence in hepatic tumours but the patterns can apply to all tumour locations. (A) Peripheral nodular recurrence on late arterial phase CT, seen in the subtotal treatment of hepatocellular carcinoma. (B) A patchy peripheral recurrence on late arterial phase CT, sometimes referred to as a 'halo' recurrence. (C) An enlarging (with reference to the ablation zone) low density lesion with increasing ill-defined treatment margin. This form of 'expanding' recurrence is seen with inadequate treatment of a colorectal metastasis. (D) Crescenteric peripheral enhancement on late arterial phase CT indicative of a subtotal treatment.

of these complex treatment modifications have diminished in practice partly through improved case selection for IGA but also through a better understanding of how the tumour pathophysiology can be modified by prior adjuvant chemotherapy bringing tumours within the scope of ablation or the use of anti-angiogenic drugs which appear to modify tumour perfusion and enhance the therapeutic effect of thermal ablation.[44] A number of studies are currently looking at the modification of tumours by agents such as adjuvant sorafenib.

In the setting of hepatocellular carcinoma thermal ablation has been combined with drug-eluting chemoembolisation with a view to enhancing the efficacy of both techniques.[45] This practice is predicated on the fact that thermal ablation most frequently fails at the margins of the tumour, yet the penumbral zone of partial thermal injury can be utilised to preferentially direct chemoembolic agents to this zone for maximum oncological benefit. The effectiveness and optimal timing of these combined approaches remains to be determined.

SPECIFICS AND CURRENT OUTCOMES

The field of interventional oncology is constantly evolving. A full discussion of the merits and limitations of these factors under each cancer type is beyond the scope of this chapter. This section focuses on some developments.

Renal Cancer

This tumour group in particular represents perhaps one of the most effective applications for IGA. Its use has been prompted by the increasing numbers of small renal tumours detected incidentally. The malignant potential of some of these smaller renal tumours remains the subject of debate with some advocating active surveillance. Yet the treatment paradigm is changed if a simple, minimally invasive and nephron-sparing intervention can be brought to bear where no simple marker of the relative potential behaviour of these tumours currently exists.

The efficacy of RFA for the treatment of sub-35-mm renal tumours has been confirmed with intermediate follow-up at 2–3 years.[46,47] Meta-analysis has suggested that cryoablation may be more effective than RFA with lower rates of local recurrence and subtotal treatment.[48] Experience to date suggests that percutaneous renal cryoablation may achieve results similar to that of surgical resection with lower morbidity.[49]

Hepatocellular Carcinoma

Hepatocellular carcinoma (HCC) is frequently a combination of two disease processes in Western society where HCC almost always arises in the setting of liver cirrhosis. There are multiple treatment options which reflect the stage of hepatocellular carcinoma at presentation but also the functional liver reserve in the setting of cirrhosis. In an attempt to clarify this decision-making process the Barcelona Clinic Liver Cancer Group published a treatment decision algorithm.[50] Chemoembolisation and systemic therapies are reserved for intermediate stage, multifocal disease. The options for more limited disease include ablation, transplantation and resection. Resection of cirrhotic livers carries significantly higher operative complications and is usually reserved for those without frank portal hypertension.

Ablation—mostly using radiofrequency or microwaves—has an increasing role in the management of paucilesional sub-5-cm hepatomas as it carries significantly lower morbidity than resection and has been shown to achieve 61% 5-year overall survival in selected Childs A patients.[51] There is increasing evidence that image-guided ablation is the treatment method of choice for nodular disease of < 2–3 cm in diameter,[52] where the patient is not amenable to transplantation or whilst on the transplant waiting list. For larger disease of 4–6 cm in diameter ablation is being combined with pre- or post-ablation chemoembolisation to good oncological effect.[45]

Colorectal Liver Metastases

Colorectal metastatic disease (MCRC) in the liver is a common problem and whilst current systemic chemotherapy is able to achieve a median survival of 14–26 months,[53] surgical resection in selected patients can achieve 50% 5-year survival.[54] There is increasing interest into whether ablation can replace surgery for isolated small volume metastases, extend the scope of surgery when combined with resection or act as an interventional oncological adjunct to systemic chemotherapy. Outcome data suggest that colorectal metastases are more difficult to ablate than HCC of similar size, with higher local recurrence rates. Most experienced practitioners confine ablation to disease of <25–30 mm in diameter. Data suggests that IGA can achieve median survival of 30–32 months in selected patients.[55,56]

Lung Tumour Ablation

Surgical resection is the preferred treatment for patient with early non-small cell lung carcinomas but is often precluded due to the poor lung function or medical co-morbidities. Conventional external beam radiotherapy is usually offered where feasible but more recently there has been increasing interest in focal stereotactic radiation therapy, percutaneous ablation and combinations of the two procedures. A recent study analysed 64 patients who underwent RFA, CRA or sublobar resection.[57] The 3-year disease-specific survival and disease-free survivals were 87.5 and 50% for RFA, 90.2 and 45.6% for CRA and 90.6 and 60.8% for sublobar resection. A number of studies are increasingly testifying to equable 3-year cancer-specific survivals and there is increasingly studies on how ablation and focal radiotherapy might be best combined.

Small volume lung metastases often occur in older patients who have already undergone previous surgery and may suffer from other medical co-morbidities. Metastases suitable for ablation are usually < 3 per hemithorax, < 35 mm in diameter and located in well-aerated lung, usually at least 2–3 cm remote form the hilar structures. Studies to date have shown radiological confirmation of complete ablation in approximately 80% of colorectal metastases.[58]

Bone Tumour Ablation

Techniques such as RFA and CRA have been increasingly used for the curative treatment of small osteoid osteomas, osteoblastomas and chondroblastomas and in the palliative pain management of larger malignant tumours such as metastases from renal carcinoma. Cryoablation, in particular, is increasingly utilised in this application where visualisation of the therapeutic iceball clearly aids treatment dosimetry. Accruing evidence suggests that cryoablation may have an increasing role in the palliative management of painful metastases.[59]

SUMMARY

Radiological imaging is demonstrating and characterising malignant disease at an ever smaller size. The detection of small volume disease in an often elderly population where organ preservation becomes increasingly more important has stimulated interest in and development of image-guided in situ tumour ablation. Many ablative technologies including RFA, MWA, CRA, IRE and stereotactic radiotherapy are continuously evolving. These minimally invasive technologies and in situ treatments will require precise radiological guidance and diligent imaging follow-up if they are to adopt a central role in the management of small volume cancers.

For a full list of references, please see ExpertConsult.

FURTHER READING

13. Hatfield MK, Beres RA, Sane SS, Zaleski GX. Percutaneous imaging-guided solid organ core needle biopsy: coaxial versus non-coaxial method. Am J Roentgenol 2008;190(2):413–17.
25. Robertson EG, Baxter G. Tumour seeding following percutaneous needle biopsy: The real story! Clin Rad 2011;66:1007–14.
28. Simon CJ, Dupuy DE, Mayo-Smith WW. Microwave ablation: principles and applications. Radiographics 2005;25(Suppl. 1): S69–83.
40. Goldberg SN, Grassi CJ, Cardella JF, et al. Image-guided tumor ablation: standardization of terminology and reporting criteria. J Vasc Interv Radiol 2009;20(Suppl. 7):S377–90.
43. Purandare NC, Rangarajan V, Shah SA, et al. Therapeutic response to radiofrequency ablation of neoplastic lesions: FDG PET/CT findings. Radiographics 2011;31(1):201–13.
44. Goldberg SN. Science to practice: Which approaches to combination interventional oncologic therapy hold the greatest promise of obtaining maximal clinical benefit? Radiology 2011;261(3):667–9.
49. Atwell TD, Callstrom MR, Farrell MA, et al. Percutaneous renal cryoablation: local control at mean 26 months of follow-up. J Urol 2010;184(4):1291–5.
52. Lau WY, Lai EC. The current role of radiofrequency ablation in the management of hepatocellular carcinoma: a systematic review. Ann Surg 2009;249(1):20–5.
58. Lencioni R, Crocetti L, Cioni R, et al. Response to radiofrequency ablation of pulmonary tumours: a prospective, intention-to-treat, multicentre clinical trial (the RAPTURE study). Lancet Oncol 2008;9(7):621–8.
59. Callstrom MR, Atwell TD, Charboneau JW, et al. Painful metastases involving bone: percutaneous image-guided cryoablation—prospective trial interim analysis. Radiology 2006;241(2):572–80.

CHAPTER 88

Image-Guided Drainage Techniques

Michael M. Maher • Owen J. O'Connor

CHAPTER OUTLINE

Image-guided drainage is an established technique with a multitude of applications. The indications, techniques and management of image-guided catheter drainage, however, continue to evolve. This chapter provides an overview of the principles of image-guided drainage. We also discuss important technical aspects of specific drainage procedures, how to care for a drainage catheter and potential complications that can arise.

INDICATIONS AND CONTRAINDICATIONS

As a general rule, image-guided drainage is indicated for treatment of an accessible collection in a suitable patient that does not require immediate surgical intervention, to obtain a fluid sample for diagnostic purposes, to relieve symptoms or to inject a sclerosant.[1] Image-guided drainage alone is sometimes sufficient for treatment of a collection, but it can also act as an adjunct or temporising measure before definitive surgical treatment.[2] Drainage of a symptomatic collection such as an abscess is performed in order to drain pus from the cavity, working in conjunction with antibiotics. Infected collections accumulate antibiotics to a limited extent, which generally precludes effective treatment with antibiotics alone unless the collection is very small (1–3 cm).[3] Antibiotic coverage is necessary for many drainage procedures, even if the collection is not infected, to reduce the chance of secondarily infecting the collection. Examples of non-infected symptomatic collections that often require drainage include hydronephrosis caused by ureteric obstruction, bowel obstruction or postoperative seroma, urinoma and haematoma. Diagnostic fluid samples help determine whether a collection is infected and may also help identify the source of a collection. Fluid should be analysed by Gram stain; culture and sensitivity analysis should also be performed. Analysis of the cell count is also useful for quantifying the number of white cells in a sample. Amylase, bilirubin, lymphocytes and creatinine content can be used to identify collections of pancreatic, biliary, lymphatic and urinary origins, respectively.[4]

There are few absolute contraindications to image-guided drainage. Profound uncorrected coagulopathy, clinical instability and lack of safe access to a collection are among the most common contraindications to image-guided drainage. In practice, many coagulopathies can be corrected to allow drainage. The authors stratify procedure-related bleeding risk into three categories: low, medium and high. Paracentesis, catheter exchange and aspiration are considered low risk. Abdominal and chest procedures are considered medium risk, whereas primary biliary or renal drainages are stratified as high risk. The authors consider correction of abnormal indices for a low-risk procedure if the platelet count is less than 30,000/μL and the international normalised ratio (INR) exceeds 2.5, or for a medium-risk procedure if the platelet count is less than 30,000/μL and the INR exceeds 1.7 or the partial thromboplastin time is 1.5 times normal. Correction is performed prior to a high-risk procedure if the platelet count is less than 50,000/μL and the INR exceeds 1.7 or the partial thromboplastin time is 1.5 times normal. These guidelines need to be tailored to the collection and the patient, taking into account the fact that an untreated abscess has a very high mortality rate, and successful drainage reduces morbidity.[5,6] Encasement by bowel loops and large blood vessels preclude drainage catheter placement. A 19–22G needle can be used to traverse the small bowel for diagnostic sampling but risks infecting a fluid collection with enteric organisms. General anaesthetic or monitored anaesthesiology care is necessary for clinically unstable patients requiring image-guided drainage catheter placement. Lack of maturation of an abscess is a potential reason for close-interval observation before drainage. Peritonitis and a large volume of intraperitoneal air in the setting of a collection are indications for surgical rather than image-guided drainage. Air localised and contained within the vicinity of a collection, generally, does not preclude image-guided drainage, and is usually caused by local gastrointestinal perforation such as from appendicitis or diverticulitis. In cases where there is uncertainty, good communication between the interventional radiologist, referring physician and patient or family is indicated in order to reach consensus.

IMAGING GUIDANCE

Ultrasound and CT are primarily used for image-guided drainage. Modern ultrasound provides excellent real-time visualisation of superficial structures, and good visualisation of viscera or collections. This facilitates careful monitoring of a catheter or needle as it is guided into a collection, irrespective of the plane of angulation. This is preferred in paediatric patients for whom radiation exposure should be minimised and can also be performed at the bedside in an intensive care unit (Fig. 88-1). It is important to maintain the needle or catheter in the plane of imaging when using ultrasound. If possible, a needle-probe angle of 55°–60° should be maintained to optimise reflection of the ultrasound beam and needle or catheter visualisation.[7] The optimal grey-scale image map for ultrasound-guided procedures is different to that of diagnostic ultrasound, and should be sought. Additionally, frequency compound imaging is an ultrasonic imaging technology which can help with needle visualisation during drainage. Compound imaging emits ultrasound at multiple incident beam angles, which increases needle conspicuity because of increased artefact. Compound imaging reduces the pulse repetition frequency, however, which can cause image discontinuity. Ultrasound is often suboptimal for catheter guidance if a collection contains air or if there are bowel loops adjacent to a collection which prevent adequate imaging and increase the risk of bowel injury. Ultrasound guidance can be used in a hybrid manner for drainage purposes (Fig. 88-2). Combined with fluoroscopy, ultrasound can guide access and catheter placement into a large or partially visualised collection before optimal catheter manipulation and positioning by fluoroscopic guidance. Fluoroscopic guidance is also beneficial for guidance of catheters placed using the Seldinger technique and reduces the risk of losing access and kinking the guidewire (Fig. 88-2).

CT-guided fluoroscopy has many proponents since it offers potential real-time guidance and excellent spatial

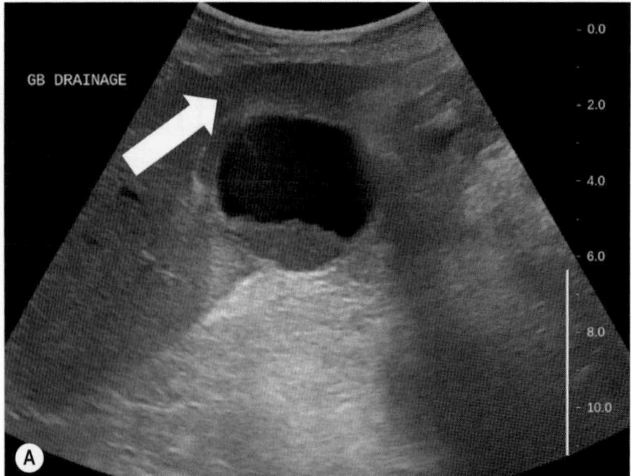

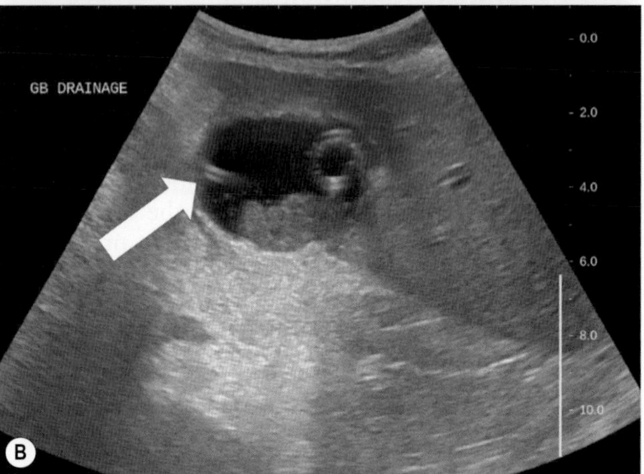

FIGURE 88-1 ■ Ultrasound-guided drainage of gallbladder for acute cholecystitis in an 85-year-old female in the intensive care unit. (A) Direct visualisation of catheter placement (arrow) through the liver into the gallbladder was provided with portable ultrasound. (B) The catheter (arrow) was released from the metal stiffener and the position confirmed before aspirating the contents of the gallbladder.

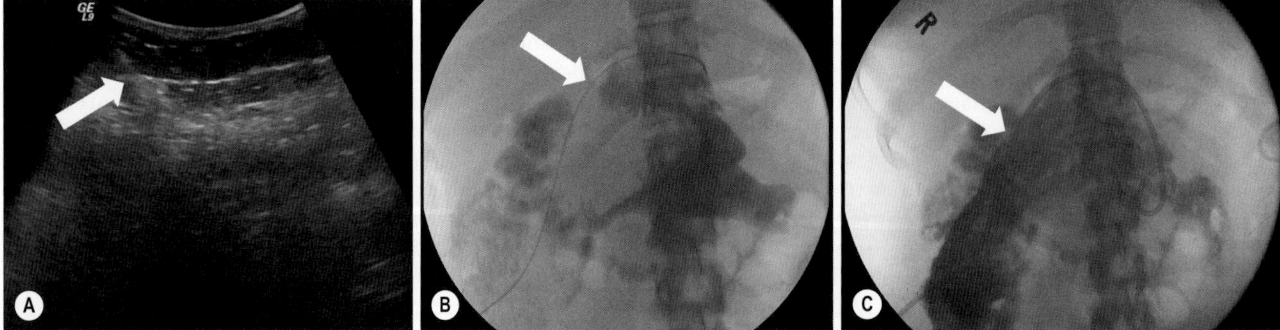

FIGURE 88-2 ■ Abdominal wall collection drainage following abdominoplasty in a 23-year-old female using ultrasound and fluoroscopy. (A) There was a large abdominal wall collection on CT. The collection was accessed through the midline with an 18G needle under ultrasound guidance (arrow). (B) A guidewire was directed into the collection using a Kumpe catheter (arrow) after contrast injection under fluoroscopic guidance confirmed position. (C) A multi-sidehole drainage catheter (arrow) was placed into the collection. The collection was successfully treated and no surgery was required.

resolution, which can reduce procedural time. One study has shown a 37% reduction in needle placement time but no significant reduction in room time using CT fluoroscopy for interventional radiology procedures.[8] CT fluoroscopy can be performed *real time* or by using a *quick-check* method. Real-time guidance involves holding the needle or catheter with a clamp and imaging as it is advanced. Quick-check CT guidance is used to image the needle tip after manipulation. Quick-check guidance considerably reduces fluoroscopic time and radiation dose compared with real-time guidance. Conventional CT guidance is favoured over ultrasound for drainage of deep collections with a difficult percutaneous access window.[9] Superior spatial resolution of CT over ultrasound often allows better localisation of the margins of a collection, the thickness of the wall, the adjacent organs and the access route. Tilting the angle of the CT gantry in a cranial or caudal direction is a useful adjunct, which can help image a safe direct route of access into a collection that is not available in the axial plane. This can create an additional level of difficulty for the interventional radiologist; the gantry laser guide is very useful for catheter direction in this circumstance. Room time, available resources, user preference and experience have a determining impact on the choice of image guidance.

PATIENT PREPARATION AND CARE

The authors recommend broad-spectrum antibiotics at least 1 h prior to abscess drainage. This does not preclude culture of material from an abscess since the rind of tissue that surrounds an abscess excludes most abscesses from the normal circulation.

Written informed consent is an important aspect of image-guided drainage. Optimal informed consent entails description of the indications for image-guided drainage, the alternatives, the procedure itself, potential complications and also the expected treatment plan after drainage. Since drainage catheters often remain in place for weeks, it is important that the patient be made aware of this so as to avoid unrealistic expectations. Effective teamwork and open communication between all those involved in the patient's care helps to reduce the risk of error and improves patient safety.[10,11] Normally, nursing sedation and continuous monitoring of vital signs is required for image-guided drainage. Patients should fast for 8 h prior to conscious sedation. The authors normally use fentanyl citrate (Elkins-Sinn, Cherry Hill, NJ, USA) and midazolam (Versed; Hoffmann-La Roche, Nutley, NJ), supplemented by antiemetics where appropriate. General anaesthesia is required for paediatric patients and severely ill or uncooperative patients. The authors advocate 4 h close observation after drainage to assess for complications.

CATHETER INSERTION

The following paragraphs provide an overview of techniques used for generic image-guided drainage. Drainage procedures which require special techniques or consideration will be discussed later in the chapter. Percutaneous aspiration is less likely to treat an abscess adequately compared with drain insertion. A collection which communicates with the bowel, biliary or urinary tracts should not be treated by aspiration. Occasionally, a small collection inaccessible to drain insertion, such as an interloop abscess in an immunosuppressed patient with Crohn's disease, may be treated by aspiration; otherwise, drain insertion is favoured.

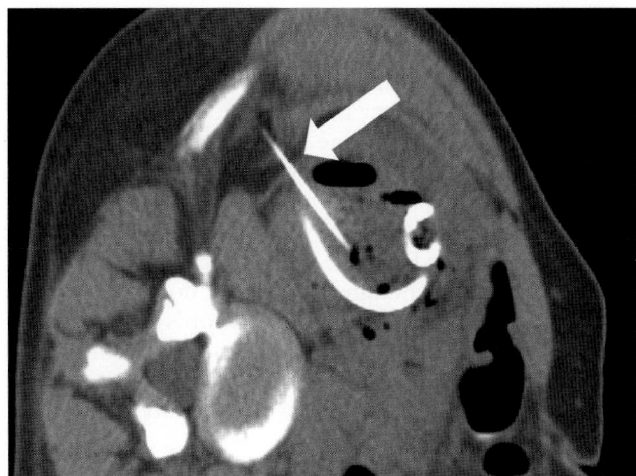

FIGURE 88-3 ■ CT-guided drainage of periappendiceal abscess using tandem-trochar technique in a 54-year-old female. A catheter was placed parallel to the guide needle (arrow) into the right lower quadrant collection with the patient in the left lateral decubitus position.

CT-guided catheter placement is generally performed by one of two methods: tandem-trochar or Seldinger. Tandem-trochar technique relies on the placement of a catheter containing a hollow stiffener and a diamond-pointed stylet, parallel to a guide needle into a collection (Fig. 88-3). Trochar catheters are available from 8 to 16Fr in size. The authors normally use a hydrophilic-coated Ultrathane catheter with a locking loop (Cook, Bloomington, IN, USA) for image-guided drainage. A CT examination, with a radio-opaque grid on the patient's skin enables a safe route for needle and catheter placement to be chosen. The distance from the skin surface to the abscess is measured and a 20G guide needle of appropriate length chosen. The portion of the needle outside the skin needs to be long enough to guide the trajectory of the catheter. Following cleansing and local anaesthetic administration, the needle is placed through the skin into the collection and a sample obtained for culture. This sample also allows assessment of the viscosity of the collection but the collection should not be aspirated further until the catheter is placed. A 10–12Fr catheter is usually necessary if the contents are frank pus; an 8–10Fr catheter may be adequate for less viscous fluid. The distance from the skin to the contents of the collection should be marked on the catheter. Following a skin incision and tissue separation adjacent to the guide needle, the catheter is introduced parallel to the guide needle, to the level of the mark on the catheter. The catheter may then be advanced over the stiffener or the stiffener withdrawn and the retention pigtail formed.

Once adequate catheter position is confirmed, the contents of the collection are evacuated, the catheter is secured to the skin with an adhesive device and a drainage bag is attached. Catheter irrigation at the time of abscess drainage using normal saline can increase drainage yield, disrupt adhesions and improve healing time. However, the volume of normal saline injected must not exceed that of the fluid drained from the collection to prevent cavity distension and reduce the risk of bacteraemia. The tandem-trochar technique is fast and does not require serial dilatation, the metal stiffener affords good catheter directionality. It should be noted that some collections have tough fibrous walls which can deflect the catheter and a malpositioned catheter will generally need to be withdrawn and replaced.

The Seldinger technique allows more controlled catheter placement, especially if there is high risk of catheter transgression of the posterior wall of a collection (Fig. 88-4) and can facilitate better drainage of large multiloculated collections by placement of a multi-sidehole catheter. A 19G ultrathin needle containing a stylet or a sheathed needle is initially placed into the collection. An 0.035-inch guidewire is advanced through the needle or sheath and, once adequate positioning is confirmed, the tract is serially dilated. The Seldinger technique is time consuming and tract dilatation can be painful, especially when traversing muscles. Dilatation also carries increased risk of content spillage during dilator exchange and before catheter placement. Manipulation of a dilator over the wire in a confined space also carries a risk of buckling the guidewire, which can hinder catheter placement.

Ultrasound-guided catheter insertion is performed under direct guidance following skin preparation (Fig. 88-1). A guide needle is not necessary unless one wishes to sample contents of the collection to assess consistency before choosing the catheter size.

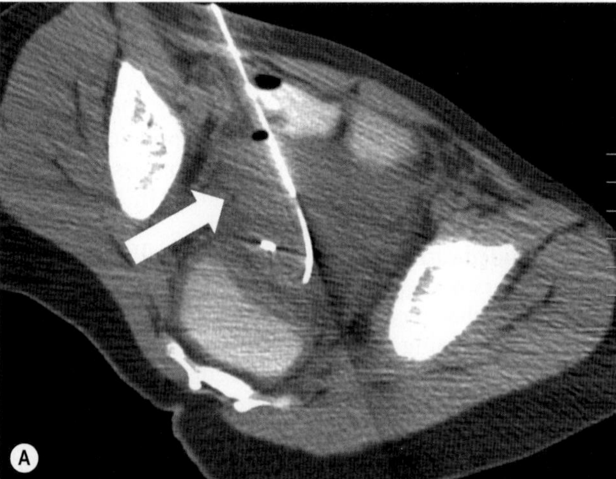

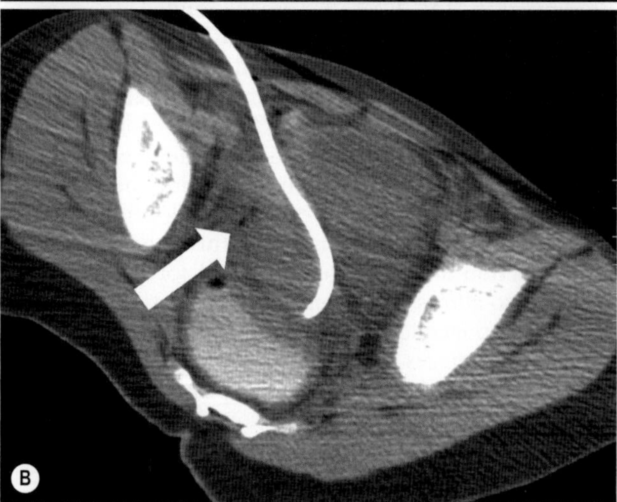

FIGURE 88-4 ■ CT-guided drainage of periappendiceal abscess using Seldinger technique in a 9-year-old girl. (A) An 18G needle was used to access the collection (arrow) and a guidewire placed. (B) A 12Fr drainage catheter (arrow) was placed over the guidewire.

CATHETER MANAGEMENT

Drainage catheters should be flushed with normal saline every 8–12 h to maintain catheter patency and optimise drainage. A flush volume of 5 cc towards the patient and 5 cc towards the drainage bag via a three-way stopcock is normally sufficient unless a collection is very small or very large. Daily catheter outputs should be monitored and the contents of the drainage bag noted. This may alert one to evolving issues such as fistulisation or bleeding. In addition, difficulty flushing the catheter, pain on flushing and catheter withdrawal can signal blockage or displacement. Contrast injection into the catheter under fluoroscopic guidance is generally indicated in these circumstances. Catheter removal is considered in a well patient when daily outputs are low, normally on the order of 10 cc or less per day. Before catheter removal it is normally necessary to confirm complete drainage of the collection by CT or ultrasound imaging and confirm that the cavity has collapsed around the catheter and that there is no fistula present by fluoroscopic-guided injection. Catheter removal at this stage should be followed by complete collapse of the cavity. Optimal drainage and complication avoidance are best achieved by active participation of the interventional radiologist in patient rounds.[12]

SPECIFIC DRAINAGE TECHNIQUES

Many image-guided drainages require technical modifications and special consideration. In this section we will discuss pertinent aspects of image-guided drainage procedures of the chest, liver, biliary system, pancreas, gallbladder, urinary tract, gastrointestinal tract, spleen, subphrenic region, peritoneum and deep pelvic territory, and organ traversal for drainage.

Chest

There are many indications for image-guided drainage in the chest, including pleural disease, lung parenchymal, pericardial and mediastinal collections. Pleural collections represent a common clinical problem for which image-guided drainage is recommended to reduce complications encountered as a result of blind drainage.[13]

Many types of pleural collections exist, and although diagnostic imaging is helpful, aspiration and drainage are often required for treatment and diagnosis. Pleural collections include effusions, haemothorax, empyema and pneumothorax. The success of image-guided drainage depends to a large extent on the contents of a pleural collection. It is, therefore, important for treatment decisions, to characterise the collection at the time of drainage, using biochemical, cytological and microbiological means. Effusions may be transudative or exudative. Light's criteria are 98% sensitive and 80% specific for an exudative effusion if the ratio of pleural fluid protein to serum protein is greater than 0.5, if the ratio of pleural fluid lactate dehydrogenase (LDH) to serum LDH is greater than 0.6 or if the pleural fluid LDH is greater than ⅔ that of the normal upper limit for serum LDH.[14]

The natural history of an exudative pleural effusion is to evolve from free-flowing fluid to fibrinopurulent material, and later develop an organised fibrous pleural peel. Drainage of an exudative pleural collection should be performed early to prevent progression. Similarly, an infected pleural fluid collection should be drained as early as feasible in order to remove infection, sterilise the cavity, obliterate the pleural space and promote lung re-expansion, which improves drainage of secretions and return of pleural elasticity. Approximately 20% of patients with pneumonia develop an effusion. Since Light's criteria are only reasonably specific for an exudative effusion, confirmation that the effusion is not a transudate is required in cases where there is discrepancy between the clinical and biochemical data. Fluid pH can be useful in these circumstances. The pH of an effusion is a strong predictor of the need for chest tube placement. Based on data from a meta-analysis, a pH less than 7.2 is an indication for chest tube placement.[15]

Image-guided pleural drainage catheters are smaller than surgical drains, measuring up to 16Fr in size, which means they are often better tolerated by patients. A smaller catheter is acceptable for treatment of free-flowing fluid but a large catheter is necessary for a complicated collection. Haemothorax caused by trauma is better treated using surgical drains (36–38Fr), although drainage of small blood-containing postoperative pleural collections may be attempted under imaging guidance. Ultrasound guidance is adequate for uncomplicated collections, but CT is usually needed for drainage of multiloculated pleural collections (Fig. 88-5). It is recommended that, where possible, the dependent portion of the collection be accessed, just above the adjacent rib, away from the paraspinal region where the neurovascular bundle lies lower in the intercostal space, and care should be taken to avoid insertion close to the scapula.[16] The authors favour suturing chest tubes to the skin in order to avoid displacement. Coughing is common as the lung re-expands. For transudative effusions thoracentesis is often preferred over chest tube placement. Aspiration is stopped and the catheter withdrawn when 1.5 L of fluid is aspirated or the patient cannot tolerate further drainage. Imaging is always performed after pleural drainage to assess response and to check for pulmonary oedema and presence of pneumothorax. Daily chest radiographs

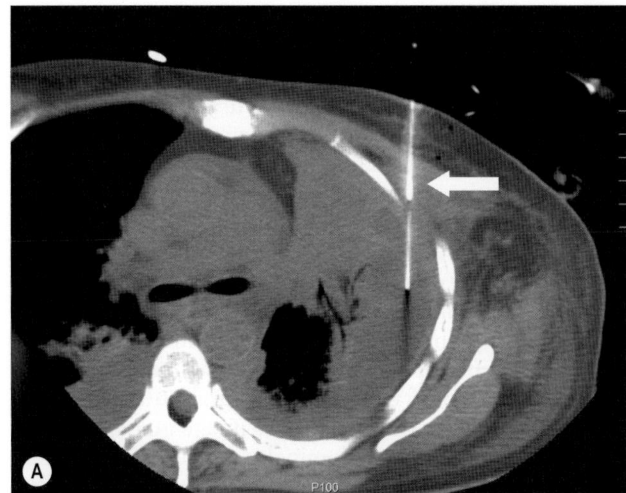

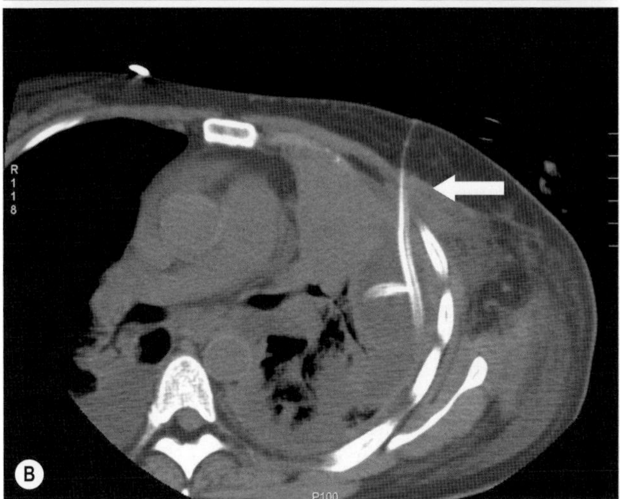

FIGURE 88-5 ■ CT-guided chest drain insertion for empyema in a 49-year-old male using tandem-trochar technique. (A) Guide needle (arrow) was placed through an anterior approach into a left chest collection. (B) Chest tube (arrow) placed parallel to guide needle.

are required and interval CT is indicated for assessment of pleural collections treated with a chest tube. It is also important to be aware of a *vacuthorax* phenomenon after pleural drainage so as to avoid unnecessary patient anxiety and harm.[17] This manifests as a pneumothorax with or without fluid on imaging following pleural drainage. Patient's generally have no symptoms from the pneumothorax and usually have an underlying diagnosis of chest malignancy. It is thought that inadequate surfactant causes non-compliance of the lung or the presence of restrictive pleural disease precipitates an asymptomatic hydropneumothorax in this setting, for which chest tube insertion is seldom required. Chest tubes inserted for parapneumonic and complicated effusions often do not drain large quantities of fluid immediately: 20 cm H_2O suction is normally sufficient and a closed underwater seal system is required.

Chest tube removal is considered when there is clinical improvement, improved imaging appearances and absence of bubbling in the one-way valve system (suggests bronchopleural fistula), and outputs have dropped below 1–1.5 cc/kg body weight per day. A chest tube placed for pneumothorax can be removed 24 h after the pneumothorax has resolved. Modified drain management is often necessary as part of pleural collection treatment. For example, air leakage from a drain should prompt search for faulty connections or exposed catheter side-holes; otherwise, a bronchopleural fistula should be suspected. The degree of suction may be carefully reduced to deter further leakage.

A partially treated pleural collection can be further treated by several means. Catheter repositioning and/or exchange for a larger catheter under fluoroscopic guidance may be helpful if the catheter is suboptimally positioned or if an appropriately positioned catheter is not functioning. A partially drained pleural effusion treated with a patent chest tube, placed by image guidance, or an inadequately draining abdominal collection, may benefit by instillation of a fibrinolytic agent, such as tissue plasminogen activator (tPA). The need for this additional measure can often be anticipated on pre-procedure imaging, by the absence of free layering or conformation, loculations, or constrictions, within a fluid collection. Four to six milligrams of tPA mixed in 25–50 cc of normal saline is a suggested dose. After tPA instillation, the patient rotates into prone, supine, right and left lateral positions, each for 15 min at a time, for 1 h, after which time the catheter is unclamped. This process is repeated twice per day for 3 days in order to complete a treatment cycle. A complete treatment cycle can adequately treat a complicated collection in 86% of cases and a repeat cycle for residual fluid is effective in 87% of patients, usually obviating the need for surgery.[18] Therapeutic anticoagulation is a relative contraindication to tPA administration. Haemorrhage has been observed in 33% (4 of 12) of patients treated with tPA receiving therapeutic anticoagulation. Prophylactic anticoagulation is not a contraindication to tPA.

Once adequate treatment of a pleural collection has been achieved, it is sometimes necessary to intervene to obliterate the pleural space, particularly in patients with recurrent pleural effusions. Pleurodesis is utilised to prevent recurrence of effusion or pneumothorax by generating pleural inflammation and fibrosis through instillation of a chemical agent which causes the pleural space to be obliterated. Bleomycin is generally suitable for this purpose. The patient rotates as above for 1 h after instillation and then 20 cm H_2O suction is applied. Mediastinal collections most often occur in the postoperative setting after lung, oesophageal, cardiac and upper abdominal surgery, or after trauma such as severe emesis. Treatment of these collections has traditionally been performed surgically. Recent data indicate that image-guided drainage is feasible and effective. One series reports 100% technical success and 96% clinical success, with avoidance of surgery.[19] Adequate patient positioning and optimum catheter trajectory are key to avoiding complications in this setting. Persistent or worsening lung abscess is another indication for image-guided drainage. Lung abscesses most often occur in the setting of aspiration or immunocompromise, and most respond to antibiotics alone.[20] Occasionally, pericardial effusions require image-guided drainage. Drainage of a pericardial effusion in the absence of tamponade is a topic of debate. Although technically feasible on almost all occasions, the incidence of cardiac arrhythmias is 26% following drainage, and so catheters should be removed as soon as possible.[21]

Hepatic Parenchyma

Hepatic abscesses generally occur when the liver is unable to sufficiently clear organisms filtered from the portal vein or the biliary tract. It is has been observed that isolated hepatic abscesses are more often of cryptogenic origin due to *Klebsiella pneumoniae*, but that multiple infected collections are usually caused by *Escherichia coli* originating from the biliary tract.[22] More than one hepatic abscess is present in approximately 46–71% of cases.[4] Potential sources of hepatic abscess include trauma, surgery, cancer, bacteraemia and super infection of a pre-existing collection such as a cyst, tumour or haematoma. Catheter-directed drainage is favoured for pyogenic collections, but for an amoebic collection only if it has failed medical management, it is greater than 6–8 cm in diameter or rupture is anticipated. Catheter drainage of an infected tumour should only be performed following careful discussion with the referring physician, surgeon and patient. A catheter placed into an infected tumour in a non-surgical candidate will likely remain permanently. CT or ultrasound guidance is generally adequate for hepatic abscess drainage. Ideally, some normal hepatic parenchyma should be traversed prior to entering the collection (Fig. 88-6). Interval CT to assess response, and interval contrast injection to assess for biliary communication, are normally recommended prior to attempting catheter removal. If possible, pleural transgression should be avoided, but, if traversed, careful observation for the accumulation of pleural fluid is necessary.

Biliary System

Image-guided biliary drainage is technically challenging. As endoscopic techniques have considerably reduced the requirement for percutaneous transhepatic cholangiography and drainage, most such procedures are complicated and are performed for patients who have failed endoscopic treatment or have altered anatomy, often due to surgery. The current indications for biliary drainage include obstructive jaundice, cholangitis, evaluation and treatment of a biliary-enteric anastomosis, access for treatment of stone disease and evaluation of suspected bile duct injury. Any available imaging must be reviewed before the procedure. It is preferable to place the patient supine on the procedure table with the right arm resting above the head and the skin over the right and left lobes of liver should be prepared in a sterile manner. If the patient is haemodynamically stable and does not require general anaesthesia, conscious sedation should be given time to work before traversing the skin, and subsequently titrated to the patient's level of discomfort. Antibiotic prophylaxis should be used, as patients with biliary obstruction are at risk of septicaemia.

Although many technical variations exist, the one- and two-stick techniques are most commonly favoured for biliary drainage. The one-stick system employs a small needle (e.g. 22G Chiba needle), microwire and dilator system to gain access to the biliary tree. Care is required to avoid kinking 0.0018-inch microwires, especially when placing the dilator; this should be directly observed using fluoroscopy. The two-stick system begins with biliary access and opacification using a small needle, followed by separate biliary access with a larger needle and conventional wire (Fig. 88-7). The lower edge of the right lobe of liver is normally accessed in the mid-axillary line and the needle directed towards the opposite shoulder under fluoroscopic guidance, in order to avoid crossing the pleura. The stylet is removed and contrast material gently injected as the needle is incrementally withdrawn. Bile duct access is indicated by observation of the so-called *dripping wax* appearance, due to contrast dissipating into bile ducts.[23] Once bile duct opacification is achieved, the location of the initial access should be studied. A second puncture, with a sheathed needle, should be made if the initial needle placement is not optimal. Biliary access on the right is preferentially through an inferior duct with a straight course to the hepatic hilum, which may better facilitate future catheter, stent or balloon placement. A fluoroscopic C arm is invaluable for the assessment of the ductal anatomy for these purposes. The proximity of the left lobe bile ducts to the anterior abdominal wall is conducive to ultrasound-guided needle placement and subsequent injection under fluoroscopic guidance. Once access has been gained, obstructions, if present, must be crossed and a catheter advanced to the duodenum. This is best achieved with a combination of an angled catheter and conventional or hydrophilic guidewires. After small bowel access is obtained, an internal–external 8 Fr biliary drain is placed across the obstruction over an Amplatz guidewire. When the patient's condition has improved, biliary stent placement may be considered for treatment of a malignant stricture or serial dilatation followed by trial of catheter clamping and subsequent removal may be considered for benign disease.

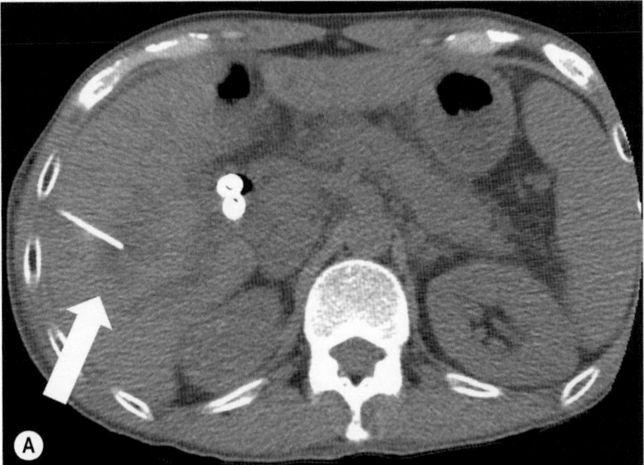

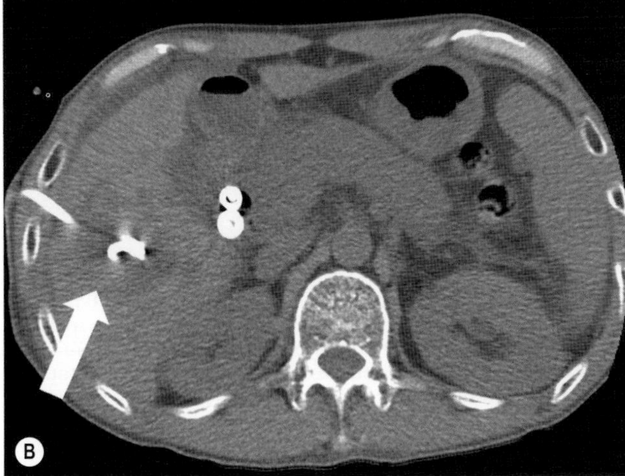

FIGURE 88-6 ■ Drainage of liver abscess in a 48-year-old male with pancreatic cancer and biliary stents. (A) A 20G needle has been placed in the collection (arrow). (B) A drainage catheter has been placed in the collection using the tandem-trochar technique (arrow).

Pancreas and Peripancreatic Region

Management of collections in the region of the pancreas can be challenging. Even the terminology used to describe pathology is this region is a topic which receives much attention. The authors recommend using the revised Atlanta criteria in order to optimise communication with referring physicians and possibly better standardise treatment.[24] Access to the region of the head of pancreas is often obtained using an anterior approach

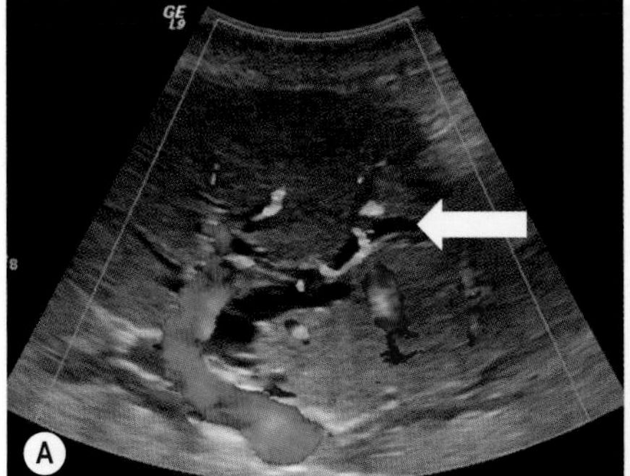

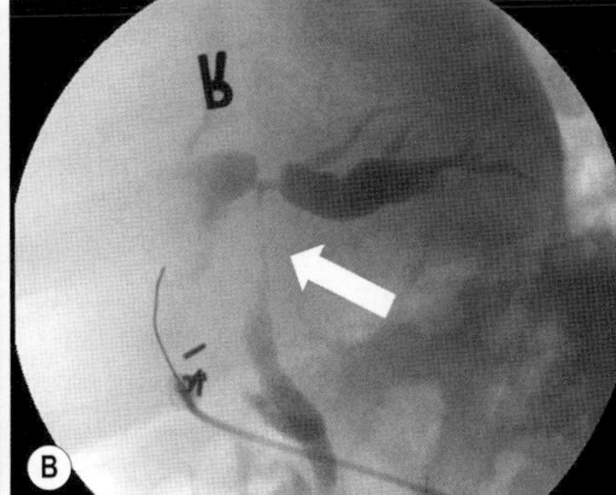

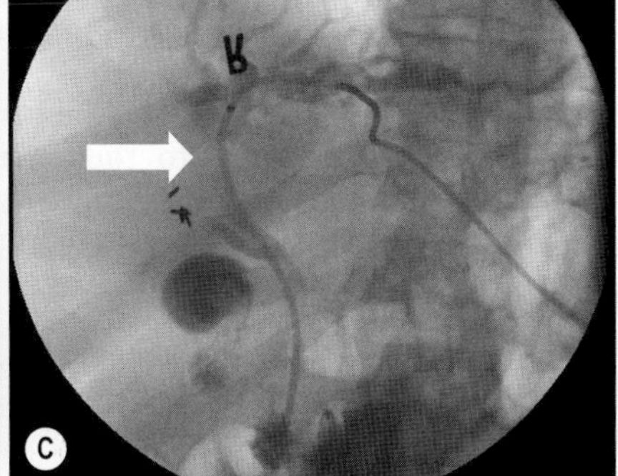

FIGURE 88-7 ■ Biliary drainage in a 63-year-old male with cholangiocarcinoma using two-stick technique. (A) Ultrasound used to confirm biliary dilatation (arrow) and guide bile duct access with a 22G Chiba needle. (B) Contrast medium was injected under fluoroscopic guidance to confirm access and demonstrate stenosis of the common hepatic duct, right and left main hepatic ducts (arrow). (C) Left-sided biliary access was obtained, the stenosis was traversed and an internal–external biliary drain was placed (arrow).

through the gastrocolic ligament. Access to the region of the tail of the pancreas is generally through the anterior pararenal space. The liver and stomach are sometimes transgressed in order to access the pancreas but the small and large bowel should not be crossed. Collections secondary to acute pancreatitis may or may not be liquefied. Differentiation can be difficult and may require CT and/or MRI imaging, as well as image-guided sampling. Interstitial oedematous pancreatitis is initially associated with acute pancreatic fluid collections and later with pseudocyst formation. Drainage of a pseudocyst may be indicated in the presence of infection, intractable symptoms such as pain, or obstruction of the gastrointestinal tract or biliary system. Acute pancreatic necrosis can be associated with a sterile acute necrotic collection in or around the pancreas, which can later become infected. Abscess formation is suggested by the presence of gas in a collection or the presence of a thick enhancing wall. Image-guided drainage of an infected acute necrotic collection is often a bridge to surgery, which is best performed after the acute phase of pancreatitis because of the high morbidity of surgery during the first 4 weeks after the onset of pancreatitis (Fig. 88-8). The merits of image-guided drainage for non-infected acute necrotic collections are debatable. The contents of acute necrotic collections are viscous. This necessitates use of large (22–24Fr) or multiple catheters, combined with irrigation, which in effect constitutes percutaneous necrosectomy. Catheter removal may take months because of disconnection of the pancreatic duct in the setting of necrosis.[25] Catheter injection under fluoroscopic guidance is important for the assessment of communication with the pancreatic duct. If ductal communication is noted, endoscopic pancreatic duct stent placement should be attempted, and if leakage persists, transcatheter embolisation may be considered.[26]

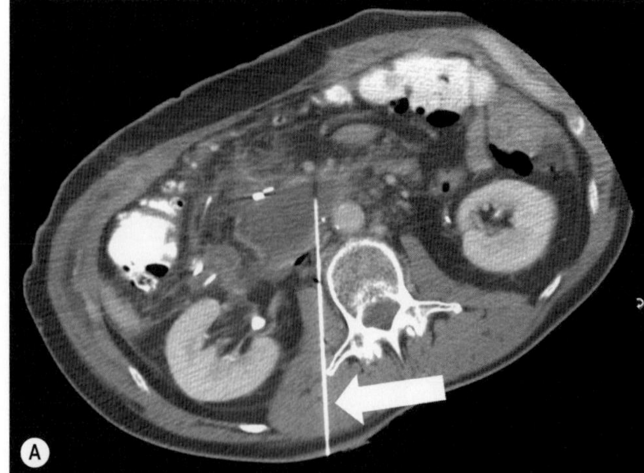

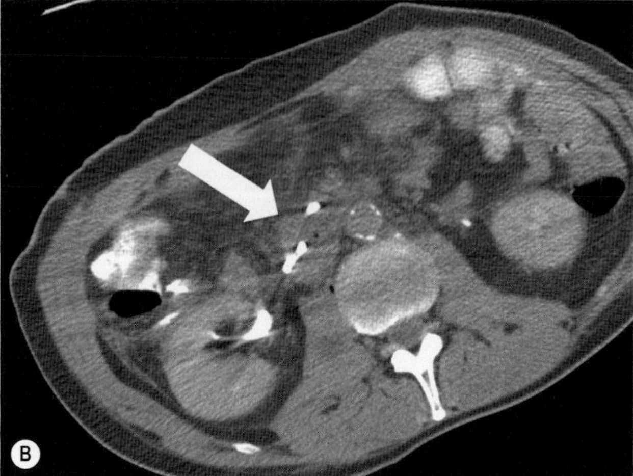

FIGURE 88-8 ■ Drainage of infected collection in a 41-year-old male with acute pancreatic necrosis. (A) Needle aspiration (arrow) through a posterior approach with the patient positioned prone confirmed the presence of pus. (B) Catheter was placed using tandem-trochar and the collection decompressed (arrow).

Gallbladder

Percutaneous cholecystostomy is used for patients with acute cholecystitis who are poor surgical candidates. It may also be employed to access the biliary tree for decompression or biliary intervention (Fig. 88-1).[27] Percutaneous cholecystostomy has a 2% mortality rate, which is much lower than the mortality of surgical cholecystectomy in very ill patients.[28] Patient selection greatly affects the results. Intensive care unit patients that require cholecystostomy catheters frequently fall into two categories: those that respond to cholecystostomy catheter and those that succumb to their underlying disease. Patients who present to the emergency department with acute cholecystitis may be very ill, but have a better likelihood of treatment response.[29] The authors favour traversing hepatic parenchyma prior to entering the gallbladder where possible to help ensure secure catheter placement and reduce the risk of peritoneal contamination. Catheters placed for calculous cholecystitis generally remain in place until surgery. Catheters placed for acalculous cholecystitis are removed after 6 weeks provided the patent is well, there are no gallstones, the cystic duct is patent and there is an established tract from the gallbladder to the skin. Recurrence rates following catheter removal are 35 and 7% for acute calculous and acalculous cholecystitis, respectively.[30,31]

Urinary Tract

Percutaneous nephrostomy is performed for urinary tract diversion, access for stone treatment or stent placement (Fig. 88-9). There are several procedure-specific points to be considered.[32] Pre-procedure antibiotics are indicated when there is infection, stones or urinary diversion, in order to help minimise procedure-related sepsis. Brodel's bloodless line of incision is a suitable posterolateral plane through which to access the collecting system. The renal parenchyma in this territory is relatively avascular since it lies at a watershed region at the junction of the anterior two-thirds and posterior third of the kidney. The central component of a lower pole posterior calyx viewed in-plane is a suitable target since this posterolateral oblique approach is orientated along the avascular plane at 20°–30° to the vertical. The procedure is usually guided using fluoroscopy or ultrasound. Direct puncture

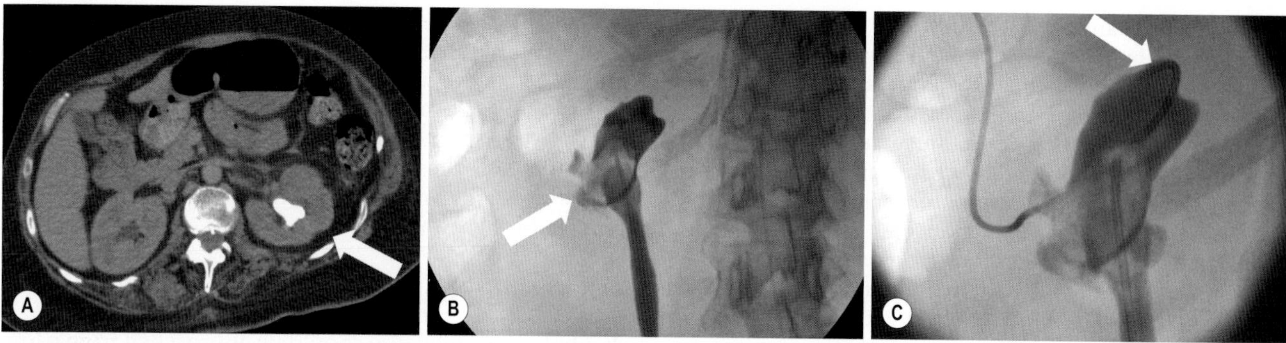

FIGURE 88-9 ■ Nephrostomy for nephrolithotripsy in a 49-year-old male. (A) CT demonstrates large left renal stone (arrow). (B) Left renal collecting system opacified using a retrograde ureteric catheter and stone is seen (arrow). (C) A lower pole calyx is traversed to access the renal collecting system and a Kumpe catheter (arrow) used to subsequently direct a guidewire into the ureter for purchase before catheter placement.

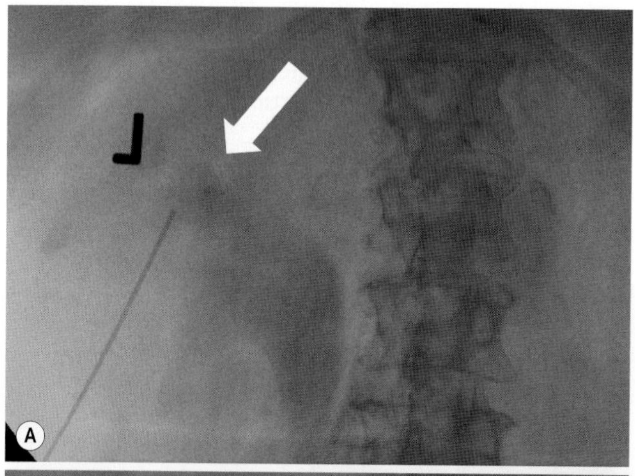

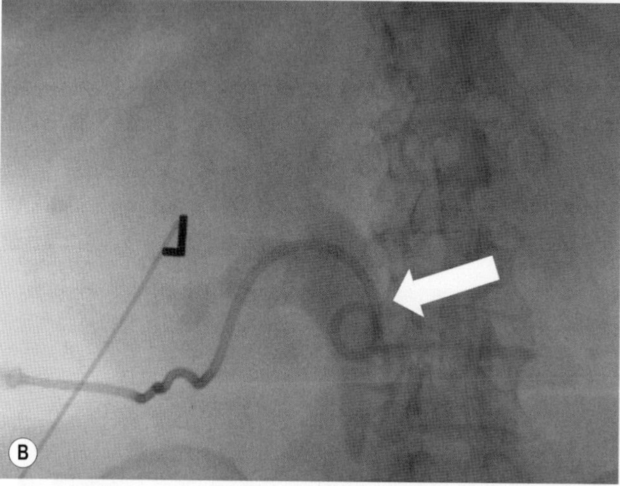

FIGURE 88-10 ■ Percutaneous nephrostomy using two-stick technique in a 77-year-old female with left renal obstruction due to ureteric stone. (A) An upper pole calyx (arrow) was accessed with a 22G Chiba needle, a small amount of urine withdrawn and a small volume of contrast injected to opacify the collecting system. (B) A lower pole calyx was traversed to place a percutaneous nephrostomy catheter (arrow).

of the collecting system under fluoroscopic guidance can be performed at the level of L1/L2, lateral to the transverse process after review of pre-procedure imaging for the location of the kidneys, colon and pleura by noting the position of the twelfth rib (Fig. 88-10). Aspiration is performed as a 22G needle is withdrawn. Once urine is aspirated, contrast material is injected to opacify the system. The first sample of urine aspirated should be sent for microbiological analysis. It is important to avoid overdistension of the collecting system, in order to reduce the risk of bacteraemia. Carbon dioxide can be used to demonstrate the posterior collecting system calyces in a prone patient. An appropriate posterior calyx may then be accessed using a thin-walled 19G needle or a sheathed 18G needle that will accept an 0.035-inch guidewire. If a ureteric stent is to be inserted, a middle or upper pole calyx should be considered, or a calyx that facilitates future intervention for stone disease if this is the indication for access. Secure wire placement in the collecting system or ureter is important prior to tract dilatation. An 8Fr catheter is normally sufficient and flushing with 10 cc normal saline every 8 h during the early post-procedure period is recommended. Colon transgression should be treated by upper and lower diversion of urine, appropriate antibiotics, withdrawal of the catheter from the kidney into the colon and subsequent removal once a colonocutaneous tract has formed. Normally, blood products clear from urine within 48 h of nephrostomy. Delayed or intermittent haemorrhage, especially after catheter manipulation or exchange can indicate pseudoaneurysm formation. This is sometimes only seen at angiography with the nephrostomy removed. It is best for this to be performed over a guidewire, which is left in place in order to allow catheter replacement for temporary tamponade before definitive treatment. The authors recommend routine nephrostomy exchange approximately every 3 months in patients who require long-term drainage.

Spleen

The American College of Radiology criteria suggest that drainage of an accessible splenic abscess with a rim of surrounding normal tissue is usually feasible.[20] Splenic collections generally occur due to haematogenous spread of infection secondary to endocarditis, sickle cell disease, immunodeficiency or trauma. Safety is a major concern in relation to splenic interventions. Good randomised data are lacking, but anecdotal experience suggests that splenic intervention is generally safe. A recent meta-analysis of splenic biopsy demonstrated sensitivity and specificity of 87 and 96%, respectively.[33] The major complication rate from core needle biopsy with an 18G needle or smaller was 2.2%, which is comparable with liver and renal biopsy. Surgical treatment of an uncharacterised lesion generally entails splenectomy with consequent risk of sepsis from encapsulated organisms and accelerated atherosclerosis.[34] Splenic aspiration or drainage can preserve the spleen and has a high success rate.[35] Peripheral, upper and mid-pole lesions are more easily treated than lower-pole lesions and ideally some normal splenic tissue should be traversed before entering a collection. One of seven patients treated with splenic catheter drainage by Lucey et al. required splenectomy as a result of post-procedural haemorrhage.[35] The remaining six patients, however, were spared splenectomy. Because of the risk of haemorrhage, patients should be admitted overnight following catheter placement. The authors favour the trochar technique, as this avoids dilatation of the tract (which is necessary with the Seldinger technique) and potential peritoneal or pleural contamination (Fig. 88-11). This is particularly important when treating hydatid disease, as contamination increases the risk of seeding. The absence of leakage can be confirmed by contrast injection and ablation of the inner lining of the cyst can be performed by instillation of alcohol. Fifty per cent of the aspirated fluid volume is replaced with 95% ethyl alcohol, the catheter is clamped for 20 min, and then the alcohol is aspirated.[36] This procedure may be repeated if necessary.

Subphrenic Collections

A subphrenic collection should be approached from a low anterior route where possible to avoid transgressing the pleura, which reduces the risk of pleural infection. The authors favour the Seldinger technique when draining subphrenic collections. Ultrasound guidance allows access into the collection and guidewire manipulation is performed under CT or fluoroscopic guidance. Sometimes the pleura must be crossed to drain a collection (Fig. 88-12). In this circumstance, follow-up chest radiographs and early chest tube insertion for new or enlarging

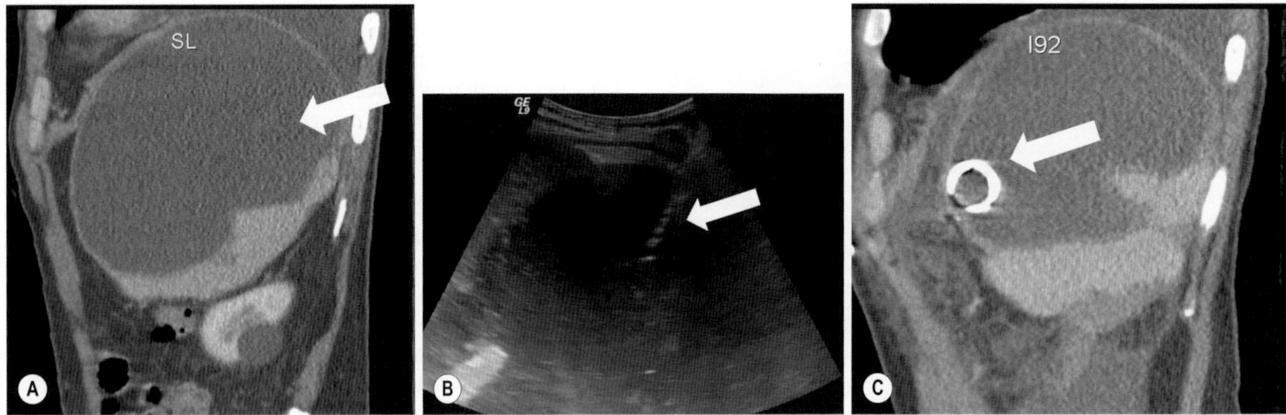

FIGURE 88-11 ■ Ultrasound-guided drainage of symptomatic splenic cyst in a 46-year-old male. (A) Large splenic cystic lesion on CT (arrow). (B) An 8Fr drain inserted (arrow) under ultrasound guidance. (C) Confirmation of drain positioning and degree of decompression after drain insertion (arrow).

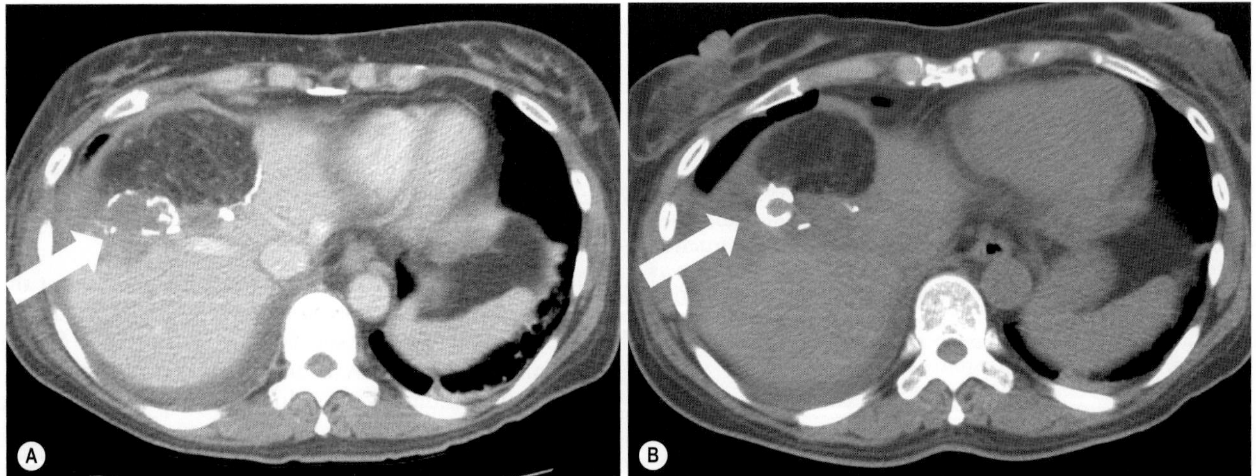

FIGURE 88-12 ■ Drainage of subphrenic abscess in a 62-year-old female following partial right hepatectomy. (A) There is a small collection in the region of the surgical material (arrow). (B) A catheter was placed by tandem-trochar technique into the collection through an anterior approach.

pleural effusions are recommended in order to avoid empyema. Right- and left-sided subphrenic collections should be sampled for bilirubin and amylase, respectively, in order to plan for further management such as biliary or pancreatic drainage.

Gastrointestinal Drainage

Gastrostomy/gastrojejunostomy (G/GJ) catheters are most commonly used to administer enteral feeding to patients with chronic malnutrition or an inability to eat or swallow, usually secondary to neurological impairment or head and neck pathology.[37] G/GJ catheters are also inserted for gastric decompression and palliation in terminal patients, allowing nasogastric tube removal.[38] Radiologic or endoscopic gastrostomy placement is favoured over surgery as these techniques are associated with higher success rates, reduced sedation requirements, fewer complications and less cost.[39] Percutaneous G/GJ requires development of a well-formed tissue tract to avoid leaks after insertion. This is usually accomplished by gastropexy, forming an adhesion of the anterior gastric wall to the anterior abdominal wall. The authors place G/GJ catheters with the patient supine using fluoroscopic or computed tomography (CT) guidance (Fig. 88-13). The stomach is inflated with air using an existing nasogastric tube or by placing a 5Fr Kumpe catheter (Cook, Bloomingdale, IN, USA) under fluoroscopic guidance through the nose into the stomach. The location of the lower left lobe liver edge is identified with ultrasound and marked on the patient's skin and the colon is identified by fluoroscopy using an on-table air or Gastrografin enema. If there is a safe fluoroscopic window to the stomach, the anterior gastric wall is fixed to the anterior abdominal wall using up to four gastropexy sutures. G/GJ catheters are placed in the stomach between the gastropexy sutures over a wire placed through an 18G hollow needle. The use of gastropexy sutures has expanded the range of patients in whom G/GJ can be attempted and, as a result, patients that would have previously been considered unsuitable, such as those with voluminous ascites, may be treated.[40]

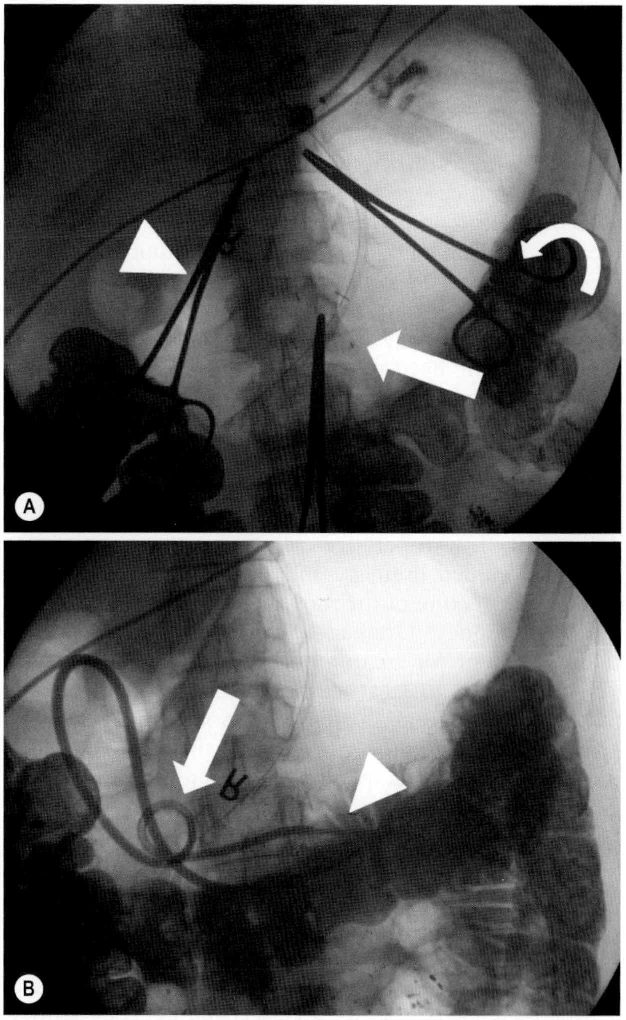

FIGURE 88-13 ■ Gastrojejuenostomy tube insertion in a 68-year-old male. (A) The stomach is inflated with air using a nasogastric tube. The colon contains barium administered the night before the procedure. Metal clamps have been placed to depict the left costal margin (curved arrow) and liver margin (arrowhead). There is a safe window to the stomach (arrow) and four 25G needles demarcate where gastropexy sutures will be placed. (B) Confirmation of tip within the small bowel (arrowhead) and locking loop in the stomach (arrow).

Peritoneum

Paracentesis is one of the most common image-guided procedures. Placement of a 7–8Fr catheter following normal preparation and local anaesthesia is generally sufficient. Portal hypertension and cirrhosis are common causes of voluminous ascites. These pathologies are associated with reduced plasma oncotic pressure. Induction of splanchnic vasodilation and an effective reduction of the circulating blood volume induces retention of water and sodium by the renin–angiotensin system and by antidiuretic hormone. Excess hepatic lymph exudes into the abdominal cavity to create ascites. Ascitic fluid should be tested for albumin content and for infection at least at the time of the first drainage. The serum albumin gradient (SAAG) is used to determine the cause of ascites. The serum-ascites albumin count on the day of paracentesis is subtracted from the ascitic albumin concentration. An SAAG greater or equal to 1.1 g/dL indicates that ascites is due to portal hypertension with 97% accuracy.[41] Causes of a SAAG of less than 1.1 g/dL include carcinomatosis, nephrotic syndrome, pancreatitis and tuberculous peritonitis. The detection of a carcinoembryonic antigen (CEA) level greater than 5 ng/mL or an alkaline phosphatase level of 240 IU/L is suggestive of perforated bowel.[42] Administration of albumin is performed in selected patients with ascites who experience circulatory disturbance following large-volume paracentesis. The authors administer up to four 12.5 g bottles of 25% albumin in the peri-procedural period for these patients. For patients with intractable malignant ascites that requires frequent paracentesis despite medical therapy, implanted peritoneal catheters offer a safe and effective palliative measure.[43]

Infected peritoneal collections are a common indication for image-guided drainage. These include perforated appendicitis, Crohn's enteritis of colitis, diverticulitis and anastomotic leakage. Drainage in the setting of perforated viscous is reasonable in the absence of free perforation or signs of peritonism. Drainage is sometimes a temporising measure before surgery. However, percutaneous catheter drainage alone is deemed sufficient by the American College of Radiology Appropriateness guidelines for periappendiceal collections (Fig. 88-3). In patients with Crohn's disease, percutaneous abscess drainage is technically successful in 96% of cases. Drainage reduces the need for surgery by 50% within 60 days of presentation and reduces the overall need for surgery by 23%.[44] Approximately 16% of patients with Crohn's disease develop metachronous collections following drainage. Postoperative collections are more successfully treated by catheter drainage than primary collections. Treatment of postoperative collections of various causes by image-guided drainage and antibiotics often suffices and represents one of the most successful applications of these techniques. Drainage catheter placement is also often sufficient for treating an anastomotic leak, which can be difficult to treat surgically due to postoperative tissue inflammation and adhesions. Sometimes upstream diversion is necessary to promote healing. Previous administration of therapeutic radiation to the perianastomotic region, such as the presacral territory for rectal cancer treatment, is associated with fibrous stiff tissues, which are often slow to collapse, and require long-term drainage before catheter removal (Fig. 88-14).

Deep Pelvic Collections

Bowel, bladder, bone, blood vessels and nerves confined in a limited space constitute a recipe for challenging drainage in the deep pelvis. A pre-procedure CT should be carefully reviewed prior to draining a deep pelvic collection. Modern intracavitary ultrasound probes provide high-resolution imaging through the rectum and vagina. Catheter placement through the vagina and rectum is often free-hand over a trochar although an improvised guide can be created using a peel-away introducer sheath. Either way, the catheter needs to be imaged throughout insertion. Care should be taken to apply gentle pressure on the probe during imaging in order to avoid compressing bowel or bladder, which can lead to inadvertent traversal. Transrectal drainage is favoured over transvaginal drainage where possible. Patients generally need to be placed in the decubitus position for intracavitary ultrasound probe insertion and image-guided drainage. Prone positioning is favoured for transgluteal drainage of deep pelvic collections, which are often performed using CT guidance. Optimal transgluteal drain insertion is at the level of the sacrospinous ligament inferior to the piriformis muscle and close to the sacrum in order to reduce pain and risk of blood vessel and nerve injury (Fig. 88-14). A CT drainage window to a high pelvic collection not accessible in an axial plane may be facilitated by tilting the CT gantry.

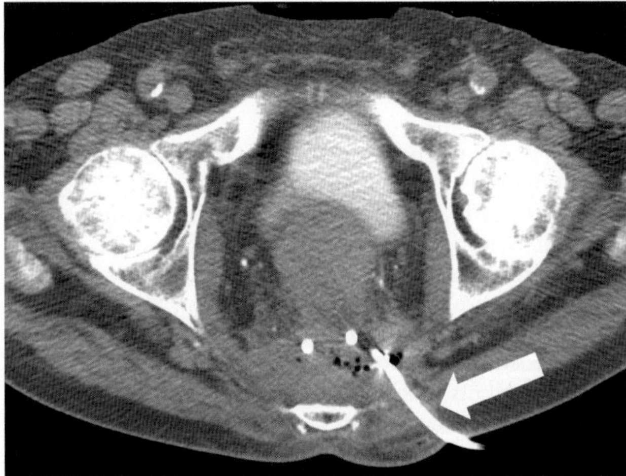

FIGURE 88-14 ■ CT-guided drainage of presacral collection in an 89-year-old male following abdominoperioneal resection of rectal cancer. Transgluteal catheter placement close to the sacrum (arrow) was performed using tandem-trochar technique under CT guidance.

Organ Traversal

A collection deep to an organ should be approached with caution. Many organs should not be traversed in order to access a collection during image-guided drainage. These include blood vessels, the spleen, the gallbladder, the pancreas, the oesophagus, the large and small bowel, the bladder, the uterus and the ovaries (Fig. 88-15). Traversal of some organs during drain insertion may be necessary, especially in an ill patient with limited surgical options. Provided the coagulation profile is acceptable, it is feasible and often safe to traverse a minimal portion of liver, avoiding the hilar vessels and the gallbladder, in order to drain a collection. Care must be taken to ensure that all catheter sideholes are within the collection in order to avoid leakage back along the catheter into the liver. The stomach is frequently traversed in order to access retroperitoneal collections, especially those of pancreatic origin. Transrectal and transvaginal approaches are feasible for drainage of a deep pelvic collection under ultrasound guidance, although catheters in these locations have a notorious propensity to fall out.

Paediatric Patients

Image-guided drainage is performed in children for collections related to acute appendicitis, inflammatory bowel disease or in the postoperative setting (Fig. 88-3). Good paediatric care requires a different approach to that of an adult. Monitoring and resuscitation equipment are tailored to age, heat loss must be minimised and sedation requirements should be undertaken by an anaesthesiologist. Ultrasound imaging should be used where possible for guidance. CT parameters should be optimised to reduce dose by shielding the gonads, minimising the range and imaging time, reducing the kilovoltage and milliamperage, using automatic tube modulation and adaptive statistical iterative reconstruction. Once planning images are obtained, greater image noise is often acceptable for catheter check images. Post-procedure

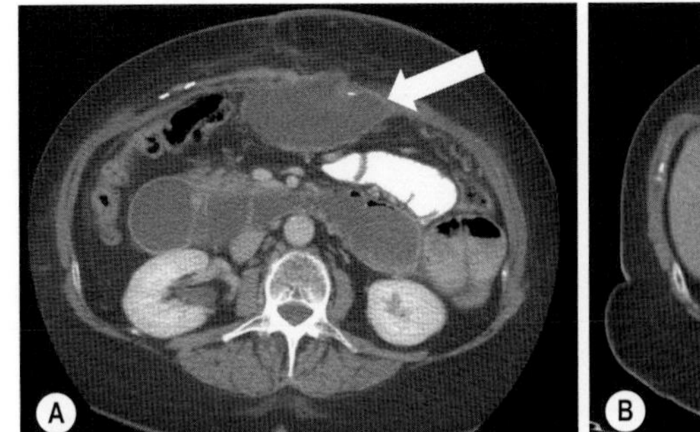

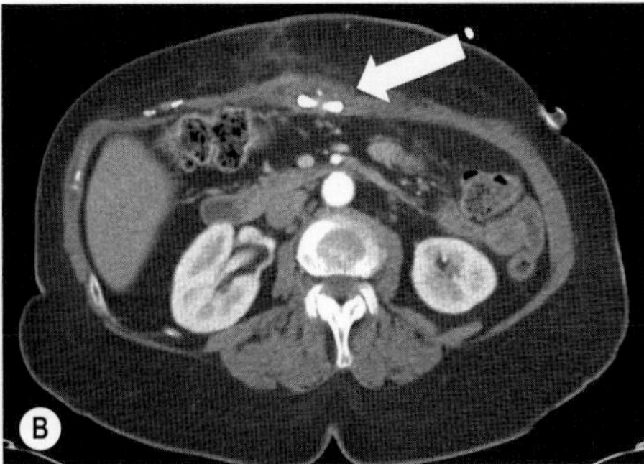

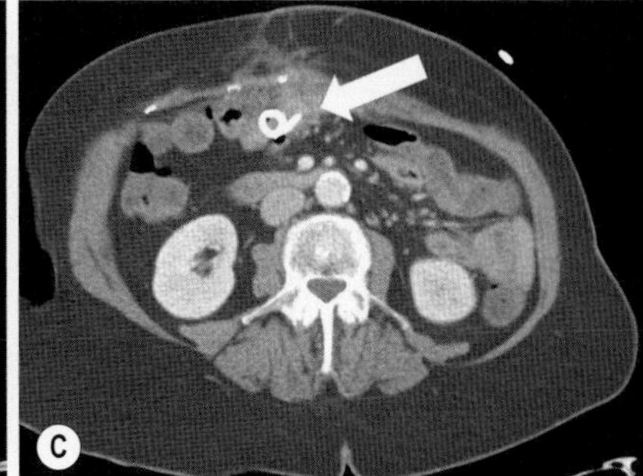

FIGURE 88-15 ■ Drainage of peritoneal collection with subsequent displacement of drainage catheter into the colon in a 76-year-old female after midline laparotomy. (A) Intra-abdominal collection present (arrow). (B) Drain placed into the collection with good decompression (arrow). (C) Interval CT demonstrated migration of the tip of the drainage catheter into the transverse colon (arrow). The catheter was withdrawn into the collection and left in place until the fistula closed.

imaging with CT should be performed sparingly and avoided altogether if possible, by relying more on clinical response, catheter outputs and ultrasound for decision making. Image-guided drainage is a safe and effective technique for treatment of appendicitis complicated by abscess formation.[45] Complications are reduced and interval appendectomy is often obviated if a perforated appendiceal abscess is treated successfully with catheter-directed drainage.

Complications

Many potential complications can occur after image-guided drainage. Some discomfort or scar formation at the site of insertion may be unavoidable. Involvement of the interventional radiologist in patient rounds is important for patient care, early detection of complications, exchange of information with referring physicians and continued learning. Although every effort is made to minimise the length of treatment, every patient is different, and catheter removal can sometimes take a long time.

There are many reasons why a collection may respond slowly to treatment, leading to prolonged drainage. Clear communication throughout the treatment process is vital to avoid misconceptions. It is important to stress from the outset what can be realistically expected. The presence of loculations, the development of a fistula and the presence of tumour can hamper catheter removal. Loculations can often be effectively treated by increasing the size of the drain or by repositioning it, or by tPA instillation as described earlier. Fistula development often results in long-term catheter placement. Diversion of upstream fluids (bile, urine, pancreatic juices, bowel content) by surgical or endoscopic means if necessary should be considered. Image-guided drainage of an infected tumour should be approached with extreme caution and should involve multidisciplinary discussion. Catheters placed into an infected tumour can rarely be removed, and often remain for life, or until surgical removal of the tumour.

Complications are uncommon following image-guided drainage of thoracic fluid collections; the National Patient Safety Agency in the United Kingdom reported 12 fatalities, and 15 instances of serious harm, caused by chest drain insertion.[46] Intraparenchymal chest tube placement, intercostal artery injury, iatrogenic infection and pneumothorax formation have been observed (Fig. 88-16). Transarterial embolisation for arterial injury, prophylactic antibiotics in some situations and aspiration of thoracentesis-related pneumothorax may be necessary (Fig. 88-17).[47] Catheter dislodgement is a frequent occurrence. It is important to adequately secure drainage catheters and educate patients regarding the risk of pulling on the catheter. The decision to reinsert a drainage catheter depends on the reason for insertion, the adequacy of treatment and need for further drainage. Long-term catheters such as a nephrostomy catheter, with an established tract, can generally be rescued within 24 h of catheter dislodgement. An established tract is formed approximately 2 to 4 weeks after catheter placement.

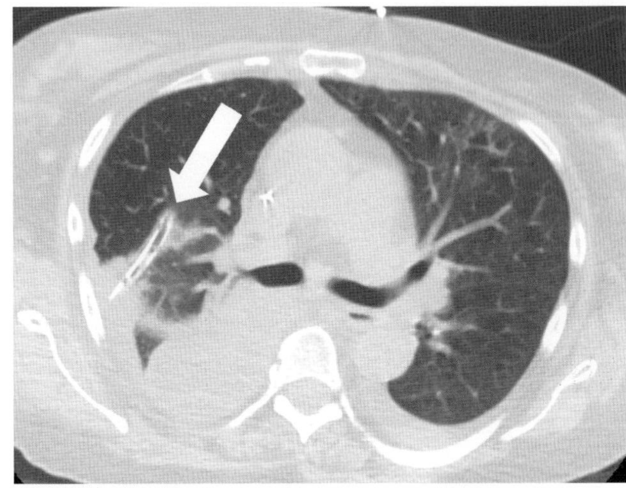

FIGURE 88-16 ■ Intraparenchymal chest tube placement in a 54-year-old female. CT demonstrates right-sided chest tube (arrow) with blood on both sides of the catheter. A new chest drain was placed and the catheter removed without further complication.

Bleeding is not uncommon after catheter placement. Bleeding from the skin site of catheter insertion may be due to the presence of altered blood in a postoperative

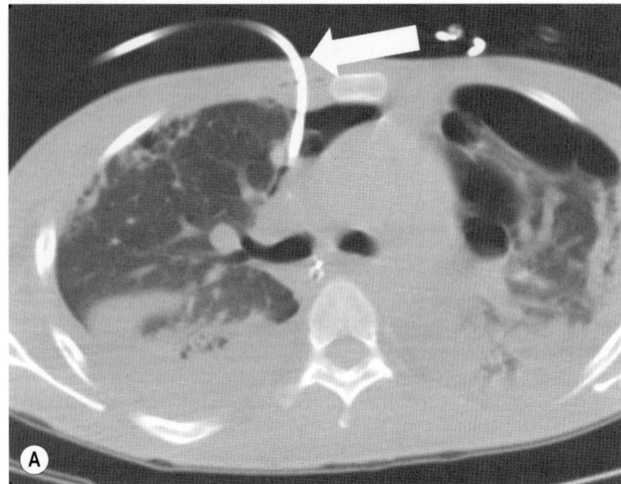

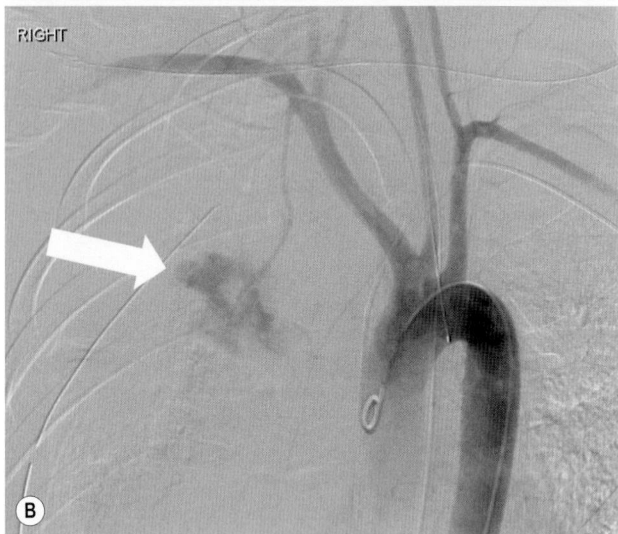

FIGURE 88-17 ■ Bleed from intercostal artery following chest tube insertion in a 23-year-old male with chronic lung disease due to a mitochondrial disorder. (A) Chest tube (arrow) was placed into the right anterior chest adjacent to the sternum for treatment of pneumothorax. (B) The patient developed haemodynamic shock after removal of the chest tube. This was due to haemorrhage from the right internal mammary artery (arrow) and was successfully treated by coil placement.

collection and is often self-limiting. However, occasionally, it can be a sign of significant injury such as pseudoaneurysm formation (Fig. 88-18). In cases of concern, it is advisable to remove a catheter over a wire, so that the catheter can be replaced to tamponade significant bleeding as a temporary measure before definitive treatment by surgery or embolization.

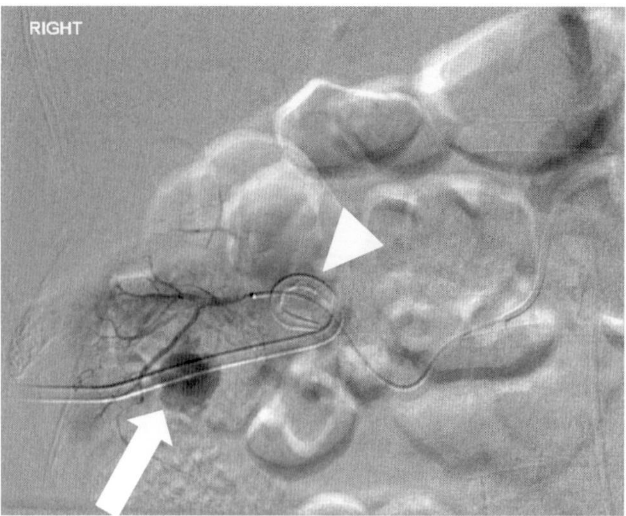

FIGURE 88-18 ■ Pseudoaneurysm in an 82-year-old male due to right percutaneous nephrostomy placement. Renal angiogram demonstrates pseudoaneurysm (arrow) over the nephrostomy catheter (arrowhead). The pseudoaneurysm was treated by coil embolisation.

CONCLUSION

Image-guided drainage can significantly contribute in a positive manner to patient management. Image-guided procedures continue to be widely used and to evolve. The principles of good image-guided drainage apply to many clinical situations. Careful patient preparation and catheter management are vital to safe practice.

For a full list of references, please see ExpertConsult.

FURTHER READING

6. Solomkin JS, Mazuski J. Intra-abdominal sepsis: newer interventional and antimicrobial therapies. Infect Dis Clin North Am 2009;23(3):593–608.
7. Bradley MJ. An in-vitro study to understand successful free-hand ultrasound guided intervention. Clin Radiol 2001;56(6):495–8.
8. Carlson SK, Bender CE, Classic KL, et al. Benefits and safety of CT fluoroscopy in interventional radiologic procedures. Radiology 2001;219(2):515–20.
9. Maher MM, Gervais DA, Kalra MK, et al. The inaccessible or undrainable abscess: how to drain it. Radiographics 2004;24(3): 717–35.
10. Miguel K, Hirsch JA, Sheridan RM. Team training: a safer future for neurointerventional practice. J Neurointerv Surg 2011;3(3): 285–7.
11. Leonard MW, Frankel A. The path to safe and reliable healthcare. Patient Educ Couns 2010;80(3):288–92.
12. Goldberg MA, Mueller PR, Saini S, et al. Importance of daily rounds by the radiologist after interventional procedures of the abdomen and chest. Radiology 1991;180(3):767–70.

CHAPTER 89

Hepatobiliary Intervention

Aoife N. Keeling • Bhaskar Ganai • Michael J. Lee

CHAPTER OUTLINE

INTRODUCTION

Biliary intervention is not as prevalent as it was 20 years ago because of the advent of endoscopic retrograde cholangiopancreatography (ERCP). Skilled endoscopists can treat the vast majority of patients with biliary obstruction with stents, stone removal and/or sphincterotomy. In addition, the days of perfoming a diagnostic percutaneous transhepatic cholangiogram (PTC) are virtually over with the advent of magnetic resonance cholangiopancreatography (MRCP). PTC is now almost always performed before a therapeutic biliary drainage. Percutaneous biliary drainage remains an important technique for managing patients with biliary obstruction where ERCP fails or is not possible. Interventional radiology (IR) also plays a significant role in treating patients with benign biliary strictures and, particularly, patients with anastomotic strictures after hepatico-jejunostomy.

Careful patient preparation is essential before any biliary procedure to avoid potentially serious complications. All patients with obstructive jaundice should be commenced on intravenous fluids during and after biliary drainage. Patients with obstructive jaundice have usually fasted for a myriad of other tests before reaching IR and are often significantly dehydrated. Any significant choleresis after biliary drainage can place patients with long-standing obstructive jaundice and high serum bilirubin levels at risk of developing hepatorenal syndrome. Coagulation screening and a serum creatinine check should be performed before all biliary drainage procedures. Correction of any bleeding diathesis should be performed before any drainage. In addition, all patients should receive broad-spectrum antibiotic coverage within one hour of the drainage procedure, or indeed any further biliary procedure, including tube change or cholangiography, to protect against biliary sepsis. The authors prefer monotherapy with piperacillin/tazobactam which has broad Gram-negative and -positive coverage and achieves high concentrations in bile. Patient preparation also includes reviewing all imaging studies, including computed tomography (CT), ultrasound (US) and magnetic resonance (MR) cholangiography, so that a full picture of the biliary procedure can be discussed with the patient during the consent process.

MANAGEMENT OF BILIARY OBSTRUCTION

Background

Biliary obstruction can arise from both benign and malignant causes. Malignant causes are more common and include obstruction from pancreatic carcinoma, cholangiocarcinoma and metastatic disease. Ultrasound is the imaging modality of choice for determining the presence or absence of dilated bile ducts. Further investigation with CT or MRI/MRCP is used to determine the cause and level of biliary obstruction, and in cases of malignancy, for staging and assessment of surgical resectability. Most malignant tumours causing biliary obstruction are not surgically resectable at the time of diagnosis and these patients have a limited life expectancy. Malignancy should be confirmed with biopsy if possible. Cross-sectional imaging will also determine the level of biliary obstruction and any atrophy/compensatory hypertrophy in a liver lobe, which can impact the proposed biliary draiange.

Mid to lower biliary obstruction is now increasingly treated endoscopically in the first instance; lesions at the liver hilum are challenging to treat at ERCP and are best dealt with by percutaneous biliary drainage.

The goal of treatment is to relieve jaundice, treat or prevent sepsis and improve symptoms of pruritus.[1]

Percutaneous Transhepatic Cholangiography

Percutaneous transhepatic cholangiography is the first step in a range of biliary interventional procedures. This is usually performed under conscious sedation or general anaesthesia. Hilar lesions may cause atrophy or compensatory hypertrophy of a liver lobe which affects the decision on whether drainage of that lobe is indicated. MRCP is important in establishing the level of the hilar obstruction and the extent of involvement of the intrahepatic ducts. For example, if the anterior and posterior sectoral ducts on the right are both involved, it may be best to drain the left lobe only (if the size of the left lobe is sufficient to provide palliation of jaundice). Puncture of the ducts in the right lobe access can be performed under either fluoroscopic or ultrasound guidance, whilst left lobe punctures are usually performed under US guidance.

A coaxial introducer system employing a 21G Chiba needle and 0.018-inch guidewire which enables upsizing to a 0.035-inch guidewire reduces the risk of haemorrhage. If fluoroscopic guidance is used on the right side, the point of entry is the mid axillary line just above the tenth rib. A peripheral duct should be selected and, after aspiration of bile, a diagnostic cholangiogram is performed with iodinated contrast material. After cholangiography, the guidewire is passed into the central ducts to maintain access for further interventions.

Biliary Drainage: External, Internal–External

In most cases an external drain (tube is left above the level of obstruction) is a temporary measure and an internal–external biliary drain from the duodenum through the biliary system to the skin surface is preferred. In patients with biliary sepsis, the goal of treatment is rapid decompression and drainage with minimal catheter manipulation and contrast material injection. In cases where a stricture cannot be crossed in the first sitting an external drainage catheter can be placed. The stricture can be negotiated during a subsequent session.

An internal–external drainage catheter will have side holes both above and below the stricture and pass into the duodenum. It can be used after biliary stenting to preserve access to the biliary tree for a few days (a safety catheter) if the procedure has been difficult or there is blood in the biliary system limiting bile drainage and is usually followed by placement of a stent in patients with malignant obstruction.

Biliary Stenting: Metal, Plastic

Two main types of biliary stents are available: plastic or metallic. Plastic stents (e.g. Cotton-Leung stents; Cook Medical, Bloomington, IN) offer lower patency rates due to encrustation of bile and often require a larger tract through the liver (10–12Fr), causing increased patient discomfort during insertion. They have the advantage that they are easily removed at endoscopy/surgery and can therefore be used preoperatively in patients who require drainage (e.g. for sepsis) before surgical resections.

Metallic stents offer better patency rates than their plastic counterparts.[2] These stents are inserted in a contracted state but when released, expand to a predefined diameter. This enables their placement though a smaller-calibre percutaneous tract (6–8Fr). Metallic stents elicit a marked fibrotic reaction; for this reason they should be avoided preoperatively and in benign disease. The larger-diameter lumen reduces the rate of occlusion from bile encrustation. Metallic stents occlude from either tumour growth through the interstices of the stent or, more frequently in hilar tumours, overgrowth at the ends of the stent. In lower common bile duct (CBD) strictures, stenting through the sphincter of Oddi may help provide better drainage with the theoretical risk of increased infection due to reflux of enteric contents.

Covered stents have been developed for the biliary system. These metallic stent grafts have a fabric covering which aims to prevent tumour ingrowth, but have the drawbacks of increased migration and coverage of side branches leading to cholecystitis or pancreatitis with cystic duct and pancreatic duct occlusions, respectively. Despite these drawbacks, early data are promising in both malignant[3] and benign[4] disease.

When stenting, the goal of treatment is to try and drain the largest volume of tumour-free liver. Careful review of pre-procedure imaging is mandatory to allow planning of the PTC approach for stent placement and the superior extent of obstruction. In a hilar obstruction, if both hepatic lobes require drainage then either a 'T' stenting configuration from a single percutaneous access site or a 'Y' configuration from bilateral access sites may be employed (Fig. 89-1). When the stent(s) have been placed, balloon dilatation can be performed to bring the stents up to nominal diameter (usually 8 mm in hepatic ducts, 10 mm in CBD), usually after administration of a further dose of analgesia as the dilatation can be very painful (Fig. 89-2).

Benign Disease

Benign strictures are often the result of iatrogenic ductal injury during laparoscopic cholecystectomy. Further causes include post-hepatic transplantation ischaemia, biliary atresia, choledochal cysts and sclerosing cholangitis.

Transhepatic drainage can be performed in benign strictures or stones to:

1. Drain an obstructed infected system not amenable to endoscopic drainage
2. Dilate benign strictures, often iatrogenic secondary to laparoscopic cholecystectomy, biliary-enteric anastamotic strictures (including post-hepatic transplant) or sclerosing cholangitis.
3. Treat intrahepatic or ductal calculi.

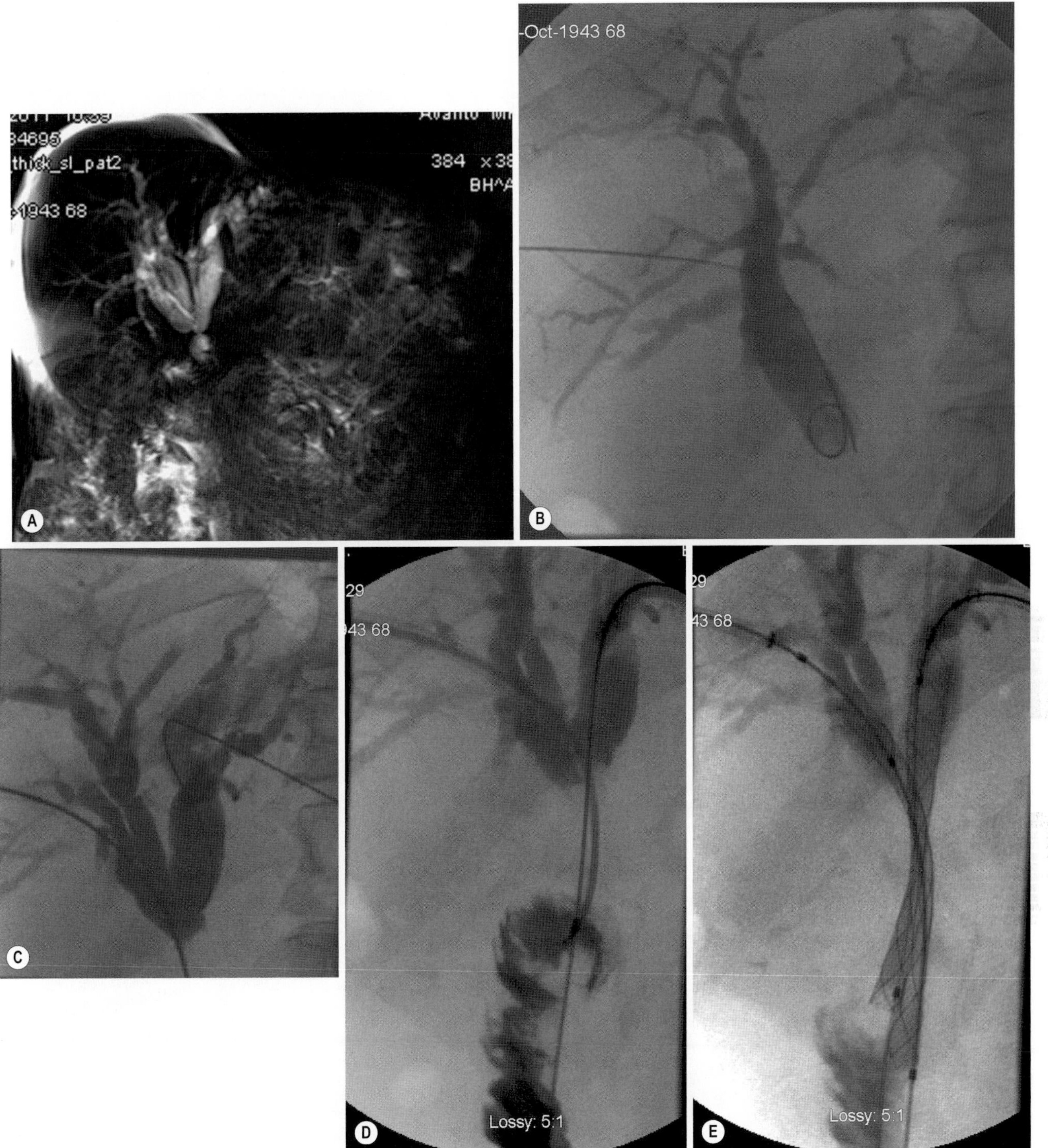

FIGURE 89-1 ■ A 68-year-old female with a background of a prior Whipple's resection for a pancreatic head cancer re-presented with jaundice and weight loss. MRCP demonstrated a tight stricture at the biliary-enteric anastomosis with a corresponding soft-tissue mass in keeping with local recurrence (A). A PTC was performed via the right side (B). The left side was then punctured (C) and the proximal tight stricture at the biliary-enteric anastomosis was elicited (D). It was elected to place metallic biliary stents from both the right and left sides in a Y configuration as the stricture was so high. Ten-millimetre metallic self-expanding stents were deployed simultaneously across the stricture (E).

Benign Strictures

PTC is performed as described above and a balloon dilatation is performed with an 8- to 10-mm balloon. Following balloon dilatation, at least 2 weeks of biliary drainage with the catheter crossing the stricture is required.

In cases of biliary-enteric anastomoses, the ERCP approach is less likely to be successful due to the formation of a Roux loop or Billroth II gastric anastomosis.

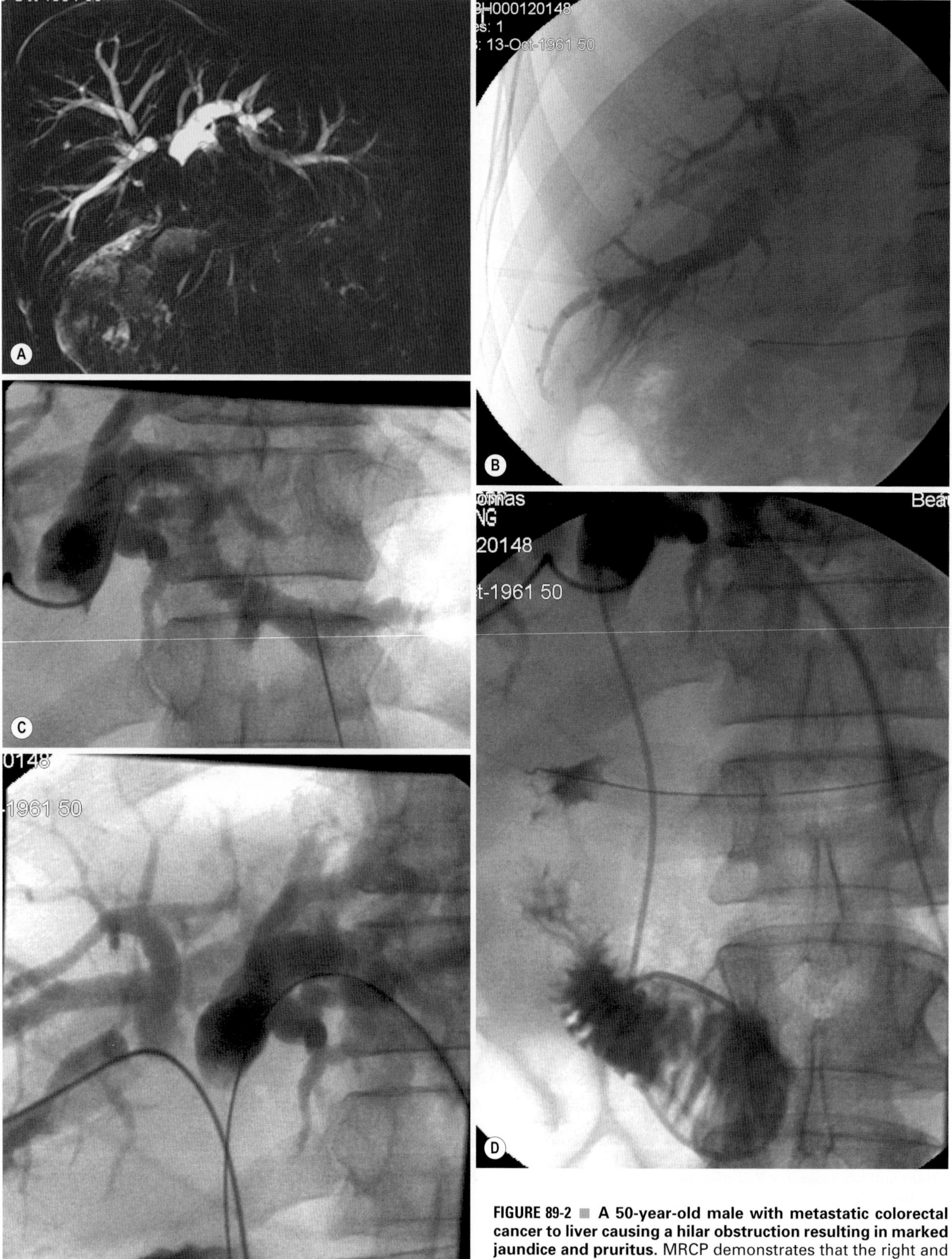

FIGURE 89-2 ■ A 50-year-old male with metastatic colorectal cancer to liver causing a hilar obstruction resulting in marked jaundice and pruritus. MRCP demonstrates that the right and left main hepatic ducts do not communicate (A). A PTC was performed via the right side (B) confirming no communication between the ducts. The left side was then punctured (C) and the long stricture within the hilum and common duct was elicited (D). Therefore it was elected to place metallic biliary stents from both the right and left sides in a Y configuration. Guidewires were placed through the stricture via both sides (E).

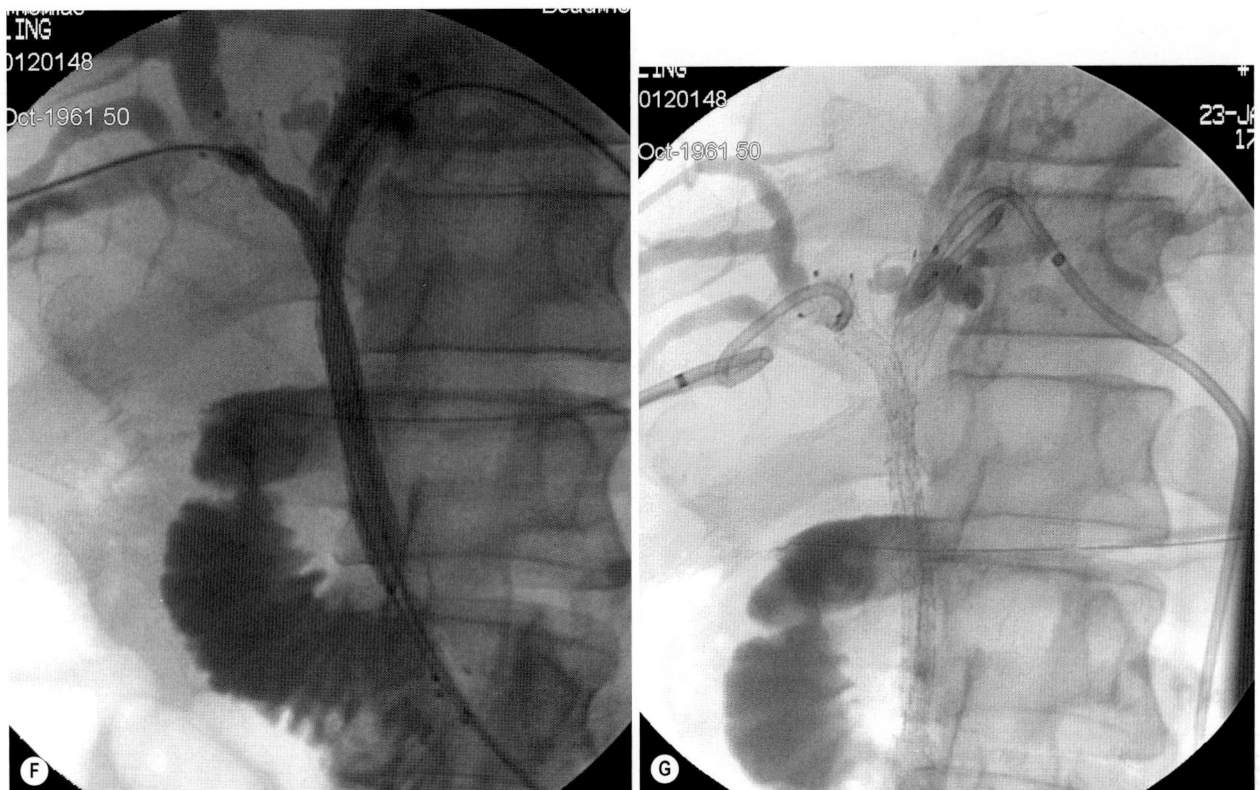

FIGURE 89-2, Continued ■ Ten-millimetre metallic self-expanding stents were deployed simultaneously across the stricture; note the tight stricture proximally within the right-sided stent which required balloon dilatation with an 8-mm balloon (F). Following balloon dilatation, the stents are widely patent, with safety external biliary drains placed for 24 hours (G).

Some surgeons advocate burying either the afferent or efferent Roux-en-Y loop during the biliary enteric anastomosis under the skin. The position of this loop is marked with surgical clips, enabling subsequent percutanous fluoroscopically guided access for stricture dilatation and stone extraction. This allows safe, well-tolerated access over many years.[5]

In patients with post-laparoscopic cholecystectomy bile duct injury or stricture, the goal is to cross the stricture or bile duct interruption and place a stent or stents to allow healing around the stent. It may be necessary to approach bile duct interruptions from both above and below so that a guidwire placed from one end can be snared in 'open space' from the other end to obtain through-and-through access.

Benign strictures should be dilated to approximately 10 mm. It is useful to leave a 4Fr access catheter in place for approximately 6 weeks, in order to facilitate redilatation if early recurrence occurs. If there is no significant restenosis, the catheter should be removed.

Percutaneous stents are not commonly used in benign strictures, as they will almost always become occluded after a few months.

Calculous Disease

Biliary obstruction secondary to distal CBD calculi is usually initially managed endoscopically. In cases where ERCP is unsuccessful or the calculi are intrahepatic, a percutaneous approach can be employed. A PTC is performed as described above and a guidewire manipulated past the calculus into the duodenum. A balloon catheter is placed over the guidewire and passed beyond the calculi and the sphincter of Oddi is dilated. The balloon is then deflated and placed above the calculus. The balloon is reinflated and then pushed forward to move the calculi into the duodenum.[6]

Post-cholecystectomy retained bile duct stones are usually removed endoscopically. If a T-tube has been placed at surgery, percutaneous removal can be performed. The T-tube tract is allowed to mature for 6 weeks and the T-tube is removed over a guidewire. A second safety guidewire is placed to maintain access and the calculi is then removed with a basket.

Percutaneous Biliary Intervention Complications

Percutaneous biliary drainage is relatively safe.[7] Procedure-related mortality is around 2% with 30-day patient mortality >10% in many series due to the underlying advanced malignant disease and co-morbid conditions.

Complications include localised pain, bile leak, bleeding including haemobilia and septicaemia. If the pleura

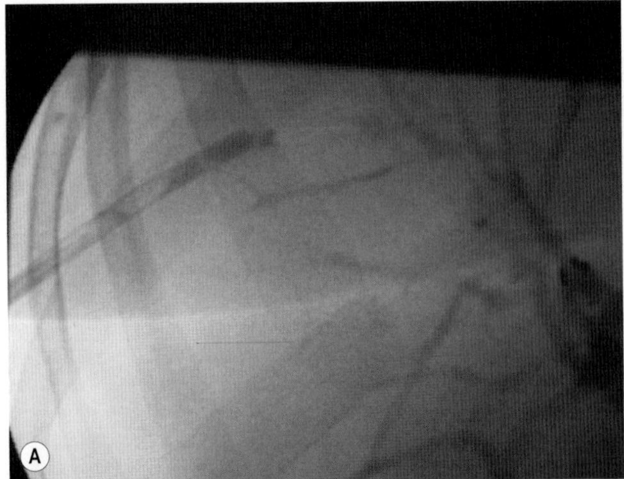

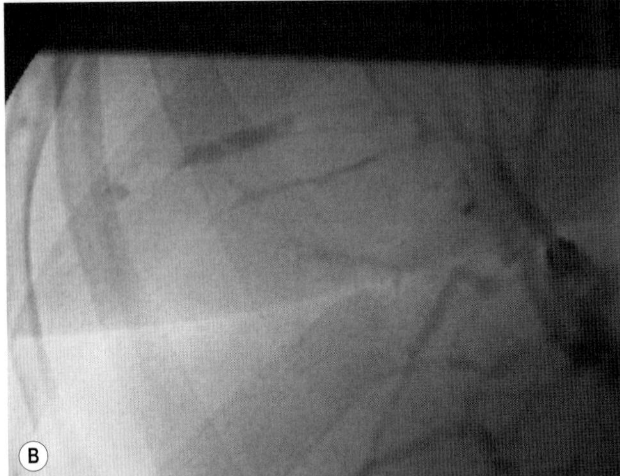

FIGURE 89-3 ■ Patient in whom biliary stent was placed and track embolised with pledgets of Gelfoam. (A) Peel-away sheath has been inserted into the hepatic track and contrast media injected to outline the track. One Gelfoam torpedo (air column in contrast-filled track) has been delivered and the second Gelfoam torpedo can be seen in the peel-away sheath. (B) Both Gelfoam torpedoes (torpedoes appear as air density tubular structures) have been delivered and the peel-away sheath removed.

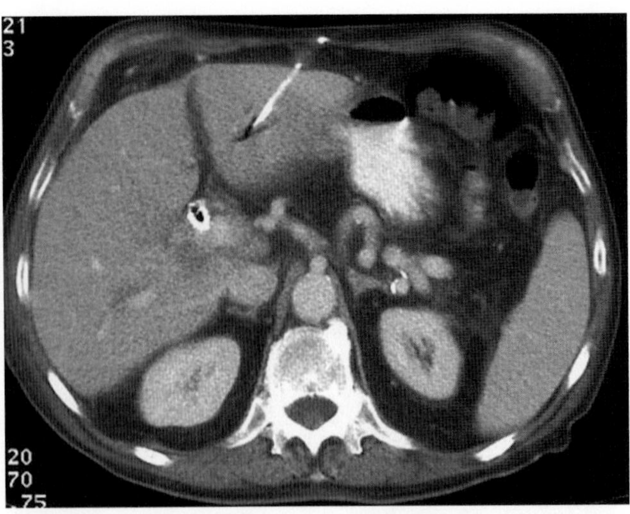

FIGURE 89-4 ■ Patient in whom a biliary stent was placed from a left-sided approach. CT was performed over the ensuing months. The CT shows the mixture of glue and lipiodol (1:1 mixture) in the percutaneous track in the left liver lobe. The glue is delivered using a fascial dilator.

is transgressed, there are additional risks or pneumothorax and haemothorax. External and internal–external drainage catheters can kink, become dislodged and exacerbate bilovenous fistulae.[8] Metallic stents can become blocked and 10–30% will require reintervention.

Track embolisation at the end of the procedure can also help to reduce the latter complications and reduce post-procedure pain. Track embolisation can be performed with pledgets of Gelfoam pushed into the peel-away sheath and left in the hepatic track as the peel-away sheath is withdrawn (Fig. 89-3). Alternatively, a 1 : 1 mixture of lipiodol : cyanoacrylate can be delivered with a dilator into the transhepatic track (Fig. 89-4).

VASCULAR INTERVENTIONAL TECHNIQUES IN THE LIVER

CHEMOEMBOLISATION

Background

Malignant tumours receive almost all their blood supply from the hepatic artery, whereas the normal liver parencyma receives blood from both the portal vein and the hepatic artery. Transarterial chemoembolisation (TACE) aims to induce tumour ischaemic necrosis by occluding the blood supply to the tumour while preserving the blood flow to the normal liver parenchyma. Both hepatocellular carcinoma (HCC) and metastases may respond to TACE. Local delivery of chemotherapy directly into the tumour bed reduces systemic chemotherapy side effects.[9]

Indications

Patients with HCC with preserved liver function and Eastern Cooperative Oncology Group (ECOG)[10] performance status of 0–1 without extrahepatic disease are most suitable for chemoembolisation.[11,12] If the aim is to prolong life, patients with metastases should be treated if the disease is confined to the liver or if there is stable extrahepatic disease. In patients with neuroendocrine tumours, TACE can control symptoms such as flushing, sweating and palpitations.

TAE/TACE may be employed to reduce tumour bulk to allow an initially unresectable tumour to become resectable or to control or reduce tumour bulk in patients with HCC until a liver becomes available for transplantation.

TACE Contraindications

Poor outcomes occur in patients with little liver reserve and therefore chemoembolisation should be avoided in patients with more than 50–75% of liver parenchyma replaced by tumour, in patients with advanced cirrhosis and in those in liver failure. Advanced or progressive extrahepatic disease is also a contraindication. Relative contraindications include portal vein thrombus, Child-Pugh Class C, hepatic encephalopathy, active gastrointestinal (GI) bleeding, refractory ascites, transjugular intrahepatic portosystemic shunt and a serum bilirubin >5 mg/dL.[13] Patients with biliary-enteric anastomosis, prior sphincterotomy or CBD stents are at higher risk of infection and liver abscess formation due to reflux of enteric contents into the biliary system; thus antibiotic prophylaxis should be extended.

Pre-Procedure Medication/Sedation/Analgesia

Intravenous antibiotics and intravenous fluids are administered prior to chemoembolisation in most centres. Local analgesia and conscious sedation are given as per operator preference.

Performing the Procedure

Thorough good-quality digital subtraction angiography (DSA) is employed prior to embolisation to map out tumour arterial blood supply, identify anatomical variants, detect arteriovenous shunts, confirm portal vein patency and guide treatment strategy. Selective digital subtraction angiography is performed with microcatheters (Fig. 89-5). Dynamic CT can help to to map out tumour arterial feeders and recruitment of arterial feeders from unsuspected locations, i.e. dome lesions supplied from inferior phrenic arteries.

Chemoembolisation should be performed as superselectively as possible (Fig. 89-5). Various chemoembolisation agents are currently available. Slow controlled injections are necessary, watching closely under fluoroscopic guidance to avoid reflux or non-target embolisation. The end point is elimination of the tumour blush but not complete arterial stasis.

Post-Procedure Complications

Embolisation is often followed by the post-embolisation syndrome (PES), as a result of cell death and the release of various cytokines. It usually develops within 12 hours and manifests as nausea, vomiting, pain, fever and general malaise for a period of 2–7 days. PES may be prevented or ameliorated by the use of analgesia, antiemetics, antipyretics and intravenous fluids during and immediately after the procedure.

The overall complication rate of TACE is quoted at 4%[11] and includes hepatic failure due to infarction, abscess, biliary necrosis leading to biliary stricture, tumour rupture and non-target embolisation, especially of the gallbladder and the bowel wall.

Imaging Post-Chemoembolisation

Cross-sectional imaging with either CT or MRI can be utilised to assess tumour response following chemoembolisation and is usually performed 6 weeks after the

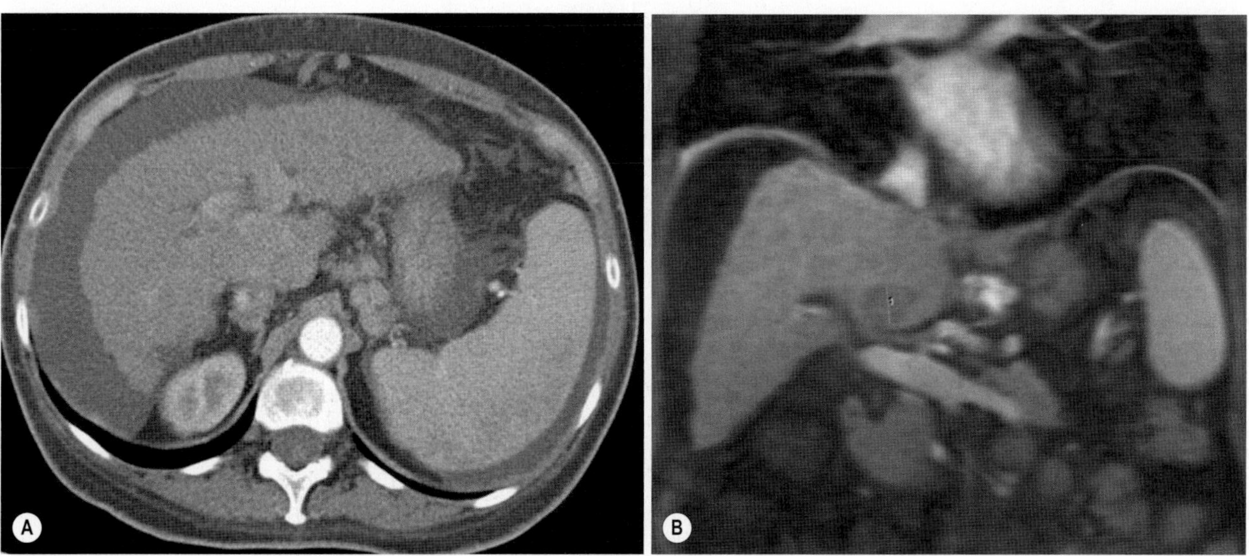

FIGURE 89-5 ■ A 59-year-old male with hepatitis C virus and long-standing cirrhosis with a raised AFP has both CT (A) and MRI (B; T1 fat-saturated post-contrast), demonstrating a caudate lobe mass lesion consistent with HCC. Note the irregular liver contour, ascites and splenomegaly.

Continued on following page

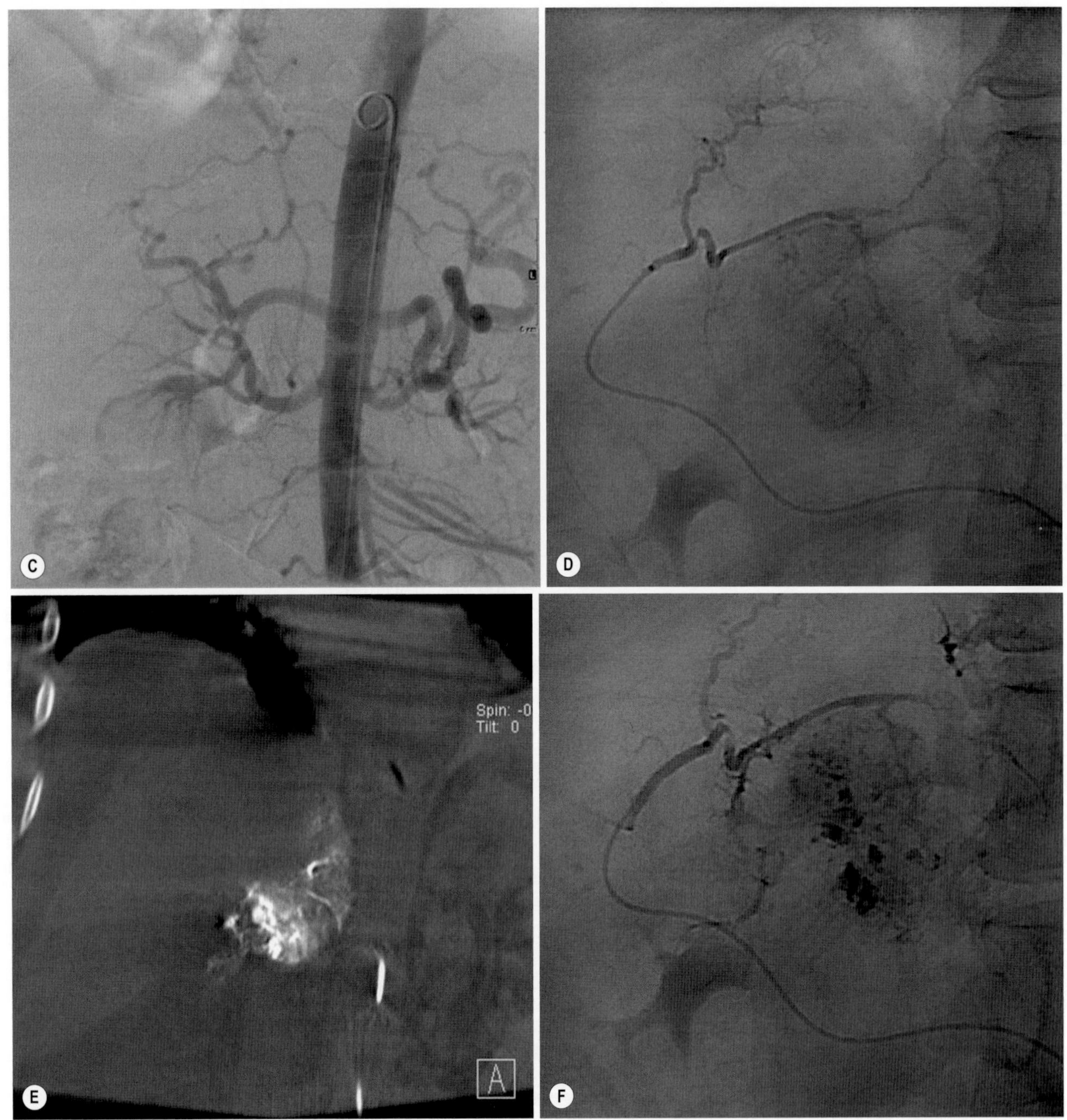

FIGURE 89-5, Continued ■ Angiography demonstrates normal mesenteric anatomy (C) and tumour blush when the left hepatic artery is selectively catheterised with a microcatheter (D). Intense focal contrast opacification of the tumour with DynaCT (E) confirms that the microcatheter is perfusing all arterial tumour feeders. Chemoembolisation (TACE) was then performed with a cisplatin, doxorubicin, mitomycin combination regimen mixed with lipiodol, administered via the microcatheter (F).

procedure. Repeat embolisation can be considered if there is any viable residual tumour. Follow-up protocols are variable, with most centres performing further imaging at 3- or 6-monthly intervals.

The method of actual individual lesion size measurement and lesion number reporting is variable. The World Health Organisation (WHO) (bidimensional perpendicular measurements of the tumour) has published guidance on the anatomical assessment of tumour response to therapy.[14] As the measuring methods and selection of target lesions are not clearly described in the WHO guidelines, assessment of tumour response is shown to be poorly reproducible between investigators.[15] In 2000 the Response Evaluation Criteria in Solid Tumours (RECIST) guidelines (unidimensional measurements of the tumour) were published.[16] The European Association for Study of the Liver (EASL) guidelines were published in 2001 and were based on the per cent change in the amount of enhancing tumoural tissue post-treatment.[17]

TACE Literature

There are two randomised controlled trials available, comparing chemoembolisation with conservative treatment for HCC and comparing bland embolisation against conservative treatment for HCC. Survival rates for patients with HCC following TACE at 1 and 2 years were 82 and 63% versus 63 and 27% for conservative treatment.[13] Survival rates for patients with HCC following TACE at 1, 2 and 3 years were 57, 31 and 26% versus 32, 11 and 3% for conservative treatment, respectively.[18] Survival rates for patients with HCC following TAE at 1 and 2 years were 75 and 50% versus 63 and 27% for conservative treatment, respectively.[13] A meta-analysis from Llovet's group demonstrated a significant 2-year survival benefit for patients with HCC treated with chemoembolisation versus conservative treatment alone.[19] There was no 2-year survival benefit for HCC patients treated with bland embolisation.[19] In the Precision V trial, Lammer et al. compared DC Bead chemoembolisation versus conventional TACE in patients with HCC and demonstrated higher rates of complete response, objective response and disease control in the DC Bead group than in the conventional TACE group (27 versus 22%, 52 versus 44% and 63 versus 52%, respectively).[20]

RADIOEMBOLISATION

Background

Also known as selective intra-arterial radiotherapy (SIRT) or selective intra-arterial brachytherapy, radioembolisation is a form of local radiotherapy. Micron-sized particles containing a radioisotope are given directly into the liver tumour via its feeding arteries in order to enable direct delivery of radiation. This technique delivers significantly higher radiation doses than external beam radiotherapy and minimises radiation dose to normal surrounding liver tissue.

Glass or resin particles impregnated with a β-emitting radio-isotope yttrium-90 (^{90}Y) are used to deliver the local tumour radiation. ^{90}Y is a pure β emitter with a half-life of 64.2 hours, which decays to stable zirconium-90. Despite the first clinical trials being conducted in the 1960s and its safety in human livers established in the 1980s, radioembolisation has only become readily available over the past decade. Two radioactive microsphere products are currently available on the market: a glass sphere known as TheraSphere (MDS Nordion, Canada) and a resin sphere known as SIR-Sphere (Sirtex Medical, Australia). TheraSphere gained FDA (Food and Drug Administration of America) approval in 1999 for use in the treatment of primary and/or metastatic HCC, with SIR-Sphere gaining FDA approval in 2002 for use in the treatment of colorectal cancer liver metastases.

Radioembolisation combines the advantages of embolisation and internal brachytherapy. It is necessary to perform detailed, pre-treatment angiography to map out tumour and liver arterial anatomy, to identify variant arterial anatomy, to delineate tumour arterial supply and to determine arterio-portal shunting.

Patient Selection

Patient selection for radioembolisation should be performed in a multidisciplinary team setting with both tumour characteristics and patient characteristics being highly important. Indications include an unresectable lesion, lack of fitness for transplantation, lesions unsuitable for thermal ablation and failed conventional chemotherapy. Patient characteristics include an ECOG performance status of 0–2 and an estimated life expectancy of greater than 12 weeks.[10]

Performing the Procedure: Planning

Pre-^{90}Y administration planning, diagnostic mesenteric angiography with meticulous technique is vital.[21] Diagnostic mesenteric angiography aims to determine hepatic arterial anatomy and variant anatomy, as 50% of the population will have aberrant hepatic arteries and 15% have aberrant arteries from the liver supplying the GI tract.[22] Salem et al. have provided an excellent description of the technique required to obtain good-quality angiography.[21] The use of a power injector pump to administer contrast, along with a base 5Fr catheter in the coeliac and superior mesenteric artery is mandatory.[21] Delayed venous imaging with the base catheter in the coeliac artery enables demonstration of a patent portal vein (Fig. 89-6).[21] A microcatheter, with an adjusted contrast flow rate on the power injector, is used to demonstrate the common, right, left and middle hepatic arteries, along with the gastroduodenal artery (GDA).[21] Dynamic CT or C-arm CT can be used to delineate tumour arterial supply via intra-arterial contrast administration during CT acquisition using a microcatheter at slow flow rates (Fig. 89-6).[21] This ensures the demontration of all arterial feeders to the lesion and avoids missing dual tumour supply, which is particularly important for dome lesions, which can parasitise flow from the inferior phrenic arteries.[22]

Non-target (normal tissue) embolisation is a greater problem with ^{90}Y than with chemoebolisation, as ^{90}Y not only causes ischaemia but also radiation injury to non-target tissue. The planning angiography procedure provides an opportunity to identify and deal with GI branches that could cause non-target ^{90}Y embolisation.[22] Coils may be used to embolise arteries to normal tissue, such as the GDA, left and right gastric artery, falciform artery and cystic artery in order to avoid non-target tissue damage, which may result in GI haemorrhage or pancreatitis. As there is a rich collateral arterial supply, proximal coils do not usually cause ischaemia and protect the bowel from ^{90}Y, thus allowing tumour-only delivery.

HCC is characterised by significant shunting, with lung shunting being of particular concern for treatment with ^{90}Y. The planning angiography procedure allows one to determine the lung shunt fraction (LSF) with a technetium ^{99m}Tc albumin aggregated (^{99m}Tc-MAA) shunt study.[22] LSF is calculated by injecting ^{99m}Tc-MAA into arteries to be treated with ^{90}Y and then imaging with a single photon emission computed tomography (SPECT) to detect shunting to pulmonary vasculature (Fig. 89-6). The size of the MAA particles is the same as the size of

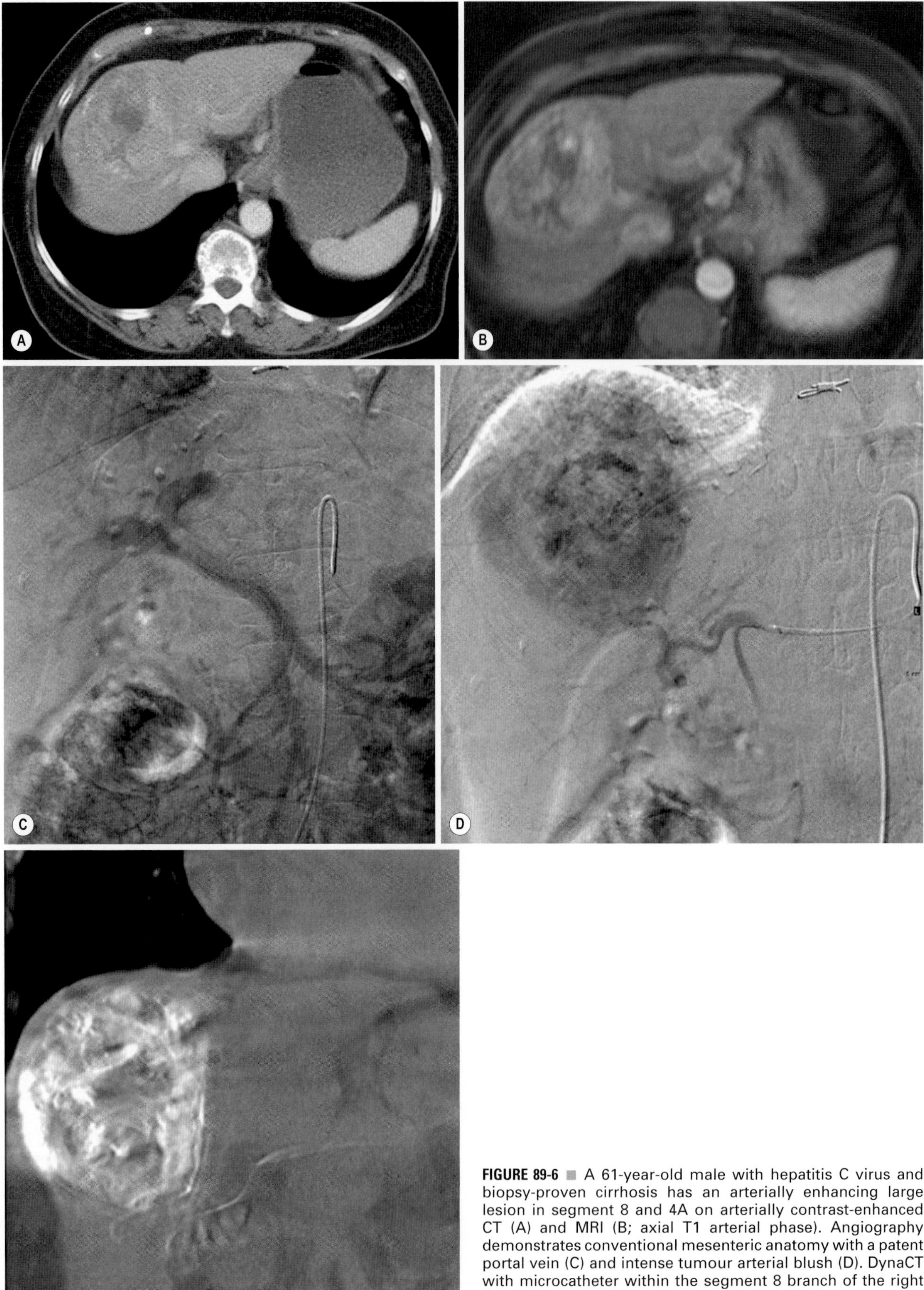

FIGURE 89-6 ■ A 61-year-old male with hepatitis C virus and biopsy-proven cirrhosis has an arterially enhancing large lesion in segment 8 and 4A on arterially contrast-enhanced CT (A) and MRI (B; axial T1 arterial phase). Angiography demonstrates conventional mesenteric anatomy with a patent portal vein (C) and intense tumour arterial blush (D). DynaCT with microcatheter within the segment 8 branch of the right hepatic artery demonstrates tumour contrast opacification only, thus no non-target enhancement (E).

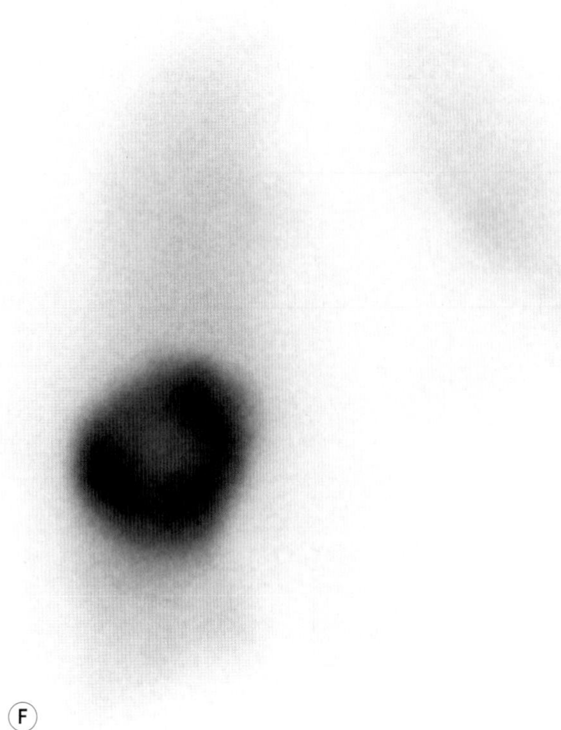

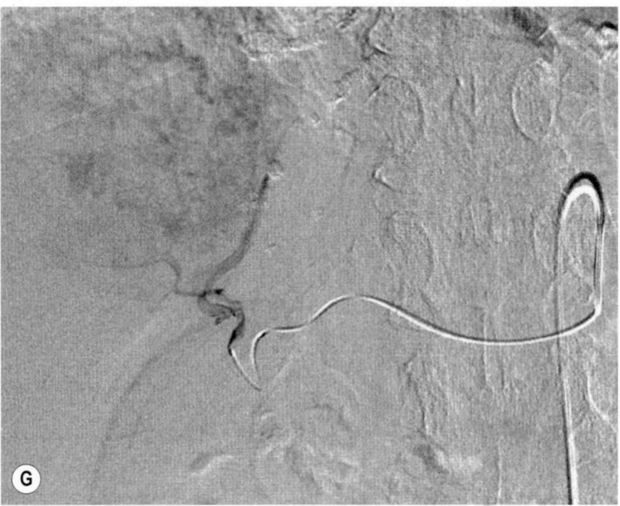

FIGURE 89-6, Continued ■ Radionuclide scan of segment 8 arterially injected MAA (F) demonstrates minimal lung shunting, thus confirming that it is safe to proceed with yttrium-90 radioembolisation. Microcatheter position for ^{90}Y injection (G).

^{90}Y; thus, the MAA shunt study can be considered a test run for the ^{90}Y. If LSF exceeds 20%, radioembolisation is not considered a safe option.[23]

^{90}Y Administration

One lobe is treated at any one time, with at least 4 weeks between lobar treatments. Repeat angiography should be performed prior to ^{90}Y administration to determine arterial flow characteristics, to detect failed coiling with reperfusion to non-target areas, thus enabling re-coiling if necessary. A slow, steady injection of ^{90}Y via a microcatheter with saline flushes and radiation monitoring should be performed (Fig. 89-6). Check angiography is performed on completion.

^{90}Y Complications

Riaz et al. provided a concise review of complications following radioembolisation with ^{90}Y.[24] Post-radioembolisation syndrome, which is similar to the usual post-embolisation syndrome, can occur and is managed conservatively. Hepatic dysfunction, radiation cystitis/biliary stricture, portal hypertension, radiation pneumonitis, GI complications from non-target embolisation and hepatic arterial injury are the main potential complications following radioembolisation.[24]

Imaging Post-Radioembolisation

The assessment of response using imaging is similar to that following TACE. Riaz et al. demonstrated that the primary index lesion concept significantly correlates with disease progression and patient survival.[25]

Radioembolisation Results

Treatment of HCC with radioembolisation has demonstrated survival rates following ^{90}Y at 1, 2 and 3 years of 84, 54 and 27%, respectively.[26] Treatment of CRC metastases with radioembolisation with ^{90}Y have yielded survival rates at 1 and 2 years of 39.1 and 22.1%, respectively, with imaging response rates quoted from 23 to 74% across a number of studies.[27] ^{90}Y is better at HCC downstaging than TACE.[28] Colorectal cancer metastases treated with ^{90}Y in combination with irinotecan produced a median progression-free survival of 6.0 months, with a median survival of 12.2 months.[29] Randomised controlled trials (RCT)s of ^{90}Y versus TACE are currently ongoing.

HEPATIC ARTERIAL EMBOLISATION FOR HAEMORRHAGE

Liver arterial haemorrhage occurs following trauma, blunt or penetrating, spontaneously from tumour or cyst

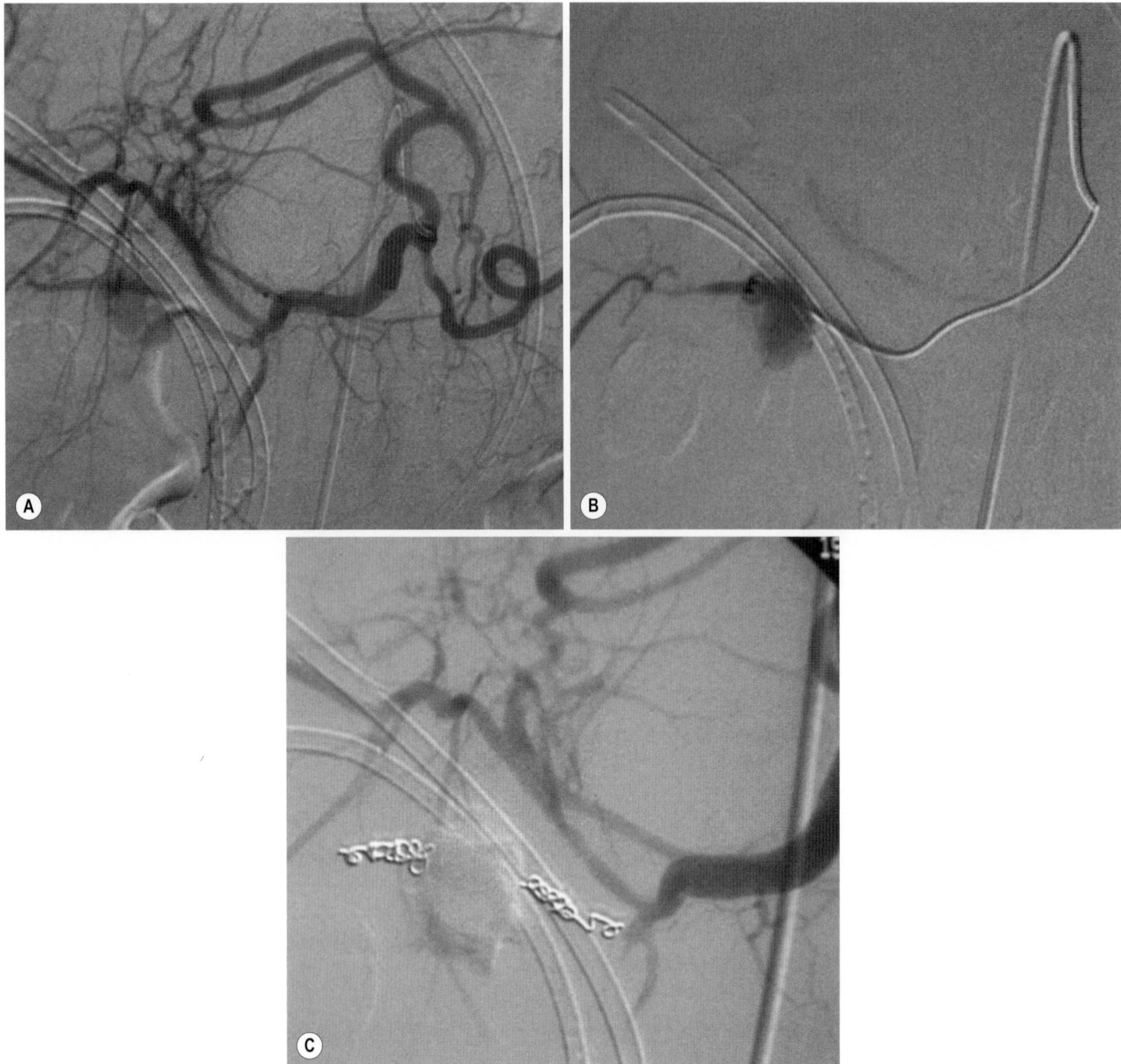

FIGURE 89-7 ■ A 74-year-old male with cholangiocarcinoma causing obstructive jaundice recently had an internal–external biliary drain placed to enable biliary decompression prior to stenting. He became hypotensive with bright red blood pouring out of his biliary drain. Digital subtraction angiography with a catheter in the coeliac artery demonstrated a large hepatic arterial pseudoaneurysm at the site of the internal–external biliary drain (A). Superselective catheterisation with a microcatheter eloquently identifies the pseudoaneurysm (B). Both the front door and the back door to the pseudoaneurysm were coil embolised to achieve haemostasis (C).

rupture or from iatrogenic causes such as following liver biopsy or biliary drainage (Fig. 89-7). Diagnosis can be made with triphasic liver CT. In the setting of an unstable patient with active arterial bleeding or a pseudoaneurysm, control of bleeding can be achieved by transcatheter embolisation. The pre-procedure planning and procedure technique is very similar to that employed for chemoembolisation or radioembolisation, with good-quality digital subtraction angiography with contrast pump injectors essential to delineate the arterial anatomy and the exact site of arterial injury. Embolisation can be performed with a variety of agents, depending on the configuration of the arterial injury: e.g. coils, particles or liquid embolic agents such as glue. The goal is to elicit a rapid diagnosis, clear demonstration of the anatomy and rapid haemorrhage control. Close liaison with surgical and anaesthetic colleagues is essential for optimum patient outcome.

TRANSJUGULAR INTRAHEPATIC PORTOSYSTEMIC SHUNT

Background

Transjugular intrahepatic portosystemic shunt (TIPSS) creates a transhepatic communication between a major intrahepatic portal vein branch (usually the right) and a hepatic vein using a needle system from the jugular vein. The transhepatic tract patency is maintained with a metallic covered stent. The creation of the shunt reduces the portal venous pressure. Accepted indications for TIPSS include variceal bleeding, both acute and refractory to endoscopic therapy,[30] refractory ascites[31] and hepatic hydrothorax. Further indications include Budd–Chiari syndrome[32] and hepatorenal/hepatopulmonary syndromes.

Imaging

Preoperative imaging is geared towards delineating hepatic vascular anatomy and confirming patency of the portal vein. Cardiovascular status should be assessed with cardiac failure contraindicating TIPSS due to the haemodynamic changes associated with the creation of a portosystemic shunt. Sepsis and biliary obstruction are further contraindications and coagulopathy should be corrected.

Pre-Procedure Evaluation

Various preoperative scoring systems are available, with the model for end-stage liver disease (MELD) scoring system developed for those undergoing elective TIPSS.[33] The prognosis according to MELD score is as follows:[34]

MELD <17: 3-month mortality: 16%
MELD >18: 3-month mortality: 35%
MELD >24: 3-month mortality: 65%.

Performing the Procedure

The procedure is generally performed under general anaesthesia. The right internal jugular vein is accessed and a vascular sheath is placed to the right atrium and the right hepatic vein is catheterised. The portal vein is deliniated by various methods: percutanous placement of portal vein guidewire before the procedure; aortoportography with delayed imaging after contrast injection from the SMA; or wedged CO_2 portography from the hepatic vein. A transhepatic trocar is advanced from the hepatic vein to the region of the portal vein, the needle withdrawn and the catheter is aspirated as it is withdrawn. Once blood is aspirated, a small amount of contrast material is injected to confirm portal venous position (Fig. 89-8). A guidewire is passed to the portal vein and pressure measurements are obtained in the portal vein and right atrium. The tract is measured with a calibated catheter from the portal vein to the confluence of the hepatic vein with the inferior vena cava (Fig. 89-8). The tract is dilated with an angioplasty balloon and a covered stent (e.g. Viatorr; Gore Medical, Flagstaff, AZ) is placed. The stent is balloon dilated. Pressure measurements are performed to ensure that adequate shunting has been established (pressure <12 mmHg or halving the portosystemic gradient). Angiography is performed at the end of the procedure. If there is continued opacification of varices, these should be embolised, if the patient has had a significant variceal bleed (Fig. 89-8).

Post-Procedure

The haemodynamic changes can lead to cardiac failure and diuretics may help reduce central venous pressure. The risk of encephalopathy ranges from 5 to 35%.[35] Periprocedural lactulose and rifaximin are effective in reducing gut flora.

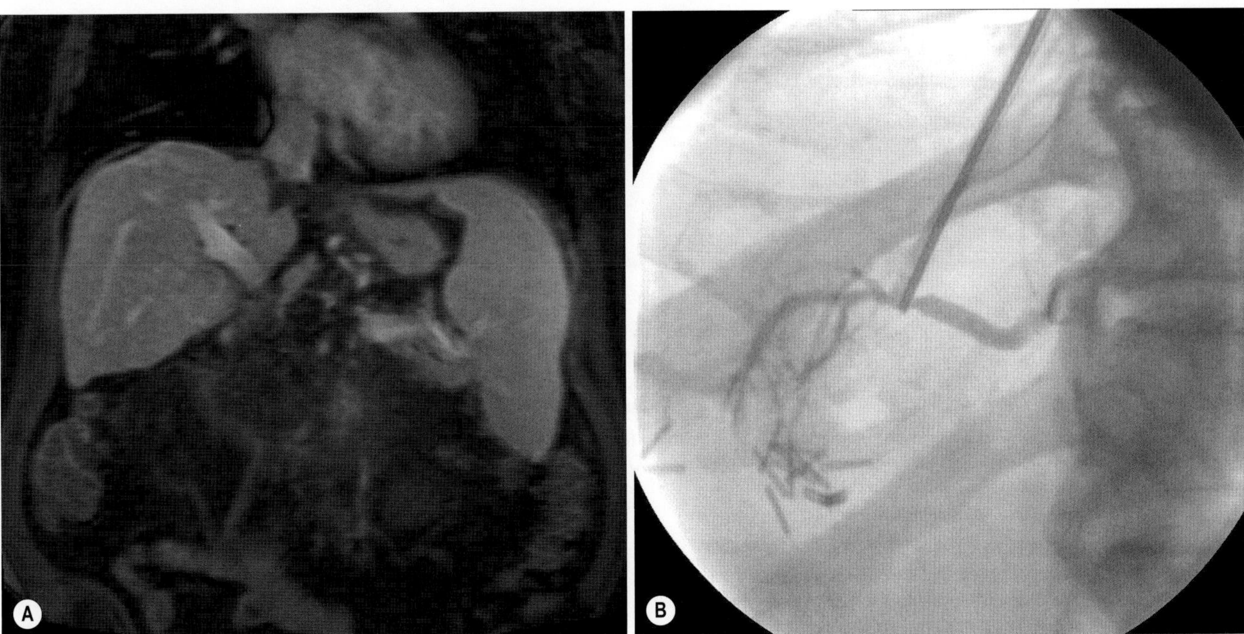

FIGURE 89-8 ■ A 55-year-old male alcoholic presented with massive upper GI haemorrhage secondary to bleeding oesophageal varices, with a MELD of 11. MRI demonstrated a patent portal vein, cirrhosis and splenomegaly (A). Due to the massive variceal bleeding it was elected to perform a TIPSS. A right hepatic vein to right portal vein approach was taken (B).

Continued on following page

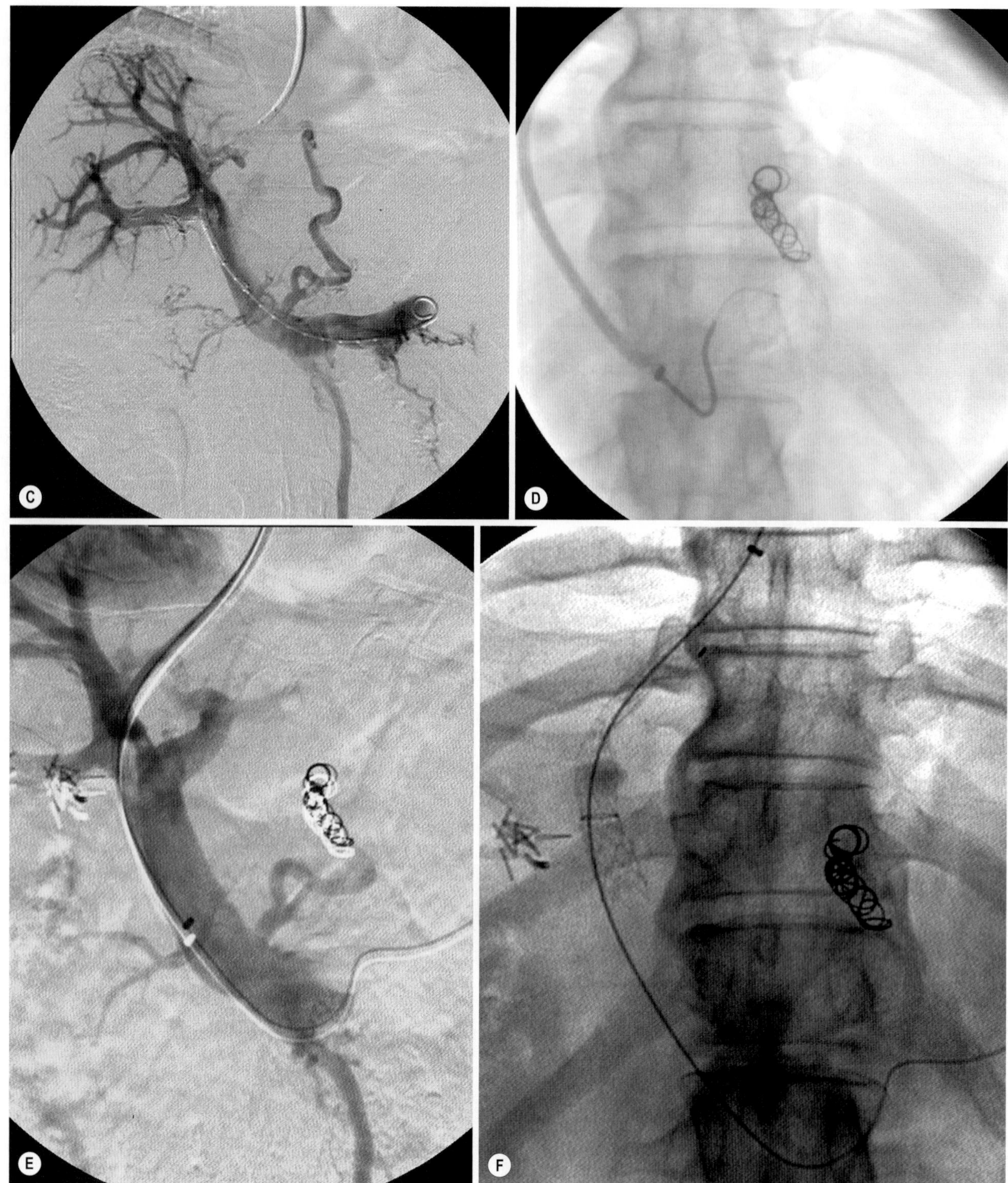

FIGURE 89-8, Continued ■ Portogram with a measuring catheter demonstrated a large left coronary vein contributing to the large oesophageal varices (C). The coronary vein was coil embolised (D). Repeat portogram demonstrated no flow within the left coronary vein following embolisation (E). A Viatorr 10 mm × 8 cm TIPSS was placed, which demonstrated some stenosis initially (F).

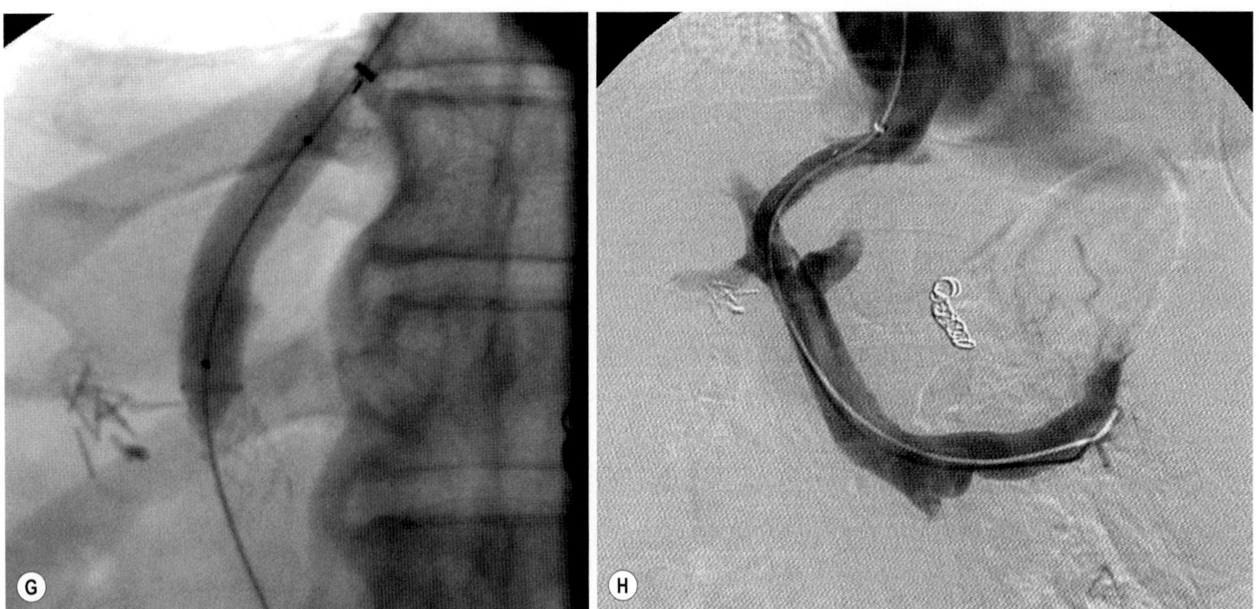

FIGURE 89-8, Continued ■ The stent was ballooned to 8 mm (G). Completion venography demonstrates a widely patent TIPSS with no variceal flow (H).

Complications

Direct procedural-related mortality is lower than 2%[35] and relates to hepatic arterial injury, capsular perforation or direct puncture of the extrahepatic portal vein with intraperitoneal haemorrhage. Right atrial perforation may occur from misplaced stents. Bile duct injury with haemobilia and intraparenchymal haematoma may occur at the time of the procedure. Further complications include heart failure and encephalopathy due to shunting. Stent occlusion and subsequent sepsis have been reduced with the advent of covered stents but remain problematic.

PORTAL VEIN EMBOLISATION

Background

Preoperative portal vein embolisation is performed in patients undergoing liver resection for localised metastases to the liver or primary hepatocellular carcinoma. It is used in cases where the future liver remnant (usually left lobe) will not provide sufficient function, and exploits the ability of the liver to regenerate. Volumetric analysis from CT is undertaken to calculate the functional liver volume required, which is related to body surface area. If the future liver remnant is less than 25% in a normal liver, or less than 40% in a cirrhotic liver, then portal vein embolisation should be considered.[36] In addition, systemic disease with diabetes mellitus may limit the degree of hypertrophy.[37] The portal vein embolisation is performed 4–6 weeks before surgical resection, and the section of liver to be resected is embolised to divert portal venous blood flow to the remaining liver to allow hypertrophy.

Performing the Procedure

US-guided percutaneous access is gained to the portal vein with a coaxial microaccess set (e.g. Neff Set (Cook)). A sheath is placed and portal venography is performed to delineate the anatomy. An angiographic catheter is placed to the branch portal vein supplying the tumour. Embolisation is performed with glue, coils, plugs or a combination of these. Specific complications of portal vein embolisation include main portal vein thrombosis, which would preclude surgery and portal hypertension resulting in variceal haemorrhage.[37]

HEPATIC VENOUS INTERVENTIONS: BUDD–CHIARI SYNDROME

Background

Budd–Chiari syndrome is a heterogeneous group of disorders characterised by hepatic venous outflow obstruction at the level of the hepatic veins, the inferior vena cava (IVC) or the right atrium.[38] Budd–Chiari syndrome is not a primary condition of the liver parenchyma; it is due to partial or complete obstruction of hepatic venous outflow. This obstruction subsequently leads to progressive sinusoidal congestion, centrilobular necrosis, fibrosis and nodular regeneration. Percutaneous therapies performed in properly selected patients can help improve liver function and arrest hepatic destruction.[39]

Diagnosis

Clinically, patients usually present with tender hepatomegaly and ascites. However, they may present in fulminant hepatic failure and rarely present with chronic liver impairment. Doppler ultrasound may demonstrate lack of flow in the hepatic veins, hepatic venous thrombus or intrahepatic venous collaterals. Flow reversal in the distal hepatic veins, a caval web, caval stenosis or occlusion may also be demonstrated. Cross-sectional imaging with CT or MRI can confirm the ultrasound findings.

Treatment

The aim is to restore normal hepatic venous drainage from the liver. In acute thrombus, direct catheter-based thrombolysis with tissue plasminogen activator (tPA) is employed. A hepatic venous or caval stenosis can then be unmasked with clot dissolution, enabling venoplasty and/or stenting. However, restenosis is common. TIPSS creation is an alternative option to maintain venous outflow drainage from the liver in Budd–Chiari. Close post-TIPSS surveillance is needed in this patient group to detect shunt restenosis and enable balloon dilatation. Liver transplantation may be necessary in some patients.

For a full list of references, please see ExpertConsult.

FURTHER READING

7. van Delden OM, Lameris JS. Percutaneous drainage and stenting for palliation of malignant bile duct obstruction. Eur Radiol 2008;18:448–56.
11. Llovet JM, Burroughs A, Bruix J. Hepatocellular carcinoma. Lancet 2003;362:1907–17.
25. Riaz A, Miller FH, Kulik LM, et al. Imaging response in the primary index lesion and clinical outcomes following transarterial locoregional therapy for hepatocellular carcinoma. JAMA 2010; 303:1062–9.
30. Garcia-Pagan JC, Caca K, Bureau C, et al. Early use of TIPS in patients with cirrhosis and variceal bleeding. N Engl J Med 2010;362:2370–9.
33. Malinchoc M, Kamath PS, Gordon FD, et al. A model to predict poor survival in patients undergoing transjugular intrahepatic portosystemic shunts. Hepatology 2000;31:864–71.
34. Ferral H, Gamboa P, Postoak DW, et al. Survival after elective transjugular intrahepatic portosystemic shunt creation: prediction with model for end-stage liver disease score. Radiology 2004;231:231–6.
39. Cura M, Haskal Z, Lopera J. Diagnostic and interventional radiology for Budd-Chiari syndrome. Radiographics 2009;29:669–81.

CHAPTER 90

Vascular Genitourinary Tract Intervention

Jonathan G. Moss • Reddi Prasad Yadavali

CHAPTER OUTLINE

KIDNEY

Renal Artery Stenosis

Background

Stenosis of the renal artery (RAS), which is usually focal, can cause a cascade of ischaemic-driven events in the kidney plus other potential insults such as cholesterol embolisation. This can lead to clinical consequences, which include secondary hypertension, impaired renal function and fluid retention (flash pulmonary oedema). Much interest has focused on correcting the anatomical abnormality, initially with angioplasty and latterly with stents in an attempt to reverse or halt the clinical manifestations.

Aetiology and Pathology

In Western populations, atherosclerosis is the leading cause in over 90% of cases. However, in younger age group, the non-atheromatous arteritides should be considered (Table 90-1) particularly in the non-Caucasian individual.

Diagnosis of RAS

Once suspected clinically, the optimal imaging modality is contrast-enhanced magnetic resonance angiography (MRA) (Fig. 90-1). However, due to a small number of reported cases of nephrogenic systemic fibrosis linked to gadolinium contrast media exposure, guidelines suggest caution if the e GFR is <30 mL/min and is contraindicated when <15 mL/min. Other imaging options include computed tomographic angiography (CTA) and newer MRI sequences, avoiding contrast media altogether. Although Doppler ultrasound and functional nuclear medicine scans can be used, they have largely fallen out of favour in recent years. Despite this, they may still play a limited role specific circumstances, however, they similarly selective renal vein sampling is seldom used nowadays.

Atheromatous Renovascular Disease (ARVD)

ARVD is by far the commonest cause of RAS and usually develops as part of a systemic inflammatory atheromatous syndrome with disease in other vascular beds (coronary, peripheral). There is a strong correlation with both smoking and type 2 diabetes. Anatomically over 90% of ARVD involves the renal ostium as a result of encroaching aortic plaques.

Clinical Presentation of ARVD. Many patients are asymptomatic and the condition is often detected whilst investigating other symptoms, e.g. lower limb ischaemia. Others present with hypertension, impaired renal function or 'flash pulmonary oedema'. The latter is a poorly understood condition where there are recurrent attacks of fluid overload with normal or near normal cardiac function but the kidney's ability to excrete fluid is impaired.

Treatment of ARVD. Treatment of the global atherosclerotic burden should be addressed with smoking cessation, aspirin, statins and optimising blood pressure control. Although intuitively contraindicated, ACE inhibitors should be given with careful monitoring of renal function. There is some evidence that this 'package of medical treatment' can stabilise atheromatous plaque and even induce regression.

Revascularisation of the stenotic artery has evolved over the years. Initially performed by open surgical repair, percutaneous transluminal angioplasty (PTA) gained rapid acceptance in the 1980s. However, high restenosis rates due to elastic recoil from the aortic plaques led to

TABLE 90-1 Non-Atheromatous Arteritides

- Fibromuscular disease
- Neurofibromatosis
- Takayasu arteritis
- Williams syndrome

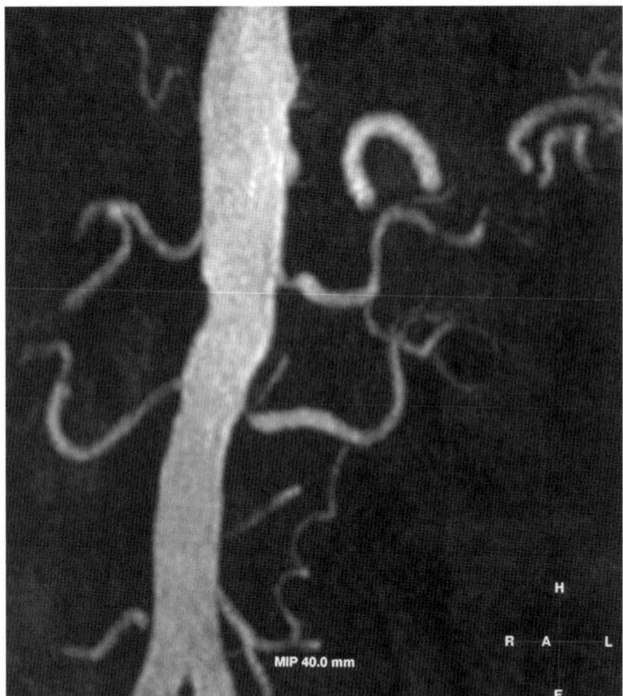

FIGURE 90-1 ■ **Renal artery stenosis.** Coronal MIP MRA shows osteal stenoses of superior and inferior left renal arteries.

disappointing anatomical and clinical results.[1] The introduction of metallic stents in the early 1990s led to a resurgence in endovascular activity and the mechanical limitations of renal PTA were overcome with a significant reduction in restenosis.[2] Almost overnight renal stenting became the dominant strategy for ARVD.

However, although stenting clearly led to improved patency it was often difficult to clearly link this with clinical benefit, e.g. blood pressure reduction or improvement in renal function. It was often said that the 'rule of thirds' applied with one-third showing some improvement, another third static and the final third deteriorating. This continuing uncertainty triggered several randomised trials which spanned both the PTA and stenting era.

Renal Revascularisation Trials. The early trials[3–5] predated stents and focussed on blood pressure outcomes. The later trials used stents exclusively and focussed on renal function.[6,7] None of these trials with meta-analyses of over 1000 patients have been able to prove any clear benefit of either PTA or stenting over medical treatment alone.[8,9] These trials, including the largest (ASTRAL n = 806), have all been criticised and the debate continues. A large ultrasound (US) trial (CORAL) is due to report in 2014 and may provide more information.[10]

Routine renal stenting for hypertension or impaired renal function is therefore difficult to justify in view of the lack of evidence. However, not all patients entered these trials and possible but unproven indications for renal stenting may include the following:

- Intractable hypertension on maximum medical treatment;
- Rapidly deteriorating renal function;
- A single kidney with a critical stenosis (>90%);
- Flash pulmonary oedema; and
- Acute renal failure with preserved renal size (>8 cm).

Careful individualised patient evaluation is necessary as complications can occur in 5–10% of procedures. These are mostly minor, e.g. groin haematoma, but can include damage to the renal artery, cholesterol embolisation and occasional loss of the kidney. Very rarely a patient will present with acute renal failure and an occluded single renal artery; stenting in these circumstances is worthwhile and can restore renal function with little to lose (Fig. 90-2).

Technique for Renal Angioplasty and Stenting

Renal Angioplasty. The angle from which the renal artery leaves the aorta will help decide between a femoral and an arm (brachial or radial) approach. Over 90% are approachable from the femoral artery. Similarly the angle at which the renal artery ostium lies in the coronal plane will determine the correct angle to place the 'C-arm', in order to project the origin of the renal artery clear of the aorta. Careful perusal of the baseline imaging is essential. Advances in guidewire and catheter technology have meant most operators now use the so-called 'low platform' systems, which use a 3–4F catheter with 0.014–0.018 guidewires. Delivered through a 6–7F guiding catheter, they are less traumatic than the old 0.035 guidewire systems. Having accessed the renal artery ostium and placed a guide catheter, the lesion is crossed and angioplastied with an appropriate sized balloon. Intraoperative heparin and a proprietary antispasmodic should be given. When dealing with non-atheromatous lesions angioplasty is usually sufficient (Fig. 90-3) but atheromatous lesions are almost always stented to overcome elastic recoil.

Renal Stenting. The procedure is similar to PTA and again uses a 'low platform' stent. The lesion is crossed as above and the stenosis pre-dilated to 3 mm and then the stent placed. Accurate C-arm positioning is critical to ensure accurate stent placement with 2–3 mm protruding out into the aorta. Most operators use balloon-expandable rather than self-expanding stents because they are easier to place accurately at the renal artery ostium (Fig. 90-4).

Fibromuscular Disease. In the West, fibromuscular disease accounts for 10% of all cases of RAS. Although it is most frequently found in the renal arteries (60%) other major vessels such as the carotid, viscerals and coronaries can be involved. There are at least five different pathological types but the most common is medial fibroplasia where there are alternating areas of stenosis

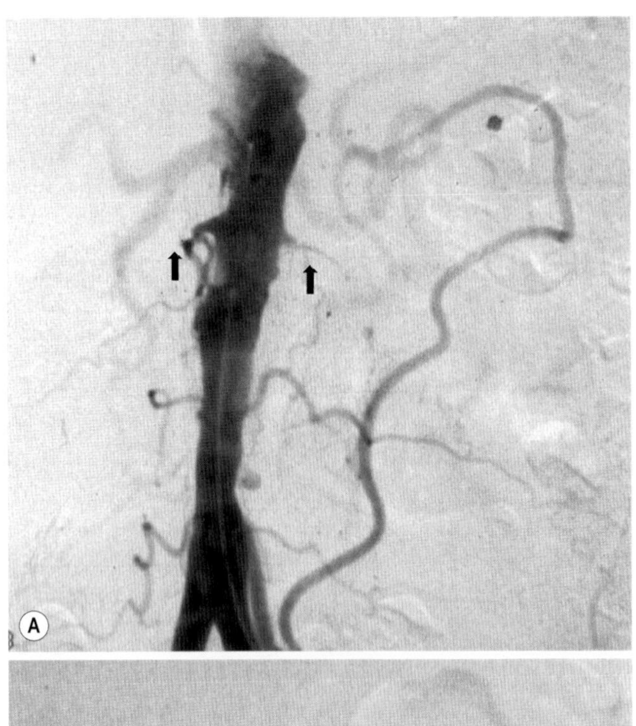

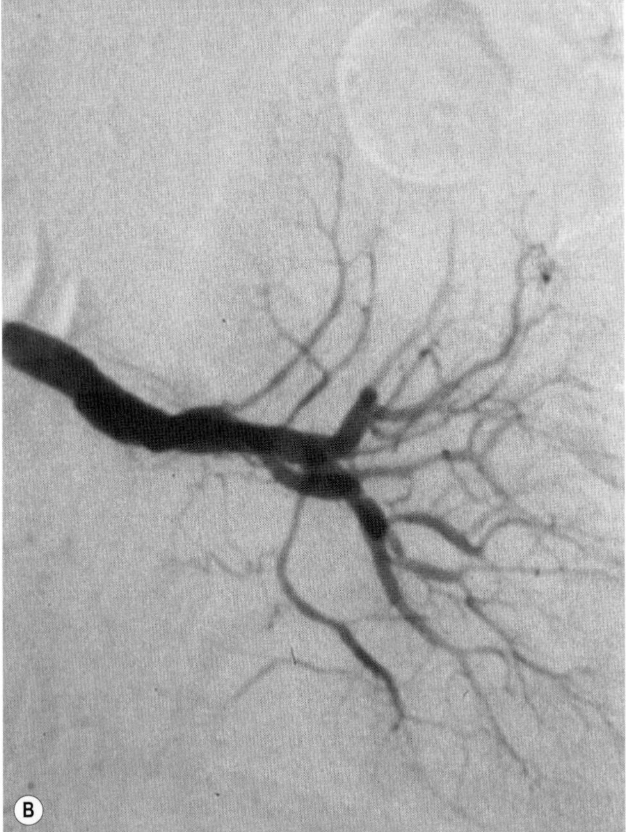

FIGURE 90-2 ■ (A) Patient presenting with acute kidney injury. Angiogram showing bilateral renal artery occlusions. (B) Selective left renal angiogram following successful recanalistion and stenting of the renal artery. Satisfactory renal function was re-established with a massive diuresis.

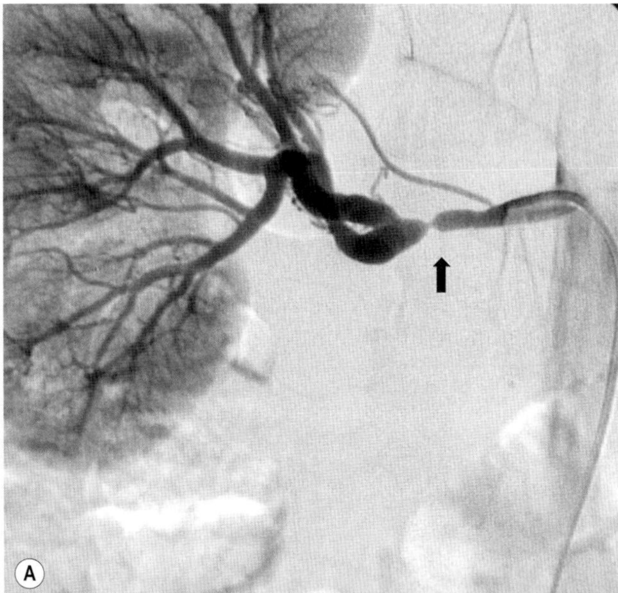

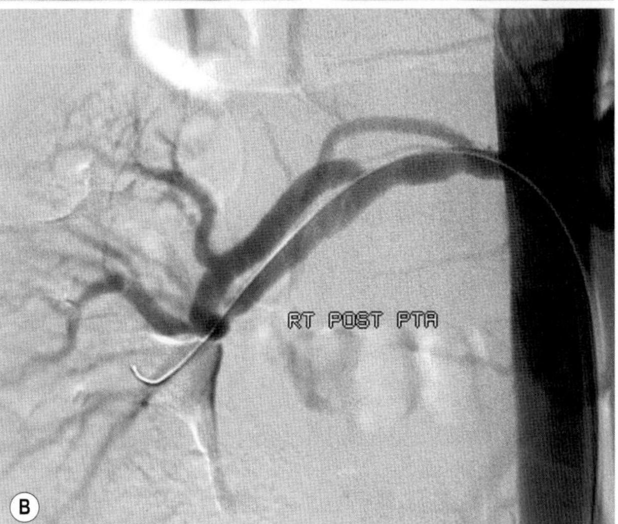

FIGURE 90-3 ■ **Female patient aged 23 years with severe hypertension.** (A) Selective right renal angiogram showing a tight focal stricture due to fibromuscular disease. (B) Aortogram showing good post angioplasty result. There was a dramatic drop in blood pressure, necessitating cessation of all antihypertensive medications.

and aneurysmal dilation leading to the classical 'string of beads' appearance (Fig. 90-5). A much rarer type leads predominantly to aneurysm formation (Fig. 90-6) and requires a different management strategy. The typical presentation is a young person, commonly female, with new onset hypertension. Renal function is usually normal and although the lesion may progress, complete vessel occlusion is rare. Although initial management with drugs is usual there is a strong case for angioplasty as the lesions respond well and there is often a good chance of 'cure' or significant improvement in blood pressure control.[11]

Takayasu Arteritis. The epidemiology of RAS is different in the Indian subcontinent and the Far East, with vasculitis, including Takayasu arteritis, said to be responsible for up to 60% of RAS cases. Although PTA can be used, this inflammatory condition can be resistant to dilation. Steroids are often successfully used to suppress the inflammatory component.

Neurofibromatosis. This rare congenital condition is known to cause a myriad of symptoms and signs. Less well recognised is the involvement of vessels, commonly the renal arteries. The pathology is usually one of stenosis and aneurysmal dilatation. Although PTA can be utilized, the lesions are often resistant to dilatation and in this young patient group surgical reconstruction of the vessel may be a better option.

Williams Syndrome. This rare congenital condition presents in childhood. Although the renal arteries are commonly involved there is almost always aortic hypoplasia and the extent to which angioplasty and stenting can help is very limited.

Renal Denervation (RDN)

Background

Essential hypertension is extremely common in Western societies where approximately one-third of adults have high blood pressure. With an ageing population, Westernisation and increasing obesity and diabetes, the prevalence of hypertension will only increase. In the USA in 2011, 69% of first heart attacks, 77% of first strokes and 74% with congestive cardiac failure had a blood pressure higher than 140/99 mmHg.[12] The costs to the global

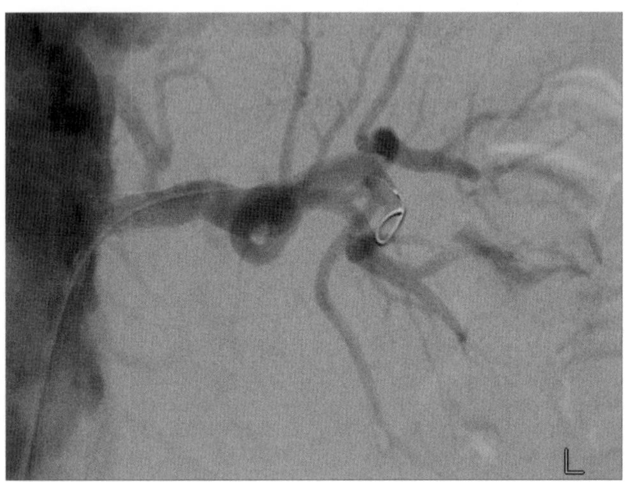

FIGURE 90-4 ■ Renal artery stent. Balloon-expandable stent in the proximal left renal artery for atheromatous osteal stenosis.

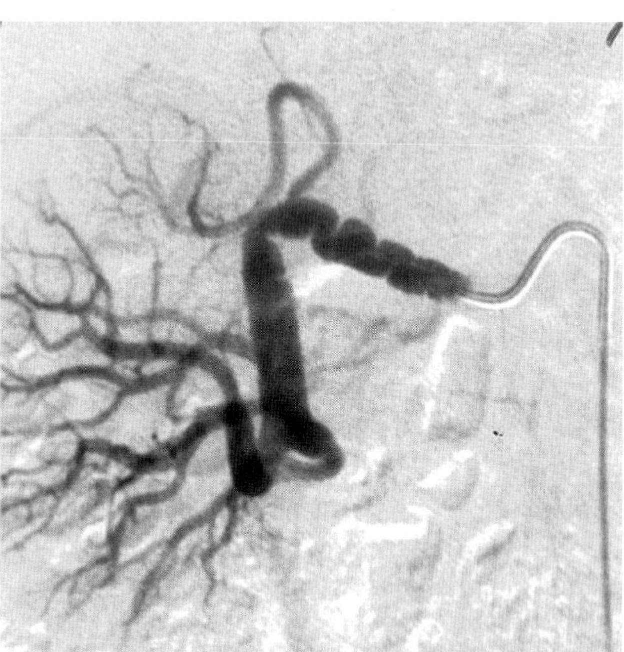

FIGURE 90-5 ■ 'String of beads'. Right renal angiogram showing multifocal stenosis secondary to fibromuscular disease.

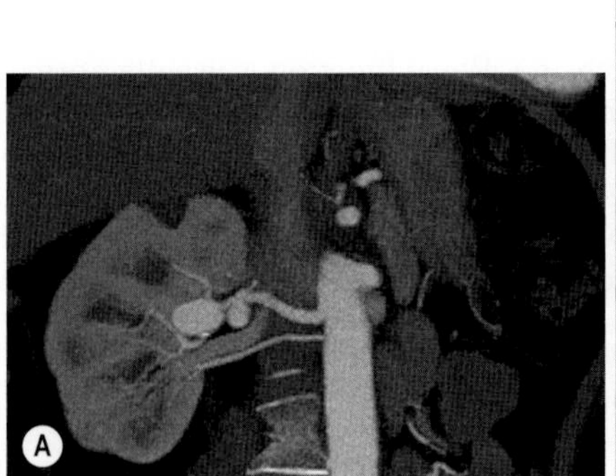

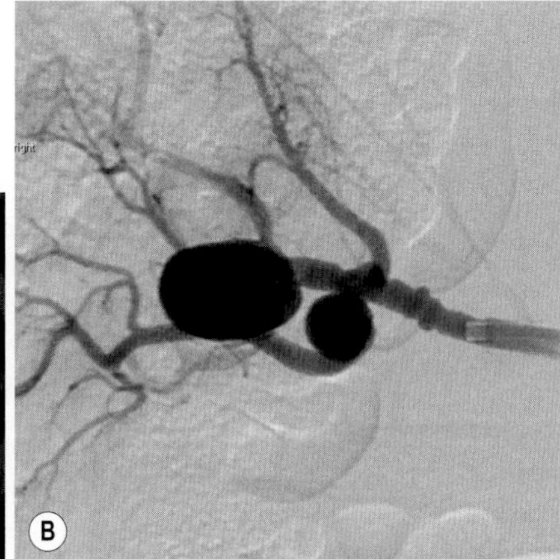

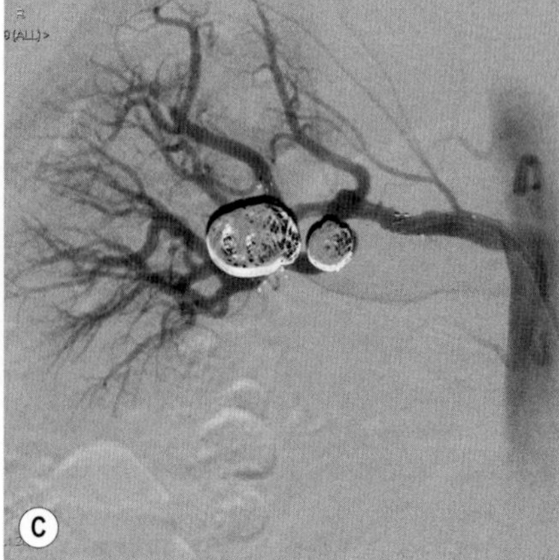

FIGURE 90-6 ■ Renal artery aneurysms. (A) CT MIP image showing two renal artery aneurysms. Both are complex with no neck and arising from branch divisions. (B) Right renal angiogram showing additional irregularity of the proximal renal artery thought to represent fibromuscular disease. (C) Completion right renal angiogram afer second embolisation. Three solitaire detachable stents were used in a stent through stent configuration to preserve blood flow to the kidney and then coils placed through the stents to gain aneurysm thrombosis. A complex case like this can take several hours and cost £15–20,000 in disposable equipment alone.

healthcare system are huge. There is a direct correlation between high blood pressure and cardiovascular risk. Although many patients can be controlled with antihypertensive drugs there is a cohort who do not achieve good control despite multiple medications. This group is estimated to be as high as 30% although in specialist centres, with drug optimisation and having excluded poor compliance and secondary causes, the figure is more likely to be 5%. In this significant minority, until very recently, there was little to offer that was effective.

History of Sympathectomy

The idea of renal denervation is not a new one. Since the 1920s open radical surgical sympathectomy had been practised mainly for malignant hypertension. Although a very invasive procedure it clearly reduced blood pressure and observation studies of over 2000 patients have been reported.[13] Carried out into the 1960s the introduction of modern antihypertensives such as beta-blockers ultimately relegated the procedure to the history books. It was not until the 1990s that interest was renewed with initially rhizotomy in rats and then selective renal denervation using an endovascular approach in pigs. The first reports of successful renal denervation in humans appeared in 2009 with a multicentre ‘proof of principle’ study.[14]

Pathophysiology

The kidneys receive an efferent sympathetic supply from preganglionic brain fibres via the thoracic and lumbar sympathetic trunks, which run through the major visceral ganglia before providing postganglionic supply to the kidneys. Efferent stimulation of the kidneys results in activation of the renin–angiotensin–aldosterone system and leads to water and sodium retention and reduced renal blood flow. In addition, the kidneys have an afferent sympathetic output from both mechanoreceptors and chemoreceptors responding to stretch and ischaemia, respectively. Via the dorsal root ganglia these afferent fibres travel to the cardiovascular centres in the brain (Fig. 90-7). Afferent activation leads to antidiuretic hormone and oxytocin secretion and also plays a role in modulation of systemic vascular resistance. Surrogate markers such as noradrenaline spillover and microneurography have demonstrated sympathetic overactivitiy in essential hypertension and this has a myriad of effects described above, all of which ultimately increase blood pressure.

Both the afferent and efferent sympathetic fibres run within the adventitia of the renal arteries and this is where they are targeted by the RDN procedure.

Technique

This technology is evolving rapidly and at the time of writing only one device is CE marked for clinical use. However, at least another six devices are at various stages of development and will be soon arriving on the market. The current device (Medtronic Inc, USA) uses a small steerable radiofrequency probe placed into the lumen of

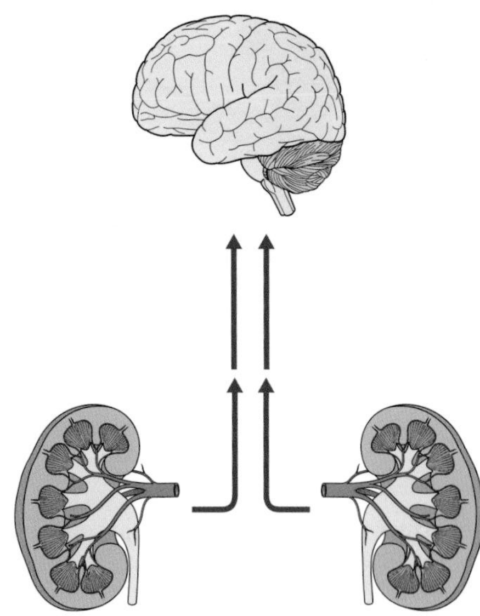

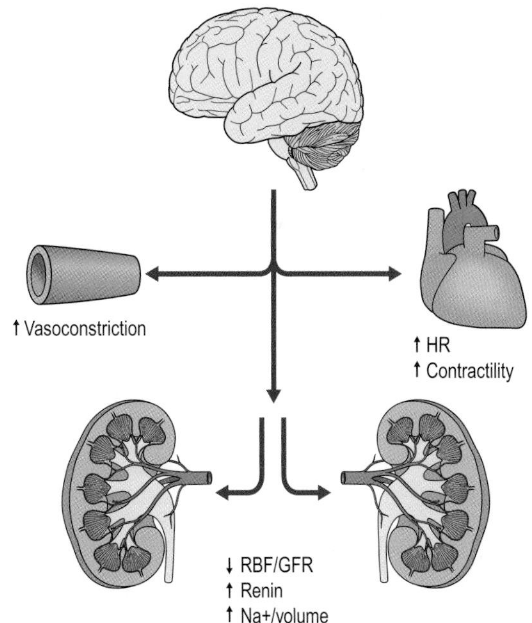

FIGURE 90-7 ■ Afferent and efferent sympathetic innervations of the kidney. (Redrawn from Papademetriou V, Doumas M, Tsioufis K 2011 Renal sympathetic denervation for the treatment of difficult-to-control or resistant hypertension. Int J Hypertens 2011: 196518, Fig. 6.)

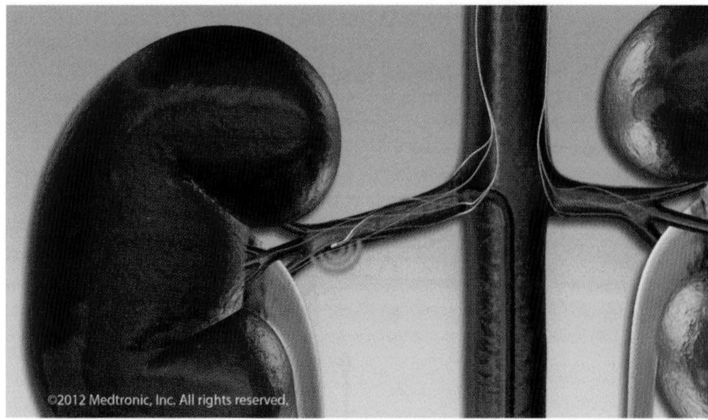

FIGURE 90-8 ■ RDN procedure showing the sympathetic nerves in the adventitia of the renal arteries being ablated with the Ardian device. (Reproduced with permission from Medtronic Inc.)

the renal artery through a guiding catheter from a transfemoral approach (Fig. 90-8). Several pulses (5–7) of energy deployed in a spiral fashion are used to heat up and destroy both the afferent and efferent renal sympathetic nerves lying in the adventitial layer. The procedure is repeated in both kidneys.

Although performed under local anaesthesia the procedure is relatively painful and an analgesic protocol is required. A regimen similar to that needed for fibroid embolisation is suggested. The procedure is commonly carried out as a day case admission.

Indications

The precise indications for RDN are not yet fully developed. The reader is directed to the recent guidance issued by the Joint UK Societies Consensus Statement and NICE in 2012.[15]

Broadly speaking, patients should have a sustained blood pressure of ≥ 160 mmHg (≥ 150 mmHg in type 2 diabetes) on three or more medications. Ambulatory blood pressure measurements should be used. As the procedure is evolving other potentially beneficial effects are being reported. These include reduced insulin resistance, and improved renal and cardiac function. Further research is ongoing in these patient groups.

Results

The early results have been very promising and a randomised controlled trial (Symplicity HTN-2) reported in 2010 showed a mean reduction in blood pressure of 32/12 mmHg in the active group compared to 1/0 mmHg in the control group.[16] This was a highly significant difference $p < 0.0001$. There were no serious procedure-related or device-related complications and occurrence of adverse events did not differ between groups. At the time of writing, further trials are underway (Symplicity HTN-3) and longer term follow-up on both safety and efficacy is needed. NICE have produced guidance for the UK, stating the procedure can be undertaken with 'special arrangements for clinical governance, consent and audit or research'.

Renal Tumours

Intervention for renal tumours is essentially limited to the control of haemorrhage. Preoperative embolisation to facilitate surgical excision although popular in the past is rarely undertaken nowadays with improvements in surgical management.

Benign

Benign renal tumours are rare. Oncocytomas are often indistinguishable from malignant tumours when small and even differentiation at pathology can be challenging. Bleeding is rare but there are case reports in the literature of embolisation being used. Angiomyolipomas are much more common and present a challenge to the interventional radiologist. Although the majority are isolated there is a well-known link with tuberous sclerosis where they are said to be the commonest cause of death. It is in this syndrome and when lesions are > 4 cm in size that the risk of bleeding increases significantly. Spontaneous bleeding occurs in 50–60% when > 4 cm and up to a third of patients present with shock.[17]

Embolisation is the procedure of choice and controls bleeding in over 90% (Fig. 90-9). Embolic agents include particles, alcohol and coils, often in combination. Although there is a potential risk of loss of renal function, this is rare or minimal. Re-bleeding is reasonably common but can be treated with repeat embolisation. Complications are uncommon but include aneurysmal rupture. The angiomyogenic component of the tumour is more sensitive to embolisation than the lipomatous elements and it is the former that is thought to bleed.[18]

Malignant

This group essentially consists of renal cell carcinoma. Spontaneous haemorrhage is not uncommon and indeed may be the initial presentation often with a history of trivial trauma. Usually hypervascular (85%) these tumours are very amenable to embolisation. Provided the other kidney is normal, embolisation of the entire kidney is the simplest approach. Although placing coils in the main proximal renal artery is tempting and easy, a more distal embolisation should be performed as parasitic supply from other vessels, e.g. lumbar arteries, is common and these in turn may need to be embolised. A careful eye should be kept for connections with other vessels such as colic arteries, particularly if liquid embolic agents are contemplated. The choice of embolic agent includes particulate matter (e.g. polyvinyl alcohol), liquids (e.g. alcohol), histoacryl glue or Onyx. When using alcohol, temporary balloon occlusion of the main renal artery will considerably reduce the peri-procedural pain.

Renal Arteriovenous Malformation (AVM)

Renal arteriovenous malformations are abnormal connections between the intrarenal arteries and veins. They are either congenital or acquired (often iatrogenic). Acquired lesions are often termed A-V fistula and are

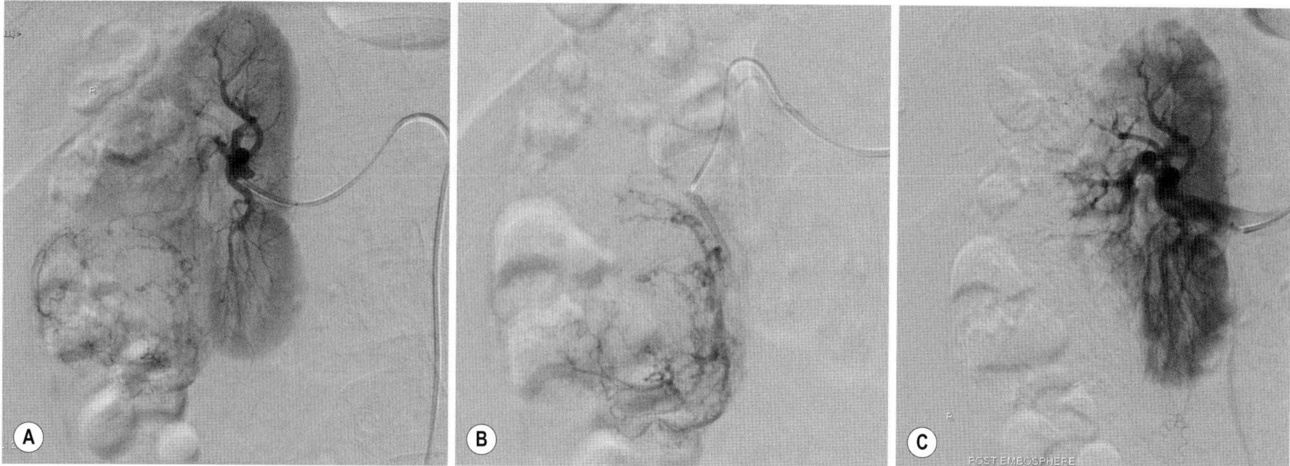

FIGURE 90-9 ■ **Renal embolization—angiomyolipoma presenting with acute loin pain and haematuria.** (A) Right renal angiogram showing abnormal mass of tissue at the lower pole. (B) Super selective angiogram showing multiple abnormal vessels supplying the angiomyolipomatous tissue. (C) Image taken following embolisation with particulate matter showing complete de-vascularisation of the AML.

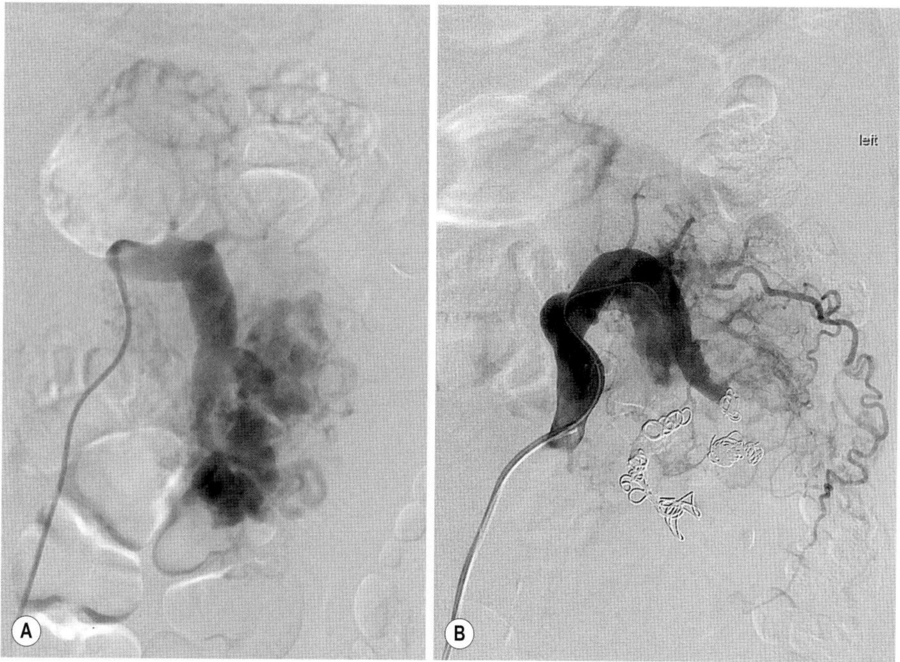

FIGURE 90-10 ■ **Renal arteriovenous malformation.** (A) Left renal angiogram showing massively enlarged left renal artery with a complex AVM involving the middle and lower pole of the kidney. A small upper pole branch is not involved. Patient presented in high output cardiac failure. (B) Renal AVM embolisation. Left renal angiogram following embolisation of the AVM with a combination of coils, alcohol and histoacryl glue.

dealt with in the section 'Trauma Embolisation'. AVMs are either detected coincidentally or present with haematuria and a renal mass. Patients are commonly hypertensive and occasionally there may be so much shunting that high output cardiac failure ensues (Fig. 90-10A). The more common cirsoid lesion has multiple feeding arteries and draining veins with a definite mass. The less common cavernous type consists of a single artery feeding a dilated chamber draining through a single vein. Embolisation has almost completely replaced surgery for these lesions and the results are good with cure being a realistic expectation. However, embolisation of any AVM is always complex and should only be undertaken by those with adequate experience and training. Referral to a tertiary centre is frequent. Embolisation is almost always from the arterial side and it may be necessary to use temporary occlusion balloons to reduce blood flow to control the embolisation process (Fig. 90-10B). Alcohol, histoacryl glue, Onyx and particles have all been used and each has their advocates.

Renal Artery Aneurysms

Visceral artery aneurysms are rare but renal aneurysms make up 22% of the group. The main aetiologies are atherosclerosis, fibromuscular disease (Fig. 90-6) and the other rarer arteritides. Usually asymptomatic and detected incidentally, they can present with hypertension, haematuria or flank or abdominal pain. Indications for treatment are size > 2 cm, symptoms and women who wish to become pregnant. Pseudoaneurysms are usually a result of trauma and dealt with in the section 'Trauma Embolisation'.

Technique

Although there may be the occasional argument for open surgical repair, advances in endovascular technology have led to embolisation being employed in the vast majority of cases. However, embolisation of these aneurysms can be technically very demanding and should be undertaken only by experienced operators. Every attempt should be made to preserve renal tissue and the only excuse for simple embolisation (closing off the vessel distal to the aneurysm) is in small intra-renal lesions where functional loss would be minimal. Loss of renal tissue or even ischaemic renal tissue may lead to troublesome post embolisation hypertension.

Treatment options include coil or liquid embolisation with either an adhesive agent, e.g. histoacryl or a non-adhesive agent such as Onyx. Although these can be used as stand alone therapy some form of protection for the distal renal vessel is often required. Examples include using an angioplasty balloon to prevent reflux of liquid Onyx or stents to 'jail in' coils. New neuroradiology systems with electrolytic released stents (Solitaire EV3, UK) allow complex branches to be preserved by stenting through stents and then using retrievable coils placed through the stent lattices. Although very expensive this technology lends itself to challenging anatomy (Fig. 90-6). There is a case for some form of continued imaging surveillance on an annual basis and smaller aneurysms not treated should also be kept under review.

TRAUMA EMBOLISATION

Haemorrhage control has recently become a major focus for interventional radiology (IR) service provision with increased recognition of its benefits over more invasive open surgery. There is reasonable evidence (although no trials) to show that embolisation can halt traumatic arterial haemorrhage with the advantage over surgery of offering a minimally invasive approach with minimal tissue or organ loss. It can often be carried out under local anaesthesia.

Kidney

Although both blunt and penetrating trauma, e.g. stabbing, is well recognised the majority of cases are iatrogenic in origin from either percutaneous nephrostomy or renal biopsy. Imaging studies have shown a high prevalence (1–10%) of traumatic pseudoaneurysm or A-V fistula following renal biopsy. The majority of these settle with simple observation and embolisation should only be considered if there is expansion of the pseudoaneurysm, persistent pain or frank haemorrhage. If treatment is deemed necessary then embolisation using coils is the procedure of choice. Care should be taken to use a superselective technique with coaxial catheters to ensure a distal embolization, minimising any loss of renal tissue (Fig. 90-11).

Occasionally following major blunt abdominal trauma the main renal artery may be either avulsed or occluded. Usually the kidney will have suffered irreversible ischaemia but on occasion it may be worth considering an

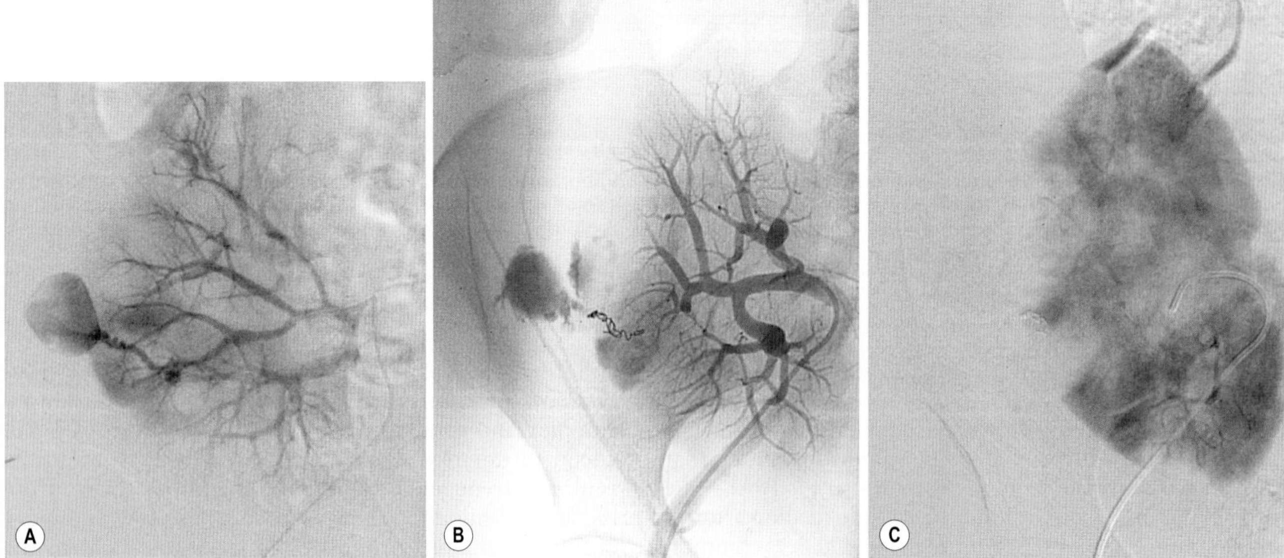

FIGURE 90-11 ■ Renal pseudoaneurysm. Patient with haematuria following biopsy of a renal transplant. (A) Angiogram shows a large pseudoaneurysm. (B) Angiogram following coil occlusion of feeding branch. (C) Late nephrogeic phase showing minimal loss of renal tissue.

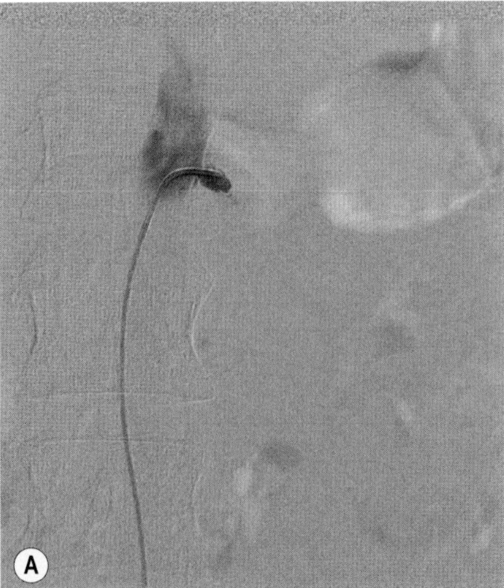

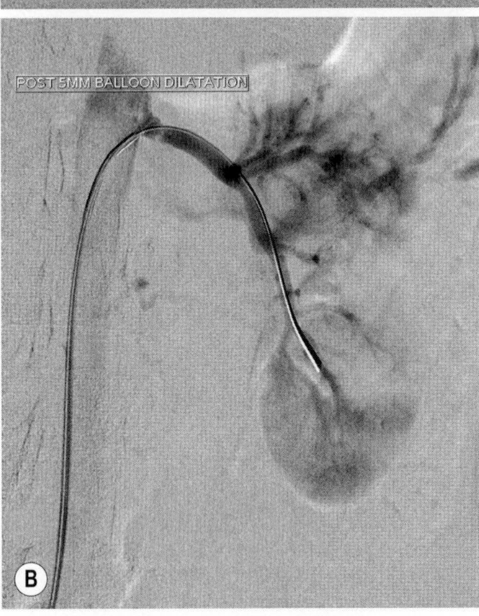

FIGURE 90-12 ■ **Renal artery traumatic occlusion.** (A) Angiogram shows occluded left renal artery with a short stump at origin. (B) Successful recanalistion and angioplasty. (Reproduced by kind permission of Dr A. Todd Raigmore Hospital Inverness.)

attempt to recanalise the vessel using angioplasty or stenting (Fig. 90-12).

Ureter

Ureteric trauma is rare and almost always iatrogenic. Rarely a fistula between the ureter and the adjacent iliac artery can develop and present with massive haematuria. The aetiology is usually related to a ureteric stent eroding through the ureter or direct invasion by cancer. Treatment involves placing an appropriate sized stent graft in the iliac artery.[19]

Bladder

Vascular damage to the bladder or prostate causing intractable haemorrhage is very rare but there are case reports of prostatic embolisation being used after prostatic surgery. Rarely chemotherapy (e.g. cyclophosphamide) can cause a severe haemorrhagic cystitis requiring embolisation.[20]

PROSTATIC ARTERY EMBOLISATION

Symptomatic benign prostatic hyperplasia (BPH) is a common condition typically presenting in the sixth and seventh decades. Over 40% of males will be symptomatic usually presenting with lower urinary tract symptoms (LUTS) such as hesitancy, frequency and urgency. Extreme cases present as an emergency with acute urinary retention. Standard treatment is usually with drugs such as 5-alpha reductase inhibitors and selective alpha-blockers. When these fail, the classical surgical procedure is transurethral resection of the prostate (TURP), although recently other options such as laser and microwave ablation have been under evaluation.

Prostatic artery embolisation is not new and has been used sporadically for haemorrhage since 1976. However, its potential use in controlling the symptoms of BPH has only recently been reported.[21]

Rather similar to fibroid embolisation it relies on occluding the blood supply to the prostate gland, thereby reducing the volume of the gland and its pressure on the urethra (Fig. 90-13). The procedure involves catheterising the prostatic arteries and embolising with a propriety embolic agent, e.g. PVA particles. Early experience to date (2012) is limited to two centres (in Brazil and Portugal) who have collectively treated about 90 patients. The procedure is technically demanding due to the size of the vessels, tortuosity and anatomical variation and failure rates of up to 30% are reported. Complications have included bladder wall ischaemia, rectal bleeding and urethral pain. Mean reduction in prostatic volume appears to be around 30% with an improvement in both quality of life and objective urinary symptom scores. Several patients using long-term catheters have been able to re-establish normal micturition. Advantages over surgery may include lack of incontinence and preserved sexual function.

Clearly an exciting new procedure, the long term outcomes and durability are unknown. Prostatic embolisation is currently undergoing assessment by NICE (2012) in the UK.

FIBROID EMBOLISATION

Uterine Artery Embolisation (UAE)

Uterine fibroids are the commonest tumour found in women of reproductive age and the prevalence increases up to the menopause where it can be as high as 80% in some ethnic groups (Afrocarribean). At least half of women with fibroids are asymptomatic and need no active treatment. Symptoms include menorrhagia, pain and pressure; the pressure symptoms commonly involve the bladder and occasionally the bowel. A further group either has problems conceiving or suffers early pregnancy loss. The pathophysiology behind all these symptoms is not clear and in particular the link between fibroids and infertility is tenuous and may only apply to submucosal locations. Women with fibroid-related menorrhagia often have more severe menstrual loss than those with dysfunctional uterine bleeding and are more resistant to standard medical care.

Treatment Options

Medical management includes drugs such as non-steroidal anti-inflammatories, anti-fibrinolytics and hormonal manipulation. Second-line treatment includes the progesterone intrauterine device (Mirena coil) and endometrial ablation. These second-line measures are only technically feasible if the uterine cavity is less than 12 cm in length and not distorted by the fibroids. Third-line management is either surgical (myomectomy or hysterectomy) or uterine artery embolisation (UAE). Current guidance states that all treatment options should be discussed with patients so that they can make an informed choice.

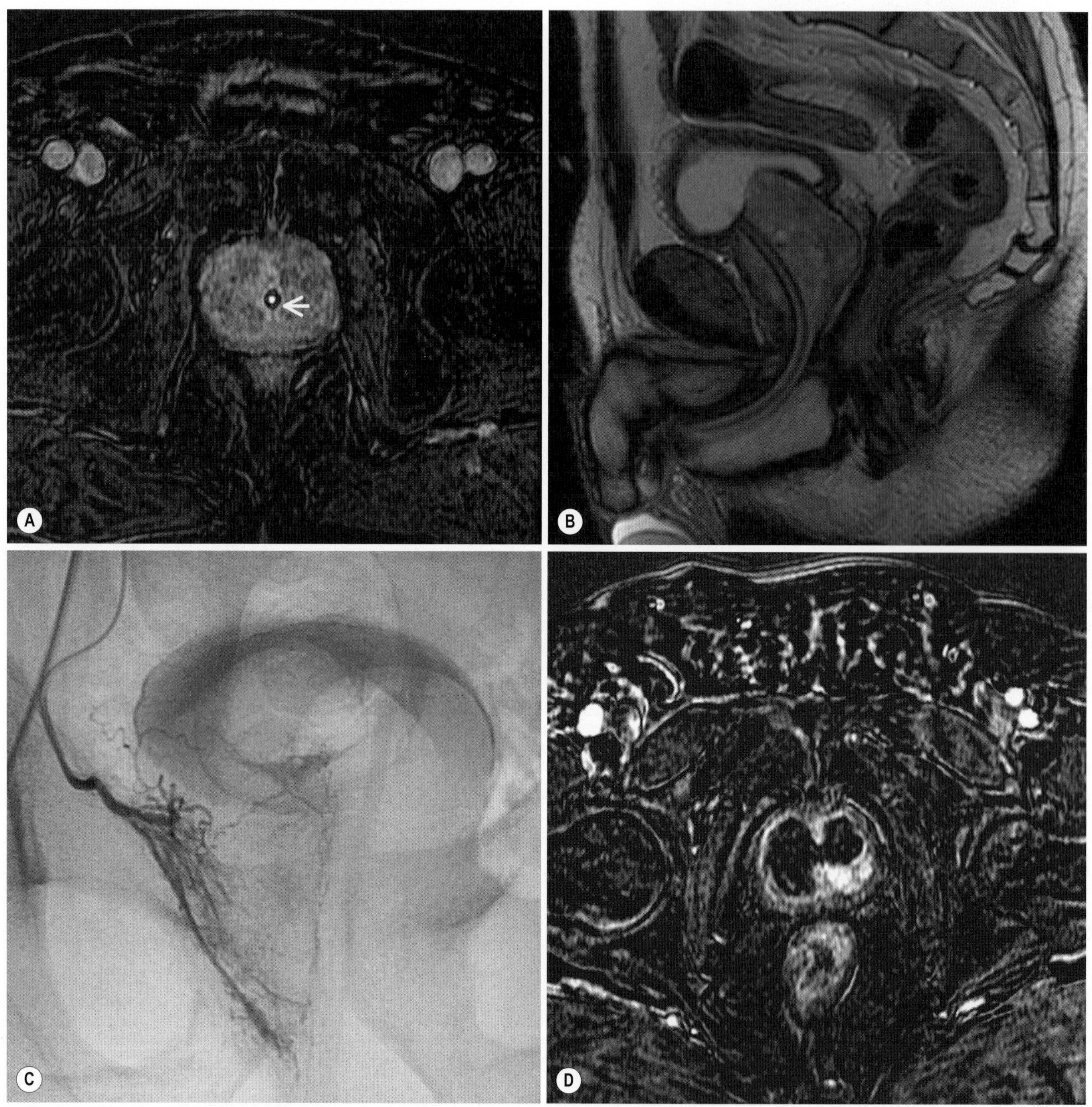

FIGURE 90-13 ■ (A) Pre-embolization MRI. Axial post-contrast T_1-weighted image depicting the enlarged prostate due to central gland nodules. Note the presence of the urethral catheter (white arrow). (B) MRI pre-embolization. Sagittal T_2-weighted image depicting an enlarged prostate due to central gland nodules protruding into the bladder neck. Note the presence of the urethral catheter. (C) Arteriogram after superselective catheterization of the right inferior vesical artery showing the right prostate arteries—urethral arteries (black arrow) and the capsular arteries (white arrow). (D) One-month post-embolization MRI. Axial post-contrast T1-weighted image depicting bilateral avascular areas (mainly on the right side) in the central gland (white arrows), and reduction of the prostate size.

Continued on following page

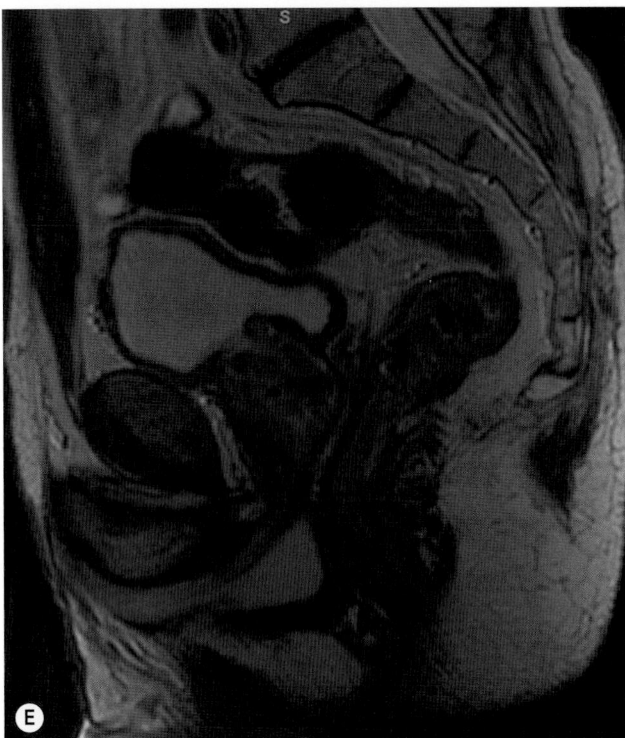

FIGURE 90-13, Continued ■ (E) MRI post-embolization. Sagittal T2-weighted image showing a reduction of the central gland size. (Reproduced with kind permission from Dr FC Carnevale, MD. PhD, Professor and Chief of Interventional Radiology, University of Sao Paulo, Brazil.)

Imaging

Some form of baseline imaging is essential prior to embarking on UAE. This is to firmly establish the diagnosis, exclude other pathologies and assess the number of fibroids and their location. Although ultrasound is inexpensive, it lacks the precision of MRI and suffers from operator expertise and poor assessment of vascularity. The general availability of MRI should make this the imaging modality of choice (Fig. 90-14A) and contrast enhancement should be used routinely. Occasionally a non-enhancing fibroid which would not be suitable for UAE is seen. Adenomyosis is a not-infrequent concomitant finding and can cause identical symptoms to fibroids. It is not a contraindication to embolisation but the outcomes are less robust than with fibroids alone. Although almost any fibroid can be embolised there are situations where surgery may be more effective, examples include a submucosal fibroid on a stalk where hysteroscopic resection is simple and effective. More controversy surrounds pedunculated subserosal fibroids and very large lesions but increasingly these are being safely embolised. Clearly UAE is not appropriate if the diagnosis of fibroids is in any doubt and it should be remembered that neither MRI nor any other imaging modality can reliably detect the very rare coincidental leiomyosarcoma unless there are signs of extrauterine spread.

It is increasingly common practice and reassuring to repeat the MR imaging at around 6 months to confirm infarction and tumour shrinkage (Fig. 90-14B).

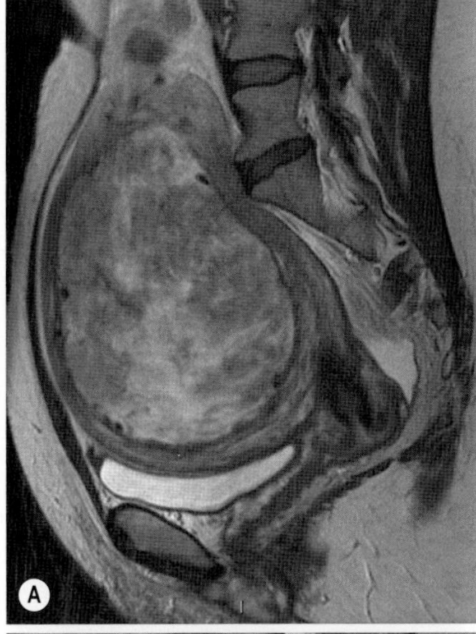

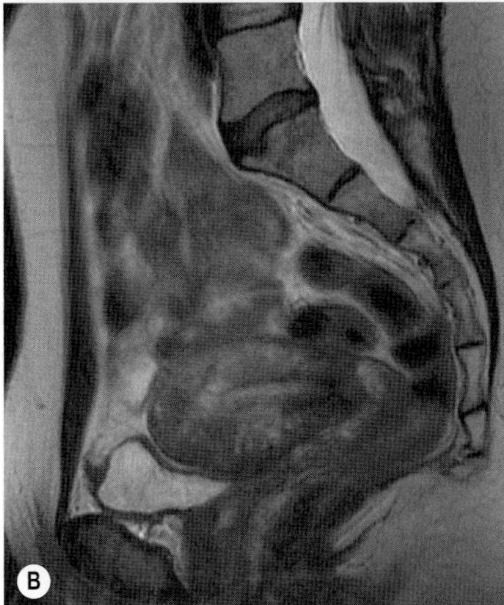

FIGURE 90-14 ■ **Fibroid uterus.** (A) Sagittal T_2-weighted image showing a large intramural fibroid. (B) Sagittal T_2-weighted image following uterine artery embolisation shows complete resolution of fibroid.

Technique

Preoperative preparation is essential for this procedure. The patient will usually be admitted on the day of the procedure and expect to be staying for one night. This is purely to manage the post embolisation pain, which if improperly controlled can be very severe. An analgesic protocol should be in place ideally agreed in liaison with the anaesthetic department. Analgesia should be administered on the ward prior to UAE, during and after the procedure. Opioid drugs are required with antiemetics and can be given using a patient-controlled pump if desired. Patients will be discharged on oral analgesia.

The procedure itself is relatively straightforward and not painful. Prophylactic antibiotics are often administered. Access is from the right common femoral artery and using a 4–5F cobra-shaped catheter the aortic bifurcation is crossed and the contralateral anterior division of the internal iliac artery selected. It is common practice

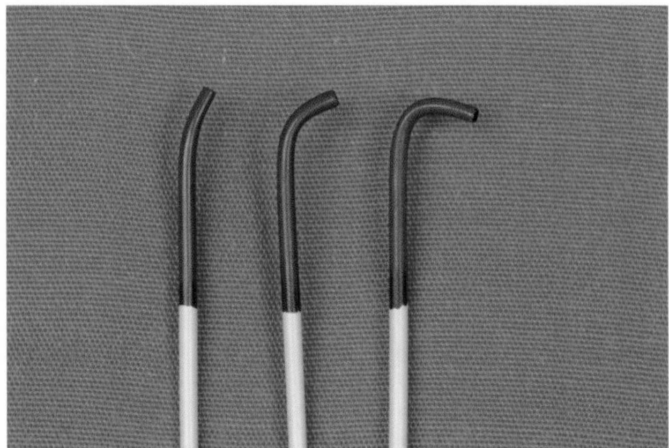

FIGURE 90-15 ■ Catheters. The various types and shapes of Vanschie catheter tips (Cook, UK) used for selective uterine artery catheterisation.

at this stage to use a coaxial catheter to select the uterine artery. This minimises the risk of spasm, allowing free flow embolisation. The choice of embolic agent is often one of operator preference and there is no evidence that any of the newer more expensive agents are superior to standard non-spherical PVA. Particle size ranges between 300 and 700 μm and a frequently used embolic end-point is complete stasis in the uterine artery. The catheter is then withdrawn and the ipsilateral internal iliac and uterine artery selected and embolised. Occasionally the anatomy can be challenging and other catheter shapes such as a reverse curve or Vanschie (Cook, Europe) are required (Fig. 90-15). A minority of operators use a bilateral femoral artery approach claiming a reduction in radiation burden.

Safety and Efficacy

NICE has recently (2011) updated its guidance on UAE, stating it can be carried out using 'normal arrangements'.[22] Complications are usually minor and include the post embolisation syndrome (pain, fever, raised inflammatory markers), vaginal discharge and infection. Major complications are less frequent and include severe infection, fibroid expulsion and premature ovarian failure. When compared with surgical options the incidence of complications is very similar, albeit the complications are different.

Long-term follow-up from several randomised trials,[23–25] a Cochrane review[26] and a meta-analysis[27] has shown a similar improvement in quality of life and patient satisfaction compared with surgery but there is a need for re-intervention in a significant minority (20–30%) after UAE due to either complications or recurrent/persistent symptoms. The advantage of UAE over surgery is a significantly faster recovery time with more rapid return to normal activities and uterine preservation. Re-intervention does not always mean hysterectomy and if there is incomplete fibroid infarction, repeat UAE can be offered and is often successful.

Questions still remain, particularly the role of UAE in women wishing to preserve their fertility. A small trial has suggested superior pregnancy outcomes with myomectomy[28] but a much larger trial (FEMME; <http://www.hta.ac.uk/project/2378.asp>) is now underway in the UK.

OBSTETRIC HAEMORRHAGE

The World Health Organisation estimates that severe bleeding complicates 10% of all live births and accounts for 24% of all maternal deaths annually.[29] However, in the developed world there has been a dramatic reduction in maternal death due to haemorrhage. Advances in blood transfusion, surgical techniques and critical care have all made major contributions. However, major obstetric haemorrhage (MOH) remains a major cause of maternal morbidity and is the leading cause in Scotland (4.3/1000 live births).[30] A wide range of clinical interventions is now available and has been proposed in the management of MOH, including:

- Pharmacological agents (recombinant activated factor VII);
- Intrauterine balloons;
- Uterine compressive suture (B Lynch suture);
- Supportive interventions (cell salvage); and
- Interventional radiological techniques (embolisation and balloon occlusion).

In 2006 the Royal College of Obstetricians and Gynaecologists recommended the early involvement of interventional radiology in the management of post partum haemorrhage (PPH).[31] One challenge for IR is to provide a deliverable 24/7 service (which is still patchy in some countries, e.g. the UK) before obstetricians will fully accept its role.

Post Partum Haemorrhage

The definition of PPH depends on the timing and blood loss. Primary PPH occurs within the first 24 hr of delivery and involves a blood loss of at least 500 cc. Secondary PPH occurs after 24 hr and is usually linked to either retained parts and/or infection.

Causes of PPH

- Uterine atony—the commonest cause > 50%
- Genital tract lacerations
- Abnormal placentation
- Post caesarean section or hysterectomy
- Rare causes, e.g. uterine AVM

Management of PPH

Embolisation is never the first-line treatment but should also not be used as a last resort. Units should develop their own agreed algorithm but a generic strategy would include standard use of uterotonics, and removal of any retained parts. If this fails then an intrauterine balloon is a simple and effective next step with reported success rates as high as 91%.[32] If the abdomen is already open then a uterine compression suture, e.g. B-Lynch, can be placed. If these measures are ineffective then embolisation should be used with the primary aim of stopping bleeding and preserving the uterus. Avoidance of maternal mortality is critical. Obstetric units can measure the effectiveness of their PPH algorithm by auditing the peri-partum hysterectomy rate.

Technique

Although CT angiography is now used routinely prior to embolisation in the gut or following trauma, it is infrequently deployed in PPH, as it is usually obvious on clinical grounds whether haemorrhage is occurring. However, it may have a role in recurrent bleeding or post hysterectomy. The embolisation technique is fairly standard and very similar to that used for fibroids. Access, however, is best from a bilateral common femoral artery approach with catheterisation of the anterior divisions of the internal iliacs and embolisation of the offending bleeding point (usually the uterine artery) with Gelfoam. A negative angiogram should prompt a search for other vessels particularly if post-caesarean section or hysterectomy (Fig. 90-16). However, a negative angiogram is not uncommon particularly with uterine atony. It has become accepted practice to carry out 'empirical embolisation' in these circumstances although there is little high quality evidence to support this strategy. Almost always bilateral embolisation will be required as there is such a good cross flow collateral circulation in the pelvis. Failure to control PPH by embolisation is rare but more likely to occur with abnormal placentation (see section below). Continued haemorrhage requires good clinical judgement and a hysterectomy may be unavoidable. Recurrent bleeding can usually be re-embolised.

Abnormal Placentation

Abnormal placentation occurs when a defect within the decidua basalis allows invasion of the chorionic villi into the myometrium. There are three types (Fig. 90-17) with the least invasive (accreta) being the most prevalent (84%). Placenta accreta refers to a placenta invading the myometrium. Placenta increta (13%) occurs when the serosa is reached and percreta (3%) when invasion occurs beyond the serosa into adjacent structures such as the bladder. Maternal morbidity is clearly related to the degree of invasion. Abnormal placentation has increased in incidence by a factor of 10 over the past 50 years and the most important risk factors are the combination of previous caesarean sections and placenta previa. Ideally this condition should be suspected and confirmed pre-natally to allow a management plan. Imaging modalities include US and increasingly MRI but the sensitivities vary from 33 to 95%. The more severe case with bladder invasion is easier to detect. This condition is the leading cause of a peri-partum hysterectomy and carries a maternal mortality of up to 7%.

Management of Abnormal Placentation. If confirmed or suspected pre-natally an organised pre-delivery strategy should be put in place involving an interventional radiologist. The plan must include the location of delivery, e.g. interventional or obstetric theatre, availability of cell salvage for blood transfusion and a decision whether to try to preserve the uterus, possibly leaving the placenta in situ or a planned caesarean hysterectomy. Whatever is decided these are complex procedures and fully informed consent should be obtained by both the obstetrician and interventional radiologist. The patient's view on caesarean hysterectomy is important and should be respected if possible. Bilateral common femoral artery access should be established. Some suggest that after establishing access, the IR should wait and see how the caesarean section progresses. If the bleeding can be controlled by surgical means no embolization may be required. However, many would be more pro-active and place at least guidewires and possibly occlusion balloons in the common iliac, internal iliacs or uterine arteries and inflate these just prior to incising the uterus or placenta. Care should be taken to correctly size the balloons and particular care taken if the uterine arteries are catheterised prior to delivery (Fig. 90-18). There are anecdotal reports of anoxia in the child where balloons have been inflated in the uterine arteries, which are sensitive to spasm. There are reports of parasitic supply to the uterus from branches arising from the common femoral artery and others and the author's preference is to use common iliac balloons, which will cater for most extrauterine supply. On occasion an aortic occlusion balloon may be useful as a last-resort life-saving manoeuvre. If balloon inflation controls the haemorrhage, and the obstetrician can suture satisfactorily, embolisation may not be needed. However, if on deflating the balloons bleeding returns then embolisation will be required. Depending on the balloon position, this may require further selective catheterisation. Embolisation should always be as targeted as possible. Gelfoam is the usual embolic agent although almost all other particle types have been reported. If the decision has been made to leave the uterus and placenta in situ, embolisation of the uterus may facilitate subsequent placental involution.

Complications of Embolisation and Balloon Occlusion

In experienced hands the complications rates should be low and this is supported by the literature. Most complications are minor and puncture site-related. However, major complications can occur and include buttock and lower limb ischaemia, small bowel, uterine, vaginal, cervical and bladder wall necrosis.[33] Neurological damage involving the sciatic and femoral nerves has occurred. Control of PPH can be challenging for the interventional radiologist; sometimes the imaging equipment is suboptimal, e.g. a mobile C-arm, plus the added pressure of needing to work quickly in an already overcrowded obstetric theatre environment.

Results of Haemorrhage Control for PPH

There is little doubt that embolisation for PPH works: a meta-analysis of nonsurgical management found a

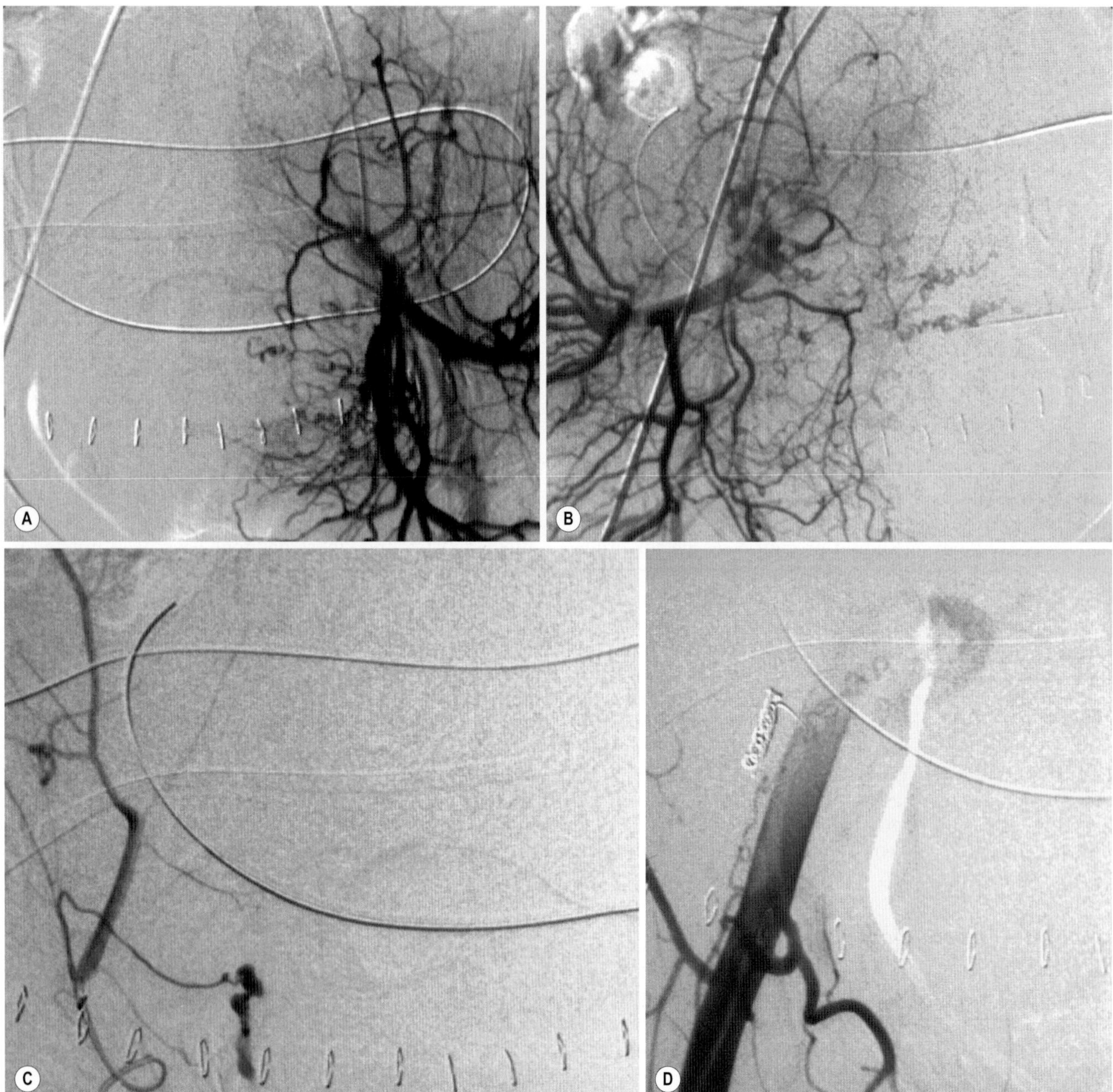

FIGURE 90-16 ■ **Patient bleeding after emergency caesarean section.** (A) Selective left and (B) right internal iliac artery angiograms show no evidence of uterine bleeding. (C) A selective angiogram of the right inferior epigastric artery shows frank extravasation of contrast from a muscular branch of the rectus muscle. (D) Initial occlusion of the distal inferior epigastric prior to particulate embolisation of the small branch.

cumulative success rate of 91%.[34] A recent national cohort study carried out in the UK (226 maternity units) identified 272 women who were treated with one or more second-line treatments, representing an estimated rate of 2.2 cases per 10,000 women delivering.[35] The success rates of the first second-line therapy were as follows: uterine compression sutures 75%, pelvic vessel ligation 36%, embolisation 86% and rFVII 31%. The overall peri-partum hysterectomy rate was 26%.

Outcomes for abnormal placentation are less clear and the literature produces conflicting results. It is likely that an invasive placenta is a predictor for embolisation failure and the more invasive the placenta, e.g. percreta, the worse the outcome. This probably reflects the aggressive blood supply from both uterine and non-uterine arteries. Clear benefit to mother and child requires further research and study.

Ectopic Pregnancy and Spontaneous Abortion

Cervical ectopic pregnancy is very rare (0.15% of all ectopics) but carries a significant haemorrhagic risk. Embolisation has been reported for both active bleeding and prior to dilation and curettage.[36] Re-bleeding is relatively frequent (25%) and may require further embolisation or a more radical surgical solution. Post abortion haemorrhage can usually be controlled medically but there are sporadic case reports of successful embolisation in the literature.[37]

PELVIC CONGESTION SYNDROME

Chronic pelvic pain is a common problem affecting women aged between 18 and 50 years. Pelvic congestion syndrome (PCS) is one of the many possible causes of this condition. Dull pelvic ache is thought to be secondary to ovarian and pelvic varicosities. Incompetent venous valves, multiple pregnancies, effect of oestrogen, retroaortic left renal vein, compression of left ovarian and renal veins by superior mesenteric artery and compression of left common iliac vein by right common iliac artery are proposed predisposing factors.[38] By the time of referral to an interventional radiologist patients will usually have already undergone extensive investigation and imaging often including laparoscopy. Cystic ovaries are seen in more than half of these women. Vulval or leg varicosities may also be present. MRI with MR venography (Figs. 90-19, 90-20) is a valuable

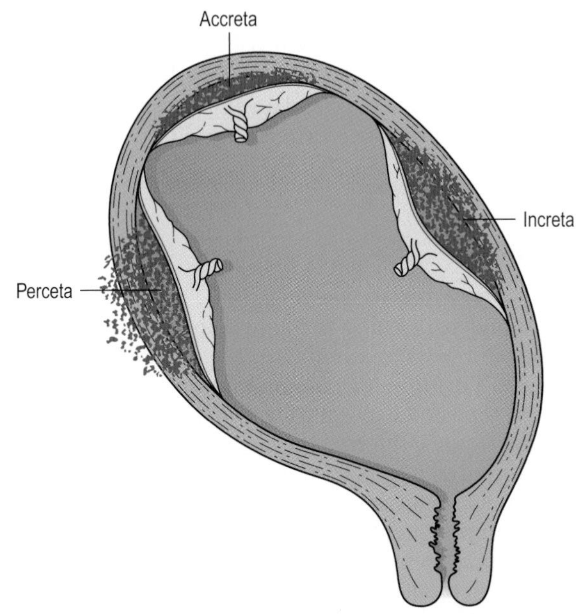

FIGURE 90-17 ■ Classification of invasive placenta. Image showing different degrees of placental invasion into the uterine wall.

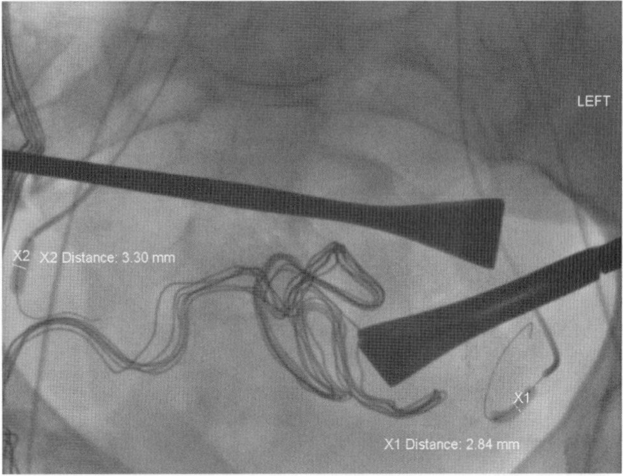

FIGURE 90-18 ■ Uterine artery balloon occlusion. Patient with an invasive placenta undergoing prophylactic balloon occlusion of both uterine arteries to minimise blood loss during caesarean section.

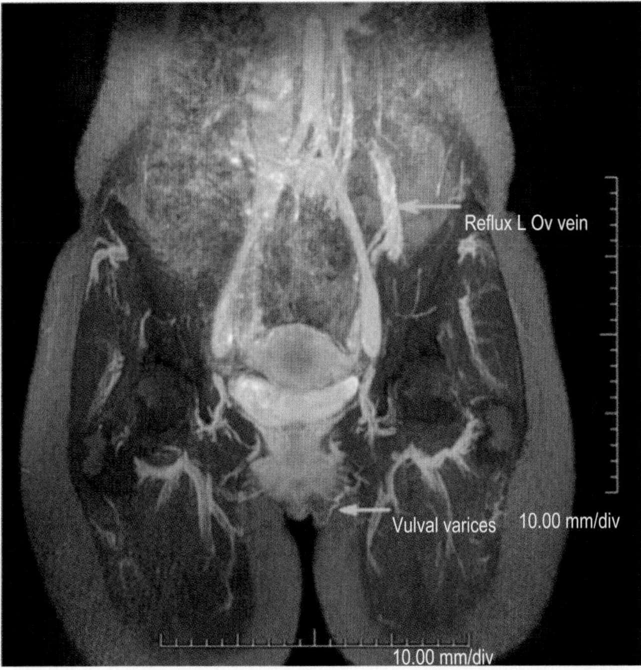

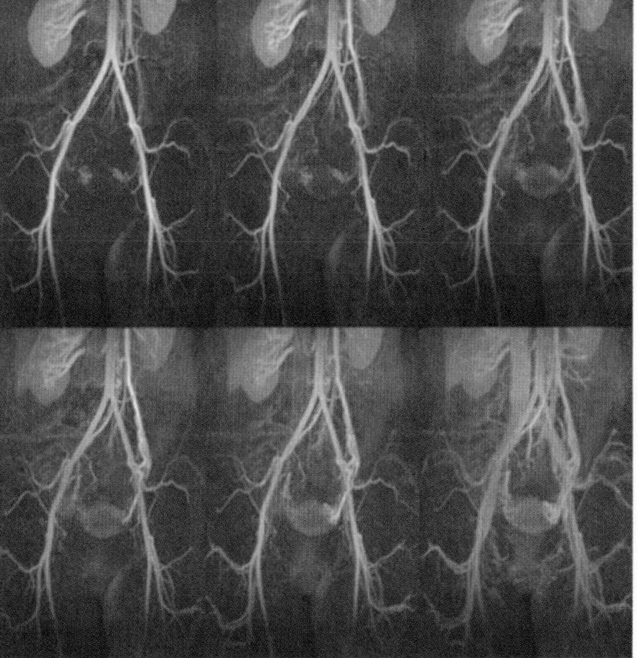

FIGURE 90-19 ■ Dynamic multiphase first-pass MIPs and subsequent steady-state phase slab MIP of contrast-enhanced MRA/V of abdominopelvic veins. Patient with vulval varicosities demonstrating rapid early reflux in incompetent left ovarian vein. (Reproduced with permission from Giles Roditi, Magnetic Resonance Venography in Clinical Blood Pool MR Imaging 2008, pp 115–130. Fig 10.16A.)

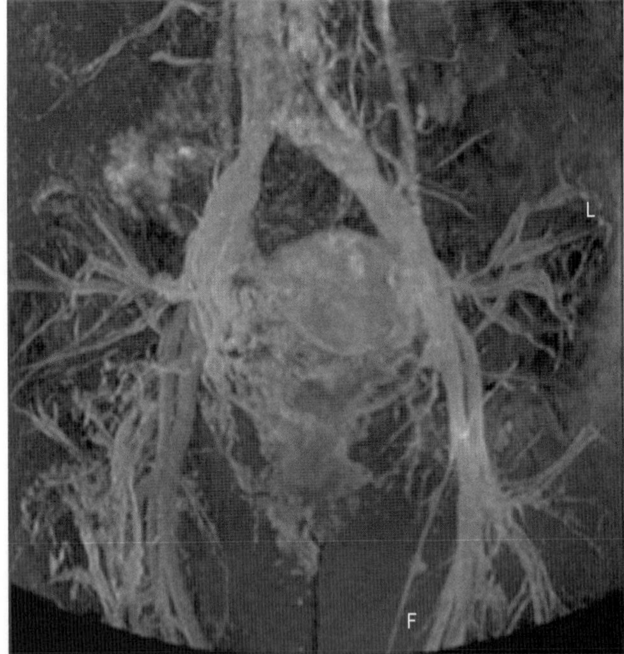

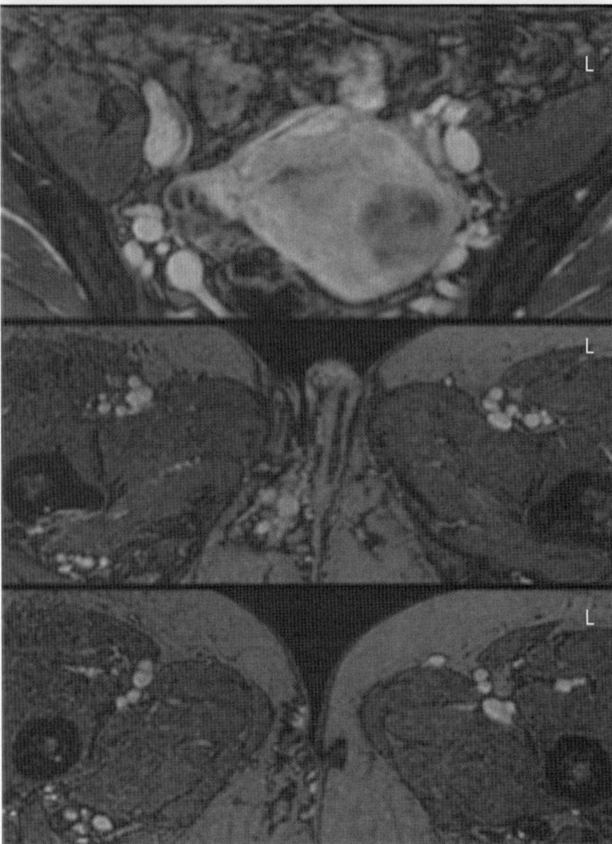

FIGURE 90-20 ■ Coronal MIP of pelvis in steady state in patient with vulval varicosities demonstrating ipsilateral deep venous varicosities in right thigh draining to internal iliac pelvic venous varicosities (incidental uterine fibroid). (Reproduced with permission from Giles Roditi, Magnetic Resonance Venography in Clinical Blood Pool MR Imaging 2008, pp 115–130.)

TABLE 90-2 Diagnostic Criteria for PCS on Venography

- 5 mm or greater diameter of ovarian vein
- Retrograde flow in ovarian or pelvic veins
- Presence of tortuous collateral veins in pelvis crossing the midline
- Delayed clearance of contrast from pelvic veins

non-invasive imaging tool. However, all non-invasive imaging suffers from potential venous collapse in the supine position and many will still perform conventional catheter ovarian vein venography with the table tilted head up to fully assess gonadal vein incompetence. Generally agreed diagnostic criteria for PCS[39] are listed in Table 90-2.

Treatment

Ovarian vein embolisation (Fig. 90-21) is usually straightforward and performed through either a right common femoral vein or increasingly a right internal jugular vein approach. This is a day case procedure and embolisation has been reported using a wide variety of embolic agents including liquids, sclerosants, gelfoam, coils and vascular plugs. It is often necessary to embolise both ovarian veins. Technical success rates are high and some have reported clinical improvement in 83% of patients.[40] Clinical failures may be due to additional incompetent internal iliac venous collaterals and more aggressive workers also target these claiming good results. Complications are rare and include venous perforation, non-target embolisation and thrombophlebitis.

Vulval varices can cause labial hypertrophy affecting one or both side. If troublesome these can be treated by direct injection sclerotherapy using sodium tetradecyl sulphate (STD). It is important in these cases always to exclude and treat any ovarian venous incompetence first.

VARICOCOELE

The male equivalent of PCS, a varicocoele, is an abnormal dilatation of the pampiniform plexus of veins draining the testes resulting from an incompetent testicular vein. A common condition said to afflict up to 10% of males it is usually asymptomatic, requiring simple reassurance. When symptomatic the discomfort is described as a dragging sensation usually in the left testicle often worse during strenuous activity. In 10–15% of cases they can be bilateral. Patients with unilateral right-sided varicocoele should be evaluated for pathology such as renal tumours, retroperitoneal lymphadenopathy and anatomical variants such as situs inversus. Ultrasound has a very high sensitivity and specificity and tortuous veins greater than 3 mm are considered diagnostic.[41] Typically, on palpation they are described as a 'bag of worms'.

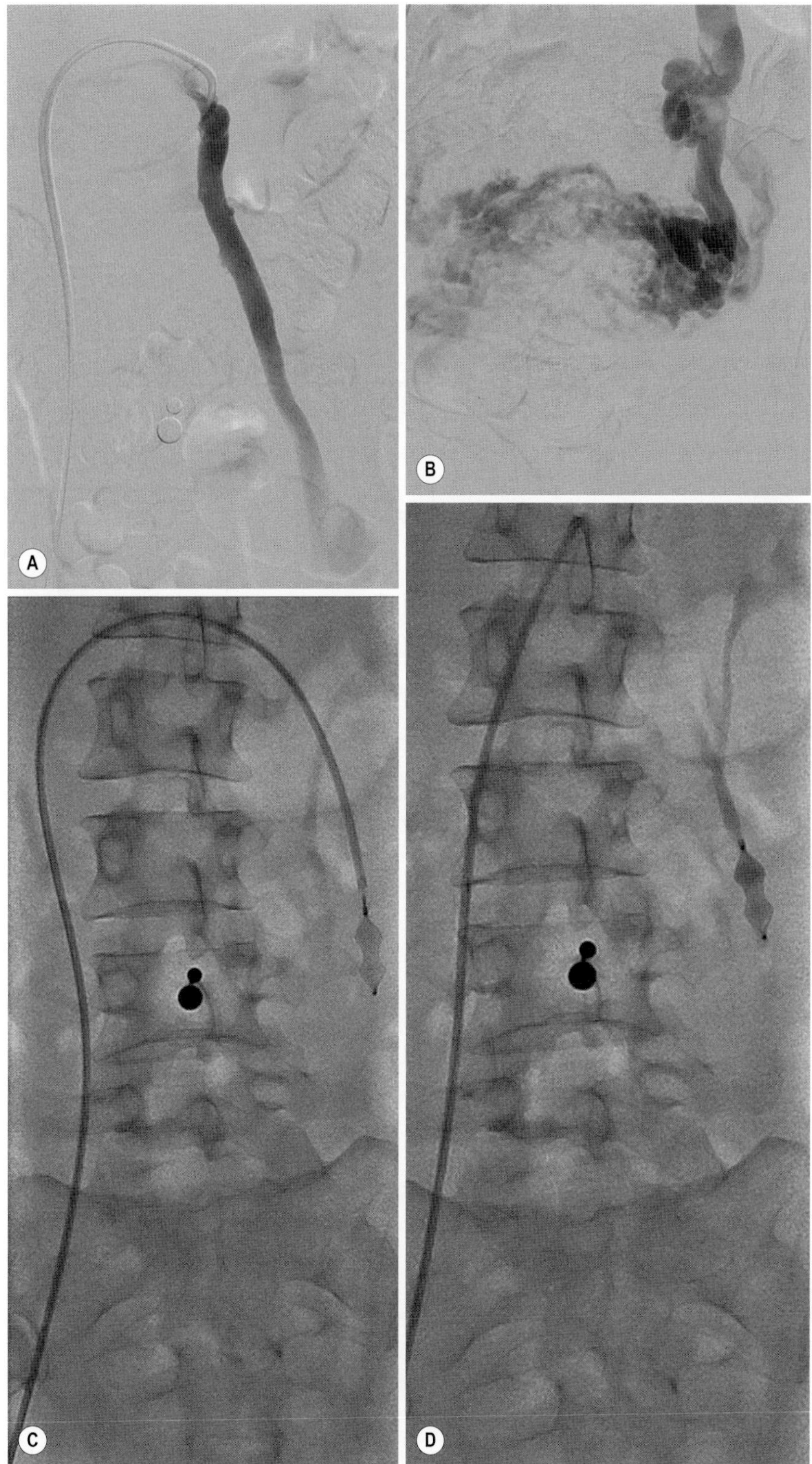

FIGURE 90-21 ■ Ovarian vein embolisation. (A) Left renal venogram shows reflux into the left ovarian vein. (B) Venogram shows enlarged left ovarian vein and tortuous pelvic veins crossing midline. (C, D) Deployment of Amplatzer vascular plug in the left ovarian vein from right femoral vein approach.

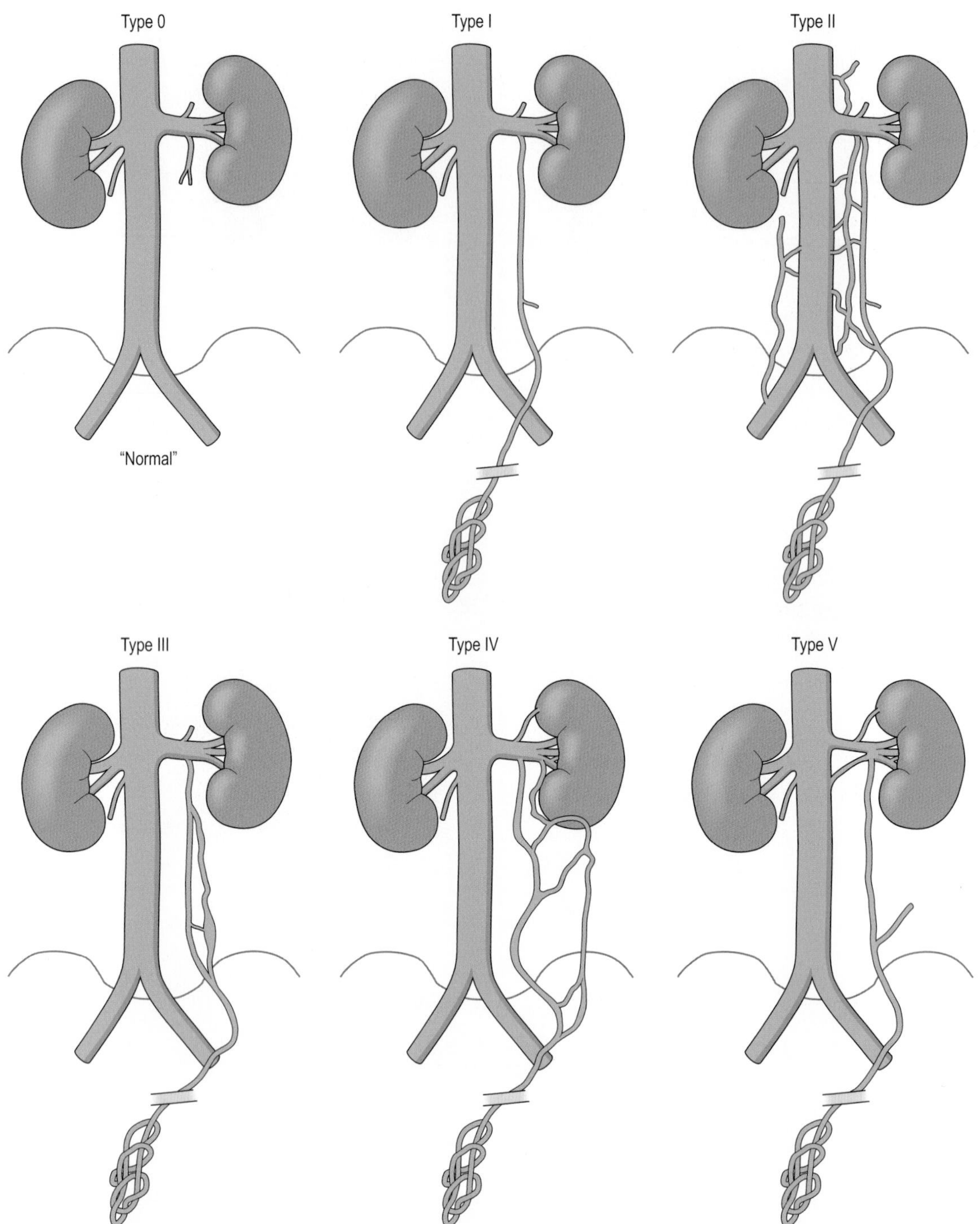

FIGURE 90-22 ■ Line diagram showing anatomical variants of testicular venous drainage. (Redrawn from Sigmund G, Bahren W, Gall H, et al 1987 Idiopathic varicoceles: feasibility of percutaneous sclerotherapy. Radiology 164(1):161–168.)

Varicocoeles are sometimes discovered during investigations for male infertility but although improvement in sperm density, motility, morphology and testicular volume after treatment have been reported, NICE guidelines currently state, 'Men should not be offered surgery for varicocoeles as a form of fertility treatment because it does not improve pregnancy rates.'[42]

There is a lot of anatomical variation in testicular venous drainage. A recognised description is presented as shown in Fig. 90-22. See also Table 90-3.

Treatment

Although the gonadal vein can be ligated in the inguinal canal or from a pre-peritoneal laparoscopic approach,

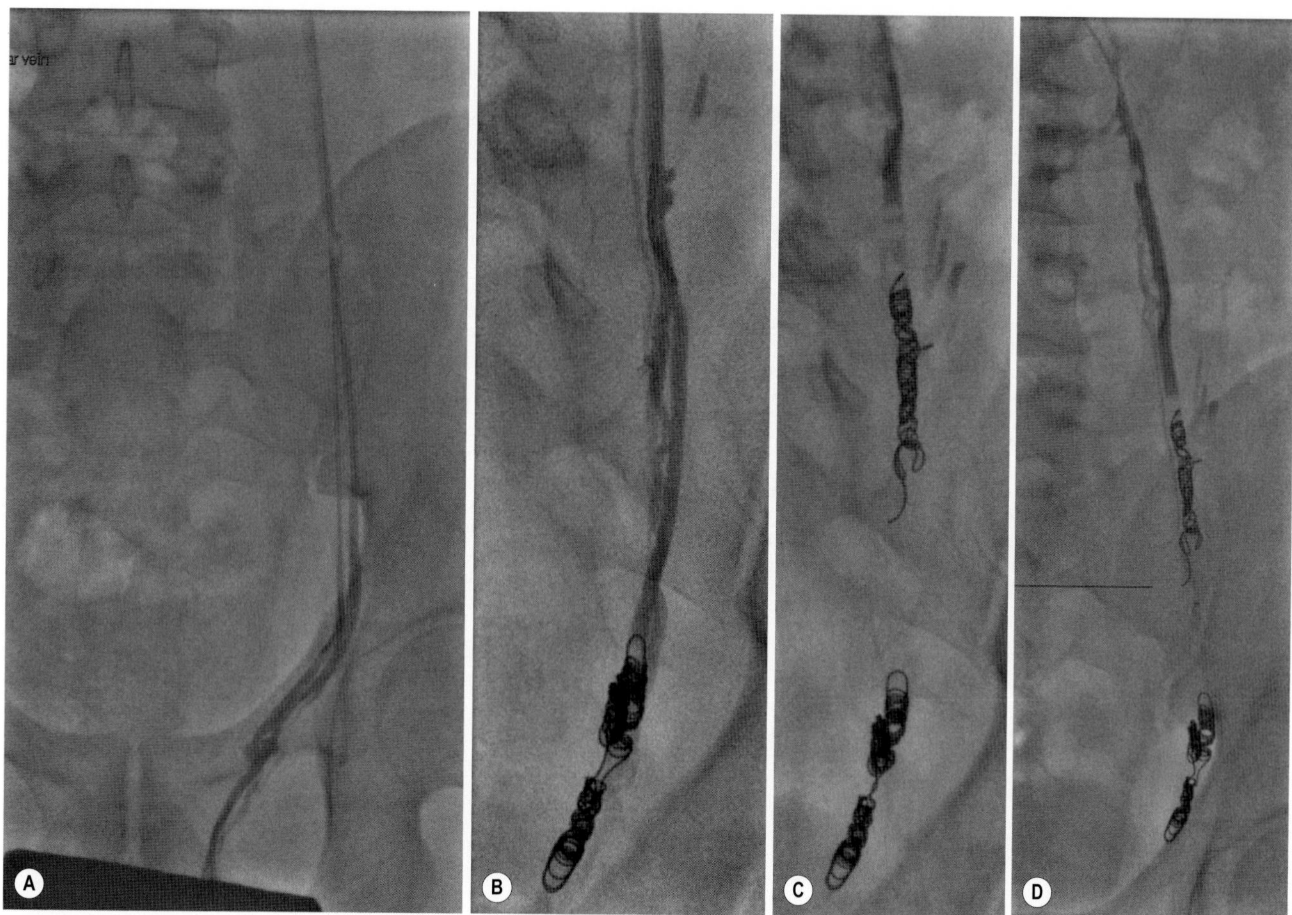

FIGURE 90-23 ■ **Left varicocoele embolisation.** (A) Venogram of left spermatic vein and (B–D) images showing embolisation with multiple coils.

TABLE 90-3 **Classification of Gonadal Vein Anatomy**

Type 0	Normal
Type I	Single testicular vein without valves
Type II	Afferent collateral medial retroperitoneal vessels to the ascending lumbar or retroperitoneal veins
(IIa	No valve)
(IIb	Valve present at entry into renal vein)
Type III	Duplicated testicular vein/internal spermatic vein
Type IV	Collateral flow from lateral renal vein and peri-renal veins to testicular vein
(IVa	No valve)
(IVb	Valve present and bypassed by insufficient collaterals)
Type V	Bifurcated renal vein with a retroaortic component

embolisation (Fig. 90-23) has become the mainstay of modern minimally invasive treatment. A simple day case procedure undertaken from either a common femoral but increasingly right jugular vein approach, the left renal vein and the left testicular vein are selectively catheterised. Venography is performed to confirm reflux and delineate the anatomy. The right testicular vein usually arises from the IVC directly around the level of the right renal vein and is more difficult to select. Almost every embolic agent manufactured has been reported in this procedure but the majority of operators will choose to use simple embolisation coils, placing these fairly distal at the level of the inguinal ligament. Embolisation is performed from distal to proximal. Complications related to the procedure include venous spasm, perforation and non-target embolisation and thrombophlebitis post procedure. Care is taken to minimise the radiation dose to the testes by using a gonadal shield.

Although the technical success rate is close to 100% the clinical results are lower at around 85%. It should be appreciated there are other causes of scrotal pain and the varicocoele may simply be coincidental.

For a full list of references, please see ExpertConsult.

FURTHER READING

1. Textor SC. Revascularization in atherosclerotic renal artery disease. Kidney Int 1998;53:799–811.
7. Wheatley K, Ives N, Gray R, et al. Revascularization versus medical therapy for renal-artery stenosis. N Engl J Med 2009;361(20): 1953–62.
11. Tegtmeyer CJ, Matsumoto AH, Angle JF. Percutaneous transluminal angioplasty in fibrous dysplasia and children. In: Novick A, Scoble J, Hamilton G, editors. Renal Vascular Disease. 1st ed. London: WB Saunders; 1995. p. 363–83.
16. Esler MD, Krum H, Sobotka PA, et al. Renal sympathetic denervation in patients with treatment-resistant hypertension (The Symplicity HTN-2 trial): a randomised controlled trial. Lancet 2010; 376:1903–9.
21. Carnevale FC, Antunes AA, Motta-Leal-Filho JM, et al. Prostatic artery embolization as a primary treatment for benign prostatic hyperplasia: preliminary results in two patients. Cardiovasc Intervent Radiol 2010;33(2):355–61.
25. Moss J, Cooper K, Khaund A, et al. Randomised comparison of uterine artery embolisation (UAE) with surgical treatment in patients with symptomatic uterine fibroids (REST trial): 5-year results. BJOG 2011;118:936–44.
26. Gupta JK, Sinha A, Lumsden MA, Hickey M. Uterine artery embolisation for symptomatic uterine fibroids. Cochrane Database Syst Rev 2012;(5):CD005073.
29. World Health Organization (WHO) Department of Reproductive Health and Research. Maternal mortality in 2000: estimates developed by WHO, UNICEF, and UNFPA. WHO, Geneva; 2004.
31. Royal College of Obstetricians and Gynaecologists. The role of emergency and elective interventional radiology in postpartum hemorrhage. Royal College of Obstetricians and Gynaecologists Good Practice Guideline No. 6. Royal College of Obstetricians and Gynaecologists, London. Available at: http://www.rcog.org.uk/womens-health/clinical-guidance/role-emergency-and-electiveinterventional-radiology-postpartum-haem; 2007.
42. NICE | Clinical Guideline 11. Fertility: assessment and treatment for people with fertility problems. Available from: http://www.nice.org.uk/nicemedia/live/10936/29267/29267.pdf.

CHAPTER 91

Non-vascular Genitourinary Tract Intervention

Uday Patel • Lakshmi Ratnam

CHAPTER OUTLINE

INTRODUCTION

The genitourinary (GU) tract is especially prone to anatomical and morphological variations and successful intervention relies on careful anatomical appreciation and planning. This chapter describes the various interventional procedures currently used in the GU tract, but commences with a review of the anatomy relevant to renal access, as this is the cornerstone of most GU interventions.

PERCUTANEOUS RENAL ACCESS—IMPORTANT ANATOMICAL FACTORS

Renal Position

The kidneys lie in the perinephric space at the level of T12 to L2/3 vertebral bodies. The upper pole is more medial than the lower, with a coronal axis tilt of about 15°. The upper pole is also more posterior facing than the lower. In the short axis the renal pelvis points anteromedially. Anatomical disposition in the 3 planes is illustrated in Fig. 91-1.

Relations of the Kidney

The important relations regarding renal access are those adjacent structures that may be inadvertently injured—the liver, spleen, diaphragm, pleura/lung and the colon. Variant anatomy should also be remembered: for example, the splenic flexure of the descending colon may be abnormally high and posterior (said to be more common in obese women). Pre-procedure ultrasound (US) will identify these hazards.

Pelvicalyceal Anatomy of the Kidney

The adult kidney has approximately 8–9 calyces. Typically, the upper and lower pole calyces are fused; and therefore larger and easier to access. Calyces will also vary in orientation, facing either relatively anterior or posterior. The posterior calyx is ideal for access, being closer to the skin surface. Posterior calyces also allow better intrarenal navigation; e.g. the route from a posterior to an adjacent anterior calyx or the renal pelvis is more or less in a straight line forward. However, access to the pelviureteric junction (PUJ) and ureter is easier from an interpolar or upper pole calyx. These points are illustrated in Fig. 91-2.

Renal Vascular Anatomy

The main renal artery divides into a (larger) anterior division and smaller posterior division, and each division further separates into segmental and lobar divisions (Fig. 91-3). Peripherally, the lobar and arcuate arteries skirt around the calyx. Thus, the safest place to puncture a calyx is its middle.[1,2] Puncture into the infundibulum or renal pelvis may lacerate larger arterial branches. A

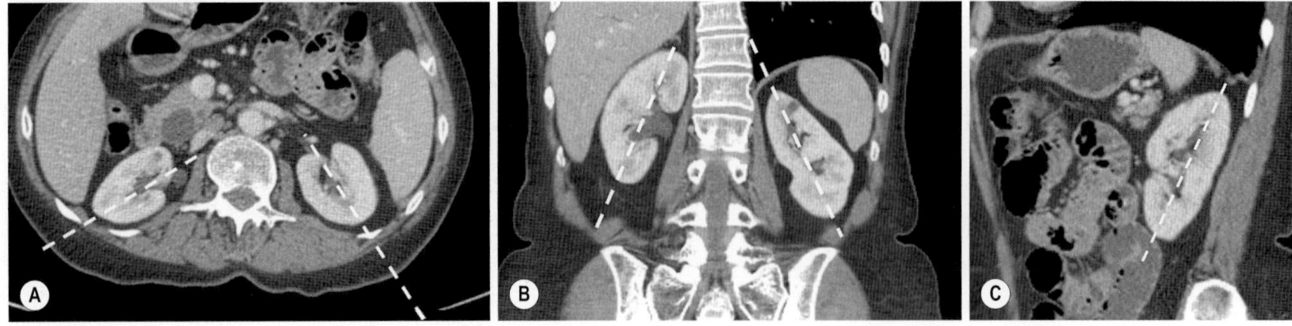

FIGURE 91-1 ■ CT images of the renal axis and disposition. CT images of the renal axis and disposition in the axial (A), coronal (B) and sagittal (C) planes. Note that the pelvis faces anteromedially and the upper pole is more medial and posterior.

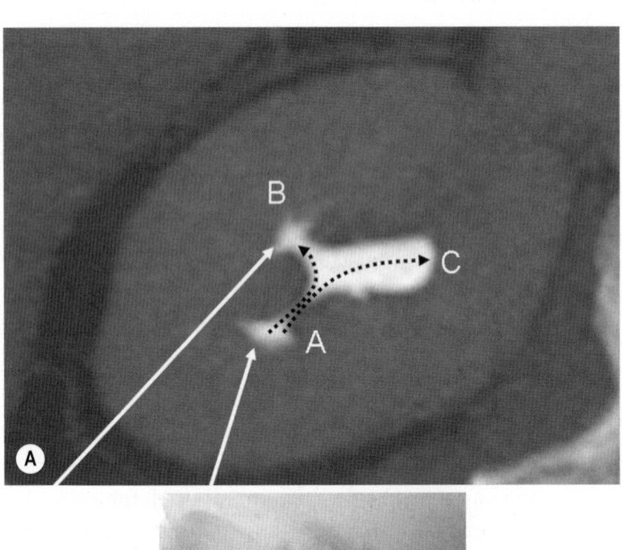

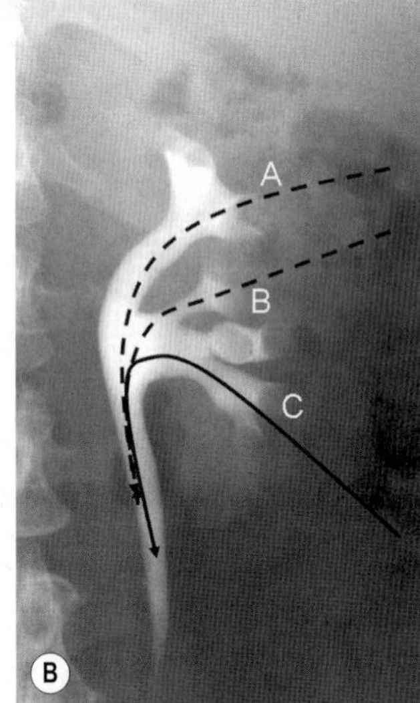

FIGURE 91-2 ■ Calyceal selection for renal access. These two images illustrate the importance of choosing the right calyx for renal access. (A) Axial CT image showing entry into a posterior-facing calyx A allows easy navigation into the anterior calyx B as well as towards the infundibulum and the renal pelvis C. Entry into an anterior calyx B would be poor for intrarenal navigation. (B) Coronal fluoroscopic image demonstrating that upper pole A or interpolar entry B is better for ureteric access. Lower pole entry C is less favourable.

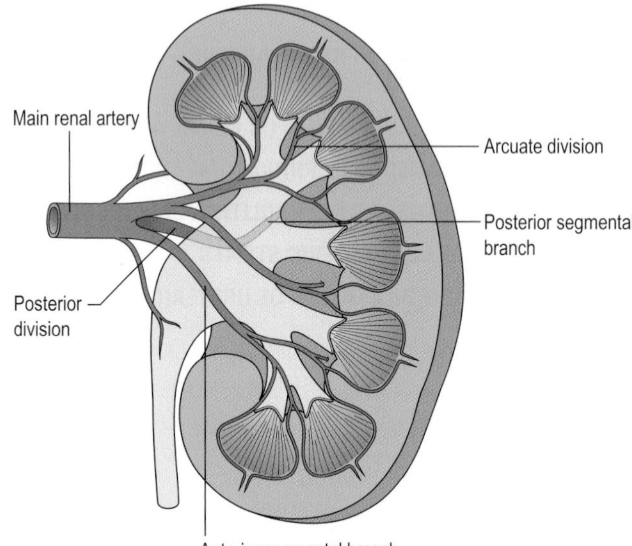

FIGURE 91-3 ■ Normal renal arterial anatomy as seen from the front. Note that the posterior division of the main renal artery lies behind the collecting system, and is vulnerable during percutaneous renal access in the prone position, especially if a more medial puncture is made.

further potential hazard is the posterior division, which is the only major renal arterial division that lies *posterior* to the collecting system. Typically it lies behind the upper renal pelvis but occasionally it is behind the upper pole infundibulum, where it may be injured if entry is misdirected towards the infundibulum rather than the upper pole calyx. Normally there is a single renal artery and vein, but up to 25% of kidneys have more than one renal artery and variant renal veins are seen in 3–17%. These do not influence access, but may explain the occasional vascular injury that occurs despite adherence to safe anatomical principles.

Other Anatomical Factors Important for Renal Access

Part of either kidney will lie above the eleventh/twelfth rib, especially the left kidney, and upper pole access may require an intercostal entry, placing the intercostal artery or pleura at risk. The intercostal artery runs in a groove

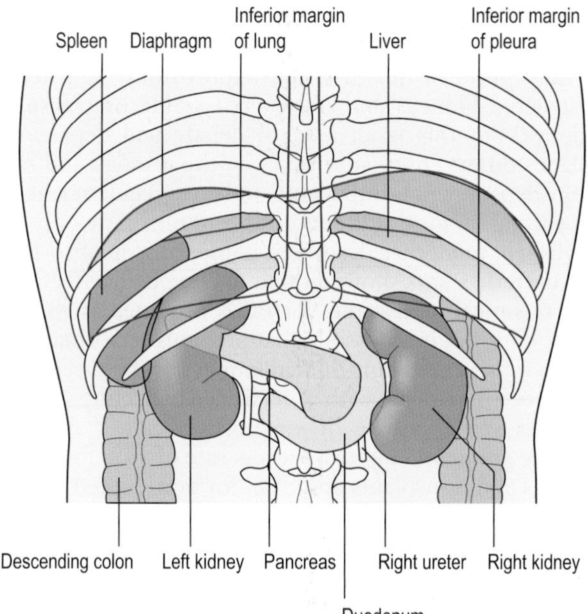

FIGURE 91-4 ■ Posterior view of the kidneys and their immediate anatomical relationships. The pleura can reach down to the twelfth rib, but veers away from the ribs laterally. Therefore, if renal access is performed above the twelfth rib, it should be laterally placed. However, too lateral a puncture may injure the liver or spleen.

underneath the rib and is vulnerable with angled cephalad needle puncture. The posterior reflection of the parietal pleura is horizontal and reflected off the lateral portions of the ribs, and puncture through the latter half of the intercostal space is theoretically safer (Fig. 91-4).

Renal Anatomy and Percutaneous Entry

From this discussion, it can be appreciated that there are numerous factors to consider when planning safe, effective percutaneous renal access. The important considerations are summarised in Table 91-1. The safest point for calyceal puncture is the centre of the calyx, approached through the relatively avascular plane (Brödel's line) between the branches of the anterior and posterior divisions of the renal artery. Puncturing the centre of the calyx avoids injury to the arcuate divisions that course around the infundibulum. This is the ideal, and is illustrated in Fig. 91-5.

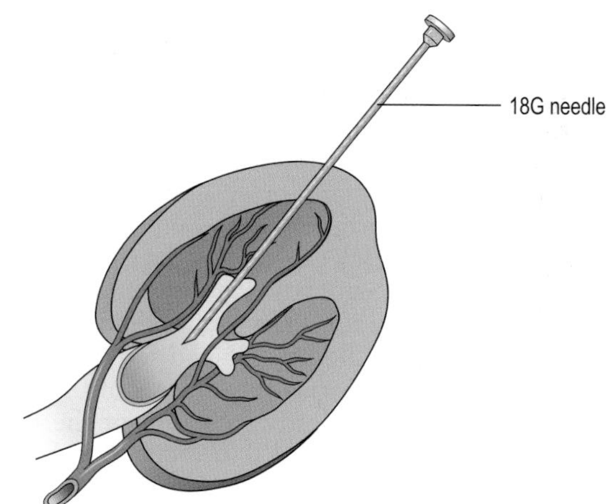

FIGURE 91-5 ■ The safest place to puncture a calyx. The safest place to puncture a calyx is its middle, (see text).

TABLE 91-1 Anatomical Considerations That Influence Renal Access in a Normally Sited Kidney

1. The Lie of the Kidney
   a. The upper pole is more posterior.
   b. The short axis lies posterolaterally.
2. The Calyces
   a. The calyces lie either anterior or posterior.
   b. Upper or lower calyces are often compound or fused and so bigger.
3. Vascular
   a. There is a theoretically 'avascular' line along the lateral margin of the kidney.
   b. The lobar branches course in a curvilinear fashion around the calyx and papilla.
   c. The posterior segmental division may lie *behind* the upper pole infundibulum.
4. Adjacent Structures
   a. Pleura lies above the 12th and 11th ribs laterally.
   b. Intercostal artery lies underneath the rib.
   c. Liver, spleen and (left) colon may overlie the upper pole.

To summarise: A lower pole, posterolateral puncture of the centre of the calyx is theoretically the safest. The upper pole is more posterior and allows for easier navigation but must be approached with due care.

GENERAL EQUIPMENT FOR RENAL ACCESS

Personal preference may determine choice of equipment, but some general principles can help guide selection.

Access Needle

The two broad choices are a one-part 21G needle system (sometimes known as a micropuncture access system) or a one-part 18G/4Fr sheath system. With the former, the puncture is with a 21G needle, through which a 0.018-inch. platinum-tipped wire is inserted, followed by a 4Fr dilator and finally a 0.035-inch. working guidewire. A one-part system is an 18G diamond point needle, over which is a 4Fr sheath and the whole is inserted as a single unit. The puncture size is smaller with the two-part system (21G vs 18G or 0.032 inch vs 0.048 inch diameter) and should be safer, but this has not been proven.[3]

Guidewires

The ideal puncture site is the centre of a calyx, but the calyx is a small structure with a usually even smaller outlet. Thus to navigate out of the calyx, a soft flexible wire with good torque is important, whereas rigidity is less vital. We favour either a straight-tipped Bentson wire or an angled-tipped hydrophilic wire. With the former wire, the floppy tip should not be too long. Once the guidewire has been manipulated out of the calyx (ideally down into the ureter, or at least into the renal pelvis), rigidity becomes more important, and a stiffer Amplatz-type wire is useful, especially if the track is being dilated for PCNL or a stent is being inserted through a malignant stricture. A stiff shaft hydrophilic wire has particular merits, being both rigid and kink resistant, whereas the other guidewires can kink. Kinks impede catheter advancement and lead to rupture of the renal pelvis.[4] The standard diameter is 0.035 inch, but thinner wires, especially with stiff inner cores, e.g. nitinol core, can be useful with tight ureteric strictures.

Catheters

Used for either navigation or drainage. For the former, a short angled-tip (e.g. Kumpe) or Cobra shape, high-torque catheter is best. Hydrophilic catheters are useful for bypassing tight ureteric strictures. For drainage, a pigtail catheter with large holes along the inner surface of the pigtail is chosen, as these are less likely to obstruct once the system decompresses. Any size > 6Fr should suffice, but the pigtail may not easily form in a small renal pelvis. The location and size of the drainage holes in the pigtail ensures good drainage. The pigtail should assist anchorage, especially with a locking system, but they do still fall out, and we routinely also further secure them in place (see below). Drainage catheters less frequently used are straight catheters or those with a Malecot-type tip, both useful with the small renal pelvis.

PERCUTANEOUS NEPHROSTOMY (PCN)

Percutaneous nephrostomy insertion is a commonly performed interventional procedure, most frequently for the relief of renal obstruction, with or without associated infection, and some further indications are listed in Table 91-2.

Ideally, a nephrostomy should be performed within working hours, on a stable, well-resuscitated and monitored patient. However, it is also important not to unnecessarily delay renal decompression, especially in those with suspected pyonephrosis or infected hydronephrosis, as these patients can rapidly deteriorate.[4] Our practice is to only perform out-of-hours nephrostomy in infected obstructed kidneys and obstructed single or transplant kidneys, but this is an area of debate and department policies differ. Discussion between the urology and radiology department is important, and an agreement reached depending on local skill sets and resources. The only two published randomised studies comparing nephrostomy and ureteric stents showed them to be equally effective.[5,6] The technical success rate for PCN is quoted as 98–99% of patients, but it is possible that previous series may have under-represented non-dilated kidneys as the success rate is reduced in patients with non-dilated collecting systems, complex stone disease or staghorn calculi.[7–9] Available practice guidelines quote a success rate of 98% for dilated systems and transplants and 85% for non-dilated systems and staghorn calculi.[10]

There are no absolute contraindications to performing a PCN. Severe coagulopathy is a relative contraindication but this can be corrected. In patients with a limited life expectancy, a nephrostomy should be inserted only if this would lead to improved quality of life and survival. In all cases a multidisciplinary approach and close liaison with referring clinicians is essential.

Techniques

Patient Preparation and Procedure

Written consent should be obtained for all PCNs. Acceptable thresholds for complications are listed in Table 91-3. Where local complication rates are known, these should inform the consent process. Intravenous access and adequate hydration should be established; metabolic acidosis and hyperkalaemia should be corrected. A normal coagulation profile, with an INR <1.3 and platelet count of >80,000/dL, should be ensured. Antibiotic prophylaxis should be given,[11] especially if there is clinical evidence of infection. A single dose of a wide-spectrum agent is sufficient for low-risk patients. In high-risk cases, (elderly, diabetic, indwelling urinary catheter, bacteriuria, ureteroenteric conduit), antibiotics may have to be continued and modified appropriately once urine culture results are known.

TABLE 91-2 Indications for Insertion of PCN

1. Urinary tract obstruction from internal or external causes: stones, malignancy, sloughed papillae, crossing vessels, retroperitoneal fibrosis, iatrogenic causes (operative damage to ureter producing oedema/ stricture)
2. Pyonephrosis or infected hydronephrosis
3. Urinary leakage or fistulas
4. Access for interventional or endoscopic procedures: ureteric stenting, PCNL, delivery of chemotherapy/ medication (stone dissolution, antibiotic therapy for fungal infection), foreign body retrieval, biopsy
5. Urinary diversion for haemorrhagic cystitis

TABLE 91-3 Accepted Thresholds for Major Complications for PCN

Complication	Incidence (%)
Septic shock requiring major increase in level of care	4
Septic shock (in setting of pyonephrosis)	10
Haemorrhage requiring transfusion	4
Vascular injury (requiring embolisation or nephrectomy)	1
Bowel transgression	<1
Pleural complications	<1
Complications resulting in unexpected transfer to an intensive care unit, emergency surgery or delayed discharge	5

From ref 10.

Insertion is usually performed in the prone or prone oblique position. A true lateral or supine/oblique position is feasible; however, this increases the technical difficulty, with a greater risk of trauma to the liver, spleen or bowel. CT guidance may help if there is concern about variant anatomy. The procedure is usually performed under monitored sedo-analgesia. In addition, a local anaesthetic agent is infiltrated down to the renal capsule. Occasionally, when dealing with a confused or restless patient it may be safer to perform the procedure with the assistance of an anaesthetist, who can maintain a deeper level of sedation with safety, whilst the interventionist focuses on performing the procedure.

Following puncture of an appropriate calyx, a small amount of urine is aspirated to confirm the position of the needle. If the urine is clear, and the patient does not demonstrate any signs of sepsis, a small volume of iodinated contrast medium (approximately 10 mL) is injected into the collecting system. Over-distension should be avoided as this greatly increases the risk of bacteraemia. If the puncture site is acceptable, a wire is inserted and the track dilated for catheter insertion (single puncture PCN—Fig. 91-6). If the puncture site is revealed to be unsuitable (i.e. entry is into an infundibulum or the renal pelvis) then a second puncture should be performed into a more suitable calyx (double puncture PCN—see below).

Single Puncture Ultrasound-Guided PCN

On ultrasound, the posterior calyces are the most superficial and medial with the patient lying prone. With advances in ultrasound equipment and technique, primary puncture of a target calyx has become more common and is usually uneventful in a dilated system,[7] allowing for a single puncture PCN.

Single Puncture Fluoroscopically Guided PCN

Intravenous iodinated contrast medium can be used to opacify and select a suitable calyx. On fluoroscopy of an opacified collecting system, the calyces that demonstrate the largest range of movement when viewed on continuous screening (with tube below couch) from +30 to −30 oblique positions are the most posterior calyces. Being non-dependent, posterior calyces will be also be the least densely opacified in a prone position. Double contrast pyelography can also be used to highlight the posterior calyces as any gas (air or CO_2), being buoyant, will preferentially gravitate into the non-dependent parts of the collecting system. Not more than 20 mL of gas should be injected slowly and under continuous fluoroscopy. Care should be taken to avoid gaseous extravasation into the surrounding tissues, vessels or the retroperitoneum. Once a suitable calyx is identified, the needle is inserted under fluoroscopic guidance (Fig. 91-7).

Double Puncture Combined Ultrasound and Fluoroscopy-Guided PCN

The collecting system is initially punctured under ultrasound guidance. Ideally the definitive calyx for PCN should be punctured and subsequent tract dilatation and catheter insertion carried out under fluoroscopic guidance. However, if definitive calyceal entry is not feasible (e.g. when the calyces are small), then any part of the collecting system visualised on ultrasound is entered with a 22G needle, a single or double contrast pyelogram performed and the pyelographic information used to select a target calyx. The chosen calyx is then punctured under fluoroscopic guidance, the tract dilated and a catheter inserted.

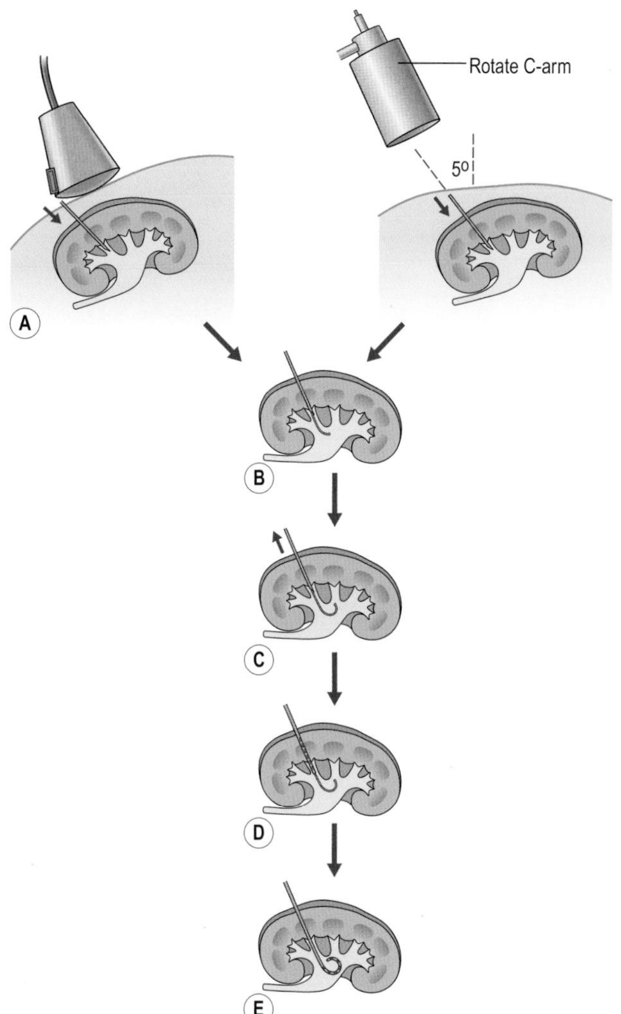

FIGURE 91-6 ■ Single puncture PCN. (A) Needle is inserted into the kidney either under ultrasound or fluoroscopic guidance. (B) Guidewire is passed through the needle (C) Needle is removed over the wire. (D) The nephrostomy is inserted over the wire. (E) The final position of the nephrostomy.

CT-Guided Nephrostomy

This technique is useful and safer when variant renal anatomy is suspected: e.g. horseshoe kidney, pelvic kidney or suspected retrorenal colon. A planning pyelographic phase CT is performed in the prone or supine/oblique position. The procedure can be performed under sole CT guidance or as a combined CT/fluoroscopy method. Needle access is gained under CT guidance and a guidewire inserted. Subsequent tract dilatation and

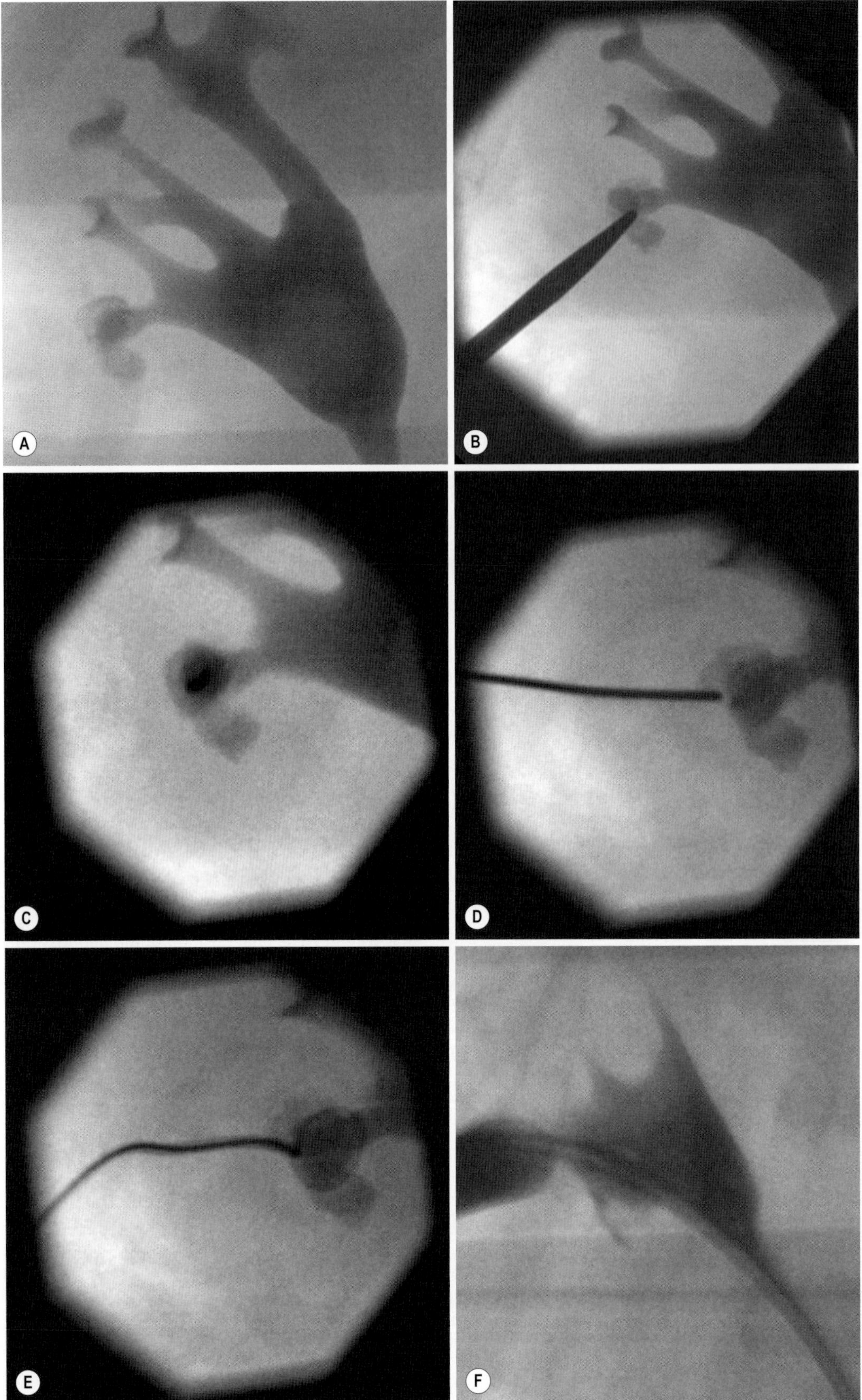

FIGURE 91-7 ■ Fluoroscopically guided single puncture for PCNL access. (A) Collecting system opacified with IV contrast medium demonstrating large stone in renal pelvis and smaller stone in lower pole calyx. (B) Tip of forceps over calyceal target used to centre image. (C) The needle centred over the target calyx 'like a dart'. (D) Angled screening once the needle is seen to move with the kidney in order to advance it to the calyx. (E) The wire coiled within the calyx. (F) Wire through calyx and into ureter with PCNL sheath in place.

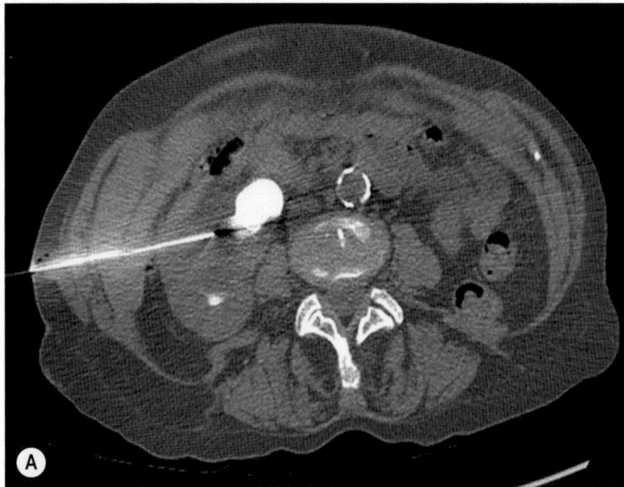

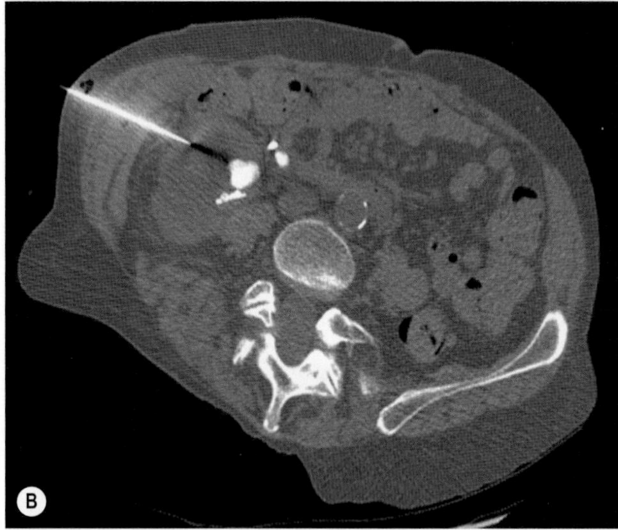

FIGURE 91-8 ■ **CT-guided nephrostomy.** (A) The procedure being performed in the supine position. (B) Puncture in the supine/oblique position. Either position is suitable, as is prone insertion. The procedure can be carried out solely under CT guidance or as a combined CT–fluoroscopic procedure (see text for details).

catheter insertion is done under fluoroscopic control. For the latter, care should be taken to ensure the access is secure before transferring the patient to the interventional suite[12] (Fig. 91-8).

Catheter Fixation and Removal

Displacement of a nephrostomy catheter is a constant hazard, particularly with long-term drainage. Definitive management (e.g. ureteric stenting) should not be delayed. The catheter should also be meticulously secured. Most nephrostomy tubes have a self-retaining suture, which once pulled forms a 'locked' pigtail within the collecting system. However, anchorage is not guaranteed and we further secure the tube to the skin (Fig. 91-9). A single anchoring suture through skin should be made close to the tube entry site. A small piece of tape is secured around the tube. The suture is then wrapped around the tube in a 'roman sandal' configuration with knots at every turn going away from the skin entry site. The suture should be firmly tightened against the catheter but not so tightly as to kink the tube. Once the top of the tape is reached, the suture is returned towards the skin entry site, as a reversed 'roman sandal' pattern. In addition we also apply a standard 'drain-fix' dressing.

Removal of a nephrostomy tube should be performed under fluoroscopic control and, using a guidewire. The pigtail should be unlocked and, if this fails, the nephrostomy tube can be cut at the hub; however, this increases the likelihood of the suture being caught in the soft tissues on withdrawal of the nephrostomy tube, leaving a fragment behind. A retained suture acts as a foreign body and a nidus for stone formation.[13] Therefore, it is preferable to unlock the catheter whenever possible and not to cut the suture.[13]

Difficult or Complicated Nephrostomy

Non-dilated Kidneys

Non-dilated calyces are not visualised on ultrasound examination and, being small, they are difficult to puncture. Also the space is too restricted for wire/catheter manipulation. The double contrast technique can be used in these cases. If the renal pelvis can be seen on US then this can be punctured with a 22G needle and a double contrast pyelogram performed to identify and distend the posterior calyces. If no part of the collecting system can be seen on US, then intravenous contrast medium is used to opacify the system and a posterior calyx selected and punctured. Using this technique, a success rate of up to 96% can be achieved in the non-dilated system.[14]

Horseshoe Kidney

Because of its anatomical disposition, the horseshoe kidney is prone to impaired drainage, infection and stone formation but the orientation of the calyces and vessels are such that percutaneous access is relatively safe. As horseshoe kidneys are located more inferiorly, the upper poles are usually well below the ribs. The lower pole and pelvis are usually more anterior facing and a lower pole lateral entry may damage large anterior division arteries or accessory branches from the iliac artery. Thus a medial lying, upper pole calyx entry should be chosen for PCN (Fig. 91-10).

Transplant Kidney

Ultrasound-guided PCN is usually relatively straightforward in a transplant kidney as it is superficial and good views can be obtained.[15] The procedure is performed with the patient supine. A lateral, upper pole entry is preferred to avoid puncturing the peritoneum. An upper pole or interpolar anterior-facing calyx is ideal as this allows more favourable access to the PUJ and ureter for subsequent ureteric stenting. Careful ultrasound technique helps reduce the risk of bowel injury or puncture of the inferior epigastric artery. Often, there is marked capsular fibrosis around the transplant and this can make dilation and catheter insertion difficult. Over-dilatation of the tract by 2Fr will facilitate catheter passage.

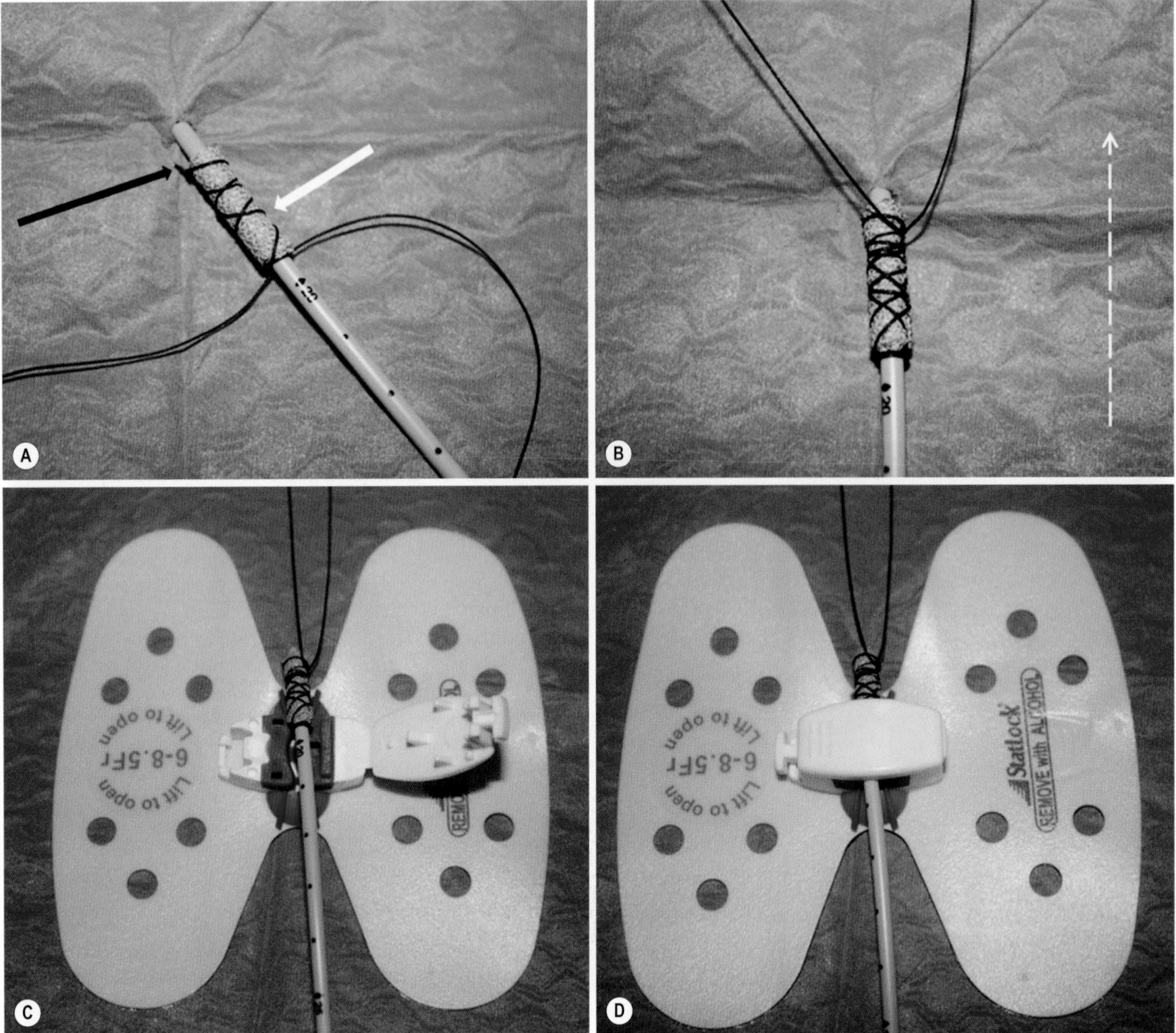

FIGURE 91-9 ■ Securing a nephrostomy catheter. (A) Small piece of tape secured onto nephrostomy tube. Anchoring suture (black arrow) is made through the skin; the suture is then wrapped around the tape in a 'roman sandal' configuration (white arrow) going away from the skin entry site. (B) 'Reversed roman sandal' knot along the tape in the direction of the dashed arrow. (C) The sutured tube is placed within a drain-fix dressing. (D) The top of the drain-fix dressing is locked in place to further secure the tube.

Paediatric Nephrostomy

Percutaneous nephrostomy in children should be performed under general anaesthesia. Ultrasound-guided PCN is technically straightforward as the collecting system is well seen, as it is superficial and usually generously dilated. However, in children the collecting system can rapidly decompress on needle entry and access may be lost. Decompression may occur because the system is under high pressure or because it is non-compliant. Therefore, the catheter must be inserted as swiftly as feasible. In straightforward cases with a dilated collecting system, initial puncture is performed with a sheathed needle, a stiff 0.035-inch. guidewire is inserted and the nephrostomy catheter advanced directly over this, as previous dilatation is not necessary. Special neonatal nephrostomy catheters (5Fr) are available; however, a standard 6Fr pigtail system works well. Care should be taken to minimise radiation dose to the patient by using low-dose techniques, good collimation and fluoroscopic image capture with minimal screening.[16]

Pregnancy

Urolithiasis is the common cause of true ureteric obstruction in pregnancy and will usually resolve with conservative measures. If this fails, nephrostomy may be required and an ultrasound-guided procedure should be performed. Fluoroscopy should be used sparingly and only if necessary. A lateral or supine/oblique approach may be used and intravenous opiates alone utilised to minimise fetal respiratory depression.

When fluoroscopy is used, radiation exposure should be minimised by lead shielding of the mother's abdomen

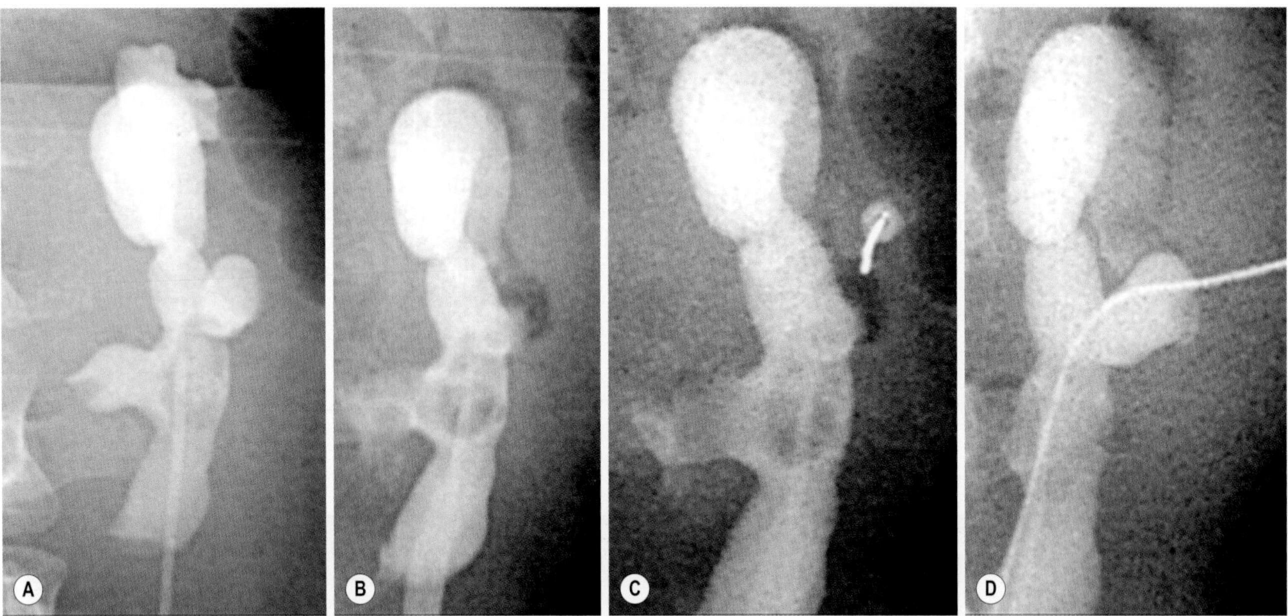

FIGURE 91-10 ■ **Fluoroscopically guided PCN of a horseshoe kidney.** (A) Ureteric catheter in situ used to perform a double contrast pyelogram. (B) The posterior-facing, non-dependent calyx is seen outlined by the introduced gas. (C, D) Percutaneous access achieved.

and by using similar safeguards as those recommended for paediatric cases.[17]

Complications of PCN and Management

The commonest serious complications following PCN insertion are sepsis and haemorrhage—Table 91-3. Patients at risk of pyonephrosis should receive pre-procedural antibiotics and nephrostomy insertion should not be delayed. Over-distension and manipulation of the collecting system should be avoided as these increase the risk of bacteraemia. In the well-dilated system, the entire procedure can be performed under ultrasound guidance, without any contrast pyelography. Performing a diagnostic nephrostogram should be delayed until the patient has recovered from the septic episode.

Haematuria, with or without clots, for a few days is not uncommon and usually resolves spontaneously but occasionally may require bladder catheterisation and washout. Major haemorrhage requires blood transfusion and/or further intervention. If the bleeding is venous in origin, continued drainage via the nephrostomy, catheter tamponade and blood transfusion, as necessary, can usually deal with the problem. Arterial bleeding can sometimes be managed in this way but more prolonged catheter tamponade, sometimes for several weeks, may be necessary. If this fails or the bleeding is not controllable with catheter tamponade, then renal angiography and embolisation should be undertaken.[18] Angiography should be performed with the catheter initially in situ and, if no bleeding point is seen, then the catheter should be withdrawn over a wire, whilst maintaining access, and repeat angiographic images are acquired in order to unmask an occult bleeding point.

Renal or pelvic injury is usually due to poor technique. Overzealous tract dilatation can rupture the pelvis. Care should be taken when inserting dilators and when advancing peel-away sheaths, particularly towards the renal pelvis and ureter. Avoidance of kinked guidewires will reduce dilator or sheath injuries. Most of these injuries are self-limiting and are treated with prolonged internal or external drainage.[19]

Bowel injuries are rare. If recognised during the procedure, the guidewire should be withdrawn out of the kidney and a drain left in the colon. A separate, second nephrostomy should be performed for renal drainage. Adequate renal drainage either via a PCN or a stent helps prevent renal-enteric fistulation. After a few days, a nephrostogram should be performed to exclude a renocolic fistula. If this is excluded, the colonic catheter can be removed. Theoretically, a mature track should minimise colonic spillage. If the patient develops signs of peritonitis, surgical intervention is required. Pleural complications include pneumothorax, empyema, hydrothorax and haemothorax. These are rare (0.1–0.2%) and are generally avoided by not performing punctures above the twelfth rib[19] and treated expectantly.

PERCUTANEOUS NEPHROLITHOTOMY (PCNL)

The indications for percutaneous endoscopic surgery are renal pelvic stones >2 cm, staghorn calculi, lower pole stones > 1 cm or stones in kidneys with poor drainage (e.g. stones in calyceal diverticula, horseshoe kidneys etc.). Hard stones (CT density > 1000 HU) and cysteine content are relative indications.[20] Less common indications are resection of transitional cell carcinoma of the renal pelvis, balloon dilatation or incision of PUJ obstruction and retrieval of foreign bodies. All these procedures require large-bore (30Fr) tract dilatation and sheath insertion.

Technique of PCNL

Leaving aside stone fragmentation, the key steps are access and tract dilatation. Regarding access, in addition to the sound anatomical principles discussed above in relation to renal puncture, the key consideration is that the entry should be well planned, in order to facilitate good intrarenal navigation and enable all/most stones to be removed.

Tract Planning

Appreciation of the intrarenal anatomy and the precise location of the stone are crucial and a good-quality IVU or 3D CT pyelogram will provide this key information (Fig. 91-11).[21] If complete stone clearance is not achievable, at the least the renal pelvis should be cleared in order to de-obstruct the kidney. If possible, the lower pole calyces should be cleared as fragments here may not drain naturally. The underlying principles regarding tract planning are summarised in Fig. 91-12.

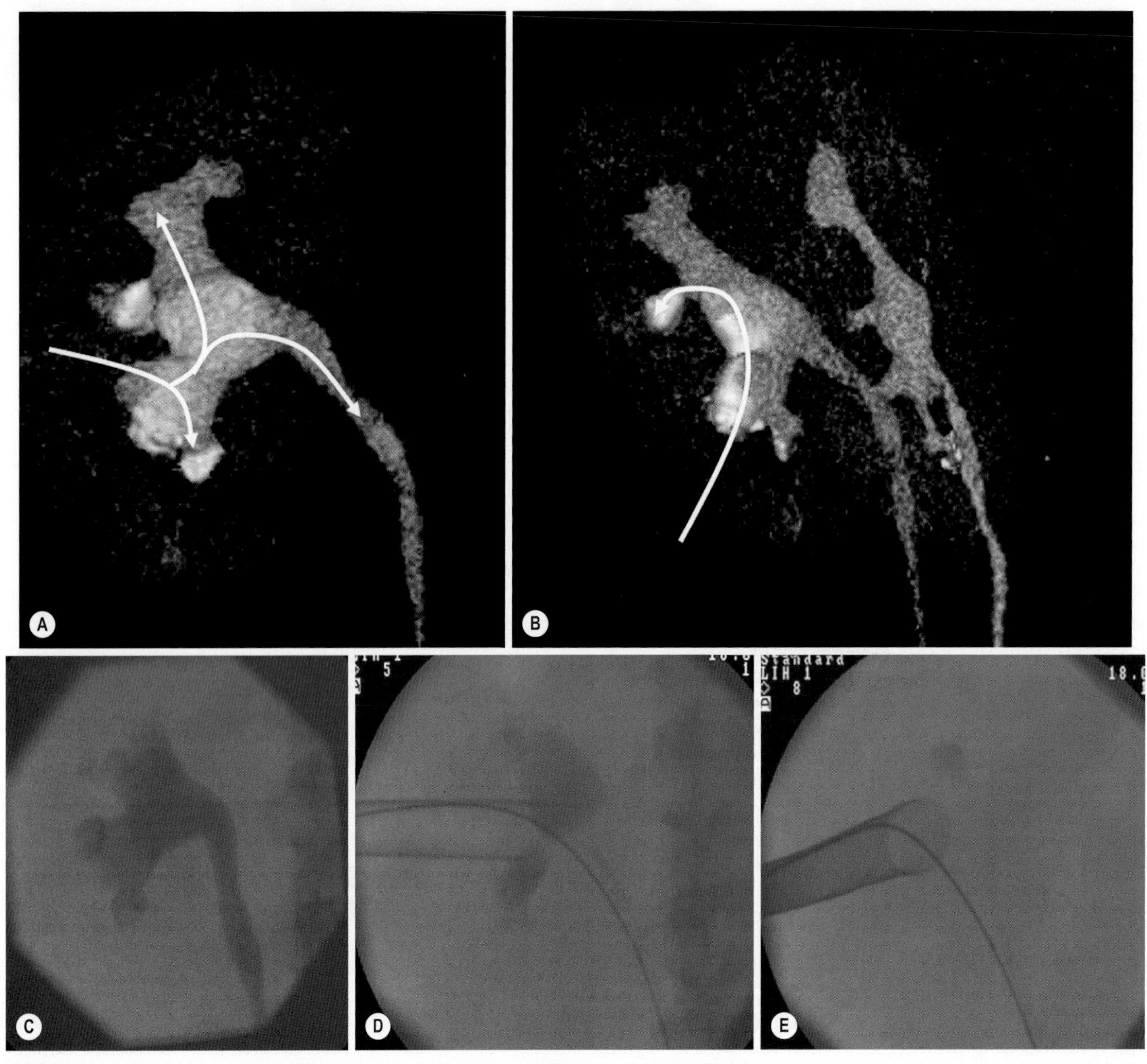

FIGURE 91-11 ■ The importance of 3D anatomical planning of PCNL tracts. The 3D CT pyelograms demonstrate a staghorn calculus with calyceal extension into the lower pole calyx and also a fragment in an interpolar calyx. As planned, a single tract will allow navigation into the lower pole calyces, pelvis and upper pole (arrow), as well as the ureter (A). However, the posterior-facing interpolar calyx presents an excessively acute angle from this access (arrow) (B). The three intraoperative images (C–E) confirm the accuracy of the pre-operative navigational map, as at the end of procedure the interpolar calyceal calculus was not retrievable. This was later treated with extracorporeal lithotripsy.

Tract Dilatation

The tract can be any size from 16Fr to 32Fr, but 30Fr is usual. Ideally, two guidewires should be inserted: a stiff wire for dilatation and a safety wire. There are three systems available for dilatation—a balloon mounted sheath system, serial plastic dilators or concentric/telescopic metal dilators. Balloons are quick, serial plastic dilators are easy to use and the metal dilators are reusable. The latter are especially useful when dilating onto a calyceal diverticulum. In a recent study,[22] bleeding and operating times were higher after balloon dilatation, but there were many uncontrollable variables in the study and other studies disagree.[23]

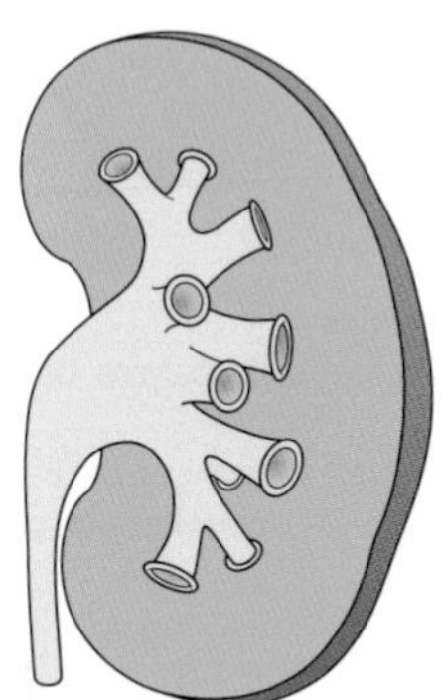

Principles of PCNL access
Aims
1. Aim for complete stone clearance
2. If complete clearance is not possible:
 • Clear renal pelvis to improve renal drainage.
 • Clear lower pole calyces as these may not respond to ESWL.
 • Residual stones in the upper/interpolar calyces can later be treated with ESWL.

Renal access
1. Posterior calyces allow access to anterior calyces.
2. Anterior calyceal entry poorer for intrarenal navigation.
3. Upper pole entry allows deep access of the PUJ/upper ureter:
 • May puncture posterior division artery.
 • May puncture pleura
4. Some interpolar calyces may be difficult with either lower or upper entry.

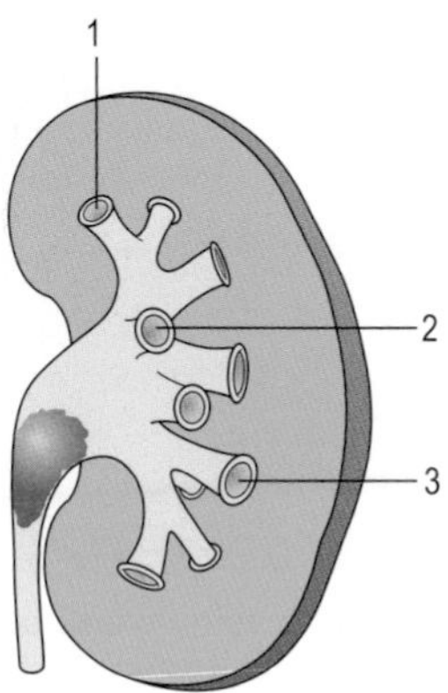

Stone in renal pelvis
Stone removed with minimal fragmentation. Ureteric fragments may be difficult to chase. Access planned according to PUJ anatomy.

1. Routes 1 and 2 are preferred with straight navigation to PUJ.
2. Route 3 may be difficult if the infundibulo-pelvic angle is acute and distal stone may be beyond reach.

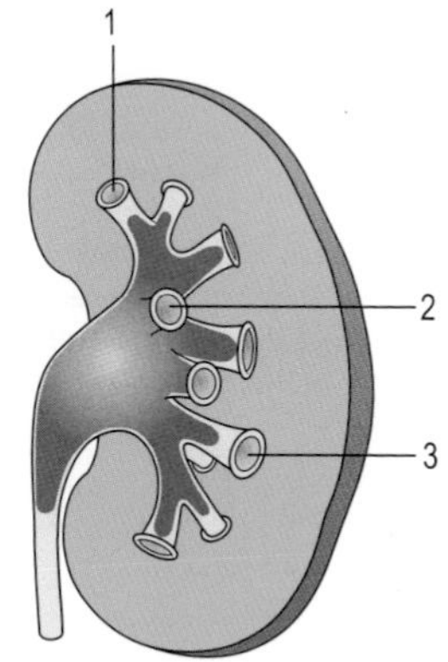

Complete staghorn
Stone clearance may be impossible with a single puncture.

1. Route 1 or 2 may be preferred—with Route 3 PUJ/ureteric clearance may be difficult.
2. With either routes some interpolar calyces may be difficult.

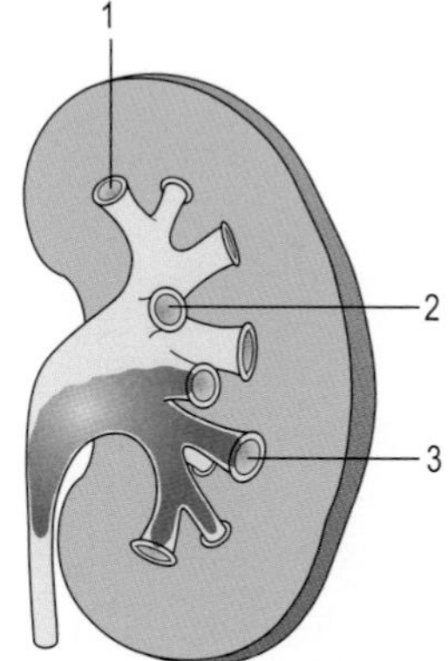

Stone in pelvis and lower calyces
Complete clearance is important (see under Principles/Aims).

1. Route 1 is often best.
2. Poor views of the interpolar calyx.
3. Poor views of upper ureter

FIGURE 91-12 ■ (A–F) The principles of tract planning for PCNL. A well-planned tract should allow for maximal/all stone removal and easy intrarenal navigation, such that most/all calyces should be endoscopically accessible.

Continued on following page

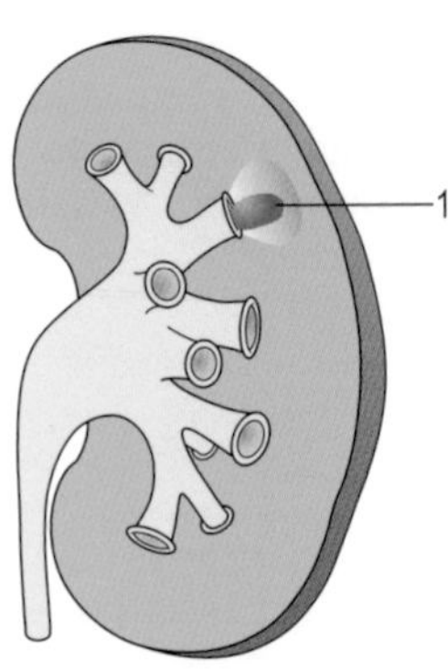

Stone in calyceal diverticulum with tight neck

Complete clearance is ideal. To decrease chances of recurrence, the neck should be dilated (thereby improving drainage) or the diverticulum should be obliterated. Direct puncture onto stone (1). Hydrophilic wire and good distension (with air/CO_2) help in searching for neck.

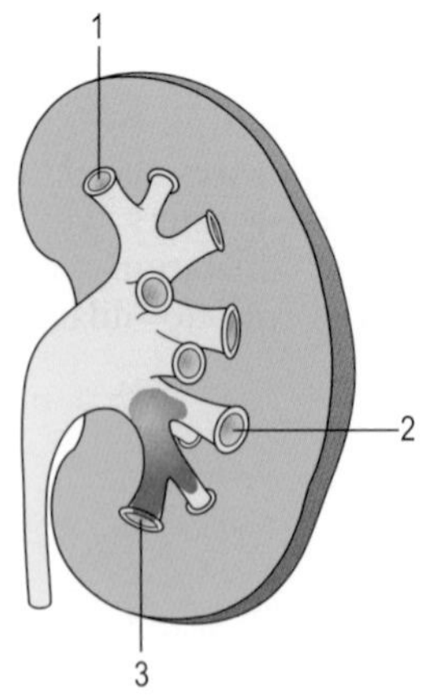

Lower-pole branched calculus

Stones in anterior and posterior parallel calyces. Complete clearance as ESWL may not work.

1. Route 1 preferred as both parallel calyces can be seen.
2. Route 2 (posterior calyx) better than 3 (anterior calyx) as navigation easier.

FIGURE 91-12, Continued

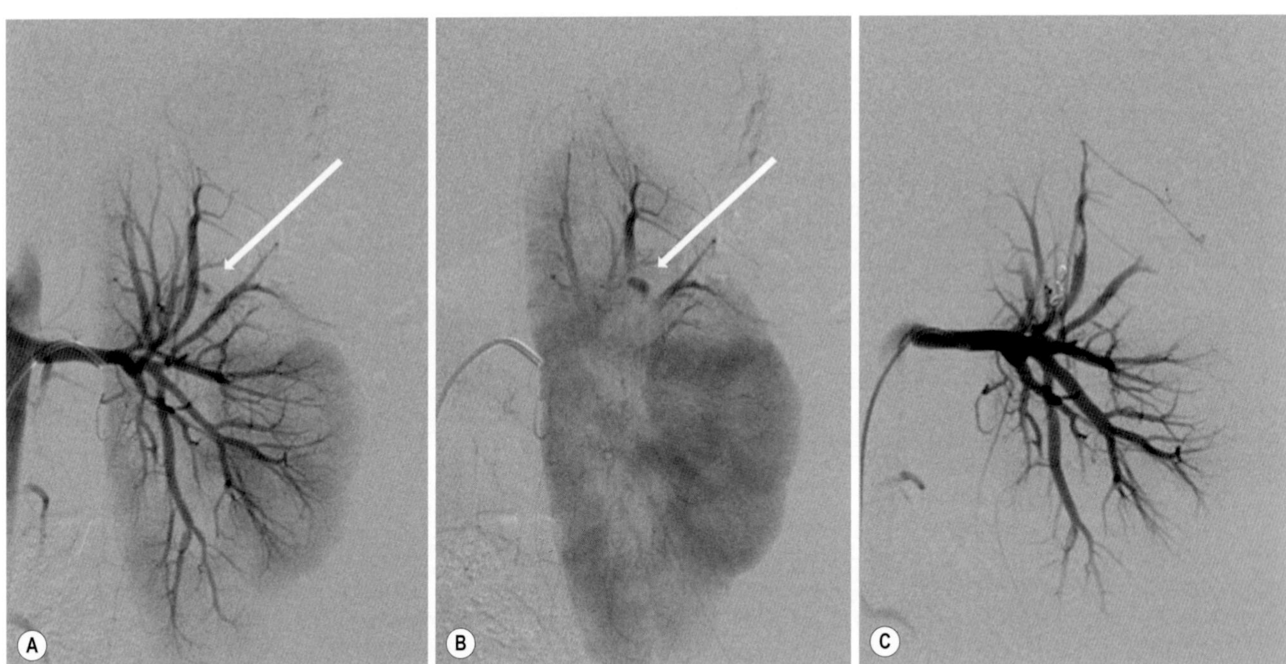

FIGURE 91-13 ■ Embolisation of pseudoaneurysm (PSA). (A) Upper pole PSA (white arrow) in early phase of contrast medium injection. (B) More prominent filling of the PSA in later stage of contrast medium injection (white arrow). (C) Post-embolisation image with coils in place. PSA is no longer seen to fill.

Complications of PCNL and Management

In a large international study, significant complications were bleeding (7.8%), renal pelvic injury (3.4%) and pleural effusion (1.8%). Bowel and visceral injury are less frequent. The principles of management are similar to those detailed under post-nephrostomy complications. Embolisation is necessary in < 1% of cases. Pneumothorax and pleural effusions should be treated on their merits. Bowel injury should be treated expectantly to let the tract mature, but may require operative correction. Delayed complications include late pseudoaneurysm, haemorrhage (Fig. 91-13) and ischaemic stricture of the collecting system (Fig. 91-14), which can occur weeks or months after the procedure.

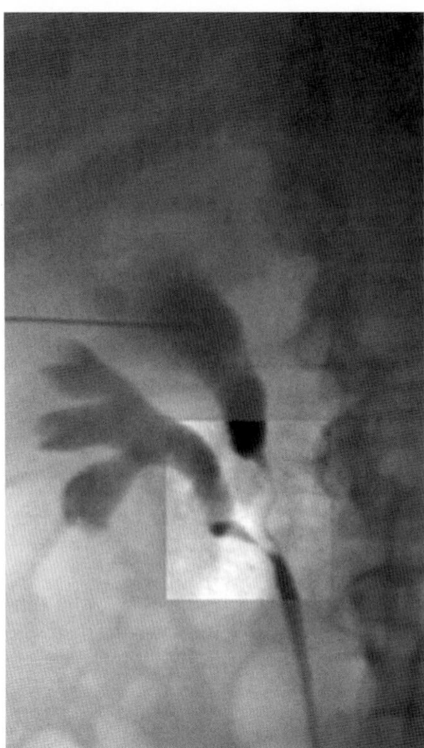

FIGURE 91-14 ■ Post-PCNL ischaemic stricture. Stricture of the renal pelvis extending into both infundibula post-PCNL. This was successfully balloon dilated.

ANTEGRADE URETERIC STENTS

A stent functions both as a splint and a conduit for natural flow. In the urinary tract, it is an alternative to a nephrostomy and although a stent is free of the complications of an external drain (external bag, leakage, skin irritation, accidental removal and infection) and better for home care, it has disadvantages.[24] The urinary tract does not tolerate artificial materials well. Stents can irritate the bladder or become infected. All stents, irrespective of their design or material of construction, will eventually become occluded, necessitating replacement.

Indications for Ureteric Stents

The common indications are relief of ureteric obstruction or leakage, and splinting of the ureter after balloon dilatation of ureteric strictures or after ureteric surgery. Stenting prior to stone therapy is now a relative indication.[25]

Ureteric Stents versus Percutaneous Nephrostomy

There are only two randomised studies comparing stents with nephrostomy (also referred to above under PCN). Both were in the setting of acute urolithiasis.[5,6] One reported no clinical difference and the other found a higher technical failure with retrograde stenting, but the numbers were small in both series. In a separate survey,[26] respondents (radiologists and urologists) favoured antegrade approaches with pelvic malignancy, and retrograde in those with uncomplicated benign disease or coagulopathy. Regarding quality of life, the two methods were rated equal in one study.[27]

Types of Ureteric Stents

Plastic Stents

The standard design is a hollow tube with a double pigtail (or double J) stent which covers the full length of the ureter. There are drainage holes in both pigtails and, in some designs, along the shafts. The earliest stents, which were made of polyethylene or polyurethane, had a high encrustation and fracture rate. Polymers are now used because of their better biocompatibility. However, these stents require regular exchange. Novel designs include a softer, narrow bladder tail, to reduce bladder irritation. A metal braided double pigtail stent is more rigid and durable and may have a role in malignant strictures.

Metal Stents

Unlike double J stents, metal ureteric stents become permanently incorporated into the wall by epithelialisation. Many metallic designs have been tried[28–30] but only one, the Memokath 051, has been specifically designed for the urinary tract.[31] Unlike the others, the Memokath does not epithelialise and can be removed even after several years. Covered metal stents have been used but they also become occluded as a result of urothelial overgrowth.

Pathological and Functional Changes after Stenting

All stents, including modern polymer stents, lead to reactive urothelial hyperplasia, thickened mucosa and periureteral inflammation.[32] In both animals and humans,[24] reduced and ineffective peristalsis is seen with stents in situ and early drainage is passive, and dependent on the renal-bladder pressure gradient. In one study, peristalsis was rarely seen before 2 months and in other studies intrapelvic pressures rose after stenting.[24,33,34] Plastic stents also develop a biofilm and eventually become encrusted and blocked. Open mesh metal stents are also not well tolerated, exciting a profuse inflammatory response with urothelial hyperplasia.[35] Stent incorporation into ureteric mucosa is also unpredictable and eventually stents will obstruct due to malignant ingrowth or overgrowth, or as a result of encrustation.

Clinical Efficacy of Current Stents

Technical success varies from 77 to 95%.[24,36–39] However, in one study, 30% were blocked at 3 months.[40] Stent material and infection all have a bearing on encrustation. Dysuria or urinary frequency affects up to one half of all patients. Stent reflux can lead to infection and loin pain.

Practical Aspects of Antegrade Stenting

Antegrade ureteric stenting may be performed either as a primary stenting procedure [36] or as a second procedure following several days of external drainage. The technical success rate for the former is around 85% and near 100% for the latter.[24] Primary stenting is contraindicated with infected obstructed systems.

Technique of Antegrade Stenting

Interpolar or upper pole renal access is better but lower pole entry can be used, though with some difficulty. A nephrostogram will confirm the level and completeness of the stricture. The stricture can be negotiated with a curved tip hydrophilic wire combined with an angled tip, high torque catheter for stricture cannulation; or with a straight tip guidewire combined with a Cobra shape catheter. Once the stricture is crossed, the catheter is advanced into the bladder and the wire exchanged for a stiff guidewire to support stent insertion. A long peel-away sheath may be used to support stent insertion, especially if the perinephric track is long and/or with lower pole access. The tract is dilated to one size larger, or to 1Fr or 2Fr larger than the chosen stent.

Stent Lumen Size

A lumen >5Fr can accommodate a flow rate of up to 10 mL/min with minimal rise of the intrapelvic pressure. The nature of the obstruction may influence choice. Stents for bypassing obstructing ureteric stones are used for relatively short periods. Benign strictures also allow drainage around the stent as the ureter dilates (so-called peri-stent drainage), whereas malignant tissue does not permit such dilatation. We tend to use 8Fr stents for malignant or ischaemic/post-surgical strictures; and 6Fr to bypass ureteric calculi or inflammatory strictures. There is no consensus regarding metal stents, but 6- to 8-mm diameter stents have been used.

Stent Length

Direct ureteric length measurement can be used: the wire tip is advanced to the ureterovesical junction and a clip placed on the wire at the skin exit site. Then the wire is withdrawn until the wire tip is just in the renal pelvis and a second clip is placed. The inter-clip distance is the length of the ureter. However, this method can be inaccurate, particularly if the ureter is tortuous. An alternative is to use the patient's height. One formula suggests <175 cm height = 22-cm-long stent; 175–195 cm = 24 cm; and >195 cm = 26 cm.[41] This is a reliable method of calculating the length of the ureter, unless there is an anatomical anomaly or the two fixed points (the PUJ and VUJ) have changed position, e.g. because of a large bladder tumour or after renal pelvic surgery. In such cases a longer stent is selected. Patients with a urostomy usually require a 22-cm stent or shorter. A 12-cm length is generally sufficient for transplant ureters. The ureteric length in children should be judged according to their height.

Type of Stent

Polymer stents offer the best combination of rigidity, lumen flow and durability but no material is of proven superiority. Hydrophilic coatings allow easier passage but are expensive. The release method is a matter of individual preference. The presence of an internal stiffener, positioning thread loops and visible markers may benefit the novice. Occasionally the stiffener and the thread loops can create their own difficulties and the simplest design has no stiffener or thread lops, and uses only a pusher. Extra care is needed with this simple design, as there is no scope for repositioning.

Insertion of a Plastic Stent

The site of obstruction can be pre-dilated with either long dilators or with a 4- to 6-mm-diameter balloon catheter. High pressures may be necessary, especially with benign strictures. The stent is advanced with short, firm thrusts over the stiff guidewire, until the distal tip lies in the bladder and the proximal tip is in the renal pelvis. If it has been advanced too far, reposition by pulling on the stent assembly—and also the thread loops, if present. The distal tip should be within the bladder, but an excessively long bladder loop increases stent-related dysuria.

The stent is released by withdrawing the guidewire (and internal stiffener if one is being used). The thread loops can then be removed under fluoroscopic control, in order to avoid pulling the proximal pigtail into the renal parenchyma. The guidewire can then be re-advanced to regain renal access, a catheter is inserted and a check nephrostogram performed (Fig. 91-15). If stent patency is confirmed and there is no substantial clot in the renal pelvis, then all access can be removed. However, if flow is poor and/or there is marked clot, then a covering nephrostomy should be inserted and left on external drainage. This can be removed after 24–48 hours if the clot has cleared and the stent is functioning normally.

Insertion of a Metal Ureteric Stent

The length and position of the stricture are carefully documented. A stent longer than the stricture is used. Overlapping stents should be avoided, as this increases the risk of encrustation. No stent is of proven superiority. The Memokath stent is made of a coiled nickel–titanium shape memory alloy, which expands to its full diameter (9Fr shaft and 17Fr proximal flange) when the ureter is flushed with water at 50°C. When flushed with cold water, it returns to its smaller size even months/years after insertion, and can be fully retrieved. With all metal stents, immediate drainage can be unreliable, perhaps because of mucosal oedema over the ends and a covering nephrostomy may be necessary. This can be removed after a 24-h trial of nephrostomy clamping.

Further Issues about Ureteric Stents

Retroperitoneal Looping of Stent/Wire

This can occur as a result of a long retroperitoneal tract or an extrarenal cavity such as an urinoma. The tract

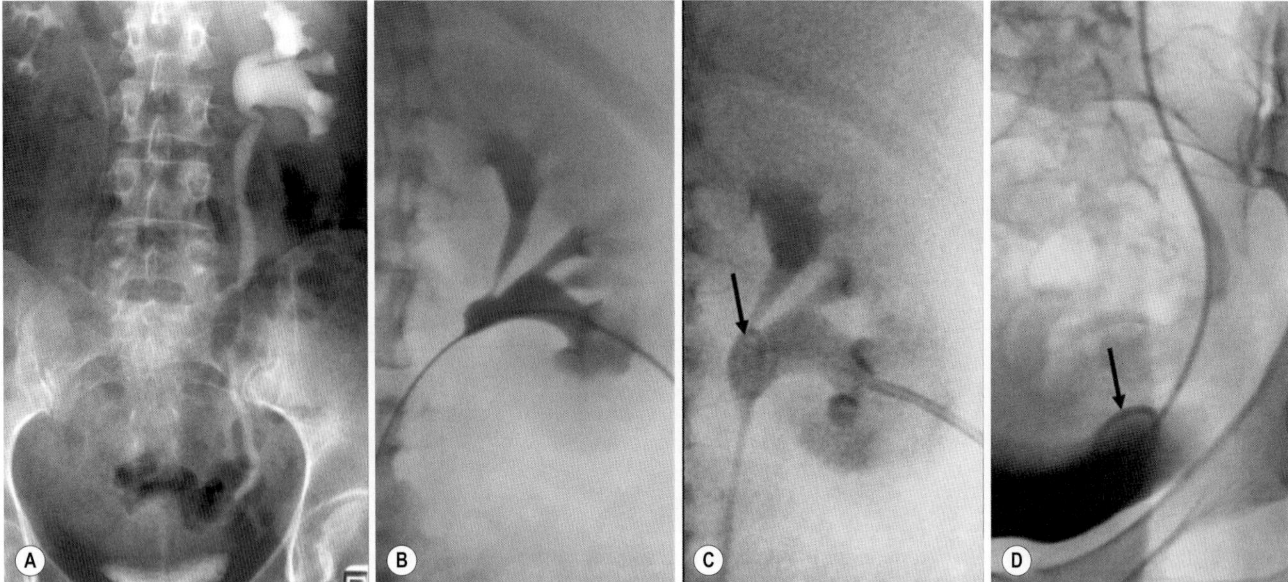

FIGURE 91-15 ■ **Ureteric stent insertion.** (A) Complete obstruction of the lower third of the ureter. (B) Renal access through a posterior-facing lower calyx. A wire was manipulated across the stricture (not shown) and a double pigtail stent was inserted. (C, D) The stent length was ideal as the upper pigtail (C) is coiled in the renal pelvis (arrow) and the lower pigtail (D) is just beyond the vesicoureteric junction (arrow) and not too long. We find the patient's height the most reliable method for choosing stent length, but there are other methods (see text).

needs to be supported using a stiff wire and a peel-away sheath. Some advocate the routine use of a sheath. We use it selectively, but the sheath should be one French size larger than the stent.

False Passage Created during Stricture Cannulation

If this complication occurs, it is best to stop, commence antibiotics and insert a protective nephrostomy catheter. Stenting can be reattempted after 3–7 days of external drainage.

Stenting of Ureteroileal or Ureterocolic Anastomosis

This can be performed by the standard antegrade route, or retrogradely under fluoroscopic guidance if the ureter can be demonstrated on loopography. Shorter stents are necessary but mucus can obstruct the stent. Use at least an 8Fr lumen stent and irrigation of the stoma may be necessary. A separate problem is the pressures generated by small bowel peristalsis. This will result in stent reflux and the urine may preferentially drain through the covering nephrostomy and stent blockage may be incorrectly assumed. A covering Foley catheter can be inserted into the urostomy or bladder to assist stent drainage. Both mucus and pressure problems can be overcome by using an extra-long stent with the distal pigtail externalised into the stoma bag. Rarely, peristalsis may expel the stent into the stoma, implying that the stricture may have resolved and stricture status should be re-evaluated on loopography.

Tortuous Ureter

The use of a high-torque, angled-tip catheter with a hydrophilic wire will facilitate navigation of most ureters. Once the wire is in the bladder, it should be exchanged for a stiff wire and a peel-away sheath should be inserted. This will improve the redundancy.

Tight or Rigid Stricture

The stiff end of a hydrophilic wire can be used to forcefully cross an unyielding stricture, but considerable force may be necessary with risk of creating a false passage. Thin stiff wires also have a role. If a subintimal passage is made, then stenting is still feasible once the true lumen has been re-entered distally. The only sure sign that a wire is in the bladder is to exchange it for a catheter and to confirm that the bladder fills with contrast medium. A hydrophilic catheter may be necessary to traverse a rigid stricture. If this fails, a long dilator or a balloon may help. In very resistant strictures, another attempt after 1 week of nephrostomy drainage is often successful.

A Stent Cannot Be Advanced across the Stricture, Even after Dilatation

In such cases, a stiff hydrophilic wire and/or a narrower stent and/or a hydrophilic coated stent should be used. If placement is still not possible, the distal tip of the hydrophilic wire can be snared in the bladder and externalised out of the urethra. This allows a push–pull manoeuvre and the stent can be forced across the unyielding stricture. Retrograde placement of a soft catheter

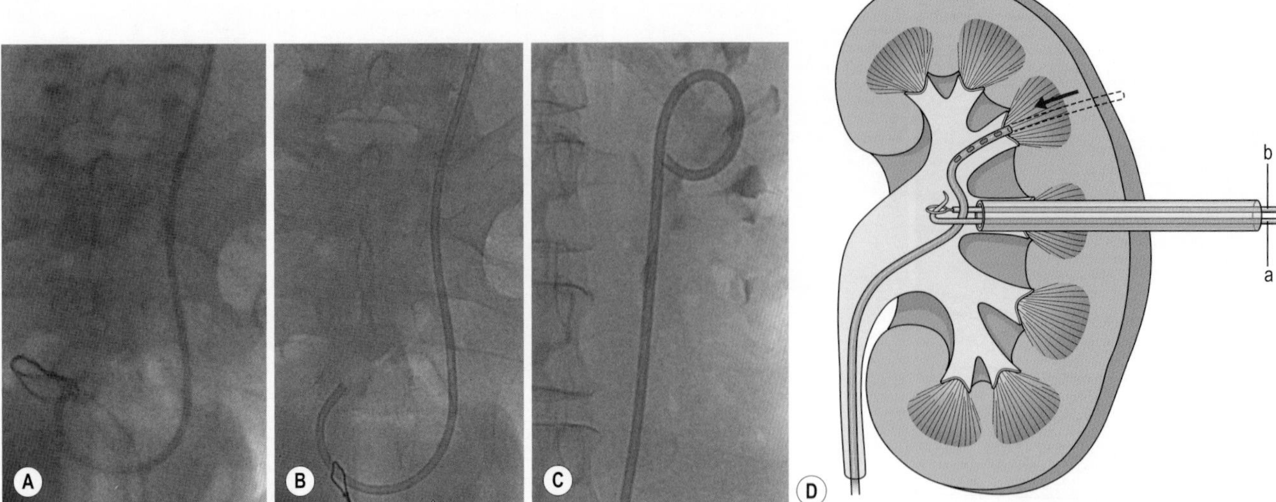

FIGURE 91-16 ■ **Repositioning of a ureteric stent that has been misplaced with the tip in the perinephric space.** A standard transurethral Foley catheter is initially inserted, after which a wire is placed into the bladder. A sheath is then placed in the bladder and bladder distended for ease of snaring. (A) Lower end of stent snared in bladder. (B) Snare loop tightened around stent. (C) Repositioned stent now within collecting system. (D) Line illustration of the antegrade method for repositioning a ureteric stent. Through a new puncture, an angled-tip catheter (a) and snare (b) are advanced to lie on either side of the shaft of the stent, and the tip of the catheter is ensnared. By pulling the catheter and snare together, the stent tip is pulled out of the perinephric space (arrow) and into the collecting system.

across the urethra and ureteric orifice during this manoeuvre protects against tissue laceration.

Improvement in Stent Position

If the stent has been released too soon and the tip is in the renal parenchyma, the simplest method of dealing with the problem is to snare the distal pigtail transurethrally and withdraw the stent (Fig. 91-16A-C). Alternatively, an antegrade approach can be employed, by snaring of the stent shaft (Fig. 91-16D).[42] If the upper pigtail is in the ureter, retraction is straightforward if the threads are still present. If a narrow PUJ makes such retraction difficult, a wire can be manipulated into the ureter and advanced past the upper pigtail, allowing a sheath (or catheter) to be inserted over it until it abuts the stent tip. Simultaneous withdrawal of the stent and sheath/catheter may allow a smooth transition across the PUJ. If there are no threads, repositioning is difficult but can be accomplished by using a snare, or more traumatically with grabbers, through a sheath.

The Thread Loops Will Not Disengage

In this situation a small (3–4Fr) dilator should be advanced over the thread (using a rotatory motion) until it abuts the stent. Pulling the thread will then allow release.

Extra-anatomical Stenting

If the stricture cannot be bypassed with a guidewire, then either a rendezvous technique or a ureteroneocystostomy[43] can be performed. The first is a combined antegrade and retrograde approach with in situ snaring of the wire. The latter can be performed if the stricture is at the level of the bladder, in which case, under lateral fluoroscopy a curved tip catheter is firmly wedged in the stricture and directed anteromedially towards the bladder. The stiff end of a hydrophilic wire is then used to puncture through the tumour/bladder wall. Both techniques are examples of extraluminal stenting and are of established safety, but the position of the wire within the bladder should be confirmed before a stent is inserted. The final option is true extra-anatomical stenting,[44] by creating a subcutaneous tunnel between the kidney and bladder. A dedicated stent system is available for this technique.

Monitoring Ureteric Stents

Intravenous urography, contrast or radionuclide cystography, renography, supplemented with diuretic renography and Doppler ultrasound measurement of resistive index or ureteric jets can all be used. None are ideal. Plain ultrasound of the collecting system can be confusing, as stent reflux can lead to upper tract distension. However, in routine practice ultrasound correlated with renal biochemistry is simplest, as progressive dilatation is seen with stent dysfunction. For patients requiring long-term stenting, it is prudent to electively change the stent at set intervals (3–6 months) rather than depend on stent patency assessments.

Exchanging or Removing Stents

Stents should be exchanged every 3–6 months. This can be accomplished retrogradely[45,46] or antegradely using a snare. Retrograde exchange is preferable. Under fluoroscopy the bladder pigtail is snared and the stent is retrieved until it just exits the urethra. A full bladder helps retrieval.

A guidewire is inserted through the exiting stent lumen to establish ureteral access. Replacement is then a simple matter, but if difficulty is encountered a peel-away sheath, ureteric dilatation and stiff wire may be helpful, especially in males. Antegrade exchange using a snare can be used, but it is important to have a safety wire in place.

BALLOON DILATATION OF URETERIC STRICTURES

Balloon dilatation of benign ureteric strictures is an alternative to surgical repair. There are many causes of ureteric strictures (Table 91-4).[47] Such strictures can be treated with balloon dilatation. The overall success rate of this procedure is quite variable and ranges between 16 and 83%. Even in cases of technical success, the results are not durable. Balloon dilatation alone has been shown to have a high recurrence rate, but failed balloon dilatation does not prevent a patient from having a surgical procedure.

An interpolar calyx is ideal for ureteric access and a nephrostogram is used to delineate the position and length of the stricture. This may be particularly useful should the patient subsequently require surgical correction. Using an angled-tip catheter and a hydrophilic guidewire, the stenosis can usually be crossed. Either repeated gentle probing or firm direct pressure with the wire tip should be tried, as either technique may succeed, although the former is less traumatic. If the stenosis is very tight, a hydrophilic coated catheter may be required to cross the stricture. A peel-away sheath helps support the catheter and wire during exchange. The hydrophilic guidewire is then exchanged for a stiff guidewire and the stricture dilated using a 6- to 8-mm balloon. High dilatation pressures may be necessary. The pressure is gradually increased until the 'waist' of the balloon disappears. Abolition of the waist with minimal contained extravasation is anecdotally believed to be a 'good' sign. Once the stricture is dilated, a stent is placed as a splint and removed after 4–6 weeks. Ureteric perforation can occur when attempting to cross a tight stricture. When this occurs the procedure should be abandoned if the leak is substantial. External drainage via a PCN should be established. Up to 1 week should be allowed for the perforation to heal before a repeat attempt can be made to cross the stricture.

Treatment of adult-onset pyeloureteric junction obstruction with balloon dilatation has shown to be successful in up to 80% of patients. However, there is a limited role for balloon dilatation in childhood pyeloureteric junction obstruction as the results are worse than antegrade and retrograde endopyelotomy or open surgery. In ureteric strictures following renal transplantation, the success rate of high-pressure balloon angioplasty is reported as 16–62%.[34,48,49] Cutting balloon angioplasty has been used for resistant ureteric strictures in the post-transplant ureter, with a primary patency rate of 55% and a secondary patency rate of 78%.[38,39,50] Early treatment of strictures improves the success rate. The best outcome is seen in strictures developing soon after percutaneous nephrolithotomy (PCNL) and ureterolithotomy, early postoperative stenosis and proximal well-circumscribed stenosis. The success rate is lower for dilatations performed at the vesicoureteric junction (VUJ)[39,51] and in ischaemic strictures. Long stenoses (≥3 cm) do not respond as well.

TABLE 91-4 Indications for Ureteric Balloon Dilatation

Post-surgical: accidental ureteric ligation, anastomotic stenoses, postrenal transplantation
Inflammatory: postradiation, TB, retroperitoneal fibrosis, calculus
PUJ obstruction
Malignancy

TREATMENT OF URINARY LEAKS AND FISTULAS

Surgical repair of urinary leaks is unsuccessful in up to 12–35% of cases and carries a significant morbidity.[52] Postoperative urine leaks (Fig. 91-17) or leaks secondary to malignant disease or after radiotherapy can all be managed percutaneously. Occasionally ureteric occlusion is performed for severe dysuria, haematuria or to treat total urinary incontinence. Small leaks will usually resolve with external drainage alone. A nephrostomy is inserted and left in place for at least 3 days (Fig. 91-18). If the leak has not resolved, then the nephrostomy should be upsized to a 12–14Fr drain to maximise external drainage. A stent may also be required to splint the ureter.

If simple drainage and splinting is unsuccessful, ureteric occlusion may be necessary. This can be achieved by several different methods and is combined with external drainage. Where the aim is to exclude flow to the bladder, bilateral occlusion may be required. The use of detachable and non-detachable balloons, large-bore occluding catheters, combination of coils and Gelfoam pledgets, plugs, adhesives, intraluminal electrocautery and retroperitoneal clipping have been described.[52] Irrespective of the type of occlusive material used, there is a high rate of dislodgement. Adequate external drainage is critical to the success of the procedure; malfunctioning nephrostomy catheters increase the rate of dislodgement.

SUPRAPUBIC BLADDER CATHERISATION

The need for long-term bladder catheterisation arises mainly in patients with bladder outlet obstruction and neurogenic bladder dysfunction. The procedure is sometimes necessary following bladder or urethral injury or fistula. Studies have demonstrated the superiority of suprapubic catheters over transurethral catheters in long-term bladder drainage[53] with reduced urinary tract infections, less need for recatheterisation, and improved comfort. Image guidance decreases the risk of bowel

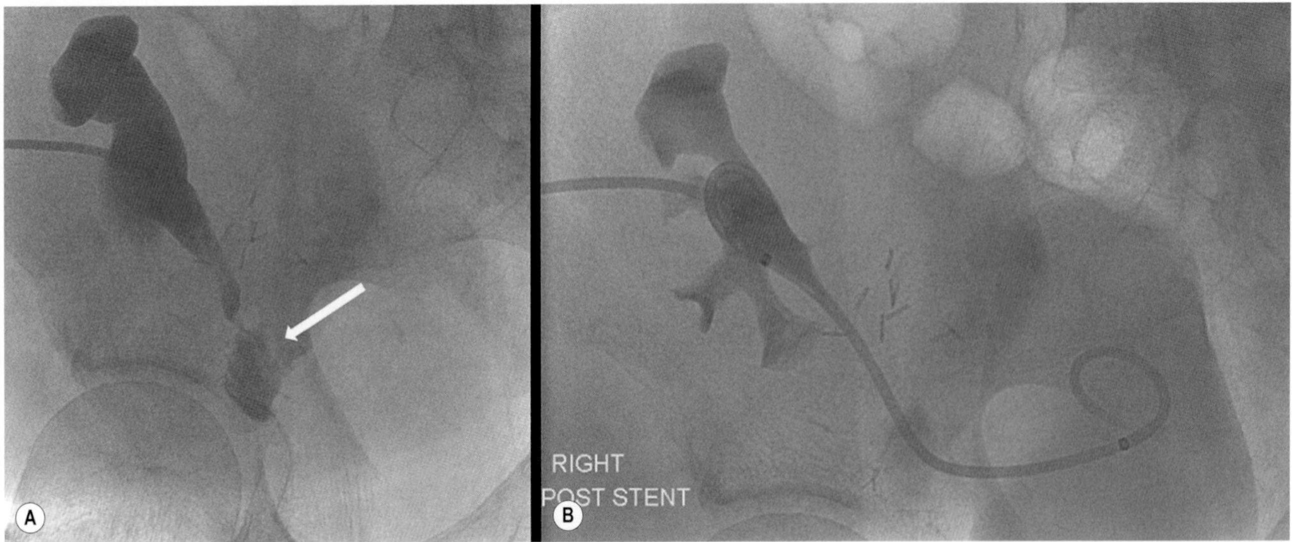

FIGURE 91-17 ■ **Post-surgical urine leak.** (A) Contrast medium injected from catheter in renal pelvis showing extravasation (white arrow) at the site of the transplant anastomosis. (B) Ureteric stent in situ after the site of the leak has been crossed.

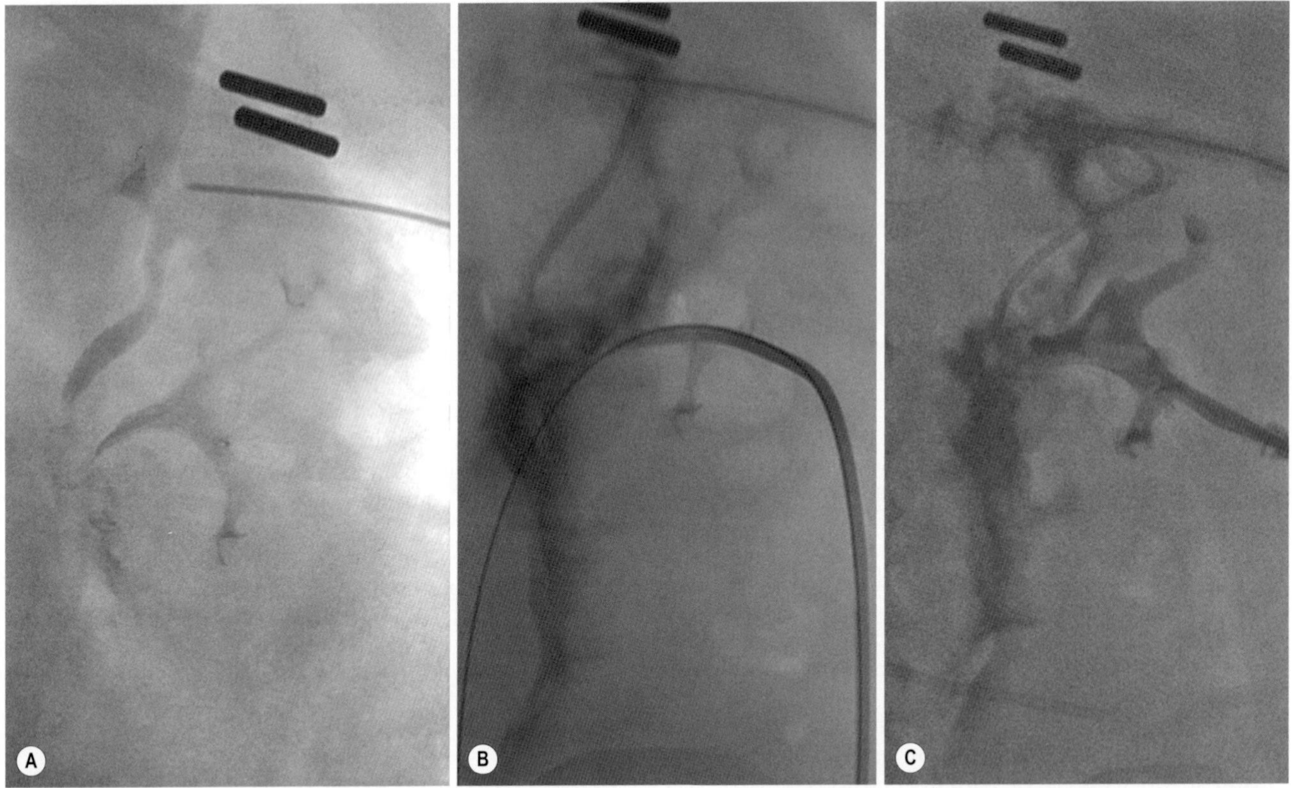

FIGURE 91-18 ■ **PCN for treatment of post-traumatic renal pelvic leak following a gunshot wound.** (A) Fluoroscopic opacification of the collecting system following initial IV contrast medium injection demonstrates a bifid collecting system with contrast medium leak seen from the pelvis. (B) Access via a lower pole calyx into the ureter. (C) Two nephrostomies sited in upper and lower pole to ensure adequate drainage of the bifid collecting system.

injury and is especially recommended when adequate bladder distension cannot be achieved, and in those with previous lower abdominal surgery.[54]

The procedure is performed using sedoanalgesia and prophylactic antibiotics in those likely to have bacterial colonisation of urine. It is important to ensure adequate bladder distension of at least 300 mL, either via an existing urethral catheter or by oral hydration and natural filling. This will displace the bowel loops superolaterally as well as making perforation of the posterior bladder wall by through-and-through puncture less likely. Adequate bladder distension is confirmed using ultrasound. If required, the bladder can be further distended via a 20G Chiba needle inserted into the bladder under ultrasound guidance, which also helps to confirm the absence of any intervening vascular structures or interposed bowel. The catheter should pass through the rectus sheath in the midline, not more than 2 cm above the pubic symphysis or along a safe tract as defined on ultrasound.

Either a Seldinger technique or a trocar (Fig. 91-19) technique can be used. The bladder is punctured under ultrasound guidance. With the trocar technique, once urine is aspirated the catheter is advanced into the bladder. When using the Seldinger technique, urine is aspirated via the puncture needle to confirm intravesical position. A stiff guidewire is inserted into the bladder and serial dilatation of the tract performed, ending with a peel-away sheath of a suitable size to accommodate the catheter. When the catheter is in place and secured by inflating the balloon, final confirmation of position within the bladder can be performed with contrast medium injection under fluoroscopy. CT-guided insertion is indicated in patients with complex pelvic anatomy caused by previous surgery or congenital abnormalities. In a large series of image-guided suprapubic catheter insertion a bowel perforation rate of 0.3% was reported.[53] This compares to a bowel perforation rate of between 2.4 and 2.7% for cystoscopically assisted suprapubic catheter insertion.[55]

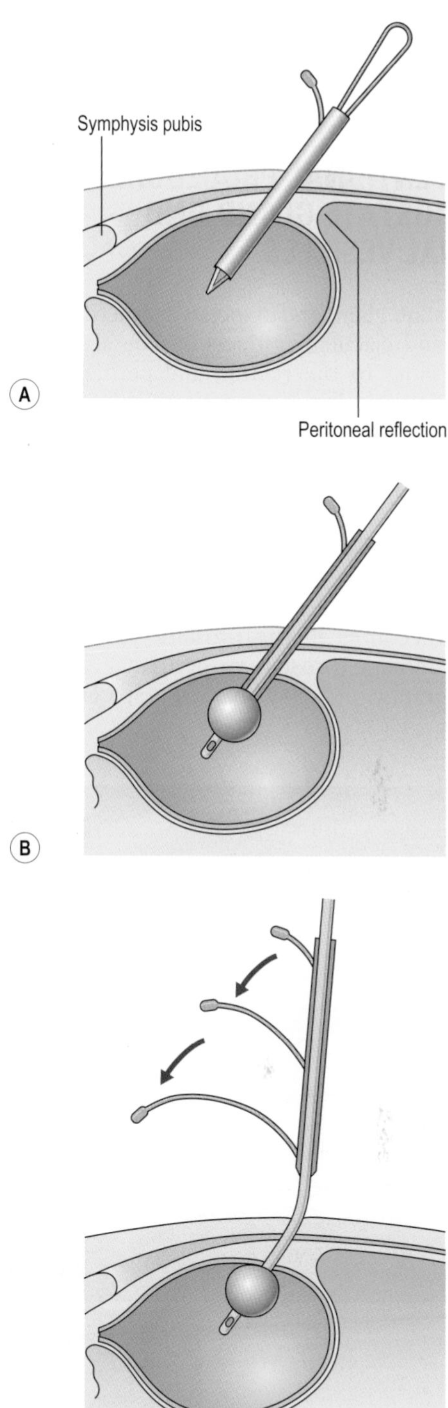

FIGURE 91-19 ■ **Suprapubic catheter insertion.** (A) The suprapubic catheter introducer (trocar and sheath) is advanced into the bladder midline at an angle of approximately 40° from the vertical until urine is seen rising up the trocar. The trocar is then removed from the sheath and the catheter inserted to its midpoint. (B) The catheter balloon is inflated and the sheath is then slid back along the catheter shaft until it is external to the abdomen. (C) The sheath is 'stripped' and removed.

MANAGING A NON-DEFLATABLE URINARY CATHETER BALLOON

The balloons of urinary catheters may fail to deflate if the balloon channel becomes obstructed by debris. The balloon can be ruptured by overinflation but this method carries the risks of bladder rupture and retained catheter fragments.[56] Injection of various liquid agents into the balloon can be used to dissolve the balloon, but may induce chemical cystitis. An elegant solution is to reopen the channel by the passage of a hydrophilic or an 0.018-inch stiff guidewire.[57] Alternatively, the sharp end of the guidewire could be used to rupture the balloon, allowing it to deflate. If this fails, the balloon can be punctured under transabdominal ultrasound guidance using a 22G needle, whilst the balloon is fixed by gentle traction per urethra. An alternative is transrectal ultrasound-guided puncture, under antibiotic prophylaxis. Either method may require multiple punctures.

PERCUTANEOUS CYSTOLITHOTRIPSY (PCCL)

Bladder stones are primarily treated by transurethral or open cystolithotripsy. PCCL is indicated when transurethral access is not feasible, e.g. in patients with urethral strictures, following bladder augmentation, and in neurogenic bladders. It is also performed in children as they have a narrow urethra, which makes more difficult the transuretheral removal of fragments. The technique is a hybrid of that described for the insertion of a suprapubic catheter and PCNL. Once guidewire access is obtained into the bladder, tract dilatation is performed as described for PCNL. A 30Fr rigid sheath is inserted, through which bladder stones are fragmented and removed.

INTERVENTIONAL PROCEDURES IN THE PROSTATE GLAND AND SEMINAL VESICLES

The prostate gland and associated structures, the seminal vesicles and ejaculatory ducts can be accessed easily, as they lie close to the rectum and perineum, and either route is feasible for intervention. Transrectal interventions can be performed as outpatient procedures in the left lateral position, under local anaesthesia. There is a risk of rectal haemorrhage and infection, both of which can be severe. The risk of major complications by the transperineal route is almost negligible but it is painful and requires a general anaesthetic or generous sedo-analgesia. Commonly performed non-vascular interventional procedures in the prostatic bed include biopsy, abscess drainage (prostate or perirectal abscess), seminal vesiculography, prostate brachytherapy and cryotherapy, and ablation with high-intensity focused ultrasound (HIFU).[58] Balloon dilatation of the prostate gland is ineffective. Insertion of prostatic stents has a high morbidity.

Drainage of Prostate and Perirectal Abscess

Abscess of the prostate may occur after prostatitis, urethral catherisation or prostate biopsy. Perirectal abscesses are seen after surgery, such as appendectomy. All these can be drained percutaneously. However, abscess secondary to colitis, especially Crohn's disease, should not be drained by this route as a fistula may develop, and are best dealt with via the transabdominal or transgluteal routes. Needle aspiration to dryness is preferred to catheter drainage, as catheter placement can be difficult and is also inconvenient for the patient. The transrectal route is technically easier but may not be tolerated because of pain. Using a prostate biopsy needle guide attached to the transrectal probe, a long 18G needle is directed into the centre of the abscess under US guidance (Fig. 91-20). The needle tip is always very easily seen,

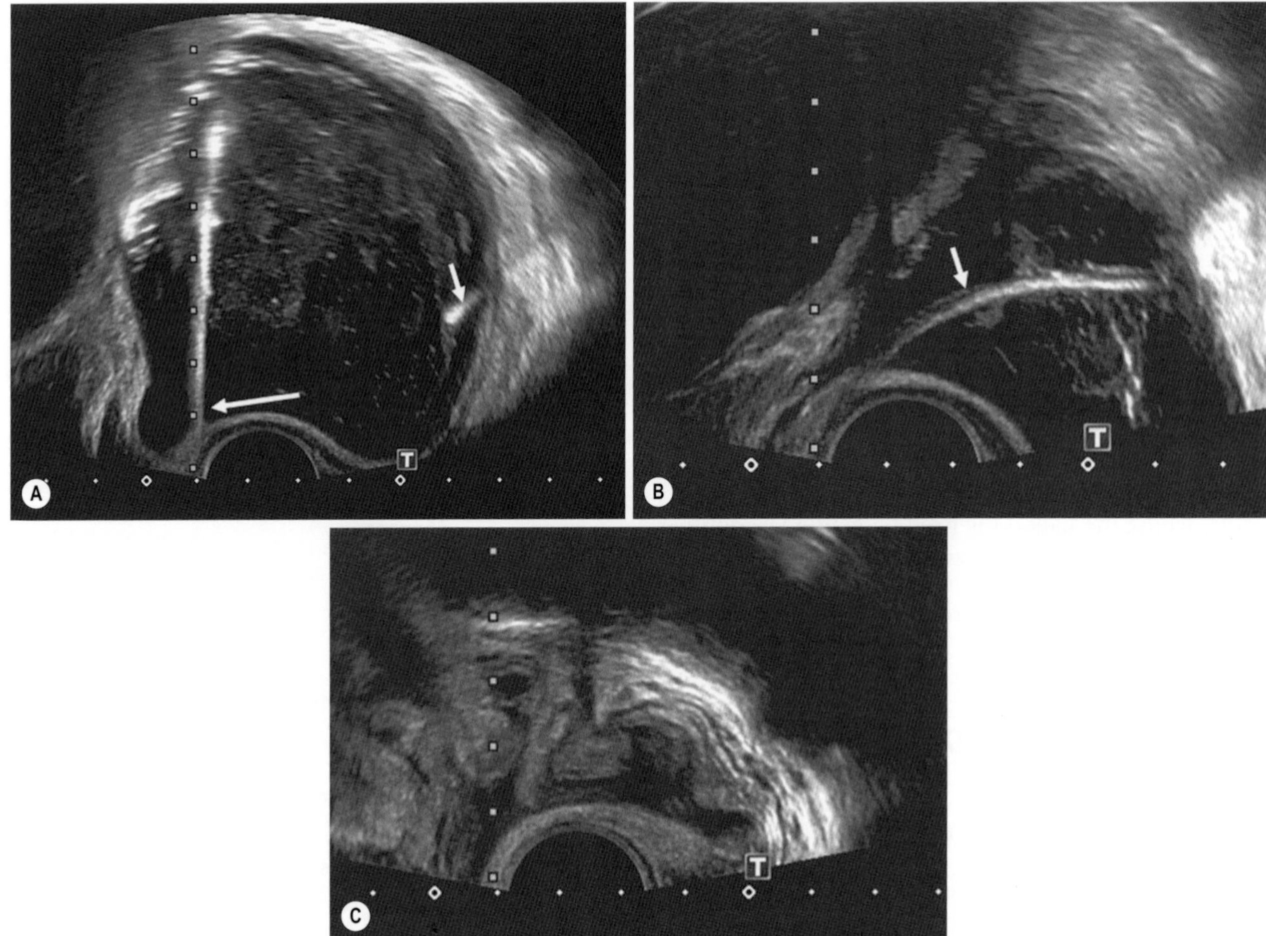

FIGURE 91-20 ■ Transrectal ultrasound (TRUS)-guided drainage of post-appendectomy pelvic abscess. (A) A wire (small arrow) has been inserted and looped within the abscess cavity through an 18G long needle (long arrow) inserted into the abscess using the biopsy attachment of the TRUS probe. (B) A catheter (arrow) has been inserted and the abscess is being drained. (C) The abscess is fully drained and the catheter was removed.

and once tip position is confirmed, the contents should be completely aspirated. If the pus is thick and difficult to aspirate, a pigtail drainage catheter is inserted into the cavity using the Seldinger technique and removed once the cavity has been thoroughly drained. Loculated collections may require multiple needle aspirations.

Seminal Vesiculography and Cyst Sampling

This is a combined ultrasound–fluoroscopic technique[59] for confirming whether seminal vesicle (SV) dilatation is due to ejaculatory duct obstruction in men with low or absent sperm count. The transperineal route is preferred as the risk of introduced infection is lower, but the transrectal route has been used safely. Initial investigations should have confirmed dilated SVs. By the transrectal route with the patient in left lateral position, the dilated vesicle is punctured using a long 22G needle, and contrast medium is injected with the C arm of the fluoroscopic unit in a horizontal position. If the duct is patent, contrast medium will be seen to flow into the bladder rather than the urethra, as the external sphincter will stop such antegrade flow. Occasionally, aspiration of a prostatic cyst, which is usually a utricle cyst, is required to exclude infection or to sample its content. In this case the transperineal route is preferred to avoid introducing infection.

Prostate Brachytherapy, Cryotherapy and HIFU Prostate Ablation

Detailed description of these techniques is outside the scope of this book, but the guiding principles are similar to those used for other prostatic interventions. Brachytherapy and cryotherapy are carried out under general anaesthesia using the grid template transperineal method. Needles are driven into the grid locations on the predetermined treatment plan, and either radioactive seeds (for brachytherapy) or cooled gases are used to ablate the prostate gland, sparing the urethra and rectum. Both can be used to treat non-metastatic prostate cancer, but only the former is an established technique. HIFU ablation is still under investigation, and uses the transrectal route to ablate the prostate in patients with prostate cancer.

ABLATION OF RENAL CYSTS OR LYMPHOCELES

The clinical indication for either procedure should be soundly established. Very few renal cysts are symptomatic and most lymphoceles are also clinically silent. If necessary, the clinical relevance of either can be established by simple needle aspiration to dryness, to see whether the symptoms improve, before embarking on ablation. Numerous ablation techniques have been tried, but none is universally successfully.[60]

Ablation is performed under combined ultrasound and fluoroscopic guidance. It is important to exclude malignancy using CT or MRI. The cyst is punctured under US guidance, and a 5–6Fr catheter is inserted using the Seldinger technique. The cyst volume is calculated by complete evacuation. The integrity of the cyst and absence of any communication with the renal parenchyma or the collecting system is excluded by filling the cavity with iodinated contrast medium under continuous fluoroscopy. The cavity should be filled to 50% of the cyst capacity (up to a maximum of 100 mL) using > 95% ethanol. The alcohol is left in situ for 1 h, and the patient is asked to change their position by rotating around 90° every 15 min, so the entire cyst wall comes in contact with the alcohol. The alcohol is then completely removed. Some pain may be experienced but is usually not very severe and systemic effects of the alcohol are rare if the 100 mL limit is not exceeded.

Pelvic lymphoceles are seen around renal transplants or after lymphadenectomy. Only a few will require ablation, which can be carried out under US/fluoroscopic or CT guidance, following otherwise similar principles. The diagnosis of a lymphocele can be established by biochemical analysis of the fluid. Lymph contains high triglyceride levels, with serum equivalent levels of creatinine and urea. It is important to ensure cavity integrity with lymphocele as inadvertent peritoneal spill may lead to long-term sequelae. With any cyst ablation, sterile technique is important to reduce the risk of introducing infection.

For a full list of references, please see ExpertConsult.

FURTHER READING

1. Sampaio FJ, Zanier JF, Aragão AH, Favorito LA. Intrarenal access: 3-dimensional anatomical study. J Urol 1992;148:1769–73.
6. Pearle MS, Pierce HL, Miller GL, et al. Optimal method of urgent decompression of the collecting system for obstruction and infection due to ureteral calculi. J Urol 1998;160:1260–4.
7. Wah TM, Weston MJ, Irving HC. Percutaneous nephrostomy insertion: outcome data from a prospective multi-operator study at a UK training centre. Clin Radiol 2004;59:255–61.
8. Farrell TA, Hicks ME. A review of radiologically guided percutaneous nephrostomies in 303 patients. J Vasc Interv Radiol 1997;8:769–74.
9. Lee WJ, Patel U, Patel S, Pillari GP. Emergency percutaneous nephrostomy: results and complications. J Vasc Interv Radiol 1994;5:135–9.
14. Patel U, Hussein F. Percutaneous nephrostomy of non-dilated renal collecting systems with fluoroscopic guidance: technique and results. Radiology 2004;233:226–33.
15. Kobayashi K, Censullo ML, Rossman LL, et al. Interventional radiologic management of renal transplant dysfunction: indications, limitations, and technical considerations. Radiographics 2007;27:1109–30.
28. VanSonnenberg E, D'Agostino H, O'Laoide R, et al. Malignant ureteral obstruction: treatment with metal stents—technique, results and observations with percutaneous intraluminal US. Radiology 1994;191:765–8.
29. Lugmayr H, Pauer W. Wallstents for the treatment of extrinsic malignant ureteral obstruction: midterm results. Radiology 1996;198:105–8.
30. Liatsikos EN, Karnabatidis D, Katsanos K, et al. Ureteral metal stents: 10-year experience with malignant ureteral obstruction treatment. J Urol 2009;182:2613–17.
48. Bachar GN, Mor E, Bartal G, et al. Percutaneous balloon dilatation for the treatment of early and late ureteral strictures after renal transplantation: long-term follow-up. Cardiovasc Intervent Radiol 2004;27:335–8.
60. Lucey BC, Kuligowska E. Radiologic management of cysts in the abdomen and pelvis. Am J Roentgenol 2006;186:562–73.

CHAPTER 92

Venous Access and Interventions

Anthony Watkinson • Richard J. Morse

CHAPTER OUTLINE

The placement and maintenance of long-term vascular access catheters accounts for a considerable percentage of the workload of any interventional radiologist, particularly one who works in a large oncology or nephrology unit.

Long-term venous access is usually required for a few, relatively distinct, groups of patients:

- Those requiring access for the instillation of irritant therapeutic agents such as chemotherapy or total parenteral nutrition (TPN), which must be delivered into a large-calibre central vein.
- Those who require access for haemodialysis.
- Patients in whom long-term venous access is required and therefore peripheral venous cannulas are inappropriate, e.g. septic arthritis requiring long courses of antibiotics.

Central access can be gained via either a central or, in certain circumstances, a peripheral vein; the latter is referred to as a peripherally inserted central catheter (PICC).

GENERAL ASSESSMENT OF PATIENTS BEFORE VASCULAR ACCESS PROCEDURES

Before approaching any vascular access case, certain haematological parameters must be checked. As the overwhelming majority of patients referred for access procedures will be elective or semi-elective, there should be time for any clotting abnormalities to be corrected before the commencement of intervention. Central venous access should not be undertaken with a platelet count of $< 50 \times 10^9$/L, and if necessary a platelet transfusion should be arranged after discussion with the local haematology unit. Correction of an international normalised ratio (INR) of > 1.5 should also be performed, ideally with an oral dose of 1–5 mg of phytomenadione (vitamin K_1). The INR measurement should be repeated 24 h later. If there are reasons why a patient cannot wait to have an abnormal INR corrected, then human fresh frozen plasma (FFP) can be administered; however, the prescription and usage of FFP must first also be discussed with the local haematology service.

There is less need to be concerned about abnormalities in clotting parameters when performing PICC lines, but common sense should be exercised. As part of the general pre-procedure, haematological and biochemical work-up, it is also good practice to know the patient's haemoglobin level and glomerular filtration rate (GFR).

Any previous cross-sectional, venographic or ultrasonographic imaging must be reviewed before central access placement. This can alert the practitioner to any unusual anatomical features, the presence of implanted cardiac devices, any previously inserted and now removed long-term vascular access catheters and the presence or absence of venous occlusions.

Informed written consent must be obtained prior to central venous access, ideally in a situation removed in time and place from the interventional suite to allow appropriate consideration of the risks by the patient. The patient should be counselled for the risk of bleeding/haematoma, infection and pneumothorax.

GENERAL PATIENT AND INTERVENTIONAL SUITE PREPARATION FOR CENTRAL VENOUS ACCESS

Strict asepsis must be observed and all staff should wear operating theatre hats and masks. Imaging requirements are a fluoroscopy suite and an ultrasound unit capable of colour Doppler imaging.

The patient should wear a hospital gown which unties at the neck and also an operating theatre hat. It is not essential that they have a peripheral cannula in situ; in many patients peripheral venous access will be very poor and the reason they have been referred for long-term vascular access. The patient should be placed supine on the fluoroscopy table with their head as close to the end of the table as possible. A pillow can be used to support the head and a wedge should also be placed under the knees, for patient comfort but also to help distend the chest and neck veins. Ultrasound examination of the preferred point of access should be undertaken. Usually, the right internal jugular vein (RIJV) is punctured, as it is easily assessed using ultrasound guidance, can be manually compressed in the event of bleeding and provides the most direct route to the superior vena cava/right atrial junction. Ultrasound imaging enables assessment of the venous anatomy and establishes whether the veins are patent and whether they contain thrombus.

The available instruments should include a standard sterile vascular procedure pack and a minor operations surgical set (including scissors, toothed and non-toothed forceps, artery forceps and a needle driver).

INSERTION OF TUNNELLED CENTRAL VENOUS CATHETER

Hickman Line

Once the interventional radiologist and any assistants have scrubbed, the patient's skin should be prepared with an effective skin decontamination agent. Skin preparation should occur from the ipsilateral hairline posteriorly, the angle of the mandible superiorly, the suprasternal notch to the manubriosternal angle anteriorly and across to the lateral border of the ipsilateral pectoralis major laterally. The skin should then be draped; it is the authors' practice to use a standard fenestrated angiographic drape. By placing the top of the fenestration 2–3 cm above the medial aspect of the right clavicle and extending the opening by 2–3 cm inferiorly it is possible to create a well-draped sterile field. The patient's head is covered by the drape; patients are asked to look to their left and the left side of the drape at the head end is elevated on a stand to create a 'tent' under which they stay for the duration of the procedure.

Local anaesthetic is drawn up: 10 mL of 1% lidocaine/1 : 100,000 adrenaline is usually sufficient. The catheter is opened and both lumens are flushed and locked with 5 mL of 0.9% sodium chloride with 1000 IU of heparin. Care should be taken at this point to avoid touching the catheter; if necessary, the non-toothed forceps can be used to handle it.

A sterile ultrasound probe cover is fitted and the RIJV reassessed prior to guided local anaesthetic infiltration of the overlying skin and soft tissues. It is advisable to aim to puncture the vein as close to the clavicle as possible in order to avoid kinking of the catheter. A 5- to 10-mm transverse incision is made and a small pocket created using blunt dissection with the back of the scissors or the needle driver. Ultrasound-guided puncture (in the transverse plane) can then be performed with a standard 18-gauge one-part needle or with a micropuncture set. It is important to ensure that the tip of the puncture needle is always visible on ultrasound in order to reduce the risk of inadvertent carotid arterial puncture or transgression into the pleural cavity. A 10-mL syringe with 3 mL of 0.9% sodium chloride is fitted to the back of the needle and when RIJV puncture has been performed, aspiration on the syringe is undertaken to confirm correct needle placement. Once the RIJV has been punctured, the left hand holding the needle must remain fixed in position; this is easiest if one or two fingers of the left hand are balanced on the patient's clavicle. The syringe can then be removed immediately followed by the insertion of an 0.035-inch J-wire. A prompt exchange reduces the risk of air aspiration into the vein. The wire is inserted and should run freely. If any difficulty is encountered when advancing the wire, the needle should be turned through 180° before another attempt is made to advance the wire. If this is unsuccessful the wire should be withdrawn and syringe aspiration on the needle should be performed to confirm correct positioning. When the wire has been inserted successfully, fluoroscopic guidance is utilised to confirm its passage through the right side of the heart into the inferior vena cava (IVC). It is not uncommon to encounter difficulty in exiting the right atrium with the wire preferentially passing through the tricuspid valve and into the right ventricle. If simple manoeuvres such as a breath-hold fail to help in exiting the right atrium, a 4 French (4Fr) multipurpose catheter can be used to guide the wire out of the heart.

Once the wire is safely in the IVC, the part outside the patient can be recoiled and fastened to the drape above the patient's right shoulder. Local anaesthetic can then be infiltrated subcutaneously, starting approximately 5–6 cm inferior to the lower border of the right clavicle and continuing superiorly to meet the puncture site. In female patients it is advisable to aim for the catheter to exit as medially as possible to help avoid soft tissues pulling it inferiorly when the patient stands up; this is a less important consideration in thin male patients. Aesthetic considerations may need to be taken into account, especially in female patients who may wish to wear a V-neck style blouse and therefore would want the line exiting more laterally.

An 8- to 10-mm incision is made at the point which the catheter is to exit and a further pocket is made aiming superiorly. The end of the line is attached to the tunnelling device by means of a screw thread at the bottom of the tunneller and the tunneller and line pushed through the subcutaneous tissue to exit at the neck incision site. Two types of tunneller are available, metal or plastic. The metal devices are stiffer and can be bent into a gentle curve. If difficulty is encountered in pushing the tunnelling device through the fascial layers or platysma, a small incision with the scalpel directly onto the device tip will usually free it. The tunneller and catheter are then pulled through the neck incision completely until the cuff of the catheter lies well within the chest wall pocket. Once the catheter is through the tunnel, it should be laid over the patient's chest, aiming to reproduce the path it will follow inside the patient and fluoroscopic screening is utilised to assess where it needs to be cut; its tip should be left near the right atrial/superior vena caval junction—usually 2–3 cm below the carina. The catheter can then be cut using scissors, and the tunneller and the removed section of catheter discarded.

A peel-away sheath one French size greater than the line diameter is inserted over the wire. Then the wire and inner dilator of the sheath are removed and the end of the catheter is advanced into the sheath with the aid of the non-toothed forceps. The patient should lie still, not talk and breathe gently during the line insertion into the peel-away sheath. With a well-hydrated individual the risk of venous air aspiration is very low.

Once the catheter is in place and the peel-away sheath removed, both lumens can be flushed and locked with heparinised sodium chloride solution. Fluoroscopy is used to check the position of the catheter. 3-0 Prolene sutures are used to close the neck incision with a mattress suture and the chest incision with a standard suture subsequently attached to the catheter. Occlusive dressings are applied to the venotomy site in the neck and the catheter exit site on the chest.

Groshong Catheter

The Groshong catheter (Bard Access Systems, UT, USA) has a three-way valve at the tip of the catheter which remains closed at neutral pressure but opens outwards during infusion and inwards during aspiration. This device aims to minimise the maintenance required for a tunnelled central catheter and helps avoid line thrombosis. Many of the principles which apply to the insertion of a Hickman line also apply to the insertion of a Groshong catheter, but there are some important technical differences.

The catheter is always placed via the subclavian vein, at the junction of the outer and middle thirds of the clavicle. The vein is punctured with a Micropuncture (COOK Medical Inc, Bloomington, IN, USA) needle and an 0.018-inch wire introduced into the IVC. After a long peel-away sheath has been inserted over the wire, the inner dilator is removed along with the wire and the catheter inserted. Once the position of the catheter tip is confirmed as satisfactory, the peel-away is removed. It is then that the cuff position is marked on the skin with the line positioned inferomedially across the chest and further local anaesthetic infiltrated and a small incision is made on the chest wall. The tunnelling device is attached to the distal end of the line and inserted through the infraclavicular incision, aiming towards the chest wall incision through which it is brought out. The cuff is left under the skin surface and the hub is then attached and secured before the incisions are closed, again with 3-0 Prolene.

PORT-A-CATH PLACEMENT

Port-a-caths consist of a self-sealing septum encased in a port made of stainless steel, titanium or plastic, attached to a silicone catheter. The port is placed subcutaneously and is accessed via specially designed needles inserted into the septum through the skin surface (Figs. 92-1 to 92-8).

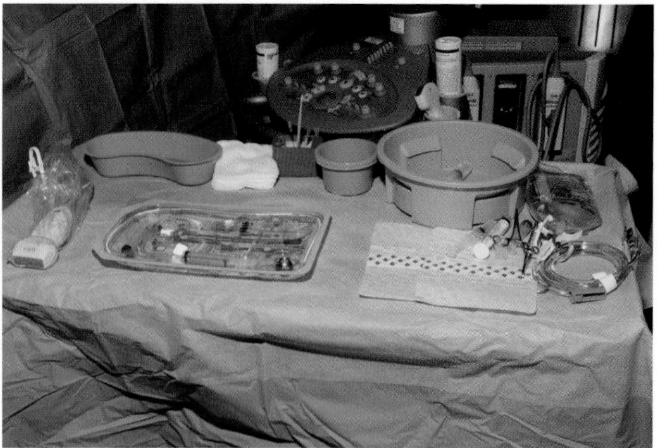

FIGURE 92-1 ■ **Trolley laid up before port-a-cath insertion.**

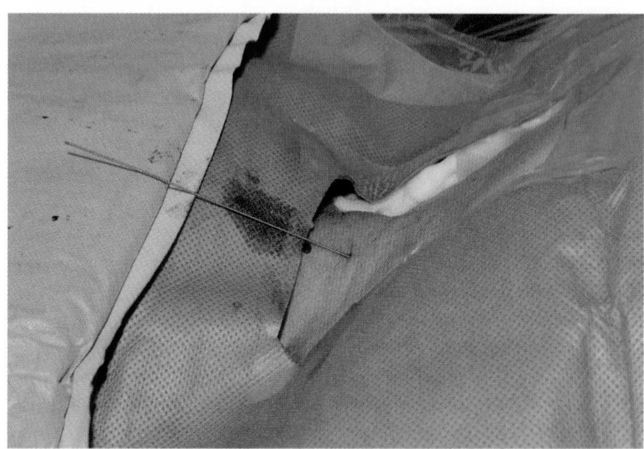

FIGURE 92-2 ■ **Guidewire inserted into right internal jugular vein.**

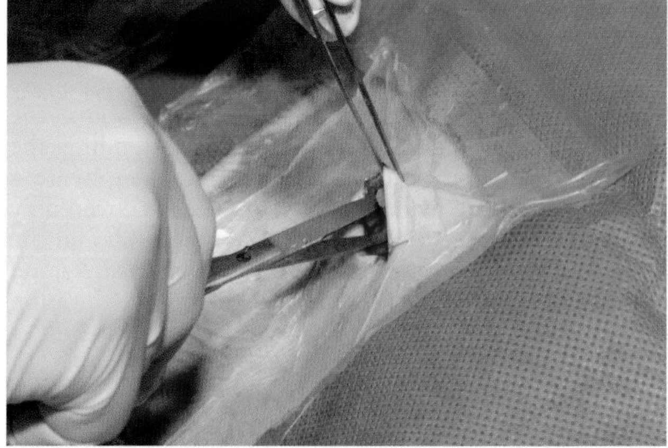

FIGURE 92-3 ■ **Subcutaneous pocket formed in anterior chest wall.**

The method of insertion of the catheter is generally the same as for other tunnelled devices. It is important to know the type of chemotherapy the patient will receive. The use of bevacizumab (Avastin, Genentech Inc., CA, USA) has been shown to delay wound healing and the manufacturers recommend an interval of 28 days after

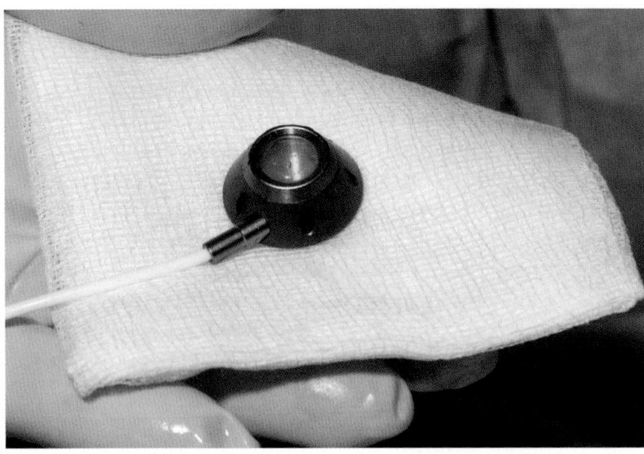

FIGURE 92-4 ■ Port-a-cath hub prior to insertion.

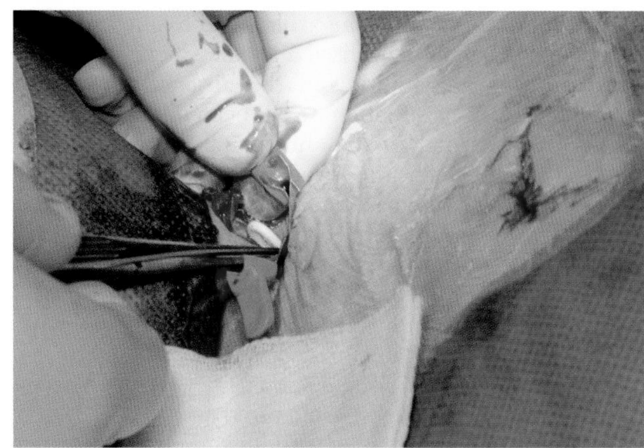

FIGURE 92-7 ■ Catheter inserted into peel-away sheath.

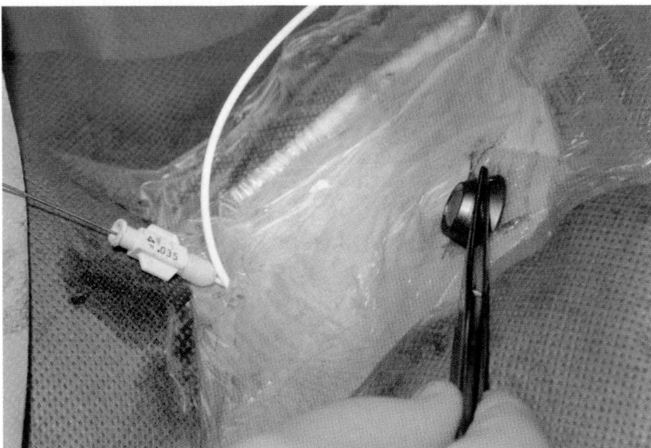

FIGURE 92-5 ■ Catheter has now been tunnelled and the hub is being inserted into the subcutaneous pocket.

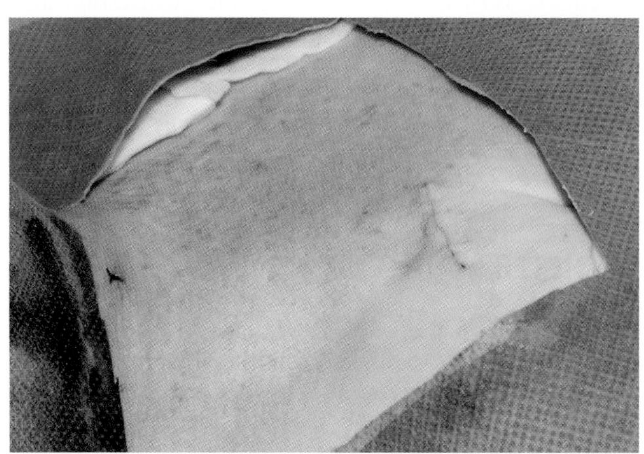

FIGURE 92-8 ■ Final result.

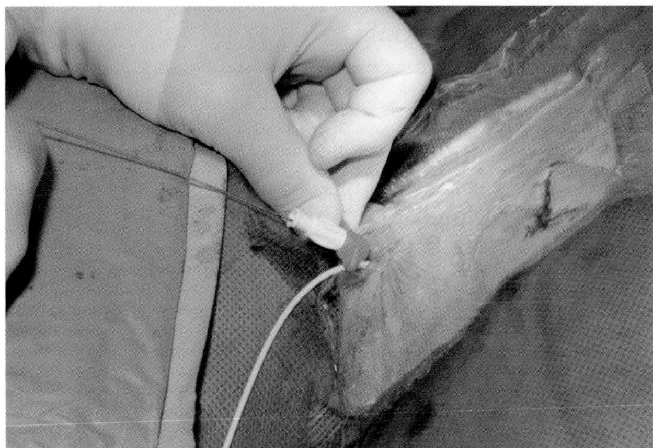

FIGURE 92-6 ■ Peel-away sheath inserted before catheter insertion.

surgery before commencement of the drug. It is also important to try and avoid placement of the port within a potential radiotherapy field as this can also adversely affect wound healing.

An internal jugular venous puncture is made, preferably on the right, and a wire is inserted into the IVC. The site of insertion of the port is generously infiltrated with a local anaesthetic agent, usually 20 mL of 1% lidocaine/1 : 100,000 adrenaline. An incision of 4–5 cm is made in line with the ipsilateral clavicle and a subcutaneous pocket formed. It is very important at this stage to ensure that the subdermal layer is well dissected as this will allow the port to lie correctly within the pocket. The port is also flushed and attached to the catheter by means of a metallic cuff. The port is then sutured to the underlying deep fascial layers by means of three 2-0 Prolene sutures with the septum facing anteriorly. The catheter is measured and cut and inserted through a peel-away sheath in the same fashion as for a Hickman catheter. Two to three 2-0 Vicryl sutures are then used to bring the subcutaneous tissues in apposition over the port before a 3-0 continuous subcuticular Vicryl suture is placed and closed with an Aberdeen knot before dressing. Fluoroscopy is used to check the final position of the catheter.

PERIPHERALLY INSERTED CENTRAL CATHETERS

Initial assessment is made of the venous suitability of the veins of the upper arms using ultrasound and a tourniquet applied high up towards the axilla. The basilic, cephalic or brachial vein can be utilised and assessment should be made for compressibility and the absence of venous thrombosis. Once a suitable site has been identified, preferably just proximal to the antecubital fossa, measurement is taken from the proposed entry site to the ipsilateral mid-clavicular line to the third intercostal space. This measurement corresponds to the desired length of the catheter. The skin is decontaminated and draped appropriately and a sterile ultrasound probe cover-fitted before infiltration of the soft tissues with 3–5 mL of 1% lidocaine under ultrasound control. A tourniquet is used to distend the veins. Using a Micropuncture needle, the vein is punctured and an 0.018-inch wire inserted. The needle is withdrawn and a peel-away sheath inserted. The wire and inner dilator of the sheath are removed and the pre-cut catheter inserted. Asking patients to turn their head to the side of insertion and lowering their chin to their chest helps avoid the catheter turning superiorly into the internal jugular vein. A chest radiograph is then performed to document the position of the catheter tip position before securing the catheter to the skin surface.

CATHETER MAINTENANCE

There is little in the way of maintenance that is usually required to keep a tunnelled central catheter or port-a-cath in good working order. When the catheter is not in use, it is standard practice to flush the lumen(s) with 0.9% sodium chloride before locking a solution of heparin sodium (50 IU/5 mL) into it to help prevent the formation of blood clots. If the catheter is not to be used for a prolonged period, regular flushing and locking of the lumen(s) every 2 weeks maintains patency.

CATHETER REPOSITIONING

It is possible for central venous catheters and port-a-caths to become malpositioned, especially if the line is left short. Malposition may be noted on chest radiography or reported by nursing staff following malfunction. Catheters may enter the contralateral or ipsilateral brachiocephalic or subclavian vein, or the azygos vein.

Repositioning is usually straightforward. Access can be gained via an ultrasound-guided puncture of a femoral vein under standard aseptic conditions. A 5Fr sheath can then be inserted to allow the passage of a guidewire and catheter into the central chest veins. A reverse curve catheter can be hooked over the malpositioned catheter, which is then moved into its correct position. If this technique fails, a snare device inserted via a sheath in the contralateral groin can be used to grasp a wire passed through the reverse curve catheter over the malpositioned catheter and, by gentle withdrawal of the snare whilst grasping the guidewire, the catheter can be pulled back into position.

TUNNELLED DIALYSIS CATHETERS

Whilst the preferred haemodialysis access method is via a surgically formed arteriovenous fistula or graft,[1] there are occasions in which a patient with established renal failure may require a tunnelled catheter for dialysis, e.g. whilst waiting for a surgically formed fistula to mature or if they have exhausted all other potential access options.

The initial patient assessment and preparation are similar to that for tunnelled venous access catheters. It is essential that previous access history is reviewed as a tunnelled dialysis catheter is often the last access option for a patient in whom all other methods have failed. It is not uncommon in this situation to find multiple areas of central venous stenotic disease which may require venoplasty prior to line insertion.

The patient is prepared and positioned as for a tunnelled venous access catheter. The right internal jugular vein is the preferred entry point. The femoral veins, whilst suitable for an urgent non-tunnelled catheter, are unsuitable for a tunnelled dialysis catheter because of the risk of infection but may be used when other venous sites are occluded.

Tunnelled dialysis catheters are available in different lengths to allow for variation in patient body habitus and site of insertion. The technical procedure for insertion of the tunnelled dialysis catheter is similar to that used to insert a Hickman catheter. The main difference is that there is no cutting and measuring of the catheter, as its length is fixed. As a general rule a 28-cm catheter is appropriate from the RIJV and a 32-cm from the LIJV. Prior to insertion of the catheter the two lumens should be gently pulled apart and separated, if appropriate, before attaching them to the tunnelling device. Separation of the catheter tips helps to minimise recirculation of blood and optimises haemodialysis. Inserting a dialysis catheter via the LIJV can be problematic; caution must be utilised when inserting the 16Fr peel-away sheath as rupture of the brachiocephalic vein has been reported. Use of a stiff guidewire can help to minimise the risk of this potentially serious complication.

A variety of alternative access approaches for tunnelled haemodialysis catheters, including the external jugular vein[2] and translumbar,[3–5] transhepatic[6] and transrenal[7] approaches to the IVC, have been described.

DIALYSIS CATHETER MAINTENANCE

Tunnelled dialysis catheters have a high propensity to form a fibrin sheath around the line tips, leading to suboptimal haemodialysis function.

'Stripping' poorly functioning haemodialysis catheters (Figs. 92-9 to 92-11) can deal with this problem. This technique involves snaring the catheter from below, having placed a 6Fr sheath in a femoral vein and stripping away the fibrin from both lumens. It is often necessary to advance a standard J-wire down each lumen in turn and into the IVC in order to grasp this with the snare, as trying to grasp the line itself in the right atrium can be very difficult. This straightforward procedure, which can be performed on an outpatient basis, usually results in

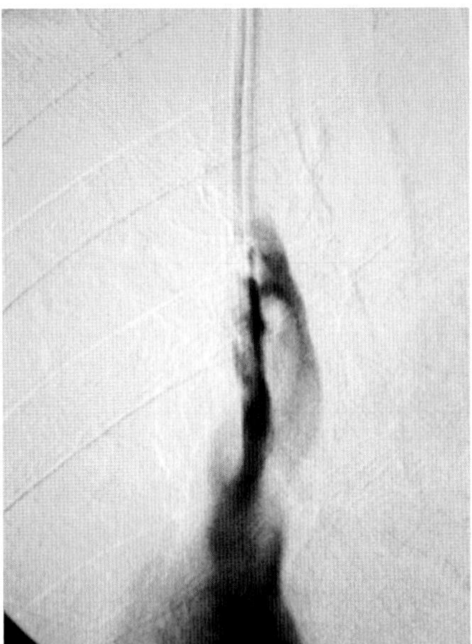

FIGURE 92-9 ■ Linogram demonstrating extensive fibrin sheath formation.

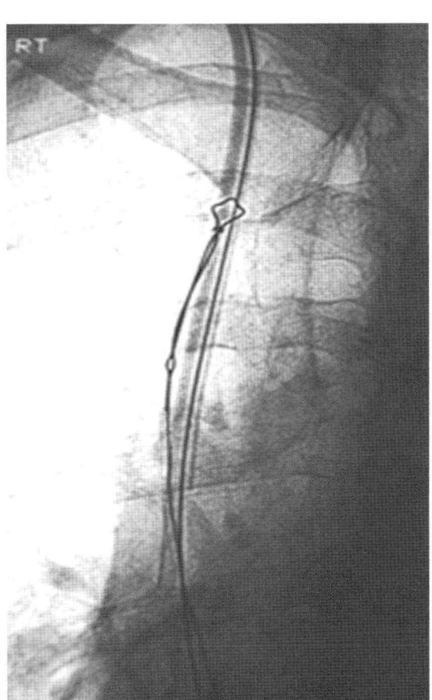

FIGURE 92-10 ■ 'Stripping' the line from below with a snare.

significantly improved dialysis flow rates.[8] The fibrin sheath stripped from the line lodges in small pulmonary arteries but this does not lead to clinical problems.

Alternatively, the catheter can be replaced using an over-the-wire technique.[9] The cuff is dissected out from the skin before a stiff guidewire is inserted through one

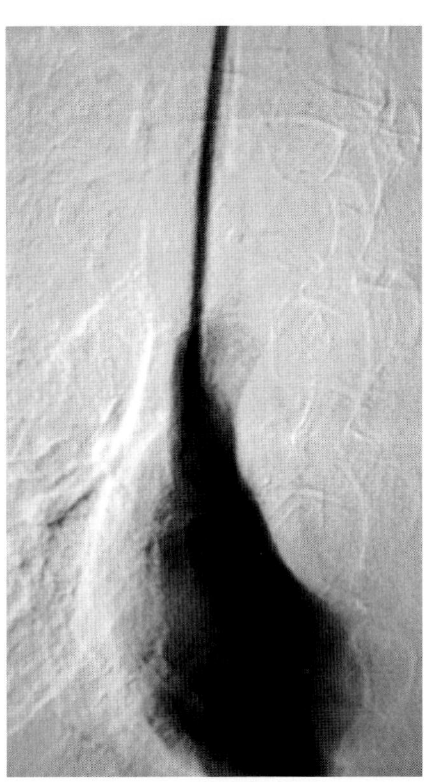

FIGURE 92-11 ■ Post-procedural linogram demonstrates removal of the fibrin sheath.

of the lumens and into the IVC. The catheter is then removed and a peel-away sheath is inserted over the guidewire. The new tunnelled catheter is inserted through the sheath.

Venoplasty can be performed to disrupt the fibrin sheath immediately prior to catheter exchange; however, this may lead to subsequent central venous stenosis.[10]

For a full list of references, please see ExpertConsult.

FURTHER READING

1. National Kidney Foundation KDOQI Guidelines. Updates clinical practice guidelines and recommendations. Am J Kidney Dis 2006;48(Suppl 1):S176–247.
2. Lorenz JM. Unconventional venous access techniques. Semin Intervent Radiol 2006;23(3):279–86.
5. Power A, Singh S, Ashby D, et al. Translumbar central venous catheters for long-term haemodialysis. Nephrol Dial Transplant 2010;25:1588–95.
6. Smith TP, Ryan JM, Reddan DN. Transhepatic catheter access for haemodialysis. Radiology 2004;232(1):246–51.
9. Merport M, Murphy TP, Egglin TK, Dubel GJ. Fibrin sheath stripping versus catheter exchange for the treatment of failed tunneled hemodialysis catheters: randomised clinical trial. J Vasc Interv Radiol 2000;11(9):1115–20.
10. Ni N, Mojibian H, Pollak J, Tal M. Association between disruption of fibrin sheaths using percutaneous transluminal angioplasty balloons and late onset of central venous stenosis. Cardiovasc Intervent Radiol 2011;34(1):114–19.

CHAPTER 93

Spinal Interventions

Konstantinos Katsanos • Tarun Sabharwal

CHAPTER OUTLINE

INTRODUCTION

Spinal interventional procedures are used in the diagnosis and treatment of various spinal pathologies of benign or malignant origin. Procedures described in the present chapter are performed by interventional radiologists, who work within a wider multidisciplinary team of clinical specialists that may include neurosurgeons, orthopedic surgeons and oncologists. Interventional radiologists are appropriately trained to carry out spinal intervention with minimal risks, and can manage any relevant procedure-related complications.

IMAGE-GUIDED VERTEBRAL BIOPSY

Vertebral bone biopsy is a minimally invasive percutaneous procedure with the advantages of low cost, low morbidity, high accuracy and repeatability and it has replaced open surgical biopsy in most cases. Fluoroscopy-guided bone biopsy was first described in the 1970s and image-guided bone biopsy is today a critical part of the management of musculoskeletal lesions, including primary tumours, bone metastases and bone infections. Spinal applications include image-guided biopsy of the vertebrae, the sacrum and the iliac bones. Disc aspiration for the investigation of spondylodiscitis is also widely practiced. Under X-ray guidance a biopsy needle can be used to access and sample small lesions in difficult anatomies, such as the vertebral body or intervertebral discs, without surgical exploration.

Patient Preparation

Before considering an image-guided spinal biopsy all relevant medical history, laboratory tests and relevant imaging findings must be analysed thoroughly and discussed with the multidisciplinary team. The multidisciplinary team usually includes the spinal neurosurgeon, the musculoskeletal radiologist, the responsible oncologist and an experienced cytopathologist. Correlation with plain films and MRI is critical to avoid unnecessary procedures in certain benign lesions with typical imaging appearances ('do not touch lesions'). Well-recognised and accepted indications and contraindications for spinal biopsies are outlined in Table 93-1. In general, spinal biopsy is indicated to identify tumour or infection. If bone metastasis is suspected, biopsy should be undertaken only if the result will influence oncologic management. Spinal biopsy may also be considered for tumour staging, or to compare histological characteristics in patients with synchronous or metachronous metastatic cancer. Primary musculoskeletal tumours require identification, grading and often cytogenetic analysis to determine appropriate treatment strategies and prognosis. Bleeding diathesis is the only absolute contraindication to spinal biopsy as it can cause severe haemorrhage or epidural haematoma that may compromise the spinal cord. Alternative options and the risk–benefit ratio should be considered in all patients with spinal lesions that are difficult to access percutaneously.

Correction of coagulopathy, informed consent and consideration regarding conscious sedation or general anaesthesia constitute key elements of preoperative assessment for all spinal biopsy procedures. Anticoagulants like warfarin and heparin must be stopped prior to the procedure per local institutional policy and a platelet count below 50,000/mL must be corrected with adequate platelet transfusion. Bleeding diathesis with an international normalised ratio (INR) higher than 1.3–1.5 may be reversed with transfusions of fresh frozen plasma or cryoprecipitate as needed. Antiplatelet agents must be stopped in all cases of spinal interventions at least 5 days prior to the procedure to correct platelet dysfunction.

Image Guidance

Image guidance may be real-time plain fluoroscopy based on bony landmarks or computed tomography (CT), which offers higher soft tissue resolution, but is not real time. There are several different routes for performing an image-guided spinal biopsy depending on lesion anatomy and size. Typically, patients are placed in a prone or lateral decubitus position. The transpedicular or posterolateral approach is often used for lumbar vertebral body biopsy (Fig. 93-1). The intercostovertebral approach is usually indicated for the thoracic spine and an anterolateral approach with manual displacement of the large vessels is recommended for the cervical spine (Fig. 93-2). Fluoroscopic guidance is the modality of choice for the majority of spinal procedures and may be supplemented by CT for cervical lesions (Fig. 93-3). Biplane fluoroscopy or rotational flat panel angiography with cone beam CT capabilities are emerging modalities for enhanced image guidance during difficult spinal procedures. CT fluoroscopy is readily available in many institutions, but is generally avoided because of the increased radiation exposure. An oropharyngeal approach is indicated for biopsy of C1 or the dens. A posterior oblique CT-guided approach is usually chosen for biopsy of the pedicles and the other posterior spinal elements or the surrounding soft tissues. The access route will also depend on the image-guidance modalities available. Beware that certain musculoskeletal tumour lesions may be eligible for curative surgical resection; thus certain anatomical compartments, not involved by the tumour, must not be breached by the biopsy needle. This is especially true for soft tissue sarcomas and osteosarcomas to limit local recurrence after resection. Nevertheless, the risk of tract seeding

TABLE 93-1 Image-Guided Vertebral Bone Biopsy: Indications and Contraindications

Indications

- Determine the nature of a non-specific solitary bone or soft tissue lesion.
- Confirm or exclude spinal metastases in patients with known primary tumour.
- Determine nature of spinal metastases in patients with unknown primary tumour.
- Exclude metastatic disease or multiple myeloma in patients with vertebral compression fractures.
- Determine causative infectious agent in spondylodiscitis or osteomyelitis.
- Before vertebroplasty or cementoplasty for medicolegal reasons.

Contraindications

- Uncorrectable coagulopathy.
- Uncooperative patient.
- Hypervascular lesion in the cervical or thoracic spine.
- Anatomical location difficult or unsafe to access.
- Risk of infection spreading to the bone.

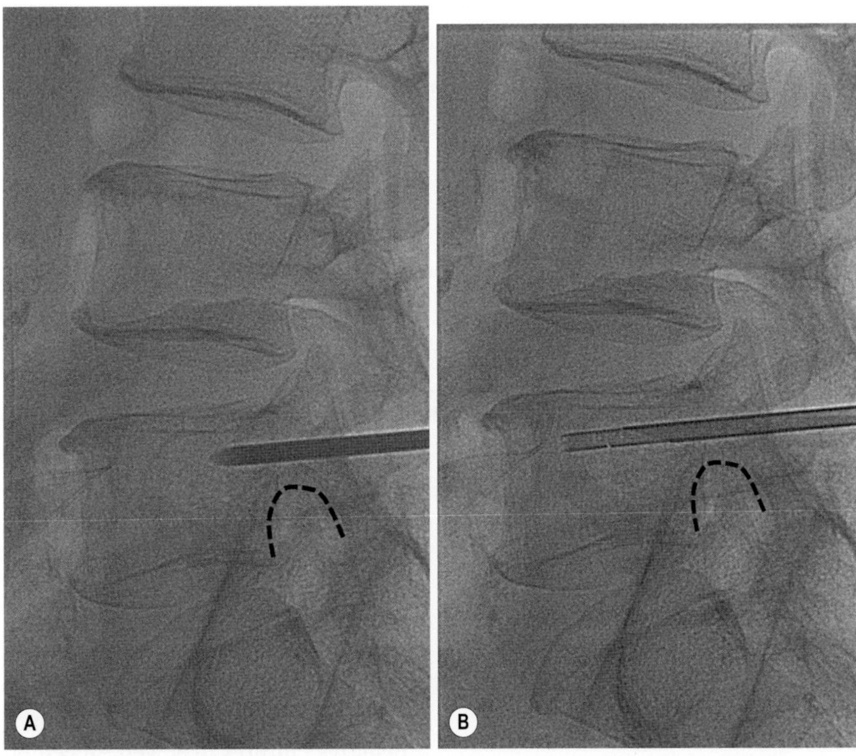

FIGURE 93-1 ■ Fluoroscopically guided transpedicular biopsy of the L5 vertebral body (lateral projection). (A) Note the advancement of a beveled 10G needle trocar across the pedicle (black dotted line denotes the superior aspect of the underlying intervertebral foramen). Needle must not breach either the underlying foramen to avoid spinal nerve injury or the medial aspect of the pedicle to avoid epidural haematoma or thecal sac injury. (B) Coaxial insertion of a 12G trephine needle to obtain a bone marrow sample of the cancellous bone of the L5 vertebral body.

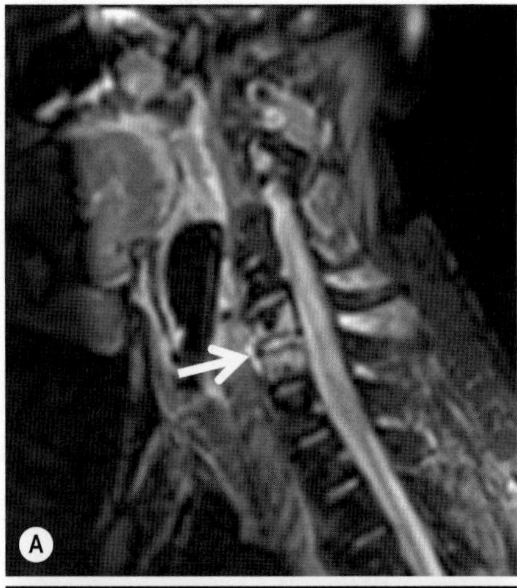

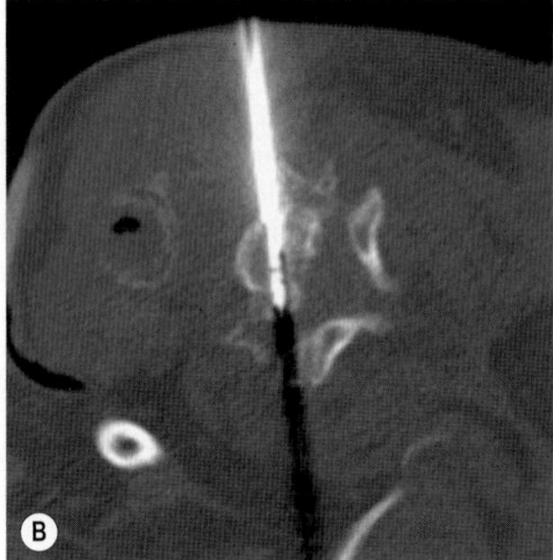

FIGURE 93-2 ■ CT-guided anterolateral biopsy of the C5 vertebral body. (A) Increased signal of the C5–C6 intervertebral disc and the adjacent vertebral bodies (white arrow) in keeping with infectious spondylodiscitis (sagittal STIR image). (B) CT-guided biopsy of the C5 vertebral body using an anterolateral approach and a beveled 10G needle trocar (axial CT image on a lateral decubitus position). A 12G trephine needle has been inserted coaxially for bone sampling. When performing cervical spine biopsies the needle must never breach the transverse foramen to avoid injuring the vertebral artery (dissection or thrombosis), which may induce a vertebrobasilar stroke.

following musculoskeletal fine needle aspiration is very low, estimated at 3–5/100,000 cases.

Performing the Procedure

Routine monitoring of vital signs is necessary during all spinal procedures. Percutaneous vertebral biopsy is a painful procedure because of osseous puncture and conscious sedation is necessary. Sedation is routinely administered using a combination of fentanyl and midazolam according to national and international guidelines. General anaesthesia may be necessary on a case-by-case basis.

In patients with multiple spinal metastatic lesions, the largest and most easily accessible lesion should be chosen. The integrity of the underlying weight-bearing bone must also be considered, although the risk of post-biopsy iatrogenic vertebral fracture is very low. In patients with painful vertebral pathologic fractures, consideration of palliative cementoplasty following successful histologic analysis is worthwhile to improve quality of life. Bone sampling may be accompanied by sampling of adjacent soft tissues, and percutaneous disc biopsy may include biopsy of the neighbouring subchondral vertebral endplates to increase diagnostic yield. When planning a vertebral biopsy, mixed sclerotic-lytic or contrast-enhancing lesions are preferred as target lesions compared to hypodense or cystic areas that often contain necrotic components. Beware of certain spinal lesions, such as renal cell carcinoma metastases and haemangiomas, which may be highly vascular and can be associated with an increased risk of haemorrhagic complications. Different specimens must be sent for histology, cytopathology and microbiology.

With regard to needle choice, the length of the needle (10–20 cm long) must be appropriate to the depth of the lesion. Spinal bone biopsies require use of 11–15G trephine needles that obtain an adequate core of bone marrow. Spinal trephine needles are inserted through a matching outer cannula that is hammered to penetrate the osseous cortex, as necessary. Routine 16–20G core biopsy cutting needles are used in patients with tumours that have a soft tissue component or extensive osteolysis. Fine needle aspiration with a 20–22G needle (Chiba needle) is usually enough for sampling intervertebral discs and aspiration of collections. Larger bore needles are preferred for percutaneous biopsy of the vertebrae because of their rigidity and ability to be hammered or drilled into the bone. Automated drilling biopsy guns have recently been made available for routine bone marrow biopsy and can be used in patients with bony lesions that have a thick overlying cortex. Depending on the indication, trephine core biopsy for histology may be combined with coaxial fine needle aspiration for cytology and microbiology.

Results

Reported diagnostic accuracy of spinal bone biopsies is above 95%, but there is always a small risk of a non-diagnostic outcome because of insufficient tissue sampling or sampling of necrotic or sclerotic areas. Diagnosis of spinal metastatic tumours is considered generally easier than primary bone tumours, but diagnostic yield also depends on lesion size and accessibility. In general, more than three needle passes are recommended to obtain an adequate volume of tissue and increase biopsy success. Multiple core biopsies are required for diagnosis of lymphoma, whereas fine needle aspiration may suffice for the diagnosis of metastasis and infection. Large core trephine biopsy is indicated for investigation of primary spinal tumours like osteoblastomas. The diagnostic accuracy of percutaneous disc biopsy for the investigation of infectious spondylodiscitis is around 50% and the rate of negative cultures may well exceed 60%, even when paravertebral or intervertebral disc fluid collections are aspirated. The most commonly isolated pathogen in infectious spondylodiscitis is blood-borne *Staphylococcus aureus*, and empirical antibiotic treatment may be initiated even

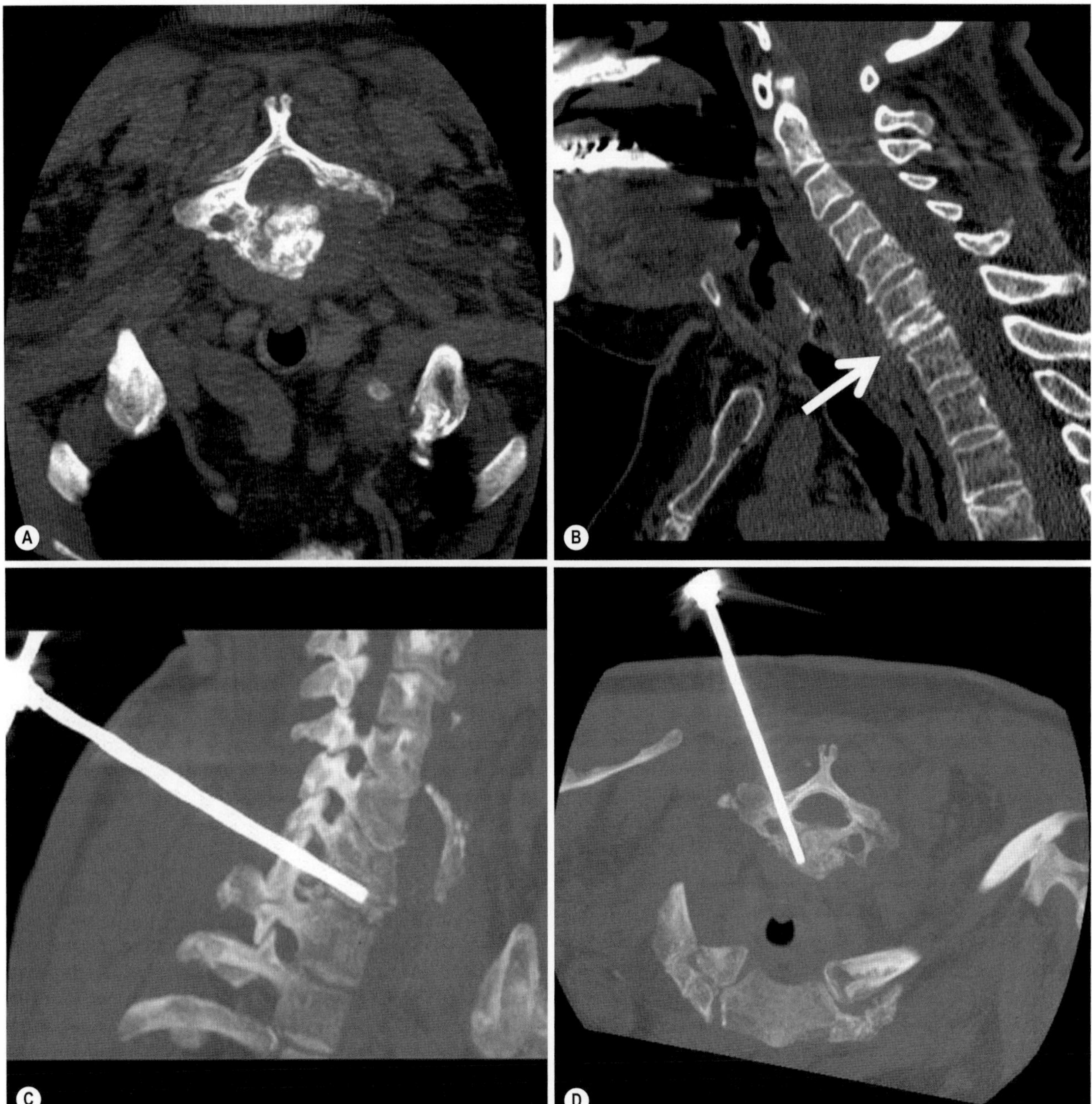

FIGURE 93-3 ■ **CT-guided transpedicular biopsy of the C7 vertebral body.** (A, B) Collapse and destruction of the C7 vertebral body (white arrow) in a patient with history of metastatic lung adenocarcinoma (A: axial CT image; B: sagittal reformatted CT image). (C, D) CT-guided transpedicular bone biopsy using a beveled 10G needle trocar with coaxial insertion of a 12G trephine needle. Note the oblique needle tract without breach of the spinal canal, the ipsilateral transverse foramen or the over- and underlying intervertebral foramen (C: sagittal CT image; D: axial volume-rendered CT image).

without definite diagnosis. Antibiotics can be stopped 24–48 h prior to tissue sampling to increase diagnostic yield from fluid cultures.

SPINAL INJECTION PROCEDURES

Lumbar Disc Herniation

Lumbosacral radicular pain is defined as pain radiating to one or more lumbar or sacral dermatomes caused by nerve root compression producing irritation and inflammation. The pathology is also known as sciatica or nerve root pain. Radiculitis (only radicular pain) should be distinguished from radiculopathy that includes objective findings of sensory or motor disturbance. Lumbosacral radicular pain is the commonest form of neuropathic pain with an annual prevalence of 9.9–25% in the general population. Pain usually resolves spontaneously in two-thirds of patients within 12 weeks of onset. However, almost a third of patients continue to suffer from radicular pain after 3 months to 1 year. Before the age of 50 the most frequent cause is disc herniation, while after the age of 50 degenerative spine changes are more prevalent. Radiating pain may be sharp, stabbing, throbbing or burning and diagnosis is based on medical history and medical examination. Dermatomal distribution, pain that increases while bending forward or coughing, and a positive Lasègue or crossed Lasègue test are the usual clinical findings. Disc herniation most commonly occurs in the L4–L5 (around 30%) and L5–S1 (around 50%) intervertebral segments and the L4, L5 and S1 roots are the ones most commonly affected. MRI may confirm the presence of a disc herniation, but the specificity of the examination is very low because incidental disc herniations are detected in 20–36% of asymptomatic individuals.

Selective segmental nerve blocks, whereby a specific nerve root is anaesthetised via an image-guided transforaminal injection of a small amount of lignocaine, may be helpful in excluding one level if negative, but positive blocks are considered non-specific because of significant overlap between innervation of adjacent segments. Transforaminal blocks may simultaneously block afferent input from the corresponding nerve root, the sinuvertebral nerve that innervates the intervertebral disc anteriorly and the dorsal ramus that innervates the facet joint and the muscles posteriorly at the same level. Therefore, differential diagnosis between true radiculitis, discogenic low back pain and mechanical facetogenic low back pain may be difficult. It is crucial that any red flags (trauma, cancer and infection) are excluded during diagnostic workup of the patient. Watch out for a previous medical history of cancer or unexplained weight loss, structural spinal deformities, symptoms appearing before the age of 20 or after 50 and acute neurological deficits that may require urgent surgical decompression. For example, a patient with acute cauda equina syndrome with saddle anaesthesia, sacral polyradiculopathy and sphincter dysfunction must be referred for emergent surgery.

Indications

Spinal epidural injections with local anaesthetic and corticosteroids are generally indicated in patients with ongoing lumbosacral radicular pain who have failed conservative therapy with non-steroidal anti-inflammatory drugs (NSAIDS), early mobilisation and physiotherapy for at least 6–12 weeks. The primary indication is local compression of a nerve root or exiting spinal nerve by intervertebral disc herniation confirmed by CT or MRI. Spinal injections are also indicated for pain relief in patients with failed back surgery syndrome (FBSS) and degenerative spinal canal stenosis and in elderly patients who are not surgical candidates. The pathophysiology of sciatica combines mechanical nerve compression and the local release of pro-inflammatory mediators such as prostaglandins, nitrous oxide, phospholipase A2 and cyclooxygenase-2. The rationale for epidural corticosteroid injections is based on their potent anti-inflammatory properties. Epidural steroid injections are contraindicated in pregnancy, active peptic ulcers and uncorrectable coagulopathy and caution should be exercised in patients with diabetes and osteoporosis.

Technique

Approaches to epidural peri-radicular injections include (1) the classical interlaminar, (2) the targeted transforaminal and (3) the caudal approach. Transforaminal epidural injection of steroids is reported to provide the best results in patients with segmental radicular symptoms. Compared to the posterior interlaminar approach, the transforaminal approach may achieve more precise delivery at the level of the inflamed root and the drugs may theoretically reach the interface between the disc hernia and the compressed nerve root at the ventral epidural space, more easily. The interlaminal approach may be chosen in posterolateral disc herniations, while the transforaminal approach is usually preferred for foraminal and extraforaminal herniations. However, transforaminal injections can be associated with rare neurological complications, including paraplegia in the lumbar spine and tetraplegia or death in the cervical spine (discussed later). Either fluoroscopy or computed tomography (CT) may be used for image guidance. The latter has the advantage of superb soft tissue contrast resolution, but fluoroscopic guidance is faster and allows for real-time control of needle advancement and drug injection to avoid complications (Fig. 93-4).

When a fluoroscopic-guided interlaminal epidural injection is used, the patient is positioned in the prone position or in the decubitus foetal position based on operator preference. The correct intervertebral segment is identified using fluoroscopic guidance and bone landmarks. Cranial angulation of the tube usually helps to

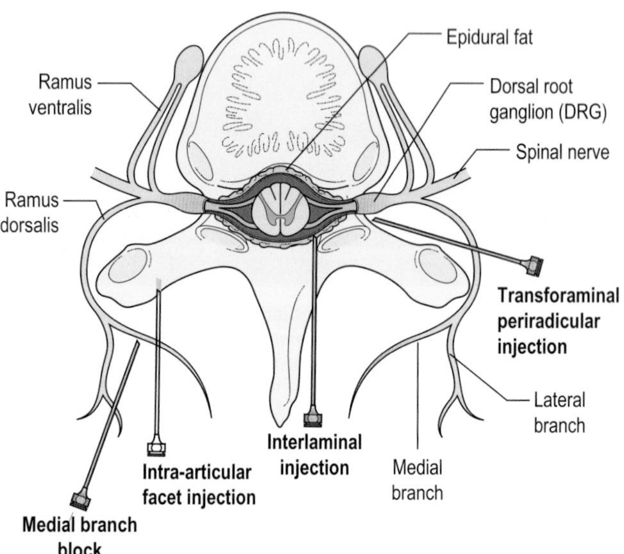

FIGURE 93-4 ■ **Spinal injections.** Schema shows the various different approaches for spinal injections to treat mechanical or radicular cervical and lumbar back pain. Transforaminal and interlaminal approaches are used for the injection of steroids and anaesthetics to the epidural space. Intra-articular injections are used for the injection of steroids into painful degenerated zygapophysial (facet) joints. Medial branch blocks are used for temporary anaesthesia or radiofrequency ablation of the medial branch of the dorsal ramus to achieve long-lasting denervation of the painful facet joints.

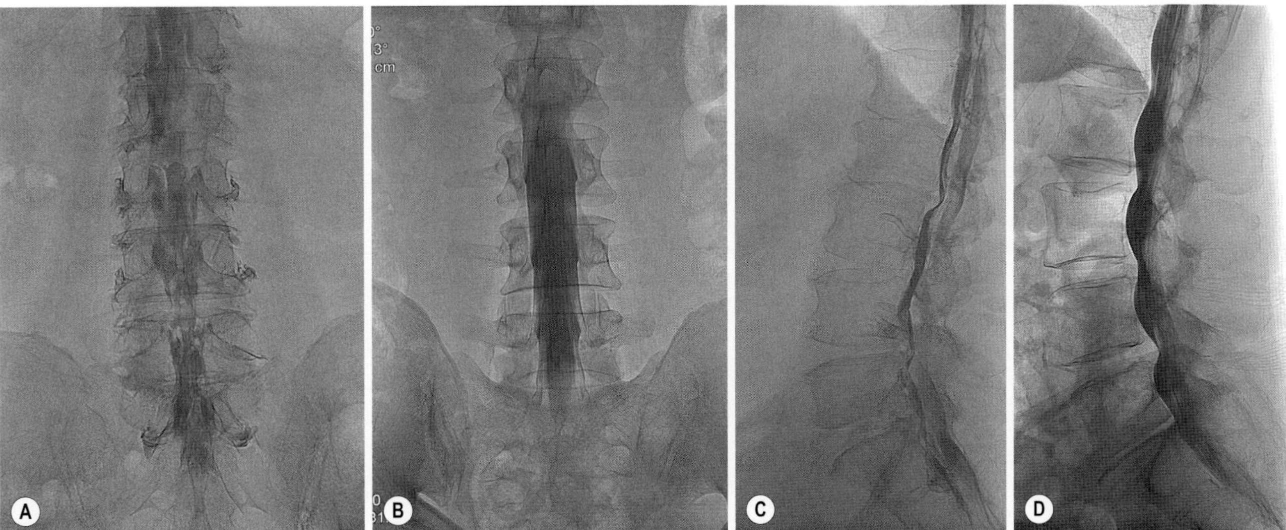

FIGURE 93-5 ■ Epidurography versus myelography. (A) Anteroposterior view after injection of iodinated contrast medium into the epidural space (dorsal interlaminal epidurographic approach). (B) Anteroposterior view after injection of iodinated contrast into the subarachnoid space (interlaminal myelographic approach). (C) Lateral projection of epidurography. (D) Lateral projection of myelography. In epidurography and spinal injections the agents are injected into the epidural fat compared to myelography that involves injection of contrast into the cerebrospinal fluid. In epidurography the contrast material outlines the epidural fat and the exiting spinal nerves beyond the intervertebral foramen (AP view), as well as the epidural space in between the thecal sac and the posterior longitudinal ligament (lateral view). In myelography the contrast material outlines the subarachnoid space and opacifies the CSF that surrounds the spinal cord denoting the root sleeves of the nerve roots inside the spinal canal.

adjust for the lordosis of the lumbosacral junction. Typically, a 22G spinal needle (alternatively an 18- to 20G Tuohy needle) is used to enter the interspinous and the flavum ligaments. The latter consists almost entirely of collagen fibres and provides the greater resistance to the needle. Entry to the dorsal epidural space is confirmed with the loss of resistance technique and may be confirmed with the injection of an aliquot of contrast agent. Operators must be familiar with the different imaging features of contrast material patterns between intrathecal (myelography) and epidural (epidurography) injections (Fig. 93-5). The paramedian interlaminal approach with the needle pointing towards the affected side is recommended for more targeted injections (Fig. 93-6). In this case a contralateral oblique projection is used to monitor advancement of the needle and the needle tip enters the epidural space when it crosses the imaginary spinolaminar line (Fig. 93-7).

When a fluoroscopic-guided transforaminal epidural injection is used, the patient is positioned prone and the C-arm is rotated to an ipsilateral oblique projection until the ipsilateral facet column is superimposed midway between the anterior and posterior wall of the vertebral bodies ('scotty dog' projection). The tube may also need to be angled cranially to align the superior and inferior vertebral endplates for the lower lumbar levels. Using tunnel collimation a 22- to 25G needle is advanced into the intervertebral foramen. The needle must slip along the lateral border of the respective facet joint and enter the dorsocranial quadrant of the intervertebral foramen (Figs. 93-8, 93-9). On scotty dog projections the needle target is actually below the junction of the pedicle and the ipsilateral transverse process ('eye of the scotty dog') and lateral to the inferior articular process of the respective facet joint. The depth of the needle is checked periodically in a lateral projection and elicitation of paresthesia (provoked by puncture of the spinal nerve) is best avoided. Some authors refer to the so-called 'safe triangle' when describing bone landmarks used for transforaminal periradicular nerve injections. On an ipsilateral oblique projection, the triangle is an imaginary triangular area formed cranially by the pedicle and transverse process, laterally by a line connecting the lateral edges of the superior and inferior pedicle and inferomedially by the spinal nerve root, which serves as the tangential base of the triangle. Once the needle tip is in the correct position, contrast medium is injected to outline the nerve sheath of the exiting root and exclude intrathecal, intra-arterial or intravenous injections (Fig. 93-10). After correct opacification of the epidural fat surrounding the spinal nerve, 1 mL of local anaesthetic is injected (bupivacaine 0.5% or lignocaine 1–2%) followed by a dose of steroid. In selective cases the caudal approach through the sacral hiatus may be chosen (Fig. 93-11).

Complications

Spinal epidural injections are generally considered very safe procedures with variable rates of pain relief (50–70%) that depend on a variety of factors (age, duration of symptoms, aetiology, etc). A time interval of at least 2 weeks is recommended between repeat steroid injections and no more than 3–4 injections per annum are allowed. The most frequent complication of a lumbar interlaminal injection is inadvertent puncture of the dura (2.5%)

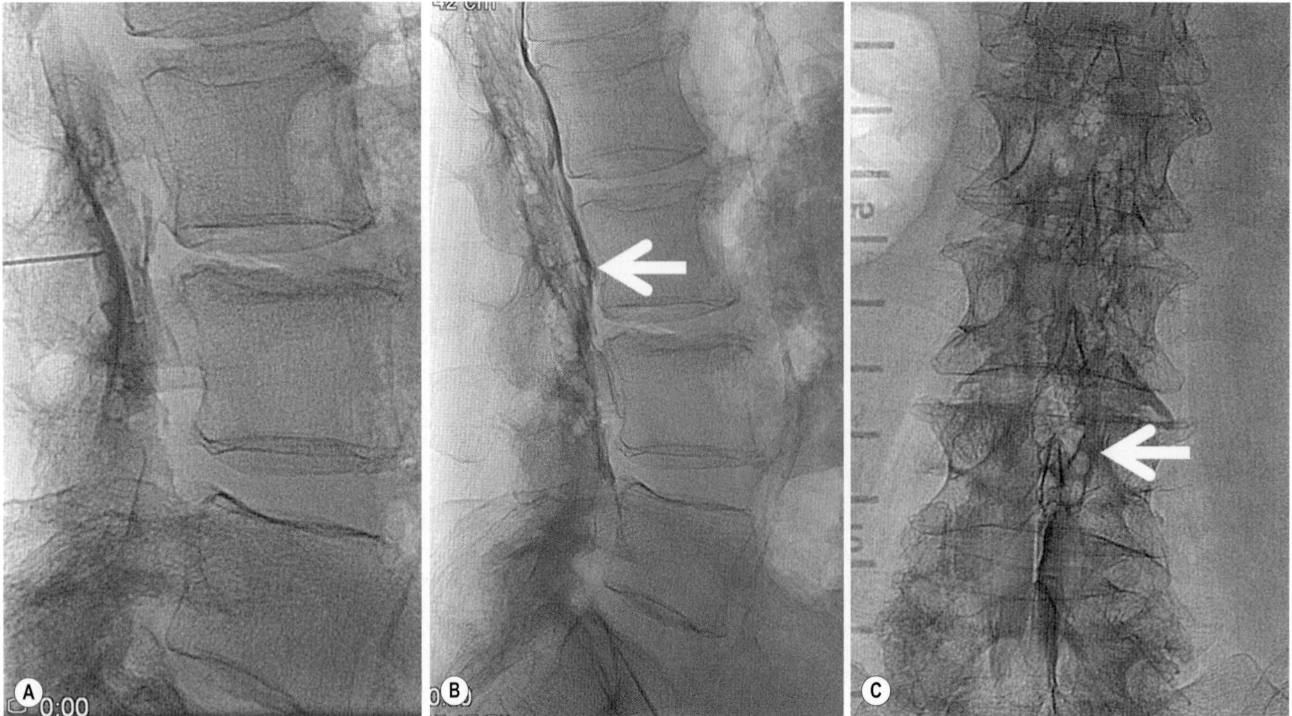

FIGURE 93-6 ■ Interlaminal spinal injection. (A) Interlaminal injection of dilute contrast material with steroids and local anaesthetic at the L3–4 dorsal epidural space in a patient with non-specific mechanical low back pain. (B) Lateral projection. Note spread of the contrast material (and the steroids) to the anterior epidural space (white arrow). (C) Anteroposterior projection after completion of the injection. Note the air bubbles accumulated at the dorsal epidural space because of air injected during application of the loss-of-resistance technique (white arrow).

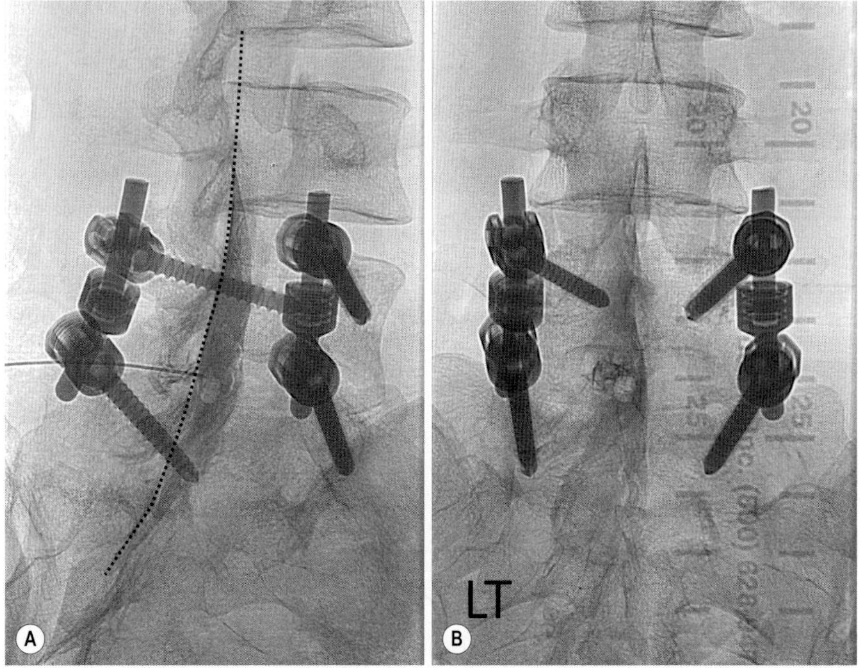

FIGURE 93-7 ■ Paramedian interlaminal injection. (A) Fluoroscopic-guided paramedian interlaminal injection at the L5–S1 level in a young patient with recurrent left-sided radiculopathy 1 year following surgery (failed back surgery syndrome, FBSS). The needle reaches the paramedian dorsal epidural space once the tip of the spinal needle breaches the imaginary spinolaminar line (black dotted line) on the contralateral scotty-dog oblique projection. (B) Anteroposterior view after the injection of the contrast material and steroids confirms selective application of the solution to the affected side.

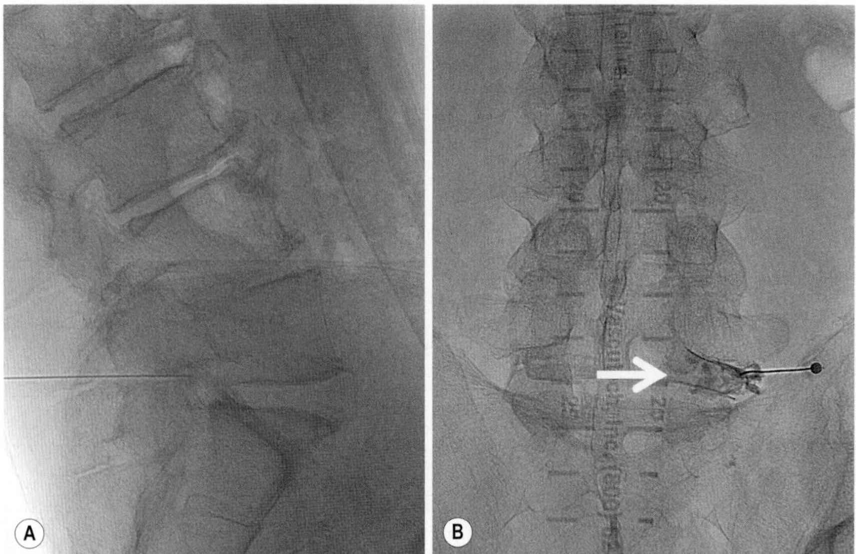

FIGURE 93-8 ■ Transforaminal periradicular injection. (A) Fluoroscopic-guided transforaminal periradicular injection of the L5 spinal nerve. Note the location of the tip of the needle at the dorsal aspect of the intervertebral foramen (lateral view). (B) Test injection of contrast material to exclude intravascular needle placement outlines the exiting L5 spinal nerve (white arrow—anteroposterior view).

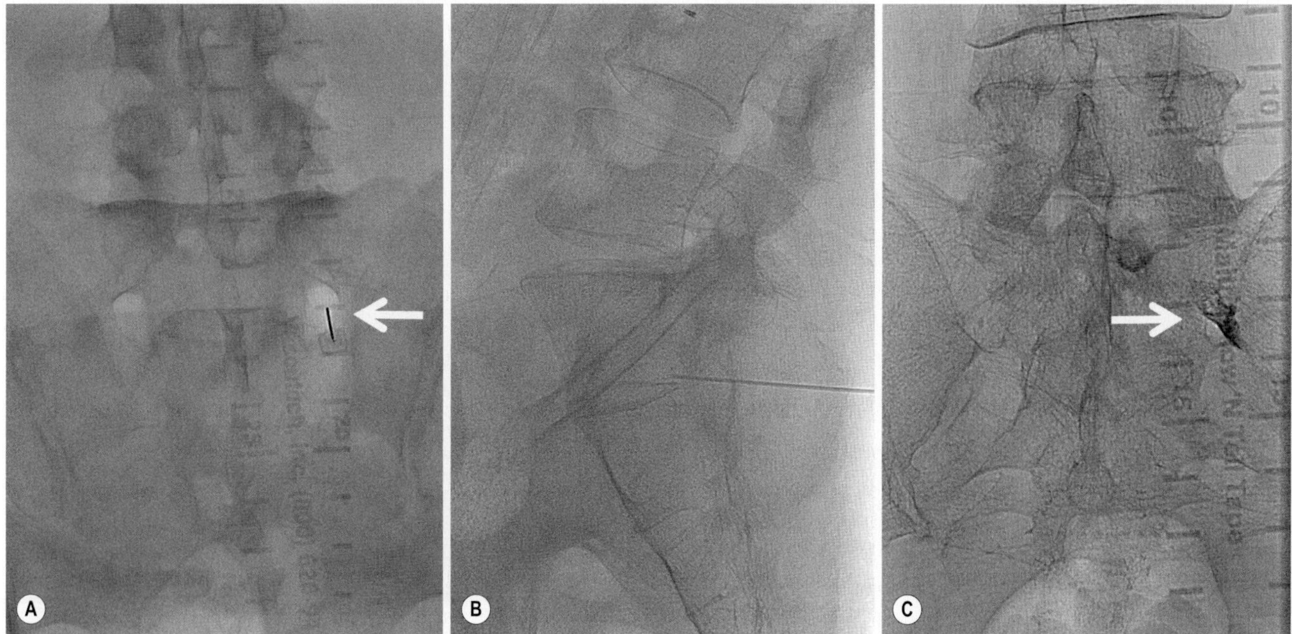

FIGURE 93-9 ■ Transforaminal periradicular injection. (A) Fluoroscopic-guided transforaminal periradicular injection of the S1 spinal nerve. The C-arm tube has been rotated cranially to align the dorsal with the ventral sacral foramen. Note the location of the tip of the needle at the superolateral quadrant of the S1 intervertebral foramen (white arrow—lateral view). (B) The needle has been advanced inside the spinal canal (anteroposterior view). (C) Test injection of contrast material to exclude intravascular needle placement outlines the descending S1 spinal nerve (white arrow—anteroposterior view).

which may produce a transient headache. Accidental subarachnoid or subdural punctures may easily be identified with a test injection of contrast agent in the lateral projection to avoid intrathecal injection of the steroid and anaesthetic agents. Radicular pain may also be exacerbated temporarily because of the local effects of the injection. Other rarely reported complications include arachnoiditis, aseptic or infectious meningitis, epidural abscess and systemic cardiovascular or gastrointestinal side effects from the steroid injection (severe adverse events <0.05%; mild reactions to steroids <5%). Of note, paraplegia is a catastrophic complication that has been

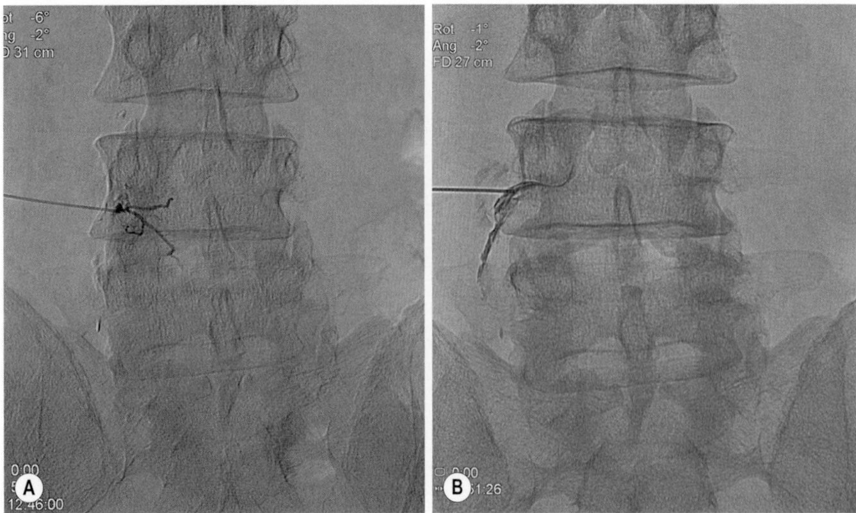

FIGURE 93-10 ■ **Intra-arterial injection.** (A) Test injection of contrast material during an L4 transforaminal injection confirms inadvertent puncture of a radicular arterial branch. Accidental injection of particulate steroids inside a spinal radiculomedullary branch may cause terminal cord ischaemia and result in a catastrophic neurological event (paraplegia). (B) Successful transforaminal periradicular injection after repositioning of the needle under fluoroscopic control. Note how the contrast material now outlines the L4 spinal nerve and diffuses medially to the epidural space.

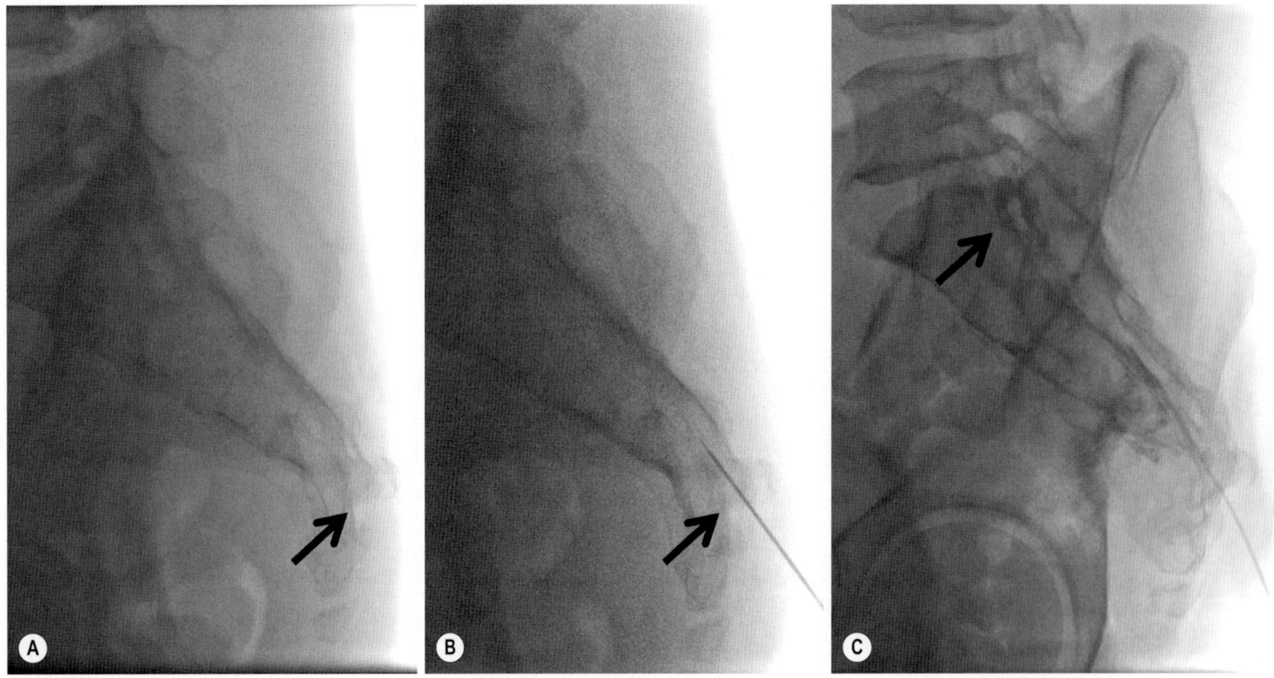

FIGURE 93-11 ■ **Caudal spinal injection (lateral views).** (A) Caudal approach for the injection of agents into the sacral epidural space. The aim is to puncture the superficial dorsal sacrococcygeal ligament (sacrococcygeal membrane) that covers the hiatus (black arrow). (B) The needle follows an oblique ascending course into the sacral epidural space. More injections can be performed at that point (black arrow). (C) Alternatively, a catheter may be advanced up to the L5–S1 level for more selective injection of the steroids (black arrow).

documented in a handful of case reports in association with lumbar transforaminal injections of particulate steroids above the level of L3. The most probable cause is inadvertent intra-arterial injection and embolisation within an unusually low dominant radiculomedullary artery. The largest radicular artery is the arteria radicularis magna (artery of Adamkiewicz), which usually enters the spinal canal on the left side in the lower thoracic level (T9–L1). Accidental injection of particulate steroids into an aberrant radicular branch may then produce terminal

TABLE 93-2 **Steroids**

	Pharmacology	Concentration (mg/mL)	Usual Dose (mg)
Triamcinolone (Kenacort, Bristol-Myers Squibb, New York, NY, USA)	Microparticulate steroid depot	40	40–80
Betamethasone (Celestone, Schering Plough, Kenilworth, NJ, USA)	Microparticulate steroid depot	6	6–12
Dexamethasone (Merck, Whitehouse Station, NJ, USA)	Non-particulate steroid depot	4–10	8–12
Methylprednisolone (Depo-medrol, Pfizer, New York, NY, USA)	Microparticulate steroid depot	40–80	40–80

spinal cord ischaemia with irreversible transverse ischaemic myelitis resulting in paraplegia. Triamcinolone, betamethazone and methylprednisolone have all been found to form aggregations acting as microparticles. Only dexamethasone is considered a particulate-free steroid and is therefore recommended as the drug of choice for all upper lumbar and cervical spinal injections (Table 93-2). No neurologic complications have been reported so far with the use of dexamethasone for spinal injections. Because of the risk of paraplegia, the latest guidelines on spine interventional procedures underline the utility of real-time high-quality fluoroscopy, ideally with digital subtraction angiography, to effectively exclude intra-arterial injections.

Pulsed Radiofrequency Ablation

Epidural corticosteroids are more effective in subacute cases of radiculitis. In chronic cases with established radiculopathy epidural corticosteroids are less effective and they may be combined with pulsed radiofrequency ablation (PRF) of the dorsal root ganglion (DRG) using a routine transforaminal approach. PRF is gaining recognition for effective treatment of persistent neuropathic pain and is applied in combination with corticosteroids. Although its exact mechanism of action remains to be fully elucidated, the rationale of PRF involves modification of transmission of pain signals at the level of the DRG after application of non-thermal pulsed radiofrequency ablation (45 V for 20 ms with a frequency of 2 Hz, for a total of 2–4 min with temperature not exceeding 42°C). No complications or side effects have been reported so far with the use of PRF on the cervical or lumbar DRG.

Adhesiolysis (with hyaluronidase and hypertonic saline) and epiduroscopy are also emerging image-guided techniques for the treatment of persistent or recurrent post-surgery radicular pain, whereas spinal cord neurostimulation is reserved for selected cases with life-disabling pain symptoms.

Facet Joint Syndrome

Axial pain originating from the lumbar zygapophysial joints (facet joint syndrome) is also a common cause of low back pain in the general population. Mechanical pain may arise from any mobile part of the inflamed degenerative facet joints, including the fibrous capsule, the hyaline cartilage and the bone. Painful inflamed facet joints may be associated with spinal canal stenosis because of hypertrophic ligamentum flavum which may also cause sciatica. Advanced age, degenerative disc disease and spondylolisthesis or spondylolysis predispose to facetogenic axial lumbar pain. Diagnosis is always difficult, but paravertebral tenderness on palpation of the facet joints is considered indicative of facetogenic mechanical pain. Intra-articular injection of local anaesthetic with or without steroids or alternatively anaesthetic blocks of the medial branch (medial branch of the dorsal ramus of the spinal nerve that innervates the facet joints) are routinely used for confirmation and treatment of facet joint syndrome (Fig. 93-12). More definite treatment with long-lasting pain relief (6–12 months) may be accomplished with facet denervation using thermal radiofrequency ablation of the medial branch, which is now considered the gold standard treatment of facetogenic pain.

Technique

The technique involves an ipsilateral oblique approach with the patient in the prone position. The needle target is the top of the transverse process, as close as possible to the superior articular process, which is where the medial branch travels. Once the tip of the electrode is in correct position, an RF ablation at 80–90°C for 60 s is performed. Superior and inferior adjacent levels must be treated also because there is significant overlap of zygapophysial joint innervation. Complications are minimal and reported rates of pain relief are well above 60%. Degenerative conditions of the sacroiliac joints may also be responsible for mechanical low back pain radiating to the buttocks and the thighs. In line with facet joint injections, intra-articular steroid injections and thermal radiofrequency denervation are routinely used for pain relief from sacroiliac joint syndrome (Fig. 93-13).

Cervical Spine

Spinal steroid injections and medial branch radiofrequency ablation are equally applicable for the treatment

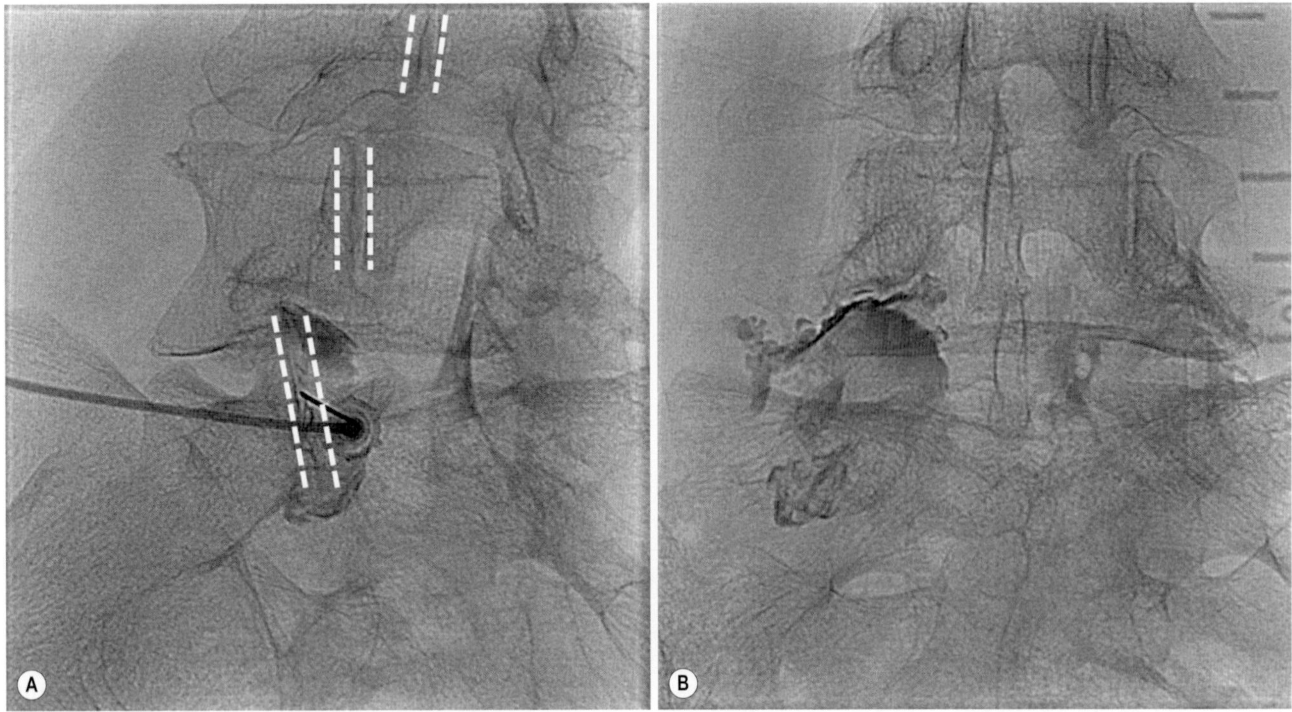

FIGURE 93-12 ■ **Lumbar zygapophysial joint injection.** (A) Intra-articular steroid injection of the L5–S1 facet joint. White dotted tram-lines denote the facet joints of the L3–L4, L4–L5 and L5–S1 levels (oblique scotty dog projection). (B) Injection of the steroid–contrast material mixture outlines rupture of the lateral and medial aspects of the facet joint capsule.

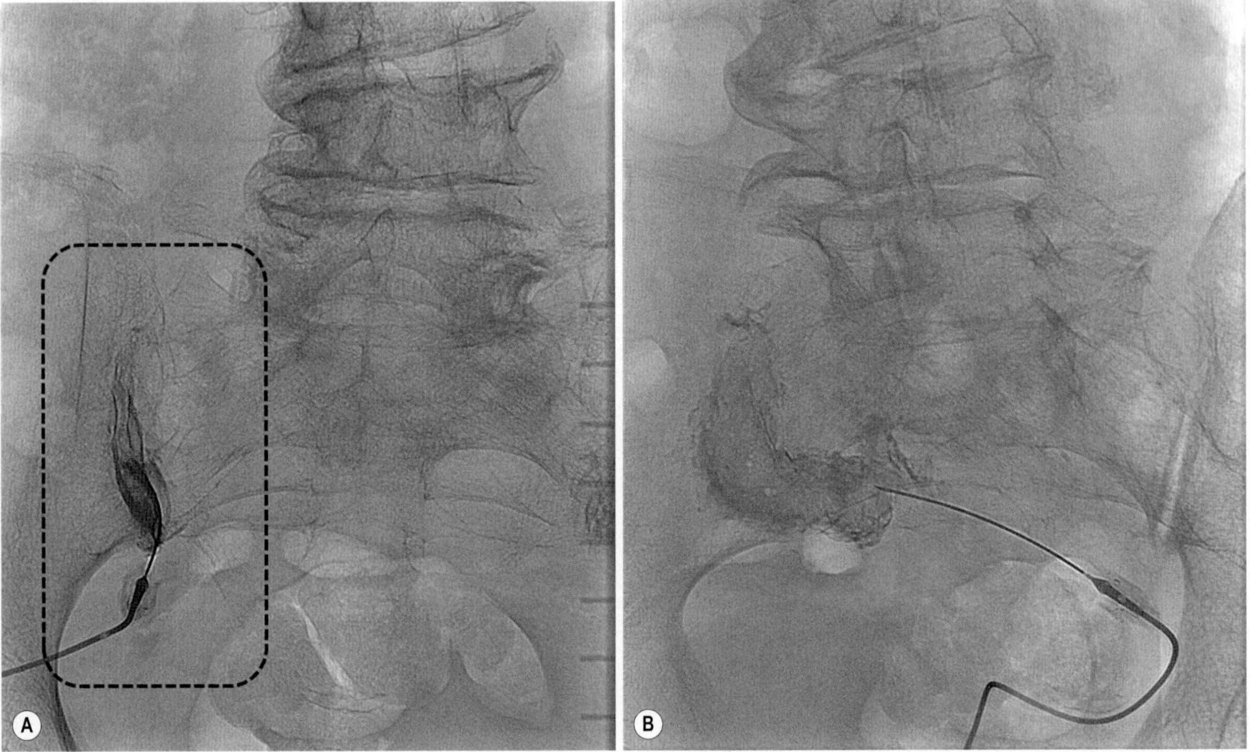

FIGURE 93-13 ■ **Sacroiliac joint injection.** (A) Fluoroscopic-guided injection of the sacroiliac joint for mechanical low back pain radiating to the buttock and the thigh. Point of needle entry should be the caudal aspect of the joint capsule (anteroposterior view). (B) Injection of contrast outlines the ear-shaped configuration of the sacroiliac joint on ipsilateral oblique projection.

of cervical radicular and axial mechanical pain. Cervical radicular pain is defined as electrical or shooting pain perceived in the upper limbs that is caused by compressive irritation of a cervical spinal nerve or its roots. The incidence of cervical radicular pain is approximately 1 person in 1,000. There is a medical history of physical exertion or trauma in 15% of the cases and almost half of the patients report a history of sciatica. The levels of C7 (45–60%) and C6 (20–25%) are affected in the majority of the cases. A detailed neurological examination is necessary to characterise pain distribution, presence of muscle weakness, sensory loss or reflex disturbances. Dermatomal distribution must be correlated with MRI findings of disc prolapse to identify the responsible level. Red flags such as infection, vascular disorders and tumours must be excluded during work-up and imaging may be supplemented by electrophysiological testing in equivocal cases. Interventional treatment of cervical radicular pain includes interlaminal and transforaminal epidural administration of corticosteroids and both approaches can achieve significant relief of pain. In line with the lumbar spine, transforaminal injections offer more accurate administration of the drugs to the affected root. Cervical injections may be performed under fluoroscopic or CT guidance based on the experience and preference of the operator. For cervical transforaminal peri-radicular injections a lateral approach is chosen and the tip of the needle enters the dorsal aspect of the intervertebral foramen posterior to the exiting spinal nerve and in contact with the anterior side of the facet joint, thereby avoiding accidental puncture of the anteriorly located vertebral artery (Fig. 93-14).

The drugs used in the cervical spine are the same as those injected in the lumbar segment, but with a clear preference for particulate-free dexamethasone. Local anaesthetic agents should not be injected in the cervical spine to avoid central nervous system depression and transient phrenic nerve palsy. Steroid injections may also be combined with pulsed radiofrequency ablation of the cervical DRG for enhanced pain relief. Although rare, complications following cervical spinal injections may be catastrophic and deserve special attention. They are divided into spinal cord lesions within the context of anterior spinal artery syndrome and central nervous system side effects involving the brain stem and the cerebellum. The first are attributed to inadvertent injection of a particulate steroid into a radiculomedullary branch feeding the anterior spinal artery and the second are attributed to accidental injection of the anaesthetic and steroid agents into the vertebral artery.

In contrast to the lumbar spine where symptoms of sciatica are more prevalent, facet-related pain is more frequent in the cervical spine. Reportedly, more than 50% of patients presenting with neck pain may suffer from facetogenic pain, usually described as unilateral pain without radiation to the arm, but with limited and painful rotation and retroflexion. Conservative treatment options for cervical facet pain such as physiotherapy, manipulation and mobilisation, although supported by little evidence, are frequently applied before considering interventional treatments. In line with the lumbar spine, interventional pain management techniques, including intra-articular steroid injections, medial branch blocks and radiofrequency ablation denervation are usually offered for the treatment of axial neck pain related to cervical spondylosis and osteoarthritis.

PERCUTANEOUS DISC DECOMPRESSION

The healthy intervertebral disc is avascular and has a complex nerve supply. The sensory innervation of the disc stems from branches of the sympathetic trunk. The dorsal circumference of the annulus fibrosus and posterior longitudinal ligament are innervated by the sinuvertebral nerve, whereas the anterolateral circumference of the annulus fibrosus and the anterior longitudinal ligament are innervated from lateral branches of the communicating ramus and direct branches of the sympathetic trunk. The sinuvertebral nerve stems from the communicating ramus, which in turn interconnects the

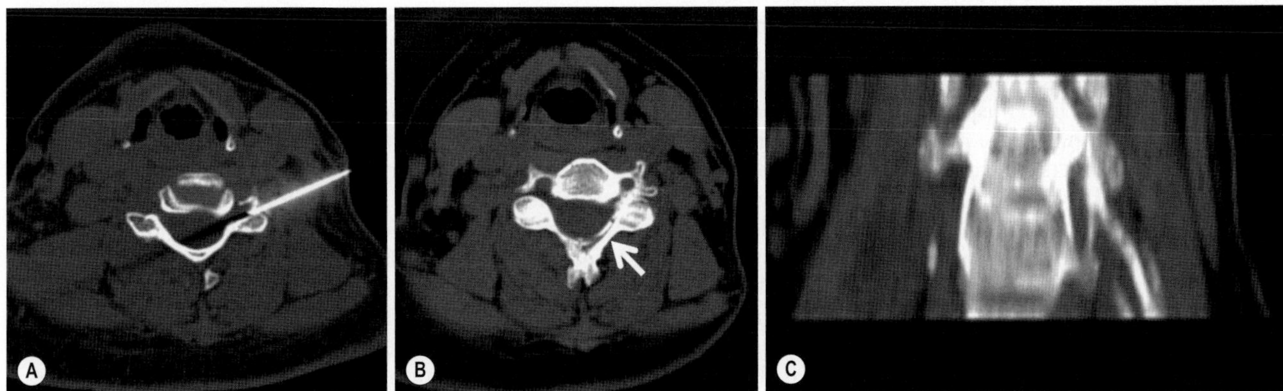

FIGURE 93-14 ■ **Cervical transforaminal injection.** (A) CT-guided transforaminal peri-radicular injection of the left C6 nerve root in a woman with radiculitis. The needle slips posterior to the nerve and in contact with the anterior surface of the facet joint. (B) Note diffusion of the contrast material around the root and into the dorsal epidural space (white arrow—axial image). (C) There is also tracking of the contrast material along the affected spinal nerve (white arrow—reformatted coronal CT image).

sympathetic trunk with the spinal nerves. This extensive nerve plexus has many horizontal and lateral connections resulting in significant overlap in the distribution and projection of painful stimuli originating from adjacent levels and/or structures. Discogenic pain is usually localised medially in the back and may share clinical signs of lumbosacral radicular pain; it is typically provoked by pressure on the spinous processes and exacerbated by coughing, and painful levels are positively correlated with findings of provocation discography.

Disc herniation is defined as local release and herniation of the disc's gelatinous nucleus pulposus because of rupture of the cartilaginous annulus fibrosus. Pain associated with intervertebral disc herniation is a complex process including physical pressure on the adjacent nerve root and local release of proinflammatory cytokines. After failure of 6–12 weeks of conservative treatment, including peri-radicular epidural steroid injections described previously, percutaneous disc decompression is indicated as the next step of treatment. Intervertebral discs constitute a closed hydraulic space. Percutaneous disc decompression aims to reverse spinal nerve compression by removing a small volume of the nucleus pulposus and reducing intradiscal pressure. Techniques of disc decompression (also known as disc nucleotomy) may be chemical (alcohol gel, oxygen–ozone mixture), mechanical (automated discectomy, radiofrequency coblation) or thermal (laser or radiofrequency disc denervation). Percutaneous disc decompression is generally indicated in symptomatic contained disc hernias, but contraindicated in extruded disc hernias and free discal fragments. Red flags should be excluded prior to treatment and acute neurological deficits should be referred for urgent neurosurgery.

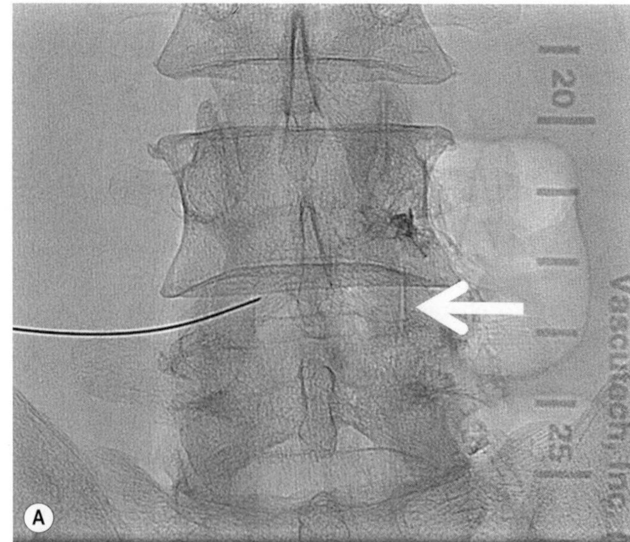

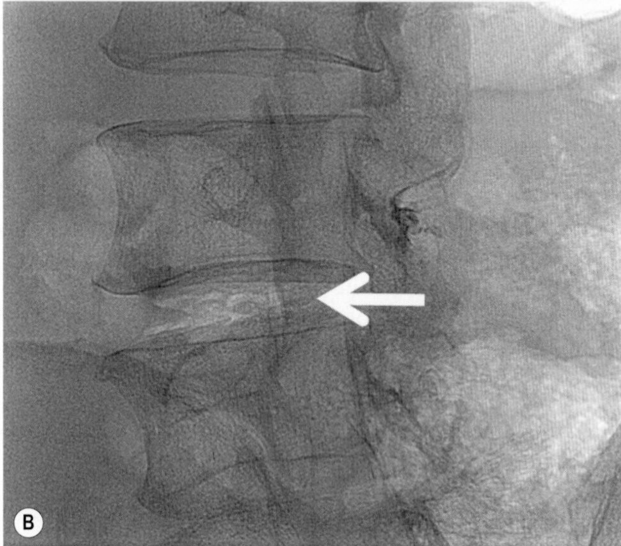

FIGURE 93-15 ■ Intradiscal ozone injection. (A) Fluoroscopic-guided injection of the L4–L5 disc (white arrow) with an oxygen–ozone mixture (ozonelysis) for treatment of radiculitis associated with posterolateral disc prolapse (AP view). (B) Note the increased intradiscal radiolucency following injection of the oxygen–ozone mixture into the nucleus pulposus (white arrow—oblique view).

Technique

Strict asepsis is required and an approach under fluoroscopic control is used for disc puncture and discectomy. For the lumbar levels the patient is positioned prone and the C-arm tube is rotated first craniocaudally to align with the intervertebral level and second laterally in an oblique 'scotty dog' projection. The needle target lies above the junction of the pedicle and the ipsilateral transverse process ('eye of the scotty dog') and lateral to the superior articular process of the respective facet joint. The needle must slip along the articular process and enter the disc at the lower aspect of the foramen to avoid puncturing the spinal nerve. Intradiscal position of the needle is then confirmed on lateral and anteroposterior projections. For the cervical levels the patient is placed supine and an anterolateral approach is used. Using manual palpation the carotid artery and jugular vein are displaced laterally and the needle is advanced to the intervertebral space travelling between the major vessels laterally and the esophagus medially. Depending on the device used, a needle of appropriate size is used (16–19G) to allow for introduction of the discectomy device from the non-affected side of the disc.

In chemical discolysis (chemonucleolysis), a small dose of an oxygen–ozone mixture or alcohol gel is injected inside the disc (Fig. 93-15). The exact mechanisms of ozone action remain unknown, but combined oxidative dehydration of the nucleus pulposus and epidural anti-inflammatory properties are claimed. Chemical nucleotomy aims to dehydrate the nucleus pulposus and decompress the hernia by accelerating disc degeneration. The principle of disc decompression with mechanical devices, laser light or radiofrequency coblation is to reduce intradiscal pressure by vaporising a small amount of the nucleus pulposus and decompress the contained herniation. Mechanical devices may use a variety of automated instruments to extract a small volume of the nucleus pulposus. Thermal energy techniques produce fusion and shrinkage of the peripheral collagen fibres along with denervation of the annulus fibrosus nociceptors responsible for pain. However, there is the risk of thermal damage to the adjacent endplates or the spinal nerves. On the other hand, radiofrequency coblation nucleotomy produces a low-temperature ionic plasma field that disintegrates molecular bonds and cavitates the disc without the risk of heat damage. The coblation electrode debulks the disc by digging multiple channels inside the nucleus pulposus.

Compared to surgical disc decompression, which may cause epidural fibrosis and is associated with a 20–30% risk of FBSS, percutaneous disc decompression with either discectomy or discolysis techniques may achieve 70–90% long-term relief of discogenic and related radicular pain with significant improvement of quality of life. Percutaneous discectomy is also associated with a minimal risk of scar tissue development. Shrinkage of the herniation on CT or MRI is only visible several months following percutaneous disc decompression. The procedure is generally safe and is performed as a day case procedure. Potential complications include infectious discitis, epidural haematoma and vascular or neural injuries (0.25–0.7%).

TABLE 93-3 **Percutaneous Vertebral Augmentation: Indications and Contraindications**

Indications

- Osteoporotic vertebral compression fractures
- Painful osteolytic lesions of the vertebrae (metastases, lymphoma, multiple myeloma)
- Insufficiency fractures of the sacrum and the acetabulum
- Aggressive vertebral haemangiomas and giant cell tumours
- Acute vertebral burst fractures
- Miscellaneous (osteonecrosis, Langerhans cell histiocytosis, vacuum phenomena)

Contraindications

- Spinal cord compression
- Responders to medical therapy
- Uncorrectable coagulopathy
- Osteomyelitis, discitis or active systemic infection
- Allergy to cement or other filler materials
- >5 or diffuse bone metastases
- Lack of neurosurgical support

PERCUTANEOUS VERTEBRAL AUGMENTATION

Percutaneous vertebral augmentation refers to a variety of interventional procedures aimed at stabilising insufficiency or pathologic fractures of the vertebrae and to some extent the pelvis. Vertebral augmentation goes beyond plain cementoplasty, i.e. percutaneous application of cement for bone consolidation, to include interventions that aim to restore the height of the collapsed vertebrae. Procedures like vertebroplasty, kyphoplasty, osteoplasty and sacroplasty are included. Bone packing with cement with or without adjunctive augmentation procedures like kyphoplasty generally aim to treat or prevent pathological fractures and pain in patients with vertebral and pelvic insufficiency fractures or neoplastic osteolytic lesions. Image-guided injection of radiopaque cement is widely used for the stabilisation of painful osteoporotic or malignant vertebral compression fractures and aggressive vertebral haemangiomas. Non-traumatic vertebral compression fractures are defined as reduction in the individual vertebral body height by more than 20% or 4 mm. Vertebral compression fractures produce debilitating back pain with poor quality of life. Most common causes include osteoporosis and bone metastases. Osteoporosis is estimated to afflict more than 10 million people resulting in more than 700,000 vertebral compression fractures per annum in the United States alone. On the other hand, spinal bone metastases, multiple myeloma and lymphoma are the predominant neoplasms associated with spinal pathologic fractures. Well accepted indications for spinal augmentation procedures after failed conservative therapies are outlined in Table 93-3. For osteoporosis the latter is defined as failure to relieve pain even with excessive doses of opiates or inadequate pain management for a period of at least 3 weeks. For metastases, it is defined as unsuccessful pain relief despite appropriate oncological treatment and radiotherapy. Patients with aggressive vertebral haemangiomas and giant cell tumours are also candidates for percutaneous vertebroplasty to achieve tumour devascularisation, lesion consolidation and pain relief. In patients with aggressive haemangiomas with anterior epidural spread and/or spinal compression, cementoplasty with adjunctive sclerotherapy may be used as a standalone treatment or as a preoperative treatment.

The ideal candidate for percutaneous vertebroplasty is a patient who presents within 3–6 weeks of a fracture not improving with conservative medical treatment, has mid-line non-radiating back pain that increases with weight bearing and which is exacerbated by manual palpation of the spinous process of the involved vertebra. Preoperative planning for vertebral augmentation involves thorough review of baseline radiographic studies, contrast-enhanced CT and MR imaging in order to identify the level(s) of the fracture, estimate its age, outline the extent of lysis, identify any involvement of the pedicles, evaluate the integrity of the posterior vertebral body wall and exclude epidural or foraminal tumour spread and retropulsed bone fragments, all of which are associated with an increased likelihood of complications. Be extremely careful in case of osteolysis or fracture of the posterior vertebral column, if the tumour extends into the spinal canal, because of a considerably higher risk of complications, including cement leak and further tissue retropulsion. Spinal cord compression with neurologic deficits should be dealt with by operative decompression and posterior spinal stabilisation.

Acute, subacute and non-healing fractures appear hypointense on T1-weighted images and hyperintense on T2-weighted and STIR images. STIR sequences suppress fat and are particularly sensitive in the detection of bone marrow oedema and metabolically active fractures, i.e. acute or chronic non-healing ones. Vertebral haemangiomas are typically hyperintense on both T1- and

T2-weighted images. Of note, an aggressive symptomatic type of haemangiomas with low signal on T1-weighted images and high on T2 has been described. A bone scan is helpful for distinguishing the symptomatic level in case of multiple contiguous fractures and for identifying additional insufficiency fractures of the sacrum and pelvis. Percutaneous vertebral augmentation is not indicated if there is bone sclerosis that suggests successful healing of the fracture of if there is no high signal intensity on STIR sequences.

Vertebroplasty is typically performed with strict asepsis either under local anaesthetic and conscious sedation or under general anaesthesia when larger bore instruments are used, such as those used in kyphoplasty or newer height restoration procedures. Good technique involves, first, proper needle placement and, second, watchful cement injection. Image guidance involves biplane fluoroscopy (Fig. 93-16), but combined guidance with a mobile C-arm placed in front of the CT gantry may be used in lesions difficult to access, such as in osteoplasty of pelvic or other extraspinal lesions. Cement injection must always be monitored in real time with high-quality fluoroscopy in the lateral projection. Biplane fluoroscopy allows simultaneous visualisation in two orthogonal planes, but CT guidance is superior in the detection of small cement leaks. Typically, the patient is placed prone and the safest needle pathway is the standard transpedicular approach in the thoracic and lumbar levels with a medial needle trajectory through the pedicle (Fig. 93-17). Alternatively, an intercostovertebral, a parapedicular or a paravertebral pathway may be followed if the vertebral pedicles are not readily visible on frontal X-ray fluoroscopy because of neoplastic infiltration or fracture and collapse. An anterolateral approach by manual lateral displacement of the carotid–jugular complex is typically followed in the cervical spine with the patient in supine position. Note that at least one-third of the vertebral body height is necessary for safe needle insertion and cement injection (Fig. 93-18).

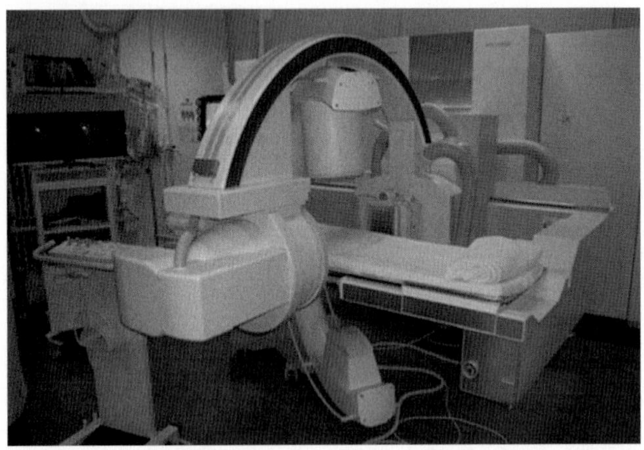

FIGURE 93-16 ■ Biplane fluoroscopy. A combination of a C-arm tube and an angiography unit may be placed in an orthogonal configuration for biplane real-time fluoroscopy during vertebroplasty and cementoplasty procedures of the spine.

A transpedicular vertebral puncture typically involves the following steps: (1) selection of a large-bore, 10- to 15G, diamond- or bevel-shaped needle, (2) localisation of the relevant pedicle under anteroposterior fluoroscopic projection, (3) local anaesthetic infiltration down to the cortex, (4) needle advancement with a surgical hammer to perforate the cortex at the upper and lateral aspect of the pedicle, (5) avoiding transgression of the medial and inferior border of the pedicle, because the needle might breach the spinal canal or the underlying intervertebral foramen, (6) continuous needle advancement with a 15°–30° angle relative to the midline coronal plane. For unipedicular procedures the needle tip should reach the anterior one-third to one-fourth of the vertebral body, as close as possible to the midline. Kyphoplasty and other vertebral augmentation procedures mandate bipedicular puncture with bilateral needle placement at the lateral aspects of the vertebral body. Such procedures may achieve more symmetrical cement distribution and stabilisation of the vertebral body.

The principle of pain relief with vertebroplasty or kyphoplasty is based on consolidation of the weakened

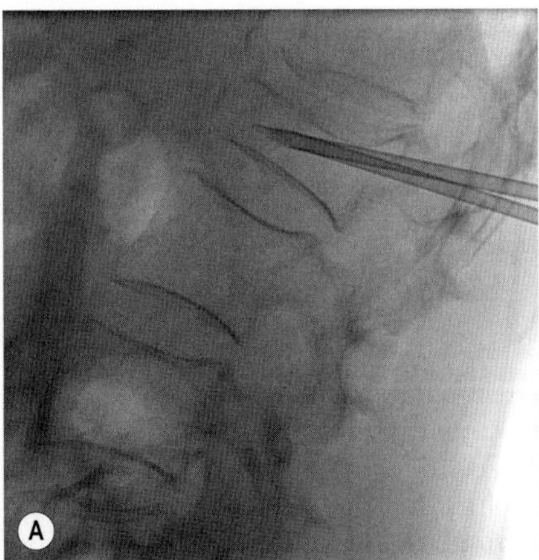

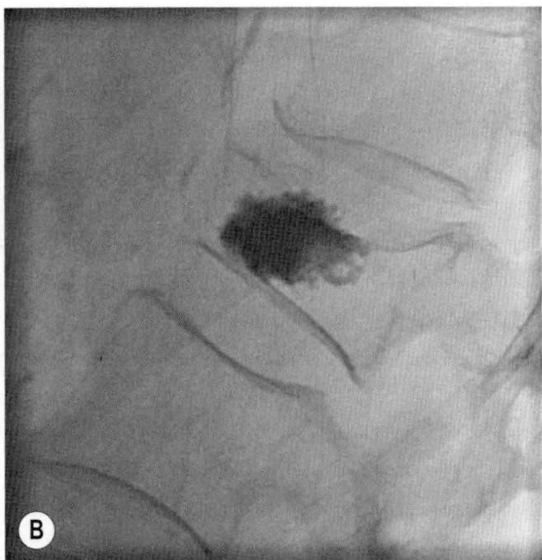

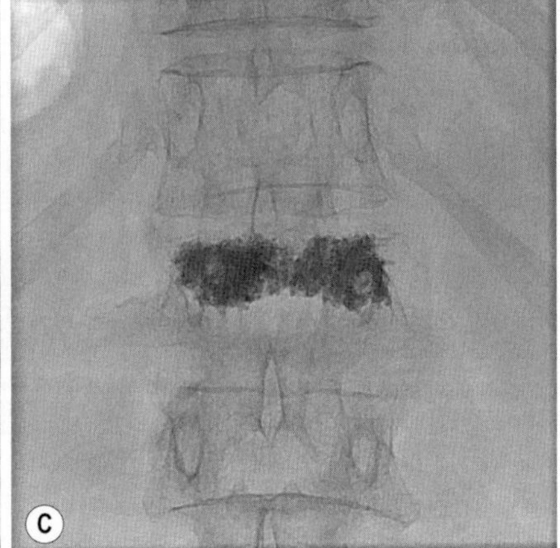

FIGURE 93-17 ■ Percutaneous vertebroplasty. (A) Bilateral transpedicular approach for percutaneous vertebroplasty of a painful L1 osteoporotic fracture (lateral projection). (B) There is sufficient cement filling of the anterior and mid-third of the vertebral body (lateral projection). (C) There is optimal cement filling across the midline of the vertebral body (anteroposterior projection).

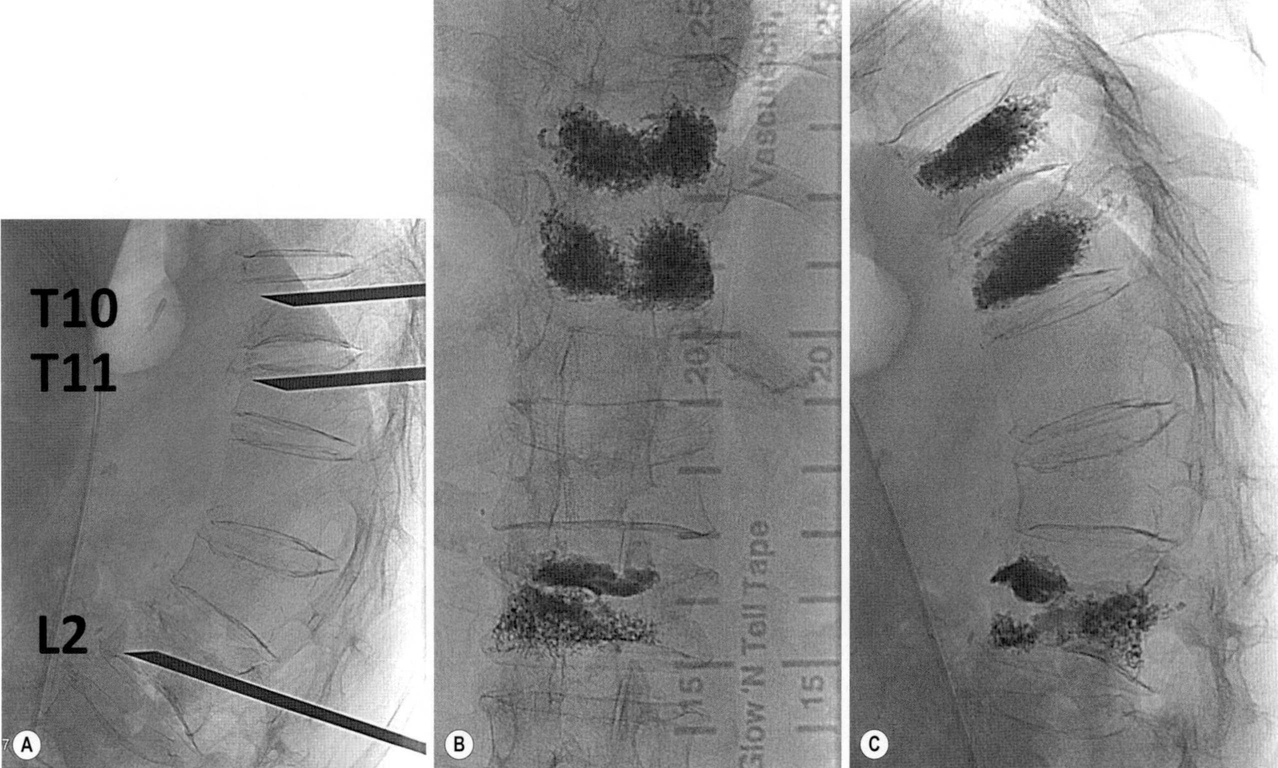

FIGURE 93-18 ■ Multilevel cementoplasty. (A) Percutaneous vertebroplasty of three levels in a multiple myeloma patient with several insufficiency fractures of the thoracolumbar spine. Transpedicular approach to the T10, T11 and L2 vertebrae (lateral projection). There is optimal cement filling of all treated vertebrae on the AP view (B) and the lateral view (C). Note the minor cement leak from the anterosuperior aspect of the L2 body towards the disc. Most intradiscal leaks are asymptomatic.

and pathologic cancellous bone. The combined chemical and thermal cytotoxic effects of cement polymerisation also contribute to pain relief. In fact, adequate pain relief may be obtained in metastasis after injection of a volume of only 2 mL of cement. Nowadays, a variety of injectable cements are commercially available. The various cement types are different in terms of chemical synthesis, polymerisation times, biocompatibility, mechanical strength, radiopacity and rheology, and may be indicated for different spinal pathologies. However, polymethylmethacrylate (PMMA) is still the most widely used cement with several decades of experience in orthopedic surgery. Within 1–3 minutes of its recommended preparation, the PMMA increases its viscosity from thin, to thick and pasty. To minimise cement leaks, PMMA must be injected while it remains in this pasty phase. Note that polymerisation of PMMA is an exothermic reaction and cement temperature reaches 80–120°C, which produces local thermocoagulation of tumoural cells, but may also damage healthy neighbouring tissues, like neural roots and the spinal cord itself, in case of extensive leak. Tissue temperatures as high as 70°C have been recorded during PMMA cementoplasty. The suggested endpoint of vertebroplasty is cement packing of the anterior half to two-thirds of the vertebral body with symmetrical cement distribution that extends across the midline to the contralateral side of the vertebra. After completion of the procedure the operator should wait for approximately 30 min for the cement to harden before transferring the patient back to his bed.

The recommended complication threshold for a specialised tertiary centre performing percutaneous vertebroplasty and cementoplasty for pain management is 2% for osteoporotic patients and 10% in malignant patients. Cement leak is the first and most fearsome complication of vertebroplasty, but it is usually asymptomatic. Cement may leak into the epidural veins or the epidural space, inside the neural foramina, towards the disk, the perivertebral venous plexus or into the paravertebral soft tissues. Cement leaks tracking into the arterial system have also been described. Urgent neurosurgical decompression is required in case of cement leak into the spinal canal with cord compression. Cement leaks into the perivertebral venous plexus may continue undetected and produce cement pulmonary embolism that may be potentially fatal. In general, vertebral augmentation procedures are expected to produce satisfactory pain relief with improved mobility and quality of life in approximately 70% of patients with painful bone metastases, 80% of vertebral haemangiomas and 90% of patients with osteoporotic fractures. After vertebroplasty, new compression fractures occur in up to a quarter of patients and almost half of those are located in levels adjacent to the initially treated ones. Kyphoplasty is a modification of vertebroplasty and aims to more effectively restore vertebral height by employing a balloon tamp to create a

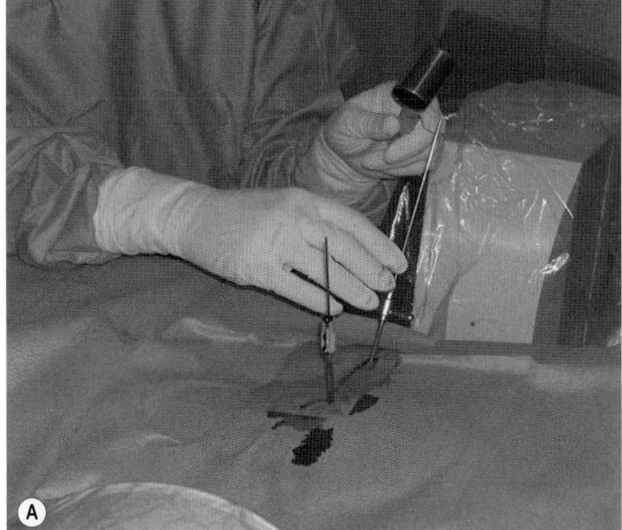

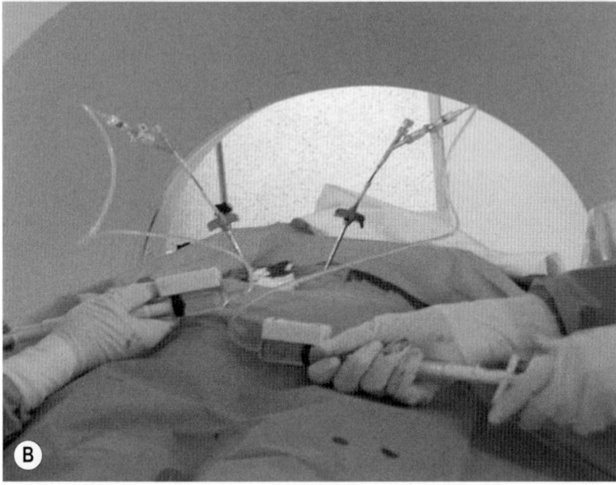

FIGURE 93-19 ■ Percutaneous kyphoplasty. (A) Bipedicular advancement of bone trocars under general anaesthesia. (B) Concomitant inflation of bilateral kyphoplasty balloon tamps to try to restore height before cement delivery. (Images courtery of Professor A. Gangi, Strasburg, France.)

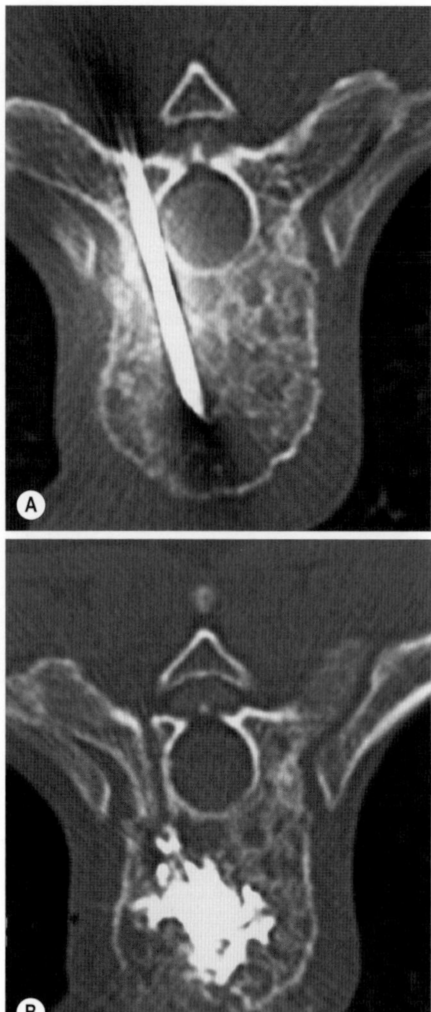

FIGURE 93-20 ■ Vertebroplasty of haemangioma. (A) CT-guided vertebroplasty of an aggressive painful haemangioma. Note the transpedicular route of the bone trocar (axial CT images). (B) Final image after successful cement injection. (Images courtesy of Professor A. Gangi, Strasburg, France.)

cavity inside the vertebral body to accommodate the injected cement (Fig. 93-19). The reported mean height restoration after kyphoplasty for compression fractures is around 3–5 mm at the centre of the vertebral body. However, recent data from randomised controlled trials of vertebroplasty or kyphoplasty versus optimal medical therapy have shown that both procedures are significantly better in terms of pain relief and remain most likely equally effective. Osteoplasty refers to radiological cement consolidation of painful insufficiency fractures or malignant osteolyses of the sacrum, the pubic rami, the ischial tuberosities and the acetabulum.

Percutaneous vertebroplasty is also a safe and effective therapy for the treatment of symptomatic vertebral haemangiomas. Its role is limited to pain relief in case of aggressive haemangiomas and in the absence of neurologic deficits (Fig. 93-20). In fact, vertebroplasty was initially described in the late 1980s by Galibert and Deramond for the treatment of a painful aggressive vertebral haemangioma. Alternatively, vertebroplasty may be used pre-operatively to consolidate the vertebral body and reduce the risk of haemorrhage during subsequent neurosurgical decompression with laminectomy and resection of the epidural extension of the haemangioma.

Latest developments include new mechanical devices for more effective restoration of vertebral height, and the introduction of osteoconductive and osteoinductive cements that may be able to promote more physiological bone healing by being gradually absorbed and substituted by normal osseous minerals. Calcium phospate cements (CPCs) are the most biocompatible and most expensive type of cement commercially available today and are promising because of their osteoconductive properties. CPC consist of calcium phosphate powders dissolved in an aqueous solution. Around room temperature apatite or brushite crystals precipitate from injectable CPC, which in turn stimulate new bone formation. Histological

TABLE 93-4 **Cement Fillers**

Polymethylmethacrylate (PMMA)	Composite Cements	Calcium Phosphate Cements
Methylmethacrylate polymers	Dimethacrylate resins	Apatite or brushite phosphates
Good radiopacity	Good radiopacity	Low radiopacity
Low cost	Moderate cost	High cost
Exothermic reaction and coagulation (80–120°C)	Abrupt setting at low temperature (<58°C)	Delayed setting at room temperature
Fibrous tissue encapsulation	Surrounding bone mineralisation	Biocompatible and bioresorbable
Recommended for osteoporosis and metastases	Recommended for osteoporosis in younger ages	Recommended for recent burst fractures

examination has shown early bioresorption of CPC after 2 weeks and abundant new bone apposition without inflammation or fibrous encapsulation. Consequently, vertebral augmentation with CPC has been proposed for repair of recent thoracolumbar burst fractures in younger populations (Table 93-4).

ABLATION OF SPINAL TUMOURS

Tumour ablation is defined as the direct application of chemical or physical therapies to a tumour with the aim of achieving complete eradication or substantial destruction. A wide range of radiological locoregional ablative techniques is now available, which induce tumourous cell death primarily through coagulative necrosis or ischaemia. They may be broadly categorised into thermal ablation, cryoablation and transcatheter embolisation. The latter obliterates the vascular supply of the target tumour and can also be combined with targeted chemotherapy.

The main indications for spinal ablation procedures are (1) palliative treatment of painful pre-terminal metastatic bone disease of the spine and pelvis and (2) selected cases of curative treatment of selected benign bone tumours like osteoid osteomas or local control of aggressive vertebral haemangiomas. Typically, thermal ablation is used for pain management in patients with bone metastases and intractable pain that have not responded to radiotherapy and opiates. Up to 85% of patients presenting with breast, prostate and lung cancer have evidence of bone metastases at the time of death. Relief of pain from these deposits is an important aspect of palliative care. Pain from bone metastases is thought to be caused by a combination of periosteal stretching by tumour expansion, cytokine release from tumour cells, osteolysis and fracture fragments that move under compressive loads, and infiltration or compression of nerves or soft tissues. External beam radiation therapy may have variable and transient results. In fact, it can take weeks to take effect and fails to relieve pain in up to 30% of patients.

Spinal tumour ablation can be performed as a day case procedure under conscious sedation and with acceptably low morbidity and mortality. Percutaneous ablation may be repeated for new or recurrent disease and has a low complication rate due to its minimally invasive nature. Pain symptoms must correlate accurately with radiological findings and informed consent must be obtained with realistic patient expectations. Spine ablation procedures are carried out under CT or X-ray guidance, or a combination thereof. If cement is to be injected, high-quality fluoroscopy is of paramount importance to enhance procedural safety. Lately, real-time open-bore MR guidance systems are available for dedicated state-of-the-art interventional oncology suites. CT guidance is generally adequate for routine procedures because it offers high tissue spatial resolution and may differentiate sensitive adjacent organs and neural structures, at the expense, however, of increased patient exposure to radiation. Conscious sedation (i.e. neuroleptanalgesia) is sufficient for radiofrequency and microwave ablation of lytic lesions, but ablation of osteoid osteomas definitely requires regional or general anaesthesia.

Percutaneous ethanol injection is the simplest and cheapest method of percutaneous tumour ablation. Alcoholisation causes tumour necrosis directly through cellular dehydration and indirectly through vascular thrombosis and tissue ischaemia. Typically, a fine needle (21–22G) is directed into the centre of the target lesion and a mixture of iodinated contrast (25%) and lidocaine 1% (75%) is first injected to assess the extent of tissue diffusion and provide local anaesthesia. Then 5–25 mL of 96% ethanol is instilled into the tumour, provided there is no vascular communication or adjacent vital organ or neural structure communication. Alcoholisation is reserved for ablation and local control of large pelvic tumours or expansile mass lesions, because of the unpredictable diffusion of alcohol which can cause irreversible neurological injury.

Radiofrequency ablation (RFA) was first applied in the early 1990s for the treatment of hepatic tumours and is today the most widely adopted and commonly employed technique for percutaneous ablation of solid organ malignancies. Nowadays, RFA has evolved into a multi-purpose tool for the skeletal system. In general, RFA applicators are available in the form of straight or expandable electrodes that are inserted under guidance into the centre of the target tumour. Then, a high-frequency alternating current (460–500 kHz) is delivered inside the tumour, which causes agitation of the tissue ionic molecules, which in turn produces frictional heat. The applied electrical current exits the body through grounding pads attached usually at the thighs. The thermal effect depends on the electrical conducting properties of the tissues treated. Local tissue temperatures approach 100°C and result in coagulative necrosis of the tumour. Ablation treatment must include a 0.5–1 cm margin of healthy tissue around the target lesion to eradicate any microscopic satellite foci and avoid early local recurrence. Note that the efficacy of RFA may be limited by adjacent high-flow vascular structures, which act as a cooling circuitry (widely known as the heat-sink phenomenon) and increased tissue impedance if tissue vaporisation and/or charring occur. In palliative ablation of bone metastases the principal aim of RF is to ablate the bone–tumour interface, where the pain source arises. Large ablation volumes are generally avoided near the spine and sacrum to minimise the risk of nerve injury. Microwave thermocoagulation is another emerging ablative technology, which depends on the application of an electromagnetic wave (around 900 MHz) through an electrode antenna. Electromagnetic microwaves travelling through tissue produce ultrahigh-frequency agitation of water molecules and production of frictional heat, which results in coagulative necrosis of the tissues. No grounding pads are necessary for the transmission of electromagnetic microwaves. Microwaves are more versatile and efficient than RFA, since they operate independently of any electrical current convection and can achieve higher temperatures and larger ablation zones more quickly than RFA. Microwaves also suffer less from heat-sink phenomena compared to RFA.

Cryotherapy is an alternative technique that freezes lesions to form an 'iceball'. Briefly, miniaturised argon-gas applicators can produce controlled percutaneous tissue freezing under CT or MR imaging (Fig. 93-21). Rapid expansion of argon gas delivered under high pressure inside a sealed cryoprobe reaches −100°C within a few seconds on the basis of the Joule–Thomson effect. Freezing then develops gradually around the cryoprobe to form an ovoid iceball. Cellular necrosis occurs below −20°C via a combination of ice formation and osmosis along tissues causing protein denaturation and rupture of cell membranes. Effective cryoablation involves a freeze–thaw–freeze cycle; i.e. high-pressure argon gas is delivered to achieve a freezing phase followed by a thawing phase with helium gas, and then a second argon gas-freezing phase. Effectiveness of cryoablation may be limited by tissue thawing from nearby high-flow vascular structures (known as the cool-sink phenomenon), which is the opposite of the heat-sink phenomenon occurring during thermoablation. Cryoablation has the added advantages of direct CT or MR visualisation and monitoring of treatment outcome with less peri- and postoperative pain. The iceball is visible in real time under CT or MR. However, cryoablation is a lot more expensive and time-consuming than traditional RFA and MW procedures.

As a general rule, severe pain from bone metastases can be treated with percutaneous ablation when conventional therapies such as opiate analgesia, chemotherapy and radiotherapy are ineffective, too slow acting or cause unacceptable side effects. Significant symptomatic improvement is expected in more than 80% of patients with sustained pain relief for more than 6 months. Ablation of weight-bearing bones must be supplemented with prophylactic cement consolidation if a pathological fracture is anticipated. Proposed criteria to identify bone lesions at a high risk of pathological fracture include cortical destruction >50%, lytic lesion with a diameter >3cm and weight-bearing pain on exertion. For example, cementoplasty of painful expansile osteolytic lesions of the acetabulum may be combined with cryo- or thermocoagulation techniques with the aim of palliative bone consolidation following tumour destruction. PMMA

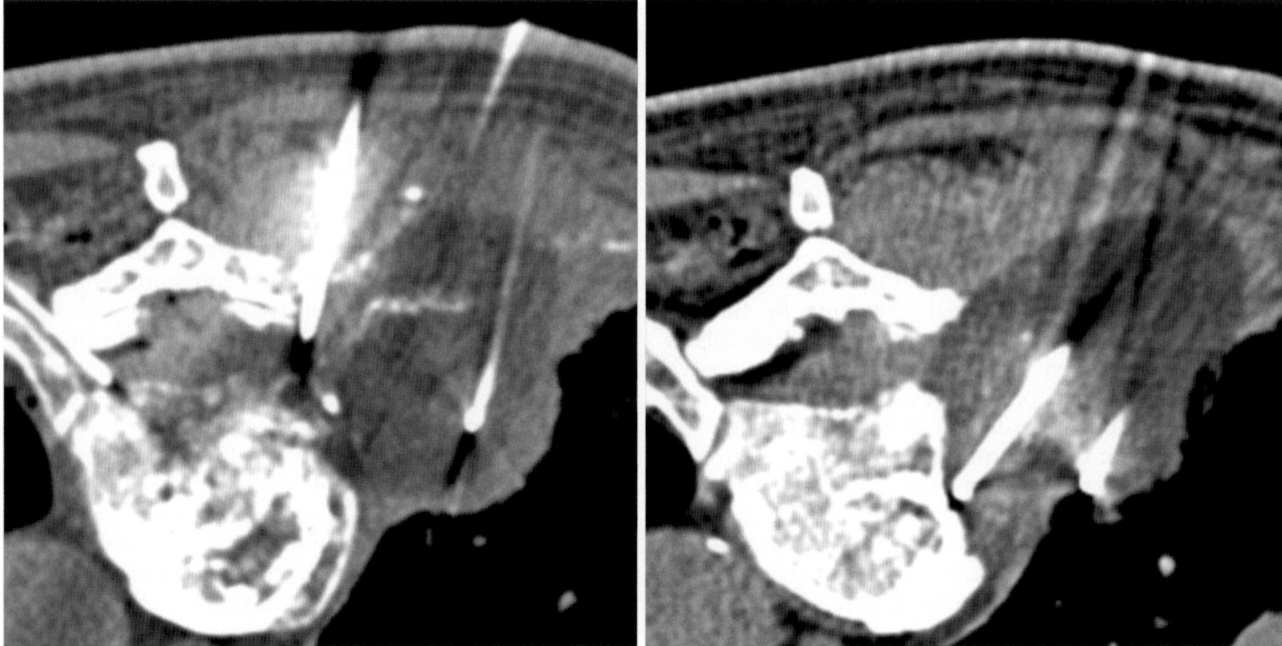

FIGURE 93-21 ■ **Cryoablation.** CT-guided percutaneous cryoablation of a painful bone metastasis of the thoracic spine. Cryoablation allows for real-time monitoring of the treatment effect (hypodense ellipsoid iceball) to avoid neurologic injury. (Image courtesy of Professor A.Gangi, Strasburg, France.)

cementoplasty, which also has inherent antineoplastic properties, may be used either as an individual therapy for painful insufficiency fractures or as adjunctive stabilisation treatment following spine and pelvic ablation therapies. Note that PMMA setting times depend on local tissue temperature. Therefore, higher ambient temperatures, such as after radiofrequency or microwave ablation, will accelerate polymerisation and hardening of the material. In contrast, lower temperatures, such as during subzero cryoablation, will significantly delay cement polymerisation reaction with increased risk of cement leak. Therefore, cement injection may be performed 1 day after ablation to allow for normalisation of tissue temperatures.

Complications

General complications of spinal bone ablation include damage to surrounding structures such as nerve roots with bowel and bladder symptoms, formation of tumour-cutaneous fistulae and pathological fractures or cement leak with the use of adjunctive cementoplasty. Use of appropriate thermosensors and insulation techniques, like carbon dioxide insufflation, may improve safety and efficacy of spinal ablation procedures. During thermal ablation, passive thermocouples, which are available as fine needles, may be inserted alongside the electrodes to monitor temperature rise in sensitive structures, such as at the level of the intervertebral foramina or in the posterolateral epidural space to protect the spinal cord and exiting nerve roots from inadvertent thermal injury. Carbon dioxide can be also very useful for displacement of vital hollow organs and protection of adjacent nerves because of its high insulation coefficient and zero risk of gas embolism.

Osteoid Osteomas

Percutaneous ablation is also considered first-line therapy for eradication of osteoid osteomas. Osteoid osteoma (OO) is a benign skeletal neoplasm of unknown aetiology consisting of both osteoid and woven bone elements that are surrounded by osteoblasts. OO represents 4% of all bone tumours and accounts for 12% of all benign cases. The lesion is usually smaller than 1.5 cm in diameter and may occur in any bone, but it is found in the posterior spinal elements in approximately 6% of patients. Patients complain of dull or aching pain, worse during the night and typically relieved by salicylates. The usual appearance of OOs is of a small sclerotic bone island with a circular radiolucent defect called a nidus. Computed tomography (CT) is the imaging method of choice for precise localisation of the OO nidus and accurate guidance during percutaneous thermal ablation (Fig. 93-22). Intervention is performed under general or spinal anaesthesia, because penetration and ablation of the OO nidus is extremely painful. Regional nerve blocks can be used if the extremities are involved. Typically, the nidus is ablated with a standard non-perfused radiofrequency electrode or with a laser optical fibre that emits near-infrared wavelength laser light (neodymium yttrium aluminum garnet Nd:YAG). Resolution of pain symptoms is reported after 24–48 h in the majority of the cases with overall clinical success rates of 80–100%. Radiofrequency ablation has also been successfully applied in the eradication of osteoblastomas, chondroblastomas, giant cell tumours, enchondromas and eosinophilic granulomas. Percutaneous ablation for cytoreduction of sacral chordomas and sarcomas, and local control of aggressive desmoid tumours has also been reported.

EMBOLISATION OF SPINAL TUMOURS

Another field of spinal interventional oncology includes arterial embolisation to pre-operatively reduce tumour vascularity or palliate patients who are poor surgical candidates but require symptom relief. The spine is the most common site of bone metastases and primary or secondary spinal tumours may produce pain, mechanical instability, and radiculopathy or compression myelopathy. Transcatheter arterial embolisation of hypervascular spinal tumours can reduce mass effect, relieve cord compression and even improve resectability during neurosurgical reconstruction and stabilisation of the spine. Operators must be skillful in microparticle and microcoil embolisation techniques and be familiar with normal and aberrant cord vascular anatomy to avoid disastrous complications of non-target embolisation. The normal spinal cord is supplied by three longitudinal arteries: one anterior spinal artery that runs anteriorly in the groove of the anterior median fissure and two posterior spinal arteries that run in parallel posterolaterally on the cord itself. Spinal arteries are supplied by terminal branches of the subclavian, vertebral, intercostal, lumbar and internal iliac arteries, the so called segmental or radiculomedullary arteries, the largest of which is the arteria radicularis magna (artery of Adamkiewicz).

Embolisation may be indicated for a variety of hypervascular benign (e.g. haemangioma, aneurysmal bone cyst, osteoblastoma), primary malignant (e.g. chordomas and sarcomas) and secondary malignant spinal tumours (e.g. renal cell carcinoma, thyroid carcinoma and hepatocellular carcinoma) (Fig. 93-23). Pre-operative embolisation is used to reduce tumour size, minimise blood loss during surgery and facilitate radical neurosurgical resection. In patients with unresectable lesions, palliative embolisation of advanced hypervascular spinal tumours may be carried out to relieve pain and improve compressive neurological symptoms. Lately, transcatheter tumour chemoembolisation has been used to combine devascularisation and ischaemia with delivery of regional chemotherapy. In selected occasions, serial arterial embolisation may be offered for curative treatment of certain primary bone tumours such as giant cell tumours and aneurysmal bone cysts.

High-resolution subtraction angiography is critical during spinal embolisation for the identification of the radiculomedullary and spinal arteries. Spinal angiography is performed using routine access from the femoral artery. Non-selective aortograms followed by selective angiograms after catheterisation of the lumbar and intercostal arteries of the affected vertebra and 1–2 adjacent

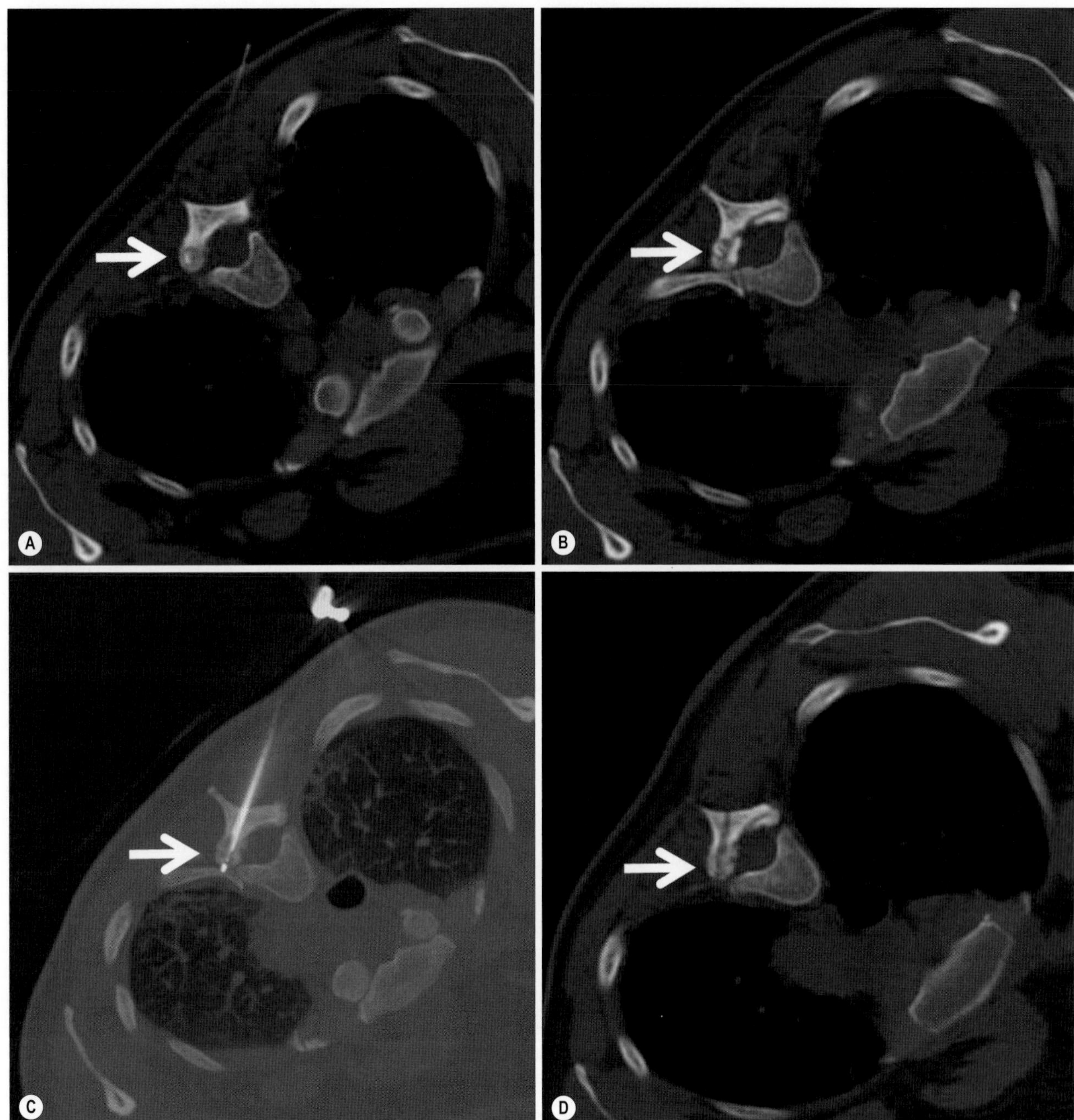

FIGURE 93-22 ■ Ablation of osteoid osteoma. (A, B) Painful osteoid osteoma located at the posterior elements of the T4 vertebra. Note the central sclerosis surrounded by a radiolucent area (nidus) (white arrows). (C) CT-guided targeting of the lesion with a beveled trocar to allow for introduction of a non-perfused radiofrequency ablation electrode with a 10-mm active tip (white arrow). (D) Note the needle tract across the lamina after completion of the procedure (white arrow).

segments above and below are obtained. The vertebral, carotid, thyrocervical and costocervical trunks may need to be evaluated in patients with cervical tumours, whereas the iliolumbar and the lateral and medial sacral arteries may provide feeding branches in patients with sacral tumours. Multiple projections may be necessary, but the spinal and radiculomedullary arteries are best identified on an anteroposterior projection. The latter are characterised by a sharp hairpin configuration as they enter the spinal canal and join the spinal arteries. Once the tumour-feeding branches have been identified and the decision for embolisation has been made, a 3-French microcatheter is advanced co-axially inside the angiographic catheter for superselective embolisation of each feeder without systemic reflux of the embolisation material. Particulate (polyvinylalcohol, PVA, or trisacryl gelatin microspheres), liquid (*n*-butyl cyanoacrylate, NBA glue) and coils (fibred or non-fibred platinum micro-coils) may be used for terminal tumour devascularisation (Fig. 93-24). Of note, liquid agents may be

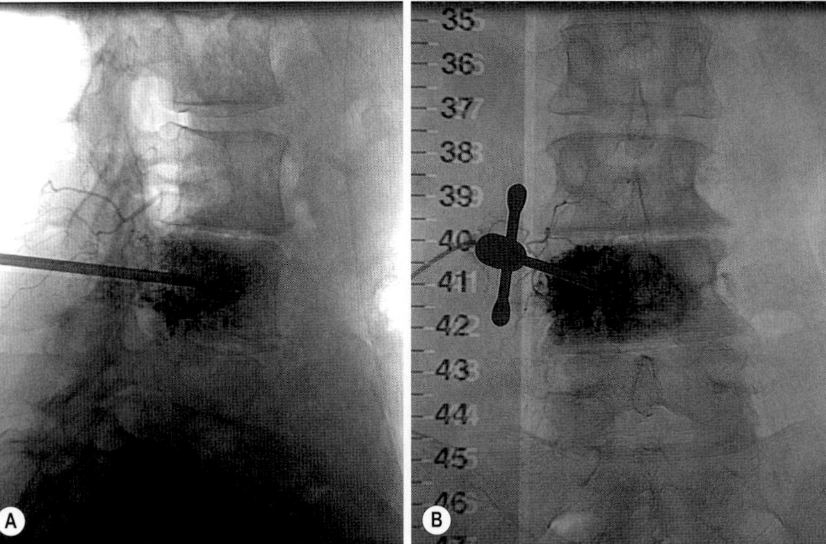

FIGURE 93-23 ■ Hypervascular tumour. Transpedicular biopsy of a hypervascular solitary lesion infiltrating the pedicle and most of the L4 vertebral body. Contrast injection through the bone trocar opacifies the extensive tumour neovascularity. Note the retrograde filling of the lumbar arteries at the same level. (A) Lateral and (B) anteroposterior projection.

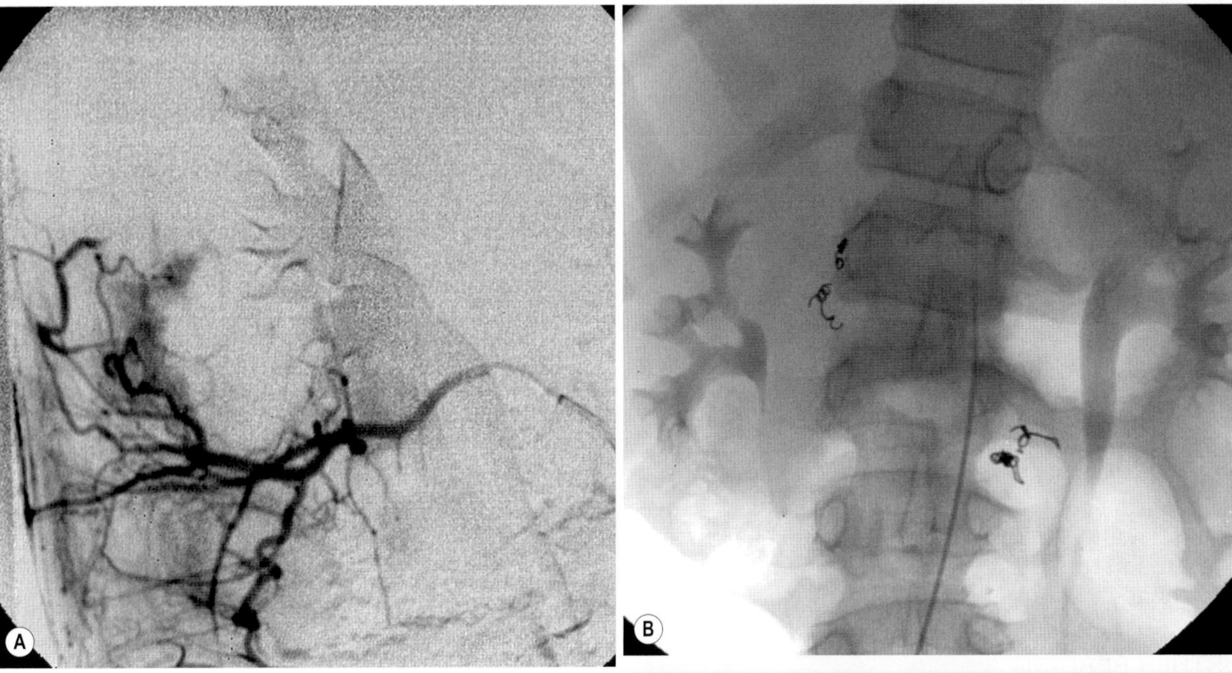

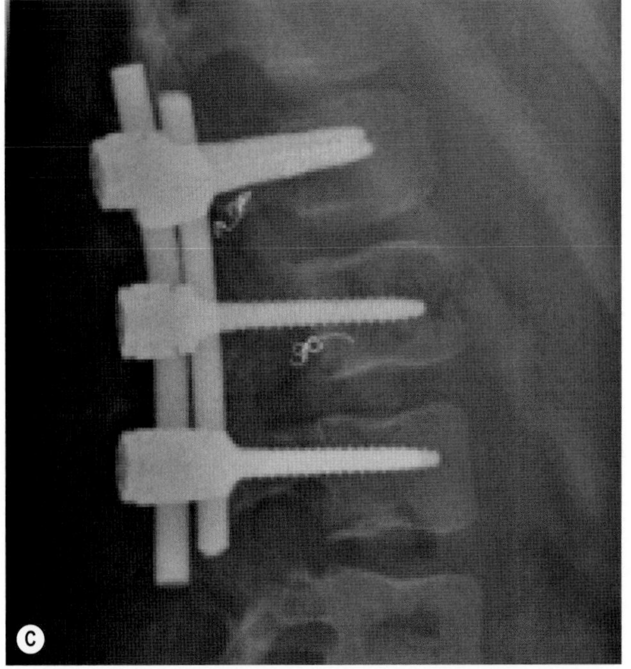

FIGURE 93-24 ■ Spinal embolisation. (A) Selective cannulation of the segmental lumbar arteries and angiography in a patient with an aggressive osteoblastoma. Note the hypervascularity of the lesion located at the posterior elements of the lumbar spine. (B) The lesion was embolised with 500 μm PVA microparticles through bilateral lumbar arteries of the same and the overlying level. Micro-coil embolisation was then performed to occlude the major lumbar feeders (anteroposterior view). (C) The patient was operated the following day with minimal blood loss. Note the final outcome after laminectomy and spine fixation of the affected segment. Micro-coils remained in situ (lateral projection).

difficult to control and coils alone are ineffective because they produce proximal occlusion of the segmental branches. However, they are usually used in conjunction with microparticle embolisation to achieve more optimal devascularisation. Coils can also be used to control normal vascular anatomy, i.e. occlude intersegmental anastomoses and prevent non-target embolisation of the cord. Nowadays, 100–500 µm spherical PVA or trisacryl microparticles are preferred because they are controlled and non-absorbable, have homogeneous shape and can penetrate deep into the tumour capillary bed. Microparticle embolisation is performed in each feeder artery under continuous fluoroscopic control applying a slow pulsatile injection until stagnation of flow (near stasis).

A neurologic examination must be performed immediately following successful embolisation to identify potential neurologic deficits. In most cases a mild post-embolisation syndrome characterised by nausea, pain, low-grade fever and elevated inflammatory markers occurs within the first few days because of tissue ischaemia. Neurosurgery should be performed within 1 day of embolisation for reduced intra-operative bleeding, because later tumours are revascularised through collaterals from adjacent levels. In general, the reported success rate of complete tumour embolisation is around 50–80% depending on the morphology of the tumour and the relevant vascular anatomy, and at least a 30–50% reduction in intra-operative blood loss is anticipated. Adequate embolisation of large unresectable spinal tumours has also been shown to provide significant and long-lasting pain relief and improvement of neurologic symptoms. Spinal embolisation is relatively safe, but it carries a low risk of catastrophic spinal cord ischaemia (or stroke when embolisation of cervical tumours is performed) if non-target embolisation of unrecognised radiculomedullary branches occurs. Detailed knowledge of the relevant vascular anatomy and meticulous analysis of subtracted intra-procedural angiograms is vital to avoid complications.

FURTHER READING

1. Katsanos K, Sabharwal T, Adam A. Percutaneous cementoplasty. Semin Intervent Radiol 2010;27(2):137–47.
2. Katsanos K, Ahmad F, Dourado R, et al. Interventional radiology in the elderly. Clin Interv Aging 2009;4:1–15.
3. Sabharwal T, Katsanos K, Buy X, Gangi A. Image-guided ablation therapy of bone tumors. Semin Ultrasound CT MR 2009;30(2): 78–90.
4. Kelekis AD, Filippiadis DK, Martin JB, Brountzos E. Standards of practice: quality assurance guidelines for percutaneous treatments of intervertebral discs. Cardiovasc Intervent Radiol 2010;33(5): 909–13.
5. Kelekis AD, Somon T, Yilmaz H, et al. Interventional spine procedures. Eur J Radiol 2005;55(3):362–83.
6. Buy X, Gangi A. Percutaneous treatment of intervertebral disc herniation. Semin Intervent Radiol 2010;27(2):148–59.
7. Gangi A, Tsoumakidou G, Buy X, et al. Percutaneous techniques for cervical pain of discal origin. Semin Musculoskelet Radiol 2011;15(2):172–80.
8. Gangi A, Dietemann JL, Ide C, et al. Percutaneous laser disk decompression under CT and fluoroscopic guidance: indications, technique, and clinical experience. Radiographics 1996;16(1): 89–96.
9. Rybak LD, Gangi A, Buy X, et al. Thermal ablation of spinal osteoid osteomas close to neural elements: technical considerations. Am J Roentgenol 2010;195(4):W293–8.
10. Gangi A, Tsoumakidou G, Buy X, Quoix E. Quality improvement guidelines for bone tumour management. Cardiovasc Intervent Radiol 2010;33(4):706–13.
11. McGraw JK, Cardella J, Barr JD, et al; SIR Standards of Practice Committee. Society of Interventional Radiology quality improvement guidelines for percutaneous vertebroplasty. J Vasc Interv Radiol 2003;14(7):827–31.
12. Ozkan E, Gupta S. Embolization of spinal tumors: vascular anatomy, indications, and technique. Tech Vasc Interv Radiol 2011;14(3):129–40.
13. Owen RJ. Embolization of musculoskeletal bone tumors. Semin Intervent Radiol 2010;27(2):111–23.
14. Van Zundert J, Huntoon M, Patijn J, et al. Cervical radicular pain. Pain Pract 2010;10(1):1–17.
15. van Boxem K, van Eerd M, Brinkhuizen T, et al. Radiofrequency and pulsed radiofrequency treatment of chronic pain syndromes: the available evidence. Pain Pract 2008;8(5):385–93.
16. van Eerd M, Patijn J, Lataster A, et al. Cervical facet pain. Pain Pract 2010;10(2):113–23.
17. Welch BT, Welch TJ. Percutaneous ablation of benign bone tumors. Tech Vasc Interv Radiol 2011;14(3):118–23.
18. Peh WC, Munk PL, Rashid F, Gilula LA. Percutaneous vertebral augmentation: vertebroplasty, kyphoplasty and skyphoplasty. Radiol Clin North Am 2008;46(3):611–35, vii.
19. Van Boxem K, Cheng J, Patijn J, et al. Lumbosacral radicular pain. Pain Pract 2010;10(4):339–58.
20. van Kleef M, Vanelderen P, Cohen SP, et al. Pain originating from the lumbar facet joints. Pain Pract 2010;10(5):459–69.
21. Benyamin RM, Manchikanti L, Parr AT, et al. The effectiveness of lumbar interlaminar epidural injections in managing chronic low back and lower extremity pain. Pain Physician 2012;15(4): E363–404.
22. Kallewaard JW, Terheggen MA, Groen GJ, et al. Discogenic low back pain. Pain Pract 2010;10(6):560–79.

Subject Index

Page numbers followed by 'f' indicate figures, 't' indicate tables, and 'b' indicate boxes.

Notes

To simplify the index, the main terms of imaging techniques (e.g. computed tomography, magnetic resonance imaging etc.) are concerned only with the technology and general applications. Users are advised to look for specific anatomical features and diseases/disorders for individual imaging techniques used.

vs. indicates a comparison or differential diagnosis.

To save space in the index, the following abbreviations have been used:

CHD—congenital heart disease
CMR—cardiac magnetic resonance
CT—computed tomography
CXR—chest X-ray
DECT—dual-energy computed tomography
DWI-MRI—diffusion weighted imaging-magnetic resonance imaging
ERCP—endoscopic retrograde cholangiopancreatography
EUS—endoscopic ultrasound
FDG-PET—fluorodeoxyglucose positron emission tomography
HRCT—high-resolution computed tomography
MDCT—multidetector computed tomography
MRA—magnetic resonance angiography
MRCP—magnetic resonance cholangiopancreatography
MRI—magnetic resonance imaging
MRS—magnetic resonance spectroscopy
PET—positron emission tomography
PTC—percutaneous transhepatic cholangiography
SPECT—single photon emission computed tomography
US—ultrasound

A

B

C

D

G

H

J

M

N

O

P

Q

R

S

U

V